D1687735

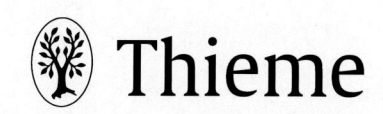

Imaging of the Head and Neck

Second edition, revised and enlarged

Mahmood F. Mafee, M.D., F.A.C.R.
University of Illinois at Chicago
Chicago, USA

Galdino E. Valvassori, M.D., F.A.C.R.
University of Illinois at Chicago
Chicago, USA

Minerva Becker, M.D.
Geneva University Hospital
Geneva, Switzerland

With contributions by:
J. S. Lewin, S. G. Nour, and A. L. Weber

3750 illustrations

Thieme
Stuttgart · New York

Library of Congress Cataloging-in-Publication Data

Mafee, Mahmood F.
  Imaging of the head and neck / Mahmood F. Mafee, Galdino E. Valvassori, Minerva Becker ; with contributions by J.S. Lewin, S.G. Nour, and A.L. Weber.—2nd ed.
    p. ; cm.
  Valvassori's name appears first on the earlier ed.
  Includes bibliographical references and index.
  ISBN 3-13-100942-X (GTV : alk. paper)—ISBN 1-58890-009-6 (TNY : alk. paper)
    1. Head—Imaging. 2. Neck—Imaging.
    [DNLM: 1. Diagnostic Imaging. 2. Head—radiography. 3. Head and Neck Neoplasms—radiography.
    4. Neck—radiography. WE 705 M187i 2005] I. Valvassori, Galdino E. II. Becker, M. (Minerva) III. Title.
  RC936.I43 2005
  617.5'10754—dc22
                                                                    2004021288
1st English edition 1995

List of Contributors

Jonathan S. Lewin, M.D.
Martin W. Donner Professor and Director
Department of Radiology
Johns Hopkins University School of Medicine
Radiologist-in-chief
Johns Hopkins Hospital
Baltimore, MD, USA

Sherif. G. Nour, M.D.
Assistant Professor of Radiology
Case Western Reserve University School of Medicine
University Hospitals of Cleveland
Cleveland, OH, USA

Alfred L. Weber, M.D.
Chief of Radiology, Emeritus
Massachusetts Eye and Ear Infirmary
Professor of Radiology
Harvard Medical School
Boston, MA, USA

© 1995, 2005 Georg Thieme Verlag,
Rüdigerstrasse 14, 70469 Stuttgart, Germany
http://www.thieme.de
Thieme New York, 333 Seventh Avenue,
New York, NY 10001 USA
http://www.thieme.com

Typesetting by primustype Hurler GmbH, Notzingen
Printed in Germany by Grammlich, Pliezhausen

ISBN 3-13-100942-X (GTV)
ISBN 1-58890-009-6 (TNY)

Important note: Medicine is an ever-changing science undergoing continual development. Research and clinical experience are continually expanding our knowledge, in particular our knowledge of proper treatment and drug therapy. Insofar as this book mentions any dosage or application, readers may rest assured that the authors, editors, and publishers have made every effort to ensure that such references are in accordance with **the state of knowledge at the time of production of the book**.
Nevertheless, this does not involve, imply, or express any guarantee or responsibility on the part of the publishers in respect to any dosage instructions and forms of applications stated in the book. **Every user is requested to examine carefully** the manufacturers' leaflets accompanying each drug and to check, if necessary in consultation with a physician or specialist, whether the dosage schedules mentioned therein or the contraindications stated by the manufacturers differ from the statements made in the present book. Such examination is particularly important with drugs that are either rarely used or have been newly released on the market. Every dosage schedule or every form of application used is entirely at the user's own risk and responsibility. The authors and publishers request every user to report to the publishers any discrepancies or inaccuracies noticed. If errors in this work are found after publication, errata will be posted at www.thieme.com on the product description page.

Some of the product names, patents, and registered designs referred to in this book are in fact registered trademarks or proprietary names even though specific reference to this fact is not always made in the text. Therefore, the appearance of a name without designation as proprietary is not to be construed as a representation by the publisher that it is in the public domain.

This book, including all parts thereof, is legally protected by copyright. Any use, exploitation, or commercialization outside the narrow limits set by copyright legislation, without the publisher's consent, is illegal and liable to prosecution. This applies in particular to photostat reproduction, copying, mimeographing, preparation of microfilms, and electronic data processing and storage.

We dedicate this edition to our spouses and children:

Mahvash, Rana, Alireza, and *Mariam Mafee;*
Eleanor, Danielle, Alex, Laura, and *Pia Valvassori;*
Christoph, Marie-Christine, and *Manuel Becker.*

Authors' Affiliations

Mahmood F. Mafee, M.D., F.A.C.R.
Professor of Radiology, School of Medicine
University of Illinois at Chicago, Chicago, Illinois, USA
Chief of Head and Neck Radiology, Eye and Ear Infirmary
Director of MR Imaging
Former Head of Department of Radiology
University of Illinois Hospital at Chicago, Chicago, Illinois, USA
Past President of the American Society of Head and Neck Radiology
Former Distinguished Scientist, Armed Forces
Institute of Pathology, Washington DC, USA
Honorary Visiting Professor of the
International Neuroscience Institute, Hanover, Germany

Galdino E. Valvassori, M.D., F.A.C.R.
Professor in the Departments of Radiology and Otolaryngology–Head & Neck Surgery, University of Illinois Hospital at Chicago, Chicago, Illinois, USA
Co-founder and First President of the American Society of Head and Neck Radiology
Honorary Member of the American Society of Neuroradiology and of the German Society of Otorhinolaryngology (Deutsche Gesellschaft für Hals-Nasen-Ohren-Heilkunde, Kopf- und Hals-Chirurgie)

Minerva Becker, M.D.
Associate Professor
Chief of Head and Neck Radiology
Division of Diagnostic and Interventional Radiology
Department of Radiology and Medical Informatics
Consulting Staff
Clinic of Otorhinolaryngology and Head and Neck Surgery
Geneva University Hospital, Geneva, Switzerland
Chairman of the Educational Committee of the European Society of Head and Neck Radiology

Preface

Remarkable advances in medical diagnostic imaging have been made during the past three decades. The development of new imaging techniques and continuous improvements in the display of digital images have opened new horizons in the study of head and neck anatomy and pathology. The American Society of Head and Neck Radiology (ASHNR) and its European and Asiatic counterparts evolved because of the emerging awareness of the roles that head and neck radiologists play in the diagnosis and management of head and neck, base of the skull, neuro-ophthalmologic and neuro-otologic diseases.

This edition continues the tradition of excellence set by the first edition of Valvassori's *Head and Neck Imaging* (which was also the first textbook in head and neck radiology), and provides a comprehensive review of the most pertinent and up-to-date knowledge in the field of head and neck imaging. The content of this edition has been organized into 12 chapters according to anatomic regions. It now includes new material on the temporomandibular joint, the lacrimal drainage system, dental scanning, fibro-osseous and cartilaginous lesions of the head and neck, MRI sialography, MR interventional technique, and thyroid and parathyroid glands. All chapters have been expanded to address new developments in the field and to stress the importance of imaging anatomy, pathologic correlation, and pertinent clinical data.

For each anatomic region, the embryology and anatomy are introduced, followed by congenital and developmental disorders, inflammatory processes, benign and malignant neoplastic diseases, trauma, and postoperative changes. The detailed reference lists in each chapter include key references and are as recent as possible. Care has been taken to include exquisitely reproduced illustrations that provide the maximum of pertinent information.

It is our hope that this textbook will be useful to students and physicians in the fields of radiology, otolaryngology, neuro-otology, rhinology, head and neck surgery, ophthalmology, neuro-ophthalmology, oromaxillofacial–temporomandibular surgery, neurology, neurosurgery, and oncology.

We are greatly indebted to Cliff Bergman M.D. and the editorial and production staff of Thieme International, particularly Stephan Konnry, Gert Krüger, and Ingrid Schöllhammer, for their patience, valuable guidance, and extreme professionalism; and finally to our secretary Mrs. Jacqueline Jamieson for her diligence in typing and organization. Without their tireless efforts, this book could not have been completed on time.

Fall 2004

Mahmood F. Mafee
Galdino E. Valvassori
Minerva Becker

Acknowledgements

Mahmood F. Mafee, M.D.
My contribution to the previous edition of this textbook and to this edition as an editor, and above all my medical training and academic career could not have been achieved without the dedication, encouragement, and continued support of many individuals. First and foremost, I thank my mother and my late father, Mostafa F. Mafee, Pharm.D., and my brothers Ali F. Mafee, M.D. and Reza F. Mafee, M.D. Their enthusiasm for the field of medicine, in general, and encouragement in my pursuing an academic career in radiology has served me significantly in my 28 years of academic endeavor in radiology. They deserve my heartfelt gratitude for their dedication in shaping all aspects of my life.

I am indebted to all of my teachers, particularly those at the School of Medicine at Tehran University in Iran, from whom I had the privilege of learning basic and clinical medicine. Special thanks go to Dr. Galdino E. Valvassori, who taught me the basics of head and neck imaging; to Dr. Glen D. Dobben, who taught me to appreciate all aspects of neuroradiology; to Dr. Velastimil Capek, my former chairman, for inspiring me to pursue academic radiology; to Drs. Arvind Kumar, Gholann Peyman, Joyce Schild, Michael Friedman, Barry L. Wenig, Michael Yao, David Calderalli, and Leslie B. Heffez, D.D.S. for teaching me the clinical knowledge and understanding of head and neck disorders and imaging appreciation of postoperative changes of head and neck surgical procedures; to Drs. Bruce M. Wenig and Dennis K. Heffner for teaching me the pathology of the head and neck during the year I spent at the Armed Forces Institute of Pathology (AFIP) as a distinguished scientist in the Department of Radiologic Pathology; to Claude Dejardins, Ph.D., Associate Dean of Research at the University of Illinois in Chicago, for his continued support in clinical research; to all of the radiology, otolaryngology, ophthalmology, neurology, neurosurgery, oncology, oromaxillofacial surgery residents, fellows, and clinical colleagues with whom I had the pleasure of working and interaction; and to all of my administrative assistants for their dedication and diligence on my behalf. I offer my sincerest gratitude to all of them.

Galdino E. Valvassori, M.D.
I would like to acknowledge the contribution of my colleague and friend Richard A. Buckingham M.D., who sectioned and photographed the temporal bones. I have spent innumerable hours with him studying and comparing tissue sections with the corresponding images. I also want to thank my wife Eleanor for all her help in preparing and reviewing the numerous versions of the manuscript.

Minerva Becker, M.D.
I acknowledge with gratitude the contributions of my colleagues and friends from the Clinic of Otorhinolaryngology and Cervicofacial Surgery, Geneva University Hospital, particularly Professor Willy Lehman, Dr. Francis Marchal, and Dr. Pavel Dulguerov, and Professor Peter Zbären, Department of Otorhinolaryngology and Head and Neck Surgery, Bern University Hospital. Many thanks to Dr. Paulette Mhawech and Dr. Anne-Marie Kurt, Department of Clinical Pathology, Geneva University Hospital, for their kind assistance.

I thank my colleagues and friends from the Radiology Department of the University Hospital in Geneva, particularly Dr. Jacqueline Delavelle, Dr. Nathalia Dfouni, Dr. Alain Keller, Dr. Romain Kohler, Dr. Haleem Khan, and Dr. Marco Palmesino, as well as Mr. Domingos Orlando and Mr. Philippe Cammarassa from the audiovisual unit for their contributions.

Finally, I would like to thank my colleagues and friends throughout Europe who have contributed US, CT, and MRI images of their cases, particularly Dr. Alexandra Borges, Dr. Jan Casselmann, Dr. David Coutinho, Dr. Nicole Freling, Dr. Guy Moulin, and Dr. Fernando Torrhina.

Contents

Section I Temporal Bone

1 Imaging of the Temporal Bone 3
Galdino E. Valvassori

Sectional Anatomy of the Temporal Bone 3
    Anatomical Notes 3
    Sectional Anatomy 3
Imaging Techniques 30
    Conventional Radiography 30
    Computed Tomography (CT) 30
    Magnetic Resonance Imaging (MRI) 32
Developmental Variations 36
    Mastoid 36
    Lateral Sinus 36
    Tegmen 36
    Jugular Fossa 37
    Carotid Artery 38
    Arachnoid Granulations 40
    Petrous Apex 40
Congenital Abnormalities of the Temporal Bone 41
    Imaging Assessment 41
    Embryology 41
    Anomalies of the Sound-Conducting System 43
    Facial Nerve Anomalies 47
    Anomalies of the Inner Ear 47
    Cerebrospinal Fluid Otorrhea 52
    Imaging Assessment for
    Cochlear Implantation 52
    Congenital Vascular Anomalies 52
    Syndromic Hearing Loss 53
Temporal Bone Trauma 54
    Classification 54
    Clinical Findings 54
    Imaging Findings 54
    Labyrinthine Concussion and Bleeding 55
    Longitudinal Fractures 55
    Transverse Fractures 56
    Comminuted Mastoid Fractures 56
    Ossicular Dislocation 58
    Projectile Injuries 58
    Traumatic Facial Nerve Lesions 59
    Iatrogenic Lesions 61
    Meningoencephalocele 61
    Cerebrospinal Fluid Otorrhea 61
Acute Otitis Media, Mastoiditis, and Malignant
Necrotizing External Otitis 62
    Acute Otitis Media and Mastoiditis 62
    Imaging Findings 62
    Imaging Technique 63
    Differential Diagnosis 65
    Acute Labyrinthitis 65
    Chronic Labyrinthitis 65
    Facial Neuritis 66
    Malignant Necrotizing External Otitis 66
    Imaging Findings 66
    Healing Stages 68

Chronic Otitis Media and Mastoiditis 68
    Clinical Findings 68
    Otoscopic Findings 68
    Imaging Techniques 68
    Imaging Findings 69
Cholesteatoma of the Middle Ear 74
    Acquired Cholesteatoma of the Middle Ear
    and Mastoid 75
    Clinical and Otoscopic Findings 75
    Imaging Techniques 75
    Diagnosis of Cholesteatoma 76
    Patterns of Imaging Findings 76
    Pars Flaccida Cholesteatomas 76
    Epitympanic Retraction Pockets 77
    Pars Tensa Cholesteatomas 78
    Combined Pars Flaccida and Pars Tensa
    Cholesteatomas 79
    Evaluation of the Extent
    of Cholesteatoma 79
    Labyrinthine Fistulas 82
    Petrous Extension of Cholesteatoma 83
    Facial Nerve 84
    Congenital Cholesteatoma
    of the Middle Ear 84
    Petrous Pyramid and Epidural Cholesteatomas 85
    Keratosis Obturans and Cholesteatoma of the External
    Auditory Canal 89
Postoperative and Postirradiation Imaging
of the Temporal Bone 90
    Simple and Radical Mastoidectomies 90
    Tympanoplasty 90
    Imaging Findings 91
Tumors 95
    Benign Tumors 95
    Malignant Tumors 105
Internal Auditory Canal and Acoustic Schwannomas 109
    Normal Internal Auditory Canal 109
    Imaging Studies 112
    Pathology of the Internal Auditory Canal 113
    Pathology within the Internal Auditory Canal 113
    Meningeal Pathology 118
    Vascular Abnormalities 118
    Heterotopic Lesion within the Internal
    Auditory Canal 120
Otosclerosis and Bone Dystrophies 122
    Otosclerosis 122
    Paget Disease 129
    Osteogenesis Imperfecta 130
    Osteopetrosis 130
    Fibrous Dysplasia 130
    Craniometaphyseal Dysplasia 130
References 132

Contents

Section II   Eye and Orbit, Base of the Skull

2 Eye and Orbit 137
Mahmood F. Mafee

Part 1: The Eye 137
Embryology 137
   Lens 137
   The Ciliary Body, Iris, and
   Suspensory Ligaments of the Lens 137
   The Vitreous 137
   The Choroid 137
   The Sclera 137
   The Cornea 137
   Vascular System 137
   Extraocular Muscles 139
   The Eyelids 139
   The Lacrimal Gland 139
   The Lacrimal Sac and Nasolacrimal Duct 139
   The Orbit 139
References 139
Anatomy 140
   Tenon's Capsule and Extraocular Muscle Sheaths
   (Sleeves) 140
   Sclera 140
   Cornea 141
   Uvea (Choroid, Ciliary Body, and Iris) 141
   Retina 142
   Vitreous 143
Imaging Techniques 143
   CT Technique 143
   MRI Technique 143
Pathology 146
   Congenital Anomalies 146
   Coloboma and Morning Glory Disk Anomaly 148
   Ocular Detachments 149
   Ocular Inflammatory Disorders 154
   Benign Reactive Lymphoid Hyperplasia 157
   Papilledema 157
   Intraocular Calcifications 157
   Leukokoria 158
   Retinoblastoma 159
   Intraocular Mass and Masslike Lesions Simulating
   Retinoblastoma 164
   Persistent Hyperplastic Primary
   Vitreous 164
   Retinal Dysplasia 168
   Norrie Disease 168
   Warburg Syndrome 168
   Retinopathy of Prematurity
   or Retrolental Fibroplasia 169
   Coats disease 169
   Ocular Toxocariasis
   (Sclerosing Endophthalmitis) 172
   Ocular Astrocytic Hamartoma
   (Retinal Astrocytoma) 174
   Combined Hamartoma of the Retinal Pigment
   Epithelium and Retina 174
   Incontinentia Pigmenti 175
   Juvenile Xanthogranuloma 175
   Ganglioneuroma 175
   Optic Nerve Head Drusen 176
   Choroidal Osteoma 176
   Retinal Gliosis 177
   Myelinated Nerve Fibers 177
   Subretinal Neovascular Membranes 177
   Vitreous Opacities 177
   Choroidal Hemangioma 177
   Malignant Uveal Melanoma 177
   Melanocytoma 182
   Uveal Metastasis 183
   Uveal Nevus 184
   Choroidal and Retinal Hemangiomas 184
   Angiomatosis Retinae and
   von Hippel–Lindau Disease 186
   Choroidal Hemorrhage and
   Choroidal Detachment 186
   Choroidal Cyst 186
   Ocular Lymphoma 186
   Ocular Leukemia 186
   Primary Ocular Schwannoma (Neurilemoma) 187
   Leiomyoma (Mesoectodermal Leiomyoma) 188
   Ocular Adenoma and Adenocarcinoma 188
   Medulloepithelioma 188
   Senile Macular Degeneration 189
   Ocular Trauma 190
   Anophthalmic Socket and
   Orbital Implant 191
References 192

Part 2: The Orbit 196
Embryology 196
Anatomy 196
   Bony Orbit 196
   Orbital Septum and Eyelids 200
   Orbicularis Oculi 200
   Tenon's Capsule (Fascia Bulbi)
   and Tenon's Space 200
   Orbital Fatty Reticulum 200
   Muscles of the Eye 201
   Innervation 202
   Vascular Anatomy 203
   Lacrimal Apparatus 204
Imaging Techniques 204
   Computed Tomography 204
   MRI Techniques 205
   Normal CT and MRI Anatomy
   of the Orbit 206
Pathology 215
   Hypertelorism, Hypotelorism,
   Exophthalmos, and Exorbitism 215
   Congenital and Developmental
   Abnormalities 215
   Anatomical and Developmental
   Considerations 215
   Acquired Orbital Cysts 222
   Parasitic Cysts 226
   Inflammatory Diseases 226
   Mycotic Infections 230
   Acute, Subacute, and Chronic Idiopathic Orbital
   Inflammatory Disorders (Pseudotumors) 230
   Painful External Ophthalmoplegia
   (Tolosa–Hunt Syndrome) 236
   Thyroid Orbitopathy
   (Graves Dysthyroid Ophthalmopathy) 237
   Sarcoidosis 239
   Sjögren Syndrome 241
   Vasculitides (Angiitides) 242

Amyloidosis	244
Miscellaneous Granulomatous and Histiocytic Lesions	244
Tumors	248
Orbital Vascular Conditions	252
Neural Lesions	263
Nontumoral and Tumoral Enlargement of the Optic Nerve Sheath	267
Fibrous Tissue Tumors of the Orbit	272
Lacrimal Gland and Fossa Lesions	278
Miscellaneous Lacrimal Gland Lesions	281
Fibro-Osseous Lesions of the Orbit	282
Ocular Motility Disorders	285
Traumatic Injury of Ocular Muscles	287
Congenital Anomalies of the Extraocular Muscles	287
Orbital Trauma	290
References	291

3 Base of the Skull ... 295
Mahmood F. Mafee

Embryology	295
Anatomy	295
The External Surface of the Cranial Base	297
The Pterygoid Processes, Pterygoid Plates, Scaphoid Fossa, Spine of the Sphenoid Bone, Foramen Ovale, and Foramen Spinosum	299
The Foramen Lacerum	299
Pterygoid (Vidian) Canal	299
The Squamotympanic Fissure	300
Foramen Magnum and Hypoglossal Canal	300
The Jugular Foramen	301
Stylomastoid Foramen	301
The Internal Surface of the Cranial Base	301
Superior Orbital Fissure, Foramen Rotundum, Tegmen Tympani, and Tegmen Antri	301
Cavernous Sinus	302
Trigeminal Cavity (Meckel's Cave), Trigeminal Cistern, and Ganglion	302
The Posterior Cranial Fossa	302
Role of Diagnostic Imaging in Skull Base Pathology and Surgery	304
Imaging Techniques	304
Angiography and Embolization	305
Imaging Anatomy of the Skull Base	305
Anatomical Variations	305
Skull Base Pathology	306
Developmental Cysts of the Skull Base	307
Tumors	318
Histiocytoses	342
Leukemia	342
Extracranial Lesions Affecting the Skull Base	344
Metastasis	345
Trauma	346
References	348

Section III Nasal Cavity and Paranasal Sinuses

4 Imaging of the Nasal Cavity and Paranasal Sinuses ... 353
Mahmood F. Mafee

Nasal Cavity: Embryology and Development	353
Paranasal Sinuses: Embryology and Development	353
Maxillary Sinuses	353
Ethmoid Sinuses	355
Frontal Sinuses	355
Sphenoid Sinuses	355
Anatomy: The Nasal Cavity	355
The Nasal Mucous Membrane	357
Nasal Cycle	357
Innervation	357
Blood Supply and Lymphatic Drainage	358
Lymphatics	358
Anatomy of the Paranasal Sinuses	358
The Frontal Sinuses	358
The Ethmoidal Sinuses and Surgical Anatomy of the Ethmoid Bone	358
Sphenoidal Sinuses	364
The Maxillary Sinuses	365
Functional Endoscopic Sinus Surgery and the Role of the Radiologist	366
Ostiomeatal Complex	367
Anatomical Variations	367
Pterygomaxillary Fissure, Pterygopalatine (Sphenopalatine) Fossa, and Palatine Bone	371
The Pterygopalatine (Sphenopalatine) Ganglion	375
Applied Anatomy	376
References	378
Imaging Techniques	379
General Considerations	379
Computed Tomography	379
Standard Film Radiography	380
Magnetic Resonance Imaging	385
Risk of Radiation from Sinus Imaging	385
References	386
Sinonasal Pathology	386
Congenital Anomalies of the Nose and Paranasal Sinuses	386
References	389
Inflammatory Diseases	390
Retention Cysts	406
Nasal Polyps	407
References	410
Tumor and Tumorlike Lesions of the Paranasal Sinuses and Nasal Cavity	412
Benign Fibro-osseous, Osseous, and Cartilaginous Lesions of the Sinonasal Region	442
Malignant Osseous and Cartilaginous Tumors of Sinonasal Cavities	457
Miscellaneous Tumors of Sinonasal Cavities	460
References	464
Traumatic and Postoperative Findings	466
References	474

Section IV Masticatory System

5 Temporomandibular Joint 477
Mahmood F. Mafee

Embryology 477
Anatomy 477
Diagnostic Imaging Techniques 481
    Nuclear Medicine (Scintigraphy) 482
    CT Technique 482
    MRI Technique 482
Normal Imaging Anatomy of TMJ 482
Anatomical Variations and Developmental Anomaly 483
    Condylar Agenesis (Otomandibular
    Dysostosis, Mandibulofacial Dysostosis, Hemifacial
    Microsomia) 483
    Condylar Hypoplasia 485
    Condylar Hyperplasia 485
Inflammation 486
    Infectious Arthritis 486
    Necrotizing External Otitis 487
Internal Derangements 487
Osteochondritis Dissecans 493
Arthritic Conditions 493
    Degenerative Arthritis
    (Osteoarthritis, Osteoarthrosis) 493
    Traumatic Arthritis 494
    Rheumatoid Arthritis 494
    Metabolic Arthritis 495
    Rheumatoid Variants (Ankylosing Spondylitis, Psoriatic
    Arthritis) 495
    Synovial Chondromatosis 497
    Neoplasms 499
    Miscellaneous 503
    Fractures 504
    Postoperative Conditions 505
References 506

6 Mandible and Maxilla 508
Alfred L. Weber
Mahmood F. Mafee

Embryology 508
    Dental Development 508
    Development of Enamel 508
    Ossification 509
Anatomy 509
    The Mandible 509
    The Maxillae 509
Dental Anatomy 510
    The Teeth 510
    Dental Blood and Lymphatic Vessels 510
    Dental Lymphatics 511
    Dental Innervation 511
    Dental Histology 511
    The Dental Pulp 511
    The Enamel, Cement, and Periodontal Ligament 511
    The Gingivae (Gums) 511
Imaging Techniques 511
    Intraoral Radiography 512
    Computed Tomography 512
    Magnetic Resonance Imaging (MRI) 512
Pathology 513
    Congenital and Developmental
    Anomalies 513
    Inflammation 514
    Osteoradionecrosis 514
    Benign and Malignant Tumors 514
References 549

Section V Suprahyoid Neck

7 Nasopharynx 555
Mahmood F. Mafee

Embryology 553
Anatomy 553
    Pharyngobasilar Fascia 556
    The Pharyngeal Tonsil and Pharyngeal Bursa 558
    Pharyngeal Isthmus, Oropharyngeal Isthmus,
    and Waldeyer's Ring 558
    Innervation 558
    Vascular Supply 558
    Lymphatics 558
    Regional Anatomy (Parapharyngeal Space) 558
    The Masticator Space 559
    Infratemporal Fossa 559
    Applied Anatomy 559
Histology 559
Imaging Techniques 559
Pathology of the Nasopharynx 560
    Congenital Anomalies 560
    Inflammations 561
    Infectious Mononucleosis 563
    Tangier Disease 563
    Benign Tumors 563
    Malignant Tumors 568
    Nasopharyngeal Carcinoma 569
References 578

8 Parapharyngeal and Masticator Spaces 580
Sherif Gamal Nour
Jonathan S. Lewin

Introduction 580
Anatomy 580
    Fascial Layers of the Neck 581
    Face and Neck Spaces 584
Normal Imaging Anatomy 589
Imaging Rationale and Techniques 592
    Computed Tomography 593
    Magnetic Resonance Imaging 593
Pathology 593
    Lesions Arising within the Pharyngeal Wall
    and Adjoining Deep Neck Spaces 594
    Suprahyoid Neck Trauma 618
    Obstructive Sleep Apnea Syndrome (OSA) 619
    Suprahyoid Neck Biopsy
    and Interventional MRI 619
References 620

9 Salivary Glands 625
Mahmood F. Mafee

Embryology 625
Anatomy 625
    Parotid Gland 625
    Submandibular and Sublingual Glands 628
    Applied Anatomy 629
Histology 630
Imaging 631
    Conventional Radiography 631
    Conventional Sialography 632
    Computerized Tomography (CT) and Magnetic
    Resonance Imaging (MRI) 633
    MR Sialography Technique
    Minerva Becker 636
    Ultrasound Technique 638
    Nuclear Medicine 638
Clinical Applications:
Pathological Conditions 638
    Congenital Lesions 638
    Inflammatory Diseases of the Major Salivary Glands ... 641
    Acquired Immunodeficiency Syndrome and Parotid
    Lymphoepithelial Lesions/Cysts 651
    Benign Lymphoepithelial Sialadenopathy
    (Autoimmune Sialosis) 654
    Neoplasms of Salivary Glands 654
References 680

10 Oral Cavity and Oropharynx 682
Minerva Becker

Introduction 682
Developmental Considerations 682
Normal Anatomy 683
Imaging Techniques 687
    CT 687
    MR Imaging 688
    Ultrasonography 688
Tumors of the Oral Cavity and Oropharynx 688
    Squamous Cell Carcinoma 688
    Non–Squamous Cell Neoplasms 703
Inflammatory Lesions of the Oral Cavity
and Oropharynx 711
Congenital Lesions 719
Miscellaneous Pathology 723
Acknowledgments 725
References 725

Section VI   Infrahyoid Neck

11 Larynx and Hypopharynx 731
Minerva Becker

Introduction 731
Developmental Considerations 731
Normal Anatomy 732
    Larynx 732
    Hypopharynx 735
    Tissue Characteristics on Sectional Imaging 737
Imaging Techniques 738
    Computed Tomography 738
    Magnetic Resonance Imaging 738
    Other Imaging Modalities 739
Squamous Cell Carcinoma 739
    Epidemiology and Rationale
    for Imaging 739
    Tumor Sites and Patterns of Tumor Spread 740
    Invasion of the Deep Paralaryngeal Spaces 747
    Cartilage Invasion 747
    Pretherapeutic T-Classification According to the TNM
    System 752
    Atypical Forms of Squamous
    Cell Carcinoma 753
Non–Squamous Cell Neoplasms 755
    Vasoformative Tumors 756
    Tumors of the Laryngeal Skeleton 757
    Tumors of the Lymphoreticular System 757
    Tumors of the Minor Salivary Glands 758
    Tumors of Fatty Tissue 759
    Metastases to the Larynx 759
    Myogenic Tumors 761
    Neurogenic Tumors 761
Morphological Changes Induced by Tumor Treatment
and Detection of Tumor Recurrence 761
    Surgical Procedures, Postoperative Changes,
    and Tumor Recurrence in the Operated Larynx 761
    Radiation-Induced Changes and Tumor Recurrence
    in the Irradiated Larynx 764
Cystic Lesions, Pouches,
Diverticula, and Webs 768
    Larynx 768
    Hypopharynx 770
Infectious and Inflammatory Conditions 772
Congenital Lesions 774
Vocal Cord Paralysis 775
Trauma 775
    Larynx 775
    Hypopharynx 775
References 777

12 Other Infrahyoid Neck Lesions 780
Minerva Becker

Introduction 780
Anatomy 780
Imaging Techniques 787
    CT Scanning 787
    MR Imaging 787
    Ultrasonography 787
    Nuclear Medicine Studies
    of the Thyroid Gland 788
    FDG-PET 788
Neoplastic Lesions 788
    Nodal Neoplasms 788
    Nonnodal Neoplasms 797
    Thyroid and Parathyroid Gland Masses 807
Imaging of the Neck after Treatment 813
    Radiation-Induced Changes in the Neck 813
    Postoperative Changes after Various Types of
    Neck Dissection and Reconstruction with Flaps .. 820
Infectious and Inflammatory Conditions 823
    Cervical Chain Nodal Inflammation and Infection . 824
    Infection of the Retropharyngeal Space 827
    Bacterial Soft-Tissue Infections 829
    Complications of Bacterial Infections 831
    Vertebral Body Spondylodiskitis 832

Inflammatory Diseases of Neck Muscles and Tendons .. 832
Inflammatory Lesions of the Thyroid Gland 833
Branchial Cleft Anomalies 834
Thyroglossal Duct Cyst 837
Vascular Malformations 839

Miscellaneous Pathology 840
Acknowledgments 842
References 842

Index 846

Abbreviations used for Imaging Techniques

2D FSE	2D fast spin-echo sequence	HU	Hounsfield unit
3D FSE	3D fast spin-echo sequence	MIP	maximum intensity projection
CECT	contrast-enhanced CT	MRA	magnetic resonance angiography
CISS	constructive interference in steady state	MRV	magnetic resonance venography
DTPA	diethylenetriaminepentaacetic acid	NCCT	noncontrast CT
DWI	diffusion-weighted image/imaging	PD	proton density
EXPRESS	extended phase symmetry rapid spin echo sequence	PET	positron emission tomography
FDG	2-(^{18}F)fluoro-2-deoxy-D-glucose	RARE	rapid acquisition with relaxation enhancement
FISP	fast imaging with steady-state precession	STIR	short tau inversion recovery
FLAIR	fluid-attenuated inversion recovery	T1W	T1-weighted
FLASH	fast low angle shot	T2W	T2-weighted
FSE	fast spin-echo	TE	echo time
FSEIR	fast spin-echo inversion recovery	TI	inversion time
GRASE	gradient and spin echo	TR	repetition time
GRASS	gradient-recalled acquisition in the steady state	US	ultrasonography/ultrasound
HASTE	half acquisition single-shot turbo spin-echo technique		

Section I   Temporal Bone

Chapter 1 Imaging of the Temporal Bone

Sectional Anatomy of the Temporal Bone 3

Imaging Techniques 30

Developmental Variations 36

Congenital Abnormalities of the Temporal Bone 41

Temporal Bone Trauma 54

Acute Otitis Media, Mastoiditis, and Malignant Necrotizing External Otitis 62

Chronic Otitis Media and Mastoiditis 68

Cholesteatoma of the Middle Ear 74

Postoperative and Postirradiation Imaging of the Temporal Bone 90

Tumors 95

Internal Auditory Canal and Acoustic Schwannomas 109

Otosclerosis and Bone Dystrophies 122

References 132

1 Imaging of the Temporal Bone

Galdino E. Valvassori

Sectional Anatomy of the Temporal Bone

■ Anatomical Notes

Mastoid

The mastoid air cells are a series of intercommunicating cavities lined by mucous membrane. The mastoid antrum is the largest air cell and communicates anteriorly with the attic through an opening called the aditus.

External Auditory Canal

The canal is approximately 2.5–3.5 cm long and 6–9 mm wide. The outer one-third is formed by an extension of the cartilage of the auricle, the inner two-thirds by the incomplete ring of the tympanic bone. The canal and the outer surface of the tympanic membrane are lined by skin.

Tympanic Membrane

The membrane separates the external auditory canal from the middle ear cavity and consists of a fibroelastic layer covered on the outer surface by the canal skin and on the medial surface by the middle ear mucosa. The circumference of the membrane is thickened and forms a fibrocartilage ring (annulus) that is open anterosuperiorly. The adjacent triangular segment of the membrane bordered by the mallear folds is devoid of fibroelastic layer, thus dividing the membrane into a small pars flaccida and a large pars tensa. The membrane is convex medially and the handle of the malleus, which is firmly attached to the inner surface of the membrane, reaches the point of greatest convexity, called the umbo.

Middle Ear

The middle ear or tympanic cavity is an air-filled irregular space bounded laterally by the tympanic membrane and above it by the lateral attic wall, medially by the capsule of the inner ear, superiorly by the tegmen tympani, and inferiorly by the hypotympanic floor. It is divided into three portions: medial to the tympanic membrane, the mesotympanum; above the epitympanic recess or attic; and below the level of the canal floor, the hypotympanum, which covers the jugular bulb. The eustachian tube and the tensor tympani canal open in the anterior wall. In the posterior wall of the mesotympanum is the pyramidal eminence, a hollowed conical bony protrusion that houses the stapedius muscle and transmits its tendon. Lateral to the pyramidal eminence is the facial recess, which covers the upper portion of the mastoid segment of the facial canal; medial is the sinus tympani, a posterior pocket of mesotypanum of variable depths.

The medial or labyrinthine wall of the middle ear presents an upper bulge formed by the horizontal semicircular canal and a lower rounded elevation (the promontory) due to the lateral aspect of the basal turn of the cochlea. Posterior to the promontory are the depression of the oval (vestibular) and round (cochlear) windows.

Within the middle ear space is an ossicular chain made up of three small ossicles. In the attic, the head of the malleus articulates with the incus body, which narrows posteriorly to form its short process. The malleus handle extends inferiorly to the tympanic membrane; the long process of the incus articulates with the head of the stapes.

Facial Nerve

The facial nerve exits the brain about 2 mm anterior to the eighth cranial nerve, crosses the cerebellopontine cistern, and enters the internal auditory canal anterosuperior to the acoustic nerve. At the fundus of the canal, the facial nerve enters the facial or fallopian canal, which runs anterolaterally to the geniculate ganglion (labyrinthine or petrous segment) where the greater petrosal nerve leaves the ganglion to join the deep petrosal nerve and thus forming the vidian nerve. At the geniculate ganglion, the nerve makes a sharp turn (anterior genu) and then follows the entire medial wall of the middle ear, passing just above the oval window (tympanic segment). At the level of the pyramidal eminence, the facial nerve turns again (pyramidal turn) and passes downward to the stylomastoid foramen (mastoid segment), where it exits the temporal bone to enter the parotid gland.

Inner Ear

The bony labyrinth, which lies within the petrous pyramid, is filled with perilymph. The smaller membranous labyrinth, which contains endolymph, lies within the bony labyrinth and floats in the perilymph. The perilymphatic space is in direct communication with the subarachnoid space via the cochlear aqueduct. The endolymph-filled spaces have no connection with the subarachnoid space and terminate in the closed endolymphatic sac, which lies under the dura of the posterior cranial fossa.

The bony labyrinth consists of the cochlea, vestibule, and semicircular canals. The membranous labyrinth includes the cochlear duct within the cochlea, the utricle and saccule within the vestibule, and the membranous semicircular canals. The overall volume of the bony labyrinth is 0.2 cm^3 or 200 µl.[3] The membranous labyrinth volume is approximately one-fifth of the bony labyrinth, namely 0.04 cm^3 or 40 µl.

■ Sectional Anatomy

The normal sectional anatomy will be illustrated by macrosections of the temporal bone obtained in the axial, coronal, 20° coronal oblique, and sagittal planes. Each section will be compared to the corresponding microradiograph and CT image.[31] However, whereas all microradiographs and sagittal CT images were obtained from the same temporal bone as the macrosections, the axial, coronal, and 20° coronal oblique CT images are from other studies on living objects. This explains why the CT sections are similar but not identical to the corresponding macrosections and microradiographs.

Axial Sections

Figure 1.1 exposes structures in a 2 mm thick axial section of a right adult temporal bone, 2 mm inferior to the arcuate eminence. The mastoid air cells occupy the lateral portion of the sec-

1 Imaging of the Temporal Bone

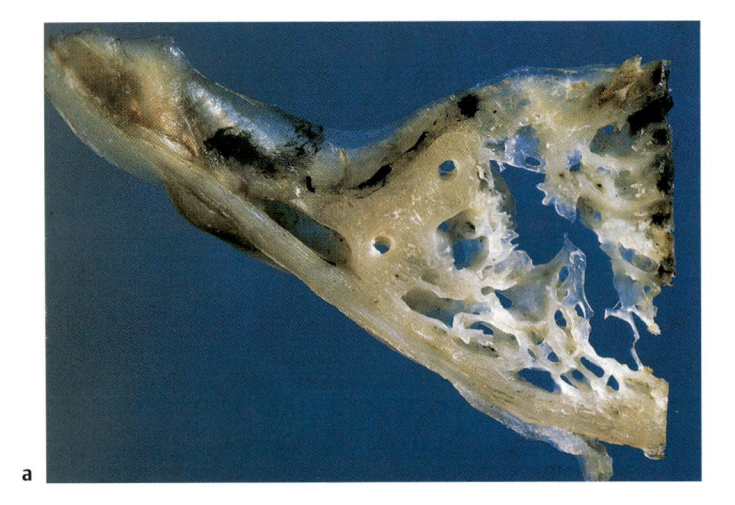

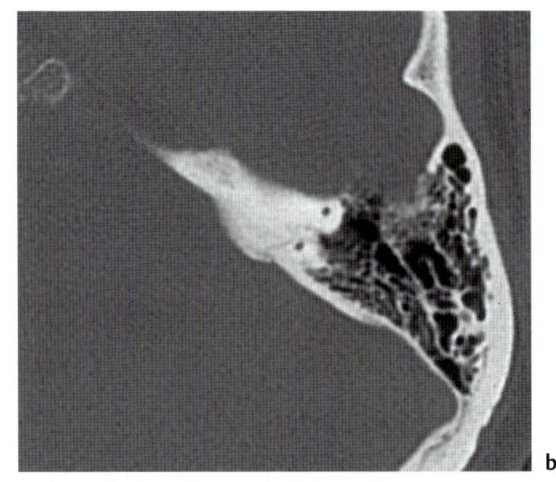

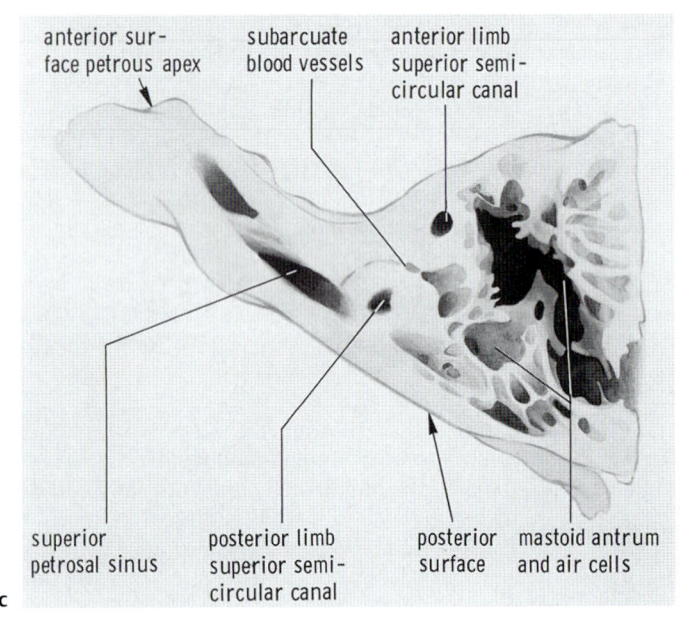

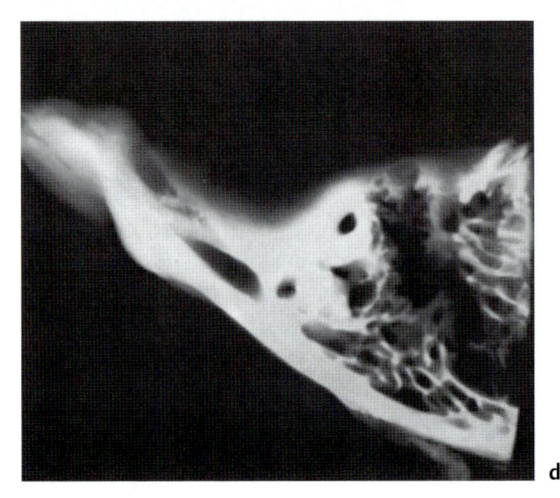

Fig. 1.1 a Axial macrosection 2 mm below the arcuate eminence.
b CT corresponding to **a**.
c Structures seen at this level.
d Microradiograph corresponding to **a, b**.

tion; the anterior and posterior limbs of the superior semicircular canal are in the center. Subarcuate vessels pass between the limbs of the superior canal. The superior petrosal sinus courses along the superior margin of the petrous apex.

Figure 1.2 shows the structures in a 2 mm thick axial section of a right adult temporal bone immediately inferior to Figure 1.1. The aditus of the mastoid antrum opens into the epitympanum. Mastoid air cells surround the epitympanum and antrum. Superior portions of the malleus head and incus body appear in the epitympanum. The nonampullated limbs of the superior and posterior semicircular canals join at the crus commune. The subarcuate vessels pass from the subarcuate fossa laterally between the limbs of the superior semicircular canal. The horizontal semicircular canal forms the medial wall of the antrum, and the ampullated portions of the horizonal and superior semicircular canals open into the superior portion of the vestibule. This section also exposes the roof of the internal auditory canal.

Figures 1.3 and 1.4 reveal the structures seen in the upper and lower surfaces of a 2 mm thick axial section of a right adult temporal bone immediately inferior to Figure 1.2. Mastoid air cells surround the antrum and extend lateral to the epitympanum. The malleus head and incus body occupy the epitympanum, and the incus short process rests in the fossa incudis. The cavity of the epitympanum assumes a somewhat triangular shape at this level. The medial and lateral epitympanic walls converge posteriorly at the aditus, while the base of the triangle lies anteriorly. The medial wall forms a 20–25° angle with the sagittal plane crossing the fossa incudis. The lateral wall forms a 10° angle lateral to the sagittal plane through the fossa incudis.

The ampullated end of the horizontal semicircular canal enters the vestibule anteriorly (Fig. 1.3), and the nonampullated end opens into the posterior portion of the vestibule (Fig. 1.4) The posterior semicircular canal extends posterolaterally from the crus commune. The macula of the utricle stretches across the upper portion of the vestibule (Fig. 1.4a). The facial and superior vestibular nerves occupy the internal auditory canal. The superior vestibular nerve arches toward the utricular macula and the ampullae of the horizontal and superior semicircular canals (Fig. 1.3a). The petrous or labyrinthine portion of the facial nerve extends from the internal auditory canal to the geniculate ganglion. At the geniculate ganglion, the facial nerve turns sharply into the horizontal portion and extends posteriorly along the medial wall of the tympanum just below the horizontal semicircular canal (Figs. 1.3a, 1.4b). Superior portions of the basal and middle coils of the cochlea appear anterior to the fundus of the internal auditory canal. The superior turn of the vestibular aqueduct passes adjacent to the posterior semicircular canal (Figs. 1.3b, 1.4b).

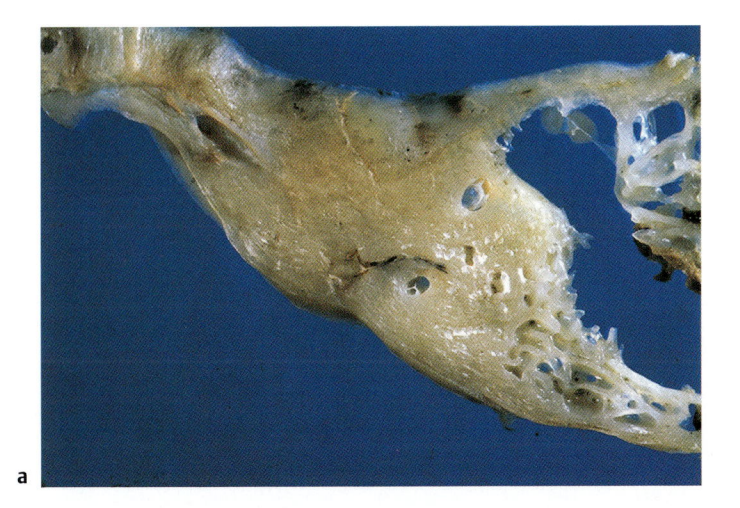

Sectional Anatomy of the Temporal Bone 5

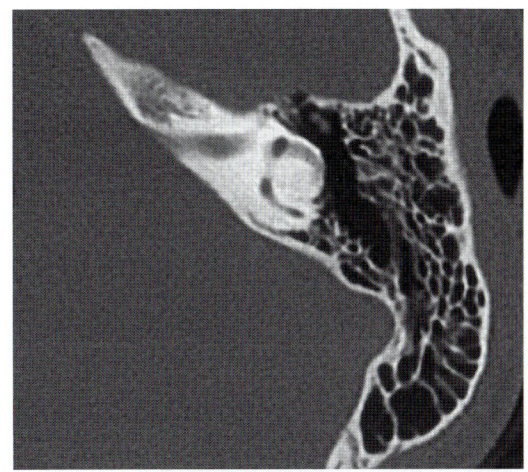

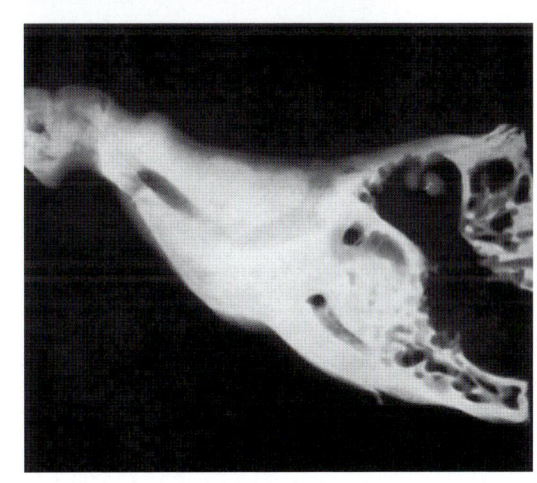

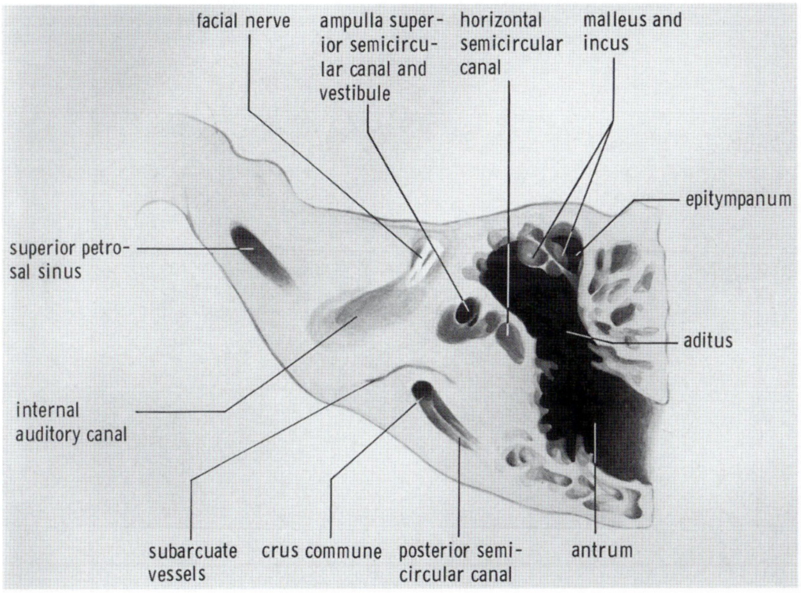

Fig. 1.2 a Axial macrosection immediately inferior to Fig. 1.1 a.
b CT corresponding to **a**.
c Structures seen at this level.
d Microradiograph corresponding to **a**, **b**.

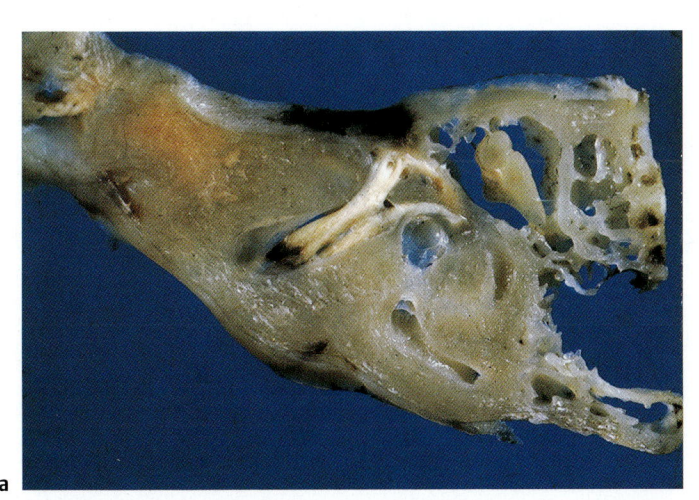

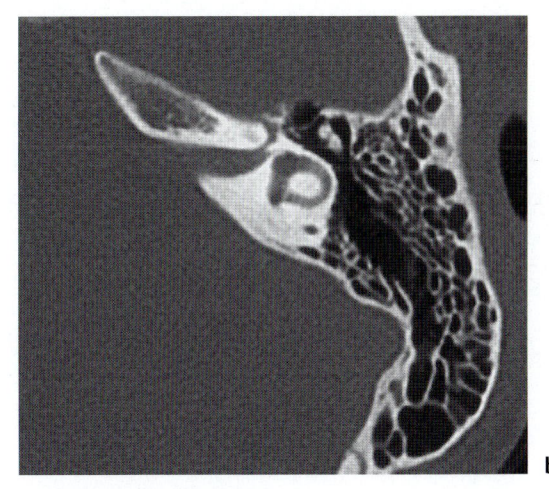

Fig. 1.3 a Upper surface of an axial macrosection immediately inferior to Fig. 1.2 a.
b CT corresponding to **a**.

Figures 1.5 and 1.6 demonstrate the structures seen in the upper and lower surfaces of a 2 mm thick axial section of a right, adult temporal bone, immediately inferior to Figure 1.4. The sections cross the mastoid antrum and the superior wall of the external auditory canal. The tendon of the tensor tympani muscle stretches from the cochleariform process to the neck of the malleus. The tensor tympani muscle appears on the inferior surface of the section (Fig. 1.6 a). In the oval window, the stapes footplate is canted slightly downward, and the incudostapedial joint lies slightly below the level of the footplate (Fig. 1.6 c). The facial nerve extends from the oval window to the second turn. The stapedius tendon and the pyramidal eminence lie anteromedial

1 Imaging of the Temporal Bone

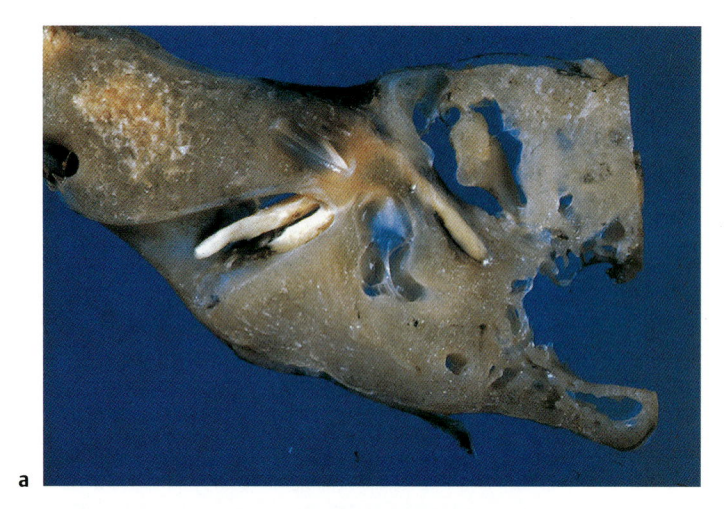

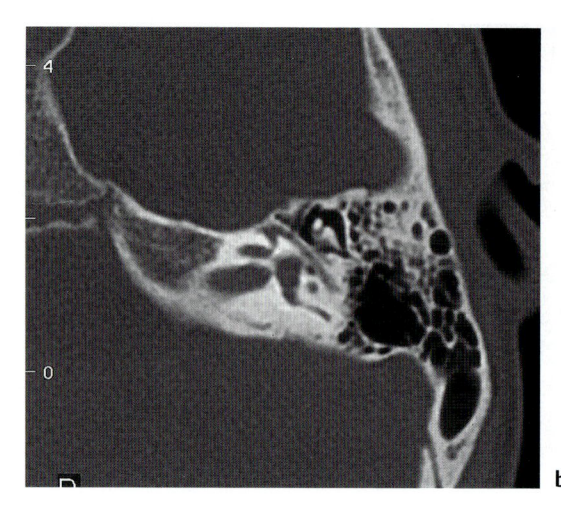

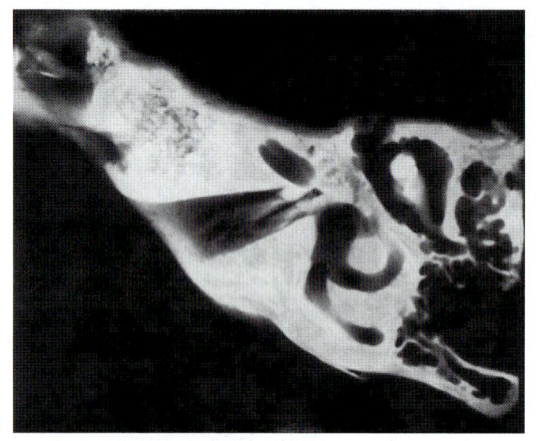

Fig. 1.4 a Lower surface of an axial macrosection 2 mm inferior to Fig. 1.2 a.
b CT corresponding to a.
c Microradiograph of macrosection corresponding to Figs. 1.3 a, 1.4 a.
d Structures seen at this level (Figs. 1.3, 1.4).

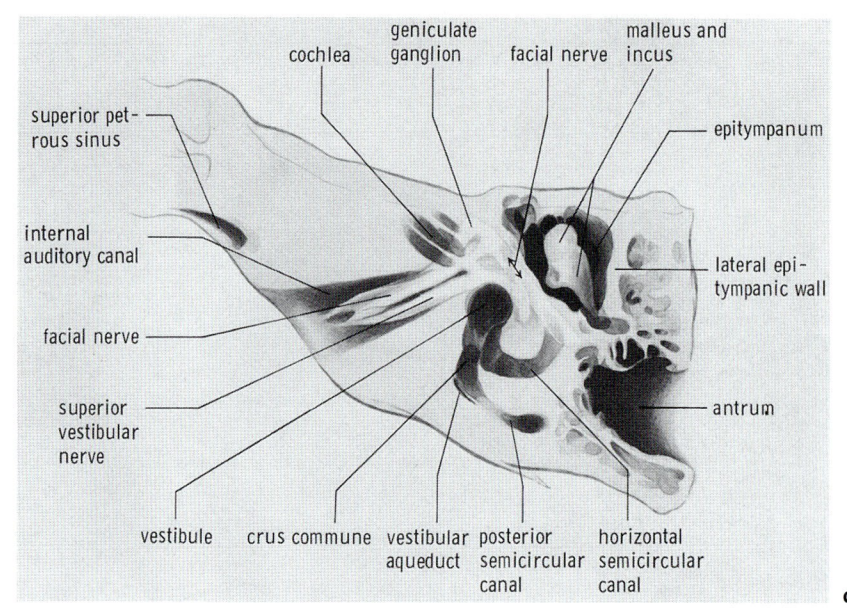

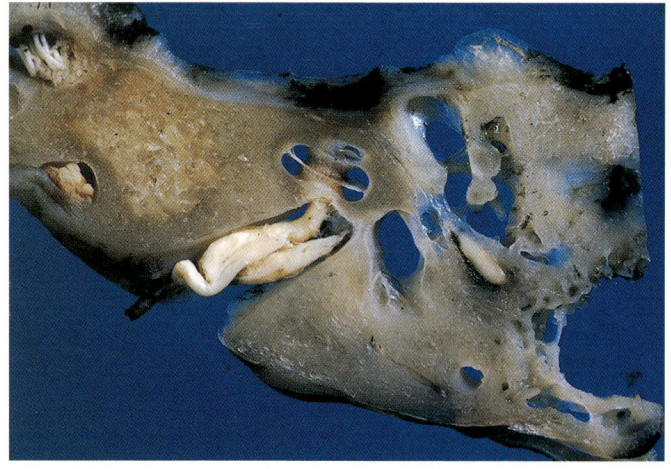

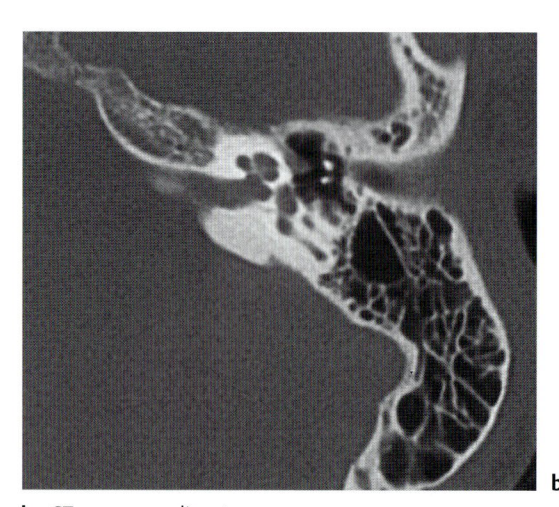

Fig. 1.5 a Upper surface of an axial macrosection immediately inferior to Fig. 1.4 a.
b CT corresponding to a.

Sectional Anatomy of the Temporal Bone

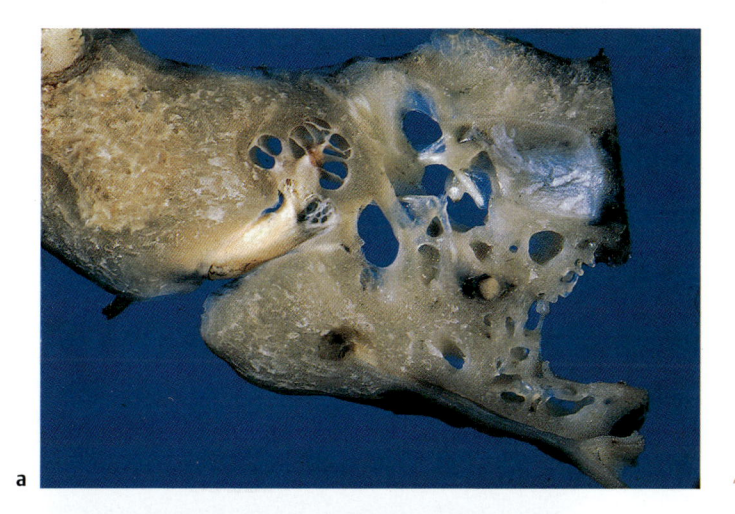

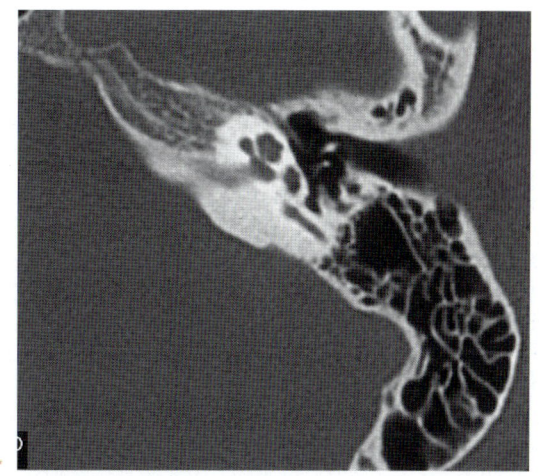

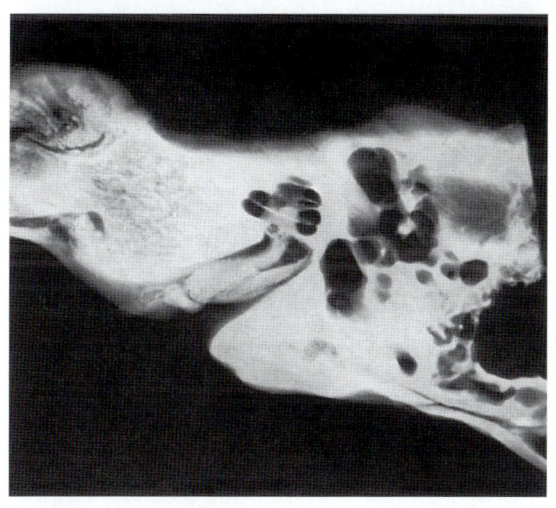

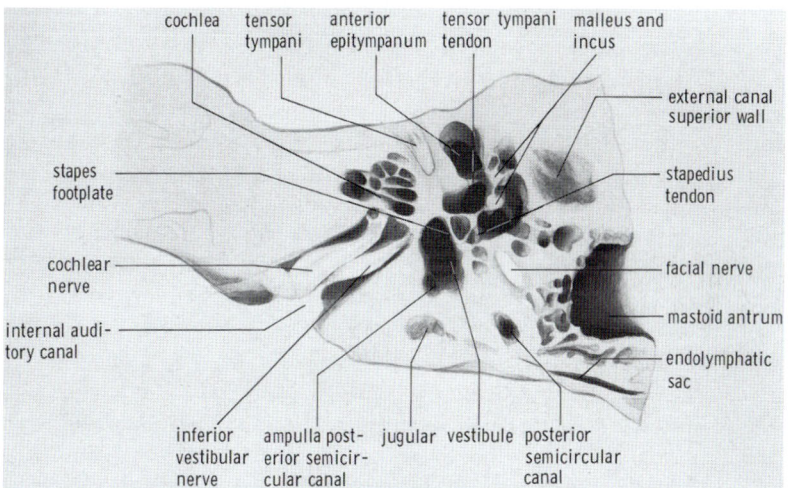

Fig. 1.6 a Lower surface of an axial macrosection 2 mm inferior to Fig. 1.4 a.
b CT corresponding to **a**.
c Microradiograph of macrosection corresponding to Figs. 1.5 a, 1.6 a.
d Structures seen at this level (Figs. 1.5, 1.6).

to the facial nerve (Fig. 1.6 a). The stapes footplate at this level forms the lateral wall of the vestibule. The membranous ampullated end of the posterior semicircular canal joins the utricle on the posteromedial margin of the vestibule (Fig. 1.6 a). The nerve to the ampulla of the posterior semicircular canal leaves the internal auditory canal at the foramen singulare (Fig. 1.6 a, b). The posterior semicircular canal lies anterior to the vestibular aqueduct. At this level the endolymphatic sac enters the vestibular aqueduct. The section passes through the modiolus and three turns of the cochlea. In the internal auditory canal, the cochlear nerve turns anteriorly into the modiolus 2 mm medial to the fundus of the canal. The cochlear and inferior vestibular nerves lie in the inferior compartment of the internal auditory canal.

1 Imaging of the Temporal Bone

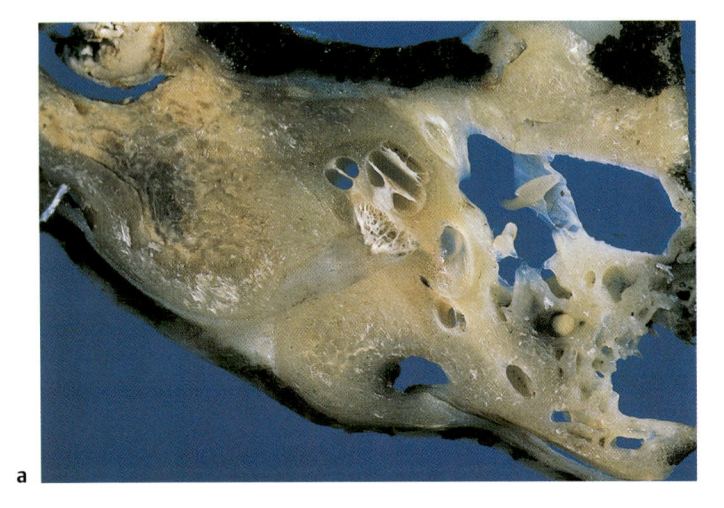

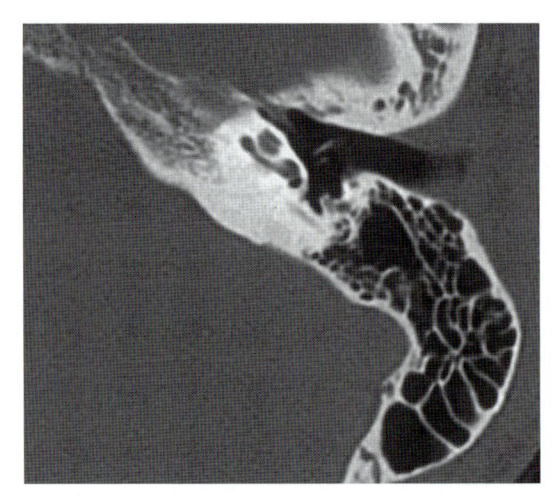

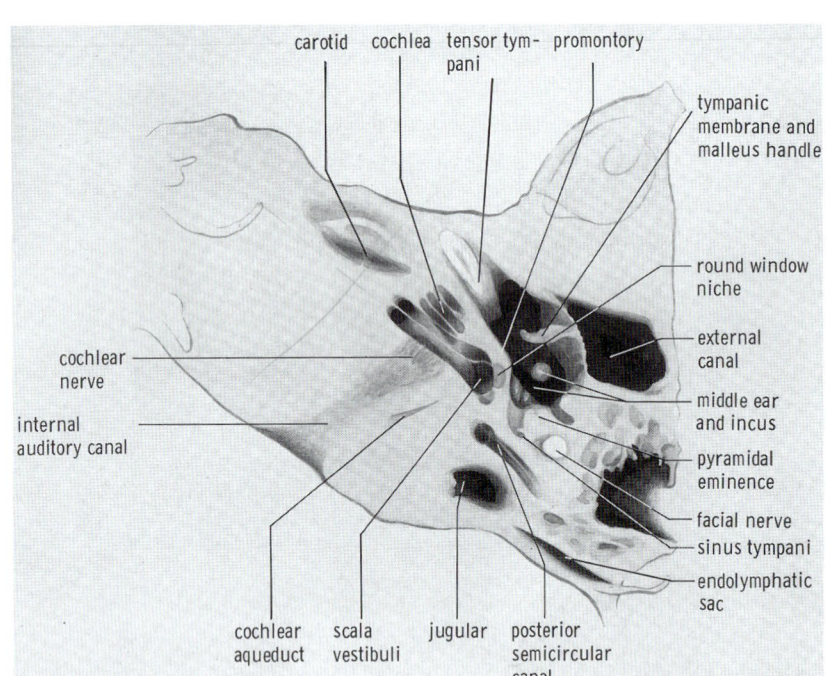

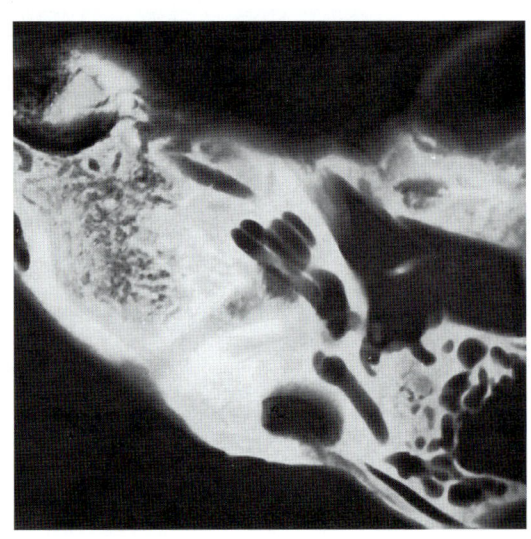

Fig. 1.7 a Axial macrosection immediately inferior to Fig. 1.6 a.
b CT corresponding to **a**.
c Structures seen at this level.
d Micrograph of macrosection corresponding to **a, b**.

Figure 1.7 shows the structures in a 2 mm thick axial section of a right adult temporal bone immediately inferior to Figure 1.6. A section of the tympanic membrane with a portion of the malleus handle separates the external canal from the middle ear. The lenticular process of the incus lies just posterior to the malleus handle. The tensor tympani canal lies on the anterior portion of the medial wall of the middle ear. The descending portion of the facial nerve lies in the posterior wall of the middle ear lateral to the pyramidal eminence and to the tympanic sinus. The proximal portion of the basal coil of the cochlea forms the promontory of the medial wall of the middle ear. All three coils of the cochlea appear. The spiral lamina separates the scala vestibuli from the scala tympani. In the niche of the round window, the round window membrane closes the scala tympani. The ampulla of the posterior semicircular canal, as it enters the inferior and posterior portion of the vestibule, lies close to the round window. The posterior semicircular canal arches posteriorly within the thickness of the tissue section between the facial canal anteriorly and the endolymphatic sac posteriorly. The dome of the jugular fossa lies medial to the middle ear. The cochlear aqueduct passes from the posterior surface of the bone to the round window area.

Sectional Anatomy of the Temporal Bone

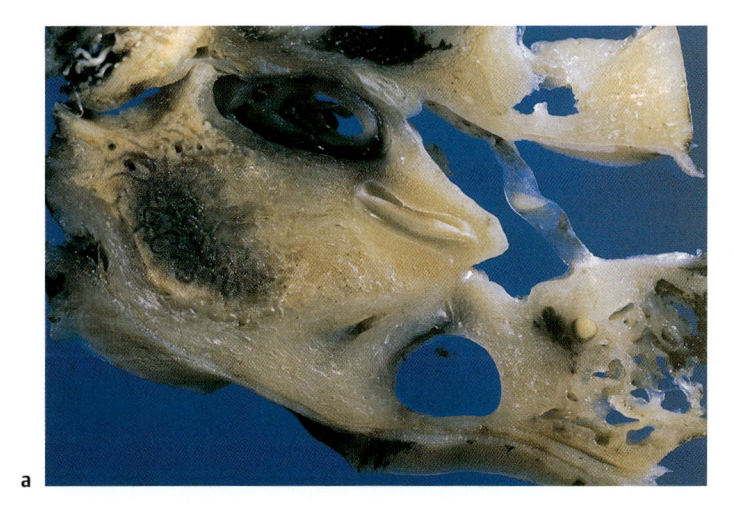

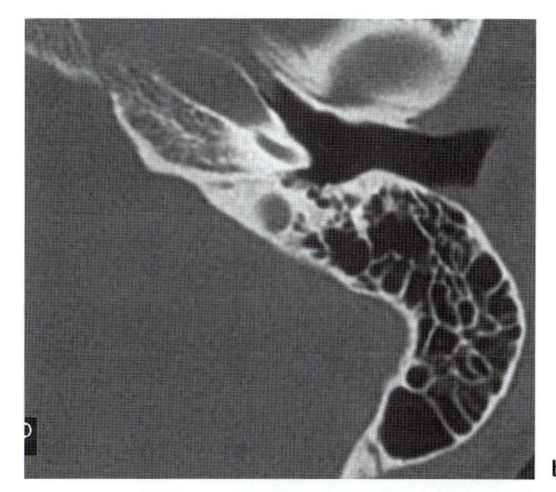

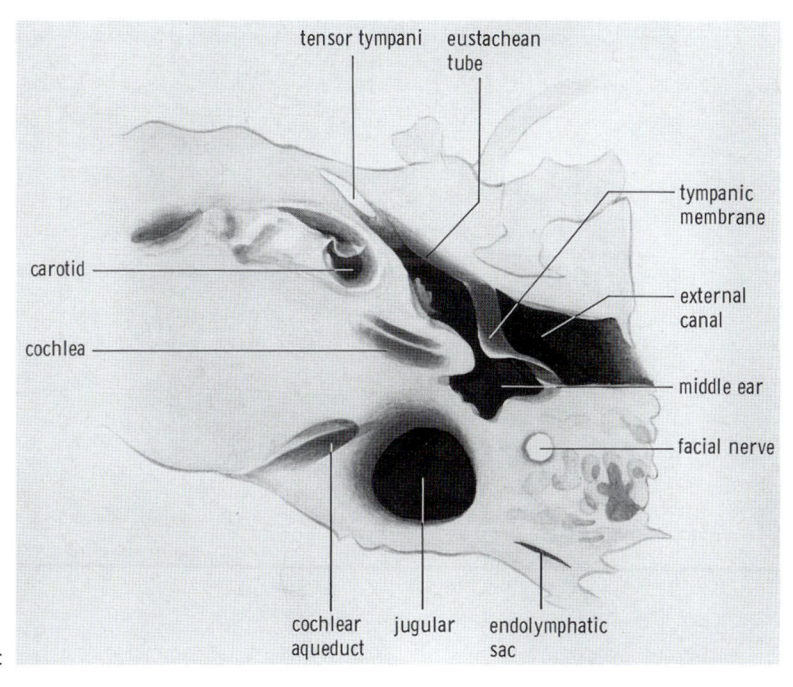

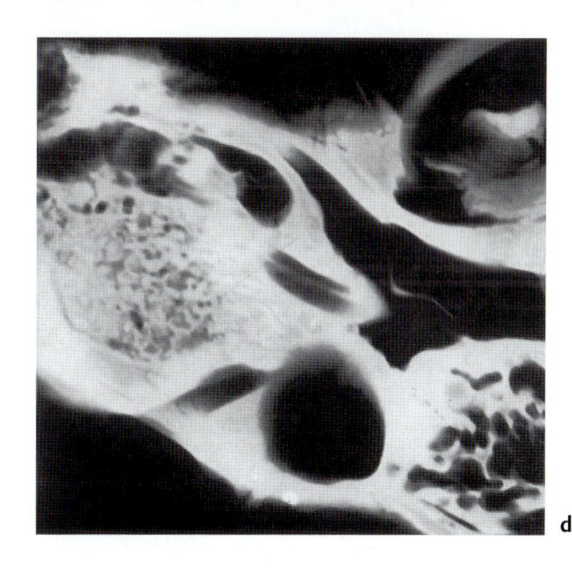

Fig. 1.8 a Axial section immediately inferior to Fig. 1.7 a.
b CT corresponding to a.
c Structures seen at this level.
d Micrograph of macrosection corresponding to a, b.

Figure 1.8 reveals the structures in a 2 mm thick axial section of a right adult temporal bone immediately inferior to Figure 1.7. The tip of the malleus handle lies at the umbo in a strip of the tympanic membrane. The tensor tympani muscle lies superior and lateral to the internal carotid artery. The carotid artery lies anterior to the basal turn of the cochlea on the medial wall of the bony eustachian tube. The descending facial nerve lies lateral to the jugular fossa. The inferior portion of the basal turn of the cochlea bounds the medial wall of the middle ear. The cochlear aqueduct lies medial to the jugular fossa and widens as it opens into the subarachnoid space.

1 Imaging of the Temporal Bone

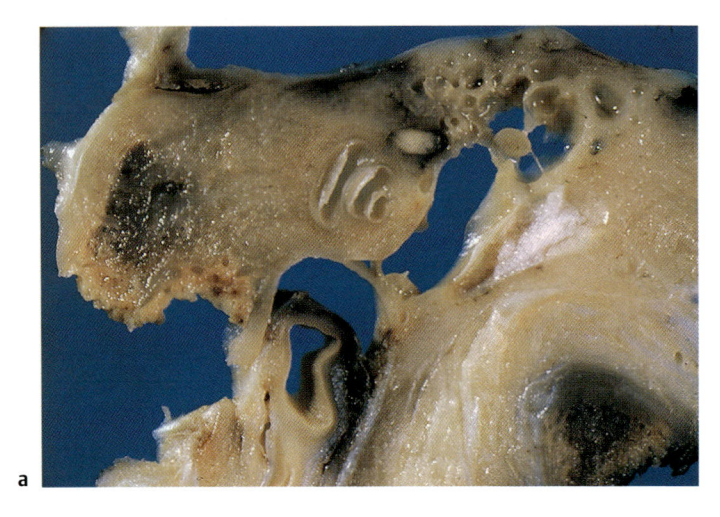

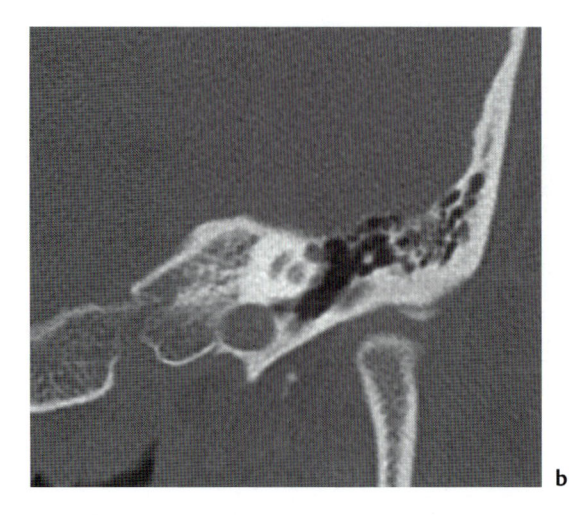

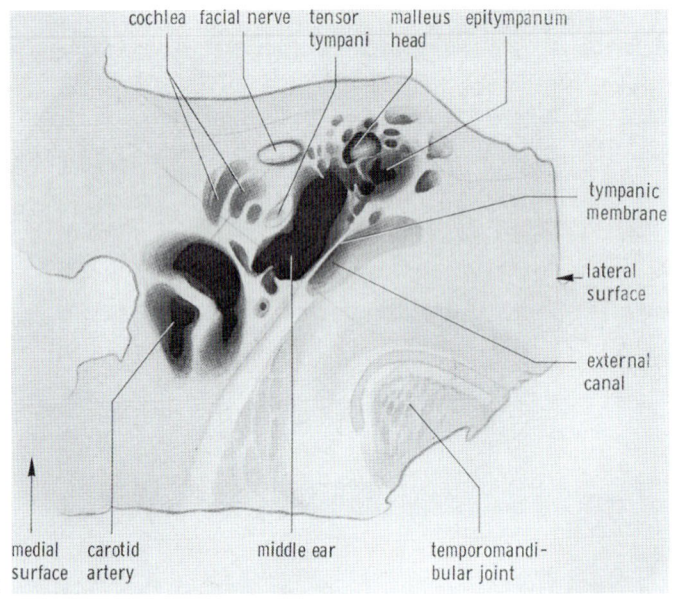

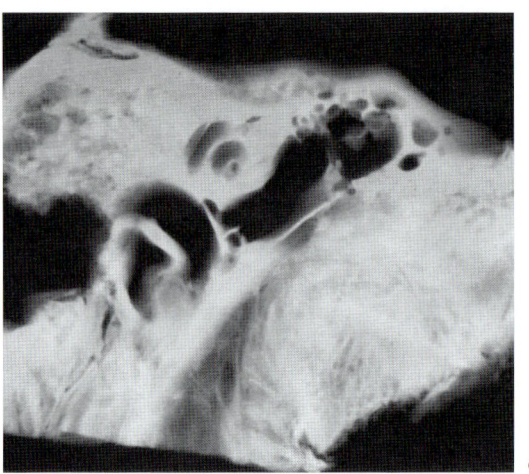

Fig. 1.9 a Coronal macrosection.
b CT corresponding to **a**.
c Structures seen at this level.
d Microradiograph corresponding to **a**, **b**.

Coronal Sections

Figure 1.**9** exposes the structures in a 2 mm thick coronal section of a left adult temporal bone at the level of the anterior wall of the external auditory canal, the most anterior portion of the tympanic membrane, and the posterior aspect of the temporomandibular joint. A small slice of the malleus head appears in the epitympanum. A thin bony septum separates the hypotympanum from the carotid canal. The geniculate ganglion of the facial nerve lies above the cochlea, while the tensor tympani canal lies on the medial wall of the middle ear.

Figure 1.**10** demonstrates the structures present in a 2 mm thick coronal section of an adult left temporal bone, immediately posterior to Figure 1.**9**. A thin section of tympanic membrane divides the external auditory canal from the middle ear. A small area of the pars flaccida is retracted above the mallear short process in the notch of Rivinus. The tendon of the tensor tympani stretches across the middle ear from the cochleariform process to the mallear neck. The lateral wall of the epitympanum joins the superior wall of the external auditory canal in a sharp edge lateral to the malleus neck. A portion of the body of the incus projects laterally from the articulation with the malleus head. This accounts for the characteristic bilobed appearance of the ossicular mass. Within the thickness of the tissue section, the facial nerve bifurcates from the geniculate ganglion into the labyrinthine and tympanic segments. In the CT image, this bifurca-

Sectional Anatomy of the Temporal Bone

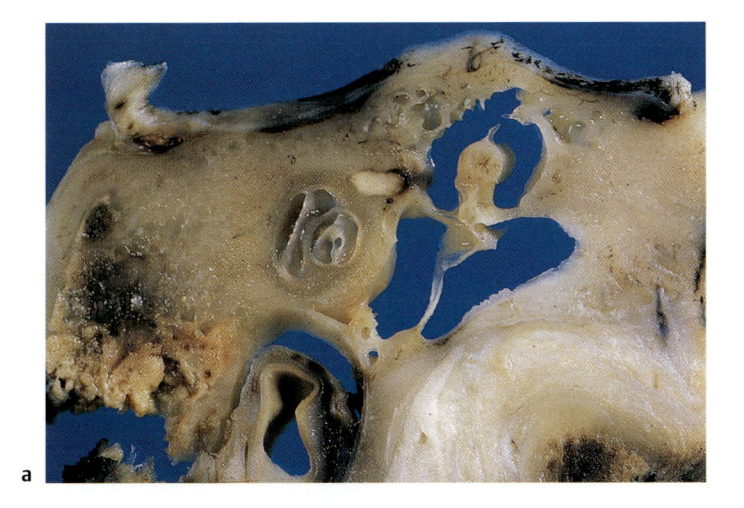

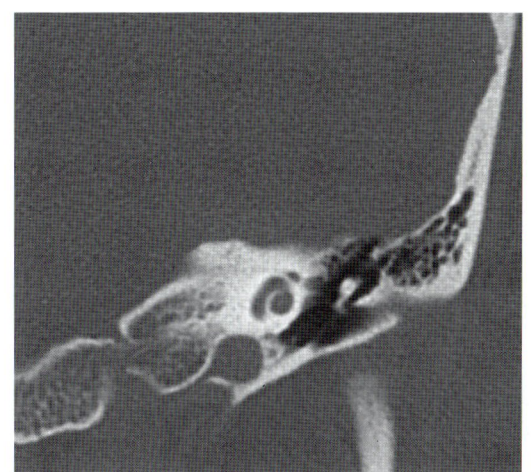

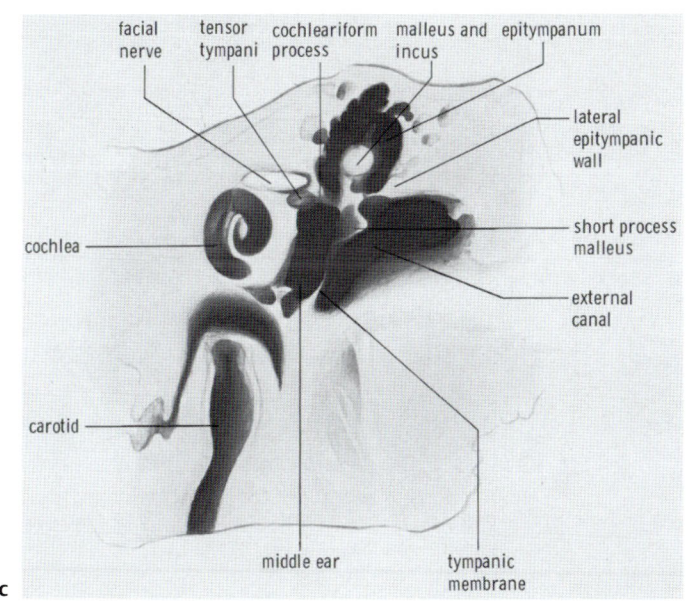

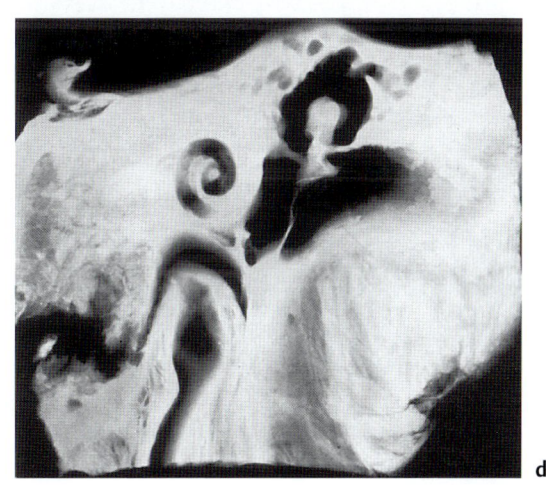

Fig. 1.**10 a** Coronal macrosection 2 mm posterior to Fig. 1.**9 a**.
b CT corresponding to **a**.
c Stuctures seen at this level.
d Microradiograph corresponding to **a**, **b**.

tion appears as paired, adjacent, circular foramina. Portions of the basal, middle, and apical coils of the cochlea lie superior to the carotid canal.

Figure 1.**11** demonstrates the structures in a 2 mm thick coronal section of a left adult temporal bone immediately posterior to Figure 1.**10**. The tympanic membrane with the malleus handle attached separates the external canal form the middle ear. The inferior margin of the lateral attic wall and the superior wall of the external canal form a triangular projection (scutum) with the apex directed medially.

Portions of the body and long process of the incus lie in the epitympanum between the prominence of the horizontal semicircular canal and the lateral epitympanic wall. The tympanic portion of the facial nerve lies below the horizontal semicircular canal and above the anterior margin of the oval window. A small anterior portion of the stapes footplate and anterior crus are in the oval window. The proximal portion of the facial nerve lies in the upper compartment of the internal auditory canal. The tissue section (Fig. 1.**11 a**) reveals the anterior wall of the vestibule, the horizontal and superior semicircular canals. Portions of the membranous labyrinth are present within the lumina of the vestibule and semicirular canals.

Below the facial nerve, the cochlear nerve enters the foraminous spiral tract of the modiolus. The proximal part of the basal coil of the cochlea forms the promontory of the medial wall of the middle ear. The carotid artery canal lies inferiorly.

1 Imaging of the Temporal Bone

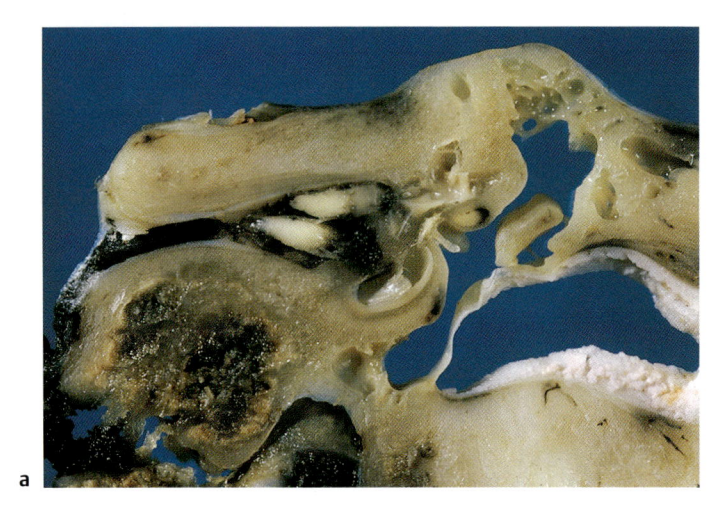

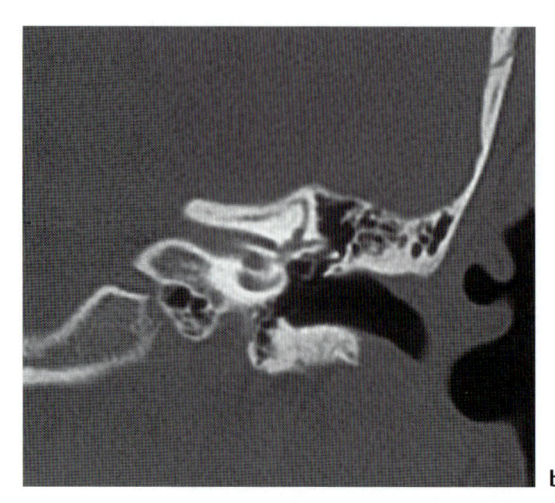

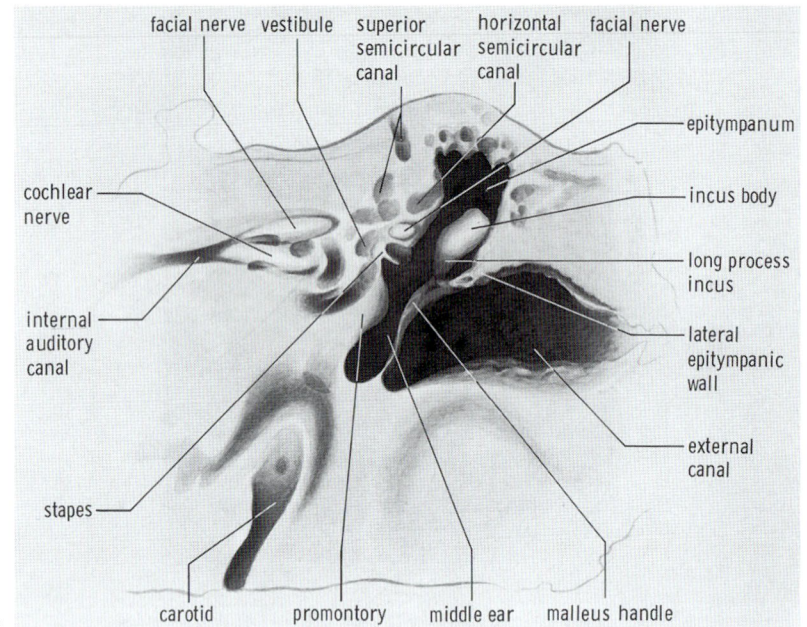

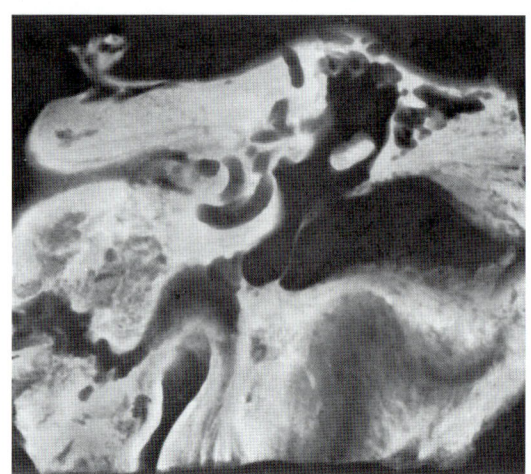

Fig. 1.11 a Coronal macrosection 2 mm posterior to Fig. 1.10 a.
b CT corresponding to a.
c Stuctures seen at this level.
d Microradiograph corresponding to a, b.

Figures 1.12 and 1.13 show the structures in the anterior and posterior surfaces of a 2 mm thick coronal section of an adult left temporal bone immediately posterior to Figure 1.11. The tympanic membrane separates the external and middle ears. The long process of the incus extends to the stapes. A portion of the long process is missing in the tissue section (Fig. 1.12 a). The tip of the short process of the incus lies in the aditus between the lateral epitympanic wall and the prominence of the horizontal semicircular canal (Fig. 1.13 a). The mastoid antrum extends superiorly and posteriorly from the aditus. The tissue sections expose the vestibule and the ampullated portions of the superior and horizontal semicircular canals. The utricle and the macula of the utricle occupy the upper portion of the bony vestibule. A portion of the saccule lies on the medial vestibular wall. The facial nerve appears between the horizontal semicircular canal and the oval window. This section includes most of the stapes footplate and superstructure. The scala vestibuli opens into the inferior portion of the vestibule, while the scala tympani extends to the round window. There are segments of the facial and acoustic cranial nerves in the internal auditory canal.

Figure 1.14 reveals the structures in a 2 mm thick coronal section of a left adult temporal bone immediately posterior to Fig. 1.13. The section exposes the external auditory canal and the posterior portion of the middle ear. The horizontal semicircular canal protrudes into the mastoid antrum. The superior semicircular canal joins the crus commune above the vestibule. The facial nerve lies inferior to the horizontal semicircular canal. The pyramidal eminence with the tendon of the stapedius muscle is below the facial nerve. The extension of the middle ear medial to the pyramidal eminence represents the sinus tympani. The facial recess lies between the facial nerve and the posterosuperior portion of the tympanic membrane. The ampullated end of the pos-

Sectional Anatomy of the Temporal Bone 13

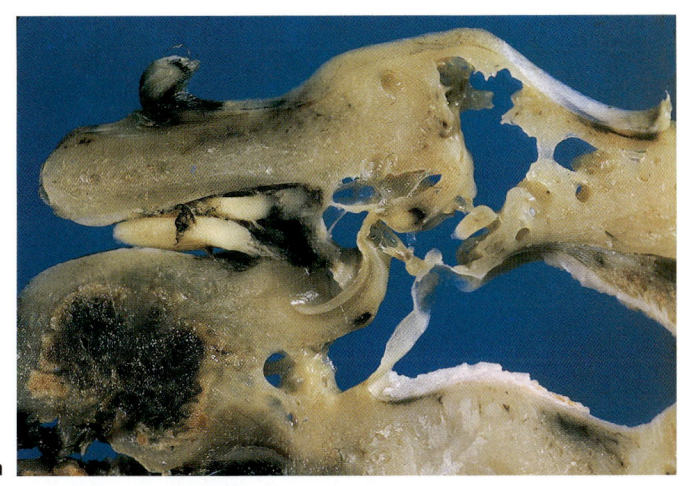

Fig. 1.**12 a** Anterior surface of coronal macrosection 2 mm posterior to Fig. 1.**11 a**.
b CT corresponding to **a**.

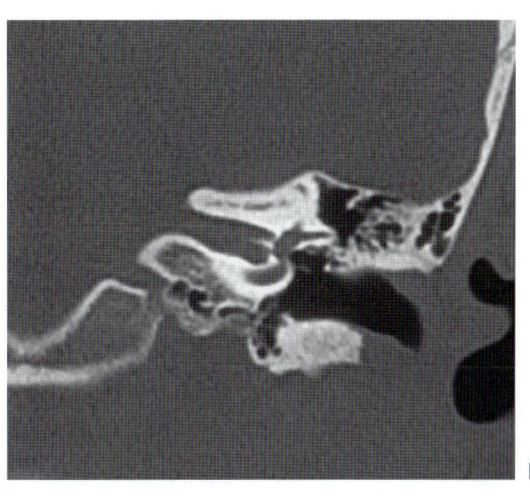

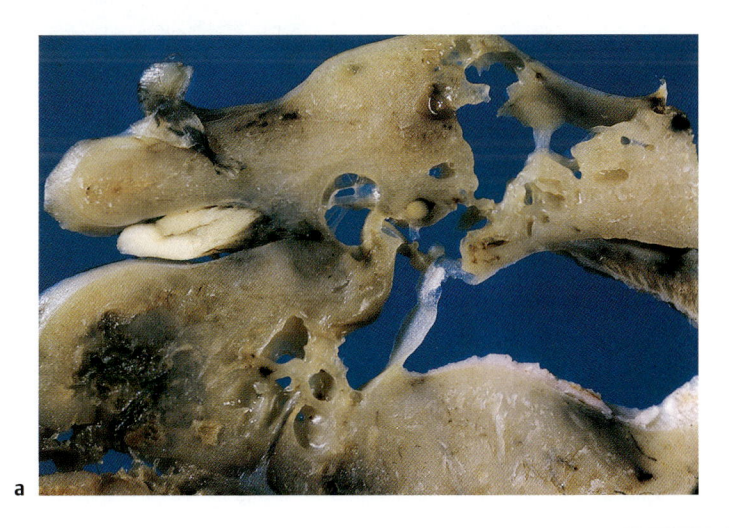

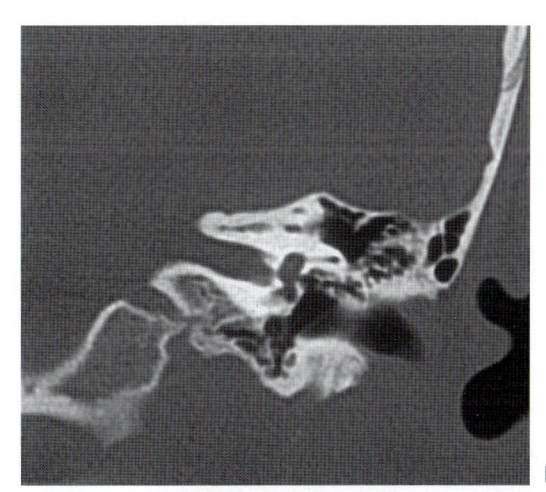

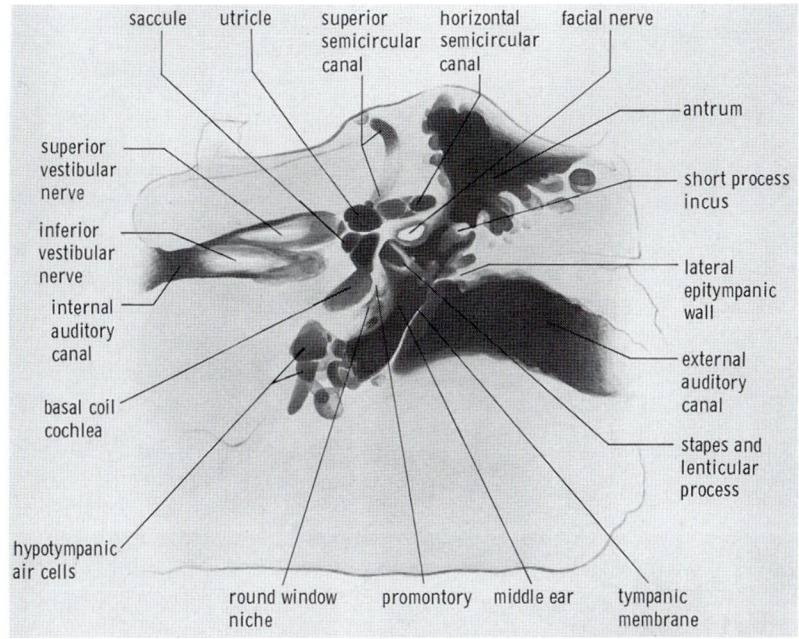

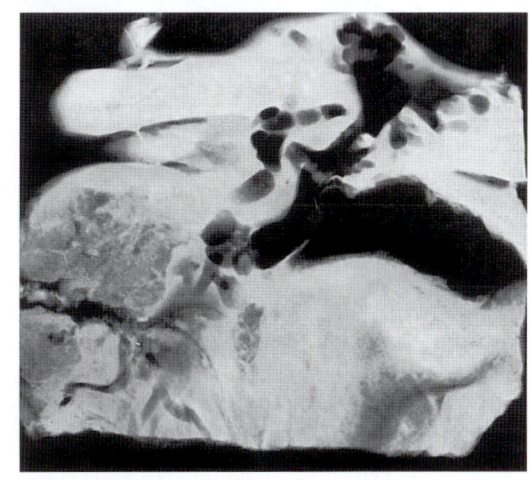

Fig. 1.**13 a** Posterior surface of coronal macrosection 2 mm posterior to Fig. 1.**11 a**.
b CT corresponding to **a**.
c Microradiograph corresponding to Figs. 1.**12 a**, 1.**13 a**.
d Stuctures seen at this level.

14   1 Imaging of the Temporal Bone

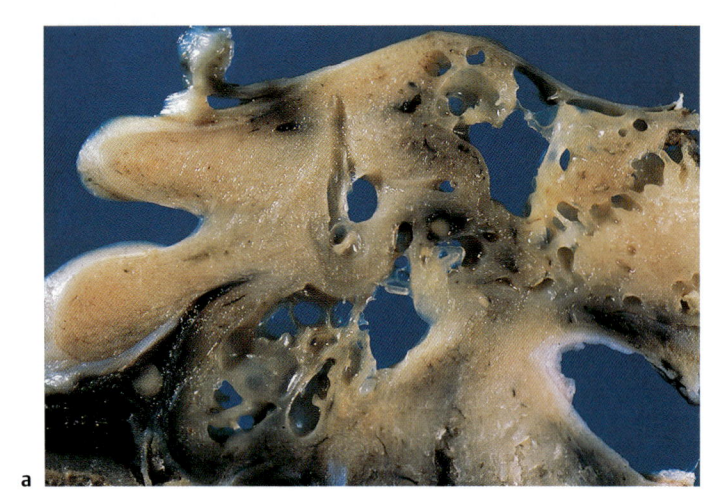

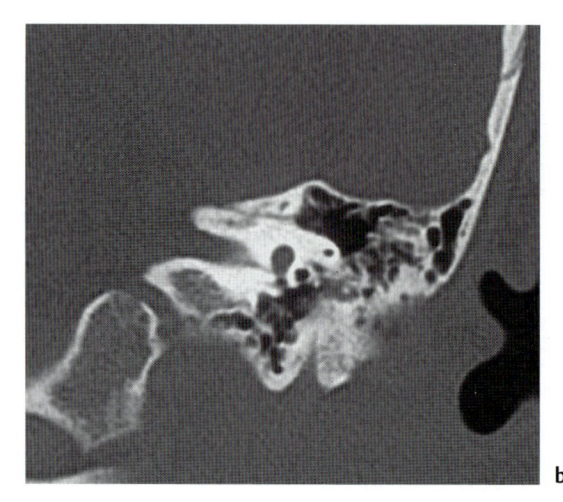

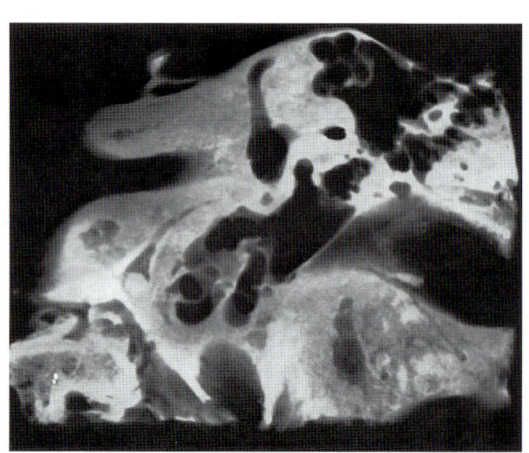

Fig. 1.**14a**   Coronal macrosection 2 mm posterior to Fig. 1.**13a**.
b   CT corresponding to **a**.
c   Stuctures seen at this level.
d   Microradiograph corresponding to **a**, **b**.

Labels in **c**: ampulla posterior semicircular canal; vestibule; superior semicircular canal; crus commune; horizontal semicircular canal; round window niche; internal auditory canal; cochlear aqueduct; IX nerve; facial nerve; facial recess; pyramidal eminence; external auditory canal; tympanic membrane; jugular; middle ear; sinus tympani.

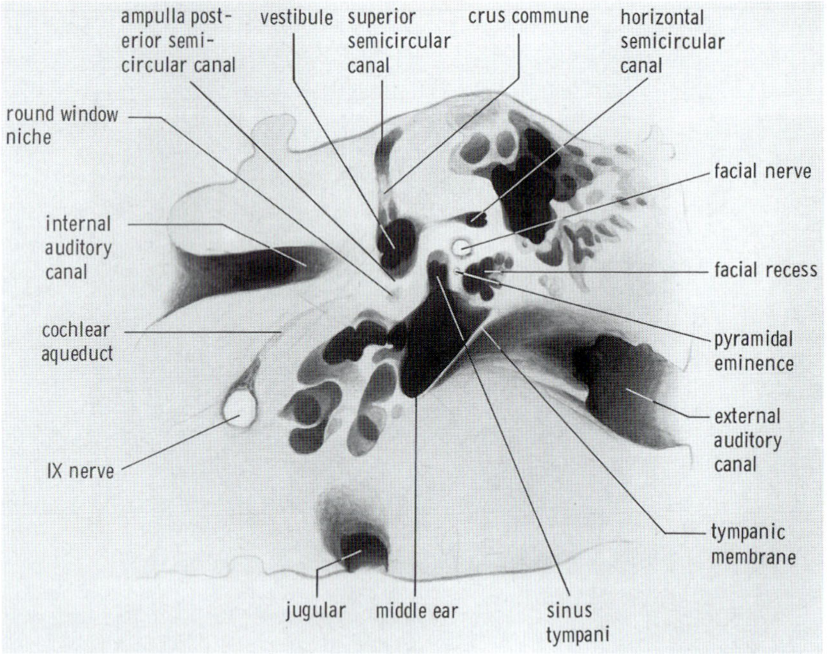

terior semicircular canal opens into the inferior portion of the vestibule. A remnant of the round window niche appears at approximately the same level. The posterior wall of the internal auditory canal is present. The cochlear aqueduct stretches inferiorly from the round window area to the jugular foramen, (Fig. 1.14a, d).

Figure 1.15 shows the structures in a 2 mm thick coronal section of a left adult temporal bone immediately posterior to Figure 1.14. The section passes through the external auditory canal and mastoid air cells. The posterior limb of the horizontal semicircular canal bulges into the mastoid antrum. The crus commune, the posterior limb of the horizontal semicircular canal, and the ampulla of the posterior semicircular canal open into the posterior portion of the vestibule. Portions of the membranous labyrinth are present within the bony canals (Fig. 1.14a). The pyramidal turn of the facial nerve lies under the horizontal semicircular canal. Air cells lie inferior to the labyrinth. The medial or jugular opening of the cochlear aqueduct lies between the porus of the internal auditory canal and the jugular fossa (Fig. 1.14a, d).

20° Coronal Oblique Sections

Figures 1.16 and 1.17 show the structures contained in the anterior and posterior surfaces of a 2 mm thick, 20°coronal oblique section of a right adult temporal bone at the level of the cochlea. The sections pass just anteriorly to the external auditory canal, through the anterior portion of the tympanic membrane, the cochlea, and the internal auditory canal. The section exposes the epitympanum, mesotympanum, and hypotympanum. The tensor

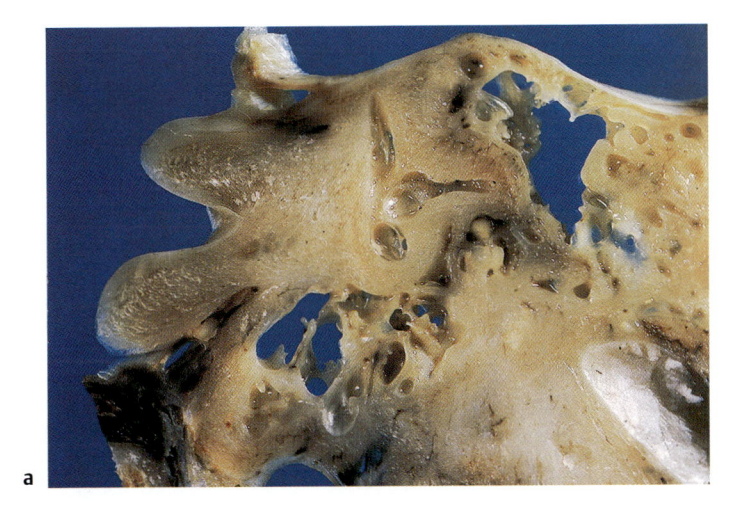

Sectional Anatomy of the Temporal Bone 15

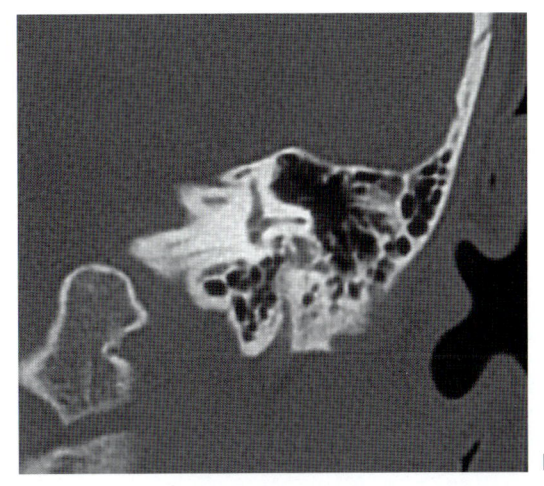

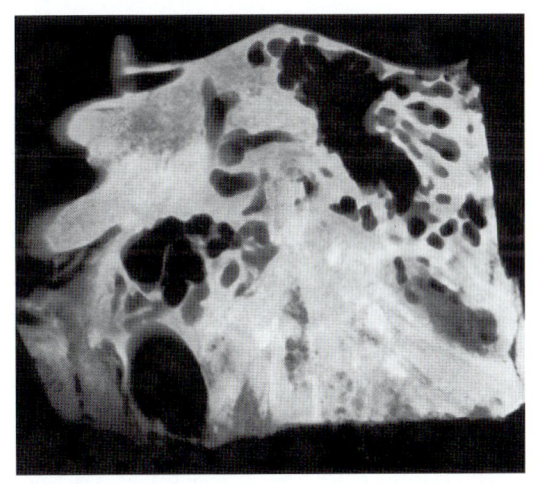

Fig. 1.15 a Coronal macrosection 2 mm posterior to Fig. 1.14 a.
b CT corresponding to a.
c Stuctures seen at this level.
d Microradiograph corresponding to a, b.

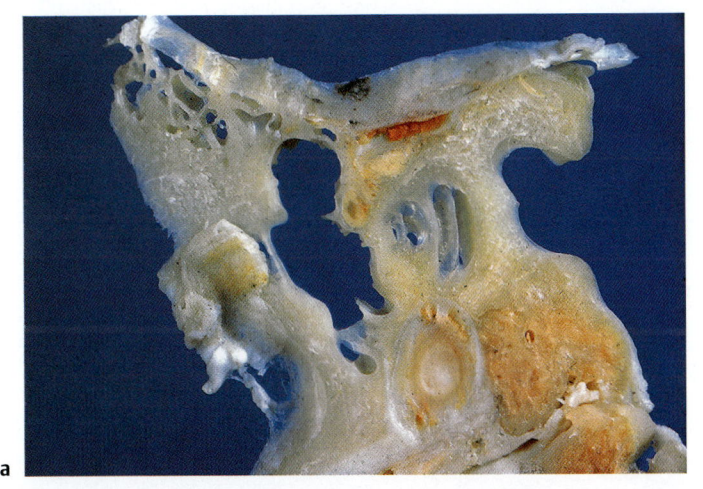

Labels in c: crus commune, superior semicircular canal, posterior semicircular canal, horizontal semicircular canal, antrum, mastoid cells, external auditory canal, facial nerve, jugular, cochlear aqueduct, internal auditory canal posterior wall, ampulla posterior semicircular canal.

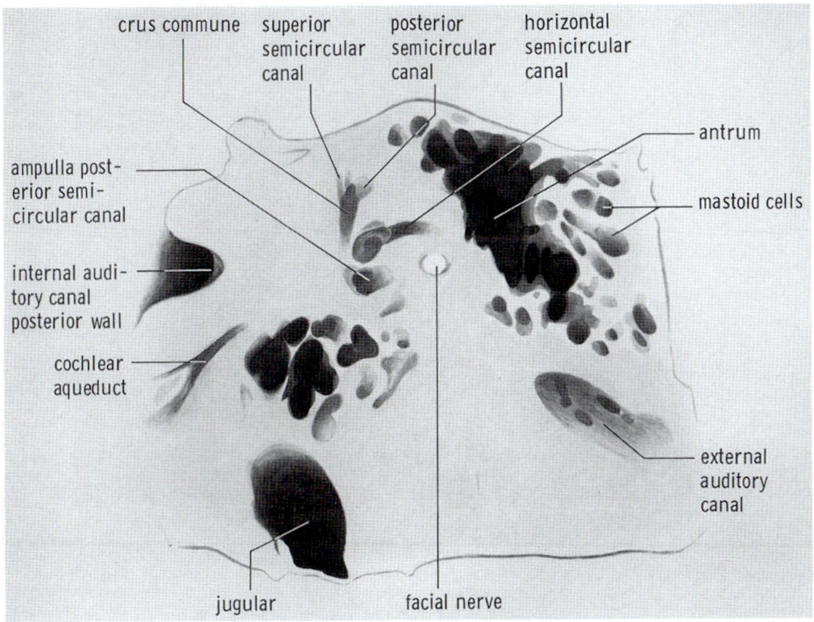

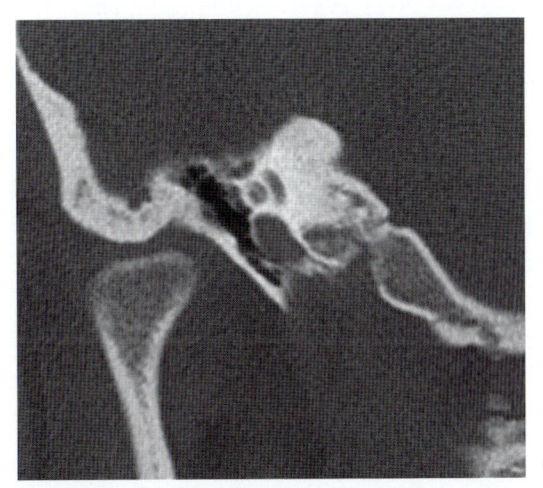

Fig. 1.16 a 20° coronal macrosection, anterior surface.
b CT corresponding to a.

1 Imaging of the Temporal Bone

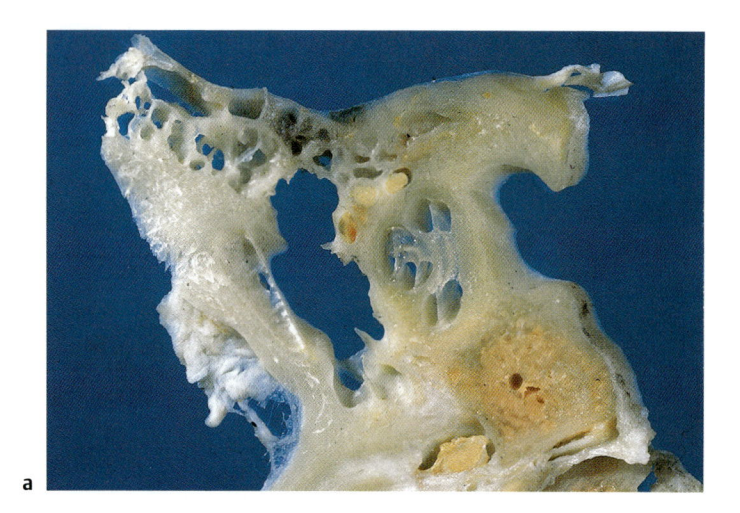

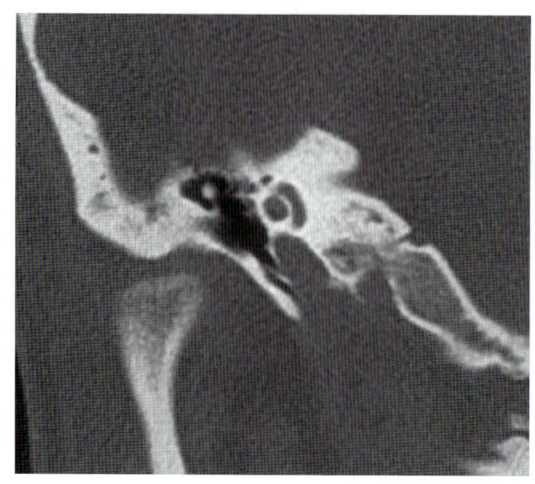

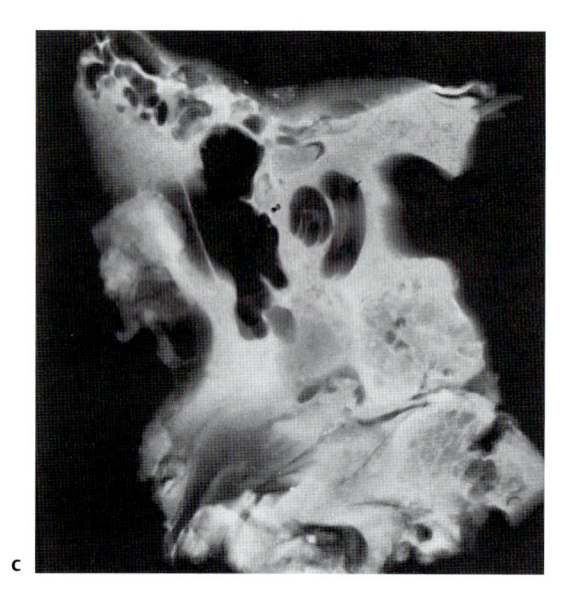

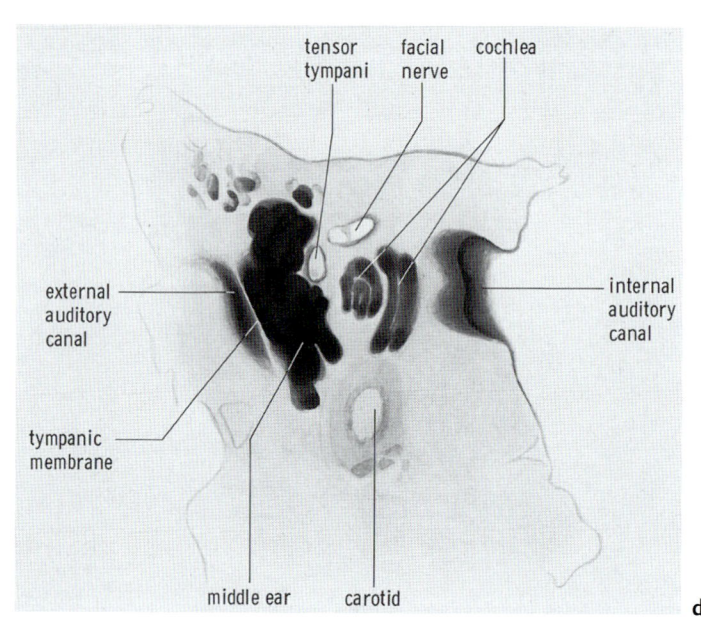

Fig. 1.17 a 20° coronal macrosection, posterior surface of Fig. 1.16 a.
b CT corresponding to a.
c Microradiograph corresponding to Figs. 1.16 a, 1.17 a.
d Stuctures seen at this level (Figs. 1.16, 1.17).

tympani muscle projects from the medial wall of the middle ear. Above the cochlea, the facial nerve bifurcates from the geniculate ganglion into its petrous and tympanic segments. Portions of three coils of the cochlea lie lateral to the internal auditory canal. The CT image shows the contour of the lumen of the spiral canal of the cochlea and the bony septa between the coils.. The carotid artery appears inferior to the cochlea.

Figure 1.18 shows the structures contained in a 2 mm thick 20° coronal oblique section of an adult right temporal bone immediately posterior to Figure 1.17. The section exposes a portion of the external auditory canal and an anterior strip of the tympanic membrane. The head and part of the neck of the malleus lie in the epitympanum. The inferior and anterior margin

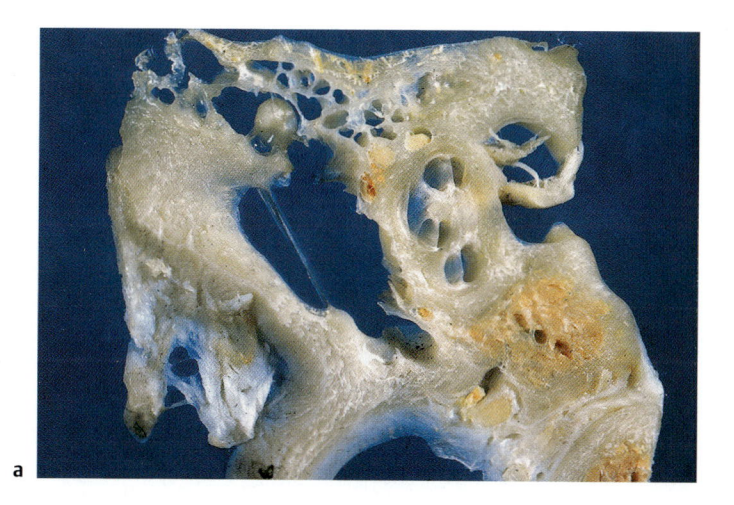

Sectional Anatomy of the Temporal Bone

Fig. 1.18 a 20° coronal macrosection 2 mm posterior to Fig. 1.17 a.
b CT corresponding to a.
c Stuctures seen at this level.
d Microradiograph corresponding to a, b.

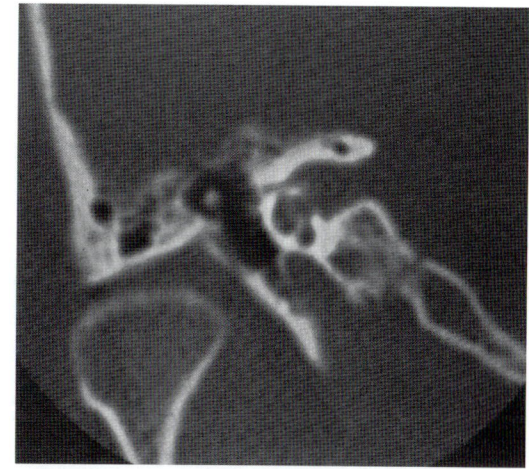

Labels in c: malleus head, lateral epitympanic wall, external auditory canal, tympanic membrane, middle ear, epitympanum, tensor tympani, facial nerve horizontal portion, facial nerve proximal portion, crista falciformis, cochlear nerve, internal auditory canal, cochlea, jugular.

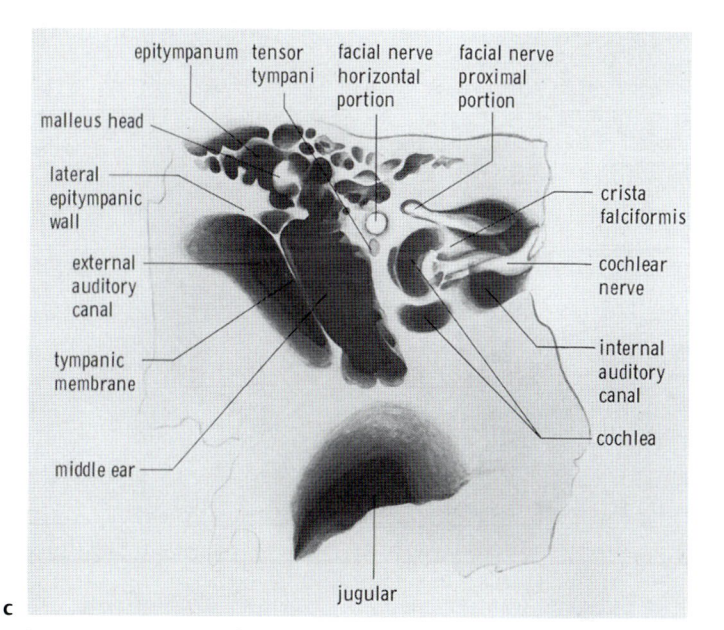

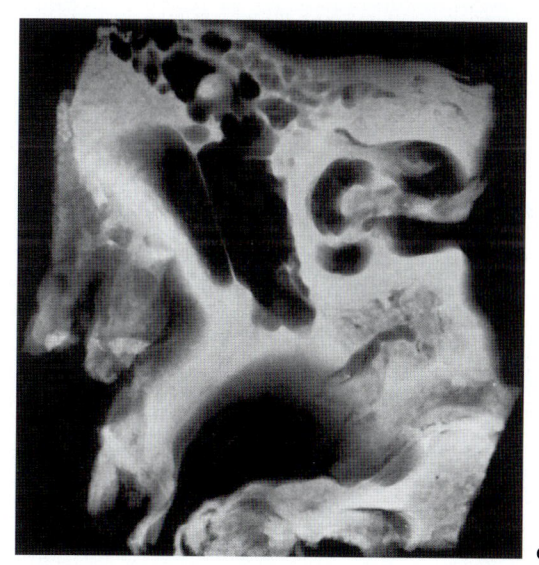

of the lateral epitympanic wall is in close relation to the malleus neck. The tensor tympani tendon lies on the medial wall of the middle ear below the horizontal portion of the facial nerve. The labyrinthine or petrous portion of the facial nerve stretches medially into the lumen of the internal auditory canal above the crista falciformis. The cochlear nerve passes into the base of the modiolus below the crista falciformis. Portions of the middle and basal coils of the cochlea lie medial to the fundus of the internal auditory canal.

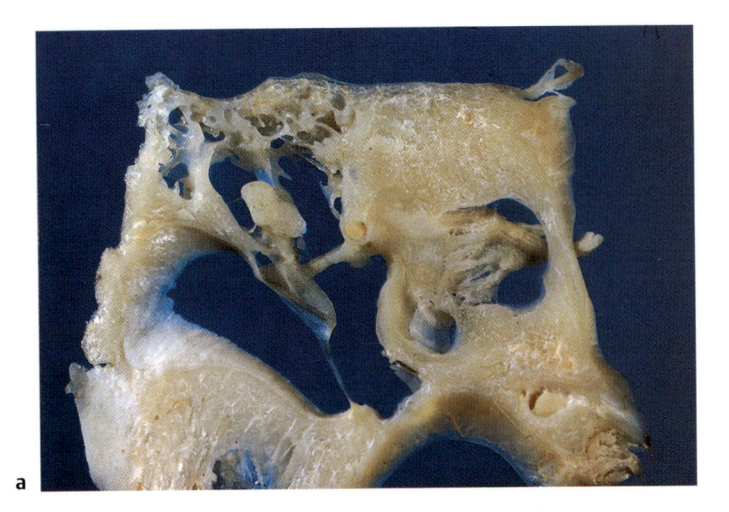

18   1   Imaging of the Temporal Bone

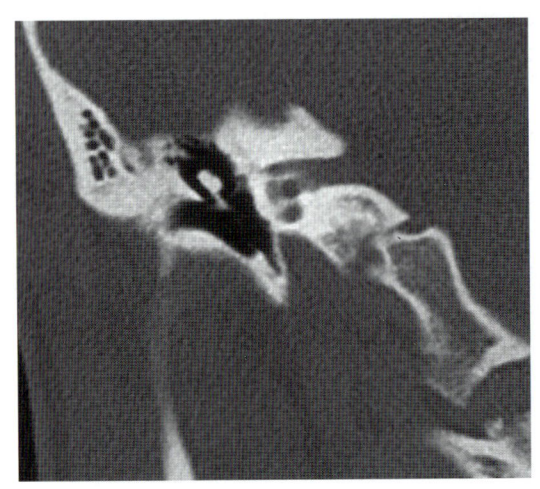

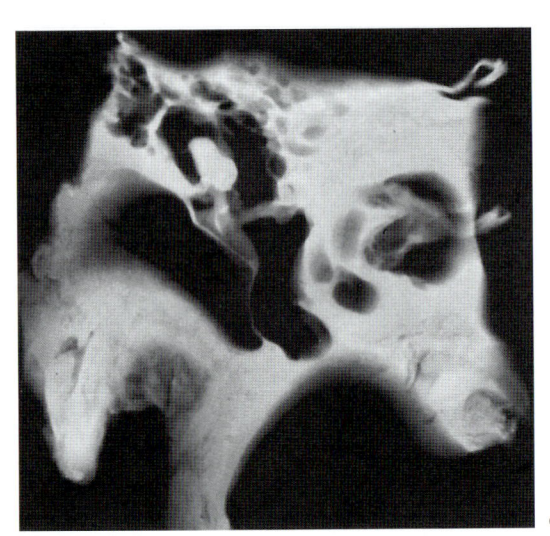

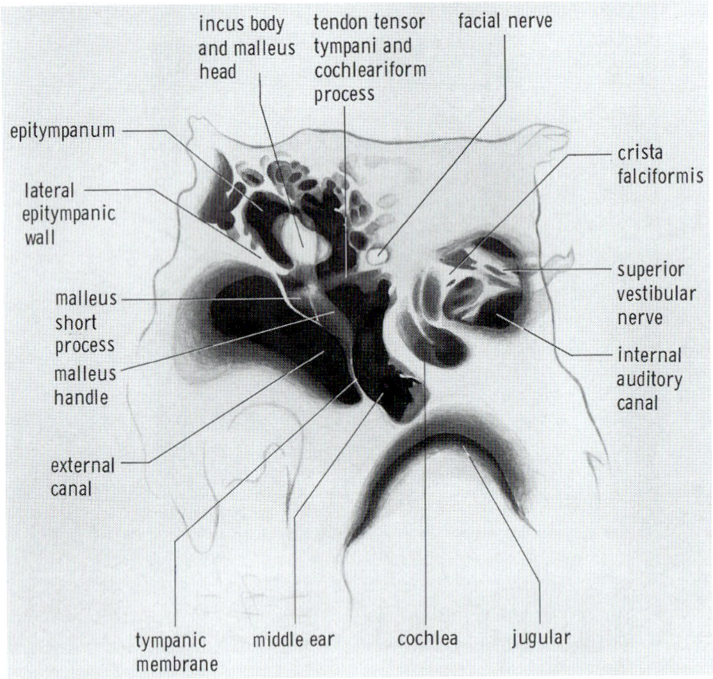

Fig. 1.**19 a**   20° coronal macrosection 2 mm posterior to Fig. 1.**18 a**.
b   CT corresponding to **a**.
c   Stuctures seen at this level.
d   Microradiograph corresponding to **a, b**.

Figure 1.**19** shows the structures contained in a 2 mm thick, 20° coronal oblique section of an adult right temporal bone immediately posterior to Figure 1.**18**. The tympanic membrane and malleus handle separate the external canal from the middle ear. The superior wall of the external auditory canal joins the inferior margin of the lateral attic wall in a sharp projection just above the short process of the malleus. In the epitympanum the body of the incus protrudes lateral from the head of the malleus (Fig. 1.**19 a**). The tendon of the tensor tympani crosses the middle ear from the cochleariform process to the malleus. The horizonal portion of the facial nerve is closely related to the cochleariform process. The promontory of the basal turn of the chochlea forms the medial wall of the tympanic cavity. The superior and inferior vestibular nerves flare at the vestibular areas in the fundus of the internal auditory canal (Fig. 1.**19 a**). The crista falciformis divides the two branches of the vestibular nerve.

Sectional Anatomy of the Temporal Bone

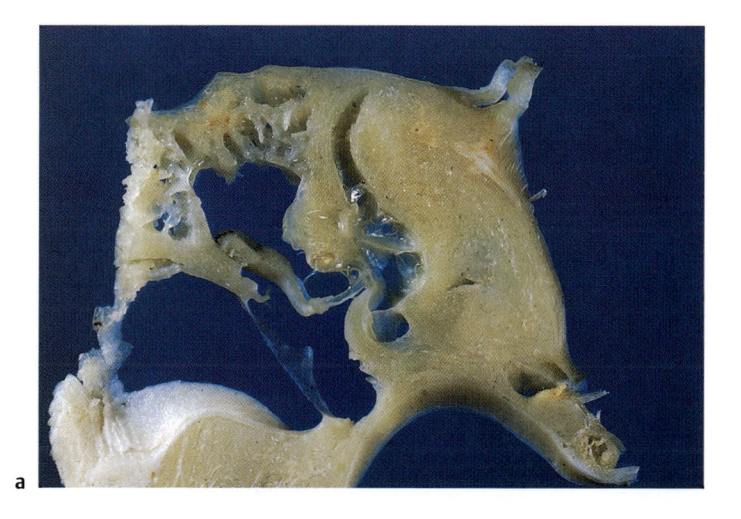

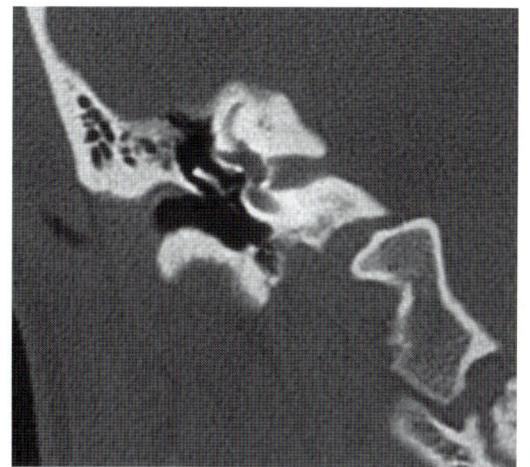

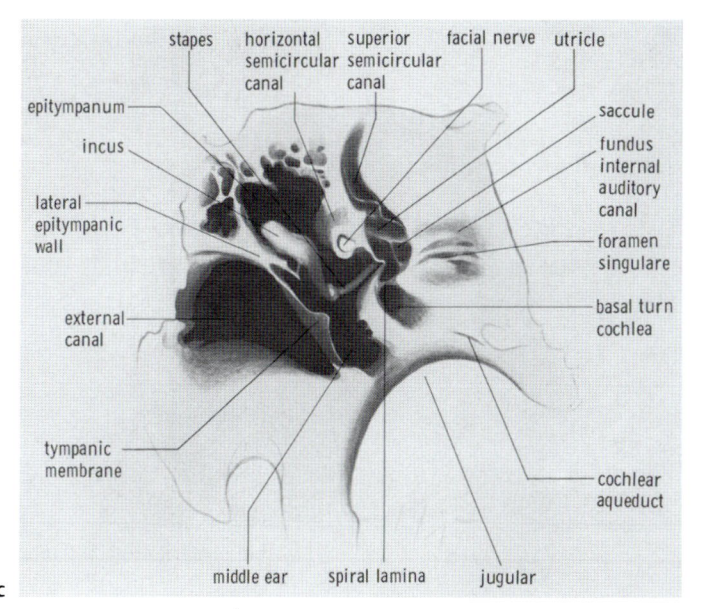

Fig. 1.20 a 20° coronal macrosection 2 mm posterior to Fig. 1.19 a.
b CT corresponding to a.
c Stuctures seen at this level.
d Microradiograph corresponding to a, b.

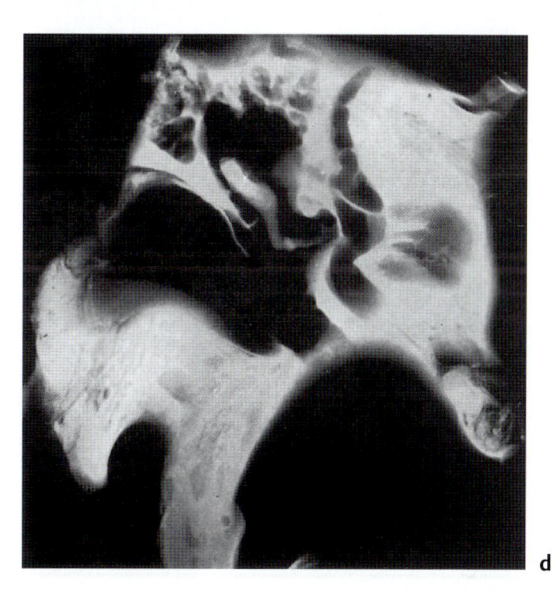

Figure 1.20 shows the structures contained in a 2 mm thick, 20° coronal oblique section of an adult right temporal bone immediately adjacent to Figure 1.19. A strip of the tympanic membrane extends from the inferior margin of the lateral epitympanic wall to the floor of the annulus tympanicus. The body of the incus lies in the epitympanum. The long process of the incus extends to articulate with the head of the stapes. The facial nerve lies in the medial wall of the middle ear below the prominence of the horizontal semicircular canal. The anterior portion of the stapes footplate closes the oval window. The anterior crus is attached to the footplate. In the lumen of the promontory, the lamina spiralis separates the scala tympani from the scala vestibuli. The scala vestibuli opens into the vestibule above the scala tympani. The ampullated ends of the superior and horizontal semicircular canals open into the vestibule. Segments of the membranous semicircular canals, the anterior portion of the utricle, the utricular macula, and the saccule occupy the lumen of the vestibule and bony semicircular canals (Fig. 1.20 a, d). Only the fundus of the internal auditory canal remains (Fig. 1.20 d). A thin bony plate covers the jugular dome.

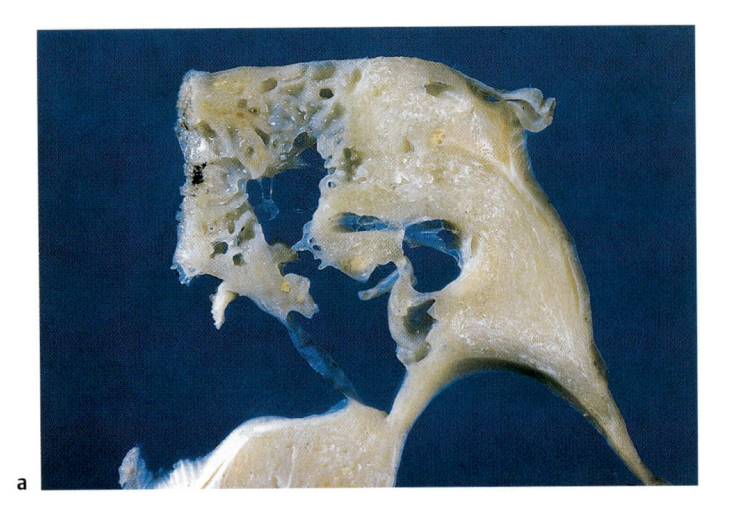

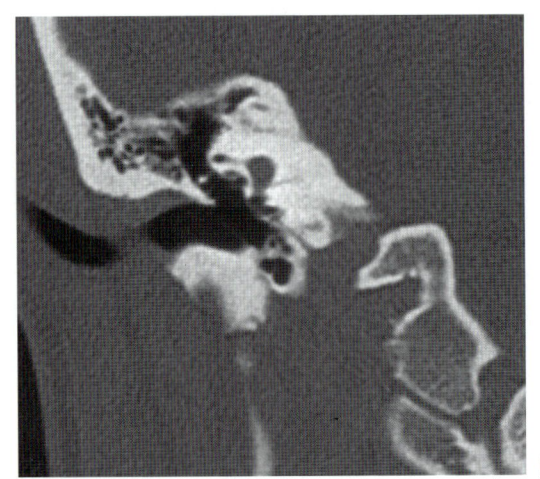

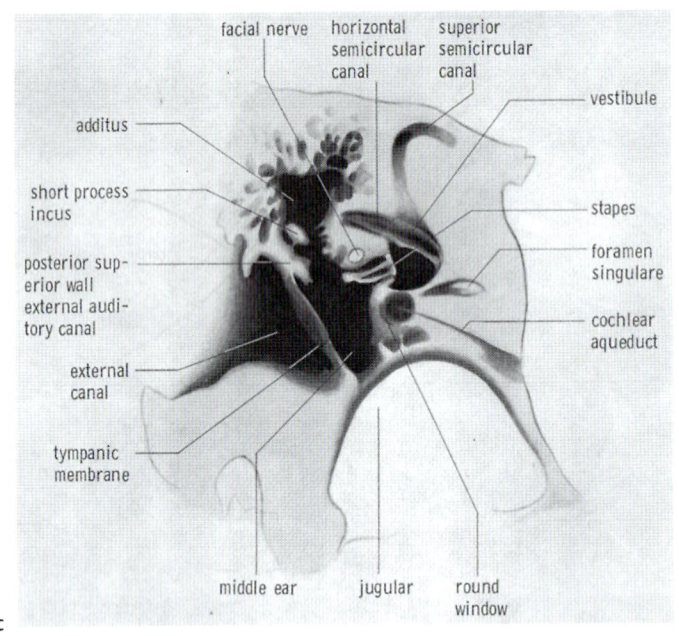

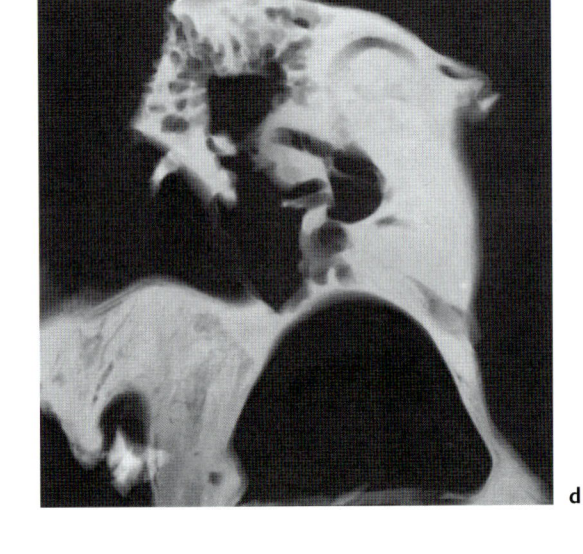

Fig. 1.21 a 20° coronal macrosection 2 mm posterior to Fig. 1.20 a.
b CT corresponding to a.
c Stuctures seen at this level.
d Microradiograph corresponding to a, b.

Figure 1.21 demonstrates the structures contained in a 2 mm thick, 20° coronal oblique section of an adult right temporal bone immediately posterior to Figure 1.20. The section includes the external auditory canal, a thin section of tympanic membrane, the middle ear, and the aditus. The short process of the incus lies above the posterosuperior wall of the external auditory canal. The horizontal semicircular canal forms the medial boundary of the aditus of the mastoid antrum. The facial nerve appears under the horizontal semicircular canal. The posterior half of the stapes footplate closes the oval window, and the posterior crus lies in the oval window niche. In the inferior aspect of the promontory, the round window membrane separates the round window niche from the scala tympani. The superior semicircular canal arches upward from the vestibule. The utricle occupies the upper portion of the bony vestibule. The cochlear aqueduct arches within the thickness of the tissue section above the jugular fossa (Fig. 1.21 c, d).

Sectional Anatomy of the Temporal Bone

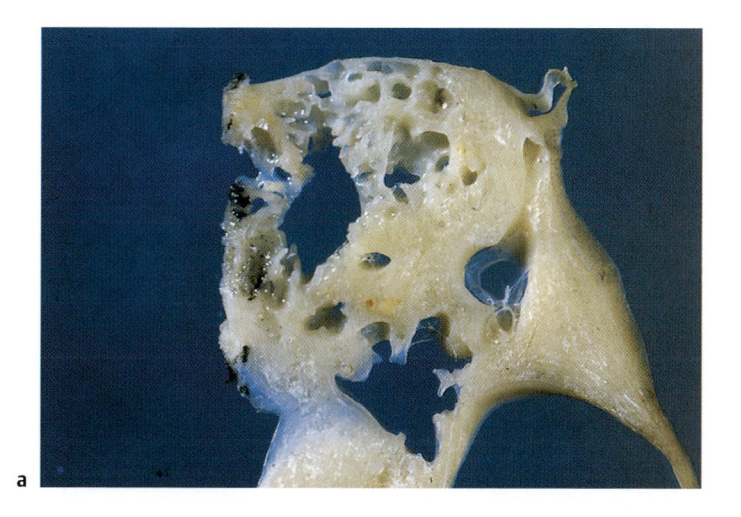

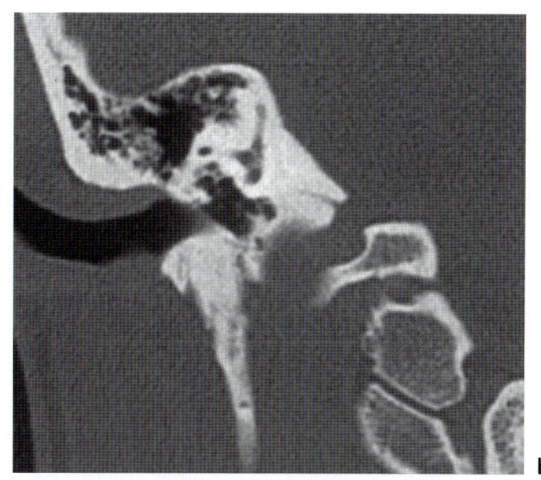

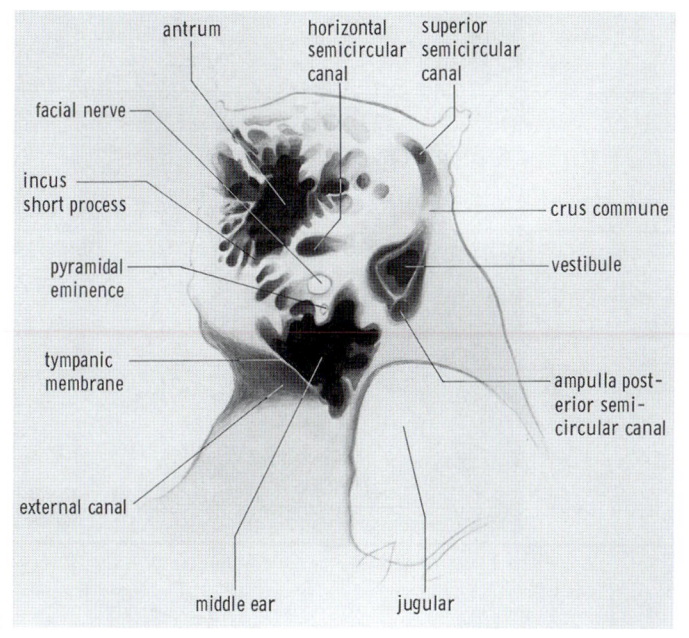

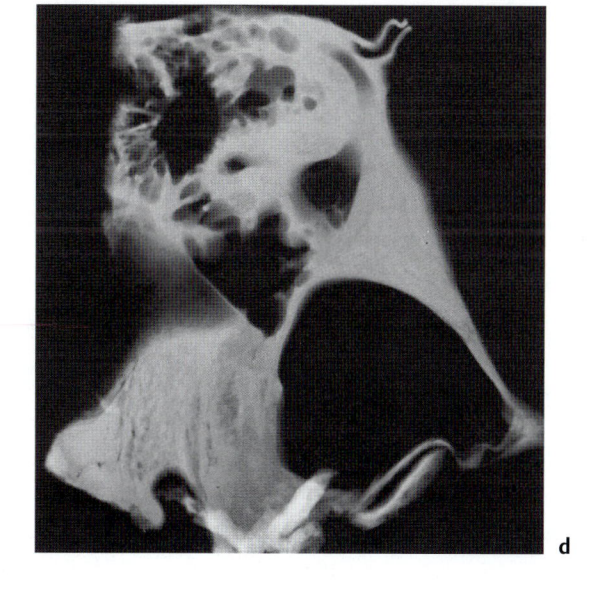

Fig. 1.**22 a** 20° coronal macrosection 2 mm posterior to Fig. 1.**21 a**.
b CT corresponding to **a**.
c Stuctures seen at this level.
d Microradiograph corresponding to **a**, **b**.

Figure 1.22 demonstrates the structures contained in a 2 mm thick, 20° coronal oblique section of a right adult temporal bone immediately posterior to Figure 1.21. The section exposes the mastoid antrum with its surrounding air cells, the posterior wall of the external auditory canal, and the posterior part of the tympanic membrane. The tip of the incus short process lies in the fossa incudis. The facial nerve and the pyramidal eminence lie in the posterior wall of the middle ear below the horizonal semicircular canal. The dome of the jugular fossa forms the floor of the hypotympanum. The horizontal semicircular canal projects into the antrum. The ampullated end of the posterior semicircular canal opens into the inferior portion of the vestibule (Fig. 1.22 a). The posterior margin of the round window lies opposite the posterior ampulla. Less than 2 mm, the thickness of this section, separates these two structures. Portions of the membranous labyrinth occupy the lumen of the vestibule.

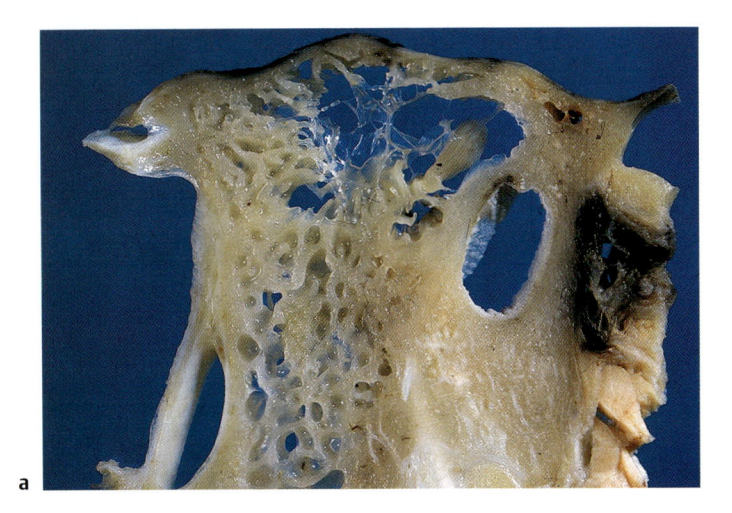

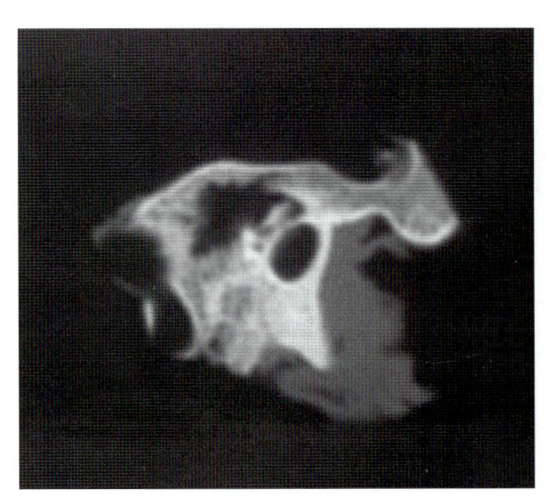

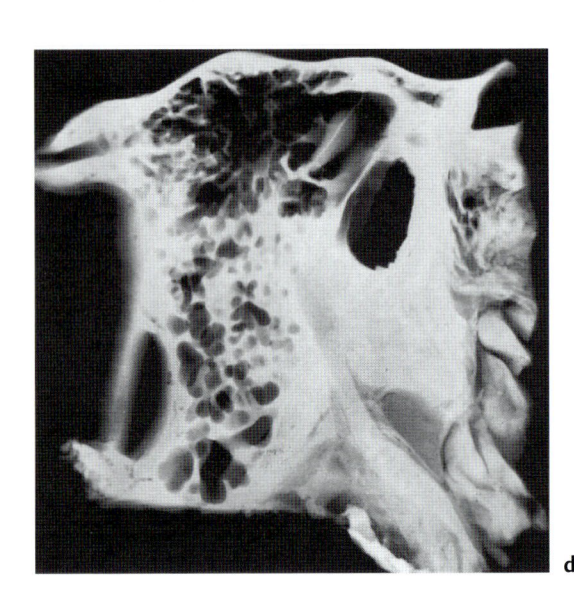

Fig. 1.23 a Sagittal macrosection at the level of the lateral portion of the epitympanum.
b CT corresponding to a.
c Stuctures seen at this level.
d Microradiograph corresponding to a, b.

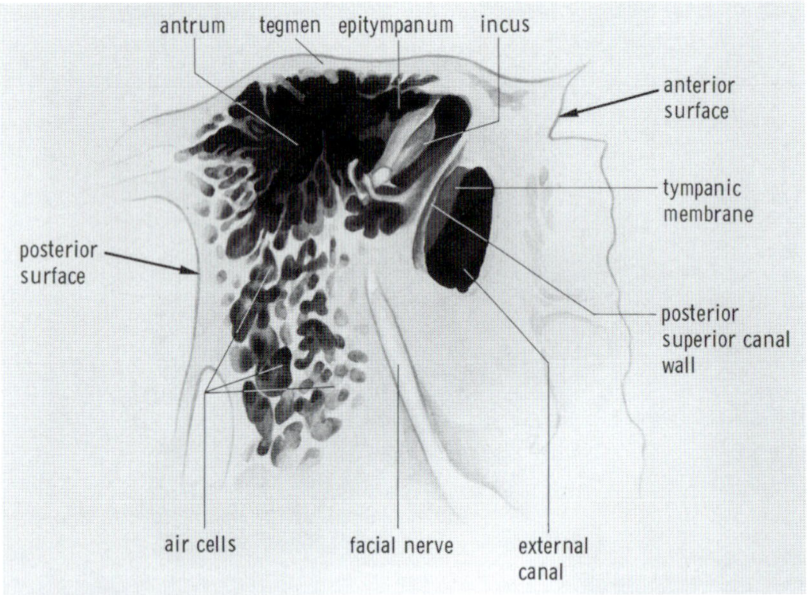

Sagittal Sections

The first sagittal section (Fig. 1.23), 2 mm thick, of this right adult temporal bone crosses the medial portion of the external auditory canal and the lateral portion of the epitympanum. A small section of the tympanic membrane is attached to the posterosuperior wall of the external auditory canal. The body of the incus is in the epitympanum and the short process in the fossa incudis. The tegmen of the middle ear and mastoid forms the upper margin of the tissue section. Mucosal strands stretch across the mastoid antrum. There are many small air cells in the mastoid. The vertical portion of the facial nerve descends inferiorly.

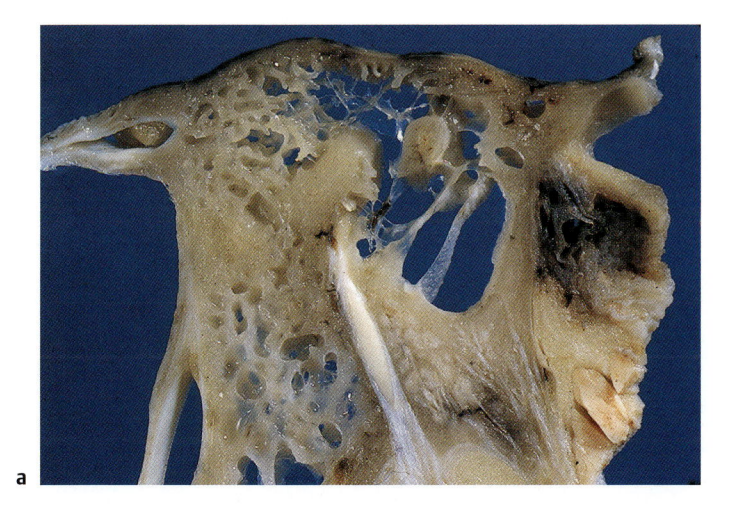

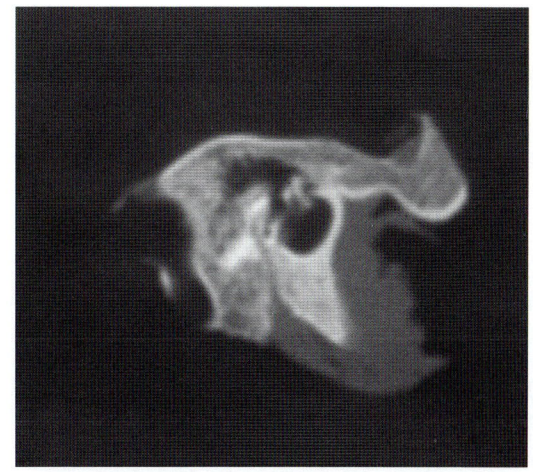

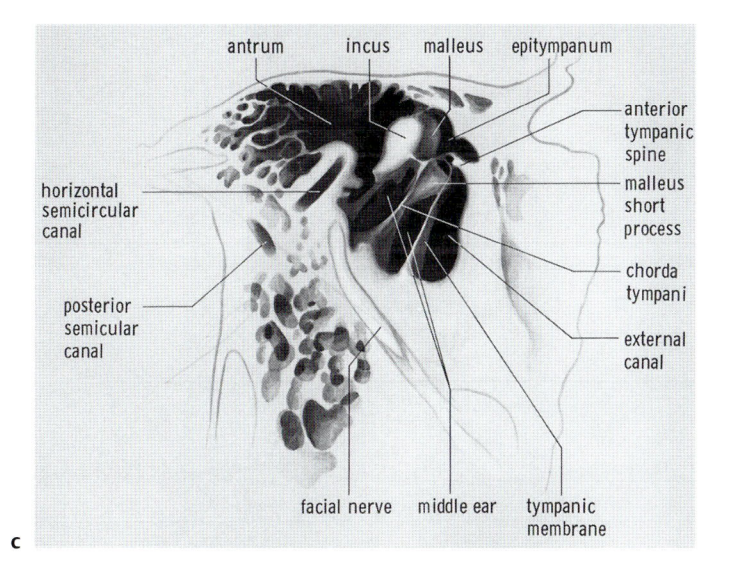

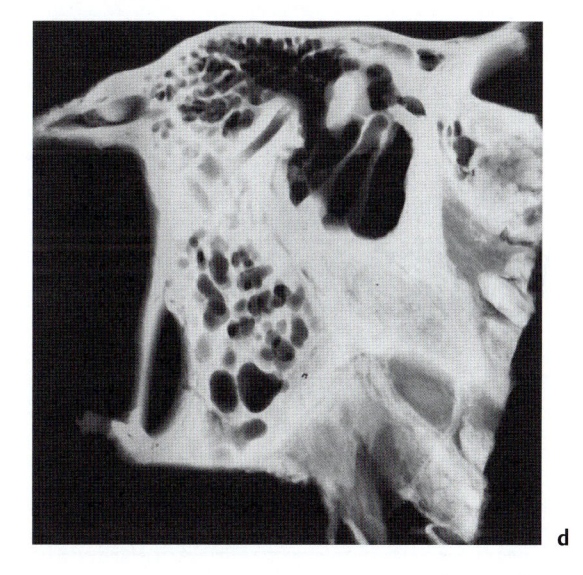

Fig. 1.24 a Sagittal macrosection 2 mm medial to Fig. 1.23 a.
b CT corresponding to **a**.
c Stuctures seen at this level.
d Microradiograph corresponding to **a**, **b**.

Figure 1.24 demonstrates the structures in the 2 mm thick sagittal section of a right adult temporal bone immediately medial to Figure 1.23. A thin strip of the tympanic membrane separates the external auditory canal anterior from the middle ear posterior. The malleus head and neck occupy the anterior portion of the epitympanum. The transected incus body articulates with the malleus head. The short process of the malleus lies in contact with the tympanic membrane. The anterior tympanic spine is just anterior to the malleus short process. A segment of the chorda tympani crosses the middle ear. The most lateral portion of the horizontal semicircular canal appears posteriorly. The facial nerve descends from the pyramidal turn toward the stylomastoid foramen.

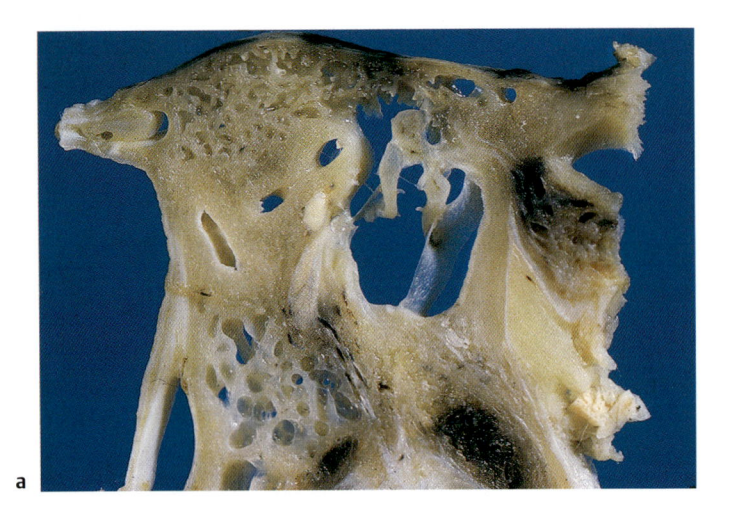

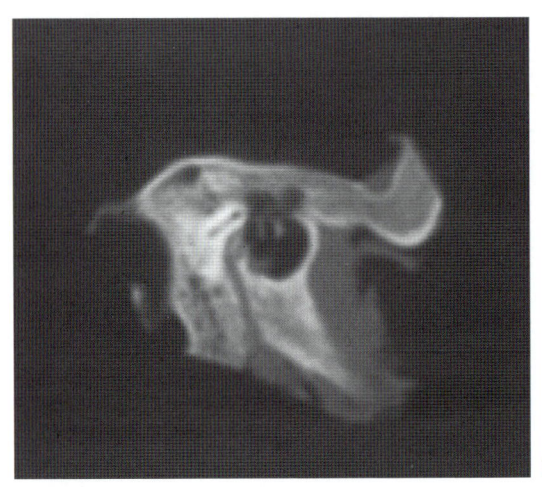

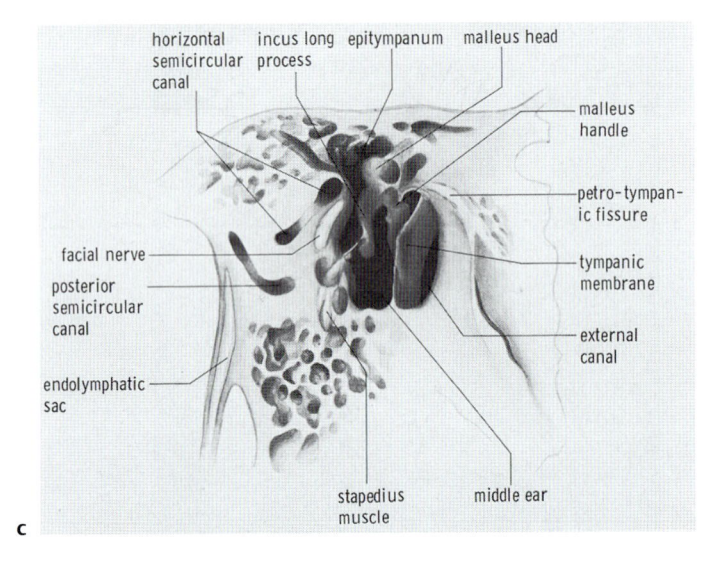

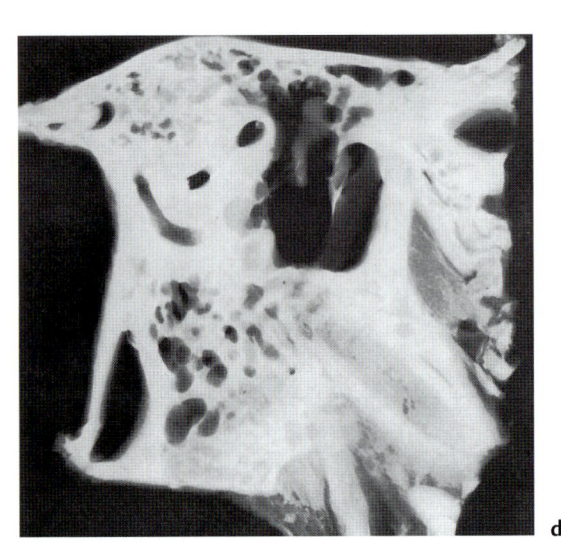

24   1 Imaging of the Temporal Bone

Fig. 1.**25 a** Sagittal macrosection 2 mm medial to Fig. 1.**24 a**.
b CT corresponding to **a**.
c Stuctures seen at this level.
d Microradiograph corresponding to **a, b**.

Figure 1.**25** demonstrates the stuctures in a 2 mm thick sagittal section of an adult right temporal bone immediately medial to Figure 1.**24**. A thin strip of tympanic membrane attached to the malleus handle separates the external canal from the middle ear. The anterior mallear ligament passes into the petrotympanic fissure above the anterior tympanic spine. The remnant of the body of the incus articulates with the malleus head. The long process of the incus extends to the lenticular process. The horizontal and posterior semicircular canals are in the bone of the petrosa. A segment of the facial nerve passes below the horizontal semicircular canal. The pyramidal eminence and stapedius muscle are inferior to the facial nerve. The endolymphatic sac lies beneath the dura of the posterior surface of the section.

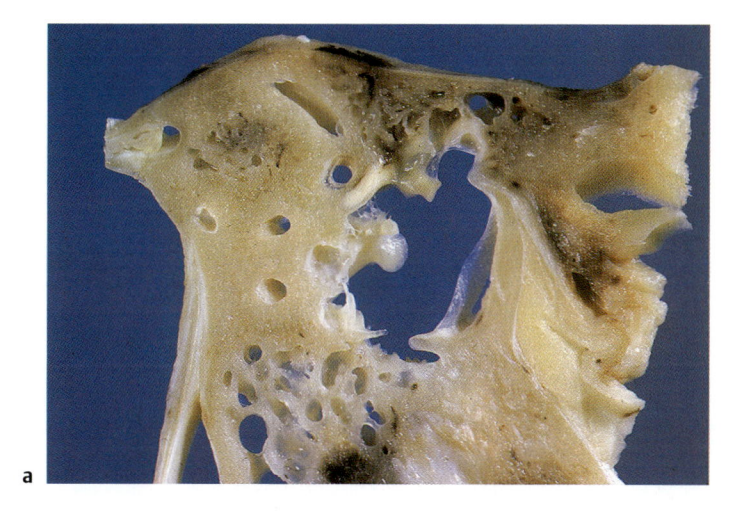

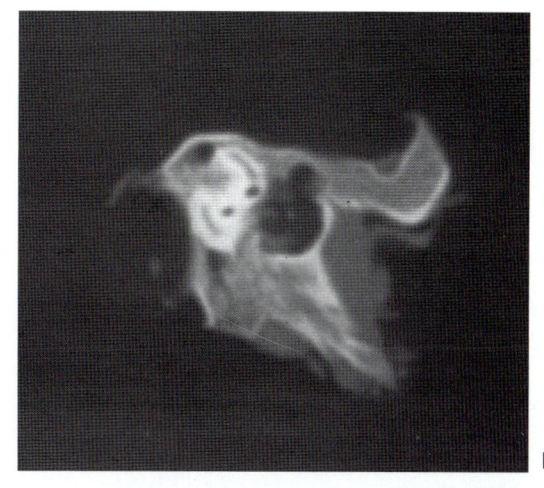

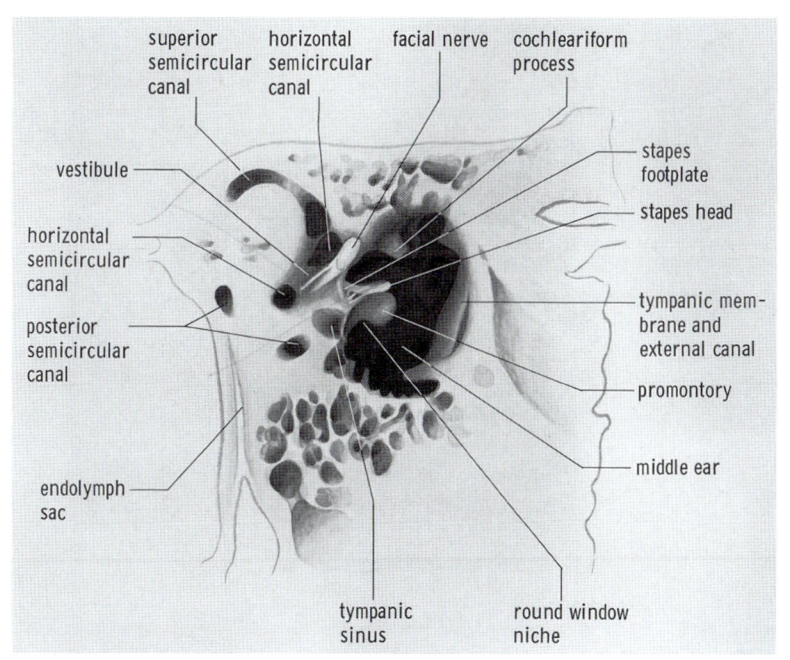

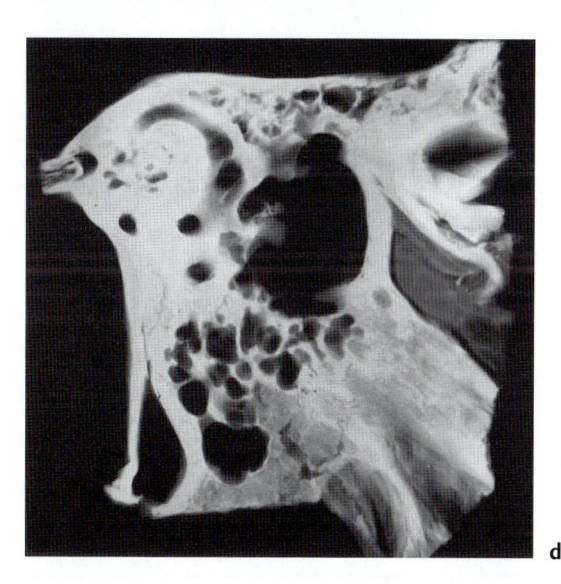

Fig. 1.26 a Sagittal macrosection 2 mm medial to Fig. 1.25 a.
b CT corresponding to a.
c Stuctures seen at this level.
d Microradiograph corresponding to a, b.

Figure 1.26 shows the structures in a 2 mm thick sagittal section of an adult right temporal bone immediately medial to Figure 1.25. The section includes the most medial portion of the external auditory canal, the anterior portion of the tympanic membrane, and a thin section of the cochlear promontory. The posterior half of the footplate, head, and posterior crus of the stapes occupy the oval window niche. The tympanic sinus extends posteriorly between the oval and round windows (Fig 1.26 a).

A section of the facial nerve is above the oval window. The cochleariform process and tensor tympani tendon are anterior to the facial nerve. The three semicircular canals occupy the petrosa posteriorly. Segments of the membranous semicircular canals including their ampullated portions lie in the canal lumina. The

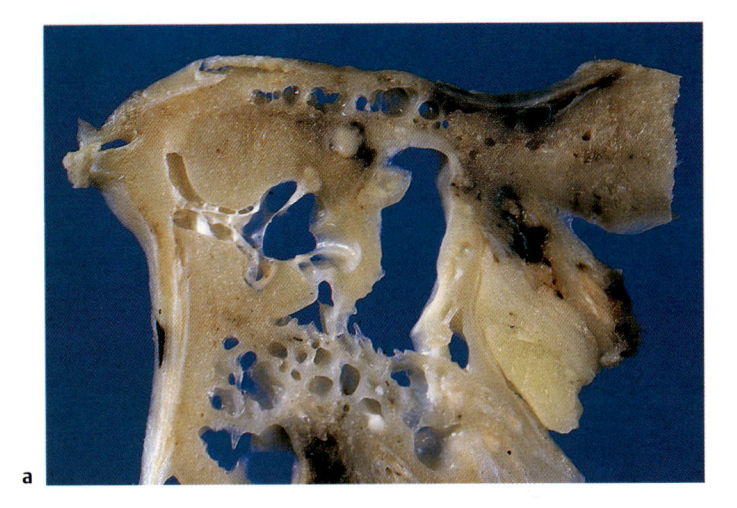

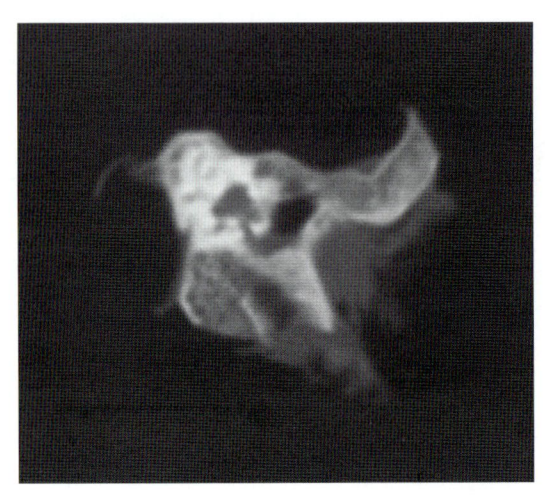

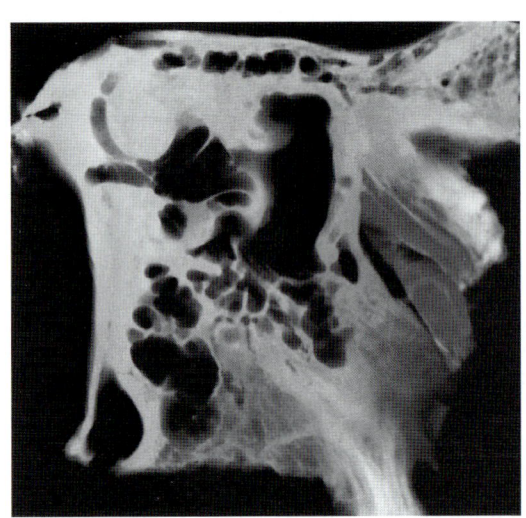

Fig. 1.27 a Sagittal macrosection 2 mm medial to Fig. 1.26 a.
b CT corresponding to a.
c Stuctures seen at this level.
d Microradiograph corresponding to a, b.

ampullated end of the horizontal semicircular canal opens into the vestibule just below the ampulla of the superior semicircular canal. Figure 1.27 reveals the structures in a 2 mm thick sagittal section of an adult right temporal bone immediately medial to Figure 1.26. The section crosses the anterior portion of the middle ear and exposes the epitympanic, mesotympanic, and hypotympanic portions of the middle ear. The tensor tympani canal protrudes into the middle ear just below the facial nerve. The anterior portion of the stapes footplate and the anterior crus lie in the anterior part of the oval window niche. The promontory with the scala vestibuli and tympani lies anterior to the vestibule. The section exposes the round window niche and membrane. The utricle stretches across the vestibule. Anterosuperiorly the utricular macula connects with the superior vestibular nerve. The utricle joins the crus commune posteriorly and the ampullated end of the posterior semicircular canal inferiorly. The bony vestibule narrows posteriorly toward the crus commune, which in turn branches to form the nonampullated limbs of the posterior and superior semicircular canals.

On the posterior aspect, the endolymphatic sac enters the vestibular aqueduct. The aqueduct extends to the vestibule medial to the crus commune.

Sectional Anatomy of the Temporal Bone

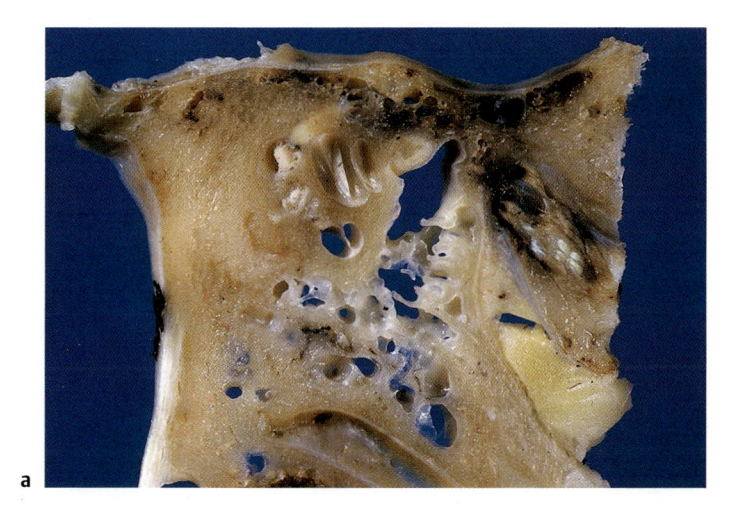

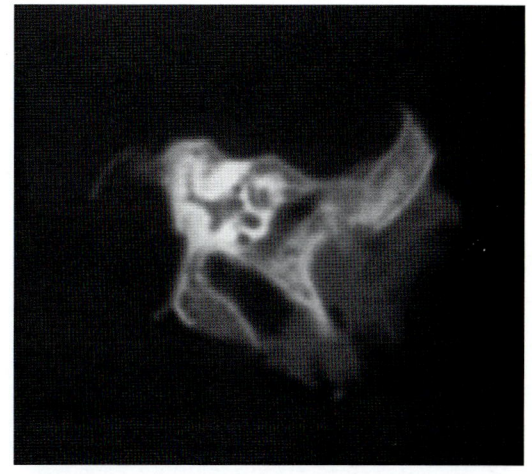

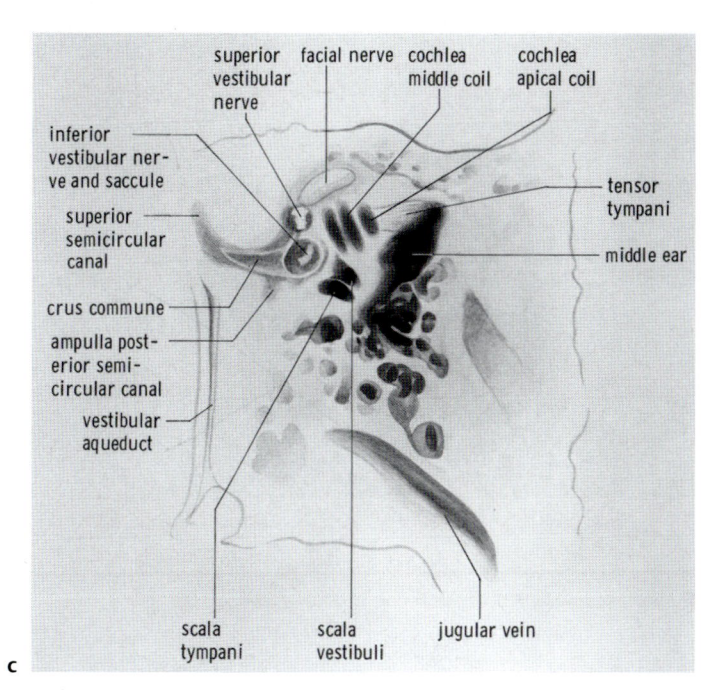

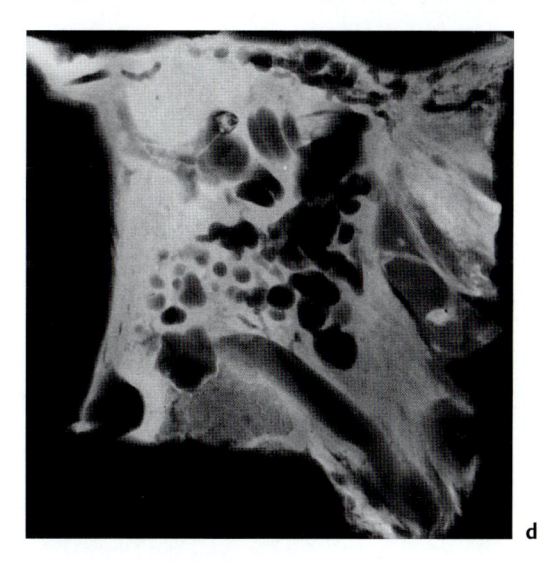

Fig. 1.28 a Sagittal macrosection 2 mm medial to Fig. 1.27 a.
b CT corresponding to a.
c Stuctures seen at this level.
d Microradiograph corresponding to a, b.

Figure 1.28 reveals the structures in a 2 mm thick sagittal section of an adult right temporal bone immediately medial to Figure 1.27. The middle ear narrows near the eustachian tube opening. The tensor tympani canal lies in the superior portion of the middle ear.

Within the thickness of the section, the facial nerve courses from the fundus of the internal auditory canal to the geniculate ganglion. The scala tympani and the smaller scala vestibuli of the first portion of the basal turn of the cochlea lie below the inferior vestibular nerve. The section exposes portions of the middle and apical coils of the cochlea. A portion of the bony superior semicircular canal passes upward from the crus commune. The vestibular aqueduct curves around the medial portion of the crus commune within the thickness of the section. The fundus of the internal auditory canal lies posterior to the cochlea. The fundus contains portions of the superior and inferior vestibular and facial nerves.

1 Imaging of the Temporal Bone

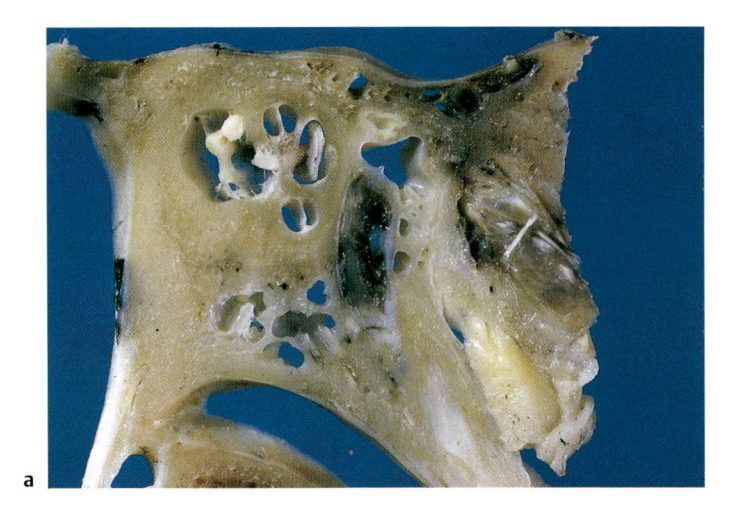

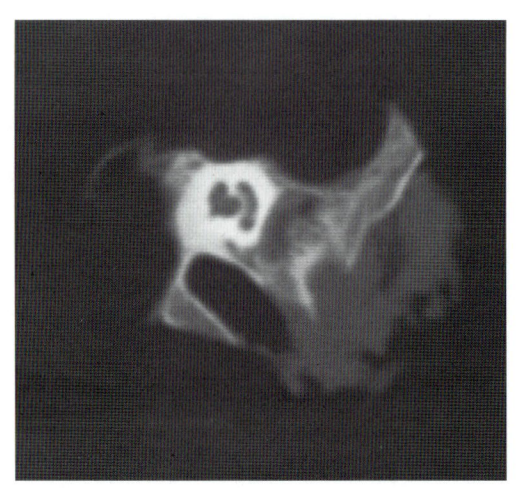

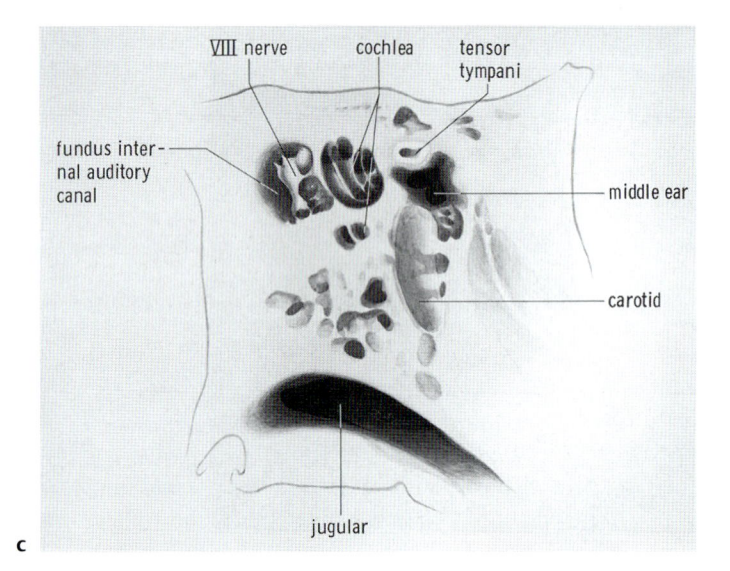

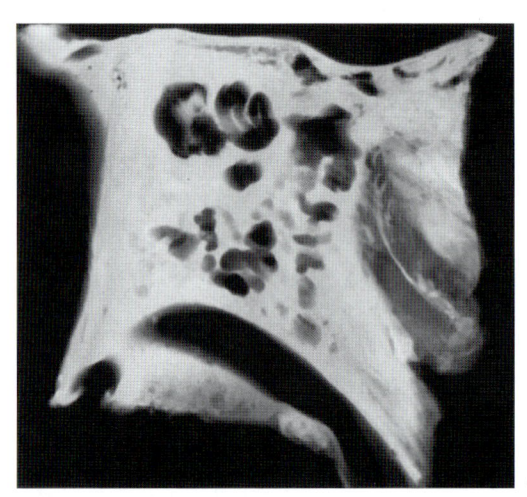

Fig. 1.29 a Sagittal macrosection 2 mm medial to Fig. 1.28 a.
b CT corresponding to a.
c Stuctures seen at this level.
d Microradiograph corresponding to a, b.

Figure 1.29 shows the structures in a 2 mm thick sagittal section of an adult right temporal bone immediately medial to Figure 1.28. The tensor tympani canal protrudes into the eustachian portion of the middle ear. The section exposes the modiolus and three turns of the cochlea. The lateral portion of the internal auditory meatus contains sections of the facial and acoustic nerves. The carotid artery lies anterior and inferior to the cochlea, while the jugular fossa passes along the inferior surface of the section.

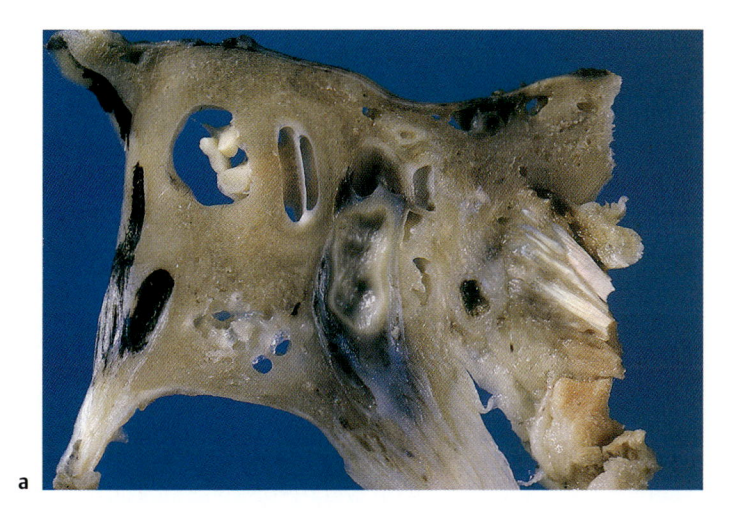

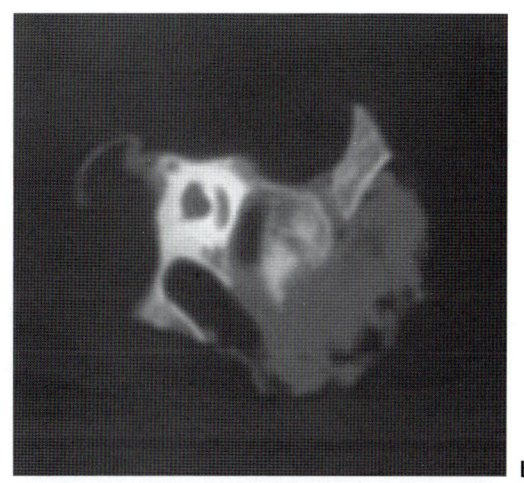

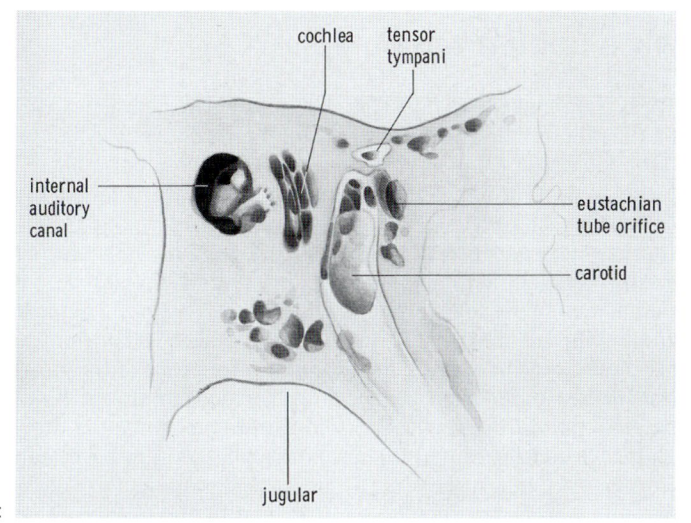

Fig. 1.**30 a** Sagittal macrosection 2 mm medial to Fig. 1.**29 a**.
b CT corresponding to **a**.
c Stuctures seen at this level.
d Microradiograph corresponding to **a**, **b**.

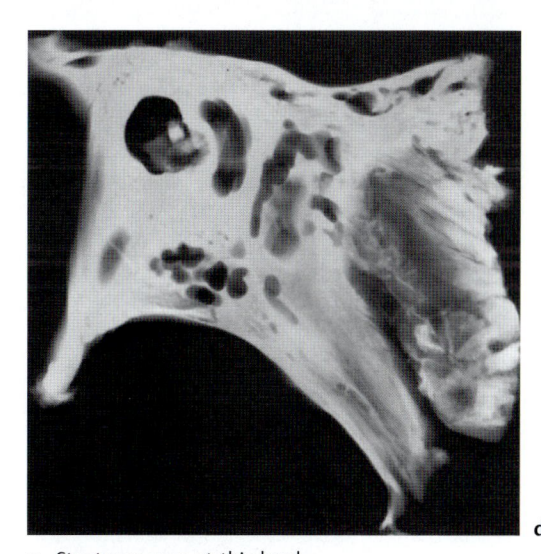

Figure 1.**30** shows the structures contained in a 2 mm thick sagittal section of an adult right temporal bone immediately medial to Figure 1.**29**. The tensor tympani is in the middle-ear portion of the eustachian tube. The carotid artery courses between the eustachian tube and the cochlea. Parts of the basal and middle coils of the cochlea lie anterior to the internal auditory meatus, while the jugular fossa forms the inferior margin of the section.

Imaging Techniques

■ Conventional Radiography

Conventional radiography is of value in screening the entire temporal bone and in determining the status of the pneumatization of the mastoid and the petrous pyramid. This method permits the recognition of large lesions that arise in or extend into the temporal bone. It is also useful in assessing the position and integrity of cochlear implant electrodes. The continuity of the wires cannot be demonstrated by tomographic techniques because segments of the electrodes are seen in several contiguous sections.

Several projections have been used in the past, but only three are of practical interest today: the lateral, or Schüller; the frontal, or transorbital; and the oblique, or Stenvers. The other projections have historical significance but no practical application.

Schüller Projection

The Schüller projection is a lateral view of the mastoid obtained with the sagittal plane of the head parallel to the tabletop and the x-ray beam rotated 30° cephalocaudad (Fig. 1.**31**).

The extent of the pneumatization of the mastoid, the distribution and degree of aeration of the air cells, and the status of the trabecular pattern are revealed in this projection. The sinus plate casts a sharp radiodense vertical line posterior to the external auditory canal. If the mastoid is well pneumatized, the sinus plate separates the superficial air cells from the deep air cells of the mastoid and of the petrous pyramid. If the mastoid is poorly pneumatized, there are no air cells posterior to the sinus plate. The vertical line of the sinus plate merges posterosuperiorly with a similar dense oblique line formed by the lateral portion of the petrous ridge. The sharp angle at the junction of the sinus and dural plates is the sinodural angle of Citelli. More anteriorly, the oblique line formed by the petrous ridge crosses the radiolucency of the external auditory canal and extends forward to reach the neck of the mandibular condyle.

Transorbital Projection

The transorbitial projection is a frontal view of the mastoid and petrous pyramid obtained with the patient either facing the film or with her or his back to the film (Fig. 1.**32**). The patient's head is flexed on the chin until the orbital–meatal line is perpendicular to the tabletop. For better details, each side should be obtained separately and the x-ray beam directed at the center of the orbit on the side under examination and perpendicular to the film.

The petrous apex is foreshortened because of its obliquity to the plane of the film. The internal auditory canal is visualized in its full length as a horizontal band of radiolucency extending through the petrous pyramid. At the medial end of the canal, the free margin of the posterior wall casts a smooth, well-defined margin concave medially. Quite often, the radiolucent band of the internal auditory canal seems to extend medially to the lip of the posterior wall into the petrous apex. This radiolucent band is, however, not due to the internal auditory canal, but rather produced by the prominence of the upper and lower lips of the porus and by the interpost groove. Lateral to the internal auditory canal, the radiolucency of the vestibule and semicircular canals is often detectable. The apical and middle coils of the cochlea are superimposed upon the lateral portion of the internal auditory canal, whereas the basal turn may be seen underneath it and the vestibule.

Stenvers Projection

For this oblique projection of the mastoid and petrous pyramid, the patient is positioned facing the film with his or her head slightly flexed and rotated 45° toward the side opposite to the side under examination (Fig. 1.**33**). Doing this, the lateral rim of the orbit of the side under investigation should lie in close contact to the tabletop. The x-ray beam is angled 14° caudad. The entire petrous apex is visualized in full length, lateral to the orbital rim. The porus of the internal auditory canal seen face-on appears as an oval-shaped radiolucency open medially and limited laterally by the free margin of the posterior canal wall. Lateral to the porus, the internal auditory canal appears quite foreshortened. The vestibule and semicircular canals, especially the posterior, which lies in this projection in a plane parallel to the film, are usually recognizable. On the outside, the entire mastoid is outlined with the mastoid process free of superimposition.

■ Computed Tomography (CT)

These days conventional CT has been replaced by helical or spiral CT that allows rapid acquisition of volumetric data of the part of the body under examination. Images are acquired at an angled plane of section and then reconstructed by interpolating the volumetric data set as 2D or high-quality 3D reformations. The continuous acquisition of images is made possible by replacing the former electric cabling of the gantry with a slip-ring design that allows continuous rotation of the source–detector assembly and by the use of high heat capacity x-ray tubes. The advantage of spiral CT includes the elimination of respiratory misregistration, decrease of motion artifact, and an obvious improvement in patient comfort due to the shortening of the examination time. This is particularly important in children whether they have been administered anesthesia or a simple sedation and in older patients who have difficulty in overextending the head.

Reconstruction of axial data in other planes produces satisfactory images, provided a collimation as small as 1 or 0.5 mm is used. A scanning time of less than one minute is sufficient to cover the mastoid and petrous portions of the temporal bone. New multidetector scanners further decrease the scanning time. The CT images provide exquisite bony details and excellent demonstration of soft-tissue density within the air spaces of the mastoids, external auditory canal, and middle ear but very limited identification of the type of substance producing the abnormal density. For instance, the density of cholesteatoma is identical to that of a tumor or granulation tissue and even of fluid.

The densitometric readings obtained with a cursor of variable size are usually unreliable because of partial volume averaging within the small cavities of the ear.

Time–density curves obtained by rapid sequential images of a preselected section after intravenous injection of a bolus of contrast material are useful for the identification of vascular masses.

At present, MR provides a far more precise identification of the type of tissue within the air spaces and abnormal cavities in the temporal bone.

3D reconstruction of the temporal bone has not added diagnostic information but is of great value in surgical planning in large lesions of the base of the skull.

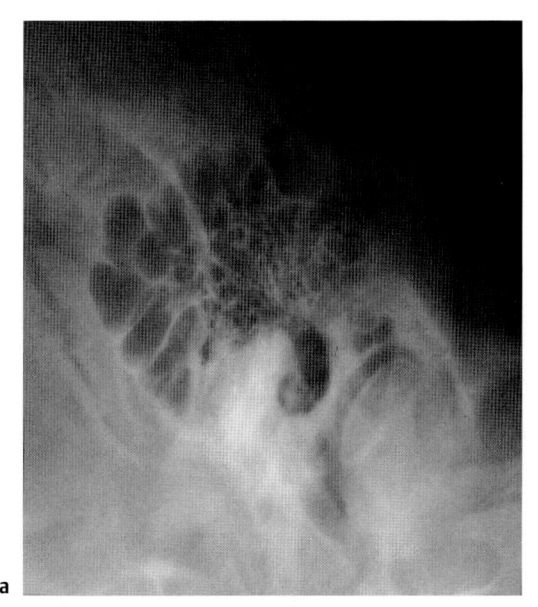

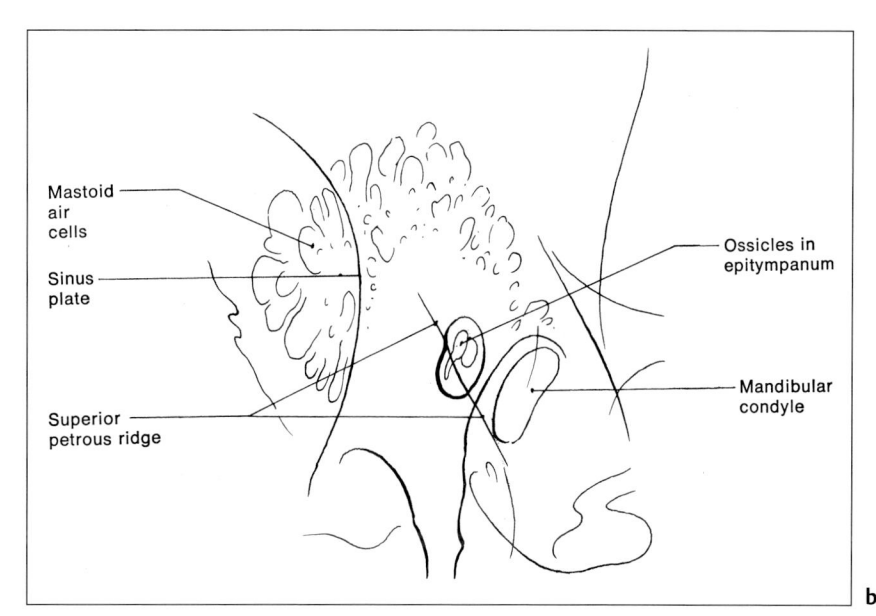

Fig. 1.**31** **a** Schüller projection. **b** Diagram of Schüller projection.

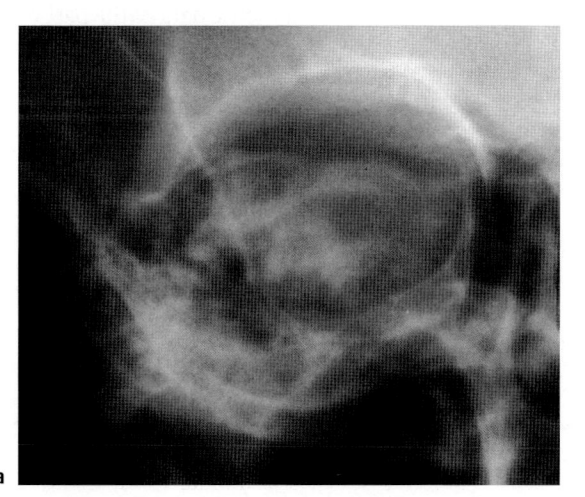

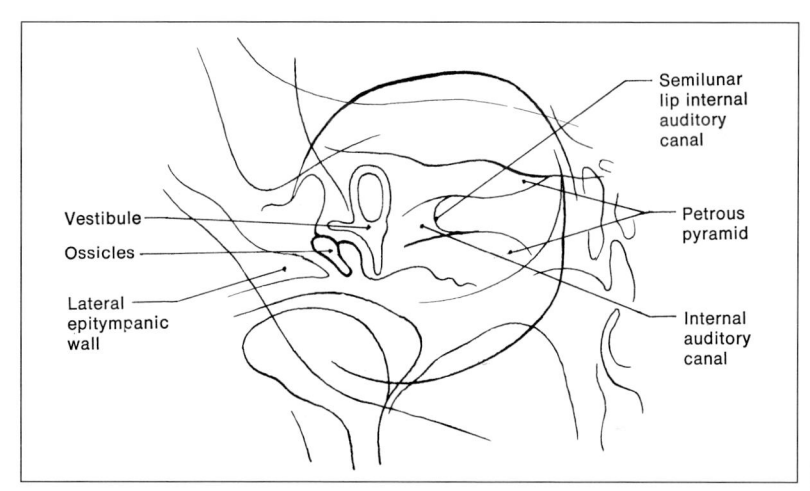

Fig. 1.**32** **a** Transorbital projection. **b** Diagram of transorbital projection.

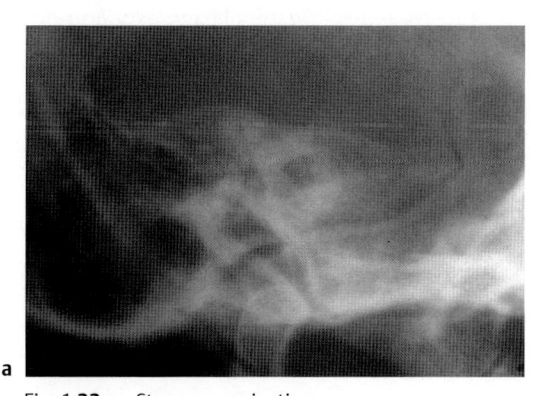

Fig. 1.**33 a** Stenvers projection.
b Diagram of Stenvers projection.

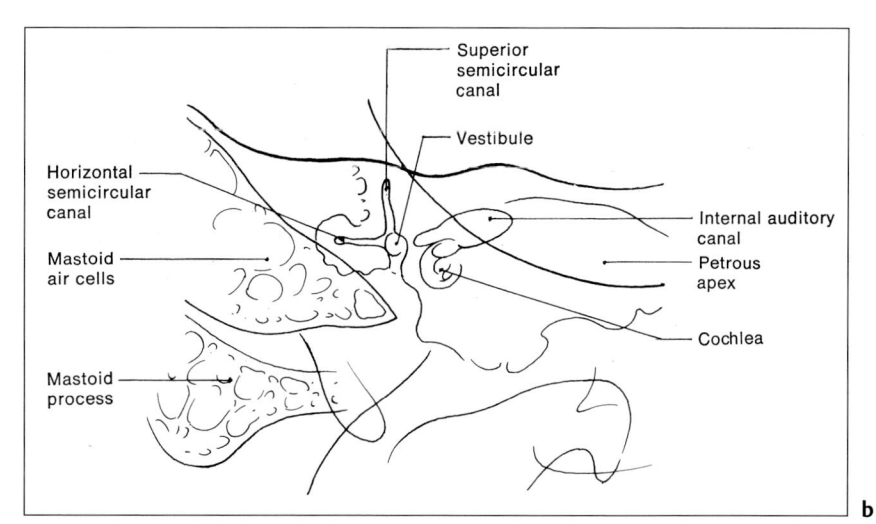

Projections

The normal temporal bone will be studied in four projections: axial or horizontal; coronal or frontal; sagittal or lateral; and 20° coronal oblique.

Axial or Horizontal Projection

Since the axial projection is the easiest to obtain, this is the standard view. The patient lies supine with the canthomeatal line perpendicular to the tabletop. Sections at 1.5 mm increments are taken, beginning at the arcuate eminence and continuing to the level of the floor of the hypotympanum and jugular fossa.

This projection delineates the anterior and posterior aspects and dimensions, but fails to demonstrate superior and inferior boundaries of the temporal bone.

Coronal or Frontal Projection

The patient lies on the table prone or supine, with the head overextended, and the gantry is tilted so that the plane of section is perpendicular to a plane passing from the tragus to the inferior orbital rim. For this projection, the gantry must tilt 15°–20°.

Sections are taken from the bony eustachian tube to the loop of the posterior semicircular canal. This projection is complementary to the axial because it demonstrates the superior and inferior boundaries and vertical dimensions of the temporal bone.

20° Coronal Oblique

This projection is obtained by rotating the patient's head from the coronal positon 20° toward the side under examination. With this rotation, the medial wall of the tympanic cavity becomes perpendicular to the plane of section. We use this projection for the study of the oval window, promontory, and tympanic segments of the facial canal. If the patient is unable to tolerate the position, reconstructed images from the axial data are obtained.

Sagittal or Lateral Projection

Direct lateral sections are difficult to obtain and can only be performed in patients with supple necks. A true sagittal projection can never be fully accomplished. At present, with spiral fast CT sagittal images almost as satisfactory as direct CT can be obtained by computer reformatting of the raw data from serial axial sections. The main reason for using this projection is to delineate the vertical portion of the facial nerve, the vestibular aqueduct, and the upper portion of the superior semicircular canal.

CT of the Facial Canal

Involvement of the intratemporal portion of the facial nerve may result in facial nerve symptoms such as partial or complete paralysis, tics, hemifacial spasms, and alterations in hearing, taste, and lacrimation. The bony canal of the facial nerve passes through the temporal bone and can be visualized by CT. The facial nerve itself can best be visualized by MR. CT sections are taken 1 mm apart, and contralateral views are obtained for comparison. The projection used in the study of the facial canal depends on the segment being examined. In the temporal bone, there are four segments of the facial canal that must be visualized.

1. First or internal auditory canal segment. Axial and coronal sections expose this segment. If an intracanalicular mass is suspected, an MR study or CT pneumocisternogram is required to determine the size and extent of the lesion.
2. Second or labyrinthine segment. This portion of the facial canal extends from the fundus of the internal auditory canal to the anterior genu. This segment is the narrowest part of the facial canal. Axial and 20° coronal-oblique sections expose the segment.
3. Third or tympanic segment. This segment extends from the anterior genu along the medial wall of the tympanic cavity to the second or pyramidal turn of the facial nerve. The axial and 20° coronal oblique sections are best to expose this segment.
4. Fourth or mastoid segment. This segment stretches from the pyramidal turn to the stylomastoid foramen, and is best visualized by sagittal or coronal sections.

■ Magnetic Resonance Imaging (MRI)

MR is an imaging technique that produces cross-sectional images in any plane without exposing the patient to ionizing radiation. MR images are obtained by the interaction of hydrogen nuclei (protons), high magnetic fields, and radiofrequency pulses. The intensity of the MR signal to be converted to imaging data depends on the concentration or density of the hydrogen nuclei in the examined tissue and on two magnetic relaxation times, T1 and T2, which are tissue-specific. One of the characteristics and advantages of MR is the feasibility of changing the appearance and information of the images by varying the relative contribution of the T1 and T2 relaxation times. This is obtained by changing the time between radiofrequency pulses (TR, or repetition time), and the time the emitted signal or echo is measured after the pulse (TE, or echo time).

The signal intensity of different tissues is directly proportional to the number of free protons present within the tissue and to the T1 and T2 relaxation times. Fat and body fluids contain large amounts of free protons and therefore yield strong MR signals. Air, cortical bone, and calcified tissue appear as dark areas, since they contain few free protons and yield a very weak MR signal. Blood vessels in which there is circulating blood appear in MR images as areas of void or no signal because the magnetized protons of the circulating blood move out of the sections before their emitted signal can be detected. A high-intensity signal will be detected from circulating blood vessels if a rapid scanning technique is used.

Pathological processes are recognizable when the proton density and relaxation times of the abnormal tissue are different from those of normal tissue. Examination is performed with the patient supine and the plane extending from the tragus to the inferior orbital rim perpendicular to the tabletop. Different projections are obtained by changing the orientation of the magnetic field gradients without moving the patient's head. Axial, coronal, and sagittal projections are usually obtained. T1-weighted images obtained by a short TR and TE offer the best anatomical delineation. T2-weighted images obtained with long TR and TE better differentiate normal from pathological tissues (see Table 1.**1**).

MR imaging technique has undergone multiple changes and refinements in order to increase the definition of the image, to decrease the acquisition time of the image and to improve the recognition and differentiation of pathological processes. First, the introduction of surface coils placed adjacent to the area of interest has increased the signal-to-noise ratio and consequently improved the image. Shorter acquisition times have been obtained:

1. By shortening the TR and using gradient pulses and flip angles smaller than 90°, a technique known as gradient-echo imaging.
2. By reducing the number of phase-encoded steps. This can be obtained by sampling or collecting only half of the raw data. This technique is known as half-Fourier imaging.
3. By increasing the data collected per excitation. Fast spin-echo (FSE) uses multiple echoes (4–16) from an excitation, therefore reducing the number of excitations necessary for forming an image. The obtained images reflect true T2 contrast, but unlike routine spin-echo T2-weighted, the fat signal remains high.

The intravenous injection of paramagnetic contrast agents (gadolinium-DTPA) has improved the recognition and differentiation of pathological processes. Normal brain does not enhance except for structures such as the pituitary gland, choroid plexus, and dura that lack a blood–brain barrier. Enhancement of brain lesions occurs whenever the blood–brain barrier is disrupted, provided there is sufficient blood flow to the lesions. Extra-axial lesions such as meningiomas and neuromas lack a blood–brain barrier and therefore undergo a strong enhancement.

The images in this chapter were obtained with a superconducting magnet, a magnetic field of 15 000 Gauss (1.5 Tesla), and two or four excitations, and were displayed on a 256 × 192 or 512 × 256 matrix.

Temporal Bone MR Imaging

Since cortical bone and air emit no signal, normal mastoid, external auditory canal, and middle ear cavity appear on MR images as black areas, and the contours of these structures are not visualized. The petrous pyramids are also dark, except for the inner ear structures and the internal auditory canals, which appear bright on the T2-weighted images from the signal emitted by the fluid within their lumina (Fig. 1.**34**). Often a strong signal is emitted from fat in the diploë bone marrow of the petrous apices (see Fig. 1.**52 b**).

Fluid and soft-tissue changes caused by trauma, infection, or tumor of the temporal bone are seen in MR as areas of abnormal signal intensity. MR is more sensitive than CT in detecting small soft-tissue lesions in the temporal bone. However, the anatomical site of the lesions and the presence and extent of bony destruction often cannot be determined by MR, since bony landmarks are absent in the MR images. Because of these factors, CT remains at present the study of choice for identification of intratemporal bone pathology.

If the lesion extends beyond the limits of the temporal bone, or arises within the internal auditory canal or jugular fossa, MR details and defines involvement more precisely than CT. This is particularly true for glomus tumors, since involvement of the jugular vein and internal carotid artery is demonstrated in MR images without need for invasive vascular studies. High-resolution images of the temporal bone can be obtained in a reasonable acquisition time by combining fast spin-echo technique and small voxel matrix (512×512). The time saved using fast spin-echo is utilized to obtain larger matrices (Figs. 1.**34**, 1.**35**, and 1.**36**). This protocol allows excellent images of the inner ear structures and internal auditory canal. Individual nerves and vascular loops are clearly demonstrated in the cerebellopontine cistern and internal auditory canal as bands of low signal (Figs. 1.**34**, 1.**35**, and 1.**36**).

Sections of the temporal bone as thin as 0.5 mm can be acquired by a three-dimensional Fourier transformation (3DFT) technique using a small receiver coil and a low flip angle (10–20°) with short TR and TE. T1-weighted images in any plane can be reformatted from the data acquired in the axial plane.[2]

Finally, three-dimensional (3D) fast spin-echo (FSE) imaging methods are used to increase the signal to noise ratio for better spatial resolution in patients selected for cochlear implant or patients with clinical suspicion for labyrinthine malformations.[5] At our institution we have applied the following technique: A dual-phase array 3 inch (75 mm) surface coil is used, with the following parameters: TR 3000 ms, TE 210 ms, 256 × 256 matrix size, 2 NEX, FOV 16–18 cm, slice thickness 0.6–0.9 mm with 0 slice overlap and ETL of 96. Either a single surface coil for imaging one side or a combination of two surface coils is used for simultaneous imaging. By using a large echo train length (ETL) we are able to decrease the scan time to approximately 8–9 minutes.

Table 1.1 MRI analysis of middle and inner ear pathology

Site/lesion	T1W	T2W	T1W and C
Middle ear			
Fluid (transudate)	0	+++	0
Cholesteatoma	+	++	0
Cholesterol granuloma	+++	+++	0
Granulation tissue	+	++	++
Jugular bulb	Mixed	Mixed	+++
Glomus tumor	+	++ (mixed)	++
Meningo-encephalocele	Brain surrounded by dark rim (fluid)	Brain surrounded by bright rim (fluid)	+/0
Petrous apex			
Congenital cholesteatoma	+	+++	0
Cholesterol granuloma	+++	+++ (mixed)	0
Mucocele	+/0	+++	+ capsule
Arachnoid cyst	0	+++	0
Petrositis-abscess	+	++	++ to +++
Inner ear			
Blood (chronic)	+++	+++	No change
Labyrinthitis	0	0/+	+ to ++
Autoimmune labyrinthitis	0	0/+	++ cochlea only
Neuroma	0	0/+	+++
Endolymphatic sac tumors	+ to ++	+ to +++	+++ (non-homogeneous)
IAC and CPA			
Vestibular schwannoma	+/0	+ to +++	+++
Meningioma	+/0	+ to +++	+++ tail sign
Lipoma	+++	Low in standard T2W	No change
Neuritis	0	+	++ thickening of nerves
Aneurysm (thrombosed)	Mixed	Mixed	++ nonhomogeneous
Hemangiomas	+	++	+++
Vascular malformations	+ (mixed)	Mixed	signal void areas due to bony spicules or calcifications
Meningeal inflammation	0	+ ++ (FLAIR)	++ linear enhancement
Facial nerve			
Bell's palsy	0	+	++ segmental
Herpes zoster (Ramsay Hunt)	0	+	+++ extending into IAC
Neuroma	+	++	+++ localized mass
Neurofibromatosis	+	++	+++ diffuse involvement
Sarcoidosis	0	+	++

T1W, T1-weighted; T2W, T2-weighted; T1W + C, T1-weighted after injection of contrast; IAC, internal auditory canal; CPA, cerebellopontine angle.
0, +, ++, +++: degree of signal intensity in T1W and T2W images and degree of enhancement in T1W + C images.

34   1 Imaging of the Temporal Bone

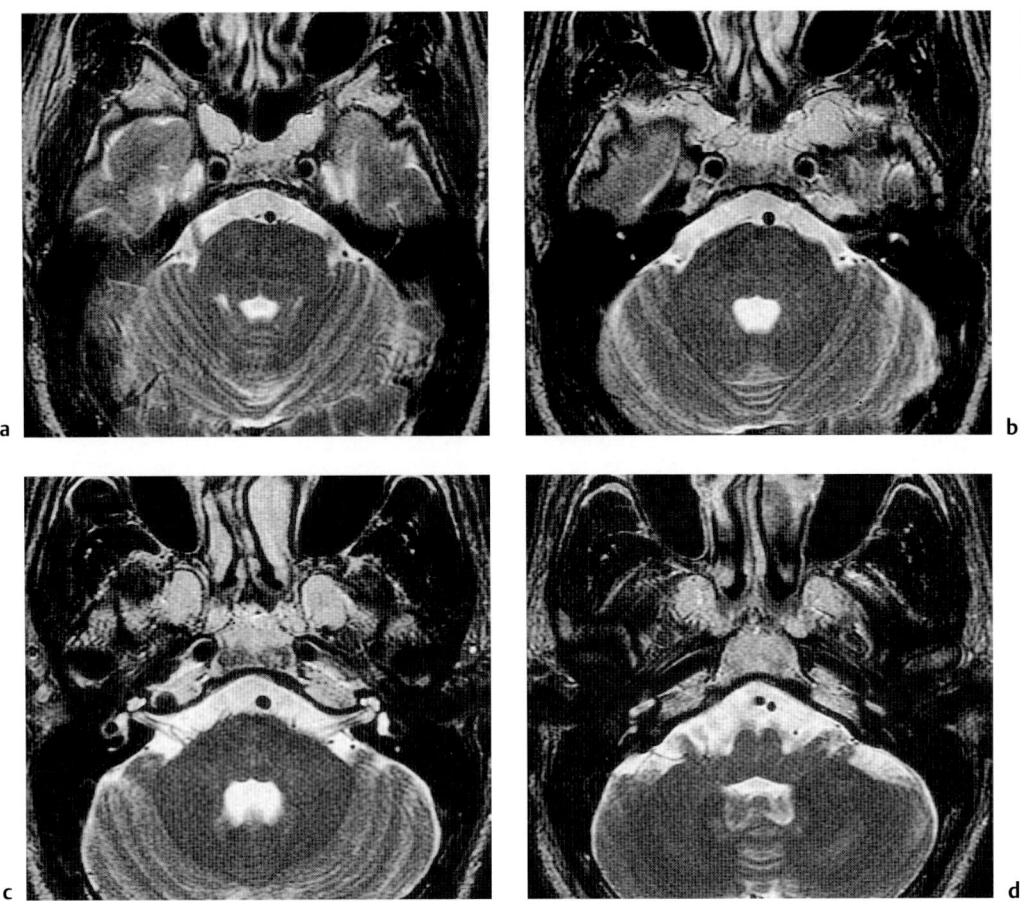

Fig. 1.34 Normal temporal bone. Axial FSE images. **a** Upper section at the level of the superior petrous ridge and fifth cranial nerve. **b** Section 3 mm caudad showing the superior semicircular canal and common crus. **c** Section 3 mm caudad to **b** exposing the cochlea, vestibule, and semicircular canals. The seventh and eighth cranial nerves course from the brainstem into the internal auditory canal. The anterior–inferior cerebellar artery loops at the porus of the internal auditory canal. **d** Section 3 mm inferior to **c** shows the inferior aspect of the basal turn of the cochlea and the posterior semicircular canal.

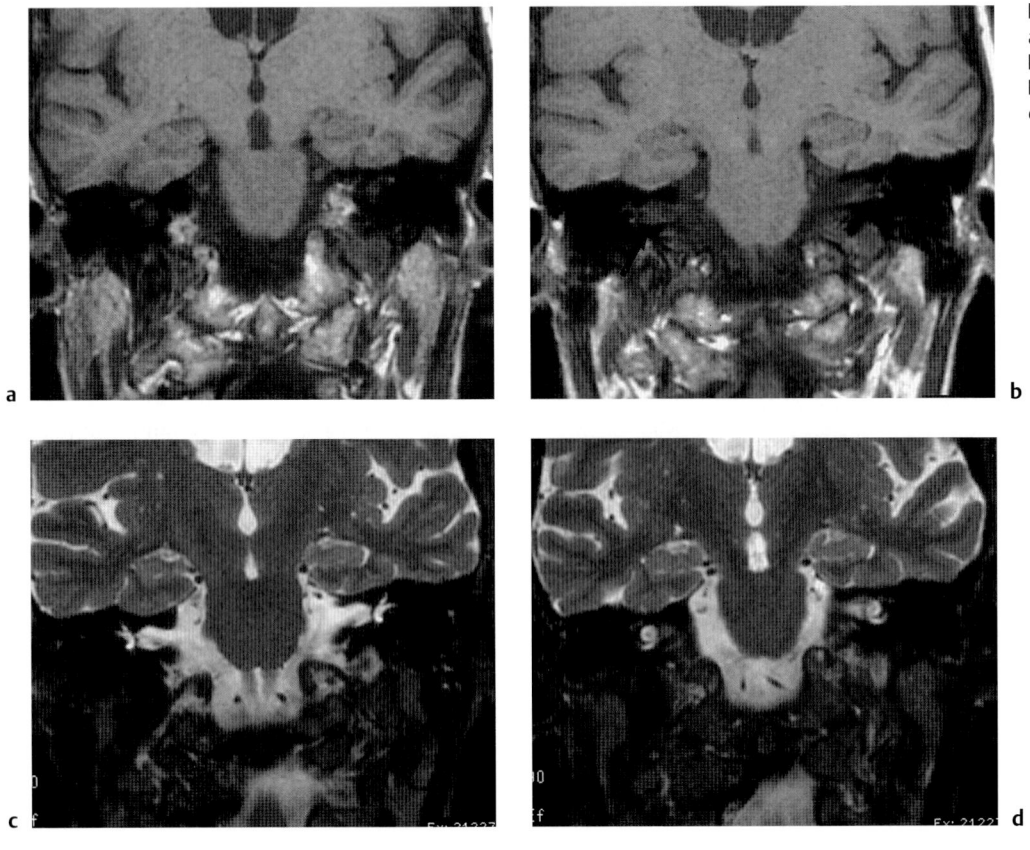

Fig. 1.35 Normal temporal bone. **a** and **b** Coronal T1. **c** and **d** coronal FSE (small arrow, cochlea; long arrow, IAC; arrow heads, vestibule and semicircular canals).

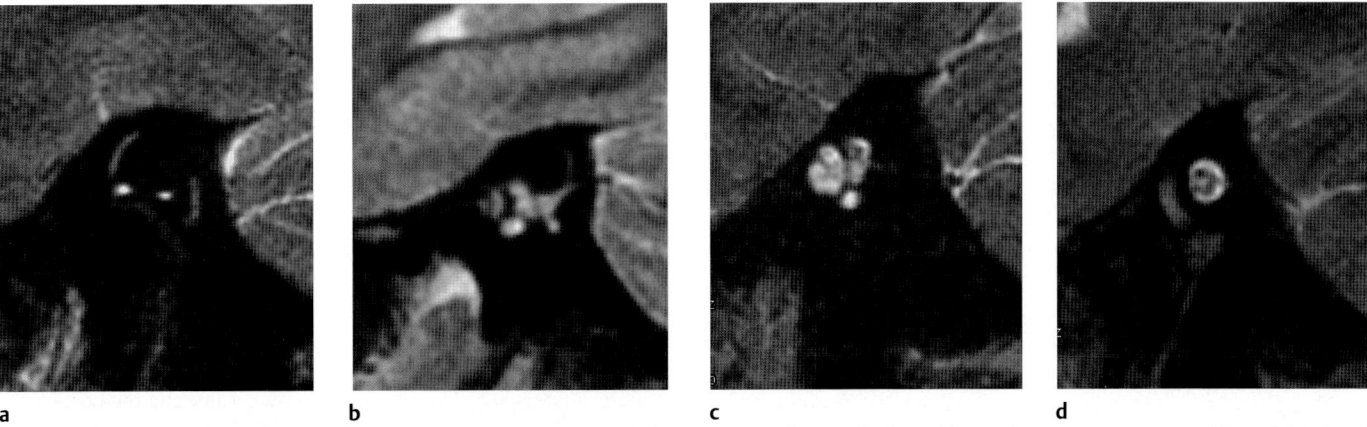

Fig. 1.36 Normal temporal bone: Sagittal FSE images showing: **a** all three semicircular canals; **b** cochlea and common crus; **c** cochlea; **d** facial and acoustic nerves within the IAC.

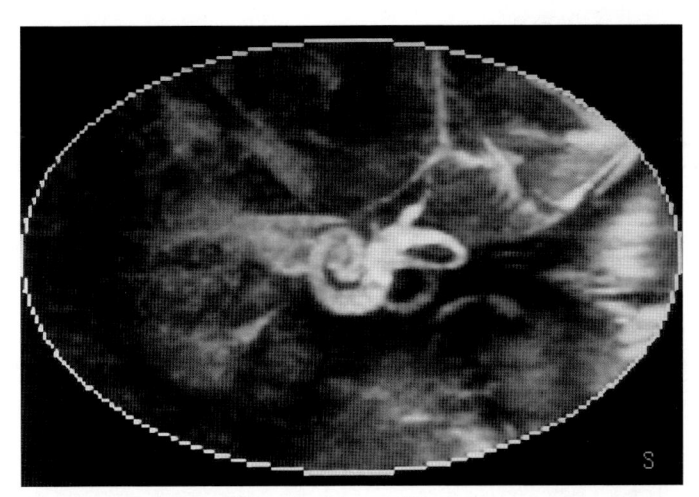

Fig. 1.37 3D image of the membranous labyrinth.

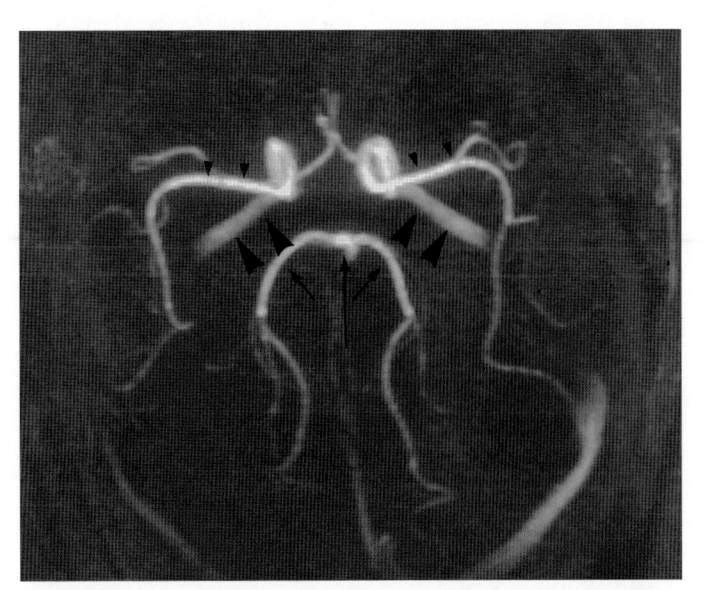

Fig. 1.38 MRA of normal intracranial vessels. Axial three-dimensional PC angiograms of the circle of Willis. Carotid arteries (large arrowheads), basilar artery (long arrow), posterior cerebral arteries (short arrows), and middle cerebral arteries (small arrowheads).

Postprocessing is performed using maximum intensity projection (MIP) software making it possible to reformat 3D images of the membranous labyrinth that can be viewed in any plane. In situations where volumetric quantitation of the membranous labyrinth is needed, a more detailed volume rendering technique may be used for reconstruction. This technique provides depth perception of the membranous labyrinth (Fig. 1.**37**).

Magnetic Resonance Angiography (MRA)

Gradient-echo techniques and flow-encoding gradients have enabled the development of MRA. Time-of-flight (TOF) angiography is a gradient-echo technique in which the stationary tissues within the imaging plane are saturated with the magnetic field so that they will not produce a signal. Blood flowing within the same plane is unsaturated and will be the only tissue to produce a signal. Phase contrast (PC) angiography is acquired somewhat differently. Instead of saturating the stationary tissues with radiofrequency pulses, a bipolar gradient of magnetization is applied to the entire slice, first with a positive value and then with a negative value. In the stationary tissues, the two opposite gradients cancel each other out. In the flowing blood, however, the two opposite gradients cannot cancel each other out because the blood will have moved to a different plane in the region before the inverse gradient is applied. With both modalities, two-dimensional or three-dimensional volume acquisitions can be obtained.

Three-dimensional MRA allows acquisition of thinner slices with a better signal-to-noise ratio than two-dimensional (Fig. 1.**38**). However, two-dimensional images have the advantage of shorter acquisition times and greater sensitivity to slow flow, and they permit imaging of large areas of interest. The slices obtained are constructed into projection images, which can be rotated in different planes to separate vessels and eliminate superimposition (Figure 1.**39**). MRA of the intracranial vasculature has been particularly useful in the demonstration of aneurysms (see Figure 1.**216**) in the region of the circle of Willis, arteriovenous malformation (AVM) (particularly a small dural AVM that may not be visible on routine spin-echo images) and vaso-occlusive pathology, including dural sinus thrombosis. MRA of the extracranial circulations provides excellent information about the patency of the carotid and vertebral arteries (Fig. 1.**40**). These vessels may be compressed or displaced by neck masses and their lumina stenosed or obstructed by thrombosis or atheromatous plaques.

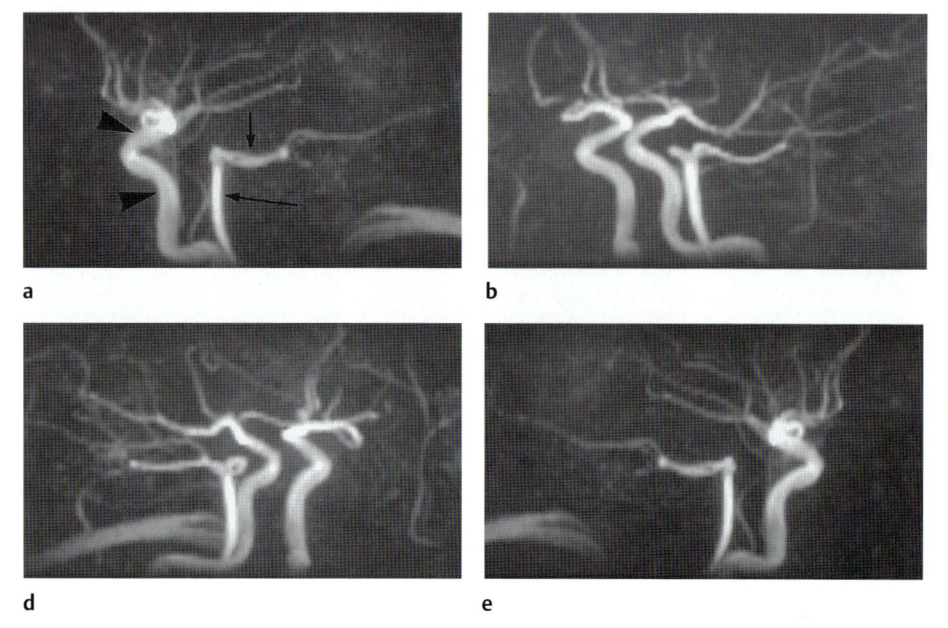

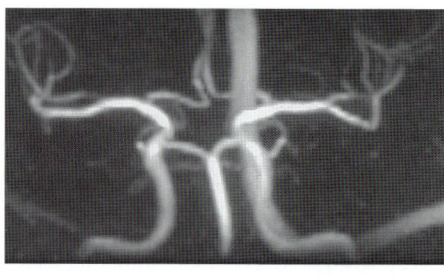

Fig. 1.39 MRA of normal circle of Willis. Three-dimensional PC angiograms. **a** Right lateral, **b** right oblique, **c** coronal, **d** left oblique, **e** left lateral views. Carotid arteries (large arrowheads), basilar artery (long arrow), and posterior cerebral arteries (short arrows).

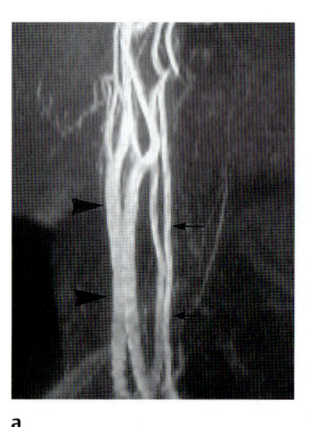

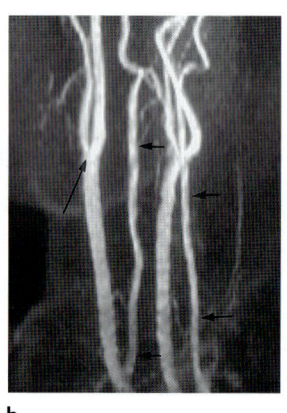

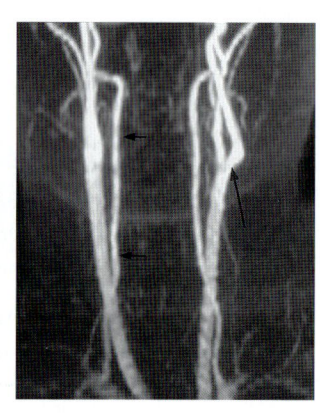

Fig. 1.40 MRA of normal large vessels of neck. Two-dimensional TOF angiograms. **a** Right lateral, **b** right oblique, **c** coronal views. Carotid arteries (large arrowheads), carotid bifurcation (long arrow), and vertebral arteries (short arrows).

Developmental Variations

Developmental variation in the size and position of several components of the temporal bone are quite common. A gray area separates developmental variation from actual anomalies and this may lead to arbitrary classification by this and other authors.

Developmental variations should be recognized by the radiologist rather than mistaken for pathological processes, but, above all, should be known to the otologists as they develop their surgical plans. Lack of appreciation of several anatomical variations may lead to serious complications and always to a more difficult and lengthy surgical procedure.

■ Mastoid

The development of the mastoids varies from person to person and, to a lesser degree, from side to side of the same individual. In some mastoids, the pneumatization is limited to a single antral cell; in others it may extend into the mastoid tip or squama of the temporal bone and invade the adjacent zygoma roots and even the occipital bone (Fig. 1.41). The nonpneumatized mastoid process may be made up of solid bone or contain spongy (diploic) spaces filled with fatty marrow. The fatty marrow produces a high signal in the T1-weighted MR sequence that decreases in the T2 and should not be confused with fluid or other pathological processes that usually have a high signal in the T2 sequence. One should also remember that it may be impossible by MR to distinguish a small mastoid containing a large aerated cell from a sclerotic mastoid since both produce an identical signal void.

■ Lateral Sinus

The lateral or sigmoid sinus forms a shallow indentation on the posterior aspect of the mastoid. Occasionally the sinus courses more anteriorly and produces a deep groove in the mastoid, best seen in the axial sections. In some cases only a thin bony plate separates the sinus from the external auditory canal (Fig. 1.42). Without this information, the otologist could enter the sinus, with consequent severe bleeding and possible complications from sinus thrombosis.

■ Tegmen

The tegmen of the mastoid and attic passes usually in a horizontal plane slightly lower than the arcuate eminence produced by the top of the superior semicircular canal. A depression of the tegmental plate is not unusual, particularly in patients with con-

Developmental Variations

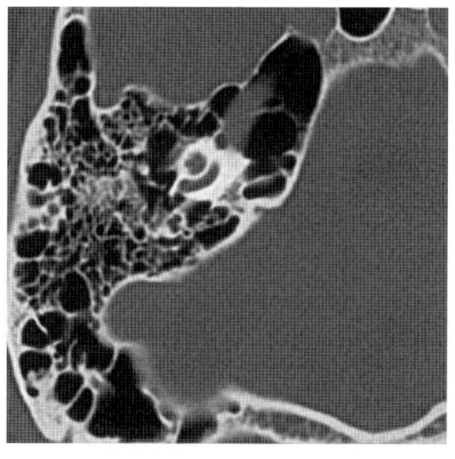

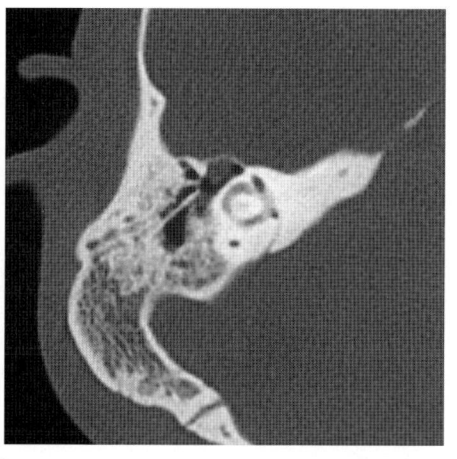

Fig. 1.41 Mastoid development: axial CT sections. **a** The mastoid and petrous pyramid are extremely pneumatized. **b** The mastoid pneumatization is limited to a small mastoid antrum.

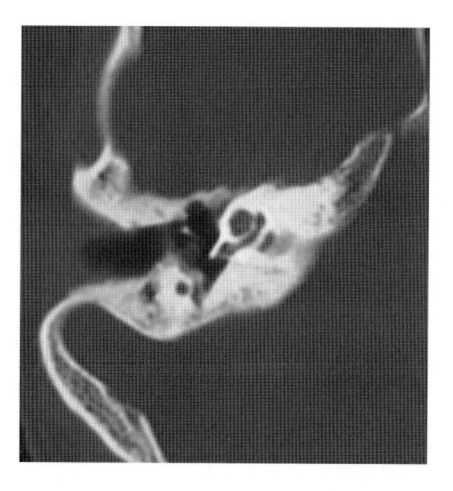

Fig. 1.42 Anterior lateral sinus: axial CT section. The sinus produces a deep groove in the posterior aspect of the mastoid and reaches the posterior wall of the external auditory canal.

Fig. 1.43 Low tegmen: **a** coronal, **b** axial CT sections. The low-lying dura covers the roof of the external auditory canal (**a**) and the middle cranial fossa deepens to form a groove lateral to the middle ear (**b**).

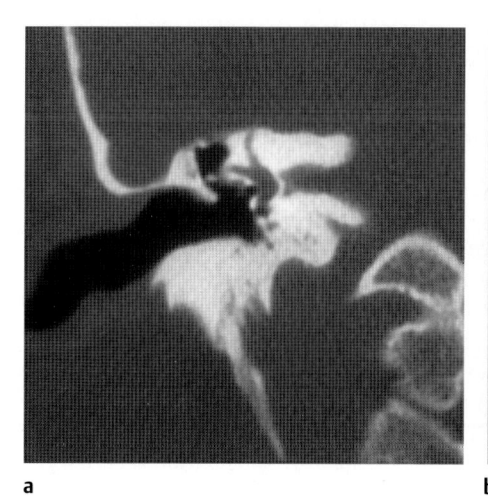

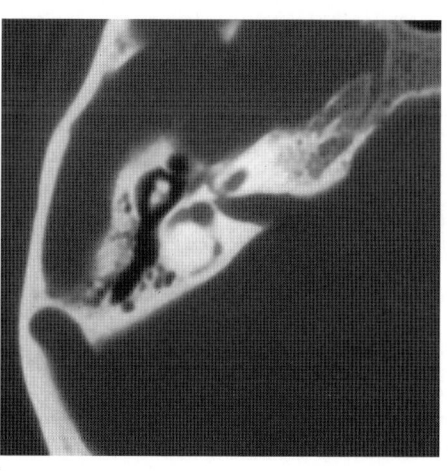

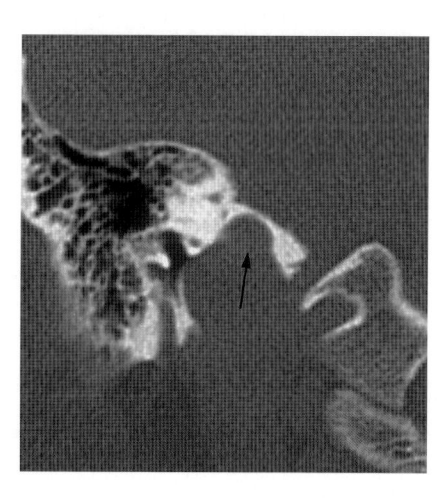

Fig. 1.44 Jugular bulb diverticulum: coronal CT section. A diverticulum extends from the dome of the large jugular bulb to the superior petrous ridge.

genital atresia of the external auditory canal. As seen in the coronal sections, the floor of the middle cranial fossa deepens to form a groove lateral to the attic and to the labyrinth. The low lying dura may cover the roof of the external auditory canal and when the canal is not developed, extend laterally to the mesotympanum (Fig. 1.43). Unless aware of this feature, the otologist will penetrate the cranial cavity during surgery.

■ Jugular Fossa

There is a tremendous variation in the size of the jugular fossa and jugular bulb. The variation occurs not only from patient to patient but from side to side on the same patient. The size of the jugular fossa is not a criterion for a pathological process. A normal jugular fossa may produce only a slight indentation on the undersurface of the petrous bone or extend upward as high as the superior petrous ridge posterior to the labyrinth and internal auditory canal (Fig. 1.44). In these instances, the jugular bulb projects so high that it blocks access to the internal auditory canal by the translabyrinthine route in acoustic neuroma surgery. Often the high venous structure is not the jugular bulb itself but rather a diverticulum arising from the dome of the bulb (Fig. 1.44).

The jugular bulb at times projects into the hypotympanum and mesotympanum. There may be a bony cover over the jugular bulb or the vein may lie exposed in the middle ear in contact with the medial surface of the tympanic membrane (Fig. 1.45). In these cases, such a high jugular bulb appears otoscopically as a blue mass, which can be misdiagnosed as a glomus tumor (Fig. 1.47).

There are three variations of high jugular bulb projecting into the middle ear:
1. The jugular fossa and the jugular vein are high and the jugular bulb is covered by a bony shell.
2. The jugular fossa and the jugular bulb are high but there is an incomplete bony shell surrounding the soft-tissue mass protruding into the middle ear.
3. The jugular fossa and the jugular bulb are not high but a diverticulum protrudes from the bulb into the middle ear through a defect in the dome of the fossa and hypotympanic floor. This variation may be confused for a glomus tumor but for the fact that the contour of the jugular fossa is intact except for the defect.

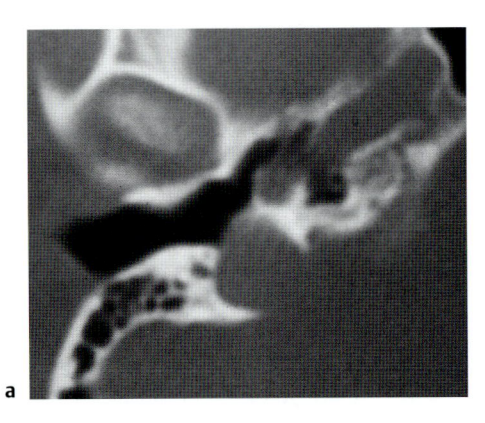

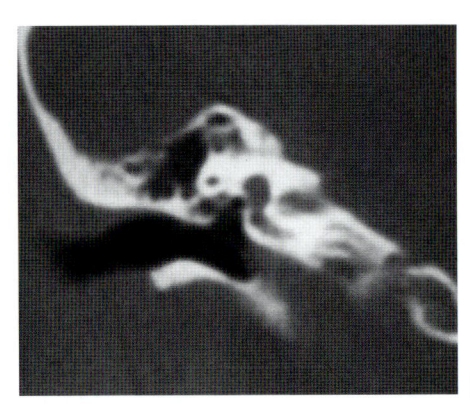

Fig. 1.45 High jugular bulb: **a** axial, **b** coronal CT. There is a large defect in the hypotympanic floor and the jugular bulb protrudes into the posteroinferior portion of the middle ear.

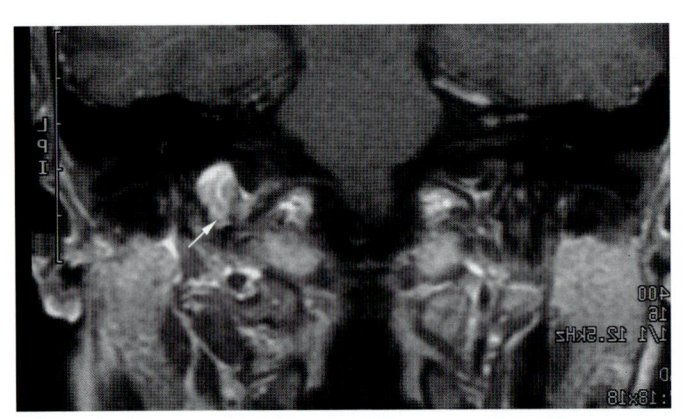

Fig. 1.46 High jugular bulb: coronal MR T1 postcontrast. The right jugular bulb appears as an enhancing mass with a vertical streak of low signal.

The MR study of a high jugular bulb may be misread as showing a glomus tumor because of the area of mixed signal within the bulb produced by turbulent flow. However, whereas a glomus contains multiple punctate areas of signal void within a mass of medium or high signal, in a high jugular bulb linear streaks of high and low signal are seen within the lumen of the bulb, usually paralleling its walls due to variations in flow velocity (Fig. 1.46). In questionable cases, an MR venogram should be performed using a 2D time-of-flight technique sensitive to slow flow or a 2D phase contrast using a short VENC (velocity encoding).

Carotid Artery

Minor variations in the intratemporal course of the internal carotid artery (ICA) are not uncommon but are of no clinical significance. The carotid artery may take an ectopic course through the middle ear. The aberrant ICA according to Moret et al occurs when the cervical portion of the artery fails to develop. The inferior tympanic artery anastomoses with the enlarged caroticotympanic artery forming the aberrant ICA. This anomaly is rare but is of clinical importance. If surgery is contemplated, the otological surgeon should be aware of the abnormal position of the artery in his surgical field. This lesion also may be misdiagnosed as a glomus or other type of middle ear tumor. We have recognized several cases of this rare vascular anomaly. All were confirmed by angiographic studies or MRA.

Microscopic otoscopy shows a pinkish or white-blue mass lying in the inferior mesotympanum in contact with the medial surface of the tympanic membrane. The mass may or may not pulsate (Fig. 1.48).

The CT findings of an ectopic intratemporal carotid artery are:
1. There is a soft-tissue mass extending throughout the entire length of the inferior portion of the middle ear cavity (Fig. 1.49a).
2. There may be a thin bony wall partially surrounding the artery.
3. Contact of the mass with the tympanic membrane causes lateral bulging of the membrane. Medially the mass may cause indentation of the promontory (Fig. 1.49c).

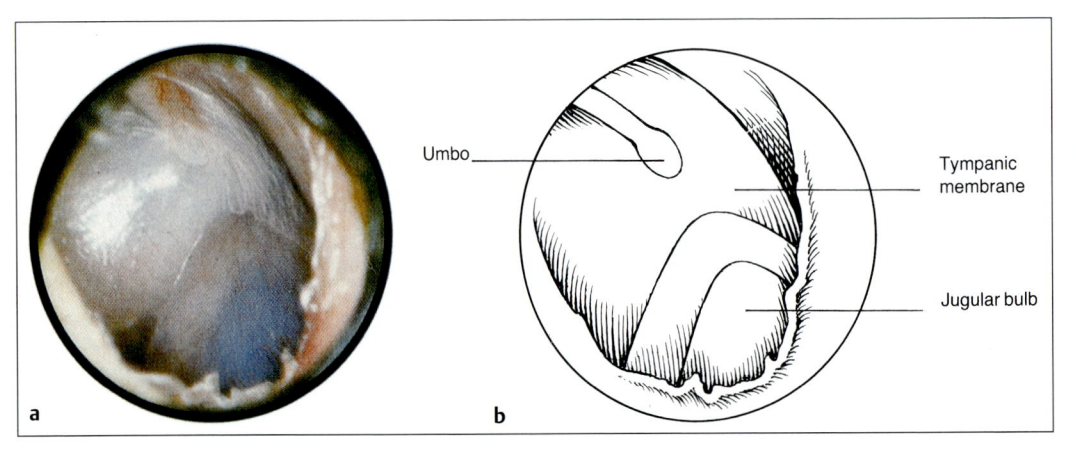

Fig. 1.47 **a** High jugular bulb, otoscopic findings, left. The dome of the jugular bulb without a bony cover protrudes into the posterior mesotympanum and lies in contact with the tympanic membrane. The jugular bulb has the characteristic blue color of venous blood. **b** Diagram of **a**.

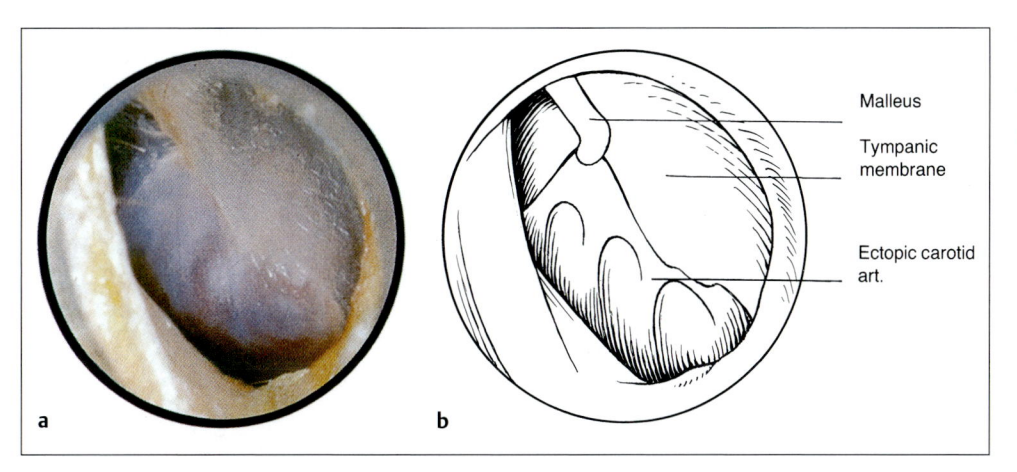

Developmental Variations

Fig. 1.48 **a** Ectopic internal carotid artery, otoscopic findings, left. A deep, red-purple mass fills the inferior middle ear and herniates the tympanic membrane slightly. This lesion did not pulsate.
b Diagram of **a**.

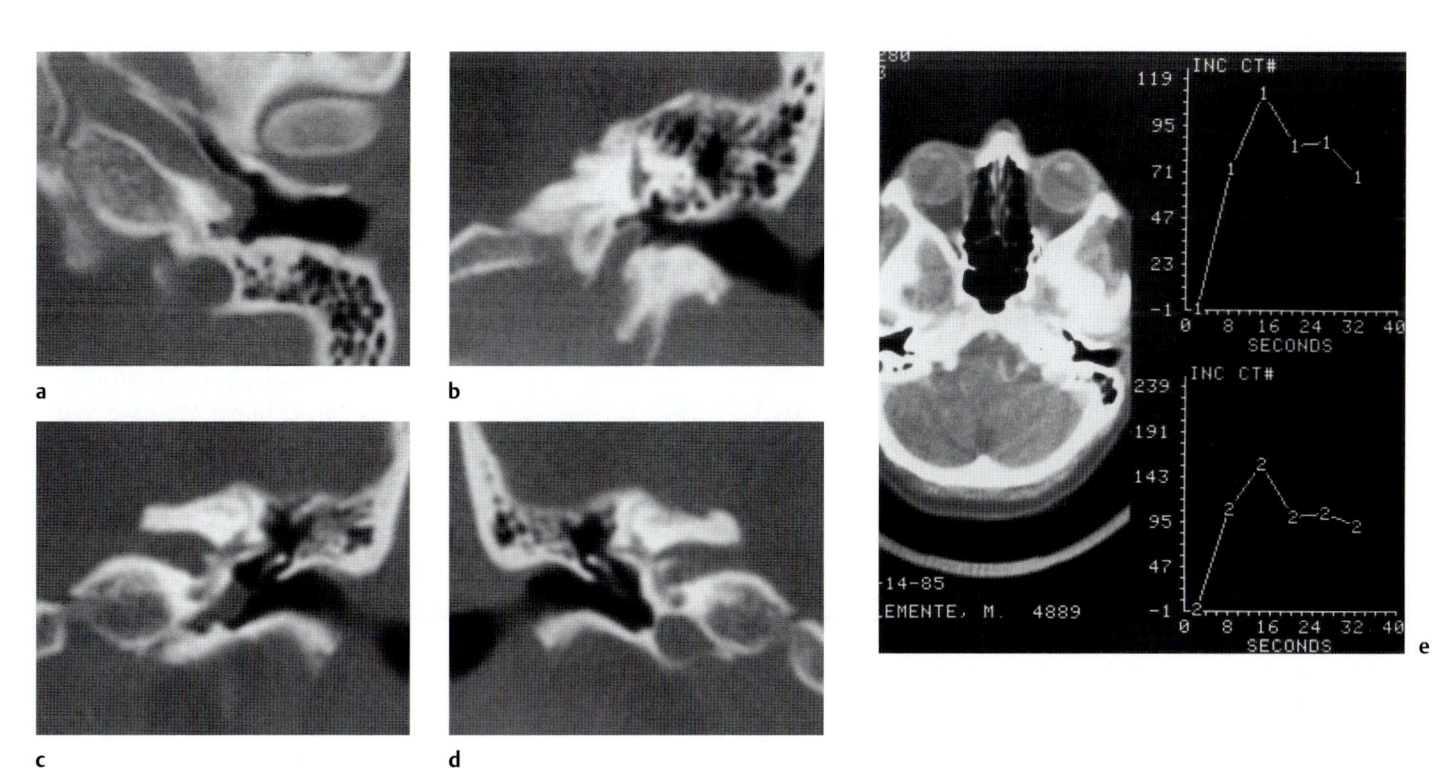

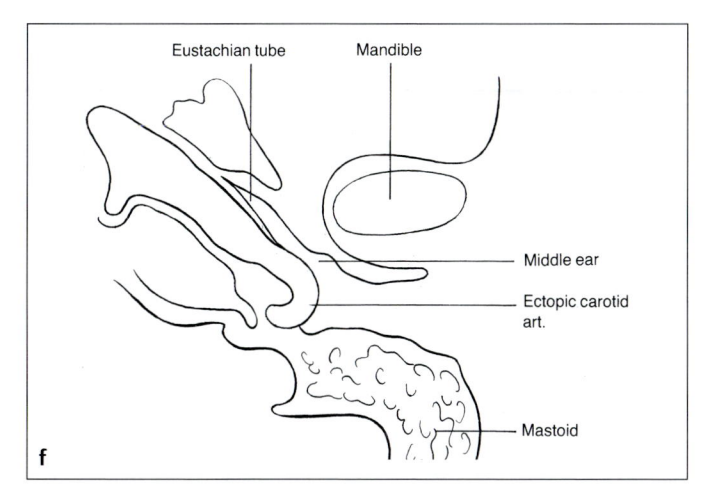

Fig. 1.49 Ectopic carotid artery. **a** Axial, **b**, **c** coronal CT sections, left; **d** coronal CT section, normal right; **e** dynamic CT study, left.
In the axial sections, the ectopic carotic artery courses throughout the entire length of the middle ear cavity. In coronal section **c**, the carotid artery appears as a well-defined soft-tissue mass in the lower mesotympanum. The proximal portion of the carotid artery, normally seen under the cochlea, is absent. Compare corresponding sections of the normal right ear (**d**), where the carotid artery is normal. The ectopic arotid artery enters the middle ear through a posteriorly displaced canal and passes into the middle ear through a defect in the hypotympanic floor (**b**). The dynamic CT study (**e**) reveals that the time–density curve of the middle ear mass (upper curve, 1) has an identical peak time to the curve obtained from the internal carotid artery in its normal position in the anterior portion at the apex of the temporal bone (lower curve, 2).
f Diagram of **a**.
g Diagram of **c**.

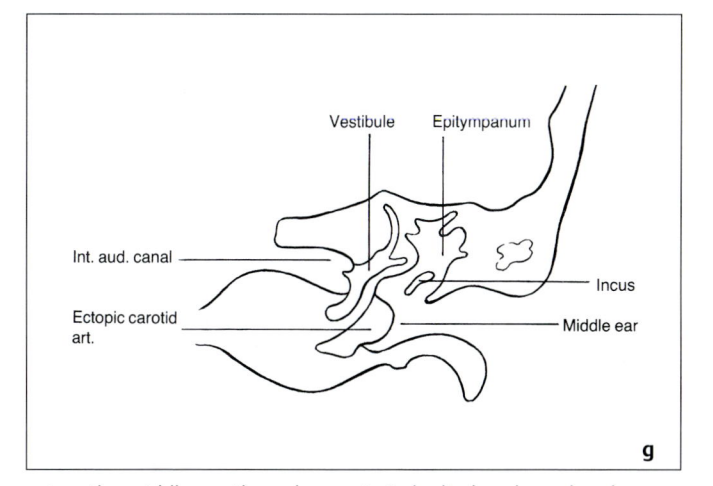

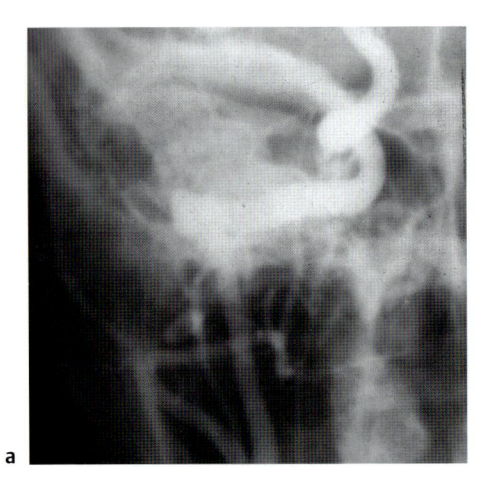

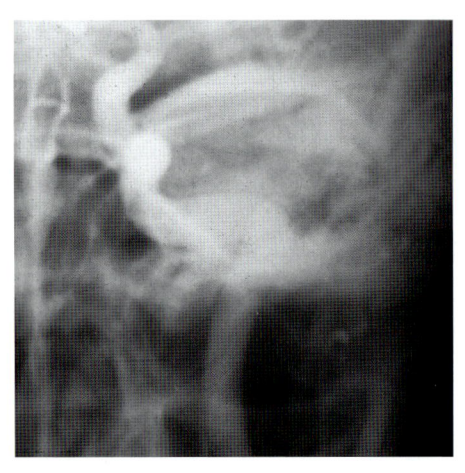

Fig. 1.**50 a** Ectopic carotid artery, arteriogram, coronal projection, right. The narrow proximal interal carotid artery enters the middle ear and courses lateral to the vestibular plane.
b Corresponding arteriogram of normal left carotid for comparison.

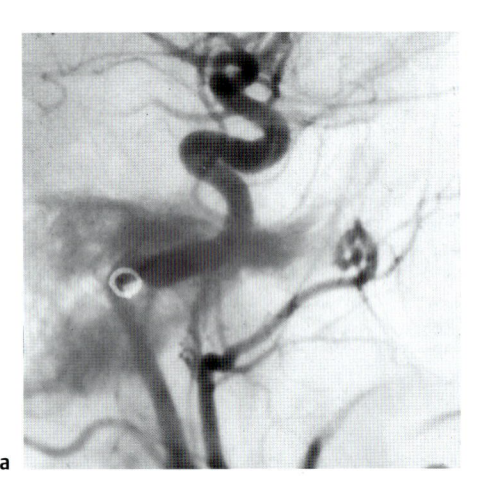

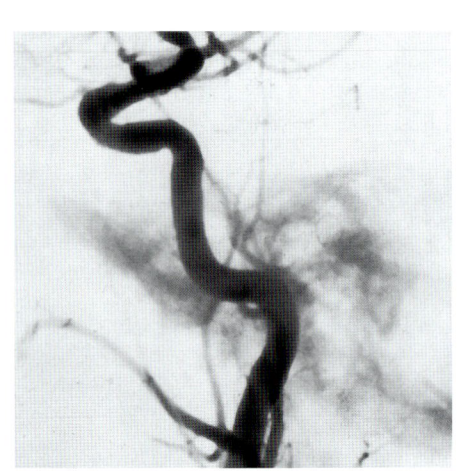

Fig. 1.**51 a** Ectopic carotid arteriogram, lateral projection, with subtraction. The ectopic carotid enters the posterior middle ear and makes a 90° turn anteriorly. The marker corresponds to the region of the vestibule.
b Corresponding arteriogram of normal left carotid for comparison.

4 The arterial tissue mass may encroach on the incudostapedial joint and cause conductive deafness.
5 The normal proximal portion of the carotid canal is absent. The normal canal is always clearly visible below the cochlea in coronal and 20° coronal oblique sections (Fig. 1.**49 c, d**).
6 The anomalous carotid artery enters the temporal bone through an enlarged tympanic canaliculus or a dehiscent area in the floor of the posterior portion of the hypotympanum between the jugular fossa medially and the vertical portion of the facial canal laterally (Fig. 1.**49 b**).

A dynamic CT study at the level showing the middle ear mass will produce a graph with a characteristic high arterial peak time (Fig. 1.**49 e**). MRA or arteriography can confirm the CT findings. The arteriographic findings are (Figs. 1.**50** and 1.**51**):
1 There is narrowing or tapering of the internal carotid artery at the site where the artery enters the base of the skull.
2 The proximal aberrant arterial segment lies at least 1 cm more laterally and posteriorly than normal. In the coronal plane, this arterial segment lies lateral rather than medial to the vertical plane, which passes through the vestibule.
3 The proximal anomalous carotid artery segment follows a straight vertical course, while the proximal segment of a normal internal carotid artery curves gently medially and anteriorly.
4 The anomalous carotid artery makes a sharp 90° turn within the middle ear cavity. The artery then runs anteriorly throughout the middle ear and exits inferior to the cochlear apex, where it usually regains the normal course in the petrous apex.

■ Arachnoid Granulations

Arachnoid granulations are villous structures that herniate through small defects in the dura and drain cerebrospinal fluid from the subarachnoid space into the venous system.
A variable number of arachnoid villi do not reach the venous target but come into contact with the intracranial surface of the middle cranial fossa and, less frequently, of the posterior surface of the temporal bone. Over a long time the pulsation of the cerebrospinal fluid may produce small areas of bony resorption and erosion. CT study will reveal small soft-tissue densities underneath the defects in the tegmen. The T2-weighted MR images show that the small masses have a high signal due to fluid. Arachnoid granulations become clinically significant when they open into an adjacent air space (attic, mastoid cells) as they may lead to spontaneous cerebrospinal fluid otorrhea and, if the mastoid and middle ear cavity are infected, to intracranial complications.

■ Petrous Apex

The petrous apex may be extensively pneumatized or made up of compact diploic bone (Fig. 1.**52 a**). In MR studies, the signal intensity of the apex varies with the bony texture: high or bright in the T1-weighted images when diploic, low or dark when highly pneumatized or compact. Often the bony texture of the two petrous apices of the same person differs, resulting in one apex being brighter than the other (Fig. 1.**52 b**).

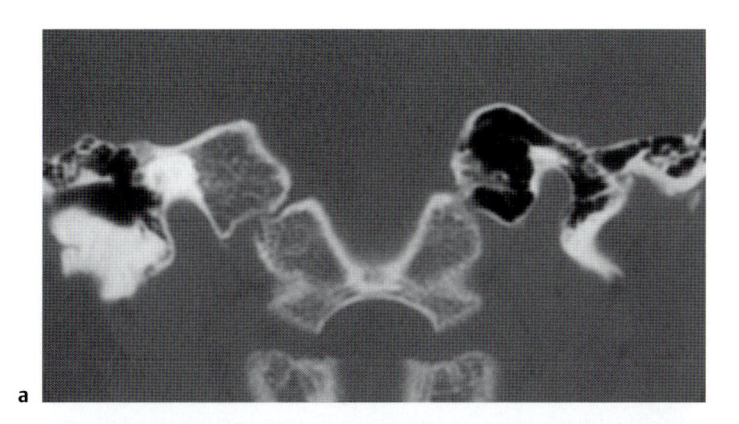

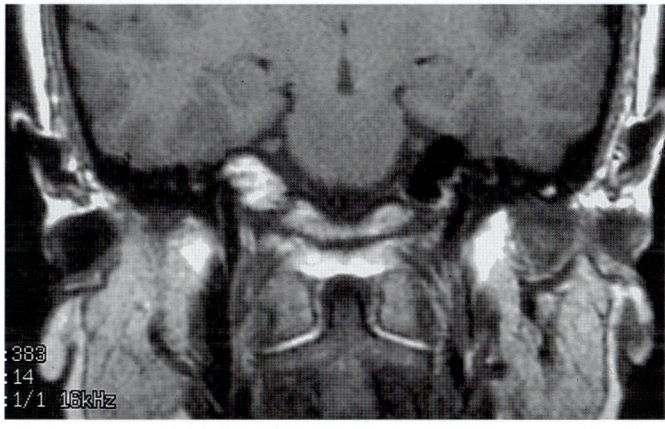

Fig. 1.**52** Petrous apex: **a** coronal CT, **b** coronal T1W MR. The right petrous apex is diploic, whereas the left is pneumatized. The right diploic apex is bright in the MR image, whereas the left pneumatized apex appears as an area of signal void.

Congenital Abnormalities of the Temporal Bone

Computed tomography has permitted the accurate evaluation of large numbers of congenital deformities of the temporal bone because the study can be made in the living patient. Prior to tomography, only a few postmortem specimens of congenital defects were available for study, and surgery was performed without the benefit of knowing the precise type and degree of anomaly present. Congenital malformations are hereditary and transmitted by genetic defects or are acquired during fetal life. The severity and degree depend on the causative factors and the age at which the fetus was affected.

Congenital malformations of the temporal bone may be divided into three groups:
1 Defects of the sound-conducting apparatus, which include the anomalies of the external auditory canal, the middle ear, the ossicles, and the labyrinthine windows.
2 Malformations of the cochleovestibular perceptive apparatus. These include anomalies of one or more structures of the inner ear.
3 Abnormalities of the facial nerve.

■ Imaging Assessment

In congenital anomalies of the ear, an imaging assessment is essential. Otoscopy is of little value in atresia and aplasia of the external auditory canal, and audiometry is unreliable in young children. A proper imaging study should demonstrate the status of the anatomical structures of the ear. Such information is of value for the otologist in determining the proper treatment for conductive and sensorineural hearing losses. Conventional radiography is of limited value except for evaluating the degree and development of pneumatization of the mastoid. CT is the study of choice and should include axial and coronal sections. In selected cases, 20° coronal oblique and sagittal images are added to evaluate the labyrinthine windows, the mastoid segment of the facial canal, and the vestibular acqueduct.

In patients with aural atresia, three-dimensional images and life-size plastic models generated from the digital data obtained in the axial CT sections are useful to the otologist for planning reconstructive surgery. The 3D images offer not only a good view of the bony surface but also, by electronically peeling away tissue layers, provide useful information about the deeper structures and, in particular, about the course of the facial nerve.

Sedation is often necessary to immobilize young, restless children during the examination. A good CT study will provide the surgeon with the following basic information about the feasibility of corrective surgery and will help in determining which type of surgery is indicated.
1 The degree and type of abnormality of the tympanic bone. These abnormalities may range from a relatively minor deformity to a complete agenesis of the external auditory canal.
2 The degree and position of the pneumatization of the mastoid air cells and mastoid antrum.
3 The position of the sigmoid sinus and the jugular bulb, and the course of the carotid canal.
4 The development and aeration of the middle ear cavity.
5 The status of the ossicular chain, the size and shape of the ossicles, and the presence of fusion or fixation.
6 The patency of the labyrinthine windows.
7 The development and course of the facial nerve.
8 The relationship of the meninges to the mastoid and superior petrous ridge. The middle cranial fossa often forms a deep groove lateral to the labyrinth, which results in a low-lying dura over the mastoid, epitympanum, and external auditory canal.
9 The degree of development and the morphology of the inner ear structures. Anomalies of the membranous labyrinth are not visible radiographically, but CT will detect abnormalities of the bony labyrinthine structures.

We studied more than 900 cases of congenital ear defects visualized by imaging. About 60% of these cases had deformities of the external auditory canal, middle ear, or both structures. Inner ear abnormalities accounted for 30% of the congenital defects, and the remaining 10% had mixed defects of the external, middle, and inner ears.

■ Embryology

A short review of the embryology of the ear is helpful in understanding the radiographic changes seen in congenital malformations.

Embryology of the Outer and Middle Ear

In the 4-week-old human embryo, three branchial arches separated by two branchial grooves appear. While the third arch and second groove disappear, the first branchial groove deepens to become the primitive external auditory meatus. Simultaneously

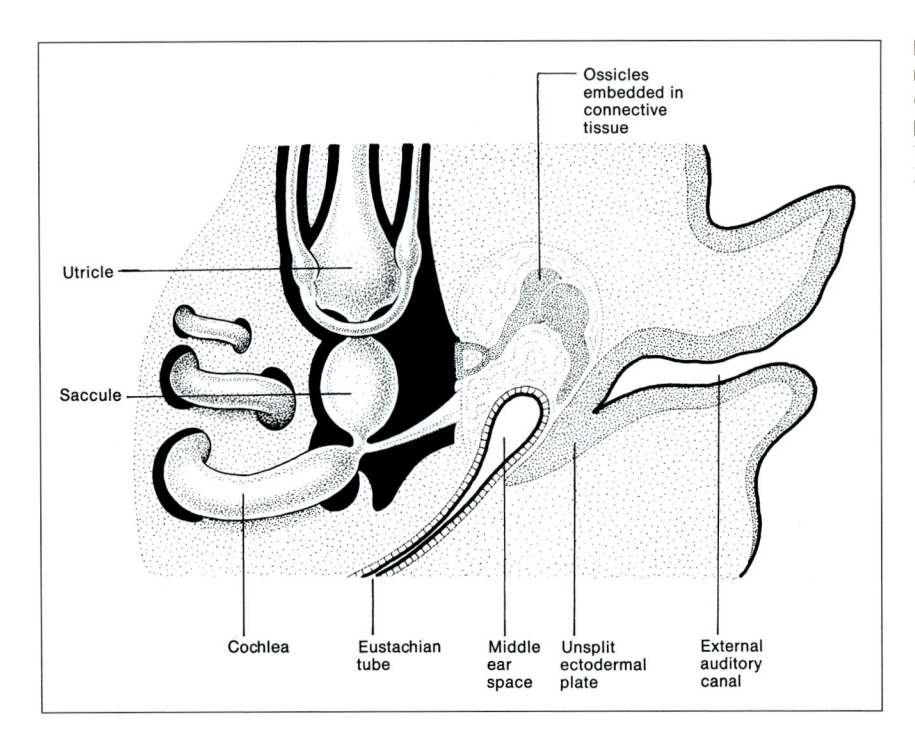

Fig. 1.53 Three-month-old fetus showing development of middle and external ears. There is a solid core of epithelial cells extending toward the first pharyngeal pouch from the primitive external acoustic meatus. (From Shambaugh GE. *Surgery of the Ear*, 2nd ed. Saunders: Philadelphia and London, 1967.)

the first pharyngeal pouch evaginates, and for a short time comes in contact with the ectoderm of the first branchial groove. Mesenchyme soon grows between and separates the layers of ectoderm and endoderm. At 8 weeks of embryonic life, a solid core of epithelial cells grows inward from the primitive external meatus toward the epithelium of the pharyngeal pouch. The thin seam of intervening connective tissue will become the fibrous layer of the definitive tympanic membrane (Fig. 1.53).

This core of epithelial tissue from the ectoderm of the first groove remains solid until the 7th month of fetal life, when the core of epithelial cells splits, beginning in its deepest portion, where it forms the epithelium of the tympanic membrane. The dissolution of this core of epithelium then proceeds externally to join the lumen of the primitive external meatus. By this time, the other structures of the outer, middle, and inner ear are well formed. This sequence of embryological events explains how in some cases of stenosis or atresia of the outer portion of the external canal, the middle ear and tympanic membrane may be well formed. The first pharyngeal pouch becomes the eustachian tube and middle ear, while the cartilage of the first and second brachial arches forms the malleus, incus, and part of the stapes. The ossicles grow only during the first half of fetal life, after which they ossify, having attained full adult size (Fig. 1.53). The air cells of the temporal bone develop as outpouchings from the tympanum, epitympanum, antrum, and eustachian tube. These outpouchings may appear in the 34-week-old fetus. When air enters the middle ear at birth, pneumatization occurs and cell development continues until early adult life, unless arrested by inflammatory processes.

Inner Ear

In the 3-week-old human embryo, a platelike ectodermal thickening occurs bilaterally near the hindbrain. This is the otic placode, which forms in a few days an otic pit. The pit becomes an otocyst by the 4th week. By 7 weeks, the otocyst has formed three semicircular canals and by the 11th week the cochlea (Fig. 1.54). The primitive labyrinth enlarges until midterm when it reaches adult form and size. The endolymphatic duct and sac are the earliest appendages of the otic vessicle. They form at $4^{1}/_{2}$

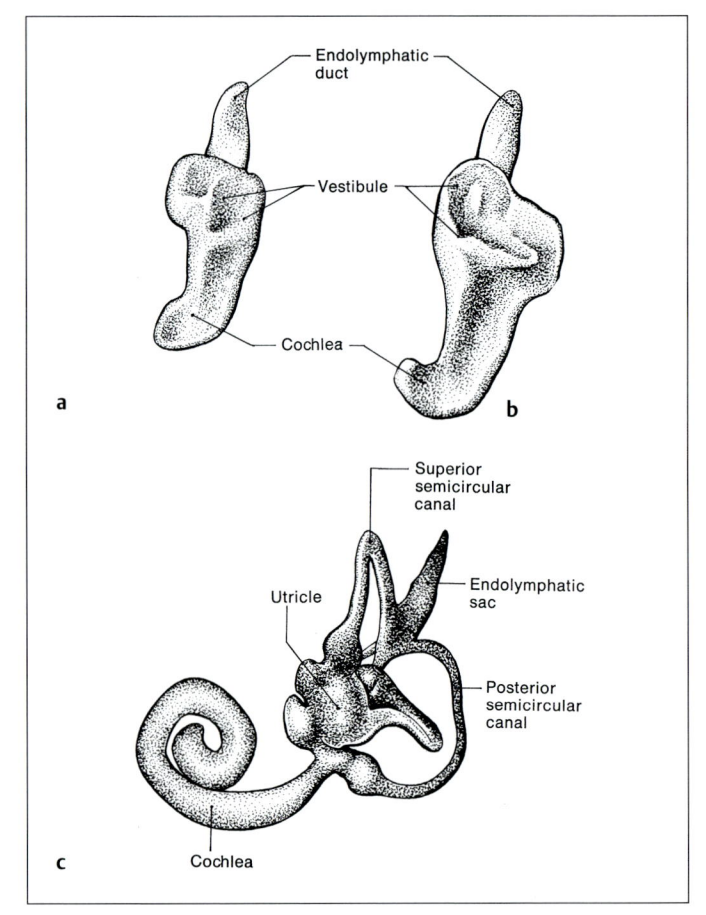

Fig. 1.54 a Development of the membranous labyrinth during a three-week period: **a** 5 weeks, **b** 6 weeks, **c** 8 weeks. (From Anson BJ. *Morris' Human Anatomy*, 12th ed. McGraw-Hill, New York, 1966.)

weeks of embryonic life when the otocyst divides into endolymphatic and utriculosaccular portions.

Throughout infancy and childhood, the endolymphatic duct and sac continue to change and enlarge to accommodate themselves with the growth of the surrounding temporal bone. Differ-

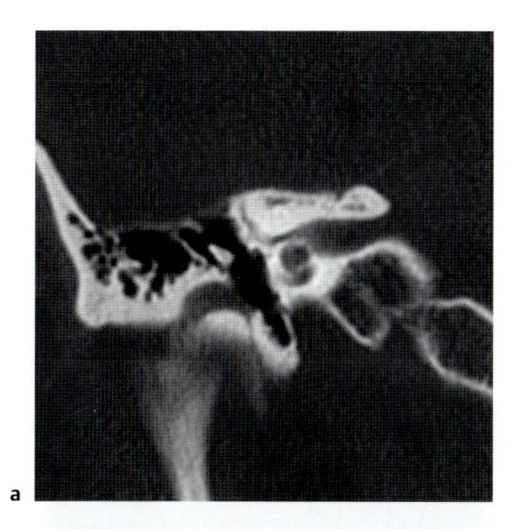

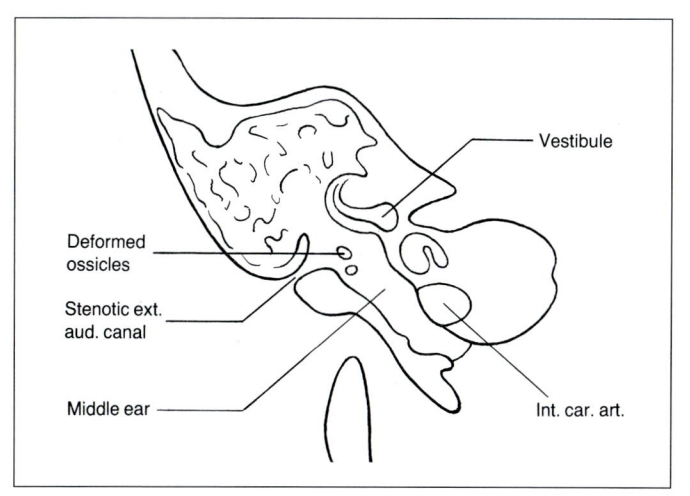

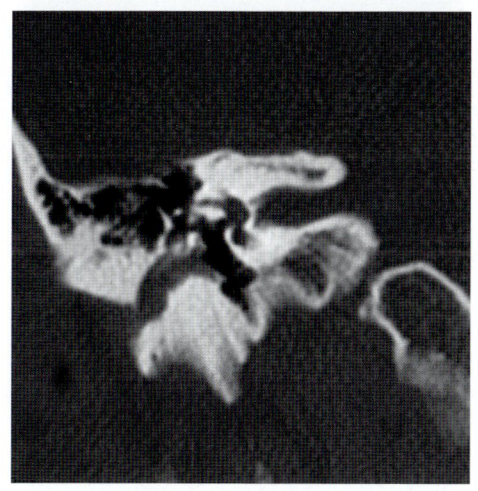

Fig. 1.55 Dysplasia of the tympanic bone. **a** and **b** Coronal CT sections, right. The external auditory canal is stenotic and closed medially by a thin bony plate. The lumen of the canal is filled by soft tissue. The middle ear is well-aerated and normal in size. Malleus and body of the incus are fused and fixed to the annulus. The oval window is normal.

entiation of the sensory cells of the semicircular canals, utricle, and saccule occurs by the eighth week, but development of sensory cells of the cochlea does not begin until the 12th week and is not complete until after midterm.

By the 8th embryonic week, the precartilage surrounding the otic membranous labyrinth changes into an outer zone of true cartilage to form the otic capsule, while the inner zone of precartilage vacuolizes to form the perilymphatic spaces. These spaces appear around the vestibule, the scala tympani and vestibuli, and the semicircular canals, and coalesce until a continuous perilymphatic space surrounds the entire membranous labyrinth. Ossification of the otic capsule does not occur until the cartilage has attained maximum growth and maturity at midterm. The endochondral layer of the bone of the otic capsule is formed from cartilage that is not removed and remodeled into periosteal haversian bone as in other bones of the body. The first ossification center of the otic capsule appears around the cochlea in the 16th week of fetal life when the cochlea has reached adult size. Ossification of the 14 centers is almost complete by the 23rd week.

■ Anomalies of the Sound-Conducting System

Anomalies of the sound-conducting system can affect the external auditory canal, the mastoid, the middle ear cavity, the ossicles, and the labyrinthine windows.

Anomalies of the Tympanic Bone

The degree and type of anomaly of the tympanic bone range from mild stenosis to complete agenesis of the external auditory canal (Figs. 1.55–1.59). Embryologically, the definitive external auditory canals begin to form medially at the level of the tympanic membrane. An arrest in this developmental process may leave an atretic plate laterally, which causes a complete external canal atresia.

Microtia

Microtia, or varying degrees of deformity of the auricle, is often associated with dysplasia of the external auditory canal. No direct relationship exists between the degree of severity of the auricular and external canal anomalies, though severe microtia is usually associated with agenesis of the canal. In agenesis of the external auditory canal, often a small tissue tag and a small pit are present in place of the normal auricle and external canal. These pits and tags usually have no topographic relationship to the mastoid and middle ear. To establish the position of the middle ear in relation to the vestigial remnant of the external ear, we tape a radiopaque pellet over the pit. CT will show the metallic marker and its relationship to the underlying structures. When the external auditory canal assumes a more vertical course than normal, CT will reveal this malposition. The origin of the external auditory canal from the first branchial groove and adjoining branchial arch explains the frequent association of abnormalities of other structures with the same derivation.

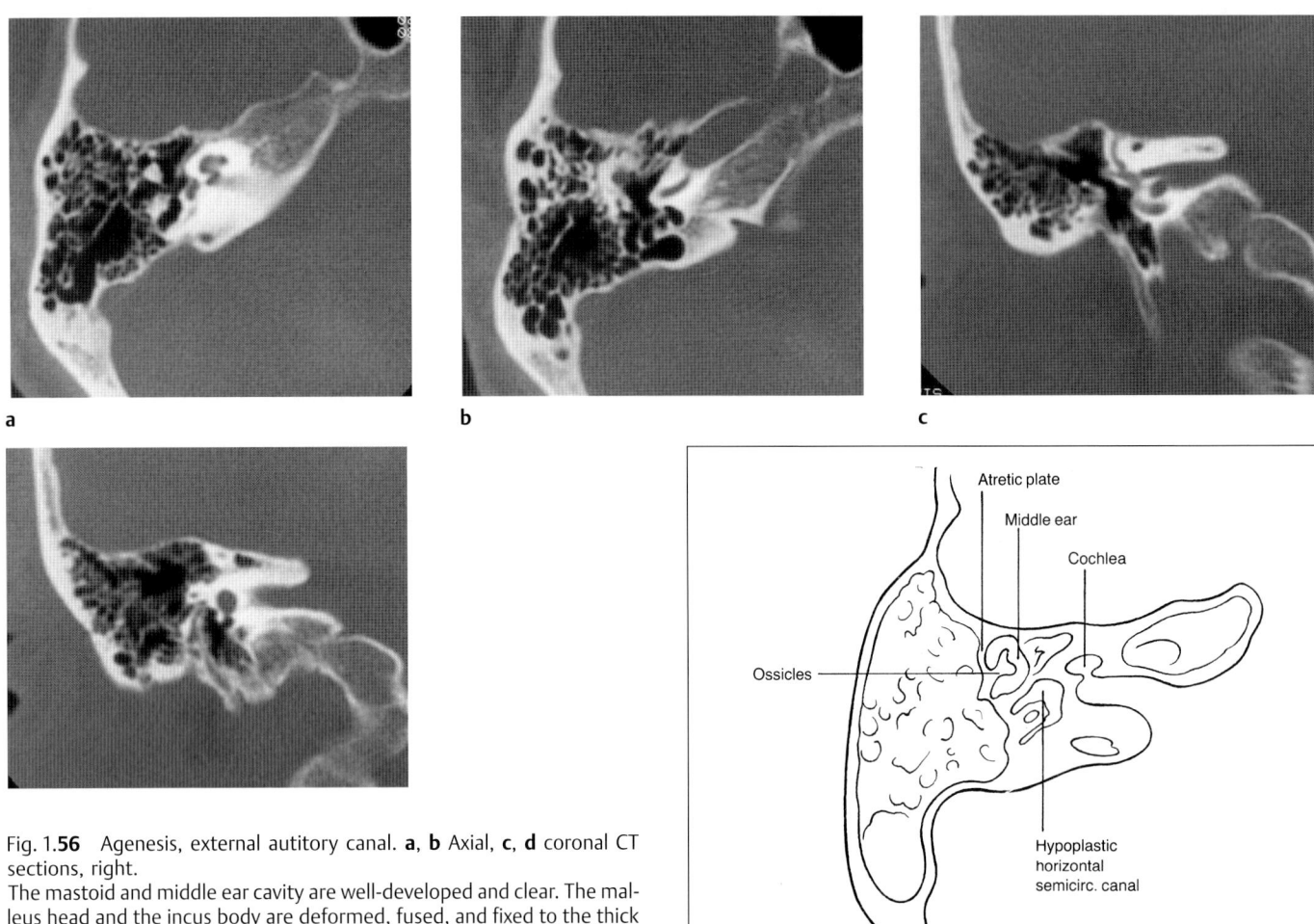

Fig. 1.**56** Agenesis, external autitory canal. **a**, **b** Axial, **c**, **d** coronal CT sections, right.
The mastoid and middle ear cavity are well-developed and clear. The malleus head and the incus body are deformed, fused, and fixed to the thick atretic plate.
e Diagram of **b**.

In many cases of congenital agenesis of the external auditory canal, the temporomandibular joint is displaced posteriorly and lies lateral to the middle ear cavity (Fig. 1.**57 b**). In some cases the mandibular condyle is hypoplastic and the temporomandibular fossa is flat.

Mastoid Pneumatization

Radiography reveals the degree of pneumatization of the mastoid. Pneumatization can be completely absent (Figs. 1.**59**, 1.**60**), limited to a small mastoid antral cell, or completely normal (Figs. 1.**56**, 1.**58**). Conventional views, and especially axial CT sections, will determine the degree of pneumatization and the position of the sigmoid sinus in relation to the external canal, antrum, and middle ear. Coronal sections are necessary to determine the relationship of the tegmental plate to the antrum and middle ear. A low-lying dura is common in congenital atresia, as the middle cranial fossa deepens to form a groove lateral to the labyrinth (Figs. 1.**59**, 1.**60**).

Anomalies of the Middle Ear

The degree of development and aeration of the middle ear is determined by axial and coronal CT sections. Malformations of the middle ear vary from minor hypoplasia to almost complete agenesis (Fig. 1.**71**.). In the majority of cases associated with atresia, the middle ear cavity is slightly hypoplastic but is usually well aerated (Figs. 1.**55**, 1.**56**).

Anomalies of the Ossicles

Anomalies of the incus and malleus occur in varying degrees. Axial and coronal sections expose the anomalies best. In cases of agenesis of the external auditory canal but relatively normal middle ear development, the malleus and incus are present but are fused together and fixed to the atretic bone plate at the level of the neck of the malleus (Figs. 1.**55**–1.**57**). In these cases, the long process of the incus is normal. If the atretic plate lies lateral to the level of the tympanic membrane, the ossicular chain may be entirely normal. When the middle ear cavity is hypoplastic, the malleus and incus exist as an amalgam of amorphous bone, and the long process of the incus is shortened or absent (Figs. 1.**58**, 1.**60**). In severe cases, the middle ear may be extremely hypoplastic, and only a rudimentary ossicular mass is present in an ectopic position (Fig. 1.**59**).

A congenital anomaly may be confined to the ossicular chain. The external auditory canal, the middle ear, and the ossicles are well formed, but the malleus or incus are fused to the epitympanic wall. The malleus is more commonly fixed than the incus (Fig. 1.**61**). CT demonstrates such an isolated fixation if there is ossified bone between the ossicle and the epitympanic wall or tegmen. In ears with a very low-lying tegmental plate, it is difficult to determine the presence of fixation, since the space between the ossicle and the tegmen is very narrow.

Congenital Abnormalities of the Temporal Bone 45

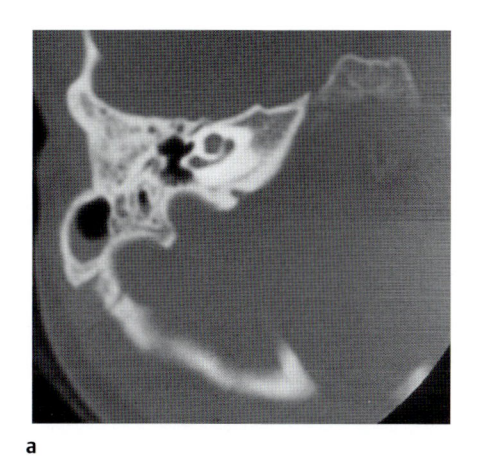

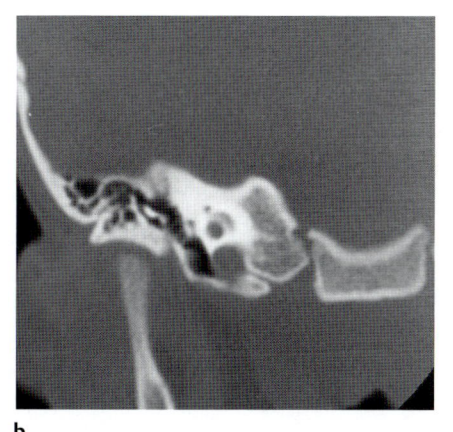

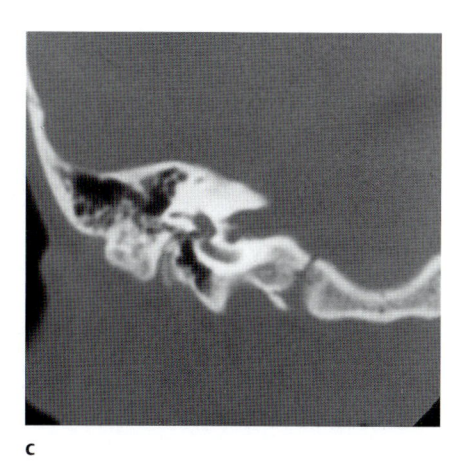

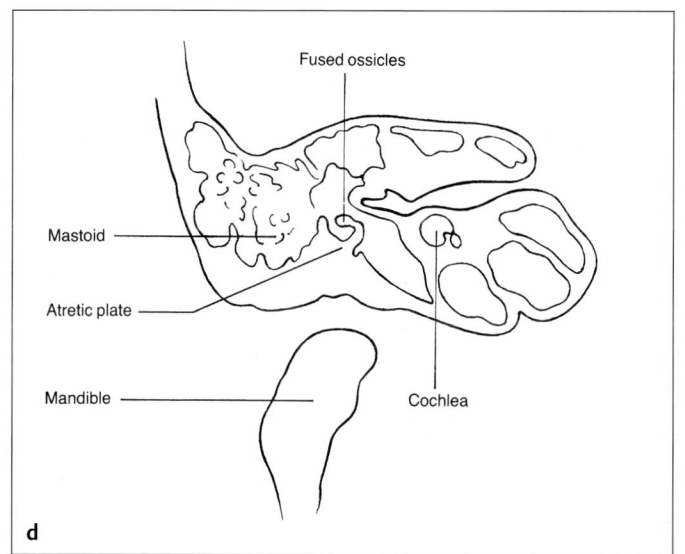

Fig. 1.**57** Agenesis, external auditory canal. **a** Axial, **b**, **c** coronal CT sections, right. The mastoid and middle ear cavity are well-developed and aerated. Malleus and incus are hypoplastic and fused. The vertical segment of the facial canal is slightly rotated outward.
d Diagram of **b**

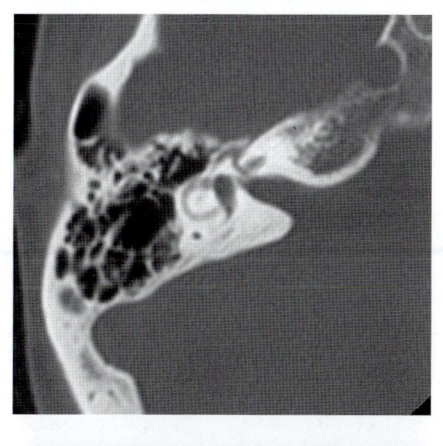

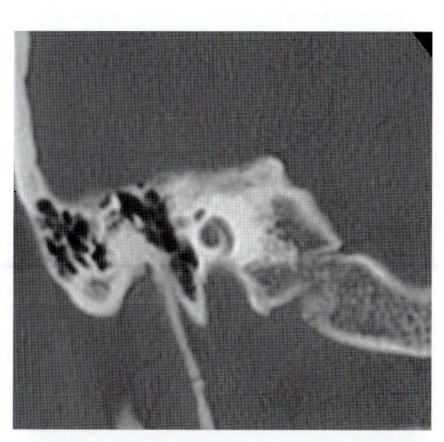

Fig. 1.**58** Agenesis of the external auditory canal. **a** Axial, **b**, **c**, **d** coronal CT sections, right. The mastoid is well developed. The middle ear cavity is aerated but small. The ossicular chain is hypoplastic. **d** The mastoid segment of the facial nerve canal is displaced anteriorly.

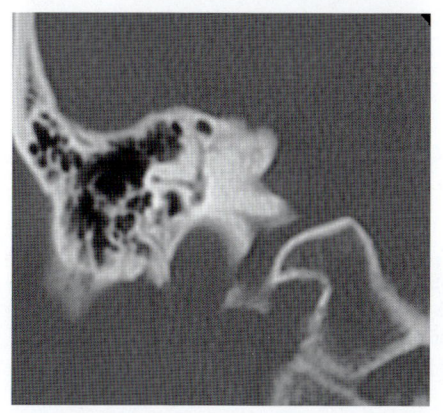

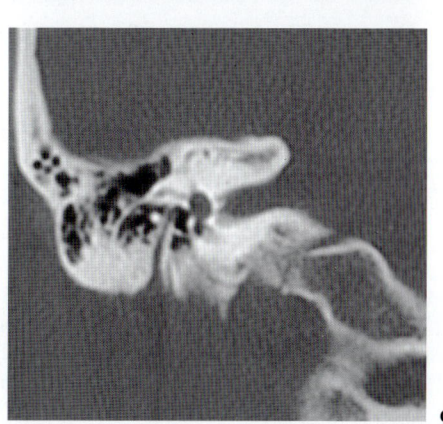

1 Imaging of the Temporal Bone

Fig 1.**59** Agenesis of the external auditory canal. **a**, **b** Axial, **c**, **d** coronal CT sections, left. The mastoid is not developed. The middle ear cavity is normal in size and the osseous segment of the eustachian tube (arrowheads) is unusually wide. The ossicles are hypoplastic and the body of the incus (short arrow) lies lateral to the malleus head. The vertical segment of the facial canal is rotated outward (long arrow).

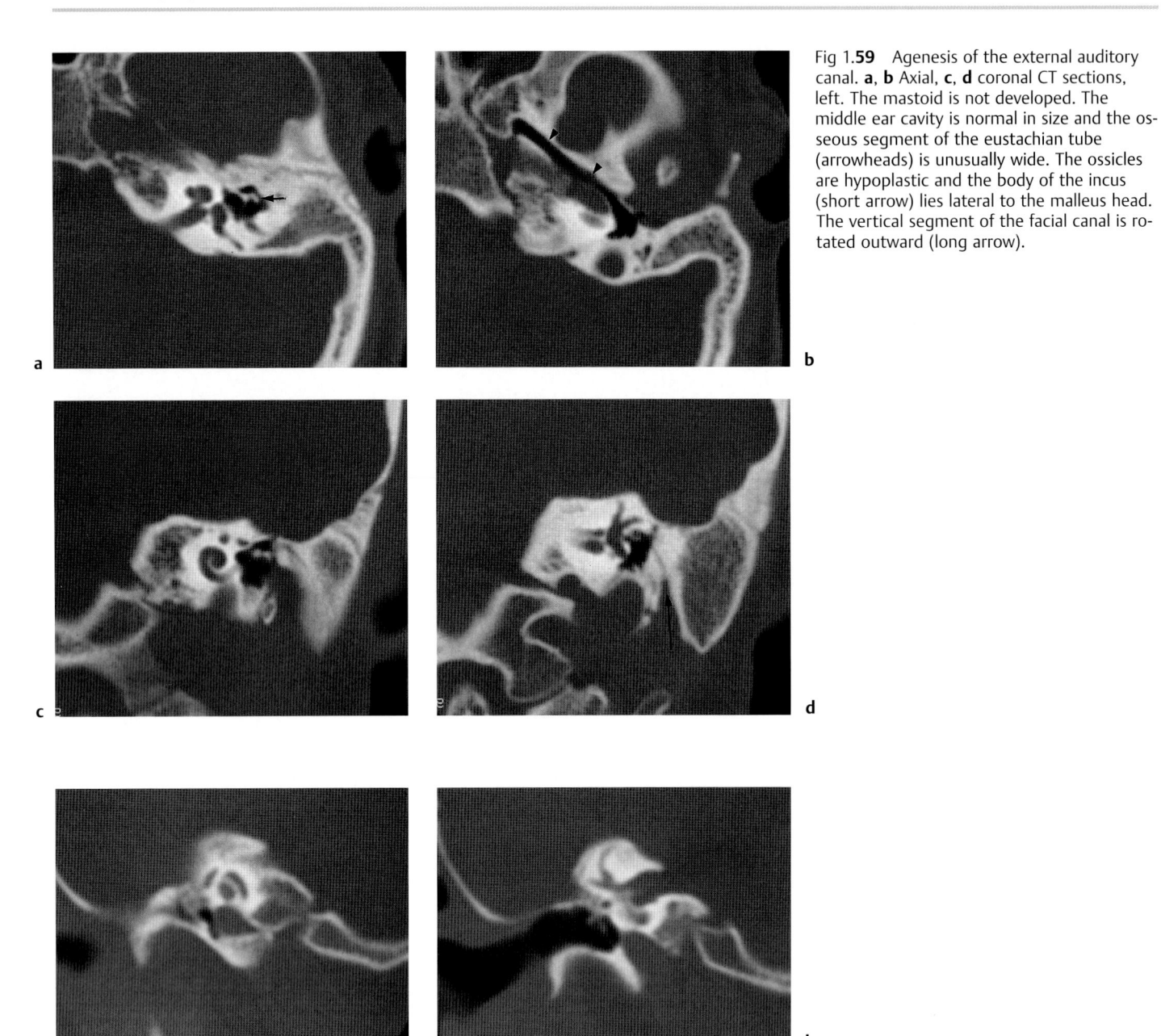

Fig. 1.**60** Hypoplasia of the mastoid and epitympanum with low dura. **a**, **b** Coronal CT sections, right. CT sections of the middle ear cavity show a small mastoid, hypoplasia of the epitympanum, a rudimentary ossicular mass and an extremely low dura lying at the level of the tympanic portion of the facial nerve.
c Diagram of **b**.

Anomalies of the Labyrinthine Windows

Anomalies of the labyrinthine windows and the stapes may be the only defect in the middle ear, or such lesions may be associated with other anomalies of the ossicles, the middle ear, and the external auditory canal. Stapes and oval window defects are more common than abnormalities of the round window. In well-developed and well-aerated middle ear cavities, 20° coronal oblique and axial CT sections will detect defects of the stapes superstructure. The most common stapes anomaly is a single, thick monopolar stapes crus. Congenital fixation of the stapes footplate is a common isolated defect, but CT can define a lesion only if the footplate is abnormally thickened and calcified. On CT, congenital fixation of the stapes resembles stapedial otosclerosis (Fig. 1.**62**).

Congenital Abnormalities of the Temporal Bone 47

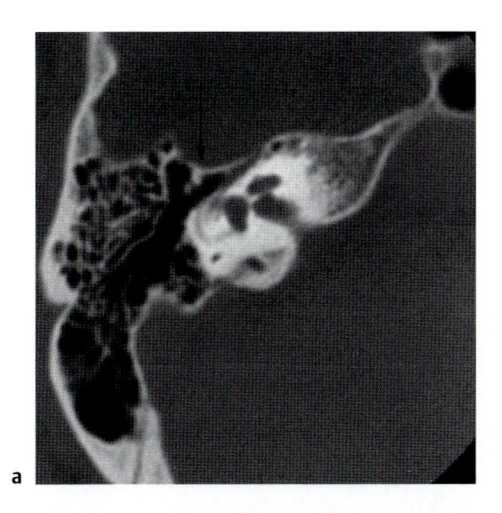

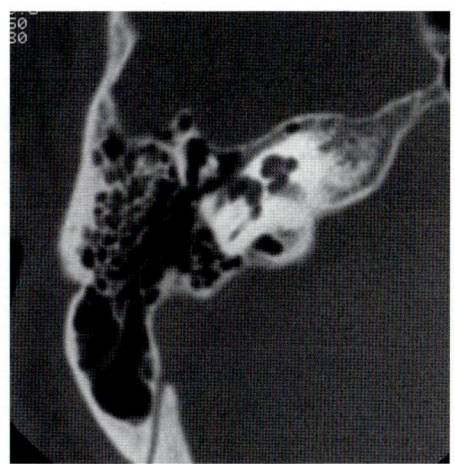

Fig. 1.**61** Congenital malleus fixation. **a**, **b** Axial CT sections, right. The head of the malleus is fixed to the anterior attic wall, which is bowed posteriorly (arrow).

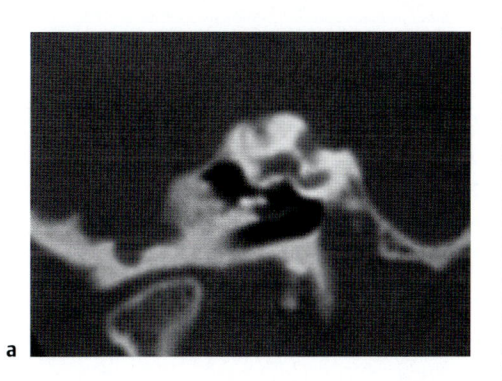

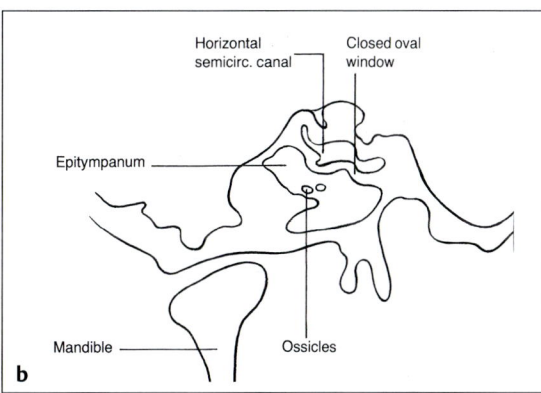

Fig. 1.**62a** Congenital closure, oval window, 20° coronal oblique CT sections, right.
The patient has a craniofacial dysplasia. The temporal bones are distorted and the dura is low. The middle ear is aerated and the malleus and incus are normal, but the thick bony plate closes the oval window. The facial canal is dehiscent above the oval window.
b Diagram of **a**.

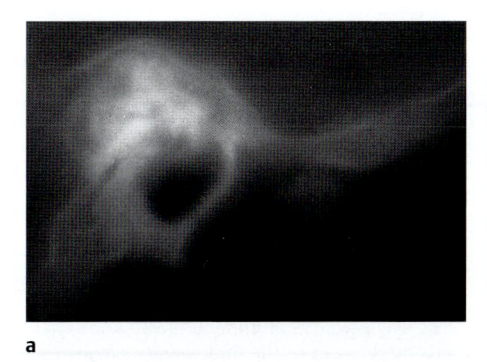

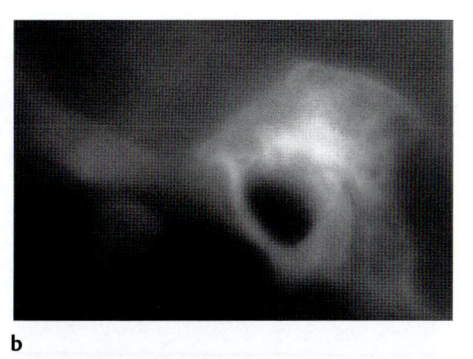

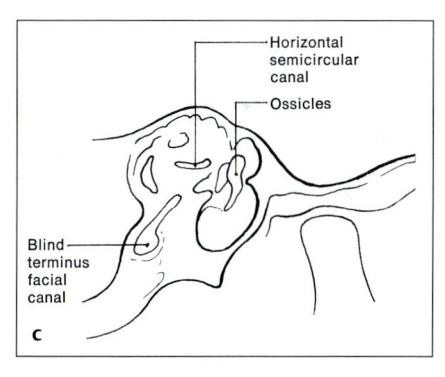

Fig. 1.**63** Congenital atresia, facial nerve canal, sagittal tomogram. **a** Right, **b** left, normal.
This 3-year-old child has congenital right facial paralysis. The facial nerve ends in a blind cul-de-sac at the mid portion of the mastoid segment (**a**). The normal facial canal appears in the tomogram **b**.
c Diagram of **a**.

■ Facial Nerve Anomalies

Congenital anomalies of the facial canal involve the size and the course of the canal. There may be complete or partial agenesis of the facial nerve with total paralysis (Fig. 1.**63**). Occasionally the facial nerve canal may be unusually narrow and hypoplastic. In these cases, intermittent episodes of facial paresis may occur. Minor variations of the course of the facial nerve are common and of no clinical or surgical significance (Fig. 1.**59**). More severe anomalies of the course of the facial nerve occur in the tympanic and vertical portions. Recognition of these anomalies is very important in planning surgical correction of ear disease. The horizontal segment at times is displaced inferiorly to cover the oval window or lies exposed over the promontory. Anomalies of the mastoid segment are common in congenital atresia of the external auditory canal. The facial canal is usually rotated laterally (Fig. 1.**59**). The rotation varies from a minor obliquity to a true horizontal course. Since facial nerve anomalies are common in congenital atresia, all such patients should have CT assessment preoperatively.

■ Anomalies of the Inner Ear

Most cases of congenital sensorineural deafness are caused by abnormal development of the membranous labyrinth. These lesions are not detectable by CT but may be seen by MRI. Defects in the otic capsule are visible by CT. Anomalies of the otic capsule may involve a single structure or the entire capsule. With recent

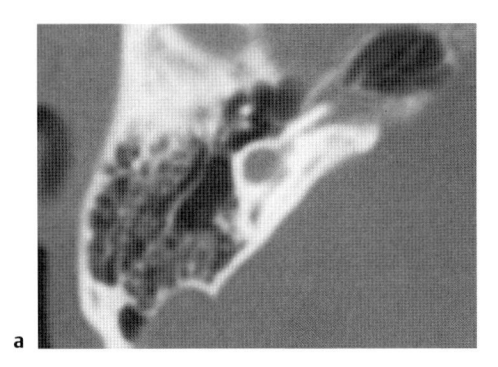

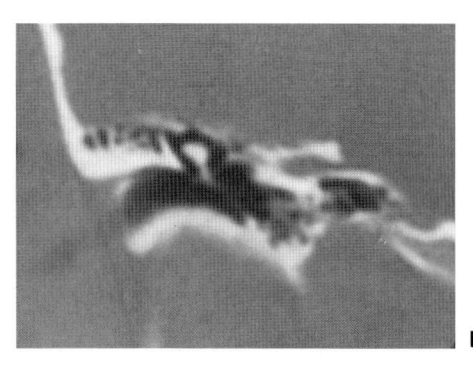

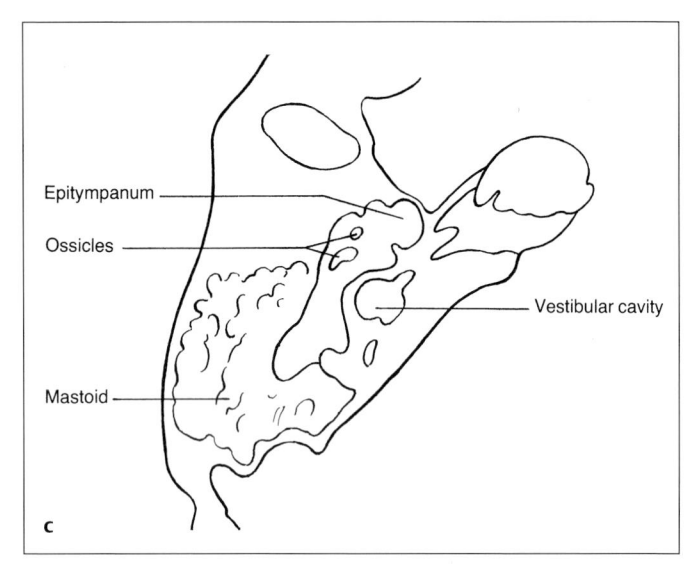

Fig. 1.**64** Michel anomaly. **a** Axial, **b** coronal CT sections, right. The mastoid and middle ear are normal, but the petrous pyramid is markedly hypoplastic. The inner ear structures are absent, except for a cavity in the region of the vestibule and horizontal semicircular canal. The internal auditory canal is very narrow and appears large enough to contain only the facial nerve.
c Diagram of **d**.

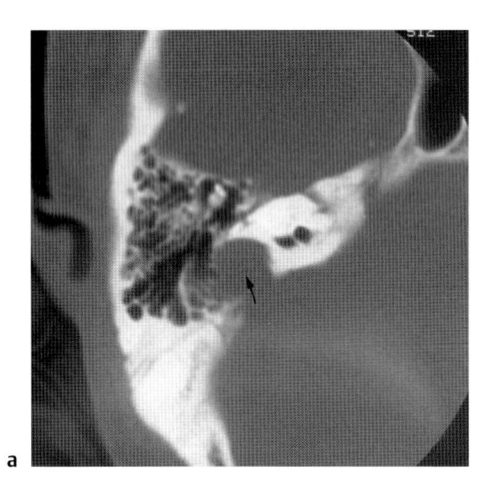

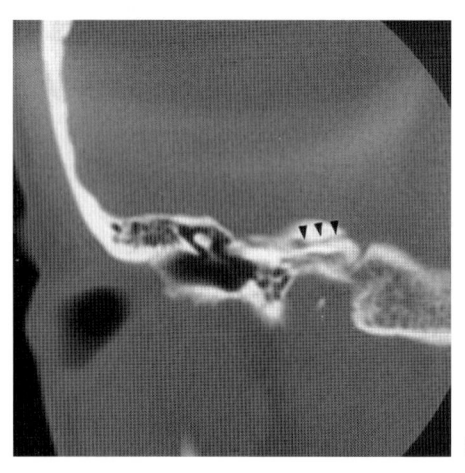

Fig. 1.**65** Michel anomaly. **a** Axial, **b** coronal CT sections, right. The petrous pyramid is hypoplastic, and the labyrinth is not developed. The internal auditory canal is markedly hypoplastic (arrowheads). The vertical segment of the sigmoid sinus is medially located and forms a large indentation on the posterior aspect of the petrous pyramid above the jugular fossa (arrow).

advances in surgical procedures for profound sensorineural deafness, CT of the labyrinth is indicated for (1) assessment of the status of the otic capsule, (2) detection of cases possibly suitable for surgery of the endolymphatic sac or other inner ear structures, and (3) selection of possible candidates for cochlear implants. The most severe anomaly of the otic capsule is the Michel type of deformity, which is characterized by a hypoplastic petrous pyramid and an almost complete lack of development of the inner ear structures (Fig. 1.**65**). There is often a single labyrinthine cavity of varying size which occupies the space normally taken by the vestibule, cochlea, and semicircular canals (Fig. 1.**64**). When facial nerve function is normal, the internal auditory canal is present, but the lumen of the canal is narrowed to the size of the facial nerve. The external auditory canal and middle ear cavity are usually normal but appear abnormally large in comparison with the small labyrinthine vestiges. The Michel deformity is usually bilateral. We have found this deformity associated with the Klippel–Feil anomaly in several cases.

A less severe deformity of the labyrinthine capsule is the Mondini type, which is characterized by an abnormal development of the cochlea and is often associated with an abnormality of the vestibular aqueduct, the vestibule, and the semicircular canals.[7] The cochlea may be hypoplastic or of normal size, but the modiolus and the bony partition between the cochlear coils are hypoplastic or absent, which gives the appearance of an "empty cochlea" (Fig. 1.**66**). The vestibular aqueduct is often shortened and dilated (Figs. 1.**66**, 1.**67**). The vestibule appears larger and the contour more globular than normal. There is often dilation of the

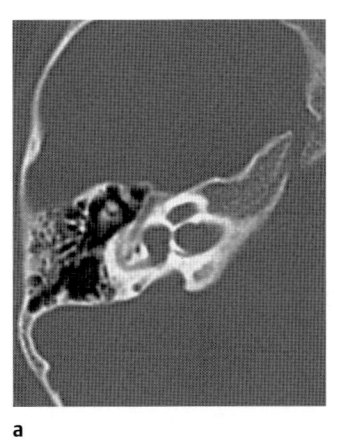

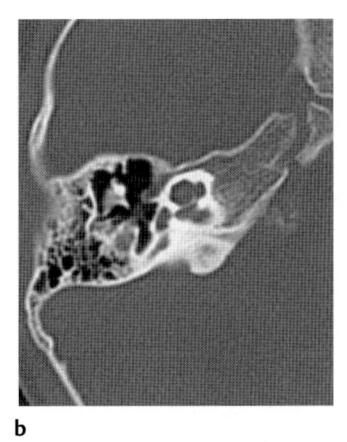

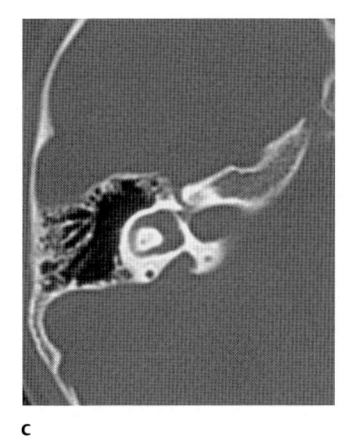

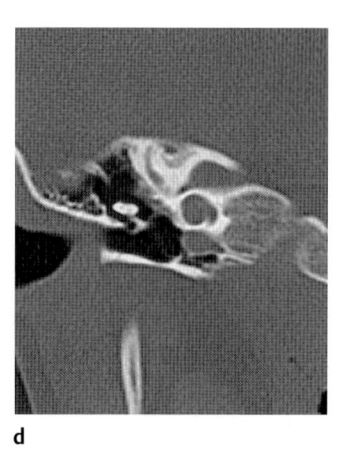

Fig. 1.66 Mondini anomaly. **a, b, c** Axial, **d** coronal CT sections, right. The cochlea is normal in size but the absence of bony partitions causes the appearance of an empty cochlea (**b, d**). The vestibule is moderately dilated (**a, c**). The vestibular aqueduct is shortened and dilated (**a, c**).

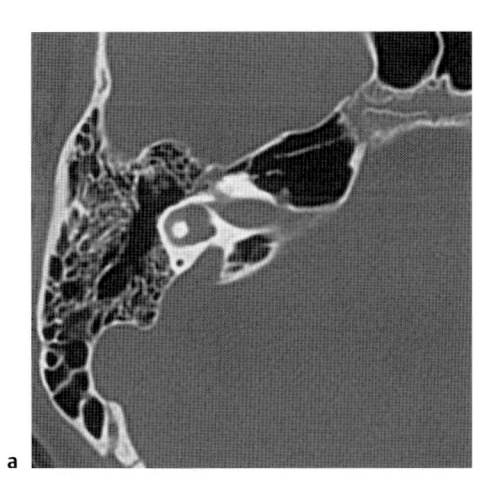

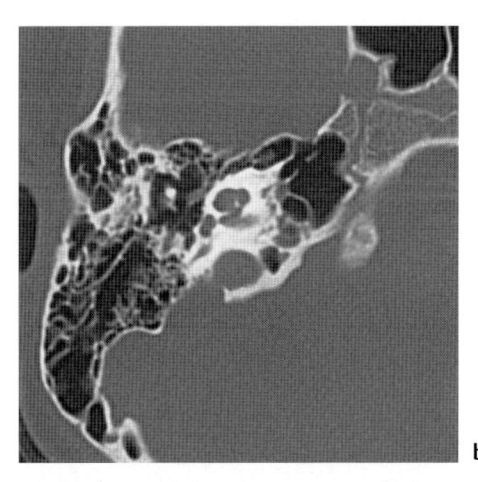

Fig. 1.67 Mondini anomaly. **a, b** Axial CT sections, right. The cochlea is normal in size but the modiolus is hypoplastic (**b**). The vestibular aqueduct is markedly enlarged and the vestibule is dilated (**a**).

ampullated ends of the horizontal and superior semicircular canals (Fig. 1.71). The Mondini deformity may be unilateral or bilateral.

Cochlea

Various anomalies of the cochlea affecting its size, the lumen, the modiolus, and the bony partitions between the coils can be visualized by CT (Figs. 1.67, 1.69). The cochlear size varies from normal to complete absence (Fig. 1.68). The lumen of the cochlea may be narrowed, obliterated, or grossly dilated. If the modiolus and the bony partitions between the cochlear coils are absent, the cochlea will appear as an empty shell (Fig. 1.66).

Vestibular Aqueduct and Endolymphatic Sac

The vestibular aqueduct is a small bony canal that extends from the posteromedial wall of the vestibule to the posterior surface of the petrous pyramid. In the adult, the shape of the aqueduct forms an inverted J. The proximal segment, the isthmus, which arches medial to the common crus, is the narrowest segment of the aqueduct and measures 0.3 mm in diameter. As the aqueduct extends inferiorly, it widens and forms a triangular slit parallel to the posterior surface of the pyramid. The outer aperture of the aqueduct measures approximately 2.0–6.0 mm in the larger diameter and 1.0 mm in the shorter.

The aqueduct contains the endolymphatic duct, which enlarges to end blindly in the endolymphatic sac lying on the posterior surface of the petrous bone and within the distal portion of the aqueduct. Axial and direct or reformatted sagittal CT sections are useful to visualize the vestibular aqueduct. The postisthmic segment is recognizable in more than 90% of the normal ears, but the isthmic segment is seen in less than 50% because of the overlying common crus and partial volume averaging. High-resolution three-dimensional MR images at 1 mm increments obtained in the axial and the sagittal or modified sagittal plane have replaced CT for the assessment of the vestibular aqueduct and endolymphatic sac. MR will show the actual content of the aqueduct and sac rather than the bony contour.

Imaging evaluation of the aqueduct is limited to the postisthmic segment. We measure the anteroposterior diameter in the sagittal sections midway between the outer aperture and the common crus. At this level, the normal aqueduct measures 0.5–1.0 mm in diameter. An aqueduct is considered abnormal when the lumen at the midpoint is wider than 1.5 mm or narrower than 0.5 mm. Occasionally an aqueduct is so narrow that it cannot be visualized in the sections. A dilated and shortened vestibular aqueduct similar in appearance to that of the Mondini deformity may occur without other radiographically visualized abnormalities.[32] In these cases the endolymphatic sac is also dilated and filled with fluid, presumably endolymph (Fig. 1.70). A narrow vestibular aqueduct is often associated with cochlear or vestibular disorders of the Ménière type and is considered a predisposing factor to these disorders. Visualization of a normal-sized aqueduct does not rule out Ménière type of otic pathology since patients with this disorder often have a normal aqueduct.

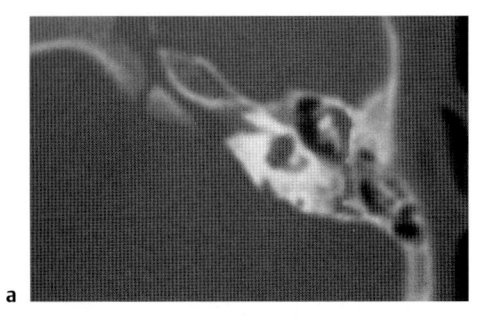

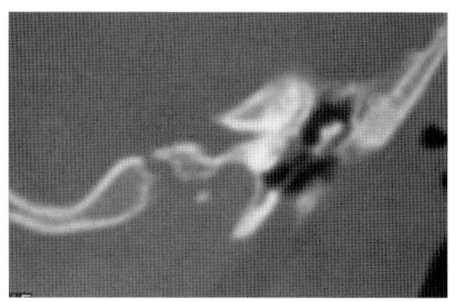

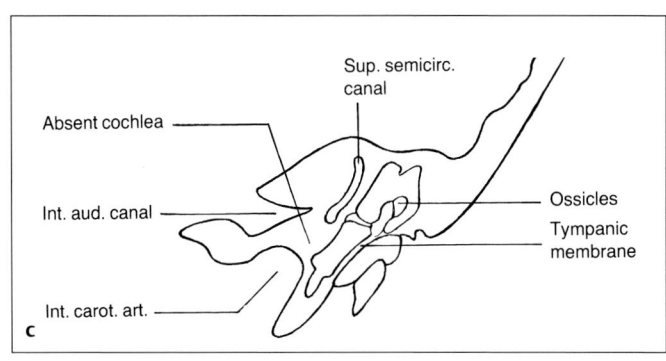

Fig. 1.**68** Agenesis, cochlea. **a** Axial, **b** coronal CT sections, left. There is severe hypoplasia of the cochlea. The horizontal semicircular canal is hypoplastic. The internal auditory canal is funnel-shaped and narrows laterally.
c Diagram of **b**.

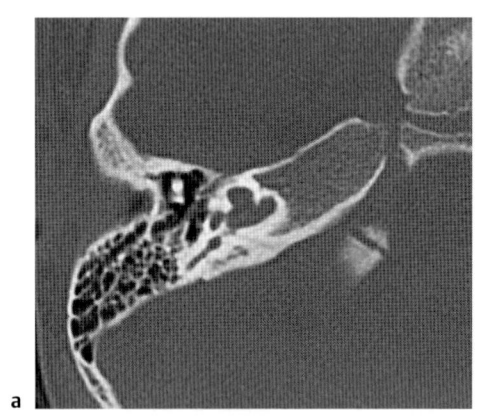

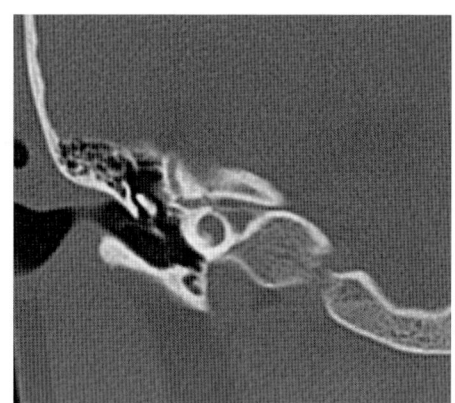

Fig. 1.**69** Cochlear malformation. **a** Axial, **b** coronal CT sections, right. The modiolus and the bony partitions between the cochlear coils are absent or hypoplastic.

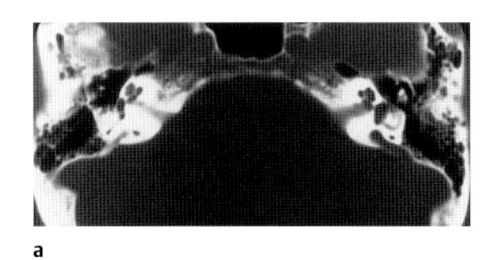

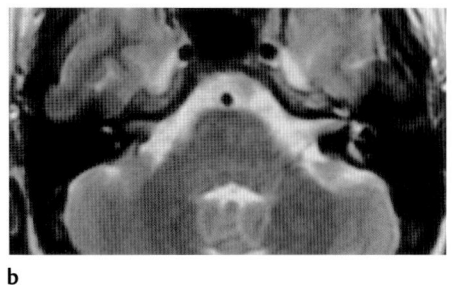

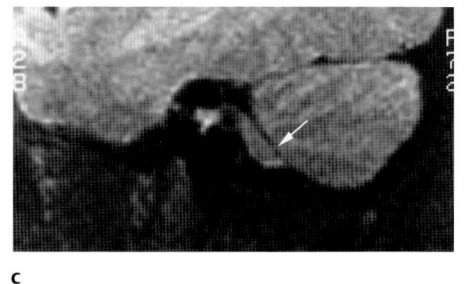

Fig. 1.**70** Large vestibular aqueduct. **a** Axial CT, **b** axial FSE MR, **c** sagittal T1W MR. The enlarged vestibular aqueduct is well seen in the CT section, whereas the MR images show the dilated fluid-filled endolymphatic sac (arrow).

Semicircular Canals and Vestibule

The semicircular canals are often congenitally deformed. This anomaly may be isolated or associated with other malformations of the bony labyrinth. The horizontal canal, which is the most commonly affected, may be shortened or dilated, or in the more severe defects exist merely as a lateral outpouching of the vestibule (Figs. 1.**68**, 1.**71**). In these cases, there is absence of the bony core around which the canal normally loops. An isolated anomaly of the horizontal canal may occur with normal cochlear and vestibular function. Hypoplasia or aplasia of the vestibule and semicircular canals can be present with or without other inner ear anomalies. This condition often occurs in association with the Waardenburg syndrome. Dilatation of the vestibule is often associated with an enlarged vestibular aqueduct (Figs. 1.**66**, 1.**67**).

Internal Auditory Canal

The most common anomaly of the internal auditory canal is hypoplasia. The hypoplasia can be isolated or be associated with other anomalies (Figs. 1.**72**, 1.**73**). Whenever a patient with bilateral involvement is a candidate for cochlear implant, an MR

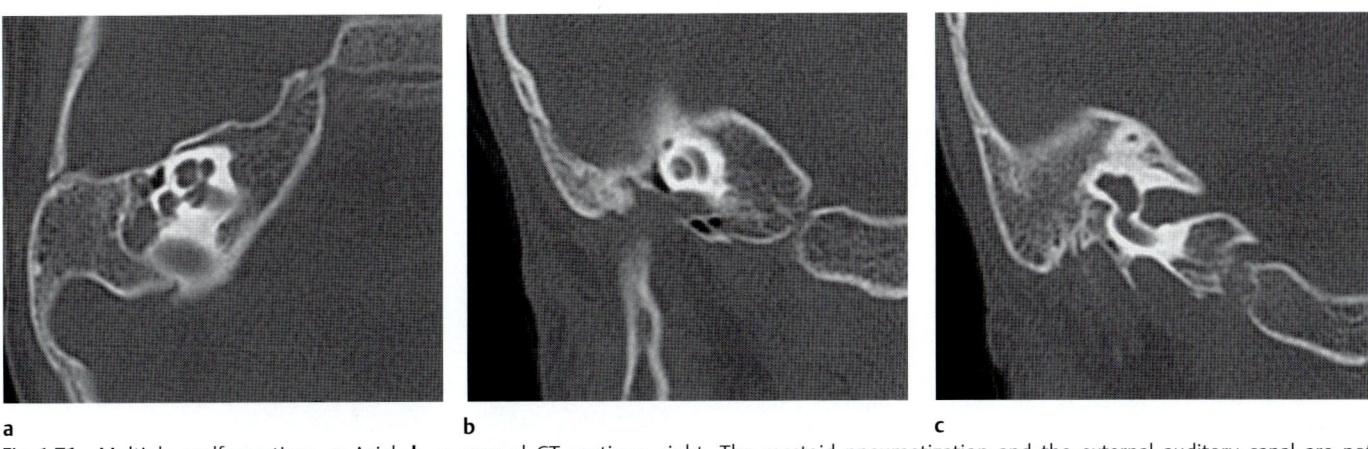

Fig. 1.**71** Multiple malformations. **a** Axial, **b**, **c** coronal CT sections, right. The mastoid pneumatization and the external auditory canal are not developed. The middle ear is small but the eustachian tube is patent. The vestibule is enlarged and the horizontal semicircular canal is malformed.

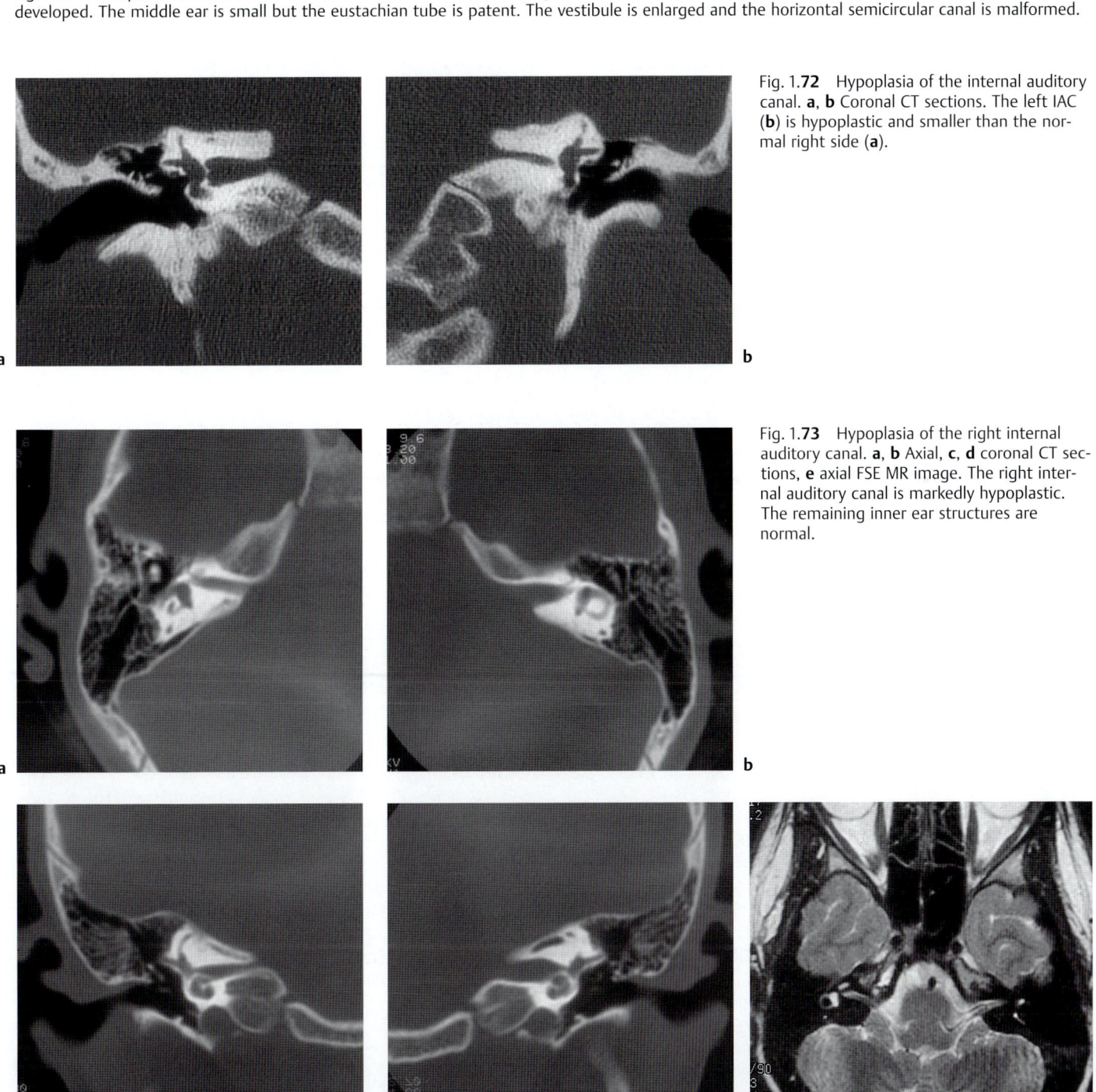

Fig. 1.**72** Hypoplasia of the internal auditory canal. **a**, **b** Coronal CT sections. The left IAC (**b**) is hypoplastic and smaller than the normal right side (**a**).

Fig. 1.**73** Hypoplasia of the right internal auditory canal. **a**, **b** Axial, **c**, **d** coronal CT sections, **e** axial FSE MR image. The right internal auditory canal is markedly hypoplastic. The remaining inner ear structures are normal.

study (T2 fast spin-echo images) should be performed to determine the presence of the cochlear nerve, which is often absent in cases of severe hypoplasia of the internal auditory canal. Rarely the canal is abnormally dilated and shortened. A dilated and shortened internal canal at times is associated with neurofibromatosis and chronic hydrocephalus. In the latter case, the dilatation is secondary to increased intracranial pressure and is not a congenital defect.

Cochlear Aqueduct

The cochlear aqueduct extends from its cochlear opening into the scala tympani medial to the round window to its outer aperture in the posteroinferior aspect of the petrous pyramid, medial to the jugular fossa. The aqueduct is 10–14 mm long, its diameter ranges from 1 mm to 5 mm at its medial aperture and tapers laterally where it becomes invisible in 90% of the cases. The cochlear aqueduct contains a loose mesh of connective tissue permeable to fluid. Enlargement of the cochlear aqueduct of over 2 mm throughout its entire course is extremely rare.

Perilymph gushers occasionally observed during manipulation of the stapes for otosclerosis or congenital footplate fixation are usually due to defects at the fundus of the internal auditory canal rather than to an enlarged or abnormally patent cochlear aqueduct.

Congenital Obliterative Labyrinthitis

A lesion acquired late in fetal life may cause bony or fibrous obliteration of the lumen of one or more of the inner ear structures, which are already well formed. This type of obliteration cannot be differentiated from obliterative labyrinthitis secondary to postnatal infections. Partial or total bony obliteration of the lumen of the inner ear structures is well demonstrated by CT. However, fibrous obliteration can only be seen in the MR images as a partial or total absence of the signal produced by the perilymph and membranous labyrinth (Fig. 1.**74**).

■ Cerebrospinal Fluid Otorrhea

Congenital defects causing cerebrospinal fluid otorrhea occur rarely and often result in repeated bouts of meningitis. The etiology is varied. In most instances, the defect in the tegmen and dura is due to arachnoid granulations. More rarely, the otorrhea is the result of defects at the fundus of the internal auditory canal and in the stapes footplate with consequent communication between the subarachnoid space and the middle ear via the internal auditory canal and the vestibule. These patients are profoundly deaf.

■ Imaging Assessment for Cochlear Implantation

Candidates for cochlear implants require a radiographic study to determine the feasibility of the procedure. CT can determine the size of the development of the mastoid, middle ear, round window, cochlea, and cochlear lumen, the position of the dura, and, of course, the facial nerve canal. The otological surgeon must know whether the mastoid and middle ear are large enough to obtain access to the promontory and round window. If an intracochlear implant is contemplated, the surgeon should know whether there is a patent round window and cochlear lumen. If the cochlea is obliterated by bone, the cochlea must be drilled or

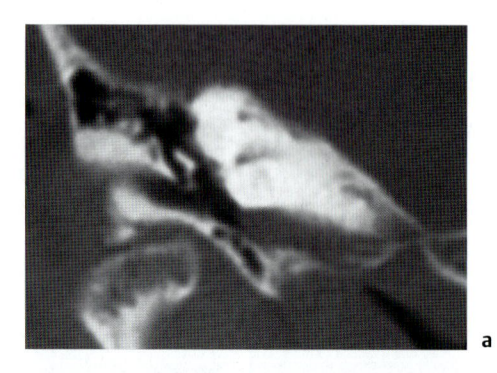

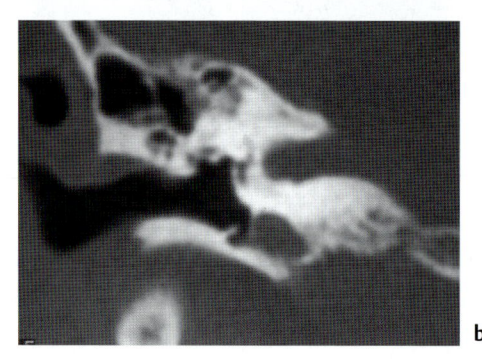

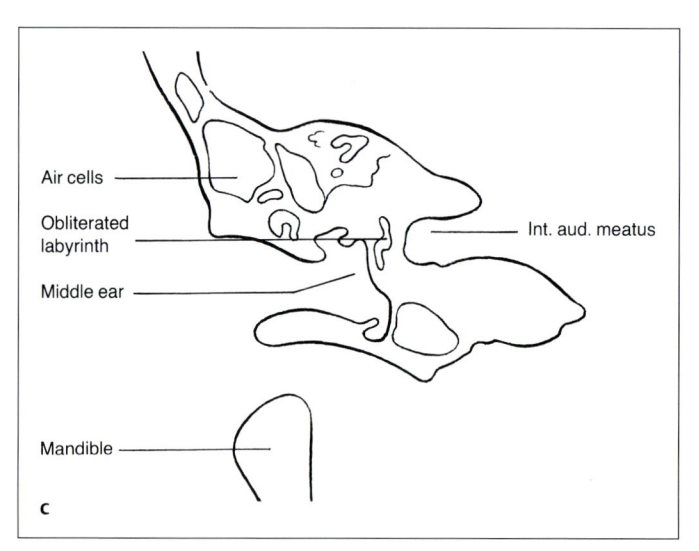

Fig. 1.**74** Obliterative labyrinthitis. **a, b** Coronal CT sections, right. The middle ear cavity and mastoid are normal. The lumen of the inner ear structures is almost completely obliterated by bone.
c Diagram of **b**.

an extra cochlear device used. Marked hypoplasia of the cochlea and internal auditory canal is often indicative of lack of development of the acoustic nerve, which will make an implant unfeasible. MR is indicated to establish the presence and status of the acoustic nerve, to rule out fibrous obliteration of the cochlear lumen that cannot be seen by CT, and to exclude the presence of central pathology affecting the auditory pathways. A postoperative transorbital or Stenver view should be obtained to determine the position of the electrodes and the integrity of the implanted wires (Fig. 1.**75**). These views will be used as a baseline for follow-up studies.

■ Congenital Vascular Anomalies

See Chapter 3.

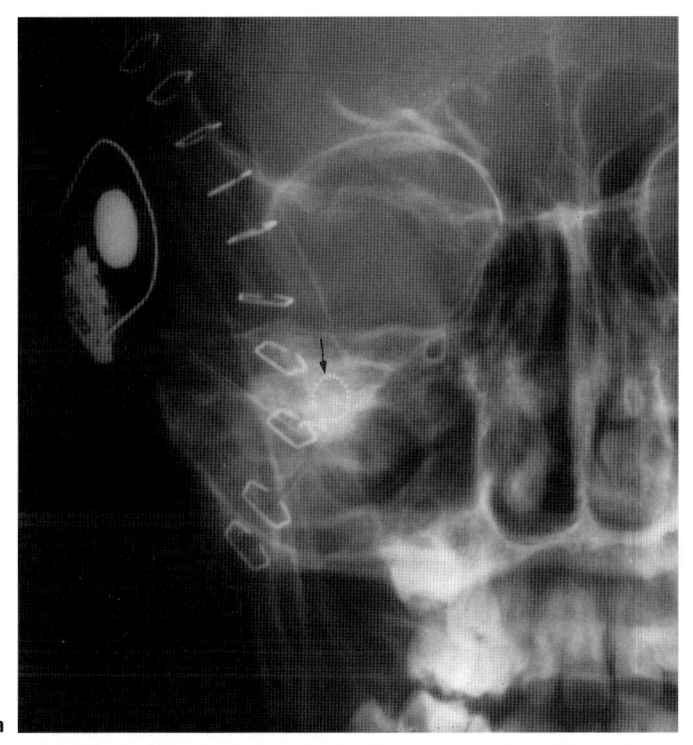

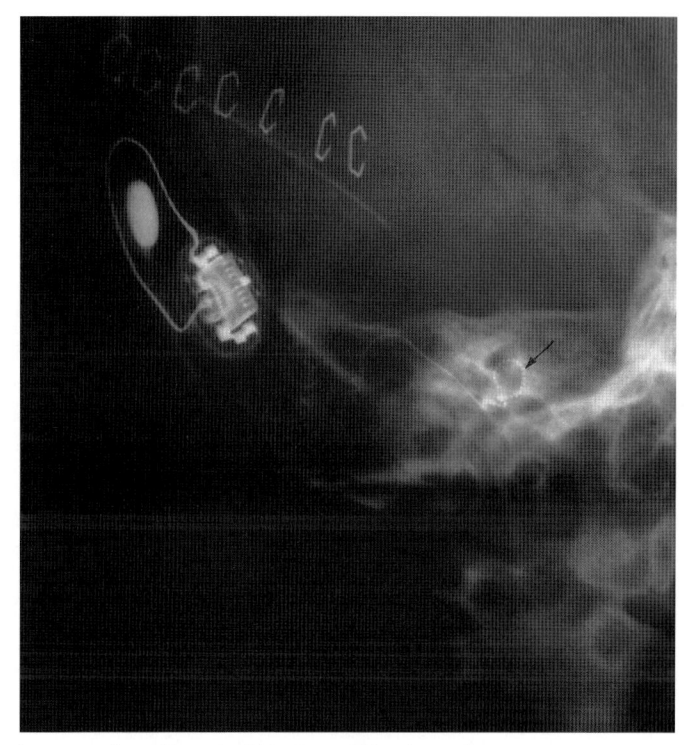

Fig. 1.75 Cochlear implant. **a** Caldwell, **b** Stenvers views. The active electrodes are well-positioned within the cochlea (arrow).

■ Syndromic Hearing Loss

Hearing loss in association with other congenital or genetic abnormalities is a frequent occurrence.[13] Approximately 50% of congenital hearing impairment discovered in children is of genetic origin. In patients with conductive hearing loss, an imaging study, usually CT, is indicated to assess the type of malformation and determine the feasibility for corrective surgery. In patients with bilateral profound sensorineural hearing loss, an imaging study should be performed whenever a cochlear implant procedure is considered.

Mandibulofacial dysostosis (Treacher–Collins syndrome) is a genetic disorder involving structures derived from the first and second branchial arches, groove, and pouch. The abnormalities are usually bilateral and symmetrical. The mandible, maxillae, and malar bones are hypoplastic; the palate is foreshortened and incomplete; the paranasal sinuses are hypoplastic; and a coloboma of the lower lid is often present. The hearing loss is usually conductive in type. The ear anomalies commonly seen are microtia or complete anotia, stenosis or atresia of the external auditory canal, hypoplasia of the middle ear, and malformation and fixation of the ossicular chain. The mastoid segment of the facial nerve may be ectopic. The inner ear structures are usually normal.

Hemifacial microsomia (oculo-auriculo-vertebral dysplasia, Goldenhar syndrome), is a sporadic craniofacial anomaly, usually unilateral, involving structures derived from the first and second branchial arches, although skeletal, pulmonary, renal, and central nervous system anomalies are not uncommon. The affected mandibular ramus, condyle, and maxilla are hypoplastic. Changes in the temporal bone are similar to the mandibulofacial dyostosis but are unilateral. Associated anomalies of the inner ear are observed in 10–15% of cases. Epibulbar dermoid or dermolipoma is a characteristic feature of Goldenhar syndrome.

Waardenburg syndrome is a genetic disorder characterized by dystopia canthorum (type I only), hypertelorism, high nasal bridge, hypoplastic nasal alae, heterochromia irides, hyperpigmentation of the ocular fundi, white forelock, and partial albinism. Sensory hearing loss is present in 20% of type I and 50% of type II syndrome and may be unilateral or bilateral. Imaging studies usually fail to show the abnormality.

X-linked hearing loss is a syndrome characterized by perilymphatic gush and a progressive mixed or purely sensorineural hearing loss. The vestibular function is normal in the carrier females but usually decreased or absent in the males. CT shows a bulbous enlargement of the lateral portion of the internal auditory canal with defects in the bony plate separating the internal auditory canal from the vestibule and in the base of the modiolus. The increased perilymphatic pressure within the vestibule is responsible for the conductive hearing loss and the perilymphatic gush if a stapedectomy is performed.

Usher syndrome is a genetic disorder that includes retinitis pigmentosa and sensorineural hearing loss. The temporal bone imaging study usually is not contributory.

Alport syndrome is a genetic disorder characterized by glomerulonephritis and progressive sensorineural hearing loss. The imaging study of the temporal bone reveals no abnormalities.

Stickler syndrome is a congenital disorder featuring flattening of the mid face, cleft palate, severe myopia, arthropathy, and hearing loss. The hearing loss is usually conductive owing to eustachian tube dysfunction.

Pendred syndrome is a genetic disorder that includes nontoxic goiter and profound sensorineural hearing loss, frequently caused by a Mondini malformation.

Branchio-oto-renal syndrome is a genetc disorder characterized by branchial cleft fistulae or cysts, renal abnormalities of various types, and otological anomalies, including malformed pinna, preauricular pits, and hearing loss, usually mixed in type.

Alagille syndrome is a congenital condition characterized by malformation of inner and outer ears, chronic cholestasis, mental retardation, and systemic abnormalities.

Temporal Bone Trauma

Imaging studies of the temporal bone following head trauma are indicated when there is cerebrospinal fluid otorrhea or rhinorrhea, hearing loss, or facial nerve paralysis. Demonstration of temporal bone fractures is important for therapeutic and medicolegal reasons. In fractures of the base of the skull, the temporal bone is usually involved. The temporal bone can also be affected by fractures of the calvaria that extend into the skull base. Temporal bone fractures are difficult to visualize radiographically. Conventional radiography is helpful in demonstrating fractures of the temporal squama and mastoid. When fractures involve the middle ear and petrous pyramid, CT is indispensible in demonstrating the extent of the lesion. In acute head trauma with unconsciousness or neurological findings, a CT or MR should be performed first to rule out the possibility of intracranial hemorrhage.

■ Classification

Temporal bone fractures are divided into longitudinal and transverse lesions depending on the direction of the fracture line. Longitudinal fractures (Fig. 1.**76**) occur more frequently than transverse fractures in a ratio of 5 : 1. Classification of temporal bone fractures into longitudinal and transverse types is somewhat arbitrary, since most fractures follow a serpiginous course in the temporal bone. Localized fractures of the mastoid and external canal are the result of direct trauma. An isolated fracture of the anterior wall of the external canal may result from indirect trauma from a blow to the mandible. The typical longitudinal fracture involves the temporal squama and extends into the mastoid. The fracture usually reaches the external auditory canal and passes medially into the epitympanum. Medial extension into the petrosa from the epitympanum may occur, and the fracture line can pursue an intralabyrinthine or extralabyrinthine course. An intralabyrinthine course of the fracture is rare since the labyrinthine bone is relatively resistant to trauma. Extralabyrinthine extension of a longitudinal fracture occurs either anterior and posterior to the labyrinth, though anterior extension is more common. A transverse fracture of the temporal bone typically crosses the petrous pyramid at right angles to the longitudinal axis of the pyramid. The fracture line usually follows the line of least resistance and runs from the dome of the jugular fossa through the labyrinth to the superior petrous ridge.

■ Clinical Findings

Clinical findings depend on the type of fracture. Hemotympanum and bleeding from the ear occur when the external auditory canal or tympanic membrane are involved. When the fracture line crosses the epitympanum, there is usually disruption of the ossicular chain with conductive deafness. Conductive deafness also occurs following displaced fractures of the anterior external canal wall and consequent canal stenosis. When the fracture runs into the petrous pyramid adjacent to but not involving the labyrinth, partial sensorineural deafness or vestibular paresis often result from labyrinthine concussion. In a longitudinal fracture with extralabyrinthine extension into the petrous pyramid, mixed hearing loss can result from simultaneous ossicular disruption and labyrinthine concussion. Facial paralysis occurs immediately or after a few hours or days following trauma. Immediate onset of facial paralysis is the result of severe direct trauma or bisection of the nerve by the fracture. Delayed facial paralysis is due to edema or hematoma of the nerve with or without fracture of the facial canal.

■ Imaging Findings

Fractures with wide separation and displacement of the fragments are easily visualized radiographically. Microfractures and fractures with minimal separation and displacement can only be recognized by CT if the plane of section passes at right angles to the plane of the fracture. For this reason, the radiographic projections vary for longitudinal and transverse fractures, and multiple projections are needed to demonstrate the contour of a serpiginous fracture. The radiographic evaluation of a temporal bone fracture should begin with conventional views including the Schüller, Towne–Chamberlain, and Stenvers views. When a fracture line is detected in the temporal squama on the Schüller view and extends into the mastoid, the fracture will be of the longitudinal type (Fig. 1.**77**). If a fracture line is seen in the occipital bone in the Towne–Chamberlain or Stenvers projection, pyramidal extension of the fracture will be of the transverse type (Fig. 1.**78**).

CT permits precise evaluation of the course of fractures into the middle ear and petrous bone. This technique shows displacement and disruption of the ossicular chain, the site of facial nerve lesions, and tegmental injuries. In longitudinal fractures, the most revealing projections are the axial and sagittal, since in these projections the plane of the fracture will be at a right angle to the section plane. Coronal and axial projections are required

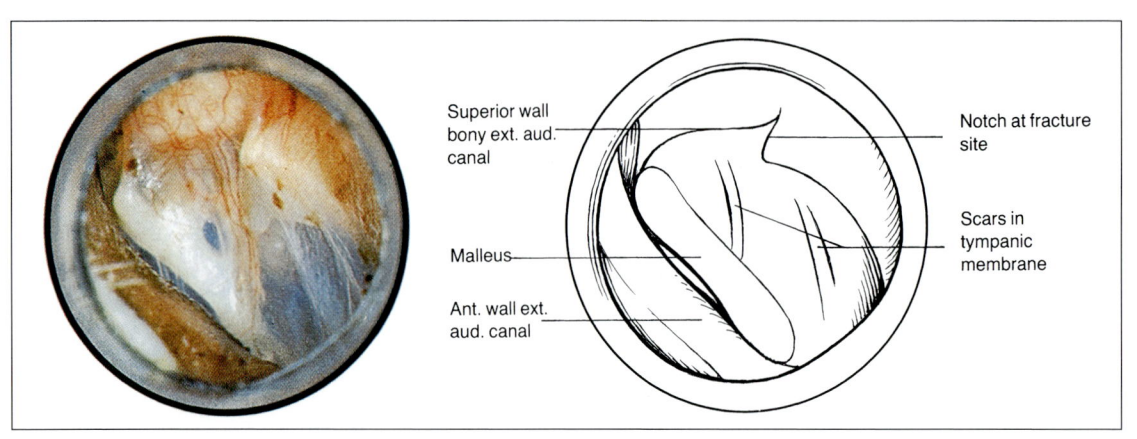

Fig. 1.**76 a** Longitudinal fracture, otoscopic findings, left. This patient suffered a longitudinal fracture 3 years previously. The notch on the posterosuperior bony margin of the external auditory canal is a result of the slight displacement of the fracture, which extended through the external auditory canal into the mastoid and ruptured the tympanic membrane.
b Diagram of **a**.

Temporal Bone Trauma

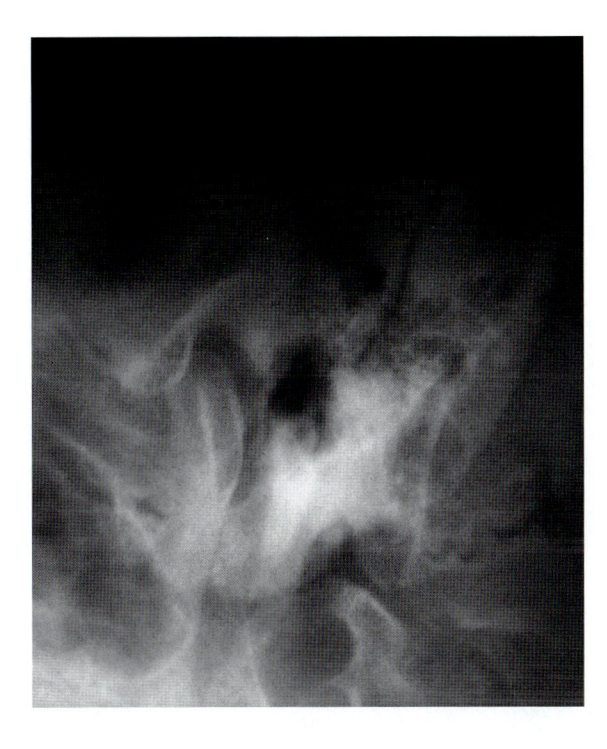

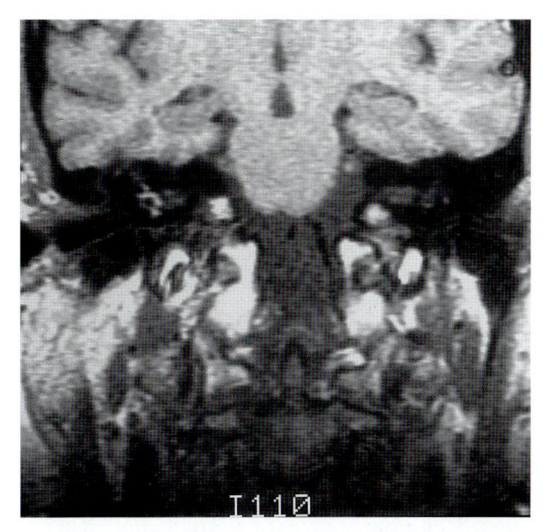

Fig. 1.79 Labyrinthine concussion. T1W coronal MR section without contrast material. The high signal intensity within the lumen of the right labyrinth is due to bleeding. No fracture was observed in the MR and CT studies.

◁ Fig. 1.77 Longitudinal fracture, temporal bone, Schüller view, left. A longitudinal fracture line extends from the temporal squama, through the mastoid, into the external auditory canal.

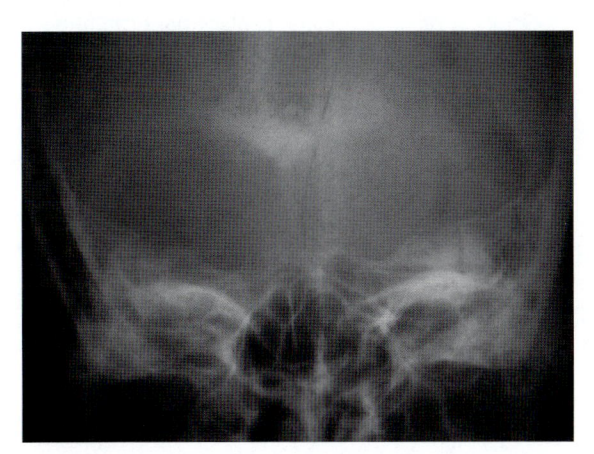

Fig. 1.78 Transverse fractures, both temporal bones, Towne view. There are fractures of both petrous pyramids and a linear fracture of the occipital bone extending to the foramen magnum.

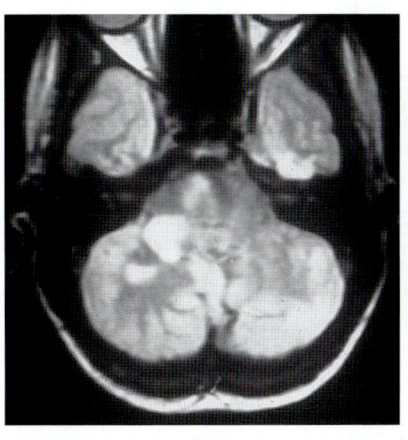

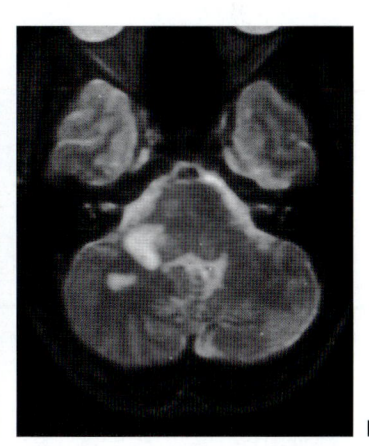

Fig. 1.80 Intracranial bleeding. **a** Proton-density-weighted, **b** T2W axial MR sections. There is bleeding in the posterior cranial fossa in the region of the right cochlear nuclei.

for demonstration of transverse fractures. A fracture line may disappear at a certain level only to reappear a few millimeters distant. This apparent gap is not due to interruption of the fracture line, but rather to the fact that the plane of the fracture changes direction and becomes invisible in some of the sections. MRI is more sensitive than CT in detecting areas of bleeding in the mastoid air cells and middle ear cavity, but fails to demonstrate the actual fractures and the status of the ossicular chain (Fig. 1.87). For this reason, CT is the primary study in temporal bone trauma.

■ Labyrinthine Concussion and Bleeding

Bleeding within the lumen of the inner ear structures may occur after trauma. If a fracture crosses the inner ear, the detection of blood is of academic value since the patient has an irreversible total deafness and vestibular paralysis, or both. If bleeding occurs by concussion without actual fracture, MR may be indicated to confirm the diagnosis. The study should be performed at least two days after the injury to allow the transformation of deoxyhemoglobin into methemoglobin, which has a bright signal in both T1- and T2-weighted images (Fig. 1.79). Intracranial bleeding in the region of the cochlear nuclei and auditory pathway may also cause transient or irreversible deafness (Fig. 1.80). Spontaneous intralabyrinthine hemorrhage has been also observed in patients with sickle cell disease due to vaso-occlusive crisis.

■ Longitudinal Fractures

Longitudinal fractures of the temporal bone involve the mastoid and extend from the floor of the middle cranial fossa and tegmen downward and often forward to the posterosuperior wall of the

1 Imaging of the Temporal Bone

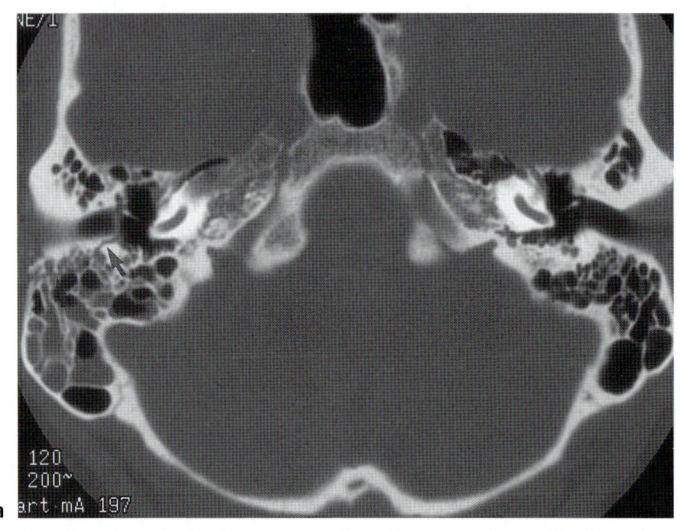

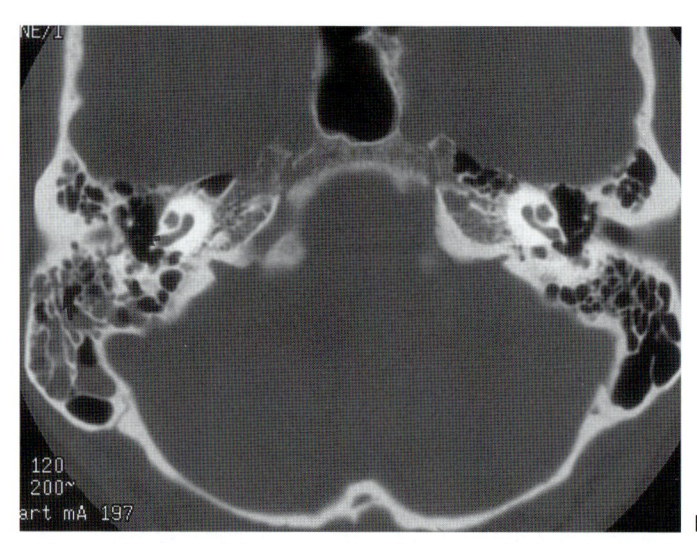

Fig. 1.81 Longitudinal fracture of the right mastoid. **a** and **b** CT axial sections. A fracture line extends from the mastoid cortex to the lateral attic wall. There is bleeding within the adjacent air cells.

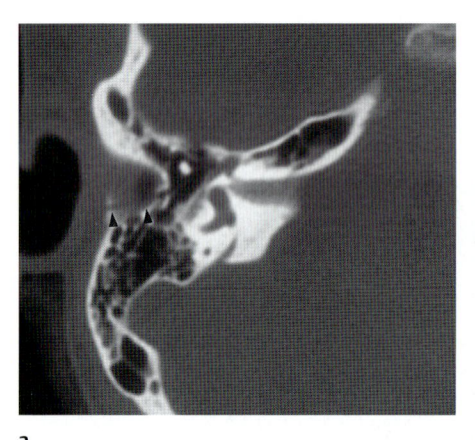

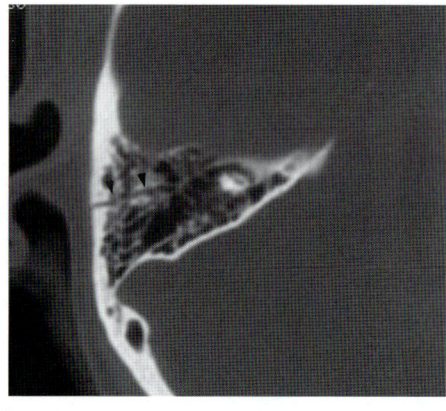

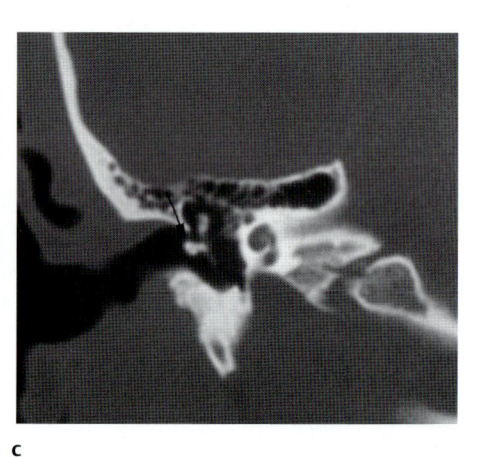

Fig. 1.82 Longitudinal fracture, right temporal bone. **a, b** Axial, **c** coronal CT sections. The longitudinal fracture reaches the attic (arrowheads). The body of the incus is displaced laterally and protrudes into the external auditory canal (arrow).

external auditory canal (Fig. 1.81). There is often an extension of the fracture to the anterior wall of the external auditory canal and temporomandibular fossa. A fracture of the posterior wall of the external auditory canal may extend medially to the facial nerve canal at or distal to the pyramidal turn of the nerve, with a resultant facial paralysis.

Medial extension of a longitudinal fracture into the epitympanum results in a disruption of the ossicular chain, a tegmental fracture, and often a cerebrospinal otorrhea (Fig. 1.82). We have observed luxation of the incus where the short process was propelled into the facial canal and paralyzed the facial nerve distal to the pyramidal turn. A longitudinal fracture may occasionally extend into the petrous pyramid through the labyrinth. Anterior petrous extension is more frequent and may involve the facial nerve at the superficial geniculate ganglion area (Fig. 1.85). Further medial extension of the longitudinal fracture may reach the carotid canal, injure the internal carotid, and lead to a post-traumatic aneurysm.

■ Transverse Fractures

Most transverse fractures of the temporal bone lie medial to the middle ear cavity and therefore involve the inner ear structures. The fractures may extend anteriorly into the floor of the middle cranial fossa and posteriorly into the occipital bone. Most commonly, transverse fractures reach from the dome of the jugular fossa to the superior petrous ridge either medial or lateral to the arcuate eminence. Laterally placed fractures involve the promontory, the vestibule, the horizontal and posterior semicircular canals, and occasionally the tympanic segment of the facial nerve. Medially situated fractures involve the vestibule, the cochlea, the fundus of the internal auditory canal, and the crus commune (Figs. 1.83, 1.84). A more unusual type of transverse fracture occurs medial to the vestibule and bisects the internal auditory canal.

■ Comminuted Mastoid Fractures

Direct mastoid trauma produces a comminuted fracture of the mastoid cortex and trabeculae and diffuse clouding of the air cells from accompanying hemorrhage (Figs. 1.86, 1.88). The fractures often extend to the external canal, the middle ear and the

Temporal Bone Trauma 57

Fig. 1.83 Transverse fracture, temporal bone. **a, b, c** Axial, **d, e** coronal CT sections, left. The fracture extends from the superior petrous ridge in the region of the arcuate eminence to the jugular fossa. The fracture involves three semicircular canals, and splits the vestibule (**b**). The facial canal is involved in the tympanic segment anterior to the oval window (**d**).

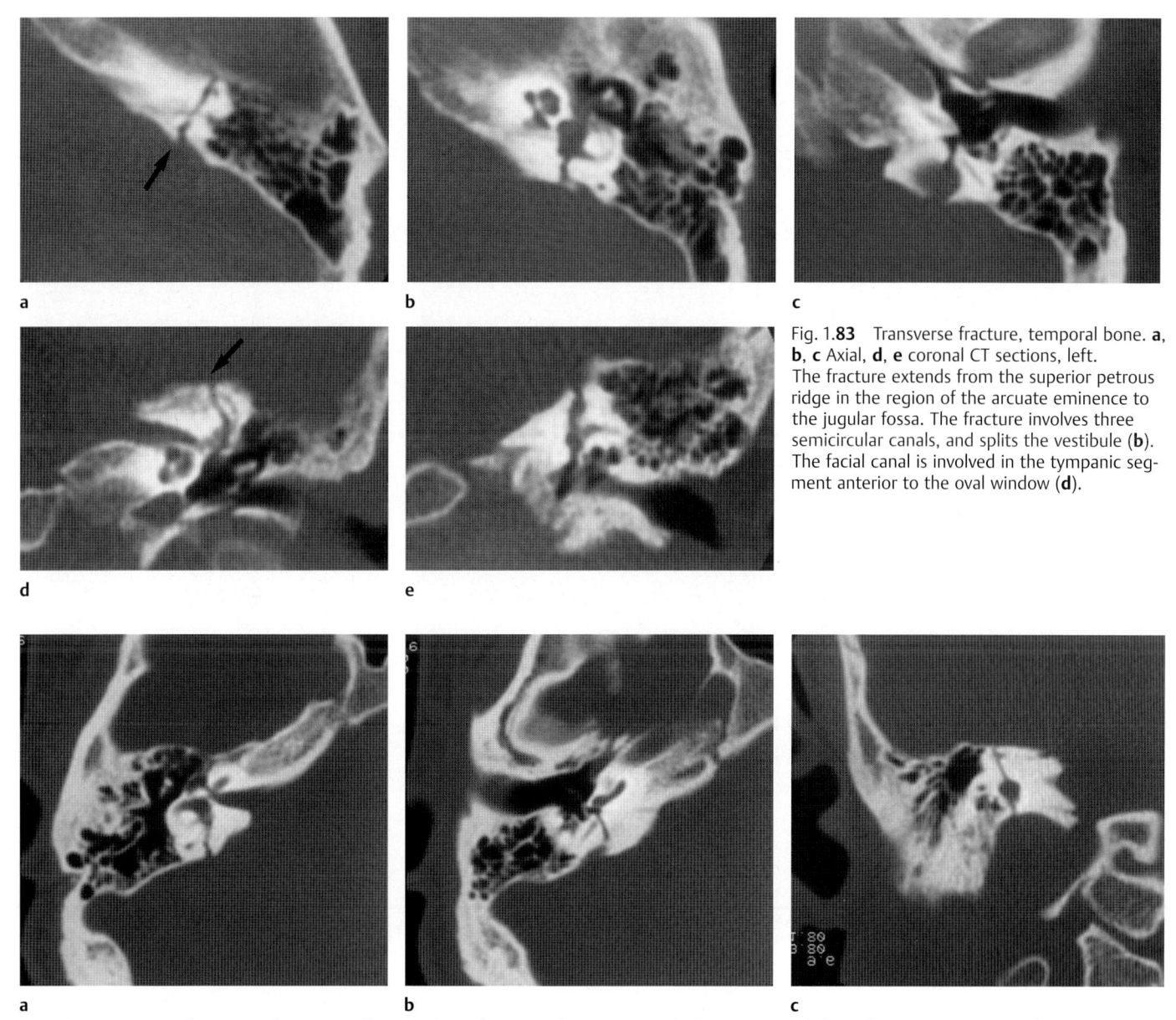

Fig. 1.84 Transverse fracture, right temporal bone. **a, b** Axial, **c** coronal CT sections. The fracture extends from the superior petrous ridge to the jugular fossa and crosses the superior posterior semicircular canals, vestibule, and basal turn of the cochlea.

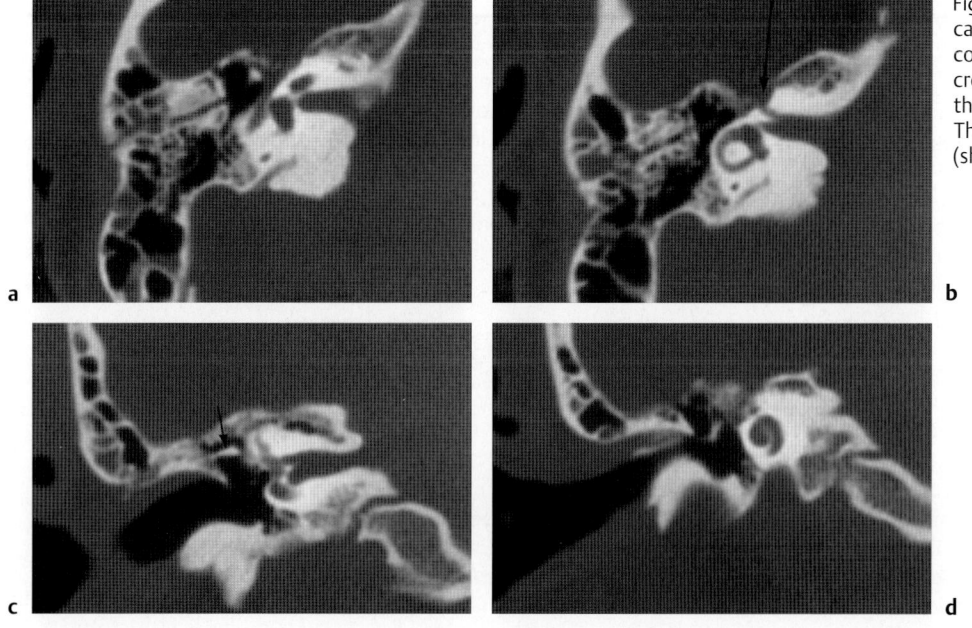

Fig. 1.85 Longitudinal fracture with incus dislocation and facial paralysis. **a, b** Axial, **c, d** coronal CT sections. The longitudinal fracture crosses the attic and reaches the facial canal in the region of the anterior genu (long arrow). The body of the incus is displaced and rotated (short arrow).

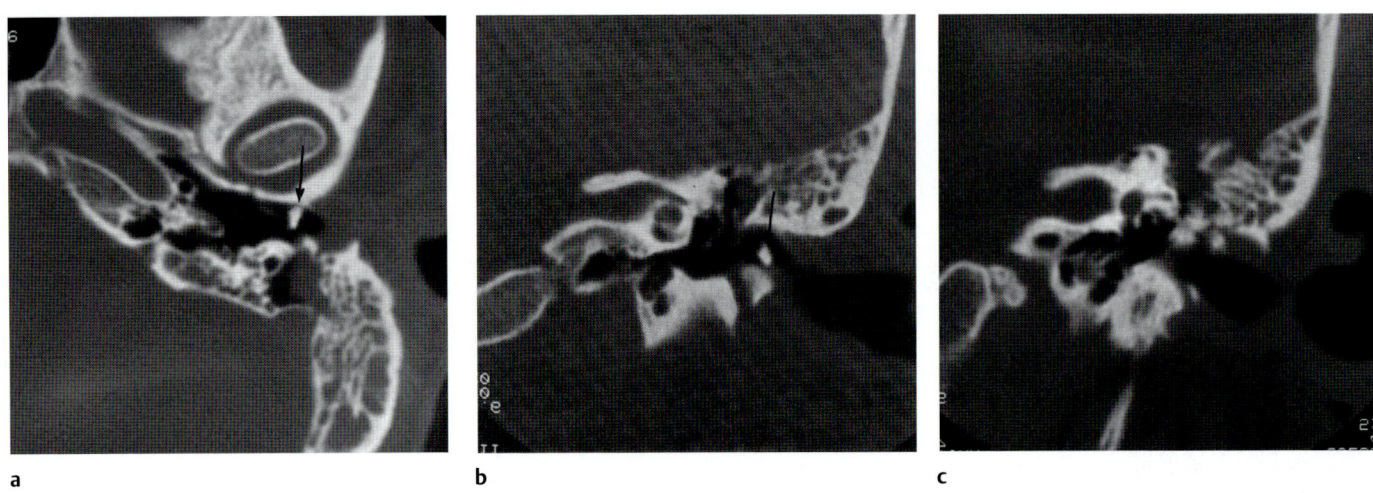

Fig. 1.**86** Comminuted fracture, left ear. **a** Axial, **b**, **c** coronal CT sections. Multiple fractures disrupt the mastoid, external auditory canal, and middle ear. The incus (arrow) is displaced in the external auditory canal.

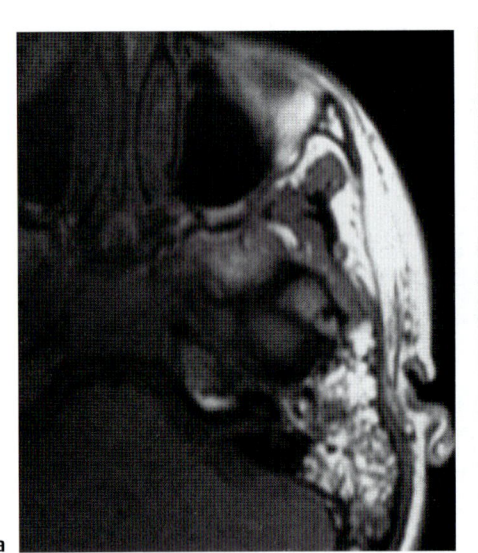

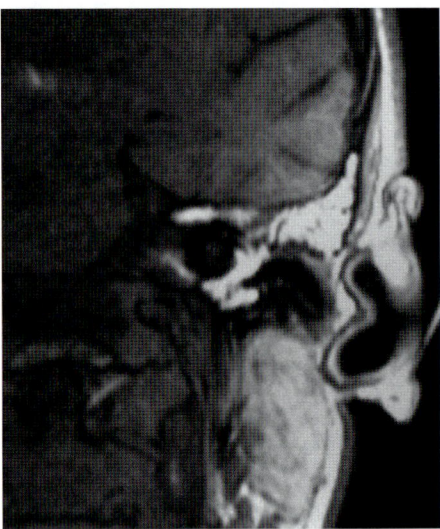

Fig. 1.**87** Cominuted fracture of the left ear. **a** Axial, **b** coronal T1W MR sections. The mastoid air cells and middle ear cavity are filled with blood. Only one fracture lateral to the attic is faintly seen.

vertical segment of the facial canal and cause facial nerve paralysis (Fig. 1.**93**).

■ Ossicular Dislocation

Following a temporal bone fracture, some patients develop a persistent conductive deafness, which is usually secondary to disruption of the ossicular chain. The disruption is associated with a fracture usually of the longitudinal type. In some cases radiographic evidence of a fracture is absent, but disruption of the ossicles is evident on CT. Ossicular disruption can also occur following direct trauma to the ear by foreign bodies perforating the tympanic membrane, from previous mastoid surgery, or by projectile missiles. Dislocation of the malleus is rare because of the firm attachment of the malleus to the tympanic membrane and the strong anterior mallear ligament. The incus is most commonly dislocated since its attachments to the malleus and stapes are easily torn (Figs. 1.**82**, 1.**85**, 1.**86**, 1.**89**). When the incudomallear joint is disrupted, the body of the incus is usually rotated and displaced superiorly, posteriorly, and laterally. More rarely the incus body is displacd inferolaterally to abut against the superior portion of the tympanic membrane. Otoscopically the dislocated incus appears as a bony mass in the upper portion of the middle ear.

The most common site of ossicular chain disruption is the incudostapedial joint area. The disruption exists as a fracture of the lenticular process of the incus, a dislocation of the incudostapedial joint, or a fracture through the stapes superstructure. Radiographic diagnosis of disruption of the incudostapedial joint area is made by detection of the separation of the incus long process from the stapes head and by recognition of displacement of the long process of the incus away from the stapes. Isolated stapes footplate fractures cannot be visualized directly. In some cases of stapes fracture or dislocation and posttraumatic perilymphatic fistula, air can be identified within the vestibular or cochlear lumina (Fig. 1.**90**).

■ Projectile Injuries

Projectiles such as bullets or metallic fragments from industrial accidents penetrate into the temporal bone and cause severe injury. A bullet injury depends on the trajectory of the bullet and the site where the bullet fragments come to rest. Following industrial accidents, we usually find radiopaque fragments lodged in the external auditory canal or middle ear (Fig. 1.**91**). Bullet wounds cause comminution of the temporal bone. There are multiple metallic bullet fragments, since bullets usually shatter

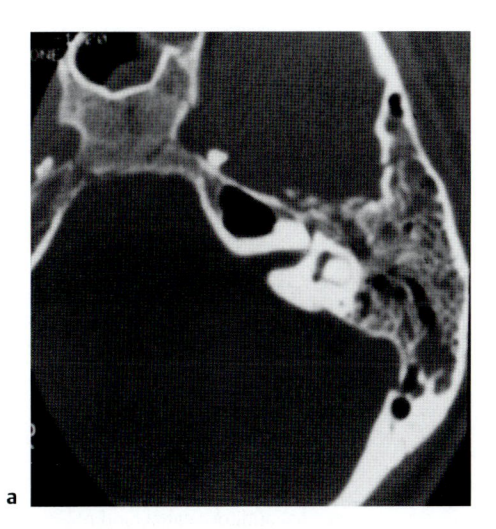

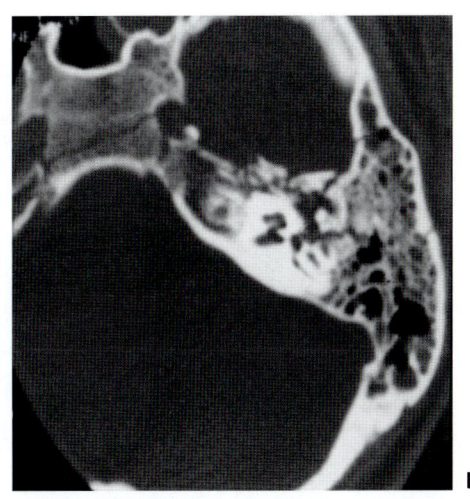

Fig. 1.88 Multiple fractures of the base of the skull. **a, b** Axial CT sections. The fractures involve the left mastoid and middle ear, and extend into the petrous pyramid anterior to the cochlea. The clivus is split and the lateral wall of the left sphenoid sinus is broken, with bleeding within the sinus cavity.

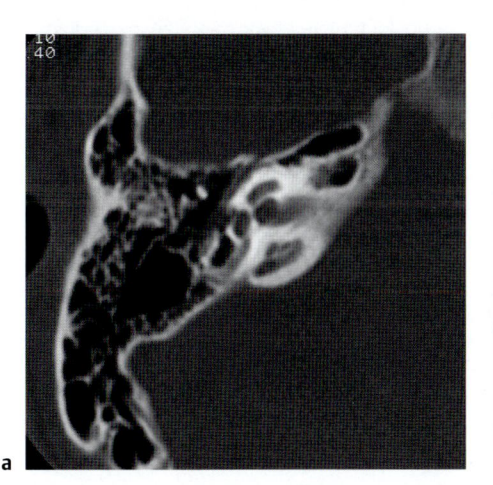

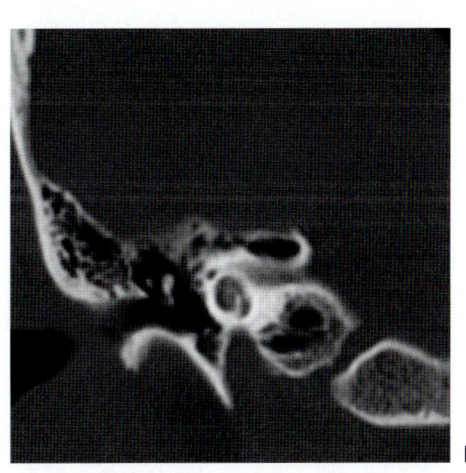

Fig. 1.89 Ossicular dislocations. **a** Axial, **b** coronal CT sections. No fracture is identified but the body of the incus is dislocated lateral to the head of the malleus.

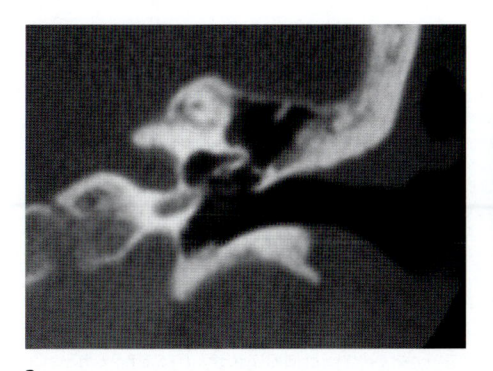

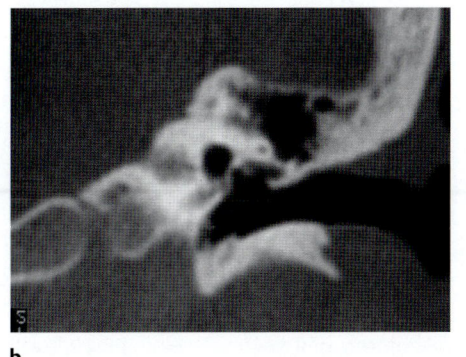

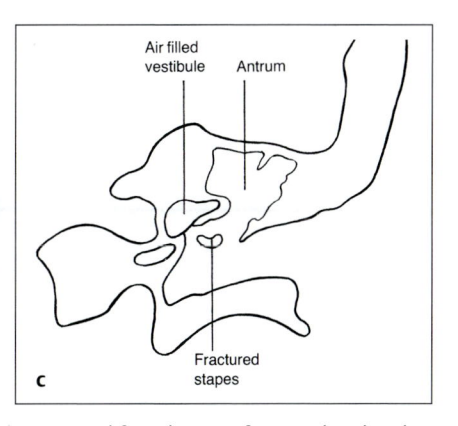

Fig. 1.90 Fracture of the stapes with pneumolabyrinth. **a, b** Coronal sections, left. The stapes superstructure and footplate are fractured and air has entered the vestibule. The lumen of the vestibule is far darker than the adjacent lumen of the cochlea. **c** Diagram of **a**.

on impact with the hard bone of the petrosa (Fig. 1.92). Bullet wounds involving the mastoid and middle ear cause cerebrospinal fluid leaks, conductive deafness, and facial paralysis. When the inner ear structures are involved there will be total sensorineural deafness and loss of vestibular function. One serious problem with CT when large metallic fragments are present is the deterioration of the image by spark artifacts. An MR study is contraindicated when there is the possibility of the presence of the ferromagnetic fragments within the temporal bone or brain.

■ Traumatic Facial Nerve Lesions

Facial paralysis due to traumatic lesions of the intratemporal portion of the facial nerve is not uncommon following head injuries of various types, especially in high-speed vehicle accidents. A CT study should be performed in these cases to demonstrate (1) the presence of a temporal bone fracture, (2) the course of the fracture, and (3) the site of involvement of the facial canal. This information is necessary if surgical decompression of the facial canal is planned.

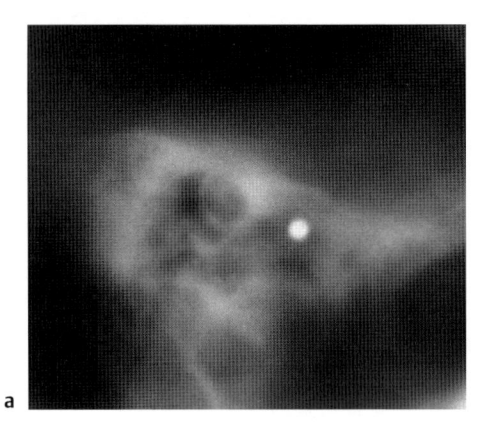

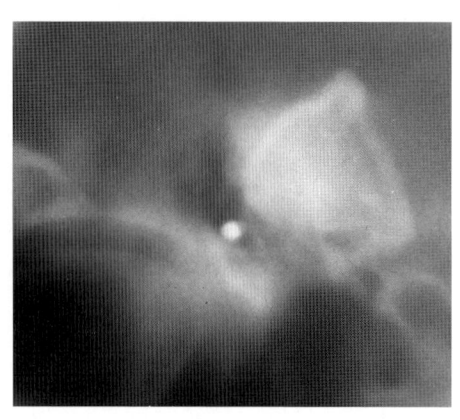

Fig. 1.**91** Metallic foreign body. **a** Sagittal, **b** semiaxial tomogram, right. A metallic foreign body, a large weld spark, lies in the eustachian tube portion of the middle ear.

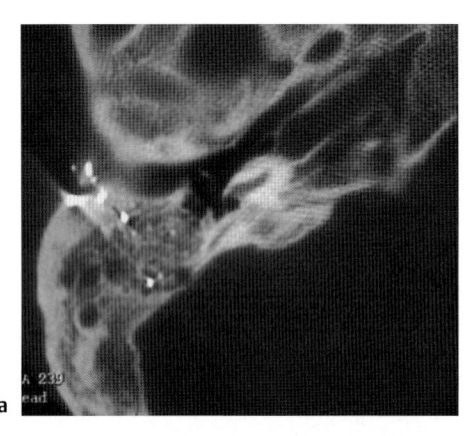

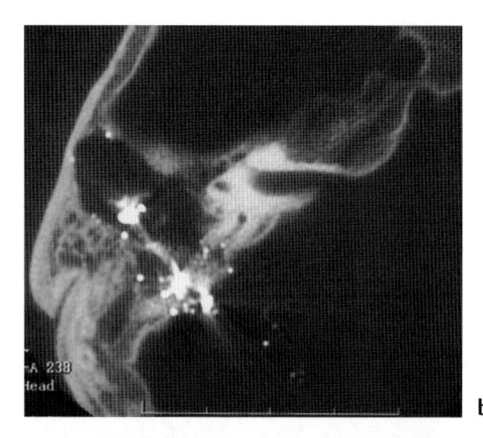

Fig. 1.**92** Bullet wound. **a**, **b** Axial, **c**, **d** coronal CT sections. The bullet has shattered the mastoid, external auditory canal, and attic. Multiple metallic fragments are noted in these and intracranial areas. The ossicular chain is disrupted at the incudo-stapedial joint. The facial nerve canal and the inner ear structures are intact.

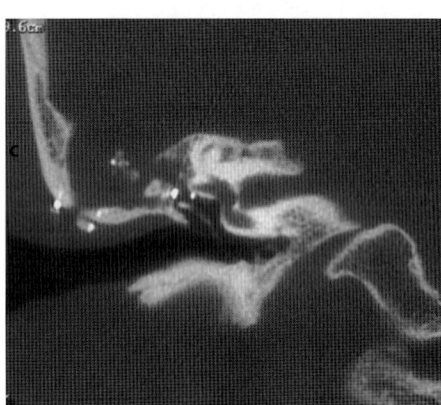

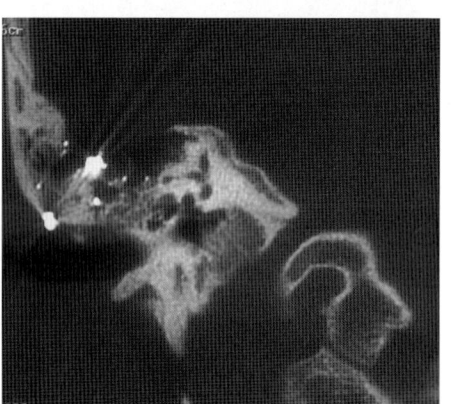

The radiographic findings are variable:
1. There may be a complete disruption of the contour of a segment of the facial canal.
2. The canal may be transected by the fracture line.
3. There may be separation and depression of a fragment of the canal wall into the facial nerve.
4. The incus may be dislocated and the short process impelled into the facial canal immediately distal to the pyramidal turn.

In some cases, the site of the involvement of the facial canal cannot be visualized by CT. However, the site of the lesion can be determined by tracing the course of the fracture line. An MR study may be useful to differentiate contusion of the facial nerve with perineural bleeding from a complete or partial tear of the nerve.

In case of contusion with bleeding, an area of high signal intensity is seen within or surrounding the nerve in T1-weighted images obtained without contrast. Perineural hematoma causes facial paralysis by compression of the nerve. Intracranial hematoma may develop by severe traction and stretching of the greater superficial petrosal nerve. In recent tears of the nerve, the facial nerve has a low-intensity signal in the precontrast T1-weighted images and may enhance following the injection of contrast due to breakdown of the blood–nerve barrier. In longitudinal fractures the most common sites of involvement of the facial nerve are the geniculate ganglion area and, less frequently, the second or pyramidal turn. In transverse fractures the nerve is usually severed within the internal auditory canal or less fequently in the proximal tympanic segment.

The facial nerve may be injured by transverse or longitudinal fractures. While the incidence of transverse fractures is less than that of longitudinal, more than 50% of transverse fractures have an associated trauma-related lesion of the facial nerve. In these cases, the nerve involvement occurs within the internal auditory canal, labyrinthine, or tympanic segments (Fig. 1.**83**). Facial para-

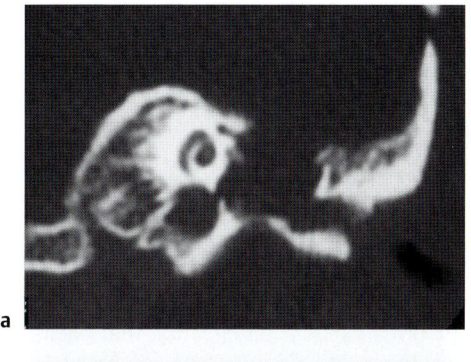

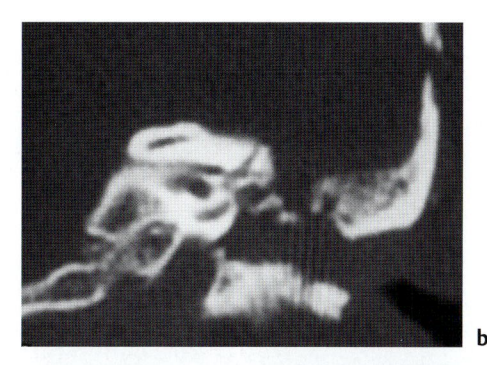

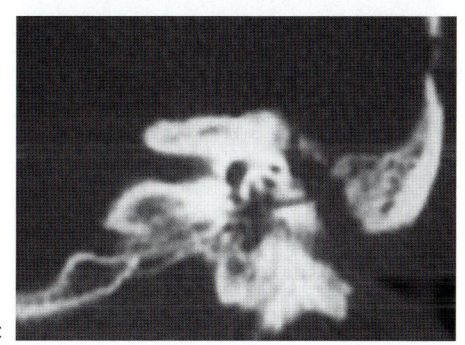

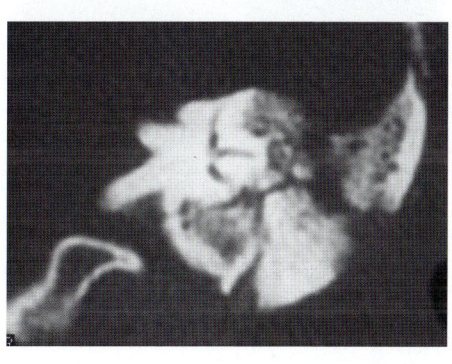

Fig. 1.**93** Multiple fractures, with immediate facial paralysis and meningoencephalocele. **a**, **b**, **c**, **d** Coronal CT sections, left.
There are fractures of the temporal squama and tegmen. A large soft-tissue mass with the same absorption coefficient as the brain extends into the middle ear through a large tegmental defect (**a**). In **b**, 3 mm posterior to **a**, there is a fracture with displacement of the lateral epitympanic wall. The incus is dislocated. The external canal and middle ear cavity are opacified by bleeding and edema. In **c**, 3 mm posterior to **b**, the fracture involves the tegmen of the antrum and crosses the posterior wall of the middle ear. In **d**, 3 mm posterior to **c**, the fracture transects the vertical segment of the facial canal.

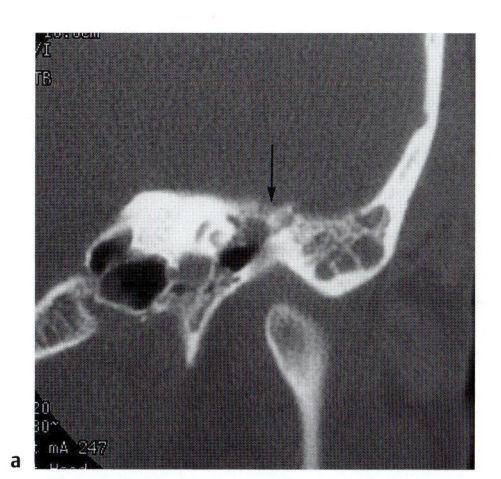

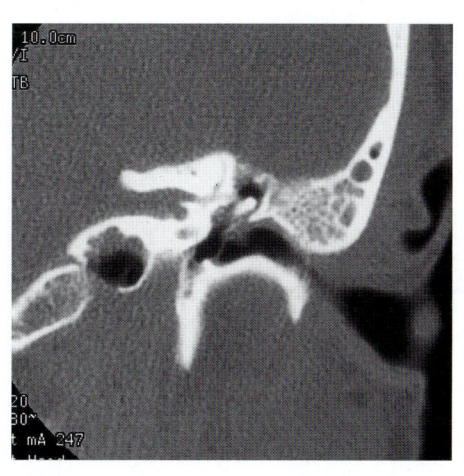

Fig. 1.**94** Cerebrospinal fluid otorrhea. **a**, **b** Coronal CT sections. The tegmen tympani is fractured (arrow) and the tegmental dura is torn. Clear fluid leaks into the external auditory canal through the ruptured tympanic membrane.

lysis occurs in approximately 20% of longitudinal temporal bone fractures.

About 40% of these lesions are located at or distal to the pyramidal turn (Fig. **1.93**) and 60% in the region of the superficial and poorly protected anterior genu (Fig. **1.85**, **1.88**).

■ Iatrogenic Lesions

Facial nerve injury may occur following mastoid surgery. In these cases, the most common involvement occurs at the pyramidal turn. The facial canal in this area is disrupted and often there is an associated defect in the horizontal semicircular canal.

■ Meningoencephalocele

Whenever the CT examination shows disruption of the tegmen or of the posterior wall of the mastoid and petrous pyramid with an underlying soft-tissue mass suggestive of a meningoencephalocele, MR should be performed to confirm this complication. If a meningocele is present, the signal of the mass is similar to cerebrospinal fluid, namely, low in T1-weighted images and bright in T2. If an encephalocele is present, the mass will have in the T1- and T2-weighted images a signal identical to that of the adjacent brain tissue. A rim of fluid usually surrounds the mass.

■ Cerebrospinal Fluid Otorrhea

When the tegmen is involved, and the tegmental dura is torn, cerebrospinal fluid otorrhea occurs if the tympanic membrane is also ruptured (Fig. **1.94**). If the tympanic membane is intact, the cerebrospinal fluid will flow into the eustachian tube and cerebrospinal fluid rhinorrhea will result.

A CT study may demonstrate the site of fracture or fractures of the tegmen but will not differentiate cerebrospinal fluid from blood or other fluid.[30] A more definite diagnosis of cerebrospinal fluid otorrhea is reached by intrathecal injection via lumbar puncture of a small amount of standard myelographic contrast that will diffuse in subarachnoid space and leak into the mastoid or middle ear (Fig. **1.95**).

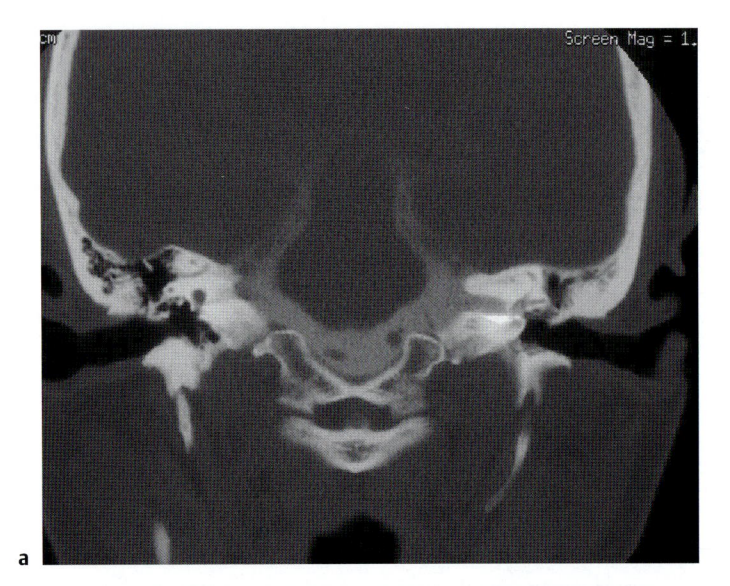

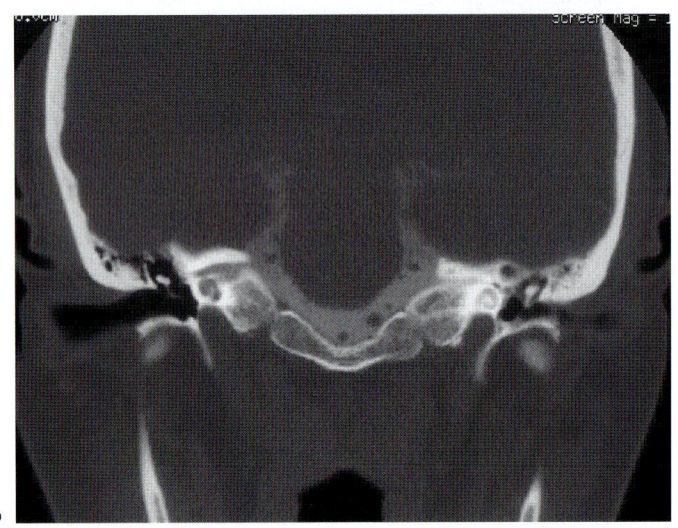

Fig. 1.**95** Metrizamide study. Patient with left profound hearing loss after head trauma and clear fluid in the middle ear cavity. The contrast fills the left internal auditory canal and passes into the inner ear structures through a nonidentifiable defect in the cribriform plate at the fundus of the internal auditory canal (**a**). The lumina of the cochlea (**b**), vestibule, and semicircular canals are opacified. At surgery the footplate of the stapes was slightly dislodged with consequent cerebrospinal fluid leak into the middle ear.

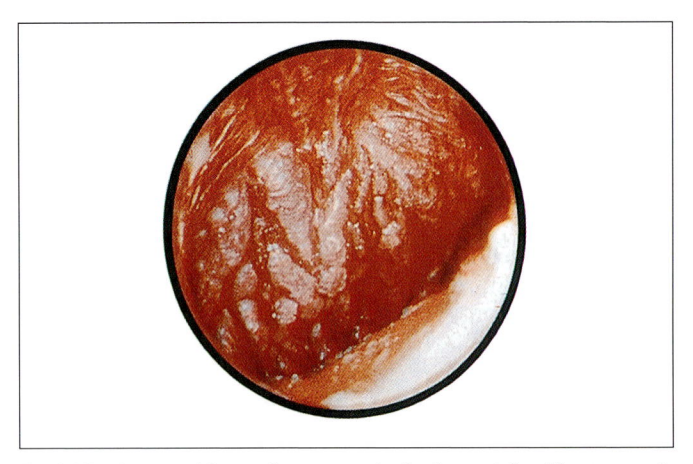

Fig. 1.**96** Acute otitis media, otoscopic findings, right. The tympanic membrane is grossly inflamed and bulges externally owing to purulent discharge in the middle ear under increased pressure. The normal landmarks are missing and the superficial epithelium in the tympanic membrane is desquamating.

Acute Otitis Media, Mastoiditis, and Malignant Necrotizing External Otitis

■ Acute Otitis Media and Mastoiditis

Acute mastoiditis occurs as a complication or extension of an acute otitis media. Acute otitis media is an infection that begins in the upper respiratory tract and nasopharynx, ascends the eustachian tube, and affects the middle ear. Probably even in the early stages of acute otitis media, the inflammatory process extends to some degree into the epitympanum and mastoid antrum. Depending on the virulence of the infecting organism, the resistance of the host, and the type of treatment, the infection may or may not extend to involve the mastoid air cells and the air cells of the petrous pyramid. Further progress of the infectious process, uncontrolled by proper therapy, leads to suppuration and destruction of air cell septa in the mastoid and petrous pyramid. This results in areas of coalescence and abscess formation.

Acute suppurative mastoiditis can extend beyond the borders of the temporal bone.[16] (This was more common in the preantibiotic era than at present.) Erosion of the posterior wall of the mastoid over the sigmoid sinus results in extradural abscess formation and septic thrombosis of the sigmoid sinus (Fig. 1.**103**). Temporal lobe and extradural abscesses may occur following erosion of the tegmen. Erosions of the cortex of the mastoid result in subperiosteal abscesses over the mastoid process and under the superior attachment of the sternocleidomastoid muscle (see Figs. 1.**101** and 1.**102**). Extension of the infection from the mastoid medially into the petrous apex leads to a petrositis with serious neurological and intracranial complications (Fig. 1.**100**). Otoscopically, the tympanic membrane in acute otitis media is inflamed, reddened, and most often bulges externally due to seropurulent fluid under increased pressure in the middle ear (Fig. 1.**96**).

In some instances, antibiotic therapy will result in improvement of the otoscopic findings, while the deep mastoid infection persists and progresses to abscess formation and intracranial complications (see Fig. 1.**103**).

Facial paralysis may occur as a complication of acute or subacute otitis media. When paralysis occurs soon after the onset of an acute otitis media, the facial nerve paralysis is usually not due to erosion of the bony canal but to edema and inflammation of the nerve within the bony canal, probably similar to Bell's palsy. MR performed after injection of contrast material often shows enhancement of the involved segment of the nerve. Recovery of facial nerve function occurs in these cases with conservative treatment.

Facial paralysis occuring two weeks or more after the onset of a persistent acute otitis media usually indicates erosion of the bony facial canal and extension of the infection. CT is indicated, and surgery may be required in cases of this type.

■ Imaging Findings

The radiographic findings of acute mastoiditis depend on the stage of the inflammatory process and the extent of pneumatization of the temporal bone. Acute mastoiditis does not occur in acellular mastoids.

The earliest finding of an acute mastoiditis is a haziness of the middle ear cavity and the mastoid air cells. As the infective process worsens, diffuse clouding of the middle ear cavity and mastoid air

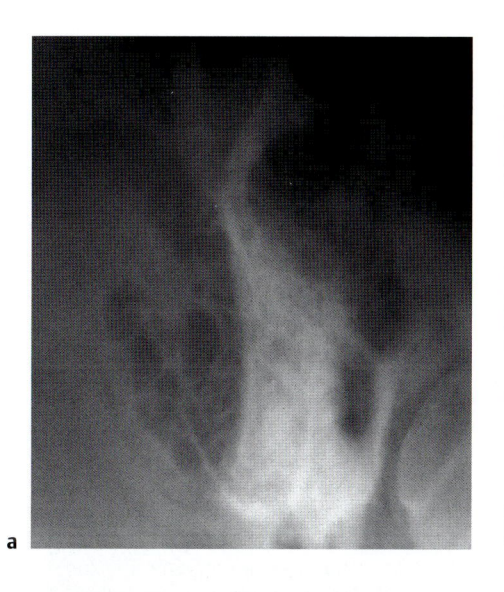

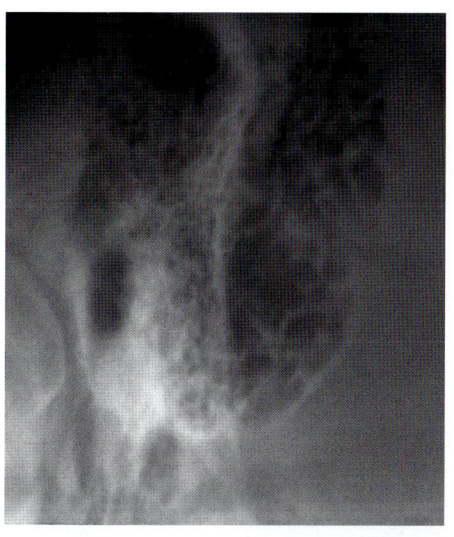

Fig. 1.**97** Acute mastoiditis. **a** Schüller view, right ear. **b** Schüller view of the opposite, normal ear. There is diffuse homogeneous clouding of the mastoid air cells with intact trabeculae (**a**). In **b**, the mastoid air cells are normal.

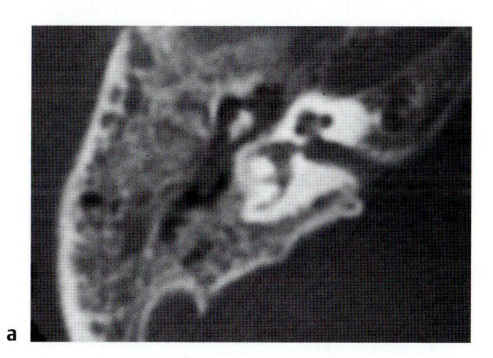

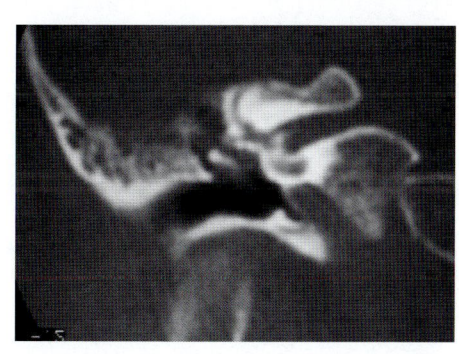

Fig. 1.**98** Acute mastoiditis and otitis media. **a** Axial, **b** coronal CT sections, right. There is a diffuse clouding of the well-pneumatized mastoid. The trabecular pattern is intact. Fluid fills the upper portion of the middle ear, and the lateral wall of the attic and the ossicular chain are normal.

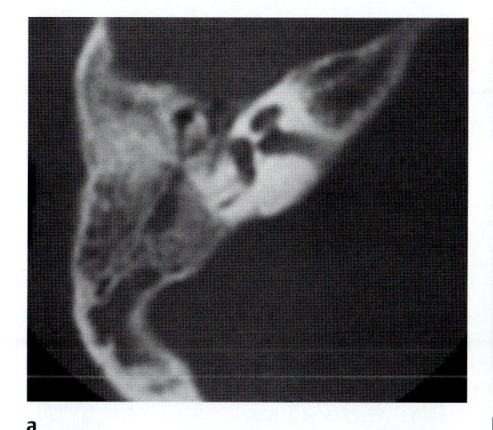

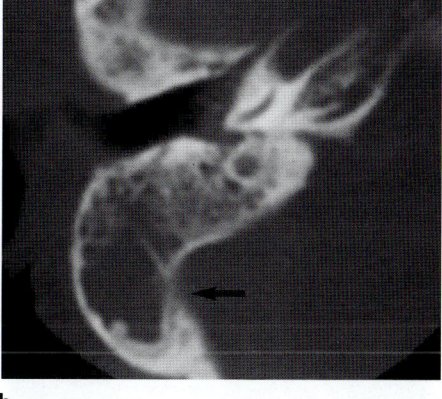

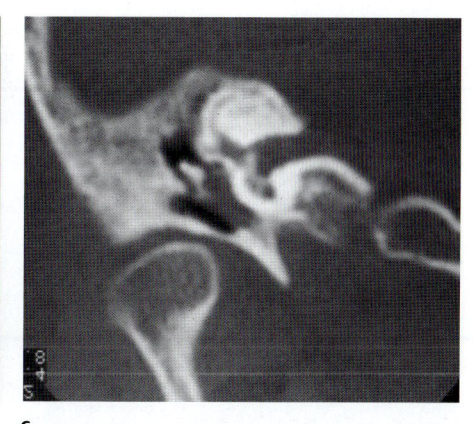

Fig. 1.**99** Acute otitis media with coalescent mastoiditis. **a**, **b** Axial, **c** coronal CT sections, right. The middle ear cavity is cloudy. The mastoid air cells are cloudy and the trabeculae are destroyed with formation of the large abscess cavity (arrow).

cells occurs. In the initial stage of the disease, the trabecular pattern of the mastoid air cells is intact (Fig. 1.**97**). However, mucosal edema and seropurulent fluid cause the trabecular pattern to be less well defined owing to lack of the normal air–bone interface (Fig. 1.**98**). A similar involvement usually occurs in the petrous air cells of well-pneumatized petrous bones.

With progression of the disease, the trabecular pattern first becomes ill-defined owing to demineralization. This phase is followed by destruction of the trabeculae with formation of coalescent areas of suppuration (Figs. 1.**99**, 1.**100**–1.**102**).[1]

When a severe coalescent mastoiditis extends posteriorly, the sinus plate becomes poorly defined and partially eroded (Fig. 1.**103**). These findings indicate possible septic thrombosis of the sigmoid sinus, which can be demonstrated by MR. Intracranial abscesses appear on CT as low-absorption areas surrounded by an enhancing margin in the epidural, intradural, or parenchymal areas (Fig. 1.**103**).

■ Imaging Technique

Conventional radiographs, such as the Schüller and Stenvers views, are usually sufficient to determine the degree of clouding of the air cells (Fig. 1.**97**) and demonstrate large areas of destruction. Axial and coronal CT sections reveal more discrete areas of mastoid or petrous coalescence and tegmental or sinus plate erosions (Figs. 1.**99**–1.**103**). When an intracranial complication is suspected, CT study of the brain with infusion of contrast material

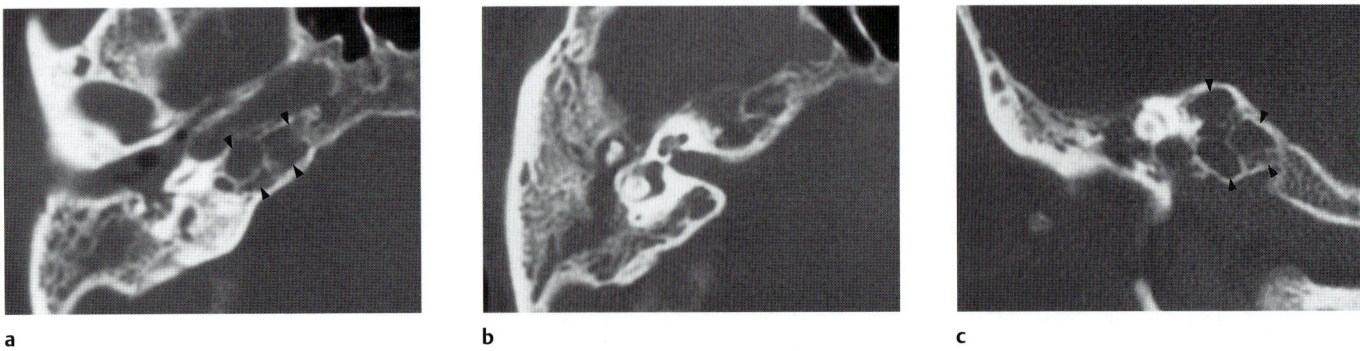

Fig. 1.100 Acute otitis media with petrositis. **a, b** Axial, **c** coronal CT sections, right. The mastoid air cells and middle ear cavity are cloudy. There is clouding of the petrous pyramid air cells with breakdown of the trabeculae in the region of the petrous apex (arrowheads).

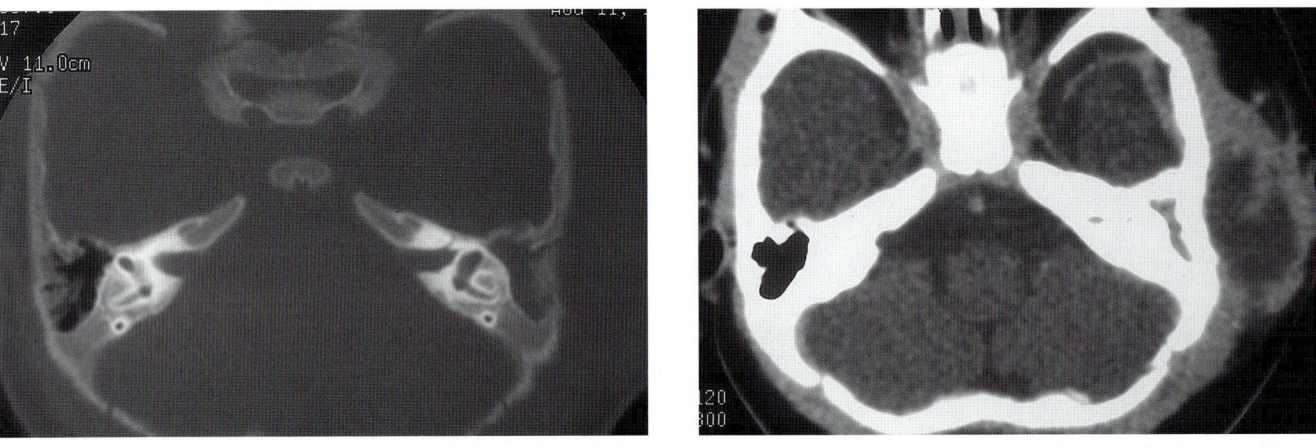

Fig. 1.101 Acute mastoiditis with subperiosteal abscess. **a, b** Axial CT sections. A coalescent cavity is noted in the left mastoid. The mastoid cortex is eroded with formation of a large subperiosteal abscess.

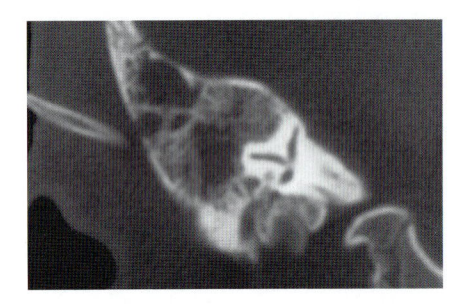

Fig. 1.102 Acute mastoiditis with subperiosteal abscess. Coronal CT section, right. The mastoid air cells are cloudy and the mastoid cortex is eroded. There is marked swelling of the soft tissues over the mastoid with a draining tube in place.

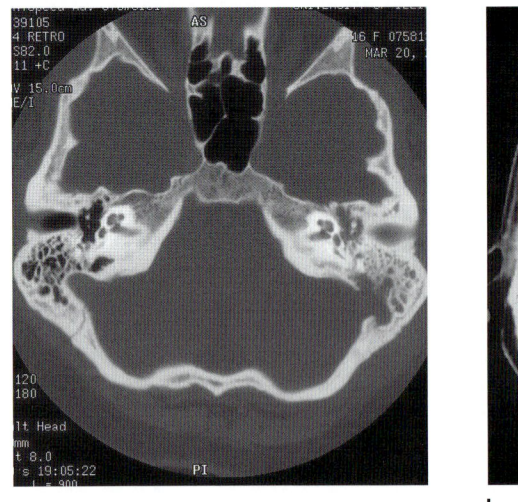

Fig. 1.103 Acute mastoiditis with intracranial brain abscesses. **a, b, c** Axial CT sections, left. In **a**, a large coalescent cavity has eroded the sinus plate and caused a septic thrombophlebitis of the lateral sinus. In **b** and **c**, a large epidural abscess extending supratentorily is visualized by contrast enhancement of the overlying dura.

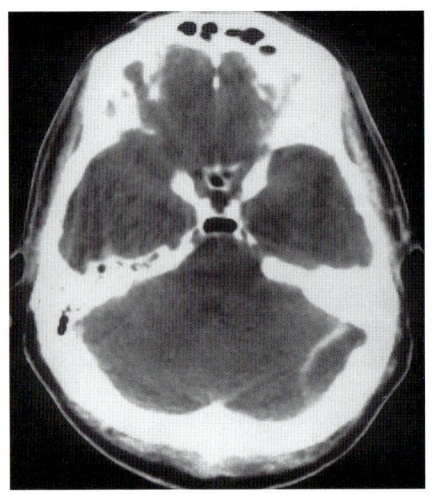

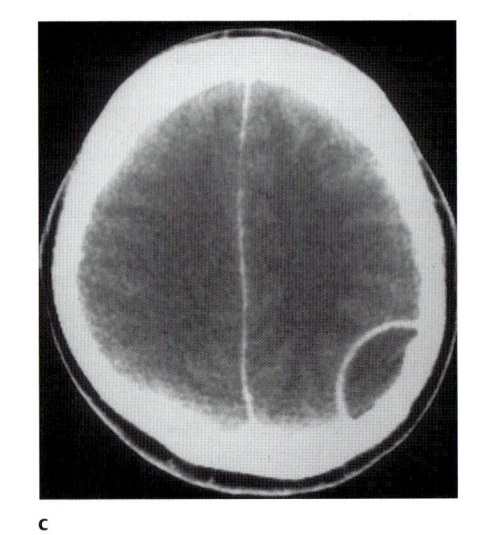

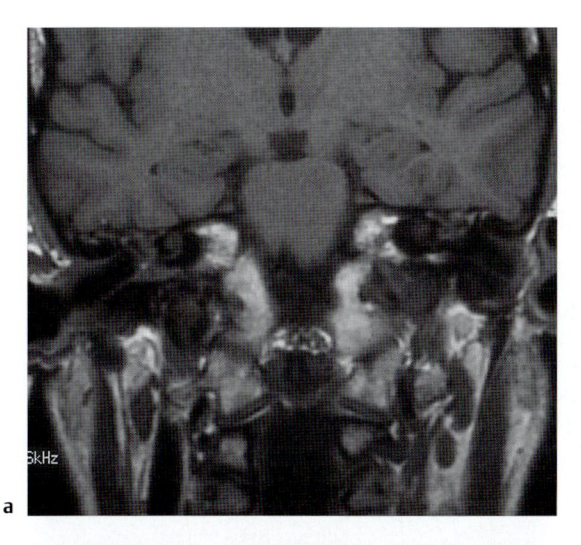

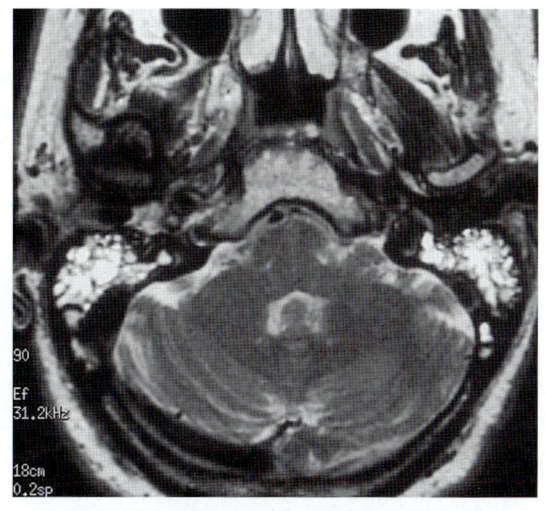

Fig. 1.**104** Acute mastoiditis with labyrinthitis. **a** Coronal T1W MR, **b** axial T2W MR, **c, d** coronal and axial T1W MR after contrast. A soft-tissue mass fills the right middle ear (**a**) and the mastoid cells are filled with pus (**b**). Following injection of contrast, there is enhancement of the granulation tissue in the middle ear (**c**) and of the right cochlea (**d**).

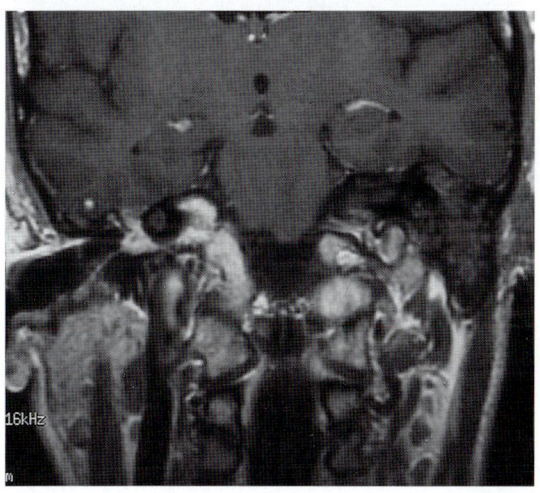

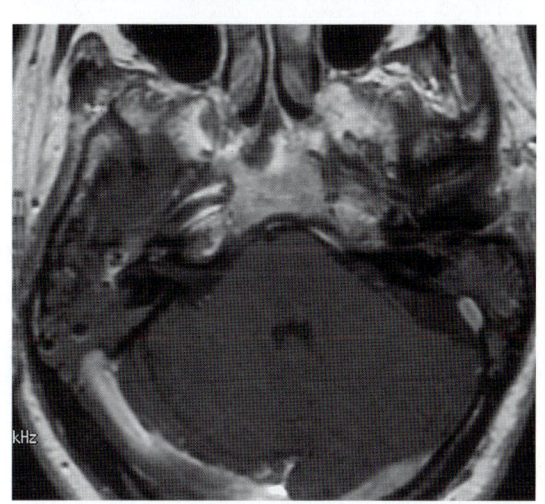

must be performed (Fig. 1.**103**). An MR study of the brain will also reveal otogenic intracranial pathology.

■ Differential Diagnosis

The early findings of acute mastoiditis may be identical to the features of serous otitis media. In serous otitis media, sterile serous fluid fills the middle ear and at times the entire mastoid air cell system. Since the clinical features of serous otitis and acute otitis media are quite different, it is imperative that the radiologist have sufficient clinical information to avoid misdiagnosis.

In a CT study, the tympanic membrane appears retracted in serous otitis but usually bulges in acute otitis media.

Langerhans cell histiocytosis (reticuloendotheliosis) in the form of eosinophilic granuloma may cause a breakdown of the trabecular pattern similar to that of acute coalescent mastoiditis or petrositis. Clinical history and otoscopic findings will enable the radiologist to diagnose this lesion correctly.

■ Acute Labyrinthitis

Enhancement within the lumen of the bony labyrinth is often observed in MR images obtained after injection of contrast material in patients with acute bacterial and viral labyrinthitis and sudden deafness.[4] Four types of acute labyrinthitis are known:
1. Acute toxic or serous labyrinthitis is caused by an irritation of the labyrinth by toxins entering the labyrinth in otitic or meningitic infections. There is no bacterial involvement of the labyrinth. The result of the MR study is negative.
2. Acute suppurative labyrinthitis is due to bacterial infection of the inner ear from contiguous meningitic or otitic infections. Both perilymphatic and endolymphatic spaces are involved and filled with pus. Further progression of the infection leads to necrosis of the membranous labyrinth. Enhancement of the inner structures is presumably due to damage of the capillaries of the endothelium, which leads to a disruption of the labyrinth–blood barrier (Figs. 1.**104**, 1.**106**).
3. Viral labyrinthitis is probably the most common cause of labyrinthine enhancement. It has been observed in patients with acute respiratory infections but, to the best of our knowledge, not in measles, mumps, and rubella. The pathological change consists of atrophy of the organ of Corti, tectorial membrane, and stria vascularis. Again the enhancement is presumably due to disruption of the labyrinth–blood barrier (Fig. 1.**105**).
4. Autoimmune labyrinthitis. The enhancement is similar to suppurative or viral labyrinthitis but is limited to the cochlea.[10]

■ Chronic Labyrinthitis

This varies from a localized reaction caused by a fistula of the bony labyrinth to a diffuse process. The lumen of the inner ear is partially or totally filled with granulation and fibrous tissues. Osteitis of the bony labyrinth occurs, which may lead to a partial or complete bony obliteration of the lumen. Whereas bony obliteration of the inner ear is readily identified by CT, fibrous oblit-

Fig. 1.**105** Acute viral labyrinthitis. MR study: **a** T1W axial section preinjection; **b** axial; and **c, d** coronal T1W sections after injection of contrast material. Following the injection of contrast material there is marked enhancement of the cochlea, vestibule, and horizontal semicircular canal (arrows).

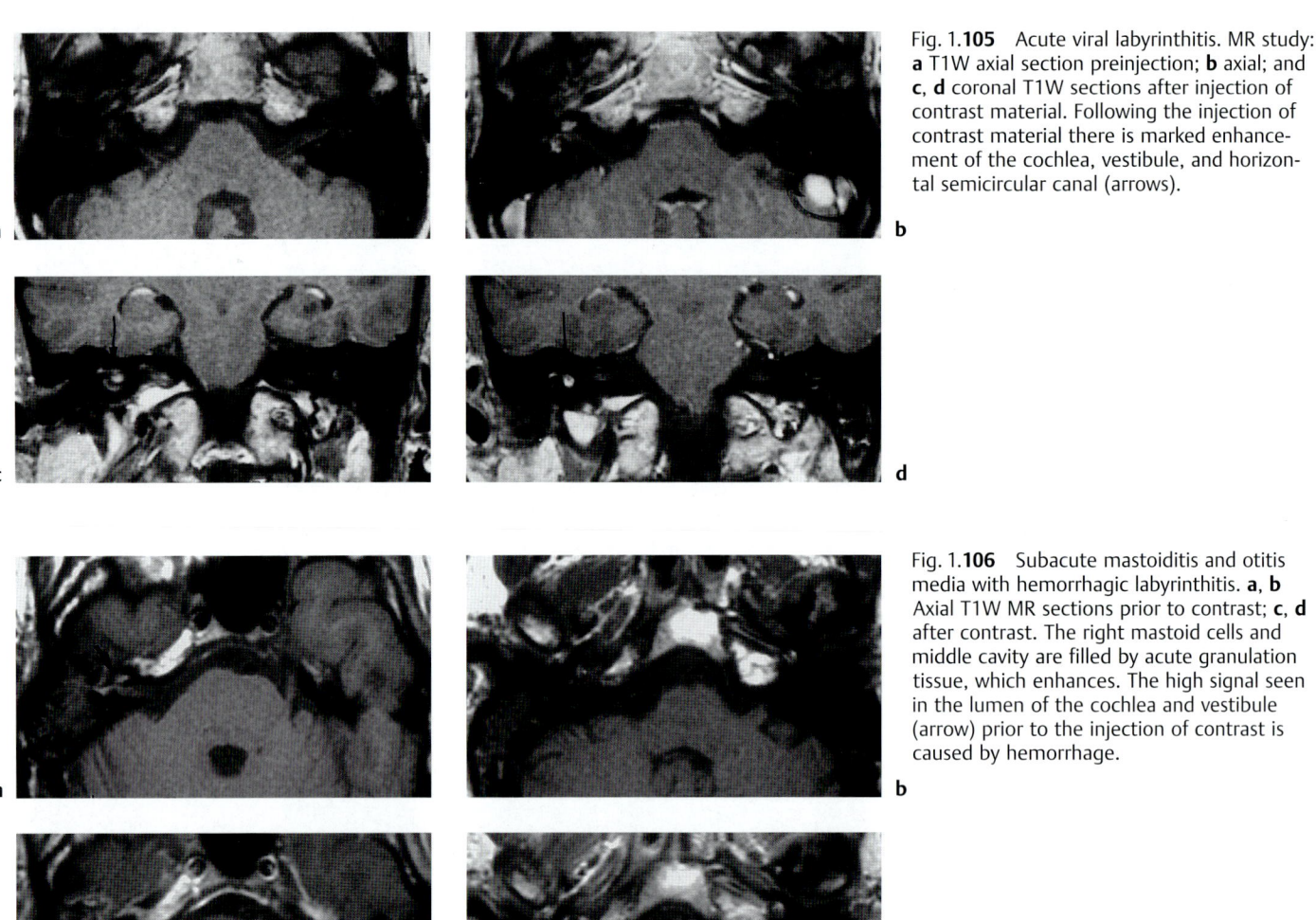

Fig. 1.**106** Subacute mastoiditis and otitis media with hemorrhagic labyrinthitis. **a, b** Axial T1W MR sections prior to contrast; **c, d** after contrast. The right mastoid cells and middle cavity are filled by acute granulation tissue, which enhances. The high signal seen in the lumen of the cochlea and vestibule (arrow) prior to the injection of contrast is caused by hemorrhage.

eration is only recognizable by MRI. In the T2-weighted images, the high signal seen within the normal inner ear structures is absent, making the involved structures no longer recognizable.

■ Facial Neuritis

Moderate bilateral enhancement of the normal facial nerve, particularly in the region of its anterior genu, is often observed in MR studies obtained after injection of contrast material. According to Gerbarski et al, this finding is due to the presence of a rich vascular plexus surrounding the facial nerve.

Asymmetric enhancement of the facial nerve more prominent on the paralyzed side is common in patients with Bell's palsy and Ramsey Hunt syndrome. The enhancement varies in intensity with the stage of the process. It is usually more prominent in the early stage and gradually decreases whether the paralysis has resolved or not.

In Bell's palsy the involvement is segmental and usually confined to the anterior genu and adjacent labyrinthine and tympanic segments. Involvement of the mastoid segment is more rare and found in the later stage (Fig. 1.**107**). In Ramsey Hunt syndrome the involvement of the herpes zoster virus is more consistent and very often extends to the nerve within the internal auditory canal (Fig. 1.**108**). In viral neuritis the nerve is usually not thickened or is only slightly swollen.

■ Malignant Necrotizing External Otitis

Malignant external otitis is an acute osteomyelitis of the temporal bone that occurs in diabetic, immunosuppressed patients and is caused by the bacterium *Pseudomonas*. The infection begins as an external otitis but spreads to involve the surrounding walls of the external canal. The process often extends into the middle ear and mastoid. The infection usually breaks through the floor of the external canal at the bony and cartilaginous junction, and spreads along the undersurface of the temporal bone to involve the facial nerve at the stylomastoid foramen. Further medial extension involves the jugular fossa and cranial nerves IX, X, XI, and XII. Anterior spread of the infection affects the temporomandibular joint.

■ Imaging Findings

CT is essential when studying malignant external otitis. Axial and coronal projections are indicated. The radiographic findings of malignant external otitis are similar to those of carcinoma of the external auditory canal. The bony canal appears eroded and partially destroyed, and the lumen is narrowed by soft-tissue edema (Figs. 1.**109**, 1.**110**).

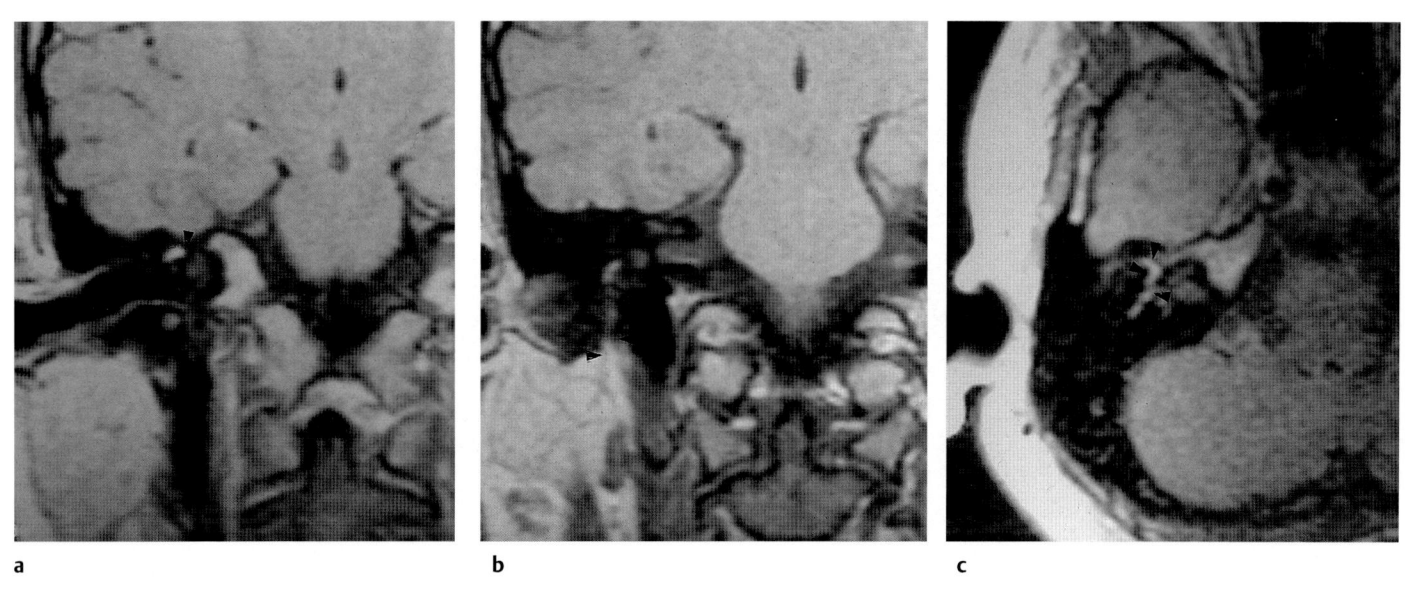

Fig. 1.**107** Facial neuritis. **a**, **b**, Coronal, **c** axial T1W MR sections obtained after injection of contrast material. The right facial nerve is enhanced throughout its intratemporal course (arrowheads).

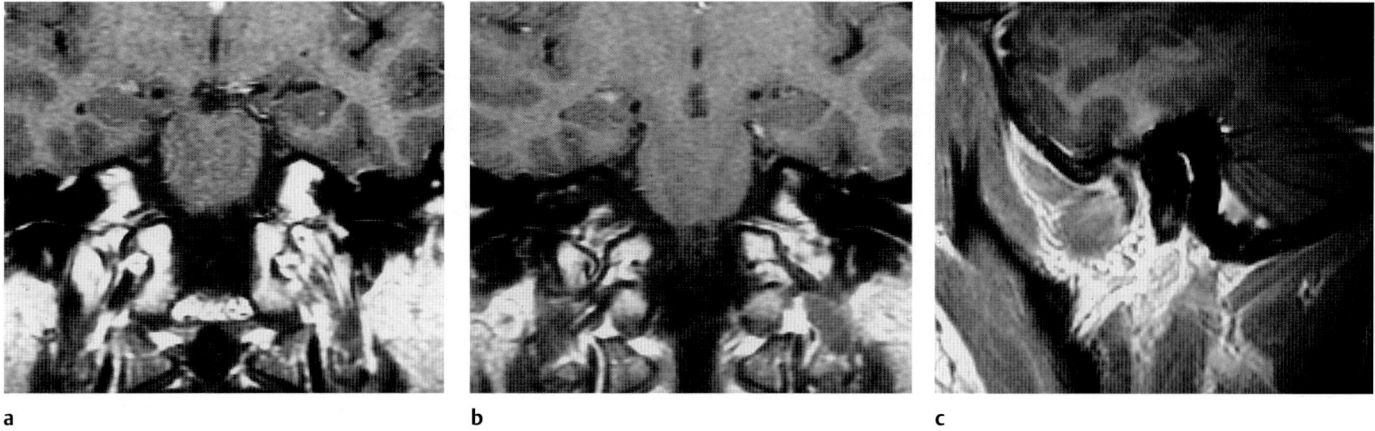

Fig. 1.**108** Ramsey Hunt syndrome. **a**, **b** Coronal, **c** sagittal T1W MR sections after contrast. There is enhancement of the right facial nerve at the anterior genu (**a**) and mastoid segment (**c**) and within the internal auditory canal (**b**).

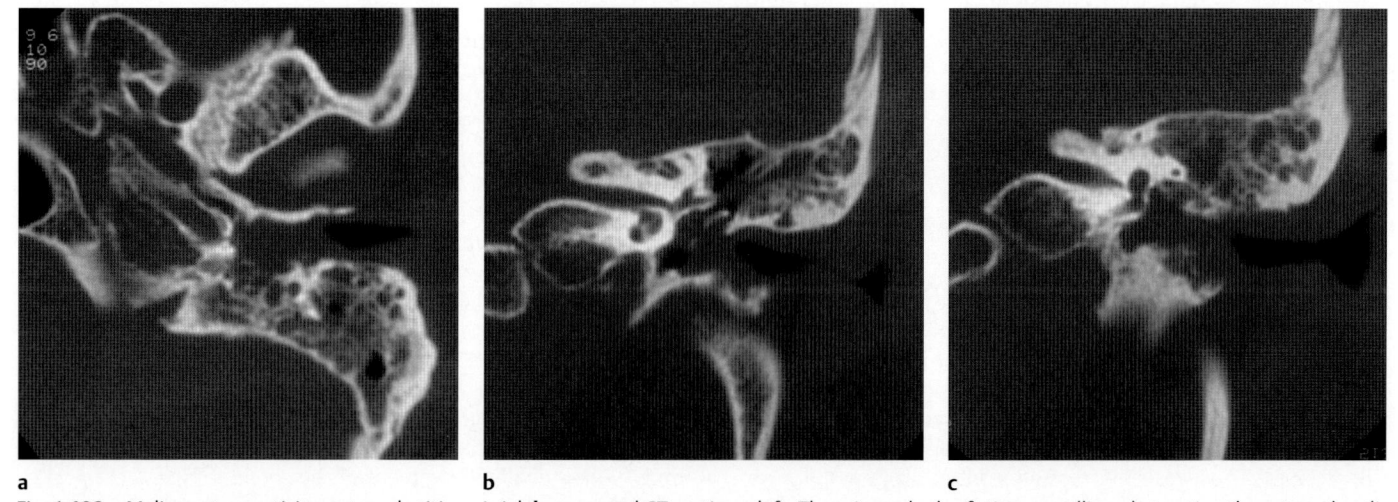

Fig. 1.**109** Malignant necrotizing external otitis. **a** Axial, **b**, **c** coronal CT sections, left. There is marked soft tissue swelling obstructing the external auditory canal of this patient with diabetes. The canal walls are eroded, and the infection extends to the mastoid and middle ear.

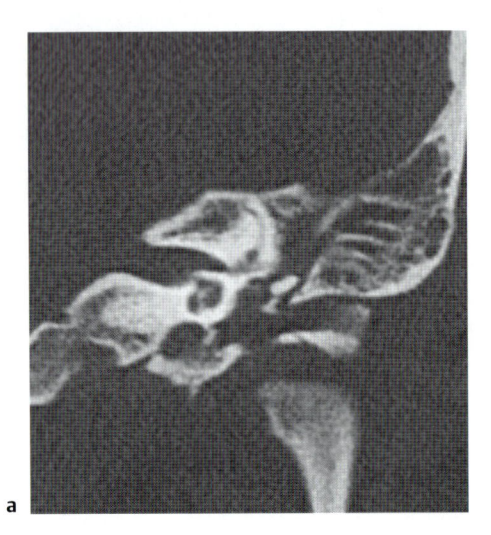

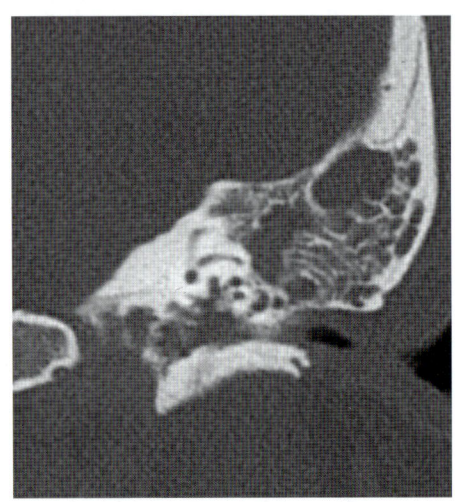

Fig. 1.**110** Necrotizing otitis externa: **a**, **b** Coronal CT sections. The lumen of the left external auditory canal is obstructed by swelling of the canal skin and the floor of the canal is partially eroded. The infection has spread to the middle ear and mastoid with formation of a coalescent cavity.

When facial nerve paralysis occurs, the facial canal is normal in the early stage. MR with i.v. injection of contrast material reveals enhancement in the mastoid segment of the facial nerve. A few days after the onset of paralysis, CT usually shows erosion of the contour of the stylomastoid foramen and of the adjacent mastoid segment of the facial canal. The lateral wall of the jugular fossa becomes eroded as the infection passes medially. If the anterior wall of the external canal is destroyed and the infection involves the glenoid fossa, the mandibular condyle is displaced anteriorly. The muscles of mastication are often swollen, and the adjacent perifascial planes obliterated. The mastoid air cells may become involved by direct posterior extension or via the middle ear (Fig. 1.**109**). The lateral attic wall and floor of the middle ear often are destroyed (Fig. 1.**110**). In advanced cases the entire petrous pyramid may be involved in a severe osteomyelitic process, which may spread to the adjacent occipital bone and cervical spine and even to the contralateral temporal bone. Whenever the infection extends outside of the confines of the temporal bone, MR becomes more precise than CT for establishing both the intracranial and extracranial extent of the process.

■ Healing Stages

If surgical and antibiotic therapy are successful in arresting the spread of and eliminating the infection, follow-up CT studies show remineralization of the petrous pyramid, mastoid, occipital bone, and other involved structures.

Chronic Otitis Media and Mastoiditis

Chronic otitis media and mastoiditis are the results of infection by an organism of low virulence or of acute infection with incomplete resolution. In the United States today, owing to improved general health, antibiotics, and vaccines, acute otitis rarely progresses to chronic otitis media. In the preantibiotic era a single severe infection by a virulent organism, associated with the decreased host resistance, often resulted in severe destruction of the middle ear and scarring, which led to chronic suppuration. Another type of chronic otitis media is the result of faulty middle ear aeration and eustachian malfunction. This is chronic adhesive otitis media and is relatively more common today in the United States.

■ Clinical Findings

The clinical findings in chronic suppurative otitis media and mastoiditis are perforation of the tympanic membrane, chronic suppurative discharge, and poor hearing in the affected ear. The mucosa of the middle ear is involved in a chronic inflammatory process, which also affects the epitympanum, mastoid antrum, and mastoid air cells.

Chronic suppurative otitis media and mastoiditis must be differentiated from chronic adhesive otitis media in which there are varying degrees of middle ear atelectasis.

■ Otoscopic Findings

In the active stage of chronic suppurative otitis and mastoiditis, there is a central type of tympanic membrane perforation and a suppurative discharge from the middle ear. The tympanic membrane is thickened and reddened, and the mucosa of the middle ear is edematous and hyperemic. There is often a granulomatous polyp of varying size that arises from the margin of the tympanic membrane perforation or from the mucosa of the medial wall of the middle ear. With subsiding of active infection, a perforation will persist without discharge and the middle ear mucosal edema resolves (Fig. 1.**111**). In chronic adhesive otitis media, there usually is a deep atelectatic, retracted pocket in a portion of the tympanic membrane that appears as a perforation. Careful microscopic otoscopy, however, will show that the atelectatic pocket is in an area of retracted and atrophic tympanic membrane and not a perforation. Chronic adhesive otitis media may evolve into a cholesteatoma, another form of chronic mastoiditis, which will be discussed separately in Chapter 8.

■ Imaging Techniques

Conventional radiography is usually sufficient to evaluate the degree of development of the mastoid, the trabecular pattern, and the degree of involvement of the air cells (Figs. 1.**112**, 1.**113**). For a more precise evaluation of the middle ear, axial and coronal CT sections are obtained. For unilateral disease, images are taken

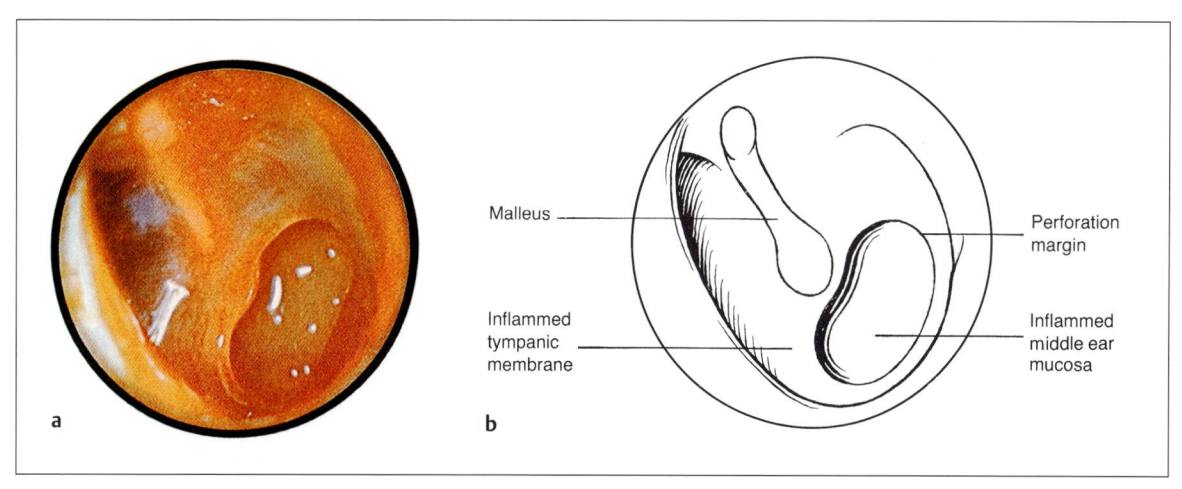

Fig. 1.**111** **a** Chronic otitis media, otoscopic findings, above. There is a posterior perforation in this chronically inflamed tympanic membrane. The middle ear mucosa is thickened and reddened. Purulent secretion was aspirated prior to photography.
b Diagram of **a**.

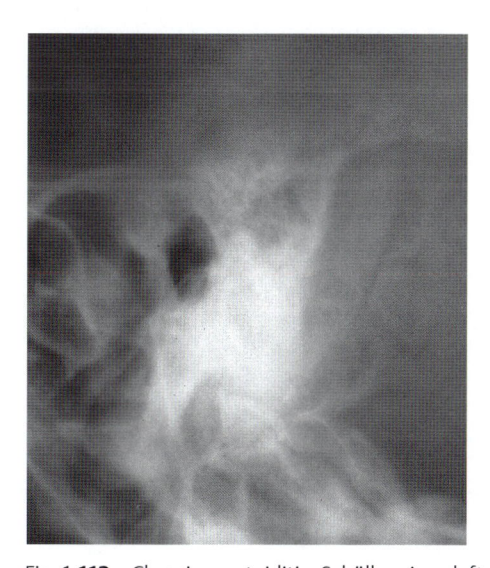

Fig. 1.**112** Chronic mastoiditis, Schüller view, left. There is a nonhomogeneous clouding of the mastoid air cells with thickening of the trabeculae. Some air cells appear constricted by reactive new bone formation.

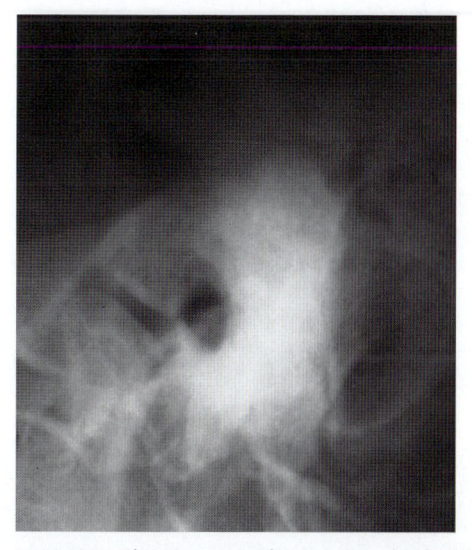

Fig. 1.**113** Chronic mastoiditis, acquired sclerotic type, Schüller view, left. The air cells are completely obliterated by reactive new bone formation.

in two projections of the involved side, but only axial sections of the uninvolved side for comparison.

Since granulation tissue enhances after the injection of paramagnetic agents, MR with contrast is useful in some cases to differentiate granulation tissue from the fluid and cholesteatoma, which have a similar density in the CT sections (Fig. 1.**117**).

■ Imaging Findings

Chronic Mastoiditis

Radiographic findings in chronic mastoiditis are a nonhomogenous clouding of the mastoid antrum and air cells with varying degrees of change in the mastoid trabeculae. Mastoid inflammation produces thickening of some trabeculae secondary to reactive new bone formation and at the same time demineralization of other trabeculae. At this stage of the process, the air cells appear cloudy and fewer than normal and the residual trabeculae are thickened (Fig. 1.**112**). As the chronic inflammatory process continues, the air cells become constricted as reactive new bone thickens the remaining trabeculae (Fig. 1.**116**). In the final stage of the process, the air cells are obliterated and the mastoid appears partially or completely sclerotic (Fig. 1.**113**). The lumen of the mastoid antrum and residual air cells are usually filled with granulation tissue and appear cloudy.

The Middle Ear

For proper evaluation of the middle ear in chronic otitis media, we use CT. The radiographic appearance of the middle ear depends on the degree of inflammatory changes in the mucosa and the aeration of the middle ear.

In chronic suppurative otitis media and mastoiditis, the residual portion of the tympanic membrane is usually thickened and visible. The middle ear is partially or completely cloudy during active suppuration (Fig. 1.**117**). If there is no active infection, the middle ear is aerated. In chronic adhesive otitis media, CT sections demonstrate thickened portions of the tympanic membrane retracted to the promontory and a contracted middle ear space (Figs. 1.**114**, 1.**115**).

Erosion of the long process of the incus commonly occurs in chronic otitis media (Figs. 1.**115**, 1.**116**) and the malleus handle is often foreshortened. Erosion of the malleus head and incus body in the epitympanum is rare unless cholesteatoma is present. In

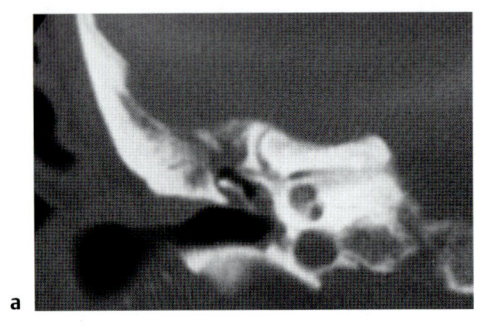

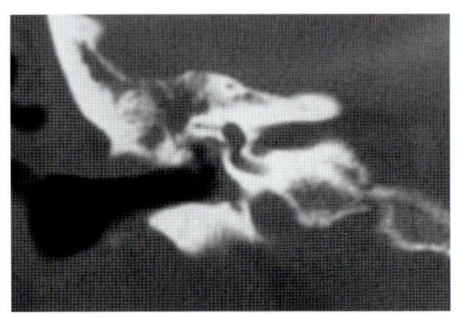

Fig. 1.**114** Chronic otitis media. **a, b** Coronal CT sections, right. The tympanic membrane is retracted on the promontory. There is a deep retraction pocket of the posterosuperior quadrant of the tympanic membrane.

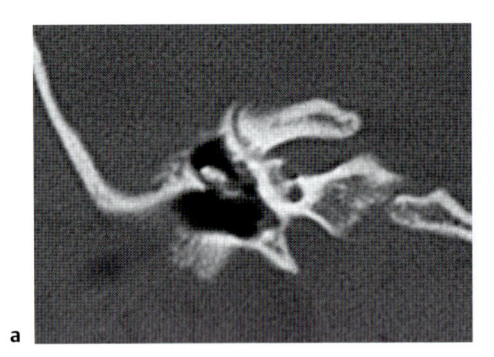

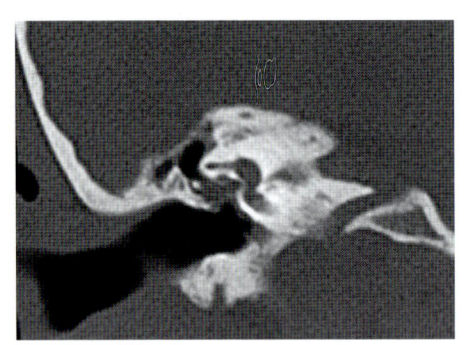

Fig. 1.**115** Chronic otitis media. **a, b** Coronal CT sections. The right tympanic membrane is thickened and retracted on the promontory. The lateral wall of the attic is intact. There is a shallow retraction pocket lateral to the neck of the malleus. Granulation tissue fills the posterosuperior quadrant of the middle ear, surrounding and eroding the long process of the incus.

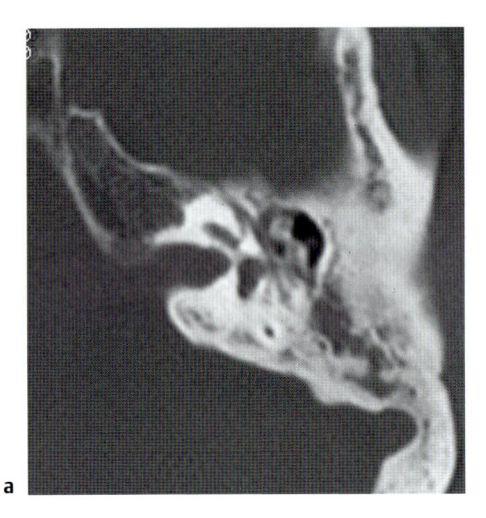

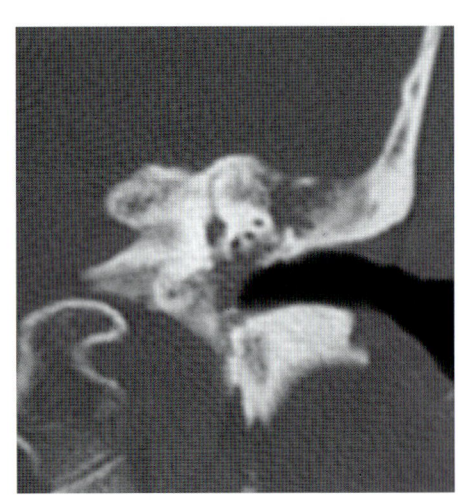

Fig. 1.**116** Chronic otitis media with tympanosclerosis. **a, b** Coronal CT. The left middle ear space is contracted owing to retraction of the tympanic membrane. Tympanosclerotic deposits in the attic surround and fix the ossicles. The mastoid trabeculae are thickened.

some ears when the long process of the incus is eroded, the tympanic membrane retracts and attaches itself to the stapes head, forming a natural myringostapediopexy.

Cholesterol Granuloma

Cholesterol granuloma is a nonspecific chronic inflammation of the middle ear and mastoid. Histologically, a cholesterol granuloma consists of a mass of chronic inflammatory tissue containing clefts of cholesterol crystals surrounded by giant cells. When a cholesterol granuloma occurs in the middle ear behind an intact tympanic membrane, otoscopically it resembles a glomus tumor. In CT the granuloma appears as a nonspecific soft-tissue mass when the middle ear is aerated. Unfortunately, the middle ear mucosa is usually inflamed, and the contour of the mass cannot be discerned. The bony walls of the middle ear are intact, but the ossicles are often eroded by the granulomatous process (Fig. 1.**118**). A more precise assessment of the type and size of the mass is accomplished with MRI. A cholesterol granuloma appears as a well-defined soft-tissue mass of high signal intensity in both T1 and T2 sequences. In the T1-weighted images the mass can be distinguished from surrounding fluid or edematous mucosa that has a low signal.

Petrous Pyramid Cholesterol Granuloma

Cholesterol granulomas are the most common primary lesions of the petrous apex. They occur in extensively pneumatized temporal bones as expansile lesions that thin and erode the surrounding bone (Figs. 1.**119**, 1.**20**). Large lesions erode the bony

Chronic Otitis Media and Mastoiditis

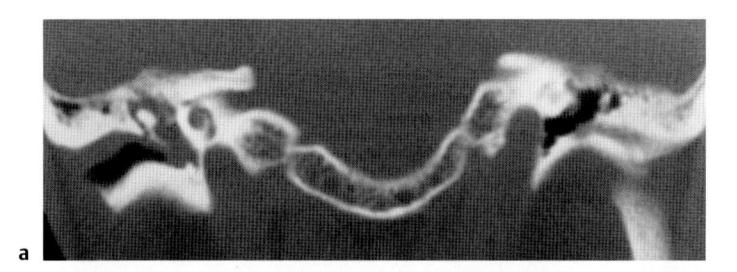

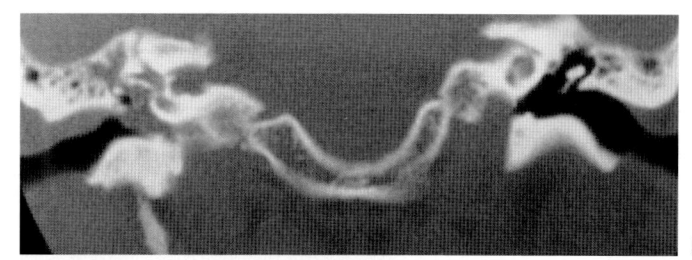

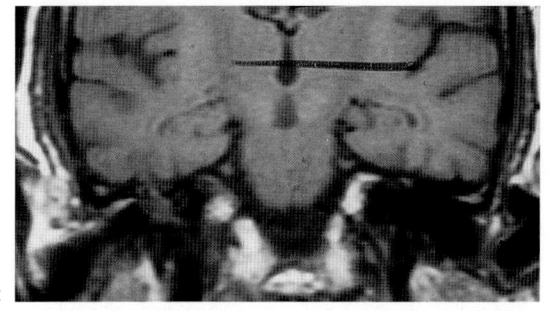

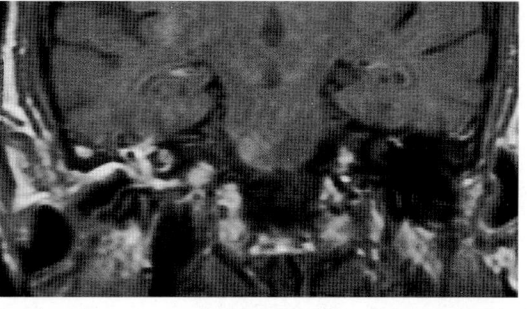

Fig. 1.117 Right chronic suppurative otitis media (tuberculosis) with labyrinthitis. **a, b** Coronal CT sections; **c, d** coronal T1W MR sections. The mastoid air cells are cloudy, and a soft-tissue mass fills the middle ear cavity. The long process of the incus is eroded. In the MR image obtained prior to injection of contrast material (**c**), the middle ear mass has a signal intensity similar to gray matter. After injection of contrast material (**d**), the middle ear mass enhances. The cochlea also enhances.

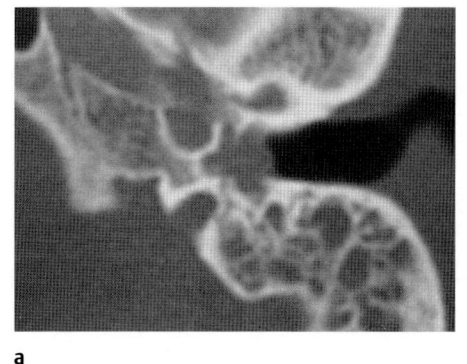

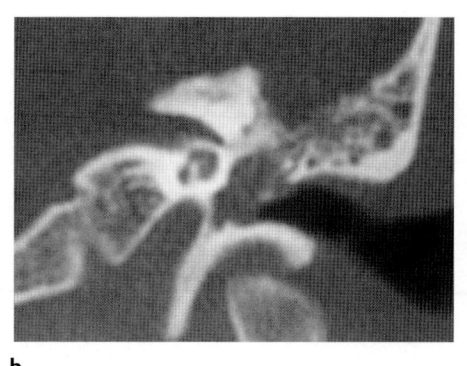

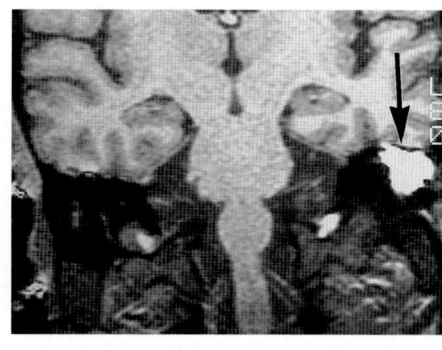

Fig. 1.118 Cholesterol granuloma, left middle ear and mastoid. **a** Axial, **b** coronal CT; **c** T1W coronal MR sections. A large soft-tissue mass fills the middle ear cavity and mastoid antrum. The ossicles are partially eroded and displaced laterally. In the T1W MR section obtained without injecting contrast material, the mass has a high signal intensity (arrow).

labyrinth. Cholesterol granulomas are indistinguishable on CT from congenital cholesteatomas and mucoceles of the petrous apex. All three lesions appear as low-density areas, which do not enhance except for a faint ring in the capsule. With MR imaging it is now possible to differentiate these three lesions. The cholesterol granuloma appears as a bright lesion characterized by a short T1 and a long T2 relaxation time (Fig. 1.119). Areas of signal void in cholesterol granulomas are produced by deposition of hemosiderin (Fig. 1.121). Congenital cholesteatomas have a signal of intermediate intensity in T1-weighted images and become brighter, in the T2-weighted sequence (see Fig. 1.152). Mucoceles have a low signal on T1-weighted and become as bright as cholesterol granulomas in T2-weighted images. Following injection of contrast material, the lesions do not enhance, but a rim of enhancement surrounding the mass is often observed in mucoceles and congenital cholesteatomas.

Tympanosclerosis

Tympanosclerosis consists of deposits of hyalinized and often calcified fibrotic granulation tissue in the middle ear, epitympanum, and tympanic membrane (Fig. 1.122). Tympanosclerosis occurs most commonly as deposits of thickened hyalinized tissue within the layers of the tympanic membrane, on the mucosa of the promontory, and in the epitympanum surrounding and fixing the ossicles (Fig. 1.116). Tympanosclerotic deposits, if large enough and calcified, are recognizable by CT. The deposits appear as punctate or linear densities within the tympanic membrane or applied to the contour of the promontory (Fig. 1.123). Large deposits of tympanosclerosis in the epitympanum appear as ill-defined calcified masses that surround the ossicles. The normal ossicular contour is lost. An isolated plaque of tympanosclerosis in the anterior or superior epitympanum may ankylose the malleus head to the tegmen (Fig. 1.124).

1 Imaging of the Temporal Bone

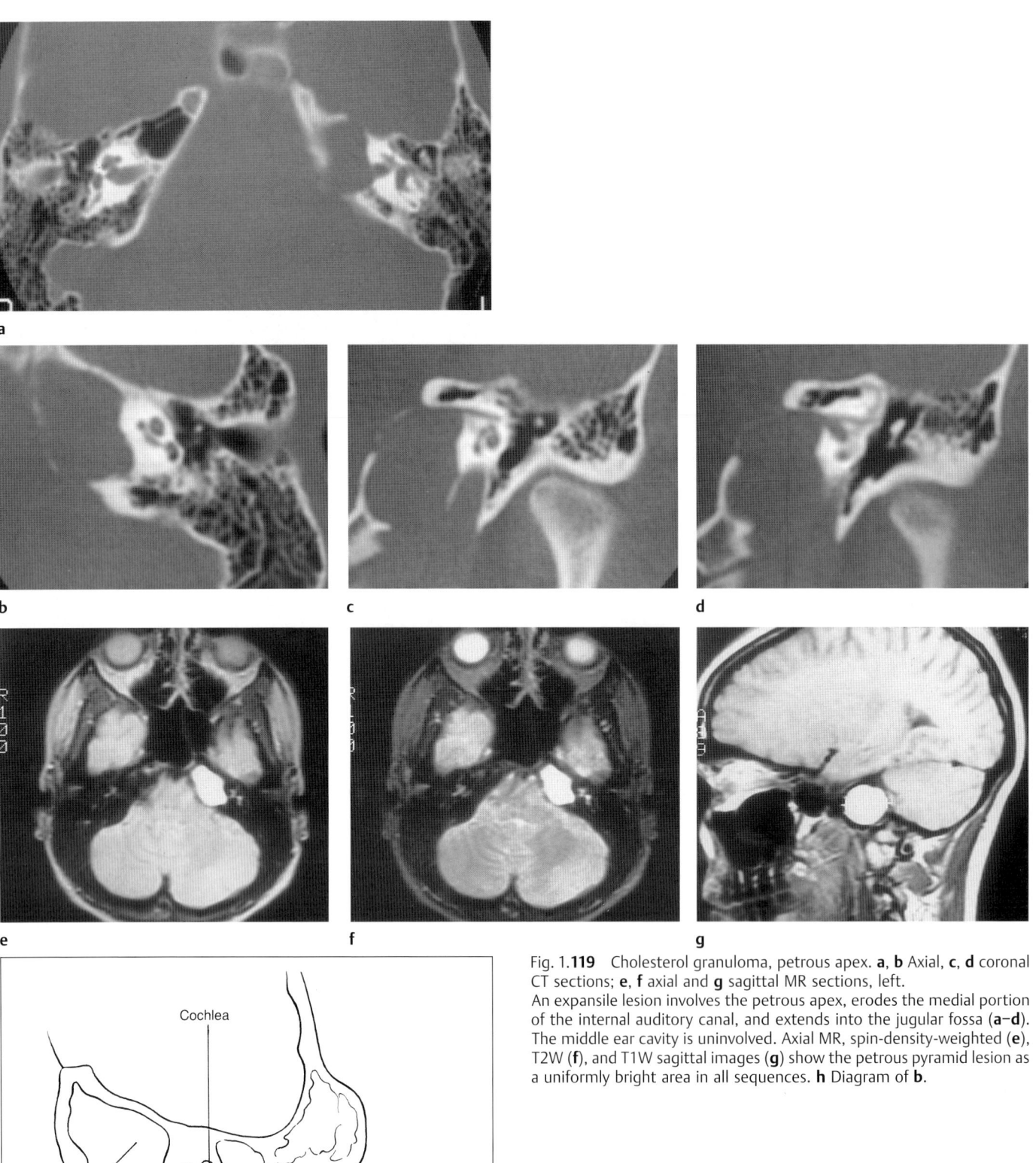

Fig. 1.**119** Cholesterol granuloma, petrous apex. **a**, **b** Axial, **c**, **d** coronal CT sections; **e**, **f** axial and **g** sagittal MR sections, left.
An expansile lesion involves the petrous apex, erodes the medial portion of the internal auditory canal, and extends into the jugular fossa (**a–d**). The middle ear cavity is uninvolved. Axial MR, spin-density-weighted (**e**), T2W (**f**), and T1W sagittal images (**g**) show the petrous pyramid lesion as a uniformly bright area in all sequences. **h** Diagram of **b**.

Chronic Otitis Media and Mastoiditis

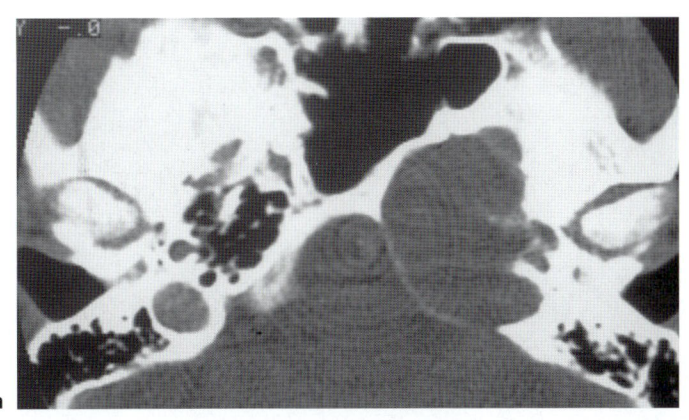

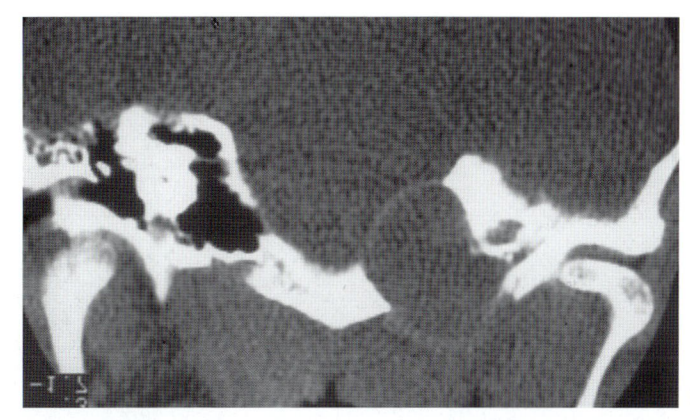

Fig. 1.**120** Cholesterol granuloma of the left petrous pyramid. **a** Axial, **b** coronal CT sections postinfusion. The lesion involves the petrous apex and adjacent base of the skull. The mass has a low density and does not enhance except for its capsule.

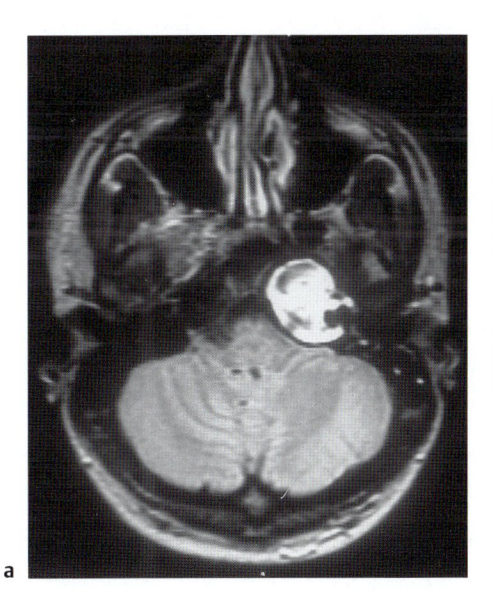

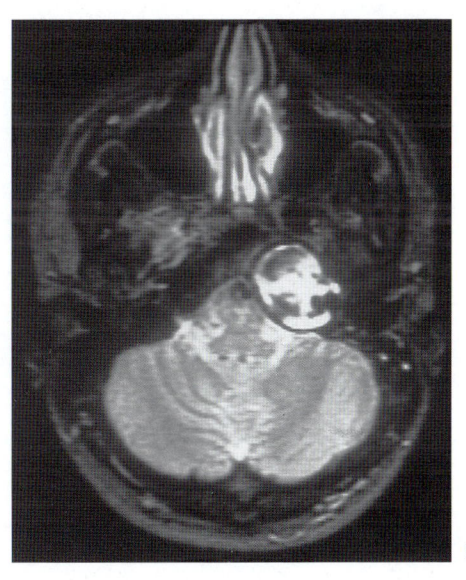

Fig. 1.**121** Cholesterol granuloma, same case as Fig. 1.**120**. MR images: **a** spin-density-weighted, **b** T2W. The mass has a high signal intensity in both sequences except for several areas of signal void due to the deposits of hemosiderin.

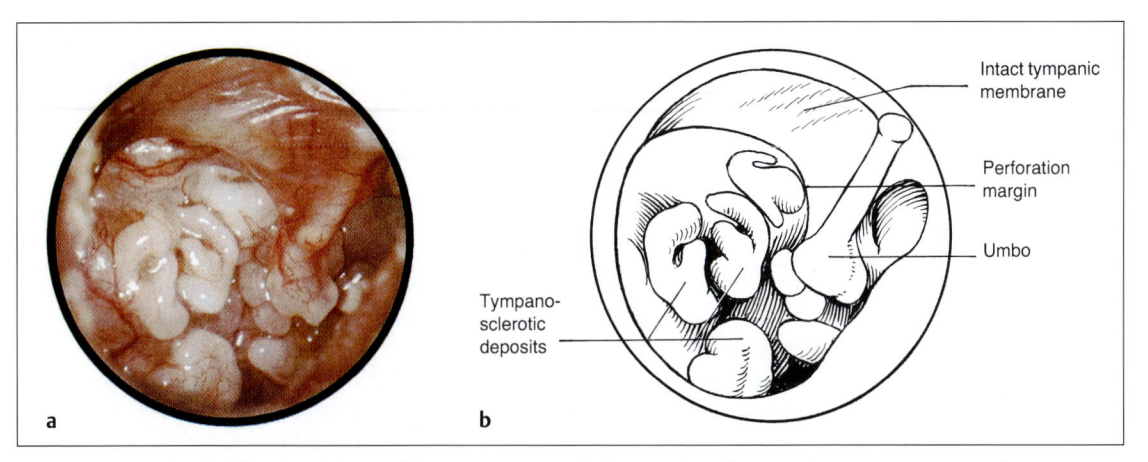

Fig. 1.**122** **a** Tympanosclerosis of the middle ear, otoscopic findings, right. There is a large tympanic membrane perforation, and white globular deposits of tympanosclerosis line the exposed medial wall of the middle ear. **b** Diagram of **a**.

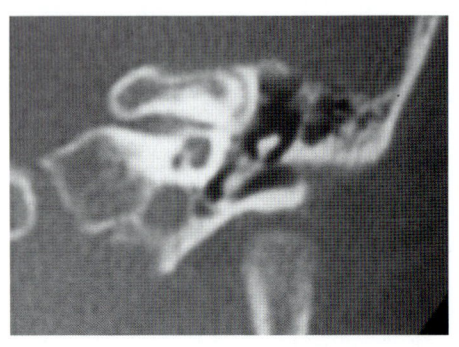

Fig. 1.**123** Tympanosclerosis. Coronal CT section, left. The tympanic membrane is thickened by a large tympanosclerotic plaque. The mastoid air cells and middle ear are aerated.

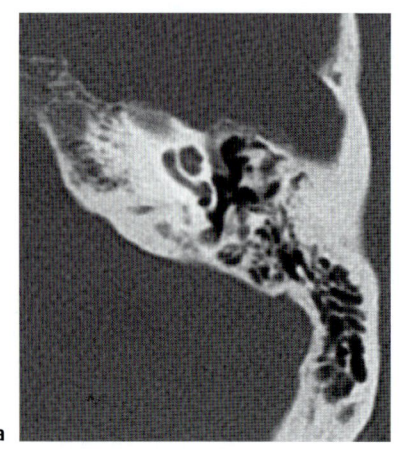

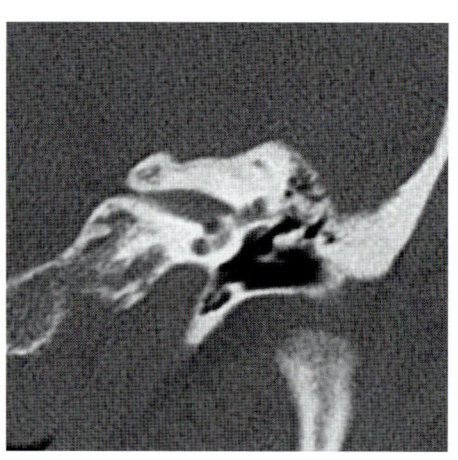

Fig. 1.**124** Chronic otitis media with tympanosclerosis. **a** Axial, **b** coronal CT sections. Tympanosclerotic deposits fix the ossicles to the attic wall. The lateral wall of the attic is blunted by a retraction pocket.

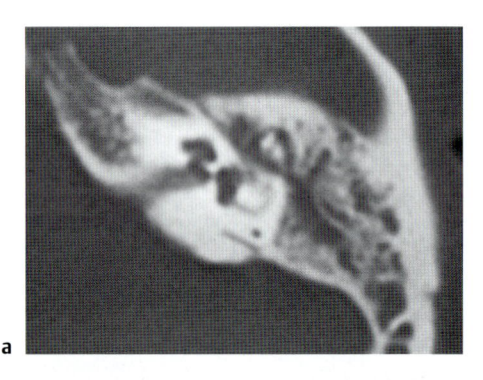

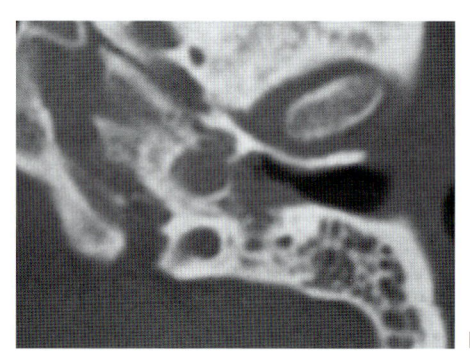

Fig. 1.**125** Tuberculosis, middle ear and mastoid. **a**, **b** Axial, **c** coronal CT sections, left. The mastoid air cells are cloudy. The middle ear cavity is filled with a soft-tissue mass surrounding, but not eroding, the ossicles. The tympanic membrane bulges externally. **d** Diagram of **c**.

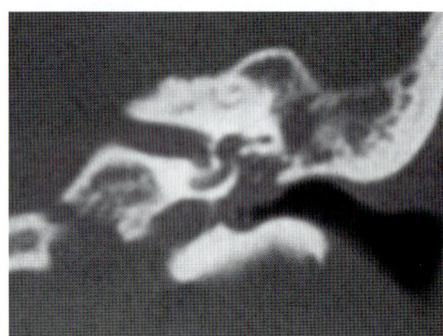

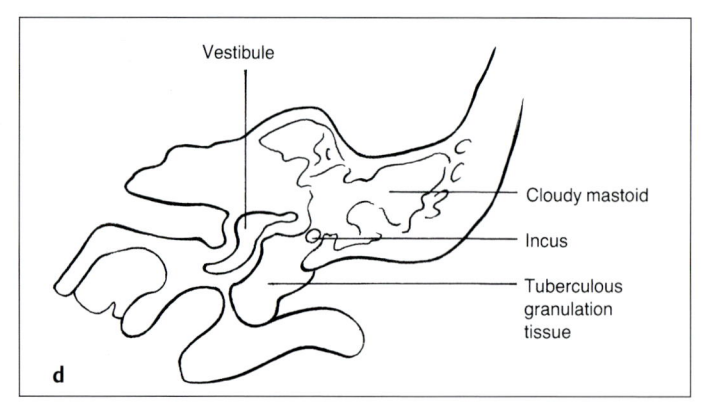

Tuberculosis

The incidence of tuberculosis in the United States has increased recently owing to the spread of acquired immune deficiency syndrome (AIDS). Infection in the ear produces a chronic suppurative otitis media characterized by multiple perforations, polyps, and granulation tissue, which may lead to abscess formation and intracranial complications. Both CT and MR findings are nonspecific and the diagnosis must be confirmed by bacteriological studies performed on the ear discharge (Fig. 1.**125**).

Cholesteatoma of the Middle Ear

A cholesteatoma is an epidermoid cyst that consists histologically of an inner layer of desquamating stratified squamous epithelium (matrix) opposed on an outer layer of subepithelial connective tissue. The lumen of the cyst is filled with desquamated epithelial debris. The subepithelial connective-tissue layer is usually involved by a chronic inflammatory process characterized by deposition of cholesterol crystals, and infiltration of giant cells and round cells.

The epithelial cyst enlarges progressively because of accumulation of epithelial debris within its lumen. As the cyst enlarges and comes into contact with contiguous bony structures of the middle ear, mastoid, and petrous pyramid, erosion of these

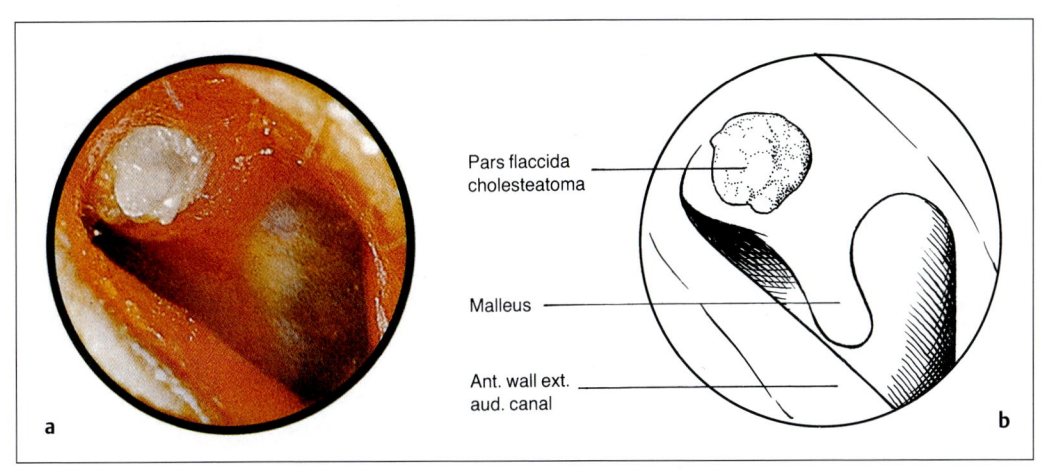

Fig. 1.**126** **a** Cholesteatoma, pars flaccida, otoscopic findings, left. There is a perforation of the pars flaccida filled with necrotic epithelial debris. The notch of Rivinus is slightly enlarged. **b** Diagram of **a**.

structures occurs owing to pressure necrosis and enzymatic lysis of bone.

Cholesteatomas may be congenital or acquired. Congenital cholesteatomas originate from epithelial rests within or adjacent to the temporal bone. Acquired cholesteatomas arise in the middle ear and extend into the mastoid and occasionally into the petrous pyramid. There is another distinct form of cholesteatoma that arises in the external auditory canal and often follows previous irradiation of the head.

■ Acquired Cholesteatoma of the Middle Ear and Mastoid

The etiology of acquired cholesteatoma is not known; four main theories attempt to explain the pathogenesis. Regardless of their etiology, acquired cholesteatomas expand slowly to erode middle ear and mastoid structures. The pathogenesis of acquired cholesteotoma may occur in one of the four following manners:
1 **Negative pressure theory**. Poor aeration of the middle ear, probably related to malfunction of the eustachian tube, results in a relative negative pressure in the middle ear. This negative pressure causes retraction in a medial direction of the pars flaccida or of atrophic areas of the pars tensa of the tympanic membrane. The retracted areas deepen to form pits, and epithelial debris collects within the lumen of the retracted pockets. When egress of the debris is impaired, encystment and cholesteatoma formation ensue. Many authors call this type of lesion occurring in the pars flaccida a primary acquired cholesteatoma.
2 **Migration theory**. This theory postulates that a previous necrotic otitis media destroys the marginal portion of the pars tensa of the tympanic membrane. Epithelium from the external auditory canal grows into the middle ear at the margin of the perforation, encysts, and forms a cholesteatoma. Most authors refer to this type of cholesteotoma as a secondary acquired cholesteatoma. Epithelium from the surface of the tympanic membrane may also migrate into the middle ear from the rim of a central perforation of the pars tensa to form a cholesteatoma.
3 **Metaplasia theory**. Following middle ear infection, the middle ear mucosa undergoes a metaplasia to desquamating stratified squamous epithelium. Encystment follows, and a cholesteatoma is formed.
4 **Papillary ingrowth theory**. This theory has been advanced by Ruedi. An inflammatory stimulus causes invasive hyperplasia of the basal layer of the stratified squamous epithelium of the tympanic membrane. The hyperplastic basal cells infiltrate into the subepithelial connective tissues, extend into the middle ear, desquamate, encyst, and form a cholesteatoma.

■ Clinical and Otoscopic Findings

Most cholestatomas originate from the stratified squamous epithelium of the tympanic membrane or external auditory canal and develop in the mesotympanum or epitympanum. As they enlarge, they destroy the ossicles and adjacent bony structures and extend into the mastoid. Acquired cholesteatomas are characterized by tympanic membrane perforation of the pars flaccida or the pars tensa or combined perforation of both pars flaccida and pars tensa. There is usually an associated chronic infection, a history of chronic aural discharge, and a conductive or mixed deafness (Figs. 1.**126**, 1.**132**).

Most perforations are of the marginal type since part of their circumference lies in contact with the bony margin of the tympanic sulcus or notch of Rivinus. Some cholesteatomas occur with central perforations of the pars tensa. The characteristic of cholesteatoma is that the lumen of the tympanic membrane perforation contains varying amounts of epithelial debris. In chronically infected cholesteatomas, granulomatous tissue and polyps accompany the epithelial debris. Otoscopically, the otologist can diagnose most cholestatomas but cannot determine the size and extent of the lesion in the epitympanum and mastoid. A small epitympanic perforation filled with epithelial debris may be the only otoscopic evidence of a large cholesteatoma (Fig. 1.**126**). On the other hand, a large tympanic membrane perforation filled with debris may be found to be associated with a relatively small lesion. Without a proper CT evaluation, the otologist has no insight into the size of the lesion, or the status of the ossicles, the labyrinth, the tegmen, or the facial nerve.

■ Imaging Techniques

CT is the method of choice because it reveals the presence of soft-tissue masses, as well as the erosion of the bony structures, such as ossicles, tegmen, and labyrinth. In cases of acute exacerbation

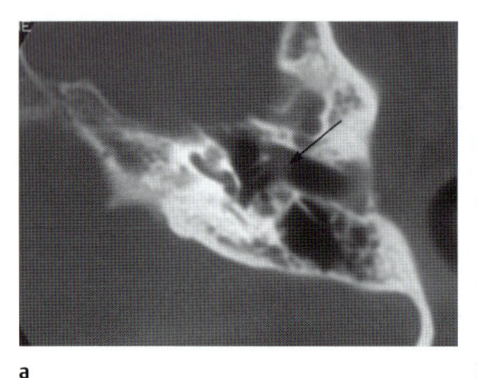

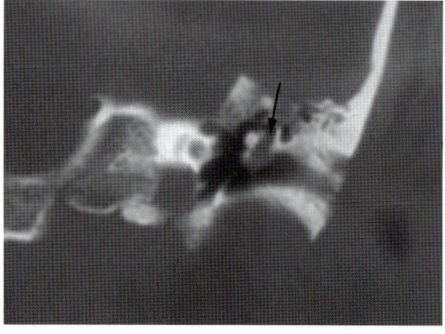

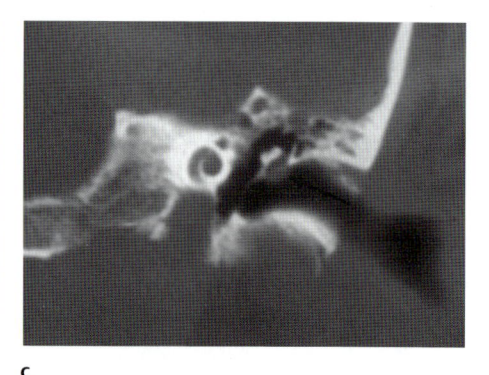

Fig. 1.**127** Cholesteatoma, pars flaccida. **a** Axial, **b**, **c** coronal CT sections, left. The inferior margin of the lateral wall of the attic is eroded by a small soft-tissue mass (arrows), which lies lateral to the ossicles. The ossicular chain is intact.

with intracranial complications, CT with infusion or MRI will demonstrate intracranial pathology such as extradural, cerebral, and cerebellar abscesses.

CT

Coronal and axial projections are required for a CT study of cholesteatoma. For the study of the tympanic segment of the facial nerve, oval window niche, and horizontal semicircular canal erosion, 20° coronal oblique sections are occasionally added.

When sagittal sections are required for the study of the mastoid segment of the facial canal, we use either reconstructed sagittal images or MRI.

Magnetic Resonance Imaging

MR images obtained with surface coils demonstrate the presence of cholesteatoma, which appears as a mass of medium signal intensity in T1-weighted and high intensity in T2-weighted images (Figs. 1.**140**, 1.**150**, 1.**152**).

The main advantage of MR is the possibility to differentiate the actual cholesteatoma mass from surrounding fluid and inflammation. The main limitations of MR are the difficulty in localizing the process due to poor visualization of bony landmarks and the lack of information concerning the status of the ossicles and other bony structures.

■ Diagnosis of Cholesteatoma

The diagnosis of acquired cholesteatoma is based on the detection of a soft-tissue mass and erosion of the lateral epitympanic wall, posterosuperior canal wall, and ossicles. Erosion of one or more of these structures is found in a great majority of cholesteatomas. Erosion of the long process of the incus occurs commonly in chronic otitis media, as well as in cholesteatoma, and is not a specific finding for cholesteatoma. The superstructure of the stapes may be eroded in cholesteatoma. The detection of stapes erosion is difficult because of the small size of the structure and because cholesteatoma and inflammatory tissue in the middle ear obscure the stapes.

The evaluation of the extent of the lesion depends on the recognition of changes in the aditus, antrum, mastoid, and petrous pyramid. With cholesteatomas, there is a soft-tissue mass in the mesotympanum or epitympanum. If the middle ear cavity is aerated, the soft-tissue mass is well outlined. When fluid or inflammatory tissue in the middle ear cavity surrounds the cholesteatoma, the mass is obscured, since the densities of the cholesteatoma, inflammatory tissue, and fluid are very similar in CT. MR may be used to differentiate the cholesteatoma mass from fluid and granulation tissue.

■ Patterns of Imaging Findings

Different patterns of radiographic findings can be observed in the study of cholesteatomas. When we analyzed these patterns, a correlation was found between the site of the tympanic membrane perforation and the radiographic findings.

Cholesteatomas of the pars flaccida, known as primary acquired cholesteatomas, have a characteristic radiographic pattern (Figs. 1.**127**–1.**130**). Cholesteatomas arising from the pars tensa, usually the posterosuperior portion, known as secondary acquired cholesteatomas, have a radiographic pattern distinct from pars flaccida lesions (Figs. 1.**134**–1.**138**).

At times, a cholesteatoma may involve both the pars flaccida and pars tensa. These lesions produce a radiographic pattern that is a combination of the two types (Fig. 1.**140**). In extensive, far-advanced cholesteatomas of either the pars flaccida or pars tensa, there is destruction of most of the structures in the mesotympanum and epitympanum and no distinct pattern remains (Figs. 1.**141**, 1.**143**, 1.**144**).

■ Pars Flaccida Cholesteatomas

Cholesteatomas arising from the pars flaccida are the easiest lesions to diagnose radiographically because the lateral epitympanic wall is eroded (Figs. 1.**127**–1.**130**). In pars flaccida cholesteatomas, the tympanic cavity is usually contracted and narrowed by retraction of the pars tensa of the tympanic membrane. Since the pars tensa is usually thickened, the retracted membrane becomes visible. The typical pattern of a pars flaccida cholesteatoma consists of one or more of the following findings:
1. There is erosion of the anterior portion of the lateral epitympanic wall.
2. There is erosion of the anterior tympanic spine.
3. A soft-tissue mass lies in the epitympanum lateral to the ossicles.
4. There is an increased distance between the lateral epitympanic wall and the ossicles. This increase is due to medial displacement of the ossicles and to erosion of the lateral epitympanic wall.
5. When the cholesteatoma fills the epitympanum and extends to the tegmen, the epitympanum acquires a smooth shell-like outline.

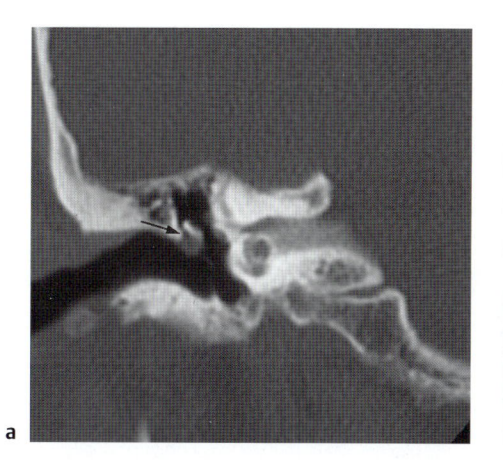

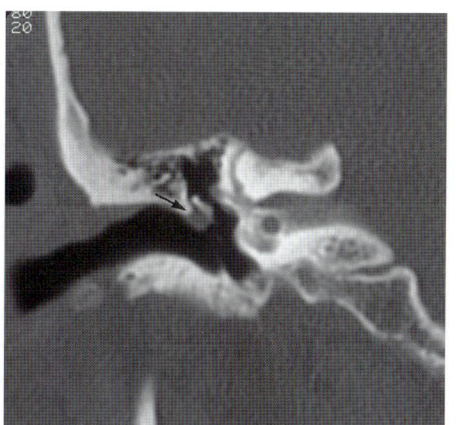

Fig. 1.**128** Cholesteatoma, pars flaccida. **a**, **b** Coronal CT sections, right. The inferior margin of the lateral epitympanic wall is eroded by a small soft-tissue mass extending into the attic lateral to the ossicles (arrows).

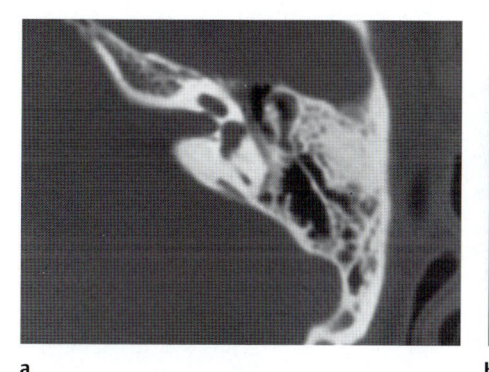

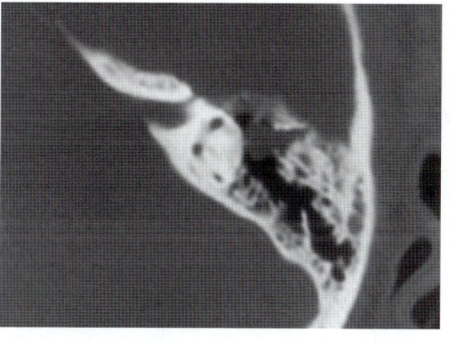

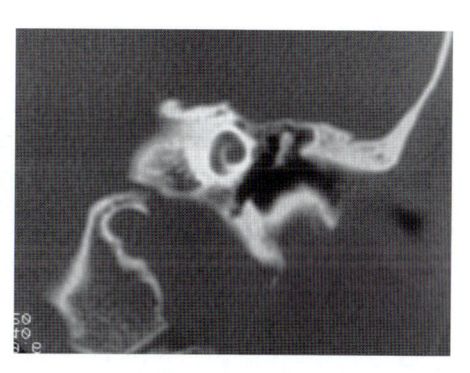

Fig. 1.**129** Cholesteatoma, pars flaccida. **a**, **b** Axial, **c** coronal CT sections. The cholesteatoma extends into the attic laterally and above the ossicles. The inferior margin of the lateral wall of the attic is blunted.

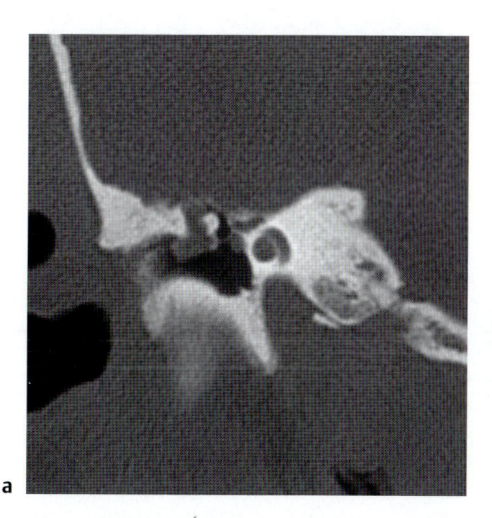

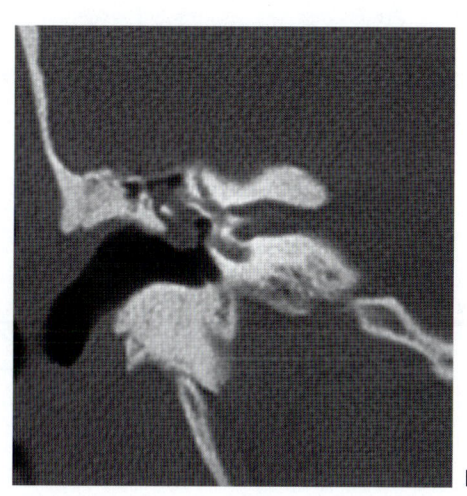

Fig. 1.**130** Cholesteatoma, pars flaccida. **a**, **b** Coronal sections, right. A polyp protrudes into the external auditory canal through a large perforation of the tympanic membrane. The anterior portion of the lateral epitympanic wall is eroded. The soft-tissue mass extends into the upper mesotympanum surrounding and eroding the long process of the incus.

When the cholesteatoma is limited to the anterior portion of the epitympanum, the adjacent aspect of the malleus head is eroded and has a concave, rather than a convex, outline. If the cholesteatoma extends into the posterior epitympanum, the body of the incus will be eroded. The long process of the incus is usually spared in pars flaccida cholesteatomas, unless the cholesteatoma sac is large and extends into the posterior middle ear. In more advanced lesions, both the malleus head and incus body are eroded (Fig. 1.**137**).

■ Epitympanic Retraction Pockets

An epitympanic retraction pocket is an invagination of the pars flaccida of the tympanic membrane without accumulation of epithelial debris. Since these lesions can be a precursor of a cholesteatoma, they must be followed carefully by the otologist. Blunting of the lateral epitympanic wall is observed in simple retraction pockets of the pars flaccida. If the pars flaccida is thickened, the membrane is clearly visible. There is no soft-tissue mass since there is no encystment of accumulated debris within the lumen of the pocket (Fig. 1.**131**). Similar pockets may also

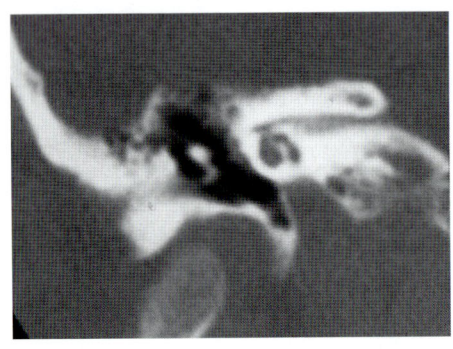

Fig. 1.**131** Attic retraction pocket. Coronal CT section. The inferior margin of the lateral epitympanic wall is eroded by an air-filled retraction pocket.

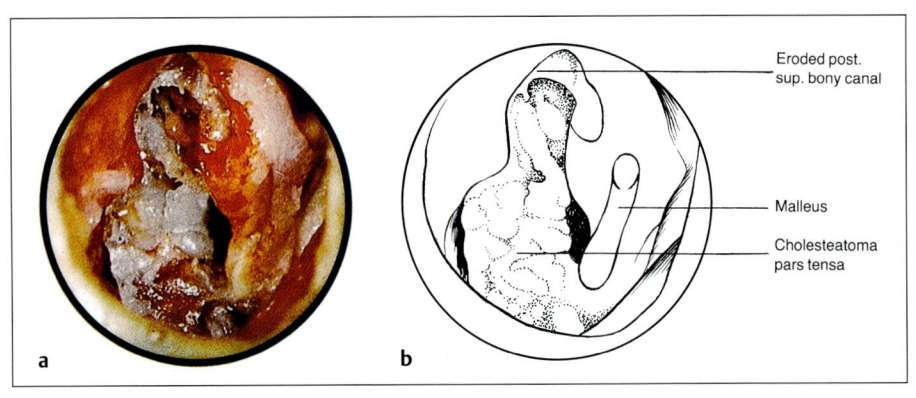

Fig. 1.**132** **a** Cholesteatoma, pars tensa. Otoscopic findings, right. There is a posterosuperior peroration filled with epithelial debris and granulation tissue. The cholesteatoma has partially eroded the posterosuperior canal wall. **b** Diagram of **a**.

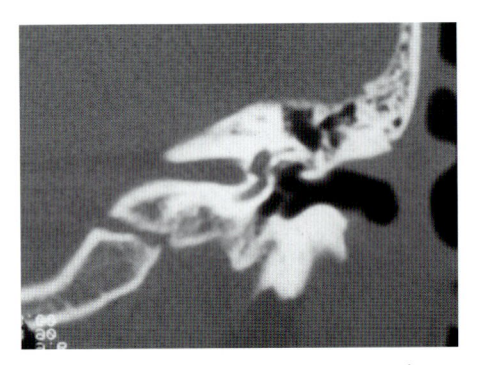

Fig. 1.**133** Posterosuperior retraction pocket. Coronal CT section. The pocket extends into the oval window niche with erosion of the long process of the incus and stapes superstructures.

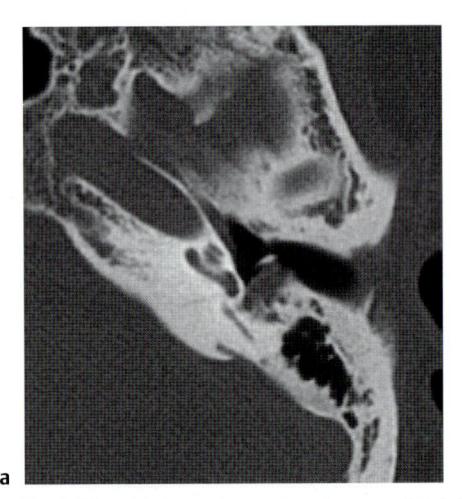

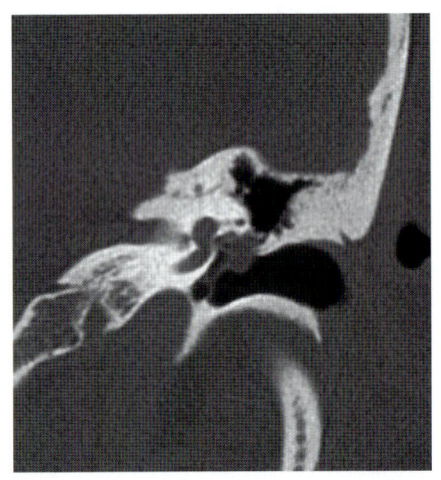

Fig. 1.**134** Cholesteatoma, pars tensa. **a** Axial, **b** coronal CT sections, left. A soft-tissue mass fills the posterosuperior quadrant of the mesotympanum and extends into the sinus tympani. The cholesteatoma surrounds and partially erodes the long process of the incus.

occur in the pars tensa of the tympanic membrane, particularly in the posterosuperior quadrant (Fig. 1.133). The long process of the incus is often eroded and the retracted membrane may become attached to the head of the stapes with formation of a myringostapediopexy.

■ Pars Tensa Cholesteatomas

Cholesteatomas of the pars tensa are more difficult to diagnose than pars flaccida lesions because the lateral epitympanic wall may be intact. In early cases, bony erosion is limited to the long process of the incus, and this is not a specific finding in cholesteatomas. The radiographic pattern for cholesteatoma of the pars tensa consists of findings common to all pars tensa cholesteatomas and of findings that depend on the site of origin of the lesion in the pars tensa. The findings common to all pars tensa cholesteatomas are one or more of the following (Figs. 1.**134**–1.**136**, 1.**138**):

1. There is a soft-tissue mass in the middle ear.
2. The long process of the incus is eroded.
3. The soft-tissue mass of the middle ear extends into the epitympanum medial to the ossicles.
4. The malleus head and incus bodies are displaced laterally by the soft-tissue mass of the cholesteatoma sac. The malleus head is usually displaced but intact while the displaced incus body is often eroded.

The most frequently occurring type of pars tensa cholesteatoma arises from the posterosuperior margin of the membrane. In these cases there is often blunting of the posterior portion of the lateral epitympanic wall and erosion of the posterosuperior bony canal wall. Cholesteatomas may arise from central or anterosuperior perforations of the pars tensa. In these cases, the posterosuperior bony wall of the external auditory canal is intact, but the other findings of pars tensa cholesteatoma are present in large lesions. Early lesions may be confined to the medial surface of the tympanic membrane. Cholesteatomas of the posterior pars tensa can extend into the sinus tympanum (Figs. 1.**134**, 1.**136**, 1.**138**). When they do, they are best visualized in axial sections. Occasionally projections of the cholesteatoma extend into the eustachian tube.

Cholesteatoma of the Middle Ear

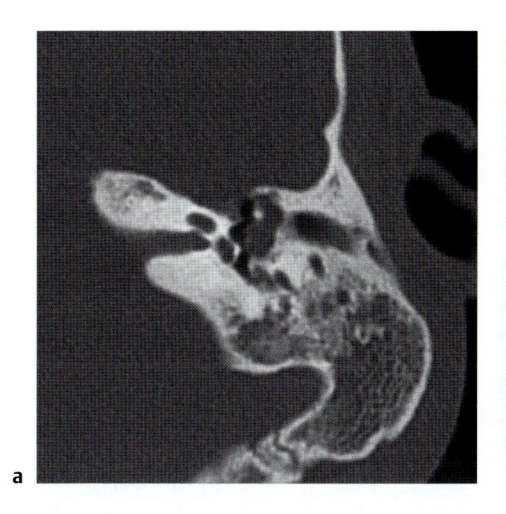

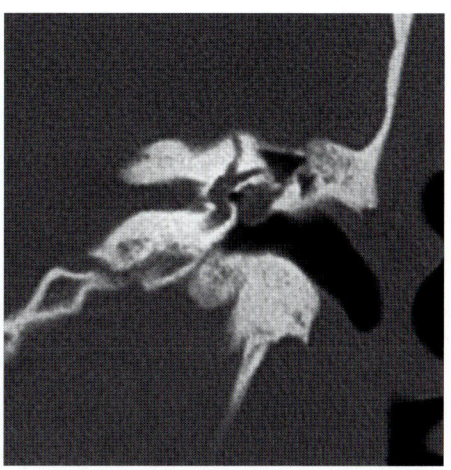

Fig. 1.**135** Cholesteatoma, pars tensa. **a** Axial, **b** coronal CT sections, left. A soft-tissue mass fills the upper mesotympanum surrounding and eroding the long process of the incus.

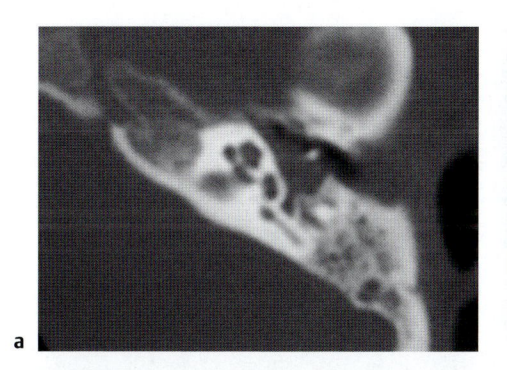

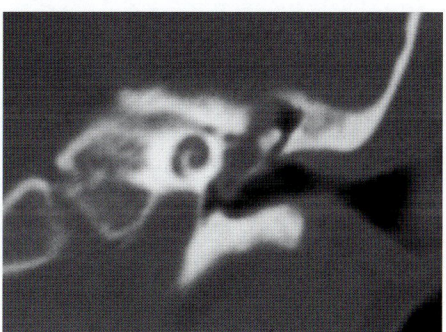

Fig. 1.**136** Cholesteatoma, pars tensa. **a** Axial, **b**, **c** coronal CT sections, left. A soft-tissue mass fills the posterior portion of the middle ear and extends into the attic medial to the ossicles. The posterosuperior bony canal wall annulus is blunted and the long process of the incus is eroded. The lesion extends into the sinus tympani (**a**). **d** Diagram of **b**.

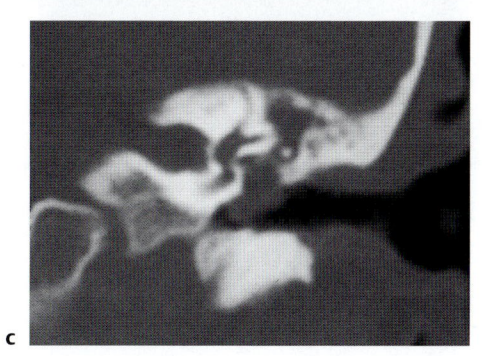

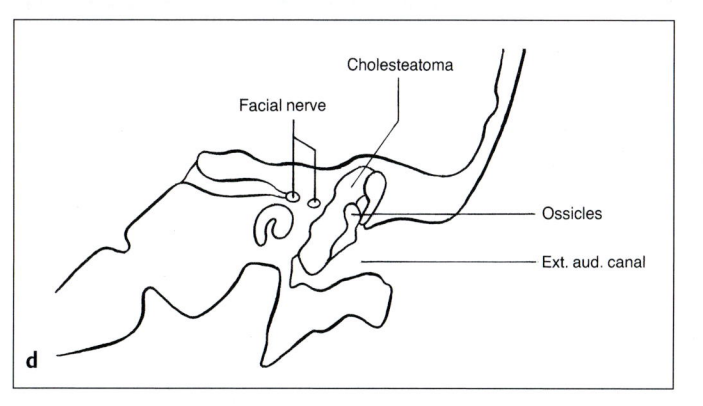

■ Combined Pars Flaccida and Pars Tensa Cholesteatomas

In cholesteatomas that arise from combined perforations of the pars tensa and pars flaccida, the radiographic findings are a combination of the two patterns (Fig. 1.**140**). At times, the entire pars flaccida and pars tensa are absent. The predominance of the findings depends on which a portion of the tympanic membrane is more extensively involved. In lesions with total absence of the tympanic membrane, the mesotympanum appears aerated and cholesteatoma matrix lines the middle ear.

■ Evaluation of the Extent of Cholesteatoma

The radiographic detection of the extent of a cholesteatoma beyond the limits of the mesotympanum and epitympanum depends on the recognition of soft-tissue and bony changes in the aditus, the antrum, the mastoid, and the petrous pyramid.

Aditus

Enlargement of the aditus is best seen in axial CT, and indicates extension of the cholesteatoma posterosuperiorly. The short process of the incus, which lies in the adjacent fossa incudis, is usually eroded (Figs. 1.**137**, 1.**138**, 1.**141**).

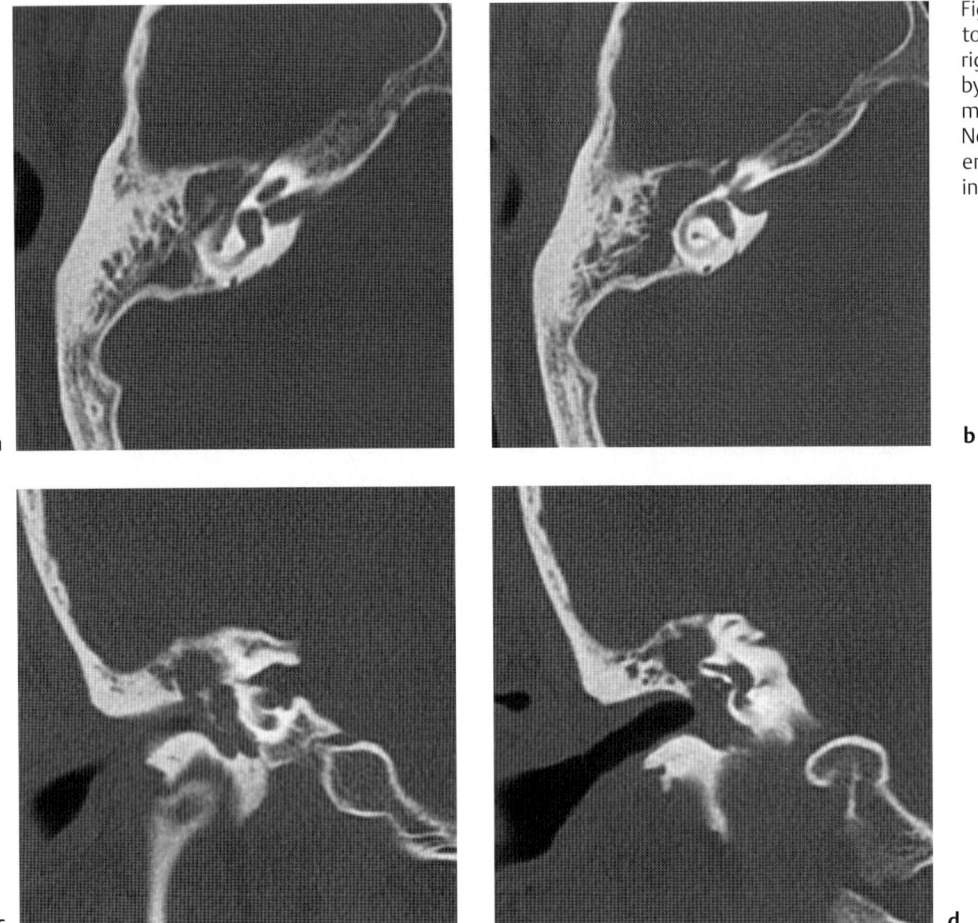

Fig. 1.137 Large pars flaccida cholesteatoma. **a, b** Axial, **c, d** coronal CT sections, right. The lateral epitympanic wall is eroded by a large soft-tissue mass filling the entire middle ear and extending into the mastoid. Note the widening of the aditus (**b**) and the erosion of the Koerner septum (**d**). Malleus, incus, and stapes superstructures are eroded.

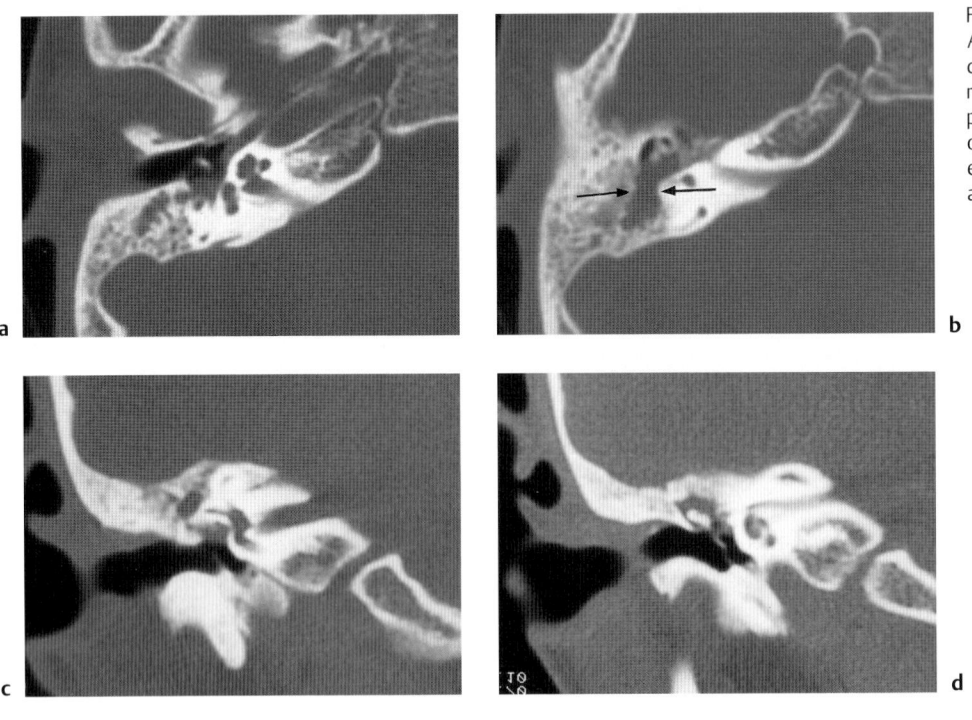

Fig. 1.138 Cholesteatoma, pars tensa. **a, b** Axial, **c, d** coronal CT sections, right. The cholesteatoma fills the posterosuperior quadrant of the mesotympanum and sinus tympani and extends into the attic medial to the ossicles. The body of the incus is partially eroded. The mass widens the aditus (arrows) and passes into the mastoid antrum.

Cholesteatoma of the Middle Ear 81

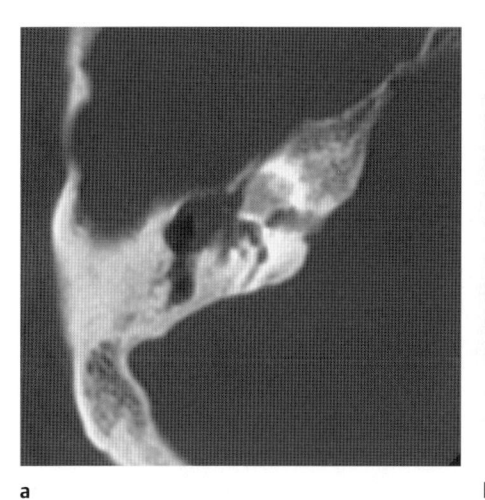

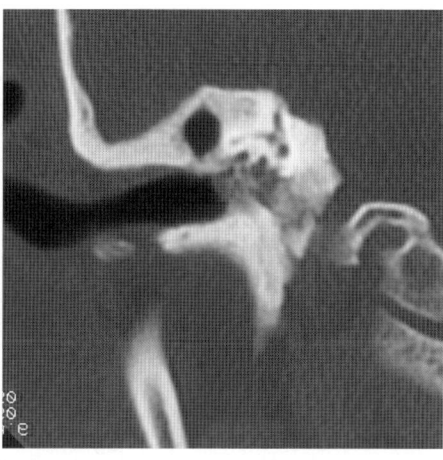

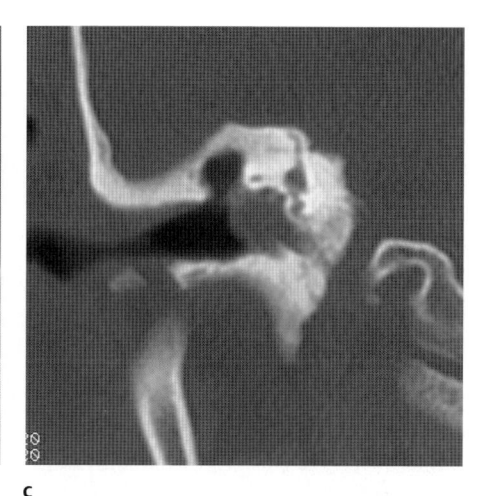

Fig. 1.**139** Cholesteatoma with fistula of the horizontal semicircular canal and labyrinthitis. **a** Axial, **b**, **c** coronal CT sections, right. The lateral attic wall and the adjacent superior canal wall are eroded. An empty cholesteatoma sac extends from the attic into the mastoid. The lateral end of the horizontal semicircular canal is eroded (**a**) and the lumen of the cochlea is partially obliterated by bone. The partially calcified soft-tissue mass in the middle ear cavity proved at surgery to be a large granuloma (**c**).

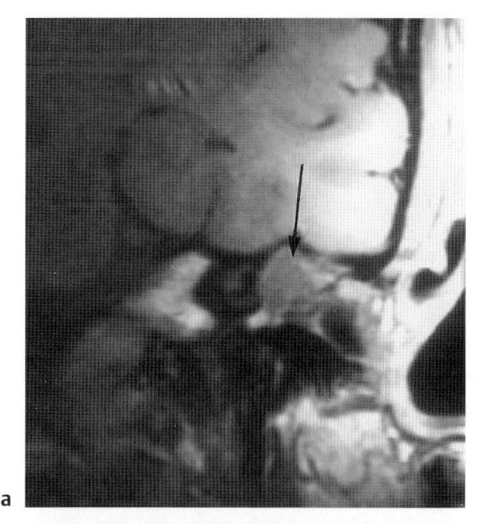

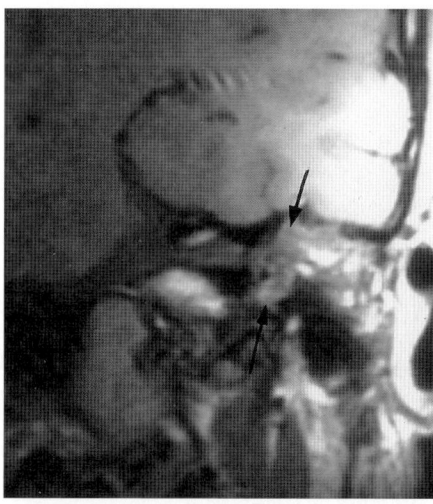

Fig. 1.**140** Cholesteatoma, pars flaccida and pars tensa combined. **a**, **b** Coronal T1W, **c** axial T2W, **d** sagittal T1W MR sections. A large cholesteatoma fills the middle ear cavity and mastoid, eroding the lateral wall of the attic and posterosuperior canal wall. There is also erosion of the horizontal semicircular canal. The mass has a signal of medium intensity in the T1W images and high intensity in the T2W image (arrows).

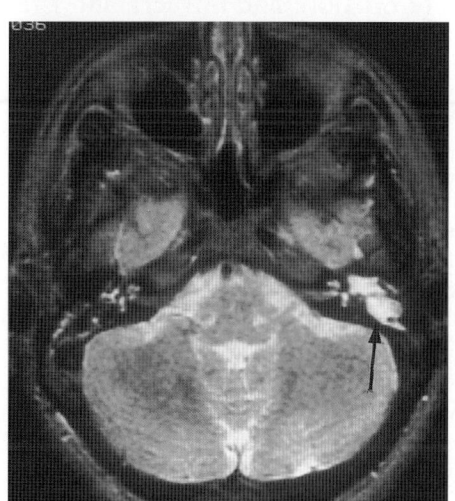

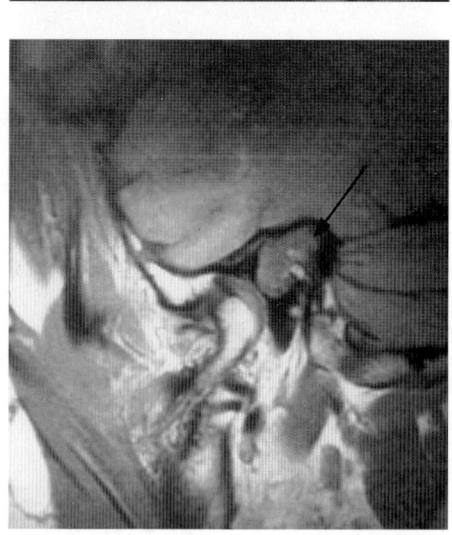

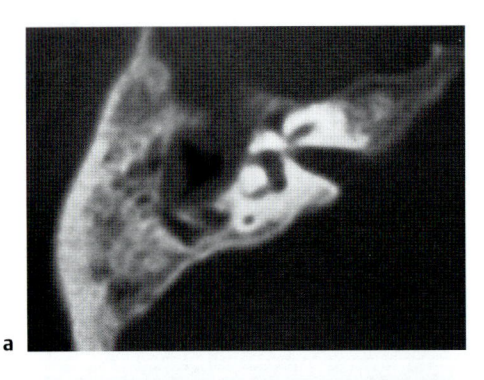

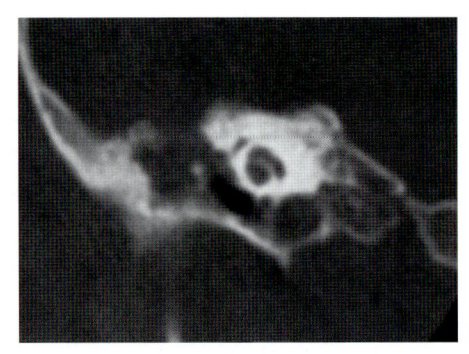

Fig. 1.**141** Cholesteatoma. **a** Axial, **b**, **c** coronal CT sections, right. A large cholesteatoma fills the epitympanum and erodes the lateral epitympanic wall. The mass extends into the mastoid antrum, enlarges the aditus and erodes and fistulizes the capsule of the horizontal semicircular canals. The tegmen tympani is eroded. The outer surface of the thickened tympanic membrane is coated with an iodine-containing therapeutic powder. **d** Diagram of **c**.

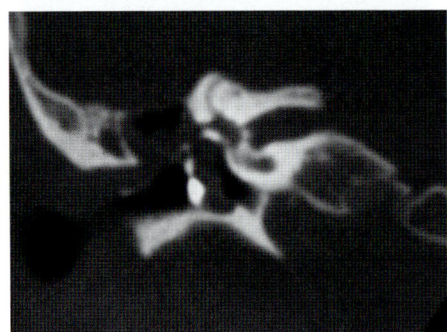

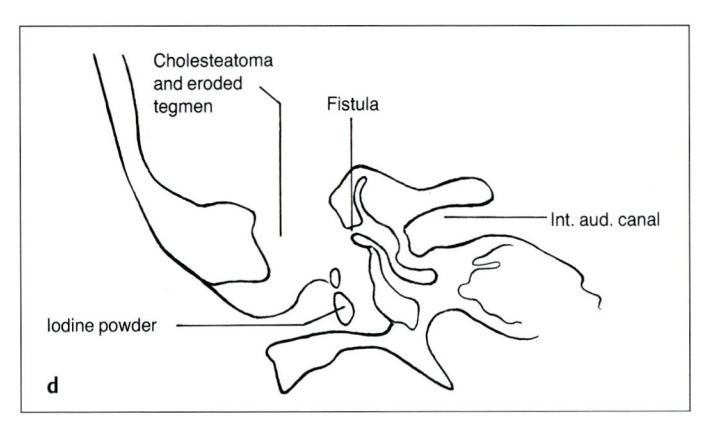

Antrum

When the cholesteatoma extends into the mastoid antrum, a mass is visible that partially or completely fills the lumen. As the cholesteatoma erodes the air cells that line the walls of the antrum, the contour becomes smooth. Further extension of the cholesteatoma results in enlargement of the antral cavity (Figs. 1.**141**–1.**144**). Superior extension of the cholesteatoma causes progressive erosion of Koerner's septum (Figs. 1.**137**, 1.**143**, 1.**144**). Koerner's septum is a rather constant landmark in pneumatized mastoids and appears as a thick, bony septum extending from the tegmen medially and inferiorly into the antrum and aditus (Fig. 1.**147**). Complete amputation of the septum indicates extension of the cholesteatoma to the tegmen of the antrum (Fig. 1.**141**).

Mastoid

Further extension of the cholesteatoma into the mastoid causes progressive destruction of the trabecular pattern and formation of a large, smooth-walled cloudy cavity (Figs. 1.**140**, 1.**144**). Occasionally, the cholesteatoma may insinuate itself into the mastoid air cells (Fig. 1.**142**) without eroding the bony trabeculae. This type of involvement, usually seen in children, causes a cloudiness of the mastoid air cells, which cannot be distinguished radiographically from simple mastoiditis.

Natural Radical

Occasionally, an extensive mastoid cholesteatoma will erode the posterior portion of the lateral epitympanic wall and the posterosuperior wall of the bony external auditory canal. The cholesteatoma exteriorizes itself into the external auditory canal and forms a "natural radical" mastoid cavity.

Complications

Complications of cholesteatomas occur when the lesion erodes the anatomical boundaries of the middle ear, antrum, and mastoid, or involves the facial nerve.
The most common complications are:
1 Erosion of the tegmen or sinus plate
2 Erosion of the labyrinthine wall with fistula formation
3 Extension of the cholesteatoma into the petrous pyramid
4 Erosion of the facial nerve canal

Tegmen, Sinus Plate Erosion, and Intracranial Complications

Erosion of the tegmen usually occurs in large cholesteatomas (Figs. 1.**141**, 1.**143**, 1.**144**). One should remember that the tegmen tympani slopes downward anteriorly and may not be visualized in conventional coronal sections. Modified coronal sections obtained with the head extended or direct or reformatted sagittal CT sections, should be obtained whenever in doubt. Meningeal and intracranial complications may occur in association with tegmental erosions, and a CT or MRI study of the brain obtained after injection of contrast material will show such lesions as otogenic abscesses (Fig. 1.**103**). Erosion of the posterior wall of the mastoid and the sinus plate occur in extensive cholesteatomas and may lead to septic thrombophlebitis of the sigmoid and lateral sinuses and to cerebellar abscess formation.

■ Labyrinthine Fistulas

Labyrinthine fistulas occur most commonly in the lateral portion of the horizontal semicircular canal, which bulges into the antrum. A fistula of the horizontal semicircular canal is characterized by flattening of the normal convex contour of the canal and by erosion of the labyrinthine capsule over the lumen of the

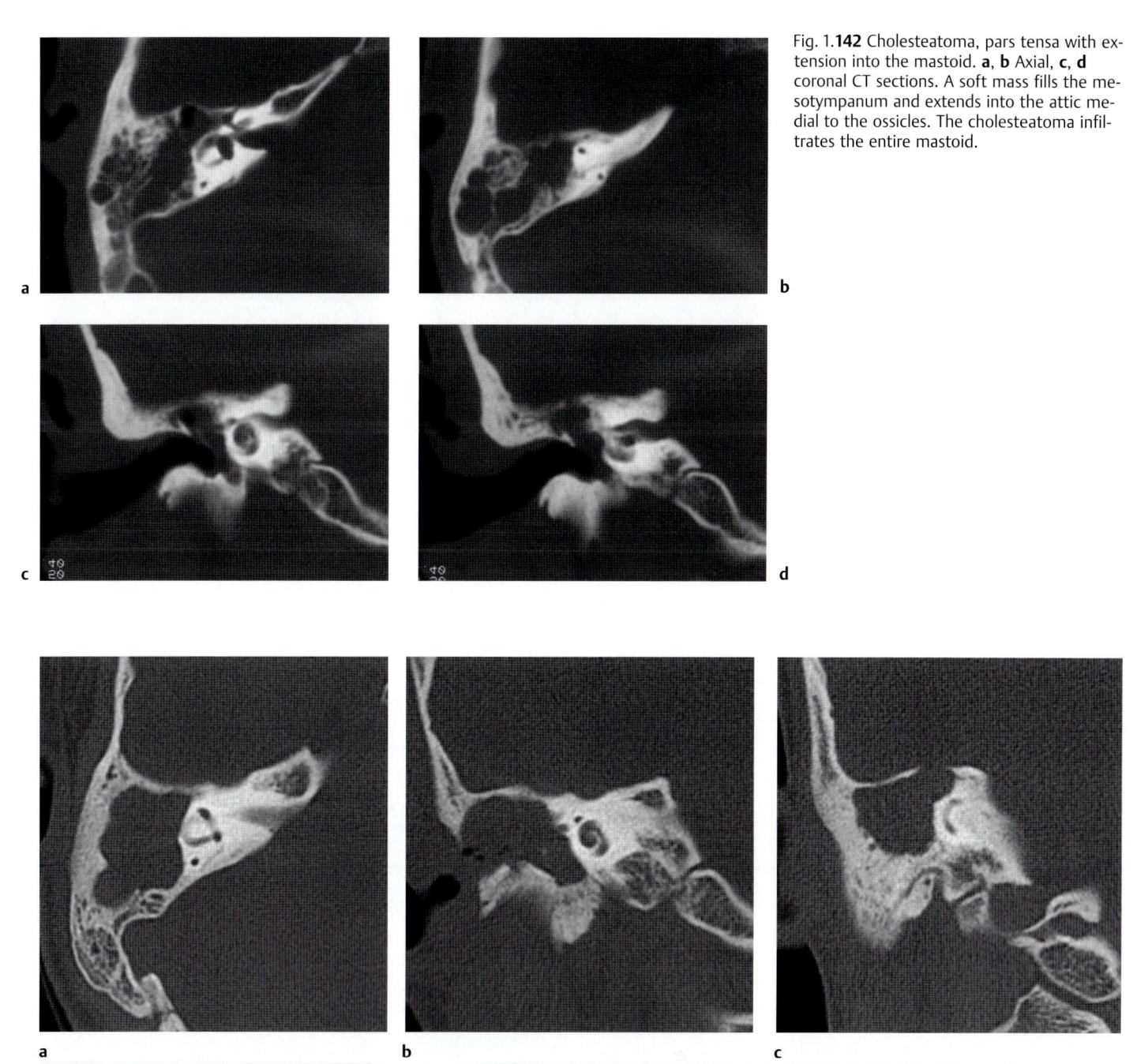

Fig. 1.**142** Cholesteatoma, pars tensa with extension into the mastoid. **a**, **b** Axial, **c**, **d** coronal CT sections. A soft mass fills the mesotympanum and extends into the attic medial to the ossicles. The cholesteatoma infiltrates the entire mastoid.

Fig. 1.**143** Cholesteatoma, extensive. **a** Axial, **b**, **c** coronal CT sections. The cholesteatoma has eroded all landmarks, with formation of a large cavity exteriorizing into the external auditory canal. The tegmen is thinned out and partially eroded (**c**).

canal. Fistulas at the lateral prominence of the horizontal semicircular canal are seen in axial and coronal CT sections (Figs. 1.**139**, 1.**140**, 1.**141**, 1.**143**, 1.**144**). Fistulas of either the anterior or posterior aspect of the horizontal canal are best exposed in axial sections. Fistulas of other areas of the labyrinth are rare and usually occur in large cholesteatomas that erode into the pyramid. Horizontal semicircular canal fistulas are rare in small or moderately sized pars flaccida cholesteatomas because the ossicles are interposed between the sac and the bony horizontal canal. In far-advanced cases, a fistula may occur in association with dissolution of the ossicles. Fistulas of the horizontal semicircular canal are not uncommon in pars tensa cholesteatoma because extension of the cholesteatoma from the middle ear is medial to the ossicles and in contact with the bony horizontal semicircular canal. If infection spreads via the fistula to the labyrinth to produce labyrinthitis, severe vertigo and deafness occur (Fig. 1.**139**).

■ Petrous Extension of Cholesteatoma

Extension of acquired cholesteatomas into the petrous pyramid occurs in large cholesteatomas that arise in well-pneumatized pertrous bone. In the medial extension, the cholesteatoma follows the course of least resistance and erodes the thin walls of the petrous air cells (Fig. 1.**144**).

The paths most commonly followed by petrous extensions are:
1. Anterosuperiorly, above the cochlea, involving the geniculate ganglion and extending to the suprameatal area of the petrous bone.
2. Posterosuperiorly, between the limbs of the superior semicircular canal to reach the fundus of the internal auditory canal. These lesions may broach the wall of the internal auditory canal.

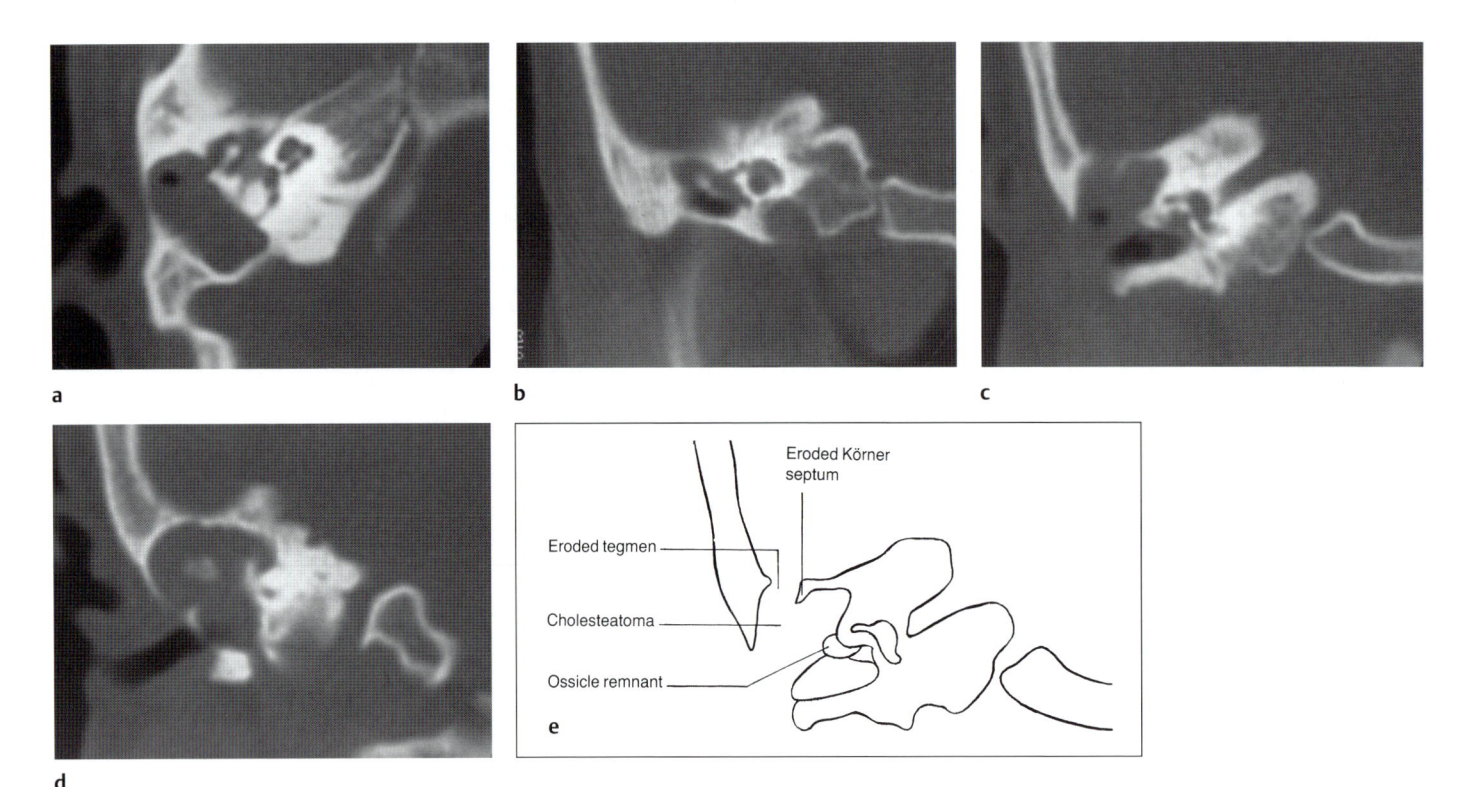

Fig. 1.**144** Cholesteatoma, extensive. **a** Axial, **b**, **c**, **d** coronal CT sections, right. An extensive cholesteatoma fills and erodes the epitympanum and the entire mastoid. The lesion has destroyed the postero- superior bony external canal wall, eroded the tegmen (**c**), and eroded and fistulized the posterior semicircular canal. The mastoid segment of the facial canal is eroded and the facial nerve is exposed. **e** Diagram of **c**.

3 Infralabyrinthine, inferior to the cochlea and internal auditory canal. Such lesions may break into the jugular fossa.

Axial CT sections demonstrate erosion of the petrous cell walls with clouding of the cavity and surrounding air cells. If bony erosion has not occurred, it may be impossible by CT to differentiate extension of the cholesteatoma from fluid. MR is used in this case to establish the extent of the lesion.

■ Facial Nerve

Facial nerve paralysis can occur if the cholesteatoma erodes the facial nerve canal and exposes the nerve. The exposed nerve must be compressed by the cholesteatoma or affected by an inflammatory process to cause paralysis. The demonstration of the facial nerve canal erosion is important to the otological surgeon, since he or she should be aware of the erosion preoperatively to avoid damage to the exposed nerve (Figs. 1.**140**, 1.**144**, 1.**149**). The most common site of facial nerve canal erosion is the area extending from the oval window to the proximal portion of the vertical segment. Erosion of the anterior portion of the tympanic segment and geniculate ganglion may occur in large epitympanic lesions. Erosion of the mastoid segment of the nerve occurs in lesions that involve the entire mastoid. Involvement of the tympanic segment of the nerve is best seen in coronal and 20° coronal oblique sections. Mastoid segment erosions are seen in sagittal and axial sections. In 50% of normal ears, the bony canal of the horizontal portion of the facial nerve is congenitally dehiscent. Therefore, evidence of defects of the bony canal of this segment of the nerve does not necessarily indicate erosion by cholesteatoma. MR sections obtained in T1 sequence after injection of contrast often show enhancement of the involved segment of the facial nerve.

■ Congenital Cholesteatoma of the Middle Ear

Congenital cholesteatomas are histologically epidermoid tumors originating from embryonic epidermoid rests located anywhere in the temporal bone or in the adjacent extradural or epidural spaces.[26] The clinical symptomatology of congenital cholesteatoma depends on the size and the site of the lesion (Fig. 1.**145**).

CT Findings

Otoscopically, congenital middle ear cholesteatomas appear as whitish globular masses lying medial to an intact tympanic membrane. There is usually no history of antecedent inflammatory ear disease. Occasionally there is an associated serous otitis media. CT sections usually show a well-defined soft-tissue mass within the aerated middle ear. Typically the mass is located in the anterior portion of the mesotympanum and the ossicular chain is intact (Figs. 1.**146**, 1.**147**). If the cholesteatoma involves the entire middle ear space or if there is an accompanying serous otitis media, the entire tympanic cavity appears cloudy and the tympanic membrane bulges laterally (Figs. 1.**146**, 1.**148**). This lateral bulging seen on coronal and axial sections enables the radiologist to differentiate the mass of the congenital cholesteatoma from serous otitis media. In both instances, the middle ear will appear cloudy, but in serous otitis media the tympanic membrane is retracted medially. The inferior margin of the lateral epitympanic wall, which is typically eroded in acquired cholesteatoma, is intact in congenital lesions. The medial aspect of the lateral epitympanic wall is often eroded from within when the congenital lesion extends into the epitympanum. In these cases the ossicular chain is eroded. Congenital cholesteatomas

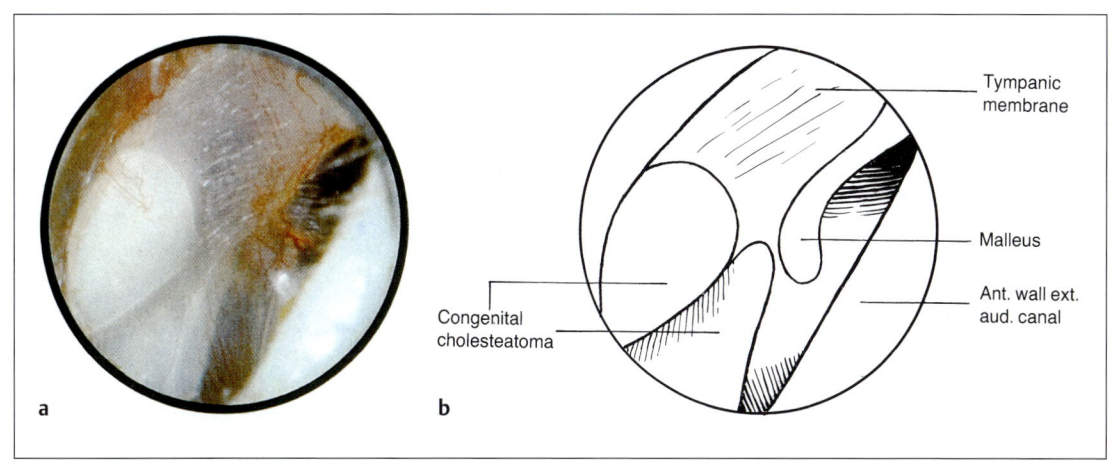

Cholesteatoma of the Middle Ear   85

Fig. 145 Cholesteatoma, congenital, otoscopic findings right ear. **a** A whitish mass of necrotic epithelial debris fills the posteroinferior portion of the middle ear medial to and in contact with an intact tympanic membrane. **b** Diagram of **a**.

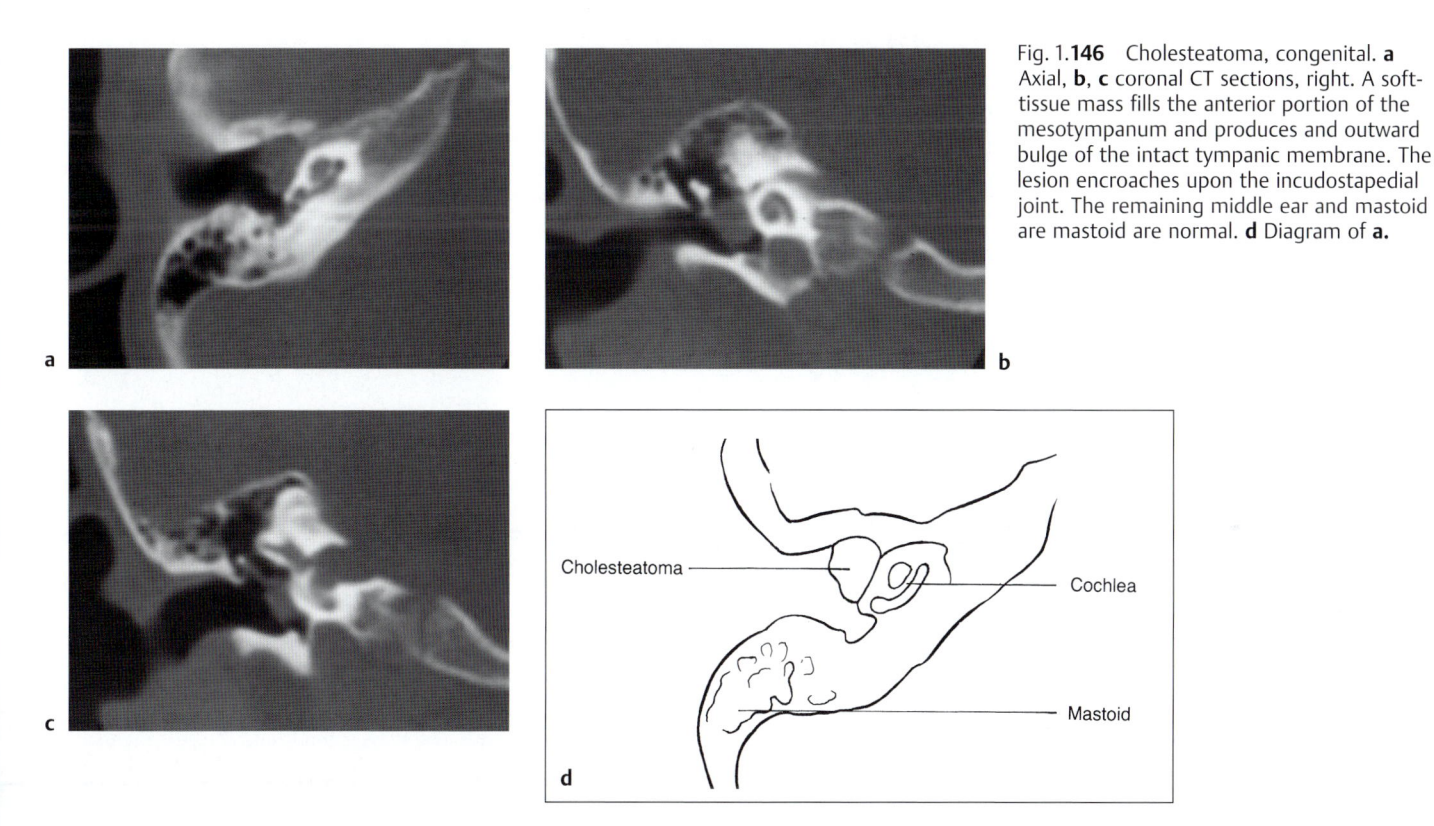

Fig. 1.146 Cholesteatoma, congenital. **a** Axial, **b**, **c** coronal CT sections, right. A soft-tissue mass fills the anterior portion of the mesotympanum and produces and outward bulge of the intact tympanic membrane. The lesion encroaches upon the incudostapedial joint. The remaining middle ear and mastoid are mastoid are normal. **d** Diagram of **a.**

arising in the mastoid are very rare and appear as areas of destruction of the trabecular pattern produced by the cystic mass in the mastoid. In such cases, the middle ear cavity is normal in contradistinction to acquired cholesteatoma where the middle ear is always involved. An MR study should be performed in these cases to differentiate a congenital cholesteatoma from a cholesterol granuloma.

■ Petrous Pyramid and Epidural Cholesteatomas

The majority of these lesions arise in the petrous apex or adjacent epidural spaces.[6] The first sign of a congenital cholesteatoma of the pyramid is often a facial paralysis of slow onset (Figs. 1.149, 1.150) followed by a sensorineural hearing loss caused by erosion of the labyrinth. In the early stages, the middle ear may be normal. Radiographic findings depend on whether the cholesteatoma arises from within the petrous pyramid or from the adjacent epidural or intradural spaces. When the cholesteatoma arises from within the petrous apex, computerized tomography will show an expansile, cystic lesion in the apex (Fig. 1.151). The involved area of the pyramid is expanded, and the superior petrous ridge is usually elevated and thinned out (Fig. 1.149). As the lesion expands, the internal auditory canal and labyrinth become eroded. Cholesteatomas arising from the epidural or intradural spaces cause a scooped-out defect on the adjacent superior aspect of the temporal bone (Fig. 1.152). The defect is caused by erosion of the pyramid from without, and there is no bony rim as in lesions arising from within the pyramid.

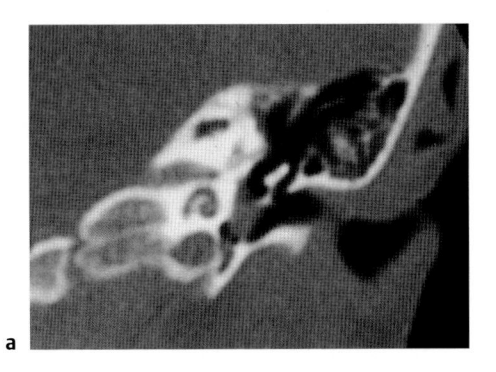

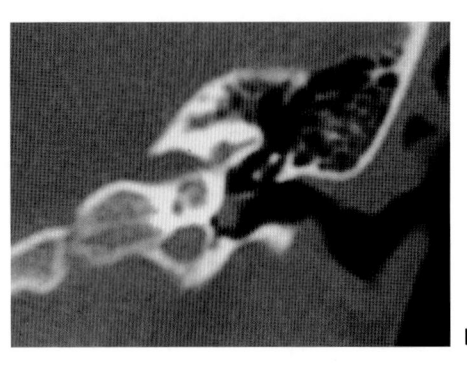

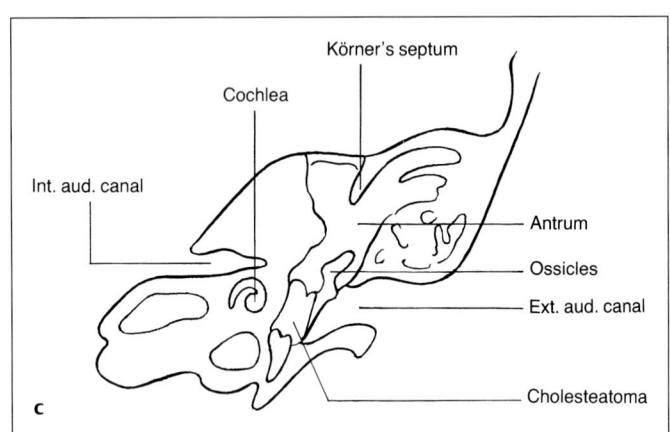

Fig. 1.**147** Cholesteatoma, congenital. **a, b** Coronal CT sections, left. A well defined soft-tissue mass lies in the mesotympanum. The mass extends from the intact tympanic membrane to the promontory. The middle ear and mastoid are well aerated. **c** Diagram of **a**.

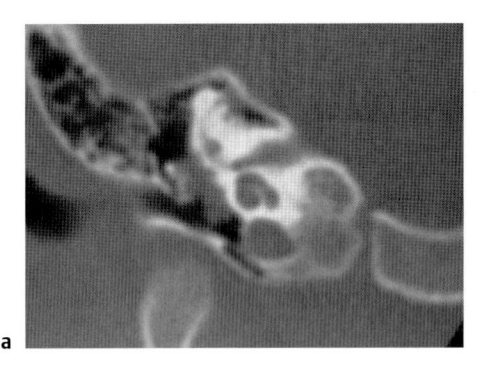

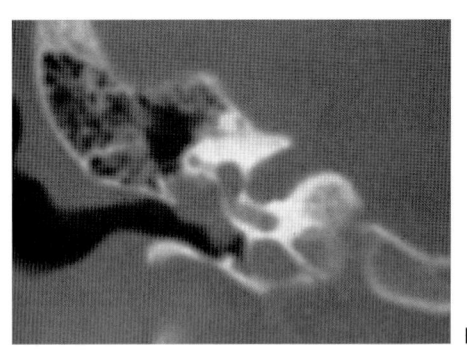

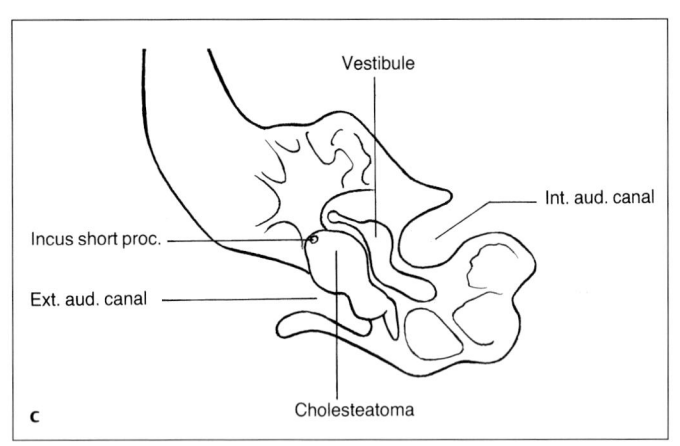

Fig. 1.**148** Cholesteatoma, congenital. **a, b** Coronal CT sections. A large soft-tissue mass fills most of the mesotympanum and displaces the intact tympanic membrane laterally. The mass extends into the epitympanum medial to the ossicles and erodes the long process of the incus. **c** Diagram of **b**.

Infusion CT shows no mass enhancement, except for a thin and often incomplete capsule. The CT findings are identical to those of a cholesterol granuloma and mucocele of the petrous apex. Cholesteatoma and cholesterol granuloma can be differentiated from each other by MRI, since in the T1 sequence the cholesterol granuloma is bright but the cholesteatoma appears less bright because of a longer T1 relaxation time (Figs. 1.**150**, 1.**152**).

Cholesteatomas originating in the jugular fossa area can cause bony changes similar to glomus jugulare tumors. Both lesions expand the jugular fossa and erode the posteroinferior aspect of the petrous pyramid and adjacent occipital bone.

Cholesteatoma of the Middle Ear   87

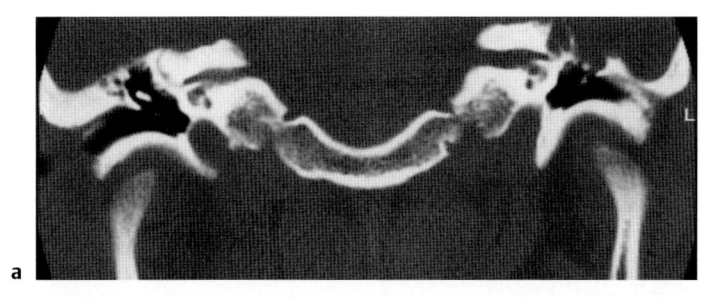

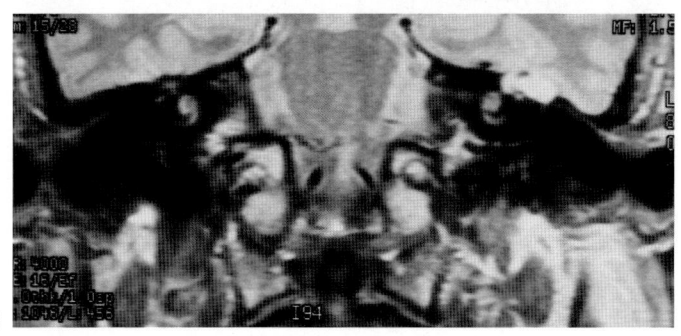

Fig. 1.**149** Congenital cholesteatoma of the left petrous pyramid. **a, b** Coronal CT sections, **c** proton density, and **d** T2W coronal MR image. An expansile soft-tissue mass erodes the superior aspect of the petrous pyramid and extends into the attic. The facial canal is involved in the region of the geniculate ganglion.

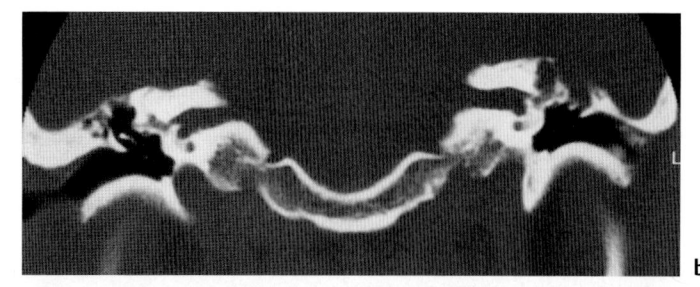

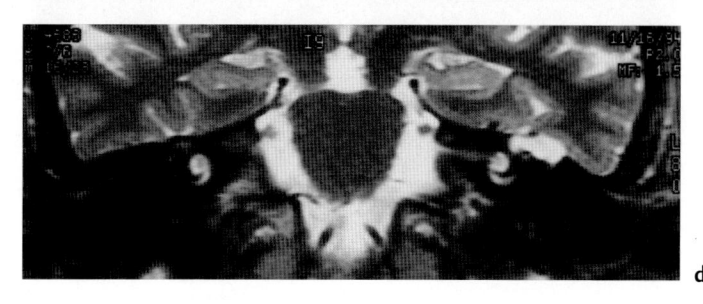

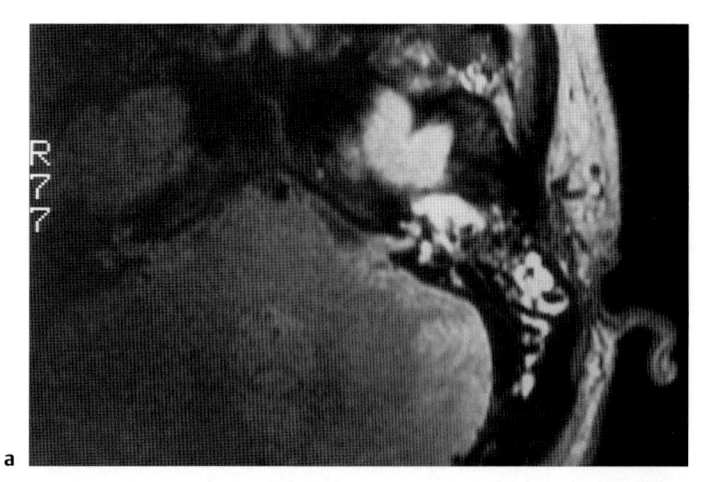

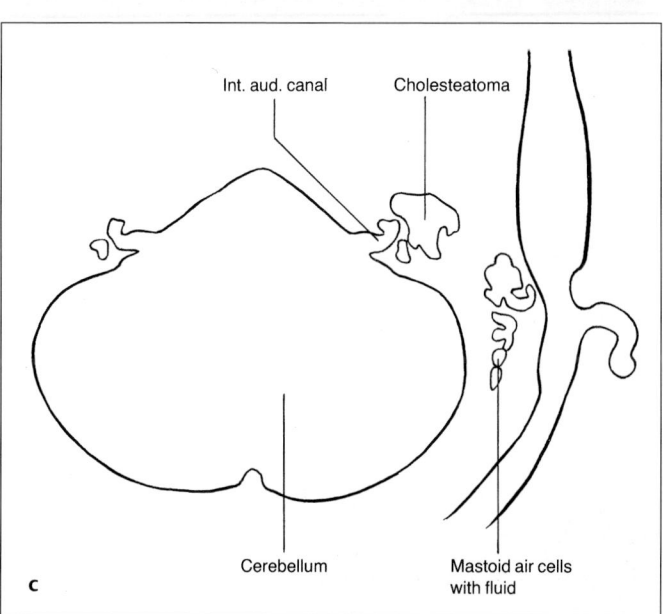

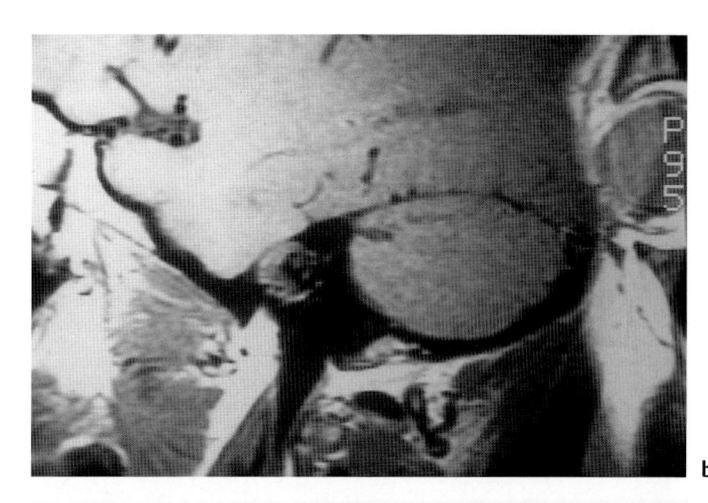

Fig. 1.**150** Cholesteatoma, congenital, petrous pyramid. **a** Axial T2W, **b** sagittal spin-density-weighted MR sections; same case as Fig. 1.**149**. The cholesteatoma appears in the T2W image as a high signal intensity mass involving the anterior aspect of the petrous pyramid and middle ear cavity (**a**). In the sagittal spin-density-weighted sections, the signal intensity is less than in T2W (**b**). In the axial T2W image, fluid in the mastoid air cells appears bright. **c** Diagram of **a**.

88   1 Imaging of the Temporal Bone

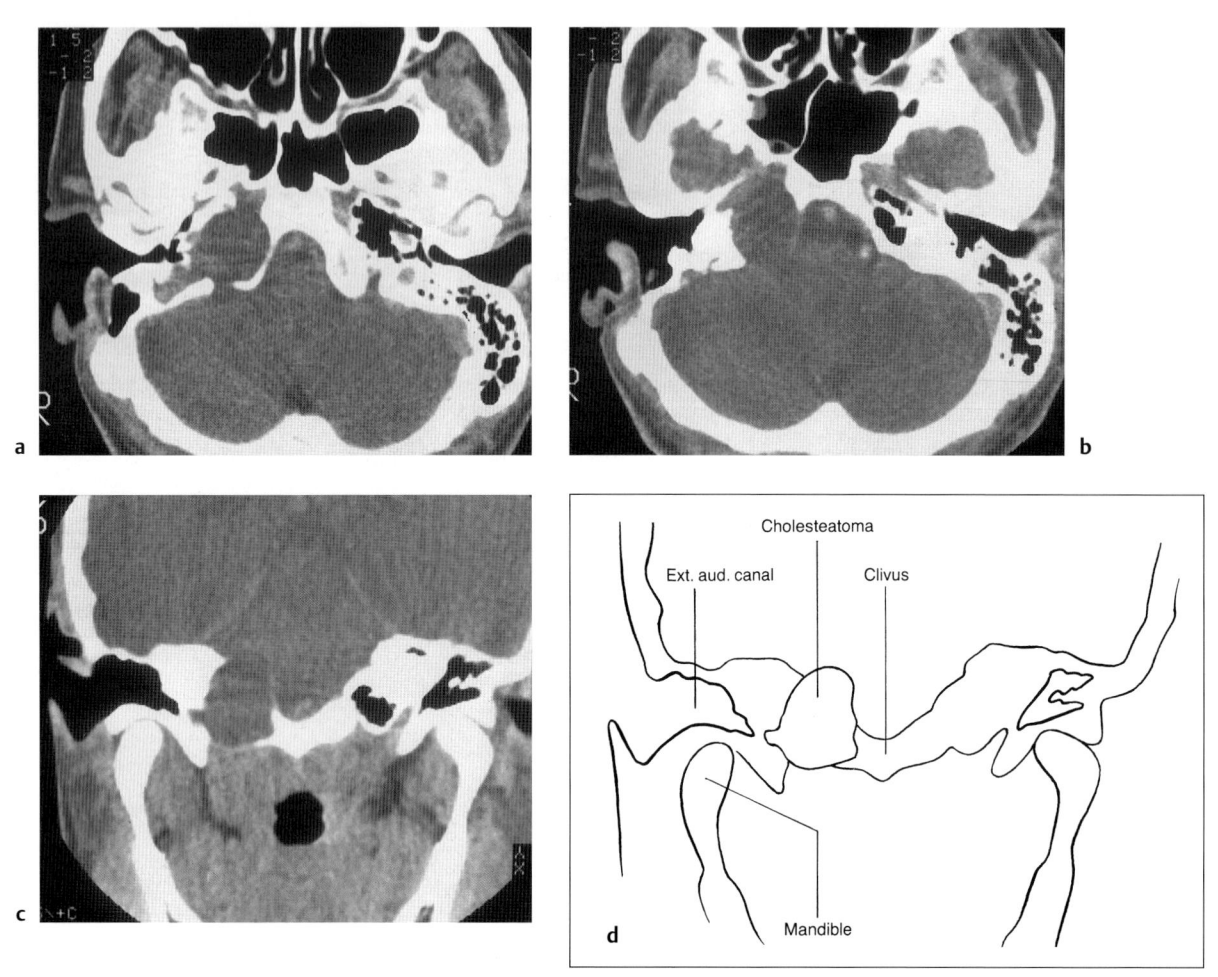

Fig. 1.**151** Cholesteatoma, petrous apex. **a**, **b** Axial, **c** coronal enhanced CT sections. The right petrous apex is destroyed by an expansile low-density lesion. Note the enhancement of the capsule. The lesion involves the clivus and occipital condyle. There is an old mastoidectomy defect. **d** Diagram of **c**.

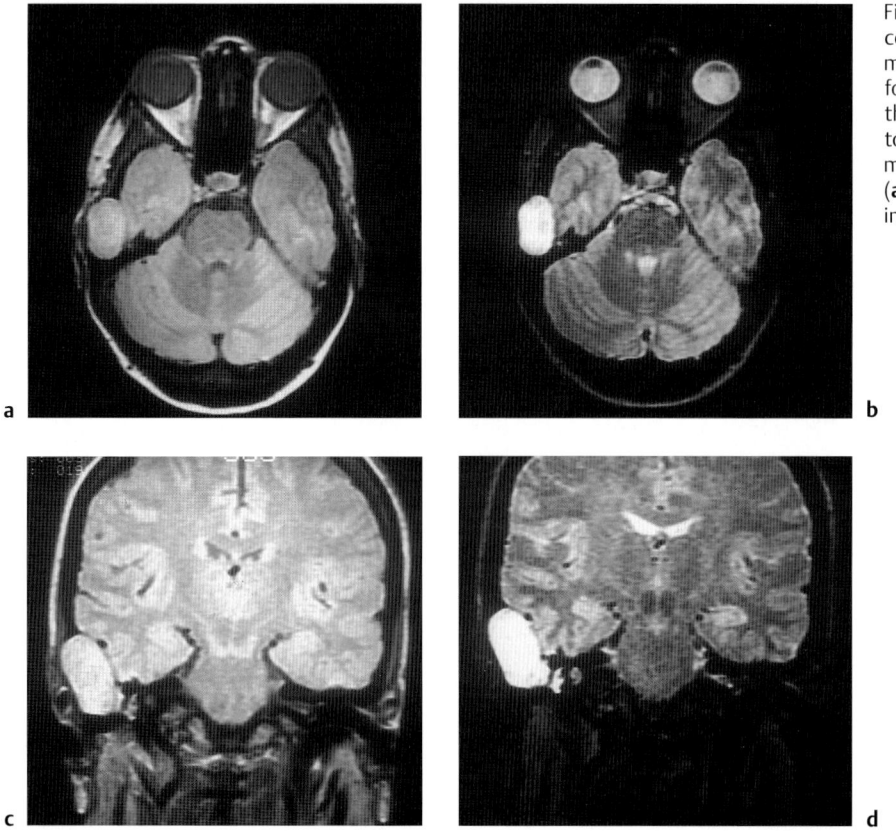

Fig. 1.**152** Congenital cholesteatoma. **a**, **b** Axial, **c**, **d** coronal MR sections, right. There is a large extradural mass in the lateral portion of the right middle cranial fossa. The mass erodes the adjacent upper aspect of the temporal bone and bulges into the external auditory canal. The lesion is characterized by a signal of medium intensity in spin-density-weighted images (**a**, **c**) and by a signal of higher intensity in the T2W images (**b**, **d**).

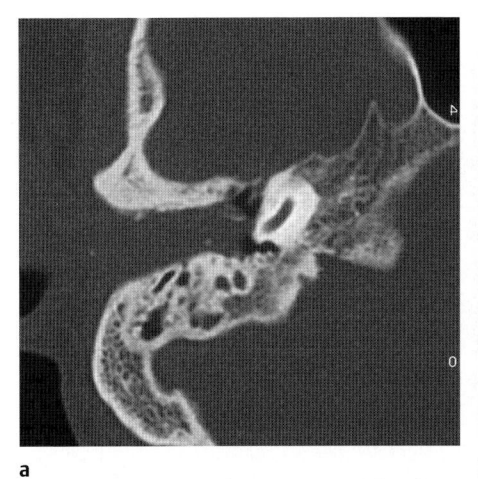

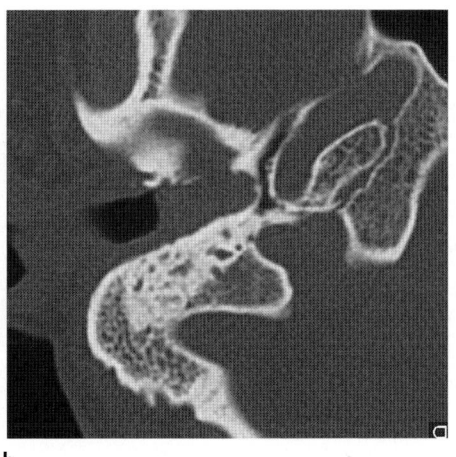

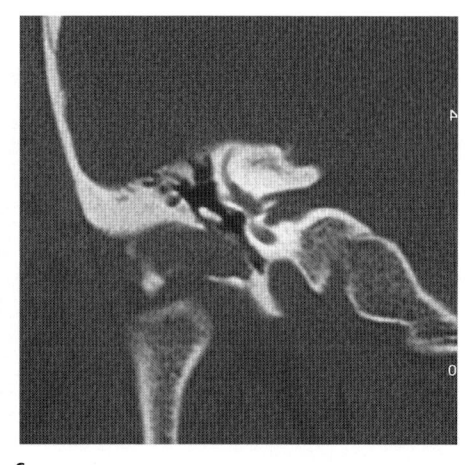

Fig. 1.**153** Keratosis obturans, external auditory canal. **a, b** Axial, **c** coronal CT sections, right. The mass fills the external auditory canal and erodes the anterior wall and floor of the canal, which appears enlarged.

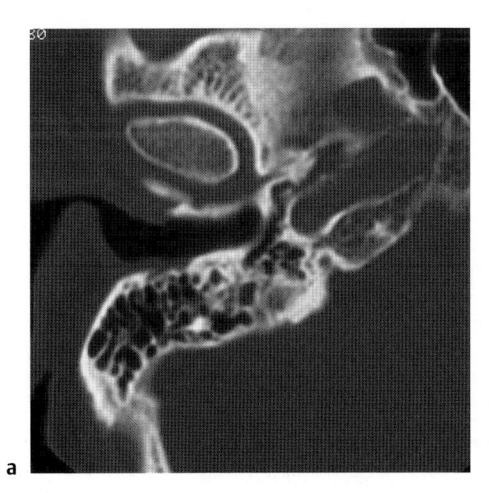

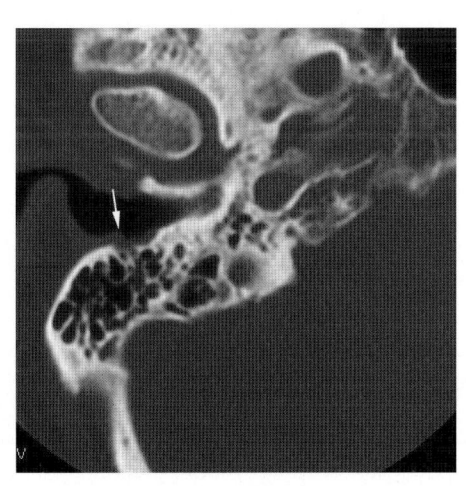

Fig. 1.**154** Cholesteatoma, external auditory canal. **a, b** Axial CT sections, right. There is a localized area of invasive keratitis in the posterior wall of the external auditory canal (arrow).

Congenital cholesteatomas of the cerebellopontine angle produce signs and symptoms similar to an acoustic neuroma. The lumen of the internal auditory canal is usually not expanded, but there is erosion and shortening of the posterior wall of the internal auditory canal. Again differentiation is easily made by MRI with contrast.

Keratosis Obturans and Cholesteatoma of the External Auditory Canal

Keratosis obturans is caused by osteomas, stenosis of the external auditory canal, or hard masses of cerumen. When it occurs in young patients, it is often associated with bronchiectasis. Blockage of the external auditory canal for a long period permits epithelial debris to accumulate in the canal and enlarge the bony contour of the external canal. CT shows concentric enlargement of the bony external auditory canal by a soft-tissue mass medial to the site of the canal stenosis or obstruction (Fig. 1.**153**).

Cholesteatoma of the external canal, also called invasive keratitis, is characterized by localized accumulations of desquamated debris in the bony canal (Figs. 1.**154**, 1.**155**). Removal of the debris reveals deep localized erosions of the bony canal wall and areas of exposed, necrotic bone. Occasionally the lesions extend and involve almost the entire circumference of the external canal. There often is a history of antecendent radiotherapy to the area of the ear. In invasive keratitis, CT shows erosion of the cortex of the involved portion of the canal. In larger lesions, there are scooped-out defects of the bony canal wall. When the lesion is diffuse, there is expansion of the involved canal segment without obstruction of the canal lumen. When the external canal cholesteatoma is large, it erodes the anulus and extends into the middle ear, attic, and mastoid.

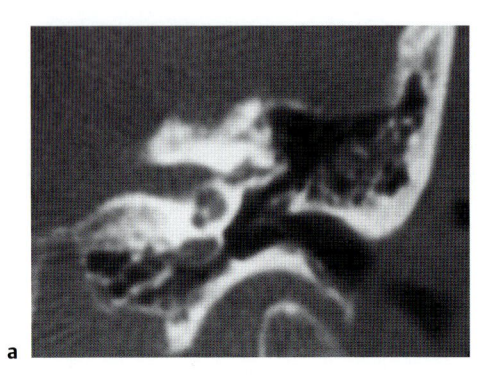

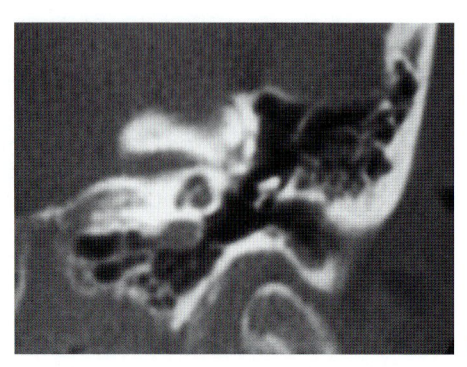

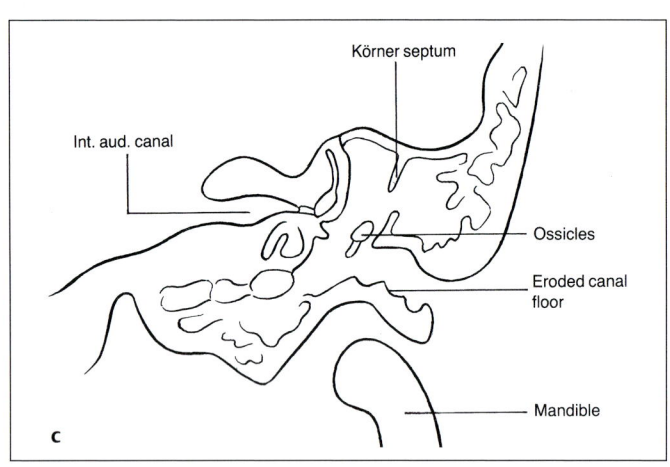

Fig. 1.**155** Cholesteatoma, external auditory canal, after radiation therapy. **a**, **b** Coronal CT sections, left. There is localized erosion of the lateral portion of the floor of the external auditory canal. Necrotic debris overlies the erosion. This patient had x-ray therapy to the head 20 years previously. **c** Diagram of **b**.

Postoperative and Postirradiation Imaging of the Temporal Bone

Postoperative radiographs of the ear are difficult to interpret. The bony landmarks are usually missing, and there is often clouding of the mastoid cavity because of recurrent pathological changes or because tissue grafts or flaps were used to fill the mastoidectomy cavity. In addition, with passage of time, new bone formation may partially fill in the surgical defects. To understand and interpret the postoperative radiographic findings of the ear, the radiologist should be acquainted with the basic techniques of middle ear and mastoid surgery.

■ Simple and Radical Mastoidectomies

Mastoid surgery may be divided into simple and radical procedures.

Simple Mastoidectomy

A simple mastoidectomy consists of drilling away the external mastoid cortex and exenterating the mastoid air cells. Air cell exenteration extends to the mastoid antrum. When indicated by the pathology, the dissection will extend to the epitympanum. The surgeon drills between the dural plate and the superior wall of the external auditory canal and leaves the inferior margin of the lateral epitympanic wall intact. At times the surgeon may explore only the antrum and epitympanum. In these cases only enough mastoid cortex and mastoid air cells are removed to expose these areas (Fig. 1.**157**).

Radical and Modified Radical Mastoidectomies

The essential feature that differentiates a simple mastoidectomy from one of the various types of radical mastoidectomies is that in the radical procedure the mastoid bridge is removed. During the surgical dissection of the mastoid, the lateral portion of the posterosuperior bony canal wall and upper portion of the lateral epitympanic wall are first drilled away. This leaves a bony arch called the mastoid bridge, which is made up of the medial portion of the posterosuperior bony canal wall and the inferior margin of the epitympanic wall. This bridge is removed during one of the last stages of the operation and converts a simple mastoidectomy into a radical mastoidectomy (canal-down mastoidectomy). Removal of the bridge transforms the mastoid cavity and the external canal into a common cavity. The modified radical mastoidectomy is the most commonly performed type of radical mastoidectomy. In the modified radical mastoidectomy, remnants of the tympanic membrane and ossicles are retained to preserve hearing. In the true radical mastoidectomy, which is rarely performed, all middle ear structures and tympanic membrane remnants are removed.

■ Tympanoplasty

Tympanoplasties are surgical procedures of the middle ear and mastoid designed to improve hearing. There are five classical types of tympanoplasties. In type I tympanoplasty a graft is used to cover defects of the tympanic membrane without altering the ossicular chain. This procedure is also known as myringoplasty.

In type II, the tympanic membrane is repaired and the continuity of the ossicular chain is restored by placing a strut between the head of the stapes and the partially eroded long process of the incus.

In type III tympanoplasty, a columella procedure is performed by:

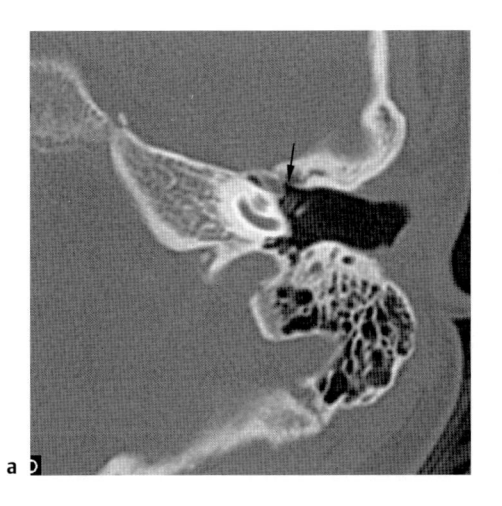

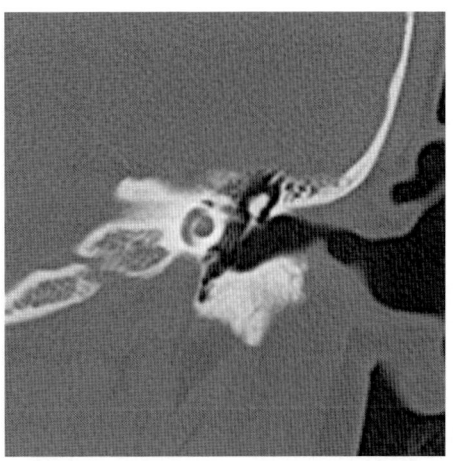

Fig. 1.**156** Displaced tympanostomy tube (arrow) into the middle ear cavity. **a** Axial, **b** coronal CT sections, left.

1. Placing the tympanic membrane or graft on the stapes (myringostapediopexy).
2. Placing a graft or partial ossicular chain replacement (PORP) between the tympanic membrane and the stapes head.
3. If the stapes crura are missing, placing a total ossicular chain replacement (TORP) between the tympanic membrane and the footplate of the stapes.

In type IV, a small closed middle ear space, including the round window and eustachian tube orifice, is created by placing the tympanic membrane graft or the remnant of the tympanic membrane on the promontory. The mobile footplate of the stapes is left exposed, covered by a thin skin graft.

Type V tympanoplasty is rarely performed and consists of a fenestration of the horizontal semicircular canal and preservation of the reduced middle ear space.

Type I and type II tympanoplasty are usually performed without mastoidectomy, types III, IV, and V in cases of canal-wall-down mastoidectomies.

Various grafting materials are used in tympanoplasty. Bone stents can be carved from the patient's removed ossicle or cortical mastoid bone (autografts). Temporal fascia is used to repair the tympanic membrane. Often the grafts come from donors and are preserved in temporal bone banks (homografts). Artificial grafting materials (allografts) are also used. Porous plastic material and biocompatible ceramics are well-tolerated and can be carved to proper size and shape.

■ Imaging Findings

Postoperative radiography of the ear is difficult and CT is essential to evaluate pathology correctly. The postoperative radiographic evaluation of the ear requires a knowledge of (1) the pathology for which the surgery was performed, (2) the type of surgery performed, and (3) the clinical and otoscopic findings that make further radiographic studies necessary. In postoperative radiography of the ear, an almost infinite spectrum of findings may occur depending on variables of the preoperative pathology, the surgical procedure, and recurrent or residual disease. Ideally, whenever the surgeon feels that at the end of the surgery there is residual disease, he or she should secure a postoperative study that can serve as a baseline for subsequent evaluations.

Mastoid Cavity

A disease-free surgical cavity appears as a well-defined and sharply outlined defect in the mastoid, epitympanum, and external canal depending on the type of surgery performed. Small defects in the tegmen produced during surgery are of no significance.

The mastoid cavity is usually clear unless some form of fibromuscular flap has been used to fill the mastoid. The radiologist must be informed about the use of such flaps. Following a radical mastoidectomy, the mastoid and external ear common cavity must be cleaned periodically to prevent accumulation of necrotic epithelial debris and cerumen. Usually the cavity is not completely filled with debris. However, if debris has been allowed to accumulate over a period of years, the cavity will appear completely cloudy. Infection and recurrent cholesteatoma will also fill and opacify the mastoid cavity, which becomes poorly defined and irregular due to osteitis of the walls, and lead to abscess formation. The trabeculae of the residual air cells become demineralized and, in long-standing infections, thickened. If recurrent cholesteatoma is filling the mastoidectomy cavity, there is expansion of the cavity and thinning of the walls, which leads to erosions in the tegmen and sinus plates (Fig. 1.**159**). Fistulae of the labyrinth may be present (Fig. 1.**160**). If a fistulized labyrinth becomes infected, partial or complete bony obliteration may occur (Fig. 1.**158**). Recurrent cholesteatoma may erode the facial canal and extend into the labyrinth (Fig. 1.**159**). Recurrent cholesteatoma should be differentiated from cholesterol granuloma cyst, which usually has a lower density and a smoother margin. In cases of doubt, MR will differentiate these lesions.

Stenosis of the External Auditory Canal

At times, following myringoplasty and tympanoplasty where the external canal is preserved, the canal becomes filled with a fibrous scar. CT will show the amount and extent of the soft-tissue stenosis of the external canal. When scar tissue fills the canal, the air column of the external canal ends in a blind sac lateral to the tympanic sulcus. After radical mastoidectomy, the external auditory canal may become stenosed or obliterated by fibrosis due to recurrent or persistent infection.

Middle Ear

The middle ear cavity may be normal in size or contracted but still aerated following successful mastoid surgery. Clouding of the middle ear cavity is evidence of recurrent infection or

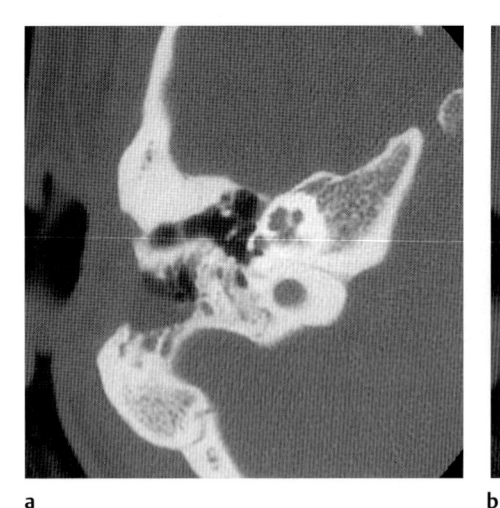

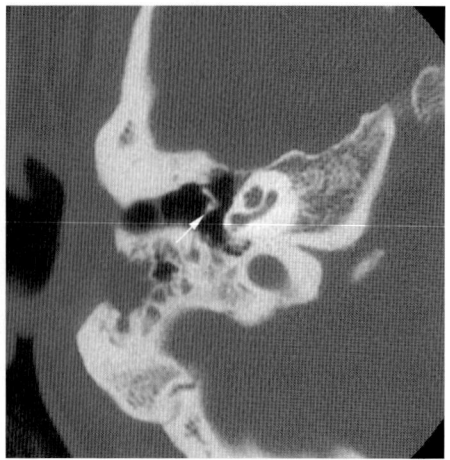

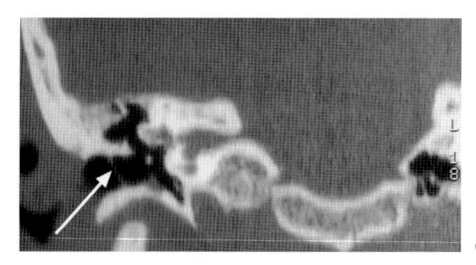

Fig. 1.**157** Post-right simple mastoidectomy and tympanoplasty. **a**, **b** Axial, **c** reformatted coronal CT sections. The tympanic membrane graft is lateralized (long arrow) and the transposed incus body appears rotated and displaced laterally (short arrow).

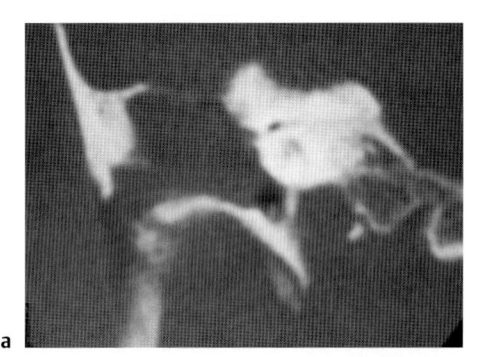

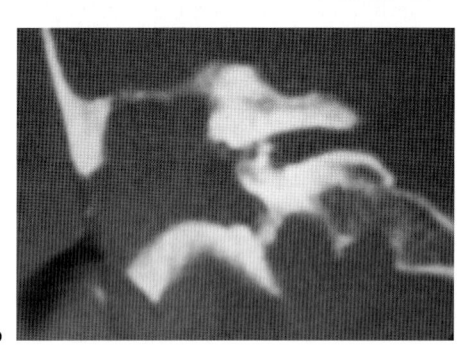

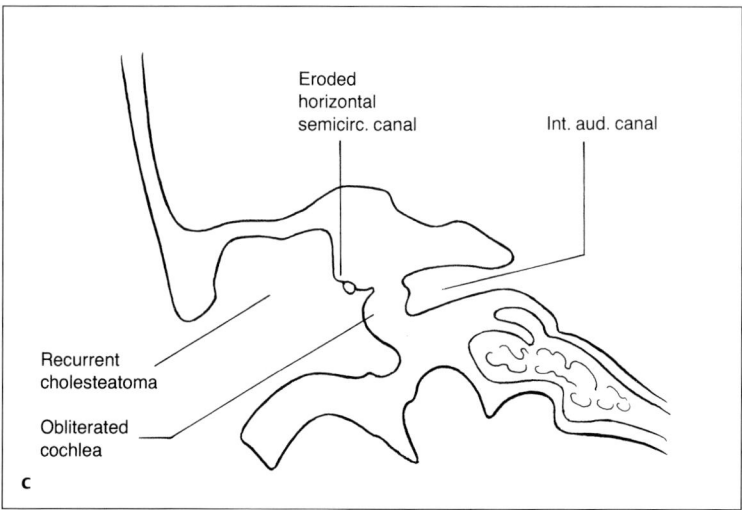

Fig. 1.**158** Cholesteatoma, recurrent, with obliterative labyrinthitis. **a**, **b** Coronal CT sections, right. There is soft-tissue stenosis of the external auditory canal, and a recurrent cholesteatoma fills the mastoidectomy cavity and middle ear. There is a horizontal semicircular canal fistula, which led to a suppurative labyrinthitis and consequent partial bony obliteration of the lumen of the cochlea, vestibule, and semicircular canals. **c** Diagram of **b**.

cholesteatoma. At times following tympanoplasty, the graft used to reconstruct the tympanic membrane becomes displaced laterally to the tympanic sulcus. Thickened, scarred, lateralized grafts are seen in axial and coronal CT sections (Fig. 1.**157**). Occasionally, radiopaque foreign bodies, such as the broken-off tip of a surgical instrument or a displaced tympanostomy tube, may be found within the middle ear cavity (Fig. 1.**156**).

Ossicles

The appearance of the ossicular chain will depend on whether the ossicles have been removed at surgery, left in place, or transposed. The body of the incus is the ossicle most often transposed. When properly transposed, the body of the incus can easily be seen lying in the posterosuperior quadrant of the middle ear between the tympanic membrane or malleus handle and the oval window region. With recurrent infection, the incus may be resorbed. Placement of the incus between the tympanic membrane or malleus handle and the stapes may fail, and the incus may migrate inferiorly, where it is visualized by CT (Fig. 1.**157**). Recurrent cholesteatoma can also displace a transposed incus inferiorly. When the ossicular chain has been eroded or has had to be removed at surgery, some form of ossicular reconstruction is usually performed. Homografts obtained from a temporal bone bank or allografts are used. Allografts are made of various materials. Metallic or ceramic (hydroxyapatite) ossicular replacement prosthesis are well visualized by CT, whereas plastic struts are often not recognizable.

Facial Canal

The appearance of the facial canal in the postoperative CT study varies with the extent of the pathology and the surgery. The facial canal may be normal and uninvolved, eroded by the original lesion, dissected, or traumatized at surgery (Fig. 1.**159**).

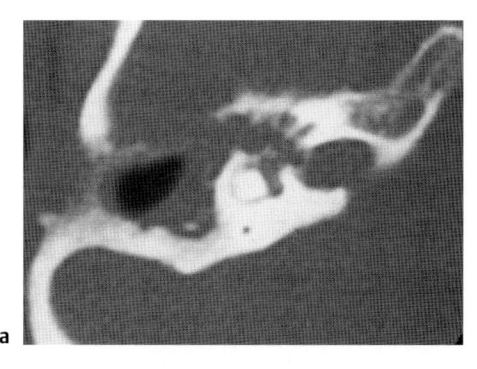

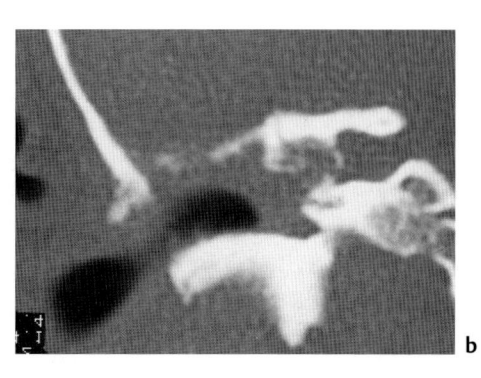

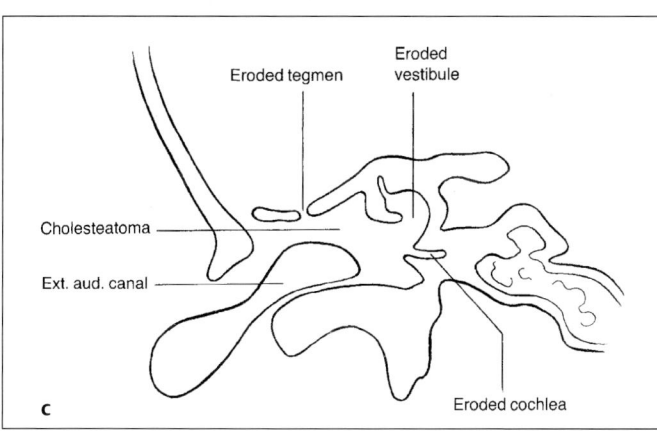

Fig. 1.**159** Cholesteatoma, recurrent, post–modified radical mastoidectomy. **a** Axial, **b** coronal CT sections, right. The recurrent cholesteatoma fills the medial portion of the mastoidectomy cavity and erodes into the cochlea and vestibule. The tegmen is eroded. The entire tympanic segment of the facial canal from the geniculate ganglion to the pyramidal turn is eroded. **c** Diagram of **b**.

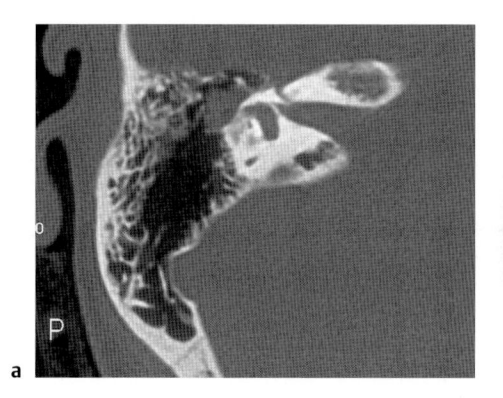

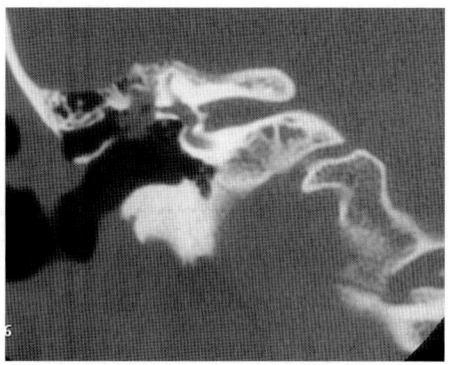

Fig. 1.**160** Cholesteatoma, recurrent, post–simple mastoidectomy. **a** Axial, **b** coronal CT sections, right. The posterosuperior canal wall is preserved. A soft-tissue mass fills the attic and erodes the horizontal semicircular canal with formation of a fistula. The head of the malleus is partially eroded; the incus was removed at surgery.

Petrous Pyramid

Follow-up MR studies are often performed in patients who have undergone removal of acoustic neuromas or other lesions of the cerebellopontine angle by a translabyrinthine approach. In these cases the large surgical tract extending from the mastoid to the internal auditory canal is usually filled, after removal of the tumor, by a large fat graft. The extent of the graft is well demonstrated by thin T1-weighted axial or coronal sections. After injection of contrast material, the same sequence is repeated using a fat-suppression mode in order to differentiate a possible enhancing mass indicative of a residual or recurrent tumor from the surrounding fat.

Meningocele and Meningoencephalocele

A soft-tissue mass contiguous to a defect in the tegmen of the mastoid suggests the possibility of a meningocele or meningoencephalocele. If the brain and meninges herniate into the relatively small space of the antrum or epitympanum, the constant pulsation of the cerebrospinal fluid is transmitted through the walls of the meningocele to cause a gradual resorption of the surrounding bony walls (Fig. 1.**161**). CT demonstrates the bony defect in the tegmen and a soft-tissue mass extending into the mastoid cavity (Figs. 1.**161**, 1.**162**). This soft-tissue lesion cannot be reliably differentiated from a recurrent cholesteatoma, since the absorption coefficients of both lesions are similar. A more definite diagnosis of meningocele by CT is reached by lumbar injection of a small amount of myelographic contrast, which will diffuse into the subarachnoid space and within the herniated mass. The differentiation between a meningocele and a cholesteatoma can best be made by MR. On MR images, cholesteatoma appears as a lesion of medium signal intensity in T1-weighted images and of higher intensity in T2-weighted images. A meningocele will have the same characteristics as cerebrospinal fluid: low signal intensity in T1-weighted images and high intensity in T2-weighted images (Fig. 1.**162**). On MR, encephaloceles have the same characteristics of the adjacent brain (Fig. 1.**161**), which are quite different from a cholesteatoma.

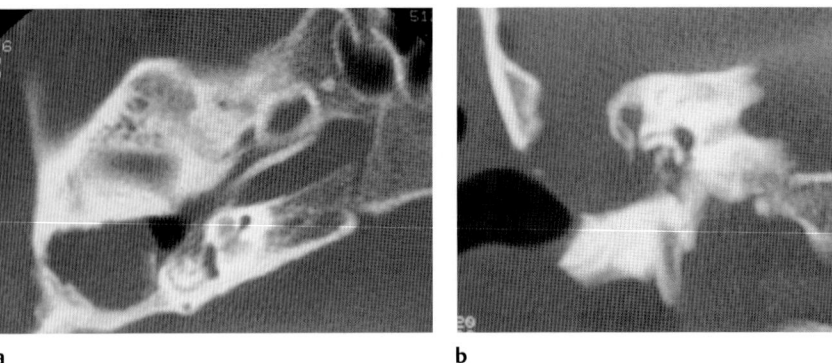

Fig. 1.**161** Meningoencephalocele, post–modified radical mastoidectomy. **a**, **b** Coronal CT images, **c** coronal T1W MR image. A large defect of the tegmen permits the herniation of a meningoencephalocele into the mastoid cavity.

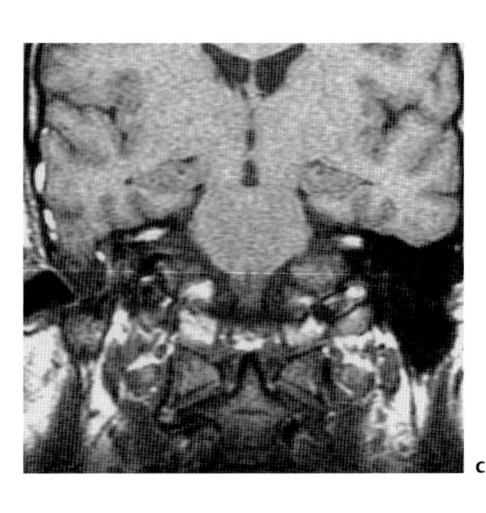

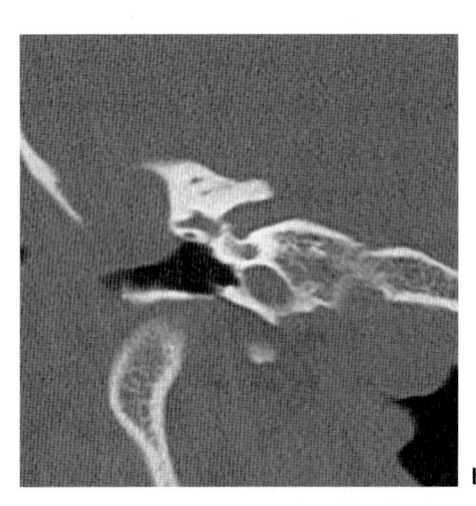

Fig. 1.**162** Meningocele, post–radical mastoidectomy. **a** Axial, **b** coronal CT images, **c** coronal T1W and **d** axial T2W MR images. There is a large defect in the tegmen with herniation of a meningocele into the mastoid cavity and external auditory canal.

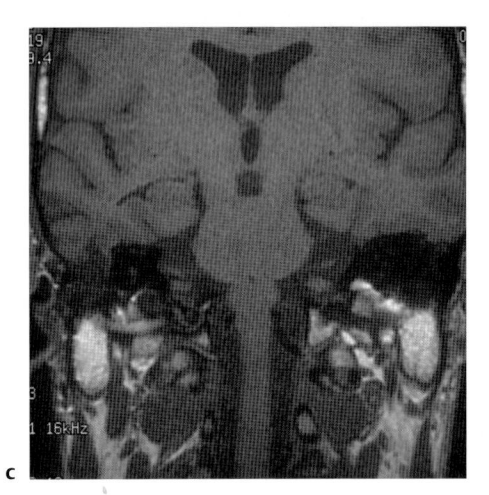

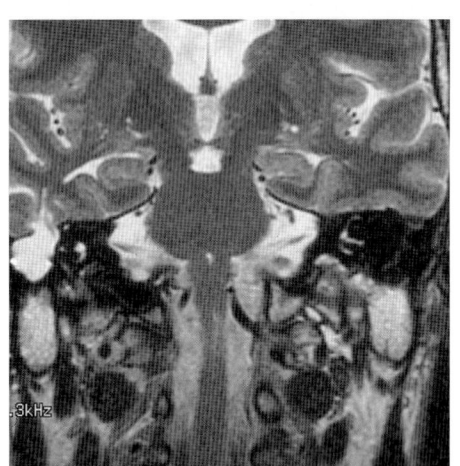

Postirradiation Changes

Radionecrosis may follow high-dose radiotherapy to the temporal bone for intracranial and extracranial malignancies. These changes occur several years after therapy and range from ulceration of the skin of the external auditory canal to extensive necrosis of the temporal squama, mastoid, and petrous pyramid (Fig. 1.**163**).

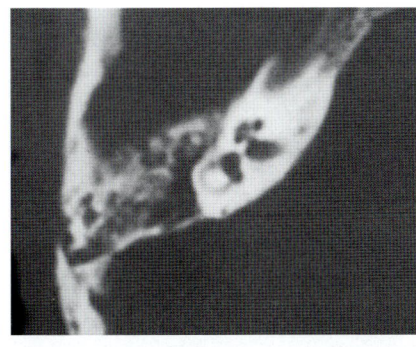

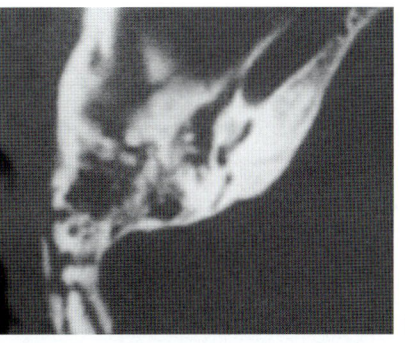

Fig. 1.**163** Osteoradionecrosis. **a**, **b** Axial CT sections, right. This patient was treated for carcinoma of the parotid 11 years previously. There is extensive dissolution and decalcification of the temporal squama and of the mastoid. The middle ear is clouded.

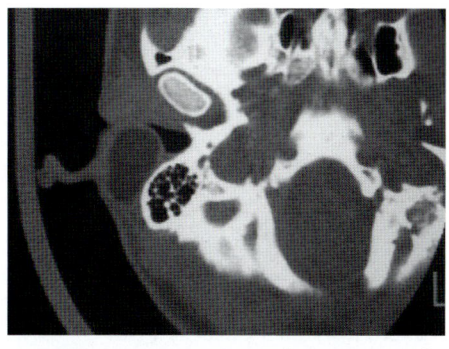

Fig. 1.**164** Lipoma retroauricular region. Axial CT section. A fat-containing mass encroaches upon and narrows the lumen of the cartilaginous portion of the right external auditory canal.

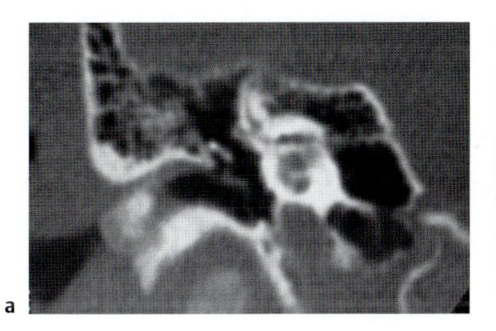

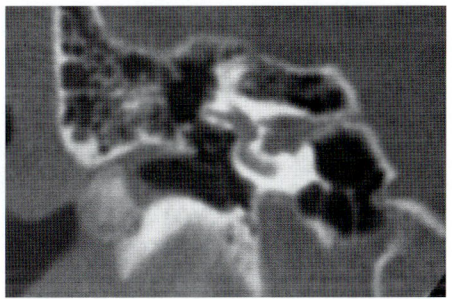

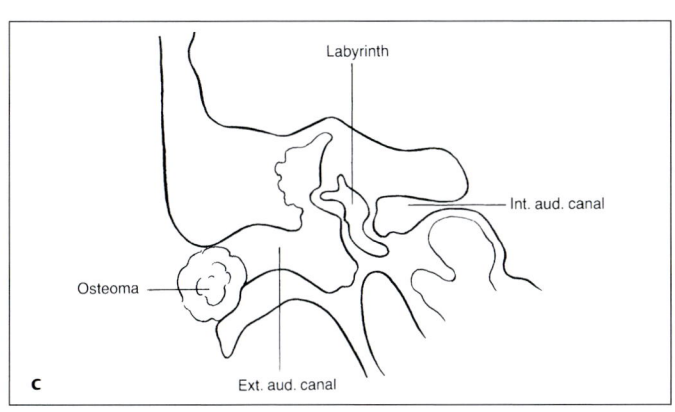

Fig. 1.**165** Osteoma, external auditory canal. **a**, **b** Coronal CT sections, right. A large concellous osteoma obstructs the lumen of the outer portion of the right external auditory canal. The middle ear cavity is normal. **c** Diagram of **b**.

Tumors

■ Benign Tumors

Benign tumors of the temporal bone originate in the squama, the mastoid, and the petrous pyramid or from adjacent structures, such as the meninges, the jugular vein, and cranial nerves. At times, benign tumors arising from adjacent structures can impinge on the temporal bone and external canal. Lipomas, and occasionally pleomorphic adenomas, of the parotid gland can become large enough to narrow or obstruct the external canal (Fig. 1.**164**). Acoustic schwannomas, because of their distinctive characteristics and diagnostic problems, will be discussed separately in Chapter 11.

Exostoses

Exostoses are the most common tumor of the external auditory canal. Exostoses represent local or diffuse areas of hyperostosis often caused by frequent swimming. They are usually multiple, may be large or small, and are often bilateral. Small lesions cause no symptoms, while large lesions obstruct the canal. Exostoses have a variable CT appearance. Small lesions appear as dense nodules protruding into the lumen of the external auditory canal. More diffuse lesions appear as dense bony ridges that stretch along the canal walls. Occasionally the entire circumference of the canal is thickened and the lumen is constricted.

Osteoma

Osteomas are benign bony tumors that are usually single and may occur anywhere in the temporal bone. There are two types: cancellous and compact. Radiographically, the compact lesion appears as a well-defined, occasionally lobulated dense bony mass. Cancellous osteomas appear as partially ossified masses. A common site is the external auditory canal, where the osteoma appears as a single bony mass occluding the lumen (Fig. 1.**165**). This lesion may cause retention of epithelial debris and cerumen, which results in cholesteatoma of the external auditory canal. Osteomas may also occur as a solitary lesion in the squama, mastoid, middle ear, and petrous pyramid. In the squama, an osteoma produces a hard mass on the surface of the bone, usually above

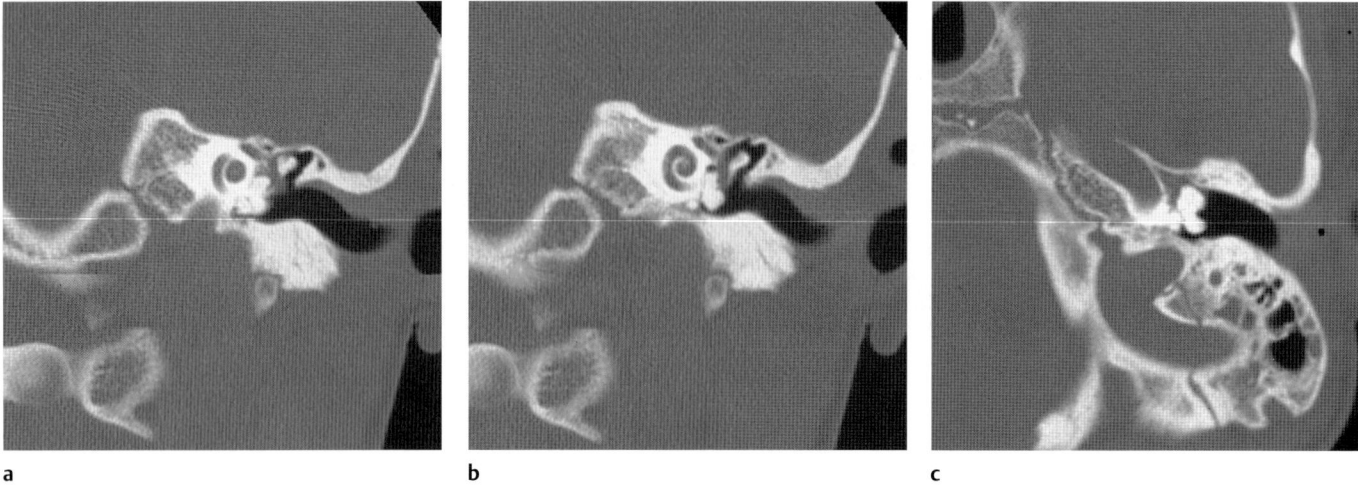

Fig. 1.**166** Osteoma of the right middle ear cavity. **a**, **b** Coronal, **c** axial CT sections. A bony mass arising from the promontory fills the inferior portion of the middle ear cavity. (Courtesy of Dr. B. Carter.)

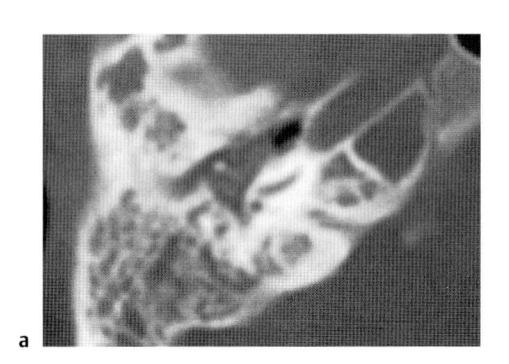

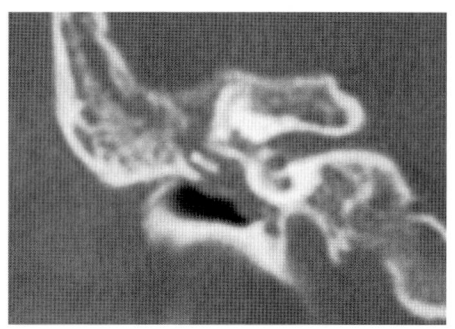

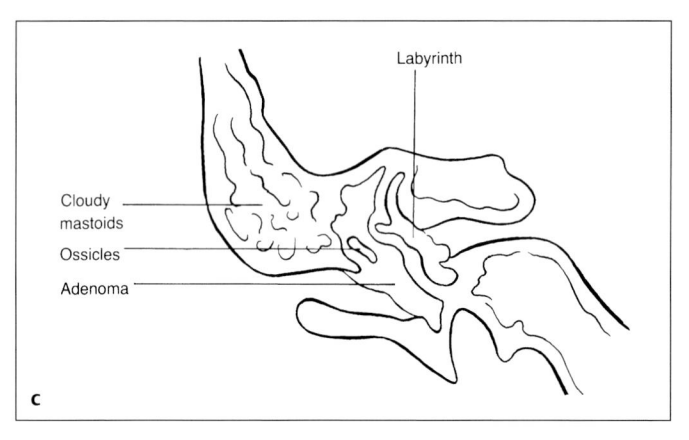

Fig. 1.**167** Adenoma, middle ear cavity. **a** Axial, **b** coronal CT sections, right. A lobulated soft-tissue mass fills most of the mesotympanum and attic, surrounding but not eroding the ossicles. The tumor extends into the sinus tympani and mastoid antrum. The lateral wall of the attic is intact. The mastoid air cells are cloudy as a result of fluid. **c** Diagram of **b**.

and posterior to the auricle. When they occur in the mastoid, osteomas are usually asymptomatic unless they encroach upon the facial nerve.

Osteomas may lie in the middle ear and cause conductive hearing loss by impinging upon the ossicular chain (Fig. 1.**166**). In the petrous pyramid, osteomas are usually situated in the region of the porus of the internal auditory canal. Rarely they may encroach on the neurovascular structures of the internal auditory canal and cause hearing and vestibular disturbances.

Adenoma

Adenomas usually arise from ceruminous glands of the cutaneous lining of the fibrocartilaginous portion of the external auditory canal. As with other benign tumors of the external canal, imaging is not indicated unless the lesion obstructs the canal and obscures the view of the tympanic membrane and middle ear. Middle ear adenomas are rare. The lesion has a tendency to recur after surgery and may degenerate into adenocarcinoma. A middle ear adenoma appears in CT sections as a diffuse or localized nonspecific soft-tissue mass (Fig. 1.**167**). There is no bony erosion unless malignant degeneration of the adenoma into adenocarcinoma has occurred.

Hemangioma

Hemangiomas are rare tumors of the temporal bone. The clinical and radiographic features depend on the anatomical location.

They may occur in the temporal squama, where they produce an area of radiolucency with typical spokelike trabeculation. A hemangioma of the external canal can fill and enlarge the bony canal. Often there are phleboliths within the lesion. Figure

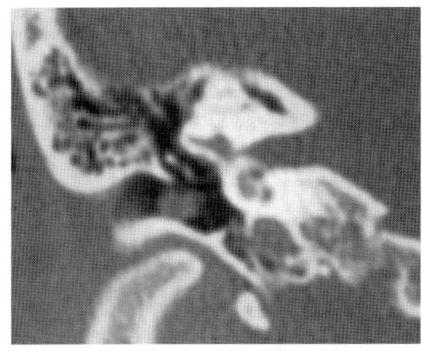

Fig. 1.**168** Capillary hemanigoma, right tympanic membrane. Coronal CT. A well-defined soft-tissue mass lies in the medial portion of the external auditory canal adjacent to the outer surface of the tympanic membrane.

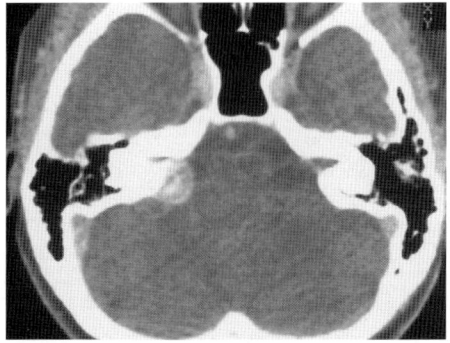

Fig. 1.**169** Meningioma, right cerebellopontine angle. **a, b** Postinfusion axial CT sections. A partially calcified soft-tissue mass protrudes from the internal auditory canal into the cerebellopontine cistern. Hyperostotic changes narrow the internal auditory canal.

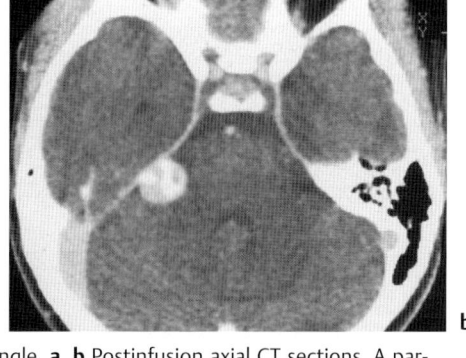

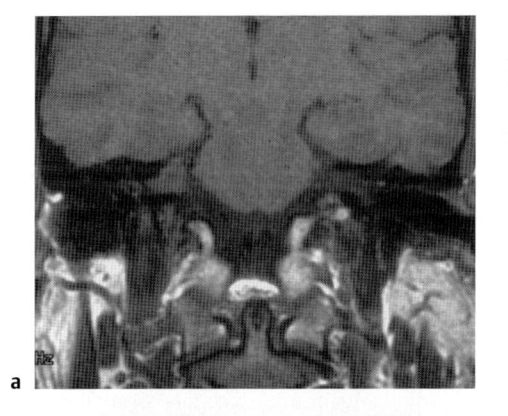

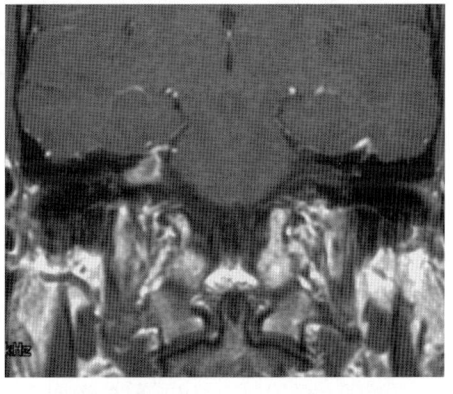

Fig. 1.**170** Meningioma, right internal auditory canal. MR images: **a** coronal precontrast, **b** coronal, **c, d** axial postcontrast. A soft-tissue mass fills the internal auditory canal and extends into the adjacent cerebellopontine cistern. The partially calcified mass undergoes a nonhomogeneous enhancement.

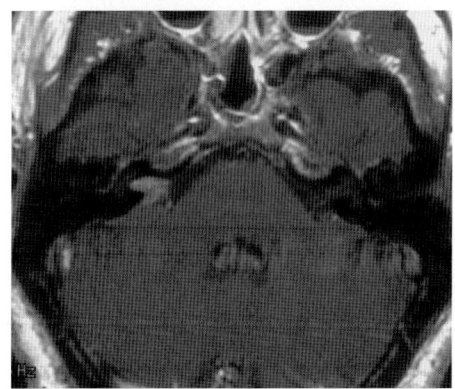

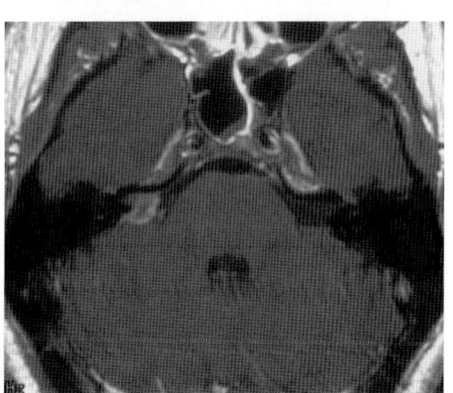

1.**168** shows a hemangioma arising from the tympanic membrane. A hemangioma of the middle ear appears on CT images as a poorly defined soft-tissue mass that may be associated with ossicular erosion. With CT, a hemangioma of the middle ear can be differentiated from a glomus jugulare tumor because the hemangioma does not erode the hypotympanic floor, but it cannot be distinguished from a glomus tympanicum. In MR, hemangiomas have a characteristic appearance; the mass has a low signal in TI-weighted images that becomes uniformly bright in T2-weighted images and undergoes a strong and uniform enhancement after injection of contrast material. Hemangiomas of the petrous pyramid produce a mottled demineralization with multiple honeycombed radiolucencies and at times bony spicules extending into the adjacent cranial cavity.

A hemangioma may lie in the internal auditory canal and cerebellopontine angle and mimic an acoustic schwannoma. Differentiation can be made by MRI or angiography including subtraction arteriography.

Meningioma

Meningiomas arise from the meningeal covering (arachnoid villi and arachnoid epithelial-type cells) of the temporal bone and from meningeal extension within the internal auditory canal.

The most common type of meningioma arises from the dura and the arachnoid covering the petrous ridge. Radiographically the findings vary from hyperostosis (Fig. 1.**169**) to moth-eaten erosion, which can progress to frank destruction of the petrous bone. Often there is a combination of these findings. Calcifications are often present within the tumor mass (Figs. 1.**169**, 1.**170**). Another form of meningioma is the en plaque lesion. Some meningiomas erode the tegmen and break into the middle ear

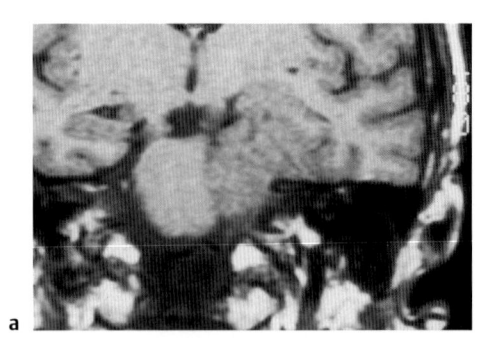

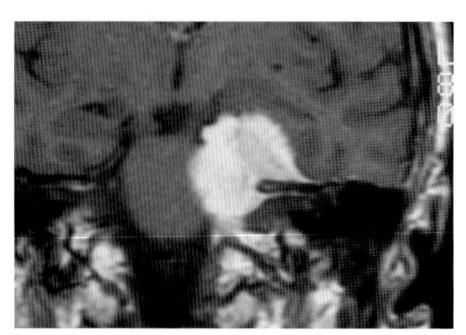

Fig. 1.**171** Meningioma, left cerebellopontine angle. Coronal T1W MR sections, **a** before and **b** after injection of contrast material. A large enhancing mass arising from the tentorial notch extends inferiorly into the cerebellopontine cistern and superiorly into the middle cranial fossa. Note the en plaque involvement (tail sign) of the meninges lining the superior wall of the internal auditory canal and the superior petrous ridge.

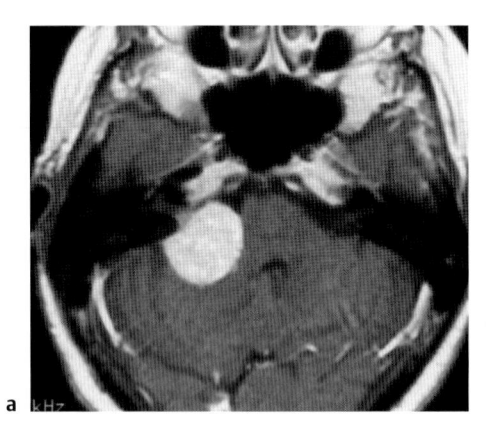

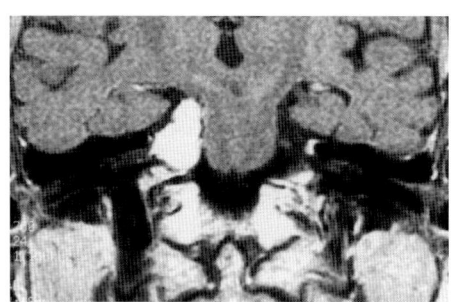

Fig. 1.**172** Meningioma, right cerebellopontine angle. MR images: **a** axial, **b** coronal T1W postinfusion. A large enhancing soft-tissue mass extends from the cerebellopontine cistern to the tentorial notch. The mass indents the brainstem and compresses the fourth ventricle. The tumor does not involve the internal auditory canal.

cavity. The occasional ectopic meningioma can involve the middle ear cavity without erosion of the tegmen or intracranial involvement. Facial nerve involvement can occur in the region of the geniculate ganglion. Erosion of the labyrinth is rare.

Precontrast and postcontrast CT and MRI are indicated in cases where a meningioma is suspected, since these techniques will demonstrate the involvement of the base of the skull and the presence of any intracranial component of the tumor (Figs. 1.**170**–1.**172**). En plaque meningiomas are frequently not recognized by CT because of lack of enhancement of the sheetlike tumor. Meningiomas arising within the internal auditory canal and cerebellopontine angle cistern mimic acoustic schwannomas clinically and radiographically (Fig. 1.**170**). Differential diagnosis can be made if there is hyperostosis of the walls of the internal auditory canal and of the crista falciformis, or if there are calcifications scattered within the mass.

On MR, meningiomas have a heterogenous appearance. The majority are isodense with the surrounding brain tissue in T1-weighted images and appear as bright masses of high signal intensity in T2-weighted images. Some tumors, however, maintain a low signal in the T2-weighted images, which is strongly suggestive of a meningioma. Following the injection of contrast material, meningiomas undergo a strong and homogeneous enhancement (Figs. 1.**171**, 1.**172**). Calcifications within the tumor produce areas of signal void (Fig. 1.**170**). En plaque meningiomas are usually recognizable on MR as areas of meningeal thickening and enhancement. A typical but not diagnostic finding of meningioma is the so-called dura tail sign produced by en plaque extension of the tumor mass or by reactive mesothelial tissue (Fig. 1.**171**).

Inflammation of the meninges as it occurs in meningitis and after surgery should not be confused with an en plaque meningioma. Both lesions enhance, but the inflamed leptomeninges are not or are only minimally thickened. In meningitis, the involvement is usually diffuse rather than localized as in meningiomas (see Fig. 1.**212**).

Schwannomas of the Facial Nerve

Intratemporal neuromas or schwannomas of the facial nerve occur rarely.

The clinical findings depend on the site of origin and size of the lesion. Lesions arising within the internal auditory canal may present symptoms mimicking an acoustic schwannoma (see Fig. 1.**207**). Schwannomas that arise within the facial canal usually cause a peripheral facial paralysis or tic. When a neuroma arises within the tympanic portion of the facial nerve canal, the first symptom may be conductive deafness due to encroachment of the tumor on the ossicular chain (Fig. 1.**173**). In our series of facial neuromas, the most common site of involvement is the geniculate ganglion region (Fig. 1.**174**).

Imaging Findings

Initially, facial nerve schwannomas cause thickening of the nerve and expansion of the lumen of the bony nerve canal (Figs. 1.**173**, 1.**175**). To detect early changes, it is necessary to compare the affected and normal sides. Enlargement of the lesion results in erosion of the bony canal and involvement of the adjacent structures of the petrous pyramid, middle ear, and mastoid (Figs. 1.**173**). When the tumor extends into the middle ear, a well-defined soft-tissue mass appears (Figs. 1.**173**).

CT shows expansion or erosion of the facial canal (Fig. 1.**175**) and, if the tumor extends into the aerated middle ear, the actual tumor mass (Fig. 1.**173**). MR is the study of choice for the assessment of the size and extension of the lesion. Initially the involved portion of the facial nerve appears thickened (Fig. 1.**175**) and will enhance following i.v. injection of contast medium. As the tumor enlarges, the MR images demonstrate both intratemporal and intracranial involvement. Postcontrast T1-weighted images should be obtained since the tumor undergoes a marked and homogeneous enhancement (Figs. 1.**174**, 1.**175**).

Tumors 99

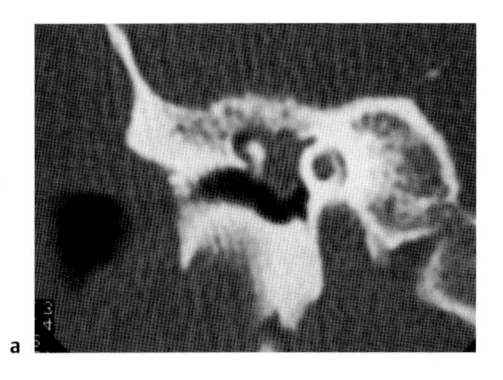

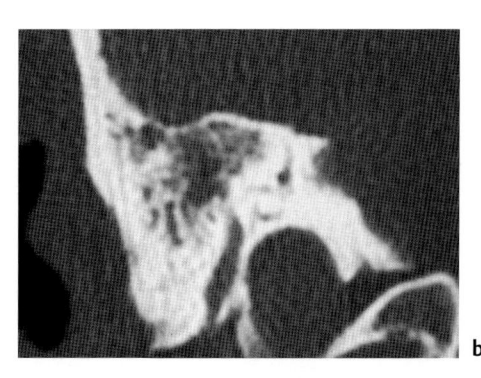

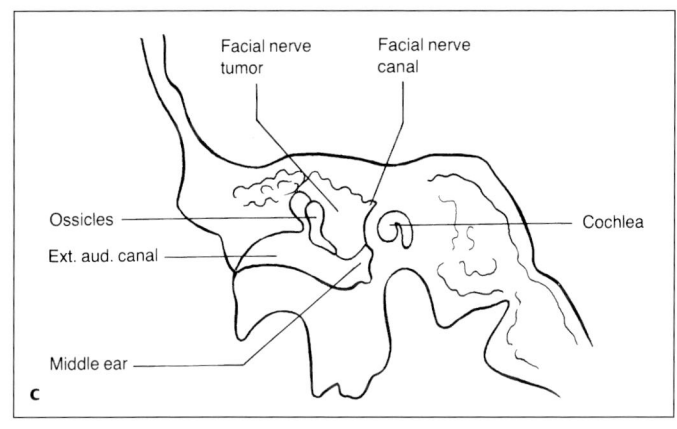

Fig. 1.**173** Facial nerve neuroma. **a**, **b** Coronal CT sections, right. A soft-tissue mass fills the middle ear medial to the malleus (**a**). In **b**, a section 6 mm posterior, the extension of the neuroma into the vertical portion of the facial nerve has produced an expansion of the bony canal. **c** Diagram of **a**.

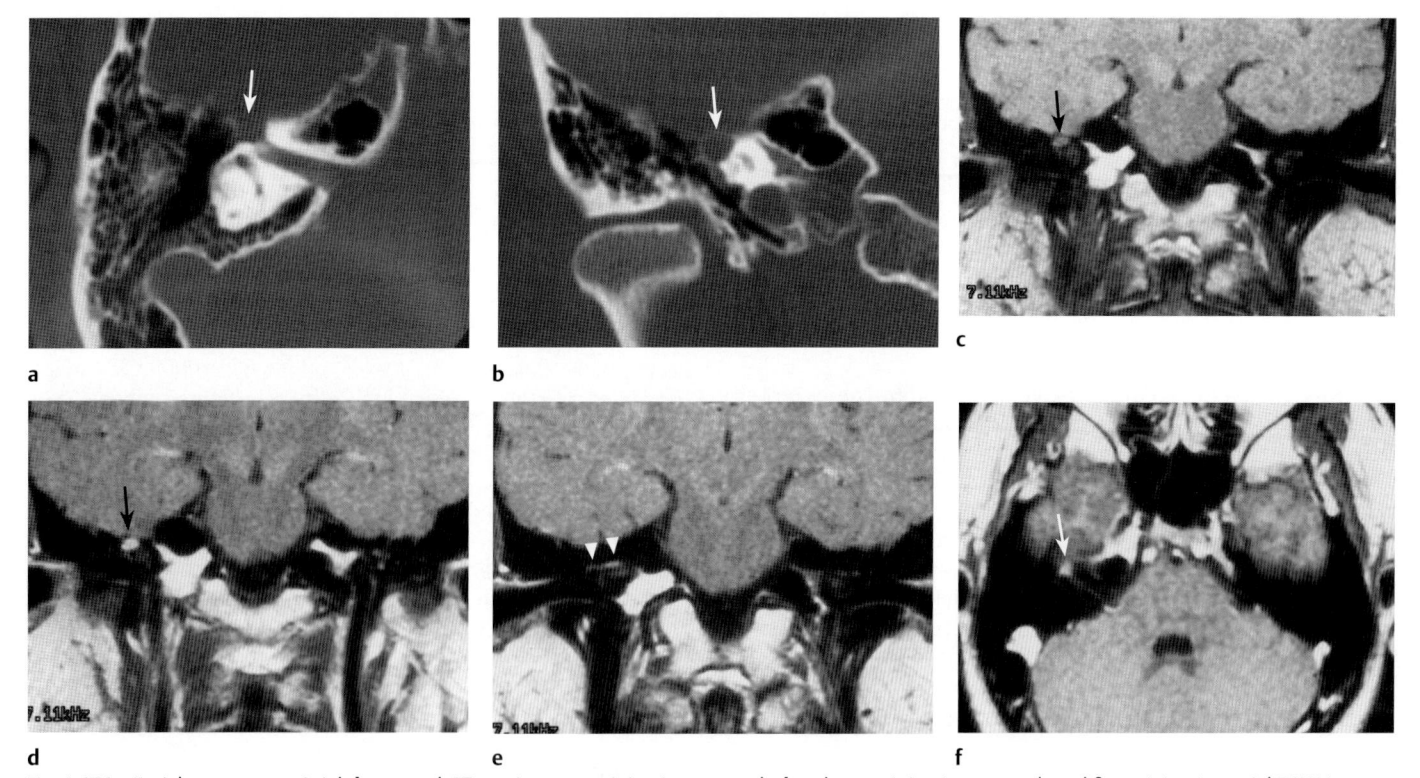

Fig. 1.**174** Facial neuroma. **a** Axial, **b** coronal CT sections; **c** preinjection coronal, **d** and **e** postinjection coronal, and **f** postinjection axial T1W images. The facial canal is expanded in the region of the anterior genu (arrow) by an enhancing soft mass. Notice in **e** the enhancement of the facial nerve within the internal auditory canal (arrowheads) owing to extension of the lesion.

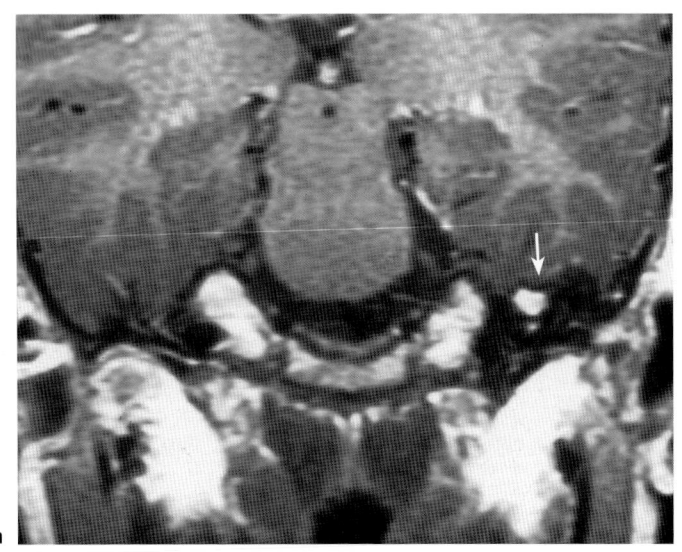

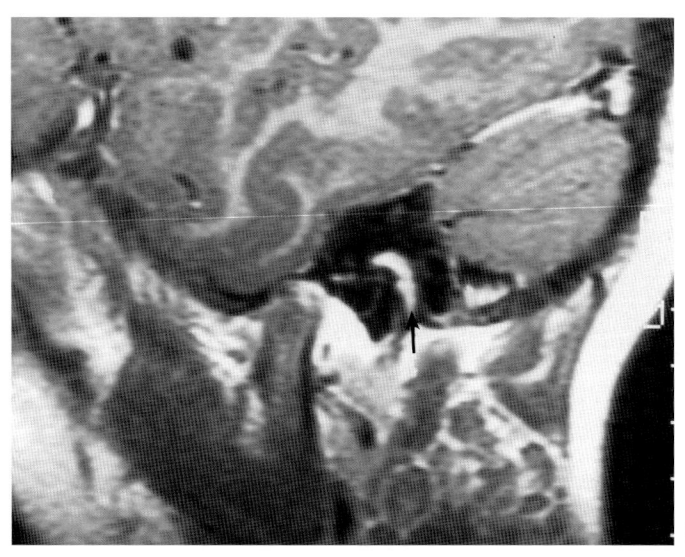

Fig. 1.175 Left facial neurofibroma. **a** Coronal, **b** sagittal T1W MR images after injection of contrast material. The entire intratemporal facial nerve is markedly thickened and enhanced (arrows).

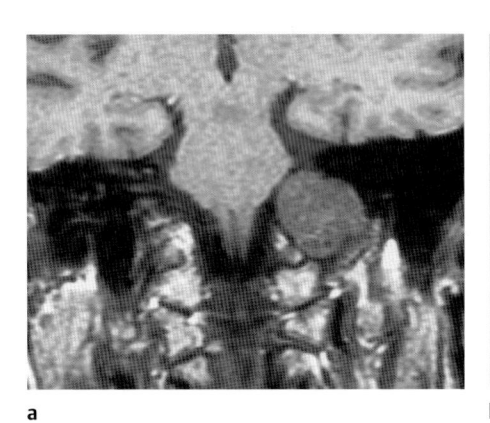

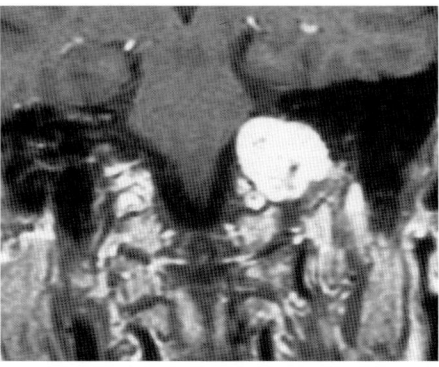

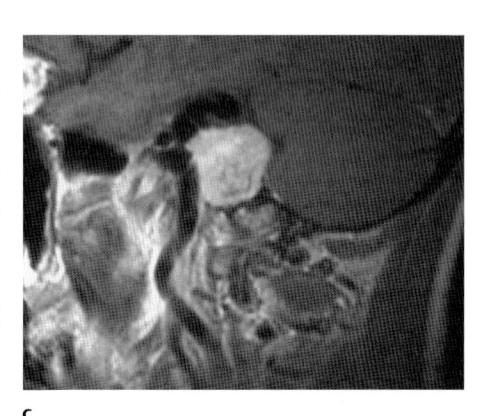

Fig. 1.176 Vagus nerve schwannoma. **a** T1W coronal precontrast MR image; **b**, **c** T1W coronal and sagittal postcontrast MR images. An enhancing soft-tissue mass erodes the posteroinferior aspect of the left petrous pyramid. The jugular fossa is enlarged, but the tumor does not extend into the middle ear cavity. The jugular bulb is compressed by the mass.

Fifth Nerve Neuromas

Neuromas of the fifth cranial nerve arising from the cisternal portion of the nerve or from the gasserian ganglion tend to enlarge superiorly into the middle cranial fossa. Occasionally these tumors cause indentation and erosion of the superior petrous ridge medial to the internal auditory canal. Axial and coronal CT sections will demonstrate the site and degree of bony involvement. The tumor mass is better demonstrated in coronal and axial MR images. The lesion varies from thickening of the nerve to masses of variable size, characterized by high signal intensity in the T2-weighted images and intense enhancement.

Ninth, Tenth, Eleventh, and Twelfth Nerve Neuromas

Neuromas of the 9th, 10th, 11th, and 12th nerves arise in the jugular fossa or in the hypoglossal canal. They produce paralytic lesions of various types. As the tumor enlarges, it produces a progressive expansion of the jugular fossa and hypoglossal canal similar to a glomus jugulare tumor (Fig. 1.176). Neuromas can also extend intracranially into the posterior cranial fossa and the foramen magnum.

In contrast to glomus jugulare tumors, neuromas of cranial nerves IX, X, XI, and XII do not extend into the middle ear unless very large, and they produce a more sharply defined expansion of the jugular fossa than do glomus tumors. The diagnosis and evaluation of the size and extent of the lesion is made by CT (including bolus infusion) or MR imaging.

Contrast CT will show an enhanced soft-tissue mass. The computer-generated time–density curve is quite different from the high peak curves and rapid washout phase of the glomus tumors. Schwannomas demonstrate slow washout phase.

MR images demonstrate a mass with a high signal intensity in the T2-weighted images, which undergoes homogeneous enhancement after injection of contrast material (Fig. 1.176).

Eosinophilic Granuloma

Eosinophilic granuloma (Langerhans cell histiocytosis) is a benign chronic granuloma related to other diseases of the reticuloendothelial system such as Letterer–Siwe, Hand–Schüller–Christian, and histiocystosis X.[12] The letter X was used to indicate the unknown origin of the histiocytes. It is now known that the hystiocytes are morphologically and immunologically identical to the Langerhans cells. The etiology is unknown, but eosinophilic granuloma is commonly classified as a benign tumor.

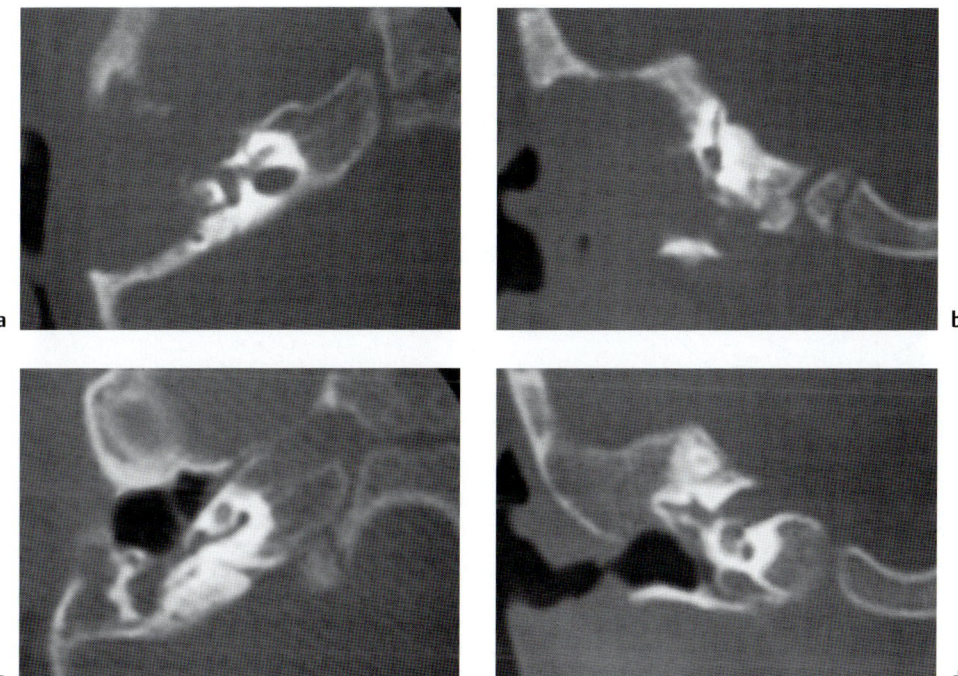

Fig. 1.**177** Eosinophilic granuloma. **a** Axial, **b** coronal CT sections, right. A large soft-tissue mass fills and erodes the bony contour of the mastoid, external auditory canal, middle ear, and the labyrinthine capsule in the region of the horizontal semicircular canal. **c, d** Coronal CT images four months following radiation therapy. There has been a dramatic improvement owing to shrinkage of the soft-tissue mass and partial remineralization of the involved portion of the temporal bone.

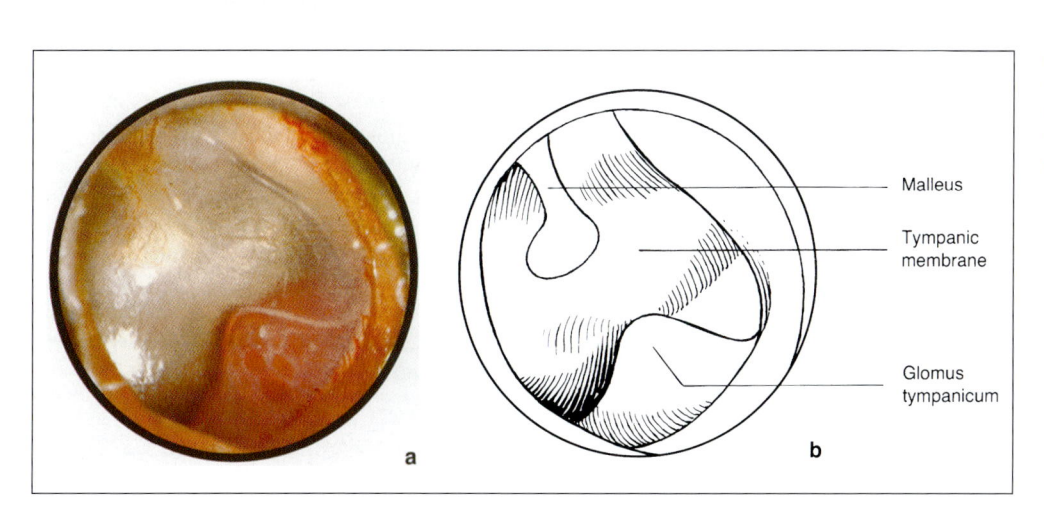

Fig. 1.**178 a** Glomus tympanicum, otoscopic findings, left. A purple-red mass lies in the inferior portion of the middle ear in contact with the tympanic membrane. **b** Diagram of **a**.

Eosinophilic granuloma of the temporal bone usually involves the mastoid. Radiographically the findings are similar to an acute mastoiditis with areas of coalescence. The involved mastoid air cells appear cloudy, and the trabecular pattern is destroyed with formation of a cavity. The mastoid cortex may be thinned, destroyed, or expanded (Fig. 1.**177**).

As the disease progresses, the external auditory canal and middle ear cavity become involved, with the destruction of their walls. Hence, the lesion may extend to the petrous pyramid and labyrinth. At this stage it may be difficult to differentiate the process from a malignant tumor, particularly from rhabdomyosarcoma in children. When the disorder affects the squama, eosinophilic granuloma causes lytic areas of variable size. There is no reactive new bone at the margins of the lesion. Following radiation therapy there is usually a partial or complete remineralization of the involved portion of the temporal bone (Fig. 1.**177**).

Glomus Tumors

Glomus tumors, also called chemodectomas and nonchromaffin paragangliomas, are benign tumors arising in the middle ear or jugular fossa from minute glomus bodies, which are found chiefly in the jugular fossa and on the promontory of the middle ear.

The symptomatology depends on the site and size of the lesion. Lesions arising in the jugular fossa, called glomus jugulare tumors, encroach upon the adjacent cranial nerves and may cause paralysis of these nerves. The tumor usually involves the middle ear, where it may cause conductive deafness by encroaching upon the ossicular chain. As the lesion enlarges, it extends into the mastoid and external auditory canal. Involvement of the labyrinth causes tinnitus, sensorineural deafness, and vertigo. Glomus tympanicum is a lesion that arises from glomus bodies along the Jacobson's nerve on the promontory. Early, these lesions are small and confined to the middle ear, where they may encroach upon the ossicles. If the lesion enlarges inferiorly and destroys the hypotympanic floor, it becomes indistinguishable from a glomus jugulare tumor.

Otoscopic Findings

The characteristic finding of a glomus tumor is the presence of a reddish purple mass in the middle ear. In the early stages, the mass lies medial to the intact tympanic membrane. Contact of the tumor with the tympanic membrane often causes a curvil-

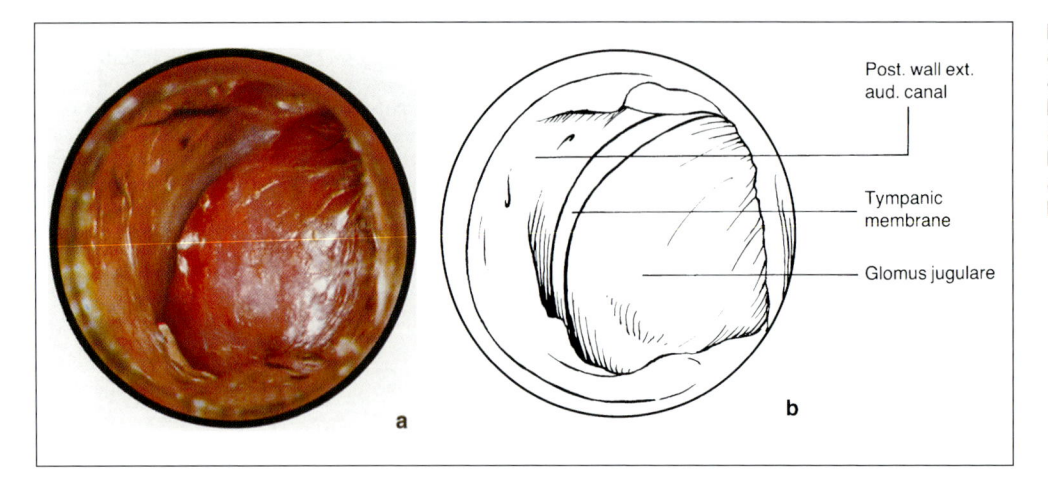

Fig. 1.**179 a** Glomus jugulare tumor, otoscopic findings, right. A large glomus jugular fills the middle ear and herniates the tympanic membrane into the external auditory canal. The lesion has a characteristic red-purple color of glomus tumors.
b Diagram of **a**.

inear air–tumor interface. Since both glomus jugular and glomus tympanicum tumors arise in the inferior portion of the middle ear, otoscopic differentiation between the two types is impossible (Figs. 1.**178**, 1.**179**).

As the lesions enlarge, the tympanic membrane is sloughed, and reddish purple polypoid masses appear in the external auditory canal. These polypoid lesions bleed easily and profusely when manipulated, while inflammatory polyps of chronic otitis media bleed only slightly. The diagnosis should be confirmed by biopsy. This procedure should be performed after radiographic evaluation to avoid obscuring the mass by hemorrhage. When the tumor is confined to the middle ear and lying behind an intact tympanic membrane, the otoscopic appearance of a glomus tumor may be confused with a high jugular bulb, an ectopic internal carotid artery (see Fig. 1.**48**), or a cholesterol granuloma of the middle ear (Figs. 1.**178**, 1.**179**).

Imaging Techniques

CT is the most useful technique for the diagnosis and evaluation of the extent of glomus tympanicum tumors. MR is indicated in larger lesions that extend outside of the confines of the middle ear. Arteriography and venography have been largely supplanted by CT and MR angiography.

CT

Axial and coronal CT sections before and after bolus injection of contrast are indicated. Images are studied for soft tissue and bone. A dynamic CT study of a preselected section showing the tumor mass will differentiate a glomus tumor from other vascular massses such as high jugular bulb. The computer-generated density–time curve reveals a high, early, quasi-arterial peak, rather than a delayed venous peak of a high jugular bulb (Fig. 1.**180**).

MR

The MR study can be performed with a surface coil to obtain better image definition. The tumor appears as a mass of medium signal intensity in both T1-weighted and T2-weighted images, containing multiple small areas of signal void produced by blood vessels (Figs. 1.**185**, 1.**186**). The mass undergoes enhancement following injection of contrast material. In order to differentiate the tumor mass from the adjacent diploic bone, the postcontrast T1-weighted images should be obtained in the fat-suppression mode. Whereas intracranial extension is well-outlined by both CT and MR with contrast, extracranial extension is far better seen in MR images because the glomus has a signal intensity different from the surrounding structures, in particular muscles. In addition, involvement of the jugular vein and carotid artery is usually seen in routine spin-echo or gradient-echo images (Fig. 1.**185**). Whenever the vessels are not well seen, a MR or CT angiogram should be performed. For MR angiography, we use the three-dimensional time-of-flight technique for the carotid artery and two-dimensional time-of-flight technique for the jugular vein.

Arteriography

Arteriography is indicated to identify the feeding vessels of the glomus tumor prior to embolization or surgical ligation and tumor removal. Common carotid artery injection is used to visualize feeding vessels, which can come from both the external and internal carotids. The ascending pharyngeal artery is the most common feeder. A vertebral arteriogram will visualize feeders from the vertebrobasal circulation.

Subtraction should be used to delineate the vascular mass and feeding vessels that are otherwise obscured by the density of the surrounding temporal bone (Fig. 1.**187**).

Retrograde Venography

Retrograde jugular venography is seldom indicated since MR images can visualize tumor extension into the vein (Fig. 1.**188**). The study is done by percutaneous puncture of the jugular vein or through the femoral vein with a Seldinger needle. The stylet is withdrawn and a guide wire is advanced through the needle lumen into the internal jugular vein to the bony roof of the jugular fossa. The needle is removed and a radiopaque polyethylene catheter is threaded into the jugular vein over the guide wire, which is in turn removed.

Imaging Findings

Glomus Tympanicum

CT and MR are important in establishing the diagnosis and are essential in determining the size and extent of the lesion.

In glomus tympanicum, CT examination shows a soft-tissue mass of variable size, usually in the lower portion of the tympanic cavity (Figs. 1.**180**, 1.**181**). When inflammation or serous fluid fills the middle ear and surrounds the tumor, the contour of the mass is obscured. A large glomus tympanicum filling the entire middle ear causes a bulge of the tympanic membrane laterally and a concave erosion of the bone of the promontory. The lesion may also extend posteriorly into the mastoid and inferiorly into the hypotympanic cells. The floor of the hypotympanum is usually intact. Should the lesion erode into the jugular fossa, the tumor becomes indistinguishable from a glomus jugulare. Jugular bulb and jugular vein are normal.

Tumors 103

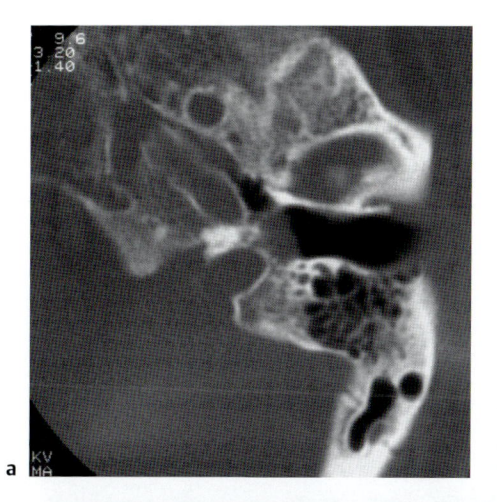

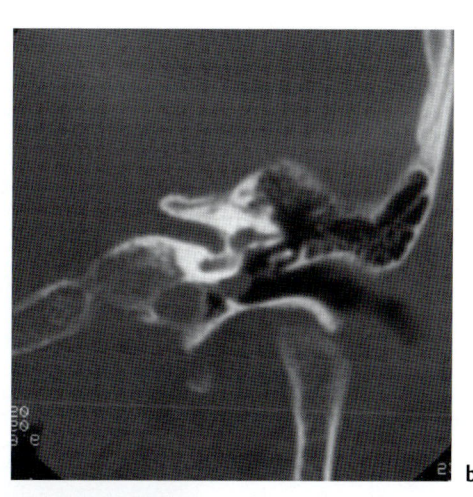

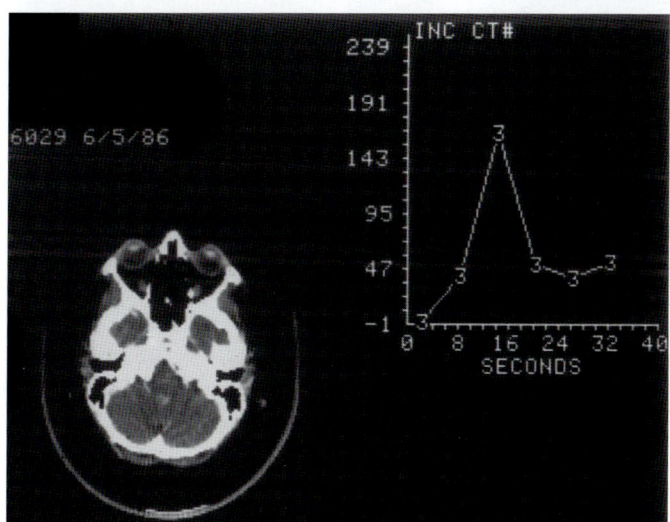

Fig. 1.**180** Glomus tympanicum. **a** axial, **b** coronal CT images; **c** time–density curve. An enhancing soft-tissue mass fills the lower portion of the middle ear cavity. The dynamic study reveals the tumor to be highly vascular with arterial peak time.

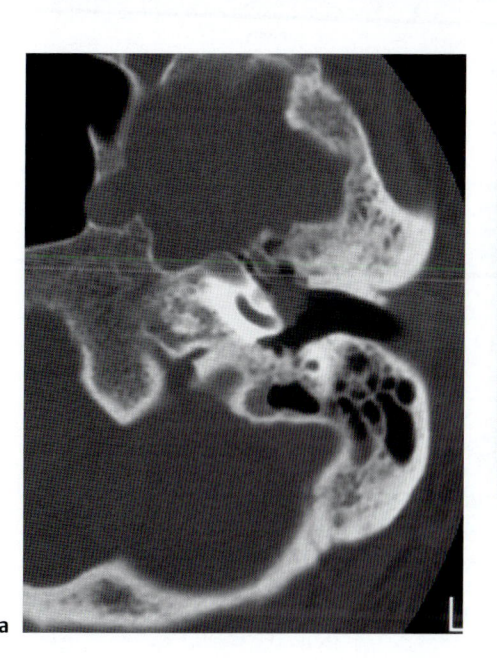

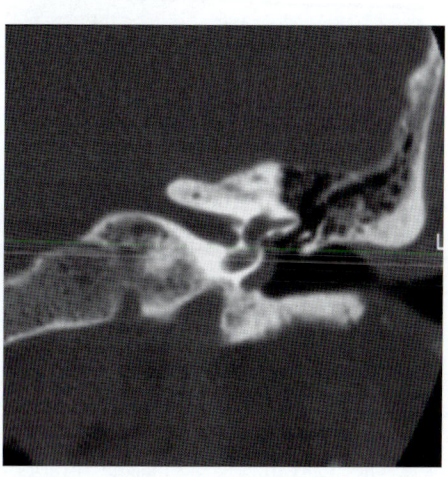

Fig. 1.**181** Left glomus tympanicum. **a** Axial, **b** coronal CT sections. A well-defined soft-tissue mass lies in the inferior portion of the mesotympanum. The remainder of the middle ear is aerated and no bony erosion is identified.

Glomus Jugulare

Typical CT findings of a glomus jugulare tumor are (Figs. 1.**182**–1.**186**):

1. Erosion of the cortical outline and enlargement of the jugular fossa. The size of the jugular fossa is extremely variable, and asymmetry of the two jugular fossae is a common finding. A large jugular fossa is not indicative of a glomus tumor unless there is associated cortical erosion.
2. Erosion of the triangular bony septum that divides the jugular fossa from the outer opening of the carotid canal. This finding appears best on sagittal images.

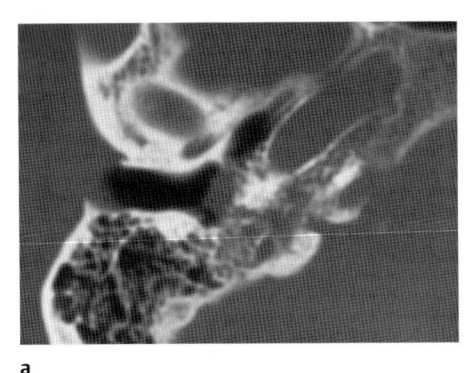

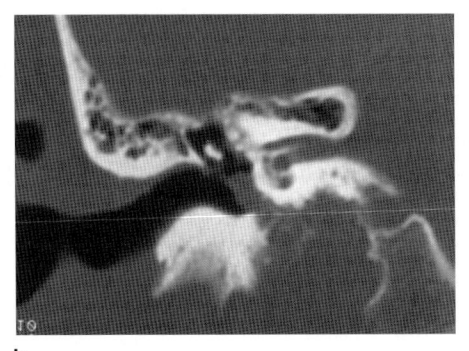

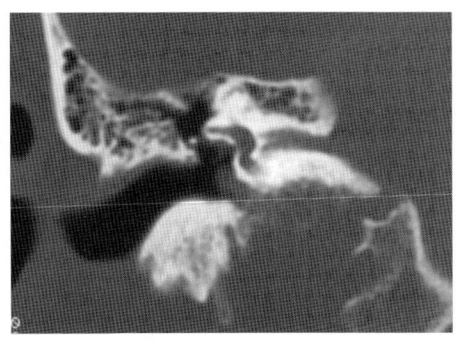

Fig. 1.**182** Glomus jugulare. **a** Axial, **b**, **c** coronal CT sections, right. The jugular fossa appears enlarged, and the hyptympanic cells and floor appear eroded. An enhancing soft-tissue mass protrudes into the mesotympanum and impinges on the incudostapedial joint.

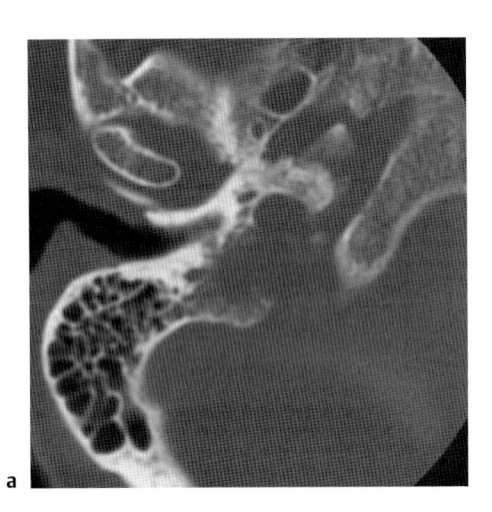

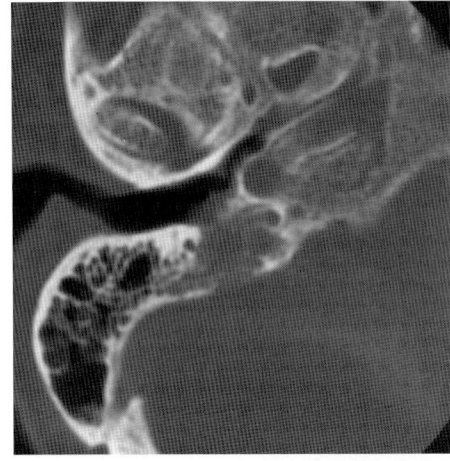

Fig. 1.**183** Glomus jugulare. **a**, **b** Axial, **c**, **d** coronal CT sections, right. The jugular fossa and the posteroinferior aspect of the petrous pyramid are eroded. The enhancing soft-tissue mass extends into the mesotympanum and envelops the long process of the incus and stapes.

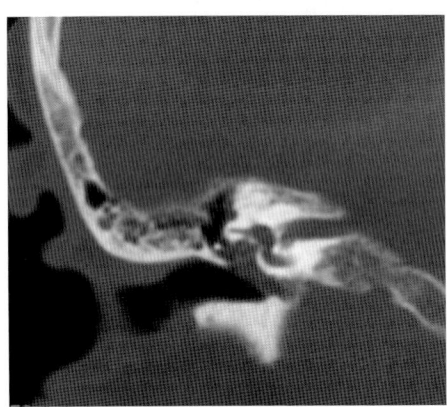

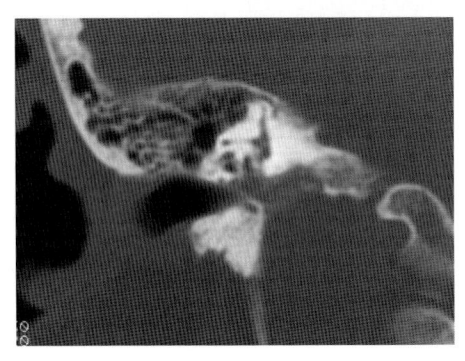

3 Erosion of the floor of the middle ear cavity.
4 An enhancing soft-tissue mass of variable size projecting into the middle ear cavity from the jugular fossa. The mass may extend superiorly to encroach upon the ossicular chain. Further extension may occur into the mastoid. Lateral extension of the mass erodes the tympanic membrane and fills the external canal.
5 Erosion of the posteroinferior aspect of the petrous pyramid. This is typical of medial extension of the glomus. The glomus first undermines the posteroinferior aspect of the petrosa and erodes the external aperture of the cochlear aqueduct. Further enlargement of the lesion leads to partial or complete destruction of the petrous apex. The labyrinth becomes skeletonized but is seldom invaded.
6 The adjacent aspect of the occipital bone is often involved and is gradually eroded in large lesions. Further medial extension involves the hypoglossal canal and reaches the foramen magnum.
7 Large tumors erode the petrous pyramid and protrude extradurally into the middle and posterior cranial fossae (Figs. 1.**183**, 1.**184**, 1.**186**).
8 Inferior extension within and along the jugular vein occurs quite often. Such extension is best visualized by MR (Fig. 1.**185**).

MR Imaging

MR is indicated for glomus jugulare tumors with large extratemporal extension. The tumor appears in both T1-weighted and T2-weighted images as a nonhomogeneous mass of medium signal intensity. Several small areas of signal void are scattered throughout the tumor mass, produced by intralesional high-flow blood vessels. The signal intensity is easily differentiated from surrounding intracranial and extracranial soft tissues (Figs. 1.**185**,

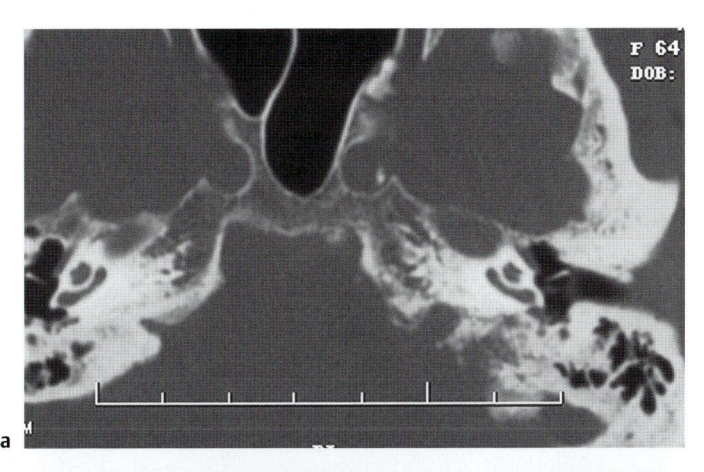

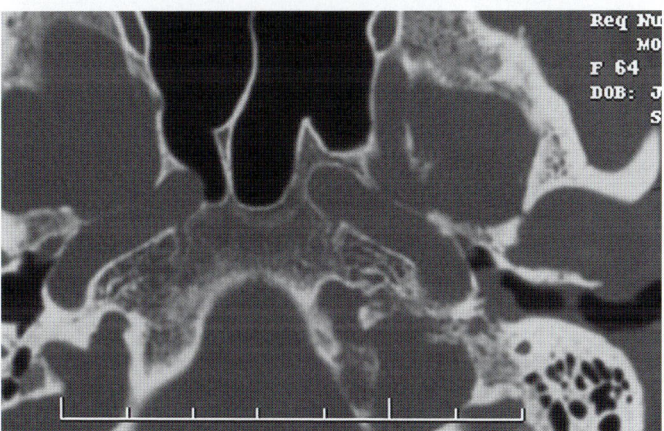

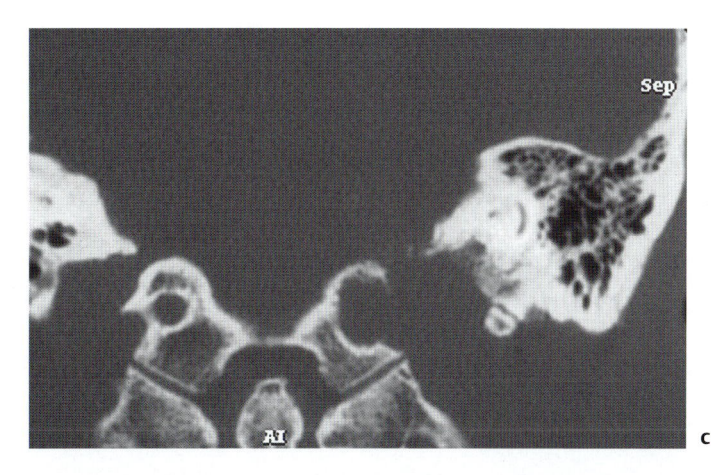

Fig. 1.**184** Glomus jugulare, left. **a**, **b** Axial, **c** coronal CT sections. The tumor erodes the contour of the jugular fossa, the posterior aspect of the petrous pyramid, and the adjacent occipital bone including the hypoglossal canal (**c**). The hypotympanic floor is also involved and the mass extends into the lower portion of the middle ear (**b**).

1.**186**). Following i.v. injection of contrast material, the tumor undergoes a moderate to intense enhancement (Fig. 1.**186b**). The main advantage of MR is that the jugular vein and the internal carotid artery are visualized without need for invasive vascular procedures. MR will demonstrate displacement, narrowing, encroachment, or obstruction, and thrombosis of these vessels (Figs. 1.**185**, 1.**186**). Extension of the tumor within the lumen of the vessels can be clearly identified. When extensive skull base surgery is contemplated, it is essential to know precisely whether the great vessels are compromised by tumor.

Venography

When MR is not available, retrograde jugular venography is the best method to demonstrate a downward extension of a glomus tumor into the neck within the lumen or along the wall of the jugular vein (Fig. 1.**188**). This information is necessary to outline the inferior margin of the radiotherapy ports.

Arteriography

Subtraction arteriography is not required to diagnose the glomus tumor but, as indicated, it identifies feeding vessels of the lesion prior to embolization or surgical ligation (Fig. 1.**187**).

Endolymphatic Sac Tumor

Endolymphatic sac tumors are locally aggressive papillary adenomatous tumors. They are often associated with Von Hippel–Lindau disease, a genetic multisystem neoplastic disorder.[19] At first, endolymphatic sac tumors involve the adjacent dura and endolymphatic duct. From there the lesion extends to the vestibule, semicircular canals, mastoid, and middle ear cavity, where it appears through an intact tympanic membrane as a bluish mass, often confused with a glomus tumor. Continuous growth leads to complete replacement by tumor of the mastoid and petrous pyramid. Axial CT images show initially a localized area of erosion of the posterior aspect of the petrous pyramid in the region of the endolymphatic sac (Figs. 1.**189**, 1.**190**).[15] As the lesion enlarges, destruction of the petrous pyramid is observed with involvement of the inner ear structures. In the MR images, the tumor has a heterogeneous appearance with areas of high signal due to cysts filled with blood or high proteinaceous fluid and multiple small areas of signal void due to calcifications and blood vessels.[22] Following i.v. administration of contrast material, the solid portion of the mass undergoes a nonhomogeneous enhancement (Fig. 1.**189**, 1.**190**).

■ Malignant Tumors

Primary Malignancies

Carcinoma

Carcinomas of the temporal bone arise chiefly from the external auditory canal. Primary carcinomas of the middle ear cavity are extremely rare since most middle ear carcinomas actually begin in the external canal at the annulus and infiltrate from there. Carcinomas of the canal tend to infiltrate and spread deep into the surrounding portions of the temporal bone. The predominant symptoms are pain and bleeding. Since there is no subcutaneous tissue between the skin and the periosteum of the external canal, carcinomas infiltrate the periosteum early, causing severe pain (Fig. 1.**192**).

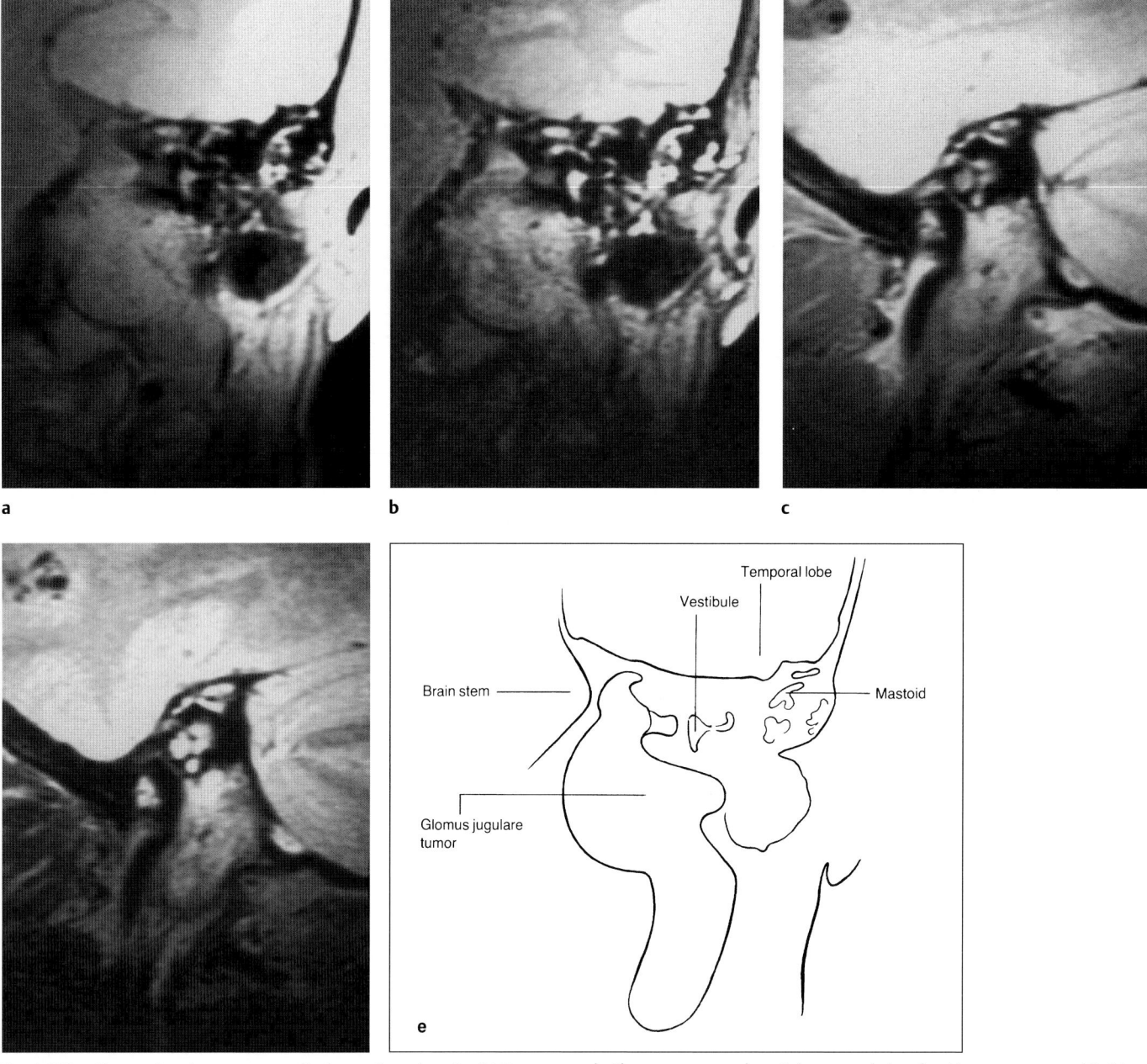

Fig. 1.185 Glomus jugulare tumor. **a**, **b** Coronal, **c**, **d** sagittal MR sections, left. **a** and **c** are spin-density-weighted and **b** and **d** are T2W images. A large soft-tissue mass extends from the jugular fossa into the petrous pyramid. The mass is characterized by mixed intensity signals in both sequences and contains several signal void areas, presumably blood vessels. The tumor obstructs the jugular bulb and reaches but does not involve the carotid artery. **e** Diagram of **a**.

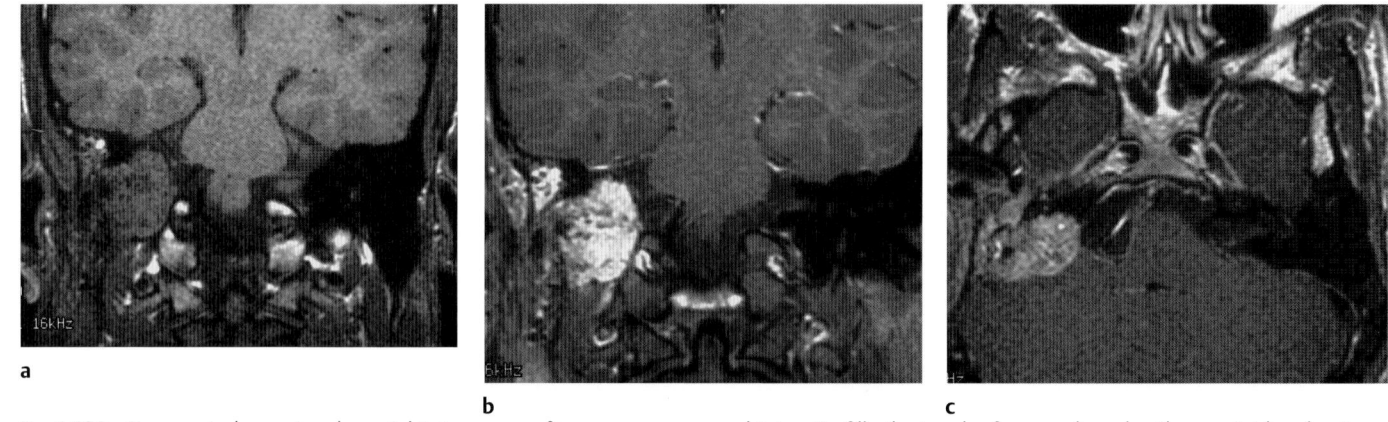

Fig. 1.186 Recurrent glomus jugulare, right, two years after surgery. **a** Coronal T1W MR image prior to injection; **b** coronal and **c** axial T1W MR images after contrast. A large soft-tissue mass of nonhomogeneous signal intensity fills the jugular fossa and erodes the mastoid and petrous pyramid (**a**). The enhancing tumor mass, which contains multiple areas of signal void, erodes the internal auditory canal (**b** and **c**).

Tumors

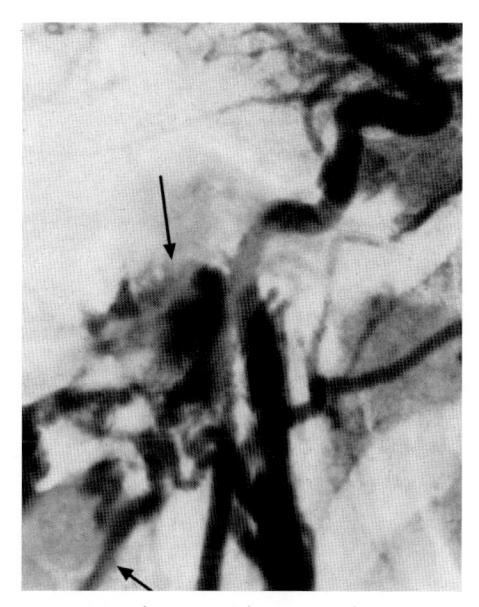

Fig. 1.**187** Glomus jugulare. carotid angiogram with subtraction, right. A vascular mass (long arrow) lies in the region of the inferior aspect of the petrous pyramid. The ascending pharyngeal artery (short arrow), which feeds the glomus tumor, is dilated.

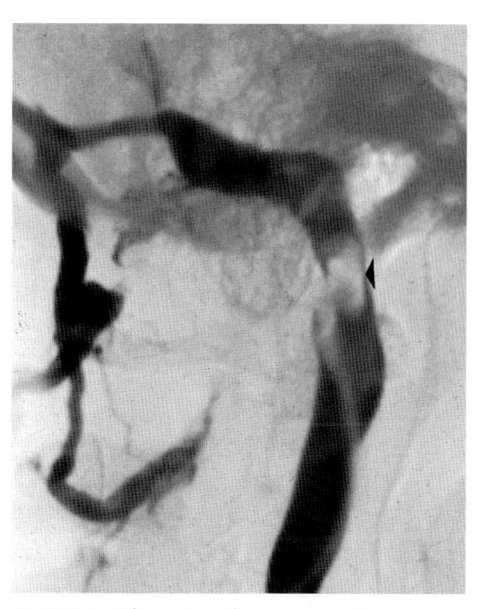

Fig. 1.**188** Glomus jugulare, retrograde venogram, right. A filling defect (arrow) is present in the jugular vein 1 cm below the dome of the jugular bulb.

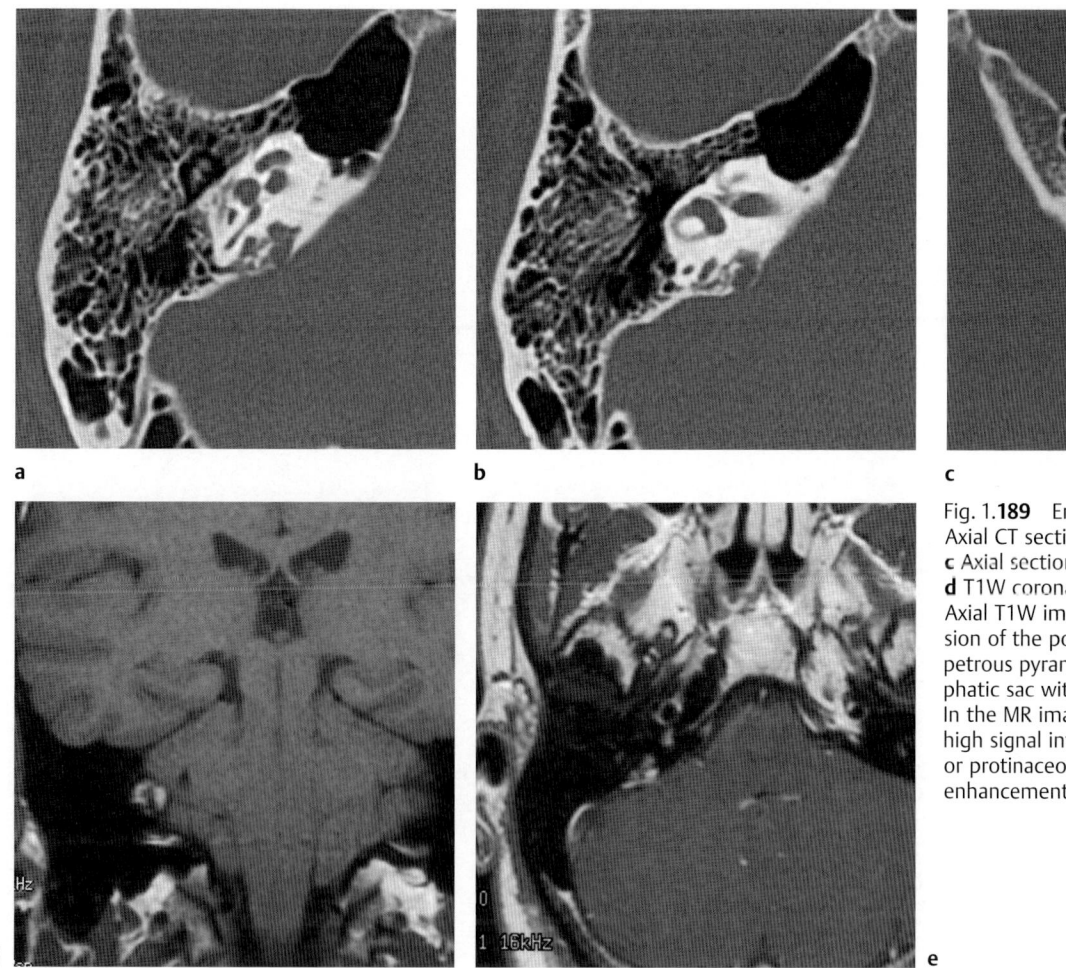

Fig. 1.**189** Endolymphatic sac tumor. **a, b** Axial CT sections of the right petrous pyramid. **c** Axial section of the left side for comparison. **d** T1W coronal MR image prior to contrast. **e** Axial T1W image after contrast. There is erosion of the posterior aspect of the right petrous pyramid in the region of the endolymphatic sac with formation of an irregular cavity. In the MR images, the tumor contains areas of high signal intensity due to blood by-products or protinaceous fluid and shows some spotty enhancement after contrast.

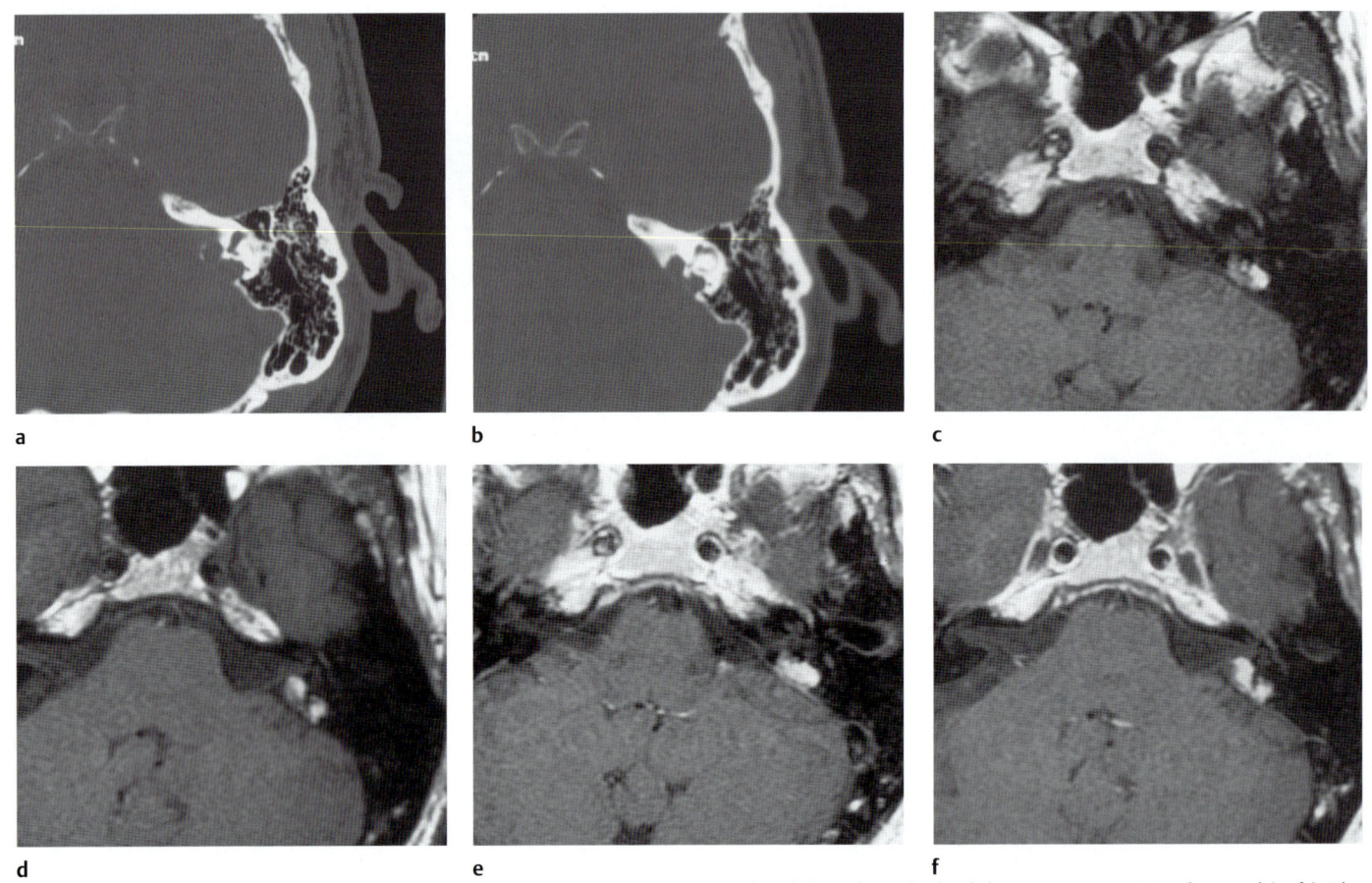

Fig. 1.**190** Endolymphatic sac tumor.
a, b Axial CT; **c, d** axial T1W MR images prior to contrast; **e, f** axial T1W images after contrast. The tumor has eroded the posterior aspect of the left petrous pyramid, including the posterior wall of the internal auditory canal and the inferior limb of the posterior semicircular canal (**a, b**). The tumor contains areas of high signal intensity due to blood by-products or protinaceous fluid and enhances after contrast.

Extension

Carcinomas of the external canal can extend anteriorly into the temporomandibular joint, posteriorly into the mastoid and facial nerve, inferiorly into the neck, and medially into the middle ear. Further medial extension involves the jugular fossa and the petrous pyramid.

Otoscopic Findings

Otoscopically in carcinoma of the external canal, there is a granular ulcerating lesion that bleeds easily on contact with an instrument. All such granular lesions of the external and middle ear should be biopsied (Fig. 1.**191**).

Imaging Assessment

The role of CT in temporal bone carcinomas is twofold: to demonstrate bony erosions characteristic of carcinomas and to delineate the extent of the lesion. This information will enable the surgeon to determine the resectability of the lesion. When radiotherapy is indicated, the radiographic evaluation will help in establishing the size of the treatment ports. In large lesions with extratemporal involvement, MR becomes the study of choice because it shows both intracranial and extracranial extension better than CT.

In an early lesion, CT will show an irregular soft-tissue mass within the external canal and erosion and destruction of portions of the bony wall (Fig. 1.**192**). Spread of tumor through the anterior canal wall will result in erosion of the temporomandibular fossa and anterior displacement of the condyle. Extension into the mastoid causes a typical moth-eaten appearance of the bone. The vertical segment of the facial canal is often involved in posterior extensions.

As the lesion extends medially there will be a soft-tissue mass in the middle ear. From the middle ear, the lesion often extends inferiorly into the jugular fossa or medially into the petrous pyramid. Petrous extension usually results in skeletoni-

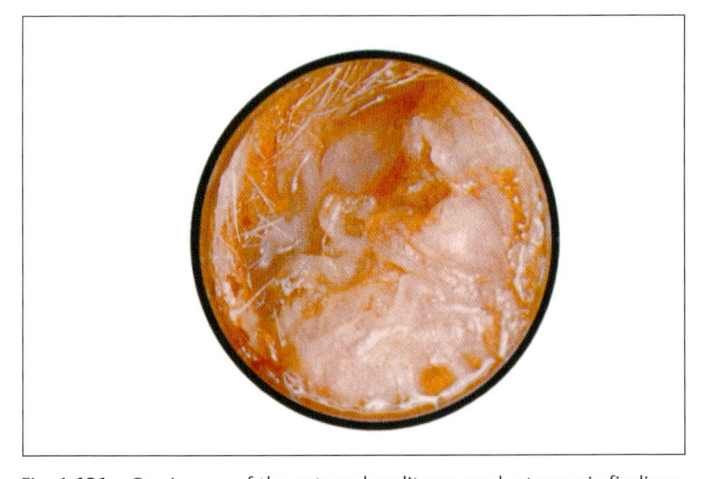

Fig. 1.**191** Carcinoma of the external auditory canal, otoscopic findings, right. A large granular squamous carcinoma fills the external auditory canal.

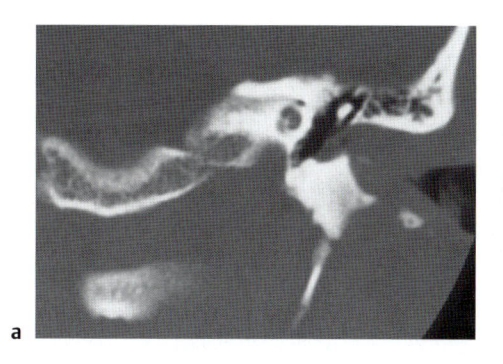

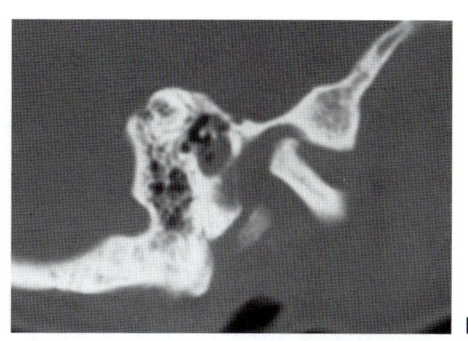

Fig. 1.**192** Carcinoma of the external auditory canal. **a** Coronal, **b** sagittal CT sections, left. A soft-tissue mass fills the lumen of the external auditory canal but does not extend into the middle ear cavity. The tumor has eroded the floor and anterior wall of the canal.

zation of the labyrinth, since the otic capsule is relatively resistant to infiltration. Far-advanced carcinomas cause massive destruction of the temporal bone and adjacent bony structures. In these cases. MR will demonstrate intracranial and neck extension of the tumor better than will CT.

Sarcoma

Sarcomas of the temporal bone are extremely rare. They usually occur in children and arise from the middle ear or petrous pyramid. Histologically they are rhabdomyosarcomas, fibrosarcomas, lymphosarcomas, osteogenic sarcomas, chondrosarcomas, and undifferentiated sarcomas (see Chapter 3).

Imaging Findings

CT studies consist of axial and coronal sections. CT infusion studies and MR will demonstrate intracranial and extracranial extensions of the lesion.

If the lesion originates in the middle ear, there will be a soft-tissue mass that often causes lateral bulging of the tympanic membrane. The mastoid air cells appear cloudy in early lesions, but they are destroyed with growth of the tumor.

The external auditory canal is usually intact. Sarcomas tend to spread into the eustachian tube. Sarcomas that arise in the nasopharynx and eustachian tube extend retrogradely to involve the middle ear and temporal bone. The pyramid is often completely destroyed either by lesions arising in the petrosa or by extension of the highly malignant tumor from the middle ear (see Chapters 3 and 7).

Secondary Malignancies

Secondary involvement of the temporal bone by malignant tumors occurs by direct extension from lesions in adjacent structures and by metastases.

Direct Extension

The most common lesion that involves the temporal bone by direct extension is carcinoma of the parotid. As the lesion extends upward from the parotid, it involves the base of the skull and the temporal bone. The floor of the external canal and the inferior surface of the mastoid are usually eroded by tumor. The lesion may obstruct the external auditory canal. Involvement of the stylomastoid foramen will cause facial nerve paralysis. Adenoid cystic carcinomas have a tendency to spread from the stylomastoid foramen along the facial nerve and erode and expand the facial nerve canal. With the growth of the tumor, the mastoid, middle ear, and petrous pyramid become involved (Fig. 1.**193**). CT will demonstrate the progressive destruction of the temporal bone. MR images show the enhancing mass involving the base of the skull (Fig. 1.**193**), as well as the perineural extension of the tumor along the facial nerve.

Metastatic Extension

The most common metastatic lesions of the temporal bone are carcinoma of the breast, lung, prostate, and kidney. Melanomas and other tumors also metastasize to the temporal bone (Figs. 1.**194**, 1.**195**). Any area of the temporal bone may be involved, and symptomatology varies depending on the location of the lesion. The lesion may be destructive, as with lung metastasis; osteoblastic, as with carcinoma of the prostate; or mixed, destructive, and sclerotic, as with breast carcinoma.

CT or MR should be performed to rule out intracranial extension of the temporal bone lesion and to establish the extent of the temporal bone involvement. They also help to rule out the presence of other intracranial metastases.

Internal Auditory Canal and Acoustic Schwannomas

■ Normal Internal Auditory Canal

The normal internal auditory canal (IAC) extends from its opening in the posteromedial surface of the petrous pyramid to the cribriform plate, which closes the canal laterally and separates the canal from the vestibule (Figs. 1.**196**–1.**198**). It measures 10–20 mm in length and has a diameter as small as 2 mm and as large as 12 mm. However, whereas the internal auditory canals of different individuals may differ greatly in size, the two canals of any person are identical or vary by no more than 1 mm. The internal auditory canal contains the acoustic nerve, which splits within the canal into its cochlear and vestibular divisons; the facial nerve; the nervus intermedius; the labyrinth artery; and, in 20–40% of the cases, a loop of the anterior-inferior cerebellar artery. There are several small openings within the canal.[9] At the fundus, the superior vestibular nerve passes through small openings in the cribriform plate to reach the ampullae of the horizontal and superior semicircular canals, as well as the macula of the utricle. Above the falciform crest in the anterior wall of the canal[9] laterally is the opening of the fallopian canal for the facial nerve and nervus intermedius. Below the falciform crest, 2–3 mm medial to the fundus of the canal, is the spiral foraminous tract, a series of small foramina in the base of the modiolus for the cochlear nerve. At the junction between the inferior and posterior walls is the opening of the singular canal, which transmits a branch of the inferior vestibular nerve to the ampulla of the posterior semicircular canal. The remaining portion of the inferior vestibular nerve passes through the cribriform plate to reach the macula of the saccule. The internal auditory canal is lined by dura and is bathed by cerebrospinal fluid. The amount of fluid within the canal is of course proportional to the size of the canal.

110   1 Imaging of the Temporal Bone

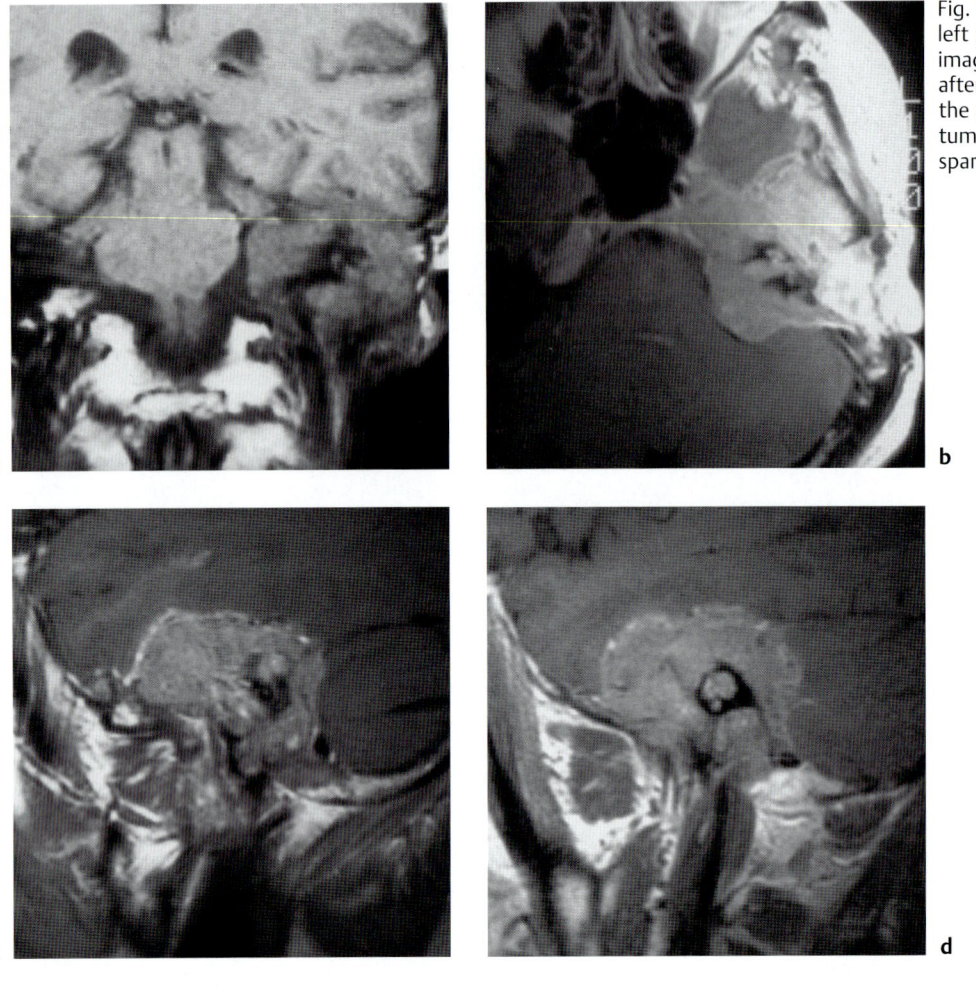

Fig. 1.**193** Recurrent adenocystic carcinoma, left parotid gland. **a** coronal T1W preinjection image; **b** axial, **c** and **d** sagittal T1W images after contrast. An enhancing tumor replaces the entire mastoid and petrous pyramid. The tumor invades the internal auditory canal but spares the labyrinth.

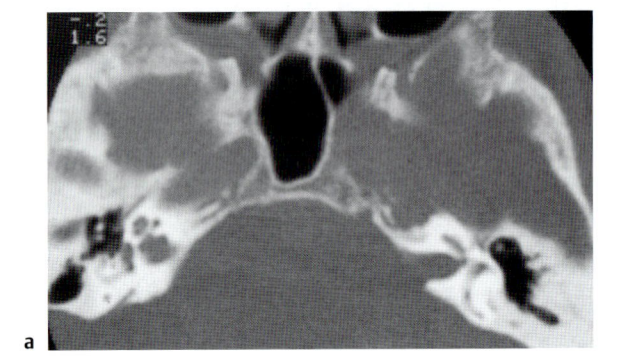

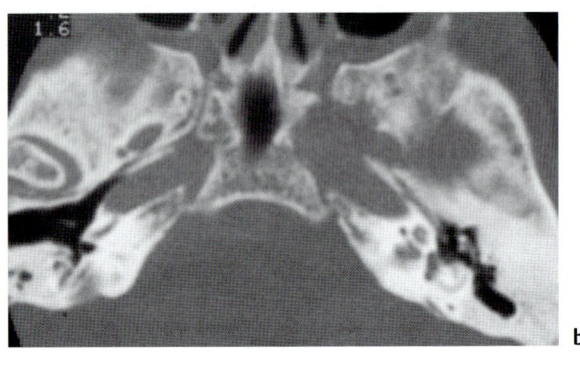

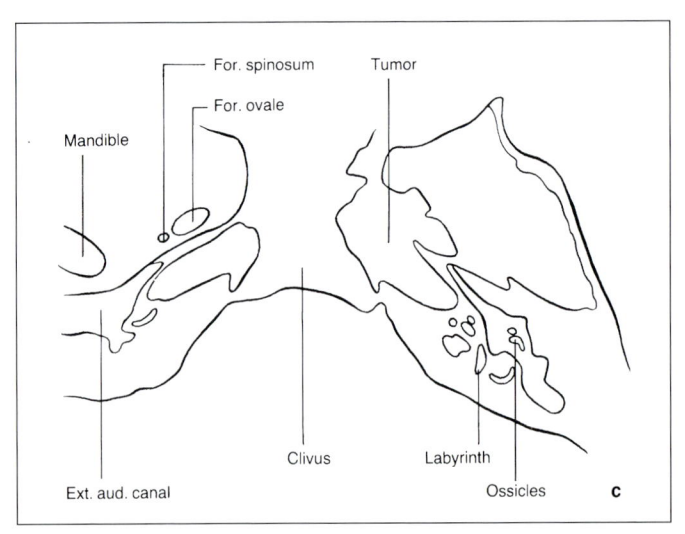

Fig. 1.**194** Metastatic carcinoma of the lung. **a**, **b** Axial CT sections. A large destructive lesion involves the left petrous apex, clivus, and floor of the middle cranial fossa including the foramen ovale. The lesion extends into the left sphenoid sinus. **c** Diagram of **b**.

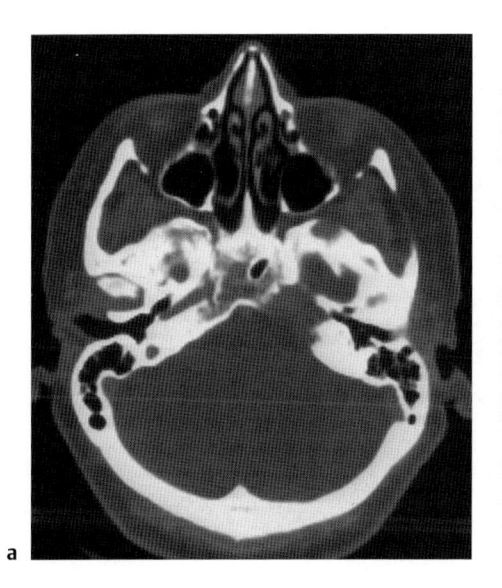

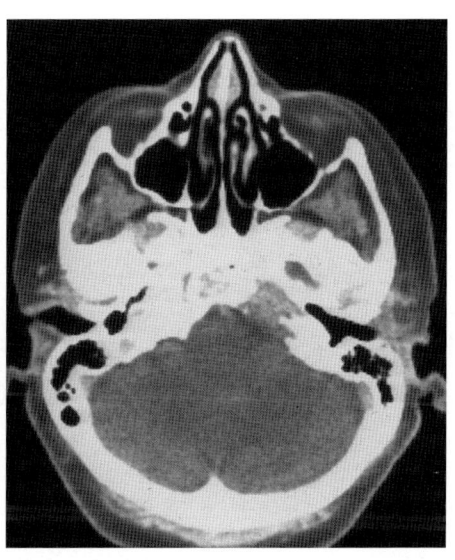

Fig. 1.**195** Metastatic carcinoma of the breast. **a, b** Axial CT sections. A large destructive lesion involves the left petrous pyramid, clivus, and adjacent floor of the middle cranial fossa. An enhanced soft-tissue mass fills the bony defect (**b**).

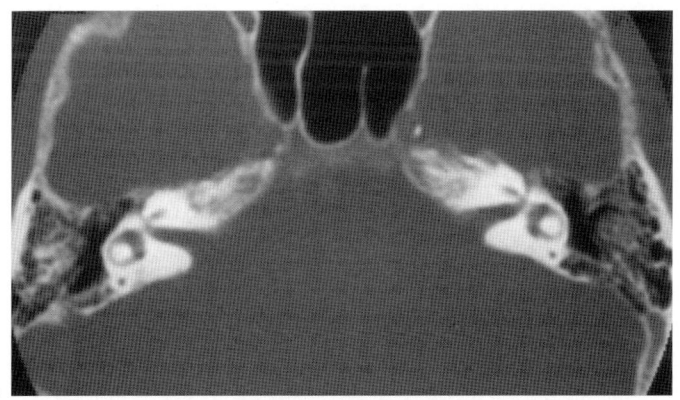

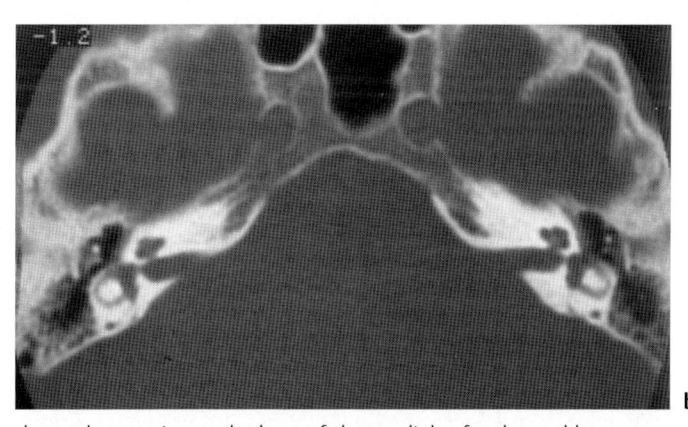

Fig. 1.**196** Normal internal auditory canal. **a, b** Axial CT sections. **a** Section through the upper compartment of the internal auditory canal. The facial nerve canal extends from the fundus of the canal to the geniculate ganglion area. **b** Section crossing the inferior compartment of the canal shows the opening at the base of the modiolus for the cochlear nerve. The opening of the internal auditory canal has a bevel shape, with the posterior wall forming a sharp margin, while the anterior margin blends smoothly with the posteromedial surface of the petrous bone.

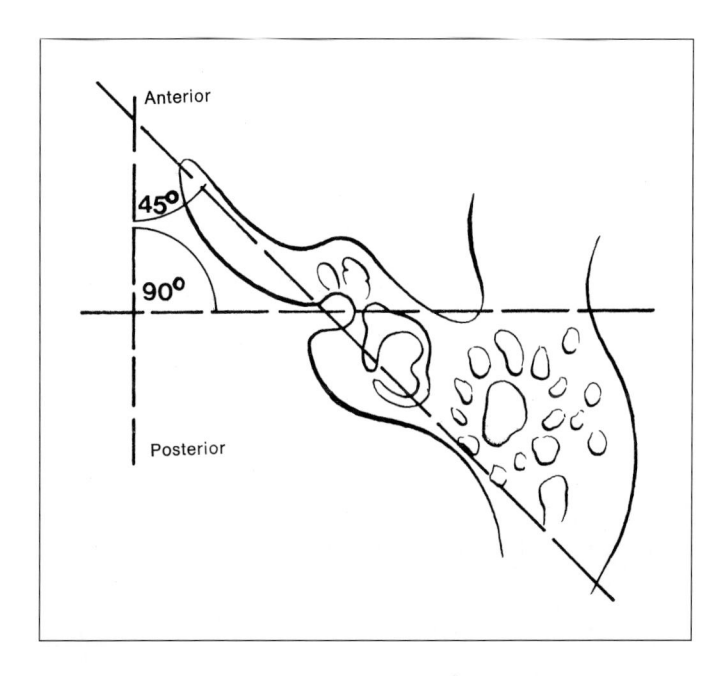

Fig. 1.**197** Diagram of internal auditory canal relationship. The long axis of the petrous pyramid forms an angle of approximately 45° with the sagittal plane. The internal auditory canal enters the pyramid at an angle of 90° to the sagittal plane.

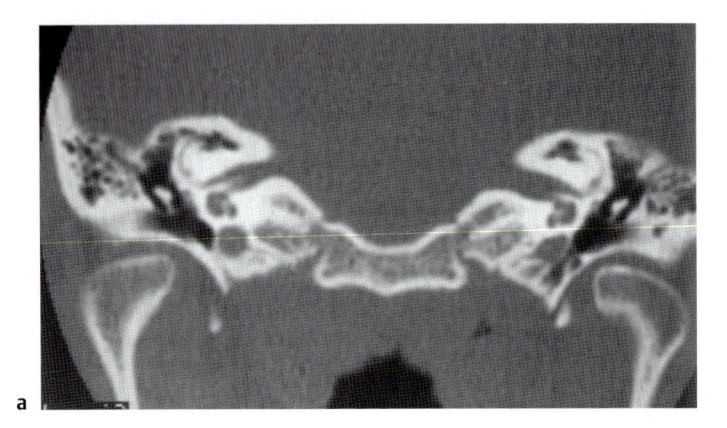

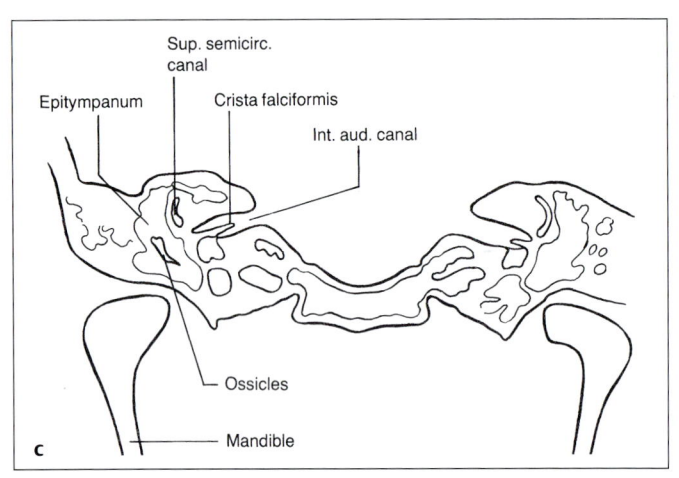

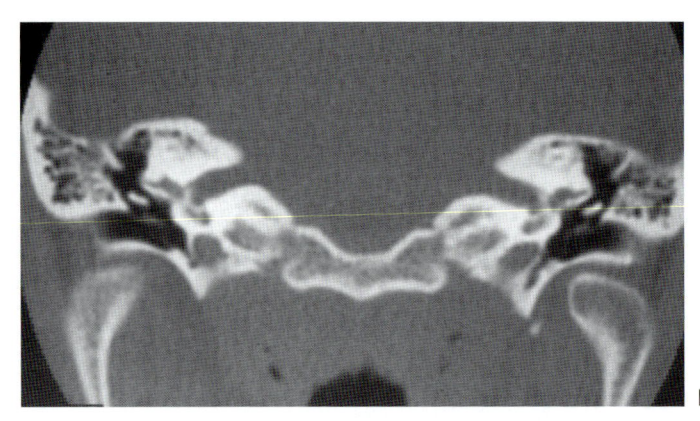

Fig. 1.**198** Normal internal auditory canal. **a**, **b** Coronal CT sections. **a** The most anterior section shows the crista falciformis dividing the lateral portion of the canals. **b** Midcanal section. **c** Diagram of **a**.

■ Imaging Studies

Imaging studies of the internal auditory canal and cerebellopontine cistern should be performed on all patients with sensorineural hearing or vestibular losses of unknown origin. Audiometric and vestibular tests have a high degree of sensitivity but cannot provide a definite diagnosis of cerebellopontine tumors. MRI is universally accepted as the study of choice. CT with infusion and pneumcisternography should be performed whenever MR equipment is not available (Figs. 1.**208**–1.**211**). Thin axial and coronal sections with bone algorithm are also very valuable in the assessment of bony dysplasias involving the internal auditory canal (Fig. 1.**200**).

Contrast-enhanced MRI has become the gold standard for the diagnosis of acoustic schwannomas and other space-occupying lesions within the internal auditory canal (Figs. 1.**202**–1.**205**). However, the cost of the examination has been a limiting factor in using the procedure as a screening test for the study of progressive sensorineural hearing loss of unknown origin. Recently, fast spin-echo (FSE) MR without contrast has been shown, according to several authors, to be "as sensitive and effective in the detection of acoustic schwannomas as contrast-enhanced MRI" (Fig. 1.**203**–1.**205**). According to the same authors, this approach has become the most cost-effective method to screen for retrocochlear pathology.[24] Fast spin-echo T2-weighted sequence produces images of superb quality where the cerebrospinal fluid within the canal behaves as a medium of high signal intensity.[34] Nerves, vessels, and space-occupying lesions appear as filling defects of various lengths and shapes. The adjacent inner ear structures are well visualized by the high signal of the fluid within them (Fig. 1.**34**). We use the fast spin-echo sequence to study the internal auditory canals prior to cochlear implant and for hemifacial spasm, but we feel that it has serious limitations in the assessment of the canals for space-occupying lesions. First of all, the fast spin-echo approach becomes questionable in narrow internal auditory canals that contain very little cerebrospinal fluid and therefore little high signal intensity medium. More importantly, small masses, less than 2 mm in diameter, may be missed or confused with filling defects produced by vessels seen end-on. Lack of specificity of the filling defect is another serious drawback. All masses within the internal auditory canal produce identical filling defects. It is therefore impossible to differentiate an acoustic neuroma from a lipoma, a small aneurysm, arteriovenous malformations, neuritis or a meningeal mass. If a schwannoma is present, fast spin-echo images will not recognize extension into the modiolus, which is instead well seen after the injection of contrast (hook sign) and are of course of poor prognostic value.[8] Finally, the spin-echo T2-weighted images will fail to diagnose inflammatory lesions involving the acoustic and facial nerves, the labyrinth, and the meninges, which are usually well identified after injection of contrast because of the enhancement. This is particularly true in the assessment of patients with sudden hearing loss since a viral labyrinthitis or neuritis is a far more frequent occurrence than an acoustic schwannoma.

Our search for cost-effective assessment of patients with sensorineural hearing loss or vestibular disturbances of unknown origin has led us to a multiform approach.

Limited Study of the IAC

As implied by the title, this is not a screening study to select patients for a more complete assessment but an accurate examination limited to the internal auditory canal and adjacent inner ear structures. Twelve T1-weighted 2 mm thick axial or coronal sections are obtained through the petrous pyramid prior to and after i.v. injection of contrast material. The total examination time is approximately 20 minutes. The preinjection T1-weighted images are mandatory to differentiate an enhancing mass from a bright lesion, such as a lipoma, bleeding, or varix. The postcontrast T1-weighted sections show the presence, size, position, and extent of the enhancing tumor. It is important to observe whether the tumor extends to the fundus of the internal auditory canal or, more rarely, within the cochlea, vestibule, or fallopian canal, because such extensions will make the removal of the tumor more difficult and increase the risk of damaging the facial nerve.

Complete Study of the IAC and Brain

This assessment is indicated in the following cases:
1. In patients with bilateral sensorineural hearing loss, since in these cases the possibility of neurofibromatosis and/or other central nervous system pathology should be entertained.
2. In patients with vertigo and abnormal vestibular findings, whether or not associated with SNHL.
3. Whenever the SNHL is associated with other neurological findings.

The examination includes, before the injection of contrast material, 2 mm fast spin-echo axial images of the posterior cranial fossa and internal auditory canal, 2 mm T1-weighted coronal sections of the internal auditory canals, and 5 mm FLAIR axial sections of the brain, particularly useful for the detection of demyelinating processes. After the i.v. injection of contrast material, 2 mm T1-weighted coronal images of the IACs and 5 mm axial sections of the brain are obtained.

No-Contrast FSE Study of IAC

Assessments of the IAC prior to cochlear implantation and for hemifacial spasm are, in our opinion, the only indications for a study limited to thin T2-weighted fast spin-echo images. Prior to cochlear implantation, particularly in cases with congenital deafness, axial and sagittal images of the IACs are obtained in order to identify the cochlear nerve. Of course, congenital absence or atrophy of the nerve are contraindications to cochlear implantation. In patients with hemifacial spasm, axial and coronal sections may demonstrate a vessel or vascular loop encroaching upon the facial nerve.

■ Pathology of the Internal Auditory Canal

Pathological conditions involving the internal auditory canal may involve the canal walls or arise from the content of the canal.

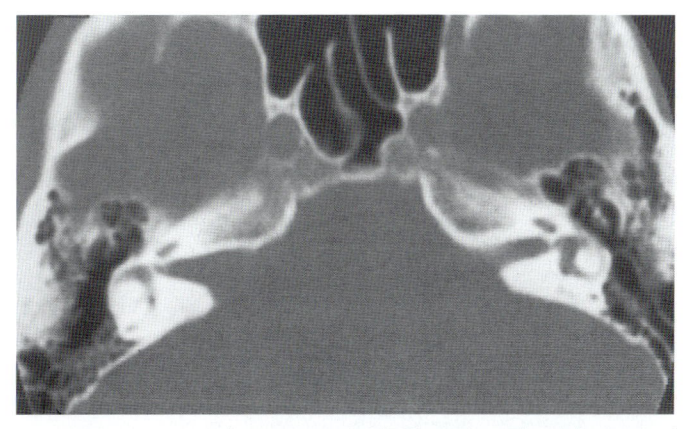

Fig. 1.**199** Acoustic schwannoma. Axial CT section. The right internal auditory canal is enlarged and wider than the left. The posterior wall of the right canal is blunted and slightly shorter than the left.

Osseous Changes

Pathological conditions, either congenital or acquired, may lead to excessive narrowing or abnormal enlargement of the canal. Congenital narrowing is usually observed in children with profound sensorineural hearing loss due to hypoplasia of the acoustic nerve. Acquired stenosis of the canal is caused by osteomas, meningiomas, fibrous dysplasia, Paget disease, osteopetrosis, and other more unusual bony dysplasia. The osseous growth or the thickening and hyperostosis of the canal walls encroaches upon the content of the canal and produces sensorineural hearing loss, or more rarely, facial nerve palsy.

Abnormal expansion of the IAC is due either to a space-occupying lesion within the canal (Figs. 1.**199**, 1.**209**) or to dural ectasia with no tumor mass within the dysplastic IAC, as is often observed in neurofibromatosis (Fig. 1.**200**).

■ Pathology within the Internal Auditory Canal

The normal internal auditory canal contains facial and acoustic nerves and vessels, and is lined by meninges. Pathological processes may arise from each of these structures and more rarely from heterotopic tissue.

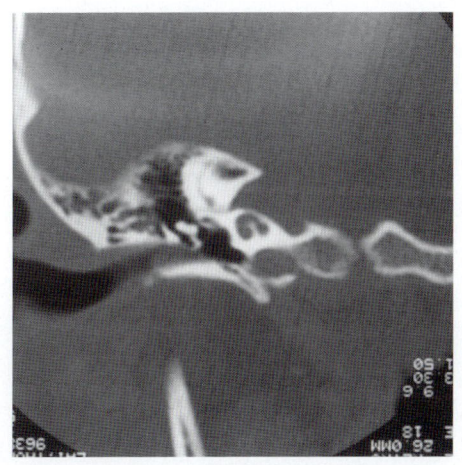

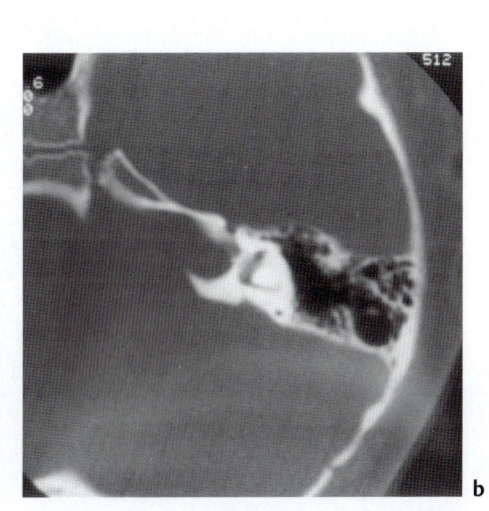

Fig. 1.**200** Neurofibromatosis. **a** Coronal, right, **b** axial, left CT images. The internal auditory canals are enlarged owing to dural ectasia but no tumor mass.

1 Imaging of the Temporal Bone

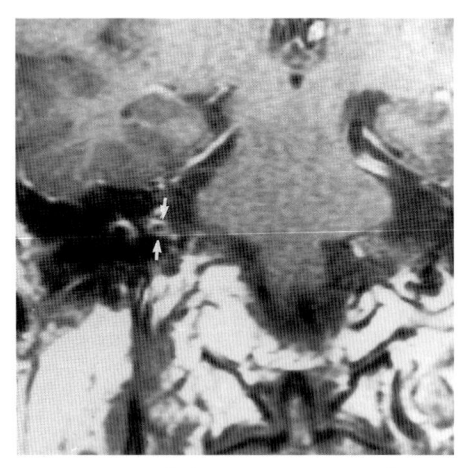

Fig. 1.**201** Vestibular neuronitis. Coronal T1W MR image after contrast. There is enhancement of the vestibule, the semicircular canals, and the vestibular nerves (arrows).

and more rarely hearing loss. In several patients, an MRI study after i.v. injection of contrast material demonstrates enhancement of the vestibular nerves (Fig. 1.**201**). Enhancement of a swollen segment of the acoustic nerve may appear as a pseudo-mass, which can be confused with a schwannoma. The following points may help in a differential diagnosis. Enhancement of neuritis is not as solid and homogeneous as an acoustic schwannoma and the margins are usually scalloped rather than smooth and concave as in a tumor. In addition, in some cases there is also enhancement within the vestibule and semicircular canals due to a labyrinthitis.

Vestibular Schwannomas

Acoustic schwannomas are the cause of progressive unilateral sensorineural hearing loss and vestibular function loss in approximately 10 % of the patients.

Acoustic schwannomas usually arise within the lumen of the internal auditory canal and, as they slowly enlarge, erode the bony margins of the meatus (Fig. 1.**199**). Erosion of the canal is visible radiographically. Acoustic schwannomas account for approximately 80–90 % of all cerebellopontine angle tumors. An acoustic neuroma is a benign, encapsulated, slowly growing tumor of one of the branches of the eighth cranial nerve. The lesion arises from proliferation of the neurilemmal or Schwann cells. Histologically, the tumors are made of up streams of elongated spindle cells with fairly large nuclei, which are often arranged in a palisading pattern. The larger tumors may undergo cystic degenerative changes within the tumor mass (Fig. 1.**208**). Most acoustic schwannomas arise from the vestibular division of the eighth nerve and only few from the chochlear division. Most acoustic nerve tumors arise within the lumen of the internal auditory canal at the junction between the neurilemmal sheaths deriving from the peripheral ganglia and the neuroglial fibers that extend peripherally from the brainstem (Figs. 1.**203**, 1.**204**).

Neurogenic Pathology

Because of the differences in clinical symptomatology and often in imaging findings, the facial and acoustic nerves will be reviewed separately. For both nerves, the pathological involvement consists of inflammatory and neoplastic conditions (schwannomas).

Acoustic Nerve Inflammatory Processes

Inflammatory processes of the acoustic nerve usually involve the vestibular components of the nerve and are the result of a viral infection. The clinical symptomatology is vertigo, nausea, vomiting,

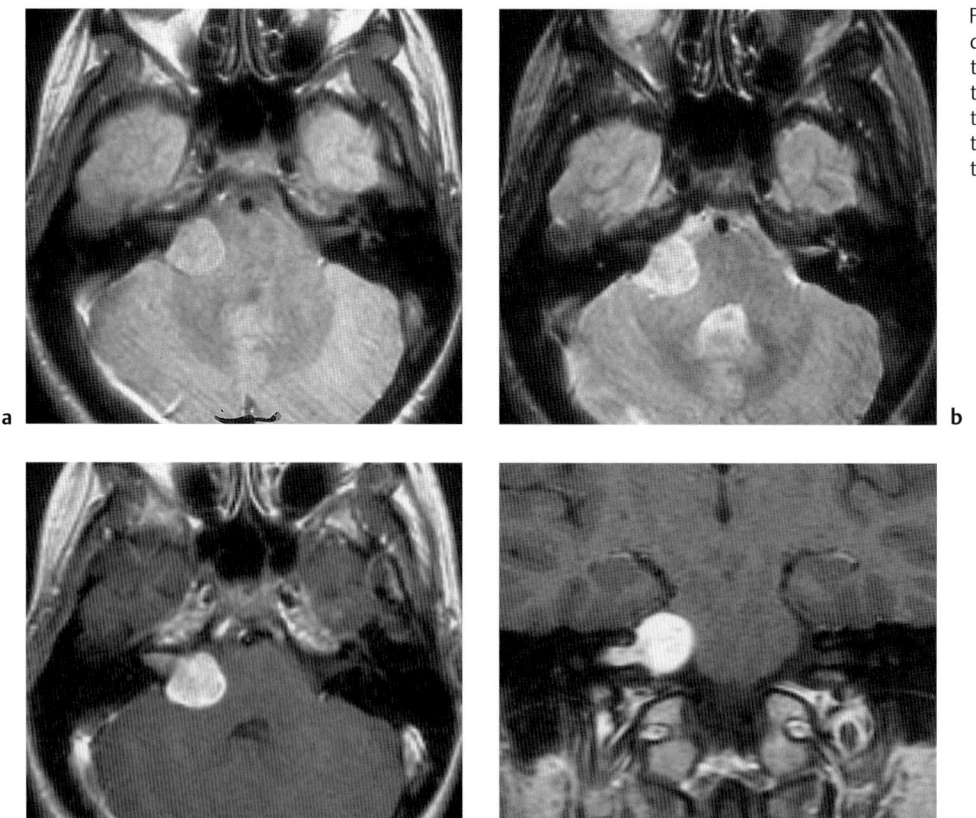

Fig. 1.**202** Acoustic schwannoma. **a** Spin-density, **b** T2W preinjection, **c** T1W postcontrast axial images. **d** T1W coronal postcontrast image. A highly enhancing tumor fills the IAC and extends into the cerebellopontine cistern. The tumor reaches and indents the brain stem.

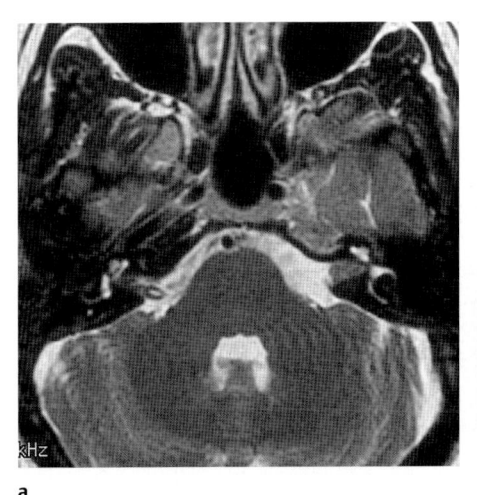

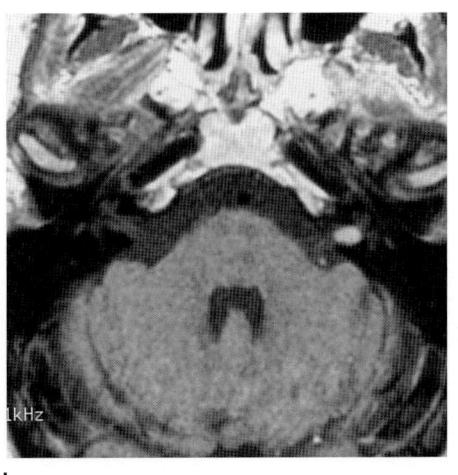

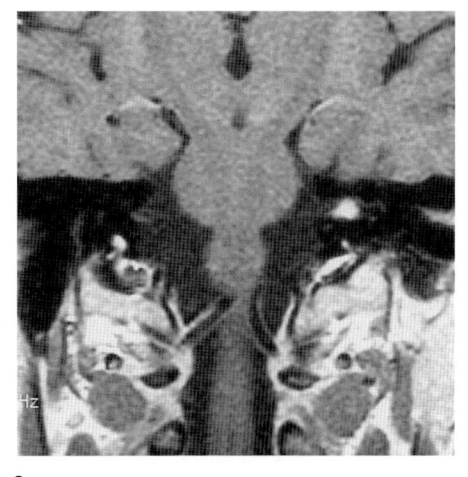

Fig. 1.**203** Acoustic schwannoma. MR images: **a** axial FSE, **b** axial and **c** coronal T1W postcontrast. An enhancing tumor fills the left internal auditory canal. The filling defect of the mass is well seen in the FSE.

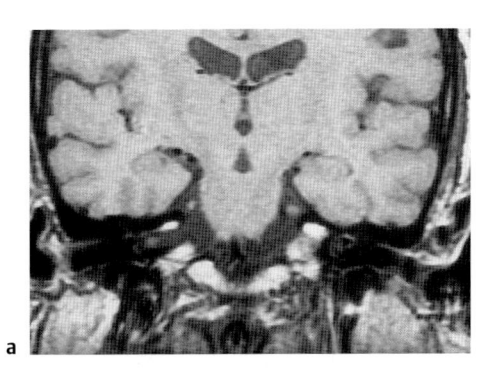

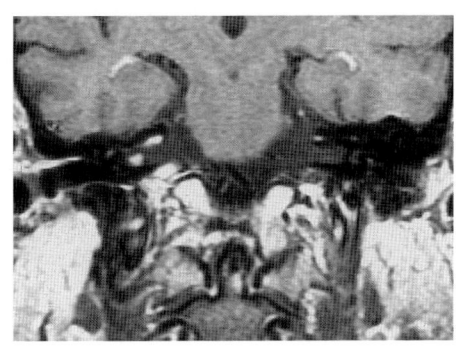

Fig. 1.**204** Acoustic schwannoma. T1W coronal MR sections: **a** before contrast, **b** after contrast. A small tumor, about 2 mm in diameter, is seen within the right internal auditory canal.

Early growth of an acoustic schwannoma occurs within the lumen of the internal auditory canal without producing significant symptoms (Fig. 1.**204**). Once the lesion has expanded to come into contact with the walls of the internal auditory canal, pressure of the growing tumor results in erosion of the walls of the internal auditory canal and consequent enlargement of the canal. A few acoustic schwannomas arise within the cerebellopontine cistern and do not extend into the internal auditory canal. Other lesions, such as meningiomas, epidermoids, and arachnoid cysts, occur in the cistern and mimic acoustic schwannomas.

Bilateral acoustic schwannomas are extremely rare except in patients with neurofibromatosis (type II).

The most common symptom of an acoustic schwannoma is slowly progressive sensorineural hearing loss; however, sudden hearing loss or normal hearing have been observed in some cases. Vestibular disturbances, such as mild dizziness and a sensation of imbalance, occasionally occur as the first symptoms. The otolaryngologist uses a series of hearing tests that help in differentiating cochlear from retrocochlear lesions and in selecting patients for referral for imaging studies. The commonly used tests are pure-tone air and bone conduction audiometry, speech discrimination tests, adaptation tests, such as the tone decay test, tympanometric stapedial reflex measurements, and brainstem evoked responses. Caloric tests and electronystagmography determine the function of the vestibular portion of the eighth nerve. Vestibular function is abnormal in over 80% of acoustic neuromas. The facial nerve is rarely involved in neuromas because of the resistance of the motor fibers of the seventh nerve to pressure. As the schwannomas grow, they extend medially into the cerebellopontine angle (Fig. 1.**202**, 1.**205**). Upward extension of the lesion causes pressure on the fifth cranial nerve. Loss of the corneal reflex on the ipsilateral side may be the first sign of pressure on the fifth nerve. Further enlargement of the tumor mass will produce encroachment on the other cranial nerves with paralytic lesions of the 5th through the 12th nerves. Encroachment on the cerebellum and brainstem likewise occurs in large lesions. Fortunately, far-advanced lesions of this severity are rarely seen today because of improved methods for early diagnosis.

With early diagnosis, increased cerebrospinal fluid pressure and papilledema occur extremely rarely. Cerebrospinal fluid proteins are elevated only in the larger tumors.

Neurofibromatosis

Bilateral vestibular schwannomas (Fig. 1.**206**) are the hallmark lesion of neurofibraomatosis II, a genetic disorder in the long arm of chromosome 22. Other lesions found in NF II are meningiomas, sarcomas, schwannomas of the fifth or other cranial nerves, ependymomas, gliomas, and juvenile posterior subcapsular cataracts. NF II should be differentiated from neurofibromatosis I, a more common genetic disorder of the long arm of chromosome 17 and characterized by the presence of multiple neurofibromas and café-au-lait spots. Other features of NF I are plexiform neurofibromas, axillary or inguinal freckling, optic gliomas, Lisch nodules (hamartomas of the iris), and dysplasia of skull and meninges.

116   1 Imaging of the Temporal Bone

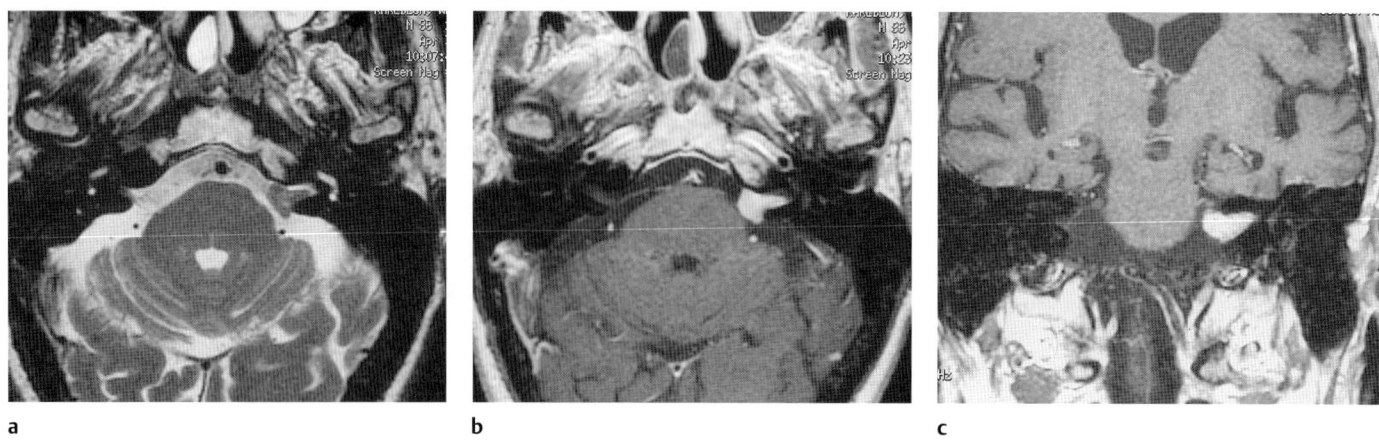

Fig. 1.**205** Acoustic schwannoma, left. MR images: **a** FSE, **b** precontrast, and **c** T1W postcontrast. Enhancing soft-tissue mass fills the internal auditory canal and extends into the cerebellopontine cistern. The tumor is well outlined in the FSE (**a**) as a filling defect within the bright cerebrospinal fluid.

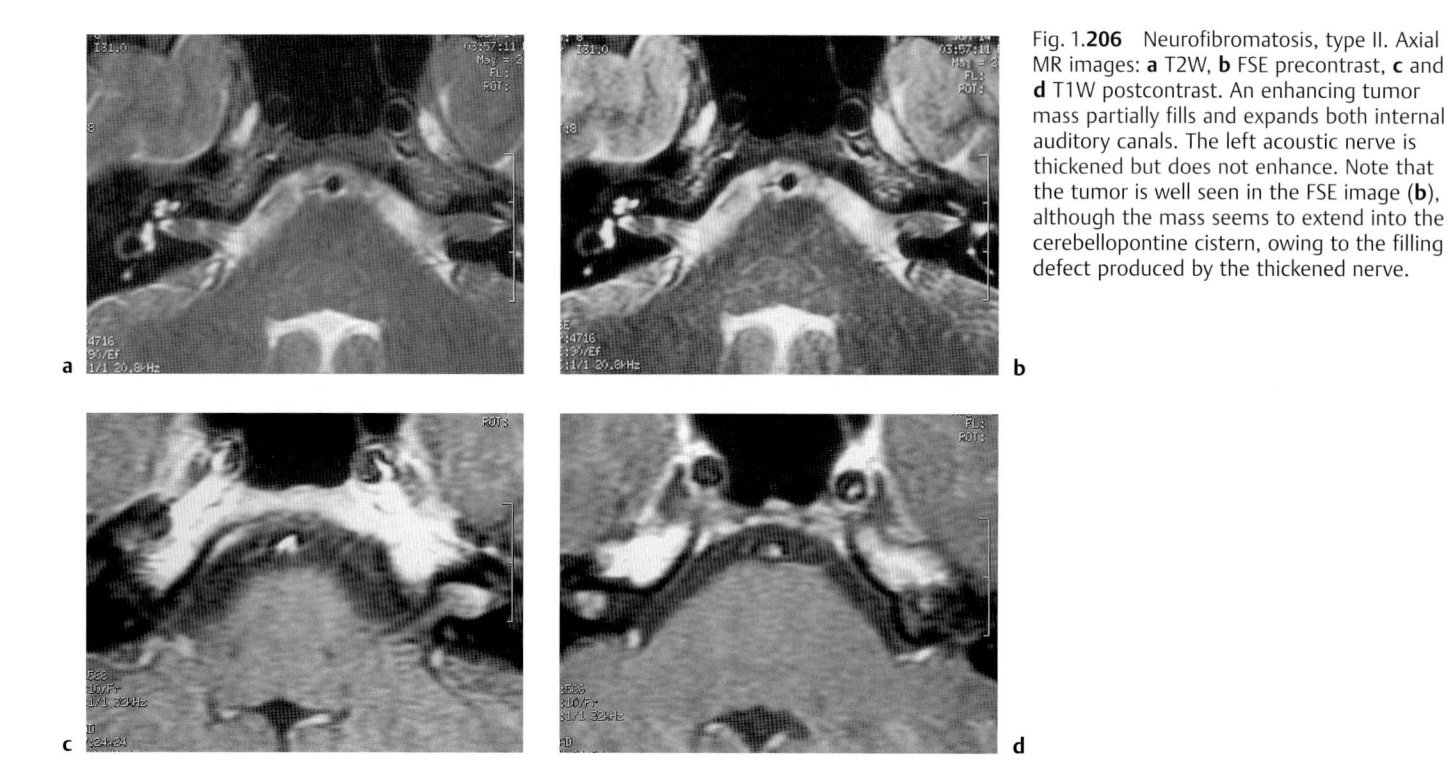

Fig. 1.**206** Neurofibromatosis, type II. Axial MR images: **a** T2W, **b** FSE precontrast, **c** and **d** T1W postcontrast. An enhancing tumor mass partially fills and expands both internal auditory canals. The left acoustic nerve is thickened but does not enhance. Note that the tumor is well seen in the FSE image (**b**), although the mass seems to extend into the cerebellopontine cistern, owing to the filling defect produced by the thickened nerve.

Bilateral acoustic schwannomas as seen in NF II present a management dilemma for the otologist since the removal of both schwannomas very often leads to complete deafness. Follow-up audiometric and MR studies should be obtained early to determine the level of hearing and rate of growth of the tumors.

Facial Nerve

The facial nerve leaves the brainstem 2–3 mm anterior to the acoustic nerve and, after crossing the cerebellopontine cistern, enters the anterosuperior quadrant of the IAC. Close to the fundus of the canal, the facial nerve passes into the fallopian canal, which follows a serpiginous course to the stylomastoid foramen.

Internal Auditory Canal and Acoustic Schwannomas

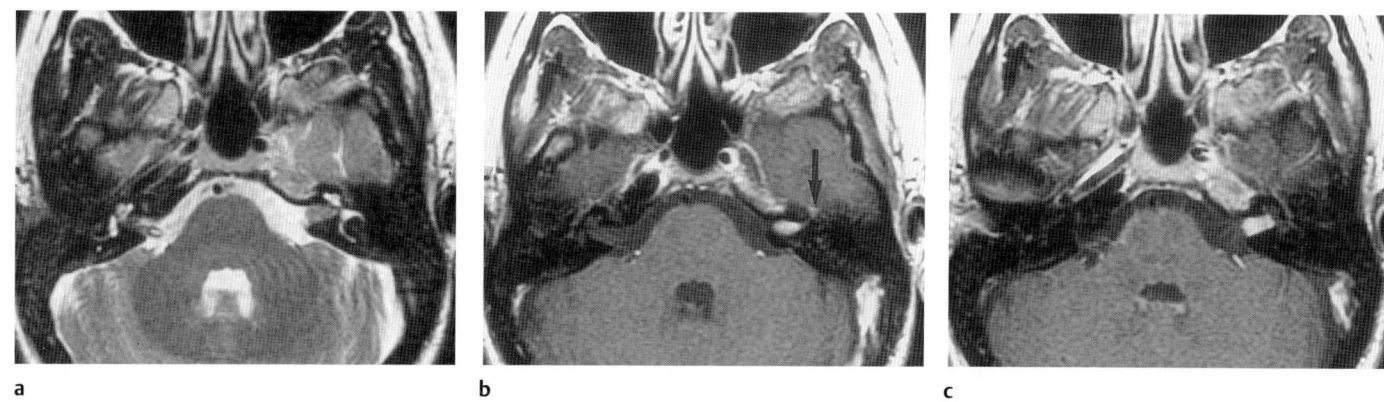

Fig. 1.**207** Facial nerve schwannoma. Axial MR: **a** FSE T2W, **b** and **c** T1W postcontrast. An enhancing soft-tissue mass fills the left internal auditory canal and extends into the facial canal, reaching the geniculate ganglion (**b** arrow). In the FSE T2W image, it is impossible to differentiate this tumor from a vestibular schwannoma since the extension into the facial nerve canal is not recognizable.

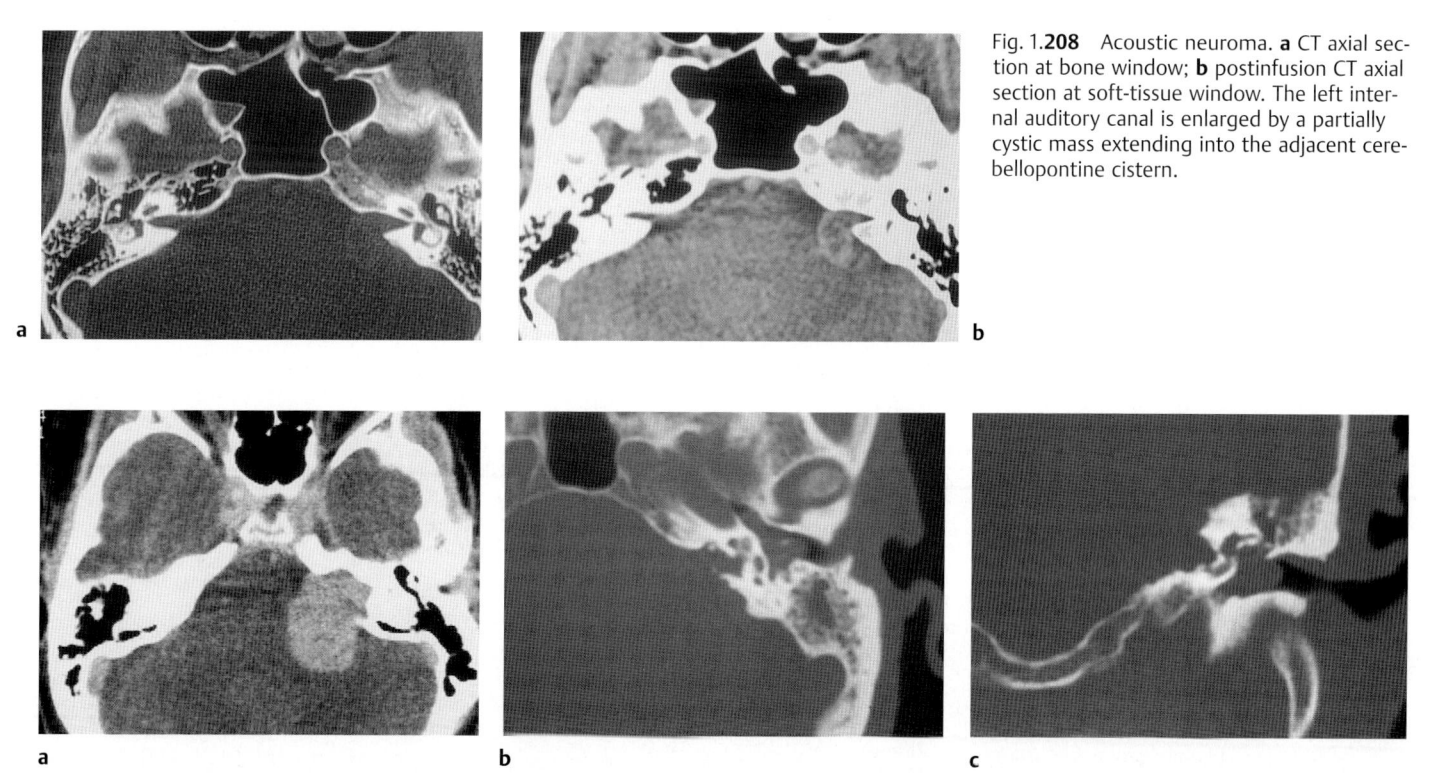

Fig. 1.**208** Acoustic neuroma. **a** CT axial section at bone window; **b** postinfusion CT axial section at soft-tissue window. The left internal auditory canal is enlarged by a partially cystic mass extending into the adjacent cerebellopontine cistern.

Fig. 1.**209** Acoustic schwannoma with middle ear extension. **a** Axial CT of the posterior cranial fossa after contrast; **b** axial and **c** coronal CT of the left ear. A large tumor mass expands the internal auditory canal and protrudes into the posterior cranial fossa. The lesion extends into the middle ear cavity and bulges into the external auditory canal.

Inflammatory Conditions

See Facial Neuritis, page 66.

Tumors

The facial schwannomas may occur within the internal auditory canal but are usually recognizable because of the extension into the fallopian canal itself (Fig. 1.**207**). A high-definition CT study usually reveals expansion of the involved segment of the canal, usually the labyrinth segment and the anterior genu. The MR study demonstrates enhancement and thickening of the facial nerve due to the enveloping tumor mass. As the lesion becomes larger, the enhancing soft-tissue mass may fill the entire internal auditory canal and break laterally into the middle ear cavity (Fig. 1.**173**) or anteriorly into the middle cranial fossa.

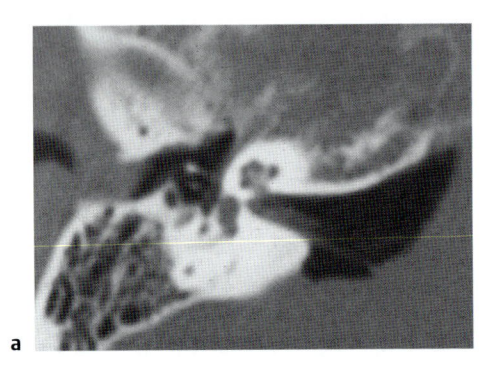

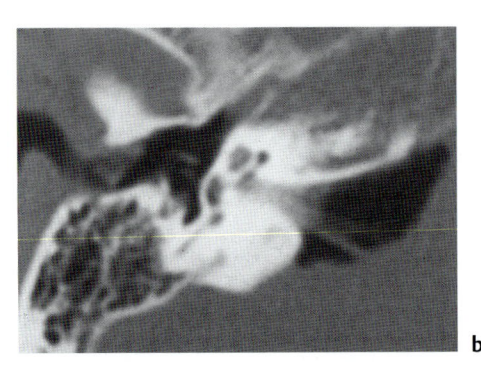

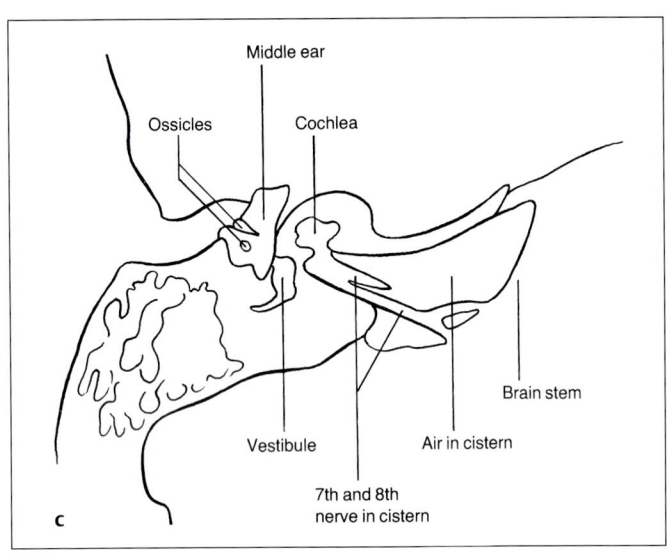

Fig. 1.**210** Normal cerebellopontine pneumocisternogram. **a**, **b** Axial CT sections, right. The gas fills the cerebellopontine cistern and the internal auditory canal. The normal seventh and eighth cranial nerves are well visualized as they stretch from the brainstem into the internal auditory canal. **c** Diagram of **a**.

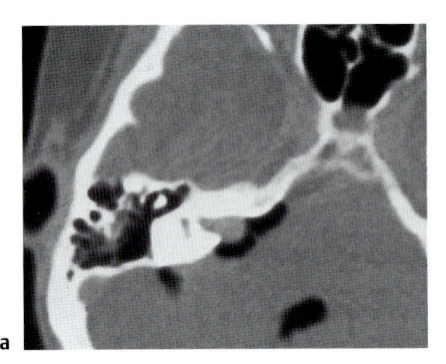

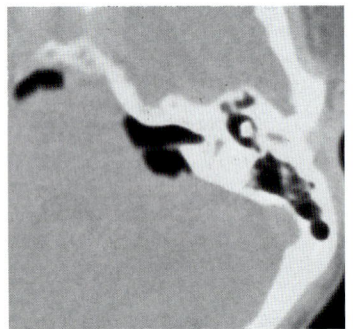

Fig. 1.**211** Acoustic neuroma CT pneumocisternography. **a** Right, **b** left axial CT sections. A small tumor mass (**a**) fills and expands the right internal auditory canal and protrudes into the cerebellopontine cistern. The proximal portion of the eighth nerve is normal and enters the medial espect of the tumor. **b** shows the normal left side for comparison.

■ Meningeal Pathology

Inflammation from bacterial meningitis, sarcoidosis, or postsurgical irritation may involve the intracanalicular meningeal extension. In the first instance, the MR study performed after i.v. injection of contrast material shows enhancement of the entire meningeal lining of the canal (Fig. 1.**212**). In postsurgical inflammation, the enhancement is usually limited and appears as a bright band at the fundus or along one of the walls of the canal.

Meningiomas

Meningiomas are the second most common tumor of the cerebellopontine angle (CPA) and usually arise outside the IAC, although they may extend within the medial portion of the canal. Meningiomas limited to the IAC are rare and mimic an acoustic schwannoma both clinically and by imaging. Meningiomas grow as a solid mass or en plaque and may cause hyperostosis (Fig. 1.**169**) or erosion of the adjacent bony structures. MR images obtained after i.v. injection of contrast material show a homogeneous enhancement of the tumor except in about 10% of the cases where small areas of signal void due to calcifications are noted within the mass (Fig. 1.**169**, 1.**170**). En plaque lesions appear as areas of enhancing meningeal thickening and are often associated with masslike tumors, thus producing a so-called tail sign, which is helpful, but not specific for the diagnosis of meningioma (Fig. 1.**171**).

■ Vascular Abnormalities

Vascular Loop

The concept of clinical symptoms produced by cross-compression of the cranial nerves by blood vessels was first introduced by

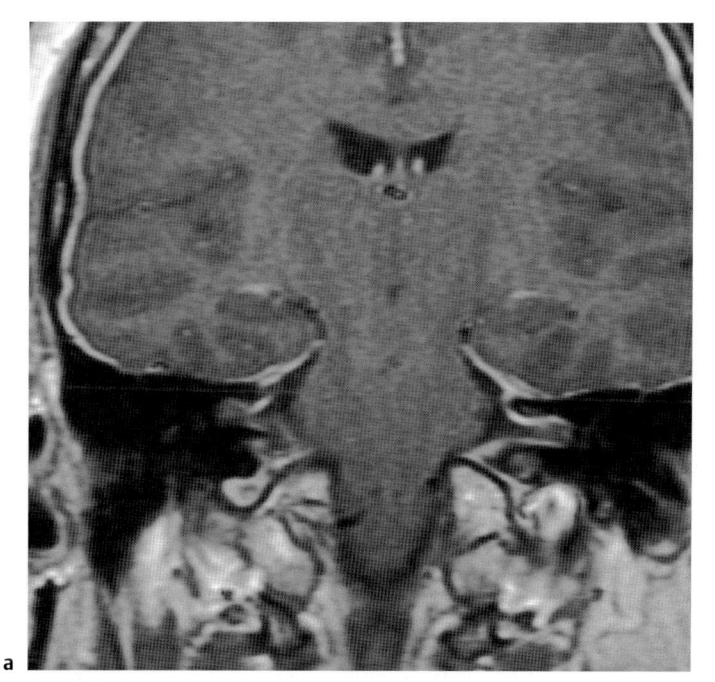

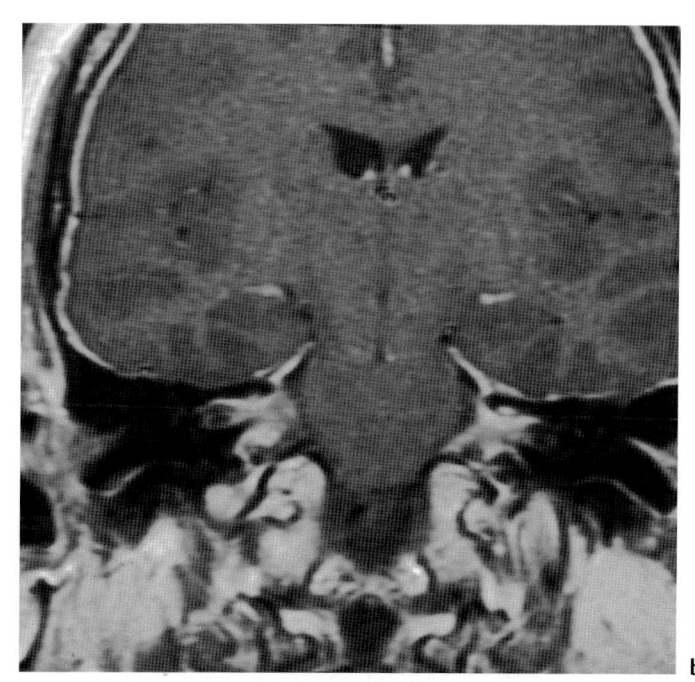

Fig. 1.212 Meningitis. **a, b** Coronal T1W MR images postcontrast. There is diffuse meningeal enhancement, including the lining of the internal auditory canals.

Dandy in 1934 for trigeminal neuralgia. Later the same concept was extended to the facial nerve to explain several cases of hemifacial spasm and more recently to the eighth cranial nerve as a possible cause of tinnitus, vertigo, and hearing loss. The anterior–inferior cerebellar artery (AICA) often loops within the cerebellopontine cisterns and in over 20% of the cases it actually enters the IAC. In addition, tortuous vertebral or basilar arteries often form prominent loops within the cerebellopontine cistern. Cross-compression of the nerve usually occurs at its exit from the brainstem owing to absence of slack of the nerve at this point, or within a narrow internal auditory canal. In the past, vascular loops were identified by CT pneumocystography (Fig. 1.213). At present we use T2 FSE MR images in both axial and coronal planes (Figs. 1.214, 1.215).

Aneurysm

An aneurysm within the internal auditory canal is extremely rare; I recall having encountered only three. Two small intracranial aneurysm were studied, one with opaque cisternogaphy and the other with CT pneumocystography. In both instances they appeared as nonspecific masses thought to represent small acoustic schwannomas. The third lesion was studied by MR imaging and appeared on T1-weighted and T2-weighted images as a small mass of high signal presumably due to thrombosis or slow flow. Following the i.v. injection of contrast material, the lesion appeared slightly larger. At surgery a small aneurysm arising from the labyrinth artery was found.

Aneurysms within the cerebellopontine cistern may compress the acoustic or facial nerve and mimic the symptomatology of a schwannoma. The MR images obtained prior to the i.v. injection of contrast material reveal a mass of nonhomogeneous high signal intensity produced by the clot. If the lumen of the aneurysm is partially patent, the flowing blood will appear as an area of signal void (Fig. 1.216).

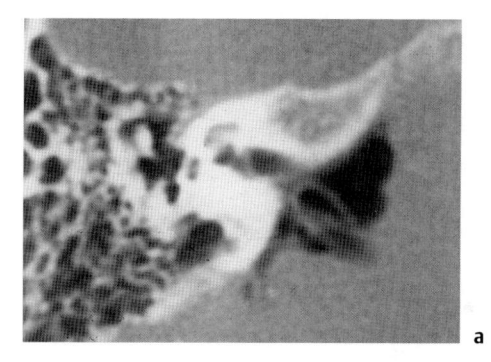

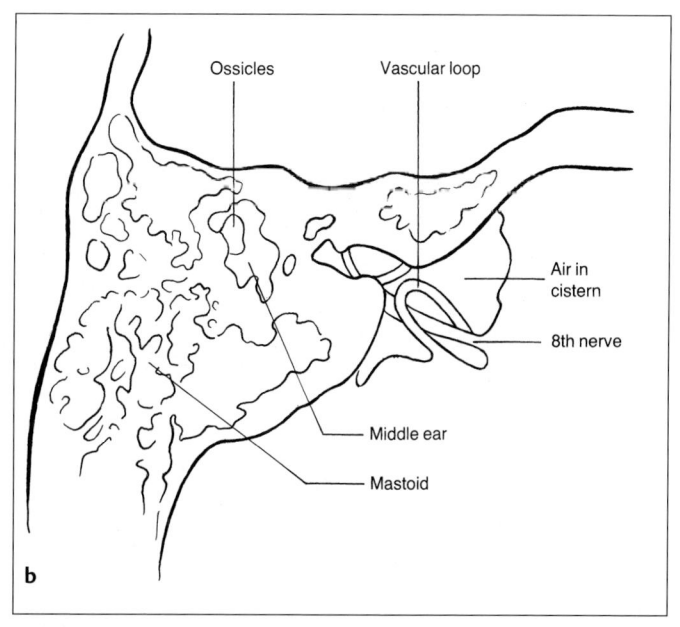

Fig. 1.213 **a** Vascular loop. Axial CT cerebellopontine pneumocisternogram, right. The gas fills the right internal auditory canal and cerebellopontine cistern. A large vessel, presumably the anterior inferior cerebellar artery, forms a large loop within the cistern. The vessel crosses and seemingly compresses the eighth cranial nerve close to its exit from the brainstem and at the porus of the internal auditory canal. **b** Diagram of **a**.

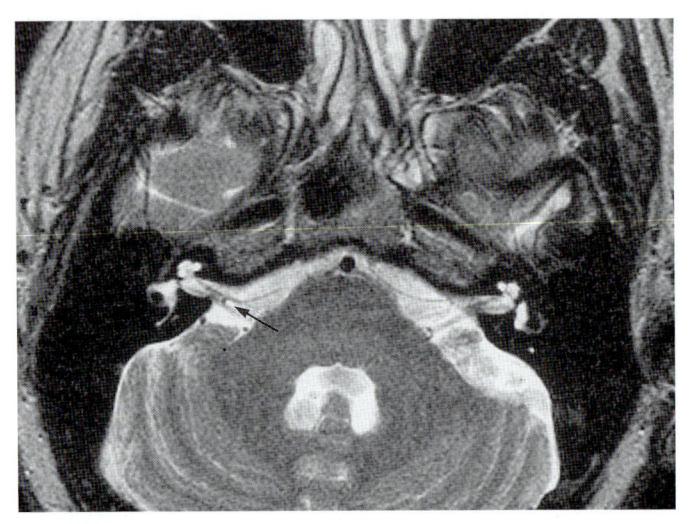

Fig. 1.**214** Vascular loop, right. Axial FSE MR image. A vascular loop passes between the cochlear and vestibular nerves (arrow). No surgical confirmation.

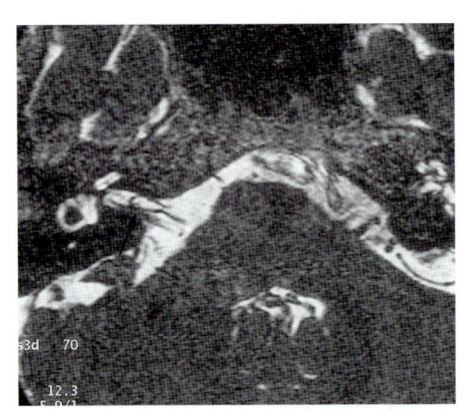

Fig. 1.**215** Vascular loop. The anterior–inferior cerebellar artery loops within the right internal auditory canal and compresses the acoustic nerve. The internal auditory canal was decompressed with relief of the imbalance and tinnitus.

Varix

In my experience, varix malformation is extremely rare. In the single case that I have seen, the CT images showed enlargement of the internal auditory canal and a ringlike calcification within the canal resembling phleboliths. The MR study revealed a high signal intensity mass within the IAC that became considerably larger and brighter following the administration of contrast.

Hemangiomas

Small hemangiomas or arteriovenous malformation limited to the lumen of the internal auditory canal are rare. They appear in the precontrast images as areas of high signal intensity due to slow flow, which become larger following the i.v. injection of contrast material. The mass has nonhomogeneous intensity and may contain signal void areas due to calcifications.[20] Larger hemangiomas involve the bone of the petrous pyramid and may extend within the internal auditory canal. These lesions are characterized by masses of medium intensity in the T1-weighted precontrast images, which contain spokelike areas of signal void due to calcifications.[27] The tumor becomes bright after i.v. injection of contrast material but maintains the same nonhomogeneous intensity (Fig. 1.**217**).

■ Heterotopic Lesion within the Internal Auditory Canal

Lipomas (Choristomas)

In all four cases that I have seen, the lipoma was located at the fundus of the IAC. The diagnosis is made either by obtaining T1-weighted and T2-weighted precontrast images or by adding fat-suppression technique whenever a bright mass is seen on postcontrast T1-weighted images (Fig. 1.**218**).[11] Lipomas may also involve the CPA region and the labyrinth.

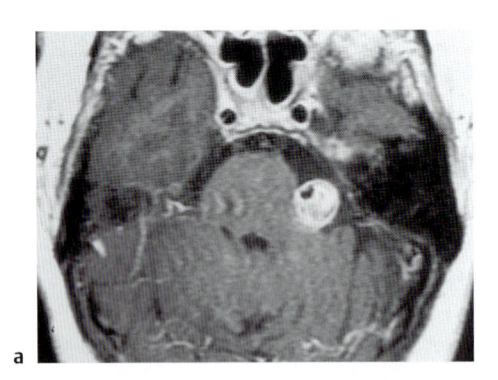

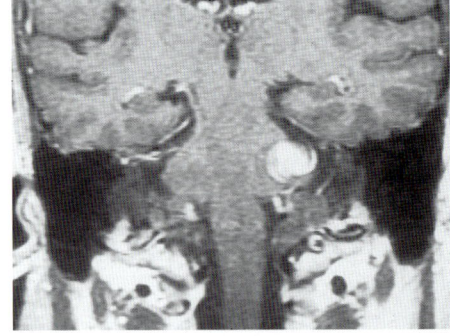

Fig. 1.**216** Aneurysm, left vertebral artery. **a** Axial, **b** coronal T1W MR sections after contrast. **c, d** Three-dimensional phase-contrast MR angiograms. An enhancing mass of uneven signal intensity is seen in the left cerebellopontine cistern. MR angiography demonstrates an aneurysm arising from the left vertebral artery.

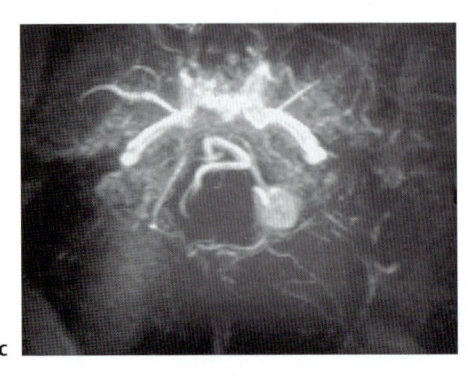

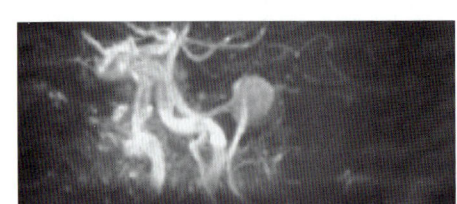

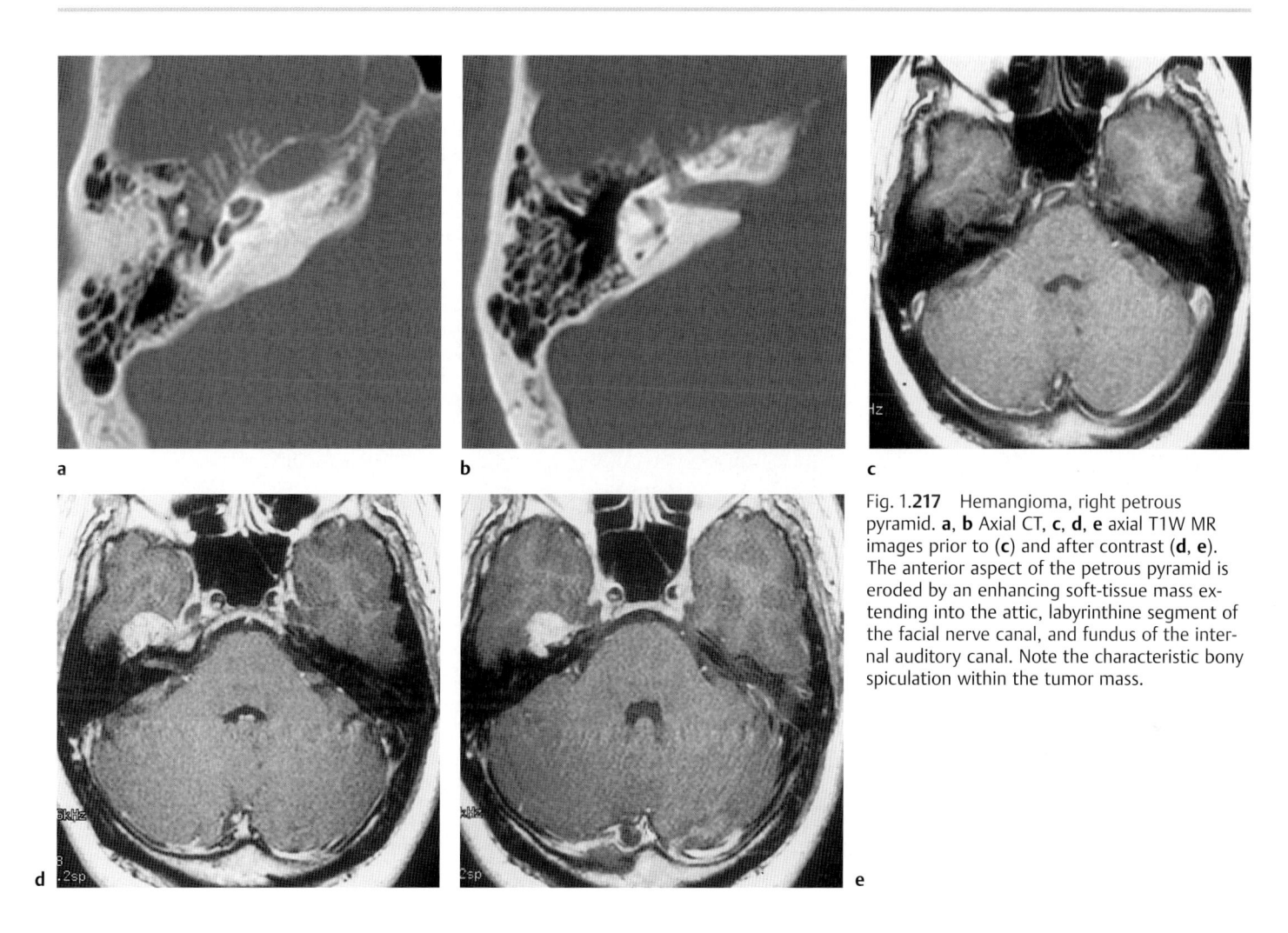

Fig. 1.217 Hemangioma, right petrous pyramid. **a, b** Axial CT, **c, d, e** axial T1W MR images prior to (**c**) and after contrast (**d, e**). The anterior aspect of the petrous pyramid is eroded by an enhancing soft-tissue mass extending into the attic, labyrinthine segment of the facial nerve canal, and fundus of the internal auditory canal. Note the characteristic bony spiculation within the tumor mass.

Epidermoid Cysts

Epidermoid cysts usually occur in the cerebellopontine cistern but are rarely seen within the internal auditory canal. The MR study shows a nonenhancing mass of low signal in T1-weighted images that becomes bright in T2-weighted images (Fig. 1.**219**). Unlike arachnoid cysts, epidermoid cysts appear hyperintense on FLAIR and diffusion-weighted MR pulse sequences.

Metastasis

In my experience of internal auditory canal metastasis, the primary is breast or lung carcinoma and melanoma (Fig. 1.**220**). Whenever there is no bone involvement, the diagnosis of metastasis is difficult, although it should be considered whenever the patient has a positive history. MRI is the study of choice. The lesion has a signal of medium intensity in the T1-weighted images that becomes brighter on T2-weighted images. Following the i.v. injection of contrast material, the mass undergoes a homogeneous or nonhomogeneous enhancement. Involvement of the IAC is usually due to leptomeningal spread of tumor.

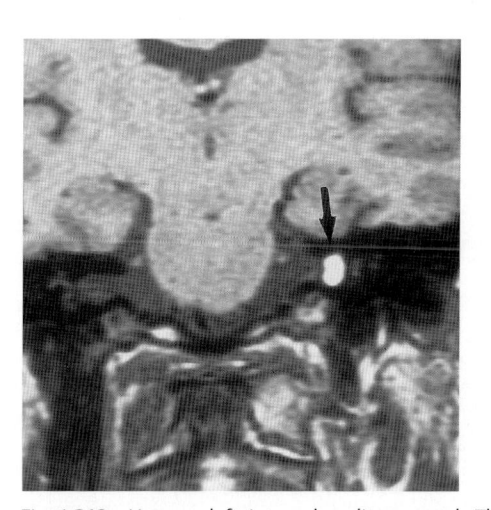

Fig. 1.**218** Lipoma, left internal auditory canal. This coronal T1W MR section, obtained without injecting contrast material, shows a high signal intensity mass (arrow) within the left internal auditory canal.

Lymphoma

Leukemic and lymphomatous infiltrations have been described as occurring within the internal auditory canal and cerebellopontine cistern. In the precontrast images, the characteristics of the lesions are similar to those of metastatic deposits. After the i.v. injection of contrast material, however, the enhancement is more prominent and homogeneous. Lymphomas are characteristically hyperintense on diffusion-weighted MR scans.

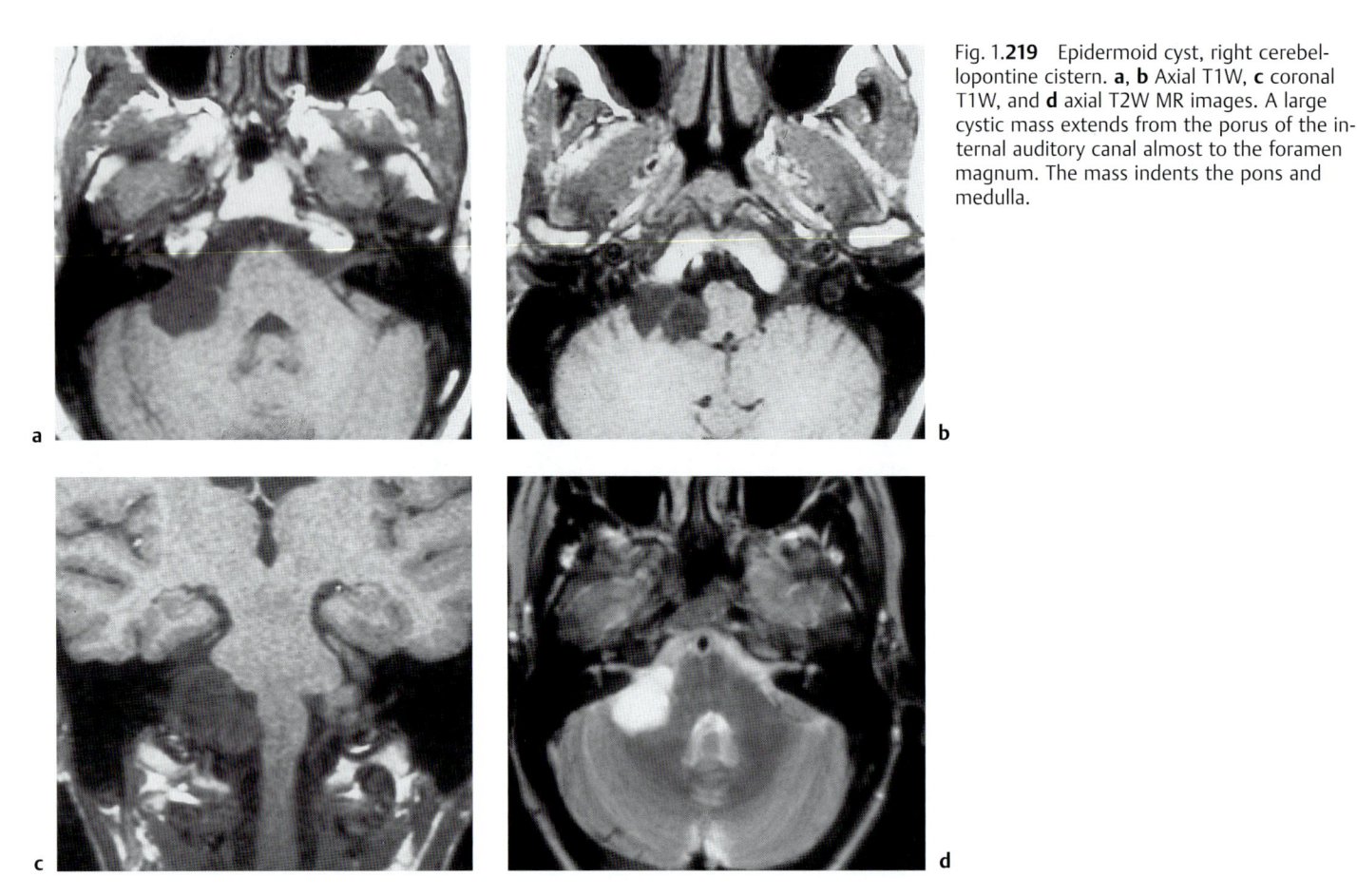

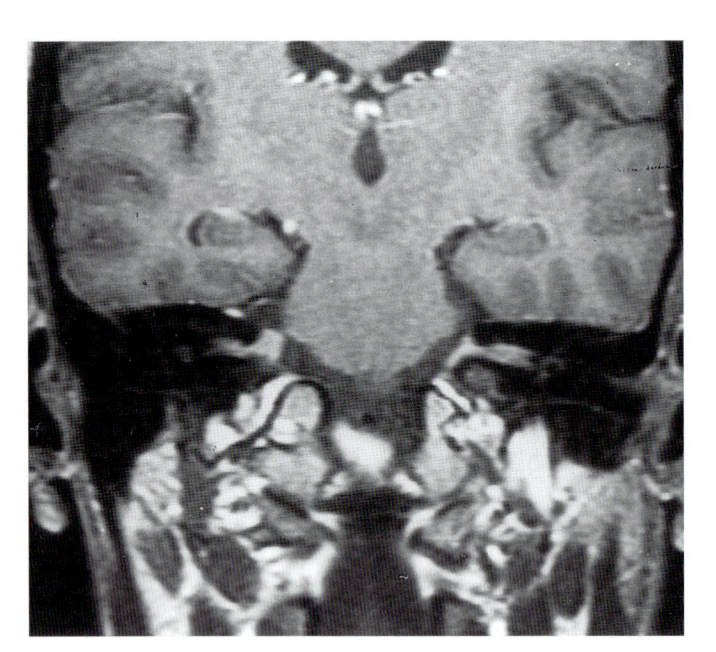

Fig. 1.**219** Epidermoid cyst, right cerebellopontine cistern. **a**, **b** Axial T1W, **c** coronal T1W, and **d** axial T2W MR images. A large cystic mass extends from the porus of the internal auditory canal almost to the foramen magnum. The mass indents the pons and medulla.

Fig. 1.**220** Metastatic melanoma. Coronal T1W postcontrast MR image. Enhancing lesions involve both cerebellopontine cisterns and extend into the internal auditory canals.

Otosclerosis and Bone Dystrophies

Otosclerosis

Otosclerosis is a primary focal disease of the labyrinthine capsule. The otosclerotic foci may be single or multiple and undergo periods of resorption and redeposition of bone at variable intervals. There appears to be a hereditary factor in the etiology. The most common site of a focus is in the labyrinthine capsule just anterior to the oval window (fisulla ante fenestram). This focus tends to extend posteriorly to fix the stapes footplate, and at times it invades and thickens the footplate. Similar foci occur in other areas of the labyrinthine capsule, particularly in the cochlea. Involvement of the oval window with fixation of the stapes causes conductive deafness. Cochlear foci produce sensorineural deafness by an unknown mechanism.

Histologically the foci that arise in the endochondral layer vary in appearance. In an active focus, there is a loose and irregular network of bony trabeculae with numerous blood vessels, osteoblasts, and osteoclasts. In a mature focus, there is a dense type of bone that is relatively avascular and contains fewer cells. These foci may progressively enlarge and extend to the endosteal and periosteal layers of the labyrinthine capsule. Periosteal involvement produces small exostotic-like protrusions into the lumen of the tympanic cavity.

The progression of otosclerosis is characterized by remission and exacerbation. The disease may be quiescent for relatively long periods, or there may be rapid progression with deterioration of hearing.

Otosclerosis and Bone Dystrophies

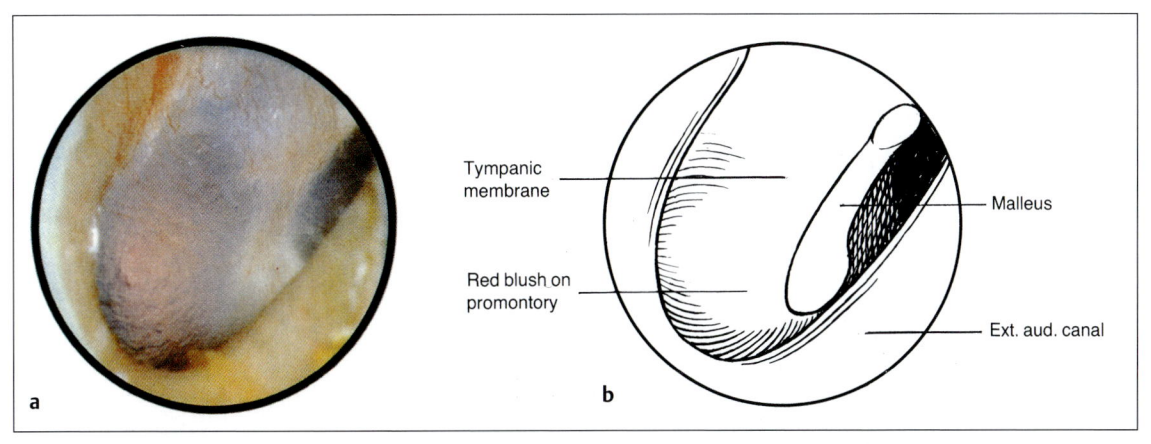

Fig. 1.**221** Otosclerosis, Schwartze sign; otoscopic findings, right. **a** A red blush of the promontory seen through the intact tympanic membrane is a sign of cochlear otosclerosis and demineralization. **b** Diagram of **a**.

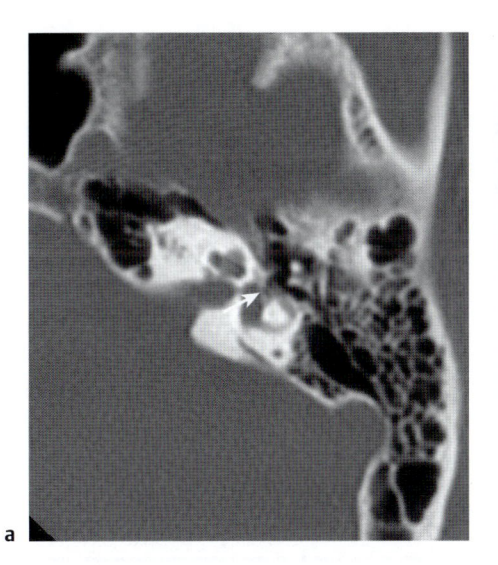

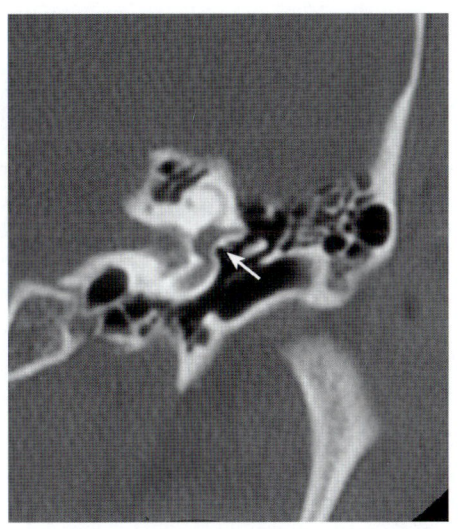

Fig. 1.**222** Left stapedial ostosclerosis. **a** Axial CT, **b** 20° coronal oblique CT images. The oval window appears closed by a thickened footplate (arrows). The cochlear capsule is normal.

Clinical Course

Otosclerosis usually begins in young adults as a gradually progressive conductive or mixed type of deafness. The hearing loss, which at the onset is usually conductive, may stabilize for relatively long periods. Progression usually occurs in bouts of exacerbations until there is maximum conductive deafness. Further deafness may then occur due to superimposed sensorineural hearing loss caused by involvement of the cochlea by the otosclerotic process.

In the usual case of otosclerosis, the tympanic membrane and the middle ear appear normal on otoscopy. When there is severe involvement of the cochlea and promontory by large, active, and vascular otosclerotic foci, the mucosa of the promontory becomes hyperemic. This hyperemia is visible through the normal tympanic membrane and causes a blush of the promontory, called the Schwartze sign (Fig. 1.**221**).

CT of the Labyrinthine Windows

CT is used to study and diagnose otosclerosis of the labyrinthine windows, the cochlea, and other inner ear structures.

The projections used for the study of the labyrinth windows and cochlear capsules are the axial and 20° coronal oblique. The first projection demonstrates the cochlear coils and the round window. For exposure of the oval window, the 20° coronal oblique is far superior to the standard coronal projection.

The oval window lies in the medial labyrinthine wall of the middle ear cavity, which forms an angle of about 20° open posteriorly with the sagittal plane of the skull. The vertical axis of the window measures 1.5–2 mm and the long axis 3–4 mm.

Beginning at the level of the anterior aspect of the cochlea, sections 1 mm apart are taken that will pass through the oval window area.

The oval window appears as well-defined bony dehiscence in the lateral wall of the vestibule below the ampullated limb of the horizontal semicircular canal. The footplate of the stapes is sectioned at right angles to the long axis. A normal footplate appears as a fine line extending across the oval window (see Fig. 1.**20**). The round window membrane closes the scala tympani and is located deep in the round window niche (see Fig. 1.**21**). On axial sections, the round window niche is well seen on the inferior aspect of the promontory below the oval window (see Fig. 1.**7**).

Radiographic Findings of Fenestral Otosclerosis

The radiographic appearance of otosclerosis of the oval window depends on the degree of maturation and the extent of the pathological process.

In mature otosclerosis, the oval window becomes narrowed or closed by calcified foci (Fig. 1.**222**). In active otosclerosis or otospongiosis, the poorly calcified foci may not be recognizable,

1 Imaging of the Temporal Bone

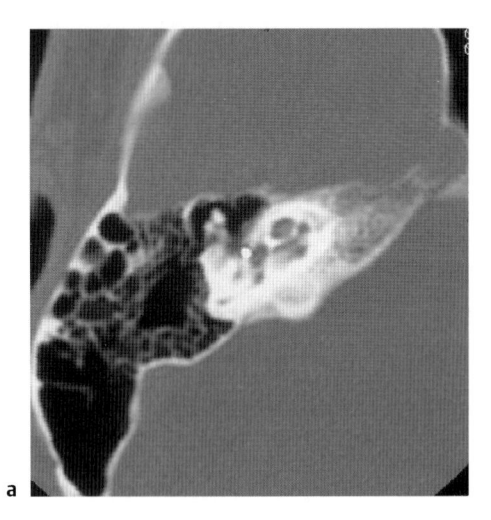

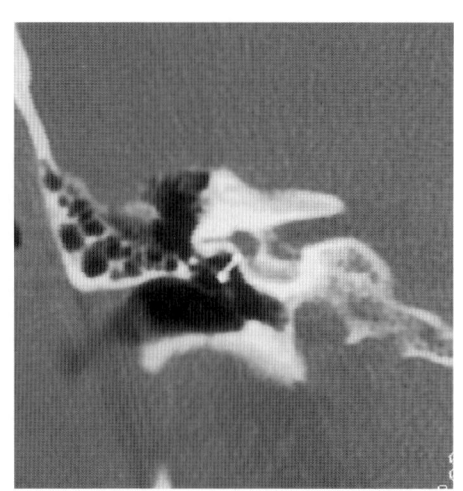

Fig. 1.**223** Stapedial otosclerosis after stapedectomy. **a** Axial, **b** coronal CT sections. A metallic prosthesis extends from the long process of the incus to the oval window. The prosthesis is in good relationship to the long process of the incus and to the oval window.

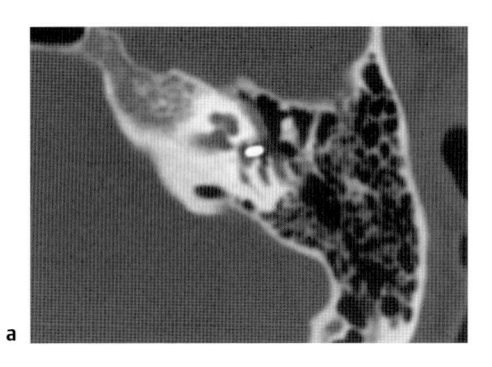

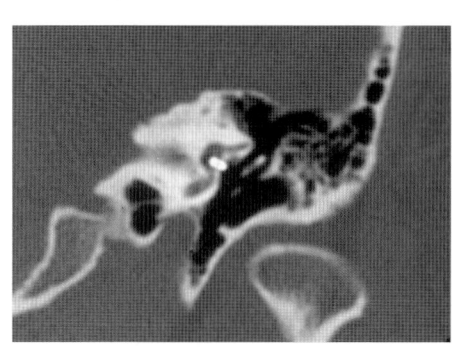

Fig. 1.**224** Left stapedial otosclerosis after stapedectomy. **a** Axial, **b** 20° coronal oblique CT sections. The oval window is patent and the medial end of the strut protrudes into the vestibule.

but the margin of the oval window becomes decalcified so that the oval window seems larger than normal (Figs. 1.**228**, 1.**232**). Occasionally the footplate of the stapes becomes greatly thickened with minimal involvement of the surrounding oval window margin. In diffuse otosclerosis, the entire footplate is involved as well as the oval window margin. In these cases the oval window appears completely obliterated by a thick bony plate.

The otosclerotic process may involve the vestibular aspect of the footplate and oval window margin to encroach upon the vestibule. The round window may be involved by an isolated focus or by extension of a large focus from the oval window area. Areas of demineralization or sclerotic foci may surround and encroach upon the round window. It is difficult to predict the functional loss of hearing from round window otosclerosis, since it is known that a minute opening in the round window is sufficient for its hydrodynamic function.

Preoperative and Postoperative Evaluation of the Labyrinthine Windows

Otosclerosis is diagnosed clinically by the otologist on the basis of otoscopy, audiometry, and tuning fork tests. The clinical evaluation cannot determine the extent or the degree of the pathological involvement of the footplate. CT can visualize the extent of the pathology of the oval window and footplate and can be used in those cases where the clinical diagnosis of otosclerosis is in doubt and in some bilateral cases for selection of the ear to be operated. CT is also indicated in patients with pronounced mixed deafness to determine the presence of capsular involvement (Figs. 1.**222**–1.**234**).

CT after Stapedectomy

CT is helpful in determining the cause of immediate and delayed vertigo and poststapedectomy hearing loss. The position of the prosthesis is usually evident in CT sections (Figs. 1.**223**, 1.**226**). Because of partial volume averaging effects, very thin metallic prostheses may not be seen, whereas thicker metallic prostheses are distorted and appear thicker than they actually are. CT can also visualize some thick plastic prosthetic struts.

In cases where severe sensorineural deafness or vertigo follow immediately after surgery, CT can demonstrate protrusion of the prosthesis into the vestibule (Figs. 1.**224**, 1.**225**).

When conductive deafness develops after an initial hearing improvement, the cause may be reobliteration of the oval window with fixation (Figs. 1.**228**, 1.**232**) or dislocation of the prosthesis (Fig. 1.**226**). If the oval window remains patent, conductive deafness can occur from separation of the lateral end of the prosthesis from the incus, or from necrosis of the long process of the incus. At times the lateral end of the strut is attached to the long process, but the medial end is dislocated from the oval window.

CT in Cochlear Otosclerosis

CT visualizes otosclerotic foci within the cochlear capsule. The normal cochlear capsule appears as a sharply defined dense bony shell outlining the lumen of the cochlear coils. When the otosclerotic foci affect the cochlear capsule, there is a variable disruption of the density and outline of the capsule (Figs. 1.**227**–1.**234**). In the interpretation of the radiographic findings of cochlear otosclerosis, three factors must be considered:

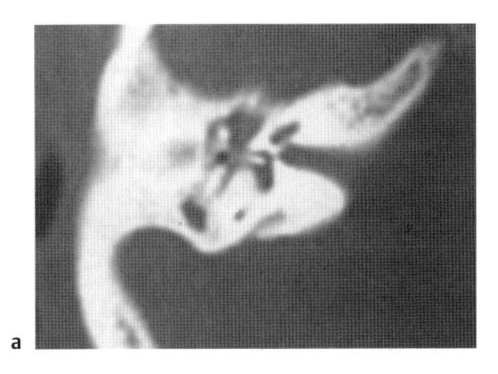

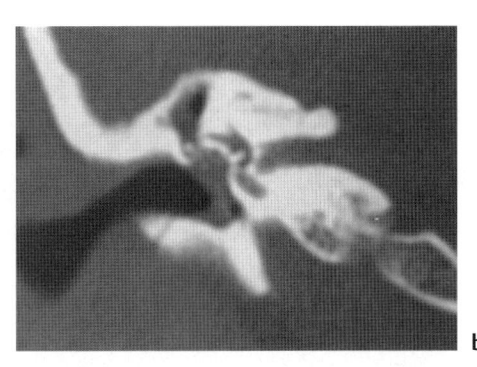

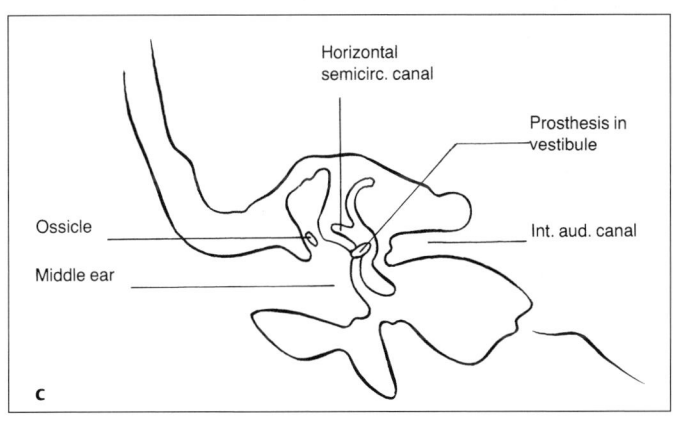

Fig. 1.225 Right fenestral otosclerosis after stapedectomy. **a** Axial, **b** coronal CT sections, right. A metallic prosthesis extends from the long process of the incus to the oval window, which appears patent. The medial end of the strut protrudes at least 2 mm into the vestibule. The changes in the middle ear cavity are due to a chronic otitis media. **c** Diagram of **b**.

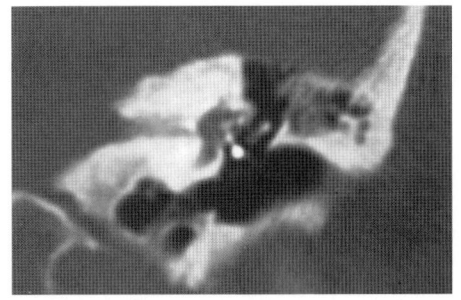

Fig. 1.226 Otosclerosis after stapedectomy. Coronal oblique CT section, left. The lateral end of the prosthesis is displaced downward and separated from the long process of the incus.

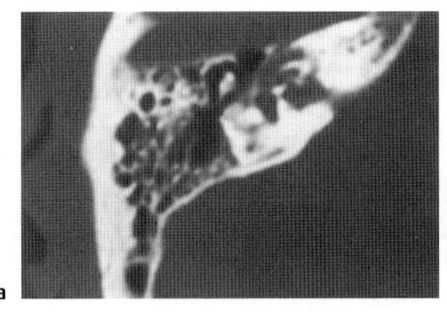

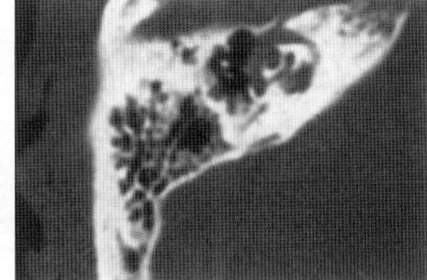

Fig. 1.227 Severe cochlear otosclerosis. **a, b** Axial CT sections. The contour of the cochlear capsule is disrupted by severe demineralization. The residual dense areas are fragments of the normal cochlear capsule.

1. The otosclerotic foci must be 1 mm or larger in diameter to be visible in the sections.
2. The density of the otosclerotic focus must be different from the density of the normal otic capsule.
3. Since the normal labyrinthine capsule is very dense, sclerotic foci can only be recognized when they are apposed to the periosteal or endosteal surfaces of the capsule.

The radiographic changes of cochlear otosclerosis are classified according to the extension of the process and maturation of the focus.

The otosclerotic process may be limited to a small portion of the basal turn of the cochlea immediately adjacent to the anterior margin of the oval window, spread into the basal turn, or involve other areas of the cochlea. Occasionally the fundus of the internal auditory canal, the semicircular canals, and the vestibule are affected. The radiographic appearance of the otosclerotic lesion varies with the stage of maturation of the disease. In the demineralizing or spongiotic stage, the normally sharp outline of the capsule becomes disrupted and may disappear completely (Fig. 1.227). The demineralization of the capsule causes loss of the normal differential density between the lumen of the cochlear coils and the capsule. A typical sign of cochlear otosclerosis is the formation of a double ring effect due to the confluence of spongiotic foci within the thickness of the capsule (Figs. 1.228, 1.231–1.234). This band of intracapsular demineralization may be limited to a segment of the capsule or follow almost the entire cochlear contour. This double ring sign is also seen in osteogenesis imperfecta and tertiary syphilis. In the mature or sclerotic stage, there are localized or diffuse areas of thickening of the capsule due to apposition of new otosclerotic bone. Such foci when seen end-on appear as areas of roughening or scalloping of the outer or inner aspects of the capsule.

When spongiotic and sclerotic changes occur simultaneously, there is a mosaic pattern characterized by a mixture of areas of decreased density intermingled with areas of increased density.

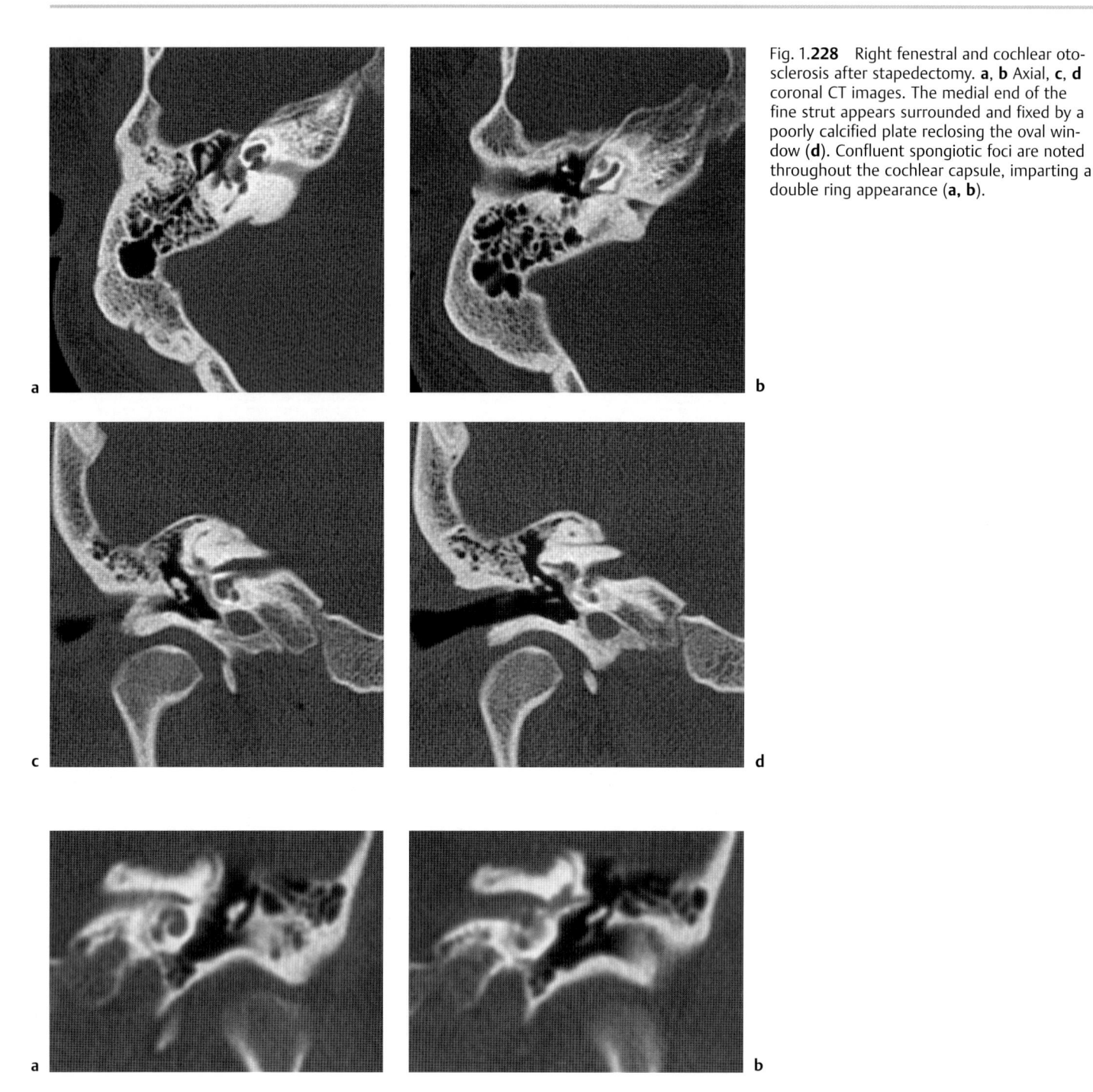

Fig. 1.**228** Right fenestral and cochlear otosclerosis after stapedectomy. **a, b** Axial, **c, d** coronal CT images. The medial end of the fine strut appears surrounded and fixed by a poorly calcified plate reclosing the oval window (**d**). Confluent spongiotic foci are noted throughout the cochlear capsule, imparting a double ring appearance (**a, b**).

Fig. 1.229 Otosclerosis. **a, b** Coronal CT sections, left. The anterior portion of the footplate is thickened. **b** Confluent spongiotic foci lie in the medial aspect of the chochlear capsule, imparting a double ring appearance. **c** Diagram of **a**.

CT Densitometry

Quantitative assessment of the involvement of the cochlear capsule by otosclerosis is made by CT densitometric studies.[33] Using the smallest cursor, the contour of the cochlear capsule is scanned and 31 densitometric readings are obtained. Readings are taken from two axial sections, the lower section passing through the basal turn and round window niche, the upper crossing the modiolus and three cochlear coils. Fifteen readings are taken from the lower section and 16 from the upper. A densitometric profile of the capsule is obtained by plotting the densitometric values against the 31 points where the readings were obtained. The topographic distribution of the 31 measured points, which begin at the prom-

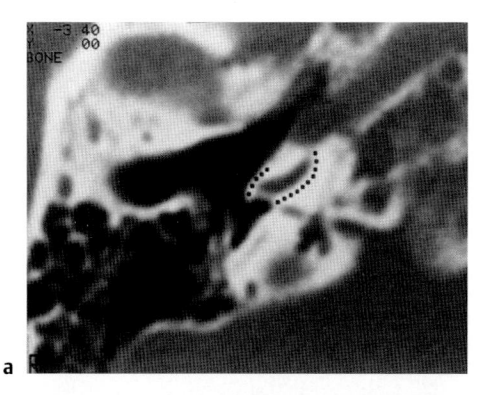

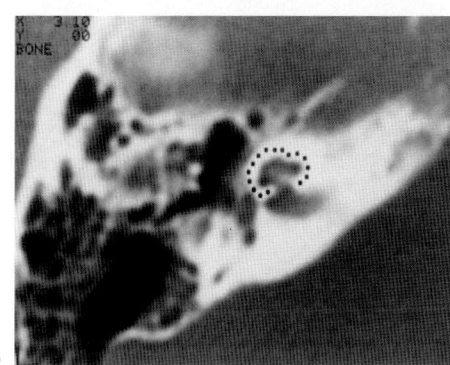

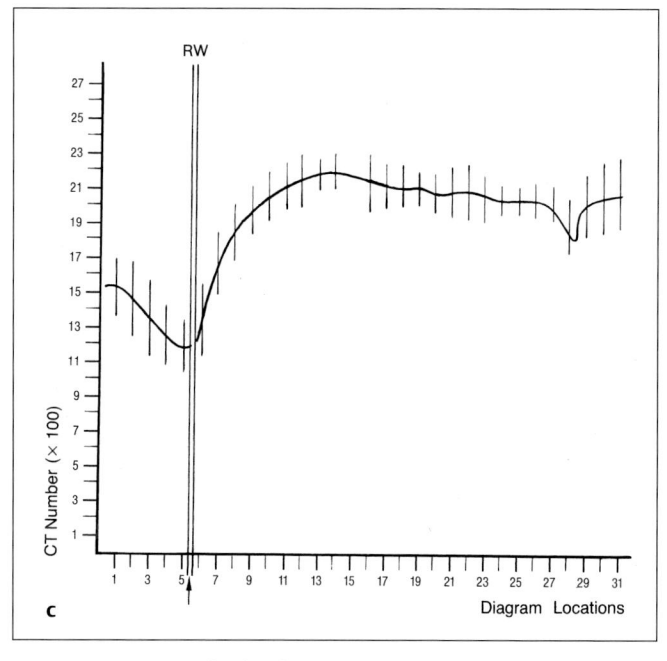

Fig. 1.**230** Topographic localization of 31 densitometric readings of the cochlear capsule. **a** Lower section crossing round window niche; **b** mid-modiolar section. Fifteen readings are obtained from the lower section, five along the promontory and ten along the medial aspect of the basil turn. Sixteen readings are obtained in the upper section following the contour of the cochlea, and the results are plotted on the graph. **c** Densitometric curve with standard deviations of the normal cochlear capsule. CT numbers are listed on the vertical axis and the sites of the cursor readings on the horizontal axis starting shortly before the round window. RW is the location of the round window niche.

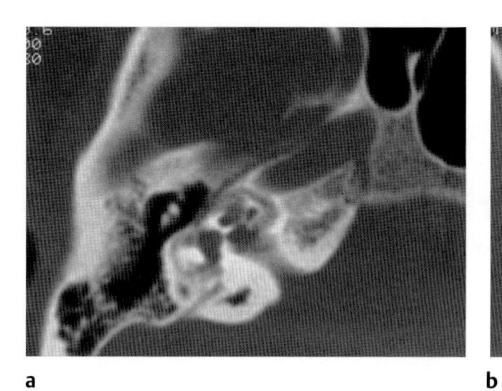

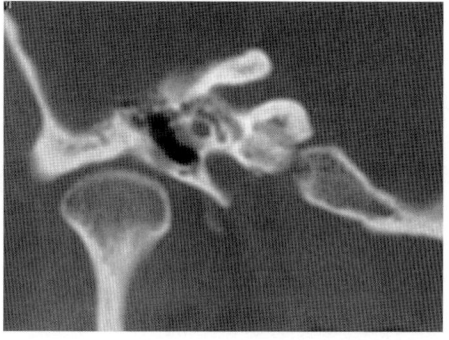

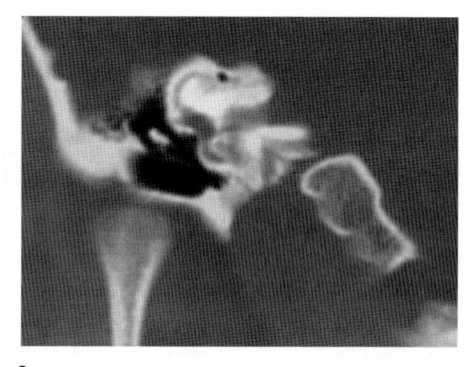

Fig. 1.**231** Right stapedial and cochlear otosclerosis. **a** Axial, **b**, **c** 20° coronal oblique CT sections; **d** densimetric profile of the cochlear capsule. The footplate of the stapes is thickened and a large band of demineralization is present within the medial aspect of the cochlear capsule. The promontory is not involved.

ontory and pass through the three cochlear coils to reach the anterior aspect of the vestibule, is shown in Figure 1.**230**. The horizontal axis of the graph indicates the areas where the measurements were taken and the vertical axis shows the density of the capsule expressed in CT numbers.

Curves from the patients are compared to previously obtained curves from normal ears. Variations of density exceeding standard deviations of 10–15 % for each point indicate cochlear involvement.

CT densitometry is an objective approach to the identification of otosclerotic foci in the cochlear capsule and determination of the degree of maturation of the disease. Densitometry is also useful in the evaluation of the progress of the disease after medical therapy and for following the natural course of the disease (Figs. 1.**231**–1.**233**).

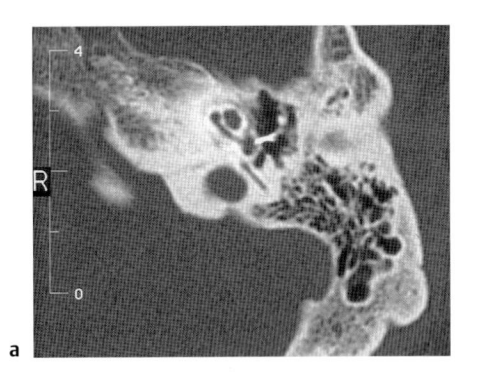

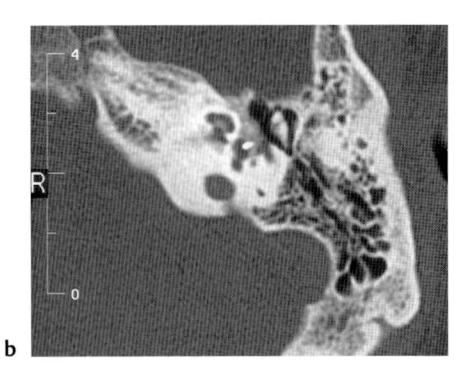

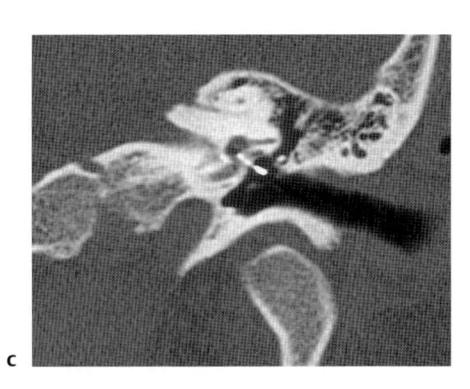

128 1 Imaging of the Temporal Bone

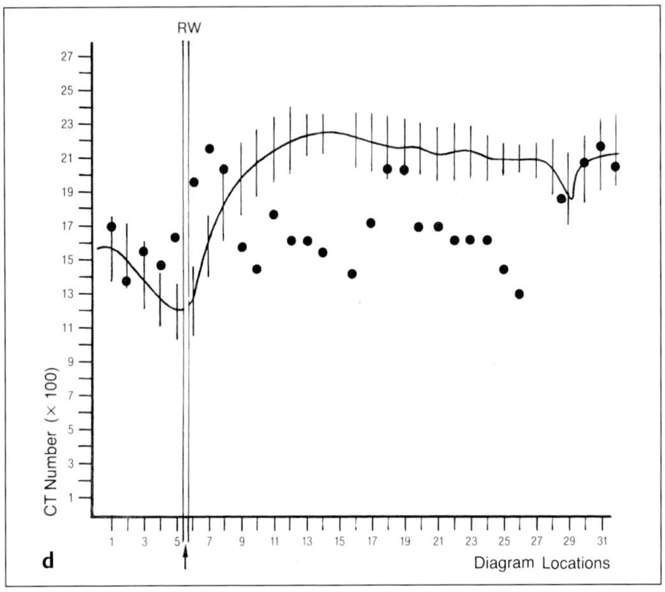

Fig. 1.**232** Fenestral and cochlear otosclerosis, after stapedectomy. **a**, **b** Axial, **c** coronal CT sections; **d** densimetric profile of the cochlear capsule. The prosthesis is in satisfactory position, but the oval window is reobliterated by a large poorly calcified plate. Spongiotic foci are noted in the cochlear capsule, sparing the promontory.

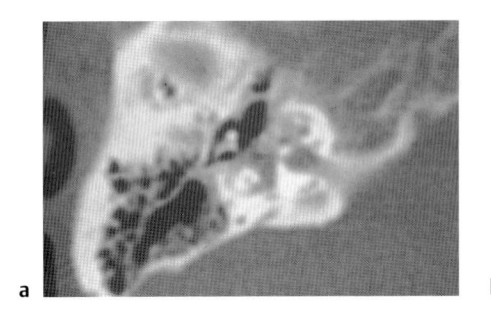

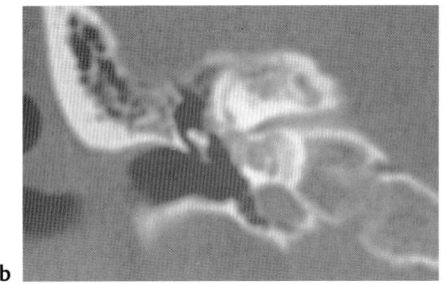

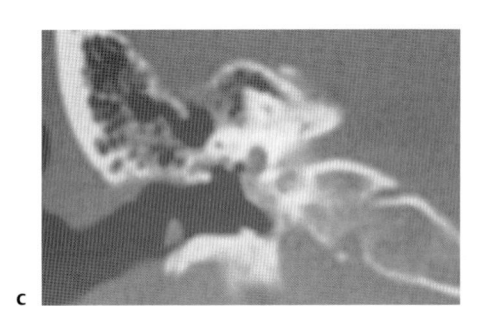

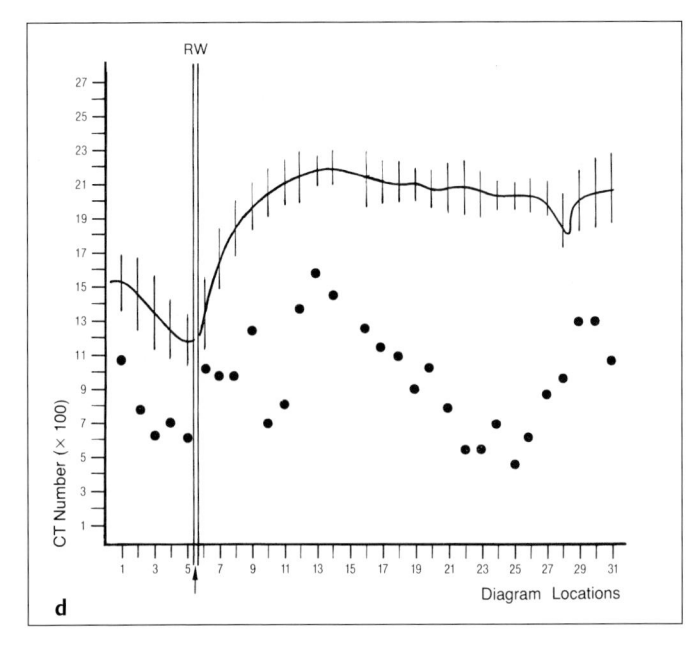

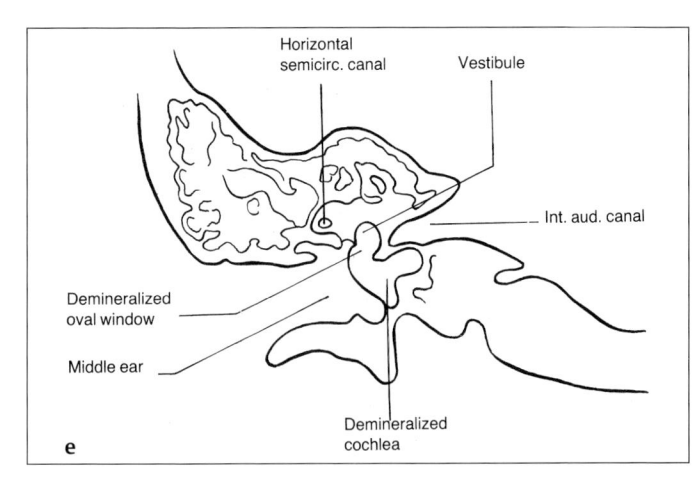

Fig. 1.**233** Cochlear otosclerosis. **a** Axial, **b**, **c** coronal CT sections; **d** densitometric profile, right. There are severe spongiotic changes throughout the cochlear capsule with formation of a double ring effect. The involvement is particularly severe in the basal turn and apical coil. The densitometric profile (**d**) (black dots), demonstrates the severity of the process. The lowest regions of the densitometric curves correspond to the areas of most severe demineralization at 3–5 and 20–27 on the horizontal axis of the graph. Normal curve above. **e** Diagram of **c**.

Densitometric curves similar to otosclerosis occur in Paget disease, osteogenesis imperfecta, and tertiary syphilis. Differentiation is made by other clinical, radiographic, and laboratory studies.

MRI of the Cochlea

We have recently started a new MR imaging protocol for patients with a positive Schwartze sign and severe spongiotic changes in the CT study. Using a three-dimensional Fourier transformation (3DFT) gradient-echo technique with very low TE and low flip angle, T1-weighted images as thin as 1.0 mm are obtained through the cochlea in axial and coronal planes. Images are acquired prior to and after injection of contrast material and then compared.

In several cases we have observed enhancement within the demineralized areas of the capsule (Figs. 1.**234**, 1.**239**). We presume that this blush is produced by pooling of contrast within the numerous blood vessels and lacunae found in young otospongiotic foci. Further investigation is necessary to confirm this observation and to establish a possible correlation between the intensity of enhancement and the activity of the process.

■ Paget Disease

Paget disease can affect the calvaria and the base of the skull, including the petrous pyramids. When the disease process extends into the otic capsule, there will be a mixed or sensorineural hearing loss that is progressive.

Radiographic Findings

Even in the absence of typical changes elsewhere in the skeleton, the diagnosis of Paget disease can be made by recognition of pathognomonic features in the skull and petrous pyramids.

In Paget disease there is an active stage with progressive bone resorption followed by a stage of irregular remineralization leading to a hypertrophied, irregularly mineralized bone (Fig. 1.**235**, 1.**236**).

The haversian bone of the petrosa is affected first, with spread of the disease from the apex laterally. At first, owing to severe

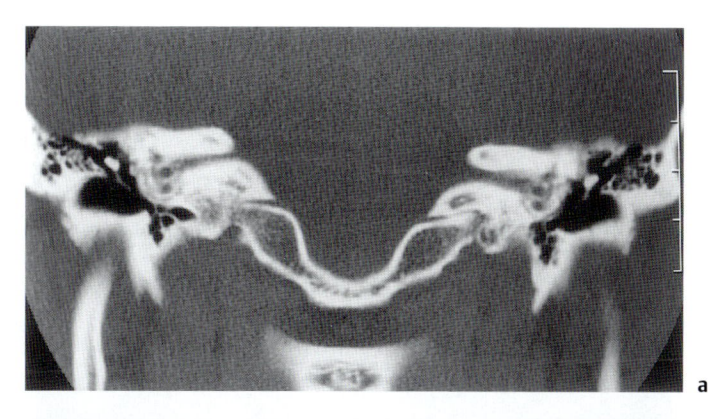

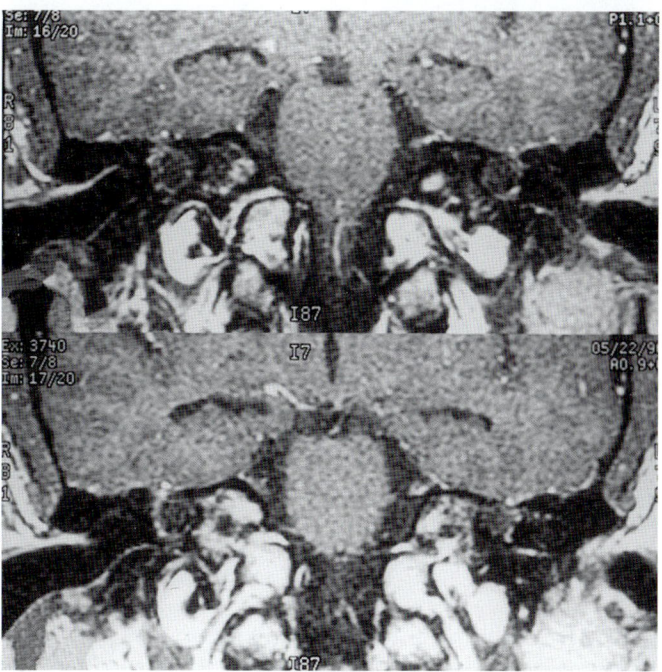

Fig. 1.**234** Cochlear otosclerosis. **a** Coronal CT image, **b** coronal T1W MR images after contrast. Severe spongiotic changes are noted throughout both cochleas (**a**). The MR images obtained after injection of contrast show enhancement of the highly vascular foci (**b**).

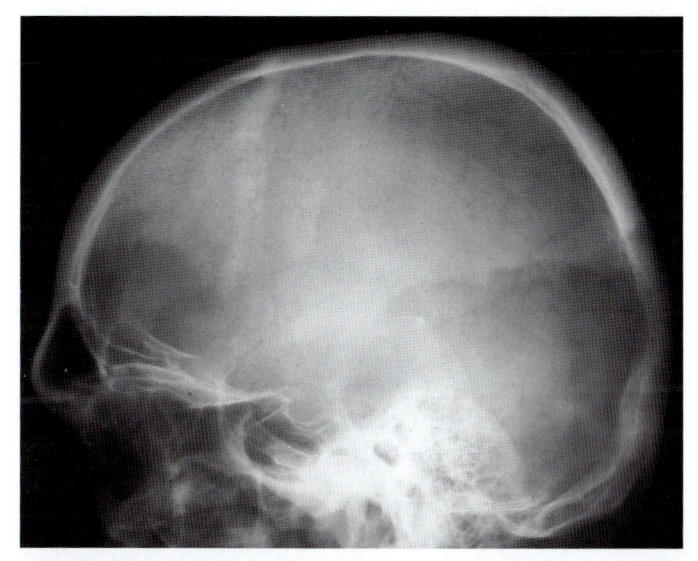

Fig. 1.**235** Paget disease, lateral skull. Two sharply defined areas of demineralization, osteoporosis circumscripta, are present in the occipital and frontal bones.

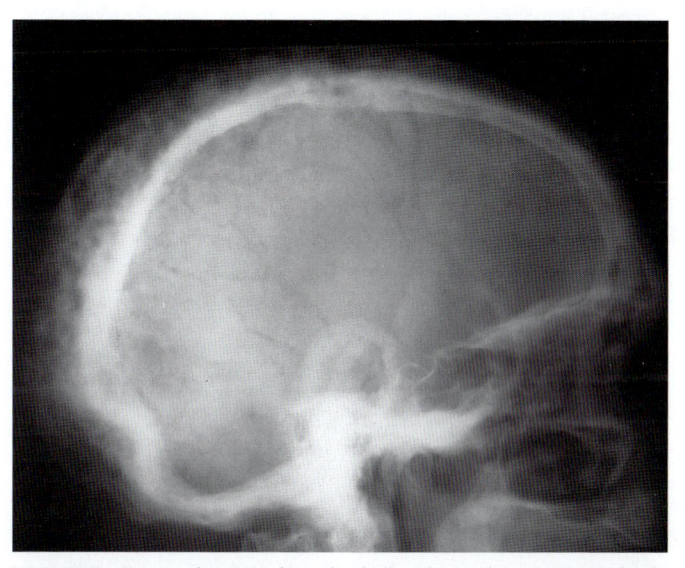

Fig. 1.**236** Paget disease, lateral skull. The calvaria is markedly thickened and the pathological remodeling of bone causes an irregular recalcification of the thickened calvaria.

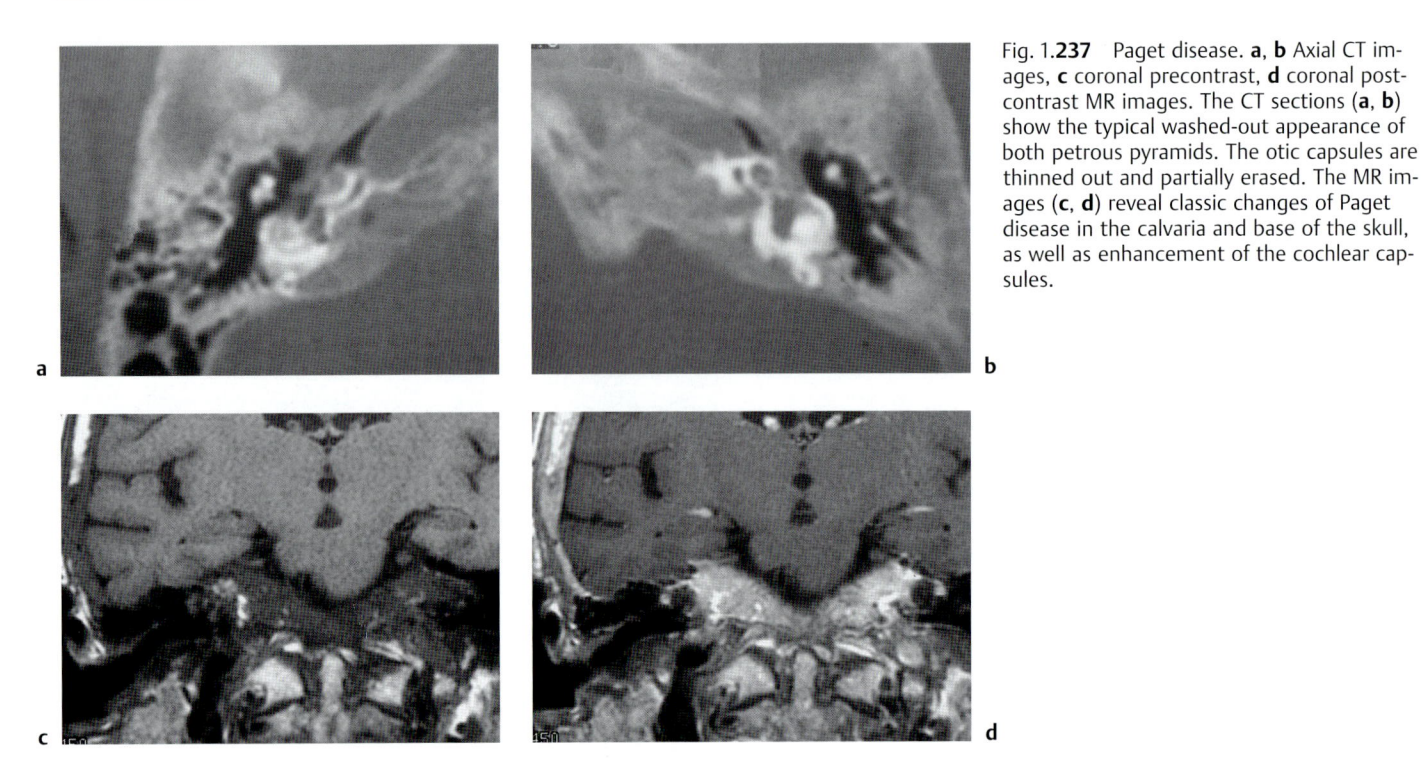

Fig. 1.**237** Paget disease. **a**, **b** Axial CT images, **c** coronal precontrast, **d** coronal postcontrast MR images. The CT sections (**a**, **b**) show the typical washed-out appearance of both petrous pyramids. The otic capsules are thinned out and partially erased. The MR images (**c**, **d**) reveal classic changes of Paget disease in the calvaria and base of the skull, as well as enhancement of the cochlear capsules.

demineralization of the petrosa, the labyrinthine capsule becomes more prominent than normal. Involvement of the otic capsule begins at the periosteal surface. Slow demineralization occurs, which produces first thinning and finally complete dissolution of the capsule. This results in a washed-out appearance of the entire petrous bone characteristic of Paget disease (Fig. 1.**237**). The internal auditory canal is usually the first structure involved, followed by the cochlea and the vestibular system (Fig. 1.**237**). In the late stage of the disease, deposition of irregular mineralized new bone occurs, which results in thickening of the petrous bone.

■ Osteogenesis Imperfecta

Osteogenesis imperfecta, or fragilitas osseum, is characterized by abnormally thin and fragile long bones with a history of multiple fractures, by a blue color of the sclera, and by severe mixed deafness. In some forms of the disease, one or more of the features may be absent. The head is large, the calvaria is abnormally thin, and the otic capsules are involved.

The CT and MR findings resemble those of active cochlear otosclerosis but are much more diffuse and involve the entire otic capsule (Fig. 1.**238**, 1.**239**).

■ Osteopetrosis

Osteopetrosis (Albers–Schonberg disease, marble bone disease) is a rare bone disease characterized by formation of new bone while resorption of bone is diminished. This results in sclerosis of bone with obliteration of the medullary cavities and diploic spaces and narrowing of the foramina of the skull. The petrous bone shows a complete lack of pneumatization and a homogenous diffuse sclerotic appearance. Progression of the disease results in narrowing of the internal auditory canals and encroachment on the neurovascular bundles. Facial paralysis may occur on the same basis. For more details, see Chapters 3 and 4.

■ Fibrous Dysplasia

Fibrous dysplasia is an osseous dystrophy of unknown etiology that may involve the skull. There are two different types of changes that occur in the skull. In the calvaria and mandible there is expansion of the affected portion by multiple cystic lesions. In the base of the skull the lesions are the result of abnormal proliferation of fibrous tissue intermixed with trabeculae of woven bone within the medullary cavity. These changes lead to increased density and thickening of the affected areas. Involvement by fibrous dysplasia is usually unilateral, which leads to asymmetry (Fig. 1.**240**). In the temporal bone, the squama becomes thickened and the pneumatic system obliterated. The external auditory canal is often stenosed by new bone formation. As the petrous pyramid becomes thickened and dense, the outline of the labyrinthine capsule becomes poorly distinguishable from the surrounding bone. Further progression may lead to narrowing of the internal auditory canal and obliteration of the lumen of the labyrinth.

■ Craniometaphyseal Dysplasia

Craniometaphyseal dysplasia is a genetic disorder characterized by alterations in the metaphyses of the long bones and by bony overgrowth of the skull, particularly the face and jaw.

The skull shows marked thickening and increased density of the calvaria with obliteration of the diploic space. The base of the skull, the maxilla, and the mandible become enlarged, thickened, and sclerotic. The paranasal sinuses are obliterated (Fig. 1.**241 a**). In the temporal bone, the external auditory canal and middle ear are gradually filled in by new dense bone formation.

The petrous pyramids are thickened and the lumen of the labyrinth becomes obliterated (Fig. 1.**241 b, c**).

The temporal bone and labyrinthine capsule are also involved in other rare congenital disorders and bony dysplasias such as cleidocranial dysostosis and Hurler syndrome.

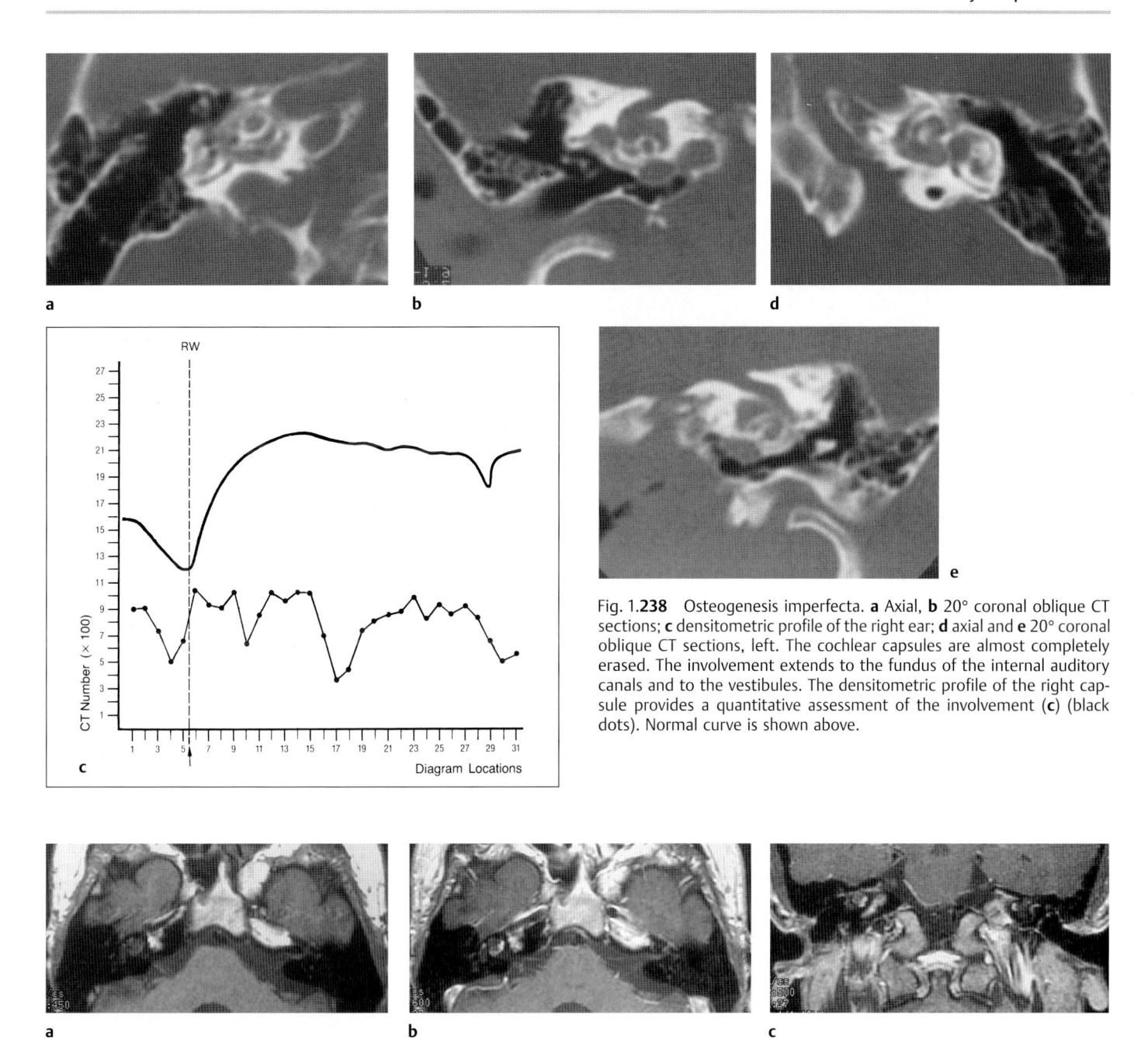

Otoscerosis and Bone Dystrophies **131**

Fig. 1.**238** Osteogenesis imperfecta. **a** Axial, **b** 20° coronal oblique CT sections; **c** densitometric profile of the right ear; **d** axial and **e** 20° coronal oblique CT sections, left. The cochlear capsules are almost completely erased. The involvement extends to the fundus of the internal auditory canals and to the vestibules. The densitometric profile of the right capsule provides a quantitative assessment of the involvement (**c**) (black dots). Normal curve is shown above.

Fig. 1.**239** Osteogenesis imperfecta, same case as Fig. 1.**238**. MR images: **a** axial T1W prior to contrast; **b**, **c** axial and coronal postcontrast. Several areas of enhancement are noted in the cochlear capsules, particularly on the right.

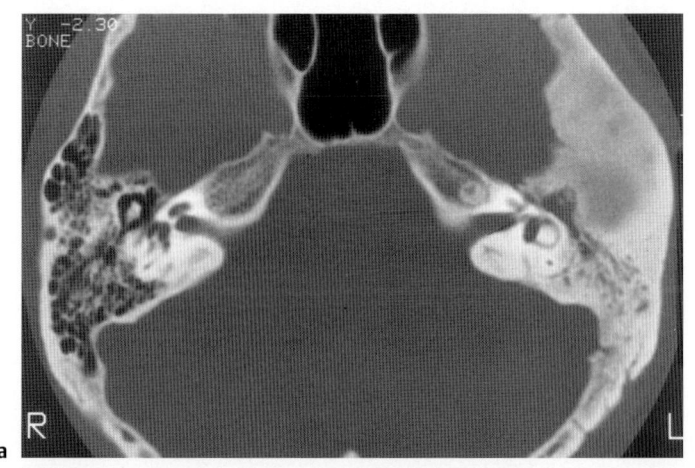

Fig. 1.**240** Fibrous dysplasia. **a**, **b** Axial, **c** direct sagittal CT sections, left. The temporal squama is markedly thickened. The disease extends to the temporomandibular fossa, which is shallow. The proliferative hyperostotic process obliterates some of the mastoid air cells and obstructs the external auditory canal. Because the external canal is obstructed, a cholesteatoma fills the middle ear.

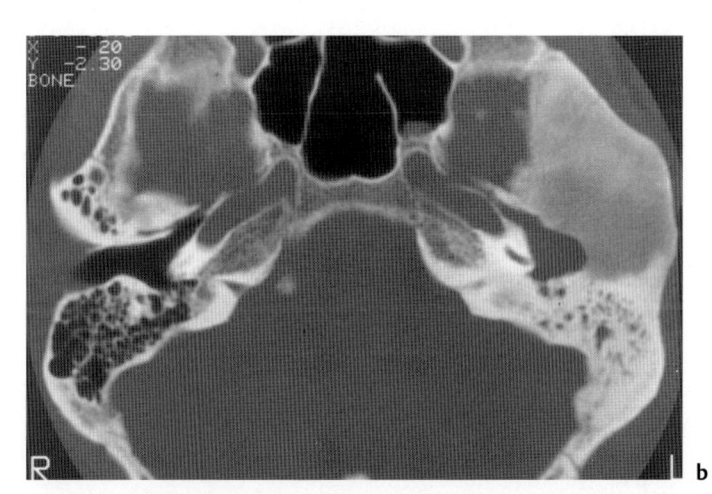

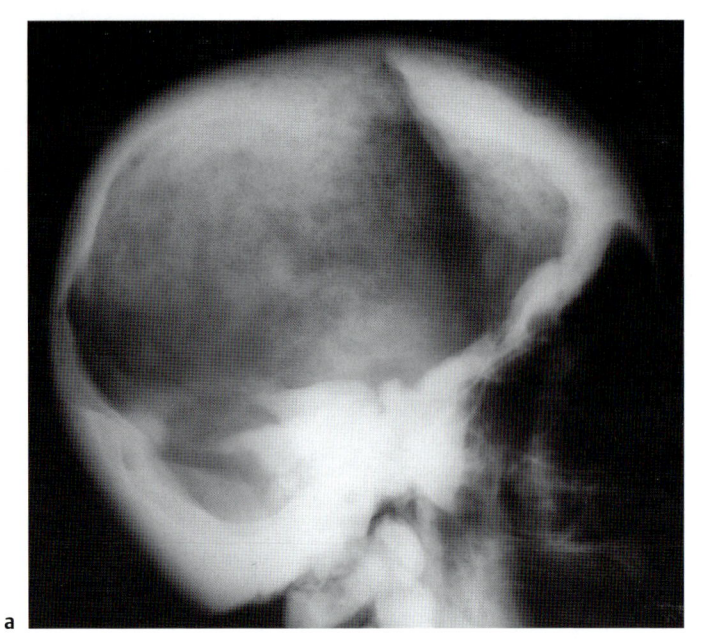

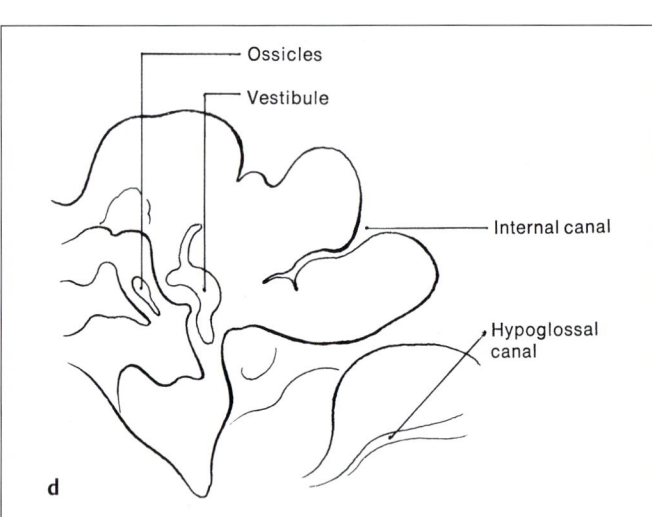

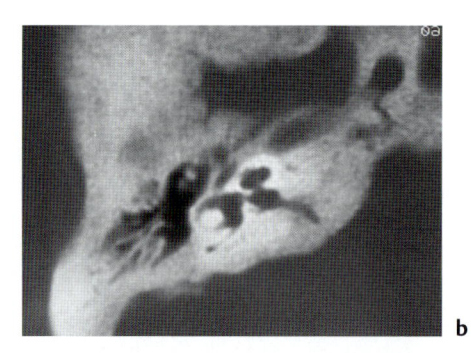

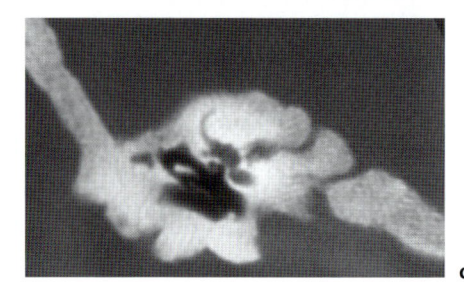

Fig. 1.**241** Craniometaphyseal dysplasia. **a** Lateral skull, **b** axial, and **c** coronal CT sections, right. The calvaria and petrous pyramid are thickened by dense sclerotic bone. The process extends to the internal auditory canal, which is markedly stenotic. **d** Diagram of **c**.

References

1. Antonelli PJ, Garside JA, Mancuso AA, Stricker ST, Kubilis PS. Computed tomography and the diagnosis of coalescent mastoiditis. Otolaryngol Head and Neck Surg 1999; 120(3): 350–354.
2. Arnold B, Jager L, Grevers G. Visualization of inner ear structures by three-dimensional high-resolution magnetic resonance imaging. Am J Otol 1996; 17(3): 480–485.
3. Buckingham RA, Valvassori GE. Inner ear fluid volumes and the resolving power of magnetic resonance imaging: can it differentiate endolymphatic structures? Ann Otol Rhinol Laryngol 2001; 110(2):113–117.
4. Casselman JW, Kuhweide R, Ampe W, Meeus L, Steyaert L. Pathology of the membranous labyrinth: comparison of T1 and T2 weighted and gadolinium-enhanced spin-echo and 3DFT-CISS imaging. AJNR 1993; 14: 59–69.
5. Casselman JW, Kuhweide R, Deimling M, et al. Constructive interference in steady state 3DFT MR imaging of the inner ear and cerebellopontine angle AJNR 1993; 14:47–57.
6. Chang P, Fagan PA, Atlas MD, Roche J. Imaging destructive lesions of the petrous apex. Laryngoscope 1998; 108(4 Pt 1):599–604.
7. Davidson HC, Harnsberger R, Lemmerling MM, et al. MR Evaluation of vestibulocochlear anomalies associated with large endolymphatic duct and sac. AJNR 1999; 20:1435–1441.
8. Dubrulle F. Ernst O, Vincent C, Vaneecloo FM, Lejeune JP, Lemaitre L. Cochlear fossa enhancement at MR evaluation of vestibular Schwannoma: correlatioin with success at hearing-presrvation surgery. Radiology 2000; 215(2): 458–462.
9. Fatterpekar GM, Mukherji SK, Lin Y, Alley JG, Stone JA, Castillo M. Normal canals at the fundus of the internal auditory canal: CT evaluation. J. Comput Assist Tomogr 1999; 23(5): 776–780.
10. Fitzgerald DC, Mark AS. Sudden hearing loss: frequency of abnormal findings on contrast-enhanced MRI studies. AJNR 1998; 19(8):1433–1436.
11. Greinwald JH Jr, Lassen LF. Lipomas of the internal auditory canal. Laryngoscope 1997; 107(3): 364–368.
12. Koch BL. Langerhans' Histiocytosis of temporal bone: role of MRI. Top Magn Reson Imaging 2000; 11: 66–74.
13. Mafee MF, Valvassori GE. Radiology of the craniofacial anomalies. Otolaryngol Clin North Am 1981; 14: 939–988.
14. Mafee MF, Lachenauer CS, Kumar A, et al. CT and MR imaging of intralabyrinthine schwannoma: report of two cases and review if the literature. Radiology 1990; 174: 395–400.
15. Mafee MF, Wee R, Lee G, Mafee RF. Imaging of vestibular aqueduct, endolymphatic duct and sac and adenocarcinoma of probably endolymphatic sac origin. Riv Neuroradiol 1995;8: 951–961.
16. Maffee MF, Singleton EL, Valvassori GE, et al. Acute otomastoiditis and its complications: role of CT. Radiology 1985; 54: 391–397.
17. Mafee MF, Aimi K, Valvassori GE. CT in the diagnosis of primary tumors of the petrous bone. Laryngoscope 1984; 94: 1423–1430.

18. Mafee MF, Raofi B, Kumar A, Muscato C. Glomus faciale, glomus jugulare, glomus tympanicum, glomus vagale, carotid body tumors, and simulating lesions: role of MR imaging. Radiol Clin North Am 2000; 38: 1059–1075.
19. Megerian CA, MCKenna MJ, Nuss RC, Manaiglia AJ, Ojemann RG, Pilch BZ, Nadol JB Jr. Endolymphatic sac tumors: histopathologic confirmation, clinical characterization, and implication in von Hippel-Lindau disease. Laryngoscope 1995; 105(8 Pt 1): 801–808.
20. Mislav Gjuric, Koester M, Paulus W. Cavernous hemangioma of the internal auditory canal arising from the inferior vestibular nerve: case report and review of the literature. Am J Otol 200; 21: 110–114.
21. Moret J, Dickens JR, Jackson CG. Vascularization of the Ear. Normal Variations, Glomus Tumors. J Neuroradiol 1982; 9: 209–260.
22. Mukherji SK, Albernaz VS, LoWW, Gaffey MJ, Megerian CA, Feghali JG, Brook A, Lewin JS, Lanzeri CF, Talbot JM, Meyer JR, Carmody RF, Weissman JL, Smirniotopoulos JG, Rao VM, Jinkins JR, Castillo M. Papillary endolymphatic sac tumors: CT, MR imaging and angiographic findings in 20 patients. Radiology 1997; 202(3): 801–808.
23. Noujaim SE, Pattekar MA, Cacciarelli, et al. Paraganglioma of the temporal bone: role of MRI versus CT. Top Magn Reson Imaging 2000; 11(2): 108–122.
24. Parlier-Cuau C, Champsaur P, Perrin E, Rabischong P, Lasau JP. High resolution computed tomography of the canals of the temporal bone: anatomical correlations. Surg Radiol Anat 1998; 20(6): 437–444.
25. Pisaneschi MJ, Langer B. Congenital cholesteatoma and cholesterol granuloma of the temporal bone: role of MRI. Top Magn Reson Imaging 2000; 11(2): 87–97.
26. Robert Y, Carcasset S, Rocourt N, Hennequin C, Dubrulle F, Lemaitre L. Congenital cholesteatoma of the temporal bone: MR findings and comparison with CT. AJNR 1995; 16(4): 755–761.
27. Rodgers GK, Appelgate L, De La Cruz A, et al. Magnetic resonance angiography: analysis of vascular lesions of the temporal bone and skull base. Am J Otol 1993; 14: 56–62.
28. Schmalbrock P, Chakeres DW, Monroe W, Saraswat A, Miles BA, Welling DB. Assessment of internal auditory canal tumors: a comparison of contrast-enhanced T1 weighted and steady-state T2 weighted gradient-echo MR imaging. AJNR 199; 20: 1207–1213.
29. Shelton C, Harnsberger HR, Allen R, King B. Fast spin-echo magnetic resonance imaging: clinical application in screening for acoustic neuroma. Otolaryngol Head Neck Surg. 1996; 114(1): 71–76.
30. Stone JA, Castillo M, Neelon B, Mukherji SK. Evaluation of CSF leaks: high resolution CT compared with contrast-enhanced CT and radionuclide cisternography. AJNR 1999; 20(4): 706–712.
31. Valvassori GE, Buckingham, RA. Tomography and cross sections of the ear. Philadelphia: WB Saunders; Stuttgart: Georg Thieme Verlag, 1975.
32. Valvassori GE, Clemis JD. The large vestibular aqueduct syndrome. Laryngoscope 1978; 88: 723–728.
33. Valvassori GE, Dobben GD. CT Densitometry of the cochlear capsule in otosclerosis. AJNR 1985; 6: 661–667.
34. Valvassori GE. The internal auditory canal revisited. Otolaryngol Clin North Am 1995; 28(3): 431–451.

Section II Eye and Orbit, Base of the Skull

Chapter 2 **Eye and Orbit**

Part 1: The Eye

Embryology 137

Anatomy 140

Imaging Techniques 143

Pathology 146

Part 2: The Orbit

Embryology 196

Anatomy 196

Imaging Techniques 204

Pathology 215

Chapter 3 **Base of the Skull**

Embryology 295

Anatomy 295

Role of Diagnostic Imaging in Skull Base Pathology and Surgery 304

Imaging Techniques 304

Imaging Anatomy of the Skull Base 305

Anatomical Variations 305

Skull Base Pathology 306

2 Eye and Orbit

M. F. Mafee

Part 1: The Eye

Embryology

The globe is formed from both ectoderm and mesoderm.

The rudimentary eyeballs appear as two ectodermal hollow diverticula (optic pits) from the lateral aspects of the forebrain (diencephalon) (Fig. 2.1). The diverticula grow out laterally and their ends become dilated to form the optic vesicles, while the proximal part of each becomes constricted to form the optic stalk[1-7] (Fig. 2.1). At the same time, a small area of surface ectoderm overlying the optic vesicle thickens to form the lens placode (lens pit)[1-7] (Fig. 2.1). The lens placode invaginates and sinks below the surface ectoderm to form a hollow lens vesicle (Figs. 2.1 b, c). In the meantime, the outer wall of the optic vesicle becomes invaginated toward the wall of diencephalon to form the double-layered optic cup (Fig. 2.1 c). For a time, a wide hiatus groove, the optic fissure or choroidal fissure (embryonic fissure), exists along the optic stalk in the inferior edge of the optic cup[1,2] (Fig. 2.1 c). Through the embryonic fissure, the mesenchyme extends into the optic stalk and cup, carrying the hyaloid artery with it.[1-7]

The retina develops from the optic cup (Fig. 2.1). For purposes of description, the retina may be divided into two developmental layers, the pigment layer and the neural layer (Fig. 2.1 d). The pigment layer is formed from the outer, thinner, layer of the optic cup (Fig. 2.1). It is a single layer of cells that become columnar in shape and develop pigment granules within their cytoplasm. The neural layer is formed from the inner layer of the optic cup.[1-7] The ganglion cells, the amacrine cells, and the somata of the sustentacular fibers of Müller are formed from the inner neuroblastic layer of the retina.[1, 2, 8, 9, 10, 11] The horizontal cells, the nuclei of the bipolar rod and cone nerve cells, and probably the rod and cone cells are formed from the outer neuroblastic layer of the retina.[1,2]

Lens

The rudimentary lens, the lens placode, invaginates below the surface ectoderm to form the lens vesicle (Fig. 2.1 c). The lens is invested by a vascular mesenchymal condensation termed the vascular capsule of the lens. The lens is supplied by the hyaloid artery, which forms a plexus on the posterior surface of the lens capsule (Fig. 2.1 d).

The Ciliary Body, Iris, and Suspensory Ligaments of the Lens

The connective tissue of the ciliary body, the smooth-muscle fibers of the ciliary muscle, and the suspensory ligaments of the lens are formed from the mesenchyme, situated at the border of the optic up. The iris sphincter and dilator smooth muscles are formed from neuroectoderm.[1] The iris vasculatures derive from the mesoderm.[1, 2]

The Vitreous

The primitive or primary vitreous body is derived partly from the ectoderm and partly from the mesoderm.[1, 2, 3] The primitive vitreous is supplied by the hyaloid artery and its branches (Fig. 2.1 d). The definitive or secondary vitreous arises between the primitive vitreous and the retina. It is at first a homogeneous gel, which rapidly increases in volume and pushes the primitive vitreous anteriorly to behind the iris. Hyalocytes, derived from the mesenchyme around the hyaloid vessels, now migrate into the secondary vitreous. Later the hyaloid vessels atrophy and disappear, leaving the acellular hyaloid canal.[2, 12-18]

The Choroid

The choroid, the posterior segment of the uveal tract, develops early and is formed from the mesenchyme surrounding the optic cup (Fig. 2.1 e). The anterior part of the choroid is modified to form the ciliary body and ciliary processes.

The Sclera

The sclera is derived from a condensation of the mesenchyme surrounding the optic cup (Fig. 2.1 e). It first forms near the future insertion of the rectus muscles.[1]

The Cornea

The surface ectoderm overlying the optic vesicle forms the corneal epithelium, and the adjacent mesenchyme forms the mesothelium of the anterior chamber.[2, 17] The substantia propria and the endothelium covering the posterior surface of the cornea are formed from mesenchyme.[1]

Vascular System

The development of the vascular system of the eye is a complex process that involves the appearance of vessels to meet the nutritional needs of the developing eye and subsequent regression of those same vessels.[3, 12-19] In the early embryo the internal carotid artery supplies a fine capillary plexus to the dorsal aspect of the optic cup (ventral and dorsal ophthalmic arteries). The hyaloid artery is a branch of the dorsal ophthalmic artery which passes through the embryonic fissure into the optic cup (Figs. 2.1 d, e).[3]

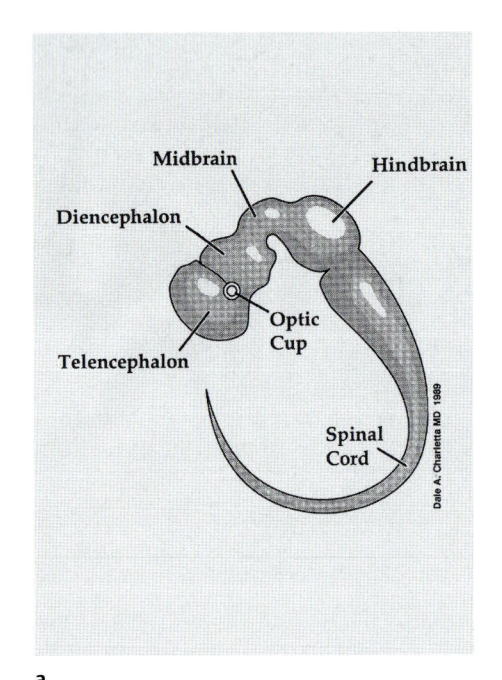

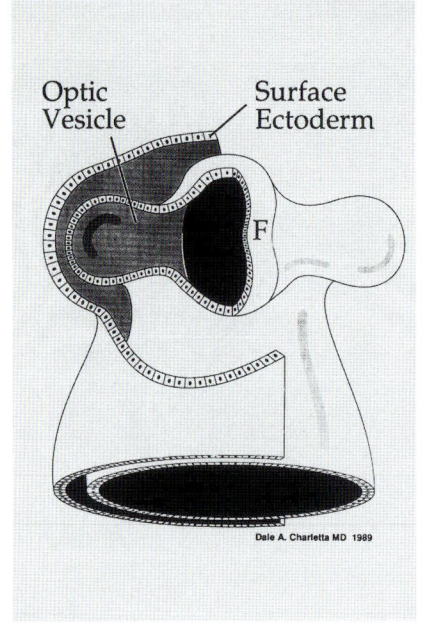

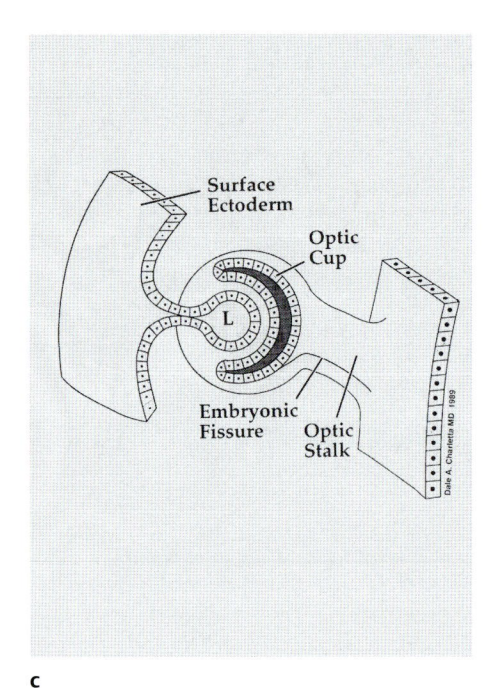

Figs. 2.1 a–c Development of the eye
a The 5 mm developing human embryo (four weeks gestation). By the third week of gestation two indentations appear, one on each side of the neural groove. These are the optic pits and they deepen to form the optic vesicles, one on each side of the forebrain. The optic vesicles give rise to an optic stalk and optic cup on each side.
b Development of the ocular structures. In the 4 mm embryo, lateral diverticula on each side of the forebrain (F) have given rise to two optic vesicles. The distal portions of the optic vesicles expand while the proximal portions become the tubular optic stalks.
c At the 5 mm stage, the external surface of each optic vesicle invaginates to form the optic cup. The inner wall of the optic cup (formerly the outer wall of the optic vesicle) gives rise to the retina, while the outer wall of the cup becomes the retinal pigment epithelium. The optic vesicle is covered by a layer of surface ectoderm, which forms the lens (L). Note the embryonic fissure, through which mesenchyme extends into the optic stalk and cup. Adapted from Brown G, Tasman W, eds. Congenital Anomalies of the Optic Disc. New York: Grune and Stratton; 1983. From Mafee MF et al. CT of optic nerve coloboma, morning glory anomaly, and colobomatous cyst. Radiol Clin North Am 1981;25:693–699. With permission.
d, e The eye at different stages of development.
d Diagram of the eye in an early stage of development. Note the inner and outer layers of the optic cup, developing lens, developing vitreous humor (body), hyaloid artery, and developing eyelids.
e Diagram of the eye in an advanced stage of development. Note the layers of the retina, choroid, sclera, cornea, vitreous body, lens, anterior and posterior aqueous chambers, conjunctival sac, and fused eyelids. The eyelids remain fused until the seventh month of gestation.
Figs. d and e Reprinted with permission from Snell R, Lemp MA. Clinical Anatomy of the Eye. Cambridge, MA: Blackwell Scientific Publications; 1989.

During the sixth week of gestation, the primitive dorsal ophthalmic artery is transformed into the definitive ophthalmic artery and the ventral ophthalmic artery regresses and transforms into the posterior nasal ciliary artery.[3-6] In the third trimester, the hyaloid system begins to regress.[4,5,14-18] Remnants of this system may sometimes be seen in the adult as a persistent papillary membrane.[6] The hyaloid artery is no longer patent and loses its connection to the disk in the seventh month of gestation. Occasionally, a connective bud may remain attached to the disk as Bergmeister's papilla.[3]

■ Extraocular Muscles

The eyeball is surrounded by a highly cellular paraxial mesoderm. This mesodermal tissue in the region of the developing eye forms the extraocular muscles of the eye.[1,17,20] The extraocular muscles during the developmental course become associated with the third, fourth, and sixth cranial nerves.[1] Eye movement can be demonstrated by fetal ultrasonography.[20]

■ The Eyelids

The eyelids develop from surface ectoderm and adjacent mesoderm. The eyelash and sebaceous glands are formed from surface ectoderm; however, the tarsus of the eyelid is developed from neural crest cells.[20] The surface ectoderm forms the conjunctival epithelium. The eyelids, as they grow, become united with each other at about the third month of gestation.[1] The lids remain fused until about the fifth month of fetal life, when the eyelids begin to separate. Separation of the eyelids is completed by the seventh month of gestation.[1] While the lids are fused, a closed space—the conjunctival sac—exists in front of the cornea.

■ The Lacrimal Gland

The lacrimal gland forms from epithelial buds, developing from the surface ectoderm, and grows superolaterally from the superior conjunctival fornix into the underlying mesenchyme (Fig. 2.1e).[1,20] The gland becomes divided into orbital and palpebral parts with the development of the levator palpebrae superioris.[17]

■ The Lacrimal Sac and Nasolacrimal Duct

The lacrimal sac and nasolacrimal duct initially develop as a solid cord of ectodermal cells that are trapped between the maxillary and lateral nasal elevations or processes. Later the central cells of the epithelial solid cord break down and the cord becomes canalized to form the nasolacrimal duct and the superior end becomes dilated to form the lacrimal sac.[1,2,17,20] Further cellular proliferation results in the formation of lacrimal ducts (inferior and superior and common canaliculi) that enter each eyelid.

■ The Orbit

The mesenchyme that encircles the optic vesicle forms the orbital bones.[1,2,17] The bony orbit is formed from a combination of membranous and cartilaginous anlage. The base of the skull, the cranial bones, and the ethmoid and sphenoid bones arise from the cartilage of the more primitive chondrocranium, and the ethmoid and sphenoid bones contribute to a large portion of the orbit. The superior portions of the orbit and calvaria develop from a membranous anlage.[1,21] The medial wall forms from the lateral nasal process. The lateral wall and inferior wall develop from the maxillary process (see Chapter 4). The bony orbit undergoes rapid changes in size and shape between six months of fetal life and eighteen months after birth.[20] It is interesting to note that early in development the eyeball develops at a faster rate than the orbit, so that in the sixth month of fetal life the anterior half of the eyeball projects beyond the orbital opening.

References

1. Warwick R, Williams PL. Gray's Anatomy, 35th British edition. Philadelphia: W.B. Saunders; 1973: 145–147.
2. Snell RS, Lemp MA, eds. Clinical Anatomy of the Eye. Boston: Blackwell Scientific; 1989: 1–15.
3. Mann IC. Developmental Abnormalities of the Eye, 2d ed. Philadelphia: J.B. Lippincott; 1957: 74–78.
4. Mann IC. On the development of the fissure and associated regions in the eye of the chick and some observations of the mammal. J Anat 1921; 55: 113–118.
5. Mann IC. The Development of the Human Eye. New York: Grune and Stratton; 1969.
6. Yanoff M, Duker JS, eds. Ophthalmology. Philadelphia: Mosby; 1999: 3.1–3.6.
7. Mafee MF, Jampol LM, Langer BC, Tso M. Computed tomography of optic nerve colobomas, Morning glory anomaly, and colobomatous cyst. Radiol Clin North Am 1987; 25: 693–699.
8. Driell D, Provis JM, Billson FA. Early differentiation of ganglion, amacrine, bipolar and Müeller Cells in the developing fovea of the human retina. J Comp Neurol. 1990; 291: 203–219.
9. Hollenberg J, Spira AW. Human retinal development. Ultrastructure of the outer retina. Am J Anat. 1973; 137: 357–386.
10. Mann IC. On the morphology of certain developmental structures associated with the upper end of the choroidal fissure. Br J Ophthalmal 1922; 6: 145–163.
11. Brown G, Tasman W, eds. Congenital Anomalies of the Optic Disc. New York: Grune and Stratton; 1983: 97–191.
12. Jack RL. Regression of the hyaloid vascular system: an ultrastructural analysis. Am J Ophthalmol 1972; 74: 261–271.
13. Renz BE, Vygantas CM. Hyaloid vascular remnants in human neonates. Ann Ophthalmol 1977; 9: 179–184.
14. Mafee MF, Goldberg MF, Valvassori GE, et al. Computed tomography in the evaluation of patients with persistent hyperplastic primary vitreous (PHPV). Radiology 1982; 145: 713–717.
15. Mafee MF. Imaging of the Globe. In: Valvassori GE, Mafee MF, Carter BL, eds. Imaging of the Head and Neck. Stuttgart: Georg Thieme Verlag; 1995: 216–247.
16. Mafee MF. Magnetic resonance imaging: ocular anotomy and pathology. In: Newton TH, Bilanuik LT, eds. Modern Neuroradiology, Vol. 4. Radiology of the Eye and Orbit. New York: Clavadel Press/Raven Press; 1990; 2.1–3.45.
17. Mafee MF. The eye. In: Som PM, Curtin HD, eds. Head and Neck Imaging. St. Louis: Mosby; 2003: 441–527.
18. Mafee MF, Atlas SW, Galetta SL. Eye, orbit, and visual system. In: Atlas SW, ed. Magnetic Resonance Imaging of the Brain and Spine. Philadelphia: Lippincott, Williams & Wilkins; 2002: 1433–1524..
19. Edward DP, Mafee MF, Garcia-Valenzuela E, Weiss RA. Coats disease and persistent hyperplastic primary vitreous. Role of MR imaging and CT. Radiol Clin North Am 1998; 36: 1119–1131.
20. Edward DP, Kaufmann LM. Anatomy, development, and physiology of the visual system. Pediatr Clin North Am. 2003; 50: 1–23.
21. Becker MH, McCarthy JG, Congenital abnormalities. In: Gonzalez CF, Becker MH, Flanagan JC (eds.). Diagnostic Imaging in Ophthalmology. New York, NY: Springer Verlag; 1985: 115–187.

Anatomy

The eyeball is made up of two segments, the anterior and posterior segments. The anterior, smaller, segment is transparent (cornea) and forms about one-sixth of the eyeball. The posterior, larger, segment is opaque (sclera) and forms about five-sixths of the eyeball[1].

The eye consists of three primary layers (Figs. 2.**2**, 2.**3**):
1. The sclera, or outer layer, which is composed primarily of collagen–elastic tissue.
2. The uvea, or middle layer of the eye, which is richly vascular and contains pigmented tissue consisting of three components: the choroid, ciliary body, and iris.
3. The retina, or inner layer, which is the neural, sensory stratum of the eye.

■ Tenon's Capsule and Extraocular Muscle Sheaths (Sleeves)

The fascial sheath of the eyeball, also called the fascia bulbi, or Tenon's capsule is a thin membrane that envelops the eyeball and separates it from the central orbital fat. It thus forms a socket for the eyeball.[1-3] The Tenon's capsule blends with the sclera just behind the corneoscleral junction and fuses with the bulbar conjunctiva (Fig. 2.**3**).[3] Tenon's capsule is perforated behind by the optic nerve and its sheath and the ciliary nerves and vessels. The capsule fuses with, and extends to, the sheath of the optic nerve and the sclera around the entrance of the optic nerve (Fig. 2.**3**).[2,3] Septa of fibrous tissue are attached to the outer surface of Tenon's capsule and, near the equator, it is perforated by the vortex (vorticose) veins (draining veins of the choroid and sclera).[2] The inner surface of Tenon's capsule is smooth and shiny and is separated from the outer surface of the sclera by the episcleral (Tenon's) space.[2] This is a potential space that is traversed by fibers of loose connective (areolar) tissue, which extend between the fascia and the sclera (Fig. 2.**3**).

The tendons of all extrinsic ocular muscles pierce the capsule to reach the sclera. At the site of perforation, the fascial sheath is reflected back along the tendons of these muscles to form a tubular sleeve on each.[2] Inflammatory and intraocular neoplastic processes are the most common lesions to involve Tenon's space. In posterior scleritis, episcleritis, Tenon fasciitis, and pseudotumor, an inflammatory effusion produces a characteristic circular or semicircular distention of Tenon's capsule (Fig. 2.**4**). Retinoblastoma (Fig. 2.**5**) and uveal melanoma also may extend into the Tenon's space.[4,5]

■ Sclera

The sclera is the globe's outer white, leathery coat. It extends from the limbus at the margin of the cornea to the optic nerve, where it becomes continuous with the dural sheath.[3,6] The external side of the sclera lies against Tenon's capsule. The internal surface of the sclera blends with the suprachoroidal tissues.[6] Posteriorly, the sclera is perforated by the vortex veins, the long posterior ciliary arteries and nerves, and the short posterior ciliary arteries and nerves. The medial rectus muscle inserts 5.5 mm posterior to the limbus; the inferior rectus 6.5 mm; the lateral rectus 6.9 mm; and the superior rectus 7.7 mm.[1] The insertions of the superior oblique and inferior oblique muscles are posterior to the scleral equator. The lamina cribrosa is where the optic nerve fibers pierce the sclera. The sclera is pierced anteriorly at the insertion of the rectus muscles by the branches of anterior ciliary arteries. Except for the lateral rectus muscle, which has only one anterior ciliary artery, each rectus muscle has two anterior ciliary arteries.[1]

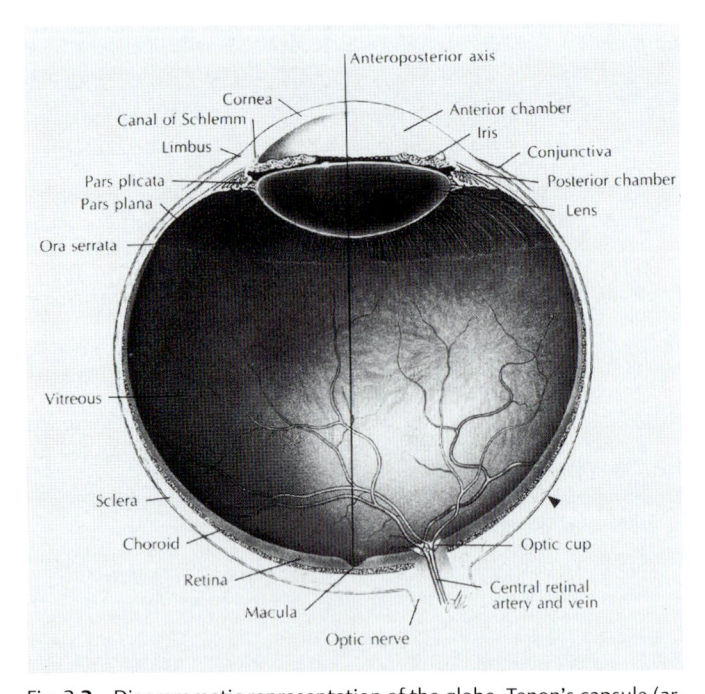

Fig. 2.**2** Diagrammatic representation of the globe. Tenon's capsule (arrowhead) envelops the eyeball and separates it from the orbital fat.

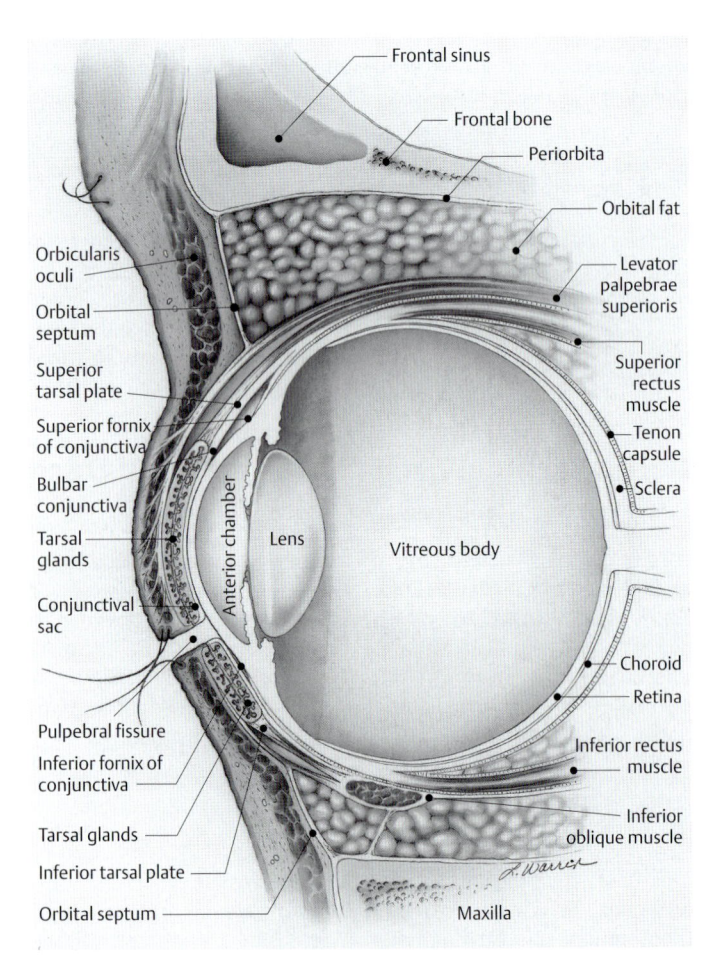

Fig. 2.**3** Diagram of a sagittal section of the gross anatomy of the eyeball and orbit at the level of the optic nerve, highlighting ocular and orbital structures.

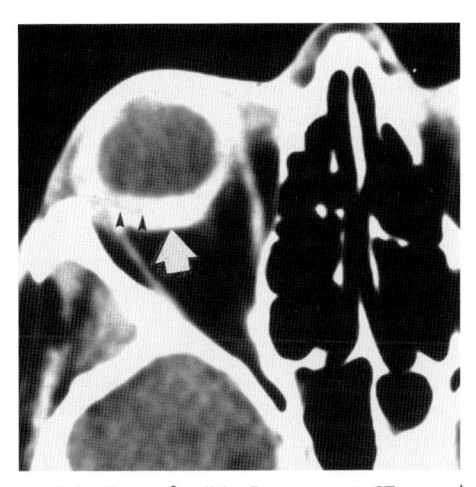

Fig. 2.4 Tenon fasciitis. Postcontrast CT scan shows increased thickening and enhancement involving the Tenon's capsule and sclera of the right globe (large arrow). Note fluid collection (arrowheads) in the potential Tenon's space.

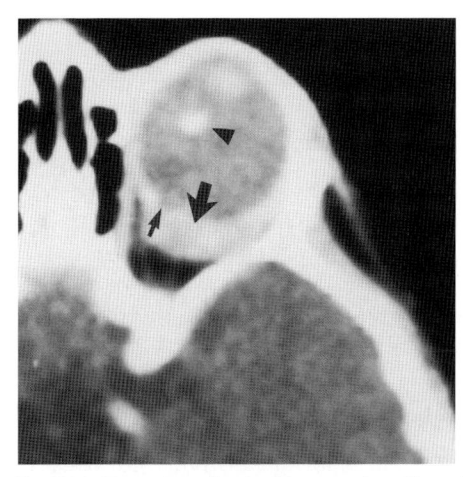

Fig. 2.5 Extension of retinoblastoma into Tenon's space. Enhanced axial CT scan. The entire left globe is filled with a retinoblastoma, which shows a focal calcification (arrowhead). Note focal invasion of the eye wall (small arrow) and marked tumor extension into the Tenon's space (large arrow).

The sclera is pierced about 4 mm posterior to the equator of the eye by the vortex veins (four or five). Anteriorly, the sclera is continuous with the cornea. Just posterior to the corneoscleral junction, and lying within the sclera, is a circularly running canal called the sinus venosus sclerae or the canal of Schlemm (Fig. 2.2).

Blood Supply and Nerve Supply of the Sclera

The sclera is a relatively avascular structure. However, anterior to the insertions of the rectus muscles, the anterior ciliary arteries form a dense episcleral plexus. The posterior sclera receives small branches from the long and short posterior ciliary arteries. The sclera is innervated by the ciliary nerves, which are a branch of the trigeminal nerve.[1,17]

■ Cornea

Microscopically, the cornea consists of five layers. From front to back, they are: (1) the corneal epithelium, (2) Bowman's layer (membrane), (3) the substantia propria, (4) Descemet's membrane, and (5) the corneal endothelium. Descemet's membrane is thicker than the endothelium. The corneal epithelium is stratified and consists of five layers of cells. The corneal endothelium consists of a single layer of flattened cells.[1]

Blood Supply and Nerve Supply of the Cornea

The cornea is avascular and devoid of lymphatic drainage. The nourishment of the cornea is established by virtue of diffusion from the aqueous humor and from the scleral and conjunctival capillaries that end at its edge. Innervation of the cornea is via the ophthalmic division of the trigeminal nerve, mainly through the long ciliary nerves.[1]

■ Uvea (Choroid, Ciliary Body, and Iris)

The uveal tract is the vascular layer of the eyeball which lies between the sclera and the retina (Figs. 2.2, 2.3). It consists of choroid, ciliary body and iris. The choroid is the section of the uveal tract that lies between the sclera and the retinal pigment epithelium (RPE), the outer layer of the retina (Fig. 2.3). It forms a membrane of predominantly vascular tissue extending from the optic nerve to the ora serrata (Figs. 2.2, 2.3), beyond which it continues as the ciliary body.[1,5,6] Its thickness varies from approximately 0.22 mm at the posterior pole to 0.10 mm near the ora, at the optic nerve, where it forms part of the optic nerve canal, and at the point of internal penetration of the vortex veins. It is firmly attached to the sclera in the region of the optic nerve and where the posterior ciliary arteries and ciliary nerve enter the eye.[7] It is also tethered to the sclera where the vortex veins leave the eyeball.[1,7] This accounts for the characteristic shape of choroidal detachment, which shows valleys at the site of the vortex veins.[7] The choroid can be divided into four layers, which are, extending from internally to externally: Bruch's membrane, the choriocapillaris, the stroma, and the suprachoroidea.[1,7,8]

Bruch's Membrane

Bruch's membrane (2–4 μm thick) is a tough, acellular, amorphous, bilamellar structure situated between the retina and the rest of the choroid.[8,9] The function of Bruch's membrane is not exactly known. When a choroidal tumor breaks through the Bruch's membrane, it results in a characteristic mushroom-shaped growth configuration (see Fig. 2.85).

Choriocapillaris

The choriocapillaris is the capillary layer of the choroid, lying immediately external to Bruch's membrane. The capillaries are drained by the vortex veins. The choriocapillaris is a visceral type of vasculature, with fenestrations (wide-bore capillaries) in the vessels, and these openings are covered by diaphragms that permit the relatively free exchange of material between the choriocapillaris and the surrounding tissues.[10,11] By contrast, the retinal capillaries show no fenestrations and present a strong barrier to the interchange of material from capillary to retinal tissue.[6] It should be noted that the density of the capillaries is greatest and the bore is widest at the macula.

Choroidal Stroma

The choroidal stroma lies external to the choriocapillaris and consists of blood vessels, nerves, fibroblasts, a collection of immunological cells, macrophages, lymphocytes, mast cells, plasma cells, and loose collagenous supporting tissue containing melanocytes. The blood vessels of the stroma are branches of the short posterior ciliary arteries and extend anteriorly. The veins are much larger and converge to join four of five vortex (vorticose) veins that drain in the ophthalmic veins.[1, 11]

Suprachoroidea

The suprachoroidea, also called perichoroidal/suprachoroidal space, is a potential space, approximately 30 μm in thickness, that lies between the choroidal stroma and the sclera.[6, 11, 12] At the optic nerve the choroid becomes continuous with the pia and arachnoid.[1, 11, 12]

Blood Supply and Venous Drainage of the Choroid

The choroid receives its blood supply mainly from the posterior ciliary arteries. A number of recurrent branches arise from the anterior ciliary arteries. All of these arteries are branches of the ophthalmic artery. The four or five vortex (vorticose) veins drain the choroid into the ophthalmic veins.[7, 8, 11]

Function

The most important function of the uvea is to provide a vascular supply to the eye and to regulate the ocular temperature.[11] The choroid is also responsible for nourishing the pigment epithelium and the outer one-third of the retina.[6]

Nerve Supply of the Choroid

Innervation of the choroid is provided by the long and short ciliary nerves.[13] The nasociliary nerve, which is a branch of the ophthalmic division of the trigeminal nerve, gives rise to long ciliary nerves. They carry sensory nerve and sympathetic fibers. The short ciliary nerves which arise from the ciliary ganglion carry sympathetic and parasympathetic fibers.[1]

Ciliary Body

The ciliary body is continuous posteriorly with the choroid and anteriorly with the peripheral margin of the iris (Figs. 2.**2**, 2.**3**) and runs around the inside of the anterior sclera. It is about 6 mm wide and extends forward to the scleral spur (a projecting ridge of scleral tissue along the internal scleral sulcus) and backward to the ora serrata of the retina.[1] On cross section, the ciliary body is triangular with its small base facing the anterior chamber of the eye. Its anterior surface is ridged or plicated and is called the pars plicata (Figs. 2.**2**, 2.**3**). The posterior surface is smooth and flat and is called the pars plana. The ciliary body is made up of (1) the ciliary epithelium, (2) the ciliary stroma, and (3) the ciliary muscle. The ciliary stroma consists of loose connective tissue, rich in blood vessels and melanocytes. The ciliary muscle consists of smooth-muscle fibers. The ciliary muscle is innervated by the postganglionic parasympathetic fibers derived from the oculomotor nerve. The nerve fibers reach the muscle via the short ciliary nerves.

Iris

The iris is a thin, contractile, pigmented diaphragm with a central aperture, the pupil (Figs. 2.**2**, 2.**3**). It is suspended in the aqueous humor between the cornea and the lens. The iris divides the space between the lens and cornea into an anterior and a posterior chamber. The aqueous humor, formed by the ciliary processes in the posterior chamber, circulates through the pupil into the anterior chamber and exits into the sinus venosus (canal of Schlemm) at the iridocorneal angle.[1, 12] The iris consists of a stroma and two epithelial layers. The stroma consists of highly vascular connective tissue containing melanocytes. The stroma also contains nerve fibers, the smooth muscle of the sphincter pupillae, and the myoepithelial cells of the dilator pupillae.[1] The arterial blood supply of the iris is from the two long posterior ciliary arteries and the seven anterior ciliary arteries.[1, 13]

■ Retina

The retina, the inner layer of the eyeball, is a thin, transparent membrane having a purplish-red color in living subjects. The external surface of the retina is in contact with the choroid, and the internal surface with the vitreous body. Posteriorly, the retina is continuous with the optic nerve. The optic nerve and the inner layer of the eye represent an anteriorly protruding portion of the brain. Grossly the retina has two layers: (1) the inner layer, which comprises the sensory retina, i.e., photoreceptors, and the first- and second-order neurons (ganglion cells) and neuroglial elements of the retina (Müller cells, or sustentacular gliocytes); and (2) the outer layer, which is the retinal pigment epithelium (RPE), consisting of a single lamina of cells whose nuclei are adjacent to the basal lamina (Bruch's membrane) of the choroid.[11, 12]

The retina is very thin, measuring 0.056 mm near the disk to 0.1 mm anteriorly at the ora serrata.[12, 13] It is much thinner at the optic disk and thinnest at the fovea of the macula. The sensory retina extends forward from the optic nerve to a point just posterior to the ciliary body. Here the nervous tissues of the retina end and its anterior edge forms a crenated wavy ring, called the ora serrata (Fig. 2.**2**, 2.**3**). The anterior, nonsensory, part of the retina at the ora serrata becomes continuous with the pigmented and nonpigmented cell layers of the ciliary body and its processes. The macula, the center of the retina, lies 3.5 mm temporal to the margin of the optic nerve (Fig. 2.**2**). The retina is attached tightly at the margin of the optic disk and at its anterior termination at the ora serrata. It is also firmly attached to the vitreous but loosely to the retinal pigment epithelium (RPE), and it is nourished by the choroid and the RPE.[12]

The RPE cells are joined to each other by tight junctions. This arrangement forms a barrier (blood–retinal barrier) that limits the flow of ions and prevents diffusion of large toxic molecules from the choroid capillaries to the photoreceptors of the retina. The neural retina consists of three main groups of neurons: (1) the photoreceptors (cone and rod cells), (2) the bipolar cells, and (3) the ganglion cells. It also possesses other important neurons, the horizontal cells and the amacrine cells, that modulate their activity.[1, 13] Supporting cells (Müller cells) are also present. The axons of the ganglion cells form the optic nerve and its fibers become myelinated after they have passed through the lamina cribrosa. The myelin sheaths of these axons are formed from oligodendrocytes rather than Schwann cells.

There are approximately 1 million ganglion cells in each retina and about 100 photoreceptor cells per ganglion cell. The axons of ganglion cells converge at the exit of the optic nerve at the optic disk. After piercing the lamina, the nerve fibers become myelinated. In some individuals the ganglion cell axons are partially myelinated; such areas are non-seeing and clinically seen as a white sheen on the retinal surface.[1]

The retinal supporting cells are similar to the neuroglial cells. One of these runs radially and is called the Müller cell. Other glial-like cells, called retinal astrocytes, perivascular glial cells, and microglial cells, have also been described.[1]

The macula lutea is an oval, yellowish area at the center of the posterior part of the retina. It measures about 4.5 mm in diameter and lies about 3 mm to the lateral side of the optic disk.

The fovea centralis is a depression in the center of the macula lutea. It measures about 1.5 mm in diameter. A rise in CSF pressure causes the optic disk to bulge into the eyeball. It is believed that the pressure on the optic nerve impedes the axon flow of its fibers and this causes the optic disk to swell.

Blood Supply of the Retina

The blood supply of the retina is from two sources. These include choroidal capillaries and the central retinal artery. The choroidal capillaries do not enter the retinal laminae, but tissue fluid exudes between these cells (cones, rods and outer nuclear layer). The retinal inner laminae are supplied by the central retinal artery. The retinal arteries are anastomotic end arteries, and there are no arteriovenous anastomoses. The retina depends on both of these circulations, neither of which alone is sufficient. The central retinal artery is the first branch of the ophthalmic artery;[1, 13] it measures about 0.3 mm in diameter and runs forward adhering to the dural sheath of the optic nerve. It enters the inferior and medial side of the optic nerve about 12 mm posterior to the eyeball. The artery is surrounded by a sympathetic plexus and accompanied by the central vein. It pierces the lamina cribrosa to enter the eyeball. Small anastomoses occur between the branches of the posterior ciliary arteries and the central retinal artery (cilioretinal artery). The central vein of the retina leaves the eyeball through the lamina cribrosa. The vein crosses the subarachnoid space and drains directly into the cavernous sinus or the superior ophthalmic vein.[14] The retina has no lymphatic vessels.[1]

■ Vitreous

The vitreous body occupies the space between the lens and retina and represents about two-thirds of the volume of the eye, or approximately 4 ml.[14-16] All but 1-2% of the vitreous is water, which is bound with a fibrillar collagen meshwork, soluble proteins, some salts, and hyaluronic acid.[1, 11, 14-16] It possesses a network of fine collagen fibrils that form a scaffolding. The vitreous is the largest and simplest connective tissue present as a single structure in the human body.[12] Any insult to the vitreous body may result in a fibroproliferative reaction (such as proliferative vitreoretinopathy), which can subsequently result in a tractional retinal detachment.[11] The vitreous body is bounded by the anterior and posterior hyaloid membranes.[1] The vitreous body is attached to the sensory retina, especially at the ora serrata and the margin of the optic disk.[1]

Within the vitreous, the hyaloid (colloquet) canal (channel) runs forward from the optic disk to the posterior pole of the lens. The vitreous body transmits light, supports the posterior surface of the lens, and assists in holding the sensory retina against the RPE.

Imaging Techniques

Computed tomography (CT) provided a major imaging advance over conventional radiography and tomography in examining the eye. The development of magnetic resonance imaging (MRI) has proved to be an even greater breakthrough in diagnostic medical imaging and biomedical research.[14-24] The anatomical detail demonstrated by an MR proton image is a representation of three physical properties of static tissue: proton (spin) density, and T1 and T2 relaxation times. Intrinsic differences in proton density, and in particular in proton relaxation times, of tissues allow excellent image contrast between various normal structures and give high sensitivity for detecting pathology states.[4, 5, 11, 16-19, 21, 24] This section discusses CT and MRI of the normal globe and the features of ocular pathology, with particular emphasis on the potential use of MRI in the practice of ophthalmology.

■ CT Technique

The CT protocol for intraocular lesions includes 1.5–3 mm axial sections of the globe. For suspected small foreign bodies, 1 mm section thickness may be used. For all foreign bodies and lesions at the 6-o'clock and 12-o'clock positions, direct 1–3 mm (depending on the size of the lesion) coronal sections may be obtained. Additional 1.5–3 mm axial sections of the eye and orbit are obtained following administration of iodinated contrast material (meglumine diatrizoate; 1 ml per pound of body weight). In cases of suspected retinoblastoma and uveal melanoma, additional 5 mm axial sections of the head are obtained to investigate the possibility of an intracranial abnormality. The major application of CT for ocular lesions includes detecting foreign bodies, eye trauma, and intraocular calcification. For intraocular tumors and other intraocular pathology, MRI is preferred to CT scanning.

■ MRI Technique

The success of MR imaging depends on cooperation of the patient and, in the case of infants and children, appropriate sedation. The procedure should be carefully explained to the patients and their families, especially if a parent or other person is required to stay with the patient in the MR scan room. For sedation in infants and children, oral chloral hydrate (75–100 mg/kg body weight) usually affords satisfactory sedation in children up to ages 2–4 years. When this proves inadequate, intramuscular diphenhydramine (Benadryl, a one-time dose of 1 mg/kg) or midazolam (Versed, 0.05–0.08 mg/kg) for children 5–8 years of age is added.[4] Other children may need intravenous medication or general anesthesia, and there may be variations between institutions regarding doses and medication used. Because of the importance of monitoring sedated patients, sedation procedures at our institution are performed by a trained dedicated MR imaging nurse. The patients are monitored during the MR imaging, using pulse oximetry, allowing evaluation of the arterial oxygen saturation. When general anesthesia is required, anesthesiologists use MR-compatible monitoring and ventilation equipment.

The majority of MRI studies in this section were performed on a 1.5 T (Tesla) Signa unit (General Electric, Milwaukee, WI, USA) with 2 mm, 3 mm, or 5 mm sections with 0 or 0.6–1.5 mm interslice gap. A complete MRI evaluation of the eye should consist of high-resolution axial, coronal, and sagittal images of the eye and surrounding structures. Evaluation of the globe can be successfully accomplished with the standard head coil. The field of view, however, should be maintained between 12 and 16 cm, with in-plane resolution of 256×192 or 256×256 or 512×256. Orbital surface coils may be used to improve the spatial resolution of MR images.[4] If they are available, they should be primarily used for lesions limited to the globe and smaller lesions that may not be detected by a head coil. For intraocular lesions that have invaded the optic nerve and retrobulbar space, we prefer to use a head coil to evaluate the entire course of the optic nerve. We recommend routine gadolinium contrast-enhanced MR imaging of the orbit and brain, using a head coil for the evaluation of children with suspected retinoblastoma and, in particular, patients with possible subarachnoid seeding of retinoblastoma and those with bilateral retinoblastoma. This allows early detection of optic nerve involvement, orbital spread, or asymptomatic pineoblastoma and suprasellar tumors.[4] Although individual examinations should always be specifically tailored to the problems of each individual patient, in general for ocular lesions our routine MR imaging examination consists of both T1-weighted and T2-weighted images and precontrast and postcontrast T1-weighted images with and without fat suppression. Our protocol for ocular MR imaging is summarized below.

Ocular MR Protocol
Head coil or surface coil
Axial view:
  TR 2000–3000 ms, TE 30/80–120 ms
  256 × 192, 3 mm slice thickness, 0.5 mm skip
  FOV 16 × 16 cm, number of excitation (NEX) = 2, no phase wrap (NP)
  This may be replaced by a fast spin echo, single echo T2-weighted fat suppression acquisition technique

Precontrast axial view:
  TR 500 ms, TE 20 ms
  256 × 192, 3 mm slice thickness, 0.5 mm skip
  FOV 14–16, NEX = 2 or 3, NP

Postcontrast axial and coronal views:
  TR 500 ms, TE 20 ms
  256 × 192, 2 or 3 mm slice thickness, 0.5 mm skip
  FOV 14–16, NEX = 3, NP

Poscontrast fat suppression axial view:
  TR 500 ms, TE 20 ms
  256 × 192, 3 mm slice thickness, 0.5 mm skip
  FOV 14–16, NEX = 3, NP

Additional postcontrast fat suppression T1-weighted sagittal view may be obtained according to the finding in axial or coronal sections.

Postcontrast axial view of the orbit and head using head coil:
  TR 500 ms, TE 20 ms
  256 × 192, 5 mm slice thickness, 1.5 mm skip
  FOV 22–24 cm, NEX = 1

The motion artifact is more pronounced on images obtained with the surface coil because of the inherent sensitivity of the surface coil.[4] A lesion is therefore sometimes better seen on images obtained with a head coil. With the surface coil, a 3 mm section thickness is used to reduce the problem of partial volume averaging. The thin section has the disadvantage of generating less signal (small volume), which may result in a decreased amount of T2-weighted information in later echoes, particularly in rapidly decaying T2 signals. In addition, structures close to the surface coil may be overshadowed by the increased signal intensity inherent to surface coil imaging. Because of these factors, at times malignant uveal melanoma or retinoblastoma may be better seen on T2-weighted images obtained with a head coil rather than with a surface coil. Fat-suppression pulse sequences are important for the detection of intraocular (small) lesions and for the evaluation of extraocular extension of eye tumors and inflammation. Fat suppression is also useful in the T2-weighted acquisitions of the optic nerve and anterior optic pathway. Fat-suppression T1-weighted pulse sequences in general result in expansion of the dynamic range of gray scale, and one can change the brightness of an image by changing the window width and window level (Fig. 2.**6**). The lacrimal gland and extraocular muscles appear hyperintense on unenhanced T1-weighted fat-suppression pulse sequences (Fig. 2.**6**). To avoid misinterpretation, it is advisable to obtain pre- and postcontrast fat-suppression T1-weighted MR sequences. The fat-suppression pulse sequences are also more prone to artifacts related to dental fillings, as well as magnetic susceptibility artifacts, generated at the bone–air interface. At times the orbital fatty reticulum on the side of dental filling or braces may not be suppressed, giving a wrong impression of abnormal enhancement (Fig. 2.**7**). Metallic (iron) artifacts due to eye make-up (Fig. 2.**8**) or lid tattoos, dental-related artifacts, and in particular magnetic susceptibility artifacts are more pronounced on images obtained using a 3 T MR scanner.

MRI and Evaluation of Intraocular Foreign Bodies

Despite the many advantages of MRI, it may not be indicated as a primary modality in the evaluation of the traumatized eye harboring a possible intraocular foreign body. This cautionary advice is based on the possibility of additional damage to the injured eye by ferromagnetic foreign bodies that are induced to move during the imaging process. A study conducted in vitro and in vivo (rabbit) experiments to examine the effects of MRI (1.5 T unit) on intraocular foreign bodies showed that diamagnetic and paramagnetic foreign bodies were imaged without artifacts and without movement during the imaging process, but ferromagnetic foreign bodies produced large amounts of artifact that prevented meaningful images being obtained.[20] For patients with a remote history of a traumatic foreign body, or in metal workers or other high-risk individuals, a high-resolution 1.5 mm thick CT scan of the orbits, and a 5–10 mm thick CT of the head is recommended to rule out the possibility of foreign bodies.

MRI appears to be safe in patients who have undergone procedures such as retinal surgery, retinal tamponade, scleral buckling, and intraocular lens (IOL) implantation. The first generation IOL was a biconvex polymethylmethacrylate (PMMA) lens. However, because of many changes in surgical techniques and IOL design and manufacture, it is our policy to check with the ophthalmologist who performed the IOL procedure, retinal surgery, or other surgical procedure to make sure there is no contraindication for MRI. Patients with stapedectomy (metallic) or other metallic prostheses that have proved to be safe for 1.5 T MR units should be carefully screened for MR study using 3 T and higher fields. There are not yet enough data available indicating that these devices will not move at field higher than 1.5 T.

MRI Artifacts

Motion artifacts may result in marked degradation of MR images. It is important to request that patients close their eyes during the examination. Artifacts may occur as a result of dental fillings, dental braces (Fig. 2.**7**), or tattooing of eyelids with iron oxide, and even from the external application of eye cosmetics (Fig. 2.**8**). Artifacts arising from tattooing or related to eye cosmetics usually appear as distortion of the skin contours in the location of the iron oxide. There also may be distortion of the shape of the globe and multiple artifacts consisting of hyperintense areas around the contour of the eyelids. Magnetic susceptibility artifacts are generated from the air–bone interface along the floor of the orbit as well as the superior ethmoid–sphenoid complex and base of the skull. These MRI artifacts are more pronounced on images obtained with 3 T MR scanners.

Normal MR Imaging Anatomy of the Eye

Regarding the anatomy and pathology of the globe, MRI is a modality that provides both excellent contrast for ocular imaging and

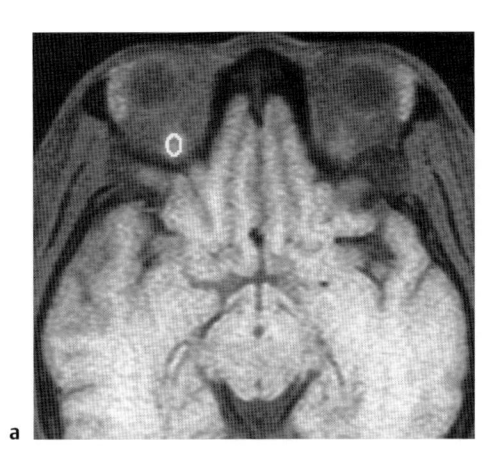

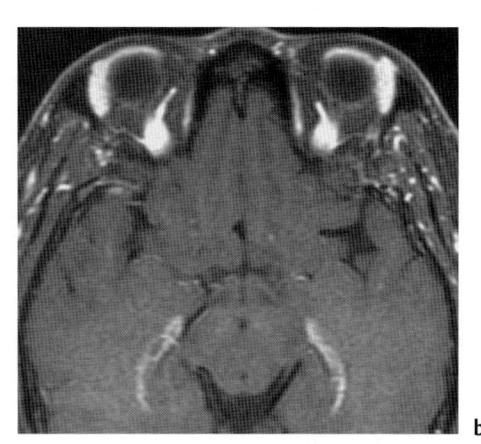

Fig. 2.6 Pre- (**a**) and postcontrast (**b**) fat-suppression T1W MR images of the orbit. Axial T1W (550/15, TR/TE) MR scans of the eye and orbit, taken at the same level. Note hyperintensity of the extraocular muscles and lacrimal glands on precontrast fat-suppression (**a**) and their intense enhancement on postcontrast fat-suppression (**b**) MR images. The images are acquired with the same pulse parameters (256 × 128/4 NEX, 16 cm FOV and 3 mm section thickness) and filmed with the same window width and window level.

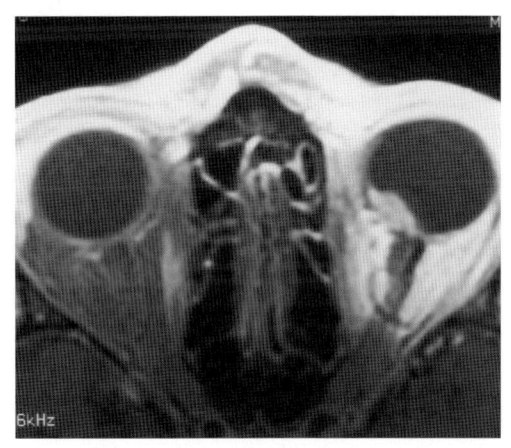

Fig. 2.7 Dental filling resulting in lack of fat suppression. Postcontrast fat-suppression T1W MR scan, showing a mass compatible with malignant uveal melanoma in the left eye. Note suppression of the retrobulbar fat on the right side and lack of suppression on the left side.

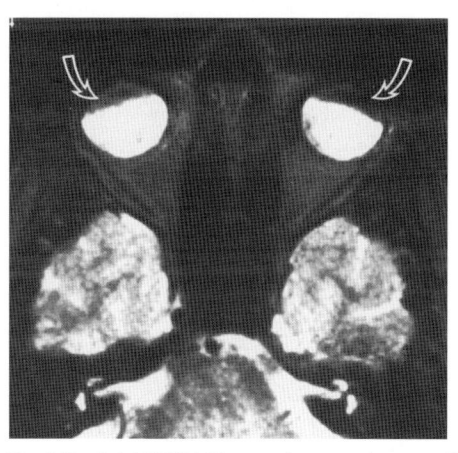

Fig. 2.8 Axial T2W MR scan shows makeup artifacts (arrows).

good sensitivity for detecting gross as well as incipient pathology.[4,14,16,18,22–24] The globe is unique in that it contains both the most (vitreous) and least (lens) water-laden soft tissues in the body.[22,23] The water content of the vitreous is 98–99%, of the cornea 80%, and of the lens 65–69%, and these differences produce different water proton relaxation times for each of these tissues.[12,18,22]

Vitreous Body

The vitreous represents about two-thirds of the volume of the eye, or approximately 4 ml.[8] The vitreous humor is a gel-like, transparent, extracellular matrix composed of a meshwork of 0.2% collagen fibrils interspersed with 0.2% hyaluronic acid, polymers, water (98–99%), and a small amount of soluble proteins.[16,17,22] Because the vitreous is a gel composed of long, fixed collagen fibrils bathed only with dilute dissolved proteins, only a fraction of its water content is in contact with macromolecules.[22] Consequently, the bulk of water in the vitreous relaxes on MRI as pure water, with only a small protein–water interaction.[14,18,22] Thus the vitreous has relaxation times that are longer than those of most tissues but are shorter than those of water.

Lens, Ciliary Body, and Ocular Coats

The lens is made up of three parts: (1) an elastic capsule; (2) a lens epithelium, which is confined to the anterior surface of the lens; and (3) the lens fibers. The lens is approximately 9 mm in diameter and 4–4.5 mm thick. Anterior to the lens is the iris and the aqueous humor; posteriorly the lens is bordered by the vitreous humor (Figs. 2.2, 2.3). On MRI the normal lens is characteristically darker than the surrounding fluid-laden tissue on T2-weighted pulse sequences, predominantly because of the dominance of its ultrashort T2 relaxation time.[22] The lens nucleus has both a lower water content and a shorter T2 relaxation time than the cortex.

MRI provides precise information regarding other ocular structures as well. The anterior chamber, just anterior to the lens, is crescent-shaped and is almost isointense to the vitreous humor on both short and long TR images.[12,22] The ciliary body may be seen on T2-weighted MR images as a hypointense area running from the edge of the lens to the wall of the globe. Differentiation by MRI of individual layers of the sclera, choroid, and retina is impossible in the normal eye.[12,18,19] The anterior chamber is a small cavity lying behind the cornea and in front of the iris (Figs. 2.3). The chamber contains aqueous humor. The aqueous fluid nourishes the corneal epithelium and the lens.[6] The iris, which is the most anterior extension of the uveal tract, lies at the anterior surface of the lens (Fig. 2.2, 2.3). The ciliary body divides the globe into two compartments (segments), the anterior segment and the posterior segment. The anterior and posterior chambers belong to the anterior segment. The anterior chamber measures about 3 mm anteroposteriorly in its central portion.[1] Its volume is about 0.2 ml.[1] The posterior chamber is a

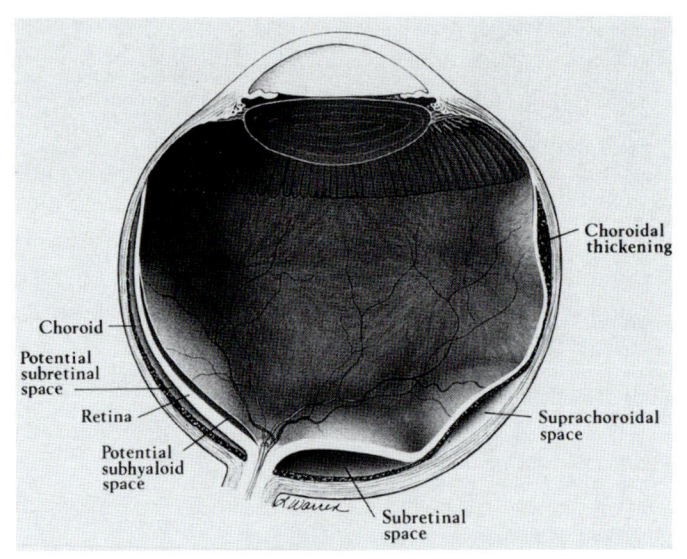

Fig. 2.9 Diagrammatic representation of intraocular potential spaces. From Mafee MF et al. Retinal and choroidal detachments: Role of MRI and CT. Radiol Clin North Am 1987; 25: 481–507. With permission.

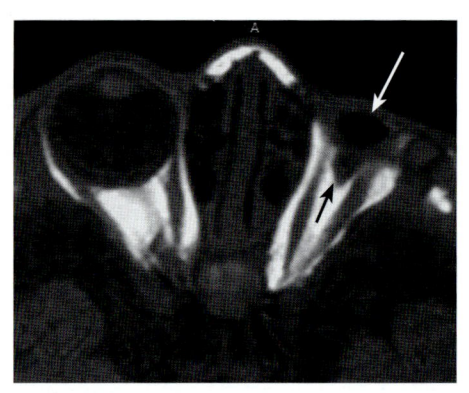

Fig. 2.10 Clinical anophthalmia. Axial T1W MR scan shows absence of the left globe. Note ocular prosthesis (long arrow) and a rudiment of the left globe (short arrow). The extraocular muscles are present.

small slitlike cavity posterior to the iris and anterior to the lens. Its volume is about 0.6 ml.[1] It is filled with aqueous fluid and communicates with the anterior chamber through the pupil. The posterior chamber is bounded anteriorly by the iris, peripherally by the ciliary processes, and posteriorly by the lens and the zonule (Figs. 2.2, 2.3).[1]

Intraocular Potential Spaces

There are basically three potential spaces in the eye that can accumulate fluid, resulting in detachment of the various coats of the globe (Fig. 2.9):[11, 12, 14, 21, 23]

1. The posterior hyaloid space, the potential space between the base (posterior hyaloid membrane) of the hyaloid (vitreous body) and the sensory retina (Fig. 2.9). Separation of the posterior hyaloid membrane from the sensory retina is referred to as posterior hyaloid detachment[11, 14, 16] (Fig. 2.9).
2. The subretinal space, the potential space between the sensory retina and the RPE. Separation of the sensory retina from the RPE is referred to as retinal detachment (Fig. 2.9).
3. The suprachoroidal space, the potential space between choroid and the sclera. The RPE and Bruch's membrane are tightly adherent to the choroid and become separated only when both layers are torn. However, the choroid is loosely attached to the sclera and can be separated, resulting in a choroidal detachment (Fig. 2.9).

Pathology

■ Congenital Anomalies

Anophthalmia

Anophthalmia denotes the complete absence of an eye as a result of a developmental defect, and is extremely rare.[25] More commonly, a small cystic remnant is seen and the term clinical anophthalmia is used (Fig. 2.10). In true anophthalmia, in addition to absence of the globes, the optic nerves and the optic chiasm may be absent. The optic tracts may be rudimentary and the lateral geniculate nuclei gliotic.[26] On CT and MRI there may be either rudimentary tissue or no globe present (Fig. 2.10). At times dystropic calcification and disorganized gliotic tissue may be present within the rudimentary tissue.

Microphthalmia

Microphthalmia (microphthalmos) refers to a congenital underdevelopment or acquired diminution in the size of the globe. Congenital microphthalmia is a continuation of a spectrum that begins with anophthalmia. The definition of microphthalmia is an eye that has an axial length less than 21 mm in an adult or less than 19 mm in a 1-year-old child.[25] In full-term infants, the globe measures 17.3 mm in axial length.[3] The size of the globe in a 2-year-old child is about 80% to 90% of an adult eye (20–22 mm).[21] Microphthalmia may be unilateral or bilateral and can occur as an isolated disorder or may be associated with other ocular, craniofacial anomalies or systemic abnormalities.[12, 14, 25, 27] Other causes of microphthalmia include the congenital rubella syndrome, persistent hyperplastic primary vitreous (PHPV), and retinopathy of prematurity (ROP). Bilateral microphthalmia and cataract may be seen in Lowe syndrome (oculocerebral renal disease).[26] Coloboma, PHPV, and congenital cataract are the most common ocular malformations associated with microphthalmia.[12, 14, 27] Microphthalmia results from an insult to the embryo after the outgrowth of the optic vesicle. The condition may be associated with an orbital cyst (Figs. 2.11 a, b).[28] The cyst may course along the optic nerve with free communication with the intraocular contents. CT and MRI in congenital microphthalmia demonstrate a small globe as well as a slightly small or poorly developed orbit. In older patients microphthalmia may occur as the result of trauma, surgery, inflammation, radiation, or other processes that result in disorganization of the eye (phthisis bulbi). In these patients, CT and MRI demonstrate a small, shrunken globe, often with extensive intraocular calcification or ossification. The principal conditions in which microphthalmia may be associated are listed in Table 2.1.

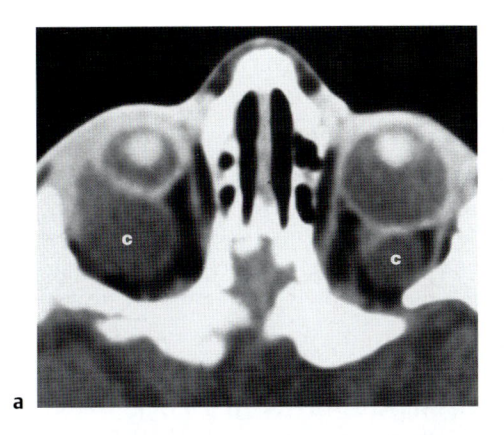

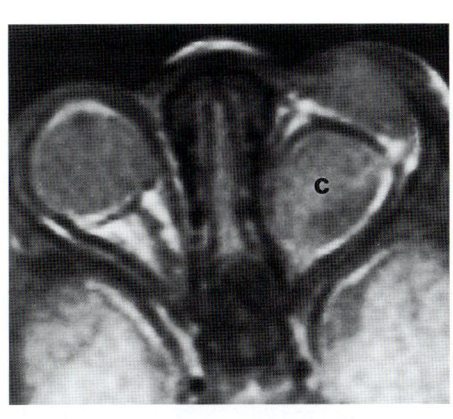

Fig. 2.11 Microphthalmia with cyst. **a** Axial CT scan shows bilateral microphthalmia with cysts (c). **b** Axial PW MR scan shows a microphthalmic left eye with a large cyst (c).

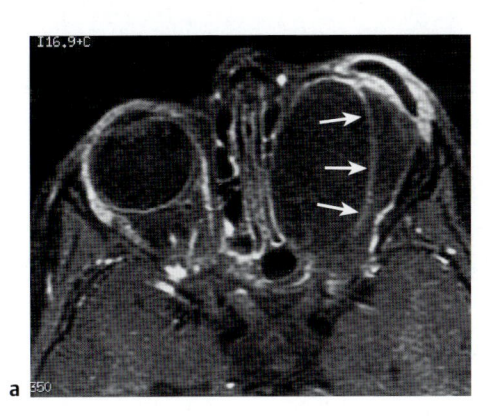

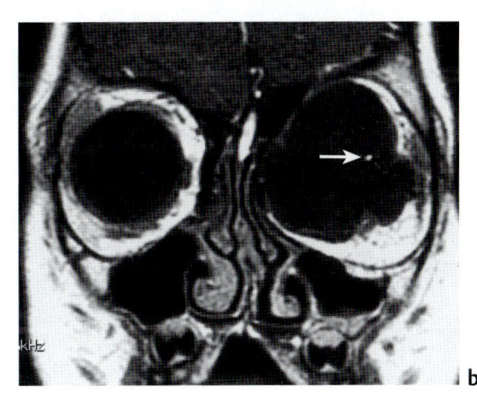

Fig. 2.12 Congenital cystic eye. Four-month-old girl with congenital cystic left eye associated with Goltz syndrome. Postcontrast axial fat-suppression T1W (**a**) and coronal enhanced T1W (**b**) MR scans through the orbit, showing a large left orbital cyst, enlarged left orbit, and no discernible normal bulbar structures on the left. Note enhancing strand (arrows), probably representing dysmorphic retinal tissue and gliosis.

Table 2.1 Microphthalmic eye, isolated, associated with other ocular disorders and some syndromes

- Isolated microphthalmia
- Microphthalmos with orbital cyst
- Persistent hyperplastic primary vitreous (PHPV)
- Retinopathy of prematurity (ROP)
- Congenital rubella syndrome
- Congenital toxoplasmosis
- Congenital syphilis
- Posttraumatic
- Postinflammation (herpes, CMV)
- Postradiation
- Hallerman-Streiff syndrome
- MIDAS syndrome (microphthalmia, dermal aplasia and sclerocornea)
- Lowe syndrome (oculocerebral-renal disease)
- Norrie syndrome
- Warburg syndrome
- Meckel syndrome
- Trisomy 13 and trisomy 18 syndromic disorders
- Other craniofacial and systemic syndromes

PHPV = persistent hyperplastic primary vitreous.
ROP = retinopathy of prematurity.
CMV = cytomegalovirus.
sclerocornea = scleral-like clouding of the cornea

Congenital Cystic Eye

Congenital cystic eye is a rare congenital anomaly resulting from failure of the optic vesicle to invaginate during the fourth week of embryogenesis.[14,28] It presents at birth as a complex cyst occupying the orbit, without any vestige of a globe evident (Fig. 2.12). The cyst wall is lined with cells derived from undifferentiated retina and retinal pigment epithelium. There may be present some remnant of an optic nerve–like structure and extraocular muscles.[28]

Macrophthalmia

Buphthalmos and Megalophthalmos

Macrophthalmia, or enlargement of the globe, is seen in patients with axial myopia, congenital glaucoma (buphthalmos), Sturge–Weber syndrome, and neurofibromatosis (see Fig. 2.**109c**). As many as 50% of patients with lid and facial involvement in neurofibromatosis exhibit glaucoma on the affected side.[14] Up to 30% of patients with Sturge–Weber syndrome have glaucoma and nearly two-thirds of these develop buphthalmos.[29] The hallmark of all forms of glaucoma in infants and young children is ocular enlargement (Fig. 2.13), which occurs because of the immature and growing collagen that constitutes the cornea and sclera in the young eye still responds to increased intraocular pressure by stretching.[25] Megalophthalmos is referred to an enlarged cornea in an overall enlarged eye that does not have glaucoma. The most common cause of macrophthalmia is axial elongation of the eye associated with high myopia (Fig. 2.14).[26] The normal adult eye has an axial length of about 24–25 mm. The axial length and width of the globe have been published on the basis of CT data,.[30] In addition to ocular elongation, CT and MRI may also demonstrate thinning of the posterior scleral–uveal rim.

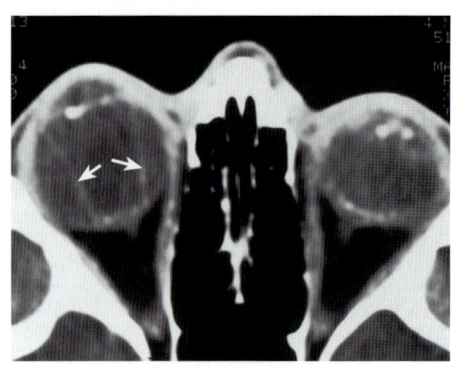

Fig. 2.13 Buphthalmos. Right macrophthalmia due to glaucoma and left microphthalmia related to complication of surgery for glaucoma. The right eye is enlarged and in addition shows serous choroidal detachment (arrows). The left eye is small and shows increased density of the vitreous as well as a few calcifications, representing a disorganized left eye (phthisis bulbi). Note dystrophic calcification of ciliary body of both eyes.

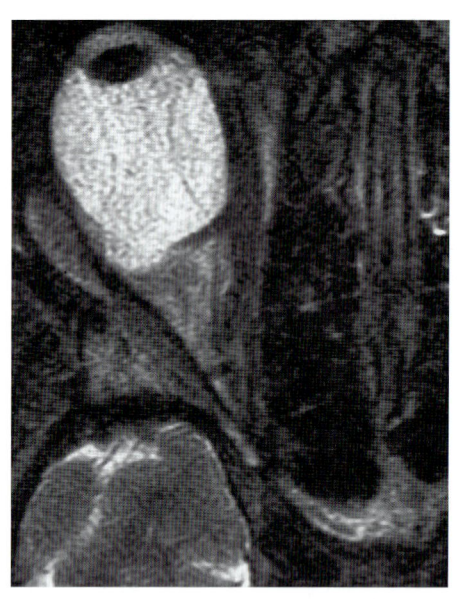

Fig. 2.14 Posterior staphyloma and myopia. Axial T2W MR scan of the right orbit. The anteroposterior diameter of the globe is enlarged. Note posterior staphyloma as indicated by the posterior bulging of the posterolateral eyeball. If the sclera gives way without involvement of uveal tissue, it is called ectasia. If the uvea is included in the ectasia, ("aneurysm"), it is termed a staphyloma.

Staphyloma

Staphyloma is referred to thinning and stretching (ectasia) of the scleral–uveal coats of the eyeball. Progressive myopia (megamyope) results in posterior staphyloma (Fig. 2.14). Staphyloma has also been reported in glaucoma, scleritis, and necrotizing infection, after surgery or radiation therapy and with trauma. All parts of the globe may stretch in response to the elevated intraocular pressure until 3–4 years of age and glaucoma-related axial myopia may be seen until the early teenage years (Fig. 2.13).[25] Anterior staphyloma also may occur as a result of inflammatory or infectious scleral-corneal thinning.[25]

Cryptophthalmos

Cryptophthalmos results due to partial or complete failure of eyelid development (eyebrow, palpebral fissure, eyelashes, and conjunctiva). Cryptophthalmos may be associated with variety of congenital ocular malformations as well as systemic anomalies, such as syndactyly and genitourinary anomalies.[14, 25]

X-linked Retinoschisis

X-linked retinoschisis is a congenital disorder in which there is splitting of the retina within the nerve fiber layer. This condition may result in retinal holes, eventually leading to full-thickness retinal detachment. The CT and MRI appearance of X-linked retinoschisis is nonspecific and compatible with retinal detachment.[4]

■ Coloboma and Morning Glory Disk Anomaly

A coloboma (Greek, "a mutilation") is a notch, gap, hole, or fissure that is congenital or acquired and in which a tissue or portion of a tissue is lacking. Ocular coloboma may involve the iris, lens, ciliary body, retina, choroid, optic nerve, or sclera.[12, 14, 28, 30] Ophthalmoscopically, optic nerve colobomas characteristically show enlargement of the papillary areas with partial or total excavation of the disk. Isolated optic nerve colobomas arise from failure of closure of only the most superior end of the embryonic fissure.[12, 14, 24, 27, 31–33] Failure of the closure of other parts of the embryonic fissure causes iridic, lenticular, ciliary body, and retinochoroidal colobomas.[34] The visual acuity in eyes with optic nerve colobomas is variable and may range from normal to light perception. Ocular colobomas may be associated with ocular or nonocular abnormalities including cardiac defects, dysplastic ears, facial palsy, and transsphenoidal encephalocele.[35] A coloboma can form in normal-sized eyes as well as microphthalmic eyes. In a small percentage of microphthalmic eyes with coloboma, a defect in the sclera allows for an extraocular herniation of the intraocular neural ectoderm to form an orbital cyst with a tunnel-like connection to the globe.[28] The relative sizes of the microphthalmic eye and colobomatous cyst, and the direction of cyst growth, are quite variable (Figs. 2.15, 2.16). Colobomatous cysts have been associated with a number of systemic syndromes, chromosomal anomalies, and familial cases (Table 2.2).[28]

Morning glory disk anomaly was first characterized by Kindler in 1970.[36] He described a unilateral congenital anomaly of the optic nerve head in 10 patients. Because of the similarity in appearance between the nerve head and a morning glory flower,

Table 2.2 Coloboma and colobomatous cysts associated with systemic and syndromic disorders

- Oculocerebrocutaneous syndrome (Dellman syndrome)
- Focal dermal hypoplasia (Goltz syndrome)
- Brachio-oculofacial syndrome
- CHARGE association
- VATER association
- Aicardi syndrome
- Proboscis lateralis
- Lenz syndrome
- Meckle syndrome
- Warburg syndrome
- Triploidy
- Trisomy 13
- Trisomy 18
- Cat-eye syndrome
- 4 p depletion
- Transethmoid and trans-sphenoid encephaloceles

Adopted from Kaufman LM, Villablanca PJ. Mafee MF, Diagnostic imaging of cystic lesions in the child's orbit. Radiol Clin North Am 1998; 36: 1149–1163.

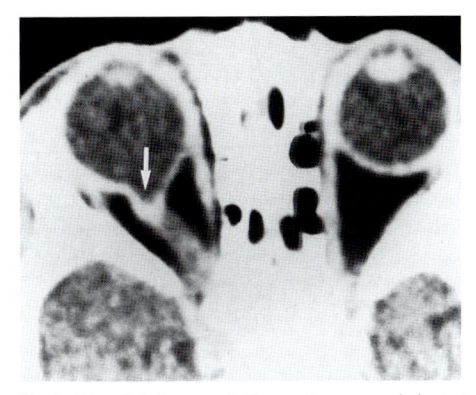

Fig. 2.15 Coloboma of the optic nerve disk. Axial postcontrast CT scan shows a large posterior global defect with optic disk excavation on the right (arrow). The defect appears surrounded by enhancing deformed sclera and seems to have a direct connection with the vitreous body. This corresponds to the ophthalmoscopic findings of a coloboma involving the right optic disk, retina, and choroid. From Mafee MF et al. CT of optic nerve: Colobomas, morning glory anomaly, and colobomatous cyst. Radiol Cin North Am 1987; 25: 693–699. With permission.

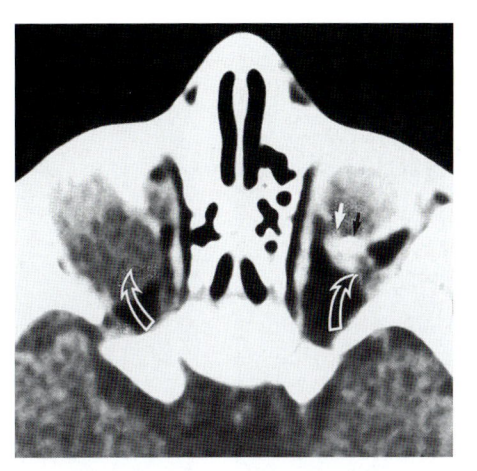

Fig. 2.16 Coloboma and colobomatous cyst and microphthalmia. Axial CT scan shows bilateral microphthalmia, colobomatous defect (white arrow), calcification (black arrow), and colobomatous cysts (curved arrows).

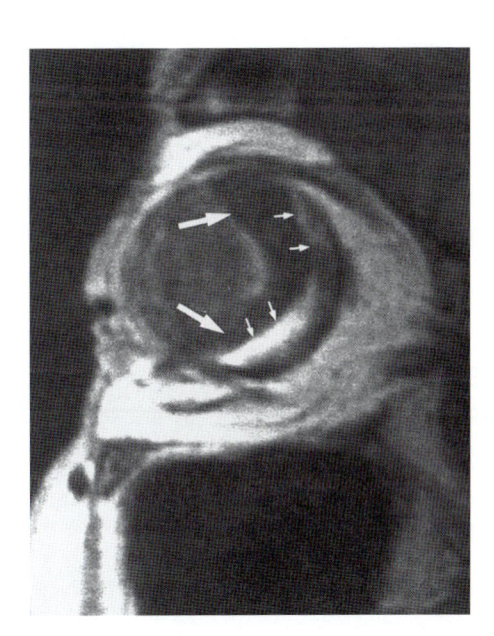

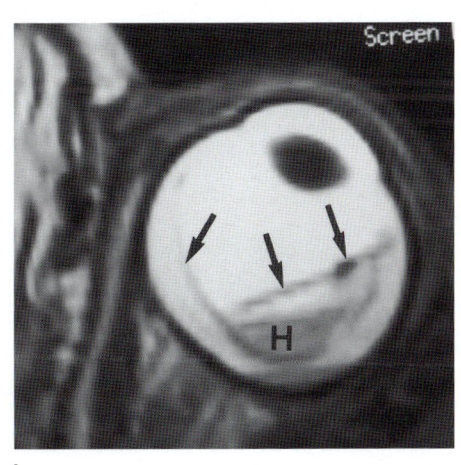

Fig. 2.17 Posterior hyaloid and retinal detachments.
a T1W sagittal MR scan. The detached posterior hyaloid membrane (large arrows) is seen anterior to the detached retina (short arrows). The hypointensity in the subhyaloid space is due to acute hemorrhage; the hyperintensity in the subretinal space is due to chronic hemorrhage. This patient had macular degeneration complicated by retinal and posterior hyaloid detachments.
b Posterior hyaloid detachment. Axial T2W MR scan in another patient, an infant with Coats disease, showing posterior hyaloid detachment (arrows) and acute subhyaloid hemorrhage (H). Note that unlike in retinal detachment, the detached posterior hyaloid membrane is separated from the optic disc.

he referred to the anomaly as the morning glory syndrome. Ophthalmoscopically the disk is enlarged and excavated and has a central core of white tissue. The disk is surrounded by an elevated annulus of light and also by variable pigmented subretinal tissue. The CT appearance of morning glory disk anomaly was first described in 1987.[32]

The CT and MRI appearance of optic disk coloboma includes a posterior global defect with optic disk excavation (Fig. 2.**15**). The imaging appearance of the morning glory anomaly is characteristic and corresponds to its clinical appearance as a large funnel-shaped disk. The colobomatous cyst associated with coloboma of the optic nerve head can be readily identified on CT and MRI (Fig. 2.**16**).

■ Ocular Detachments

Posterior Hyaloid Detachment

Posterior hyaloid detachment usually occurs in adults over the age of 50 years, but may occur in children with persistent hyperplastic primary vitreous (PHPV).[12,14,16,25] In the elderly population, the vitreous tends to undergo degeneration and liquefaction. This process may lead to posterior vitreous detachment and predispose to retinal detachment.[1,11,12,14] Posterior hyaloid detachment in adults may be associated with macular degeneration (Fig. 2.**17**).

The posterior hyaloid membrane is very thin and is invisible on MRI or CT, but it can be made visible when blood or other fluid fills the posterior hyaloid space, causing thickening of this membrane (Figs. 2.**17**–2.**19**). Fluid in the retrohyaloid space is seen on CT and MRI as a layered abnormality that shifts location in the lateral decubitus position. The retrohyaloid-layered fluid is

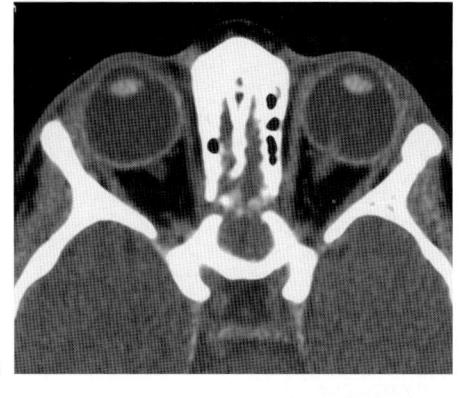

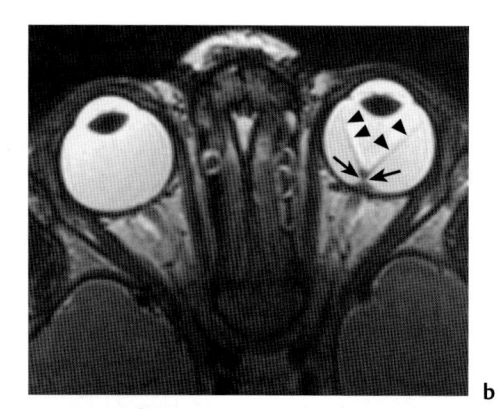

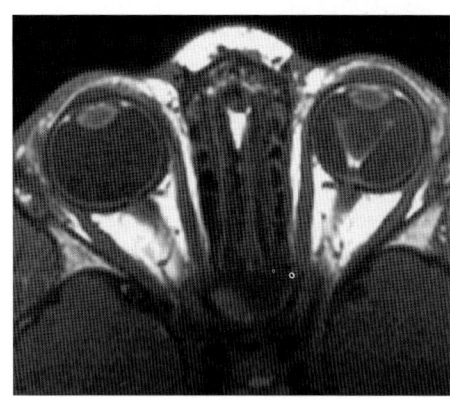

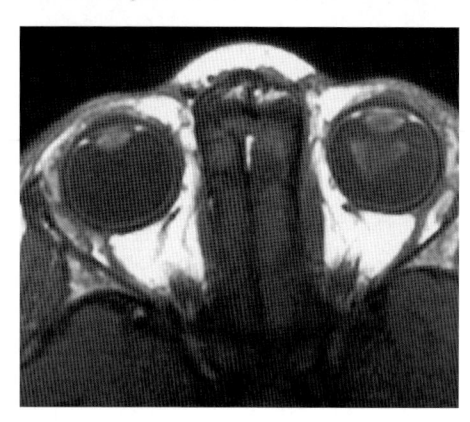

Fig. 2.18 Presumed posterior hyaloid detachment. An 18-month-old child with leukokoria of the left eye. Retinoblastoma could not be excluded on clinical evaluation.
a Axial CT scan shows a noncalcified lesion, presumed to be hematoma at the left optic disk. Note a faint V-shaped linear image, extending toward the optic disk.
b Axial T2W MR scan. Note a hypointense V-shaped image (arrowheads), with the apex of the V, connected to the disk by a very faint ill-defined linear tissue (arrows), representing the attached part of the vitreous to the retina at the edge of the optic disk.
c Axial unenhanced and d axial enhanced T1W MR scans, showing the detached posterior hyaloid membrane. There is no enhancing mass; retinoblastoma is therefore unlikely.

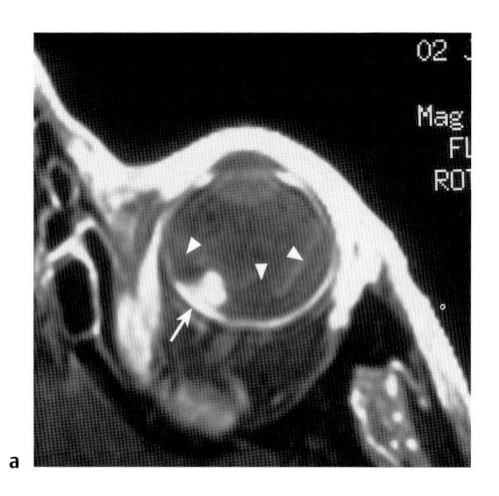

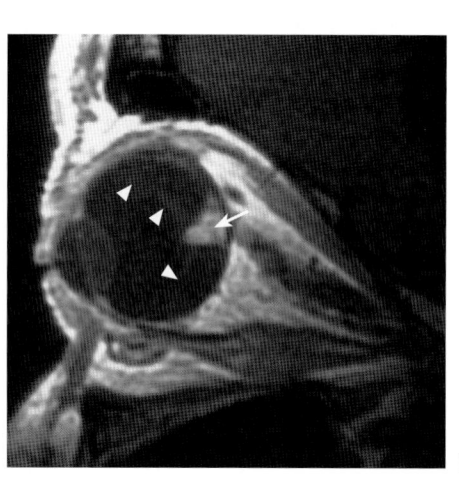

Fig. 2.19 Uveal melanoma and associated posterior hyaloid detachment.
a Postcontrast axial T1W MR scan with fat-suppression shows a choroidal melanoma (arrow). Note a curvilinear image (arrowheads) that does not extend toward the optic disk, compatible with posterior hyaloid detachment.
b Postcontrast sagittal T1W MR scan shows choroidal melanoma (arrow) and posterior hyaloid detachment (arrowheads).

shifted in the decubitus position because it is not within the substance of the vitreous. Hemorrhage within the vitreous mixes with the vitreous humor, which is a gel-like extracellular material, and therefore does not show intragel layering. Fluid in the retrohyaloid space and fluid in the subretinal space may not be differentiated from each other on CT and MRI.[21]

Retinal Detachment

Retinal detachment occurs when the sensory retina is separated from the RPE. The RPE has a barrier function; once this is damaged, fluid leaks into the potential subretinal space.[5,12,14,21] Rhegmatogenous retinal detachment refers to detachment due to a hole or a tear in the retina. The sensory retina is part of the central nervous system so, if there is a tear, the sensory retina cannot heal. On the other hand, retinal pigment epithelium has healing potential. In laser treatment for retinal detachment, the energy of the laser beam is absorbed by RPE at the site of retinal detachment, and the resultant heat heals and closes the tear. Fluid in the subretinal space can be detected by CT and MRI (Fig. 2.20). Retinal detachment usually is the result of elevation of the retina by a mass such as malignant choroidal melanoma, or of retraction of the retina, caused by a mass, a fibroproliferative disease in the vitreous such as vitreoretinopathy of prematurity, or vitreoretinopathy of diabetes mellitus; it may also occur with an inflammatory process such as the larval granuloma of toxocara endophthalmitis.[5,21] Retinal detachment may also occur because of retinal vascular leakage, which is seen in patients with Coats disease. Retinal detachment is sometimes the result of subretinal hemorrhage and occurs following trauma, senile macular degeneration, or persistent hyperplastic primary vitreous. Any choroidal lesions can cause retinal detachment (Fig. 2.21). The

Pathology 151

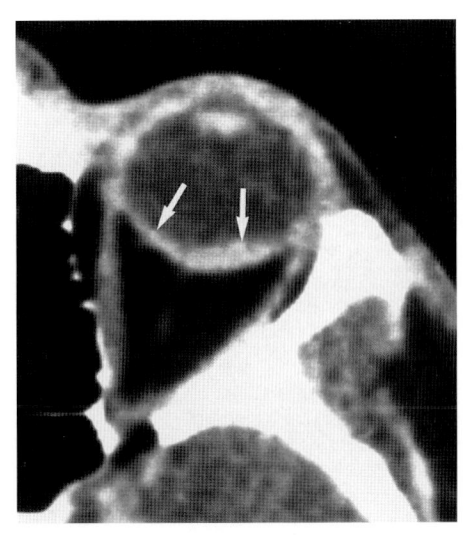

Fig. 2.20 Retinal detachment. CT scan shows a shallow retinal detachment (arrows). Note that the leaves of the detached retina converge at the optic disk. The subretinal exudate appears dense.

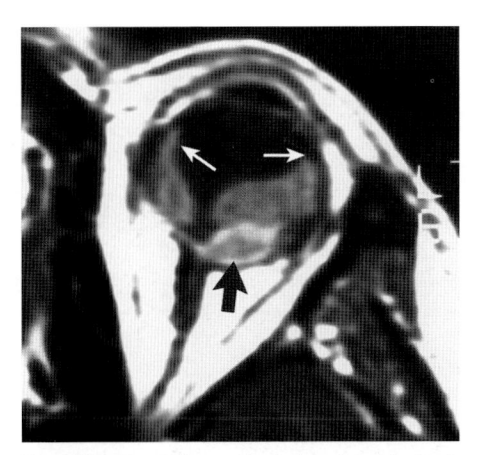

Fig. 2.21 Exudative retinal detachment. Postcontrast T1W MR scan shows characteristic appearance of a retinal detachment. The detached sensory retina extends from the optic nerve head toward the ora serrata (white arrows). Note a mass (black arrow), which has caused retinal detachment. The mass shows marked enhancement and is thought to be a choroidal hemangioma. The patient was lost to follow-up.

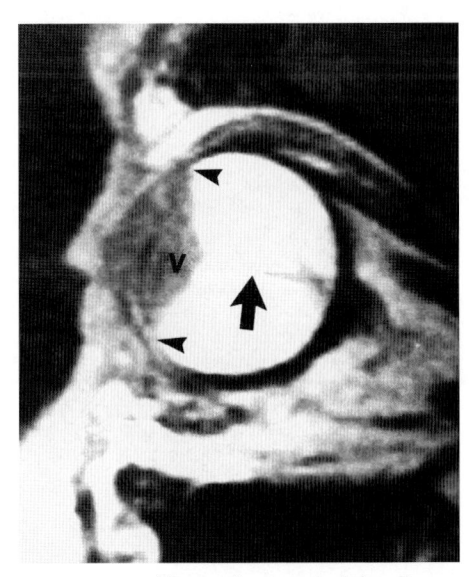

Fig. 2.22 Total hemorrhagic retinal detachment. Sagittal T1W MR scan, showing folded leaves of the detached retina (arrow), which extends toward the ora serrata (arrowheads). V = contracted vitreous body.

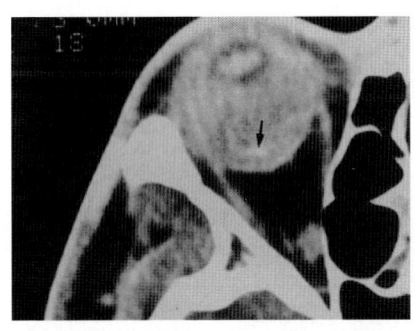

Fig. 2.23 Chronic total retinal detachment associated with calcification. Axial CT scan in a patient with known chronic retinal detachment, showing increased density of the globe due to subretinal exudate, related to total retinal detachment. Note the small calcification (arrow). This may be due to metaplastic calcification ("bone") formation by retinal pigment epithelium (RPE).

appearance of the retinal detachment varies with the amount of exudation (Figs. 2.21, 2.22) and organization of the subretinal materials, as well as presence or absence of hemorrhage.

In a section taken at the level of the optic disk, retinal detachment is seen with a characteristic indentation at the optic disk (Figs. 2.21, 2.22). When total retinal detachment is present and the entire vitreous cavity is ablated, the leaves of the detached retina may not be clearly detected. In an axial CT or MRI scan taken below or above the lens, the total retinal detachment appears as a homogeneous increased density/intensity of the globe (Fig. 2.23). Retinal detachment is seen on coronal MRI as a characteristic folding membrane (Fig. 2.24). The subretinal fluid of an exudative retinal detachment is rich in protein, giving higher CT numbers (density) and stronger MR signal intensities (on T1-weighted MR images) than those seen in the subretinal fluid (transudate) of a rhegmatogenous detachment. A rheg-

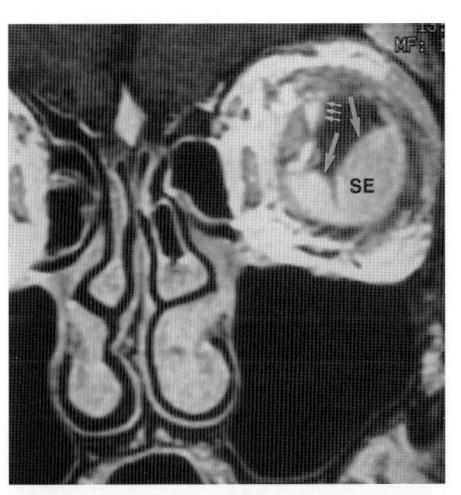

Fig. 2.24 Retinal detachment. Coronal enhanced T1W MR scan shows characteristic appearance of a totally detached retina (arrows). SE = subretinal exudate.

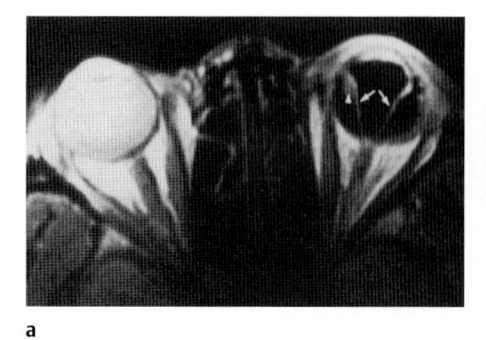

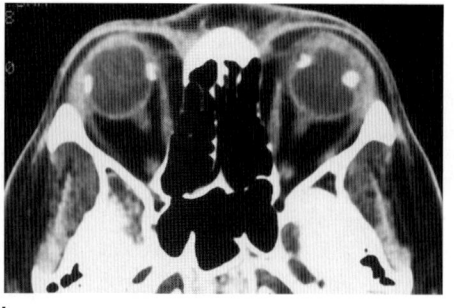

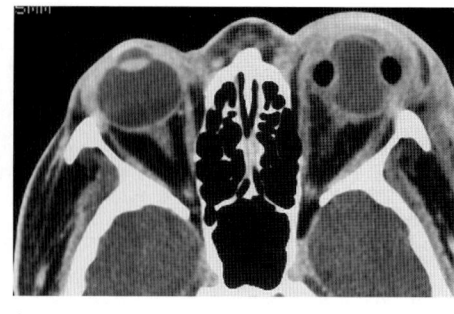

Fig. 2.25 a Retinal detachment and intravitreal silicone oil for retinopexy in a patient with retinal detachment. T2W axial MR section shows detached leaves of the retina (arrows). The hypointensity of the vitreous is due to the injection of silicone oil for retinopexy. However, the silicone has entered into the subretinal space. The hyperintense area (arrowhead) is due subretinal effusion that is not replaced by silicone oil. The retina remains detached.

b Scleral banding (buckling). Axial CT scan shows bilateral scleral banding, performed for retinopexy in this patient with bilateral retinal detachment. The silicone band appears hyperdense.

c Axial CT scan in another patient, showing scleral silicone sponge banding of the left eye that appears hypodense owing to air contained in the silicone sponge.

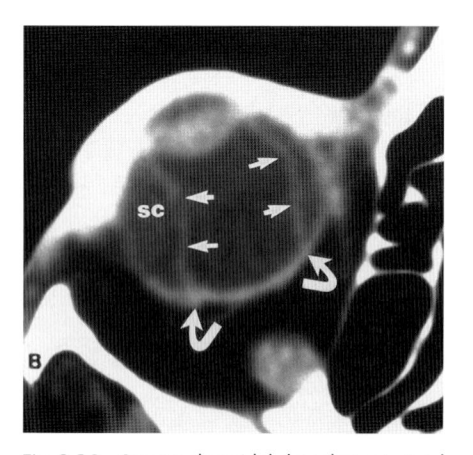

Fig. 2.26 Serous choroidal detachment. Axial CT scan. Note the detached choroid (straight arrows). At the expected region of the vortex veins (curved arrows), the detached choroid is characteristically limited by the anchoring effect of the vortex veins. Note the hypodensity of fluid in the suprachoroidal space (SC), indicative of serous fluid collection. Unlike the detached retina, the detached choroid extends toward the ciliary body and may be associated with the detachment of the root of the ciliary body.

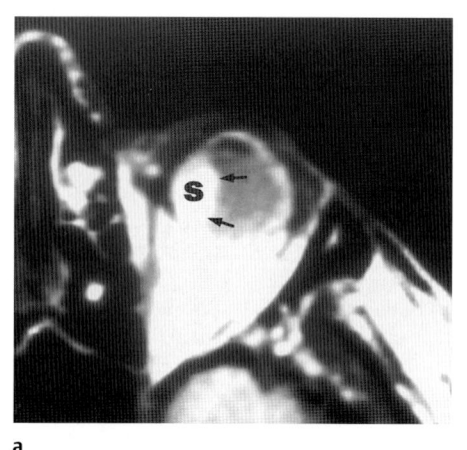

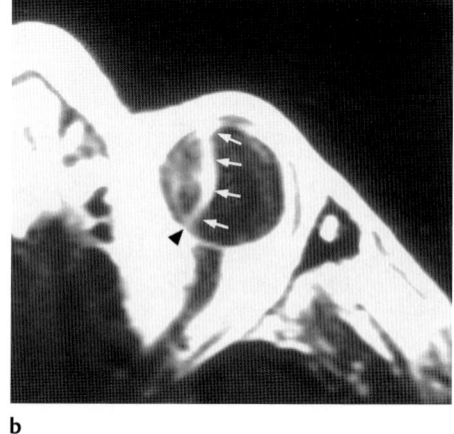

Fig. 2.27 Serous choroidal detachment. a PW MR scan showing a choroidal detachment (arrows). Note hyperintense fluid in the suprachoroidal space (s). b Postcontrast axial T1W MR scan, showing the enhanced detached choroid (arrows). Note that the detached choroid is restricted at the expected location of the vortex vein (arrowhead). From Mafee MF. Uveal melanoma, choroidal hemangioma, and simulating lesion. Role of MR imaging. Radiol Clin North Am 1998; 36: 1083–1099. With permission.

matogenous retinal detachment is produced by a retinal tear and subsequent ingress of vitreous fluid into the subretinal space.[5, 11, 12] In many cases of shallow retinal detachment the MRI and, in particular, the CT scans may not show the detached retina. In these patients, ultrasonography is superior to MRI and CT. Retinal detachment is characteristically seen on CT or MRI as a V-shaped image, with its apex at the optic disk and its extremities toward the ciliary body (Figs. 2.**21**, 2.**25**). This appearance of retinal detachment may be confused with the appearance of choroidal detachment. However, choroidal detachment, in the region of the optic disk and macula, involves detachment of the choroid that is restricted by the anchoring effect of the vortex veins, short posterior ciliary arteries, and nerves. This restriction usually results in a characteristic appearance of the detached choroid, which, unlike the detached retinal leaves, do not extend to the region of the optic disk (See Figs. 2.**26**, 2.**27**).[5, 11]

Malignant melanomas and choroidal hemangiomas are the most common choroidal neoplasms producing retinal detachment in adults (see Figs. 2.**88**, 2.**103**).[5, 11] These tumors produce various degrees of subretinal fluid accumulation, depending on the size and location of the tumor (Figs. 2.**21**, 2.**22**).

Choroidal Detachment, Choroidal Effusion, and Ocular Hypotony

Choroidal detachment is caused by the accumulation of fluid (serous choroidal detachment) or blood (hemorrhagic choroidal detachment) in the potential suprachoroidal space.[5, 37–42] Serous choroidal detachment (Figs. 2.**26**, 2.**27**) may occur following intraocular surgery, penetrating ocular trauma, or inflammatory choroidal disorders.[39] Hemorrhagic choroidal detachment often occurs after a contusion, after a penetrating injury, or as a complication of intraocular surgery.

Ocular hypotony is the essential underlying cause of serous choroidal detachment.[39] Ocular hypotony may be the result of inflammatory diseases (uveitis, scleritis), accidental perforation of

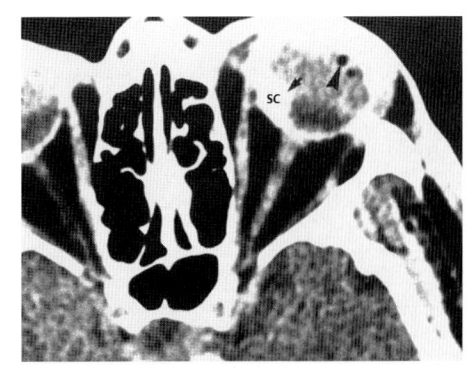

Fig. 2.28 Acute posttraumatic hemorrhagic choroidal detachment. Axial unenhanced CT scan shows detached choroid (arrow). The increased density of the suprachoroidal space (SC) is due to hemorrhage that is a few days old. Note small intravitreal air bubble (arrowhead). From Mafee MF. The eye. In: Som PM, Curtin HD, eds. Head and Neck Imaging. St. Louis: Mosby; 2003: 441–521. With permission.

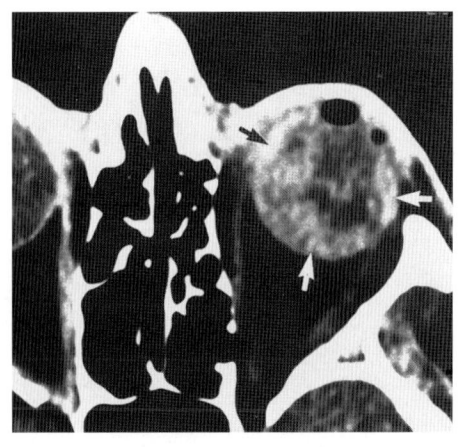

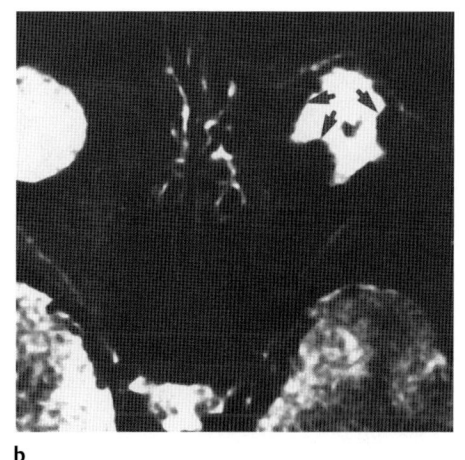

Fig. 2.29 Acute hemorrhagic choroidal detachment. **a** Axial CT scan showing multiple choroidal hematomas (arrows). **b** T2W MR scan showing hypointense acute choroidal hematomas (arrows). From Mafee MF et al. Retinal and choroidal detachments: Role of MRI and CT. Radiol Clin North Am 1987; 25: 481–507. With permission.

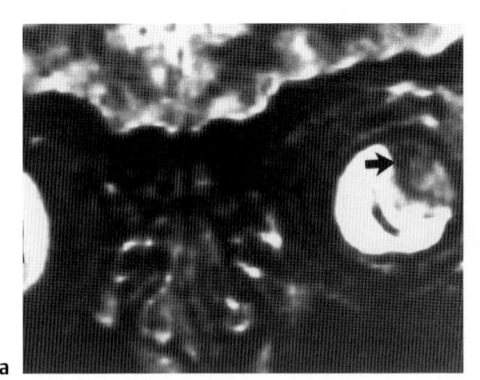

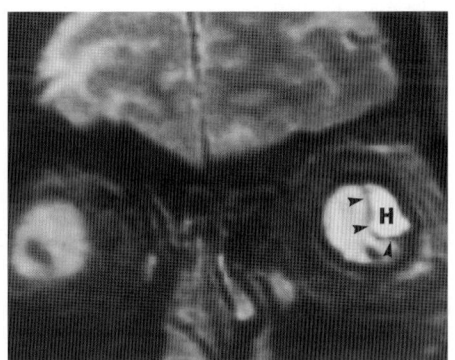

Fig. 2.30 Acute hemorrhagic choroidal detachment.
a T2W coronal MR scan shows a hypointense acute choroidal hematoma (arrow).
b Coronal T2W MR scan, obtained 10 days later, shows the hyperintense choroidal hematoma (H). Note the detached choroid (arrowheads). The MRI characteristic of acute or subacute hemorrhage as seen in **a** can be mistaken for choroidal melanoma.

the eyeball, ocular surgery, or intensive glaucoma therapy.[39–42] Ocular hypotony causes increased permeability of the choroidal capillaries. This increased permeability leads to the transudation of fluid from the choroidal vasculature into the uveal tissue and causes diffuse swelling of the entire choroid (choroidal effusion). As the edema of the choroid increases, fluid accumulates in the potential suprachoroidal (epichoroidal) space, resulting in serous or exudative choroidal detachment.[38, 39, 41, 43] Choroidal effusion, like choroidal hematoma, may be preceded by surgery or other types of trauma to the eye.[11, 39, 40, 44, 45–47] In fact, choroidal effusion may be a common, albeit transient, occurrence after intraocular surgery.[40, 46]

On CT scans, choroidal detachment appears as a semilunar or ring-shaped area of variable attenuation. The degree of attenuation depends on the cause but is generally greater with inflammatory disorders of the eyeball (Figs. 2.26, 2.27). Inflammatory diseases of the choroid (uveitis) seldom appear as a localized mounding of the choroid; they generally produce a diffuse thickening with no localized area of mounding unless there is a choroidal abscess (see Fig. 2.37).[5]

Hemorrhagic choroidal detachments appear as either a low or a high moundlike area of high density on CT, which can be quite large and irregular (Fig. 2.28). In a fresh hemorrhagic choroidal detachment, the choroid and hemorrhage in the potential suprachoroidal space are isodense. However, in a patient with chronic choroidal hematoma or a serosanguineous choroidal detachment, it may be possible to separate the detached choroid and suprachoroidal fluid accumulation (Figs. 2.26, 2.28).[39]

Choroidal hematoma is seen on MR images as a focal, well-demarcated, lenticular mass in the wall of the eyeball (Fig. 2.29). This characteristic configuration usually is not changed, but signal intensity will change as the hematoma ages.[40] Multiple lesions may occasionally be seen (Fig. 2.29). The signal intensity of the choroidal hematoma depends on its age. Within the first 48 hours or so, the hematoma (using a 1.5 T MR unit) is isointense to slightly hypointense relative to the normal vitreous body on T1-weighted and PW MRI but is markedly hypointense on T2-weighted images (Fig. 2.30a). Usually after five days, its signal intensity characteristics will alter, becoming increasingly relatively hyperintense on T1-weighted and PW images and only slightly hypointense on T2-weighted images.[5, 11, 39, 40] At this stage, the choroidal hematoma may be mistaken for a choroidal melanoma.[40] The hematoma usually continues to increase in signal intensity on T1-weighted, PW, and T2-weighted images (Figs. 2.30b, 2.31, 2.32) and usually becomes markedly hyperintense by 2 or more weeks on all MR sequences (Figs. 2.31, 2.32).[5, 39, 40]

Serous choroidal detachment (Figs. 2.26, 2.27) and choroidal effusion (Fig. 2.33) have a different appearance on CT and MRI from that of a choroidal hematoma (Figs. 2.29, 2.30). Serous

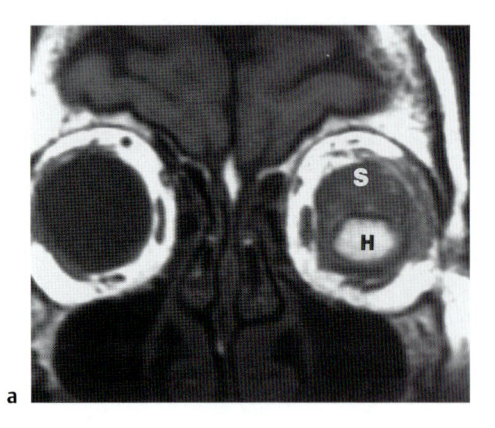

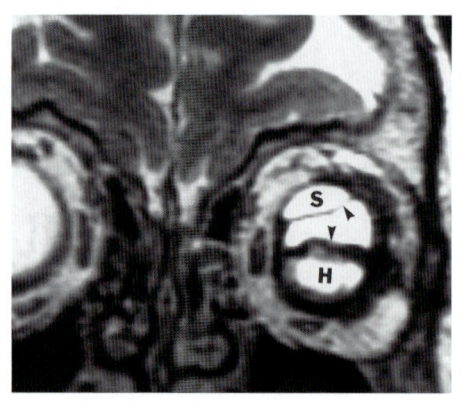

Fig. 2.**31** Serous and chronic hemorrhagic choroidal detachment.
a Coronal T1W MR scan showing serous (S) and chronic hemorrhagic (H) choroidal detachments.
b Coronal T2W MR scan. The serous (S) and hemorrhagic (H) choroidal detachments appear hyperintense. Note detached choroid (arrowheads). From Mafee MF. Uveal melanoma, choroidal hemangioma, and simulating lesions. Role of MR imaging. Radiol Clin North Am 1998; 36: 1083–1099. With permission.

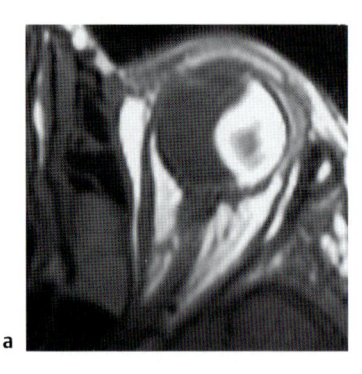

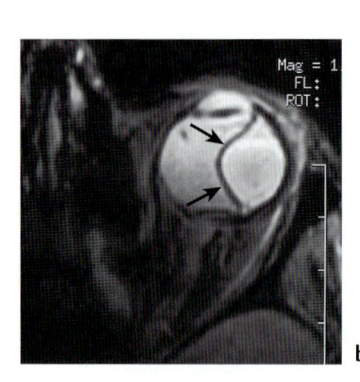

Fig. 2.**32** Subacute hemorrhagic choroidal detachment. **a** Axial T1W and **b** T2W MR scans showing a detached choroid (arrows). The detached choroid extends from the expected position of the vortex vein toward the ciliary body. Note hyperintense suprachoroidal hemorrhage.

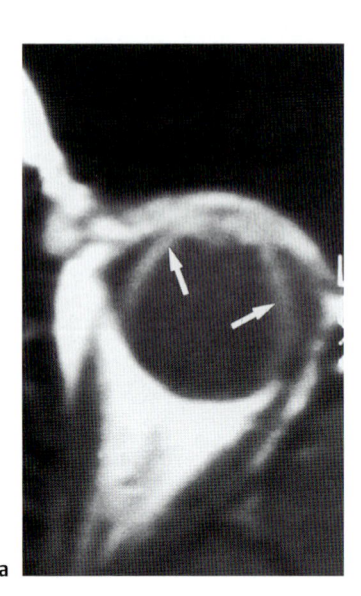

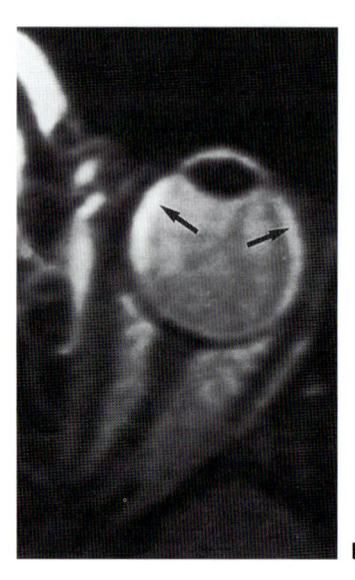

Fig. 2.**33** Choroidal effusion. **a** Axial PW, and **b** T2W MR scans show fluid collection (arrows) within the choroid, extending into the ciliary body. Fig. 2.**33 a** from Mafee MF. Uveal melanoma, choroidal hemangioma, and simulating lesions. Role of MR imaging. Radiol Clin North Am 1998; 36: 1083–1099. With permission.

choroidal detachment is caused by a nonhemorrhagic accumulation of fluid in the suprachoroidal potential space. The choroidal detachment appears as a smooth elevation of the choroid (Figs. 2.**26**, 2.**27**), the fluid in the suprachoroidal space is often hypodense on CT (Fig. 2.**26**), and its MR appearance is that of a transudate (Fig. 2.**27**). A choroidal effusion usually is seen as a crescentic or ring-shaped lesion on both CT and MRI (Figs. 2.**33**).[5,39,40] It does not resemble the lenticular appearance of a choroidal hematoma or choroidal abscess.

■ Ocular Inflammatory Disorders

The eye may be affected by either known systemic or idiopathic ocular inflammatory processes. A host of infectious diseases may affect the globe (Figs. 2.**34**–2.**40**). Viral diseases include herpes simplex (Fig. 2.**34**), cytomegalovirus (Figs. 2.**35**, 2.**36**), rubella, rubeola, mumps, variola, varicella, and infectious mononucleosis. Bacterial diseases include common pathogens (Fig. 2.**31**) and other inflammatory conditions, such as syphilis, brucellosis, tuberculosis (Fig. 2.**39**), sarcoidosis (Fig. 2.**40**) and leprosy. In immunocompromised patients and diabetic patients, fungal infections, particularly candidiasis may involve the globes.[26] Chronic

Pathology

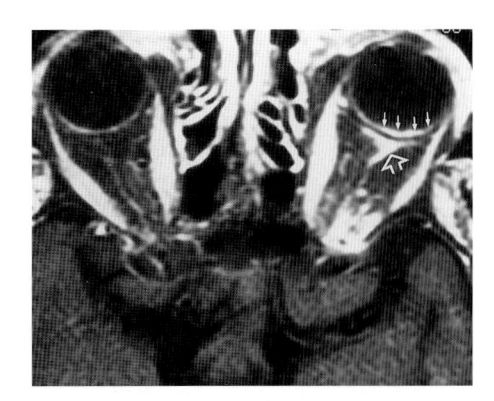

Fig. 2.**34** Herpes simplex virus ophthalmicus (HSO). A 67-year-old man with a history of diabetes and end-stage renal disease developed HSO (keratitis, trigeminal neuralgia, and left ophthalmoplegia). In this postcontrast axial fat-suppression T1W MR scan, the retina and perhaps the choroid of the left eye appear thickened and show increased contrast enhancement (small arrows). Note abnormal contrast enhancement of the Tenon's capsule as well as increased contrast enhancement along left optic nerve sheath (hollow arrow), indicating that the disease is not limited to the globe.

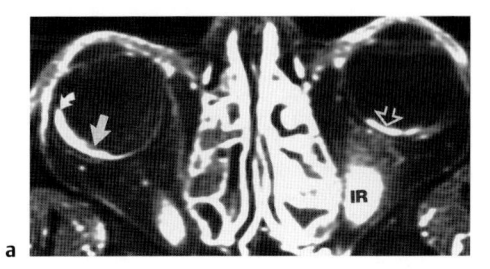

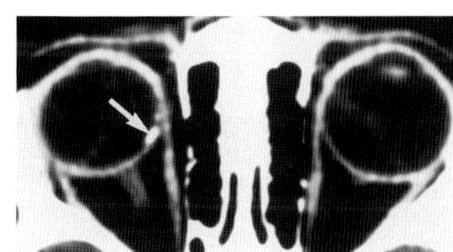

Fig. 2.**35** CMV retinitis.
a Axial postcontrast fat-suppression T1W MR scan, in an adult patient with AIDS. The retina of both globes appear thickened and show increased contrast enhancement (arrows). Note that the enhancement does not extend beyond the ora serrata (curved arrow), indicating a retinal process rather than a choroidal/uveal process. IR = inferior rectus.
b Axial CT scan shows calcification (arrow) in this 3-year-old immunocompromised child with CMV retinitis.

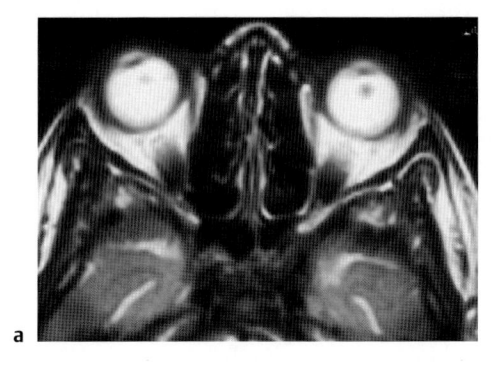

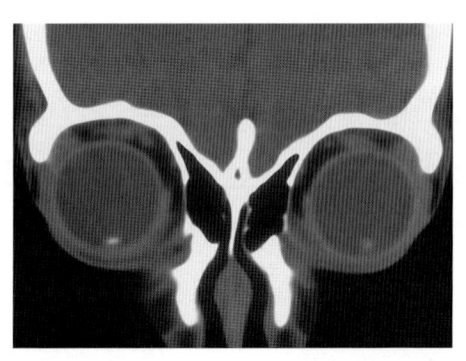

Fig. 2.**36** Chronic CMV retinitis in a 10-year-old girl with aplastic anemia and immuno-insufficiency that has brought her to a chronic CMV infection. a Axial T2W MR scan shows small hypointense images behind the lens, compatible with ganciclovir implants. b Coronal CT scan. The ganciclovir implants appear hyperdense. The implants are used for drug treatment.

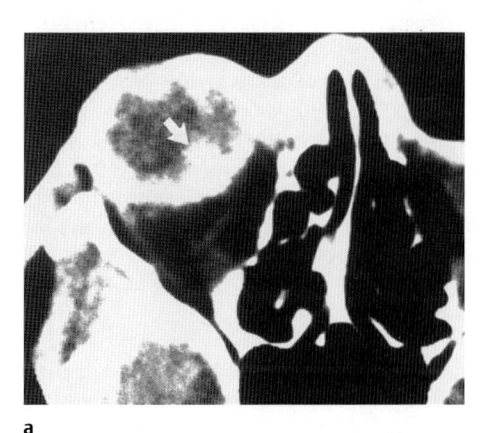

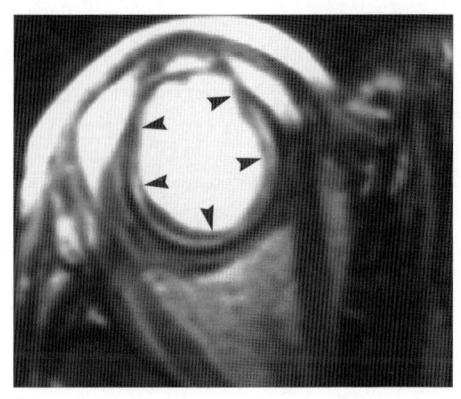

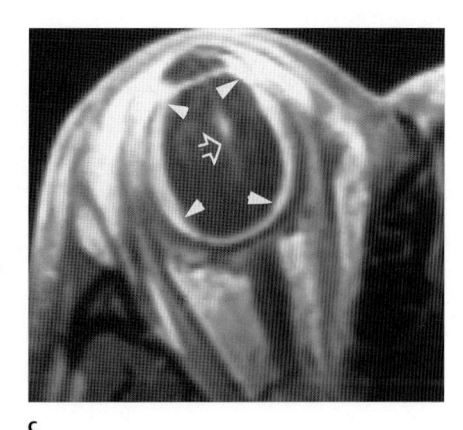

Fig. 2.**37** Endophthalmitis.
a Endophthalmitis and choroidal abscess. Postcontrast axial CT scan shows marked enhancement of the thickened uveoscleral coat. Note an area of induration (arrow), representing a choroidal abscess. From Mafee MF et al. Retinal and choroidal detachments: Role of MRI and CT. Radiol Clin North Am 1987; 25: 487–507. With permission.
b Axial T2W and c postcontrast T1W MR scans in another patient with endophthalmitis. The uveal tract appears thickened and shows increased contrast enhancement (arrowheads). Note intravitreal enhancement along the hyaloid canal as well (hollow arrow), indicating that the patient also has vitritis, and therefore the findings are more consistent with endophthalmitis. Rather than with uveitis.

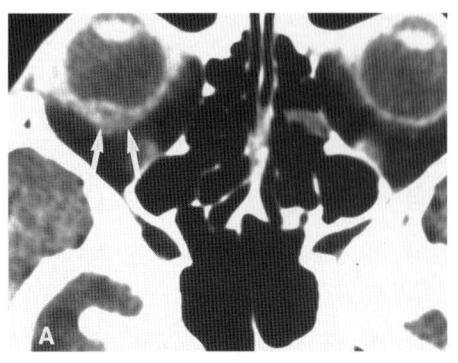

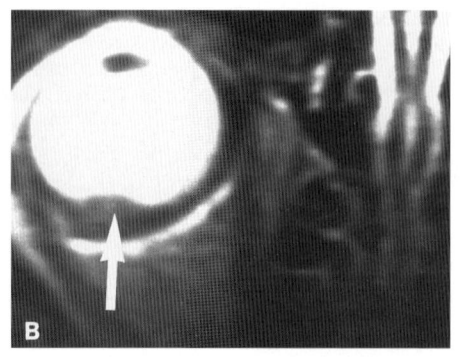

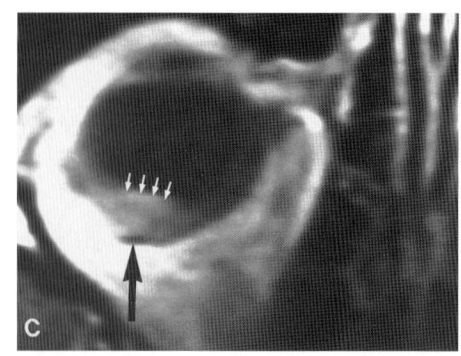

Fig. 2.**38** Posterior nodular scleritis. **a** Postcontrast CT scan shows increased thickening of the right sclera with increased contrast enhancement and focal masslike lesion (arrows). **b** Axial T2W MR scan. The lesion (arrow) appears hypointense, simulating a choroidal melanoma. The lesion was barely recognized on T1W MR images (not shown). **c** Postcontrast axial T1W MR scan. The lesion (arrows) shows moderate contrast enhancement. Patient improved and his symptoms resolved following a short course of steroid therapy. The mass was no longer present on follow-up imaging study. Figs. 2.**38 a, b** From Mafee MF. Uveal melanoma, choroidal hemangioma, and simulating lesions. Role of MR imaging. Radiol Clin North Am 1998; 36: 1083–1099. With permission.

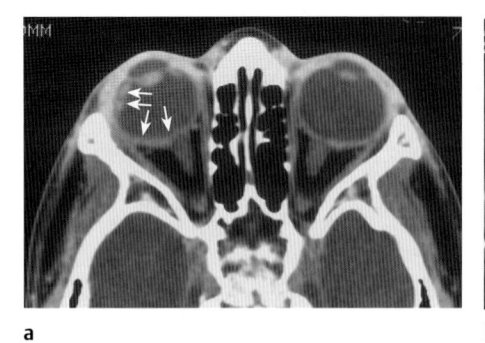

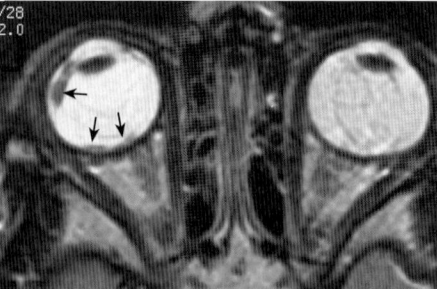

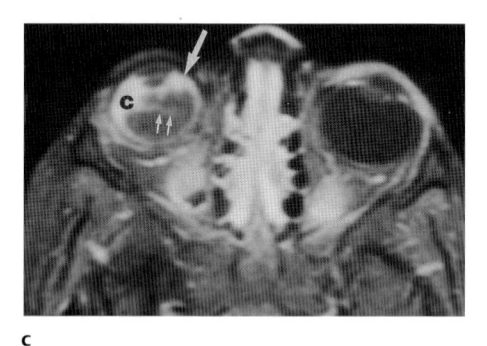

Fig. 2.**39** Granulomatous uveitis in a 3-year-old boy with leukokoria. Retinoblastoma could not be excluded on the basis of clinical evaluation.
a Postcontrast axial CT scan shows moderate thickening with increased enhancement of the right choroid and ciliary body (arrows).
b Axial T2W MR scan. Hypointense lesions (arrows) are seen within the right globe, involving the choroid and ciliary body.
c Axial fat-suppression enhanced T1W MR scan. There is marked contrast enhancement within the vitreous body (small arrows), and along the markedly thickened choroid (C) and ciliary body (large arrow) of the right eye. Figs. 2.**39 b** From Kaufman LM, Mafee MF, Song CD. Retinoblastoma and simulating lesions. Role of CT, MRI and use of Gd-DTPA contrast enhancement. Radiol Clin North Am 1998; 36: 1101–1117. With permission.

inflammatory processes may cause calcification of the sclera, choroid, and lens. Extensive disease may result in irregular calcific intraocular masses and a small deformed and disorganized globe (phthisis bulbi) (see Fig. 2.**42**).

Episcleritis

Episcleritis is a an idiopathic inflammation of the thin layer of tissue lying between the conjunctiva and the sclera. Episcleritis may be associated with deeper inflammation (scleritis). Imaging evaluation is not needed in episcleritis.

Scleritis

Scleritis can occur either as an idiopathic disease or in association with systemic diseases.[14, 25, 26, 48] The process may be unilateral or bilateral. Scleritis may be caused by collagen-vascular disorders, granulomatous diseases, metabolic disorders, infections, and trauma. Scleritis may be bacterial, fungal, or viral in origin.[14, 48] It may be caused by metabolic disease (gout) or by a group of autoimmune disorders. Sarcoidosis and Cogan syndrome also can be associated with scleritis. Cogan syndrome is a rare idiopathic autoimmune inflammatory multisystem disease that affects the eye (deep nonsyphilitic interstitial keratitis) and the ear (vestibulocochlear dysfunction) and which is also associated with vasculitis.

Scleritis is classified as anterior or posterior scleritis. Scleritis may be acute or chronic. Posterior scleritis results in thickening of the sclera and choroid.[12, 26, 48] There may be associated thickening of the Tenon's capsule, as well as secondary serous or exudative retinal detachment (see Fig. 2.**4**).[12, 48] Histopathologically, posterior scleritis is classified into two forms: nodular and diffuse. Posterior nodular scleritis may mimic uveal melanoma (Fig. 2.**38**). Diffuse posterior scleritis appears as diffuse thickening of the uveoscleral coat with variable degrees of contrast enhancement on both CT and MRI scans (Figs. 2.**4**, 2.**38**).[12, 26, 48]

Uveitis

Uveitis is an inflammatory process of the intraocular contents, often prominently involving the uveal tract.[26] The etiology of uveitis is often unknown. Vogt–Koyanagi–Harada syndrome, also known as VKH disease, is a bilateral granulomatous panuveitis of unknown cause. The entity is seen more frequently in Asians. The disease is often associated with extraocular involvement, including meningitic manifestations, fever, headache, vertigo, tinnitus and hearing loss. Uveitis may be caused by a specific organism such as tuberculosis (Fig. 2.**39**) toxoplasmosis and cytomegalovirus.

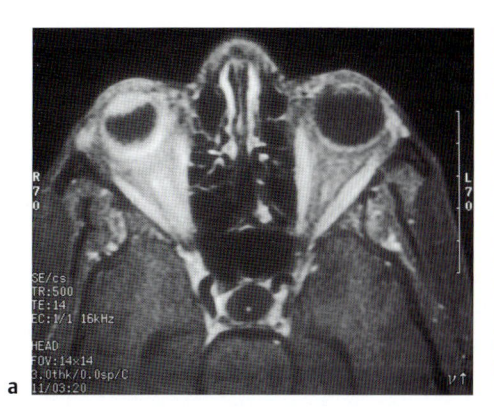

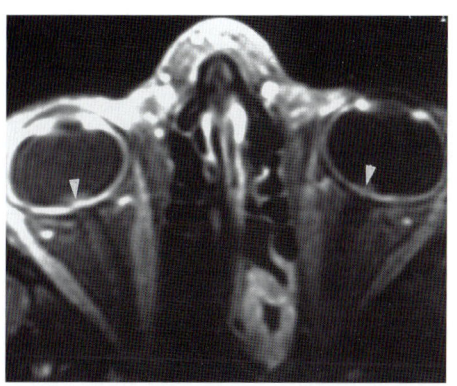

Fig. 2.40 Ocular sarcoidosis (panuveitis).
a Axial postcontrast fat-suppression T1W MR scan. There is nodular enhancement of the entire uveal tract of the right eye.
b Axial enhanced fat-suppression T1W MR scan in another patient, a 12-year-old child with bilateral idiopathic panuveitis. Note increased thickening of the uveal tracts and enhancing nodules (granuloma) at the optic nerve head (arrows).

Uveitis is a common presentation of sarcoidosis (Fig. 2.**40**). If there is uveitis, with involvement of the lacrimal gland along with fever, parotid gland enlargement, and occasional facial nerve palsy, the condition is termed Heerfordt syndrome or uveoparotid fever.

Papillitis

Papillitis, inflammation of the optic nerve head, has multiple causes including ischemia, infections, and autoimmune diseases. If the inflammatory process is severe, the optic disk can be massively enlarged and hemorrhagic so as to resemble retinoblastoma.[4]

Parasitic Infections

Larval granulomatosis usually affects children between 2 and 8 years of age. The process causes uveitis resulting from ingestion of the eggs of the nematodes *Toxocara canis* or *Toxocara cati* (see Figs. 2.**75**–2.**77**).[6, 12, 14, 26] Three clinical patterns occur: a unilateral localized granuloma which may mimic retinoblastoma, and other patterns that include endophthalmitis and pars plana disease.[26]

■ Benign Reactive Lymphoid Hyperplasia

Benign reactive lymphoid hyperplasia (BRLH) is characterized by a polymorphous infiltration of small, round lymphocytes and plasma cells. BRLH of the orbit often follows a benign course, presenting with subtle symptoms and signs with no significant change in visual acuity. BRLH of the orbit often involves lacrimal gland and conjunctiva. It may involve the Tenon's capsule and causes thickening of the posterior wall of the globe, a CT or MRI finding that can simulate posterior scleritis, uveitis, and uveal melanoma. Lymphoma and leukemic infiltration of the globe may also simulate uveitis and posterior scleritis clinically, as well as on diagnostic imaging studies (see Figs. 2.**107**, 2.**108**).

■ Papilledema

Increased intracranial pressure may result in papilledema with elevation of the optic disks. On CT and MR scans, if papilledema is significant, elevation of the optic disk bulging into the posterior aspect of the globe may be observed (Fig. 2.**41**). The diameter of the optic nerve sheath complex may be increased. On postcontrast T1-weighted MR scans, there may be increased enhancement of the optic disks (Fig. 2.**41**).

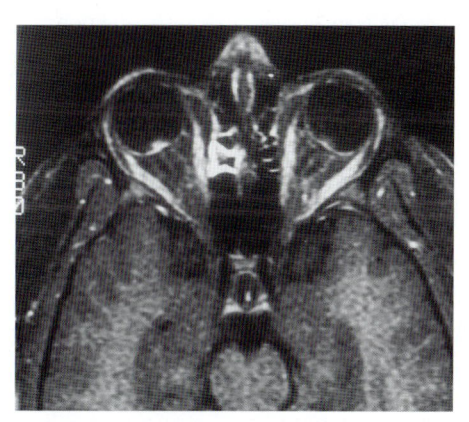

Fig. 2.**41** Increased intracranial pressure with papilledema. Axial postcontrast fat-suppression T1W MR scan. The optic disks are elevated, protruding into the vitreous, and show increased contrast enhancement.

■ Intraocular Calcifications

Deposition of calcium in ocular tissues is a complex process, the pathophysiology of which depends on the specific site of calcification. Intraocular calcifications may be metastatic (hypercalcemic states) or dystrophic, and arise in association with diverse degenerative ocular conditions (neoplasia, inflammation, congenital dysplasias, and senescent or traumatic degeneration).[26, 49] Calcifications in neoplasms may be a result of tumor necrosis. Such neoplasms include retinoblastoma and astrocytic hamartomas seen in tuberous sclerosis or neurofibromatosis type 1. Fifty percent of patients with tuberous sclerosis may develop retinal hamartomas, which often calcify. Ocular calcification or ossification may also occur in congenital vascular lesions such as Sturge–Weber syndrome, von Hippel–Lindau disease, and advanced stage of Coats disease.[14, 26] Chronic posttraumatic degeneration is probably the most common cause of dystrophic intraocular calcification (Fig. 2.**42**). Choroidal osteoma, episcleral choristoma, and optic disk drusen are other causes of intraocular calcification.[6, 12, 14, 26, 49] Retinopathy of prematurity also may cause delayed unilateral or bilateral ocular calcification.[14, 49] Scleral calcification may be seen in the elderly at or anterior to

Table 2.3 Causes and sites of calcium deposition in intraocular tissue and optic nerve

Site of Calcification	Description	Causes
Cornea	Basement membrane of corneal epithelium, Bowman's membrane; anterior stromal lamellae	Chronic iridocyclitis
Sclera	Focal, near insertion of rectus muscles	Idiopathic sclerochoroidal calcification Hypercalcemia* Rheumatoid arthritis* Microphthalmia with cyst* Metastatic calcification* Linear sebaceous nevus syndrome
Lens	Focal or diffuse, in the subcapsular or equatorial region (especially in hypermature cataracts)	Any condition that causes hypermature cataract
Ciliary body	Focal	Trauma Medulloepithelioma (teratoid)* Myopia
Choroid/RPE	Focal or diffuse (from RPE metaplasia or choroid osteoma)	Trauma Uveitis, Toxocara granuloma* Sturge–Weber syndrome* Choroidal osteoma*
Retina	Focal, scattered or diffuse	Retinoblastoma Drusen Phthisis bulbi Subretinal membrane Periretinal membrane PHPV* ROP* Coats disease* Astrocytoma* CMV retinitis* Tuberous sclerosis* von Hippel–Lindau disease* Chronic organized retinal detachment Medulloepithelioma*
Optic nerve	Focal, near the surface of the optic nerve	Drusen Astrocytoma* Medulloepithelioma* Optic nerve sheath dural idiopathic calcification* • optic nerve sheath meningeoma • AVM involving optic nerve sheath • idiopathic dural calcification of optic nerve sheath

Modified from Yan X, Edward DP, Mafee MF. Ocular calcification, radiologic-pathologic correlation and literature review. Int J Neuroradiol 1998; 4: 81–96.
* Uncommon causes.
RPE = retinal pigment epithelium.
PHPV = persistent hyperplastic primary vitreous.
ROP = retinopathy of prematurity.
CMV = cytomegalovirus.
AVM = arteriovenous malformation

Table 2.4 Common ocular disorders of children

- Retinoblastoma—most common malignant ocular cancer in children
- Persistent hyperplastic primary vitreous (PHPV)
- Retinopathy of prematurity (ROP)
- Congenital cataract
- Coats disease
- Microphthalmia with or without orbital cyst
- Coloboma of the optic disk and choroid
- Ocular trauma
- Ocular inflammatory, including granulomatous conditions (sarcoidosis, tuberculosis)
- Toxocara larval granulomatosis

the sites of insertions of the horizontal extraocular muscles (Fig. 2.43).[49] Calcification may be present at the trochlea (Fig. 2.43d). Ocular calcification may be seen in patients with hyperparathyroidism or hypoparathyroidism (Fig. 2.44). At times ocular calcification may be idiopathic (Fig. 2.45). Phthisis bulbi refers to calcification or ossification within a shrunken or atrophic globe (Fig. 2.42). Phthisis bulbi may be the result of any ocular insult with subsequent degeneration. It is most commonly a result of trauma or infection.[5, 14, 49] Table 2.3 lists the most frequent causes of intraocular calcifications.

Leukokoria

Leukokoria is a white, pink-white, or yellow-white pupillary reflex (cat's eye). The major diagnostic considerations in patients with leukokoria are retinoblastoma (Rb), persistent hyperplastic primary vitreous (PHPV), retinopathy of prematurity (ROP), congenital cataract, Coats disease, toxocariasis, retinal astrocytoma (tuberous sclerosis), medulloepithelioma, total retinal detachment, coloboma of the choroid or optic disk, uveitis, retinal storage disease, vitreous hemorrhage and a variety of other nonspecific diseases.[5, 12, 14, 16, 25] Common ocular disorders in children are listed in Table 2.4.

Leukokoria is the most common presenting sign of retinoblastoma,[50] the highly malignant primary retinal cancer. The

Pathology   159

identification of the cause of the leukokoria is critical to ensure prompt recognition and appropriate treatment, and diagnostic accuracy is particularly important because retinoblastoma is one of the few human cancers in which definitive treatment is carried out without a confirmed histopathological diagnosis.[12]

■ Retinoblastoma

Retinoblastoma (Rb) is the most common intraocular tumor of childhood.[50] It is a highly malignant, primary retinal tumor that arises from neuroectodermal cells (nuclear layer of the retina) that are destined to become retinal photoreceptors.[51,54] To ensure appropriate therapy, retinoblastoma must be differentiated from a host of ocular lesions that simulate it (Table 2.5).[4] This diagnosis must be established rapidly to permit maximum ocular sal-

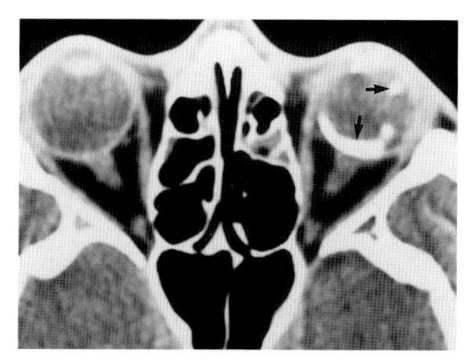

Fig. 2.42 Phthisis bulbi. CT scan shows a slightly smaller left globe, associated with increased density of the vitreous, and extensive dystrophic calcifications (arrows). This represents a nonfunctioning disorganized globe, the so-called phthisis bulbi.

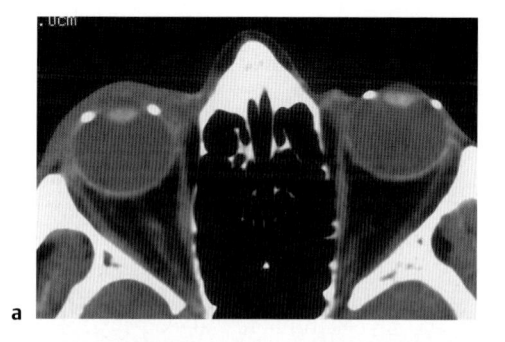

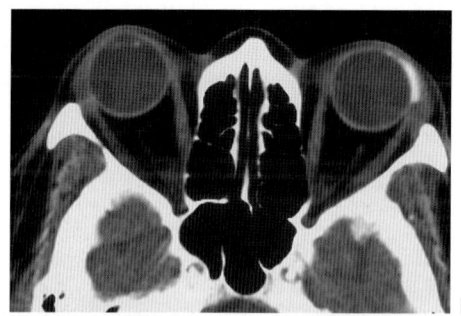

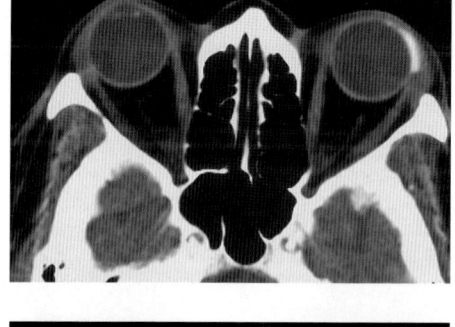

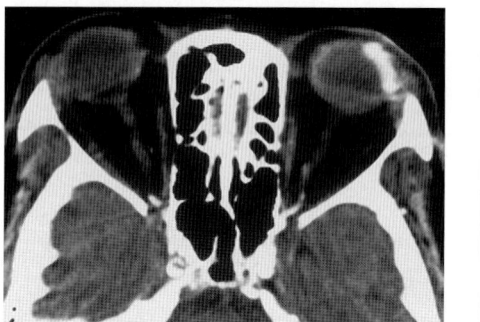

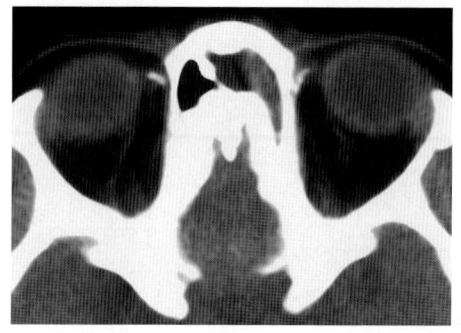

Fig. 2.43 Ocular calcification.
a Axial CT scan in an 85-year-old woman shows dense senile calcifications of the sclera at the sites of insertion of horizontal rectus muscles of both eyes.
b Axial CT scan in a 70-year-old woman shows dense calcification of the sclera along the arch of contact of the left lateral rectus muscle. Note also calcification of the right ciliary body. The patient had cataract surgery on both eyes.
c Axial CT scan shows marked calcification adjacent to the left eye. This may be idiopathic, however, possibility of an episcleral osteoma may also be considered.
d Axial CT scan shows calcification of the trochlea and part of the reflected portion of the superior oblique tendon of both orbits.

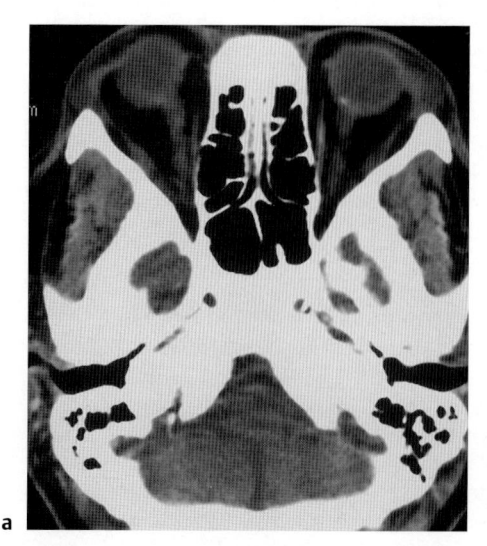

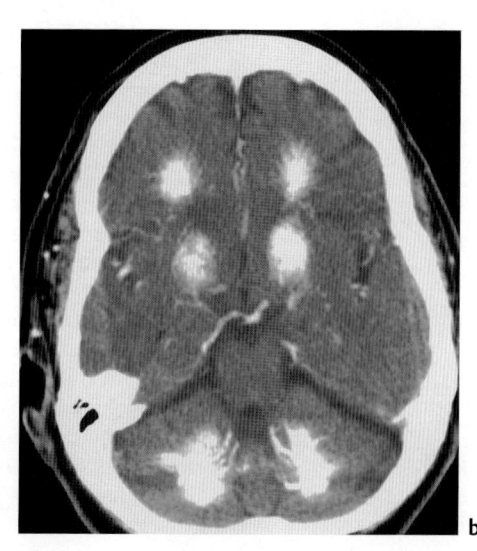

Fig. 2.44 Hypoparathyroidism and ocular calcification.
a Axial CT scan shows a small calcification involving the posterior aspect of the left globe.
b Axial CT scan shows marked calcification of the cerebellar dentate nuclei and supratentorial basal ganglia.

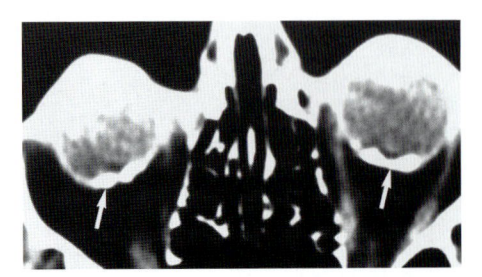

Fig. 2.**45** Idiopathic ocular calcification. CT scan shows bilateral intraocular calcifications (arrows). The patient had carcinoma of the prostate. The initial clinical diagnosis was ocular metastatic calcified deposits. Follow-up study showed no evidence for metastases.

Table 2.**5** Intraocular mass and masslike lesions simulating retinoblastoma

- Persistent hyperplastic primary vitreous (PHPV)
- Retinopathy of prematurity (ROP)
- Congenital cataract
- Coats disease
- Toxocariasis
- Medulloepithelioma
- Retinal astrocytoma
- Combined hamartoma of retinal pigment epithelium and retina
- Choroidal osteoma
- Incontinentia pigmenti
- Juvenile xanthogranuloma
- Mesoectodermal leiomyoma
- Papillitis
- Optic nerve head drusen
- Retinal gliosis
- Myelinated nerve fibers
- Chorioretinal coloboma
- Optic disk coloboma (morning glory disk)
- Walker–Warburg syndrome
- von Hippel–Lindau retinal angiomatosis
- Choroidal hemangioma
- Subretinal neovascular membrane
- Vitreous opacities
- Uveitis
- Vitreous hemorrhage
- Endophthalmitis
- Organized vitreous
- Retinal detachments
- X-linked retinoschisis
- Retinal dysplasia
- Retinal storage disease
- Norrie disease
- Developmental retinal cyst
- Falciform fold
- Familial exudative vitreoretinopathy
- Trauma
- Myopia
- Stickler's syndrome
- Congenital glaucoma
- Myiasis

Modified from Kaufman LM, Mafee MF, Song CD. Retinoblastoma and simulating lesions: role of CT, MR imaging and use of Gd-DTPA contrast enhancement. Radiol Clin North Am 1998; 36: 1101–1117.

vage and to minimize tumor-associated mortality.[12,55] When the disease extends beyond the eye, mortality approaches close to 100%.[55] With earlier diagnosis, the five-year survival rate with the tumors limited to the globe is greater than 90%.[12,56] Useful vision in the treated eye is attained in 90% of group I patients, and overall in about 75% of eyes that are not enucleated.[56]

Virchow was the first to postulate that retinoblastoma was of glial origin.[12] Bailey and Cushing divided retinoblastomas into two types: medulloblastoma and neuroepithelioma.[12] It is now well known that retinoblastoma is derived from primitive embryonal retinal cells (either photoreceptor or neuronal retinal cells).[57] This tumor can be undifferentiated or well-differentiated.[51,58] The tumor comprises small round or ovoid cells with scant cytoplasm and relatively large nuclei (blue cells).

The occurrence of a second cancer arising at or outside the treatment radiation field was pointed out by Jensen and Miller[59] and Abramson et al.[60] The worldwide incidence of retinoblastoma has been reported to be 1 in 18 000 to 30 000 live births.[61] Although the tumor is congenital in origin, it usually is not recognized at birth.[12,62] However, ocular involvement and metastasis may be present at birth.[12,14,62] In the United States the average age of the child at diagnosis is 13 months.[63] In other countries, the disease is often not detected until the fourth year of life, when it is usually far advanced.[64] Over 90% of all diagnoses are made in children younger than 5 years of age.[65] Retinoblastoma results when an individual retinal cell has an inactivation or loss of both alleles of the *Rb1* gene on chromosome.13 q14.[66–70] Retinoblastoma occurs in two distinct patterns: (1) a nonfamilial sporadic form; and (2) a familial, hereditary form that appears at the clinical level to be autosomal dominant.[12] In both forms, the biology of retinoblastoma tumor is identical. All of the patients with nonfamilial retinoblastoma have unilateral solitary tumors. With familial retinoblastoma, 85% of the cases are bilateral and 15% unilateral.[4] Overall, approximately one-third of patients with retinoblastoma have bilateral disease.[4,62,65]

The association between retinoblastoma and deletion of the q14 band of chromosome 13 (13q14) has been convincingly documented.[68–75] Esterase D, an electrophoretically polymorphic human enzyme, has also been mapped to chromosomal band 13q14.[72] In several families with hereditary retinoblastoma without apparent chromosomal deletion, the gene for retinoblastoma has been shown to be closely linked to that for esterase D and assigned to chromosome band 13q14.[72,73] Patients with familial retinoblastoma are highly susceptible to development of other nonocular cancers, usually osteogenic sarcoma as well as other neoplasms at the site of external beam radiation (see Fig. 2.**59**).[12,14,60] Second neoplasms may also arise outside the field of radiation.[14]

Trilateral retinoblastoma. The occurrence of ectopic retinoblastoma in the pineal body or in a parasellar region—"trilateral retinoblastoma"—stemmed from reports of Jakobiec et al.[76] and Bader et al.[77,78] The association of retinoblastoma–pinealoblastoma (trilateral retinoblastoma) suggests that these tumors may be related (see Fig. 2.**55**).[79] In addition to their sharing a common neuroectodermal origin, it is well known that in lower vertebrates the pineal gland has photoreceptor functions (similar to those seen in their retinas) and endocrine functions.[79] It is postulated that, because of their similar origin, the same mutations may be cancerogenic for both retinoblasts and pinealoblasts. The failure of pineoblastomas to develop in all patients with heritable retinoblastoma may be due to a smaller cell population in the pineal gland or to other unrecognized factors.[80]

Tetralateral retinoblastoma. Trilateral retinoblastoma describes the syndrome of bilateral retinoblastoma with a solitary midline intracranial tumor in the pineal gland, suprasellar region, or parasellar region.[76,77] El-Nagger et al.[81] reported an 11-month-old infant with bilateral Rbs and two distinct partially calcified intracranial tumors: a large mass in the area of the pineal gland and a second tumor in the suprasellar region. The pineal mass biopsy was compatible with a neuroblastic tumor

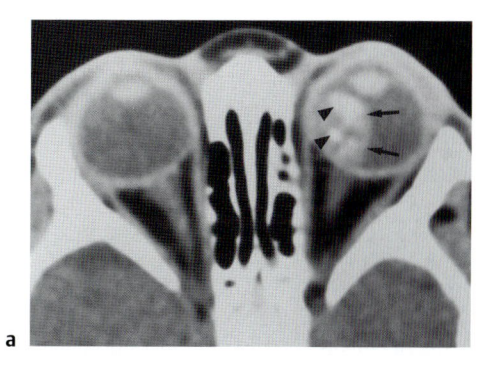

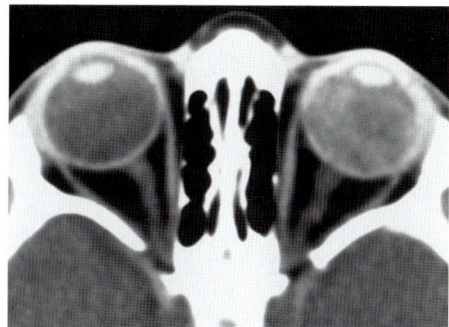

Fig. 2.46 Retinoblastoma.
a CT scan shows a retinoblastoma with multiple calcifications of varied sizes (arrows).
b CT scan shows a noncalcified retinoblastoma.

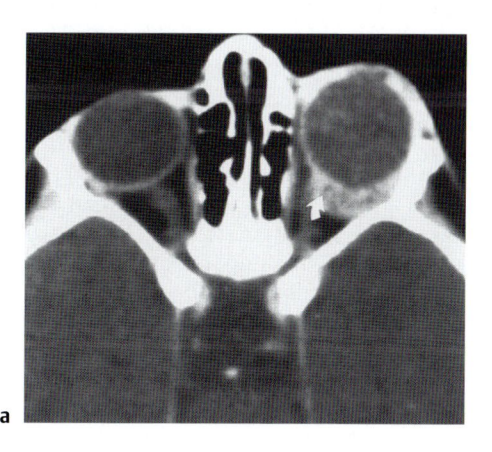

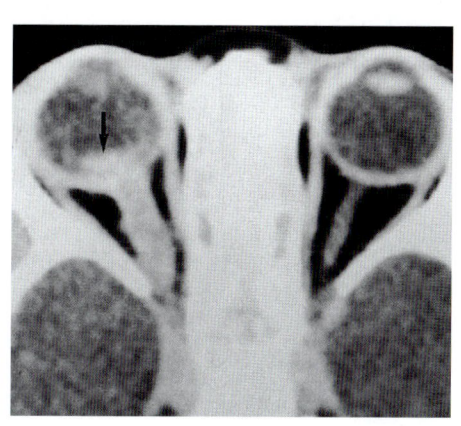

Fig. 2.47a Retinoblastoma with extension into Tenon's space. Postcontrast CT scan shows the extension of a retinoblastoma into Tenon's space (arrow). The left globe is diffusely involved, but shows no significant enhancement. The enlarged left globe is probably due to secondary glaucoma.
b Retinoblastoma with extension along the optic nerve. Postcontrast CT scan shows retinoblastoma (black arrow). Note marked involvement of the optic nerve.

(pinealoblastoma). The authors coined the term "tetralateral retinoblastoma" for their case having two distinct midline intracranial neuroblastic tumors associated with bilateral retinoblastomas.

Clinical Diagnosis

Retinoblastoma accounts for about 1% of all deaths from childhood cancer in the United States.[82] The diagnosis of retinoblastoma usually can be made by an ophthalmoscopic examination. However, the detection and clinical differentiation of retinoblastoma from a host of benign simulating lesions may be difficult.[12, 14, 62, 82–86] The most common sign associated with retinoblastoma is leukokoria, which is present in 60% of patients.[4, 12, 65] Strabismus (deviation of the eye) is the second most common sign. Pain caused by secondary glaucoma, often with heterochromia (differently colored irides), is the next most common symptom and sign, which leads to ophthalmological evaluation. The ophthalmological recognition of retinoblastoma is quite reliable. Small lesions are seen as gray-white intraretinal foci. Other characteristic ophthalmoscopic findings include tumor calcification and vitreous seeding. As tumors grow in size, they often assume a convex configuration and produce three forms of growth patterns.

1. In the endophytic retinoblastoma, the tumor projects anteriorly, breaks through the internal limiting membrane of the retina, and grows into the vitreous.
2. In the exophytic retinoblastoma, the tumor arises intraretinally and subsequently grows into the subretinal space, causing elevation of the retina;[4, 12, 62] with continued tumor growth, there is an associated exudation and rarely a subretinal hemorrhage, which progressively cause retinal detachment. Ophthalmoscopically the exophytic tumors can simulate a traumatic retinal detachment.
3. In the diffuse retinoblastoma, the tumor grows along the retina, appearing as a placoid mass. This diffuse form represents a perplexing diagnostic difficulty because of its atypical ophthalmoscopic feature (which simulates inflammatory or hemorrhagic conditions), its characteristic lack of calcification, and its occurrence usually outside of the typical age group.[12, 62]

Diagnostic Imaging

Ultrasonography, CT, and MRI are the most useful imaging techniques in the evaluation of Rb and simulating lesions. The tumor and calcification can be diagnosed by ultrasonography; however, the accuracy of ultrasonography for this condition is only 80%.[14] Diagnosis of tumor extension to the medial and lateral aspects of the orbit and extraocular extension are particularly limited with ultrasound.

High-resolution, thin-section (1.5 mm) CT can detect tumor and calcification within it with a high degree of accuracy.[4, 12, 62, 86] More than 90% of retinoblastomas show evidence of calcification on CT.[86] Calcifications may be small and single, large and single, multiple and punctate, or diffuse (Fig. 2.**46a**), or may be a few fine, speckled foci.[62] At times no calcifications may be present (Fig. 2.**46b**). The DNA released from necrotic cells in retinoblastoma has a propensity to form a DNA retinoblastoma–calcium complex. It is the frequent presence of this calcified complex that allows the intraocular tumor to be identified by funduscopic, ultrasonic, and CT imaging.[12, 14, 62, 86–88] In the extraocular component of retinoblastoma, calcification is rarely present (Fig. 2.**47a**).[62] The presence of intraocular calcification in children under 3 years of age (98% of cases present prior to age 6 months) is highly suggestive of retinoblastoma because none of the simulating lesions, except patients with CMV endophthalmitis (Fig. 2.**35b**), and patients with microphthalmia and colobo-

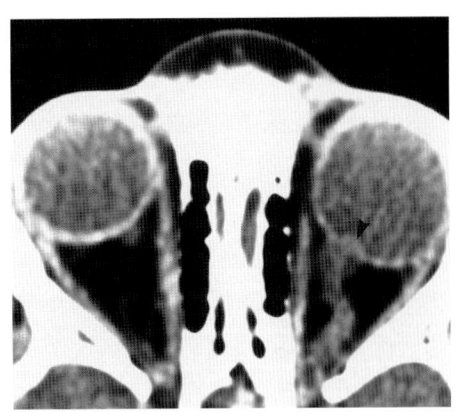

Fig. 2.**48** Myelinated nerve fiber. Axial CT scan shows an ill-defined lesion with increased density at the left optic nerve disk (arrow).

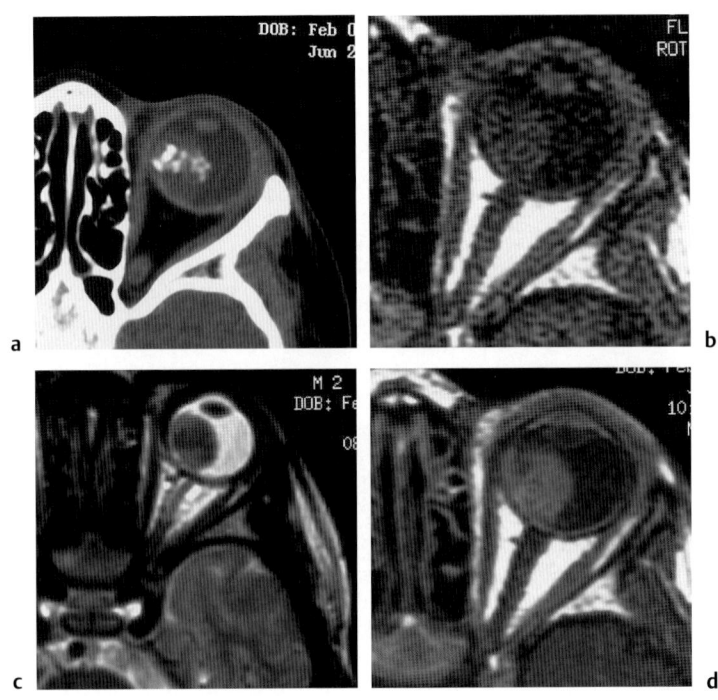

Fig. 2.**49** Retinoblastoma.
a CT scan shows a partially calcified retinoblastoma, involving the left eye.
b Axial T1W MR scan. The retinoblastoma appears slightly hyperintense to remaining normal vitreous.
c Axial T2W MR scan. The tumor appears markedly hypointense.
d Axial enhanced fat-suppression T1W MR scan. Note tumor enhancement as well as enhancement of the anterior segment of the eye.

matous cyst, contain calcification (see Fig. 2.**16**).[12,62] Retinoblastoma in the microphthalmic eye is extremely rare. In children over 3 years of age, some of the simulating lesions, including retinal astrocytoma, retinopathy of prematurity (ROP), toxocariasis, and optic nerve-head drusen can produce calcification.[12,14,62] The diffuse infiltrating form of retinoblastoma is rare and may have no calcification (see Fig. 2.**53**).[25,72] Extraocular extension of retinoblastoma and intracranial subarachnoid extension can be detected particularly on enhanced CT scans (Fig. 2.**47b**).

A retinal astrocytoma (astrocytic hamartoma) may initially appear like a retinoblastoma,[12,14,63] and the retinal astrocytoma may be present before any of the neurological or dermatological manifestations of tuberous sclerosis appear (see Fig. 2.**78**).[62] The CT appearance of myelinated nerve fibers may also be similar to noncalcified retinoblastoma (Fig. 2.**48**).[62]

MRI has been used to evaluate retinoblastoma and other simulating lesions.[4,12,14,62,82,85,89–91] In the diagnosis of retinoblastoma, MRI is not as specific as CT (Fig. 2.**46**) because of its lack of sensitivity in detecting calcification. However, the MRI appearance of retinoblastoma may be specific enough to differentiate retinoblastoma from simulating lesions (Figs. 2.**49**–2.**53**).[91] Retinoblastomas appear slightly or moderately hyperintense in relation to normal vitreous on T1-weighted (Fig. 2.**49b**) and PW images. On T2-weighted images, they appear as areas of markedly (Fig. 2.**49c**) to moderately low signal intensity in relation to the signal intensity of the vitreous. Rbs appear isointense to white matter on MR pulse sequences. Tumors elevated 2–3 mm in height may not be definitely identified on MRI,[62,91] and lesions less than 2 mm in height are not confidently recognized by present MRI technology. Calcifications on MRI may be seen as varied degrees of hypointensity in all pulse sequences including gradient-echo sequence (Fig. 2.**49b**). In contrast to CT scanning, which is highly specific for calcification (Fig. 2.**49a**), MRI may be nonspecific. In many cases a calcification may not be recognized on MRI, and thus in the diagnosis of retinoblastoma, CT is more specific because of its superior sensitivity for detecting calcifications. Calcifications as small as 2 mm can be reliably detected by CT.[91] MRI, however, has superior contrast resolution to CT, and MRI provides more information for differentiation of leukokoric eyes.[4,91] The use of paramagnetic gadolinium contrast material has improved the sensitivity of MRI. Retinoblastomas show moderate to marked enhancement on postcontrast T1-weighted MR scans (Figs. 2.**49**–2.**54**). In some of the cases, abnormal enhancement of the anterior chamber may be recognized on enhanced T1-weighted MR scans (Fig. 2.**54c**). This is nonspecific and can be seen in other ocular pathology such as PHPV.

Of the various imaging modalities, MR imaging has become the most useful in evaluating the challenging retinoblastoma patient.[4,12] As stated, CT is valuable to demonstrate calcification, but both ultrasound and CT are of lesser value in showing local

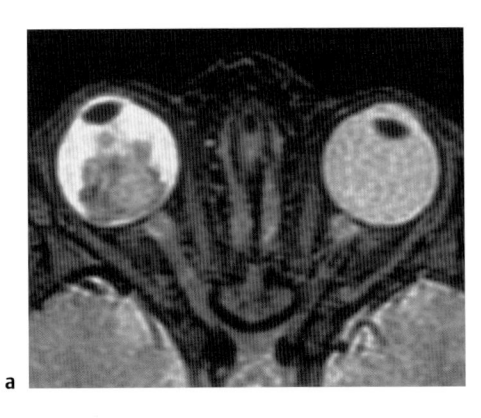

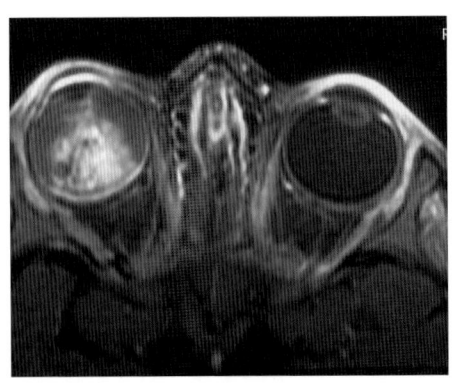

Fig. 2.**50** Retinoblastoma in an 11-year-old boy. **a** Axial T2W and **b** postcontrast fat-suppression T1W MR scans, showing a large retinoblastoma, involving the right eye. Note enhancement of the anterior segment of the involved right eye, which is related to impairment of the ocular blood barrier. The enlargement of the right eye is due to glaucoma, secondary to massive intraocular tumor.

Pathology 163

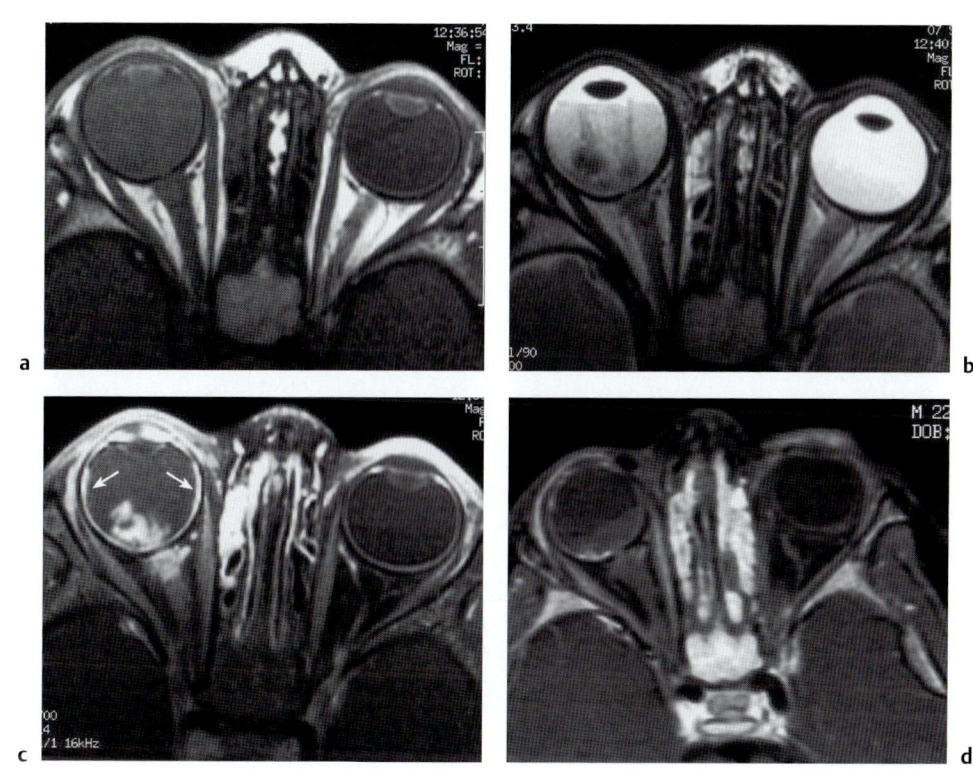

Fig. 2.**51** Retinoblastoma with optic nerve involvement. **a** Axial unenhanced T1W, **b** axial T2W, and **c** axial enhanced fat-suppression T1W MR images, showing a retinoblastoma of the right eye associated with extension into the right optic nerve. Note increased thickening and increased enhancement of the entire right retina (arrows), which may be due to tumor infiltration or reactive gliosis. Note also enhancement of the anterior segment of the right eye due to loss of ocular blood barrier. **d** Axial enhanced fat-suppression T1W MR scan following a full course of chemotherapy. There is reduction in tumor size. Note subretinal exudate. The right optic nerve remains thickened with abnormal contrast enhancement. The enucleated eye showed no tumor within the eye, but there was active tumor within a small portion of the resected optic nerve. Several months later, the patient developed diffuse subarachnoid metastasis.

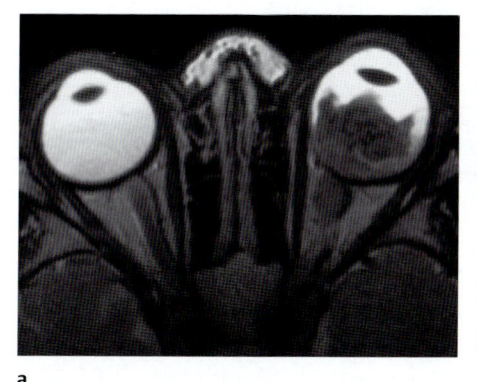

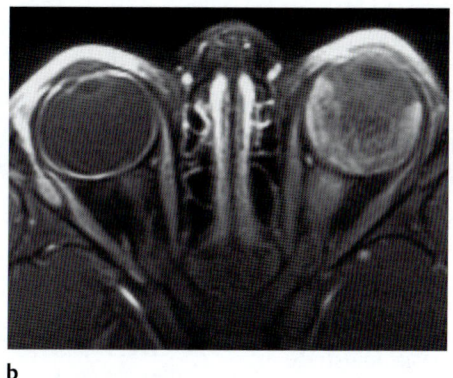

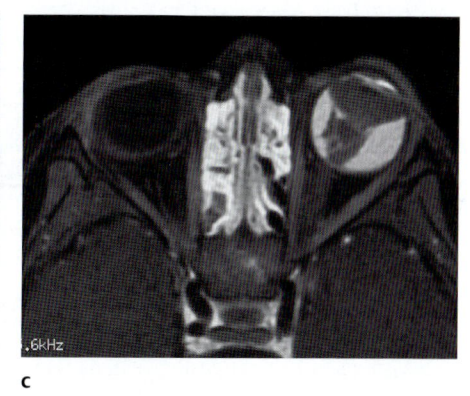

Fig. 2.52 Retinoblastoma with optic nerve involvement. **a** Axial T2W and **b** axial enhanced fat-suppression T1W MR images, showing a retinoblastoma of the left eye with extension into the left optic nerve. The tumor is very hypointense on the T2W MR image (**a**) and the retina is detached (**b**). **c** Axial enhanced fat-suppression T1W MR scan, taken following a full course of chemotherapy. The tumor has significantly reduced in size and the retina remains detached. The subretinal exudate appears hyperintense on this T1W MR image. The abnormal enhancement of the optic nerve, seen prechemotherapy in **b**, is no longer present. Following completion of chemotherapy, the left eye was enucleated. No vital tumor cell could be identified in the eye and resected optic nerve. The hypointensity seen between the detached leaves of the retina in **c** is due to scar and gliotic folded retina.

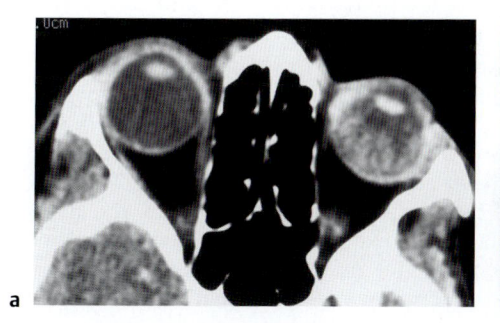

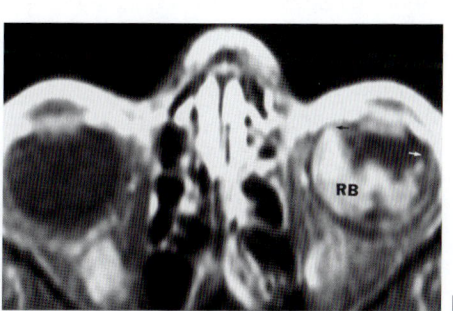

Fig. 2.53 Noncalcified diffuse retinoblastoma.
a CT scan shows a diffuse noncalcified retinoblastoma involving the left eye.
b Axial enhanced fat-suppression T1W MR scan, showing a markedly enhancing diffuse retinoblastoma (RB). The enhancement appears not to extend beyond the expected level of the ora serrata (arrows), an indication that the pathological process involves the retina, and hence retinoblastoma is the most likely diagnosis.

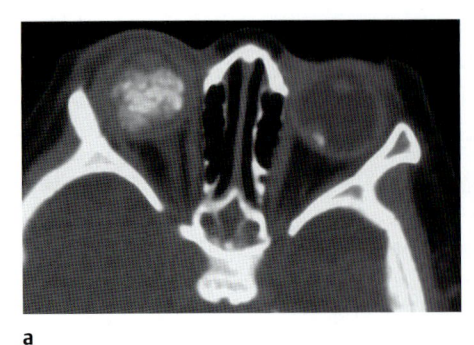

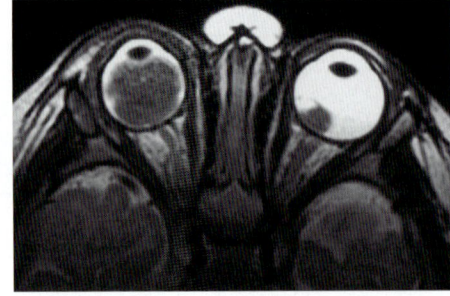

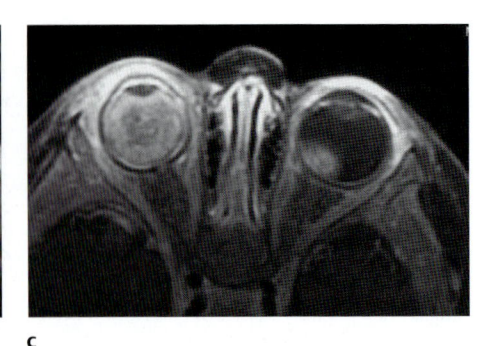

Fig. 2.54 Bilateral retinoblastoma. **a** Axial CT scan shows bilateral calcified retinoblastomas. **b** Axial T2W and **c** postcontrast fat-suppression axial T1W MR scans. The tumors appear hypointense on T2W MR imaging and demonstrate marked contrast enhancement. Note enhancement of the anterior segment of the right eye (**c**), related to impairment of the ocular blood barrier. The enhancement appears to be more along the peripheral portion of the tumor along with the detached retina.

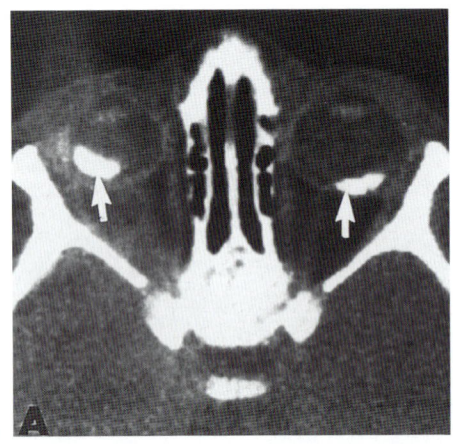

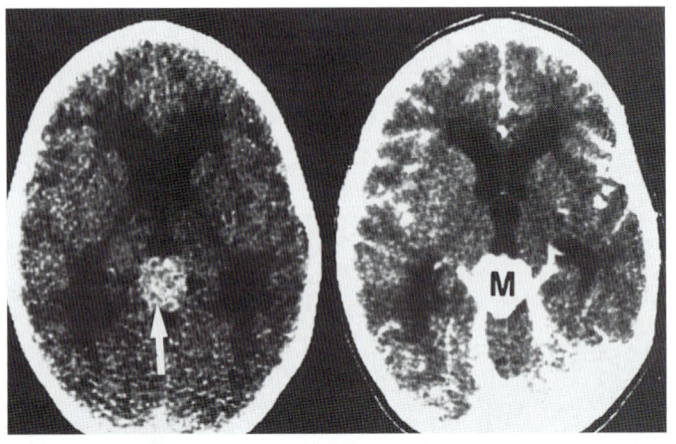

Fig. 2.55 Trilateral retinoblastoma. **a** Precontrast and **b** pre- and postcontrast axial CT scans show bilateral calcified retinoblastomas (short arrows) and partially calcified pineal mass (long arrow) with marked enhancement of the pineal mass (pineoblastoma) (M). From Mafee MF et al. Retinoblastoma and simulating lesions. Role of CT and MRI. Radiol Clin North Am 1987; 25: 667–692. With permission.

spread of retinoblastoma (Figs. 2.51, 2.52), or to distinguish retinoblastoma from stimulating lesions (Fig. 2.53). In the study of eyes with suspected retinoblastoma, our protocol includes plain axial CT (1.5–3 mm section thickness) scan of the eyes and MRI of the eyes and brain, because optic nerve (Figs. 2.51, 2.52) and intracranial involvement may be better evaluated by MRI than CT scanning. CT scanning and MRI are excellent for evaluating patients with trilateral or tetralateral retinoblastoma (Figs. 2.55, 2.56), recurrent retinoblastoma (Fig. 2.57) and metastasis from retinoblastoma (Fig. 2.58). Patients with familial retinoblastoma are highly susceptible to development of other nonocular cancers, usually osteogenic sarcoma as well as other neoplasms at the site of external beam radiation (Fig. 2.59). Second neoplasms may also arise outside the field of radiation. [4, 12] In some of our patients with bilateral retinoblastoma, following treatment, we have noticed a prominent size of the enhanced pineal gland on postcontrast T1-weighted MR scans. This appearance of the pineal gland remained unchanged on follow-up (2 years) MR studies.

■ Intraocular Mass and Masslike Lesions Simulating Retinoblastoma

There are other pediatric intraocular disorders that may clinically simulate retinoblastoma by presenting as a retinal or subretinal mass or masslike lesions, retinal detachment, or a vitreous opacity.[4, 12] Retinal detachments may undergo organization and contracture so as to resemble an intraocular mass.

■ Persistent Hyperplastic Primary Vitreous

Persistent hyperplastic primary vitreous (PHPV) needs to be differentiated from retinoblastoma. This condition is clinically characterized by a unilateral leukokoria in a microphthalmic eye of a full-term baby. At times, PHPV may be bilateral. PHPV is caused by the failure of the embryonic hyaloid vascular system to regress normally. The basic lesion is caused by a persistence of various portions of the primary vitreous and tunica vasculosa lentis with hyperplasia and extensive proliferation of the associated embryonic connective tissue. The nosology of PHPV is extremely complex.[91–94] The ocular malformation can reflect

Pathology 165

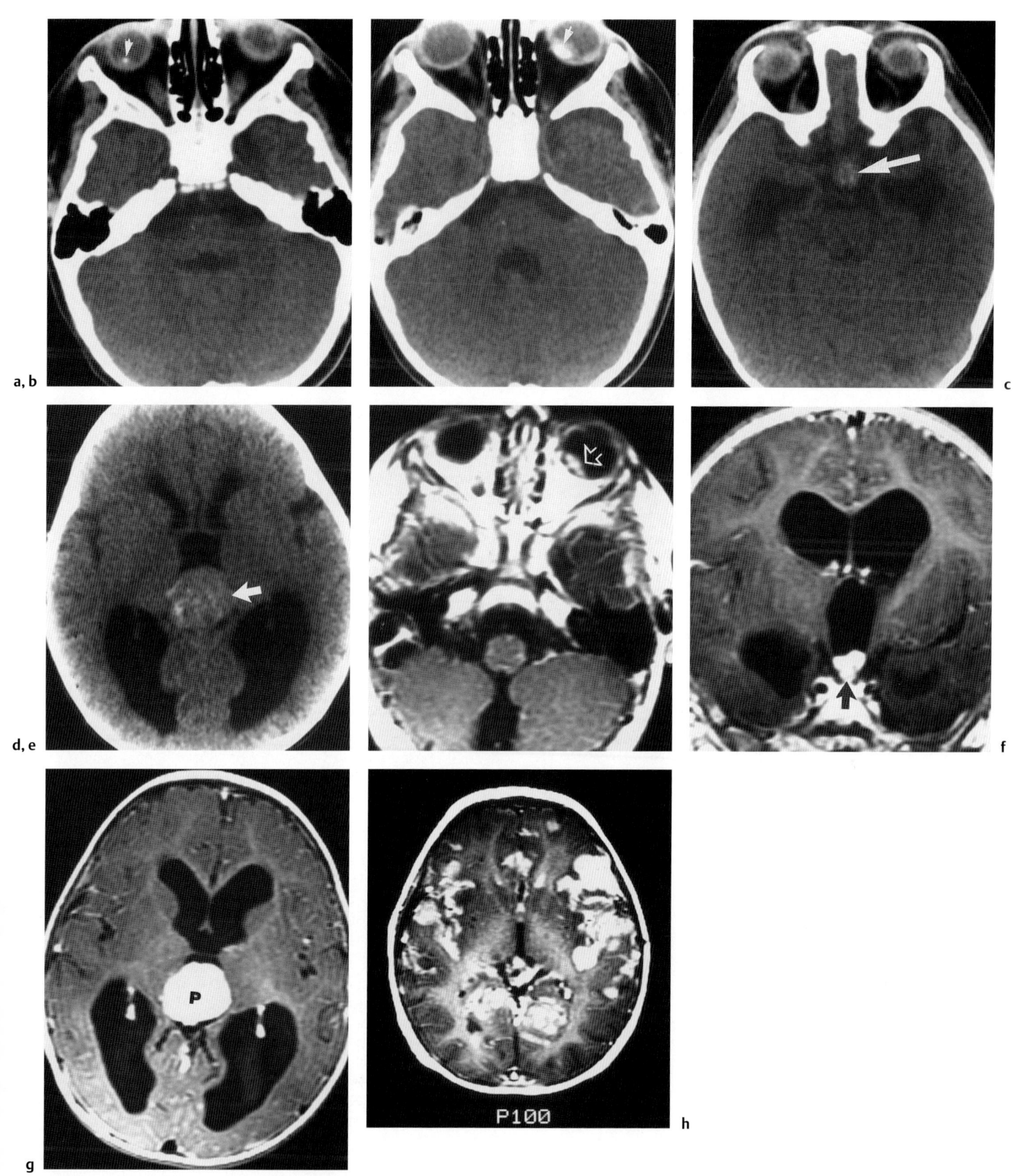

Fig. 2.**56** Tetralateral retinoblastoma. An 11-month-old-infant, presented with symptoms and signs of increased intracranial pressure. **a, b** Axial CT scans show bilateral partially calcified retinoblastoma (arrows). **c** Axial CT scan shows a calcified suprasellar mass (arrow). **d** Axial CT scan shows a large pineal tumor (arrow) with several small calcifications. Note marked hydrocephalus. **e** Axial enhanced T1W MR scan shows an enhancing retinoblastoma (arrow) of the left eye. **f** Coronal enhanced T1W MR scan shows a suprasellar enhancing mass (arrow) and marked hydrocephalus. **g** Axial enhanced T1W MR scan shows a large enhancing tumor of the pineal gland. Biopsy of the pineal tumor was consistent with primitive neuroectodermal (PNET) tumor. A few months later, this patient developed diffuse subarachnoid involvement of the entire neural axis (seen in **h**). **h** Axial enhanced T1W MR scan shows diffuse leptomeningeal enhancement due to subarachnoid spread of tumor.

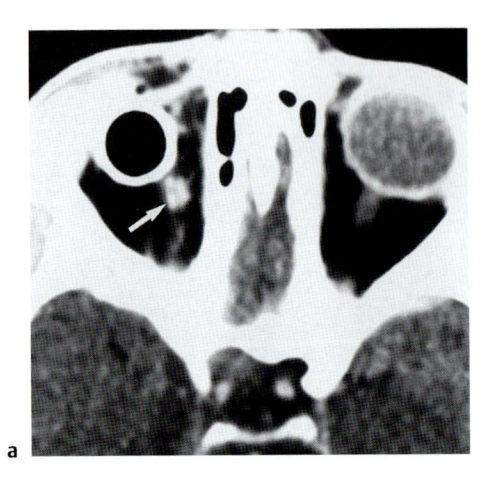

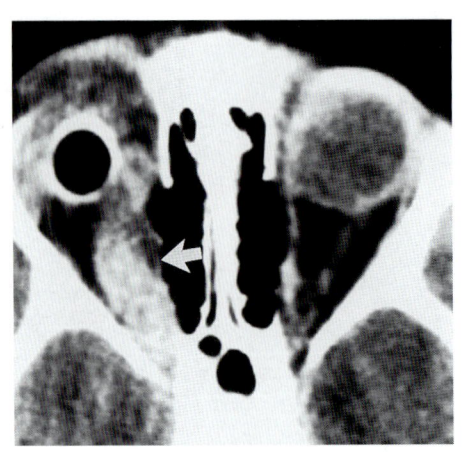

Fig. 2.57 Recurrent retinoblastoma.
a Axial enhanced CT scan following enucleation of the right eye, showing an orbital implant as well as an enhancing soft-tissue mass (arrow) posterior to the implant, which is suspicious for tumor recurrence. Had there been a baseline study available, it would have been easier to further characterize this enhancing soft-tissue lesion behind the implant.
b Axial enhanced CT scan, obtained a few months later, showing massive tumor recurrence (arrow) along the remaining part of the right optic nerve.

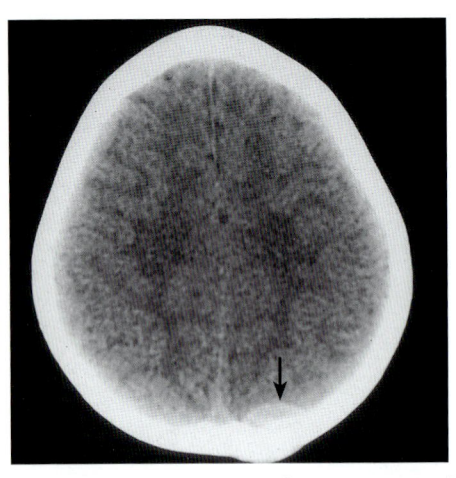

Fig. 2.58 Retinoblastoma with metastasis. Axial CT scan shows a metastatic deposit from retinoblastoma to the left occipital bone. Note involvement of the epidural space (arrow).

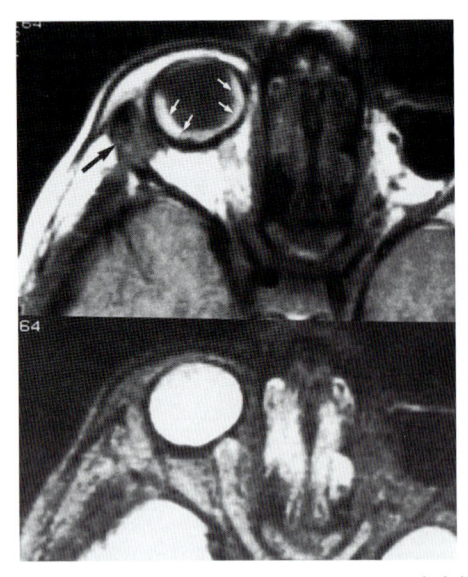

Fig. 2.59 Orbital sarcoma in a patient with bilateral retinoblastomas. Axial PW (top) and T2W (bottom) MR scans show chronic retinal detachment (arrows). There is complete regression of the retinoblastoma following radiation therapy. Note the false left eye and a mass involving the lateral aspect of the right orbit (arrow). There was destruction of bone on the CT scans. The mass is presumed to be an osteogenic sarcoma.

either an isolated congenital defect or a manifestation of more extensive ocular or systemic involvement.

The embryonic intraocular vascular system may be divided into two components: an anterior system in the region of the iris, and a posterior (retrolental) component within the vitreous. The anterior system is composed of the pupillary membrane, which is formed by small vascular buds that grow inwardly to vascularize the iris mesoderm anterior to the lens.[8] The posterior system includes the main hyaloid artery, the vasa hyaloidea propria, and the tunica vasculosa lentis.[8,16] The first vessels to undergo regression are the vasa hyaloidea propria, followed by the tunica vasculosa lentis, and eventually the main hyaloid artery.[8,16,94] During the first month of gestation, the space between the lens and the retina contains the primary vitreous. It consists of two parts: mesodermally derived tissue, including the hyaloid vessel and its branches, and a fibrillar meshwork that is of ectodermal origin.[95] In the second month of embryonic development, collagen fibers and a ground substance or gel component consisting of hyaluronic acid are produced. They form the secondary vitreous and begin to replace the vascular elements of the primary vitreous. By the 14th week, the secondary vitreous begins to fill the vitreous cavity.[16,95] By the fifth to the sixth month of development, the cavity of the eye is filled primarily with the secondary vitreous that represents the adult vitreous.[16] The primary vitreous is thus reduced to a small central space, Cloquet's canal, which runs in an S-shaped course between the optic nerve head and the posterior surface of the lens.[16,21] The Cloquet's canal cannot be visualized by CT or MRI in normal subjects.

Clinical Diagnosis

Diagnosis of PHPV is often made difficult by its extremely broad array of clinical manifestations, etiological heterogeneity, and frequently opaque ocular media.[92,94,96] Complete inspection of the interior of the eye may be precluded not only by cataract but also by vitreous hemorrhage or by opaque retrolental fibrovascular tissue. This condition usually manifests clinically as unilateral leukokoria in a microphthalmic eye. At birth, the lens is clear with a white to pinkish fibrovascular mass behind it; later the lens usually becomes swollen and cataractous.[97] In the natural course of untreated PHPV, the eye often develops glaucoma and eventually buphthalmos or phthisis, sometimes leading to loss of the globe.[97]

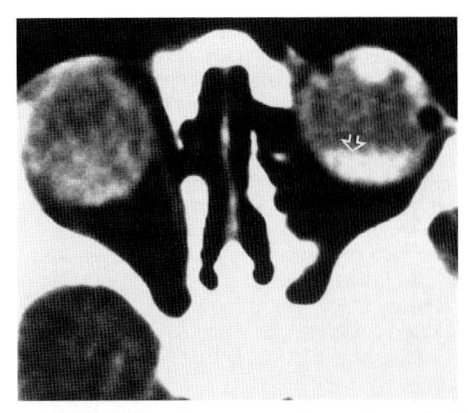

Fig. 2.**60** Bilateral PHPV. Axial unenhanced CT scan shows increased density of both globes. There is layered fluid (arrow), compatible with hemorrhage in the subretinal space or subhyaloid space. From Mafee MF et al. Persistent hyperplastic primary vitreous (PHPV): Role of CT and MRI. Radiol Clin North Am 1987; 25: 683–692. With permission.

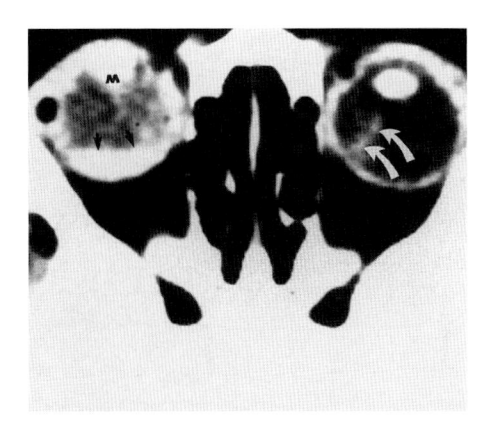

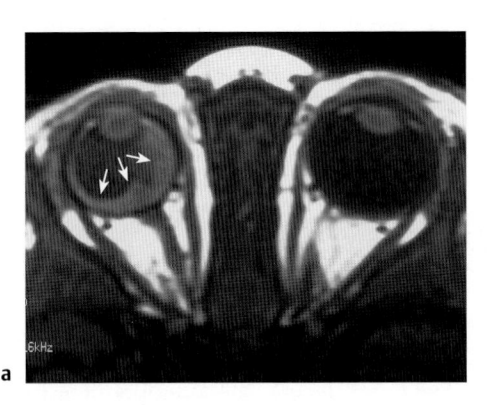

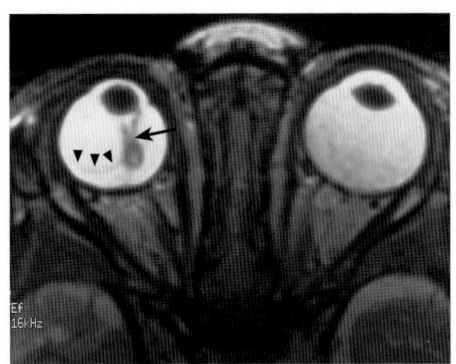

Fig. 2.**61** Bilateral PHPV. Axial unenhanced CT scan. There is increased density of the right globe with layered fluid (black arrows), compatible with hemorrhage in the subretinal space or subhyaloid space. Note increased soft-tissue mass (M) behind the right lens, related to remnant of primary vitreous. There is a tubular structure within the left eye (white arrows), compatible with remnant of primary vitreous along the hyaloid (Cloquet) canal or related to congenitally nonattached retina. From Mafee MF et al. Persistent hyperplastic primary vitreous (PHPV): Role of CT and MRI. Radiol Clin North Am 1987; 25: 683–692. With permission.

Fig. 2.**62** PHPV.
a Axial T1W MR scan shows microphthalmic right eye, slightly deformed right lens, and shallow anterior chamber as compared with normal left eye. The increased signal intensity is due to chronic hemorrhage in the subhyaloid space rather than the subretinal space, as the detached structure (arrows) (posterior hyaloid membrane) does not converge at the optic disk.
b Axial T2W MR scan shows hypointense tubular structure (arrow), related to remnant of primary vitreous and the detached posterior hyaloid membrane (arrowheads).

Diagnostic Imaging

CT Findings

The CT findings of PHPV were first reported by Mafee and Goldberg.[16,94] Maximum information was derived from the use of CT following intravenous contrast media and repeated scanning in the lateral decubitus position (Figs. 2.**60**, 2.**61**).[16]
The CT findings include the following:
1 Microphthalmia is usually detectable, although it may be minimal or absent, and other deformities in the globe configuration, which may have been undetectable by physical examination or ultrasonography.[94]
2 Calcification is absent within or around the globe.
3 Generalized increased density of the entire vitreous chamber may be visible (Figs. 2.**60**, 2.**61**), although minimally affected cases may show normal attenuation values in the vitreous chambers.
4 Enhancement of abnormal intravitreal tissue may be seen after intravenous administration of a contrast medium.
5 Tubular, cylindrical, triangular, or other discrete intravitreal densities suggest the persistence of fetal tissue in Cloquet's canal, or congenital nonattachment of the retina (Fig. 2.**61**).
6 Decubitus positioning may show a gravitational effect on a fluid level within the vitreous chamber, reflecting a serosanguineous fluid in either the subhyaloid space or the subretinal space.
7 The lens may be small and irregular and the anterior chamber may be shallow.

In more severe cases, the optic nerve on the involved side may be hypoplastic. At times, the process is mild and CT or MR scans may show no abnormal finding.[21] Occasionally the involved eye may be affected with axial myopia, and in such cases, the affected eye will not be microphthalmic.[21]

MR Findings

The MRI appearance of the different types of PHPV may be different. Early experience with MRI in patients with PHPV has revealed marked hyperintensity of the vitreous chamber on T1-weighted, PW, and T2-weighted images.[21] The MRI appearance of eyes with retinopathy of prematurity (ROP) may be identical to PHPV. The appearance of retinal detachment in PHPV has two forms: (1) retinal elevation into the vitreous from the optic nerve, resembling acquired forms of retinal detachment (Fig. 2.**61**), and (2) retinal elevation from a point in the wall of the eye that is eccentric to the optic nerve, suggesting a falciform fold or congenital nonattachment of the retina (Figs. 2.**61**–2.**63**).[92,94] Contrast-enhanced CT or MRI may demonstrate an enhanced retrolental mass, and there may be increased enhancement in the anterior segment of the involved eye (Fig. 2.**62**). PHPV is often associated with severe malformations of the optic nerve and retina.[94]

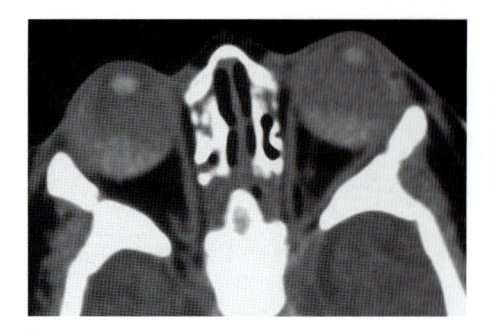

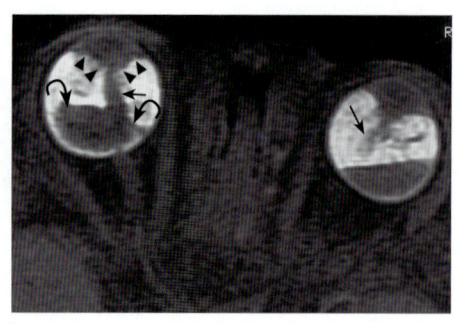

Fig. 2.63 Bilateral PHPV. **a** Axial unenhanced CT scan. There is increased density of both globes with layered fluid. Note shallow anterior chambers. **b** Axial unenhanced fat-suppression T1W MR scan, taken using a 3 T MR unit, showing layered subretinal acute hemorrhage (curved arrows) in both eyes. Note an intravitreal tubular structure (straight arrows) compatible with congenitally nonattached retina, or remnant of primary vitreous along the Cloquet (hyaloid) canal. The increased intensity of the globes is most likely related to chronic or subacute subretinal hemorrhage. The arrowheads are pointing at the detached sensory retina.

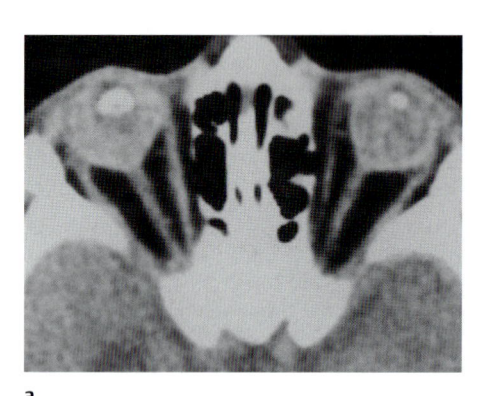

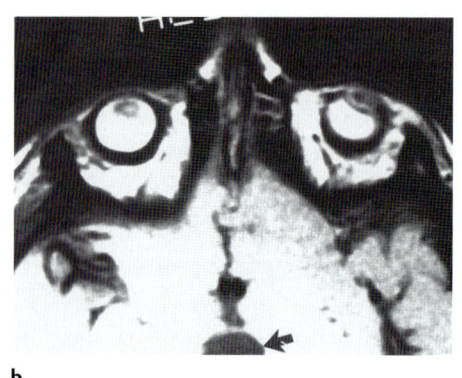

Fig. 2.64 Norrie disease.
a Axial CT scan shows bilateral microphthalmia with dense globes, most likely representing bilateral retinal detachment, due to underlying disease, which is retinal dysplasia. Note increased density as well as irregular outline of the lenses. The optic nerves are rather attenuated in appearance. In Norrie disease, the optic nerve may be very hypoplastic. From Mafee MF et al. Persistent hyperplastic primary vitreous (PHPV): Role of CT and MRI. Radiol Clin North Am 1987; 25: 683–692. With permission.
b Axial PW MR scan showing bilateral microphthalmia. Note the hyperintensity of the globes compared to CSF in the dilated anterior portion of the third ventricle (arrow).

■ Retinal Dysplasia

Retinal dysplasia includes a group of disorders such as Norrie disease and Walker–Warburg syndrome, in which abnormal proliferation and folding of the developing outer retina leads to congenital retinal detachment.[4] PHPV is manifested with more severe malformation in diseases such as Norrie disease and Warburg syndrome and in patients with retinal dysplasia (Fig. 2.63).

■ Norrie Disease

Norrie disease, or congenital progressive oculoacousticocerebral degeneration, is a rare X-linked recessive syndrome consisting of retinal malformation, deafness, and mental retardation or deterioration.[98-103] Warburg established that Norrie disease has an X-linked recessive pattern of inheritance, affects only males, and has ophthalmologically completely unaffected female carriers.[102] The affected males can exhibit ocular changes, including partial or complete retinal detachments; vitreoretinal hemorrhage, which can be present in the early neonatal period;[98] retrolental mass; cataract; glaucoma; optic nerve atrophy; choroidal hypercellularity; and phthisis bulbi. After varying periods of time these lead to bilateral blindness.[98]

The pathogenesis of Norrie disease is unknown. Histopathologically, in the early stage the condition is characterized by absence of retinal ganglion cells and the absence of normal nerve fiber layer structures in the retina.[104, 105]

The CT findings of Norrie disease were first reported by Mafee and Goldberg.[16, 21, 94] These include bilaterally dense vitreous chambers (Fig. 2.64a), retrolental mass, retinal detachment, microphthalmia,[21] optic nerve atrophy, shallow anterior chamber, and small, highly dense lens.[21] There was no evidence for intraocular or extraocular calcification, nor was there any evidence for gravitational layering of intravitreal fluid. The MRI findings of Norrie disease include bilateral microphthalmia with hyperintense vitreous, caused by chronic vitreous or subretinal hemorrhage (Figs. 2.64b); persistence of the primary vitreous may be present; the optic nerves may be hypoplastic; and there may be associated developmental anomalies of the brain.

■ Warburg Syndrome

Complex syndromes with congenital malformations of the central nervous system, microphthalmia, and congenital unilateral or bilateral retinal nonattachment have been described in a number of disorders such as Meckel syndrome, an autosomal recessive disorder with malformations of the central nervous system (encephalocele), cleft palate, polydactyly, cysts of the liver and polycystic kidneys, genital malformations, and microphthalmia.[106]

In 1971, Warburg[107] suggested that such patients might suffer from a nosologically distinct syndrome.[107] She described an autosomal recessive disorder consisting of profound mental retardation with death in infancy, hydrocephaly, microphthalmia, and congenital nonattachment of the retina.[107] Subsequent postmortem studies confirmed these clinical observations and noted the coexistence of lissencephaly in these patients.[108, 109]

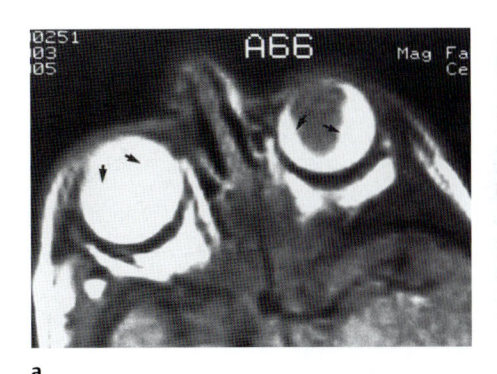

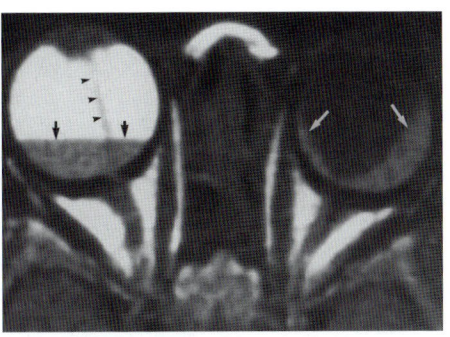

Fig. 2.**65** Warburg disease. **a** T1W axial MR scan showing bilateral chronic hemorrhagic retinal detachments (arrows). **b** Follow-up axial PW MR scan. The detached retina on the left side appears unchanged (white arrows). Note fluid–fluid level on the right side (black arrows), related to recent subretinal hemorrhage. Note the detached folded retina (arrowheads). A congenitally nonattached retina or a remnant of fetal hyaloid vascular system along the hyaloid (Cloquet) canal may have similar tubular appearance. Fig. 2.**65 b** From Mafee MF et al. Persistent hyperplastic primary vitreous (PHPV): Role of CT and MRI. Radiol Clin North Am 1987; 25: 683–692. With permission.

The syndrome was redescribed by Pagen et al.[110] and the mnemonic HARD±E was coined to point out the following characteristic features: hydrocephaly, agyria, and retinal dysplasia (detachment), with or without encephalocele.[110] The HARD±E, or Warburg, syndrome, is a congenital oculocerebral disorder, caused by a genetic defect that simultaneously affects ocular and cerebral embryogenesis and specifically involves the retina and the brain.[14,111] It is characterized by congenital bilateral leukokoria. The ophthalmic findings associated with this syndrome include microphthalmia and retinal dysplasia, associated with retinal detachment or congenitally nonattached retina.[14,110,112] Associated anomalies may include vitreous hemorrhage, a large intravitreal vessel, opaque retrolental tissue, persistent hyperplastic primary vitreous, and a hypoplastic optic disk.[111]

Microphthalmia and hydrocephaly seen in patients with Warburg syndrome may be seen in children with congenital toxoplasmosis, rubella syndrome, congenital syphilis, and herpesvirus and cytomegalovirus (CMV) infections. In toxoplasmosis, there may be characteristic chorioretinal scars and a positive serological test. The presence of significant serum antibody titers against rubella, CMV, herpesvirus, and syphilis should serve to distinguish Warburg syndrome from these simulating disease entities.[17]

The CT and MRI findings of the eyes of patients with Warburg syndrome include bilateral retinal detachment (Fig. 2.**65**), subretinal hemorrhage, vitreous hemorrhage, and gravitational intravitreal fluid (Fig. 2.**65**). Persistence of the primary vitreous also may be present.[12,14,16,21] The congenital nonattached retina or the totally detached retina exhibits a characteristic narrow funnel shape, or a triangular intravitreal mass adjacent to Cloquet's canal (Fig. 2.**65 b**).

■ Retinopathy of Prematurity or Retrolental Fibroplasia

In contrast to PHPV, retinopathy of prematurity (ROP), or retrolental fibroplasia or retinal fibroplasia, is seen in premature, low birth weight infants. ROP is usually bilateral and fairly symmetric. The essential feature of ROP appears to be prematurity. The smaller the infant, the greater the risk of developing this disease. ROP usually develops as a response to prolonged exposure to supplemental oxygen therapy. Eller et al.[113] noticed that 14 patients had an associated persistent hyaloid vascular system. A massive persistent hyaloid vascular system was found in seven of their patients.

Clinical Diagnosis

In ROP, proliferation of abnormal peripheral retinal vessels occurs with subsequent hemorrhage and cicatrization, which may organize and contract, leading to tractional retinal detachment in the advanced stages. The ophthalmoscopic findings of ROP have been divided into active, regressive, and cicatricial phases. The initial active phase is characterized by arteriolar narrowing caused by a spastic response of the vessels to hyperoxia.[114] Gradually, strands containing new vessels pass into the vitreous from the retina. There may be vitreous hemorrhage, which may be massive, and the retina may become partially or completely detached.[115]

Regressive phase. A characteristic of the disease is that during the early stage there is a tendency to spontaneous regression with disappearance of the neovascularization and even reattachment of the retina.[115] The detached retina, however, may not always become reattached. About 85–90% of cases show spontaneous regression.[115]

Cicatricial phase. Finally a dense membrane or a gray-white vascularized mass will be left as permanent evidence of the active phase. The lens always remains clear. The retina is detached, with associated retinal scars. The growth of the eye is often inhibited with microphthalmia as the final outcome.

Diagnostic Imaging

The early stage of ROP may have no specific CT and MRI findings except that the eyes may be microphthalmic. In the more advanced cases, the CT and MRI differential diagnosis between ROP (Fig. 2.**66**) and PHPV, retinoblastoma, endophthalmitis, or a number of pathological conditions wherein retinal detachment is a common feature may be difficult.[14,16,21,62,112,115] Calcification is rare in ROP. However, in the more advanced stage, calcification may be present (Fig. 2.**67**). Calcification in a microphthalmic eye is less in favor of retinoblastoma, although rarely retinoblastoma has been reported in microphthalmic eyes with and without ROP or PHPV.

■ Coats disease

In 1908 George Coats[116] described six cases of end-stage ocular disease with massive subretinal exudations, containing cholesterol clefts, with the following features: frequent occurrence in young boys; unilateral in presentation; congenital but nonfamilial; presence of retinal vascular anomalies (telangiectasis, aneurysms, arteriovascular shunts, hemorrhage, perivasculi-

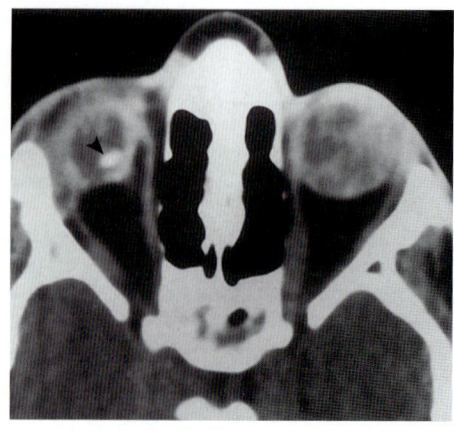

Fig. 2.**67** Advanced retinopathy of prematurity (ROP). Axial CT scan shows microphthalmic eyes and a dystrophic calcification (arrowhead). The increased density of the eyes is due to chronic retinal detachment and proliferative vitreoretinopathy and scar formation.

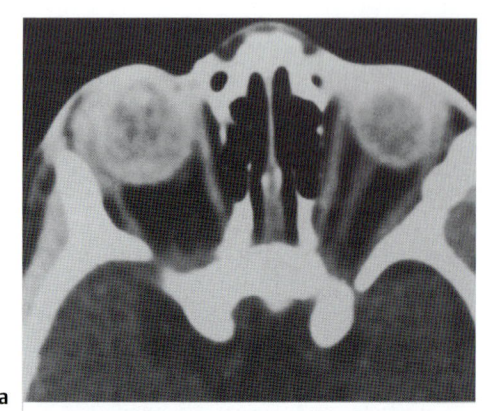

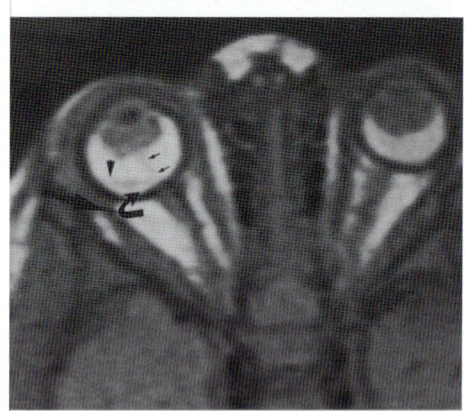

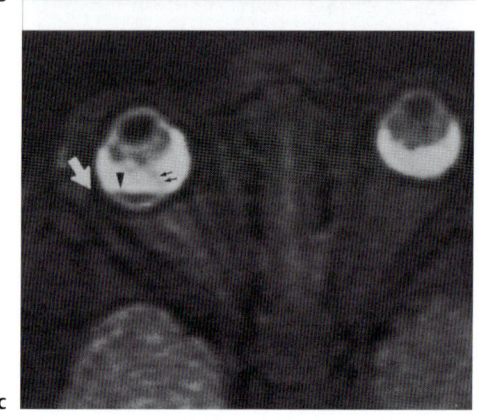

Fig. 2.**66** Retinopathy of prematurity (ROP). **a** CT scan, **b** PW MR scan and **c** T2W MR scan, showing bilateral microphthalmia. Note the retinal detachment (short arrows in **b** and **c**) and layered fluid (blood, arrowhead in **b** and **c**). The subretinal blood appears less hypointense on PW (**b**, curved arrow) than on T2W (**c**) MR images. The chronic subretinal hemorrhage or exudate appears as hyperintense as fat in the retrobulbar or peripheral fat (straight arrow in **b**) on the PW MR scan and more hypointense on the T2W MR scan (**c**).
The imaging findings in this case cannot be differentiated from a case of bilateral PHPV and retinal dysplasia syndromes such as Norrie disease and Warburg disease. The diagnosis should be made according to the appropriate clinical setting. From Mafee MF. The eye. In: Som PM, Curtin HD, eds. Head and Neck Imaging. St. Louis: Mosby; 2003: 441–527. With permission.

tis, vascular sheathing); exudation containing cholesterol; and intraretinal/subretinal infiltration by lipid-laden macrophages.[116] The disease that now bears his name, Coats disease (primary retinal telangiectasis), is a primary vascular anomaly of the retina characterized by idiopathic retinal telangiectatic and aneurysmal retinal vessels with progressive deposition of intraretinal and subretinal exudates that leads to massive exudative retinal detachment (exudative retinopathy).[6, 12, 116–123] The condition occurs more frequently in juvenile males than in females. However, the condition is also seen in adults, where it is almost always unilateral.[12, 116–118] The formation of retinal telangiectasia and the breakdown in the blood–retinal barrier with leakage of a lipoproteinaceous exudate at the telangiectasia are the essential underlying causes for the pathological changes that occur in Coats disease.[12, 119, 120] The vascular anomaly of Coats disease, although present at birth, usually does not cause symptoms until the retina detaches and central vision is lost.[121]

Clinical Diagnosis

Coats disease usually occurs in young boys, with the onset of symptoms in most patients occurring before the age of 20 years. Although the incidence peaks between 6 and 8 years,[120] cases have been reported ranging from 4 months to the seventh decade.[120] The modes of presentation include leukokoria, strabismus, failed school screening test, or painful glaucoma (11%)[123] secondary to neovascularization and angle closure.

Diagnostic Imaging

The ophthalmoscopic and biomicroscopic features of eyes with advanced Coats disease may closely resemble findings in eyes with exophytic retinoblastoma and leukokoria.[119, 122] In advanced Coats disease, a chronically detached retina with gliosis could simulate an intraocular mass.[119, 122] It is important to distinguish retinoblastoma from Coats disease. Many eyes with advanced Coats disease were enucleated because retinoblastoma could not be excluded.[119a, 123]

The CT and MRI findings in Coats disease vary with the stages of progression of the disease. At early stages, both techniques may yield little information. In later stages of the disease, retinal detachment accounts for all the pathological findings in CT and MRI. Sherman, McLean, and Merritt[121] reported two children with Coats disease. They concluded that CT could not differentiate between Coats disease and unilateral noncalcifying retinoblastoma. Haik et al. reported the CT findings in 14 patients with Coats disease, and total retinal detachment (Fig. 2.**68a**) was routinely seen in advanced Coats disease.[85] Calcification is not a feature of Coats disease; however, in advanced Coats disease, in up to fifth of all cases, there is a fibrous submacular nodule that occasionally is calcified or ossified (Fig. 2.**69a**).[119, 120, 123, 123a] These nodules might represent exuberant proliferation and

Pathology

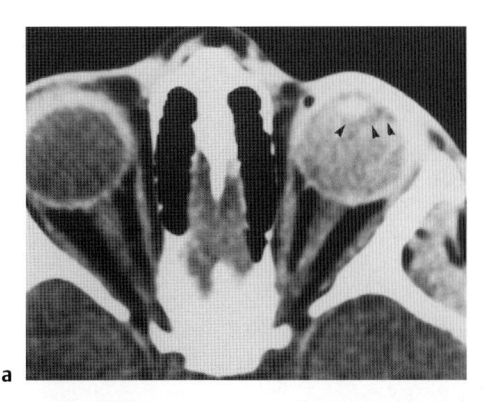

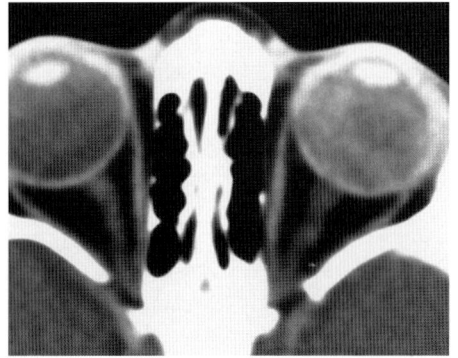

Fig. 2.**68** Coats disease.
a Axial CT scan shows diffuse increased density of the left globe. This is due to total exudative retinal detachment. The detached leaves of the retina can be seen (arrows), extending toward the ora serrata. A noncalcified retinoblastoma as seen in **b** cannot be excluded on the basis of this CT scan.
b Axial CT scan shows increased density of the left globe. This is due to noncalcified retinoblastoma and associated retinal detachment.

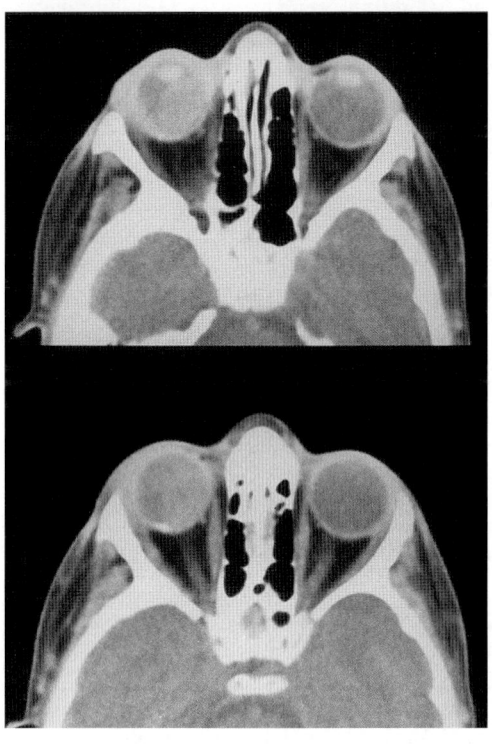

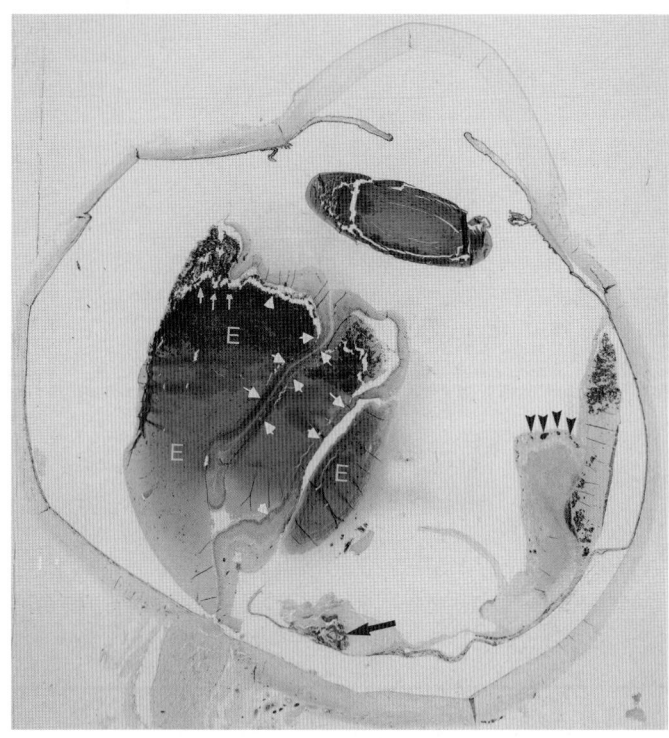

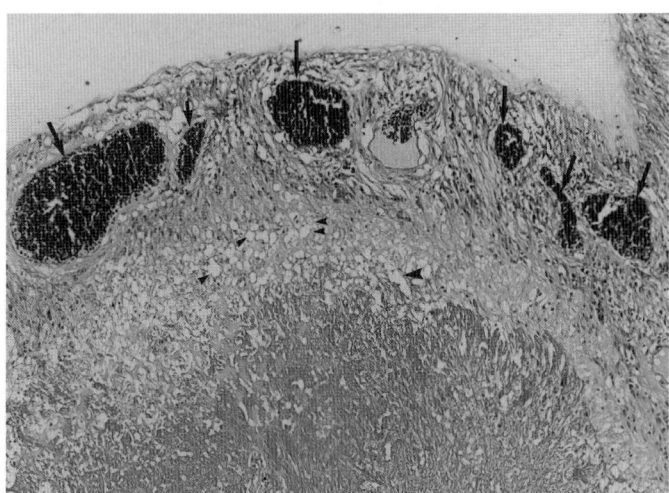

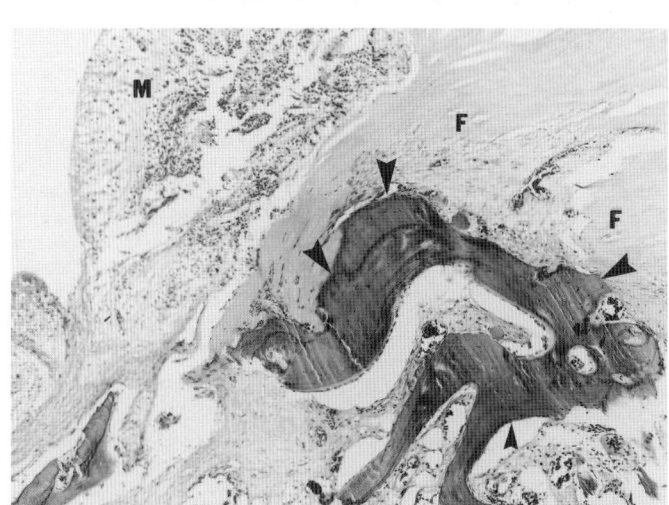

Fig. 2.**69** Coats disease.
a Enhanced CT scans demonstrate increased density of the right eye, related to total retinal detachment. Note calcification adjacent to the expected area of the right ocular macula.
b Whole of the enucleated right eye. The retina is detached, folded (white arrows), and pushed forward by massive hemorrhagic subretinal exudates (E). Within one of the retinal folds, telangiectatic retinal blood vessels are seen peripherally (arrowheads). Posteriorly, near the macular area, a fibro-osseous nodule (black arrow) is present at the level of the retinal pigment epithelium. The choroid is artificially detached. (Hematoxylin–eosin.)
c There are many telangiectatic vascular channels (arrows) present in one of the retinal folds, characteristic of Coats disease. Underneath the retina, there is proteinaceous exudate containing cholesterol clefts (arrowheads). (Hematoxylin–eosin.)
d Underneath the retina, in the macular area (M), there is a fibro-osseous nodule composed of bony trabeculae (arrowheads) and dense fibrous tissue (F).
Case Courtesy of Ahmed Hydayat, MD, AFIP, Washington, DC, USA.

metaplasia of the RPE.[120] Pe'er[123a], reported an eye with Coats disease enucleated because of suggestion of retinoblastoma. On histopathological examination, calcifications were found in the center of the detached, disorganized retina, with accompanying hemorrhage and no demonstrable connection to the RPE.[123a] Calcification and bone formation may also occur in eyes with phthisis bulbi, angiomatosis retinae, hemangioma, and astrocytic hemartoma.[119] MRI is superior to CT in differentiating Coats disease from retinoblastomas and other leukokoric eyes (Fig. 2.**70**).[91, 120] The subretinal exudation of Coats disease is usually seen as mild to moderate hyperintense signal on T1-weighted, PW, and T2-weighted MR images (Figs. 2.**70**, 2.**71**–2.**74**). In retinoblastomas, MRI characteristically shows a mass that can be differentiated from an associated subretinal exudate. The MRI findings in patients with Coats disease are often compatible with retinal detachment without the presence of an intraocular mass (Figs. 2.**70**–2.**74**).

At times in advanced Coats disease, where reactive gliosis or metaplastic (RPE) fibro-osseous nodules may be present, CT and MRI may show a calcified or noncalcified mass, particularly at the level of the macula. Posterior calcification near the macular area should not exclude Coats disease in cases of leukokoria.[119] However, a small posterior calcification due to small retinoblastoma is unlikely to cause significant or total retinal detachment. Therefore in a leukokoric eye, in appropriate clinical setting, the MRI findings of total or massive retinal detachment, associated with a small posterior calcified lesion, seen on CT scan, should raise the question of advanced Coats disease or retinal dysplasia rather than the retinoblastoma (Fig. 2.**69**).

In Coats disease the detached retina may show enhancement following intravenous injection of Gd-DTPA contrast medium (Figs. 2.**70b**, 2.**73c**). Frequently, the most characteristic and prominent telangiectatic retinal vessels are located in a retinal fold peripherally as seen in Figs. 2.**70b**, 2.**71d** and 2.**73c**. This finding may explain difficulty in implicating Coats disease clinically because of where the intraretinal telangiectatic vessels are hidden.[119] In the early stage of the disease, the CT and MRI appearance of Coats may not be differentiated from noncalcified retinoblastoma (Fig. 2.**74**), because the lesion in Coats disaease may also appear hypointense on T2-weighted MR images (Fig. 2.**74**). In this situation one may use a flow sensitive pulse sequence such as gradient-echo technique. If the lesion proves to be very vascular, then the MRI findings in appropriate clinical setting should favor Coats disease. Finally, in many cases with early-stage Coats disease, the CT and MRI findings are negative. In some cases, the affected eye on CT or MRI scans may be slightly smaller than the normal fellow eye (Fig. 2.**70**).

■ Ocular Toxocariasis (Sclerosing Endophthalmitis)

Ocular toxocariasis is a chorioretinitis caused by an inflammatory response to the nematode *Toxocara canis*.[12, 14, 124–126] Infected puppies excrete worm ova (eggs) that may survive in soil for years. The infection results from ingestion of the ova in contaminated soil. In these patients the death of the larva results in a wide spectrum of intraocular inflammatory reactions,[124–126] the more severe of which has a characteristic pathological appearance of sclerosing endophthalmitis.[125, 126] Ocular toxocariasis is usually unilateral and is seen in older children.

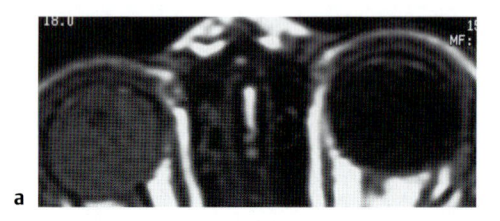

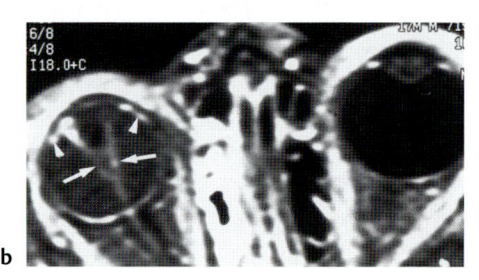

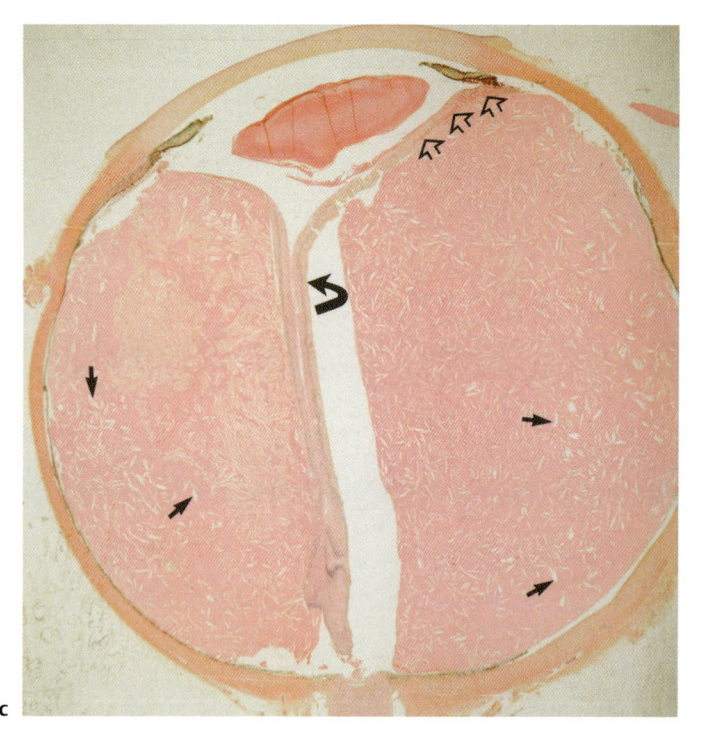

Fig. 2.**70** Coats disease.
a Axial unenhanced T1W MR scan. There is slight increased signal of the right eye.
b Axial enhanced fat-suppression T1W MR scan. There is total retinal detachment (arrows). Note enhancement of detached sensory retina (arrows) as well as enhancement at the ora serrata (arrowheads). These enhancements are related to telangiectasia and microaneurysm of sensory retina, the underlying pathology in Coats disease. The thickening of detached sensory retina is related to intraretinal exudate, also seen in **c**.
c Lower-power photomicrograph of the enucleated eye. Note detached retina (curved arrow), massive subretinal exudate, numerous cholesterol clefts (short arrows) in the subretinal exudate, and hemangioma of the peripheral retina (hollow arrows). Note intraretinal exudate, resulting in thickened detached sensory retina. From Edward DP, Mafee MF, Garcia-Valenzuela E, Weiss RA. Coats' disease and persistent hyperplastic primary vitreous. Role of MRI and CT. Radiol Clin North Am 1998; 36: 1119–1131. With permission.

Pathology 173

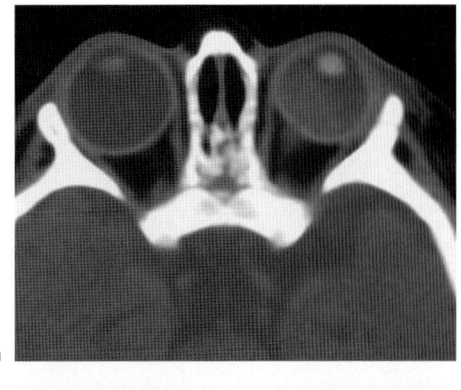

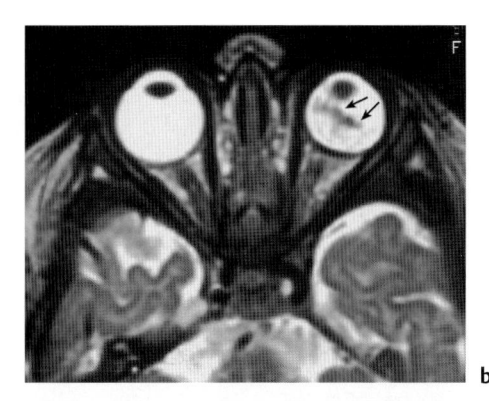

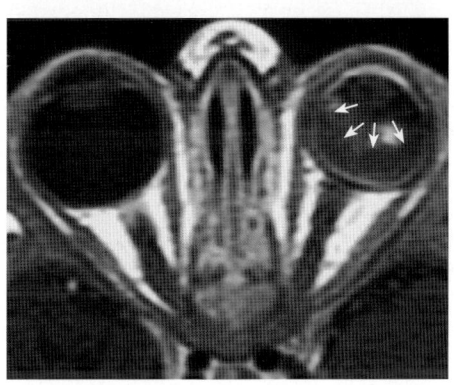

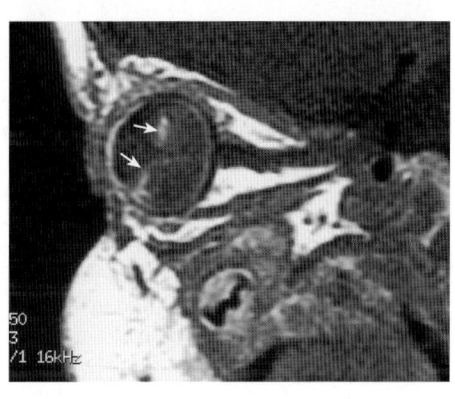

Fig. 2.71 Coats disease vs. PHPV. A 4-month-old girl with leukokoria of the left eye.
a Axial unenhanced CT scan shows a slightly microphthalmic left eye with increased density, related to retinal detachment, better identified on MR scans.
b Axial T2W MR scan. There is an irregular hypointense mass (arrows), related to funduscopic finding of a retrolental white vascularized mass, a finding most compatible with PHPV. No retinal details could be appreciated behind the retrolental mass on detailed funduscopic examination.
c Axial enhanced T1W and sagittal enhanced T1W (**d**) MR scans. There is marked enhancement of an irregular mass (arrows) compatible with white vascularized mass, seen on funduscopic examination. This is most likely related to a remnant of primary vitreous. Note enhancement of the anterior chamber of the affected eye and signal change of the left lens.

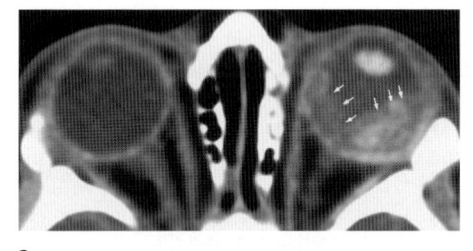

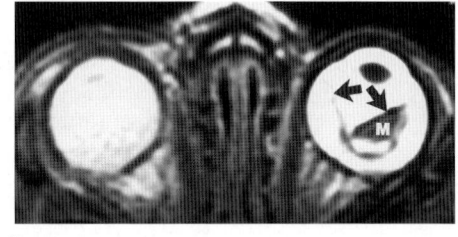

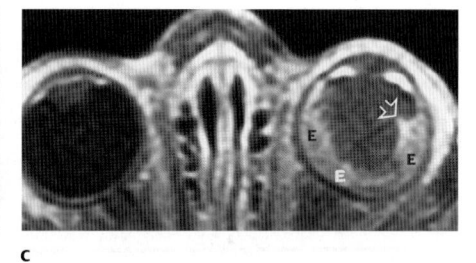

Fig. 2.72 Coats disease.
a Axial unenhanced CT scan shows what appears to be a nonspecific retinal or posterior hyaloid detachment (arrows). Retinoblastoma cannot be excluded.
b Axial T2W MR scan, showing posterior hyaloid detachment (arrows) seen in front of optic nerve head. Note a masslike image (M), which is due to hemorrhage in subhyaloid space.
c Axial enhanced fat-suppression MR scan showing exudate (E) in the subretinal space. The signal intensity of subretinal exudate was the same on unenhanced T1W MR scan, not shown here. Note enhancement of detached sensory retina (arrow), due to telangiectasia of the retina, the underlying pathology in Coats disease. From Edward DP, Mafee MF, Garcia-Valenzuela E, Weiss RA. Coats' disease and persistent hyperplastic primary vitreous. Role of MRI and CT. Radiol Clin North Am 1998; 36: 1119–1131. With permission.

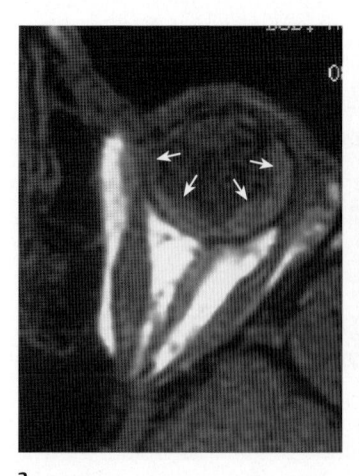

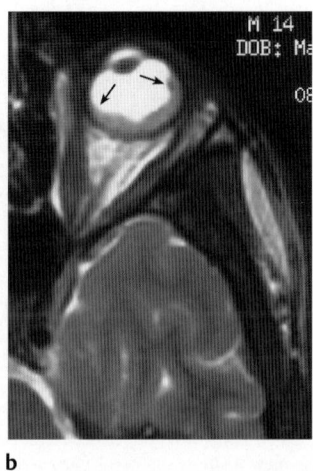

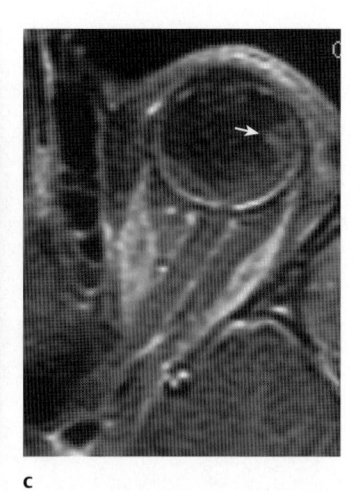

Fig. 2.73 Coats disease in 14-year-old boy with leukokoria of left eye.
a Axial T1W MR scan shows a retinal detachment (arrows).
b Axial T2W MR scan shows a retinal detachment (arrows). The hypointense subretinal image may be due to dense exudate or hemorrhage. Without an enhanced T1W MR scan, a diffuse retinoblastoma cannot be ruled out.
c Axial enhanced fat-suppression T1W MR scan. There is a focus of enhancement (arrow) along the peripheral portion of the detached sensory retina, characteristic of Coats disease. There is no enhancement of subretinal space, confirming exudate/hemorrhage rather than a diffuse retinoblastoma.

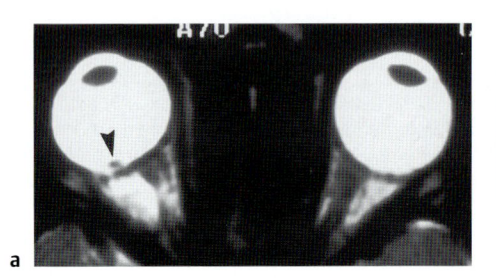

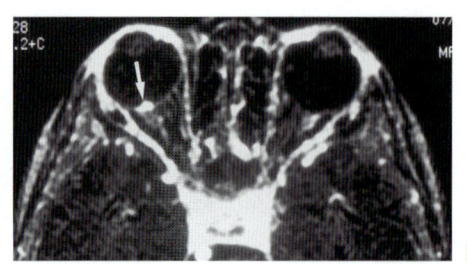

Fig. 2.74 Localized Coats disease.
a Axial T2W MR scan. There is a small hypointense lesion (arrow) at the posterior aspect of the right eye.
b Axial postcontrast FSPGR-20° MR scan, showing that the mass (arrow) is likely to be hypervascular, a finding in keeping with the diagnosis of Coats disease or other ocular vascular disease. Clinical diagnosis of Coats disease is this patient was considered most likely on the basis of ophthalmoscopic and MRI results.

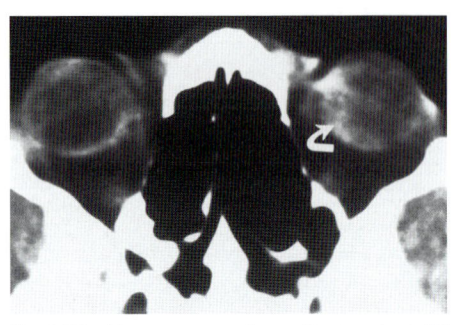

Fig. 2.75 Toxocara granuloma. Postcontrast CT scan shows an irregular mass (arrow) with slight enhancement.

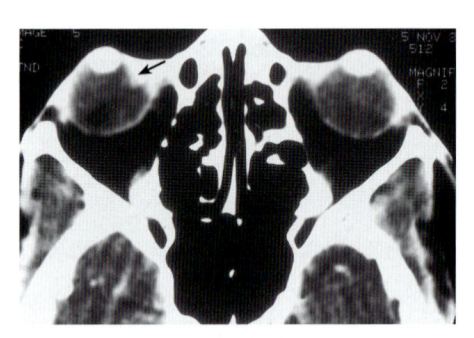

Fig. 2.76 Ocular granuloma in a middle-aged woman. Axial CT scan shows a mass in the anterior nasal aspect of the right eye. There is small calcification present (arrow). Because clinically malignant melanoma could not be excluded, the eye was removed. The histopathological finding was consistent with chronic granuloma.

Clinical Diagnosis

Clinically, ocular toxocariasis may present as endophthalmitis with vitreous haze from a profound inflammatory response, or as posterior or peripheral retina granuloma.[12] The granuloma appears as a white, elevated lesion in the retina, and may have associated adherent vitreous bands, vitreous traction, tractional retinal detachment, and dragging of the retina and optic disk.[12] The histological changes of the globe are characterized by an infiltration with lymphocytes, plasma cells, eosinophils, and giant cells. Retinal, subretinal, and vitreous hemorrhages may frequently occur. Remnants of the secondary larval stage of *Toxocara canis* are often difficult to find. A diagnostic enzyme-linked immunosorbent assay (ELISA) for *Toxocara* is now available.

Diagnostic Imaging

Margo et al.[124] reported the CT findings in three cases of histopathologically proven sclerosing endophthalmitis. These findings consisted of a homogeneous intravitreal density that corresponded to a detached retina, organized vitreous, and inflammatory subretinal exudate. These investigators concluded that the findings are similar to those seen in Coats disease and non-calcified retinoblastoma. Three cases of toxocariasis in young adults appeared on CT as a localized or diffuse ill-defined mass with no significant enhancement (Fig. 2.**75**).[62] The inflammatory process (chronic abscess) is seen on CT as an irregularity of the uveoscleral coat with a diffuse or locally thickened, slightly enhanced uveoscleral coat (Fig. 2.**76**).

In the appropriate clinical setting, the CT findings of the granuloma of *Toxocara canis* should be relied on to establish a presumptive diagnosis.[62] The MR images of a patient with a presumptive diagnosis of toxocariasis are shown in Fig. 2.**77**. In general the proteinaceous subretinal exudate produced by the inflammatory response to the larval infiltration is seen as variably hyperintense on T1-weighted, PW, and T2-weighted scans (Fig. 2.**77**). The postcontrast MR appearance of multiple toxocara abscesses in a patient with positive ELISA test is shown in Figures 2.**77c, d**. It should be noted that at times it may be very difficult to differentiate the MR and CT appearances of chronic retinal detachment and organized vitreous from toxocara granuloma, Coats disease, and even ROP, PHPV, and noncalcified retinoblastoma.[62]

■ Ocular Astrocytic Hamartoma (Retinal Astrocytoma)

Retinal astrocytoma is a benign, yellow-white rare retinal tumor that occurs in association with tuberous sclerosis or neurofibromatosis or in isolation.[127] Early retinal astrocytoma (astrocytic hamartoma) may look exactly like early retinoblastoma and may be present before any neurological or dermatological manifestations of tuberous sclerosis appear.[14,65] These tumors may appear in the retina or in the optic nerve. The usual appearance is that of a single nodule or of multiple nodules elevated 1 or 2 mm above the surface of the retina, and, at this stage, CT and MRI cannot visualize the lesions. Tumors elevated more than 3 mm can be demonstrated on CT and MRI. The CT appearance of astrocytic hamartomas is similar to retinoblastoma (Fig. 2.**78**). If typical features of tuberous sclerosis are not present, the differentiation between astrocytic hamartomas and other ocular lesions may be very difficult.

■ Combined Hamartoma of the Retinal Pigment Epithelium and Retina

Combined hamartoma of the retinal pigment epithelium and retina is a rare, congenital ocular tumor. This benign proliferation of mature cells involving the retinal pigment epithelium leads to an elevated lesion in the posterior pole or optic disk, and occurs with varying pigmentation. The less-pigmented lesions simulate retinoblastoma clinically and on CT and MR scans.[4]

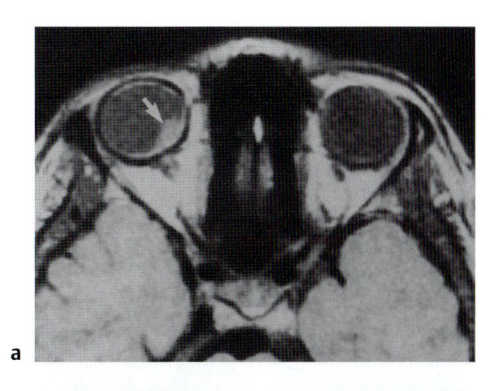

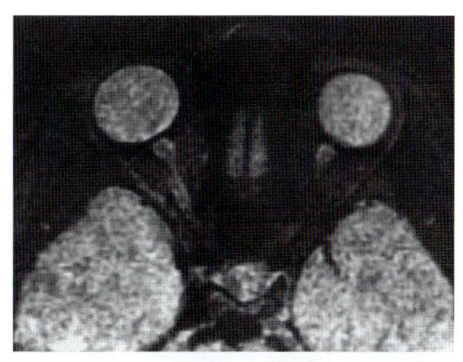

Fig. 2.77 Toxocara granuloma in a 6-year-old girl with leukokoria. **a** PW and **b** T2W MR scans showing an irregular intraocular mass (arrow). The mass appears isointense on T2W MR image. Retinoblastoma appears hypointense on T2W MR images. Figs. 2.77 **a, b**. From Mafee MF. The eye. In: Som PM, Curtin HD, eds. Head and Neck Imaging. St. Louis: Mosby; 2003: 441–527. With permission.
c, d Ocular toxocariasis in a 60-year-old woman. Axial enhanced T1W MR scans, showing intravitreal band (arrows) and chronic ocular abscesses (arrowheads).

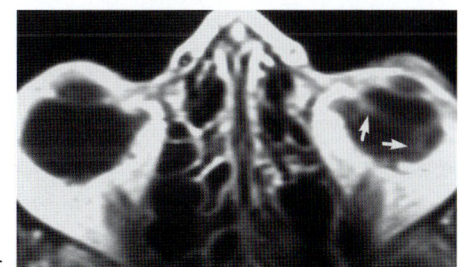

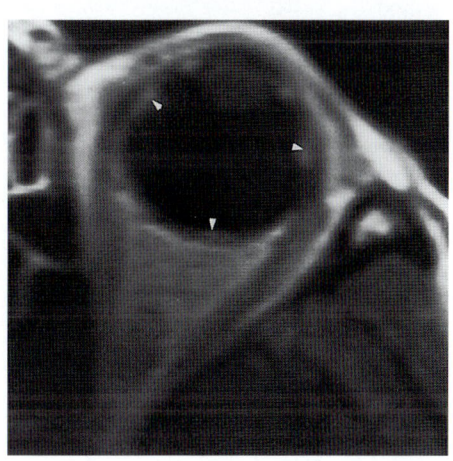

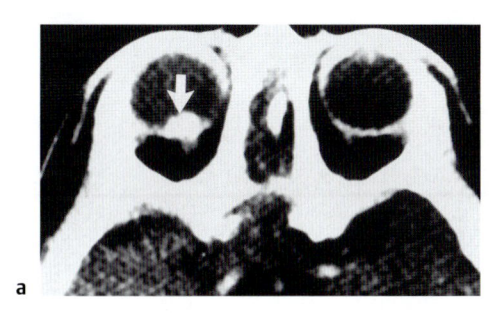

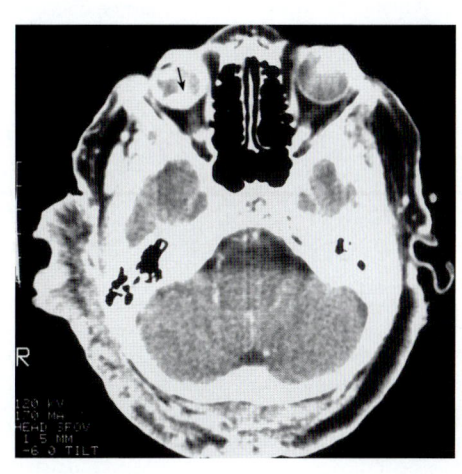

Fig. 2.78 Astrocytic hamartoma of the retina.
a Axial enhanced CT scan shows an enhancing mass (arrow) in this patient with tuberous sclerosis. Courtesy of Barett G. Haik, MD, Memphis, Tennessee, USA.
b Axial enhanced CT scan shows a calcified mass (arrow) in the posterior pole of the right eye in this patient with neurofibromatosis type 1. Note plexiform neurofibromatosis involving the right auricular region.

■ Incontinentia Pigmenti

Incontinentia pigmenti is a disorder associated with abnormalities of the skin, eye, and skeletal system.[4] Ocular involvement is bilateral, but often asymmetric. Retinal vascular abnormalities, pigmentary changes, and proliferation of retinal pigment epithelium lead to an intraocular nodular mass (pseudoglioma), usually seen in the first year of life.

■ Juvenile Xanthogranuloma

Juvenile xanthogranuloma (non-Langerhans cell histiocytosis) is a benign idiopathic multifocal cutaneous eruption affecting infants and young children.[4, 14] The cutaneous lesions are yellow-orange granulomatous nodules composed of histiocytes. It is a granulomatous inflammatory response that frequently shows Touton giant cells. In addition to involving the skin, the disease may involve the eye and orbit (Figs. 2.79). This condition usually affects the iris and ciliary body (anterior uveal tract),[128–130] but lesions in the choroid, retina, or optic nerve have been reported.[129] Juvenile xanthogranuloma has also been noted to present as a solitary or diffuse orbital mass.[130] Infiltration of the iris can cause spontaneous hyphema, glaucoma, and uveitis.

■ Ganglioneuroma

The ganglioneuroma is a rare ocular neoplasm that arises from neuroepithelial cells of the embryonic optic cup.[131] The lesion usually appears at birth or in early childhood as a yellow or pink mass in the iris. Histopathologically, the ganglioneuroma is composed of an admixture of glial cells and neurons.[131]

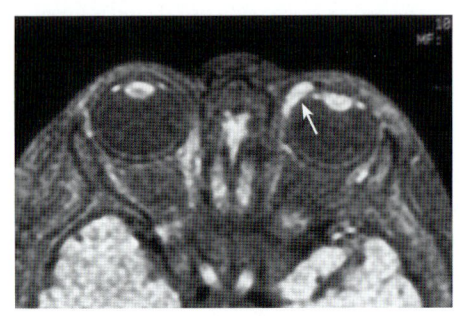

Fig. 2.79 Juvenile xanthogranuloma. Axial enhanced fat-suppression T1W MR scan. There is a mass (arrow) involving the left globe. The mass showed moderate contrast enhancement. Courtesy of Ahmad Hydayat, MD, AFIP, Washington, DC, USA.

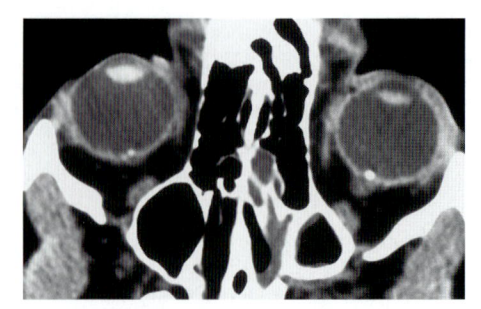

Fig. 2.80 Drusen in a 9-year-old boy with a history of pseudopapilledema. The patient was referred to an ophthalmologist because of unusual visual phenomena that he has been reporting continuously for at least several years; described as "reddish-purple blobs that can occlude the visual field and move slowly." Axial unenhanced CT scan shows bilateral calcified optic nerve head drusen.

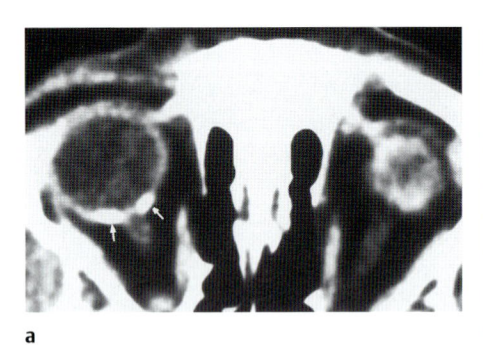

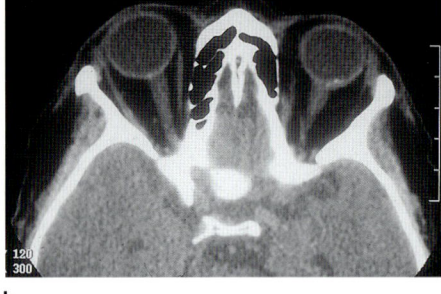

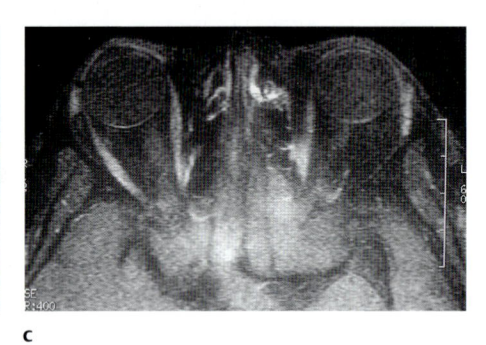

Fig. 2.81 Choroidal osteoma.
a Axial CT scan shows a peripapillary calcification compatible with a choroidal osteoma.
b Axial CT scan shows an area of increased density lateral to the left optic disk, presumed choroidal osteoma.
c Axial enhanced fat-suppression T1W MR scan, taken on a 3 T MR unit, showing an ill-defined enhancing lesion, corresponding to lesion seen in b.

■ Optic Nerve Head Drusen

Optic nerve head drusen is a benign, usually bilateral, cause of pseudopapilledema, and is occasionally inherited as an autosomal dominant condition.[132, 133] Disk drusen or hyaline bodies are spherical, acellular, laminated concretions from an unknown source, often partially calcified and possibly related to accumulation of axoplasmic derivatives of degenerating retinal nerve fibers.[132, 133] Drusen are buried within the substance of the nerve head, usually anterior to the lamina cribrosa. Drusen contain sialic acid, cerebrosides, calcium, carbohydrate, mucopolysaccharides, and iron. Optic disk drusen may vary in size (to 59–750 μm in diameter) and number; often, smaller drusen appear to coalesce to form larger aggregates. Once their calcified component is more than 1–1.5 mm, they should be recognized on thin-section (1–1.5 mm) CT scans.[132] Although optic disk drusen are rarely seen in early childhood, most drusen are believed to be present at birth.[132, 133] They become more apparent in later life as they enlarge and approach the disk surface, becoming ophthalmologically visible as "hyaline" or "colloid" bodies.[132]

Drusen are rarely detected by CT scanning in early childhood (Fig. 2.80). Careful evaluation of the optic disk may reveal a small area, slightly more dense than the rest of the disk. Some of these children and adults with drusen of optic disk may have a number of diagnostic studies including cranial CT and MRI to exclude an intracranial process. When drusen are located well beneath the surface of the disk, they may blur the disk margin and may lead to misdiagnosis of papilledema.

■ Choroidal Osteoma

Choroidal osteoma is a benign tumor that is typically found unilaterally in young, white girls.[12, 14, 49] Histopathological evaluation reveals mature bone with marrow spaces containing loose fibrovascular tissue.[49] Choroidal osteoma was originally classified as a choristoma (a benign congenital tumor composed of normal tissue elements that do not normally occur at that site), but it is currently regarded by some as an acquired benign choroidal neoplasm of unknown etiology.[131]

Patients with choroidal osteoma present with painless progressive loss of vision over several months or years or with abrupt recent blurring of central vision. Some lesions are detected initially on routine eye examination.[131] If the lesion involves the macular choroid, the visual acuity can be impaired on the basis of degeneration of the overlying RPE and neurosensory retina.[131]

Ultrasound and CT are useful in detecting choroidal osteoma. On CT scan, choroidal osteomas appear as platelike calcified thickening of the posterior ocular wall, typically in the juxtapapillary region, in which unlike drusen, typically calcification does not involve the optic disk center (Fig. 2.81). The most important lesions in the differential diagnosis of choroidal osteoma are listed in Table 2.6.

Retinal Gliosis

Retinal and optic nerve astrocytes are analogous to fibroblasts in the body.[14] Retinal gliosis refers to reactive proliferation and hypertrophy of astrocytes in the retina, especially occurring in response to injury. Gliotic tissue growth may appear masslike, simulating intraocular tumors, or cause tractional retinal detachment.

Myelinated Nerve Fibers

Oligodendrocytes and myelin are not usually present in human retina.[4] Approximately 1% of eyes have myelinated nerve fibers within the retina, but usually in a peripapillary distribution. This myelination results in a slightly elevated, white retinal plaque and, if extensive, can produce leukokoria. The CT appearance of myelinated nerve fibers may be similar to noncalcified retinoblastoma (see Fig. 2.**48**).

Subretinal Neovascular Membranes

Subretinal neovascular membrane is an acquired abnormality in which growth of new blood vessels from the choriocapillaris occurs beneath the neurosensory retina, usually in response to some retinal injury. These new vessels may hemorrhage or leak, leading to serous retinal detachment. The lesion may organize, resulting in a gliotic, elevated retinal scar and retinal traction.[4]

Vitreous Opacities

Any disease, such as uveitis, vitreous hemorrhage, endophthalmitis, or organized vitreous, associated with cells in the vitreous can simulate retinoblastoma with vitreous seeding (see Fig. 2.**39**).[4, 12] Vitreous opacities often obscure the view of the retina, causing more difficulty for the clinician in differentiating the etiology of the vitreous cells.

Choroidal Hemangioma

Choroidal hemangiomas are congenital vascular hamartomas of the choroid that are typically seen in middle-aged individuals. Normal retinal vessels overlie the mass. Choroidal hemangioma in children can simulate retinoblastoma (see Fig. 2.**106**).[4, 12, 14] The CT and MRI characteristics of choroidal hemangioma are described elsewhere in this chapter (p. 184).

Malignant Uveal Melanoma

Most primary and metastatic ocular neoplasms in adults involve the choroid, and the most common tumor is malignant melanoma.[134] Malignant melanomas of the uvea are unusual in black subjects, with the white-to-black ratio being about 15:1.[135] Those melanomas involving the ciliary body and choroid are thought to originate from preexisting nevi.[134] The neoplasm has a capacity to metastasize hematogenously; its favored metastatic site is the liver. The incidence of malignant melanoma of the choroid has been estimated to be 5.2–7.5 cases per million per year.[136] The incidence of uveal melanoma increases with age. Less than 2% of tumors are seen in patients less than 20 years of age.[5] Congenital melanosis, ocular melanocytosis, oculodermal melanocytosis, and uveal nevi are predisposing lesions that precede the development of uveal melanoma.[5]

Callender's classification of melanotic lesions, which is based on cellular features, offers the best indication of prognosis.[137, 138] The spindle-A tumors, which are comprised of spindle cells with elongated nuclei, characteristically lacking nucleoli, have the best prognosis. The next best prognoses are the spindle-B tumors, whose cells have the same shape as spindle-A lesions, but they are slightly larger and have a nucleus containing a prominent nucleolus. The next worst prognosis is the epithelioid-cell tumors, which are composed of larger, more pleomorphic cells than the spindle-cell tumor. Finally, there are mixed-cell tumors made of both spindle and epithelioid cells.[134, 138] Some of the tumors may be amelanotic, especially the spindle-cell tumors.

Clinical Diagnosis

An iris melanoma is seen as a visible spot on the iris or as a discoloration of the iris in one eye. The typical ciliary body melanoma appears as a highly elevated, nodular, dark brown lesion in the peripheral field.[139] The typical choroidal melanoma appears as a dark brown solid tumor in the fundus and has a biconvex, lenticular cross-sectional shape.[139] The tumor initially grows flat within the choroid, later elevates Bruch's membrane, and finally ruptures through it so that the melanoma assumes a characteristic mushroom shape, growing toward the vitreous cavity (Fig. 2.**82**). The retina over the surface of the tumor becomes elevated and detached (solid retinal detachment). This detachment gradually extends as a serous detachment over the slopes of the tumor. Ophthalmoscopically the lesion is seen as a circumscribed mass of varied pigmentation along with a solid retinal detachment, and the retinal vessels over the surface of the mass are elevated. The retina is usually attached to the mass and does not float easily as seen in rhegmatogenous retinal detachments. In some cases, the subretinal fluid extends only around the base of the lesion, in others, it accumulates to the extent that the retina is extensively or even totally detached (Fig. 2.**82**).[139] In some cases, the subretinal fluid is bloody, almost exclusively in eyes that have tumor eruption through Bruch's membrane.[139]

If the tumor is not treated, it may cause secondary glaucoma and eventually break through the eye into the retrobulbar region. Metastases occur primarily to the liver. Management of clinically suspected choroidal melanomas has been the subject of some controversy in recent years.[140-147] Enucleation has been a standard treatment for more than a century.[141] Some advocate early enucleation of all melanomas to prevent metastasis.[147] Radiation

Table 2.**6** CT and MRI differential diagnosis of choroidal osteoma

- Choroidal hemangioma
- Amelanotic choroidal nevus or melanoma
- Regressed retinoblastoma
- Metastatic carcinoma to choroid (prostate)
- Idiopathic or dystrophic sclerochoroidal calcification
- Posttraumatic or postinflammatory ocular calcification
- RPE metaplastic calcification or bone formation
- Bone formation in phthisical eyes
- Neurilemoma or neurofibroma of choroid
- Intraocular foreign body
- Calcification related to macular degeneration
- Vascular calcification in patients with end-stage renal disease
- Peripapillary choroidal calcification in chronic retinal detachment
- Metabolic calcification

Adopted from Mafee MF. The eye. In: Som PM, Curtin HD, eds., Head and Neck Imaging. St. Louis: Mosby; 2003: 441–527.

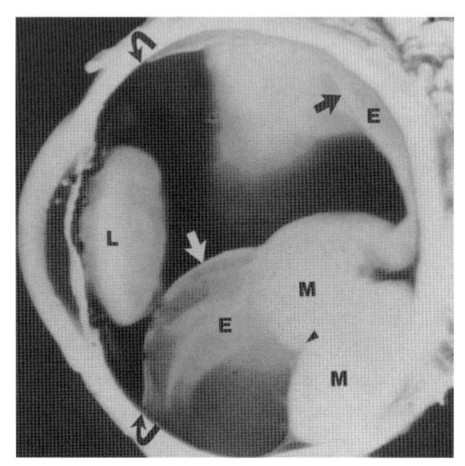

Fig. 2.82 Malignant choroidal melanoma. Gross eye specimen shows a choroidal melanoma (M) that has caused total retinal detachment (straight white and black arrows). Penetration through Bruch's membrane (arrowhead) has given the tumor a mushroomlike appearance. Note the subretinal exudate (E), ora serrata (curved arrows), and lens (L). From Mafee MF. The eye. In: Som PM, Curtin HD, eds. Head and Neck Imaging. St. Louis: Mosby; 2003: 441–527. With permission.

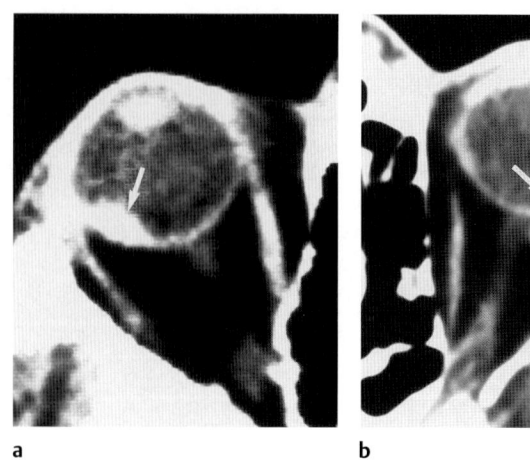

Fig. 2.83. Malignant uveal melanoma.
a Axial unenhanced CT scan shows a discoid choroidal melanoma (arrow).
b Axial enhanced CT scan shows a discoid choroidal melanoma (arrows) with an extraocular extension (arrowhead).

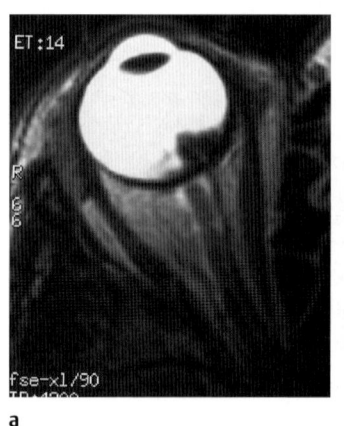

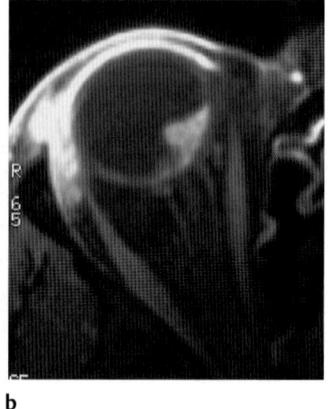

Fig. 2.84 Malignant uveal melanoma. a Axial T2W and b axial enhanced fat-suppression T1W MR scans. There is a choroidal melanoma, which appears hypointense on T2W (a). The tumor demonstrated moderate contrast enhancement (b) when compared with unenhanced T1W MR scan (not shown here).

therapy is frequently used for the treatment of uveal melanomas. Metastatic sites of primary uveal melanoma include liver, lung, bone, kidney, and brain in order of decreasing frequency, and a thorough search for metastasis is important to spare the patient an unnecessary enucleation.[143]

Diagnostic Imaging

Although uveal melanomas can be accurately diagnosed by ophthalmoscopy, fluorescein angiography, or ultrasonography, misdiagnosis continues to occur, particularly when opaque media preclude direct visualization.[122, 148–150] CT has proven to be a highly accurate method for demonstrating large (more than 3 mm in thickness) uveal melanoma, and dynamic CT can provide information about the vascularity and perfusion of intraocular lesions and can help distinguish uveal melanomas from other lesions such as choroidal hemangiomas. Most uveal melanomas are seen on CT as an elevated, hyperdense, sharply marginated lenticular or mushroom-shaped lesion (Fig. 2.83).

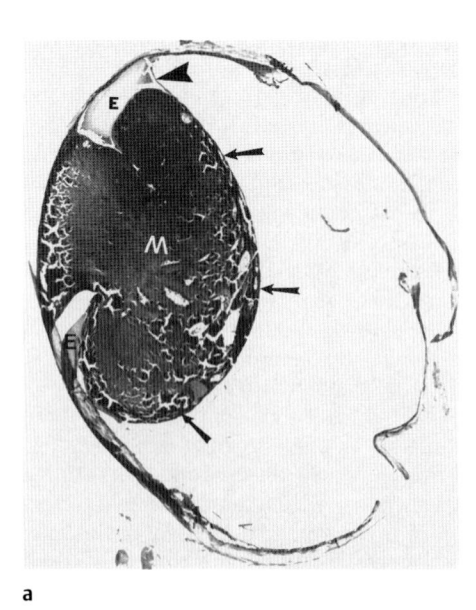

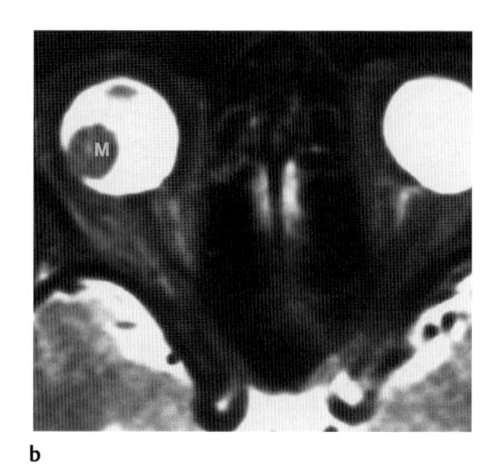

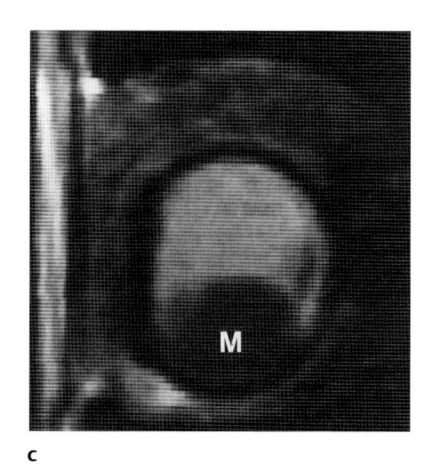

Fig. 2.85 Malignant uveal melanoma.
a Tissue section of an enucleated eye shows a mushroom-shaped choroidal melanoma (M). The retina over the mass is elevated (arrows) and is detached over the slope of the tumor (arrowhead). Note exudate (E) in the subretinal space. Penetration through the basal membrane (Bruch's membrane) of the choroid results in a characteristic mushroomlike appearance.
b Axial T2W MR scan shows a mushroom-shaped choroidal melanoma (M).
c Axial T2W MR scan of an enucleated eye of an 18-year-old African-American woman, showing a large malignant uveal melanoma.

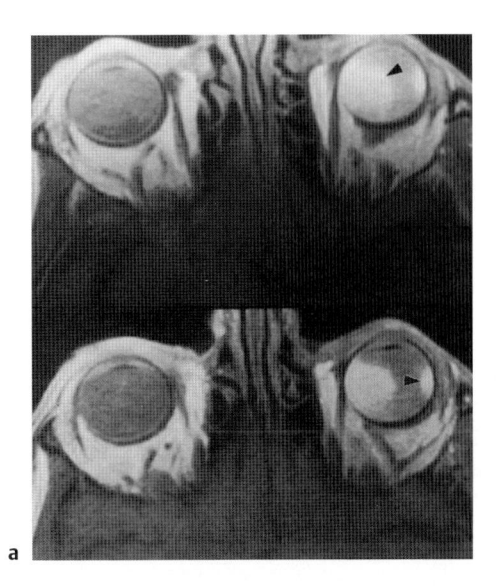

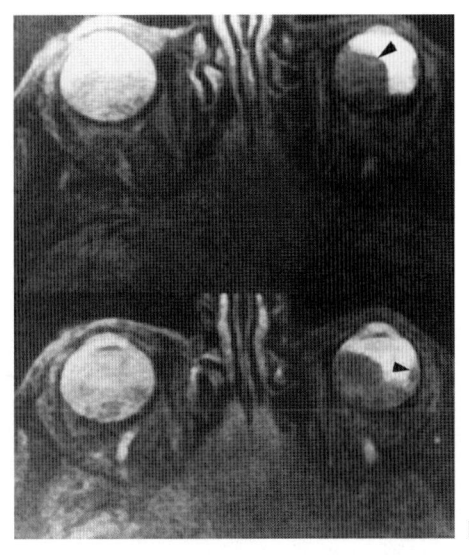

Fig. 2.86 Retinal detachment associated with chronic organized subretinal exudate and hemorrhage simulating uveal melanoma.
a Axial PW MR scans show well-defined hyperintense masses (arrowheads).
b Axial T2W MR scans show that the masses seen in **a** now appear homogeneously hypointense (arrowheads). The eye had to be enucleated, and all of these findings were confirmed to be due to organized subretinal hemorrhage. The retinal detachment was related to complication of radiation therapy for a uveal melanoma. Retinal or choroidal hemorrhages may at times be difficult to differentiate from uveal melanomas. Repeat MR study is needed to see progressive signal intensity changes in case of hematoma.

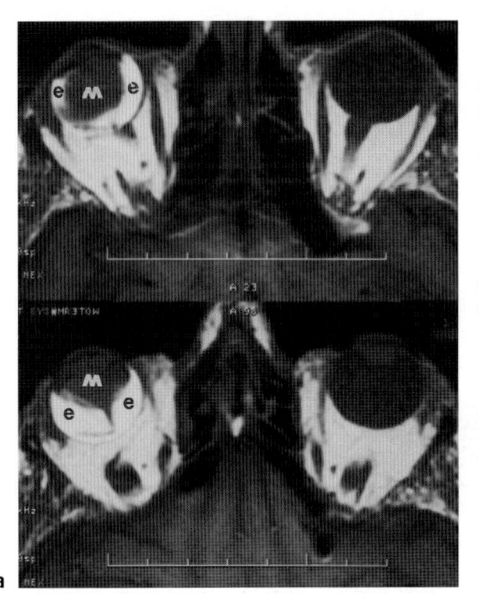

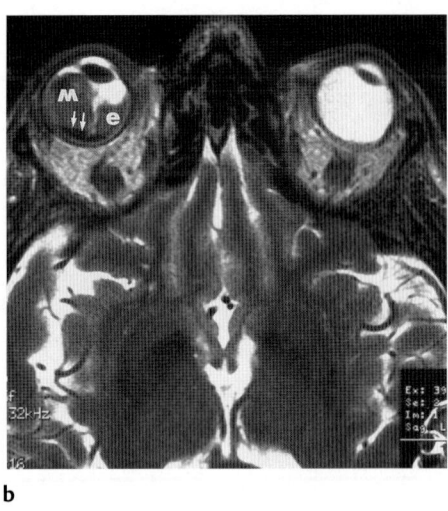

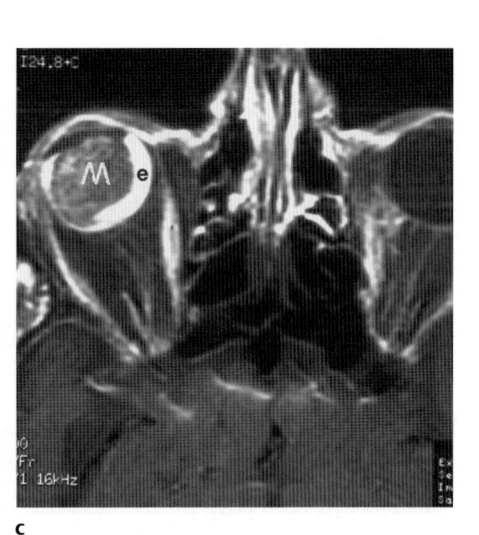

Fig. 2.87 Malignant uveal melanoma. **a** Axial unenhanced T1W, **b** axial T2W, and **c** axial enhanced fat-suppression T1W MR scans, showing a large melanoma (M), associated with retinal detachment. Note subretinal exudate (e) and layered hemorrhage (arrows in **b**). All the MR images were obtained using a 3 T MRI unit and a head coil. The clinical diagnosis in this patient was choroid hematoma and shifting subretinal hemorrhage. Because of enhancement of the mass (M), the MRI interpretation was in keeping with the diagnosis of choroidal melanoma rather than hematoma. Follow-up MRI studies did not show any change in signal characteristic of the mass (M), confirming the presence of a mass rather than hematoma. Malignant melanoma was confirmed following enucleation.

Several reports have proven the effectiveness of MRI in the diagnosis of intraocular lesions.[5,18,19,152] On T1-weighted and proton-density-weighted (PW) images, uveal melanomas are seen as areas of moderately high signal (greater signal intensity than vitreous) (Fig. 2.84a). On T2-weighted images, melanomas are seen as areas of moderate to marked low signal (less intensity than vitreous) (Figs. 2.84b, 2.85b). These MRI characteristics of uveal melanomas are very similar to those of retinoblastomas. Retinal and choroidal hemorrhage may simulate choroidal melanoma (Fig. 2.86). Associated retinal detachment is better visualized by MRI than by CT (Figs. 2.87, 2.88). Exudative retinal detachment is usually depicted on MRI as a dependent area of moderate to very high signal intensity in T1-weighted, PW, and T2-weighted images (Fig. 2.87a). Organized subretinal exudate, acute and subacute subretinal hemorrhage may appear hypointense on T2-weighted MR images (Fig. 2.89b). Chronic retinal detachment and hemorrhagic subretinal fluid have varied MRI appearances. Most uveal melanomas appear as a well-defined solid mass (Fig. 2.84, 2.85). However, atypical features of ocular melanoma may be present (Fig. 2.89). When necrotic or hemorrhagic foci are present within the uveal melanoma, the inhomogeneity present within the tumor can be problematic. Some melanomas may be seen better in T1-weighted images; discoid melanomas or ring melanomas may be difficult to detect if they are flat. Additionally, organized subretinal exudate, with or without associated hemorrhage, may have similar MRI characteristics to uveal melanoma (Figs. 2.86, 2.89). Tumor invasion of the sclera, optic disk, Tenon's capsule, extraocular orbital extension, and distant metastases can be best detected by MRI (Fig. 2.90–2.92). Intravenous administration of paramagnetic contrast material is very useful in the diagnosis of uveal melanomas; certain ocular pathology; and, in particular, for evaluation of optic nerve, as well as retrobulbar extension of ocular tumors (Fig. 2.90).

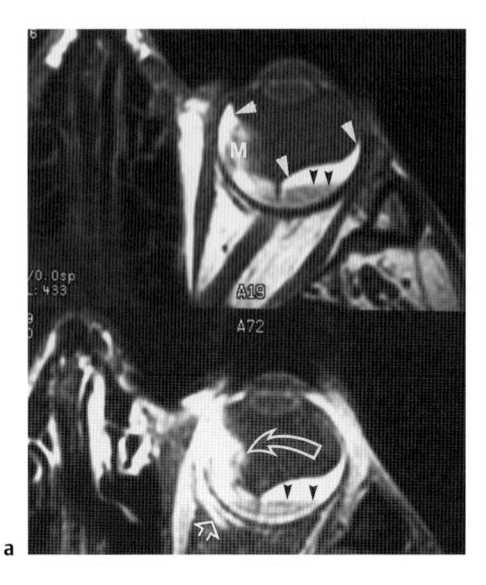

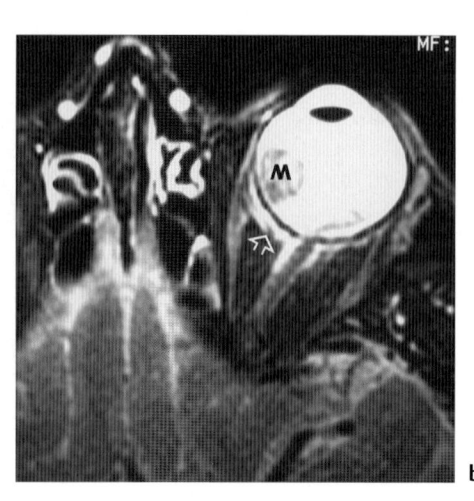

Fig. 2.88 Malignant uveal melanoma and hemorrhagic retinal detachment.
a Axial unenhanced (top) and enhanced (bottom) T1W MR scans, showing a choroidal melanoma (M), with associated hemorrhagic retinal detachment (white arrowheads). Note layered acute hemorrhage (black arrowheads) in the subretinal space. Note enhancement of choroidal melanoma (curved arrow).
b Axial T2W MR scan, showing choroidal melanoma (M). Note hyperintense fluid in the Tenon's space (hollow arrow) with increased contrast enhancement (hollow arrow in **a**) in the Tenon's capsule. There was no tumor extension into the Tenon's capsule. This is probably reactive in nature. We have seen similar changes in Tenon's capsule/space following laser treatment.

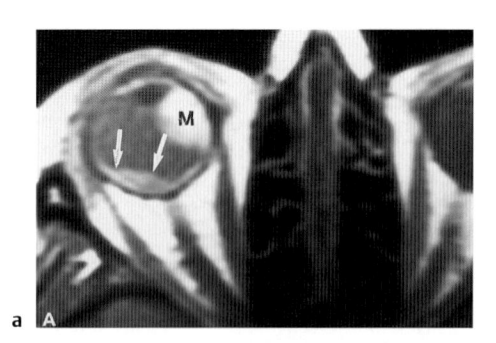

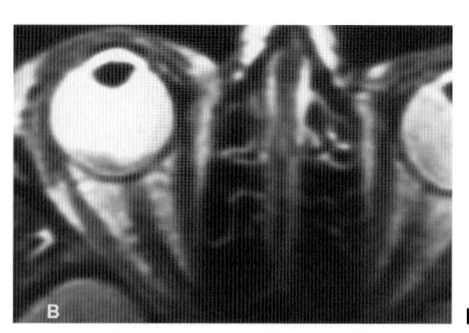

Fig. 2.89 Malignant uveal melanoma with atypical T2 signal characteristic. **a** Axial PW and **b** axial T2W MR scans. This uveal melanoma (M) appears hyperintense on both images. The subretinal hemorrhage (arrows) appears hypointense on the T2W image (**b**). The hypointensity is due to hemorrhage or dense exudate.

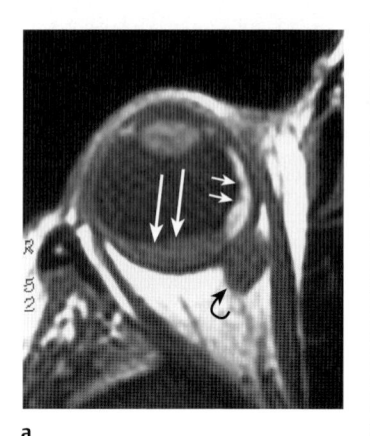

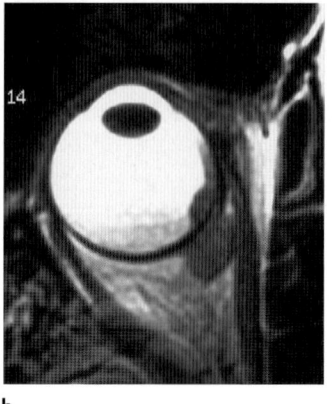

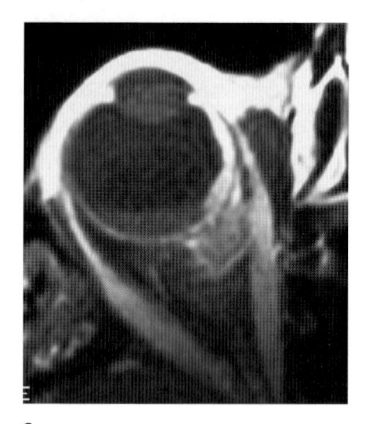

Fig. 2.90 Malignant uveal melanoma with extraocular extension. **a** Axial unenhanced T1W, **b** axial T2W, and **c** axial enhanced fat-suppression MR scans. Note a choroidal melanoma of the right eye (small arrows in **a**), which appears hyperintense on T1W (**a**) and hypointense on T2W (**b**) MR images. Note associated retinal detachment with subretinal exudate (long arrows in **a**). There is a large extraocular extension into the retrobulbar space (curved arrow in **a**).

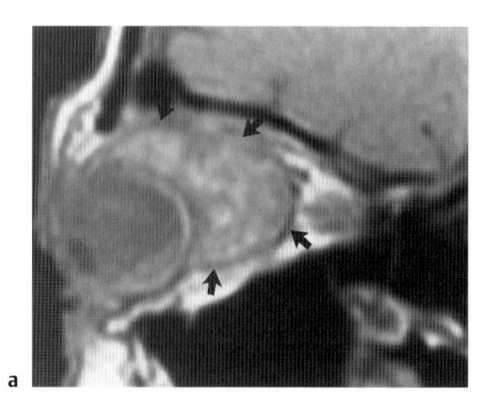

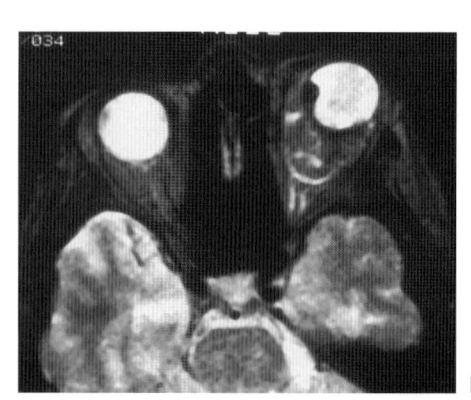

Fig. 2.91 Malignant uveal melanoma with massive retrobulbar extension. **a** Sagittal PW MR scan showing a large retrobulbar mass (arrows) due to extension of a choroidal mass, not seen in this sagittal section. **b** Axial T2W MR scan same patient as in **a** shows a hypointense choroidal melanoma along the nasal aspect of the left globe, along with a large retrobulbar extension. From Mafee MF. Uveal melanoma, choroidal hemangioma, and simulating lesions. Role of MR imaging. Radiol Clin North Am 1998; 36: 1083–1099. With permission.

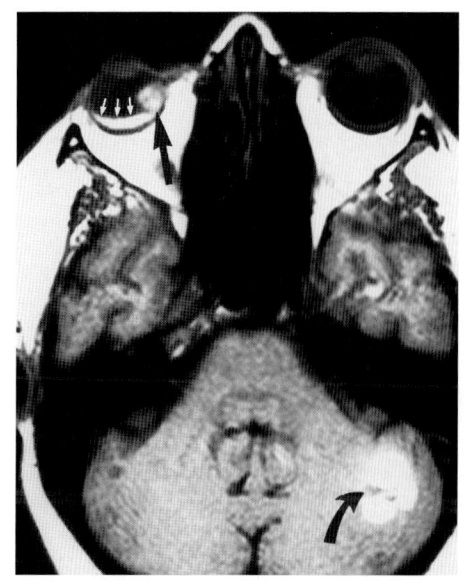

Fig. 2.92 Malignant uveal melanoma with brain metastasis. Axial unenhanced T1W MR scan showing a choroidal melanoma (black straight arrows), subretinal exudate (white arrows), and cerebellar metastasis (curved arrows). The patient had multiple liver metastases, not shown here.

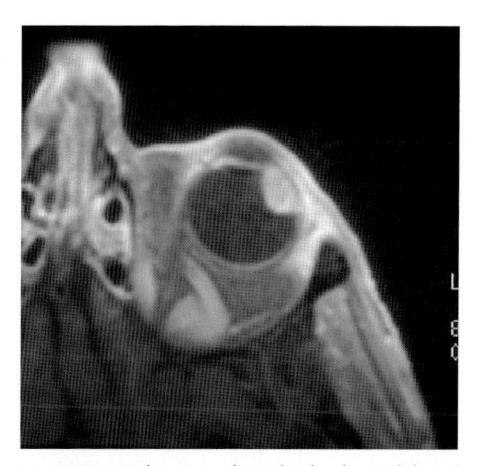

Fig. 2.93 Malignant ciliary body-choroidal melanoma. Axial enhanced fat-suppression T1W MR scan showing a ciliary body-choroidal melanoma.

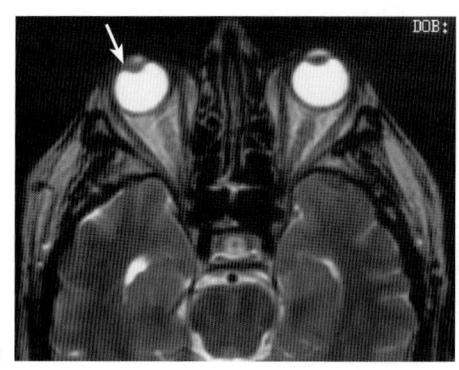

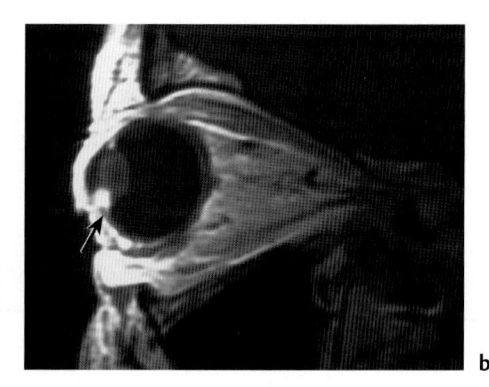

Fig. 2.94 Ciliary body presumed amelanotic tumor. a Axial T2W and b sagittal enhanced fat-suppression T1W MR scans showing a ciliary-iris mass involving the right eye (arrow in a). There is marked enhancement of tumor (arrow in b). The mass was amelanotic and yet appears hypointense on the T2W image (a). The differential diagnoses on the basis of MRI include ciliary body melanoma, ciliary body adenoma (adenocarcinoma), and metastasis.

Uveal melanomas demonstrate moderate enhancement on postgadolinium T1-weighted MR images (Figs. 2.87–2.90). On fat suppression, the T1-weighted MR images demonstrate marked expansion of gray scale with apparent increased signal intensity of the extraocular muscles and lacrimal gland. Therefore, on enhanced fat-suppression T1-weighted MR images, one should take care in evaluation of tumor extension adjacent to the arch of contact of extraocular muscles with the globe. Fat-suppression T1-weighted MR images are very prone to artifacts related to dental fillings or other foreign bodies around the orbit (see Fig. 2.7). Choroidal lesions elevated more than 3 mm are usually well visualized on MRI. Any lesion less than 3 mm is better studied with ultrasound.[4, 5, 12]

The MR characteristics of melanotic lesions are believed to be related to the paramagnetic properties of melanin.[153–155] Damadian et al.[153] reported that, unlike other tumors, melanomas have short T1 relaxation times, which the authors attributed to paramagnetic proton relaxation by stable radicals in melanin.[153] Electron spin resonance (ESR) studies have shown that melanin produces a stable free radical signal under all known conditions, and these stable radicals cause a proton relaxation enhancement that shortens both T1 and T2 relaxation time values.[154] A recent study[156] using synthetic models has shown that the content of free radicals in melanin (10^{18} spins per gram or one free radical per 3000 subunits), at the average concentration of melanin estimated within melanoma tissue (15 mg/ml), is too low to substantially affect the tissue T1 relaxation time.[156] It has been shown that melanin has a high affinity and binding capacity for metal ions,[5, 14, 156] and natural melanin contains a wide variety of bound metals in vivo (iron, copper, manganese, and zinc).[5] This indicates that melanin may have a cytoprotective function as an intracellular scavenger of free metals. The work of Enochs and associates[156] revealed that it is the binding of paramagnetic metals (paramagnetic metal scavenging) that is responsible for the high signal intensities of melanomas on T1-weighted MR images. Uveal melanomas are therefore rather unique in that both T1 and T2 relaxation values are relatively shortened. Hence on T1-weighted images, the lesion should be relatively hyperintense, the opposite of what is predicted for T2-weighted images, and these signal intensities have been observed in the overwhelming majority of uveal melanomas. At times, uveal melanomas may have mixed signal intensity or high signal intensity on T2-weighted scans (Fig. 2.89). The CT and MRI appearance of amelanotic uveal melanoma cannot be differentiated from pigmented melanoma. Ciliary body melanomas appear as nodular lesions with signal characteristics similar to choroidal melanoma (Figs. 2.93, 2.94).

The MRI diagnosis of uveal melanomas and other ocular tumors is greatly enhanced by the use of gadolinium contrast material (Fig. 2.94). Extension of a primary ocular melanoma into

2 Part 1: The Eye

Table 2.7 Differential diagnosis of iris melanomas

- Nevus of iris
- Medulloepithelioma (dictyoma)
- Metastasis
- Juvenile xanthogranuloma
- Adenoma and adenocarcinoma of ciliary epithelium
- Cyst of the iris
- Inflammatory granuloma (sarcoidosis, TB, toxocariasis)
- Leiomyoma of iris and ciliary body
- Choristoma, teratoma
- Ganglioneuroma
- Foreign body

Modified from Mafee MF. The eye. In: Som PM, Curtin HD, eds. Head and Neck Imaging, St. Louis: Mosby; 2003: 441–527.

Table 2.8 Differential diagnosis of choroidal and ciliary body melanomas

- Choroidal nevus including ocular melanocytosis
- Melanocytoma of optic disk
- Melanocytoma of choroid
- Metastasis (often bilateral)
- Choroidal hemangioma
- Choroidal osteoma
- Inflammatory granuloma of the uvea (tuberculosis, sarcoidosis)
- Nodular posterior scleritis
- Choroidal detachment
- Localized choroidal–suprachoroidal hematoma
- Localized subretinal or sub-pigment epithelium hematoma (senile macular degeneration)
- Medulloepithelioma
- Choroidal lymphoma (almost always bilateral)
- Primary ocular adenoma and adenocarcinoma of ciliary epithelium
- Hemangiopericytoma (ciliary body)
- Leukemic infiltration of uvea
- Pseudotumor of uvea
- Massive gliosis of retina
- Astrocytoma of retina
- Uveal neurilemoma/neurofibroma
- Ganglioneuroma
- Granuloma
- Phakomas (phakomatoses)
- Senile macular degeneration (retinal gliosis and hemorrhagic mass)

Modified from Mafee MF. The eye. In: Som PM, Curtin HD, eds. Head and Neck Imaging. St. Louis: Mosby; 2003: 441–527.

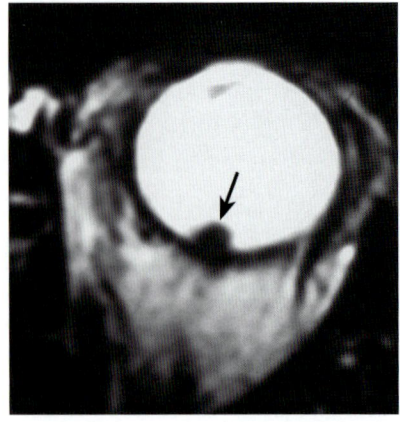

Fig. 2.95 Melanocytoma of the optic disk. T2W MR scan showing a melanocytoma of the optic disk (arrow). The lesion cannot be differentiated from a peripapillary malignant melanoma. From Mafee MF. Uveal melanoma, choroidal hemangioma, and simulating lesions. Role of MR imaging. Radiol Clin North Am 1998; 36: 1083–1099. With permission.

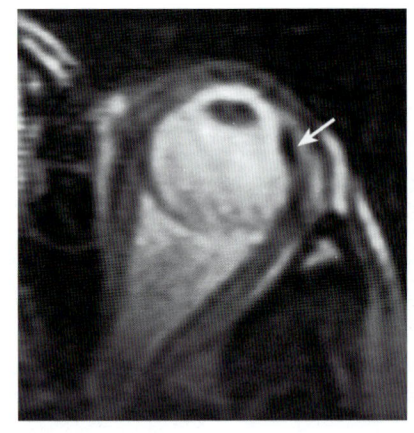

Fig. 2.96 Melanocytoma. Axial T2W MR scan showing a melanocytoma involving the temporal aspect of the left eye. This cannot be differentiated from a discoid malignant uveal melanoma.

the orbit is not common. The size of the extraocular extension is independent of the size of the ocular tumor. Extraocular involvement can be best evaluated on postcontrast fat-suppression T1-weighted MR scans (Fig. 2.90) (see also Fig. 2.97).

Differential Diagnosis

A number of benign and malignant lesions of the eye may be confused with malignant uveal melanomas, and these conditions include choroidal detachment, choroidal nevi, choroidal hemangioma, choroidal cyst, neurofibroma and schwannoma of the uvea, leiomyoma, choroidal lymphoma, uveal metastasis, adenoma of the ciliary body, medulloepithelioma, retinal detachment, and disciform degeneration of the macula.[4,151,157] The most important lesions in the differential diagnosis of iris melanomas and choroidal and ciliary body melanomas are listed in Tables 2.7 and 2.8.

■ Melanocytoma

Melanocytoma is a deeply pigmented benign tumor that usually occurs at the optic disk but may arise anywhere in the uvea. Approximately 50% of melanocytomas develop in blacks, whereas the incidence of malignant uveal melanoma in blacks is less than 1%.[5,14,136] The MRI appearance of melanocytoma is similar to malignant uveal melanoma (Figs. 2.95, 2.96). Melanocytomas appear homogenously very hypointense on T2-weighted MR images (Figs. 2.95, 2.96). Primary malignant melanoma of the optic nerve head is an exceedingly rare tumor.[158] Most melanoma of the optic nerve head is related to extension of a peripapillary choroidal melanoma.[159] Figure 2.97 shows a clinicopathologically proven primary malignant melanoma of the optic disk without choroidal involvement. The clinical appearance simulated a melanocytoma so precisely that the proper diagnosis was delayed. MRI demonstrated a discoid mass with involvement of the optic nerve (Fig. 2.97), and the patient underwent enucleation of the right eye. Even though 17 mm of nerve was obtained, tumor was present at the point of surgical resection. Later, the patient underwent right frontotemporal craniotomy to remove the remainder of the optic nerve to the chiasm.

Pathology 183

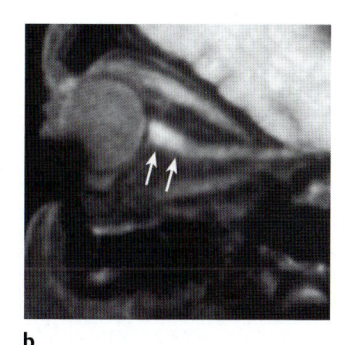

Fig. 2.**97** Malignant melanoma invading the optic nerve.
a Axial T1W MR scan shows an ill-defined mass at the right optic disk. There is increased thickening of the optic nerve (arrows).
b Sagittal enhanced fat-suppression T1W MR scan, showing abnormal enhancement of the right optic nerve. Histological study of enucleated right eye revealed malignant uveal melanoma. There was a 12 mm extension into the optic nerve. From Mafee MF. Uveal melanoma, choroidal hemangioma, and simulating lesions. Role of MR imaging. Radiol Clin North Am 1998; 36: 1083–1099. With permission.

■ Uveal Metastasis

Uveal metastasis can be confused with uveal melanoma both clinically and on imaging. Metastatic lesions of the uvea extend mainly in the plane of the choroid, usually with relatively little increase in thickness. Unlike uveal melanomas, which tend to form a protuberant mass, the metastatic lesions have a mottled appearance and diffuse outline, causing relatively little increase in its thickness.[5, 155] The malignant cells (emboli) gain access to the eye via the bloodstream by means of the short posterior ciliary arteries, and this may be the reason why the site of the majority of metastases occurs in the posterior half of the eye. The most common source of secondary carcinoma within the eye is from the breast or lung. MRI has been shown to be superior to CT in differentiating uveal metastasis from uveal melanoma.[14, 160] However, uveal metastases may have similar signal characteristics to uveal melanomas (Figs. 2.**98**–2.**102**). Gd-DTPA has increased the sensitivity of MRI for detection of uveal metastasis (Figs. 2.**98**–2.**102**).

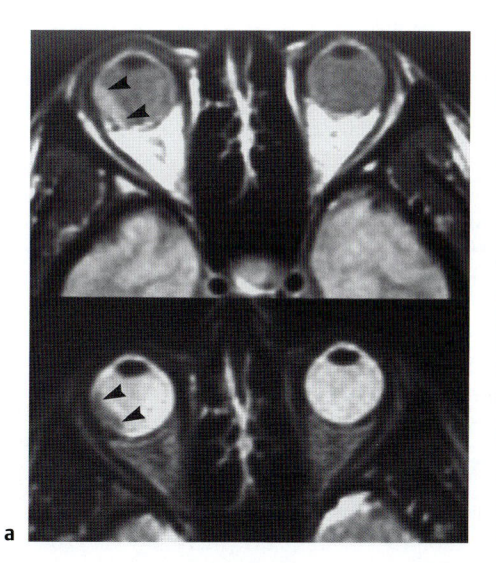

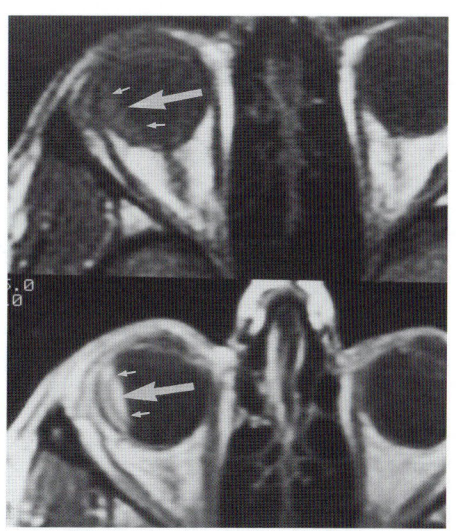

Fig. 2.**98** Choroidal metastasis from primary breast cancer.
a Axial PW (top), and axial T2W (bottom) MR scans showing choroidal metastasis (arrowheads) from primary breast carcinoma.
b Axial unenhanced T1W (top) and enhanced T1W (bottom) MR scans. Note marked enhancement of choroidal metastasis (arrows). From Mafee MF. Uveal melanoma, choroidal hemangioma, and simulating lesions. Role of MR imaging. Radiol Clin North Am 1998; 36: 1083–1099. With permission.

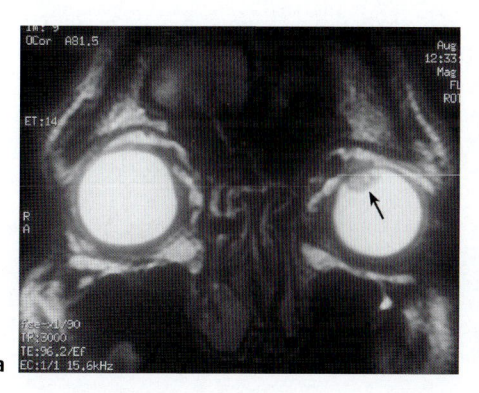

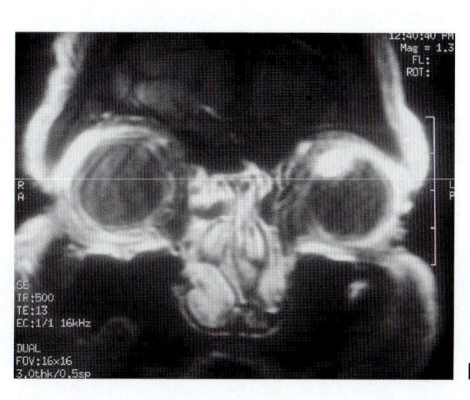

Fig. 2.**99** Choroidal metastasis from hypernephroma.
a Coronal T2W MR scan shows a hypointense mass (arrow) involving the superior medial aspect of the left eye.
b Enhanced coronal T1W MR scan shows marked enhancement of the right ocular tumor. Biopsy confirmed metastasis. Follow-up MRI after proton beam therapy showed complete resolution of the metastasis.

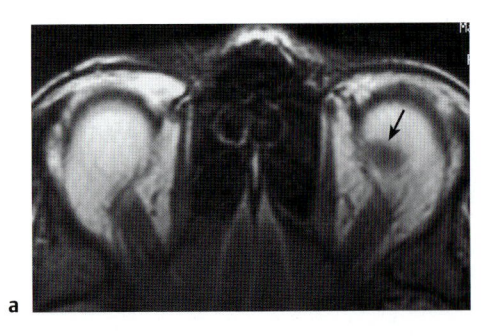

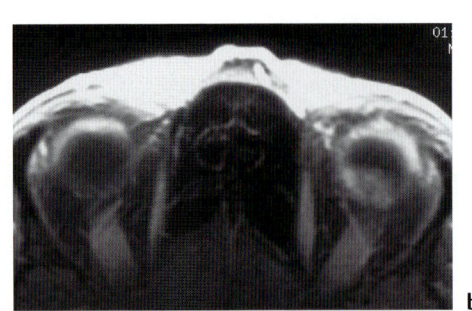

Fig. 2.**100** Choroidal metastasis from thymic carcinoma. **a** Axial T2W and **b** enhanced fat-suppression axial T1W MR scans. There is a mass involving the superior aspect of the left globe (arrow). The lesion was isointense on T1W (not shown here) and hypointense on T2W MR images and showed moderate enhancement on enhanced MR images (**b**).

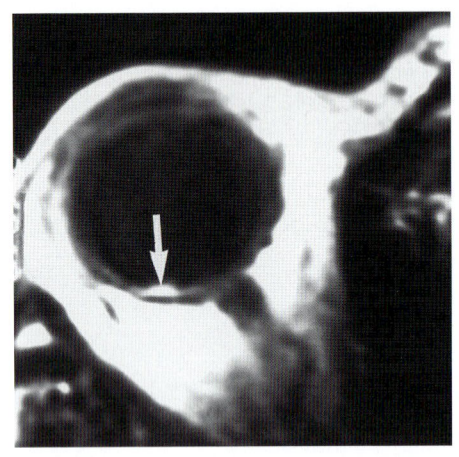

Fig. 2.**101** Choroidal metastasis from prostate carcinoma. Axial enhanced T1W MR scan showing a small metastasis (arrow) involving the posterior aspect of the right globe.

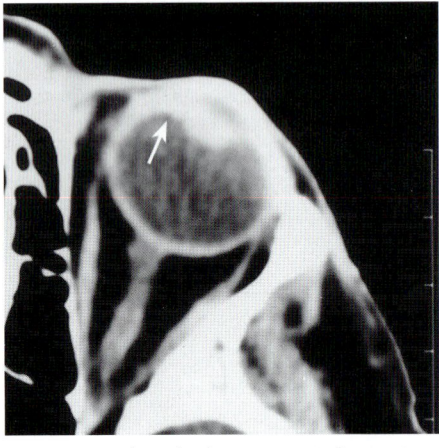

Fig. 2.**102** Ciliary body metastasis from primary lung cancer. Axial enhanced CT scan shows a ciliary body metastasis (arrow).

Table 2.**9** Differential diagnosis of uveal nevi

- Melanoma of iris, ciliary body, and choroid
- Uveal metastasis
- Inflammatory granulomas
- Leiomyoma of iris and ciliary body
- Juvenile xanthogranuloma
- Circumscribed choroidal hemangioma
- Choroidal osteoma
- Choroidal neurilemoma
- Subretinal hematoma
- Suprachoroidal hematoma
- Foreign body in iris

Uveal Nevus

Uveal nevi are congenital lesions, usually recognized late in the first decade of life and most frequently located in the posterior one-third of the choroid.[5] Most choroidal nevi are less than 5 mm in basal diameter and less than 1 mm in thickness, but occasionally lesions of this type attain a basal diameter of 10 mm or more and a thickness of 3 mm or more.[25] Occasionally, choroidal nevi may be associated with shallow serous retinal detachment with or without subretinal neovascularization.[155, 161, 162] The choroidal nevus is one of the most commonly misdiagnosed lesions to be enucleated under the misdiagnosis of malignant melanoma.[149-151] It is sometimes extremely difficult to differentiate these two lesions, with long-term follow-up being the only possible solution.[162] Most of the important lesions in the differential diagnosis of uveal nevi are listed in Table 2.**9**.

Most uveal nevi cannot be visualized by CT and MRI, because of their small sizes. Of two uveal nevi seen on CT scans and MRI, the appearance was identical to uveal melanoma. Both of these patients underwent internal eye wall resection of the lesions, and the result of histopathological study revealed a diagnosis of choroidal nevus.

Choroidal and Retinal Hemangiomas

Choroidal hemangiomas (CH) are usually seen in association with Sturge–Weber disease (encephalotrigeminal syndrome). Retinal angiomas (angiomatosis retinae), on the other hand, are seen in patients with von Hippel–Lindau disease. The diagnosis of choroidal hemangiomas on clinical grounds presents some difficulty. In the majority of cases, the lesion was discovered in the course of a pathological examination; in cases where an ophthalmoscopic examination had been made, the tumor was concealed by the detachment of the retina.[163] The diagnosis of angiomatosis retinae of von Hippel–Lindau is, on the other hand, chiefly dependent on the ophthalmoscopic appearance.

Sturge–Weber disease consists of capillary or cavernous hemangiomas that have a cutaneous distribution along the trigeminal nerve and of a predominantly venous hemangioma of the leptomeninges.[163, 164] The ophthalmic changes consist of an angioma of the choroid, buphthalmos, or chronic glaucoma with atrophy and cupping of the optic nerve.[5, 16, 163] The glaucoma may be explained by the angiomatous changes in the ciliary body or the angle of the anterior chamber.

Two different forms of choroidal hemangioma have been reported: (1) a circumscribed or solitary type not associated with other abnormalities, and (2) a diffuse angiomatosis often associated with facial nevus flammeus or variations of Sturge–Weber syndrome.[5, 14, 163]

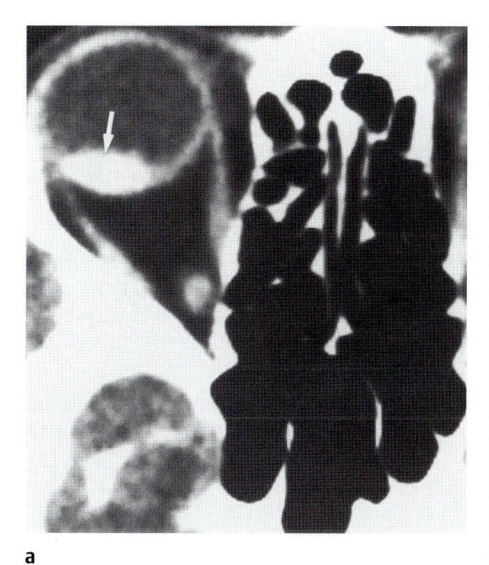

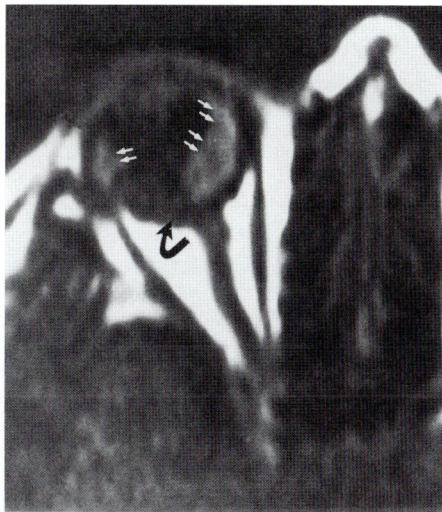

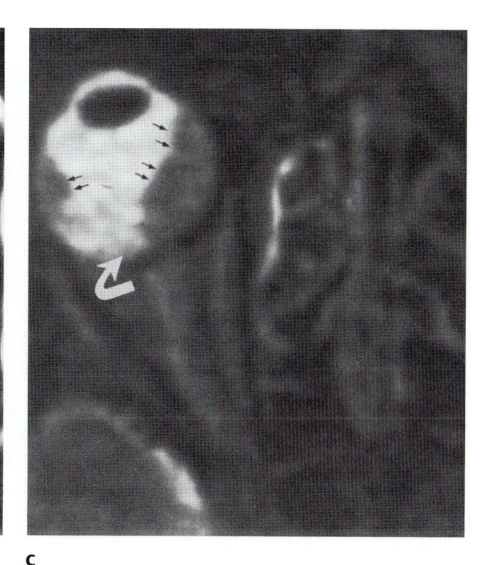

Fig. 2.103 Choroidal hemangioma.
a Postcontrast CT scan shows an intensely enhanced mass compatible with a choroidal hemangioma (arrow).
b Axial T1W MR scan, which was obtained when the patient developed chronic retinal detachment, showing the hemangioma as an isointense image (curved arrow) compared to the vitreous and brain. The subretinal fluid appears hyperintense (short arrows).
c Axial T2W MR scan shows that the hemangioma (curved arrow) now appears hyperintense compared to the brain and isointense compared to vitreous. The chronic subretinal fluid appears hypointense (short arrows). This case, like the case in Fig. 2.**86**, again exemplifies the possibility of misdiagnosing a chronic retinal detachment as a malignant uveal melanoma. Note characteristic anterior limit of detached retina at ora serrata. From Mafee MF. The eye. In: Som PM, Curtin HD, eds. Head and Neck Imaging. St. Louis: Mosby; 1999: 695–812. With permission.

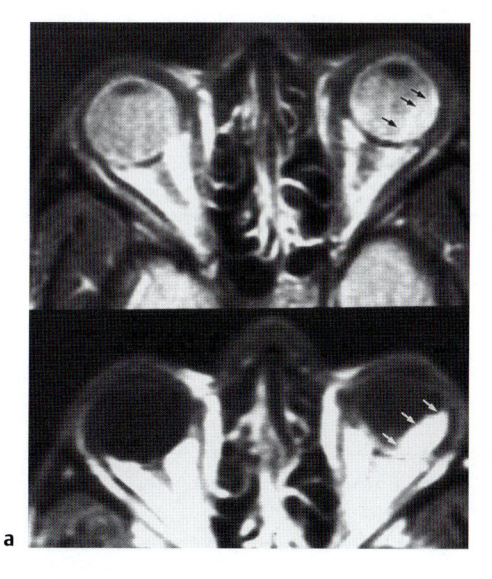

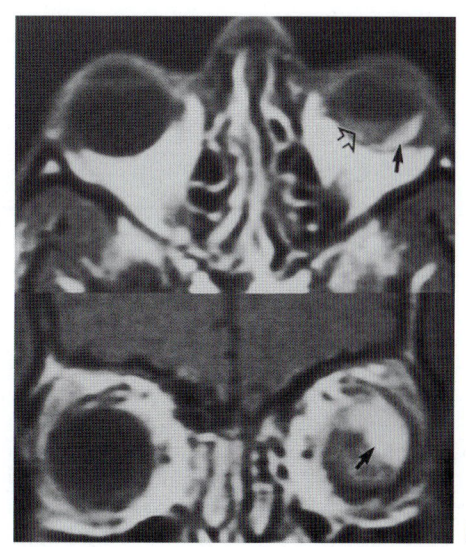

Fig. 2.104 Choroidal hemangioma.
a Axial PW (top) and post-Gd-DTPA contrast T1W (bottom) MR scans showing a slightly hyperintense mass (black arrows). Note the intense enhancement (white arrows).
b Post-Gd-DTPA axial T1W (top) and coronal (bottom) MR scans, same patient as in 2.**104a**, showing enhancement of the choroidal hemangioma (solid arrows). Note the associated dependent subretinal effusion (open arrow).

Clinical Diagnosis

The solitary CH is confined to the choroid, shows distinct margins, and characteristically lies posterior to the equator of the globe.[5,14,163] It is typically seen as a focal reddish orange choroidal tumor located in the juxtapapillary or macular regions of the fundus. In contrast, the hemangioma associated with Sturge–Weber syndrome is a diffuse process that may involve the choroid, ciliary body, iris, and occasionally, other nonuveal tissues, such as the episclera, conjunctiva, and limbus.

Diagnostic Imaging

Although uveal hemangiomas can be diagnosed by ophthalmoscopy, fluorescein angiography, or ultrasound, the clinical diagnosis may present difficulty.[5,18,19,163] A choroidal hemangioma is seen on plain CT as an ill-defined mass, which demonstrates marked enhancement with contrast infusion (Figs. 2.**103a**), and on dynamic CT scanning. In some cases the choroidal angioma may be concealed by the detachment of the retina. On MRI a choroidal hemangioma may be seen as a hypointense area on T1-weighted (Fig 2.**103b**) and hyperintense area on T2-weighted MR images (Figs. 2.**103c**, 2.**104a**). Choroidal hemangiomas demonstrate marked contrast enhancement (Figs. 2.**104**–2.**106**). They are characteristically lenticular in shape because they cannot penetrate the Bruch's membrane to become mushroom in shape. Some choroidal hemangiomas are seen as a moderately intense area in T1-weighted, PW, and T2-weighted images (Figs. 2.**104**, 2.**106**). In some cases, choroidal angioma may be concealed by the detachment of the retina (Fig. 2.**105a**).

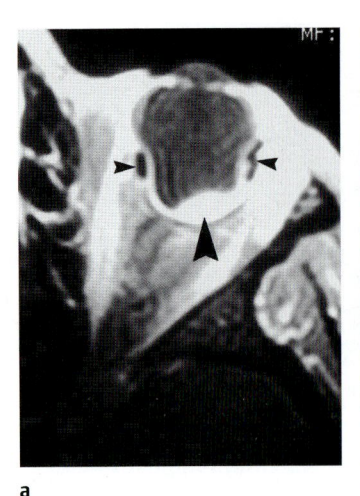

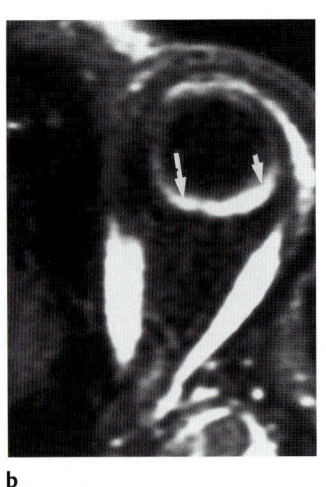

Fig. 2.**105a** Choroidal hemangioma resulting in retinal detachment. Axial enhanced fat-suppression T1W MR scan showing a choroidal hemangioma (large arrowhead). Note scleral banding for the treatment of associated retinal detachment (small arrowheads).
b Axial enhanced fat-suppression T1W MR scan shows a diffuse choroidal hemangioma (arrows) in a patient with Sturge–Weber syndrome.

■ Angiomatosis Retinae and von Hippel–Lindau Disease

Angiomatosis retinae and von Hippel–Lindau disease are interchangeable names for the phakoma of the retinal angioma.[6] This syndrome consists of a vascular malformation of the retina and cerebellum. The retinal lesion usually has the characteristics of a malformation (hamartoma), and the cerebellar lesion consists of a slowly growing cystic vascular tumor. Aside from ocular findings. These patients may develop cerebellar hemangioblastoma, optic nerve or optic chiasm hemangioblastoma, renal cell carcinoma, pheochromocytoma, or cysts in the kidneys or pancreas. The diagnosis of angiomatosis retinae of von Hippel–Lindau disease is chiefly dependent on the ophthalmoscopic appearance. Because of the small size of the lesion (1.5–2 mm), the retinal angiomas are rarely identified on CT and MRI scans. The lesions tend to enlarge progressively, and frequently lead to exudative or tractional retinal detachment complications that lead to phthisis bulbi.[14] Even at this stage the CT and MRI may not show the retinal angioma.

■ Choroidal Hemorrhage and Choroidal Detachment

In discussing the differential diagnosis of uveal melanoma, choroidal hemorrhage and choroidal detachment must be considered because they may be mistaken for a choroidal tumor. A massive choroidal hemorrhage that has failed to rupture the lamina of Bruch may simulate the ophthalmoscopic, CT, and MRI appearances of a choroidal tumor because it forms a round, even globular, dark-brown prominence that is opaque to transillumination. Serous choroidal detachment can be mistaken for choroidal melanoma. Choroidal effusion (uveal effusion) is another pathological entity that can be confused with a ring melanoma.[40, 41] The CT and MRI characteristics of choroidal hemorrhage (Fig. 2.**28**), choroidal detachment (Figs. 2.**26**–2.**32**), and uveal effusion (Fig. 2.**33**) have been discussed earlier in this chapter.

■ Choroidal Cyst

Choroidal cysts are very rare. However, they can be mistaken for a choroidal tumor. They may be bilateral, and they may give rise to retinal detachment.[5, 14]

■ Ocular Lymphoma

The increase in the number of primary lymphomas of the retina and CNS is related to acquired immune deficiency syndrome (AIDS) and other causes of immunodeficiency.[5, 14, 25] In contrast to primary ocular lymphoma, secondary ocular involvement by a systemic malignant lymphoma manifests itself mainly as a uveal tumor. Most often, the disease presents initially with signs of uveitis. Primary lymphoma of the eye is typically bilateral. Ocular lymphoma can be mistaken for choroidal tumor.[5] On MRI ocular lymphomas may have similar signal characteristics to uveal melanomas (Fig. 2.**107**). They are often bilateral. Bilateral melanomas are extremely rare.

■ Ocular Leukemia

Leukemic intraocular infiltration may involve the uvea, retina, optic disk, or vitreous. This is an uncommon ophthalmic disorder and unfortunately is a poor prognostic sign for survival.[5, 14, 25] Leukemic intraocular infiltrates can present in one eye or both eyes. On MRI, leukemic infiltrates may have similar signal characteristics to uveal melanomas, metastasis, and intraocular inflammation (microbial and nonmicrobial) (Fig. 2.**108**).

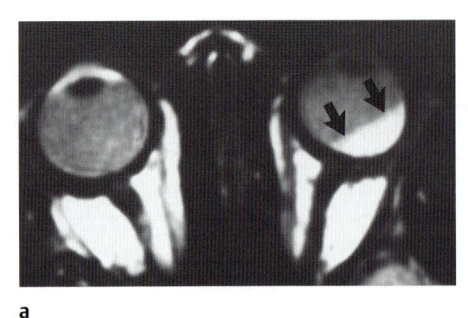

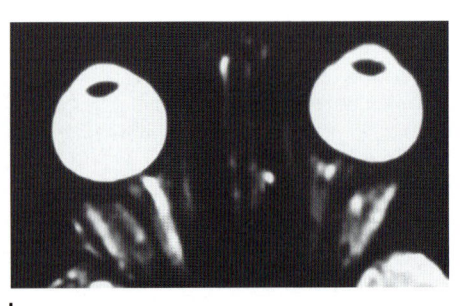

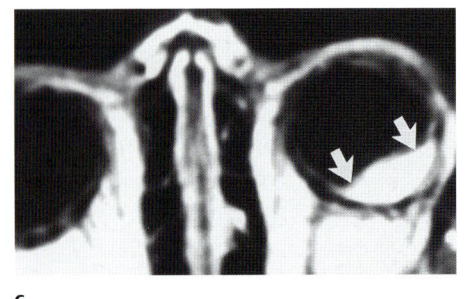

Fig. 2.**106** Choroidal hemangioma in a 5-year-old girl. **a** Axial PW, **b** axial T2W, and **c** axial enhanced T1W MR scans showing a large choroidal hemangioma (arrows). The lesion is hyperintense on PW and isointense to vitreous on T2W MR images.

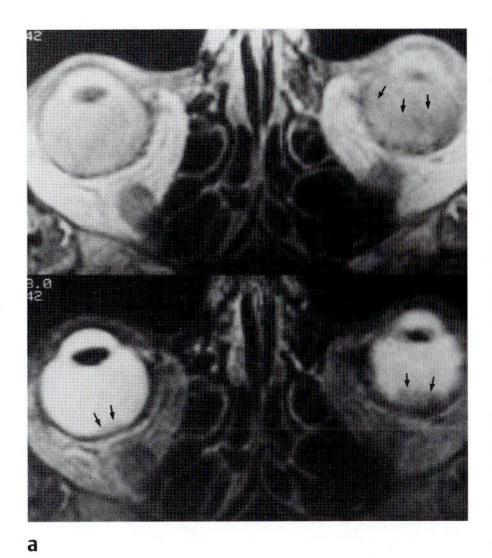

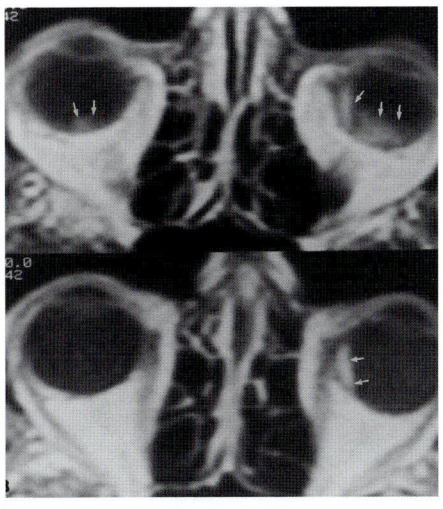

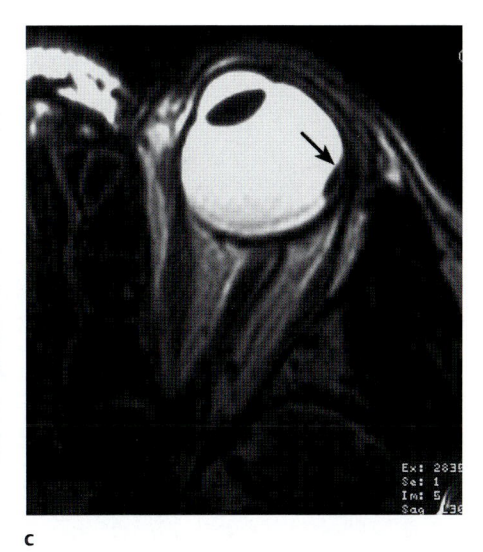

Fig. 2.107 Ocular lymphoma.
a Axial PW (top) and T2W (bottom) MR scans showing an ill-defined masses (arrows) involving both eyes. The lesions appear hypointense on T2W MR images.
b Axial enhanced T1W MR scans. There is moderate enhancement of bilateral ocular lymphoma (arrows).
c Axial T2W MR scan in another patient with ocular lymphoma involving the left eye (arrow). As seen, the MRI characteristics of ocular lymphoma are identical to malignant uveal melanoma. Ocular lymphoma is often bilateral (**a, b**). Bilateral ocular melanoma is extremely rare.

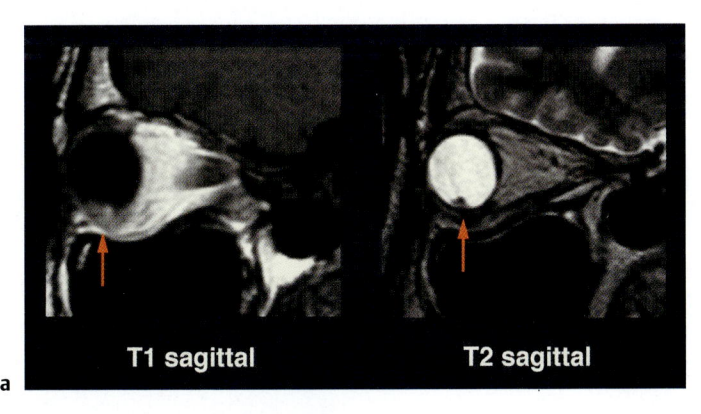

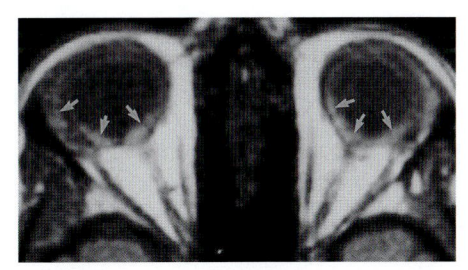

Fig. 2.108 Leukemic infiltration of the eyes. Axial enhanced T1W MR scan showing irregular nodular lesions with enhancement (arrows) compatible with leukemic infiltration. From Mafee MF. Uveal melanoma, choroidal hemangioma, and simulating lesions. Role of MR imaging. Radiol Clin North Am 1998; 36: 1083–1099. With permission.

◁ **Fig. 2.109** Uveal schwannoma.
a Sagittal T1W and T2W MR scans showing a lesion (arrows) involving the inferior aspect of the globe compatible with a uveal schwannoma.
b Gross eye specimen shows uveal schwannoma. Case Courtesy of Yuichi Inoue, MD. Ikedo, Osaka, Japan.
c Axial enhanced T1W MR scan in another patient, known to have neurofibromatosis (NF1), showing plexiform neurofibroma involving the left eyelid, lateral orbit, and left temporal fossa. The left globe is enlarged. The enhancement of the posterior segment of the left eye was due to diffuse neurofibroma of the uvea. Case courtesy of Ahmed Hydayat, MD, AFIP, Washington DC, USA.

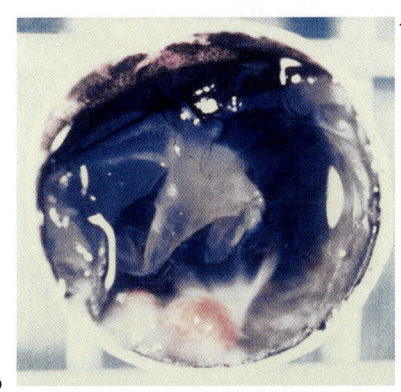

■ Primary Ocular Schwannoma (Neurilemoma)

Primary ocular Schwannoma (POS) is an extremely rare lesion that can cause diagnostic confusion with uveal melanoma. This benign neoplasm arises from the Schwann cells of the peripheral nerves in the uvea or sclera. POS occurs in patients that have neurofibromatosis type 1 or those that do not have this condition. POS usually presents itself as an amelanotic mass in the choroid or ciliary body, indistinguishable clinically, by fluorescein angiography, and by ocular ultrasonography from a uveal melanoma.[25] The CT and MRI appearance of POS (Fig. 2.**109 a, b**) cannot be distinguished from uveal melanoma.[5] At times in patients with neurofibromatosis type 1, the entire choroid may become thickened owing to diffuse neurofibroma (Fig. 2.**109 c**).

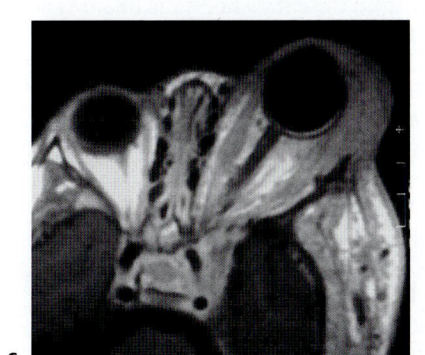

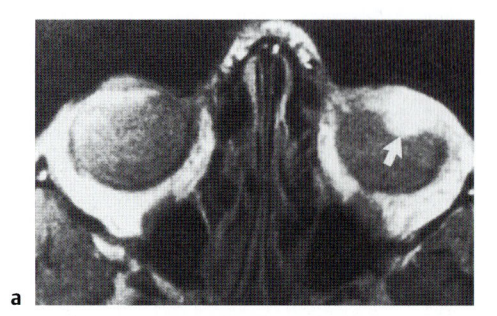

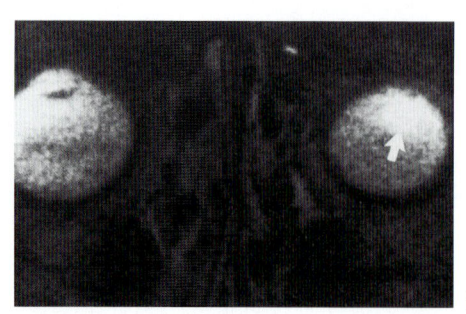

Fig. 2.**110** Mesoectodermal leiomyoma. **a** Axial PW and **b** T2W MR scans show a hyperintense ciliary body mass (arrows). Leiomyomas show marked enhancement on enhanced MR and CT scans, not shown here.

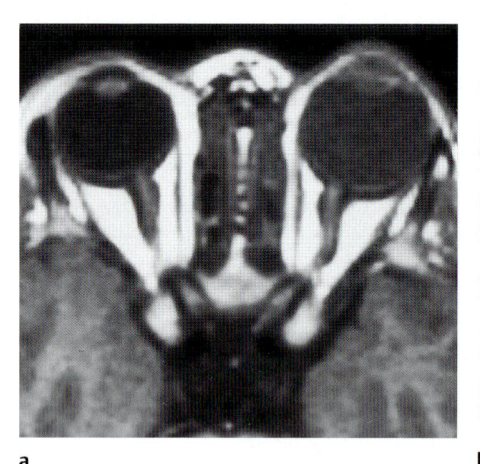

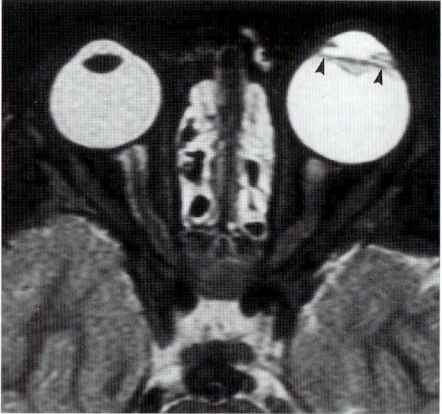

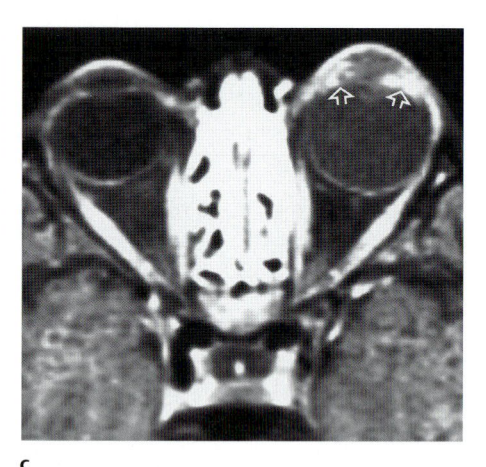

Fig. 2.**111** Medulloepithelioma of the ciliary body. **a** Axial T1W, **b** axial T2W, and **c** axial enhanced T1W MR scans in a child, showing an infiltrative process, compatible with medulloepithelioma, involving the ciliary body (arrows) of the left eye. The enlarged size of the left eye is due to secondary glaucoma. Courtesy of Sattam Lingawi, MD, Saudi Arabia.

▪ Leiomyoma (Mesoectodermal Leiomyoma)

Smooth-muscle tumors of the ciliary body are extremely rare and must be distinguished from other spindle-cell tumors, especially the more common amelanotic spindle-cell melanoma.[165,166] Jakobiec et al.[166] reported two benign tumors of the ciliary body (one in a 37-year-old woman and another in a 20-year-old woman) that were diagnosed as neurogenic tumors by light microscopy but which on electron microscopic examination were composed of smooth-muscle cells with unusual morphological features. They concluded that myogenic and neurogenic characteristics reside in the neural crest origin of smooth muscle of the ciliary body (mesoectoderm) and that these tumors constituted a new nosological entity of myogenic neoplasia. They offered the term mesoectodermal leiomyoma of the ciliary body because the cells of the neural crest that contribute to the formation of bone, cartilage, connective tissue, and smooth muscle in the region of the head and neck have been called mesoectoderm.[166] The MRI appearance of a mesoectodermal leiomyoma of the ciliary body has been reported.[62,91] The lesion appeared as a well-defined, noninfiltrative mass that demonstrated hyperintensity in T1-weighted, PW, and T2-weighted MR images (Fig. 2.**110**). The lesion may be hypointense to vitreous on T2-weighted MR images. There will be marked enhancement on enhanced T1-weighted MR images.[166a] The CT and MRI appearances of ocular leiomyoma and leiomyosarcoma cannot be confidently distinguished from uveal melanoma, uveal neurogenic tumors, and medulloepithelioma.

▪ Ocular Adenoma and Adenocarcinoma

Ocular adenoma and adenocarcinoma may arise from the pigment epithelium of the iris, ciliary body, or retina. Ocular adenoma and primary adenocarcinoma are extremely rare tumors and cannot be differentiated from ocular melanoma by CT and MR imaging (see Fig. 2.**94**).

▪ Medulloepithelioma

Medulloepithelioma, or dictyoma, is a rare primary intraocular neoplasm derived from neuroectoderm, which characteristically arises from the primitive nonpigmented epithelium of the ciliary body.[4,5,167] Medulloepithelioma is usually seen in young children, although it can be seen in adults.[5,167] In the eye, medulloepitheliomas usually arise from the ciliary body and on rare occasions arise in the iris, retina, or optic nerve. To date only six cases at the optic nerve have been reported.[167a] Histologically the tumor resembles embryonic retina and neural tissue. This tumor has been classified as teratoid and nonteratoid types. The nonteratoid type (dictyoma) is pure proliferation of cells of the medullary epithelium. Teratoid medulloepithelioma is distinguished by the additional presence of heteroplastic elements, particularly cartilage, skeletal muscle, and brain tissue. Although most medulloepitheliomas are cytologically malignant, distant metastasis is uncommon.[5] From its point of origin on the ciliary body, the tumor may spread forward along the surface of the iris or backward along the surface of the retina (Figs. 2.**111**, 2.**112**).

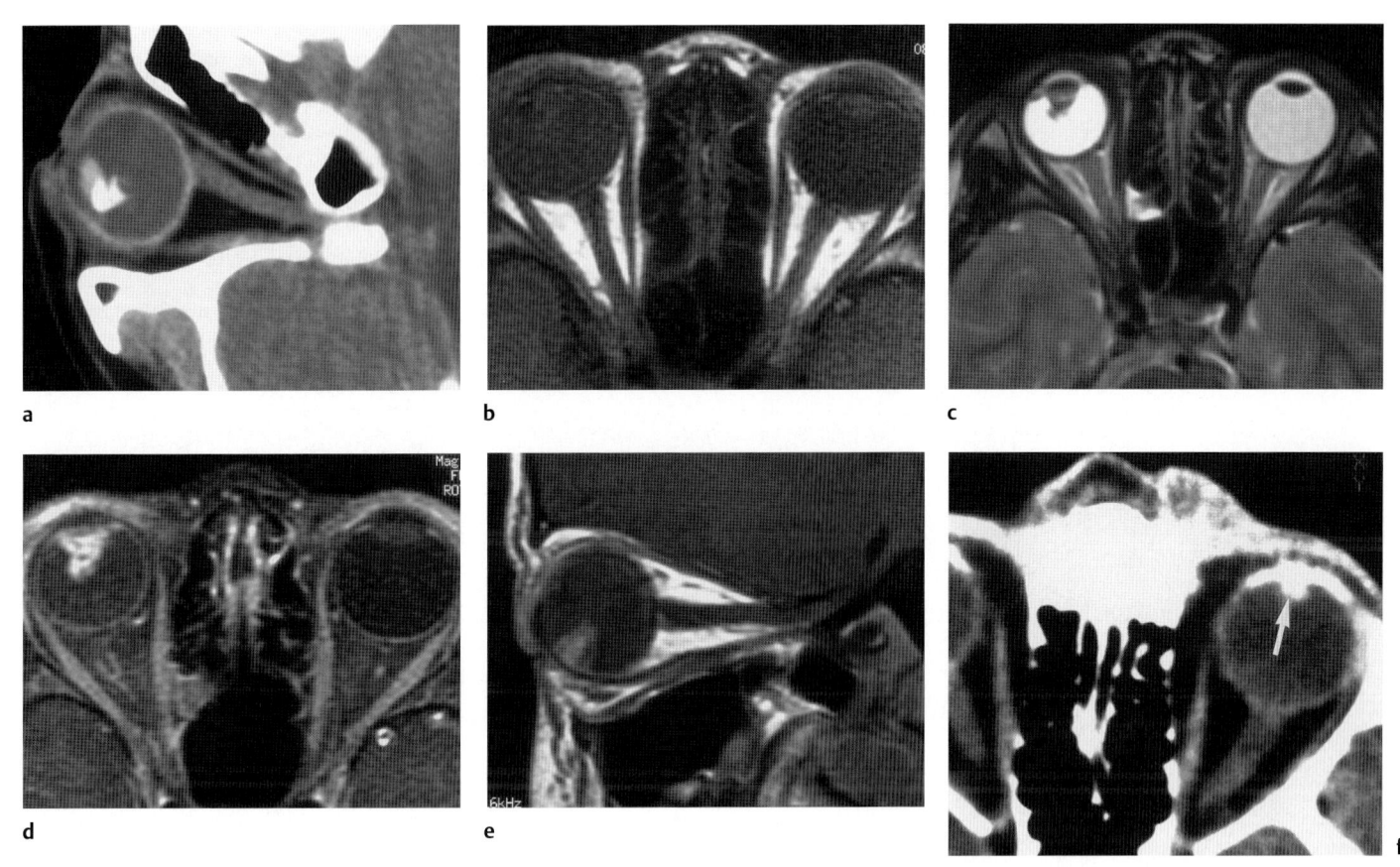

Fig. 2.**112** Medulloepithelioma of the ciliary body with calcification in a 21-month-old boy with leukokoria.
a CT scan shows a calcified mass adjacent to the lens, compatible with a calcified medulloepithelioma. **b** Axial T1W MR scan. **c** Axial T2W MR scan. **d** Axial enhanced fat-suppression MR scan. **e** Sagittal enhanced T1W MR scan.

The medulloepithelioma is hypointense on T2W MR image (**c**) and demonstrates intense enhancement (**d** and **e**).
f Axial enhanced CT scan in a 28-year-old man, showing a medulloepithelioma of the ciliary body (arrow).

Medulloepithelioma of the optic nerve may present a diagnostic challenge (Fig. 2.**113**). The diagnosis of optic nerve medulloepithelioma requires histological examination. Figure 2.**113** shows a malignant teratoid medulloepithelioma.

Medulloepithelioma generally occurs in the first decade of life as a nonpigmented ciliary body mass. In children, medulloepithelioma should be considered in the differential diagnosis of retinoblastoma, granuloma, and juvenile xanthogranuloma. Calcification may be present in medulloepithelioma (Fig. 2.**112a**). In adults, this tumor may simulate amelanotic uveal melanoma and leiomyoma of the ciliary body on ophthalmoscopic evaluation, fluorescein angiography, ultrasonography, CT (Fig. 2.**112f**) and MRI.[21]

■ Senile Macular Degeneration

Macular degeneration in the elderly is a leading cause of legally defined blindness. Arteriosclerosis of the choriocapillaries, dysfunction of the pigment epithelial cells, and loss of neuroepithelial cells are the fundamental causes of the macular degeneration syndrome in the elderly.[6] One of the serious possible complications is hemorrhage, which is limited at first to the subpigment epithelial space but later extends into the subretinal space, eventually forming an organized fibrous scar with consequent loss of almost all function of the involved macula.[5, 12, 14] The CT appearance of senile macular degeneration when associated with subretinal changes may be similar to that of uveal melanoma (Fig. 2.**114a**). However, there may be no ap-

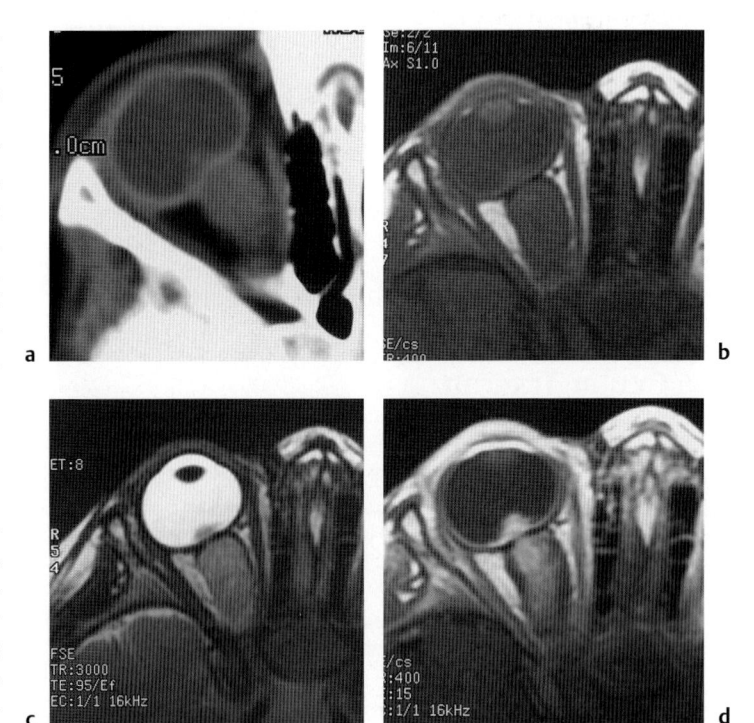

Fig. 2.**113** Medulloepithelioma of optic nerve. **a** Axial unenhanced CT scan shows marked enlargement of the right optic nerve, as well as a mass at the optic disk. **b** Axial T1W, **c** axial T2W, and **d** axial enhanced fat-suppression T1W MR images. The tumor is isointense to brain on T1W and T2W MR Images (**b, c**) and demonstrates marked enhancement (**d**).

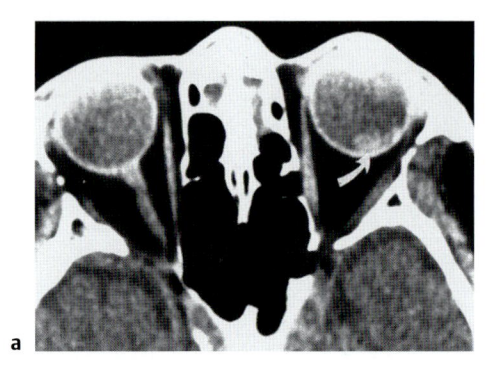

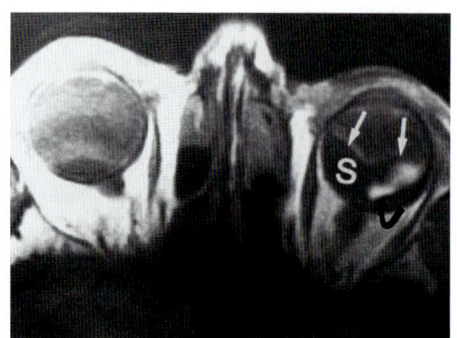

Fig. 2.**114** Macular degeneration associated with intraocular hemorrhage.
a Axial postcontrast CT scan shows an ill-defined mass (arrow).
b Axial T1W MR scan shows changes that are not easily identified on CT (**a**). Note the posterior hyaloid detachment (white arrows). The mass seen on CT is hyperintense (black arrow) and extends to the level of the optic nerve, a finding that suggests this should be in the subretinal space. At surgery this was found to be due to subretinal blood and reactive changes. The hypointensity in the subhyaloid space (S) was related to acute subhyaloid hemorrhage.

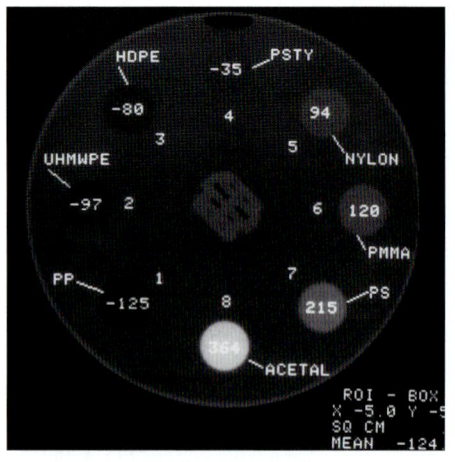

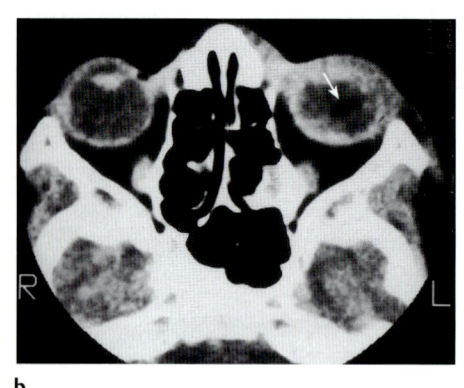

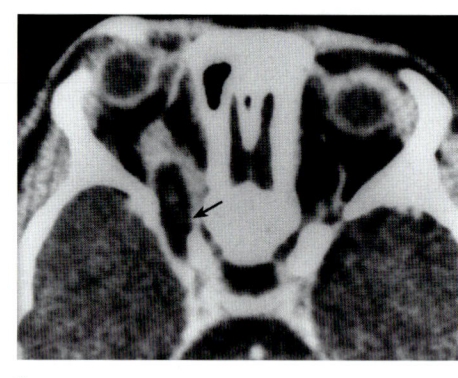

Fig. 2.**115** CT of plastic materials.
a CT scan showing varied computed tomographic densities of different types of plastic materials.
b Ocular plastic foreign body. Axial CT scan shows a hypodense plastic foreign body (arrow) in the left eye. This can easily be mistaken for an artifact.
c Orbital foreign body. CT scan shows a hypodense foreign body (arrow) at the apex of the right orbit, compatible with a piece of a pencil. Case courtesy of Dr. Tan, Taiwan.

parent lesion on unenhanced CT scans, but marked focal linear contrast enhancement in the macular region, related to leaking vessels. The MRI appearance of macular degeneration varies, depending on the stage of the disease. The lesion may show hyperintensity on all pulse sequences because of fluid in the subretinal space, or there may be varied MRI characteristics if there is associated hemorrhage and other complications such as posterior hyaloid detachment and reactive retinal gliosis (Figs. 2.**114b**).

■ Ocular Trauma

Intraocular foreign bodies (IOFBs) constitute a large percentage of ocular traumas and require the use of advanced diagnostic and surgical techniques to successfully manage them.[171–174] Factors that have impacts on prognosis of IOFBs include the size, material, location, trajectory, reactivity, inflammatory response, degree and type of tissue damage, and length of time since injury. The natural course of a retained IOFB varies widely. Siderosis bulbi may develop in an eye with a retained iron-containing IOFB. The siderotic changes may stabilize or regress.[176–177, 178] Retained IOFBs are associated with endophthalmitis in approximately 7–13% of cases.[179]

Optimal CT evaluation of intraocular pathology including IOFBs, in our experience, is with contiguous 1.5 mm axial sections parallel to the canthomeatal line. Thin sections are particularly valuable when evaluating small foreign bodies. Coronal and sagittal reconstructions are helpful in confirming the intraocular location of a foreign body, especially when it is peripherally located. Direct coronal scanning is the best means of evaluating suspected foreign bodies at the 6-o'clock or 12-o'clock positions in the globe. Unfortunately, there are limitations to the sensitivity of CT in the detection of foreign bodies. As an example, a minute copper foreign body, not demonstrated by CT, may cause irreparable retinal damage with progressive loss of vision.[26]

Plastic intraocular foreign bodies are better demonstrated at a narrow window width as described for intraorbital wood fragments.[180, 181] Plastics have a wide range of CT attenuation values (−125 to +364) (Figs. 2.**115**).[182] CT scanning may fail to detect retained nonmetallic foreign bodies, especially when they are composed of organic material such as plastic[183, 184] or wood.

Ultrasound has the disadvantage of being technically difficult to perform; it is usually contraindicated in an open globe and poorly identifies intraocular foreign bodies when more than one is present.[183]

MRI is contraindicated in the presence of a metallic foreign body.[183] Williamson et al.[186] inserted a variety of magnetic and nonmagnetic intraocular foreign bodies into 15 eyes. MRI (performed with a low-field MRI unit) was accurate in locating 11 of the 15 nonmagnetic foreign bodies. The two foreign bodies not detected were located in the suprachoroidal space, suggesting that, as with CT scanning, foreign bodies located near the sclera are hard to detect. In general, MRI is contraindicated in traumatized eyes with suspected ferromagnetic foreign bodies. For

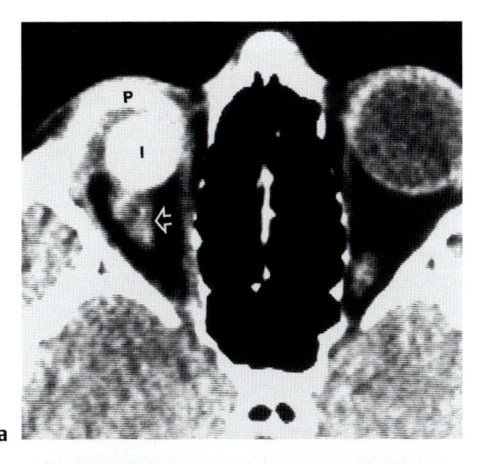

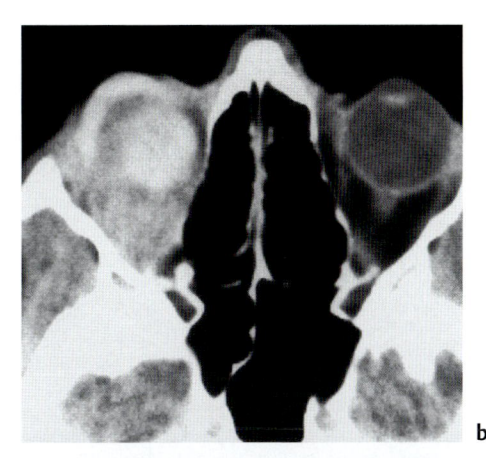

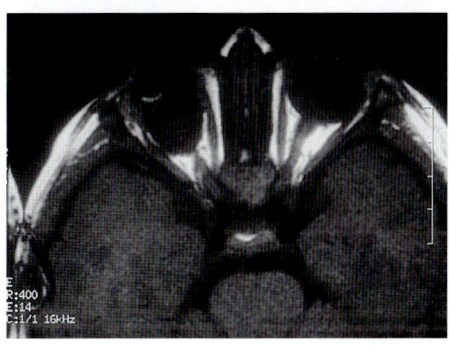

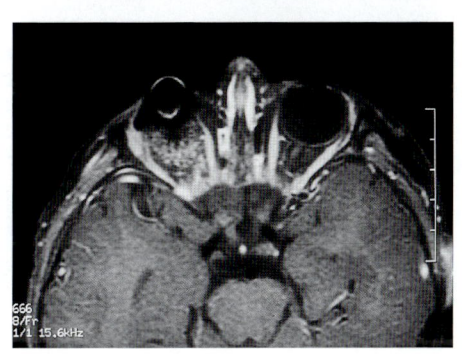

Fig. 2.**116** Migration of an orbital implant due to recurrence of retinoblastoma.
a CT scan shows enucleation of the right eye with placement of an orbital spherical implant (I) and position of the overlying prosthesis (P). Note increased soft tissue (arrow), related to recurrence of tumor.
b CT scan obtained three months later shows massive tumor recurrence. Note medial displacement of the orbital implant.
c, d Enucleation with porous implant. Axial unenhanced T1W (**c**) and axial enhanced fat suppression T1W (**d**) MR scans. Fig. 2.**116d** was taken 3 months after Fig. 2.**116c**. Note the ocular implant and the position of the overlying ocular prosthesis. There is normal enhancement of the right extraocular muscle, consistent with a favorable blood supply. Note enhancement of orbital implant consistent with satisfactory vascularization of the implant.

those with remote history of traumatic foreign bodies, metal (industrial) workers, or other suspected individuals, a high-resolution 1.5 mm thick CT scan of the orbits and 5–10 mm thick CT study of the head is recommended to rule out the possibility of foreign bodies.[188] MRI may be recommended after CT has ruled out the presence of a metallic foreign body.

Lagouros and associates[185] conducted in vitro and in vivo experiments to study MRI of intraocular foreign bodies. Diamagnetic and paramagnetic foreign bodies were imaged without artifact and without movement during the imaging process, while ferromagnetic foreign bodies, as expected, produced large amounts of artifact that prevented meaningful imaging.

The CT appearance of various plastics has been described by Henrikson and associates.[182] The authors concluded that plastics may not be readily apparent on a CT scan when they are small and in the negative CT number range (<–30 Hounsfield units). Using MRI, Lagouros and associates[185] were able to image polystyrene, which had a CT density of –35 Hounsfield units in the study by Henrikson et al.[182] It would seem that all plastics, being relatively hydrogen-poor, would be seen as signal void images in a relatively hydrogen-rich vitreous.[185]

The detection of an intraorbital wooden foreign body is difficult, particularly in cases of apparently minor trauma.[190-194] Orbital radiograhy rarely detects wooden fragments (Fig. 2.**115c**).[193] CT has been shown to detect intraorbital wood associated with metallic paint[195] or a granuloma.[196] Wooden orbital foreign bodies are seen on CT scans as an image of low density; they are often mistaken for air or partial volume averaging of orbital fat (Fig. 2.**115c**). Both experimental[196] and clinical[197] studies have shown that CT has little value in detecting dry wood alone. Tate and Cupples[197] found that the high-resolution CT scanner could not detect small pieces of wood. Myllyla et al.[197] reported that CT scanning did not detect intraorbital wood in their two patients. They noted that wood ranged from –618 to +23 Hounsfield units. Orbital ultrasound also has some limitations in detecting intraorbital wood.[198] Intraorbital wooden foreign bodies are seen on MRI as an image of low signal intensity in T1-weighted, PW, and T2-weighted images. They are particularly well-delineated in T1-weighted MR images.[190] The usefulness of MRI in detecting orbital wooden foreign bodies was first reported by Green et al.[190] These authors recommended that MRI should be done in all cases where orbital penetration by wooden foreign body is suspected and CT scan has not shown a foreign body.

■ Anophthalmic Socket and Orbital Implant

CT and MRI play an important role in the examination of the anophthalmic socket and orbital implant.[168, 200-202] There are two types of orbital implants: (1) spherical orbital implants, used following enucleation; and (2) reconstructive orbital implants, which are used to repair nonsurgical and surgical trauma.[168] The spherical orbital implant is sutured within the intraconal space (Fig. 2.**116**). An external custom-fit, ocular prosthesis is then worn on the ocular surface (Fig. 2.**116**). Spherical orbital implants can be made of nonporous materials, such as silicone and polymethylmethacrylate, or of porous materials, such as porous polyethylene or hydroxyapatite (Fig. 2.**116**).

Postenucleation imaging studies are done to evaluate porous spherical orbital implant vascularization (Fig. 2.**116**), migration, exposure, and orbital recurrence.[168] Enhanced T1-weighted MR imaging has proven to be very valuable in determining the vascularization of hydroxyapatite implants following enucleation (Fig. 2.**116**).[200, 201] Based upon the MRI enhancement within the implant, decision will be made with regard to the appropriate time to surgically integrate the spherical orbital implant with an overlying external ocular prosthesis.[168, 200, 201] The process of integration involves drilling a hole through the overlying soft tissues into the spherical orbital implant and placing an integrational peg.[168] The peg, which is positioned inside the conjunctiva-lined hole, couples with the ocular prosthesis in order to improve motility. Sufficient blood supply to the orbital implant must be present to support a conjunctival lining of the drilled interface. Surgeons may request an MRI study prior to placement of a peg. MRI documentation of fibrovascular ingrowth has broad clinical importance. The rate of fibrovascular ingrowth is both patient-dependent and surgical technique-dependent.[168, 201, 202]

References

1. Snell RS, Lemp MA, eds. Clinical Anatomy of the Eye. Boston, MA: Blackwell Scientific; 1989.
2. Reeh MF, Wobij JL, Wirtschafter JD. Ophthalmic anatomy: a manual with some clinical applications. San Francisco, CA: Am Acad Ophthalmol 1981; 11–54.
3. Edward DP, Kaufmann LM. Anatomy, development, and pathology of the visual system. Pediatr Clin North Am 2003; 50: 1–23.
4. Kaufman LM, Mafee MF, Song CD. Retinoblastoma and simulating lesion: role of CT, MR imaging and use of GD-DTPA contrast enhancement. Radiol Clin North Am 1998; 36: 1101–1117.
5. Mafee MF. Uveal melanoma, choroidal hemangioma, and simulating lesions: Role of MR imaging. Radiol Clin North Am 1998; 36: 1083–1099.
6. Siegelman J, Jakobiec FA, Eisner G, eds. Retinal Diseases, Pathogenesis, Laser Therapy and Surgery. Boston: Little Brown; 1984: 1–66.
7. Rutmin U. Fundus appearance in normal eye. I. The choroid. Am J Ophthalmol 1967: 64: 821–857.
8. Anderson H, Apple D. Anatomy and embryology of the eye. In: Peyman GA, Sanders DR, Goldberg MF, eds. Principles and Practice of Ophthalmology, Vol. 1. Philadelphia: W.B. Saunders; 1980: 3–68.
9. Nakaizumi Y. The ultrastructure of Bruch's membrane. II. Eyes with a tapetum. Arch Ophthalmol 1964; 72: 388–394.
10. Wudka E, Leopold IM. Experimental studies of the choroidal blood vessels. Arch Ophthalmol 1956; 55: 857–885.
11. Mafee MF, Peyman GA. Retinal and choroidal detachments: role of MRI and CT. Radiol Clin North Am 1987; 25: 487–507.
12. Mafee MF: Magnetic resonance imaging: Ocular anatomy and pathology. In: Newton TH, Bilanuik LT, eds. Modern Neuroradiology, Vol. 4. Radiology of the Eye and Orbit. New York: Clavadel Press/Raven Press; 1990: 2.1–3.45.
13. Warwick R, Williams PL, eds. Gray's Anatomy. 35th British Edition. Philadelphia: W.B. Saunders; 1973.
14. Mafee MF. The eye. In: Som PM, Curtin HD, eds. Head and Neck Imaging. St. Louis: Mosby; 2003: 441–527.
15. Balaz EA. Physiology of the vitreous body. In: Schepens CL, ed. Importance of the vitreous body in retinal surgery with special emphasis on reoperations. St. Louis: Mosby 1960: 29–48.
16. Mafee MF, Goldberg MF, Valvassori GE, et al. Computed tomography in the evaluation of patients with persistent hyperplastic primary vitreous (PHPV). Radiology 1982; 145: 713–714.
17. Aguayo JB, Glaser B, Mildvan A, et al. Study of vitrous liquifaction by NMR spectroscopy and imaging. Invest Ophthalmol Vis Sci 1985; 26: 692–697.
18. Mafee MF, Peyman GA, Grisolano JE, et al. Malignant uveal melanoma and simulating lesions: MR imaging evaluation. Radiology 1986; 160: 773–780.
19. Mafee MF, Puklin J, Barany M, et al. MRI and in vivo proton spectroscopy of the lesions of the globe. Semin Ultrasound CT MR. 1988; 9: 59–71.
20. Lagouros PA, Langer BG, Peyman GA, et al. Magnetic resonance imaging and intraocular foreign bodies. Arch Ophthalmol 1987; 105: 551–553.
21. Mafee MF, Goldberg MF. CT and MR imaging for diagnosis of persistent hyperplastic primary vitreous (PHPV). Radiol Clin North Am 1987; 25: 683–692.
22. Penning DJ, et al. MRI imaging of enucleated human eye at 1.5 Tesla. J Comput Assist Tomogr 1986; 10: 55.
23. Aguayo JB, Blackband SJ, Schoeniger J, et al. Nuclear magnetic resonance imaging for a single cell. Nature 1986; 322: 190–191.
24. Mafee MF, Mafee RF, Malik M, Pierce J. Medical Imaging in pediatric ophthalmology. Pediatr Clin North Am 2003; 50: 259–286.
25. Yanoff M. Duker JS. Ophthalmology. Philadelphia: Mosby; 1999.
26. Char DH, Unsold R. Computed tomography: ocular and orbital pathology. In: Newton TH, Bilanuik LT, eds. Modern Neuroradiology, Vol. 4. Radiology of the Eye and Orbit. New York: Clavadel Press/Raven Press; 1990: 9.1–9.64.
27. Levin AV. Congenital eye anomalies. Pediatr Clin North Am 2003; 50: 55–76.
28. Kaufman LM, Villablanca PJ, Mafee MF. Diagnostic imaging of cystic lesions in the child's orbit. Radiol Clin North Am. 1998; 36: 1149–1163.
29. Zion VM. Phakomatoses In: Tasman W, Jaeger EA, eds. Duane's Clinical Ophthalmology, Vol. 5, Chapter 36. J.B. Lippincott, Philadelphia 1990: 1–12.
30. Mafee MF, Pruzansky S, Corrales MM, et al. CT in the evaluation of the orbit and the bony interorbital distance. AJNR 1986: 7:265–269.
31. Brown G, Tasman W, eds. Congenital anomalies of the optic disc. New York: Grune and Stratton; 1983: 97–191.
32. Mafee MF, Jampol LM, Langer BG, et al. Computed tomography of optic nerve colobomas, Morning glory anomaly, and colobomatous cyst. Radiol Clin North Am 1987; 25: 693–699.
33. Mann I. Developmental Abnormalities of the Eye, 2d ed. Philadelphia: J.B. Lippincott; 1957; 74–78.
34. Savell J, Cook JR. Optic nerve colobomas of autosomal dominant heredity. Arch Ophthalmol 1976; 94: 395–400.
35. Pollock JA, Newton TH, Hoyt WF. Transsphenoidal and transethmoidal encephaloceles. Radiology 1968; 90: 442–453.
36. Kindler P. Morning glory syndrome: unusual congenital optic disc anomaly. Am J Ophthalmol 1970; 69: 376–384.
37. Weiter JJ, Ernest JT. Anatomy of the choroidal vasculature. Am J Ophthalmol 1974; 78: 583–590.
38. Capper SA, Leopold IH. Mechanism of serous choroidal detachment. Arch Ophthalmol 1956; 55: 101–113.
39. Mafee MF, Peyman GA. Choroidal detachment and ocular hypotony: CT evaluation. Radiology 1984; 153: 697–703.
40. Mafee MF, Linder B, Peyman GA, et al. Choroidal hematoma and effusion: evaluation with MR imaging. Radiology 1988; 168: 781–786.
41. Peyman GA, Mafee MF, Schulman JA. Computed tomography in choroidal detachment. Ophthalmology 1984; 91: 156–162.
42. Iijima Y, Asanagi K. A new Bscan ultrasonographic technique for observing ciliary body detachment. Am J Ophthalmol 1983; 95: 498–501.
43. Wing GL, Schepens CL, Trempe CL, et al. Serous choroidal detachment and the thickened choroid sign detected by ultrasonography. Am J Ophthalmol 1982; 84: 499–505.
44. Archer DB, Canavan YM. Contusional eye injuries: retinal and choroidal lesions. Aust J Ophthalmol 1983; 11: 251–164.
45. Gole GA. Massive choroidal hemorrhage as a complication of krypton red laser photocoagulation for disciform degeneration. Aust N Z J Ophthalmol 1985; 13: 37–38.
46. Maumenee AE, Schwartz MF. Acute intraoperative choroidal effusion. Am J Ophthalmol 1985; 100: 147–154.
47. Schepens CL, Brockhurst RJ. Uveal effusion. I. Clinical picture. Arch Ophthalmol 1963; 70: 189–201.
48. Chaques VJ, Lam S, Tessler HH, Mafee MF. Computed tomography and magnetic resonance imaging in the diagnosis of posterior scleritis. Ann Ophthalmol, 1993; 25: 89–94.
49. Yan X, Edward DP, Mafee MF. Ocular calcification, radiologic-pathologic correlation and literature review. Int J Neuroradiol 1998; 4: 81–96.
50. Howard GM, Ellsworth RM. Differential diagnosis of retinoblastoma: a statistical survey of 500 children. I. Relative frequency of the lesions which stimulate retinoblastoma. Am J. Ophthalmol 1965; 60: 610–618.
51. Popoff NA, Ellsworth RM. The fine structure of retinoblastoma: in vivo and in vivo observations. Lab Invest 1971; 25: 389–402.
52. Tso MOM, Fine BS, Zimmerman LE, et al. Photoreceptor elements in retinoblastoma: a preliminary report. Arch Ophthalmol 1969; 82: 5;7–59.
53. Tso MOM, Fine BS, Zimmerman LE. The nature of retinoblastoma. I. Photoreceptor differentiation: a clinical and histopathologic study. Am J Ophthalmol 1970; 69: 339–349.
54. Tso MOM. Clues to the cells of origin of retinoblastoma. Int Ophthalmol Clin 1980; 20(2): 191–210.
55. Kodilyne HC. Retinoblastoma in Nigeria: problems in treatment. Am J Ophthalmol 1967; 63: 467–481.

56 Abramson DH, Ellsworth RM, Tretter P, et al. Treatment of bilateral groups I through III retinoblastoma with bilateral radiation. Arch Ophthalmol 1981; 99: 1761–1762.

57 Kyritsis AP, Tsokos M, Triche TJ, et al. Retinoblastoma: origin from a primitive neuroectodermal cell? Nature 1984; 307: 471–473.

58 Tso MOM, Zimmerman LE, Fine BS, et al. A cause of radioresistance in retinoblastoma: photoreceptor differentiation. Trans Am Acad Ophthalmol Otolaryngol 1970 b; 74: 959–969.

59 Jenson RD, Miller RW. Retinoblastoma: epidemiologic characteristics. N Engl J Med 1971; 285: 307–311.

60 Abramson DH, Ellsworth RM, Kitchin DF, Tung G. Second nonocular tumors in retinoblastoma survivors. Ophthalmology 91: 1351–1255, 1984.

61 Pendergrass TW, Davis S. Incidence of retinoblastoma in the United States. Arch Ophthalmol 1980; 98: 1204–1210.

62 Mafee MF, Goldberg MF, Greenwald MJ, et al. Retinoblastoma and simulating lesions: role of CT and MR imaging. Radiol Clin North Am 1987; 25: 667–681.

63 Ellsworth RM. The management of retinoblastoma. Trans Am Ophthalmol Soc 1969; 67: 462–534.

64 Lennox EL, Draper GJ, Sanders BM. Retinoblastoma: a study of natural history and prognosis of 268 cases. Br Med J 1975; 3: 731–734.

65 Abramson DH. Retinoblastoma: diagnosis and management. Cancer J Clin 1982; 32: 130–140.

66 Kundson AG. Retinoblastoma: a prototype heredity neoplasm. Semin Oncol 1978; 5: 57–60.

67 Kundson AG, Jr. Mutation and cancer: a statistical study of retinoblastoma. Proc Natl Acad Sci USA 1971; 68: 820–823.

68 Lele KP, Penrose LS, Stallard HB. Chromosome deletion in a case of retinoblastoma. Ann Hum Genet 1963; 27: 171–174.

69 Kundson AG Jr., Meadows AT, Nichols WW, et al. Chromosomal deletion and retinoblastoma. N Engl J Med 1976; 295: 1120–1123.

70 Yunis JJ, Ramsey N. Retinoblastoma and subband deletion chromosome 13. Am J Dis Child 1978; 132: 161–163.

71 Cavenee WK, Murphree AL, Shul MM, et al. Prediction of familial predisposition to retinoblastoma. N Engl J Med 1986; 314: 1201–1207.

72 Sparkes RS, Sparkes MC, Wilson MG, et al. Regional assignment of genes for human esterase D and retinoblastoma to chromosome band 13 q14. Science 1980; 208: 1042–1044.

73 Sparkes RS, Murphree Al, Lingua RW, et al. Gene for hereditary retinoblastoma assigned to human chromosome 13 by linkage to esterase D. Science 1983; 219: 971–973.

74 Motegi T. High rate of detection of 13 q-14 deletion mosaicism among retinoblastoma patients (using more extensive methods). Hum Genet 1982; 61: 95–97.

75 Seidman DJ, Shields JA, Augsburger JJ, et al. Early diagnosis of retinoblastoma based on dysmorphic features and karyotype analysis. Ophthalmology 1987; 94: 663–666.

76 Jakobiec FA, Tso MOM, Zimmerman LE, et al. Retinoblastoma and intracranial malignancies. Cancer 1977; 39: 2048–2058.

77 Bader JL, Miller RW, Meadows AT, et al. Trilateral retinoblastoma. Lancet 1980; 2: 582–583.

78 Bader JL, Meadows AT, Zimmerman LE, et al. Bilateral retinoblastoma with ectopic intracranial retinoblastoma: trilateral retinoblastoma. Cancer Genet Cytogenet 1982; 5: 203–213.

79 Judisch GF, Patil SR. Concurrent heritable retinoblastoma, pinealoma and trisomy X. Arch Ophthalmol 1981; 99: 1767–1769.

80 Stefanko SZ, Manschot WA. Pineaoblastoma with retinoblastomas differentiation. Brain 1979; 102: 321–332.

81 El-Naggar S, Kaufman LM, Chapman LI, Miller MT, Mafee MF. Tetralateral retinoblastoma. Ann Ophthalmol 1995; 27(6): 360–363.

82 Schulman JA, Peyman GA, Mafee MF, et al. The use of magnetic resonance imaging in the evaluation of retinoblastoma. J Pediatr Ophthalmol Strabismus 1986; 23: 144–147.

83 Robertson DM, Campbell RJ. Analysis of misdiagnosed retinoblastoma in a series of 726 enucleated eyes. Mod Probl Ophthalmol 1977; 18: 156–159.

84 Char DH. Current concepts in retinoblastoma. Ann Ophthalmol 1980; 12: 792–804.

85 Haik BG, Saint Louis L, Smith ME, et al. Magnetic resonance imaging in the evaluation of leukokoria. Ophthalmology 1985; 92: 1143–1152.

86 Char DH, Hedges TR, Norman D. Retinoblastoma: CT diagnosis. Ophthalmology 1984; 91: 1347–1350.

87 Goldberg BB, Kotler MN, Ziskin MD. Diagnostic Uses of Ultrasound. New York: Grune and Stratton, 1975; 100.

88 Danziger A, Price MI. CT findings in retinoblastoma. AJR 1979; 133: 695–702.

89 Daniel AF, Shurin SB, Bardenstein DS. Trilateral retinoblastoma: two variations. AJNR 1995; 16: 166–170.

90 Provenzale JM, Weber AL, Klintworth GK, et al. Radiologic-pathologic correlation. Bilateral retinoblastoma with coexistent pineaoblastoma (trilateral retinoblastoma). AJNR 1995; 16: 157–165.

91 Mafee MF, Goldberg MF, Cohen SB, et al. Magnetic resonance imaging versus computed tomography of leukokoric eyes and use of in vitro proton magnetic resonance of retinoblastoma. Ophthalmology 1989; 96(7): 965–976.

92 Warburg M. Retinal malformations: aetiological heterogeneity and morphological similarity in congenital retinal non-attachment and falsiform folds. Trans Ophthalmol Soc UK 1979; 99: 272–283.

93 Ohba N, Watanabe S, Fujita S. Primary vitreoretinal dysplasia transmitted as an autosomal recessive disorder. Br J Ophthalmol 1981; 65: 631–635.

94 Goldberg MF, Mafee MF. Computed tomography for diagnosis of persistent hyperplastic primary vitreous (PHPV). Ophthalmology 1983; 90: 442–451.

95 Peyman GA, Sanders DR. Vitreous and vitreous surgery. In: Peyman GA, Sanders DR, Goldberg MF, eds. Principles and Practice of Ophthalmology, Vol. 2. Philadelphia: W. B. Saunders; 1980: 1327–1401.

96 Katz NNK, Margo CE, Dorwart RH. Computed tomography with histopathologic correlation in children with leucocoria. J Pediatr Ophthalmol Strabismus 1984; 21: 50–56.

97 Caudhill JW, Streeten BW, Tso MOM. Phacoanaphylactoid in persistent hyperplastic primary vitreous. Ophthalmology 1985; 92: 1153–1158.

98 Liberfarb RM, Eavey RD, DeLong GR, et al. Norrie's disease: a study of two families. Ophthalmology 1985; 92: 1445–1451.

99 Norrie G. Causes of blindness in children: twenty-five years experience of Danish Institutes for the blind. Acta Ophthalmol 1927; 5: 357–386.

100 Warburg M. Norrie's disease: a new hereditary bilateral pseudotumour of the retina. Acta Ophthalmol 1961; 39: 757–772.

101 Warburg M. Norrie's disease (atrofia bulborum hereditaria): a report of eleven cases of hereditary bilateral pseudotumour of the retina, complicated by deafness and mental deficiency. Acta Ophthalmol 1963; 41: 134–146.

102 Warburg M. Norrie's disease: a congenital progressive oculo-ocoustico cerebral degeneration. Acta Ophthalmol 1966; suppl 89.

103 Holmes LB. Norrie's disease: an X-linked syndrome of retinal malformation, mental retardation, and deafness. J Pediatr 1971; 79: 89–92.

104 Apple DJ, Fishman GA, Goldberg MF. Ocular histopathology of Norrie's disease. Am J Ophthalmol 1974; 78: 196–203.

105 Blodi FC, Hunter WS. Norrie's disease in North America. Doc Ophthalmol 1969; 26: 434–450.

106 Mecke S, Passarge E. Encephalocele, polycystic kidneys and polydactyly as an autosomal recessive trait simulating certain other disorders: the Meckel syndrome. Ann Genet 1971; 14: 97–103.

107 Warburg M. The heterogeneity of microphthalmia in the mentally retarded. Birth Defects 1971; 7: 136–154.

108 Chemke J, Czernobilsky B, Mundel G, et al. A familial syndrome of central nervous system and ocular malformation. Clin Genet 1975; 7: 1–7.

109 Chan CC, Egbert PR, Herrick MK, et al. Oculocerebral malformations: a reappraisal of Walker's "lissencephaly." Arch Neurol 1980; 37: 104–108.

110 Pagon RA, Chandler JW, Collie MR, et al. Hydrocephalus, agyria, retinal dysplasia, encephalocele (HARD±E) syndrome: an autosomal recessive condition. Birth Defects 1978; 14(6B): 233–241.

111 Levine RA, Gray DL, Gould N, et al. Warburg syndrome. Ophthalmology 1983; 90: 1600–1603.

112 Warburg M. Hydrocephaly, congenital retinal nonattachment, and congenital falciform fold. Am J Ophthalmol 1978; 85: 88–94.

113 Eller AW, Jabbour NM, Hirose T, et al. Retinopathy of prematurity: the association of a persistent hyaloid artery. Ophthalmology 1987; 94: 444–448.

114 Ashton N, Ward B, Sperpell G. Role of oxygen in the genesis of retrolental fibroplasia: a preliminary report. Br J Ophthalmol 1953; 37: 513–520.

115 Michaelson IC. Retrolental fibroplasia. In: Michaelson IC, ed. Textbook of the Fundus of the Eye. New York: Churchill Livingstone; 1980: 303–315.

116 Coats G. Forms of retinal disease with massive exudation. Royal London Ophthalmologic Hospital Reports 1908; 17: 440–525.

117 Mafee MF, Inoue Y, Mafee RF. Ocular and orbital imaging. Neuroimaging Clin North Am 1996; 6: 29–318.

118. Woods AC, Duke JR. Coats disease. I. Review of the literature, diagnostic criteria, clinical findings, and plasma lipid studies. Br J Ophthalmol 1963; 47: 385–412.
119. Senft SH, Hidayat AA, Cavender JC. Atypical presentation of Coats disease. Retina 1994; 14: 36–38.
119a. Silodor SW, Augsburger JJ, Shields JA, et al. Natural history and management of advanced Coats disease. Ophthalmic Surg 1988; 19: 89–93.
120. Edward DP, Mafee MF, Valenzuela EG, Weiss RA. Coats disease and persistent hyperplastic primary vitreous: role of MRI and CT. Radiol Clin North Am. 1988; 36: 1119–1131.
121. Sherman JL, McLean IW, Brallier DR. Coats disease. CT pathologic correlation in two cases. Radiology 1983; 146: 77–78.
122. Shields JA, Shields CL. Intraocular Tumors: A Text and Atlas. Philadelphia: W.B. Saunders; 1992.
123. Chang M, McLean IW, Merritt JC. Coats disease: a study of 62 histologically confirmed cases. J Pediatr Ophthalmol Strabismus 1984; 21: 163–168.
123a. Pe'er J. Calcifications in Coats disease. Am J Ophthalmol 1988; 106: 742–743.
124. Margo CE, Katz NN, Wertz FD, et al. Sclerosing endophthalmitis in children: computed tomography with histopathologic correlation. Pediatr Ophthalmol Strabismus 1983; 20: 180–184.
125. Wilder HC. Nematode endophthalmitis.Trans Am Acad Ophthalmol Otolaryngol 1950; 55: 99–104.
126. Zinkham WM. Visceral larva migrans: a review and reassessment indicating two forms of clinical expression, visceral and ocular. Am J Dis Child 1978; 132: 627–633.
127. Reesner FH, Aaberg TM, VanHorn DL. Astrocytic hamartoma of the retina not associated with tuberous sclerosis. Am J Ophthalmol 1978; 86: 688–698.
128. Zimmerman LE. Ocular lesions of juvenile xanthogranuloma. Trans Am Acad Ophthalmol Otolaryngal 1965; 69: 412.
129. Wertz FD, Zimmerman LE, McKeown CA, et al. Juvenile xanthogranuloma of the optic nerve, disk, retina, choroid. Ophthalmology 1982; 89: 1331–1335.
130. Shields CL, Shields JA, Buchanon HW: Solitary orbital involvement in juvenile xanthogranuloma. Arch Ophthalmol 1990; 108: 1587.
131. Augsburger JJ, Guthoff R. Benign intraocular tmors. In: Yanoff M, Duker JS, eds. Ophthalmology. St. Louis: Mosby; 1999: 9.9.1–9.14.2.
132. Mafee MF. Calcifications of the eye. Head and Neck Disorders (Fourth Series) Test and Syllabus. Am College Radiol, Reston, VA 1992: 70–116.
133. Friedman AM, Henkind P, Gartner S. Drusen of the optic disk: a histopathological study. Trans Ophthalmol Soc UK 1975; 95: 4–9.
134. McMahon RT. Anatomy, congenital anomalies, and tumors. In: Peyman CA, Sanders DR, Goldberg MF, eds. Principles and Practice of Ophthalmology. Philadelphia: W.B. Saunders; 1980: 1491–1553.
135. Yanoff M, Fine BS. Ocular Pathology. A Text and Atlas. Hagerstown, MD: Harper and Row, 1975; 831.
136. Depotter P, Shields JA, Shields CL, eds. MRI of the Eye and Orbit. Philadelphia: J.B. Lippincott; 1995: 35–92.
137. Callender GR. Malignant melanotic tumors of the eye: a study of histologic types in III cases. Trans Am Acad Ophthalmol Otolaryngol 1931; 36: 131–142.
138. McLean JW, Foster WU, Zimmerman LE. Prognostic factors in small malignant melanomas of choroidal and ciliary body. Arch Ophthalmol 1977; 95: 148–58.
139. Augsburger JJ, Damato BE, Bornfeld N. Malignant intraocular tumors. In Yanoff M, Duker JS, eds. Ophthalmology. St. Louis: Mosby; 1999: 9.3.1–9.8.4.
140. Peyman GA, Juarez CP, Diamond DG, et al. Ten years experience with eye wall resection for uveal melanomas. Ophthalmology 1984; 91: 1720–1725.
141. Donders PC. Malignant melanoma of the choroid. Trans Ophthalmol Soc UK 1973; 93: 745–751.
142. Zimmerman LE, McLean IW, Foster WD. Does enucleation of the eye containing a malignant melanoma prevent or accelerate the dissemination of tumor cells? Br J Ophthalmol 1978; 62: 420–425.
143. Duffin RM, Straatsma BR, Foos RY, et al. Small malignant melanoma of the choroid with extraocular extension. Arch Ophthalmol 1981; 99: 1827–1830.
144. Char DH. The management of small choroidal melanomas. Surv Ophthalmol 1978; 22: 377–387.
145. Canny CLB, Shields JA, Kay ML. Clinically stationary choroidal melanoma with extraocular extension. Arch Ophthalmol 1978; 96: 436–439.
146. Ruiz RS. Early treatment in malignant melanomas of the choroid. In: Brockhurst RJ, Boruchoff SA, Hutchinson BR, et al, eds. Controversy in Ophthalmology. Philadelphia: W.B. Saunders; 1977: 604–610.
147. Manschot WA, VanPeperzeel HA. Choroidal melanoma: enucleation or observation? A new approach. Arch Ophthalmol 1980; 98: 71–77.
148. Mauriello JA Jr., Zimmerman LE, Rothstein TB. Intrachoroidal hemorrhage mistaken for malignant melanoma. Ann Ophthalmol 1983; 15: 282–284.
149. Ferry AP. Lesions mistaken for malignant melanoma of the posterior uvea: a clinicopathologic analysis of 100 cases with ophthalmoscopically visible lesions. Arch Ophthalmol 1964; 72S: 463–469.
150. Shields JA, Zimmerman LE. Lesions simulating malignant melanoma of the posterior uvea. Arch Ophthalmol 1973; 89: 466–471.
151. Zimmerman LE. Problems in the diagnosis of malignant melanomas of the choroid and ciliary body. Am J Ophthalmol 1973; 75: 919–929.
152. Peyster RG, Augsburger JJ, Shields JA, et al. Intraocular tumors: evaluation with MR imaging. Radiology 1988; 68: 773–779.
153. Damadian R, Zaner K, Hor D, et al. Human tumors by NMR. Physiol Chem Phys 1973; 5: 381–402.
154. Gomori JM, Grossman RI, Shields JA, et al. Choroidal melanomas: correlation of NMR spectroscopy and MR imaging. Radiology 1986; 158: 443–445.
155. Mafee MF, Peyman GA, McKusick MA. Malignant uveal melanoma and similar lesions studied by computed tomography. Radiology 1985; 156: 403–408.
156. Enochs SW, Petherick P, Bogdanova A, et al: Paramagnetic metal scavenging by melanin: MR imaging. Radiology 1997; 204: 417–423.
157. Depotter P, Shields JA, Shields JA, Shields CL: Computed tomography and magnetic resonance imaging of intraocular lesions. Ophthalmol Clin North Am 1994; 7: 333–346.
158. Erzurum SA, Jampol LM, Territo C, O'Grady R. Primary malignant melanoma of the optic nerve simulating a melanocytoma. Arch Ophthalmol 1992; 110: 684–686.
159. Deveer JA. Juxtapapillary malignant melanoma of the choroid and so-called malignant melanoma of the optic disk. Arch Ophthalmol 1973; 51: 147–751.
160. Mafee MF, Peyman GA, Peace JH, et al. Magnetic resonance imaging in the evaluation and differentiation of uveal melanoma. Ophthalmology 1987; 94: 341–348.
161. Naumann G, Yanoff M, Zimmerman LE. Histogenesis of malignant melanomas of the uvea: histopathologic characteristics of nevi of the choroid and ciliary body. Arch Ophthalmol 1966; 76: 784–796.
162. Gonder JR, Augsburger JJ, McCarthy FF, et al. Visual loss associated with choroidal nevi. Ophthalmology 1982; 89: 961–965.
163. Mafee MF, Ainbinder DJ, Hidayat AA, Friedman S: MRI and CT in the evaluation of choroidal hemangioma. Int J Neuroradiol 1995; 1: 67–77.
164. Adams RD, DeLong GR. Developmental and other congenital abnormalities of the nervous system. In: Harrison's Principles of Internal Medicine. New York: McGraw-Hill; 1974: 1849–1863.
165. Meyer SI, Fine BS, Font RI, et al. Leiomyoma of the ciliary body: electron microscopic verification. Am J Ophthalmol 1968; 66: 1061–1068.
166. Jakobiec FA, Font RL, Tso MOM, et al. Mesectodermal leiomyoma of the ciliary body: a tumor of presumed neural crest origin. Cancer 1977; 39 (5): 2102–2113.
166a. Park SW, Kim HJ, Chin HS, et al. Mesoectodermal leiomyosarcoma of the ciliary body. AJNR 2003; 24: 1765–1768.
167. Apt L, Heller MD, Moskovitz M, et al. Dictyoma (embryonal medulloepithelioma): recent review and case report. J Pediatr Ophthalmol 1973; 10: 30–38.
167a. Chavez M, Mafee MF, Castillo B. et al. Medulloepithelioma of the optic nerve. J Pediatr Ophthalmol Strabismus 2004; 41: 48–52.
168. Ainbinder DJ, Haik BG, Mazzoli RA. Anophthalmic socket and orbital implants: role of CT and MR imaging. Radiol Clin North Am. 1998; 36: 1133–1147.
169. Munk PL: Uveal melanoma (letter). Radiology 1997; 204: 874–875.
170. Raizman MB, Haas JJ: Case records of the Massachusetts General Hospital: A 32-year-old-man with vitreous hemorrhage and mediastinal lymphadenopathy. N Engl J Med 1998; 338: 313–319.
171. Coleman DF, Lucas BC, Rondeau MJ, et al. Management of intraocular foreign bodies. Ophthalmology 1987; 94: 1647–1653.
172. Benson WE, Machemer R. Severe perforating injuries treated with pars plana vitrectomy. Am J Ophthalmol 1976; 81: 728–732.
173. De Juan E Jr, Stemberg P Jr, Michels RG. Penetrating ocular injuries:; types of injuries and visual results. Ophthalmology 1983; 90: 1318–1322.

174 Cridland N. Intraocular foreign bodies. Proc R Soc Med 1967; 60: 598–600.
175 Begle HL. Perforating injuries of the eye by small steel fragments. Am J Ophthalmol 1929; 12: 970–977.
176 Scott RS, Weigeist TA. Management of siderosis bulbi due to a retained iron containing intraocular foreign body. Ophthalmology, 1990; 97: 375–379.
177 Braendstrup P. Two cases of temporary siderosis bulbi with spontaneous resorption and without impairment of function. Acta Ophthalmol 1944; 22: 311–316.
178 Ambler JS, Sanford F, Meyers M. Management of intraretinal metallic foreign bodies without retinopexy in the absence of retinal detachment. Ophthalmology 1991; 39: 391–394.
179 Mieler WF, Ellis MK, Williams DF, et al. Retained intraocular foreign bodies and endophthalmitis. Ophthalmology 1990; 97: 1532–1538.
180 Grove AS. Orbital trauma and computed tomography. Ophthalmology 1980; 403–411.
181 Grove AS, Jr. Computed tomography in the management of orbital trauma. Ophthalmology 1982; 89: 433–440.
182 Henrickson GC, Mafee MF, Flandery AE, Kriz RJ, Peyman GA. CT evaluation of plastic intraocular foreign bodies. AJNR 1987; 8: 378–379.
183 Lobue TD, Deutsch TA, Lobick J. et al. Detection and localization of nonmetallic intraocular foreign bodies by magnetic resonance imaging. Arch Ophthalmol 1988; 106: 260–261.
184 Duker JS, Fisher DH. Occult plastic intraocular foreign body. Ophthalmic Surg 1989; 20: 169–170.
185 Lagouras PA, Langer BG, Peyman GA, et al. Magnetic resonance imaging and intraocular foreign bodies. Arch Ophthalmology 1987; 105: 551–553.
186 Williamson THE, Smith FW, Forrester JV. Magnetic resonance imaging of intraocular foreign bodies. Br J Ophthalmol 1989; 73: 555–558.
187 Kelly WN, Paglen PG, Pearson JA, et al. Ferromagnetism of intraocular foreign body causes unilateral blindness after MR study. AJNR 1986; 7: 243–245.
188 Zheutlin JD, Thompson JT, Shofner RS. The safety of magnetic resonance imaging with intraorbital metallic objects after retinal reattachment or trauma (Letter) Am J Ophthalmol 1987; 103: 831.
189 Sears FW, Zenansky MW (eds.). University Physics, 4th ed. Reading, MA: Addison-Wesley; 1970.
190 Green BF, Kraft SP, Carter KD, et al. Intraorbital wood: detection by magnetic resonance imaging. Ophthalmology 1990; 97: 608–611.
191 Ferguson EC III. Deep, wooden foreign bodies of the orbit: a report of two cases. Trans Am Acad Ophthalmol Otolaryngol. 1970; 74: 778–787.
192 Macrae JA. Diagnosis and management of a wooden orbital foreign body: case report. Br J Ophthalmol 1979; 848–851.
193 Brock L, Tanenbaum HL. Retention of wooden foreign bodies in the orbit. Can J Ophthalmol 1980; 15: 70–72.
194 Reshef DS, Ossoinnig KC, Nerad JA. Diagnosis and intraoperative localization of a deep orbital organic foreign body. Orbit 1987; 6: 3–15.
195 Weisman RA, Savino PJ, Schut L, et al. Computed tomography in penetrating wounds of the orbit with retained bodies. Arch Otolaryngol 1983; 109: 265–268.
196 Tate E, Cupples H. Detection of orbital foreign bodies with computed tomography: current limits. AJR 1981; 137: 493–495.
197 Mylyla V, Pyhtinen J, Pajvansalo M, et al. CT detection and location of intraorbital foreign bodies: experiments with wood and glass. Rofo Fortschr Rontgenstr Neuen Bilgeb Verfahr 1987; 146: 639–643.
198 Coleman DJ. Reliability of ocular and orbital diagnosis with B-scan ultrasound orbital diagnosis. Am J Ophthalmol 1972; 74: 704–718.
199 Macrae JA. Diagnosis and management of a wooden orbital foreign body: case report. Br J Ophthalmol 1979; 63: 848–851.
200 DePotter P, Shields CL, Shields JA, et al. Role of magnetic resonance imaging in the evaluation of the hydroxyapatite orbital implant. Ophthalmology 1992; 99: 824.
201 Shields CL, Shields JA, DePotter P. Hydroxyapatite orbital implant after enucleation: Experience with initial 100 consecutive cases. Arch Ophthalmology 1992; 110: 333.
202 Rubin PA, Green JP, Keur C, et al. Medpur motility coupling post: Primary placement in humans. Am Soc Ophthal Plast Reconstr Surg 28th Annual Symposium 1997.

Part 2: The Orbit

Embryology

The orbital bones develop from the mesenchymal capsule of the forebrain surrounding the optic vesicle. The orbit is formed from a combination of densely collagenous membranous and cartilaginous anlage. The ethmoid and sphenoid bones, which contribute to a large portion of the orbit, arise from the cartilage of the more primitive chondrocranium (enchondral bone). The superior portions of the orbit and adjacent calvaria develop from a membranous anlage (membranous bone). The medial wall forms from the lateral nasal process. The lateral and inferior walls develop from the maxillary process (see also discussion of embryology in Chapter 4). The superior wall forms from the mesenchyme encircling the optic vesicle.[1,2] The extraocular muscles are formed from the mesenchyme in the region of the optic vesicle (see also discussion of embryology in Part 1 of this chapter).

Anatomy

The orbits are two recesses that contain the globes, extraocular muscles, blood vessels, lymphatics, nerves (cranial nerves II, III, IV, V, VI and sympathetic and parasympathetic nerves), adipose and connective tissues, and most of the lacrimal apparatus. The orbit is bordered by the periosteum of seven bones (frontal, sphenoid, ethmoid, lacrimal, maxilla, zygoma, and the palatine), and is separated from the globe by Tenon's capsule.[1-3] Anteriorly are the orbital septum and the lids. The orbital cavity is pyramidal in shape, with its apex directed posteromedially and its base, the orbital opening, directed anterolaterally. Its bony walls separate it from the anterior cranial fossa superiorly; the ethmoid air cells, sphenoid sinus, and nasal cavity medially; the maxillary sinus inferiorly; and the lateral face and temporal fossa laterally and posteriorly. The volume of the orbit in adults is about 30 ml.[2,4,5] The orbital entrance averages about 35 mm in height and 45 mm in width.[2,6] The maximum width occurs about 1 cm behind the anterior orbital margin. In adults, the depth of the orbit varies from 40 to 45 mm from the orbital entrance to the orbital apex.[2]

■ Bony Orbit

Each orbit presents a roof, floor, medial wall, lateral wall, base, or orbital opening, and an apex (Figs. 2.**117**, 2.**118**). The orbital margin forms a quadrilateral spiral. The superior margin is formed by the frontal bone, which is interrupted medially by the supraorbital notch. The supraorbital foramen (notch) transmits blood vessels and the supraorbital nerve, a branch of the ophthalmic division of the trigeminal nerve. The medial margin is formed by the frontal bone above and the lacrimal crests of the maxillary bone and lacrimal bone below. The inferior margin forms from the maxillary and zygomatic bones. The lateral margin forms from zygomatic and frontal bones.

Orbital Roof

The orbital roof is formed from the orbital plate of the frontal bone and most of the lesser wing of the sphenoid bone (Figs. 2.**118**, 2.**119**). Anteromedially is the floor of the frontal sinus, and anterolaterally is the lacrimal fossa, in which lies the orbital part of the lacrimal gland. Posteriorly, at the junction of the roof and the medial wall, is the optic canal and optic foramen (Figs. 2.**118**, 2.**119**) which establish communication between the orbit and the middle cranial fossa. This canal contains the optic nerve, ophthalmic artery, and sympathetic fibers. Medially, the fovea (fossa) trochlearis, located approximately 4 mm from the superior orbital margin, forms the pulley of the superior oblique muscle. The trochlea is a curved plate of hyaline cartilage, which is attached to the trochlear fossa of the frontal bone. Calcification of trochlea is not uncommon in the elderly population.

Medial Orbital Wall

The medial wall is exceedingly thin, except at its most posterior part. This wall is formed by a small portion of the frontal process of the maxilla, the lacrimal bone, ethmoid bone, and the body of sphenoid (Figs. 2.**117**–2.**119**). The medial wall slopes gently downward and laterally into the floor. Anteriorly is the lacrimal groove for the lacrimal sac (Fig. 2.**117**). The groove communicates below with the nasal cavity through the nasolacrimal canal, which is about 1 cm long and contains the nasolacrimal duct, which opens into the inferior meatus of the nasal cavity. Also in the medial wall are two canals for the anterior and posterior ethmoidal nerves and vessels. These canals are situated at the level of the floor of the anterior cranial fossa. The anterior ethmoidal foramen is located at the frontal–ethmoidal suture and transmits the anterior ethmoidal vessels and nerve (Fig. 2.**119**). The posterior ethmoidal foramen lies at the junction of the roof and the medial wall of the orbit (Fig. 2.**119**) and transmits the posterior ethmoidal vessels and nerve through the frontal bone.[1-6]

Orbital Floor

The inferior wall, or floor of the orbit, is relatively thin and, in most of its extent, is also the roof of the maxillary antrum or sinus (Figs. 2.**118**, 2.**119**). The floor actually is made up of the orbital part of the maxilla, the orbital process of the zygomatic bone, and the orbital process of the palatine bone (Figs. 2.**118**, 2.**119**). The orbital process of the palatine bone forms a small triangular area in the posteromedial corner of the orbital floor, where the floor meets the medial wall (Fig. 2.**119**). Anteriorly, for about 1.0–1.5 cm, the floor is continuous with the lateral orbital wall. However, posterior to this area, the floor and lateral wall are separated by the inferior orbital fissure (Fig. 2.**118**). This fissure connects the orbit posteriorly with the pterygopalatine fossa, and anteriorly with the temporal fossa. The medial lip of the fissure is notched by the infraorbital groove, or fissure (Fig. 2.**118**), which passes forward in the orbital floor, sinks into the orbital floor about 1 cm behind the orbital rim, and becomes the infraorbital canal that opens on the anterior face of the maxilla as the infraorbital foramen, about 1 cm below the inferior orbital rim (Figs. 2.**118**, 2.**119**).[1] The groove, canal, and foramen transmit the infraorbital nerve, the continuation of the maxillary nerve (V2).[1-6] The inferior oblique muscle arises from the floor of the orbit just

Anatomy 197

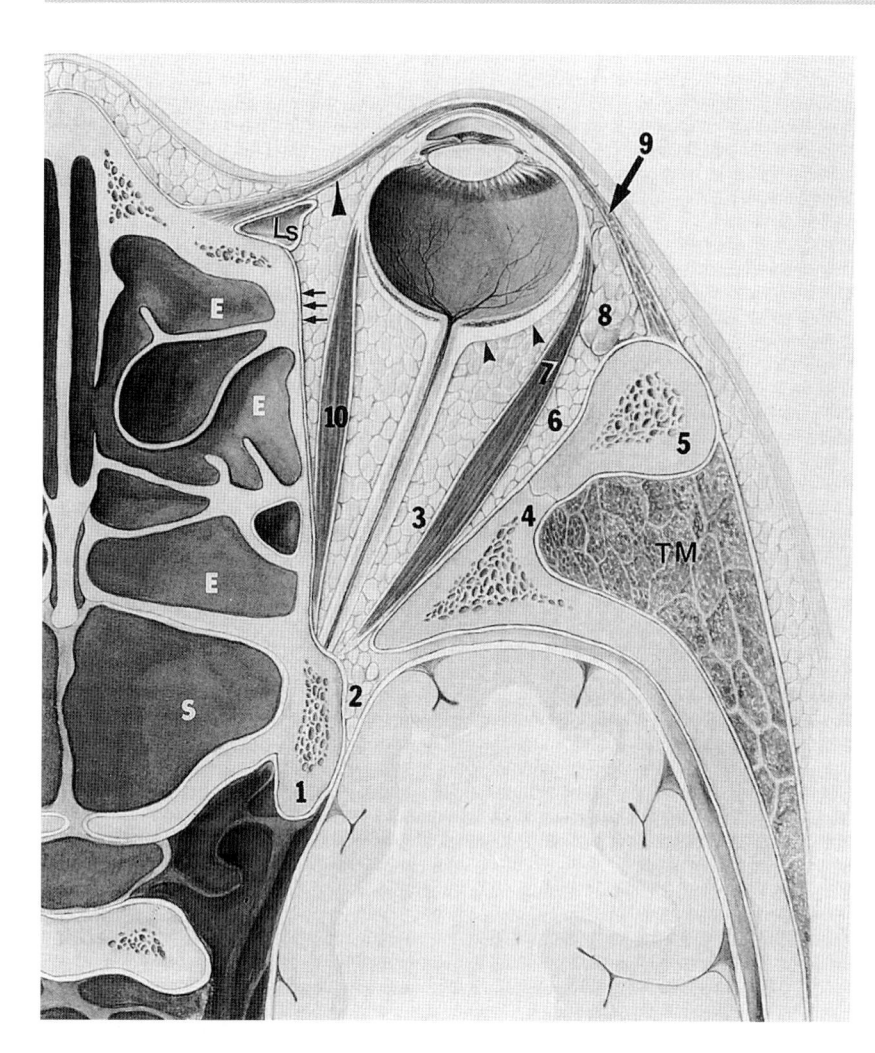

Fig. 2.**117** Diagram of an axial section of the left orbit at the level of the optic nerve. Note the periorbital periosteum (three black arrows). The periorbita (periosteum) splits at the level of lacrimal sac (Ls) and then forms the orbital septum (large arrowhead). Note Tenon's capsule (arrowheads).

 1 = anterior clinoid
 2 = superior orbital fissure
 3 = central orbital fat
 4 = greater wing of sphenoid
 5 = zygomatic bone
 6 = peripheral orbital fat
 7 = lateral rectus muscle
 8 = lacrimal gland
 9 = fibers of orbicularis oculi
10 = medial rectus muscle
 E = ethmoid air cells
Ls = lacrimal sac
 S = sphenoid sinus
TM = temporalis muscle

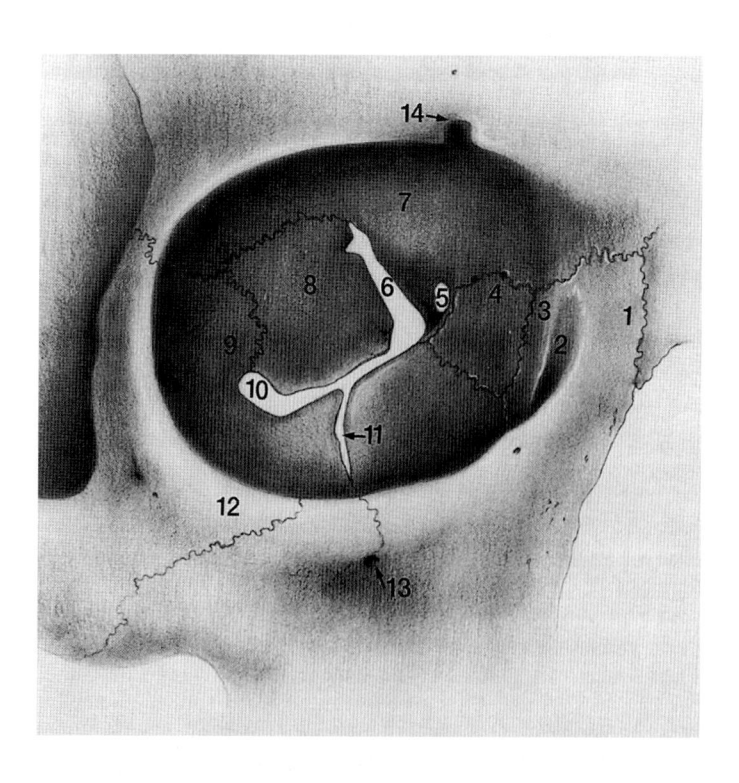

Fig. 2.**118** Schematic drawing of bony orbit.
 1 = frontal process of maxilla
 2 = lacrimal groove
 3 = lacrimal bone
 4 = lamina papyracea
 5 = optic canal (foramen)
 6 = superior orbital fissure
 7 = frontal bone
 8 = greater wing of the sphenoid
 9 = orbital plate of zygomatic bone
10 = inferior orbital fissure
11 = infraorbital groove
12 = zygoma
13 = infraorbital foramen
14 = supraorbital foramen

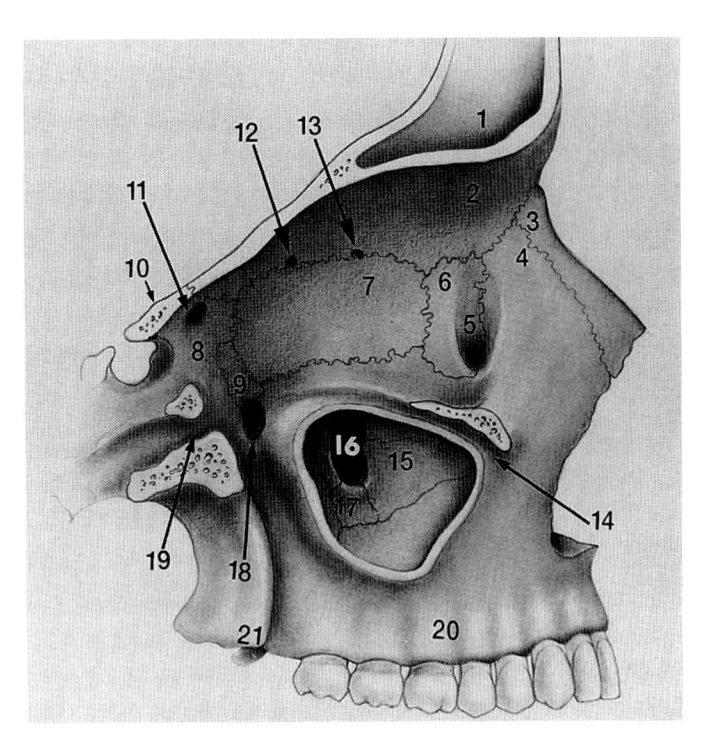

Fig. 2.**119** Schematic drawing of the orbital maxillary region.
1 = frontal sinus
2 = orbital plate of frontal bone
3 = nasal bone
4 = frontal process of maxilla
5 = lacrimal groove
6 = lacrimal bone
7 = lamina papyracea
8 = sphenoid bone
9 = palatine bone
10 = lesser wing of the sphenoid
11 = optic canal
12 = posterior ethmoid foramen
13 = anterior ethmoid foramen
14 = infraorbital canal (foramen)
15 = inferior concha
16 = maxillary hiatus
17 = palatine bone
18 = sphenopalatine foramen opening into pterygopalatine fossa
19 = vidian canal, opening into pterygopalatine fossa
20 = alveolar process of maxilla
21 = pterygoid plate

lateral to the opening of the nasolacrimal canal.[2] It is the only extraocular muscle that does not originate from the orbital apex.

Lateral Orbital Wall

The lateral wall of the orbit is the thickest wall, and it is formed by the orbital surface of the greater wing of the sphenoid bone behind, and the orbital surface of the frontal process of the zygomatic bone in front (Figs. 2.**117**, 2.**118**). The two bones meet at the sphenozygomatic suture. This aspect of the zygomatic bone presents the openings of two minute canals, one for the zygomaticofacial nerve and artery (near the junction of the floor and lateral walls), and the other for the zygomaticotemporal nerve and artery, which is slightly higher on this wall.[1,2,5,6] The lateral orbital tubercle, a small elevation of the orbital margin of the zygoma, lies approximately 11 mm below the frontal–zygomatic suture. This important landmark is the site of attachment for (1) the check ligament of the lateral rectus muscle, (2) the suspensory ligament of the eyeball, (3) the lateral palpebral ligament, and (4) the aponeurosis of the levator muscle.[5,6]

Orbital Apex

The apex of the orbit is basically formed by the optic canal and the superior orbital fissure. The optic canal and the superior and inferior orbital fissures allow various structures to enter and exit the orbit. The optic canal, having virtually no length at birth, becomes 4 mm long by 1 year of age and is up to 9 mm long in adults.[1,3] The optic canal is directed forward, laterally, and somewhat downward and has orbital and intracranial openings (foramina). The optic canal, forming an angle of about 45° with the sagittal plane of the head, is bounded medially by the body of the sphenoid bone (Figs. 2.**118**–2.**120**), superiorly by the superior root of the lesser wing of the sphenoid bone, and inferiorly and laterally by the inferior root (optic strut) of the lesser wing of the sphenoid bone.[2,3] Attached to the orbital wall close to the superior, medial, and lower margins of the orbital opening of the optic canal is the common tendinous ring of Zinn, which encircles the optic nerve and gives origin to the inferior, medial, lateral, and superior rectus muscles (Fig. 2.**120 b**).[1] The optic canal contains the optic nerve, ophthalmic artery, and sympathetic fibers from the carotid plexus.

Superior Orbital Fissure

Just inferolateral to the optic canal, and separated from it by the optic strut, is the superior orbital fissure, located between the greater and lesser wings of the sphenoid bone (Figs. 2.**118**, 2.**121**). This fissure is approximately 22 mm long and is somewhat comma-shaped, with the bulbous or wider portion inferomedially and the thin portion superolaterally. The superior orbital fissure communicates with the middle cranial fossa and transmits the oculomotor, trochlear, and abducens nerves and the terminal branches of the ophthalmic nerve and the ophthalmic veins. The lacrimal, frontal, and trochlear nerves traverse the narrow, lateral part of the fissure, which also transmits the meningeal branch of the lacrimal artery and the occasional orbital branch of the middle meningeal artery. The trochlear nerve is situated more medially and lies just outside the common tendinous ring of Zinn.[1] The two divisions (superior and inferior) of the oculomotor nerve, the nasociliary nerve (a branch of the ophthalmic nerve), the abducens nerve, and the sympathetic plexus, pass within the tendinous ring and therefore traverse the wider, medial part of the fissure.[2] They may be accompanied by the superior and inferior ophthalmic veins, but the superior ophthalmic vein may also accompany the trochlear nerve, and the inferior ophthalmic vein may pass through the medial end of the fissure below the ring.[1]

Inferior Orbital Fissure

At the posterior aspect of the orbit, the inferior and lateral walls of the orbit are separated by the inferior orbital fissure (Figs. 2.**118**, 2.**121**). The fissure lies just below the superior orbital fissure and is bounded above by the greater wing of the sphenoid, below by the maxilla and the orbital process of the palatine bone, and laterally by the zygomatic bone (the zygomaticomaxillary suture) (Fig. 2.**118**). The inferior orbital fissure extends obliquely as a gently curving continuation of the more medial pterygopalatine fossa (Figs. 2.**120**, 2.**121**). The maxillary nerve is the most important structure traversing the inferior orbital fissure. The inferior orbital fissure also transmits the infraorbital vessels, the zygomatic nerve, and a few minute twigs from the pterygopalatine ganglion. Through the anterior part of the inferior orbital fissure, a vein passes to communicate the inferior ophthalmic vein with the pterygoid plexus in the infratemporal fossa.[1] The inferior ophthalmic vein passes through its lower portion before entering the cavernous sinus.[6]

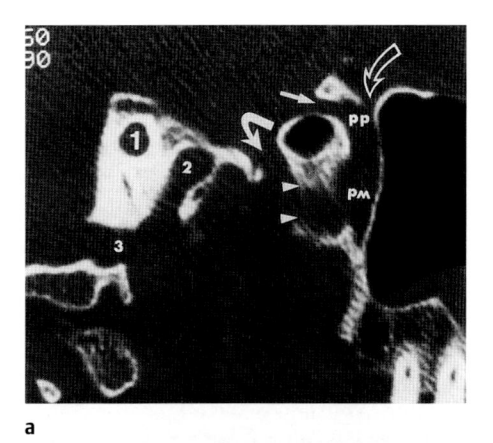

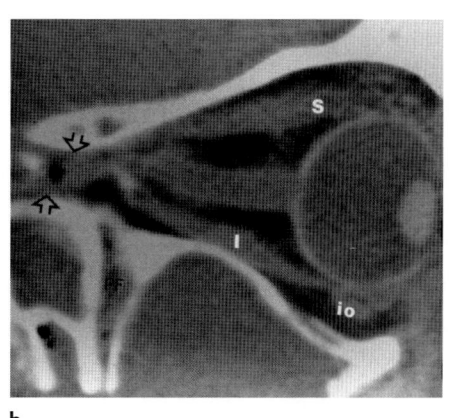

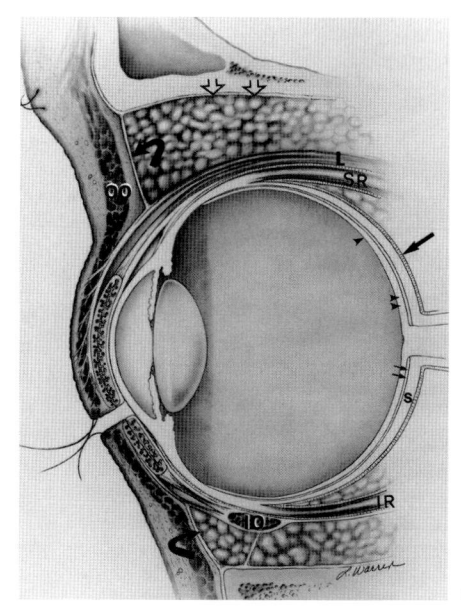

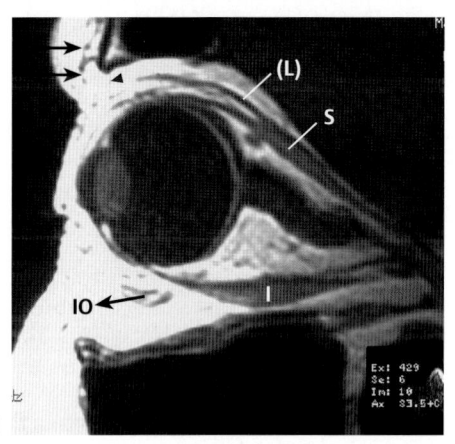

Fig. 2.**120 a** Pterygopalatine fossa. Direct parasagittal CT scan shows the pterygopalatine fossa (pp), inferior orbital fissure (hollow curved arrow), foramen rotundum (solid straight arrow), foramen ovale (solid curved arrow), pterygoid plate (arrowheads), pterygomaxillary fissure (PM), carotid canal (2), jugular fossa (3) and internal auditory canal (1).
b Orbital CT anatomy. Parasagittal CT scan of a cadaver head shows globe; optic nerve; superior rectus muscle (S), inferior rectus muscle (I), inferior oblique muscle (IO); common tendon of Zinn (arrows); and pterygomaxillary fissure (PF). The orbital periosteum, the so-called periorbita, lines the bony orbit as orbital fascia and is relatively loosely attached to the bony orbit. The periosteum is connected with the dura mater and sheath of the optic nerve at the optic canal. Normally, periosteum cannot be differentiated from adjacent soft tissues. The periosteum is continuous with the periosteum of the bones of the face and is continuous with the periosteal layer of dura at the superior orbital fissure. Note continuity of the periorbita with the periosteum of the pterygopalatine fossa and pterygomaxillary fissure (PF). CT scan courtesy of FW Zonneveld, PhD. Reproduced from Mafee MF, et al. Orbital space-occupying lesions: role of CT and MRI: an analysis of 145 cases. Radiol Clin North Am 1987; 25:529. With permission.
c Sagittal cut-away view of the gross anatomy of the eye and orbit, highlighting the periorbita (hollow arrows); orbital septum (black curved arrows); levator palpebrae superioris muscle (L); superior rectus muscle (SR); inferior rectus muscle (IR); inferior oblique muscle (IO); Tenon's capsule (single black arrow); sclera (S); choroid (double small arrows); retina (double arrowheads); and vitreous base (single arrowhead). Note the palpebral portion of the orbicularis oculi (OO), which lies in front of the orbital septum.
d Sagittal T1W MR scan shows globe; optic nerve; levator palpebrae superioris muscle (L); superior rectus (S); inferior rectus muscle (I); inferior oblique muscle (IO); orbital septum (arrowhead); and orbicularis oculi (arrows).

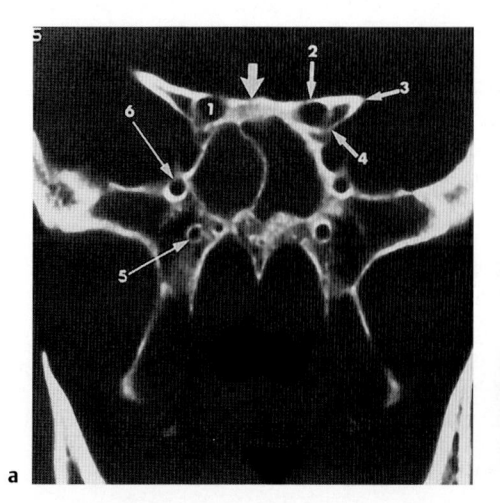

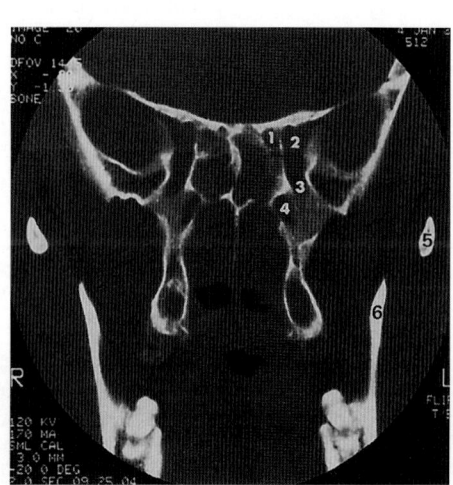

Fig. 2.**121 a** Coronal CT scan shows the optic canal (1), superior (posterior) root of lesser wing of the sphenoid (2), anterior clinoid (3), inferior (anterior) root of lesser wing of the sphenoid (4), pterygoid (vidian) canal (5), foramen rotundum (6), and planum sphenoidale (arrow).
b Coronal CT scan 6 mm anterior to **a**, showing the optic canal (1), superior (2) and inferior (3) orbital fissures, pterygopalatine fossa (4), zygomatic arch (5), and mandible (6). Note prominent adenoidal tissue.

Pterygopalatine Fossa

The pterygopalatine fossa (PPF) is a small, narrow, pyramidal space situated below the apex of the orbit and tapering inferiorly[7] (Figs. 2.**119**, 2.**120 b**, 2.**121 b**). It is bounded above by the body of the sphenoid, in front by maxilla, behind by pterygoid processes and greater wing of sphenoid, and medially by the palatine bone (Figs. 2.**119**, 2.**120**, 2.**121 b**). It communicates with the infratemporal fossa through the pterygomaxillary fissure. The five foramina that open into this fossa are the foramen rotundum, the pterygoid (vidian) canal, the pharyngeal (palatovaginal) canal (Figs. 2.**119**, 2.**120 a**, 2.**121**), the sphenopalatine canal, and the pterygopalatine canal. The most important contents of the fossa are the maxillary nerve, the pterygopalatine (sphenopalatine) ganglion, and the terminal part of the maxillary artery. The maxillary nerve (V2) runs from the inferior aspect of the cavernous sinus and exits the skull base through the foramen rotundum. The nerve then runs through the upper part of the pterygopalatine fossa just above the pterygopalatine ganglion, enters the inferior orbital fissure, and passes forward and lateral to reach the posterior end of the infraorbital groove in the floor of the orbit. The nerve finally exits on the face through the infraorbital foramen. Further anatomical details of the PPF can be found in Chapters 3 and 4.

Periorbita

The periosteum of the bony orbit is known as the periorbita or the orbital fascia.[8] The periosteum is a specialized connective-tissue structure that covers the bones. It consists of two strata: a superficial fibrous mantle and an active inner layer known as the cambium. Duhamel is credited with the first scientific investigation of the osteogenic properties of the periosteum.[9] The periorbita (orbital fascia) is generally loosely adherent to the surrounding bones except at the anterior orbital margin, trochlear fossa, lacrimal crests, and the margins of the fissures and canals.[1,3,4,8] Anteriorly, it is continuous with the periosteum of the orbital margins (Figs. 2.**117**–2.**121**). Posteriorly, it is continuous with the dura of the optic nerve and that surrounding the superior orbital fissure. Thus posteriorly located surgery or trauma may result in cerebrospinal fluid leaks.[3] The dura matter is composed of a meningeal layer and a periosteal layer. These two layers are so closely bound together that they can only be separated with difficulty.[2,4,8] After these layers pass through the optic foramen, however, they become separate. The meningeal layer continues as the sheath of the optic nerve, and the periosteal layer lines the bony orbit as the orbital fascia or periorbita. Numerous septa and fascial bands from various structures in the orbit are attached to the inner surface of the periosteum.[4] In front, the periorbita is fused with the orbital septum along the margins of the base (anterior rims) of the orbit.[6] The orbital septum is the continuation of the periosteum.[4,8]

■ Orbital Septum and Eyelids

The orbital septum is a thin sheet of fibrous tissue that forms the fibrous layer of the eyelids and is attached to the margins of the bony orbit, where it is continuous with the periorbita. In the upper lid, it fuses with the levator aponeurosis. In the lower eyelid, the orbital septum fuses with the capsulopalpebral fascia approximately 3–5 mm below the inferior tarsal border.[5] The palpebral portion of the orbicularis oculi muscle lies in front of the orbital septum (Fig. 2.**120 c**, **d**).[5] Moving from the skin inward toward the orbit, in general, each eyelid or palpebra consists of skin, subcutaneous areolar tissue, fibers of the orbicularis oculi, the tarsus and orbital septum, tarsal glands (meibomian), and conjunctiva (Figs. 2.**120 c**, **d**). The conjunctiva is the transparent vascularized mucous membrane that covers the inner surfaces of the eyelids, and is reflected over the front part of the sclera and cornea.[1,5] The line of reflexion of the conjunctiva from the eyelids on the eyeball is called the conjunctival fornix. The palpebral conjunctiva is highly vascular and its deeper part contains a considerable amount of lymphoid tissue, especially near the fornices. It is intimately adherent to the tarsi.[1] The ocular conjunctiva is loosely connected to the eyeball. On reaching the cornea, the ocular conjunctiva continues as the corneal epithelium.[1] The palpebral conjunctiva is covered by a nonkeratinized epithelium that contains the mucin-secreting goblet cells and the accessory lacrimal glands of Krause and Wolfring.[2,5] Secretions from these accessory glands form the major components of the lacrimal secretion in contrast to the reflex tear secretion from the parasympathetically innervated main lacrimal gland.[2,5] Within each eyelid, the orbital septum is thickened to form a tarsal plate. The levator palpebrae superioris is attached to the upper edge of the superior tarsal plate. A few fibers of the inferior rectus muscle are attached to the lower edge of the inferior tarsal plate.[4,5] Posteriorly, each plate is covered by conjunctiva, and has meibomian glands (modified sebaceous glands) embedded in its deep surface.

The tarsal plates consist of dense connective tissue that serves as the skeleton of the eyelids. They are attached to the orbital margin by the lateral and medial palpebral ligaments. The length (22 mm) and thickness (1 mm) of the upper and lower tarsal plates are similar.[2,6] The upper tarsus is more than twice as wide (11 mm) as the lower tarsus.[2,6] The tarsal (meibomian) glands are modified sweat glands. Their oily secretion passes through small orifices into the tear film.

■ Orbicularis Oculi

The orbicularis oculi muscle is a flat, elliptical muscle that surrounds the orbital margin, extending onto the temporal region and cheek (orbital part); it also extends into the eyelids (palpebral portion) and farther, behind the lacrimal sac (lacrimal portion) (Figs. Figs. 2.**117**, 2.**120 c**, 2.**120 d**).

■ Tenon's Capsule (Fascia Bulbi) and Tenon's Space

Tenon's capsule is a fibroelastic membrane that envelops the eyeball from the optic nerve to the level of the ciliary muscle. Tenon's capsule is also called the ocular fascial sheath, the fascia bulbi, and the bulbar fascia of the eyeball. This fibroelastic socket, which encloses the posterior four-fifths of the eyeball, separates it from the central orbital fat (Figs. 2.**117**, 2.**120 c**, **d**).[2,4,8] Movement of the eyeball is facilitated by the fascia bulbi, which invests but does not adhere to the sclera. The bulbar fascia was discussed earlier in the first part of this chapter on the eye.

■ Orbital Fatty Reticulum

Within the orbit, all structures are embedded in a fatty reticulum. The fibroelastic tissue that makes up the reticulum divides the fat into lobes and lobules.[2,8] The fatty reticulum is divided into (1) peripheral orbital fat, which is outside the muscle cone and its intermuscular membranes (Figs. 2.**117**, 2.**120 b**, 2.**120 d**, 2.**122**), and (2) central orbital fat, which is within the muscle cone (Figs. 2.**117**, 2.**120b–d**). Connective-tissue septa are present between the orbital walls, the muscles, and the globe. These fine septa can be shown on high-resolution MRI within the fat cushion of the orbit (Fig. 2.**122**).

■ Muscles of the Eye

Extraocular Muscles

The six striated extraocular muscles, including the four rectus and two oblique muscles, control eye movement (Figs. 2.**120**, 2.**122**). The rectus muscles arise from the annulus of Zinn, which is a funnel-shaped tendinous ring that encloses the optic foramen and the medial end of the superior orbital fissure, where it is continuous with the dural sheath of the optic nerve and periorbita.[2,8,10,11] The annulus has an upper portion, called the superior orbital tendon or the upper common tendon of Lockwood, and a lower portion, called the lower common tendon of Zinn.[11] Because of this intimate relationship, apical disease frequently affects all of these structures simultaneously. The inferior rectus muscle originates from the common tendon of Zinn below the optic foramen. It inserts into the inferior sclera 6.5 mm from the limbus. The superior rectus (the longest of the four recti) originates from the common tendon of Lockwood above the optic foramen and from the sheath of the optic nerve. It passes below the levator aponeurosis and inserts into the upper sclera 7.7 mm from the limbus. The medial rectus muscle (the thickest of the recti) arises from the upper tendon of Lockwood, the lower tendon of Zinn, and the sheath of the optic nerve and inserts 5.5 mm from the limbus.[2,10,11] The lateral rectus originates from the lower common tendon of Zinn and the upper common tendon of Lockwood and inserts 6.9 mm from the limbus.[2,11] The superior oblique (the longest and thinnest of the extraocular muscles) originates from the periosteum of the body of the sphenoid bone, above and medial to the annulus of Zinn and the origin of the medial rectus.[2,10,11] It passes anteriorly along the upper part of the medial orbital wall as a slender tendon and enters the trochlea, a fibrocartilaginous ring lined with a synovial-type sheath.[12] The tendon slides through the trochlea, and then turns sharply posterolaterally and downward beneath the superior rectus muscle to insert in the lateral sclera, behind the equator of the eye. The inferior oblique muscle originates from a shallow depression posterolateral to the orifice of the nasolacrimal duct. It passes under the inferior rectus and runs posteriorly, laterally, and superiorly before inserting into the inferolateral aspect of the globe.[13] All extraocular muscles are about 40 mm in length except for the 37 mm inferior oblique.[14] The inferior oblique muscle contains essentially no tendon, and the superior oblique has 20 mm of tendon.[14]

Muscles of the Eyelid

The retractors of the upper eyelid are the levator muscle, the levator aponeurosis, and the sympathetically innervated superior tarsal muscle (Müller's muscle). In the lower eyelid, the retractors are the capsulopalpebral fascia and the inferior tarsal muscle (Müller's muscle).[5]

The levator palpebrae superioris muscle originates in the apex of the orbit from the periorbita of the lesser wing of the sphenoid, just above the annulus of Zinn.[2,5] The body of the levator muscle overlies the superior rectus as it travels anteriorly toward the lid (Fig. 2.**120c, d**). The levator muscle and its tendon in adults is 50–60 mm long. The muscle portion, which is approximately 40 mm long, is innervated by the superior division of the oculomotor nerve and elevates the upper lid.[2] The levator

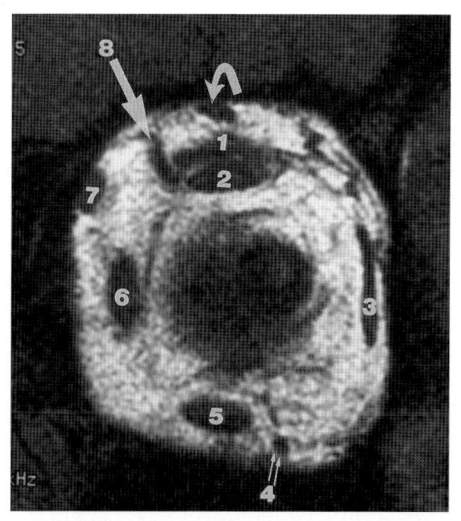

Fig. 2.**122** Coronal T1W MR scan, taken with 3 inch surface coil (450/28, TR/TE, FOV: 8 × 8, 256 × 256, 3 mm slice thickness, 0.0 spacing), showing the levator palpebrae superioris (1), superior rectus muscle (2), lateral rectus muscle (3), inferior ophthalmic vein (4), inferior rectus muscle (5), medical rectus muscle (6), superior oblique muscle (7), superior ophthalmic vein (8), and frontal nerve (curved arrow). Note numerous connective-tissue septa within the fat cushion of the orbit, giving the appearance of a fatty reticulum. As seen, the connective-tissue septa are present within the central orbital fat as well as between the orbital walls, the muscles, and partially volumed globe.

palpebrae is often called the seventh extraocular muscle. The superior transverse ligament (Whitnall's ligament) is a condensation of the sheath of the levator muscle located in the approximate area of the transition from levator muscle to levator aponeurosis.[2,5] Whitnall's ligament functions primarily as a suspensory support for the upper eyelid and the superior orbital tissues.[5] Its analogue in the lower eyelid is Lockwood's ligament.[5] As the levator aponeurosis continues forward, it inserts into the anterior surface of the tarsus (Fig. 2.**120c**) and by medial and lateral horns into the canthal tendons.[5,6] The lateral horn of the levator aponeurosis is strong, and it divides the lacrimal gland into orbital and palpebral lobes, attaching firmly to the orbital tubercle.[5] The superior tarsal muscle (Müller's muscle) inserts on the superior tarsal border.[5] This muscle provides approximately 2 mm of lift for the upper eyelid and if it is interrupted, as in Horner syndrome, a mild proptosis will result.

The capsulopalpebral fascia is the lower eyelid analogue of the levator palpebrae muscle and aponeurosis.[5]

Movements of Eyelid and Eyeball

The levator palpebrae superioris is the main, striated voluntary muscle that elevates the upper eyelid. It is opposed by the orbicularis oculi.[2,6] When the smaller, inferior stratum of nonstriated muscle, Müller's muscle, is denervated, it is responsible for the ptosis in Horner syndrome. Within its fascial sheath, the eyeball is rotated by the extraocular muscles, which displace the gaze upward (elevation), downward (depression), medially (adduction), and laterally (abduction). Rotation about an anteroposterior axis (torsion) may also occur.[10,11,13,14] The actions of the medial and lateral recti are adduction and abduction respectively. They are antagonists, and by reciprocal adjustment of their lengths the visual axis can be swept through a horizontal arc. The superior rectus muscle's primary action is elevation. This muscle also has a secondary, less powerful action of medial rotation (adduction).[1,11] Its primary antagonist is the inferior rectus, which depresses and adducts the eyeball. The superior oblique muscle acts on the eyeball from the trochlea. Its antagonist is the inferior oblique muscle.[2] The inferior oblique muscle elevates the gaze and the superior oblique depresses it. Both oblique muscles produce adduction.[1, 2, 11]

The muscular branches of the ophthalmic artery, the lacrimal artery, and the infraorbital artery provide blood supply for the extraocular muscles. Except for the lateral rectus muscle, each rectus muscle receives two anterior ciliary arteries that communicate with the major arteriole circle of the ciliary body. The lateral rectus is supplied by a single vessel derived from the lacrimal artery.[2]

■ Innervation

Optic Nerve

The optic nerve is not a nerve but actually a nerve fiber tract of the central nervous system formed by over one million axons that originate in the ganglion cell layer of the retina. The nerve has a similar organization to the white matter of the brain. Its fibers are surrounded by glial and not Schwann cell sheaths.[2, 6, 15] The optic nerve (Figs. 2.**117**, 2.**120 b, d**), along with the ophthalmic artery, traverses the optic canal, and passes forward and laterally within the cone of rectus muscles to enter the eyeball just medial to its posterior pole. The optic nerve is about 3.5–5.5 cm long and about 4 mm in diameter.[3, 6] It is divided into four portions: intraocular (1 mm), intraorbital (3 cm), intracanalicular (5–6 mm), and intracranial (1 cm).[3] The intraocular portion can be divided into 3 parts: (1) prelaminar, (2) laminar, and (3) retrolaminar. The surface of the prelaminar portion is visible ophthalmoscopically. It is a 1.75 × 1.5 mm oval with a disk-shaped depression (the physiological cup) located slightly temporal to its geometric center.[5, 6] The optic nerve head (optic disk) comprises nonmyelinated axons from the retinal ganglion cells, blood vessels, and astrocytes which form a thin basal lamina on its inner surface.[2]

The laminar portion of the optic disk is composed of astrocytes, elastic fibers, collagenous connective tissue from the scleral lamina, and small blood vessels. The lamina cribrosa of the sclera functions as a scaffold for the optic nerve axons. The retrolaminar portion extends from the lamina cribrosa to the apex of the orbit. From the lamina cribrosa centrally, the retinal ganglion cell axons become myelinated as the cross-sectional diameter of the nerve increases to approximately 3 mm. After passing through the optic canal, the optic nerves lie above the ophthalmic arteries, and above and medial to the internal carotid artery. The anterior cerebral arteries cross over the optic nerves and are joined by the anterior communicating artery. The optic nerves then pass posteriorly to join in the optic chiasm.

Meningeal Sheaths (Dura, Arachnoid, Pia)

The dura, the outer layer of the optic nerve sheath, is composed of collagenous connective tissue. The arachnoid is made up of fine collagenous fibers arranged in a loose meshwork lined by endothelial cells. The innermost layer, the pia, is made up of fine collagenous and elastic fibers and is highly vascularized. Elements from both the arachnoid and the pia are continuous with the optic nerve septa. The pial septa, which originate in the region of the posterior lamina cribrosa, enclose all neurofascicles. The septa continue throughout the orbital and intracanalicular portion of the nerve and end in the intracranial portion. The arachnoid mater is continuous with the subarachnoid space. It ends at the level of the lamina cribrosa. It is composed of collagenous tissue, small amounts of elastic tissue, and meningothelial cells. The dura mater encases the optic nerve. It is 0.3–0.5 mm thick and consists of dense bundles of collagen and elastic tissue fused anteriorly with the outer layers of the sclera and tenon capsule. The meninges of the optic nerve are supplied by sensory fibers, which accounts for the pain experienced by patients with inflammatory optic nerve diseases.

Blood Supply of the Optic Nerve

The prelaminar and the lamina cribrosa regions of the optic nerve are supplied by branches of the posterior ciliary arteries, while the surface of the optic disk is supplied by retinal arterioles that are branches of the central retinal artery, or from branches of small cilioretinal arteries.[2, 6, 15] The intraorbital part of the optic nerve is supplied by intraneural branches of the central retinal artery and multiple recurrent pial branches arising from both the peripapillary choroid and the central retinal and ophthalmic arteries.[2, 5] The intracanalicular portion of the optic nerve is supplied almost exclusively by the ophthalmic artery. The intracranial portion of the optic nerve is supplied primarily by branches of both the internal carotid artery and the ophthalmic artery. The actual distance from the back of the globe to the orbital apex is 20 mm. Thus from the optic foramen, the optic nerve takes a tortuous, S-shaped course to the back of the globe. This longer length of the optic nerve allows movement of the eye without tension on the nerve. The optic nerve is fixed to the apex of the orbit by approximation of the pia mater and the arachnoid membrane, and by fusion of the dura mater to the periosteum at the optic canal.[16] At the optic canal, the dural sheath of the nerve fuses to the periosteum so that the nerve is completely immobilized.[5] The ophthalmic artery is encased by dura in the optic canal where it lies inferolateral to the nerve. At the orbital end of the canal, it loses the dural coat and crosses medially in the intraconal space.[16]

Peripheral Nerves

Several nerves reach the orbit from the middle cranial fossa and the pterygopalatine fossae. The optic nerve traverses the optic canal. Other nerves gain access to the orbit through the orbital fissures.

Sensory Innervation

The major sensory innervation of the orbit is via the ophthalmic (V1) and maxillary (V2) divisions of the trigeminal nerve. The trigeminal nuclear complex extends from the midbrain to the upper cervical segments, often as caudal as C4.[4, 5] The ophthalmic nerve, before entering the orbit, divides into lacrimal, frontal, and nasociliary nerves, each of which enters the orbit through the superior orbital fissure.[3, 6] The frontal (largest branch) and lacrimal (smallest branch) branches of the ophthalmic nerve enter the orbit outside of the annulus of Zinn and run forward between the periorbita and the levator complex to supply the forehead and lacrimal gland. The nasociliary branch is intraconal, crosses medially over the optic nerve, continues forward along the medial wall of the orbit below the superior rectus and superior oblique muscles, and terminates as the ethmoidal (anterior and posterior) and infratrochlear nerves.[2, 6] Its branches include one to the ciliary ganglion and two long ciliary nerves.[3, 6] The long ciliary nerves carry sympathetic vasoconstrictor fibers to supply vessels within the eyeball.[6]

Motor Innervation

Oculomotor nerve (III). The nucleus of the oculomotor nerve is in the midbrain tegmentum. The nerve appears in the interpeduncular fossa, courses above the other nerves in the most cephalic, lateral wall of the cavernous sinus (see Fig. 2.**134 b, c**), and enters the orbit through the superior orbital fissure. It has superior and inferior divisions, which are often formed before entering the orbit.[2,6] The nerve enters the muscle cone within the annulus of Zinn as a superior division (supplying the levator and superior rectus) and an inferior division (supplying the medial and inferior recti and the inferior oblique). Just lateral to the optic nerve, about 1.5–2 cm behind the globe, is the ciliary ganglion.[3,6] It is chiefly a ganglion where the parasympathetic fibers from the inferior division of the oculomotor nerve form a synapse. Sympathetic fibers to the smooth muscle in the levator palpebrae superioris (Müller's muscle) and the inferior rectus Müller's muscle (arising from the capsulopalpebral head of the inferior rectus in the lower lid) enter the oculomotor nerve in the cavernous sinus and travel with its branches to these muscles.[5]

Trochlear nerve (IV). The nucleus of the trochlear nerve is in the midbrain tegmentum. Its fibers leave the central nervous system through the anterior medullary velum dorsally, cross to the opposite side, and pass rostrally and caudally to run in the lateral wall of the cavernous sinus between the oculomotor (III) and ophthalmic (V1) nerves (see Fig. 2.**134b, c**). The trochlear nerve then crosses the oculomotor nerve, and passes through the superior orbital fissure above the other nerves to supply the superior oblique muscle.[2,5,6]

Abducens nerve (VI). The nucleus of the abducens nerve is in the tegmentum of pons. Its fibers leave the central nervous system in the ventral groove between the medulla and pons, and pass through the cavernous sinus between the internal carotid artery and the ophthalmic nerve (V1) (see Fig. 2.**134b, c**). The abducens nerve then enters the orbit through the superior orbital fissure and passes forward on the inner surface of the lateral rectus, which it supplies.[2,5,6]

Other nerves. The seventh cranial nerve is the motor supply for the orbicularis oculi; its sensory division, the nervus intermedius, gives the parasympathetic supply to the lacrimal gland. The facial nerve enters the parotid gland and then divides into upper temporal facial and lower cervical facial branches. It innervates the orbicularis via the upper division, which forms the temporofrontal and zygomatic branches.[15]

Autonomic Nerves

The ciliary ganglion lies 1.5–2 cm behind the eyeball, lateral to the optic nerve. It receives sensory fibers from the nasociliary nerve, parasympathetic fibers from the oculomotor nerve, and sympathetic fibers from the internal carotid plexus in the cavernous sinus (via the superior orbital fissure).[2,3,6] Only the parasympathetic fibers synapse in the ganglion. The sensory root subserves the cornea, iris, and ciliary body through short ciliary nerves that pass from the anterior part of the ciliary ganglion into the eyeball.[2,6] The parasympathetic fibers supply the ciliary muscle and iris sphincter (which constricts the pupil). The preganglionic fibers of the parasympathetics to the sphincter muscle arise in the Edinger–Westphal nucleus of the midbrain, travel with the oculomotor nerve, and run into its inferior division to end by synapsing in the ciliary ganglion. The postganglionic fibers arise from cells of the ciliary ganglion and leave the ganglion by short ciliary nerves that pierce the sclera and run to the ciliary muscle and iris. The sympathetic fibers supply ocular vessels, the iris dilator (by means of ciliary nerves), the lacrimal gland, and the sympathetic muscles (Müller's muscle) of the upper and lower lids. The sympathetic fibers to the dilator pupillae muscle pass through the ciliary ganglion without synapse, and run with the short ciliary nerves.[2,3] The preganglionic fibers of the sympathetics to the dilator pupillae arise in the intermediolateral gray column of the upper thoracic cord, enter the sympathetic trunk, and ascend in the cervical sympathetic trunk to end by synapses in the superior cervical ganglion.[3,5] The postganglionic fibers arise in cells of the superior cervical ganglion, and ascend through the carotid and cavernous nervous plexuses. Some fibers join the ophthalmic nerve to continue in its nasociliary branch and are carried to the eye with the long ciliary branches of this nerve. Other fibers from the cavernous nerves plexus enter the sympathetic "root" of the ciliary ganglion, pass through this ganglion without synapse, and run with the short ciliary nerves.[2,5] Still other intraorbital sympathetic fibers travel with the oculomotor nerve to the smooth-muscle component of the levator palpebrae superioris and inferior recti (Müller's muscles).[3,5]

The preganglionic parasympathetic fibers of the lacrimal gland arise from cells in the superior salivatory nucleus of the pons and run in the nervus intermedius, with the facial nerve. They then leave the facial nerve, at the geniculate ganglion, as the greater superficial petrosal nerve, which becomes part of the nerve of the pterygoid (vidian) canal, to enter and synapse in the pterygopalatine ganglion. The postganglionic fibers arise from the cells of the pterygopalatine ganglion, pass through the pterygopalatine nerves to the maxillary nerve, and then through the zygomatic branch of the maxillary nerve.[2,5] These fibers then enter the zygomaticotemporal branch of the zygomatic nerve in the orbit and communicate with the lacrimal branch of the ophthalmic nerve to reach the lacrimal gland. The preganglionic sympathetic fibers of the lacrimal gland arise in the intermediolateral gray column of the upper thoracic cord, enter the sympathetic trunk, and ascend in the cervical sympathetic trunk, to end by synapses in the superior cervical ganglion.[5] The postganglionic sympathetic fibers arise in cells of the superior cervical ganglion, pass through the carotid plexus, and continue rostrally in the deep petrosal nerve, to join the superficial greater petrosal nerve to become the pterygoid (vidian) nerve. Then the fibers pass through the pterygopalatine ganglion, without synapse, and are distributed in a similar manner to the postganglionic parasympathetic fibers to reach the lacrimal gland.[2,5]

■ Vascular Anatomy

Aterial Supply

The major arterial supply to the orbit is from branches of the ophthalmic artery. This artery usually arises from the distal end of the cavernous sinus segment of the internal carotid artery. Rarely it may arise from the middle meningeal artery and enter the orbit through the superior orbital fissure.[3] In the optic canal, it runs under and lateral to the optic nerve within the dural sheath, and at the orbital apex it leaves the dura. In 82.6% of subjects, it crosses to the medial orbit over the optic nerve; in the remaining 17.4% of subjects, the artery runs under the nerve.[3] The branches of the ophthalmic artery, considering certain variations in origin, are the lacrimal, supraorbital, anterior and posterior ethmoidal, nasofrontal, and dorsonasal arteries.[2] The branches for the eyeball include the central artery of the retina and ciliary arteries. The central artery of the retina is the first branch of the ophthalmic artery.[6] It crosses the optic nerve, pierces it, and runs in its center to spread over the retina. The ciliary arteries are arranged in three groups: short posterior ciliary, long posterior ciliary, and anterior ciliary arteries. The posterior ciliary arteries supply the globe via 15–20 short branches (to the choroid and ciliary processes and the optic nerve head) and two long branches (to the ciliary muscle, iris, and the anterior choroid).[2] The lacrimal artery branches into the recurrent meningeal, zygomatic, glandular, and lateral palpebral arteries (which form the arcades of the lid). The ophthalmic artery frequently has anastomotic branches to the external carotid system, by means of the middle meningeal and lacrimal arteries, which pass through the superior orbital fissure.

Venous Drainage of the Orbit and Eyeball

The venous blood from the eyeball and adjacent structures drains into the valveless inferior and superior ophthalmic veins. The superior ophthalmic vein drains into the cavernous sinus via the superior orbital fissure. The inferior ophthalmic vein passes through the inferior orbital fissure, anastomosing with the superior ophthalmic vein and the pterygoid venous plexus.[1,3,6] Both the superior and inferior ophthalmic veins communicate with the veins of the face.[1,6]

The superior ophthalmic vein is the larger of these two veins and arises behind the medial part of the upper eyelid by the union of a branch of the supraorbital vein and a branch from the facial vein (angular vein). The superior ophthalmic vein receives tributaries that correspond to most of the branches of the ophthalmic artery. It communicates with the central vein of the retina and near the apex of the orbit it commonly receives the inferior ophthalmic vein. The superior ophthalmic vein also receives the two vorticose veins from the upper part of the eyeball (the vorticose veins correspond to the posterior ciliary veins). The more variable inferior ophthalmic vein arises from a venous plexus on the anterior part of the floor of the orbital cavity. It communicates with the facial vein over the inferior orbital margin and with the pterygoid venous plexus through the inferior orbital fissure. It passes posteriorly in the orbital fat on the inferior rectus muscle and receives muscular branches and the two inferior vorticose veins from the lower part of the eyeball.

The inferior ophthalmic vein anastomoses with the superior ophthalmic vein and has a similar branch that connects with the pterygoid plexus through the inferior orbital fissure.[3] It may pass through the lower part of the superior orbital fissure and empty directly into the cavernous sinus.

■ Lacrimal Apparatus

The lacrimal gland lies in the superolateral angle of the orbit, in a shallow fossa (lacrimal fossa) behind the upper eyelid, and is deeply indented by the lateral border of the tendon of the levator palpebrae superioris (Fig. 2.117).[1,16] The gland weighs about 78 g and measures 20 mm by 12 mm by 5 mm. It is divided into palpebral and orbital (larger) lobes by the lateral border of the levator aponeurosis.[1-3] The orbital lobe is superior to the palpebral lobe. Small ducts (10–12) open from the deep surface of the gland into the conjunctival sac. The lacrimal gland is a serous gland. The gland has a nodular surface with a fine connective-tissue pseudocapsule. The gland is supported by Whitnall's ligament and by septal attachments to the superior periorbita. The lacrimal artery penetrates it posteriorly, and the vein from it drains into the superior ophthalmic vein. Its lymphatic drainage is by means of the lid and conjunctiva to the preauricular nodes.[2,3]

In addition to the main lacrimal gland, there are accessory glands (of Krause and Wolfring) in the lids and conjunctiva.

Tears produced by the gland pass medially toward the lacrimal puncta across the surface of the cornea, assisted by blinking of the eyelids. Tears are drained into the lacrimal sac through the lacrimal canaliculi of the upper and lower lids. The canaliculi originate at the puncta and have a 2.0 mm vertical portion and an 8.0 mm horizontal portion, which join into a common canaliculus. The common canaliculus enters the lateral wall of the lacrimal sac by means of the valve of Rösenmuller, which prevents reflux.[3] The lacrimal sac lies in the lacrimal groove, which is formed by the lacrimal bone and the frontal process of the maxillary bone.[1] The lacrimal canaliculi are lined by squamous epithelium, whereas the sac and nasolacrimal duct are lined by columnar epithelium, goblet cells, and ciliated cells. The lacrimal sac is 13–15 mm in vertical length. The tears drain through the nasolacrimal duct just beneath the inferior turbinate through a fold in the duct (called the valve of Hasner) in the lateral wall of the nasal cavity.[2,3]

Imaging Techniques

CT and MRI are the two modalities most commonly used for imaging the orbit. Each has advantages and disadvantages. In general, CT is the modality of choice for bony detail and for detecting calcifications and foreign bodies, but irradiation of the orbital structures is a disadvantage. MRI, on the other hand, has no known biological side-effects and is superior to CT when evaluating the pathology of the eye. MRI is generally considered equivalent to or better than CT when evaluating the orbital soft tissues.

■ Computed Tomography

A routine CT examination of the orbits includes contiguous axial and coronal sectioning with 5 mm slice thickness. When there is a suspicion of a smaller lesion, thinner sections (3 or 1.5 mm) should be obtained. Sections of 3 mm or 1.5 mm are essential for optimal demonstration of the optic nerve anatomy and pathology. The radiologist should always tailor the examination according to the clinical information and the preliminary diagnosis. For foreign bodies, it is important to obtain 1.5 mm axial sections to increase the sensitivity for detection of smaller objects. It is often unnecessary to obtain additional direct coronal sections for the localization of foreign bodies because the use of computer reformatting is helpful in producing images in other planes, provided there is no patient motion in axial sections. For foreign bodies or lesions at the 6-o'clock or 12-o'clock positions, it is always advisable to obtain direct coronal sections. For lesions of the globe, thin sectioning (1.5 mm) is exceedingly important, because one can easily miss an ocular lesion on routine 5 mm sections.[16] For bony lesions, or orbital fractures, in addition to the routine study, retrospective high-resolution, extended bone scale images should be obtained (4000 window width, 700–800 window level).[16]

For orbital CT scanning, the need for intravenous (iv) contrast media administration should be determined by the clinical information and is best left to the discretion of the radiologist. Contrast material uniformly increases the density of most intraorbital soft-tissue structures.[2,16] Although it is not always an easy task to discriminate between orbital lesions on the basis of their patterns of enhancement, contrast material is often necessary to evaluate their vascular characteristics and more importantly for the evaluation of any intracranial extension of an orbital lesion. Not uncommonly, an apical orbital mass may be an extension of an intracranial lesion such as a meningioma, which can easily be missed on a noncontrast CT study. In general, contrast medium is not used when evaluating for foreign bodies, uncomplicated orbital fractures, uncomplicated thyroid ophthalmopathy, morphological changes or variations of the extraocular muscles, dermoid cyst (noninfected and unruptured), and bony lesions such as osteoma, osteoid osteoma, fibrous dysplasia, and Paget disease. Contrast-enhanced CT, however, is necessary in patients with osteogenic or chondrogenic sarcomas, or metastatic bone disease.

Technique

Axial sections are normally obtained roughly parallel to the infraorbital–meatal line.[16–18] This can easily be determined by obtaining a lateral digital scout view (scanogram). The inferior section should include the upper portion of the maxillary sinuses, and the upper section should include the sella and the entire frontal sinuses. For all orbital and ocular tumors, additional postcontrast 10 mm axial sections of the remainder of the head are usually obtained. Although brain metastasis from orbital and ocular tumors is uncommon, the additional sections may provide information about unsuspected lesions (meningioma, aneurysm, and arteriovenous malformation [AVM]).[16]

Coronal sections are obtained roughly perpendicular to the infraorbital–meatal line. However, in many instances the angle of the coronal sections is made more oblique (semicoronal) when the patient has many dental fillings or other metallic prostheses. Patient positioning for the coronal plane can be in either the prone or the supine positions and, as for the axial sections, the coronal plane study can be determined easily by obtaining a lateral digital scout view of the orbit. The coronal examination of the orbits should be tailored according to the clinical information and the findings on the axial sections. In patients suffering from visual loss and when evaluating the intracranial extension of an apical lesion, the coronal sections should be extended posteriorly to include the optic chiasm. For lesions involving the anterior ethmoid air cells or nasal cavity, and for lesions arising from the nasolacrimal sac and duct, coronal sections should be extended anteriorly to include the nasal bones.

Sagittal plane. Almost all CT scanners are capable of performing computer reformatting of compiled data from axial sections into coronal, sagittal, or oblique planes. Although the quality of images is inferior to direct scanning, in many instances additional information can be obtained, particularly if high-quality thin (1.5–3 mm) direct axial or coronal sections are available. Direct sagittal plane scans of the craniofacial structures can be achieved by laying the patient on a separate support and using a special head holder, which is fitted to the standard tabletop.[19] With new ultrafast spiral-helical CT scanners, reformatted sagittal images can be obtained with excellent details, eliminating the need for direct sagittal imaging.

■ MRI Techniques

Almost all MR images presented in this section were performed with a 1.5 Tesla (T) Signa unit (General Electric, Milwaukee, WI). Using a head coil, single echo spin-echo (SE) T1-weighted (T1W) pulse sequences were obtained with a repetition time (TR) of 400–800 ms and an echo time (TE) of 20–25 ms (TR/TE, 400–800/20–25 ms). Multiecho SE proton-weighted (PW) and T2-weighted (T2W) pulse sequences were obtained with a TR of 2000–2800 ms and a TE of 20–100 ms. Multiecho SE pulse sequences in our recent protocol have been replaced by fast spin-echo T2W pulse sequence, using the following imaging parameters: 2500–4200/90–102 ms (TR/TE), echo train length of 14, 256×256 data acquisition matrix, 20–22 cm field of view; two excitations are acquired.

Although each examination should be specifically tailored to the patient's problem, our routine MRI examination of the orbit included short TR, short TE sagittal images, 5 mm in thickness with 1–1.5 mm intersection spacing, using the routine head coil. These studies were most often performed with one excitation, a 256×192 or 256×256 matrix size, and a 20–24 cm field of view. Following the sagittal T1-weighted pulse sequence, an axial multiecho SE sequence (TR/TE 2000–2800/20, 80 ms) was obtained to include the entire orbital structures. For this multiecho SE pulse sequence, a section thickness of 5 mm with a 1.5–2.5 mm intersection gap was used, with a matrix size of 256×192 and a 20 cm field of view. Additional single-echo T1W or T2W fast SE pulse sequences in the coronal plane were obtained according to the findings on the sagittal and axial sections. For optic nerve lesions, additional parasagittal images were obtained by using a head coil. The orbital fat remains hyperintense on fast SE T2W pulse sequences. Because of this, we prefer to obtain fast SE T2W fat-suppression pulse sequences.

Paramagnetic contrast material, a gadolinium complex with diethylenetriaminepentaacetic acid (Gd-DTPA), should be used for suspected orbital inflammatory processes and orbital masses. Contrast-enhanced T1-weighted studies were obtained with an axial SE (600–800/20 TR/TE) pulse sequence with four excitations, a 16–20 cm field of view, and a 256×128 matrix size. Section thickness was 3 mm with a 0.5 mm intersection gap. A precontrast T1-weighted axial SE pulse sequence was always obtained. The pulse sequence parameters for this were identical to those for the postcontrast T1-weighted sequence, except that two rather than four excitations were used.

T1-Weighted Fat-Suppression Technique

Fat-suppressed T1-weighted images may be obtained using various techniques.[2,20–22] In this chapter, fat-suppressed T1-weighted images were obtained by means of a presaturation technique. Before imaging, the spectral fat peak was first determined in each patient. Subsequently, an RF pulse was applied, centered at the resonant frequency of fat. The RF pulse was followed by a spoil gradient. This fat-suppression technique (chemsat) is a standard feature on the Signa system and can easily be applied in the same time required for a standard T1-weighted pulse sequence. After the postcontrast fat-suppressed images were acquired, an immediate standard T1-weighted sequence in either the axial or coronal plane was obtained with identical parameters to the fat-suppressed T1-weighted pulse sequence. This was done because the fat-suppression pulse sequences are more sensitive to magnetic susceptibility artifacts.[20,21,22] In addition, the enhancement of the extraocular muscles, and in particular the lacrimal glands, is exaggerated on the fat-suppressed images. There is thus the possibility of misinterpreting a lesion if it is adjacent to the lacrimal gland, the extraocular muscles, or the walls of the sinuses (air–bone–soft tissue interface).[16]

Inversion Recovery Pulse Sequence and Application of Fat-Suppression Technique

Short tau inversion recovery (STIR) images result in very high lesion conspicuity by suppressing the signal from fat and by adding T1-weighted and T2-weighted information together. Because most pathology has long T1 and T2 relaxation times, pathology appears with a high signal intensity on STIR images. The lower fat signal intensity further makes any pathology stand out. The optimal TI (time of inversion) for fat suppression may vary from one individual to another, depending on coil loading and fat composition. The optimal TI for fat suppression at 1.5 T is in the 145–170 ms range. Usually the STIR image is obtained with a TR of 2000 ms, a TI of 150–160 ms, and a TE of 20 ms. STIR sequence is often used for metastatic orbital diseases.

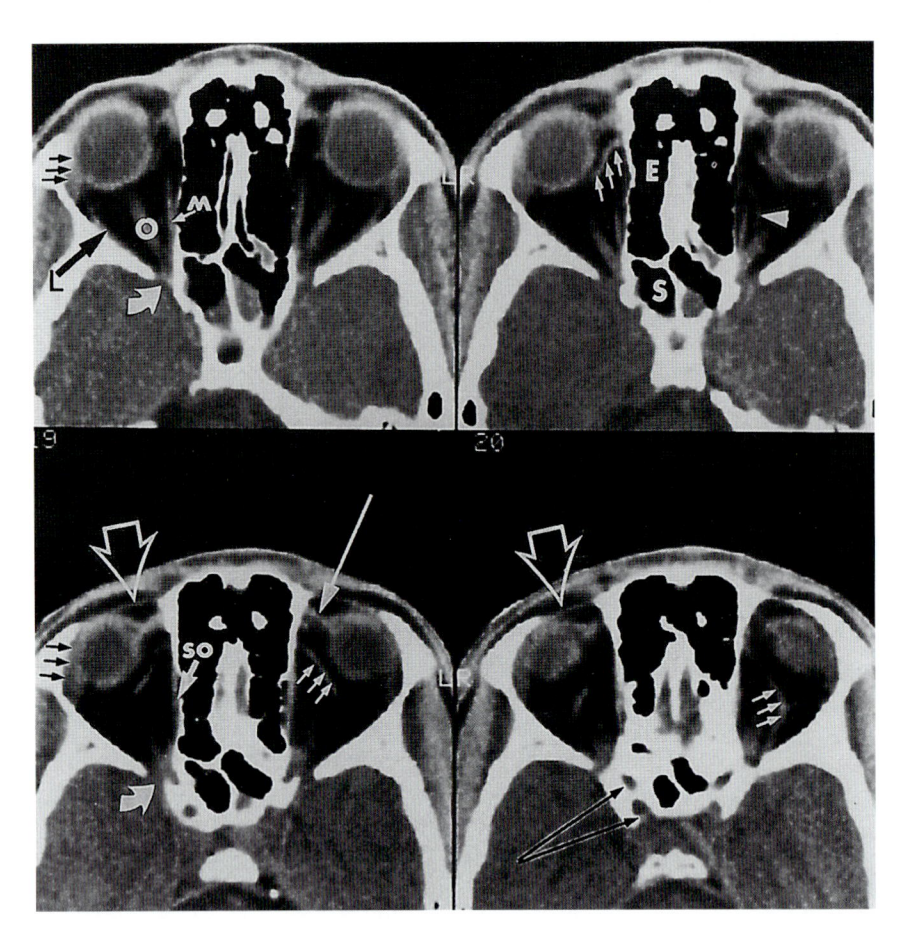

Fig. 2.123 Serial axial CT scans show the lacrimal gland (black short arrows), superior orbital fissure (curved arrows), superior ophthalmic vein (white short arrows), ophthalmic artery (arrowhead), orbital septum (hollow arrows), reflected portions of superior oblique tendon (long arrow), and optic canal (crossed arrows).
E = ethmoid sinus
L = lateral rectus muscle
M = medial rectus muscle
O = optic nerve
S = sphenoid sinus
SO = superior oblique muscle

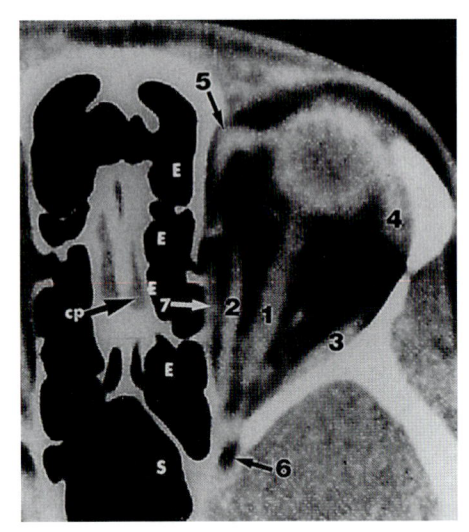

Fig. 2.124 Axial CT scan shows the optic nerve (1), medial (2) and lateral recti (3), lacrimal gland (4), reflected portion of superior oblique tendon (5) and superior orbital fissure (6), superior oblique muscle (7), ethmoid air cells (E), sphenoid sinus (s), and cribriform plate (cp).

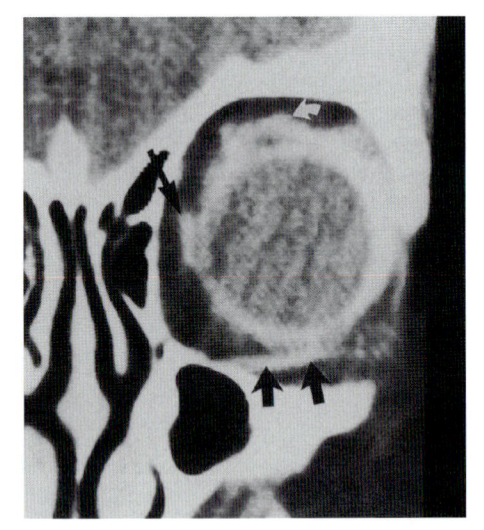

Fig. 2.125 Coronal CT scan shows inferior oblique muscle (black arrows), superior rectus levator palpebrae tendon complex (white arrow), and the tendon of medial rectus muscle (black arrow).

■ Normal CT and MRI Anatomy of the Orbit

The bony landmarks can be visualized best on CT with the aid of the bone extended scale and bone window technique. The optic canal can be seen on both axial and coronal scans. The lateral and medial bony orbital margins, the superior and inferior orbital fissures, the lacrimal fossa, lacrimal sac groove, nasolacrimal canal, infraorbital canal, and the paranasal sinuses are also equally well seen on axial or coronal scans (Figs. 2.123–2.126). Coronal scans are best for assessing the floor and roof of the orbits.

Extraocular Muscles

The extraocular muscles are well visualized on CT, and they are uniformly enhanced on postcontrast CT scans (Figs. 2.123–126). These muscles are best seen on MRI (Figs. 2.127–2.133). The ex-

Imaging Techniques 207

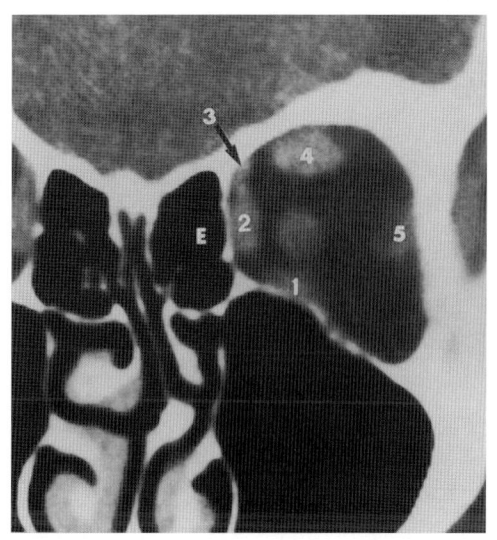

Fig. 2.**126** Coronal CT scan shows the inferior (1), medial (2), superior oblique (3), superior (4), and lateral rectus (5) muscles. E = ethmoid bulla.

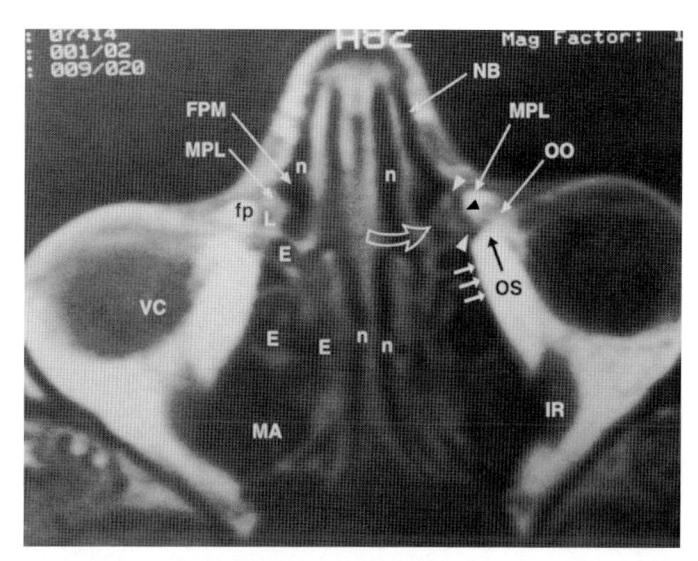

Fig. 2.**127 a** Normal MRI anatomy of the orbit. Axial T1W MR scan, obtained with surface coil, shows ethmoid air cells (E), fat pad (fp), frontal process of maxilla (FPM), inferior rectus (IR), lacrimal sac (L), superior medial portion of maxillary sinus (MA), medial palpebral ligament (MPL), nasal cavity (n), nasal bone (NB), lacrimal portion of orbicularis oculi (OO), orbital septum (OS), vitreous chamber (VC), lacrimal groove formed by lacrimal bone and frontal process of maxilla (hollow curved arrow), periorbita (periosteum) (three short arrows), and lacrimal fascia (black arrowhead). The lacrimal sac is about 12 cm long, situated in the lacrimal fossa, and is enclosed by lacrimal fascia (black arrowhead), which is attached behind to the posterior lacrimal crest of the lacrimal bone and in front to the anterior lacrimal crest of the maxilla (white arrowheads). The fascia is formed from the periorbita (three white arrows). The lacrimal fascia separates the sac from the medial palpebral ligament (MPL) anteriorly and the lacrimal part of orbicularis oculi (OO) posteriorly). The medial palpebral ligament covers only the upper part of the anterior aspect of the lacrimal sac. The upper half of the sac is related medially to the anterior ethmoid cells (E). The lower half is related medially to the anterior part of the middle meatus of the nasal cavity. The orbital septum (OS) is a fibrous membrane, attached to the orbital margin, where it is continuous with periorbita (three short arrows). The orbital septum separates the eyelids from the contents of the orbital cavity. The orbital septum lies posterior to the medial palpebral ligament. The MPL attaches the medial ends of the tarsi to the lacrimal crest and the frontal process of the maxilla.

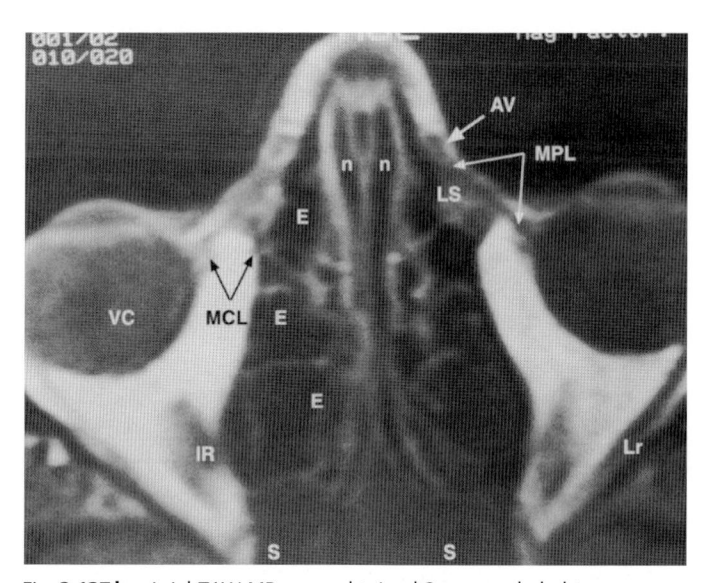

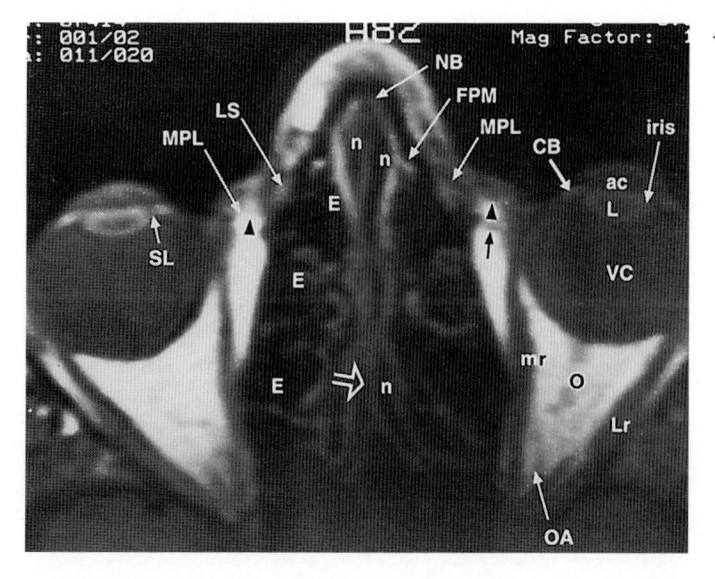

Fig. 2.**127 b** Axial T1W MR scan, obtained 3 mm cephalad to **a**.
AV = presumed angular vein
E = ethmoid air cells
IR = inferior rectus
Lr = lateral rectus
LS = lacrimal sac
MCL = medial check ligament
MPL = medial palpebral ligament
n = nasal cavity
S = sphenoid sinus
VC = vitreous chamber

◁ Fig. 2.**127 c** Axial T1W MR scan, obtained 3 mm cephalad to **b**. Note the expansion of the fascial sleeve of medial rectus as it forms the medial check ligament (black arrow). The medial check ligaments are attached to the lacrimal bone. The orbital septum (arrowheads), is seen anterior to the medial check ligament. The orbital septum at the level of the lacrimal groove splits to enclose the lacrimal sac and continues inferiorly to the periosteum of the nasolacrimal canal (see also **a**). The medial palpebral ligament (MPL) is anterior to the lacrimal sac, and the ligament attaches the medial ends of the tarsi to the lacrimal crest and the frontal process of the maxilla. The MPL is about 4 mm long and 2 mm wide and is attached to the frontal process of the maxilla in front of the nasolacrimal groove. It is separated from the lacrimal sac by the lacrimal fascia (see **a**).
ac = anterior chamber
CB = ciliary body
E = ethmoid air cells
FPM = frontal process of maxilla
L = lens
Lr = lateral rectus
LS = lacrimal sac
MPL = medial palpebral ligament
mr = medial rectus
n = nasal cavity
NB = nasal bone
O = optic nerve (partially volumed)
OA = ophthalmic artery
SL = suspensory ligament of lens, and nasal septum (hollow arrow)

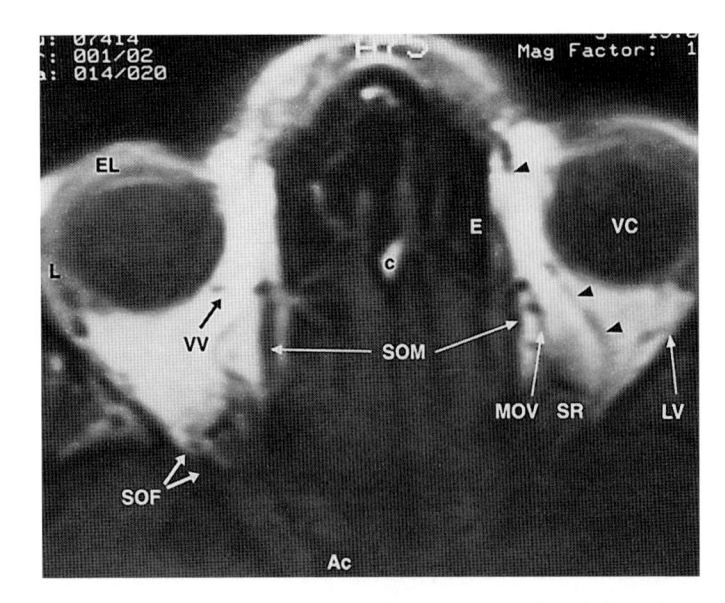

Fig. 2.127 d Axial T1W MR scan obtained 9 mm cephalad to **c**.
AC = anterior clinoid
C = crista galli
E = ethmoid air cell
EL = eyelid
L = lacrimal gland
Lv = lacrimal vein
mov = medial ophthalmic vein
SOM = superior oblique muscle
SR = superior rectus
SOF = superior orbital fissure
VC = vitreous chamber
VV = presumed vortex (vorticose) vein or medial collateral vein
Arrowheads = superior ophthalmic vein

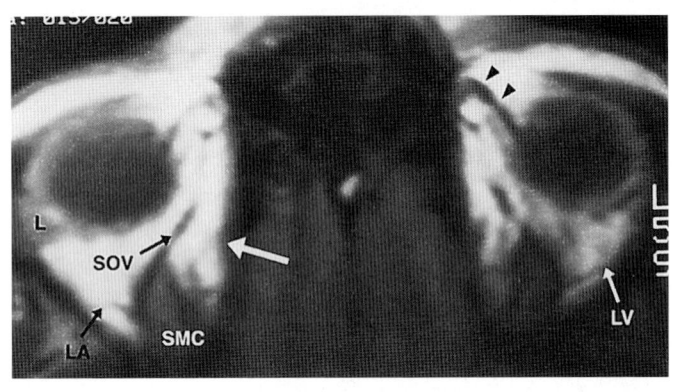

Fig. 2.127 e Axial T1W MR scan obtained 3 mm cephalad to **d**.
L = lacrimal gland
LA = lacrimal artery
LV = lacrimal vein
SMC = superior rectus levator palpebrae muscle complex
White arrow = presumed nasociliary nerve
Arrowheads = reflected portion of superior oblique muscle

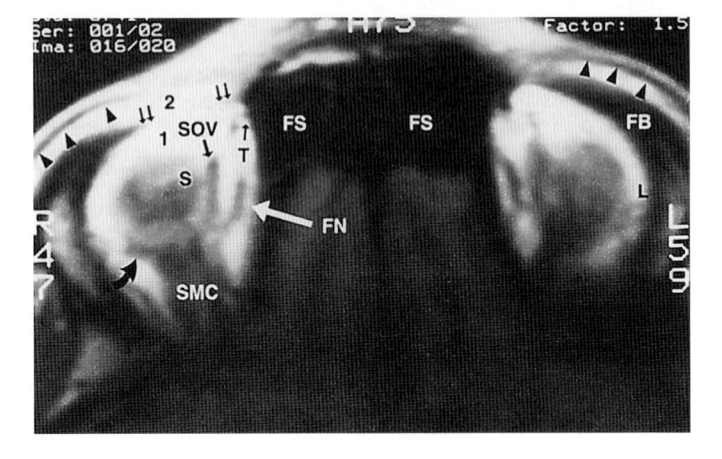

Fig. 2.127 f Axial T1W MR scan, obtained 3 mm cephalad to **e**. The orbital septum (small double arrows) separates the preaponeurotic fat pad (1) from the fat pad (2) underlying the orbicularis oculi: The orbital septum is in continuity with the periosteum. The frontal nerve (FN) lies outside the fibrous ring of Zinn and passes forward beneath the roof of the orbit on the upper surface of the levator palpebrae superioris muscle and divides into the supraorbital branch and supratrochlear branch.
1 = preaponeurotic fat pad
2 = fat pad underlying the orbicularis oculi (arrowheads)
FB = frontal bone
FS = frontal sinus
FN = frontal nerve
L = lacrimal gland
S = sclera
SMC = superior rectus-levator palpebrae complex
SOV = superior ophthalmic vein
T = trochlea
Small double arrows = orbital septum
Arrowheads = orbicularis oculi

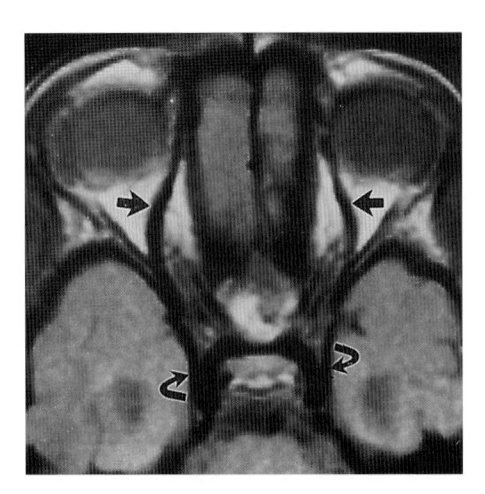

Fig. 2.128 Axial proton density-weighted (PW) MR scan, obtained with the head coil shows the superior ophthalmic veins (arrows) entering into the cavernous sinuses (curved arrows).

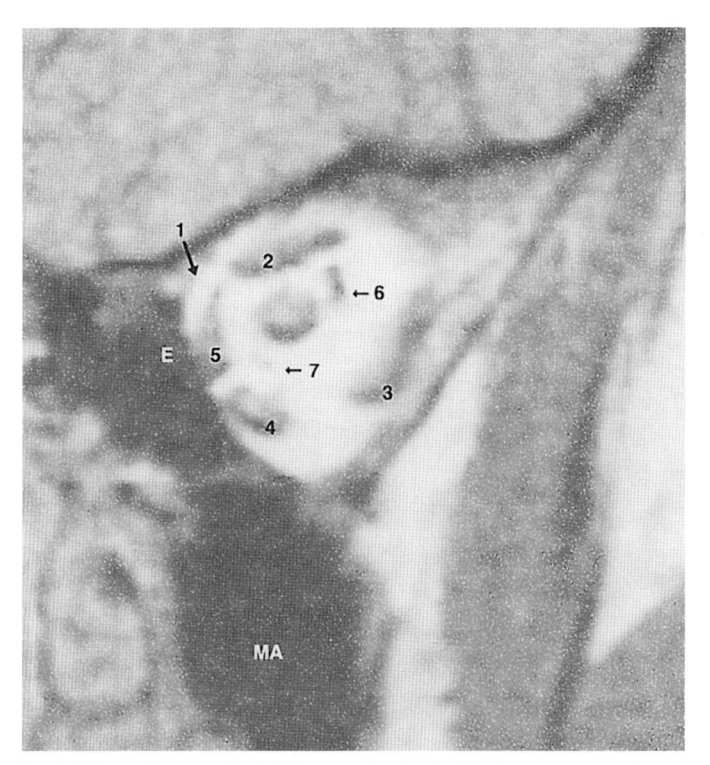

Fig. 2.**129a** Coronal T1W MR scan obtained with the surface coil
1 = superior oblique muscle
2 = superior rectus muscle
3 = lateral rectus muscle
4 = inferior rectus muscle
5 = medial rectus muscle
6 = ophthalmic artery and its muscular branch
7 = oculomotor nerve
E = ethmoid sinus
MA = maxillary antrum

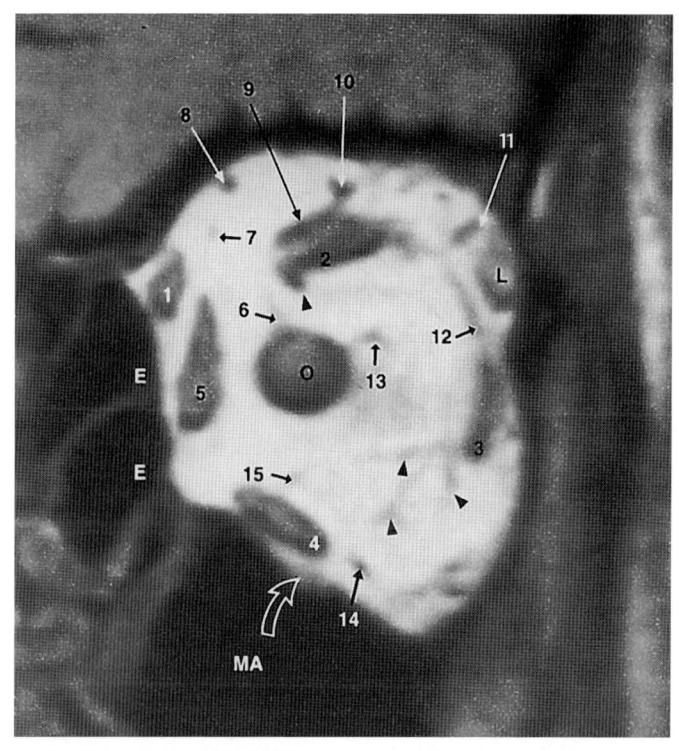

Fig. 2.**129b** Coronal T1W MR scan obtained 3 mm anterior to **a**.
1 = superior oblique muscle
2 = superior rectus muscle
3 = lateral rectus muscle
4 = inferior rectus muscle
5 = medial rectus muscle
6 = presumed posterior ciliary artery and or ciliary ganglion
7 = nasociliary nerve
8 = supratrochlear nerve
9 = levator palpebrae superioris
10 = frontal nerve
11 = lacrimal nerve, artery, and vein
12 = intermuscular septum
13 = presumed posterior ciliary artery
14 = oculomotor nerve (inferior ramus)
15 = medial orbital vein or inferior muscular artery
E = ethmoid sinus
MA = maxillary antrum
Single arrowhead = superior ophthalmic vein
Arrowheads = lateral collateral veins
Hollow curved arrow = infraorbital nerve

traocular muscles generally have a course parallel to the adjacent orbital wall. Consequently, only the horizontal recti (lateral and medial) may be seen in their entirety in an axial plane (Fig. 2.**127**). Likewise, the vertical recti (inferior and superior) may be seen best in the parasagittal (oblique) plane (Figs. 2.**120d**, 2.**130**). The tapering of these muscles in their tendinous portions and their origins at the annulus of Zinn are seen well in the parasagittal (vertical recti) and axial (horizontal recti) scans (Figs. 2.**120d**, 2.**127**, 2.**130**). The superior and inferior recti are only partially visualized in any section of the axial plane (Fig. 2.**127**). On coronal scans, all of the rectus muscles are seen in an oblique section (Fig. 2.**129**) related to their slanted orientation to the coronal plane as the walls of the orbit slant toward the orbital apex. For accurate determination of the cross-sectional size of these muscles, reformatted images or direct oblique MRI scans would have to be done separately for each muscle. This is obviously not practical, nor is it necessary, unless there is a critical situation requiring the precise size of a particular muscle.[14] The levator palpebrae superioris is closely approximated to the superior rectus muscle, and it is only identified as a separate muscle on anterior coronal images (Fig. 2.**129b**, **c**), where it diverges from the superior rectus. These two muscles can both be visualized as separate muscles on sagittal and parasagittal (oblique) MRI (Fig. 2.**120d**). The muscle portion of the superior oblique muscle can be visualized best on coronal scans, and its ten-

dinous portion is seen best on axial scans (Figs. 2.**124**, 2.**129b**). The trochlear portion of the superior oblique muscle tendon and its reflected portion are seen best on axial scans (Figs. 2.**124**). The trochlea is seen well on axial scans, and is occasionally calcified. The inferior oblique muscle is seen best on coronal, sagittal, and parasagittal scans (Fig. 2.**120d**, 2.**125**). On axial CT scans the inferior oblique muscle belly is usually poorly seen. At times the inferior oblique muscle and inferior rectus muscle can be well visualized on axial MR scans (Figs. 2.**131**, 2.**132**).

Lacrimal Gland

The lacrimal glands are readily identified in the superolateral extraconal space (Fig. 2.**129**). The gland is adjacent to the tendons of the superior and lateral rectus muscles and is separated from the globe by the lateral rectus muscle (Figs. 2.**127**, 2.**129b**, **c**).[23]

Vascular and Neural Structures

Although the vascular structures in the orbit can frequently be seen on noncontrast CT, they are highlighted with contrast. On MRI, the larger vessels usually have low signal intensity (signal void). The ophthalmic artery can be seen in the apex of the orbit on the inferior aspect of the optic nerve and then as it swings laterally before looping around and over the optic nerve to its su-

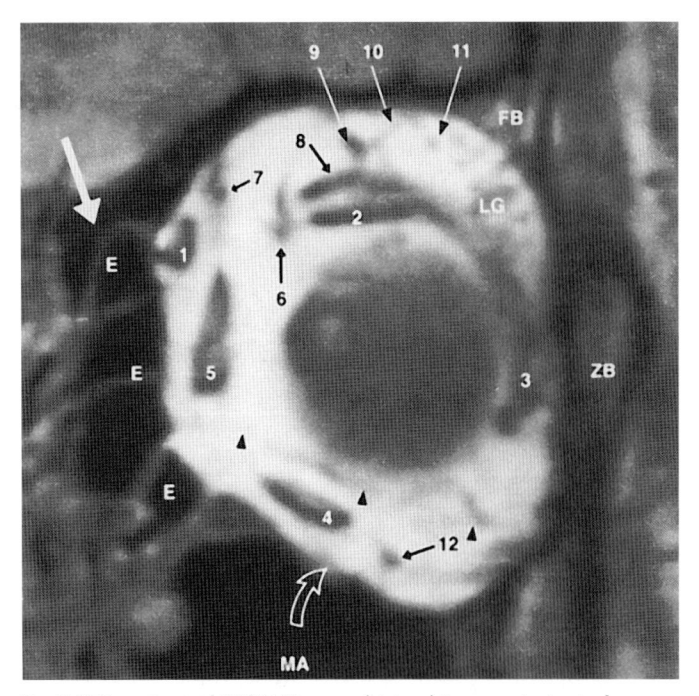

Fig. 2.**129 c** Coronal T1W MR scan obtained 3 mm anterior to **b**.
1 = superior oblique muscle
2 = superior rectus muscle
3 = lateral rectus muscle
4 = inferior rectus muscle
5 = medial rectus muscle
6 = ophthalmic artery and superior ophthalmic vein
7 = medial ophthalmic vein
8 = levator palpebrae superioris
9 = frontal nerve
10 = supraorbital nerve
11 = lacrimal nerve
12 = presumed inferior branch of oculomotor nerve
E = ethmoid air cells
FB = frontal bone
LG = lacrimal gland
MA = maxillary antrum
ZB = zygomatic bone
Arrowheads
 = presumed collateral veins
Hollow curved arrow
 = infraorbital nerve
Solid arrow = fovea ethmoidalis

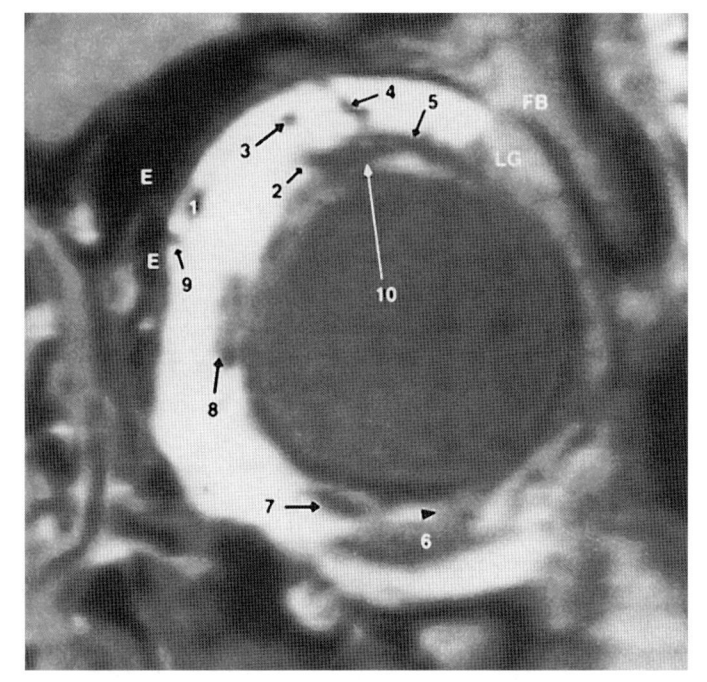

Fig. 2.**129 d** Coronal T1W MR scan obtained 3 mm anterior to **c**.
1 = tendon of superior oblique muscle
2 = reflected tendon of superior oblique muscle, under the tendon of superior rectus muscle
3 = presumed superior ophthalmic vein
4 = frontal nerve
5 = tendon of levator palpebrae superioris
6 = inferior oblique muscle
7 = tendon of inferior rectus muscle
8 = tendon of medial rectus muscle
9 = ethmoid artery
10 = tendon of superior rectus muscle
E = ethmoid air cells
FB = frontal bone
LG = lacrimal gland
Arrowhead
 = presumed suspensory ligament of Lockwood

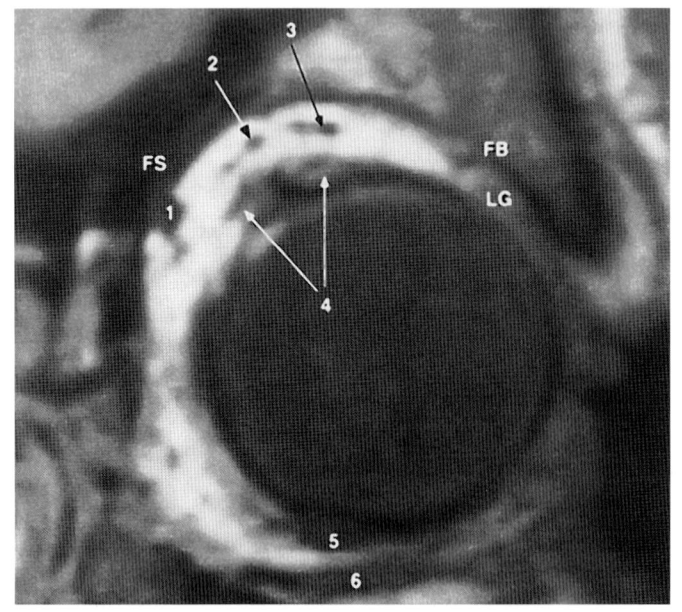

Fig. 2.**129 e** Coronal T1W MR scan obtained 3 mm anterior to **d**.
1 = tendon of superior oblique muscle
2 = presumed superior ophthalmic vein
3 = frontal nerve
4 = complex tendons of superior rectus and levator palpebrae superioris
5 = tendon of inferior rectus muscle
6 = inferior oblique muscle
FB = frontal bone
FS = frontal sinus
LG = lacrimal gland

perior medial aspect (Figs. 2.**129 a**, **c**). Several of its branches, including the anterior and posterior ethmoidal and posterior ciliary branches, may be identified.[3, 24, 25]

The superior ophthalmic vein originates in the extraconal space, in the anteromedial aspect of the orbit. It then courses near the trochlea to pass through the muscle cone beneath the superior rectus muscle and above the optic nerve. It then exits the intraconal space through the superior orbital fissure (Figs. 2.**127 f**, 2.**128**). This vein is routinely identified in axial, coronal, sagittal, and parasagittal images. The inferior ophthalmic and connecting veins are seen inconsistently.[2]

The intraconal and extraconal components of the small nerves of the orbit, particularly the frontal, supraorbital, and inferior divisions of the third nerve, as well as the infraorbital nerve, may be identified on CT and MR scans. These nerves are identified better on MRI (Fig. 2.**133**). The position of these nerves may be variable.[3] The frontal nerve can be seen between the levator palpebrae superioris muscle and the orbital roof (Fig. 2.**133**). Most of these small nerves can be seen on coronal scans of the orbital apex.[25]

Optic Nerve

The orbital segment of the optic nerve is 3–4 mm in diameter and 20–30 mm long and is best seen on axial or sagittal scans (Figs. 2.**120 d**, 2.**130**). The intracanalicular and prechiasmatic portions of the optic nerve are particularly well demonstrated by MRI.

Generally, on T1-weighted, proton density, and T2-weighted images the optic nerve has signal intensities similar to those of

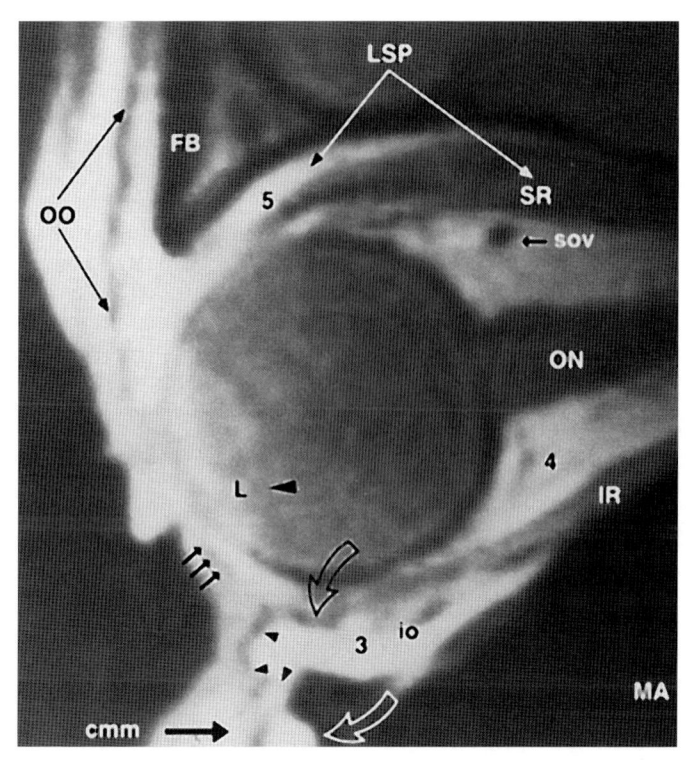

Fig. 2.130a Sagittal PW MR scan showing the following:
OO = fibers of orbicularis oculi
FB = frontal bone
5   = extraconal fat
LSP = levator palpebrae superioris
SR = superior rectus muscle
sov = superior ophthalmic vein
ON = optic nerve
4   = intraconal fatty reticulum
IR = inferior rectus
IO = inferior oblique
3   = extraconal fat
cmm = complex muscles of the mouth
L   = lens
Black curved arrow = presumed suspensory ligament of Lockwood
White curved arrow = anterior border of maxillary antrum (MA)
Three arrowheads = orbital septum
Three arrows = inferior tarsal plate
Arrowhead = posterior capsule of lens

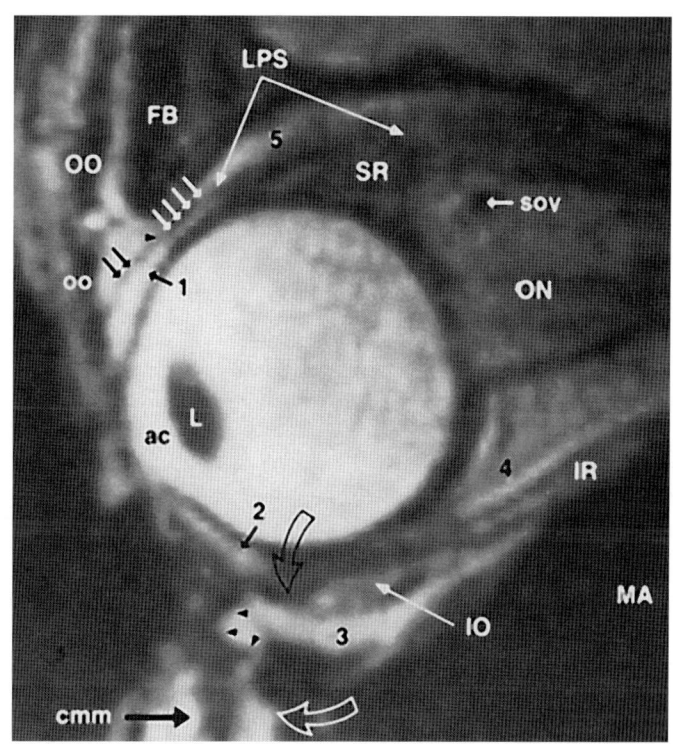

Fig. 2.130b Sagittal T2W MR scan shows fibers of orbicularis oclui (OO), frontal bone (FB), levator palpebrae superioris (LPS), extraconal fat (5), superior rectus muscle (SR), superior ophthalmic vein (sov), optic nerve (ON), intraconal fatty reticulum (4), inferior rectus muscle (IR), maxillary antrum (MA), inferior oblique muscle (IO), extraconal fat (3), anterior wall of maxillary sinus (white hollow arrow), complex muscles of the mouth (cmm), orbital septum (arrowheads), presumed suspensory ligament of Lockwood (black hollow arrow), inferior (2) and superior fornices (1), anterior chamber (ac), lens (L), superior tarsal plate (black arrows) and the tendon of insertion of levator palpebrae superioris (white arrows). This tendon is an aponeurosis that descends posterior to the orbital septum (the orbital septum is depicted as an ill-defined image [arrowhead] in this section). The tendinous fibers then pierce the orbital septum and become attached to the anterior surface of the superior tarsal plate. Some of its fibers pass forward between the muscular bundles of the orbicularis oculi (OO) to attach to the skin.

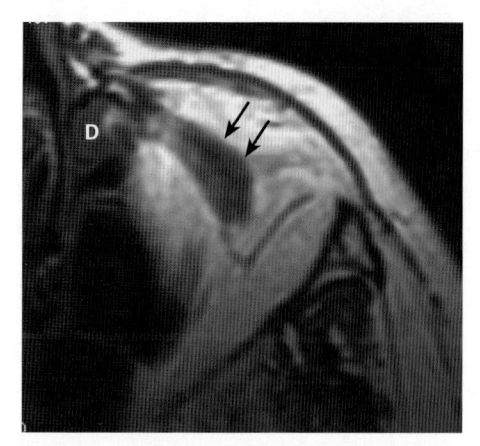

Fig. 2.131 Inferior oblique muscle. Axial T1W MR scan, taken with surface coil (550/13, TR/TE, FOV: 14×14, 3 NEX, 256×192, 2.0 mm section thickness and 0.5 mm spacing), showing the inferior oblique muscle (arrow). Note its origin adjacent to the nasolacrimal duct (D).

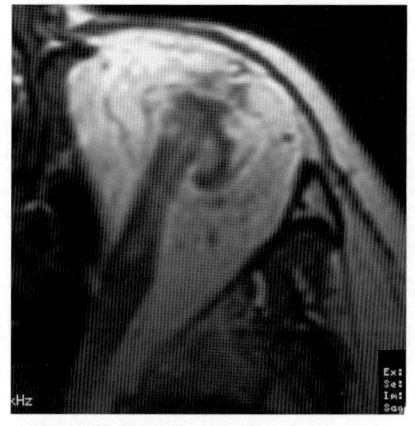

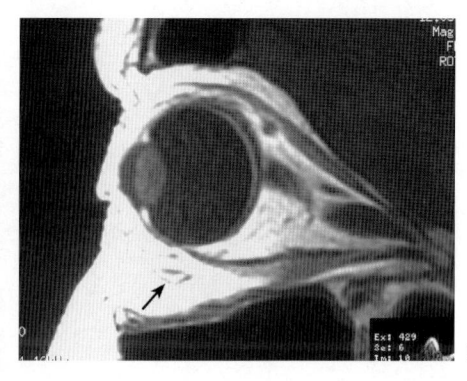

Fig. 2.132a Inferior rectus muscle. Axial T1W MR scan, taken 2.5 mm superior to Fig. 2.131, showing the inferior rectus muscle.
b Inferior and superior rectus muscles. Sagittal T1W MR scan, same individual as in a, showing the inferior oblique muscle (arrow) as well as the insertion of the inferior and superior rectus muscles.

212　2　Part 2: The Orbit

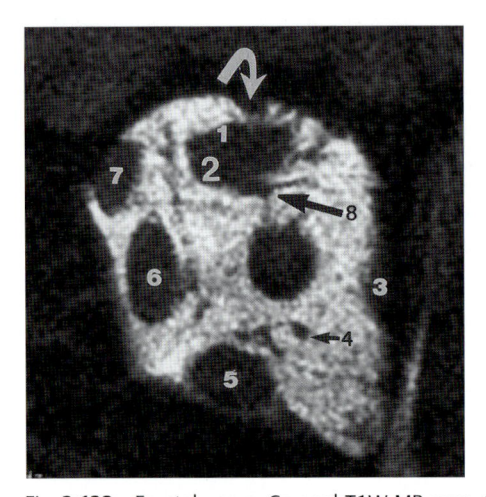

Fig. 2.**133**　Frontal nerve. Coronal T1W MR scan, taken with 3-inch surface coil (450/28, TR/TE, FOV: 8×8, 256×256, 3 mm slice thickness, 0.0 spacing), showing the frontal nerve (curved arrow), levator palpebrae superioris (1), superior rectus muscle (2), lateral rectus muscle (3), inferior ophthalmic vein (4), inferior rectus (5), medial rectus (6), superior oblique muscle (7), and superior ophthalmic vein (8). Note numerous connective-tissue septa within the fat cushion of the orbit, giving the appearance of a fatty reticulum.

Table 2.**10**　Conal lesions

Common causes of enlarged extraocular muscle include:
Graves myositis, thyroid orbitopathy (autoimmune process)
Inflammatory myositis, including cysticercosis (rare)
Granulomatous myositis (less common)
Pseudotumor (myositic type)
Lymphoma
Vascular lesions (hemangioma, AVM, carotid cavernous fistula)
Acromegaly
Pseudorheumatoid nodule (rare)
Metastasis (breast, lung)

normal white matter.[26] A ring of T1-weighted hypointensity and T2-weighted hyperintensity, representing cerebrospinal fluid (CSF) within the nerve sheath, is frequently seen on coronal sections. This should not be confused with well-defined areas of hypointensity bordering the nerve, which are caused by chemical shift artifact.

Cavernous Sinus

The cavernous sinus is directly related to the orbital apex and to the side of the body of the sphenoid bone. It carries in its lateral wall the third and fourth cranial nerves and the ophthalmic and maxillary divisions of the fifth cranial nerve (Fig. 2.**134**). The internal carotid artery and abducent nerve pass forward through the sinus. Numerous trabeculae cross the cavernous sinuses, giving them a spongy appearance (hence the name). Each sinus extends from the superior orbital fissure in front to the apex of the petrous apex. The internal carotid artery and the nerves are separated from the venous blood by endothelial covering.[2, 15] The internal carotid artery, surrounded by its sympathetic nerve plexus, runs forward through the cavernous sinus. The tributaries are the superior and inferior ophthalmic veins, the cerebral veins, the sphenoparietal sinus, and the central vein of the retina. The sinus drains posteriorly into the superior and inferior petrosal sinuses, and inferiorly into the pterygoid venous plexus.[15] The two sinuses communicate with each other by means of the anterior and posterior intercavernous sinuses, which run in the diaphragm sellae. Each sinus has an important communication with the facial vein through the superior ophthalmic vein.[2]

Orbital Compartments

In descriptive terms the orbit has been divided into the extraperiosteal, subperiosteal, extraconal, conal, and intraconal spaces (Figs. 2.**117**, 2.**129**). The intraconal space is separated from the other spaces by the rectus muscles and their intermuscular septa, which are denser in the anterior orbit and are seen best on coronal scans (Fig. 2.**129**). Because certain lesions have a predilection to present in a specific orbital space, the concept of the orbital spaces serves some practical value (Tables 2.**10**–2.**13**). It is useful for radiological differential diagnosis and for surgical planning, and these lesions are discussed later in this chapter. The distinction of intraocular and extraocular locations within the orbit is also useful when evaluating metastatic and dystrophic orbital calcifications (Tables 2.**14**–2.**15**).

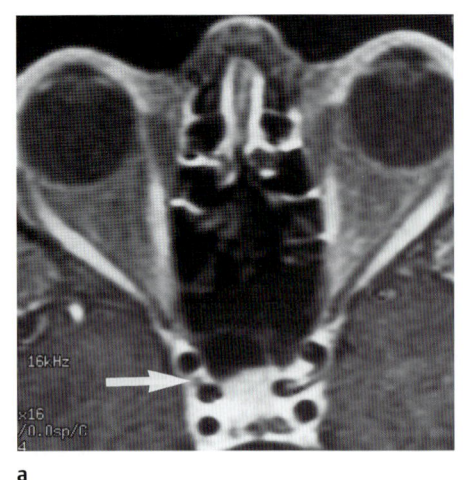

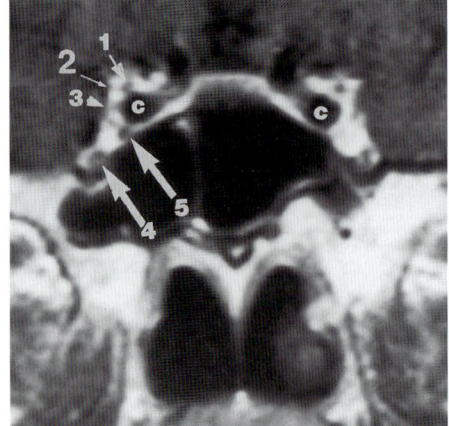

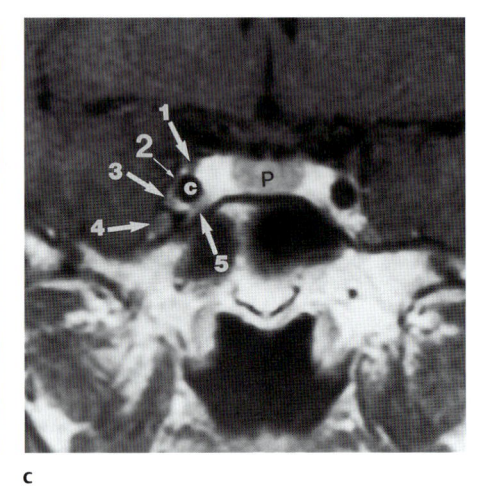

Fig. 2.**134**　Cavernous sinus, MRI anatomy.
a　Axial enhanced fat-suppression T1W MR scan showing normal intense enhancement of the venous structures of the cavernous sinuses. Note the signal void of the internal carotid arteries. The ophthalmic division of the trigeminal nerve can be recognized on the right side (arrow).

b, c　Coronal enhanced T1W MR scans showing oculomotor nerve (1), trochlear nerve (2), ophthalmic division of trigeminal nerve (3), maxillary division of the trigeminal nerve (4), and abducent nerve (5). Note internal carotid artery (C) and normal pituitary gland (P).

Table 2.11 Intraconal (central orbital) lesions

Common	Less common
Cavernous hemangioma	Capillary hemangioma
Optic nerve meningioma	Peripheral nerve tumors
Optic nerve glioma	Neurofibroma
Optic nerve granulomatous disease (sarcoid)	Schwannoma
Optic neuritis (MS)	Leukemia
Lymphoma	Hematocele
Pseudotumor	Optic nerve sheath cyst
Lymphangioma	Colobomatous cyst
Venous angioma	Hemangioblastoma (optic nerve)
Varix	Chemodectoma (ciliary ganglion)
AVM	Necrobiotic xanthogranuloma (rare)
Carotid cavernous fistula	Lipoma (rare)
Hemangiopericytoma	Amyloidosis (rare)
Fibrous histiocytoma	Sclerosing hemangioma
Rhabdomyosarcoma	
Orbital cellulitis and abscess	
Metastasis	

Table 2.12 Extraconal peripheral orbital lesions

Capillary hemangioma	Langerhans histiocytosis
Dermoid and epidermoid cysts	Lipoma
Fibrous histiocytoma	Lymphangioma
Sclerosing hemangioma	Orbital encephalocele
Hemangiosarcoma (rare)	Peripheral nerve tumors
Hemangiopericytoma	Plasmacytoma
Hematic cyst	Rhabdomyosarcoma
Amyloidosis (rare)	Sarcoidosis
Lacrimal gland lesions	Wegener granulomatosis (rare)
A Inflammation	Metastasis
B Lymphoma	
C Pseudotumor	
D Sarcoidosis	
E Epithelial tumors	

Table 2.13 Subperiosteal lesions

Common orbital subperiosteal lesions include:

Subperiosteal cellulitis	Lacrimal gland tumors spread
Subperiosteal abscess	Dermoid and epidermoid cysts
Subperiosteal infiltration of sinonasal neoplastic lesions	Hematoma and hematic cyst
	Cholesterol granuloma
Infiltration by meningiomas (en plaque meningiomas)	Fibrous histiocytoma
	Primary osseous or cartilaginous tumors
Lymphomas	
Plasmacytomas	Metastasis (neuroblastoma)
Langerhans histiocytosis	

Table 2.15 Differential diagnosis of dystrophic orbital calcification

Intraocular
Cataract
Endophthalmitis (chronic stage)
Granulomas (toxocara, sarcoidosis)
Hyaline plaques
Idiopathic sclerochoroidal calcification (senile)
Optic nerve drusen
Phthisis bulbi
Chronic retinal detachment (metaplastic calcification or bone formation by RPE)
Retinal detachment (post-scleral buckling procedure)
Retinal dysplasia, Coats disease (chronic stage)
Retinoblastoma
Retinopathy of prematurity (late stage)
Tuberous sclerosis, neurofibromatosis (hamartoma of the retina)
von Hippel–Lindau disease (chronic retinal detachment)
Choroidal osteoma

Extraocular
Within the lacrimal gland fossa
  Amyloidosis
  Choristoma
  Dermolipoma
  Malignant tumors of the lacrimal gland
  Plasmacytoma
  Pleomorphic adenoma*
  Varix
Extrinsic to the lacrimal gland fossa
  Amyloidosis
  Arteriovenous shunt or malformation
  Calcified trochlea
  Cartilaginous tumors
  Glioma*
  Hemangioma*
  Hemangiopericytoma*
  Hemorrhage
  Idiopathic inflammatory "pseudotumor"*
  Lymphangioma
  Lymphoma*
  Melanoma*
  Meningioma
  Metastatic colonic carcinoma
  Mucocele
  Neuroblastoma
  Neurofibroma*
  Orbital bone fragment after trauma
  Teratoma
  Trichinosis
  Varix

Table 2.14 Differential diagnosis of metastatic orbital calcification

Congenital
Fanconi syndrome
Milk-alkali syndrome
Renal tubular acidosis

Endocrine
Hyperparathyroidism, primary or secondary
Hypoparathyroidism
Pseudohypoparathyroidism
Pseudopseudohypoparathyroidism

Idiopathic—sarcoidosis

Infectious
Cytomegalovirus
Leprosy
Osteomyelitis
Syphilis
Toxoplasmosis
Tuberculosis
Foreign body granuloma

Toxic
Excessive ingestion of calcium phosphate or alkali
Vitamin D intoxication

Traumatic—immobilization

Neoplastic
Bronchogenic carcinoma
Metastatic involvement of bone (prostate)
Multiple myeloma
Parathyroid adenoma
Parathyroid carcinoma
Post radiation

Modified and adopted from Froula PD et al. The differential diagnosis of orbital calcification as detected on computed tomographic scans. Mayo Clin Proc 1993; 68: 256–261.

Modifieded and adopted from Froula PD et al. The differential diagnosis of orbital calcification as detected on computed tomographic scans. Mayo Clin Proc 1993; 68: 256–261.

* rarely shows calcification

Table 2.16 CT orbital measurements in 400 adults

Line, description	Measurement (cm)					
	Minimum		Maximum		Mean	
	Male	Female	Male	Female	Male	Female
aa, Approximates interpupillary distance	6.26	6.21	7.51	7.50	6.78	6.63
bb, BID measured at posterior border of frontal processes of maxillae	2.29	2.29	3.21	3.20	2.67	2.56
cc, BID measured posterior or at the level of orbital equator (useful orbits)	2.63	2.56	3.50	3.30	2.80	2.83
dd, Distance between anterior margin of frontal processes of zygomatic bones at the level of the plane of optic nerves	9.18	8.29	10.13	11.00	9.73	9.97
ee, Distance between optic nerves where they enter eyeballs	5.16	4.78	6.40	6.00	5.43	5.27
ff, BID measured at the level of posterior poles of eyeballs	2.87	2.56	3.70	3.51	3.10	2.97
gg, BID measured at its widest part (usually posterior to FF line)	3.16	2.93	4.10	3.67	3.37	3.20
hh, BID measured at its most posterior part (apex of bony orbit)	2.16	2.43	3.37	3.23	2.73	2.80
ii, Distance between superior orbital fissures at apex of bony orbit	2.90	2.70	3.83	3.63	3.10	3.00
jj, Distance between central portion of cranial opening of optic canals	2.20	2.01	2.73	2.70	2.30	2.20
kk, Distance between tips of anterior clinoid processes	2.31	2.43	3.21	3.16	2.80	2.83
ei, Length of intraorbital part of optic nerve						
Right	2.70	2.40	3.80	3.23	3.10	2.90
Left	2.60	2.40	3.80	3.21	3.20	2.80
ap, Anteroposterior diameter of eyeball						
Right	2.50	2.39	2.90	2.70	2.80	2.50
Left	2.40	2.40	2.80	2.80	2.70	2.63
tt, Transverse diameter of eyeball						
Right	2.50	2.40	2.80	2.90	2.70	2.71
Left	2.50	2.50	2.90	2.90	2.80	2.83
Angle between optic nerve axes (in degrees)	35	36.5	50	51.5	41	42.3

BID = bony interorbital distance.
From Mafee MF, Pruzansky S. Corrales MM, et al. CT in the evaluation of the orbit and the bony intraorbital distance. AJNR 1986;7:265–269. With permission.

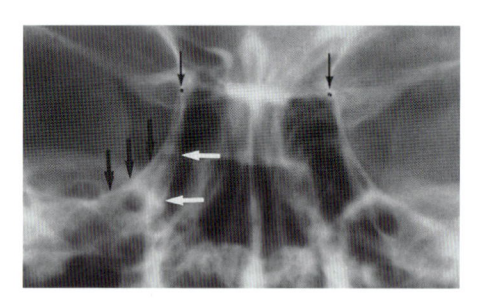

Fig. 2.135 Caldwell projection showing the anterior (triplet black arrow) and posterior (double white arrows) portions of the medial wall of the orbit. The interorbital distance can be measured where these two lines merge (black dots shown by arrows).

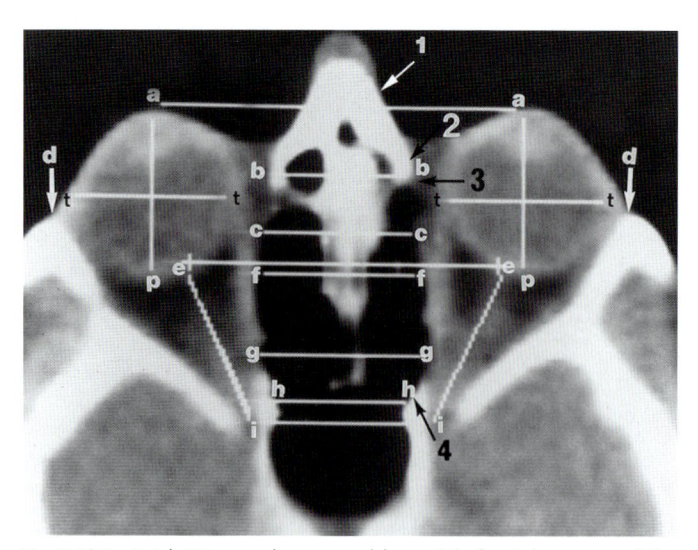

Fig. 2.136 Axial CT scan shows nasal bone (1), frontal process of the maxilla (2), lacrimal bone (3), apex of the orbit (4), and the locations of linear measurements shown in Table 2.16. From Mafee MF et al. CT in the evaluation of the orbit and the bony interorbital distance. AJNR. 1986; 1:265. With permission.

Bony Interorbital Distance

The distance between the orbits and their individual dimensions are important in the diagnosis of craniofacial anomalies. The orbits are often involved in craniofacial malformations, which include orbital clefts and orbital hypotelorism and hypertelorism. Measurement of the bony interorbital distance (BID) is useful in establishing the severity of hypertelorism. This distance is commonly measured at the interdacryon level, the dacryon being the point of junction of the nasal bone, the lacrimal bone, and the maxilla.[18] Before the advent of CT, most observers relied on standard radiographs (Fig. 2.135) for measuring the BID, and normal values for adults and the younger age groups are available.[27–31]

Hansman, using radiographs of the skull and paranasal sinuses in a large group of healthy subjects, presented measurements of the interorbital distance and the thickness of the skull.[31] According to him, from infancy to adulthood, the bony interorbital distance for girls is consistently narrower than for boys. Starting at 1 year 6 months, there is gradual increase in the size of the measurements for both sexes. At about 13 years of age, the girls' growth began to level off. Since the boys' continues to increase to the age of about 21 years, the measurements in girls fall more markedly below the boys' as growth is completed. The average adult measurement in women is 25 mm and in men 28 mm.[31]

On CT the lacrimal bones and the orbital plates of the ethmoid (lamina papyracea) are seen as a thin line of bone, and the BID can be measured at any desired point.[18] From CT studies of 400 adults (200 male aged 18–82, average age 52 years; 200 female aged 17–88, average age 54 years), the BID was measured at different points between the medial walls of the orbits (Fig. 2.136), along with certain other linear and angular measurements; these data are given in Table 2.16.

The distance between the medial walls of the bony orbits at various points and other linear and angular measurements are illustrated in Fig. 2.136. As seen in Table 2.16, the normal BID, measured at the posterior border of the frontal processes of the maxilla on nonrotated CT scans, in the plane of the optic nerve, ranges from 2.29 to 3.21 cm (average, 2.67 cm) in men, and 2.29 to 3.20 cm (average 2.56 cm) in women. The widest interorbital distance lies behind the posterior poles of the globes. This ranges from 3.16 to 4.10 cm (average 3.37 cm) in men, and 2.93 to 3.67 cm (average, 3.20 cm) in women. A line joining the lateral orbital margins in the axial plane (DD line in Table 2.**16**, Fig. 2.**136**) normally intersects the globe near its midportion, with at least one-third of the globe posterior to this line.

Pathology

■ Hypertelorism, Hypotelorism, Exophthalmos, and Exorbitism

Orbital hypertelorism describes the anatomical situation in which the medial walls of the orbits are farther apart than normal.[32–34] Patients with orbital hypertelorism almost always have eyes that are spaced more widely apart than normal. In telecanthus, a condition that may clinically mimic orbital hypertelorism, the distance between the apices of the medial canthal ligaments is increased, and the eyes appear to be spaced more widely apart than normal. However, the BID is not increased: Orbital hypotelorism refers to a decrease in the BID.

Exophthalmos describes abnormal prominence of the globe and the term proptosis emphasizes abnormal protrusion of the globe: however, exophthalmos and proptosis are commonly used as synonyms. Exorbitism, on the other hand, refers to a decrease in the volume of the orbit. The orbital contents are greater in volume than the orbital capacity and generally protrude anteriorly (proptosis), causing the globe to be unusually prominent (exophthalmos).

■ Congenital and Developmental Abnormalities

There are many hereditary and sporadic abnormalities that involve the orbits, globe, adjacent orbital tissues, and other craniofacial and skeletal structures.[35] It is beyond the scope of this chapter to list all of the congenital malformations or syndromes; many excellent books give detailed descriptions of these disorders.[33–38]

■ Anatomical and Developmental Considerations

Congenital abnormalities of the orbit and eyes result from faulty development of the embryo and fetus; the eighth week of gestation is the last week of true embryonic development.[35,43–45] By the third week of gestation, the optic pits appear, one on each side of the forebrain. Disturbance of the prosencephalic organizing center (prechordal mesoblast) can cause cyclopia, synophthalmia, or arhinencephaly. Anophthalmia occurs as a result of failure of the neuroectoderm of the optic pit to develop from the anterior portion of the neural plate. A variety of ocular and systemic abnormalities may be seen with an optic nerve coloboma. These conditions have been described in the part of this chapter on the eye. Craniosynostosis is due to abnormal development of the blastemic stage of the skull bone, including the basicranium. Mandibulofacial dysostosis and hemifacial microsomia probably are due to inhibition of mesodermal differentiation of the facial structures derived from the first and second branchial (visceral) arches.[35]

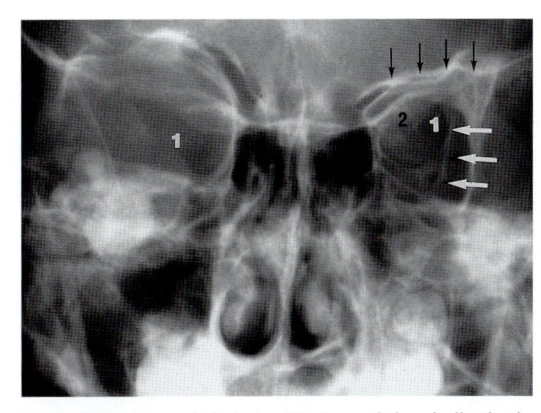

Fig. 2.**137** Microphthalmia. PA view of the skull. The lesser wing of the sphenoid (2) and the maxillary sinus are hypoplastic; Superior orbital fissures are asymmetric (1). Note the difference between the oblique lines (white arrows), which represent cortices of the temporal surface of the greater wings of the sphenoid bone. Note the hypoplasia of the roof of the left orbit (black arrows). From Mafee MF, et al. CT in the evaluation of the orbit and the bony interorbital distance. AJNR 1986; 7: 265. With permission.

Under normal conditions, the eye directs orbital growth. During the first year of life, the eye practically doubles in volume and attains more than 50% of its adult volume.[46] By the end of the third year, 75% of the adult volume is achieved (similar to neural growth).[46] The shape of the orbital cranial junction is also influenced by the development of the brain and skull.[46] When the brain is underdeveloped but the eye is normal, the orbital plate of the frontal bone is usually elevated into the anterior fossa of the skull.[18] In microcephaly, the orbits are usually circular and the roofs are highly arched.[47] When the eye is underdeveloped but the brain is normal, the orbital plate of the frontal bone appears hypoplastic and the vertical or cranial part is usually normal (Fig. 2.**137**). Enucleation of the globe in infancy and early childhood, if untreated with a prosthesis, leads to arrested development of the orbit, resulting in a small orbit.[35] In coronal suture synostosis, the orbit on the side of the fusion is elongated superiorly and laterally, imparting a harlequin appearance. Correction of the cranial deformity can lead to spontaneous correction of the orbital deformity in some instances.[48,49] In mandibulofacial dysostosis, the orbits may be defective inferolaterally because of malar bone hypoplasia. In cases of severe malar hypoplasia, the lateral wall of the orbit is formed by the greater wing of the sphenoid and the zygomatic process of the frontal bone.

Bony Abnormalities

Anomalies of ossification may result in accessory sutures and supernumerary ossicles in the orbital walls.[35] On rare occasions, congenital absence of bone in the frontal, maxillary, and orbital regions may result in deformity of the bony orbit. Asymmetric enlargement of one bony orbit may be due to eccentrically located lesions such as neurofibroma, hemangioma, lymphangioma, teratoma, dermoid cyst, epidermoid cyst, and other slow-growing processes. A small orbit is seen in anophthalmia, microphthalmia, and postenucleation of the globe in infancy, if not followed by prompt prosthetic treatment.

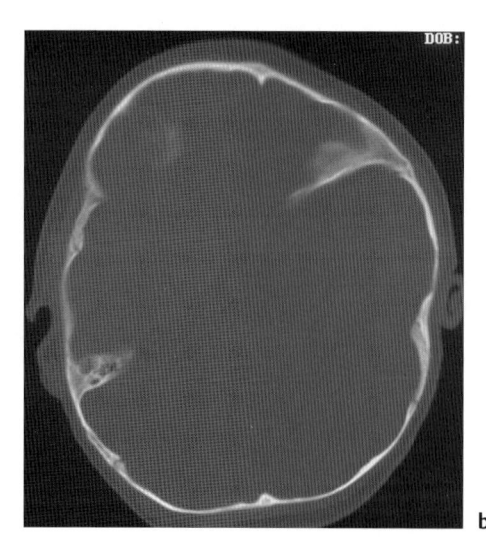

Fig. 2.**138** Plagiocephaly.
a Axial CT scan shows normal right coronal suture and nonvisualization of the left coronal suture. Note lateral displacement of the left greater wing of the sphenoid, expansion of the left middle cranial fossa, foreshortening of the lateral wall of the left orbit and tilting of the ethmoid complex toward the left side.
b Axial CT scan shows normal right coronal suture and complete fusion of the left coronal suture. Note flattening of the left frontal bone.

Bony Orbit in Craniofacial Dysostosis

Craniofacial dysostosis and developmental anomalies may result in profound orbital abnormalities. Orbital malformations in craniofacial dysostosis result chiefly from coronal synostosis. Premature closure of one or more cranial sutures, termed craniosynostosis or craniostenosis, is the common denominator of many patients with craniofacial anomaly.[50–57]

Primary Congenital Isolated Craniosynostosis

Any cranial suture may undergo premature closure, but several patterns are recognizably more common than others.[49] The incidence of congenital suture synostosis reported by Harwood-Nash, derived from a composite of his experience and from two large series reported by Anderson and Geiger and Shillito and Matson is as follows: sagittal 56%; single coronal 11%; bilateral coronal 11%; metopic suture 7%; lambdoid 1%; and three or more sutures 14%. Depending on the suture that is prematurely closed, the skull and orbit, including the interorbital distance, have a characteristic shape. These can be grouped as follows:
1. Metopic: trigonocephaly (triangular head); hypotelorism is a constant feature of the trigonocephaly.[47]
2. Sagittal: scaphocephaly (dolichocephaly), in which the anteroposterior diameter of the bony orbit is usually increased and the vertical and transverse diameters of the bony orbit are usually decreased.
3. Unilateral coronal or lambdoid: plagiocephaly, in this condition, if the coronal suture is involved, there is characteristic deformity of the bony orbit, which will be discussed later.
4. Bilateral coronal or lambdoid results in brachycephaly.
5. Coronal and sagittal: oxycephaly or acrocephaly (turricephaly).
6. Coronal, lambdoid, and sagittal: cloverleaf skull (kleeblattschädel).

Primary craniosynostosis may be associated with congenital syndromes. These conditions include the following:[38, 47, 49]
- Crouzon disease (craniofacial dysostosis)
- Apert disease (acrocephalosyndactyly, type I)
- Saethre–Chotzen syndrome (acrocephalosyndactyly, type II)
- Carpenter syndrome (acrocephalopolysyndactyly)
- Chondrodystrophia calcificans congenita (Conradi syndrome, or punctate epiphyseal dysplasia)
- Brachmann–de Lange syndrome
- Laurence–Moon–Biedl–Bardet syndrome
- Treacher Collins syndrome (mandibulofacial dysostosis)

The Orbit in Plagiocephaly

Plagiocephaly is due to unilateral closure of one of the paired sutures of the skull, frequently the coronal or lambdoid but rarely the temporosquamous sutures. Each produces a characteristic deformity of the skull. In practice, most of the time, plagiocephaly is seen in patients with hemicoronal premature synostosis, in which there is an ipsilateral elevation of the lesser wing of the sphenoid associated with upward extension of the superior lateral portion of the orbit, imparting a harlequin appearance to the orbit (Fig. 2.**138**).[49] The flattening of the ipsilateral frontal bone is also characteristic of premature coronal synostosis (Fig. 2.**138**). The volume of the anterior cranial fossa on the side of fusion is decreased. The greater wing of the sphenoid is expanded and displaced forward and downward, and forms a relatively large middle cranial fossa (Fig. 2.**138**). This occurs in addition to upward elevation of the roof of the orbit, which produces a shallow orbit. The ethmoidal plate (roof of the ethmoidal sinus) also is elevated on the side of fusion (Fig. 2.**138**). The nasal septum, crista galli, and the ethmoidal complex are tilted to the side of fusion.

Premature fusion of both coronal sutures may occur with or without any other associated abnormality. This may result in marked shortening of the anterior cranial fossa and orbital depth, and the brain impressions become more prominent on the inner table of the frontal bone. Both a harlequin appearance of the orbit and the bony changes of the unilateral coronal synostosis are duplicated in this bilateral form of premature fusion (Fig. 2.**139**). Lombardi noted a connection between sagittal or lambdoid synostosis, or both, in half the reported cases of coronal suture synostosis.[54]

The Orbit in Crouzon and Apert Diseases

Crouzon disease, also known as craniofacial dysostosis, is an autosomal dominant disorder with considerable variability in expression.[49] Apert disease, also known as acrocephalosyndactyly type I, is transmitted as an autosomal dominant disorder. The cranial and facial characteristics of Crouzon disease are somewhat similar to Apert syndrome, including brachycephaly, hypertelorism, bilateral exophthalmos, parrot-beaked nose, maxillary

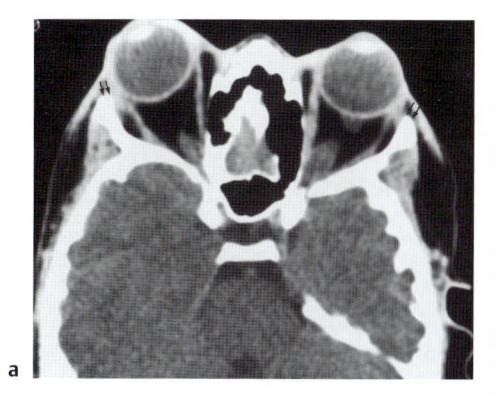

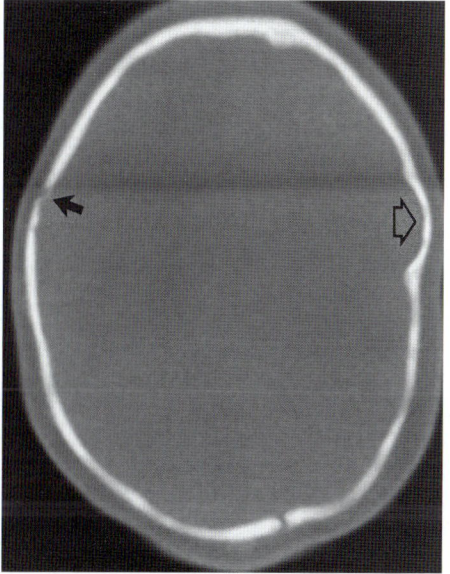

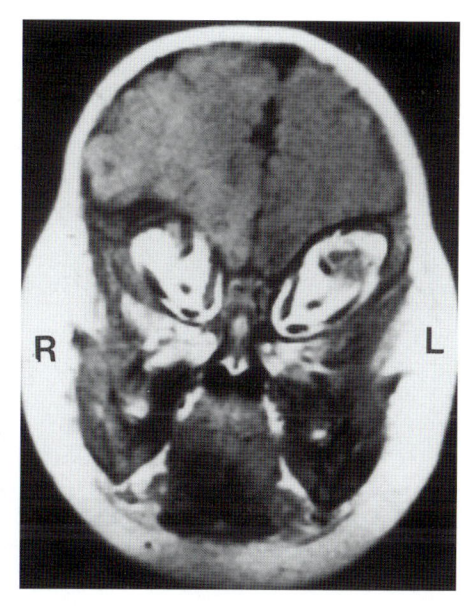

Fig. 2.139 Crouzon disease.
a Axial CT scan shows lateral displacement of the greater wings of the sphenoid, ballooning of the ethmoid complex, and recession of the lateral wall of the orbits (arrows). Note increased convolutional markings along the lateral aspect of both temporal fossae.

b Axial CT scan and **c** coronal MR image of another patient with Crouzon disease. Note marked narrowing of the right coronal suture (solid arrow in **b**) and fusion of the left coronal suture (hollow arrow in **b**), elevation of orbits (harlequin appearance), and abnormal orientation of extraocular muscles (**c**).

hypoplasia, relative prognathism, and a drooping lower lip that produces a half-opened mouth. Bilateral exophthalmos is essentially a consequence of exorbitism, which in turn is a consequence of several factors that combine to produce a decrease in orbital volume. Crouzon and Apert diseases cannot be distinguished on the basis of the skull shape alone.[49] In any large series of patients with Crouzon disease, there is no regular pattern of calvarial deformity. Oxycephaly, brachycephaly, scaphocephaly, and trigonocephaly may be present. There is too much heterogeneity to allow for a simplistic description. Generally, in Crouzon disease, brachycephaly or oxycephaly is most often observed. Apert disease is characterized by irregular craniostenosis with an acrobrachycephalic skull and syndactyly of hands and feet. Associated skeletal abnormalities such as ankylosis of the elbow, hip, and shoulder and malformations of the cardiovascular, gastrointestinal, and genitourinary systems may be present.[49]

The orbital malformation in Crouzon and Apert diseases is due mainly to premature coronal synostosis. A striking harlequin appearance of the orbits is seen that results because of the elevation of the roofs and lateral walls of the orbits (Fig. 2.**139**). The supraorbital rim is recessed, and the infraorbital rim is hypoplastic. The orbital depth is markedly reduced as the result of verticalization of the roof (upward tilt of the lesser wing and orbital plate of the frontal bone). Displacement of the greater wing of the sphenoid into a more coronal orientation, which is referred to as frontalization of the greater wing of the sphenoid, and ballooning of the ethmoid are other factors contributing to exotropia (Fig. 2.**139**). Hypoplasia of the maxilla and the intermaxillary component contributes in part to the exophthalmos and relative prognathism. Hypoplasia of the maxilla causes recession of the infraorbital rim and foreshortening of the orbital floor.[49] The optic canal in Crouzon and Apert diseases is usually narrow. This may lead to optic atrophy.[3] Patients with craniosynostosis syndromes may have marked extraocular muscle anomalies ranging from an apparent absence of ocular muscles to abnormally inserted muscles or very small extraocular muscles (Fig. 2.**140**).

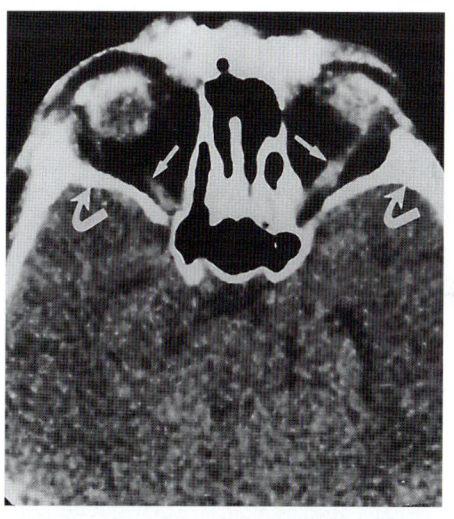

Fig. 2.140 Crouzon disease. Axial CT scan shows lateral displacement of the greater wings of the sphenoid (curved arrows), foreshortening of the lateral walls of the orbit and deformity and thinning of the superior rectus muscles (straight arrows).

Saethre–Chotzen Disease (Acrocephalosyndactyly Type II)

Saethre–Chotzen disease was described by Saethre in 1931 and in 1932 by Chotzen.[49, 54–56] The first family with this disease to be reported in the United States was described in 1970 by Bartsocas et al.[57] Saethre–Chotzen disease is characterized by synostotic malformation of multiple sutures, facial asymmetry, mild midface hypoplasia, ptosis of the eyelids, an antimongoloid slant of the palpebral fissures, a beaked nose, a low-set frontal hairline, variable brachycephaly, and variable cutaneous syndactyly, particularly of the second and third fingers. Other associated abnormalities include a high-arched palate, cleft palate, and deformity of the external ear. The orbital abnormalities in these patients are similar to those in Crouzon and Apert diseases.[49]

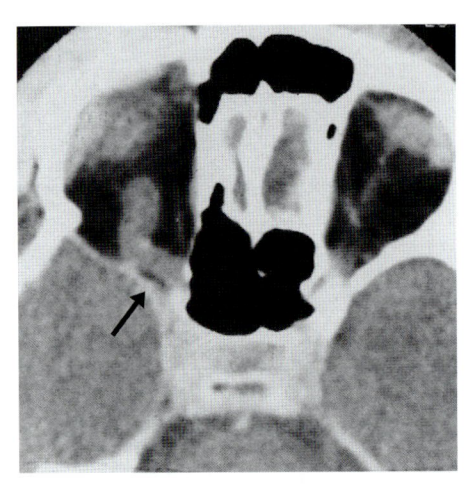

Fig. 2.**141** Neurofibromatosis (NF1). Axial CT scan shows dysplasia of the greater wing of the sphenoid (arrow), characteristic of NF1. Enlargement of the optic nerve is due to optic nerve glioma.

Neurofibromatosis

The classic description of neurofibromatosis was published by Friedrich Daniel von Recklinghausen in 1882. Clinical criteria for diagnosing neurofibromatosis include: (1) six or more café-au-lait spots, each greater than 1.5 cm in diameter; (2) axillary or other intertriginous freckles; (3) cutaneous neurofibromata; and (4) one or more unequivocally affected parents or siblings.[58] The disease itself is characterized by abnormalities of both ectodermal and mesodermal origin. It is transmitted as an autosomal dominant disorder of variable penetrance.[32] The incidence of neurofibromatosis is approximately 1 in 3000 live births.[59] About 50% of these patients have a positive family history of the disease, whereas the other 50% are the result of a spontaneous mutation.[60] The incidence of central nervous system tumors, including acoustic (vestibular) neuromas, gliomas, meningiomas, and ependymomas, is six times that of the general population.[61] Often multiple central nervous tumors are present. Although 25–35% of neurofibromas occur in the head and neck region, orbital abnormalities are relatively uncommon.[59] Orbital abnormalities are often associated with exophthalmos, which may be pulsatile and generally can be classified into one of four categories: (1) orbital neoplasms; (2) plexiform neurofibromatosis (see Fig. 2.**276**); (3) orbital osseous dysplasia (Fig. 2.**141**); and (4) congenital glaucoma.[59] The most common orbital neoplasm seen in association with neurofibromatosis is optic glioma (Fig. 2.**141**). Both optic gliomas and meningiomas may occur bilaterally. Bilateral optic nerve gliomas are pathognomonic of neurofibromatosis type 1 (NF1) (see Fig. 2.**299**), whereas bilateral optic nerve sheath meningiomas are only suggestive of neurofibromatosis. Orbital schwannoma, neurofibroma, and neurofibrosarcoma also can be seen in these patients.

Orbital (Mesodermal) Defects

Osseous dysplasia of the cranial bones, in particular the bony orbit, may be part of the abnormality associated with von Recklinghausen disease (NF1). The orbital defect is a consequence of partial or complete absence of the greater or the lesser wing of the sphenoid bone, or both (Fig. 2.**141**). The body of the sphenoid bone may also be involved, producing an abnormal and dysplastic sella turcica.[32,59] These osseous abnormalities allow the adjacent temporal lobe of the brain and its overlying, often thickened, dural membrane to herniate anteriorly into the posterior aspect of the orbit, which causes anterior displacement of the globe. The normal CSF pulsations are transmitted to the globe, resulting in pulsatile exophthalmos. Associated findings include hypoplasia of the ipsilateral frontal and maxillary sinuses and hypoplasia of the adjacent ethmoid air cells.[32,59]

Orbit in Mandibulofacial Dysostosis

The malformation known as mandibulofacial dysostosis (MFD) was first reported in 1889 by the ophthalmologist G. A. Berry.[62] Treacher Collins,[63] whose name is attached to the disease of mandibulofacial dysostosis, described the disease and noted the characteristic malar hypoplasia and the associated flattening of the cheeks. In 1923 Pires deLima and Monteior[64] stated that MFD is probably due to a developmental defect that affects the branchial arches. (The hallmark of MFD is its varied expressivity.) Franceschetti and Klein,[65] who coined the name MFD, classified the syndrome into five separate categories: complete, incomplete, abortive, unilateral, and atypical. Gorlin and Pindborg[66] stated that there is no unilateral form of the syndrome and that such cases are better classified as hemifacial microsomia. Poswillow[67] in his experimental study of a teratogenically induced phenocopy of MFD in an animal model showed that the disorder results from disorganization of the preotic neural crest about the time of cell migration to the first and second branchial arches.

Bony Orbit in Mandibulofacial Dysostosis

In MFD, the maxillae and malar bones are usually poorly developed with small antra and shallow or incomplete orbital floors.[49] The malar bones are hypoplastic, and the zygomatic arches are usually incomplete. The development of the zygomatic process of the maxilla varies among the cases described, and it may not be developed. The radiographic orbital characteristics in MFD are the downward sloping floors of the orbits in line medially with a beaklike bony nasal contour. The lateral and lower rim of the orbit is often defective. CT shows the deficiency of the lateral orbital floor, representing an orbital cleft that varies considerably in degree. The greater wings of the sphenoid may be hypoplastic, and therefore the lateralorbital wall may be defective. Herring[68] reported a patient with MFD with hypoplasia of the greater wing of the sphenoid where the temporal squamous bone extended anteriorly beyond its usual boundaries to replace the very hypoplastic greater wing of the sphenoid.

Bony Orbit in Craniofacial Microsomia

Craniofacial microsomia is known by many names, including first and second branchial syndrome, otomandibular dysostosis, and oculoauriculovertebral dysplasia.[66,49] The term hemifacial microsomia was advocated by Gorlin et al[66] to refer to patients with unilateral microtia, macrosomia, and failure of formation of the mandibular ramus and condyle. They included such malformations as the Goldenhar syndrome and oculoauriculovertebral dysplasia, previously described as separate entities, as a variant of this complex.[66] About 10 percent of the patients have bilateral involvement, but the disorder is nearly always more severe on one side.[66] The associated eye findings that are considered to be variable features of this syndrome include epibulbar dermoids or lipodermoids, microphthalmia, coloboma of the choroid and iris, and deformity of the bony orbit similar to MFD as a result of hypoplasia of the maxilla and malar bone.

Developmental Orbital Cysts

The most frequent developmental lesions involving the orbit and periorbital structures are the dermoid and epidermoid cysts, choristomas and teratomas (Table 2.**17**).[3, 8, 16, 69–71] Choristoma is a focus of tissue histologically normal for an organ or part of an organ other than the site at which it is located.[5, 6, 72] A dermoid or epidermoid cyst is a choristoma that may be found in several locations in the orbit. Lipodermoids are solid tumors that are usually located beneath the conjunctiva over the lateral surface of the globe.[2, 72] A conjunctival lipodermoid is a true choristoma, since (adipose) fatty tissue is usually not found in this region. Conjunctival choristomas are relatively common congenital lesions that possess little growth potential. They contain both dermal and epidermal elements that are not normally found in the conjunctiva.[73]

Three types of conjunctival choristomas are found—the solid limbal dermoid, the more diffuse dermolipoma, and the complex choristoma. The solid limbal dermoids typically occur unilaterally, at the inferotemporal limbus. Dermolipomas (lipodermoids) are less dense than solid dermoids and contain more adipose tissue. Dermolipomas consist of collagen tissue and adipose tissue lined by stratified squamous epithelium. They are usually devoid of hair follicles. They are typically found on the superior temporal bulbar conjunctiva near the levator and extraocular muscles (Fig. 2.**142**).[5, 6, 73] Bilateral limbal dermoids or dermolipomas are found in children who have Goldenhar syndrome. Complex choristomas consist of variable combinations of ectopic tissues such as ectopic lacrimal gland, respiratory, eyelid glands, or brain tissues. Epibulbar osseous choristomas are solitary nodules that resemble dermoids. They are composed of mature, compact bone along with other typical choristomatous elements such as pilosebaceous units and hair follicles.[2, 6] Dermoid and epidermoid cysts are choristomas that are among the most common orbital tumors of childhood. Both may be found in several locations in the orbit, most frequently superior and temporal. The tumor is congenital but may not be noted at birth. Many become evident only in the second and third decades.[6] Both result from the inclusion of ectodermal elements during closure of the neural tube. The dermal elements that are pinched off along the suture lines, diploë, or within the meninges or scalp in the course of embryonic development, give rise to these cysts.[2, 6, 16, 70] Both have a fibrous capsule of varying degree of thickness. The epidermoid has a lining of keratinizing, stratified squamous epithelium. The dermoid contains one or more dermal adnexal structures such as sebaceous glands and hair follicles. Some dermoid cysts may also contain lobules of fat.

Teratomas are choristomatous tumors that contain tissues representing two or more germ layers. Endodermal derivatives such as gut or respiratory epithelium, ectodermal tissues such as skin and its appendages, and neural and mesodermal tissues such as connective tissues, smooth muscles, cartilage, bone, and vessels may be present. Developmental orbital cysts represent 24% of all orbital and lid masses, 6–8% of deep orbital masses, and 80% of cystic orbital lesions.[74] These cysts may contain fluid or solid components.[72, 75] Teratomas are evident at birth as grossly visible cystic/solid orbital masses.[7, 70] Orbital teratomas may arise from pleuripotential stem cells delivered to the orbit hematogenously, or from stem cells displaced during their migration.[72] The tumors can be either solid or cystic or mixed. However, they are usually cystic and can cause dramatic exophthalmos at birth. Although teratomas in other sites such as testes are commonly malignant, teratomas within the orbit are only rarely malignant.[72] The dermoid and epidermoid cysts favor the upper portion of the orbit for their growth (Figs. 2.**143**–2.**147**). They normally grow slowly, but at times these cysts can grow rapidly, particularly in adults.[71] They are most frequently located at the superior temporal quadrant of the orbit, where they are fixed to the periosteum near the frontozygomatic suture line (Fig. 2.**148**).[69, 70, 71] Occasionally, they can be found at the frontothmoidal or frontonasal sutures and can simulate an encephalocele (Fig. 2.**146**).[2, 6, 16]

Table 2.**17** Common orbital disorders of children

Orbital cellulitis; most common cause of proptosis in children
Dermoid and epidermoid cysts; most common orbital masses
Capillary hemangioma and lymphangioma; most common vascular masses
Optic nerve glioma; most common optic nerve tumor in children
Rhabdomyosarcoma; most common primary malignant orbital tumor in children
Leukemia
Pseudotumor
Neurofibroma
Metastatic neuroblastoma—most common metastatic cancer to orbit in children
Subperiosteal hematoma

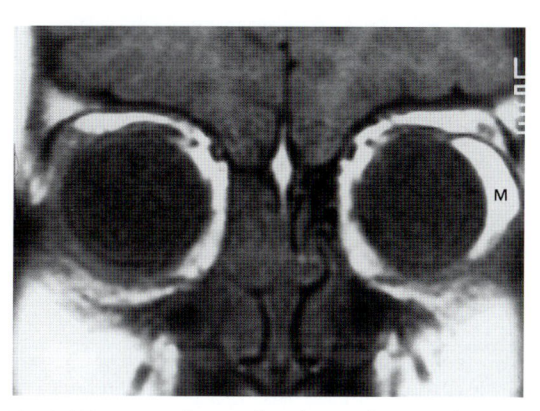

Fig. 2.**142** Dermolipoma (lipodermoid). Coronal T1W MR scan shows a hyperintense mass (M) compatible with a dermolipoma.

Diagnostic Imaging

The imaging modality of choice depends on the entity being considered. When a prominent feature of the suspected lesion is bone remodeling (Fig. 2.**143a**), bone destruction, bone or calcium deposition, or intralesional fat, CT scanning is indicated (Fig. 2.**147**). MRI may provide information about the characteristics of fluid and tissues within the cystic lesion (Fig. 2.**148**). Both epidermoid and dermoid cysts appear on CT as unenhanced, well-circumscribed, smoothly marginated, low-density masses (Figs. 2.**143a**, 2.**144**, 2.**147**). If a dermoid cyst contains fatty tissues, it has a fat density on CT (Figs. 2.**144**, 2.**147**). Similarly, calcifications may be seen within these dermoid cysts (Figs. 2.**144**, 2.**147**). Calcification is not a feature of epidermoid. Although it is rare, we have seen calcification in intracranial epidermoid but not in orbital epidermoid cysts. Fat–fluid levels may be present in dermoid cysts. A ruptured dermoid/epidermoid cyst shows surrounding inflammatory changes (Fig. 2.**144**). Rarely, some of the dermoid cysts may appear moderate to markedly hyperdense on CT scans. On MRI, dermoid and epidermoid cysts have low signal intensity on T1-weighted (Fig. 2.**143b**) and high signal intensity on T2-weighted, FLAIR, as well as diffusion-weighted MR images (see Chapter 3). A dermoid cyst that contains significant fatty tissue demonstrates the MRI characteristics of fat (Figs. 2.**146**, 2.**148**, 2.**149**). Both dermoid and epidermoid cysts may demonstrate marginal enhancement of their wall on postcontrast CT and MR scans (Fig. 2.**149**).

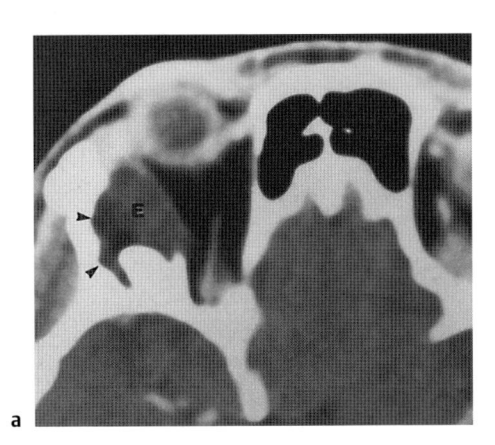

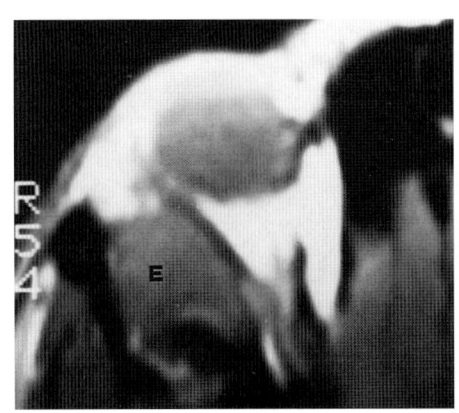

Fig. 2.143 Epidermoid cyst. **a** Axial postcontrast CT scan shows an epidermoid (E). Note the scalloping of the lateral wall of the orbit (arrowheads). **b** Axial PW MR scan, at a slightly lower level than **a**, showing isointense (to brain) epidermoid (E).

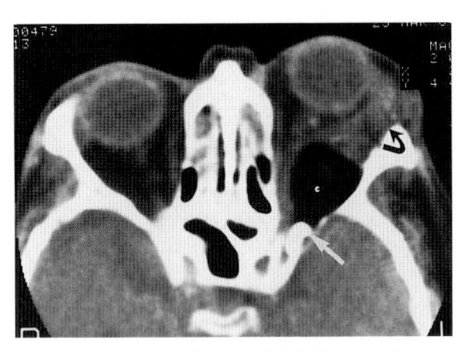

Fig. 2.144 Dermoid cyst. Axial CT scan shows a dermoid cyst (c). Note the calcification (white arrow). There is increased soft tissue anterior to the dermoid cyst (curved arrow). This was related to soft-tissue reaction due to rupturing of the dermoid cyst.

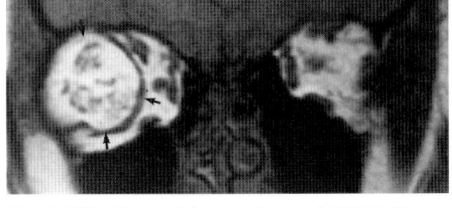

Fig. 2.145 Dermoid cyst. Coronal T1W MR scan shows a large dermoid cyst (arrows).

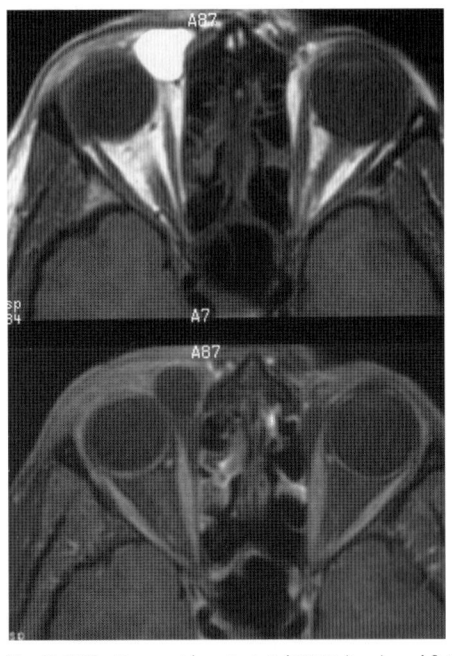

Fig. 2.146 Dermoid cyst. Axial T1W (top) and fat-suppression T1W (bottom) MR scans showing a dermoid cyst in the medial aspect of the right orbit.

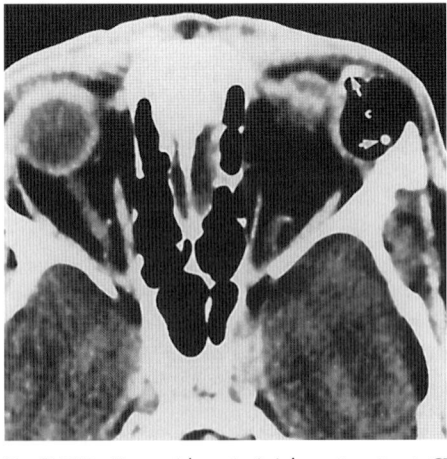

Fig. 2.147 Dermoid cyst. Axial postcontrast CT scan shows a fat-containing cyst compatible with dermoid cyst (c). Note calcifications (arrows). There is no bone erosion as compared to Fig. 2.**148**.

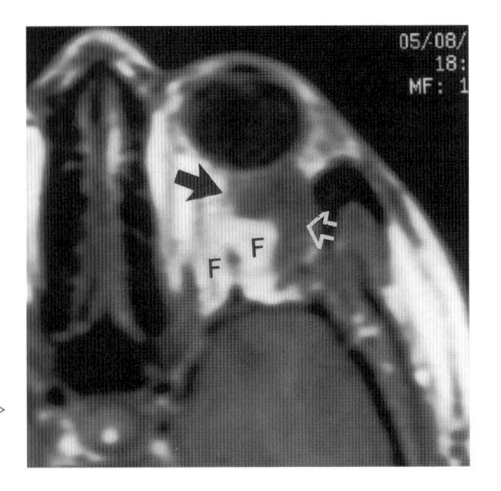

Fig. 2.148 Dermoid cyst. Axial enhanced T1W MR scan shows a large dermoid cyst that contains fat (F) and a nonenhancing component (arrows). Note significant erosion of the lateral wall of the orbit.

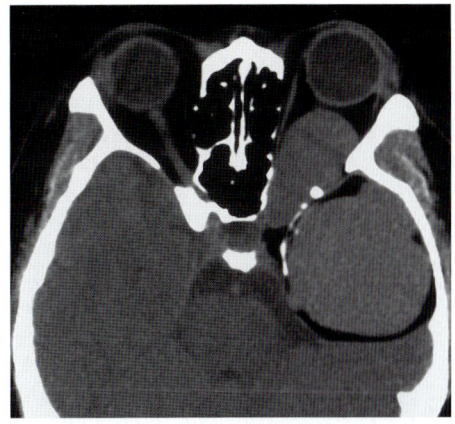

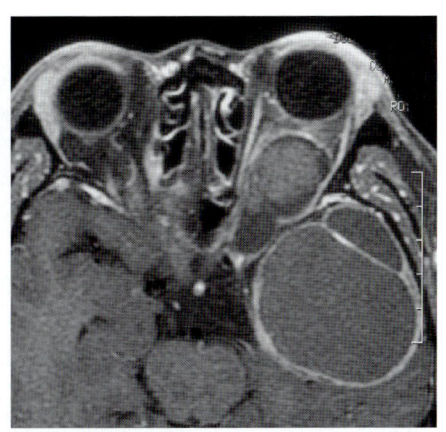

Fig. 2.**149** Presumed dermoid cyst. **a** Axial CT scan and **b** axial enhanced fat-suppression MR scan, showing a large orbital-middle cranial fossa dermoid cyst. Note enhancement of its capsule.

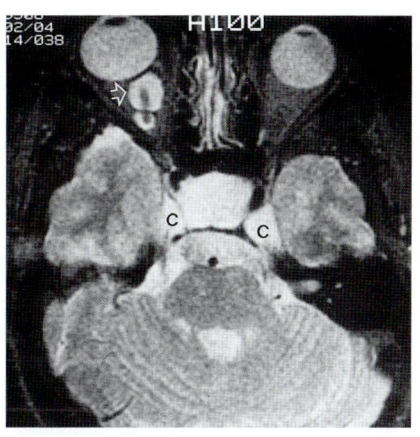

Fig. 2.**150** Perioptic nerve dural ectasia. Axial T2W MR scan shows saccular dilatation of the meninges surrounding the right optic nerve (arrow). Note an empty sella and increased size of gasserian cisterns (C).

Other Less Common Congenital Anomalies and Acquired Cysts of the of Orbit and Optic System

The orbit develops from mesodermal tissues, and the globe and optic pathway develop mainly from ectodermal tissues. Developmental defects of the eyeball may result in a small orbit. The majority of orbital changes are found in association with deformities of the skull and skeleton.[35] Cyclopia, synophthalmia, clinical anophthalmia, and microphthalmia are developmental anomalies of the globe that are seen in the fetal central system anomalies associated with problems in forebrain differentiation (holoprosencephaly). MRI is particularly noteworthy in the detection of these anomalies. In general, a variety of cyst and cystlike lesions involve the orbit (Figs. 2.**150**, 2.**151**–2.**154**); these include developmental anomalies as well as acquired lesions arising in the orbit or in adjacent structures.[72] A cyst is defined as a closed sac with a membranous or cellular lining, and a luminal space containing air, fluid, semifluid, or solid materials. Cysts typically result from developmental anomalies, from obstruction of ducts, or from parasitic infections or trauma as listed in Table 2.**18**.

Congenital Cystic Eye

Congenital cystic eye is a rare congenital anomaly resulting from failure of the optic vesicle to invaginate during the fourth week of embryogenesis.[2,72] It presents at birth as a complex cyst occupying the orbit, without any vestige of a globe evident. The cyst wall is lined with cells derived from undifferentiated retina, and retinal pigment epithelium. There may be present some remnant of an optic nervelike structure and extraocular muscles.[72] CT and MRI scans generally shows an enlarged orbit containing a rounded or ovaloid, septated cyst. Congenital cystic eye and orbital colobomatous cysts have been described in part 1 of this chapter.

Optic Nerve Sheath Meningocele

Optic neural sheath meningocele (optic nerve sheath cyst, arachnoid cyst, perioptic hygroma, and dural ectasia, among others) is a saccular dilatation of the meninges surrounding the orbital portion of the optic nerve.[76] These meningoceles may occur primarily or secondarily in association with other orbital processes, such as meningioma, optic nerve pilocytic astrocytoma, and hemangioma.[2,16] Clinically, these meningoceles may present with changes in the visual acuity, visual field, and optic nerve appearance. The CT and MRI appearance of optic nerve meningocele or ectasia is that of a prominent focal or segmental enlargement of the dural arachnoid sheath around the optic nerve (Fig. 2.**150**). The optic nerve dural ectasia may be associated with empty sella and enlarged subarachnoid cisterns, such as gasserian cisterns (Fig. 2.**150**).

Enterogenous Cysts

Enterogenous cysts are rare, congenital choristomatous cysts of the central nervous system. They contain a single layer of mucin-secreting epithelial cells that resemble gastrointestinal epithelium. The lower cervical and cervicothoracic regions are the more common sites for the lesion. An orbital location is extremely rare.[2,77] Occasionally these cysts may be seen in the anterior cranial fossa, and extending into the orbit (see Chapter 3).

Table 2.**18** Orbital cyst

I	**Developmental** Choristoma (epidermoid, dermoid, dermolipoma) Teratoma Colobomatous cyst Congenital cystic eye Optic nerve sheath meningocele Congenital dacryocele (mucocele)
II	**Adjacent structure cysts** Cephalocele (meningocele, encephalocele, meningo-encephalocele, porencephalic cyst) Enterogenous cyst Dentigerous cyst
III	**Acquired orbital cyst** Mucocele Mucopyocele Dacryocele Cystic vascular lesions (lymphangioma, orbital varix) Chocolate cyst (hemorrhagic cyst) Epithelial and appendage cysts Epithelial implantation cysts Lacrimal gland cyst Lacrimal sac cyst (dacryocele), mucocele Hematic cyst (subperiosteal) Cholesterol granulomatous cyst "Aneurysmal bone cyst" Cystic myositis Orbital abscess Parasitic cyst (hydatid cyst, cysticercoses)

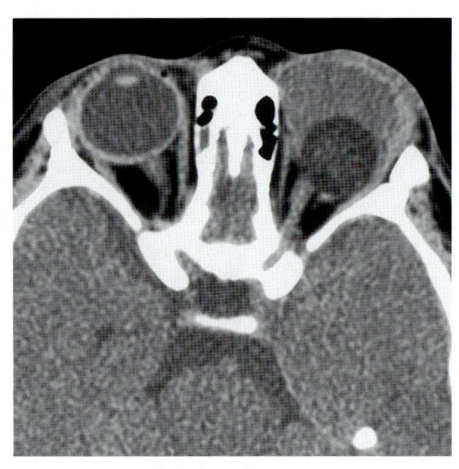

Fig. 2.**151** Epithelial implantation cyst. CT scan shows a left orbital implant. Note a mass anterior to the implant presumed to be an epithelial implantation cyst.

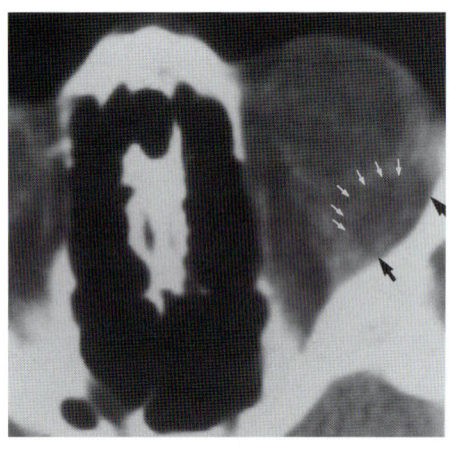

Fig. 2.**152** Lacrimal gland duct cyst. Axial enhanced CT scan shows a low-density mass (arrows) compatible with a lacrimal gland duct squamous cyst.

Dentigerous Cysts

Dentigerous cysts, fluid-filled and lined with keratinizing (keratogenic cysts) or nonkeratinizing, stratified squamous epithelium, arise from the jaw. Infrequently, the cyst can enlarge into the maxillary sinus and erode into the orbit. These cysts appear as a nonenhancing, low-density image on CT scans. On MRI they appear with a low to intermediate signal on T1-weighted images and hyperintense on T2-weighted MR images. The signal characteristics on T1-weighted MR images depend on the cyst's protein content (see Chapters 4 and 6).

■ Acquired Orbital Cysts

Cystic Vascular Lesions: Lymphangioma, Varix, Chocolate Cyst

Lymphangioma and varix will be described later in this chapter. Lymphangiomas contain numerous and variable sized cystic spaces. Acute hemorrhage into these cystic spaces, whether spontaneous or after minor trauma, results in the so-called chocolate cysts. A varix is a venous anomaly and may include a single smooth-contoured dilated vein. Intralesional hemorrhage in an orbital varix may result in formation of a "hematic cyst" or chocolate cyst.[72] Hematic cysts may develop as a result of prior trauma.

Epithelial and Appendage Cysts

Various acquired cysts involving the eyelids or superficial orbit may derive from the skin of the eyelids, the skin appendages (glands and cilia), or conjunctiva.[2, 16, 72] Chalazion, a cystic expansion of the meibomian sebaceous gland due to a blockage of its excretory duct, is common in children. Other cysts include apocrine hidrocystoma (sudoriferous cyst), originating from a blocked excretory duct of Moll's apocrine sweat gland; eccrine hidrocystoma, derived from lid eccrine sweat gland; sebaceous cyst (pilar cyst, retention cyst of the pilosebaceous structure); milia (cystic expansion of the pilosebaceous structure due to obstruction of the orifice); epidermal inclusion cyst (cutaneous or subcutaneous cyst lined by stratified squamous epithelium with a keratin-filled lumen); pilomatrixoma (calcifying epithelioma of Malherbe, a solid or cystic mass derived from hair matrix cells); and conjunctival inclusion cyst (thin-walled, fluid-filled cyst lined by stratified, nonkeratinizing, cuboidal epithelium containing mucous-secreting goblet cells). Because most epithelial and appendage cysts remain small (less than 1 cm) and limited to the eyelid and superficial orbit, medical imaging studies are only rarely ordered by the ophthalmologist.

Epithelial Implantation Cysts

Epithelial implantation cysts are derived from cells of the cutaneous epithelium, conjunctival epithelium, or respiratory epithelium that are traumatically displaced under the skin of the eyelid or into the orbit. The CT and MRI appearance of these cysts is nonspecific and similar to any simple cyst (Fig. 2.**151**). A nonenhanced cystic orbital mass following orbital surgery and enucleation should raise the question of the presence of an epithelial implantation cyst.

Lacrimal Duct Cyst

Cysts of the lacrimal glands can be acquired as a result of blockage of the gland's excretory ducts.[2, 16, 72] The cyst is then located in either the orbital or palpebral lobe of the main lacrimal gland, or in the conjunctival fornices due to blockage of the accessory lacrimal glands of Krause and Wolfring.[72] The CT and MRI appearance of lacrimal gland cysts is similar to any simple cyst (Figs. 2.**152**, 2.**153**).

Dacryocele

A dacryocele (lacrimal sac mucocele) is a cystic expansion of the nasolacrimal sac or a diverticulum of the sac. The expansion is caused by a proximal or distal block of the nasolacrimal duct. Dacryoceles are considered a congenital anomaly of the lacrimal drainage system, and are usually apparent in the first few days of life. On CT and MRI, dacryocele appears as well-circumscribed, rounded lesions centered in the nasolacrimal sac region. On CT scans, the density of the lesion is homogeneous when not infected. On MRI, a dacryocele appears hypointense on T1-weighted and hyperintense on T2-weighted images. If it is infected, there may be a rim of contrast enhancement (Fig. 2.**154**; see also Figs. 2.**359**, 2.**360**).

Hematic Cyst and Cholesterol Granuloma

Most orbital hematomas, like other localized collections of blood, resolve within days. The hematic cyst (organizing hematoma, hematocele), is a cystlike mass that slowly develops as an acute orbital hemorrhage, is incompletely absorbed and undergoes organization.[2, 16, 70, 72, 78] There may be a fibrous cyst wall with a

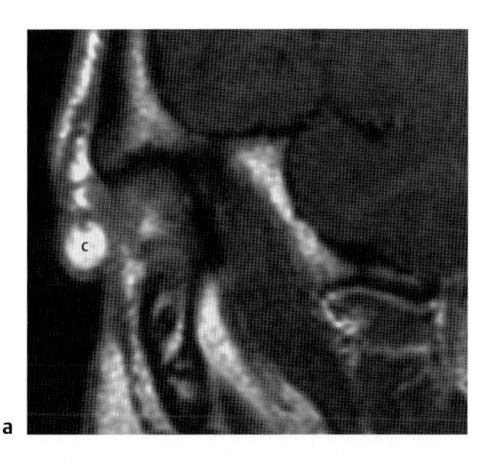

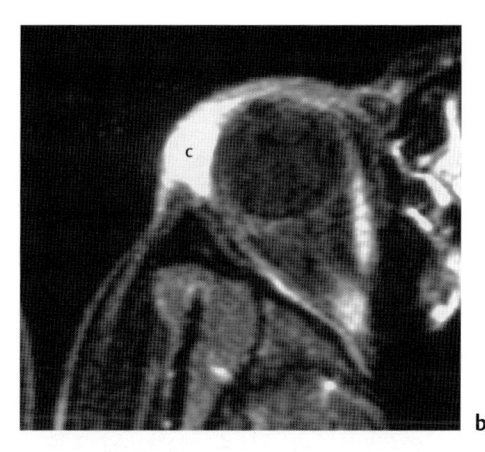

Fig. 2.153 Lacrimal gland duct hemorrhagic cyst. **a** Sagittal T1W and **b** axial fat-suppression T1W MR scans show a hyperintense lacrimal gland duct cyst (c). The cyst contained blood by-products.

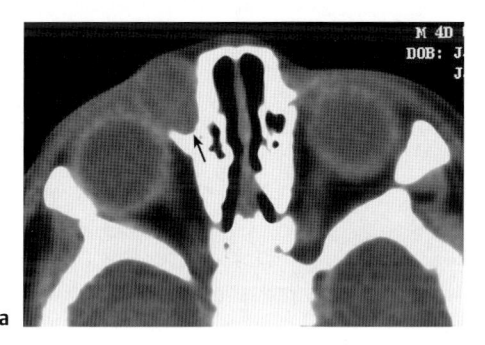

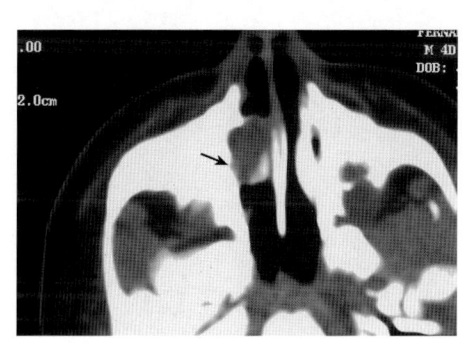

Fig. 2.154 Dacryocele (mucocele). **a**, **b** Axial CT scans showing a congenital mucocele of the right lacrimal sac and duct (arrows) in this 4-day-old boy.

lumen comprised of degraded blood products, cholesterol, hemosiderin, hematoidin crystals, erythrocytes, histiocytes, giant cells, and granuloma tissue. The hematic cyst may occur anywhere in the orbit, including the superiosteal space.[2, 16, 70]

The etiology of subperiosteal hematomas is either traumatic or spontaneous. Traumatic hemorrhage is most common, but the time interval between the traumatic episode and the clinical manifestation may vary from immediate to months or years.[16, 78] Spontaneous hemorrhage can occur as a complication of leukemia, thrombocytopenia, blood dyscrasia, hemophilia, and other hemorrhagic systemic diseases, including patients with sickle cell anemia.[2, 78]

Subperiosteal hematomas can be of several varieties. Acute subperiosteal hematoma is rare but, as a complication of trauma, can present as painful unilateral proptosis.[78] It may also develop so insidiously as to defy explanation, especially when there is no definite history of injury. It is usually the result of damage to the subperiosteal blood vessels. It may also develop as an extension of a subgaleal hematoma. At times, it is continuous with an epidural hematoma after head trauma. In cases of trauma there is a predilection for blood to collect in the subperiosteal location superiorly. The frontal bone is the largest continuous concave surface of the orbit and has a loose periosteal attachment.[78]

Diagnostic Imaging

CT is an excellent diagnostic method for evaluating subperiosteal hematomas. Coronal sections, either direct or reformatted images, are essential for accurate diagnoses. The CT appearance of acute and subacute subperiosteal hematoma is a sharply defined, extraconal, homogeneous, high density, nonenhancing mass with a broad base abutting the bone and displacing the peripheral orbital fat toward the center of the orbit (Figs. 2.**155**, 2.**156**). The mass, like other subperiosteal lesions, is fusiform or biconvex, and if limited to the superior orbit, it is confined by the fron-

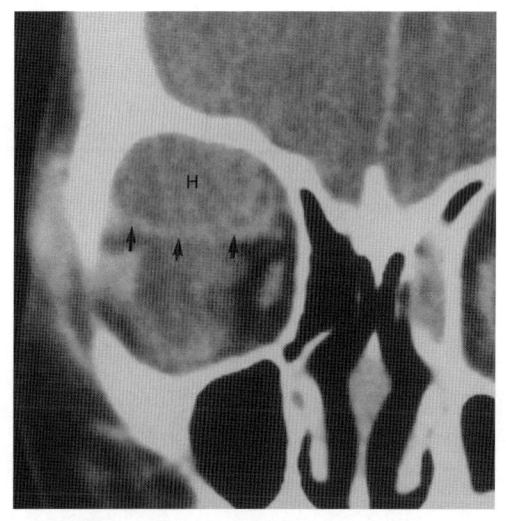

Fig. 2.155 Orbital subperiosteal hematoma. Coronal CT scan shows a large subperiosteal hematoma (H). Note displaced periosteum (arrows). The detached periosteum is often limited by the frontozygomatic suture as well as the frontoethmoid suture.

tozygomatic and frontoethmoid sutures; it is best seen in direct coronal and coronal or sagittal reformatted images (Figs. 2.**155**, 2.**156**). A chronic subperiosteal hematoma appears on CT scan as a heterogeneous, mostly relatively hypodense, sharply defined extraconal mass with a broad base (Fig. 2.**157**). Long-standing (chronic) hematic cysts, so-called cholesterol granulomas, appear as a cystic lesion, associated with compression bone atrophy as well as expansion and erosion of adjacent bone (see Fig. 2.**160**). Chronic hematic cysts on CT scan may not be differentiated from epidermoid or dermoid cyst. However, they can be easily differentiated by MRI.

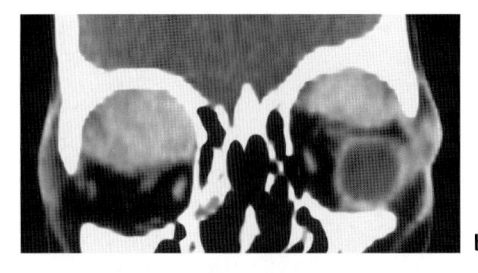

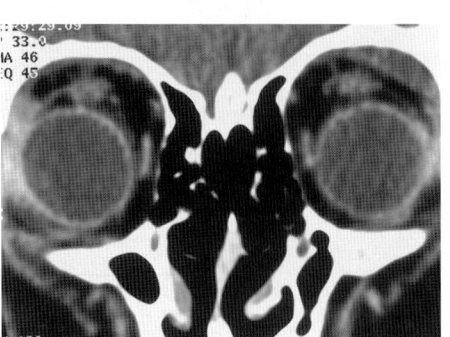

Fig. 2.**156** Acute bilateral subperiosteal hematoma. A 13-year-old boy with sickle cell anemia suddenly developed bilateral proptosis. **a** Axial CT scan shows bilateral subperiosteal hematoma (H). **b, c** Reformatted coronal (**b**) and sagittal (**c**) CT images showing characteristic appearance of subperiosteal hematoma. **d** Coronal CT scan following surgical treatment, showing minimal subperiosteal increased density on the left side. Case courtesy of Ayman Elsayed, MD, Jeddeh, Saudi Arabia.

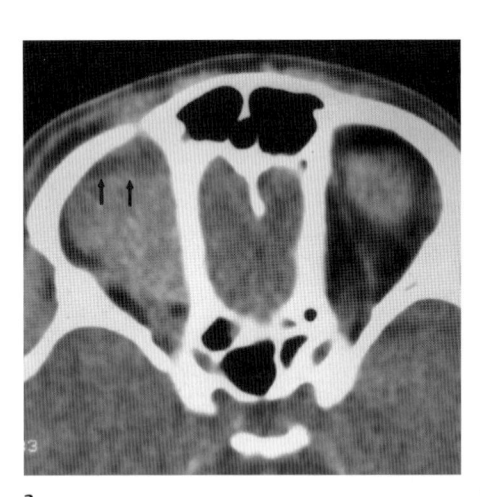

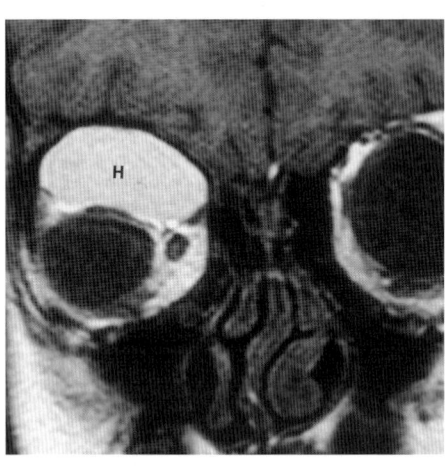

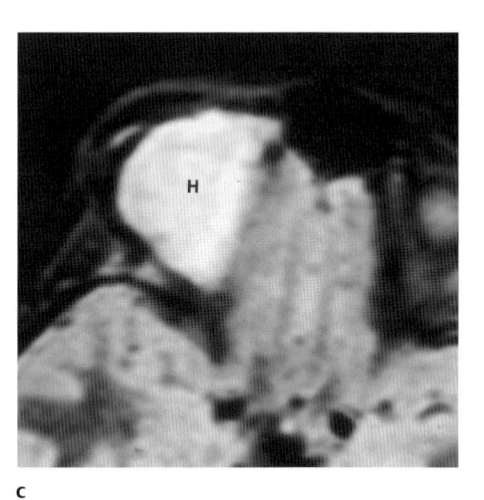

Fig. 2.**157** Subacute and chronic subperiosteal hematoma. **a** Axial CT scan shows a 9-day-old subperiosteal hematoma with fluid–fluid level (arrows). **b** Coronal T1W and **c** axial T2W MR scans. The subperiosteal hematoma (H) appears hyperintense on both T1W and T2W MR images.

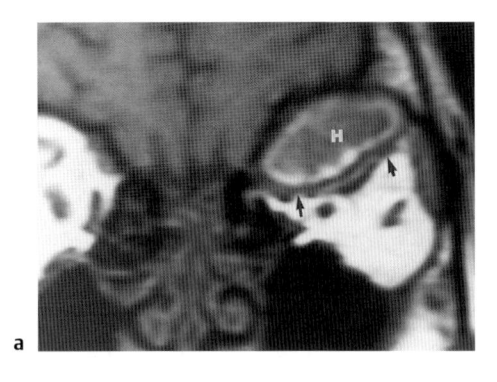

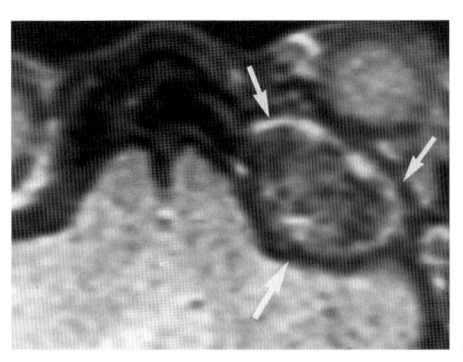

Fig. 2.**158** Acute subperiosteal hematoma. **a** Coronal T1W MR scan shows a large subperiosteal hematoma (H). Note displaced periosteum (arrows). **b** Axial T2W MR scan shows hypointense subperiosteal hematoma (arrows).

The diagnosis of hematoma is greatly aided by MRI, which can characterize all stages of blood degradation. The iron atoms of hemoglobin have different magnetic effects depending on the physical and oxidative state of hemoglobin itself.[79] Using a high-field (1.5 T) MRI unit, fresh (hyperacute) oxygenated blood (hemorrhage not older than a few hours) has the same MRI characteristics as water, being hypointense on T1-weighted and hyperintense on T2-weighted images. Acute hemorrhages (1–7 days), because of the paramagnetic effect of deoxyhemoglobin, have low signal on both T1-weighted and in particular T2-weighted images (Fig. 2.**158**). With progressive oxidation of deoxyhemoglobin to methemoglobin, hemorrhages older than 7 days become hyperintense on T1-weighted images (Fig. 2.**159**). The signal on T2-weighted MR images remains low if the

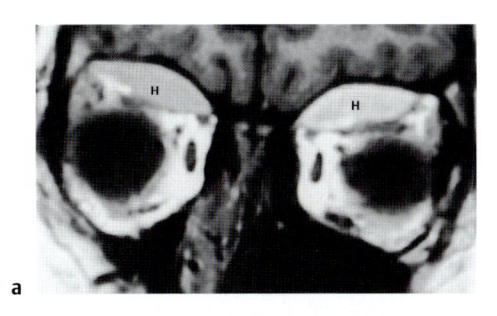

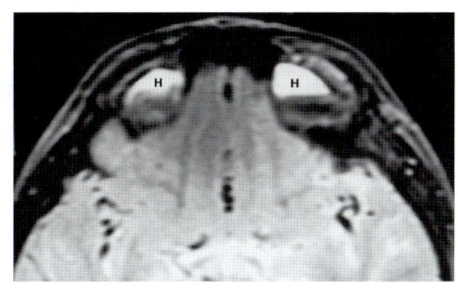

Fig. 2.**159** Subacute/chronic bilateral orbital subperiosteal hematoma. **a** Coronal T1W and **b** axial T2W MR scans showing bilateral orbital subperiosteal chronic hematoma (H). Note fluid–fluid level in **b** due to hemorrhage of different ages. Courtesy of Kyu Choi, MD, Seoul, Korea.

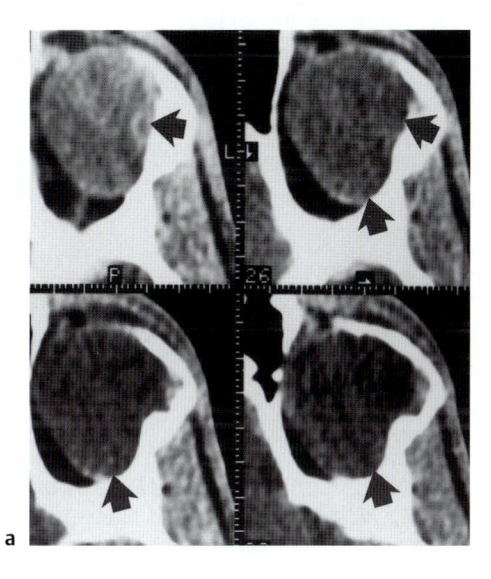

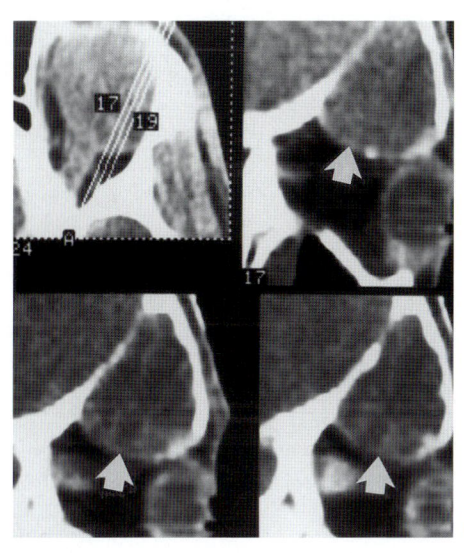

Fig. 2.**160** Cholesterol granuloma. **a** Axial CT scans show a large mass (arrows) compatible with a cholesterol granuloma. **b** Reformatted parasagittal CT images showing an expansile mass (arrows) compatible with a cholesterol granuloma.

Table 2.**19** MRI staging of orbital hematoma

	Stage				
	Hyperacute	Acute	Subacute	Subacute-chronic	Chronic
Time	Few hours	1–3 days	3–7 days	7 days–weeks	Months–years
Type	Fresh blood	Early clot	Before cell lysis	After cell lysis	Organized/scars
Content	Oxyhemoglobin	Deoxyhemoglobin	Intracellular methemoglobin	Extracellular methemoglobin	Hemosiderin
T1W MR image intensity	Low–high	Low–isodense	High	High	Low
T2W MR image intensity	High	Low	Low	High	Low

From Dobben CD, Philip B, Mafee MF, et al. Orbital subperiosteal hematoma, cholesterol granuloma, and infection. Evaluation with MR imaging and CT. Radial Clin North Am 1998; 36: 1185–1200. With permission.

methemoglobin is still intracellular. The signal is high if the methemoglobin has become extracellular (Figs. 2.**157b**, 2.**159b**). Hemosiderin, which causes a low signal on both T1-weighted and T2-weighted sequences, is encountered in scars or organized hematoma.[79] The MRI characteristics of orbital hematoma are listed in Table 2.**19**.

Orbital Cholesterol Granuloma

Cholesterol granulomas are bone-pushing and bone-destroying lesions characterized by granulomatous infiltration surrounding cholesterol crystals. Cholesterol granuloma may be etiologically related to loss of aeration of normally pneumatized bone, such as petromastoid bone. Negative pressure develops, leading to tissue edema and hemorrhage. Rupture of red blood cell membranes results in precipitation of cholesterol and membrane phospholipids. This crystallized cholesterol in turn acts as foreign body and elicits a giant-cell granulomatous reaction. There are no epithelial elements histologically in the cholesterol granuloma. Histologically, the tissues consist of foci of reactive xanthogranulomatous infiltrates, cholesterol crystals, giant cells, and hemosiderin surrounded by a fibrous capsule. The initiating factors must be different in the lesions arising in nonpneumatized bone, as in the orbital region. In the orbit, cholesterol granulomas are secondary lesions that are formed owing to post-traumatic, postsurgical, or postinflammatory events.

On CT scanning, cholesterol granulomas are seen as lytic lesions with ragged bone destruction, and invariably extend extraperiosteally into the orbit, causing proptosis (Fig. 2.**160**). Extension into the anterior and middle cranial fossae occurs less frequently.[78] On CT scans, the density of cholesterol granuloma is approximately isodense with the brain. Unlike epidermoid cyst, no sclerotic margin is seen between the mass and normal diploic bone. The lesion demonstrates no enhancement on postcontrast

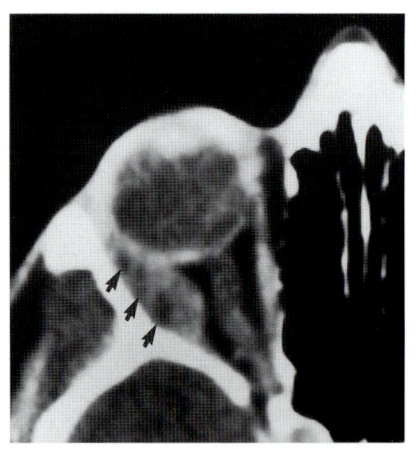

Fig. 2.**161** Cystic myositis. Axial enhanced CT scan shows enlargement of right lateral rectus muscle compatible with a pseudotumor myositic type. Note low-density cystic changes (arrows) within the enlarged muscle.

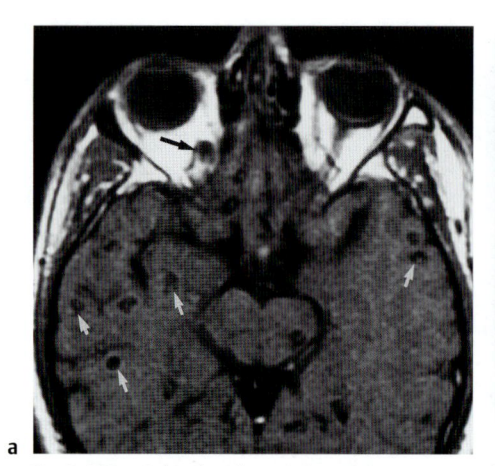

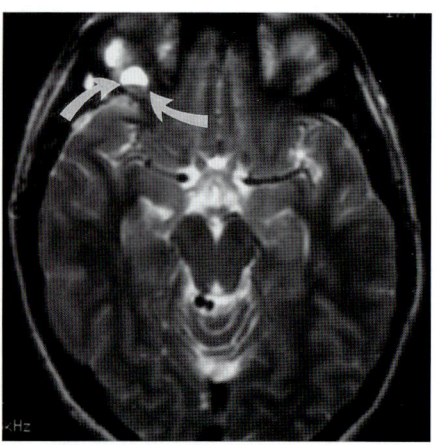

Fig. 2.**162** Orbital and cranial cysticercosis. **a** Axial T1W MR scan shows a retrobulbar mass (black arrow) compatible with orbital cysticercosis. Note several intracranial parasitic cysts (white arrows). **b** Axial T2W MR scan shows fluid–fluid level (arrows) within the orbital cyst.

CT scans. The differential diagnosis on the basis of CT scanning is limited to epidermoid and dermoid cysts or "aneurysmal bone cyst." Aneurysmal bone cysts occur almost exclusively in children.[2, 78] The MR imaging can be of most value in the diagnosis of cholesterol granuloma. These lesions give rise to high signal on T1-weighted and T2-weighted sequences, characteristic of chronic hemorrhage (Figs. 2.**157 b**, **c**; 2.**159**).[78]

Aneurysmal Bone Cyst

The term aneurysmal bone cyst (ABC) is a misnomer, because the lesion is histologically neither an aneurysm nor a cyst. Infrequently, ABC of the facial bones may involve the orbit of children.[72] ABC has been described as a benign lesion of bone characterized by a blood-filled cystlike expansion within the bone. The expansion may be complex and multilobular, with septa of bony trabeculae, fibrous tissues, and stromal giant cells. The ABC is not an entity by itself but is always secondary to an underlying bony or fibro-osseous condition such as nonossifying fibroma, ossifying fibroma, fibrous dysplasia, juvenile psammomatous active (aggressive) ossifying fibroma (see Chapter 4), chondroblastoma, chondromyxoid fibroma, osteoblastoma, giant-cell tumor (osteoclastoma), fibrosarcoma, osteochondrosarcoma, hemangioendothelioma, and hemangioma.[72]

Cystic Myositis

Infrequently, nonspecific orbital myositis may result in cystlike changes in an extraocular muscle.[72] These cysts may respond to treatment with oral corticosteroids, suggesting that the cysts do not have a parasitic origin, and probably represent edema in the muscles (Fig. 2.**161**).[72]

Orbital Abscess (Inflammatory Orbital Cyst)

Orbital abscesses are cystlike pus pockets that develop subperiosteally, or in the orbit or lids, in association with orbital or preseptal cellulitis almost always associated with sinonasal infections (see Fig. 2.**165**). The CT and MRI of orbital abscesses will be described in the following section.

■ Parasitic Cysts

Hydatid, Cysticercus Cellulosae

The occurrence of parasitic orbital cysts is limited to regions with poor sanitation where they are endemic. The hydatid cyst is related to infection by the larval form of a parasitic tapeworm, *Echinococcus granulosus*. The adult worm lives in the intestines of carnivores (usually dogs, but not humans). The infected carnivore passes the worm's ova in its feces. Grazing animals, acting as intermediate hosts, ingest the ova, which develop into larval forms in the hosts' muscles. Humans are infected by eating the undercooked meat of an infected grazing animal. Via the bloodstream, the hydatid can lodge in the orbit, resulting in a well-defined cystic mass, with or without a fluid–fluid lumen, containing the parasite. Clinically, patients present with slowly progressive, painless orbital signs.[72, 80] We have seen a large hydatid orbital cyst in a 9-year-old girl in the region of the lacrimal gland and lacrimal fossa.

Cysticercosis is a disease due to infestation by *Cysticercus cellulosae*, the larval form of the parasitic tapeworm *Taenia solium*. Clinically, patients present with either a visible subconjunctival cyst or orbital signs due to an extraocular muscle cyst that is unresponsive to treatment with oral corticosteroids.

The CT and MR imaging characteristics of most parasitic cysts are nonspecific. There may be some degree of enhancement around the cyst wall.[72, 80] Nearly all cases of orbital cysticercosis examined by CT show a cystic lesion near or within an extraocular muscle. An intraocular mass or cyst may be present.[81] A scolex can usually be identified within the cystic lesions in nearly one-half of patients by CT or MRI and is diagnostic (Fig. 2.**162**). Concurrent neurocysticercosis and orbital cysticercosis appear uncommon (Fig. 2.**162**). Neurocysticercosis is generally associated with more morbidity than orbital cysticercosis.[72] The CT and MRI features of orbital cysts are listed in Table 2.**20**.

■ Inflammatory Diseases

The frequency of orbital pathology by major diagnostic group and the age distribution of common orbital diseases are shown in Tables 2.**21** and 2.**22**. Orbital infections account for about 60% of primary orbital disease processes.[3] The infection may be acute,

Table 2.20 CT and MRI features of orbital cysts

Diagnostic group	CT characteristics	MRI characteristics
Epidermoid cyst	Nonenhancing mass with or without bone erosion. Scalloping with sclerosis of the adjacent bone may be present. No calcification. Minimal enhancement of the capsule may be present.	Hypointense on T1W and hyperintense on T2W, FLAIR, and DWI MR images. Minimal enhancement of capsule may be present. Associated orbital inflammatory changes when cyst is ruptured.
Dermoid cyst	Nonenhancing mass with or without bone erosion. Scalloping with sclerosis of the adjacent bone may be present. Calcification, if present is a characteristic feature. Hypodensity (fat), if present is characteristic (adipose tissue). Fat-fluid may be present and is characteristic. Minimal enhancement of the capsule may be present.	Hypointense on T1W and hyperintense on T2W images. Those containing fat demonstrate signal characteristics of fatty tissue. Minimal enhancement of capsule may be present. Associated orbital inflammatory changes, when cyst is ruptured.
Conjunctival choristoma (dermolipoma)	Density of adipose tissue.	Intensity of adipose tissue.
Cholesterol granuloma (chronic hematic cyst)	Nonenhancing mass with or without bone erosion. Lytic lesion with ragged bone destruction. Often isodense to brain. No sclerotic margin.	High signal on T1W and T2W images. Often homogeneous in signal characteristics. Heterogeneous signal, particularly on T2W, related to hemosiderin plaques.
Enterogenous cysts	Isodense or hyperdense, depending on the mucous content of the cyst.	Hypointense or hyperintense on T1W depending on the mucous content of the cyst and hyperintense on T2W images.
Other orbital epithelial and appendage cysts, including implantation cysts	Nonenhancing low-density mass.	Nonenhancing, hypointense on T1W and hyperintense on T2W images.
Congenital cystic eye	Nonenhancing low-density mass.	Hypointense on T1W and hyperintense on T2W images. Non-enhancing mass.
Dacryocele	Nonenhancing (unless infected) low-density mass.	Hypointense on T1W and hyperintense on T2W images. Non-enhancing mass, unless infected.
Parasitic cysts (hydatid, cysticercosis)	Cystic lesions within or near an extraocular muscle. Some degree of enhancement around the cyst wall. Scolex can be identified. Diffuse myositis may be present. Cystic lesion within or near lacrimal gland or other part of the orbit.	Cystic lesions within or near an extraocular muscle, lacrimal gland, or other portion of the orbit. Hypointense on T1W and hyperintense on T2W images. Some degree of enhancement around the cyst wall. Scolex can be identified. Diffuse myositis may be present.

From Mafee MF. The eye, orbit: Embryology; anatomy and pathology. In: Som PM, Curtin HD, eds. Head and Neck Imaging. St. Louis: Mosby; 2003: 441–654. With permission.

Table 2.21 Frequency of orbital lesions by major diagnostic group

Diagnostic group	Frequency (%)
Thyroid orbitopathy	47
Cystic lesions	8
Inflammatory lesions	8
Vascular lesions	5
Lacrimal gland lesions	4
Lymphoproliferative lesions	4
Secondary tumors	4
Myxomatous and adipose lesions	3
Mesenchymal lesions	2
Metastatic tumors	2
Optic nerve tumors	1
Fibrous and connective-tissue lesions	1
Osseous and fibro-osseous lesions	1
Histiocytic lesions	<1
Other and unclassified	17

From Dutton J. Orbital diseases. In: Yanoff M, Duker JS, eds. Ophthalmology. St. Louis: Mosby; 1999: 7; 14.1–14.18.

Table 2.22 Age distribution of common orbital diseases

Diagnostic group	Frequency (%)		
	Childhood and adolescence (0–20 years)	Middle life (21–60 years)	Later adult life (61+ years)
Thyroid orbitopathy	10	59	40
Infectious process	7	3	3
Inflammatory lesions	6	5	9
Cystic lesions	12	3	4
Vascular neoplastic lesions	15	2	1
Other vascular lesions	7	2	3
Trauma	7	4	2
Secondary orbital malignancies	1	2	9
Metastatic malignancies	1	1	8
Mesenchymal lesions	9	1	1
Lymphangiomas	6	1	0
Lymphoproliferative diseases	1	3	12
Optic nerve lesions	5	1	1
Other neurogenic lesions	5	3	2
Lacrimal gland fossa	1	1	1
Other	7	8	4

From Dutton J. Orbital diseases. In: Yanoff M, Duker JS, eds. Ophthalmology. St. Louis: Mosby; 1999: 7; 14.1–14.18.

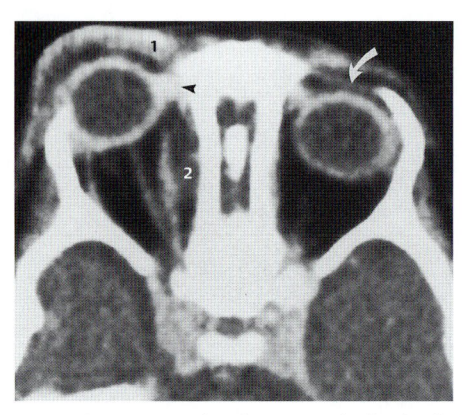

Fig. 2.**163** Preseptal and postseptal orbital inflammation. Axial postcontrast CT scan shows normal orbital septum (white arrow) and eyelid on the left side. Note edema of the right eyelid (1), thickening of the reflected portion of the superior oblique tendon (arrowhead), and retroseptal subperiosteal fluid (edema) formation (2). The right orbital septum is not delineated because it is displaced anteriorly and effaced due to edema of the subcutaneous tissues of the eyelid.

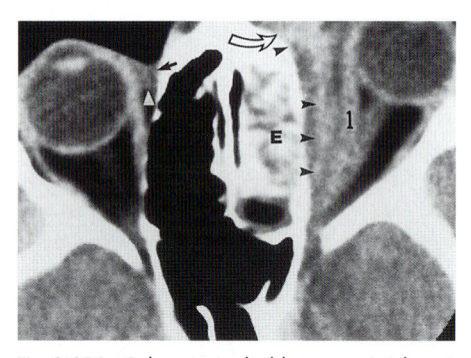

Fig. 2.**164** Subperiosteal phlegmon. Axial postcontrast CT scan shows opacification of ethmoid air cells (E) and subperiosteal infiltration (granulation tissue) (arrowheads), resulting in lateral displacement of the medial rectus muscle (1). Note the right medial check ligament (white arrowhead) and medial palpebral ligament (black arrow). The orbital septum at this level may not be seen as a discrete structure due to partial volume averaging of the lacrimal sac. The orbital septum is anterior to the medial check ligament and posterior to the medial palpebral ligament. Note the thickened left orbital septum (curved arrow).

Table 2.**23** Staging of orbital cellulitis

State	Clinical findings
Inflammatory edema	Eyelid swelling and erythema
Preseptal cellulitis	Eyelid swelling and erythema associated with inflammatory soft-tissue thickening of the orbit anterior to the orbital septum Chemosis may be present
Postseptal cellulitis	Edema of the orbital contents; proptosis, chemosis and decreased extraocular movement Visual loss (unusual)
Subperiosteal abscess	A collection of inflammatory infiltrates and pus between the periorbita and the involved sinus Globe proptotic and displaced by abscess Visual loss with progression of the disease
Cavernous sinus thrombosis	Proptosis and ophthalmoplegia with development of similar signs on the contralateral side associated with cranial nerve palsies (III, IV, V, VI) and visual loss

subacute, or chronic. The majority of acute inflammatory disorders are of paranasal sinus origin. However, the infection may develop from infectious processes of the face, oral cavity (dental) or pharynx, from trauma or foreign bodies, or it may be secondary to septicemia. The bacteria most commonly involved are staphylococcus, streptococcus, pneumococcus, pseudomonas, Neisseriaceae, haemophilus, and mycobacteria.[82,83] Herpes simplex and herpes zoster are the major virus infections of the orbit.

Acute inflammation is characterized by rapid onset associated with soft-tissue swelling and infiltration, loss of the normal soft-tissue planes, local soft-tissue destruction, and abscess formation. The location of the process is clinically important because a preseptal infection (Fig. 2.**163**) rarely affects orbital functions. On the other hand, a retroseptal infection (Fig. 2.**164**) may have a profound and sudden effect on optic nerve and orbital motility function.

Orbital Cellulitis and Sinusitis

Sinusitis is the most common cause of orbital cellulitis. Even though antibiotics have reduced the incidence of complicated sinusitis with orbital involvement, it still occurs and may be the first sign of sinus infection in children.[70,82,83] In the preantibiotic era, morbidity and mortality from orbital cellulitis were significant, with 17% of cases resulting in death and 20% resulting in blindness. Orbital cellulitis is probably the most common cause of proptosis in children.[6] The classification of orbital cellulitis includes five categories or stages of orbital involvement: (1) inflammatory edema; (2) subperiosteal phlegmon and abscess; (3) orbital cellulitis; (4) orbital abscess; (5) ophthalmic vein and cavernous sinus thrombosis.[3,70,83] It is often difficult to limit a particular inflammatory lesion to one of these categories because they tend to overlap (Table 2.**23**).[70,83]

Bacterial Orbital Cellulitis Classification

Orbital complications of paranasal sinusitis are relatively common in children but are uncommon in adults. Predisposing factors for the spread of infection to the orbit include congenital, surgical, or traumatic dehiscence in the common bony walls, the anterior and posterior ethmoid neurovascular foramina, and the valveless sinonasal and orbital veins and diploic veins, which are avenues of septic thrombophlebitic spread of sinus disease to the orbit.[84] The classification of the orbital complications of sinus infections by Chandler et al.,[85] based on the anatomy and the presumed pathogenesis of orbital cellulitis, is recognized as useful in clinical situations. The Chandler classification was devised prior to the advent of newer orbital imaging techniques and modifications that make use of information obtained from these imaging techniques are indicated. We therefore recommend the classification scheme of periorbital infections[84] outlined in Table 2.**23**.

Bacterial Preseptal Cellulitis and Preseptal Edema

Preseptal cellulitis describes infections limited to the skin and subcutaneous tissues of the eyelid anterior to the orbital septum.[84] Preseptal edema is the first stage of infection secondary to sinusitis. It is often clinically misdiagnosed as orbital or periorbital cellulitis; the infection in this early stage is actually still confined to the sinus.[83] There is swelling of the eyelids with mild orbital edema, usually involving the upper eyelid, especially medially. This reflects congestion of venous outflow. Without treatment, preseptal cellulitis develops. CT or MRI demonstrates the eyelid edema and the inflammatory paranasal sinus disease (Fig. 2.**163**).[8] Clinically, the patient has erythema and swelling of the eyelids. There is no proptosis, chemosis, or limitation of ocular motility.[84]

Pathology   229

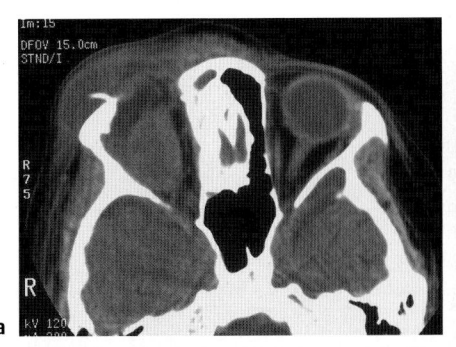

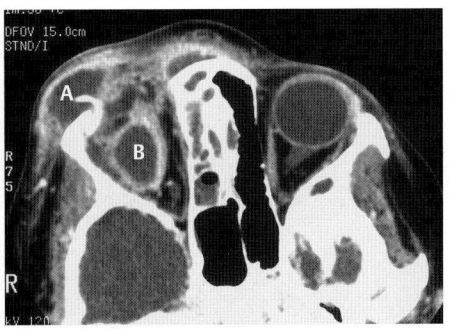

Fig. 2.**165** Sinogenic orbital abscess in a 10-year-old girl with acute sinusitis and proptosis of the right eye. **a** Axial precontrast and **b** axial postcontrast CT scans showing an eyelid abscess (A) and a large retrobulbar abscess (B). Note a drain in the eyelid abscess.

Fig. 2.**166** Subperiosteal abscess. Axial PW MR scan shows opacification of bilateral ethmoid air cells, edema (E) of right eyelid, and a large subperiosteal abscess (arrow) with air (A) and fluid collection within the abscess cavity.

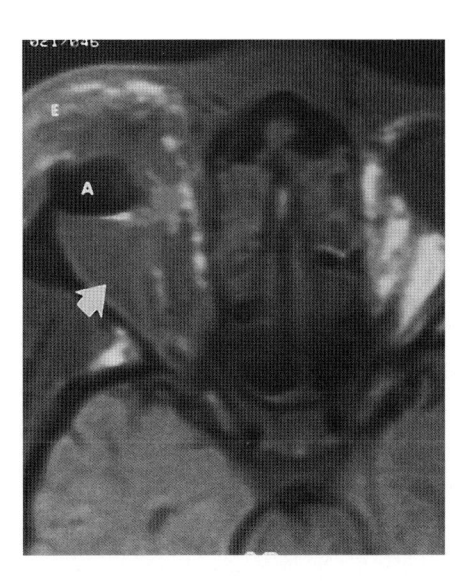

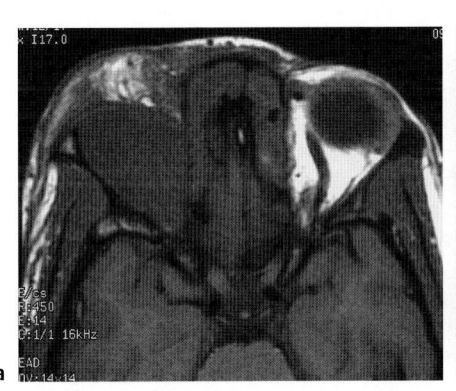

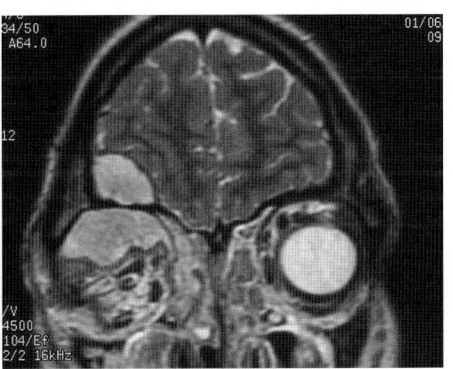

Fig. 2.**167** Subperiosteal abscess. **a** Axial T1W and **b** coronal T2W MR scans showing a large orbital subperiosteal abscess as well as a large epidural (subperiosteal) abscess (**b**). Note bilateral ethmoid mucosal changes due to acute sinusitis.

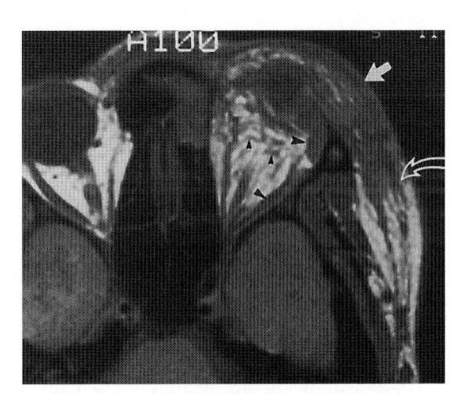

Fig. 2.**168** Orbital cellulitis. Axial PW MR scan shows marked diffuse cutaneous and subcutaneous interstitial soft-tissue thickening and edema (white arrows). There is subperiosteal phlegmon along the lateral wall of the orbit (large arrowheads). Note the increased reticulation of the retrobulbar fatty reticulum due to edema.

Postseptal Orbital Cellulitis

Postseptal orbital cellulitis describes an infectious process that occurs within the orbit proper, behind the orbital septum, and within the bony walls of the orbit. Inflammatory edema is used to describe the earliest stage of postseptal orbital infection.[84]

Diagnostic imaging can be useful in cases in which clinical differentiation of preseptal and postseptal cellulitis is impossible or when the diagnosis is unclear.[84] CT and MRI findings include soft-tissue thickening of the eyelids. Usually the process is diffuse and a localized eyelid abscess cavity is not seen. In clinically suspected postseptal orbital cellulitis, orbital imaging is indicated. Contrast-enhanced study is necessary to differentiate inflammatory edema, cellulitis, orbital phlegmon, and orbital abscess (Figs. 2.**163**–2.**165**).

Subperiosteal Phlegmon and Abscess

As the reaction of the orbital periosteum begins and gradually advances, the edema of the eyelids and conjunctivae becomes more generalized and the eye begins to protrude. Inflammatory tissue and edema collect beneath the periosteum to form a subperiosteal phlegmon (Fig. 2.**164**), which may subsequently develop into a subperiosteal abscess (Figs. 2.**166**, 2.**167**). As the disease progresses, the inflammatory process infiltrates the periorbital and retro-orbital fat, giving rise to a true orbital cellulitis (Fig. 2.**168**). The subperiosteal abscess and orbital cellulitis frequently coexist.[70,83] At this stage, extraocular motility becomes progressively impaired. With severe involvement, visual disturbances can result from optic neuritis or ischemia. Progression of intraorbital cellulitis or spread from the subperiosteal space leads to intraconal or extraconal loculation and abscess formation (Fig. 2.**165**).[3,70,83] Progression of disease may lead to ophthalmic vein thrombosis (Fig. 2.**169**) and cavernous sinus thrombosis and associated mycotic aneurysm of the internal carotid artery (Fig. 2.**170**), which are dire complications of orbital and sinonasal infections. Cavernous sinus thrombosis is heralded by central nervous system deficit and orbital functional impairment. It is an acute thrombophlebitis from an infection in an area having venous drainage to the cavernous sinus.[2,82] The general symptoms consist of headache, fever, and chills, with an elevated white count and a positive blood culture. The ophthalmological findings include edema of the lids, exophthalmos, chemosis, paralysis of the eye muscles, engorgement of the retinal veins, and papilledema.[2]

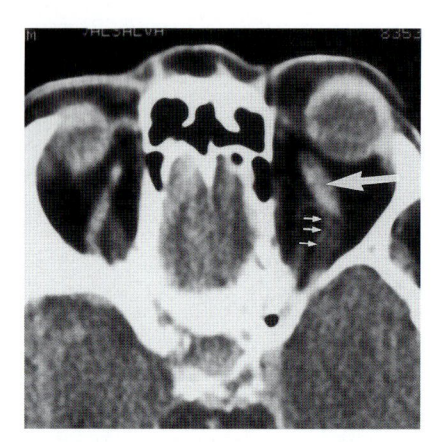

Fig. 2.**169** Superior ophthalmic vein thrombosis. Axial enhanced CT scan shows enlargement of left superior ophthalmic vein (large arrow). Note a filling defect along its posterior portion (small arrows).

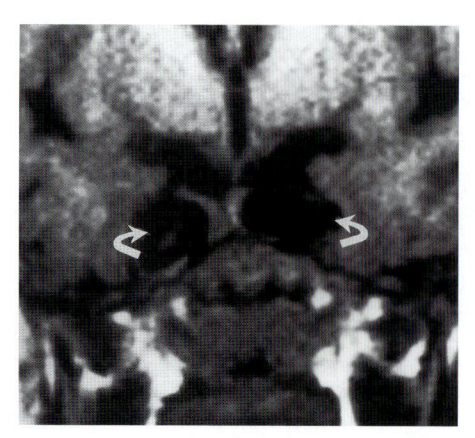

Fig. 2.**170** Bilateral mycotic aneurysm of internal carotid arteries. Coronal T1W MR scan shows hypointense masses within the cavernous sinuses (arrows), compatible with mycotic aneurysms, related to superior orbital-frontal cellulitis. Case courtesy of Jose Mondonca, MD, Sao Paulo, Brazil.

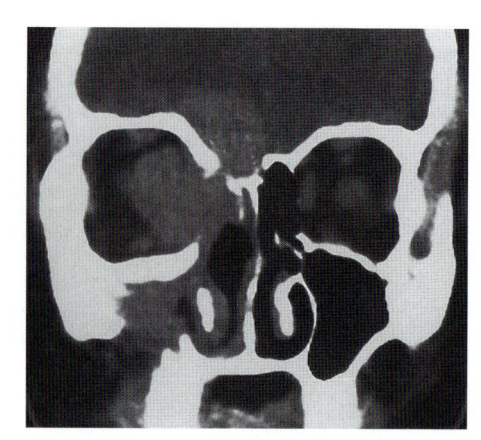

Fig. 2.**171** Mucormycosis. Coronal CT scan shows mucormycosis of the sinonaso-orbit, extending into the anterior cranial fossa. Note postsurgical changes of the maxillary, ethmoid, and nasal cavity on the involved side. Case courtesy of Dr. Hary Sherif, Cairo, Egypt.

Cavernous Sinus Thrombosis

Cavernous sinus thrombosis (CST) results from the spread of infections of the sinonasal cavities and the orbit, and from infection of the middle third of the face.[84] CST originates from a septic thrombophlebitis arising in the ophthalmic vein (Fig. 2.**169**). In thrombosis, the cavernous sinus is of low attenuation, and the contrast-enhanced internal carotid arteries stand out as contrast-enhanced tubular structures. On contrast-enhanced CT scans, filling defects are seen in the cavernous sinus. Usually, the superior ophthalmic vein is markedly enlarged. False-negative CT scans are common until late in the course of the disease.[84] Thrombosis of the superior ophthalmic vein (SOV) is seen on MRI as an enlarged vein that appears less hypointense than the normal opposite side. On T1-weighted and T2-weighted MR images, the thrombosed SOV may be seen as a hyperintense area within the lumen of the vein.[86-88] Thrombosis of the cavernous sinus results in engorgement of the cavernous sinus and ophthalmic veins, and usually, engorgement of the extraocular muscles.[84] MR imaging and MR venography are more sensitive than CT for revealing CST.[87] On MRI there is deformity of the cavernous portion of the internal carotid artery. The signal from the abnormal cavernous sinus is heterogeneous and an obvious hyperintense signal of thromboses in the vascular sinus may be seen on all pulse sequences. Mycotic (septic) aneurysm of the internal carotid artery is a serious complication of orbital infection. This can be suspected on CT or MRI scans and confirmed by MR angiography or standard angiography (Fig. 2.**170**).

■ Mycotic Infections

Orbital fungal infections are often seen in patients with a history of uncontrolled diabetes mellitus and in immunocompromised patients, such as those with AIDS. Immunocompromised patients are particularly susceptible to infection by fungi, such as *Candida* species, *Histoplasma capsulatum*, *Coccidioides immitis*, *Mucor*, and *Aspergillus* species.[84] By far, *Mucor* and *Aspergillus* are the most common fungal organisms incriminated.

The fungi responsible for mucormycosis are ubiquitous and normally saprophytic in humans; they rarely produce severe disease, except in those with predisposing conditions.[70, 82, 89] There are four major types of mucormycosis: rhinocerebral, pulmonary, gastrointestinal, and disseminated.[89] The most common form is the rhinocerebral form. The infection usually begins in the nose and spreads to the paranasal sinuses; it then extends into the orbit and cavernous sinuses (Fig. 2.**171**).[70, 89] Orbital involvement results in such orbital signs as ophthalmoplegia, proptosis, ptosis, loss of vision, and orbital cellulitis.[2, 16, 70]

The pathological hallmark of mucormycosis is invasion of the walls of small vessels. Because of this, when the cavernous sinus is invaded, particularly in patients with mucormycosis and aspergillosis, rapid brain infarction may develop.[90] *Aspergillus* is a ubiquitous fungus found primarily in agricultural dust. It may produce rhinocerebral disease and orbital involvement similar to mucormycosis, although hematogenous spread from the lungs to the brain is more common.[89] This fungus also has a well-known propensity for invading blood vessels, including the internal carotid artery.[70] One important but not pathognomonic MRI finding of mycotic infections is the hypointensity of mycotic infection on T2-weighted MR imaging scans (Fig. 2.**172**). This is thought to be due to paramagnetic materials produced by the fungi. The main contribution of CT and MRI is their clear demonstration of the relationship between sinonasal, orbital, and intracranial disease (Fig. 2.**171**, 2.**172**). One should realize that the CT and MRI findings of invasive aspergillosis are indistinguishable from those of mucormycosis. Advanced sino-orbital mucormyosis and invasive aspergillosis mimic aggressive tumors on CT and MR scans (Fig. 2.**171**, 2.**172**). At times, fungal infection begins in the eye and spreads into the Tenon's capsule and then into the retrobulbar space (Fig. 2.**173**).

■ Acute, Subacute, and Chronic Idiopathic Orbital Inflammatory Disorders (Pseudotumors)

Idiopathic inflammatory syndromes usually are referred to as orbital pseudotumors, a clinically and histologically confusing category of lesions.[2, 3, 16] In general, orbital pseudotumors represent a nongranulomatous inflammatory process in the orbit or eye with no known local or systemic causes.[91] At times, pseudotumor may display an idiopathic granulomatous pattern. It is a

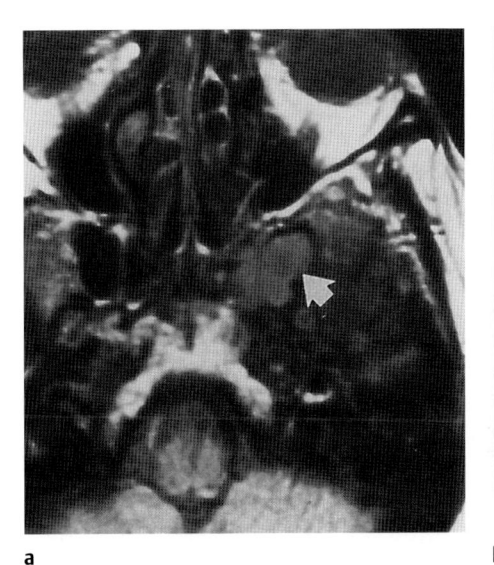

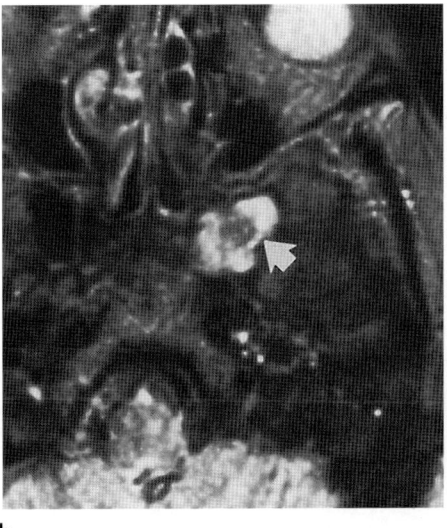

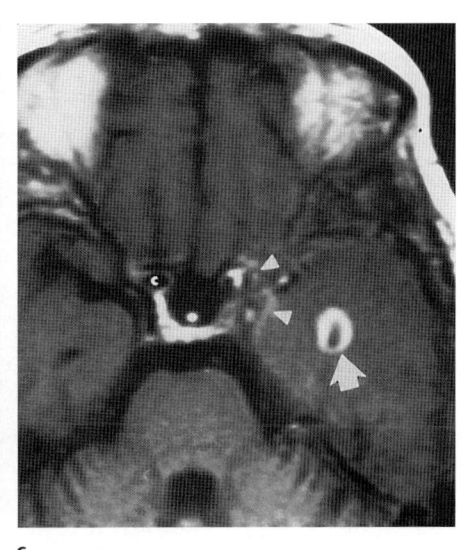

Fig. 2.172 Aspergillosis (invasive).
a Axial PW MR scan shows opacification of left sphenoid sinus (arrow).
b Axial T2W MR scan shows hyperintensity of the left sphenoid sinus (arrow) due to edema and inflammatory changes. Note a hypointense focus in the center.
c Axial post-Gd-DTPA T1W MR scan shows a temporal lobe abscess (arrow) and involvement of the left cavernous sinus (arrowheads). Note the normal right internal carotid artery (c) and constriction of the left internal carotid artery due to arteritis.

diagnosis by exclusion based on history, clinical course, response to steroid therapy, laboratory tests, and biopsy in a number of cases.[3,16,91] There is a group of diverse disease entities that can mimic pseudotumors, such as lymphoma, sarcoidosis, collagen-vascular disease such as systemic lupus erythematosus, and other granulomatous diseases. Orbital pseudotumor is defined as a nonspecific, idiopathic inflammatory condition for which no local identifiable cause or systemic disease can be found.[92,93] By definition, this excludes orbital inflammatory disease caused by entities such as Wegener granulomatosis, retained foreign bodies, "sclerosing hemangioma," trauma, and sinusitis.

In adults, after Graves orbitopathy, pseudotumor is a common orbital disorder, accounting for 4.7–6.3% of orbital disorders.[91] The disease usually affects adults but may also affect children; in children, there is a higher incidence of bilateral orbital involvement. Bilateral orbital pseudotumors in adults should suggest the possibility of systemic disease such as systemic vasculitis or a systemic lymphoproliferative disorder.[5,6] Patients with pseudotumor typically present with the acute onset of orbital pain, restricted eye movement, diplopia, proptosis, and impaired vision from perioptic nerve involvement or compression of the optic nerve. Conjunctival vascular congestion and edema, and lid erythema and swelling are common.[3,16] Pain is an important feature of pseudotumors, but not all patients with pseudotumors present with pain. Some may have minimal proptosis or may even present with a totally scarred lesion (sclerosing pseudotumor) within a single muscle or in the retrobulbar fat pad.[3,5,6,16]

Histopathology

Pseudotumor was first described in 1905 by Birch-Hirschfield[94] and has remained something of an enigma in the ophthalmology, radiology, and pathology literature.[93] The histopathology can vary from polymorphous inflammatory cells and fibrosis, with a matrix of granulation tissue, eosinophils, plasma cells, histiocytes, lymphoid follicle with germinal center, and lymphocytes, to a predominantly lymphocytic form (lymphoid hyperplasia), embedded in a loose fibrous stroma. Many cases have been reported of lymphocytic pseudotumor that, over a period of time,

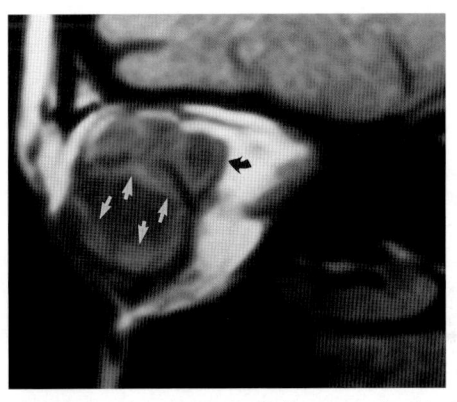

Fig. 2.173 Blastomycosis of the eye and orbit. Enhanced sagittal T1W MR scan shows marked thickening and enhancement of the uveal tract (white arrows), along with a retrobulbar mass (black arrow) compatible with endophthalmitis and an orbital abscess.

are found to harbor a malignant lymphoma without any evidence of systemic lymphoma. The presence of germinal follicles and increased vascularity are indicative of a reactive lesion, often associated with a favorable prognosis and responsiveness to steroids. An association has been noted between diffusely distributed lymphoblasts, steroid unresponsiveness, and a probable neoplastic lymphoid lesion.[93] Not all steroid-resistant pseudotumors are destined to become lymphomatous. The peculiar behavior of pseudotumor has led some authors to speculate that some forms of pseudotumor are the result of an autoimmune process.[93,95]

Pseudotumors are often multicentric, presenting myositis, dacryoadenitis, sclerotenonitis (Tenon fasciitis), and inflammation of the dural sheath of the optic nerve and surrounding connective tissue.[3,5,6,16] They may be classified as (1) acute and subacute idiopathic anterior orbital inflammation; (2) acute and subacute idiopathic diffuse orbital inflammation; (3) acute and subacute idiopathic myositic orbital inflammation; (4) acute and subacute idiopathic apical orbital inflammation; (5) idiopathic dacryoadenitis; and (6) perineuritis. Tolosa–Hunt syndrome

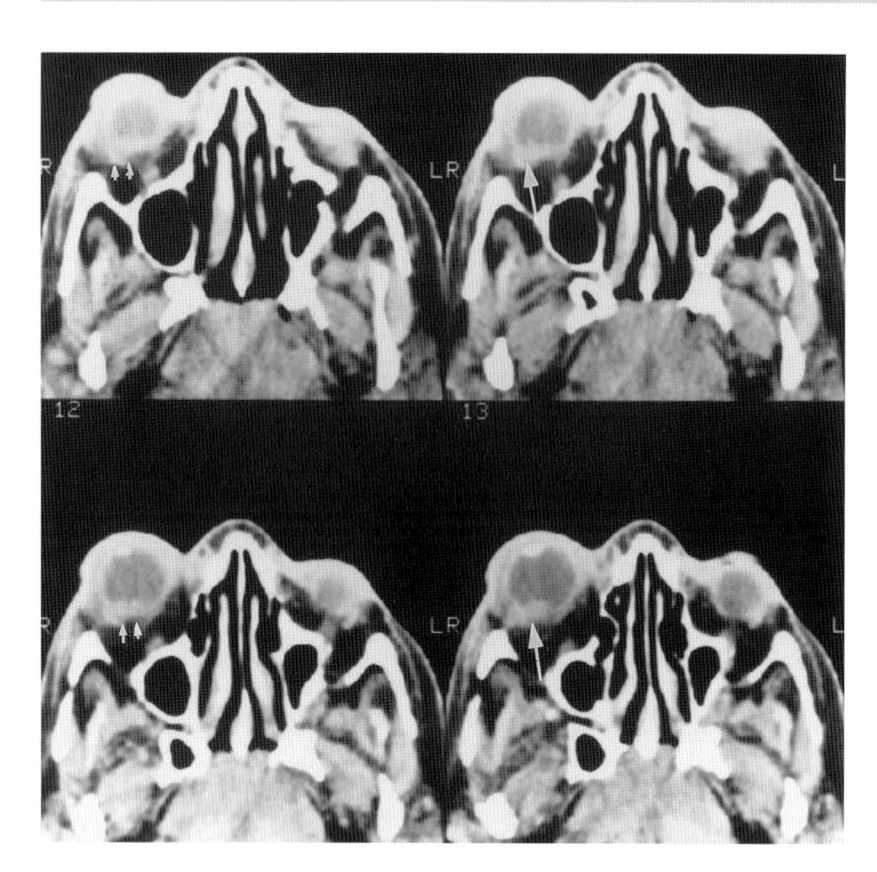

Fig. 2.**174** Pseudotumor (posterior scleritis type). Axial enhanced CT scans show proptosis, lid thickening (swelling), and increased enhancement of the posterior sclera and Tenon's capsule of the right eye compatible with sclerotenonitis. The nodular enhancement (arrows) is suggestive of posterior nodular scleritis.

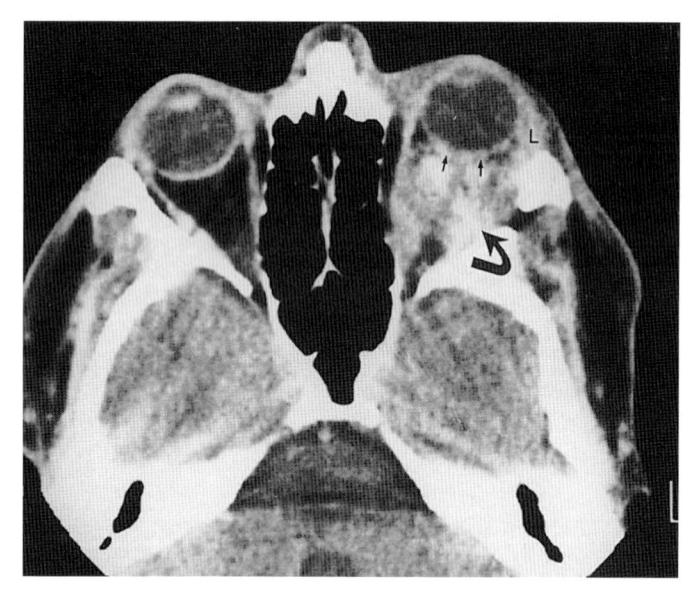

Fig. 2.**175** Pseudotumor. Axial postcontrast CT scan shows an infiltrative process involving the lacrimal gland (L), Tenon's space (arrows), and retrobulbar space (curved arrow). Note the osteotomy defect, the site for biopsy.

(painful ophthalmoplegia) is a variant of pseudotumor in which inflammatory process is restricted to the vicinity of superior orbital fissure and the optic canal, or to the cavernous sinus.[3,5,6,16]

Anterior Orbital Inflammation

In the anterior orbital pseudotumor group, the main focus of inflammation involves the anterior orbit and adjacent globe.[2,3,16] The major features at presentation are pain, proptosis, lid swelling, and decreased vision. Other findings may be ocular and include uveitis, sclerotenonitis (Tenon's capsule), papillitis, and exudative retinal detachment. The extraocular muscle (EOM) motility is usually unaffected. CT and MRI show thickening of the uveal–scleral rim with obscuration of the optic nerve junction, which enhances on CT with contrast infusion (Fig. 2.**174**).[93] These findings are due to leakage of proteinaceous edema/fluid into the interstitium of the uvea and Tenon's capsule secondary to the inflammatory reaction.[93] Fluid in the Tenon's capsule has been well documented with ultrasound (the T sign). Patients with posterior scleritis can develop retinal detachment and fundal masses, which simulate intraocular tumors (Fig. 2.**174**, see also Fig. 2.**38**).[2,93]

Diffuse Orbital Pseudotumor

Diffuse orbital pseudotumor is similar in many respects to acute and subacute anterior orbital inflammation, with a greater severity of the signs and symptoms.[2,3] The diffuse, tumefactive, or infiltrative type of pseudotumor may fill the entire retrobulbar space and mold itself around the globe, while respecting its natural shape. Even the largest mass usually does not invade or distort the shape of the globe or erode bone (Figs. 2.**175**, 2.**176**). This type of disease can be very difficult to differentiate from lymphoma. These large, bulky masses can be intraconal or extraconal or can involve both spaces.

Orbital Myositis

Idiopathic orbital myositis is a condition in which one or more of the EOMs are primarily infiltrated by an inflammatory process (Figs. 2.**177**, 2.**178**). Myositis can be acute, subacute, or recurrent. The patient usually presents with painful extraocular movements, diplopia, proptosis, swelling of the lid, conjunctival chemosis, and inflammation over the involved EOM.[3,93] The disorder may be bilateral. The most frequently affected muscles are the superior

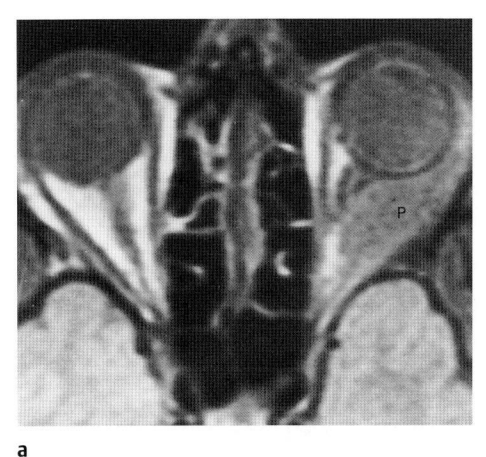

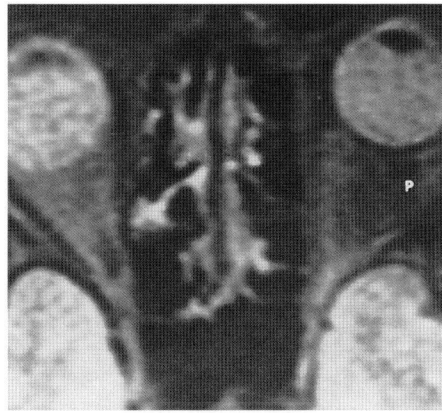

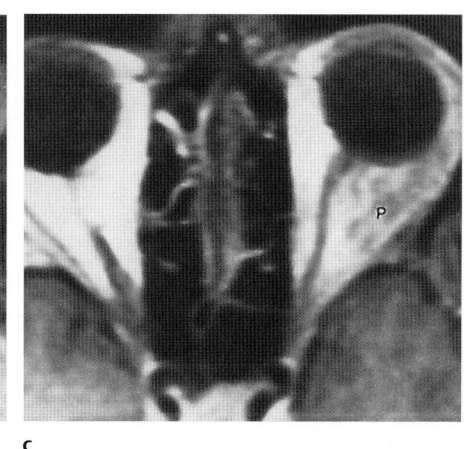

Pathology   233

Fig. 2.176 Pseudotumor.
a Axial PW MR scan shows an infiltrative process due to pseudotumor (P).
b Axial T2W MR scan shows orbital pseudotumor (P). The process appears hypointense as compared to normal retrobulbar tissue on the right side.
c Axial postcontrast T1W MR scan shows moderate enhancement of the pseudotumor (P).

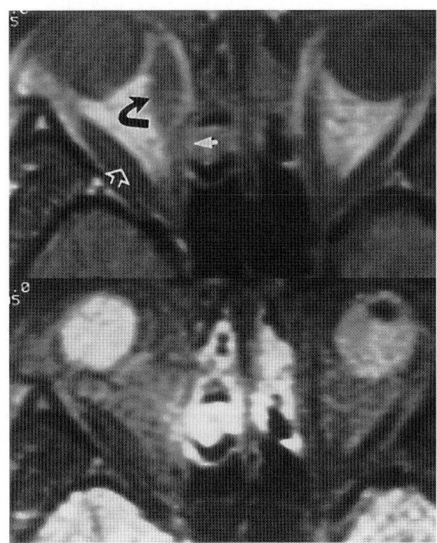

Fig. 2.177 Myositic orbital pseudotumor. Axial PW (top) and T2W (bottom) MR scans show enlargement of the right medial (curved arrow) and lateral (open arrow) rectus muscles. The medial rectus shows marked increased signal intensity on the T2W image. Note inflammatory changes in the ethmoid sinuses. This myositic pseudotumor may be due to hypersensitivity reaction to sinus infection. The edema of right medial rectus is more at the site where the medial wall of the orbit is poorly defined (white solid arrow).

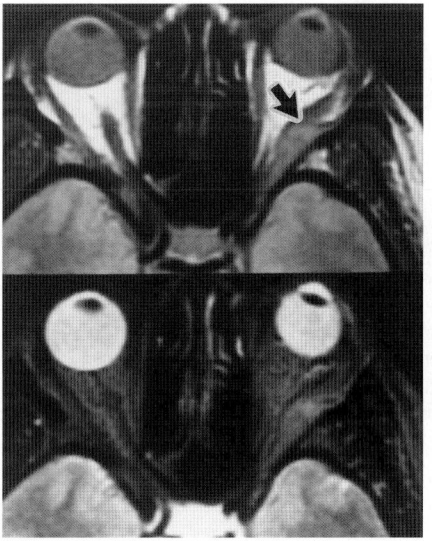

Fig. 2.178 Myositic orbital pseudotumor.
a Axial PW (top) and T2W (bottom) MR scans showing thickening of the left lateral rectus muscle (arrow).
b Axial enhanced fat-suppression MR scans, showing marked enhancement of the left lateral rectus muscle (arrow). Note extension of the inflammatory process along its tendon (arrowheads).

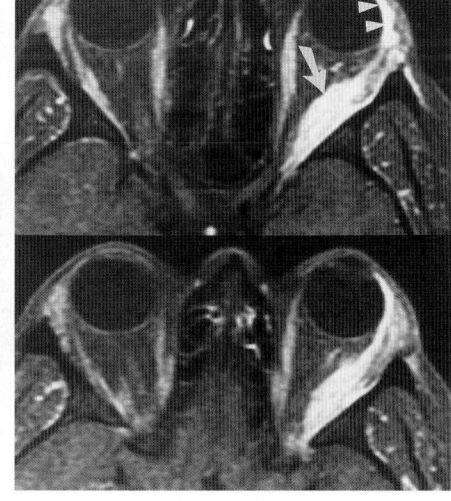

complex and the lateral and medial rectus muscles (Fig. 2.**177**). The major differential diagnosis is Graves or dysthroid orbitopathy. However, dysthyroid myopathy is usually painless in onset, fairly symmetric, slowly progressive, and associated with a systemic diathesis.[3] Trokel and Hilal[96] state that the typical CT finding in orbital myositis is enlargement of the EOMs, which extends anteriorly to involve the inserting tendon (Figs. 2.**177**, 2.**178**). Other helpful indicators of inflammatory orbital myositis include a ragged, fluffy border of the involved muscle, with infiltration and obliteration of the fat in the peripheral orbital space between the periosteum of the orbital wall and the muscle cone.

Also observed is an inward bowing of the medial contour of the muscle belly, forming a shoulder as it passes around the globe (Fig. 2.**177**). All these findings can be attributed to local tendinitis, fasciitis, and myositis of the involved muscle. In contrast, the fusiform appearance of an enlarged muscle in thyroid myopathy is produced by a myositis without involvement of the muscle tendon insertion. The muscle borders are sharply defined and the fat in the peripheral surgical space is preserved and may be expanded. Less common causes of EOM enlargement include arteriovenous fistula (e.g., carotid–cavernous fistula and dural AVM) and neoplasm (primary or metastatic).[93]

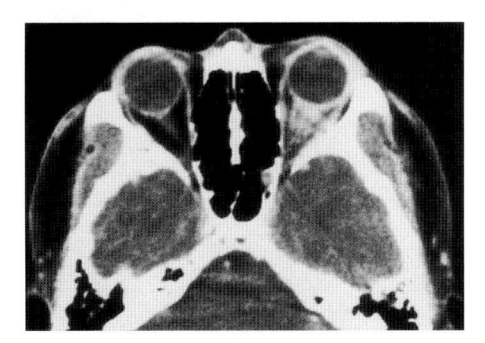

Fig. 2.179 Perineuritic orbital pseudotumor. Axial postcontrast CT scan shows perioptic nerve infiltration. Lymphoma may have an identical CT appearance.

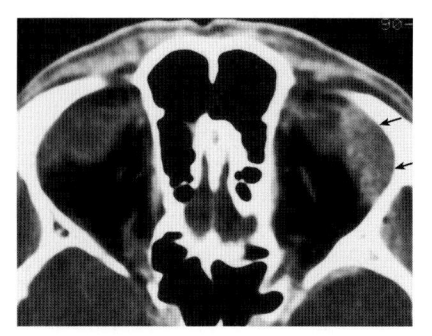

Fig. 2.180 Pseudotumor. Axial enhanced CT scan shows diffuse enlargement of left lacrimal gland compatible with an idiopathic inflammatory pseudotumor (arrows).

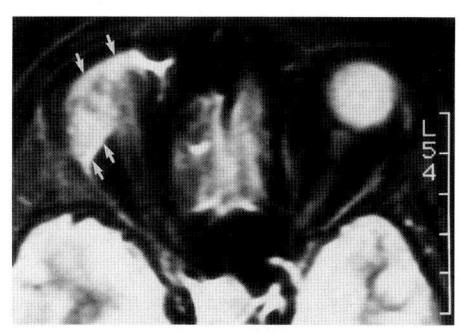

Fig. 2.181 Idiopathic lacrimal adenitis. Axial short inversion time inversion recovery (2500/40/170, TR/TE/TI) MR scan shows enlargement, as well as increased signal intensity of the right lacrimal gland (arrows).

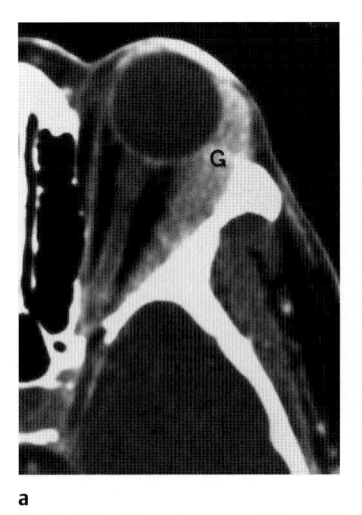

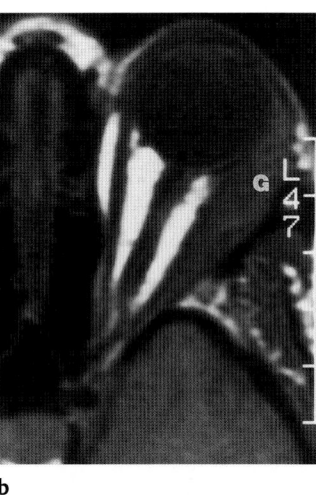

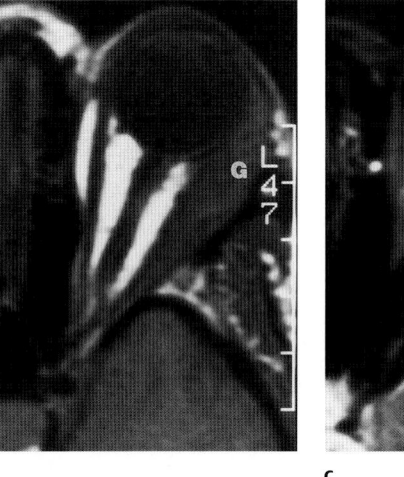

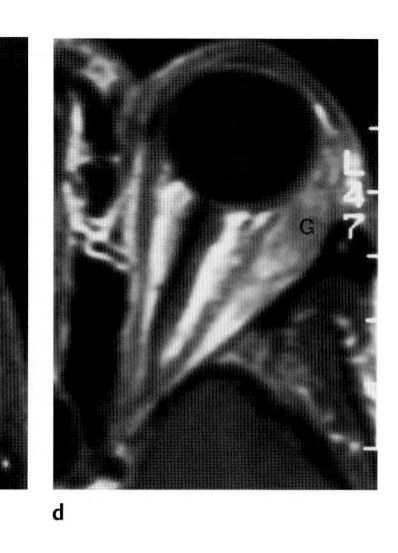

Fig. 2.182 Pseudotumor (idiopathic lacrimal adenitis).
a Enhanced CT scan shows diffuse enlargement of the left lacrimal gland (G).
b Axial unenhanced T1W MR scan shows diffuse enlargement of left lacrimal gland (G).
c Axial T2W MR scan. The left lacrimal gland pseudotumor appears predominantly hypointense.
d Axial enhanced T1W MR scan. There is moderate contrast enhancement of enlarged left lacrimal gland (G).

Perineuritis and Periscleritis

Idiopathic perineuritis (inflammation of the sheath of the optic nerve) can simulate optic neuritis by presenting with orbital pain, pain with extraocular motility, decreased visual acuity, and disk edema. In contrast to optic neuritis, pain is exacerbated with retrodisplacement of the globe, and there is mild proptosis.[93] CT and MRI show a ragged, edematous enlargement of the optic nerve sheath complex (Fig. 2.179). Periscleritis involves the tissue immediately contiguous with the sclera (Fig. 2.179).

Lacrimal Adenitis

Acute idiopathic lacrimal adenitis (pseudotumor) presents with tenderness in the upper outer quadrant of the orbit in the region of the lacrimal gland.[23,93] Viral dacryoadenitis may present in a similar fashion and is commonly associated with an etiology such as mumps, mononucleosis, or herpes zoster. Adenopathy and lymphocytosis can be present in these cases. The differential diagnosis of nonspecific lacrimal adenitis includes viral and bacterial dacryoadenitis, rupture of a dermoid cyst in the lacrimal gland region, specific lacrimal gland inflammations such as sarcoidosis and Sjögren disease, lymphoproliferative disorders, cysts, and neoplasia in this region. Because of the wide variety and incidence of pathology that can involve the lacrimal gland, biopsy of this accessible site may be necessary to obtain a definitive diagnosis.[2,16] The CT and MRI apperances of pseudotumor of lacrimal gland are shown in Figs. 2.180–2.183.

Apical Orbital Inflammation

Pseudotumor may be diffuse (Fig. 2.184) or it may present with infiltration of the orbital apex. Patients present with a typical orbital apical syndrome consisting of pain, minimal proptosis, and restricted EOM movements. The CT and MRI findings include an irregular infiltrative process of the apex of the orbit, with extension along the posterior portion of the EOMs or the optic nerve. Sarcoidosis (Fig. 2.185) and other granulomatous processes including Wegener granulomatosis may be responsible for clinical presentation of apical orbital syndrome.

Pseudotumor in Children

Pediatric pseudotumor encompasses 6–16% of orbital pseudotumors.[91] In children, approximately one-third of pseudotumors are bilateral and are rarely associated with systemic disease. Children with pseudotumor may also exhibit papillitis or iritis.[5,6] The process may be localized (Fig. 2.186) or diffuse (Fig. 2.187).

Pathology 235

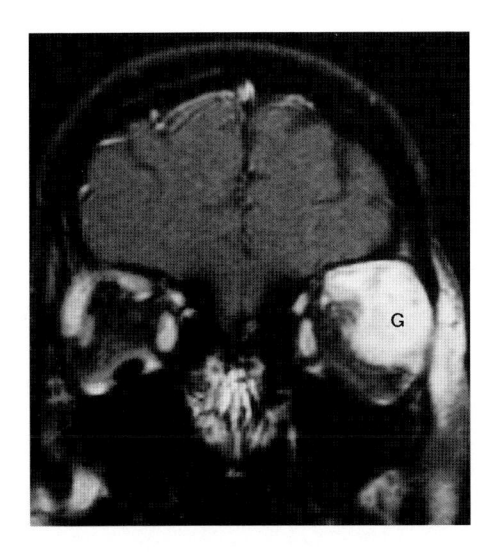

Fig. 2.**183** Pseudotumor. Coronal enhanced fat-suppression T1W MR scan shows marked diffuse enlargement of the left lacrimal gland (G), compatible with pseudotumor. This MR appearance cannot be differentiated from sarcoid involvement of the lacrimal gland.

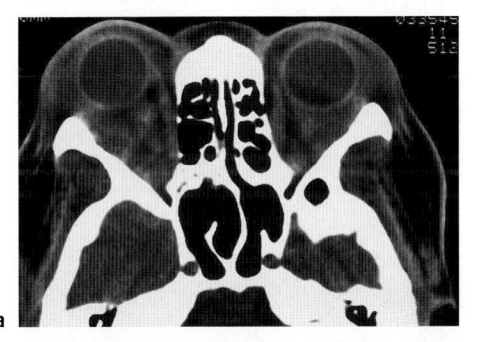

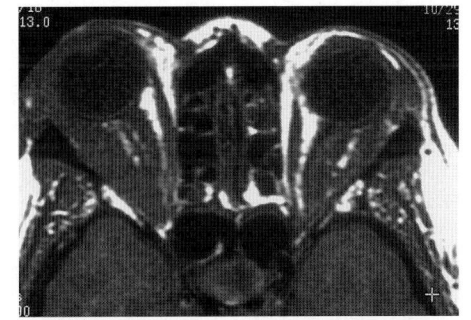

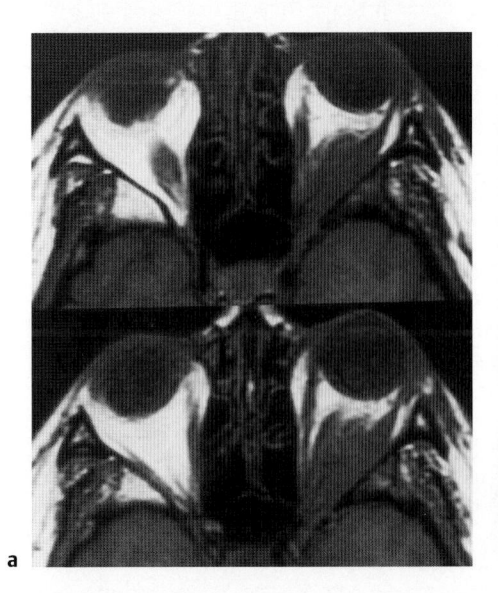

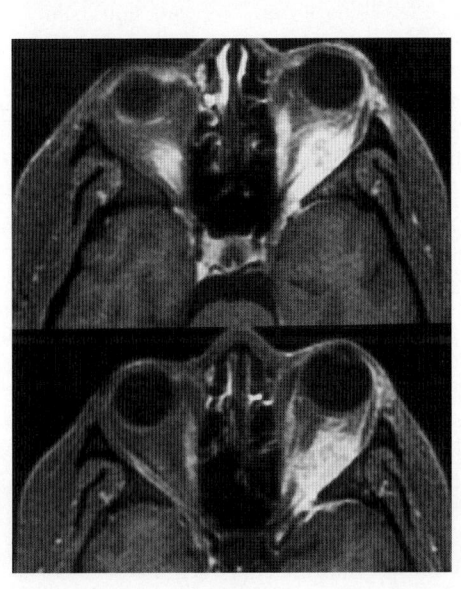

Fig. 2.**184** Bilateral diffuse orbital pseudotumor. **a** Axial unenhanced CT scan and **b** axial T1W, **c** axial enhanced T1W, and **d** axial T1W fat-suppression MR scans showing an infiltrative process involving both orbits, compatible with pseudotumor. Lymphoma, vasculitis, systemic lupus erythematosis, and orbital histiocytic disorders such as Erdheim-Chester disease and xanthogranuloma may have similar CT and MRI findings (see also Figs. 2.**204** and 2.**205**).

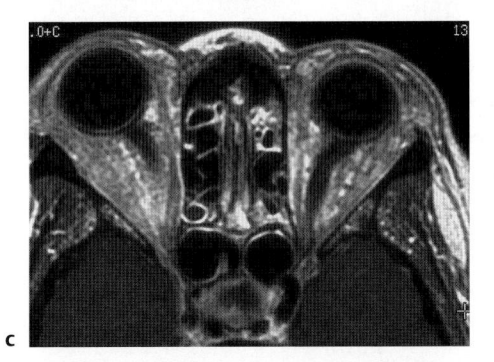

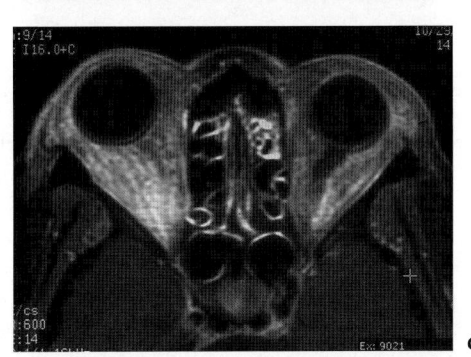

Fig. 2.**185** Sarcoidosis.
a Axial T1W MR scans show an infiltrative process involving the apex of the left orbit.
b Axial enhanced fat-suppression T1W MR scan, showing marked enhancement of the apical infiltration. Sarcoidosis was proven by biopsy.

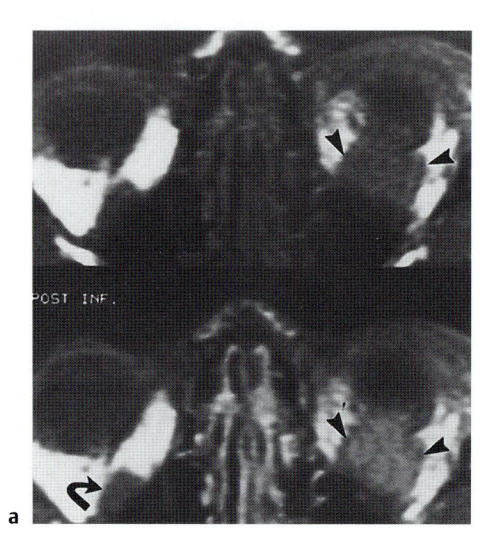

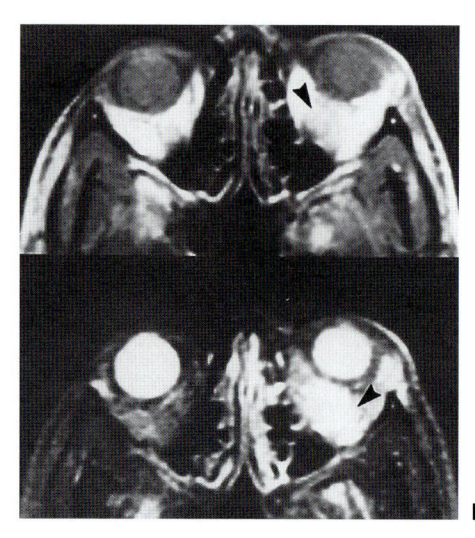

Fig. 2.**186** Myositic orbital pseudotumor in a 12-year-old girl.
a Axial T1W precontrast (top) and postcontrast (bottom) MR scans show enlargement as well as moderate enhancement of the left inferior orbital rectus muscle (arrowheads). Note normal right inferior rectus muscle (curved arrow).
b Axial PW (top) and T2W (bottom) MR scans show marked hyperintensity of this pseudotumor (arrowheads).

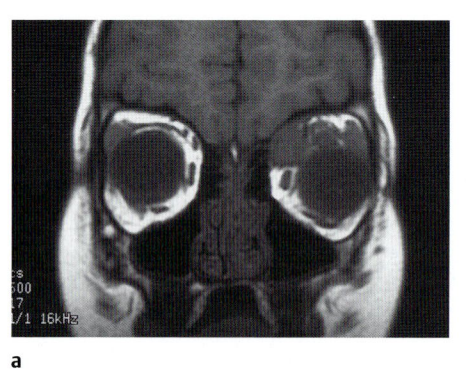

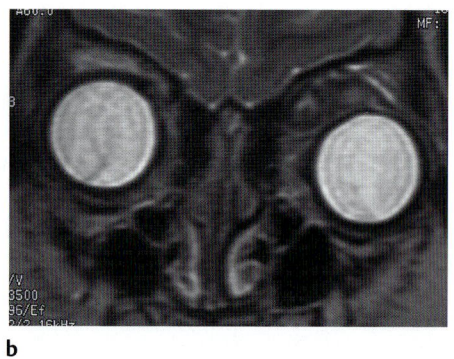

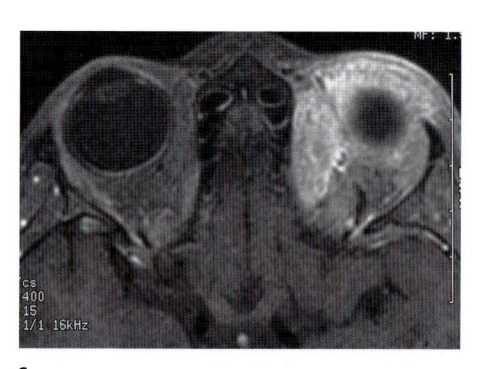

Fig. 2.**187** Pseudotumor in a 6-year-old boy with two days' history of left eye swelling with pain. **a** Coronal T1W, **b** coronal T2W, and **c** axial enhanced fat-suppression T1W scans, showing a pseudotumor of the left orbit. The process resolved following a short course of steroid therapy.

■ Painful External Ophthalmoplegia (Tolosa–Hunt Syndrome)

In 1954, Tolosa described a patient with unilateral recurrent painful ophthalmoplegia involving cranial nerves III, IV, VI, and V1.[97] Carotid arteriography in this case showed segmental narrowing in the carotid siphon. The patient died after surgical exploration, and a postmortem study showed adventitial thickening in the cavernous carotid artery surrounded by a cuff of nonspecific granulation tissue that also involved the adjoining cranial nerve trunks. In 1961, Hunt et al.[98] reported six patients with similar clinical symptoms and signs. After reviewing Tolosa's slides, these authors proposed a low-grade, nonspecific inflammation of the cavernous sinus and its walls as the cause of the syndrome. They also emphasized that angiography was essential to rule out an aneurysm or neoplasm.[98] In 1966, Smith and Taxdal applied the term Tolosa–Hunt syndrome to this entity.[99] They described five additional cases and stressed the diagnostic usefulness of the dramatically rapid therapeutic response to corticosteroids. In 1973, Sondheimer and Knapp[100] reported three patients with Tolosa–Hunt syndrome on whom orbital venography was performed. These investigators observed that the superior ophthalmic vein on the affected side was occluded in the posterior portion of the muscle cone in each case and that there was partial or complete obliteration of the ipsilateral cavernous sinus.

Painful external ophthalmoplegia, or Tolosa–Hunt syndrome, is now considered an idiopathic inflammatory process and a regional variant of idiopathic orbital pseudotumors that, because of its anatomical location (superior orbital fissure, cavernous sinus or both), produces typical clinical manifestations.[97,101] The disease manifests as recurrent attack of a steady, dull, retro-orbital pain, palsies of third, fourth, or sixth cranial nerves, and the first or second division or both of the trigeminal nerve. It is usually unilateral, but bilateral cases do occur.[91] Immediate relief of symptoms following high doses of steroid therapy differentiates pseudotumor of the orbital apex and cavernous sinus from other lesions causing Tolosa–Hunt syndrome. Pathologically there is an infiltration of lymphocytes and plasma cells along with thickening of the dura mater. The condition generally responds to systemic corticosteroid therapy. It is important to exclude the possibility of a neoplastic, inflammatory (particularly mycotic) (Fig. 2.**188**) or vasculogenic lesion. Carotid angiography and MRI are most useful in excluding aneurysm as a cause of the clinical signs and symptoms.[102] Certain cavernous sinus, orbital apex, and parasellar lesions such as lymphoma, including Burkitt lymphoma, leukemic infiltration, granulomatous diseases, pituitary adenomas, meningiomas, craniopharyngiomas, neurogenic tumors, dermoid cysts, orbital sinonasal, and nasopharyngeal carcinomas, invasive mycotic infections, aneurysm, and metastatic lesions (melanoma, lung, breast, kidney, thyroid, prostate) may produce similar symptoms.[102]

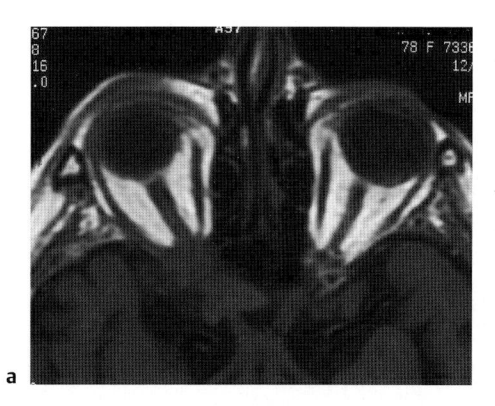

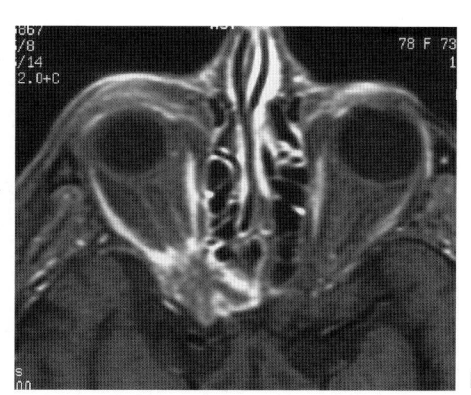

Fig. 2.**188** Tolosa–Hunt syndrome related to aspergillosis of the orbital apex. **a** Axial unenhanced T1W and **b** enhanced fat-suppression T1W MR scans, showing an infiltrative process involving the right orbital apex compatible with invasive aspergillosis.

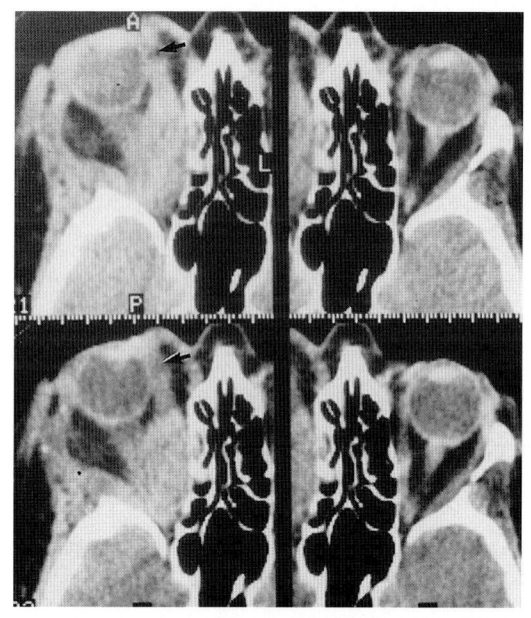

Fig. 2.**189** Thyroid opththalmopathy. Serial axial CT scans show marked enlargement of the belly of the right medial rectus muscle. Note that its tendinous portion is also thickened (arrows). The involvement of the tendinous portion of the muscles is uncommon in thyroid myositis. Note changes of lateral orbital bone resection for the compression of the optic nerve. Unilateral involvement is very uncommon in thyroid orbitopathy.

■ Thyroid Orbitopathy (Graves Dysthyroid Ophthalmopathy)

Thyroid orbitopathy, or Graves dysthyroid ophthalmopathy, is the most common cause of unilateral and bilateral exophthalmos in the adult population. The disease usually has its onset between the ages of 20 and 45 years.[6] Graves disease is a multisystem disease of unknown cause, characterized by one or more of the three pathognomonic clinical entities: (1) hyperthyroidism associated with diffuse hyperplasia of the thyroid gland; (2) infiltrative ophthalmopathy; and (3) infiltrative dermopathy.[2,6,16] Thyroid orbitopathy (Graves disease) includes any of the orbital and eyelid manifestations of this disorder. Among these clinical features are upper and lower eyelid retraction, exophthalmos, limitation of eye movements, eyelid edema, and epibulbar vascular congestion. Although the majority of patients with thyroid orbitopathy have hyperthyroidism, the orbital manifestations of the disease may occur in individuals who are hypothyroid or euthyroid. Occasionally, Graves ophthalmopathy occurs in patients with Hashimoto thyroiditis.[102]

Pathology

Immunopathology

Thyroid orbitopathy is presumed to be an autoimmune disease. It is postulated that the immune complexes (thyroglobulin and antithyroglobulin) reach the orbit via superior cervical lymph channels that drain both the thyroid and the orbit.[6,102] These complexes bind to extraocular muscles and stimulate acute inflammation characterized by an influx of lymphocytes, plasma cells, and mast cells; fibroblast proliferation; glycosaminoglycan overproduction; and orbital congestions.[6,102,103]

Histopathology

Early in Graves ophthalmopathy, the extraocular muscles are infiltrated by lymphocytes and contain an increased amount of hyaluronic acid, which binds to water and accounts for some of the orbital congestion. In chronic stages of the disease, the extraocular muscles undergo degeneration of the muscle fibers and replacement fibrosis.[6,102] Restrictive myopathy is caused by this fibrosis.

Diagnosis

The diagnosis of thyroid orbitopathy is made primarily on the basis of patients' symptoms and clinical findings. Laboratory testing including imaging studies is often valuable in confirming the diagnosis.[2,6] Exophthalmos, lid retraction, lid lag, prominence of the episcleral vessels, and lid edema are important clinical findings. In some patients, the disease is characterized by the gradual onset of diplopia, usually the vertical gaze.[10] Exophthalmos results from enlargement of extraocular muscles or increased orbital fat volume. Exophthalmos is almost always bilateral and usually relatively symmetric, though occasionally it may be quite asymmetric. The inferior rectus muscle is involved most commonly, followed by the medial rectus and the superior rectus muscles.[102]

Diagnostic Imaging

CT and MRI in the early stage of the disease (congestive stage) often display the enlarged extraocular muscles, and the coronal view is especially valuable in evaluating the enlarged muscles. Initially, in the acute congestive phase, the muscles and retrobulbar orbital contents are markedly swollen. At this stage, CT and MRI demonstrate enlargement of the extraocular muscles. The increased orbital fatty reticulum results in anterior displacement of the orbital septum and at times prolapse of lacrimal glands. Strangulation of the optic nerve is seen best on axial and sagittal CT and MRI scans.[3,10]

About 90% of patients with thyroid orbitopathy have bilateral abnormalities on CT or MRI scans (Figs. 2.**189**–2.**193**), even if the clinical involvement is unilateral.[2,3] Typically, enlargement

238 2 Part 2: The Orbit

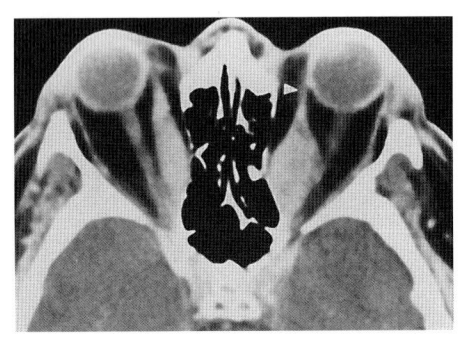

Fig. 2.**190** Thyroid ophthalmopathy. Axial CT scan shows marked enlargement of both medial rectus muscles. Note that the tendinous part of the involved muscles is normal (arrowhead).

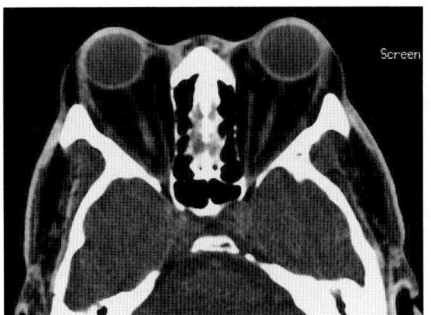

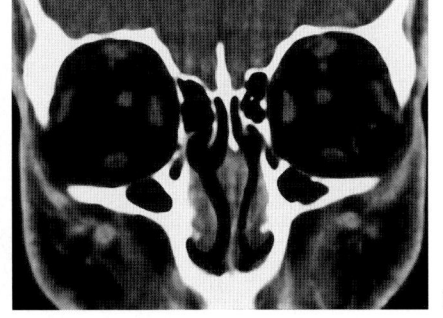

Fig. 2.**192** Thyroid ophthalmopathy. **a** Axial and **b** coronal CT scans show bilateral proptosis due to increased volume of the orbital fatty reticulum. Note attenuated extraocular muscles secondary to fibrosis.

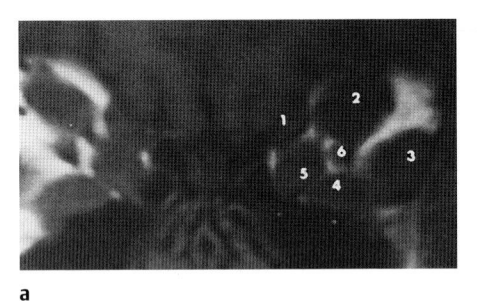

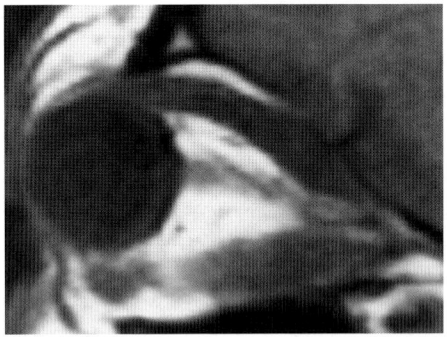

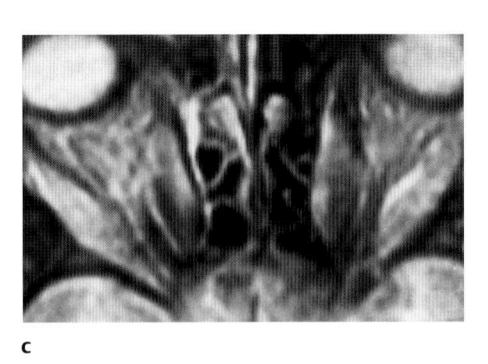

Fig. 2.**191a** Thyroid ophthalmopathy. Coronal T1W MR scan shows marked enlargement of superior oblique (1), superior (2), lateral (3), inferior (4), and medial (5) rectus muscles. The optic nerves (6) are not compressed at this level; however, they were strangulated at the apex by marked enlargement of the apical segments of the rectus muscles.

b Sagittal T1W MR scan shows marked enlargement of the vertical rectus muscles. Note strangulation of the optic nerve at the orbital apex due to enlarged rectus muscles.
c Axial T2W MR scan shows marked enlargement of the horizontal rectus muscles. There is moderate hyperintensity of the rectus muscles due to edema.

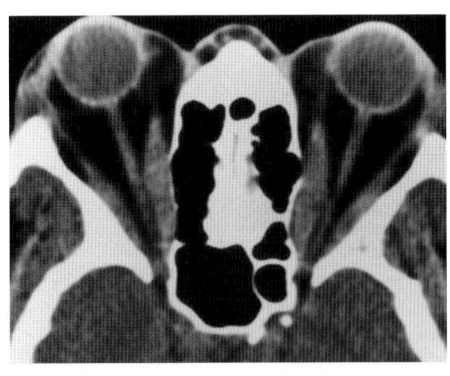

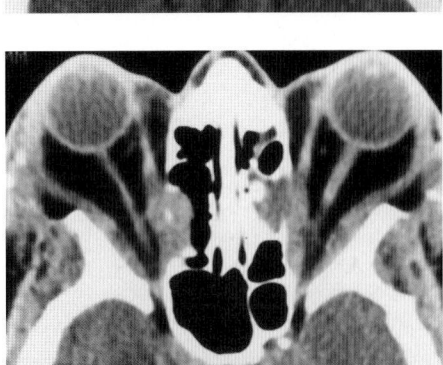

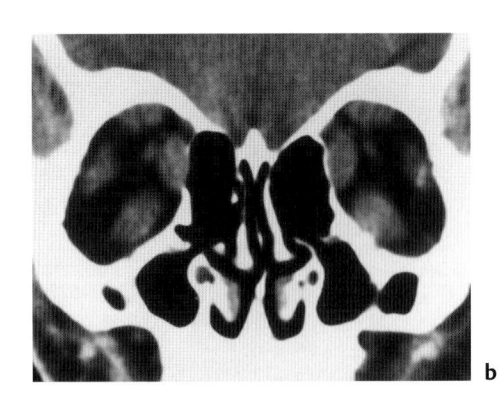

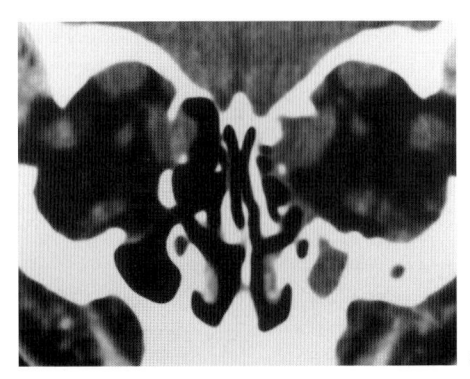

Fig. 2.**193** Thyroid ophthalmopathy. **a** Axial and **b** coronal CT scans show increased volume of the orbital fatty reticulum, along with marked enlargement of the extraocular muscles. **c** Axial and **d** coronal CT scans, showing changes of bilateral orbital decompression.

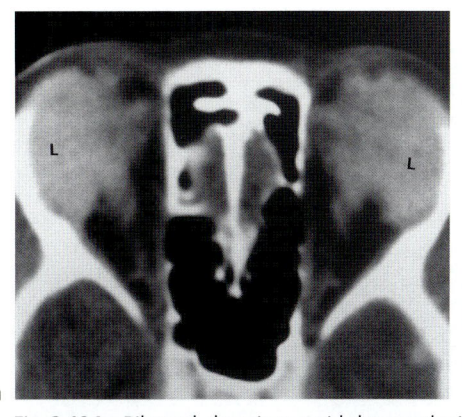

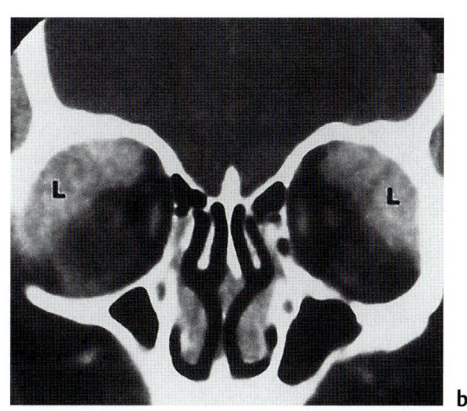

Fig. 2.**194** Bilateral chronic sarcoid dacryoadenitis.
a Axial CT scan shows marked diffuse enlargement of lacrimal glands (L).
b Sarcoidosis. Coronal CT scan shows marked bilateral enlargement of the lacrimal glands (L).

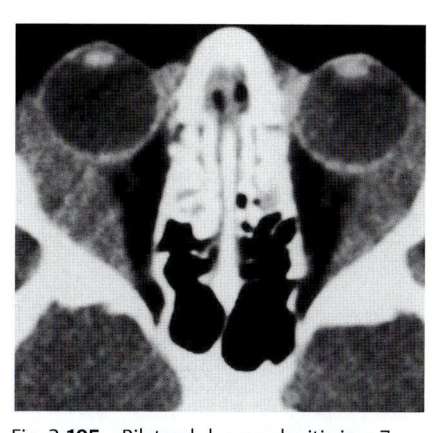

Fig. 2.**195** Bilateral dacryoadenitis in a 7-year-old African-American child with bilateral painless proptosis. Axial CT scan shows marked diffuse enlargement of the lacrimal glands (arrows), presumed to be due to sarcoidosis. Juvenile xanthogranuloma and Erdheim–Chester disease may have similar CT appearance.

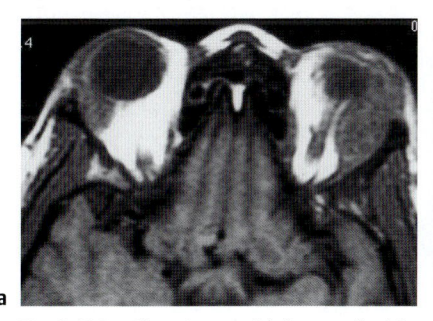

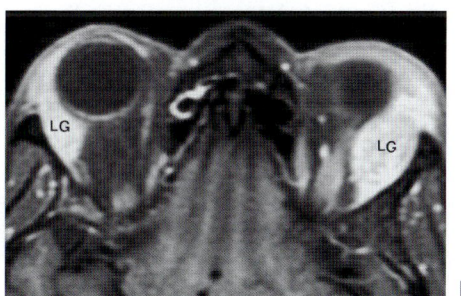

Fig. 2.**196** Chronic sarcoid dacryoadenitis. **a** Axial unenhanced T1W and **b** enhanced fat-suppression T1W MR scans showing bilateral lacrimal gland sarcoidosis (LG).

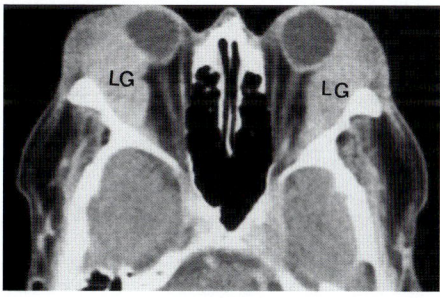

Fig. 2.**197** Pseudotumor of the lacrimal glands in an 80-year-old patient with proptosis of both eyes. Axial CT scan showing marked lobular enlargement of both lacrimal glands (LG).

involves the muscle belly, sparing its tendinous portion. However, there are rare patients who show thickening of the tendinous portion of the muscle (Fig. 2.**189**).[3] Another helpful finding in thyroid myopathy is the presence of low-density areas within the muscle bellies. These are probably the result of focal accumulation of lymphocytes and mucopolysaccharide deposition.[3] Other CT and MRI findings in thyroid orbitopathy are increased orbital fat, enlargement (engorgement) of the lacrimal glands, edema (fullness) of the eyelids, proptosis, anterior displacement of the orbital septum, and stretching of the optic nerve with or without associated "tenting" of the posterior globe. On T2-weighted MR images, areas of high signal intensity may be present within the involved muscle (Fig. 2.**191 c**). These areas presumably represent inflammation/edema, and these patients usually have a good clinical response to a trial of steroids. Later, a more chronic, noncongestive phase follows, in which a restrictive type of limited eye movement often develops, secondary to fibrosis of the extraocular muscles and to subsequent loss of elasticity.[10] At this stage, CT and MRI may show fatty replacement of the extraocular muscles (Fig. 2.**192**), or a stringlike appearance of extraocular muscles (Fig. 2.**192**). Although the muscles may be moderately to markedly attenuated, at this stage, the orbital fatty reticulum volume appears increased as may be evidenced by exophthalmos, anterior displacement of orbital septum, and prolapse of lacrimal glands.

■ Sarcoidosis

Sarcoidosis is a granulomatous systemic disease of unknown etiology characterized by subacute or chronic inflammation involving multiple systems, including orbital and ocular structures,[2, 3, 16, 104] and by its hallmark, the noncaseating granuloma. It is an immunologically mediated disease affecting delayed hypersensitivity.[3] Sarcoidosis is 10–20 times more common in African-Americans than it is in whites. Virtually any part of the globe or orbit may be involved in sarcoid. There may be uveitis, choroidoretinitis, keratoconjunctivitis, conjunctival inflammatory nodules, orbital myositis, and optic neuritis.[3, 104] The most common form of orbital involvement in sarcoidosis is chronic dacryoadenitis. This may be unilateral and can easily mimic a lacrimal gland tumor (Fig. 2.**194**). Involvement of the lacrimal glands may also be very extensive (Figs. 2.**194**–2.**196**) and, when it occurs bilaterally in the lacrimal and salivary glands, it causes a Mikulicz-like syndrome of dry eyes and xerostomia.[16, 104] Sarcoid may also involve the optic nerve; when this occurs, it may clinically resemble a primary neoplasm of the optic nerve.[105, 106] Orbital pseudotumor and lymphoma could simulate sarcoidosis (Figs. 2.**197**, 2.**198**).

Pathological and Immunological Features

Sarcoidosis is a disorder mediated by excess helper T-lymphocyte activity at sites of disease activity. The noncaseating granulomas consist of mononuclear inflammatory cells, histio-

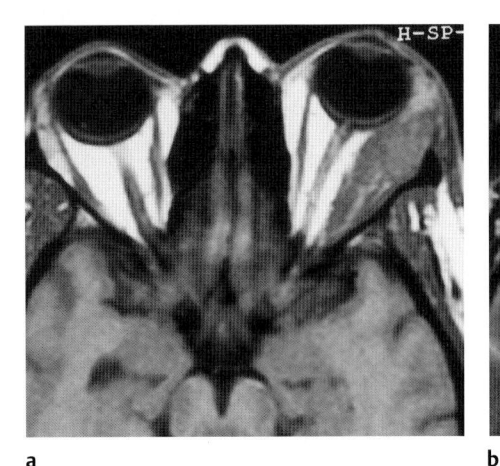

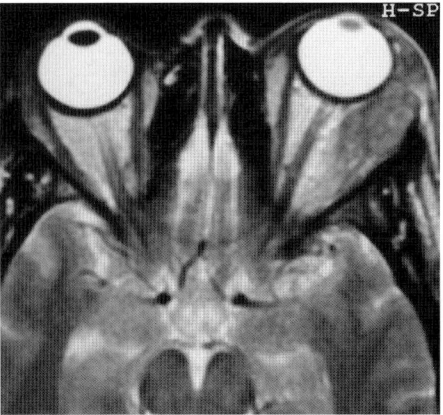

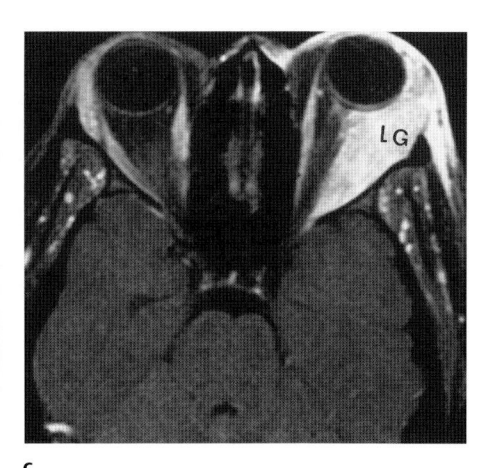

Fig. 2.198 Pseudotumor of the lacrimal gland. **a** Axial T1W, **b** T2W, and **c** enhanced fat-suppression T1W MR scans, showing marked enlargement of the left lacrimal gland (LG), compatible with pseudotumor.

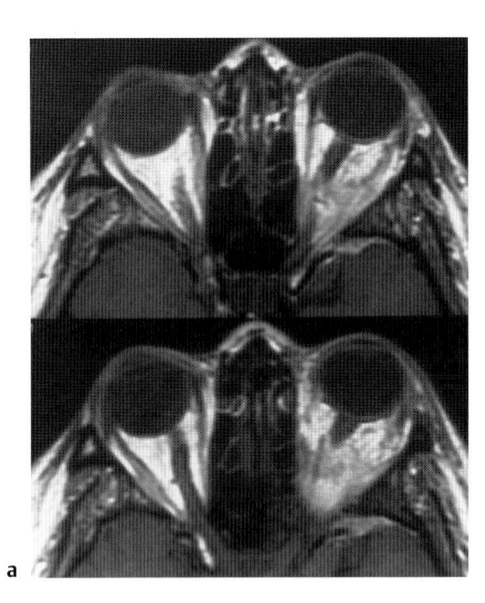

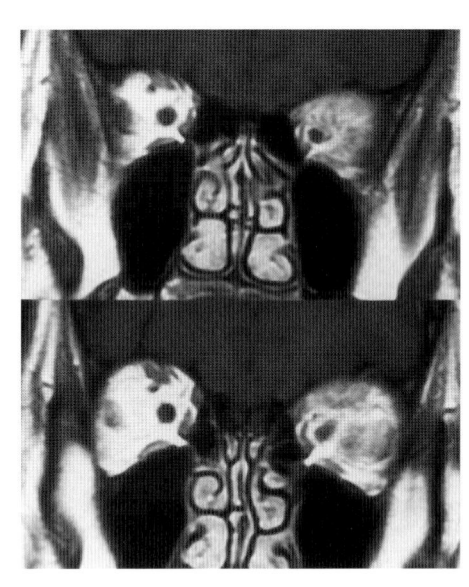

Fig. 2.199 Orbital sarcoidosis simulating pseudotumor. **a** Axial enhanced T1W and **b** coronal enhanced T1W MR scans, showing involvement of the left lateral and superior rectus muscles, as well as infiltration of the apical orbital fatty reticulum.

cytes, lymphocytes, plasma cells, and multinucleated giant cells.[104] Some of the granulomas may have necrotic centers. Significant CD4 (helper-inducer) T cells are interspersed among these inflammatory cells.

Clinical Features

The clinical presentation of sarcoidosis may range from widespread disease to involvement of only one organ system at a time. Many asymptomatic cases are discovered as part of screening chest radiography that may or may not progress to a clinically symptomatic disease. Lofgren syndrome is referred to as the constellation of erythema nodosum, bilateral hilar adenopathy, and polyarthralgias. Uveitis and parotiditis are referred to as uveoparotid fever or Heerfordt syndrome. Lupus pernio is referred to as nasal sarcoidosis.[104] An elevated angiotensin-converting enzyme (ACE) level helps to establish a presumptive diagnosis of sarcoidosis. Ophthalmic lesions develop in approximately 25% of patients. These include uveitis, infiltration of the lids, optic nerve, orbit, and extraocular muscles (Fig. 2.199), granulomatous infiltration of lacrimal glands (Figs. 2.194–2.196), retinal vasculitis, uveitis, uveoretinitis, and vitreitis. Dykhuizen and associates[107] reported a case of sarcoidosis that presented with recurrent headaches, transient right hemiparesis, and left-sided ophthalmoplegia. An excised left retrobulbar lesion demonstrated sarcoid granulomatosis. Twelve years later, the patient developed a mass in the right lung. The excised lung mass showed similar histology to the previously removed left orbital mass. Idiopathic orbital inflammation may display a granulomatous inflammatory pattern that may mimic sarcoidosis. Raskin and associates[108] reported 12 patients with a diagnosis of sarcoidosis or other noninfectious granulomatous process involving the orbit. Five of these patients were diagnosed with sarcoidosis on histological examination. In these patients, systemic evaluation failed to reveal evidence of systemic involvement. The authors suggested that clinicians should be aware of the existence of granulomatous idiopathic orbital inflammation not associated with systemic sarcoidosis as a distinct clinicopathological entity. Monfort-Gouraud and associates[109] reported an inflammatory pseudotumor of the orbit and suspected sarcoidosis in a 13-year-old boy who had uveitis and symptoms of unilateral orbital inflammation. Mombaerts and associates[110] reported seven patients with unilateral idiopathic granulomatous orbital inflammation. Histopathological analysis showed a spectrum of granulomatous inflammation, admixed with nongranulomatous inflammation and fibrosis. They concluded on the basis of their study and review of the literature that idiopathic granulomatous orbital inflammation is more related to orbital pseudotumor than to orbital sarcoidosis.

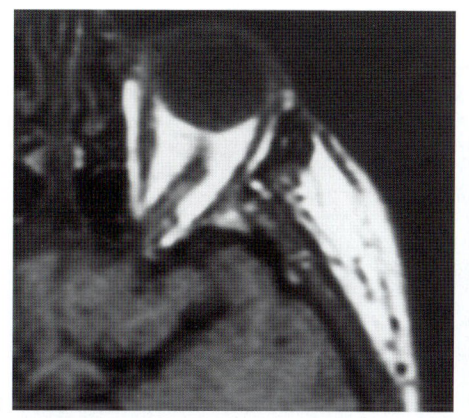

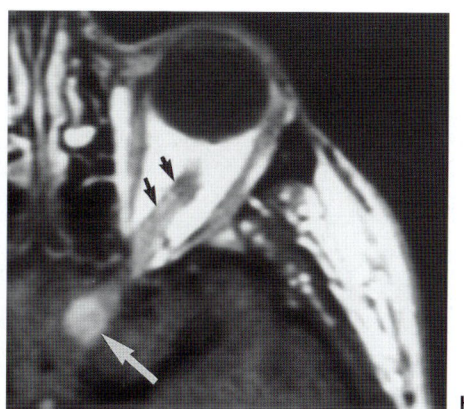

Fig. 2.**200** Optic nerve sarcoidosis. **a** Axial unenhanced T1W and **b** enhanced T1W MR scans showing sarcoidosis of the left optic nerve (arrows).

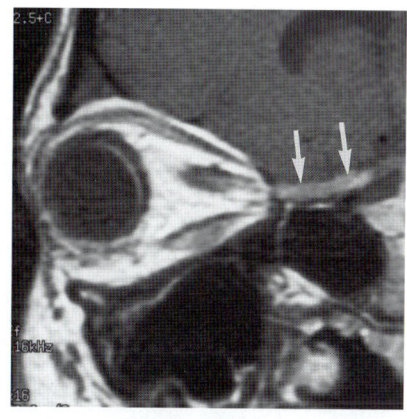

Fig. 2.**201** Optic nerve sarcoidosis. Sagittal enhanced T1W MR scan shows enhancement of intracanalicular and intracranial segments of the optic nerve (arrows), compatible with sarcoidosis.

Carmody et al[111] reported the MRI scans of 15 patients, 3 with presumed and 12 with proven orbital or optic pathway sarcoidosis. Eight patients had MR imaging evidence of optic nerve involvement by sarcoid granuloma. Perineural enhancement was seen in four cases and optic atrophy in one. Nine patients had optic chiasmal involvement. One patient had increased T2 signal in the optic radiations. Three patients had orbital masses that had MRI signal characteristics similar to idiopathic pseudotumor. Five patients had periventricular white-matter abnormalities closely resembling multiple sclerosis. Ing et al[112] reported a 22-year-old white woman with optic nerve sarcoidosis without evidence of systemic or ocular disease. The authors found 17 cases similar to theirs with the diagnosis proved by optic nerve biopsy reported in the English-language literature. In all of them, extensive prospective investigations revealed no systemic sarcoidosis. Most of these were mistaken for optic nerve sheath meningioma.

Optic Nerve Sarcoidosis

Sarcoidosis may involve the nervous system, including the optic nerve, and can present as abrupt or chronic visual loss, with or without disk changes. In one series of 11 cases of sarcoidosis of the optic nerve in patients ranging in age from 16 to 48 years, only two patients were previously known to have the disorder.[113] Four patients showed disk granulomas, four had optic nerve granulomas, and five had posterior uveitis and retinitis. In this series, chest radiographs were characteristically abnormal in 8 of 11 patients.[113] Only one-third had elevated serum levels of ACE. CT scans in these 11 patients infrequently showed enlarged nerves or other findings. Although classically sarcoidosis is believed commonly not to involve the optic nerves, we have seen increasing numbers of cases of presumed optic nerve sarcoidosis on MR images and CT scans, some of them with histological confirmation.

Although neuroimaging does not distinguish optic nerve sheath meningioma from sarcoid of the optic nerve, in the absence of uveitis and systemic sarcoid disease, certain imaging features should raise the possibility of optic nerve sarcoidosis, prompting a trial of corticosteroid therapy before proceeding to biopsy. In our experience imaging features that should favor sarcoidosis of the optic nerve include the following:

1. Enhancement of the optic nerve associated with prominent enlargement of the intracranial segment of the optic nerve (Figs. 2.**200**, 2.**202**).
2. Enlargement of the intracranial segment of the optic nerve (sharply defined), associated with contrast enhancement (Fig. 2.**201**).
3. Abnormal enhancement of the optic nerve, associated with abnormal dural and leptomeningeal enhancement or enlargement of the lacrimal gland.
4. Bilateral optic nerve enlargement along with abnormal enhancement was not seen in any of our sarcoid patients. This finding should favor optic nerve sheath meningioma, demyelinating disease, optic glioma, lymphoma, leukemic infiltration, and pseudotumor.
5. Calcification of the optic nerve was not seen in any of our patients with sarcoidosis.

Optic nerve sarcoidosis under the age of 16 years is extremely rare.[104] Enlargement and enhancement of the optic nerve in children is seen with optic nerve glioma, extension of retinoblastoma along optic nerve, and leukemic infiltration, and in very rare cases of optic nerve sheath meningioma and optic nerve medulloepithelioma.[104]

In patients with ocular, orbital, and optic nerve sarcoidosis as well as neurosarcoidosis, MR imaging remains the imaging study of choice. Gadolinium-enhanced T1-weighted pulse sequences are the most informative part of an MR imaging study (Figs. 2.**200**, 2.**201**). Enhanced fat-suppression T1-weighted MR images are essential for the diagnosis of optic nerve sarcoidosis or simulating lesions. Gadolinium-enhanced T1-weighted MR images are also essential for the diagnosis of neurosarcoidosis (meningovascular and parenchymal).[104] Neurosarcoidosis can mimic meningioma and aneurysm (Fig. 2.**202**).

■ Sjögren Syndrome

Sjögren syndrome is an autoimmune disorder characterized by keratoconjunctivitis sicca and xerostomia. Patients may have an associated autoimmune disease such as rheumatoid arthritis, systemic lupus erythematosus, polymyositis, scleroderma, or vasculitis. The lacrimal and salivary glands are initially infiltrated by periductal lymphocytes; eventually, atrophy of the acini with hyalinization and fibrosis occurs. The early disappearance of lysozymes from the tears in Sjögren syndrome may help in distinguishing it from sarcoidosis, a disease in which the lysosomes in the tears are actually increased. Orbital manifestations of

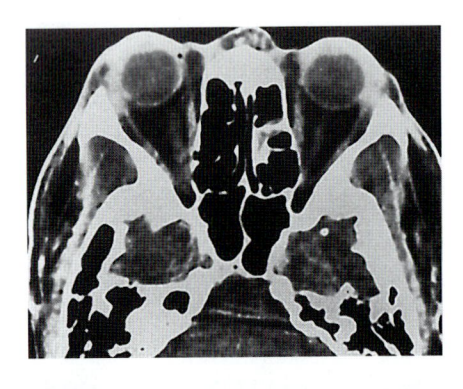

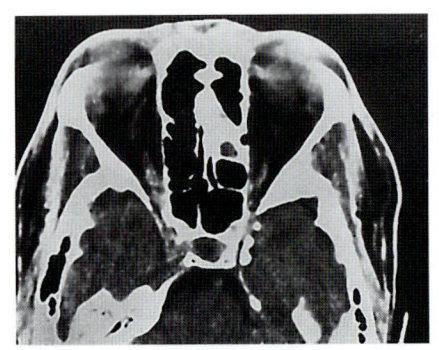

Fig. 2.**202** Sarcoidosis of the optic nerve. Serial postcontrast CT scans show enhancement of the intracanalicular and intracranial segments of the right optic nerve (white arrow), as well as an enhancing granuloma (black arrow) along the anterior aspect of the chiasmatic cistern. At surgery, sarcoid granuloma was found. Reproduced from Mafee MF. Case 25, Optic nerve sheath meningioma. Head and Neck Disorders (Fourth Series) Test and Syllabus. Reston VA: American College of Radiology, 1992. With permission.

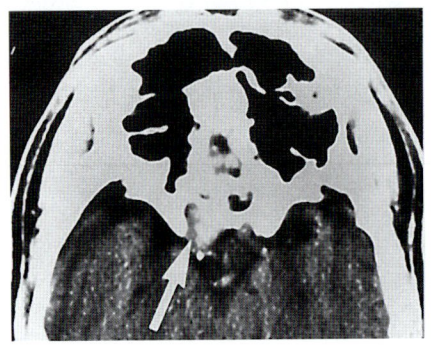

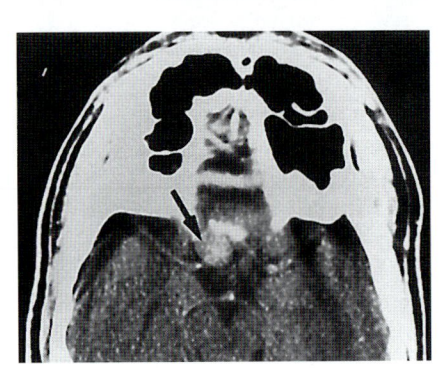

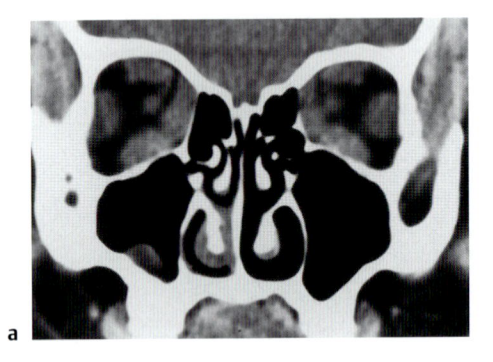

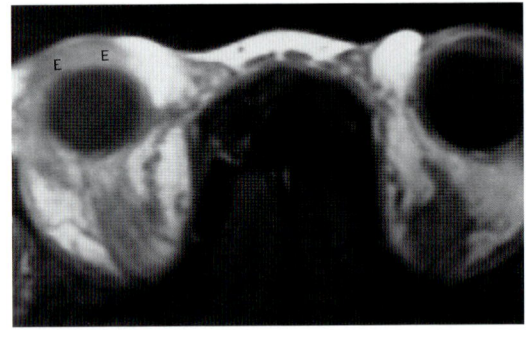

Fig. 2.**203** Sjögren syndrome.
a Coronal CT scan shows enlargement of extraocular muscles of both eyes.
b Axial T1W MR scan, same patient as in **a**, showing enlargement of superior rectus muscles, as well as thickening of the right eyelid (E).

patients with Sjögren syndrome may be similar to pseudotumor (Fig. 2.**203**).

■ Vasculitides (Angiitides)

The vasculitides (vasculitis) are an immunological complex-mediated group of diseases that include a variety of inflammatory angiodestructive processes. Clinically the vasculitides may show features of acute, subacute, and chronic inflammatory and vasoobstructive signs and symptoms.[2, 3, 16] The major diseases include polyarteritis nodosa, Wegener granulomatosis, idiopathic midline destructive disease (malignant midline reticulosis or polymorphic reticulosis), giant-cell arteritis (temporal arteritis), hypersensitivity (leukocytoclastic) angiitis, and connective-tissue disease, including systemic lupus erythematosus, rheumatoid arthritis, scleroderma, and polymyositis.

Wegener Granulomatosis

Wegener granulomatosis is a multisystem disease characterized by a triad of necrotizing granulomas in the upper and lower respiratory tract, necrotizing vasculitis (focal necrotizing angiitis of small arteries and veins) of the lung, upper respiratory tract and other sites, and glomerulonephritis.[3, 106] If left untreated, the disease is often fatal. The introduction of combined corticosteroid–cyclophosphamide treatment has proven very successful.[3] Characteristically, ocular and orbital involvement is bilateral (Figs. 2.**204**, 2.**205**) and either nonresponsive or transiently responsive to corticosteroids, often providing a clue to the diagnosis.[3] Involvement of the ocular adnexa includes lacrimal gland enlargement, nasolacrimal obstruction, and eyelid fistula formation.[3, 16]

Orbital involvement with Wegener granulomatosis should be differentiated from idiopathic pseudotumors, lymphoreticular proliferative disorders, and metastatic carcinoma.[106] The CT and MRI appearance of Wegener granulomatosis is similar to pseudotumor and lymphoma (Figs. 2.**204**, 2.**205**). Nasal and paranasal sinus involvement is present in the majority of cases. A high titer of serum antineutrophil cytoplasmic antibodies (ANCA) is highly indicative of Wegener granulomatosis.

Idiopathic Midline Destructive Granuloma (Lymphomatoid Granuloma)

Idiopathic midline destructive disease (malignant midline reticulosis or polymorphic reticulosis), formerly called lethal midline granuloma, is a clinical entity characterized by extensive de-

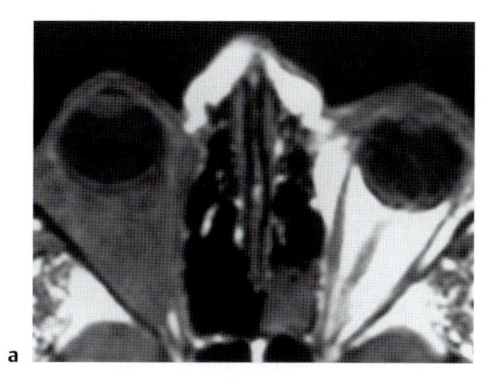

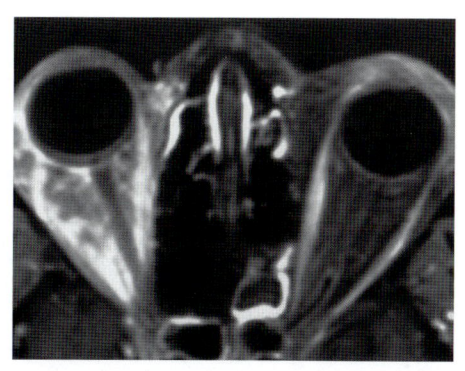

Fig. 2.**204** Wegener granulomatosis. **a** Axial unenhanced T1W and **b** enhanced fat-suppression T1W MR scans showing an infiltrative process involving the right orbit compatible with Wegener granuloma. Case courtesy of Pablo Villablanca, MD, UCLA, CA, USA.

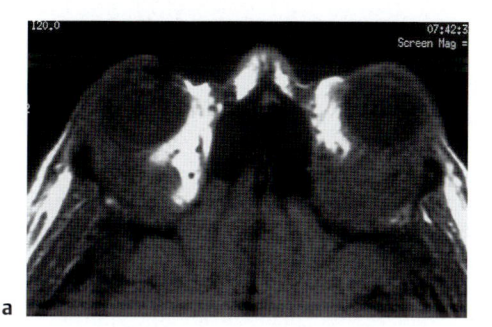

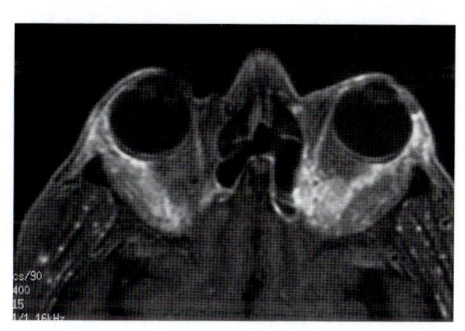

Fig. 2.**205** Wegener granulomatosis. **a** Axial T1W and **b** axial enhanced fat-suppression T1W MR scans show bilateral orbital involvement by Wegener granulomatosis.

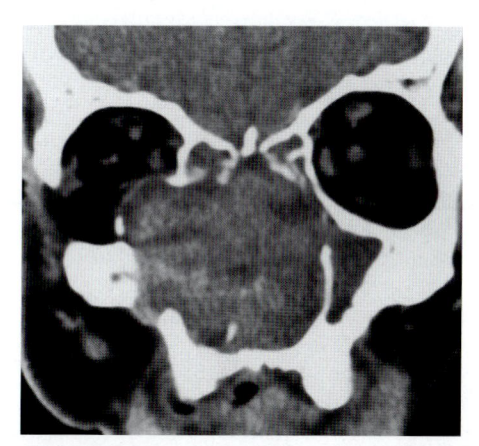

Fig. 2.**206** Midline destructive granuloma (lymphomatoid granulomatosis). Coronal CT scan shows a large mass within the nasal cavities, associated with destruction of the nasal septum as well as involvement of the right orbit.

structive lesions of the nose, sinuses, and pharynx, often with associated involvement of the orbit and central facial bones (Fig. 2.**206**). It has some similarity to Wegener granulomatosis, but pulmonary disease is rare and renal involvement is absent.[106] Although the pathogenesis is unknown, some cases may be due to a central facial lymphomatoid process. This disease, which is not necessarily midline,[101, 114] is characterized by progressive, unrelenting ulceration and necrosis, with destruction of the nasal septum. Most of these tumors are classified as T-cell lymphomas and are associated with Epstein–Barr virus infection.[101, 114] The term lymphomatoid granulomatosis, or polymorphic reticulosis, has also been applied to this type of disease.

Periarteritis Nodosa (Polyarteritis Nodosa)

This condition is a vasculitis of the medium and small arteries, adjacent veins, and occasionally arterioles and venules. The disease is segmental and leads to nodular aneurysms. The major ophthalmological manifestations are retinal and choroidal infarcts leading to exudative retinal detachment. Orbital inflammation has been described. Proptosis may occur secondary to severe inflammation of the orbital arteries, often leading to necrosis of the orbital connective tissues.[3, 106]

Hypersensitivity (Leukocytoclastic) Angiitis

This condition resembles periarteritis nodosa microscopically, but it affects smaller vessels. Pathologically the arterioles, venules, and capillaries are usually, but not necessarily, necrotic, or they may simply have perivascular infiltration with neutrophils undergoing karyolysis (leukocytoclasis). The spectrum of clinical disease varies from widespread multisystem involvement to primary dermatological lesions.[2, 106]

Lupus Erythematosus

Any of the connective-tissue disorders may be associated with systemic vasculitis. The most common include systemic lupus erythematosus, rheumatoid arthritis, and dermatomyositis. Systemic lupus erythematosus is an autoimmune disease that affects many organs. It has a female-to-male ratio of 9:1 and occurs primarily in the second and third decades of life.[2, 3, 16] Histologically the vasculitides in the connective-tissue diseases resemble hypersensitivity angiitis.[2, 3, 106] Evidence of antinuclear antibodies (ANA) is universally present in this syndrome. Twenty percent of patients have ocular involvement, primarily affecting the retinal vessels.[2, 3] Orbital involvement is rare, and is believed to be secondary to severe orbital vasculitis.[106] The CT and MR appearance of orbital lupoid disease may resemble that of the pseudotumors and lymphoreticular proliferative disorders.

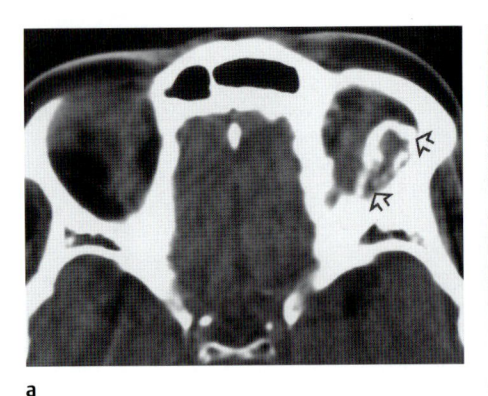

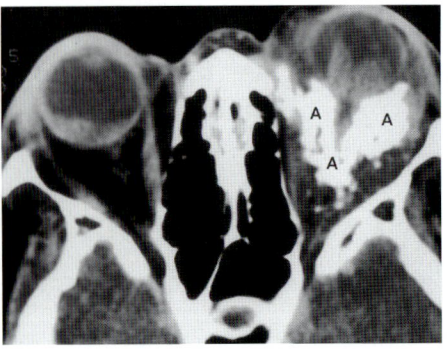

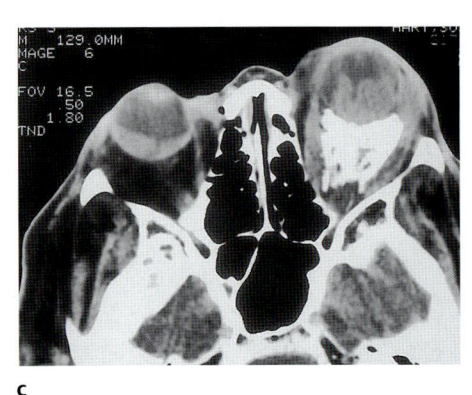

Fig. 2.**207** Primary amyloidosis of lacrimal gland and orbit.
a Axial CT scan shows irregular calcification of left lacrimal gland (arrows).
b Axial CT scan shows irregular castlike calcification involving the retrobulbar space, caused by amyloidosis (A). Note bilateral exudative retinal detachment.
c Axial CT scan of the orbit at a different level, showing diffuse left retrobulbar calcification related to primary orbital amyloidosis. Note bilateral retinal detachment.

■ Amyloidosis

Amyloidosis is caused by deposition of an amorphous hyaline material (amyloid) in various tissues such as muscle, skin, nerve, submucosa, adrenal gland, and orbit. Involvement of the orbit and ocular adnexa may occur as part of primary hereditary systemic amyloidosis, as part of secondary amyloidosis, or as a localized isolated process.[2, 16, 82, 106] Clinical features of orbital and adnexal amyloidosis include blepharoptosis caused by infiltration of the levator muscle of the upper eyelid, and oculomotor palsies resulting from involvement of multiple extraocular muscles. When the lacrimal gland is involved, the disease resembles a lacrimal gland tumor. On CT, amyloid deposits (homogeneous eosinophilic protein) simulate pseudotumors, vascular malformation, and other mass lesions, and the deposits can occasionally calcify (Fig. 2.**207**).[82] On MRI, the amyloid deposits have similar signal intensities to muscle on all imaging sequences (Fig. 2.**207**). Localized amyloid infiltrations may afflict the paranasal sinuses, and bone destruction has been reported.[82]

■ Miscellaneous Granulomatous and Histiocytic Lesions

A number of pathological entities are recognized that, except for fibrous histiocytoma, rarely involve the orbit. These include histiocytosis-X (Langerhans cell histiocytosis), Erdheim–Chester disease, juvenile xanthogranuloma, pseudorheumatoid nodules, necrobiotic xanthogranuloma, and fibrous histiocytoma.[2, 3, 16] All of these lesions bear a common feature based on local or systemic infiltration by histiocytes. Fibrous histiocytoma is the most common tumor in this category.[5]

Langerhans Cell Histiocytosis

A granulomatous disease that occurs in children more often than sarcoidosis or Wegener granulomatosis is Langerhans cell histiocytosis; the disease has a predilection for children between 1 and 4 years of age.[101]

Historical Background and New Classification

In 1953, Lichtenstein[115] introduced the term histiocytosis-X for a group of diseases that include eosinophilic granuloma, Hand–Schüller–Christian, and Letterer–Siwe diseases. He believed that the pathological common denominator of all three conditions was a distinctive and specific inflammatory histiocytosis. The letter X was used to underscore the unknown nature of the disease. Using the Birbeck granule as a marker, Nezelof et al.[116] in 1985 reported that the lesions of histiocytosis-X were the result of inappropriate proliferation and infiltration of various tissues with abnormal histiocytic cells that are morphologically and immunologically similar to Langerhans cells of the Langerhans cell system. Consequently, the name of the disease was changed to Langerhans cell histiocytosis (LCH).[117-119] This is a disease of unknown etiology. Some investigators suggested that LCH may be a disorder of immune regulation; however, recently some investigators have provided strong evidence that all forms of LCH are a clonal proliferative disease.[118, 120]

The histiocytic disorders can be divided into two general categories: (1) X histiocytic (Langerhans cell), Langerhans cell histiocytosis (LCH); and (2) non-X histiocytic (monocyte-macrophage type) proliferation, including juvenile xanthogranuloma (JXG).[117] These disorders are characterized by localized proliferation of histiocytes. However, their morphology, histochemical and immunohistochemical staining patterns, and electron-microscopic features are different. The Histiocyte Society has recently redefined the classification of the histiocytoses of childhood. Class I includes LCH; class II includes all the histiocytoses of the mononuclear phagocytes other than Langerhans cells, such as JXG; and class III includes the malignant histiocytic disorders. Orbital histiocytic disorders are classified into LCH (histiocytosis-X); sinus histiocytosis with massive lymphadenopathy (Rosai–Dorfman syndrome); JXG; Erdheim–Chester disease; necrobiotic xanthogranuloma (NXG); pseudorheumatoid nodule; and sarcoidosis.[117]

Clinical Features of Langerhans Cell Histiocytosis

The disease has a predilection for young children 1–4 years old.[101, 118] Lesions in children are most commonly located in bone or bone marrow. Although LCH is a rare disease, orbital involvement is not uncommon in patients with LCH, and with few exceptions is usually seen in the chronic form of the disease, especially eosinophilic granuloma. The overall incidence of orbital involvement in a large series of 76 children with LCH was 23%.[117] The most common signs and symptoms of orbital LCH were unilateral or bilateral proptosis, edema, erythema of the eyelid, and periorbital pain. Other signs and symptoms were ptosis, optic nerve atrophy, and papilledema. The frontal bone was most commonly involved by LCH and the lesions were usually seen in the superior or superolateral wall of the orbit in a rather anterior lo-

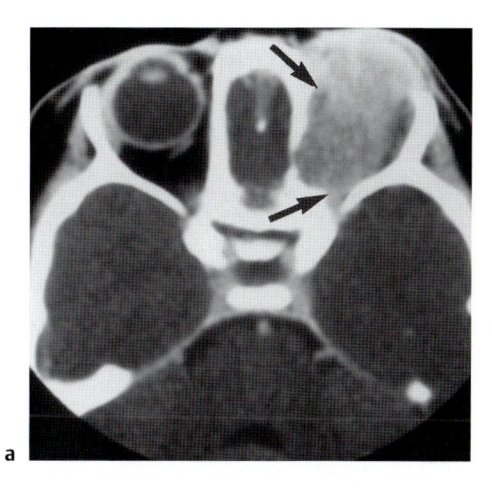

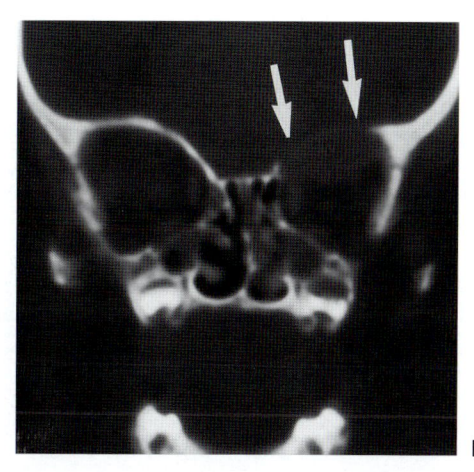

Fig. 2.208 Langerhans cell histiocytosis.
a Axial enhanced CT scan shows a large infiltrative mass involving the left superior orbital region (arrows).
b Coronal CT scan shows lytic lesion (arrows) involving the roof of the left orbit. Case courtesy of Bernadett Cook, MD, University of Cincinnati, OH, USA.

cation. On rare occasions the tumor may be noticed in the orbital apex and superior orbital fissure with or without bone involvement. Classic cases of Hand–Schüller–Christian disease (chronic disseminated form of LCH) with bilateral proptosis, diabetes insipidus, and bony defects of the skull are very rare.[117] Letterer–Siwe disease is seen in children under 2 years of age and is characterized by an acute disseminated form of LCH, associated with hepatosplenomegaly, adenopathy, fever, thrombocytopenia, anemia, and cutaneous lesions.

Ocular Manifestations

Intraocular involvement by LCH is rare and usually occurs as part of an acute disseminated form (i.e., Letterer–Siwe disease). In these cases, the uveal tract, particularly the choroid, was affected.[3]

Histopathological Features

Grossly, the lesions are usually described as soft, friable, hemorrhagic, tan-yellow tissue. Histologically, the tumors are composed of sheets of large histiocytes with interspersed eosinophils, lymphocytes, and few multinucleated giant cells.

Immunohistochemistry

LCH cells are usually positive for the following immunological markers: S-100 protein, peanut lectin, and CD1 a (OKT-6).[117]

Diagnostic Imaging

CT and MRI provide the most diagnostic assistance. Most lytic bony defects seen on standard plain film radiographs have been described as irregular, serrated, beveled, and with or without a narrow zone of sclerosis. Orbital involvement may vary, but the most common orbital manifestation is a solitary lesion. In the typical case of orbital involvement, CT and MRI show an osteolytic lesion, commonly in the superior or supertemporal orbital region (Figs. 2.**208**–2.**210**). There is a fairly well-defined or diffuse soft-tissue mass, encroaching on the lacrimal gland, the lateral rectus, other orbital structures, or even the globe. There may be extension of the soft tissue into the epidural space, as well as in the temporal fossa. There may be marked infiltration of the temporalis muscle (Fig. 2.**209**). At times multiple lesions may be present, resulting in multiple bony defects, particularly in the superolateral and orbital roof regions (Fig. 2.**210**). Similar osseous lesions may be seen in sphenoid, ethmoid, temporal, occipital and parietal, as well as facial bones. Rarely, the lesion may be totally extraosseous. On postcontrast CT and MRI scans, lesions demonstrate moderate to marked enhancement (Figs. 2.**209 c, d**).

The differential diagnosis of LCH from an imaging viewpoint includes granulomatous disease such as sarcoidosis and tuberculosis (Fig. 2.**211**), rhabdomyosarcoma, juvenile fibrosarcoma, aggressive fibromatosis, lacrimal gland tumors, lymphoma, pseudotumor, leukemic infiltration, granulocytic sarcoma or chloroma, sinus histiocytosis, metastatic neuroblastoma, metastatic Wilms tumor, and metastatic Ewing sarcoma.

Juvenile Xanthogranuloma (JXG)

JXG (nevoxanthoendothelioma)[120] is a benign, usually self-healing disorder of infants, children, and occasionally adults. Its etiology is not known. It represents proliferation of non-Langerhans (monocyte-macrophage) cells. The term juvenile xanthogranuloma was first introduced in 1936, but recognition of the entity did not occur until 1954.[117] Recently, the Histiocyte Society has redefined the classification of the histiocytoses of childhood and included JXG among class II.[117]

Clinical Features

Characteristically, the disease affects children, particularly infants, and is sometimes noted at birth. Orbital involvement with JXG is very rare. Ocular involvement is more common in the iris and ciliary body.[117] The retina, choroid, and optic nerve are rarely involved.

Histopathological Features

Histologically, the lesions demonstrate foamy histiocytes, epithelioid monocytes, lymphocytes, plasma cells, eosinophils, Touton giant cells, and spindle cells.[117] Touton giant cells are multinucleated cells with the nuclei grouped in a wreathlike arrangement around a small central island of nonfoamy cytoplasm.

Histologically, the differential diagnosis of orbital JXG includes Erdheim–Chester disease, particularly in adult patients. In both conditions, there are Touton giant cells and foamy histiocytes. Hyperlipidemia, chronic lipogranulomatous pyelonephritis, and retroperitoneal xanthogranuloma in Erdheim–Chester disease are extremely important for the correct diagnosis.[122, 123] Inflammatory pseudotumor does not show xanthoma or Touton giant cells histologically.

Diagnostic Imaging

Radiologically, the most common ocular finding is involvement of the anterior portion of the eye (see Part 1 of this chapter). It is important to know that the orbit including its bony walls may be involved (Fig. 2.**212**). Those cases with bone involvement cannot be distinguished from LCH radiologically. Recently, we have en-

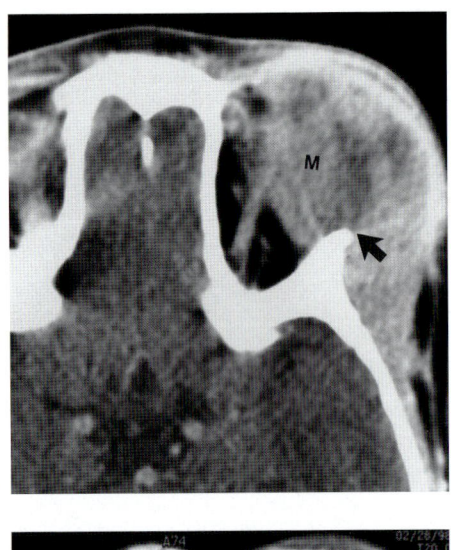

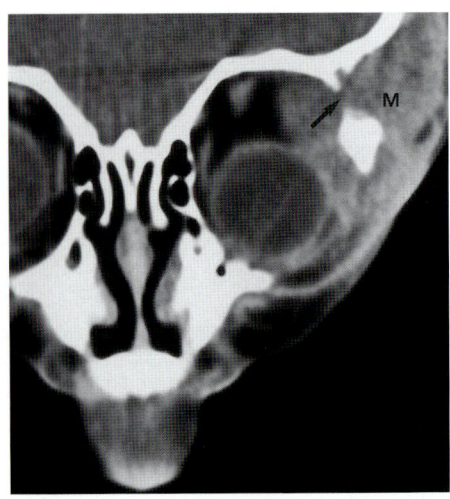

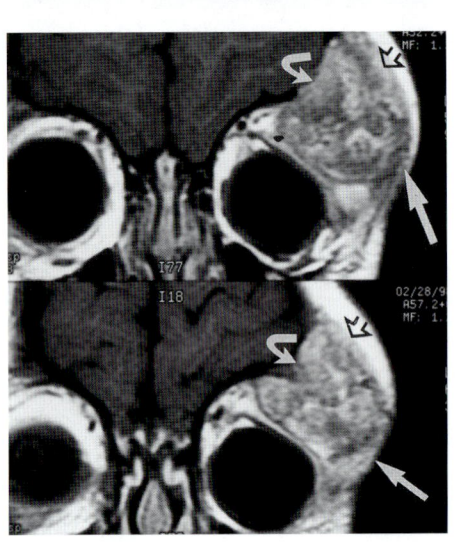

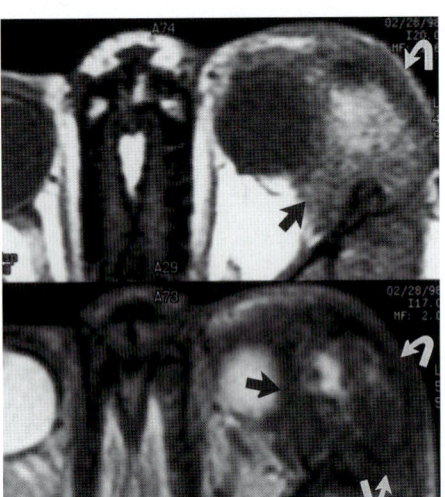

Fig. 2.209 Langerhans cell histiocytosis.
a Axial enhanced CT scan shows a large soft-tissue mass (M) associated with destruction of orbital wall (arrow).
b Coronal enhanced CT scan shows a large mass (M), associated with bone erosion (arrow), involving the superior lateral aspect of the left orbit.
c PW (top) and T2W (bottom) MR images show the mass (arrows).
d Coronal enhanced T1W MR images show marked enhancement of the lesion (arrows). The tumor showed some hemorrhage at surgery.

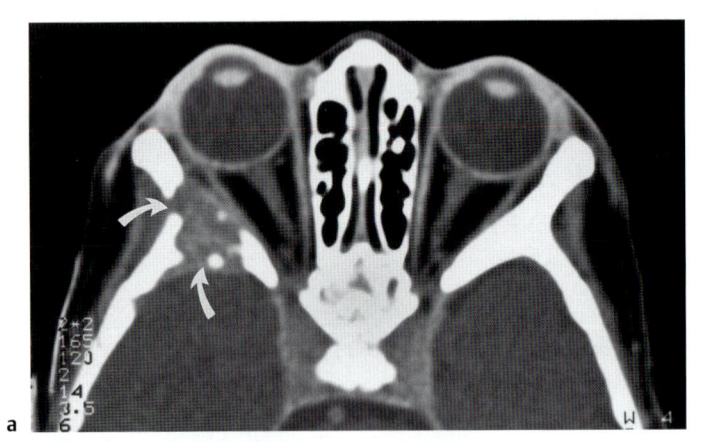

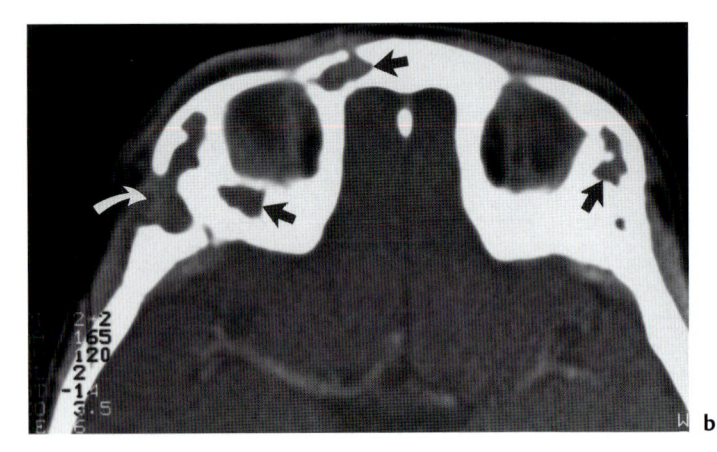

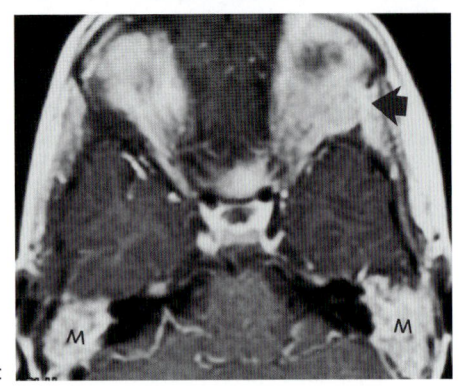

Fig. 2.210 Langerhans cell histiocytosis. **a**, **b** Axial enhanced CT scans showing lytic lesions involving both orbits (arrows), compatible with Langerhans cell histiocytosis. Case courtesy of Samir Noujaim, MD, Royal Oak, MI, USA. **c** Axial enhanced T1W MR scan in another patient shows an enhancing lesion involving the superolateral aspect of the left orbit (arrow) compatible with Langerhans cell histiocytosis. There is also involvement of both mastoid bones (M). Case courtesy of R. Schamschula, Sydney, Australia.

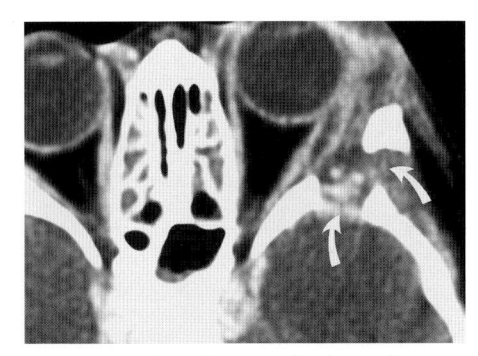

Fig. 2.211 Tuberculosis. Axial enhanced CT scan shows a destructive lesion involving the lateral aspect of the left orbit (arrows). Case courtesy of G. Markson, MD, Sydney, Australia.

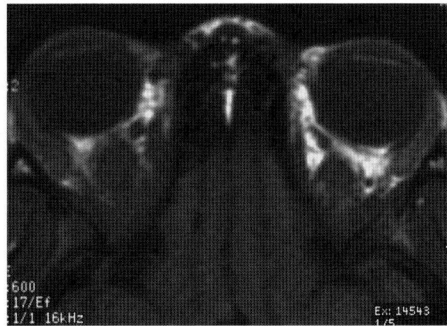

Fig. 2.212 Presumed juvenile xanthogranuloma in an 8-year-old girl.
a Axial T1W MR scan shows an infiltrative process involving both orbits.
b Axial enhanced fat-suppression T1W MR scan shows marked enhancement of presumed orbital xanthogranuloma.

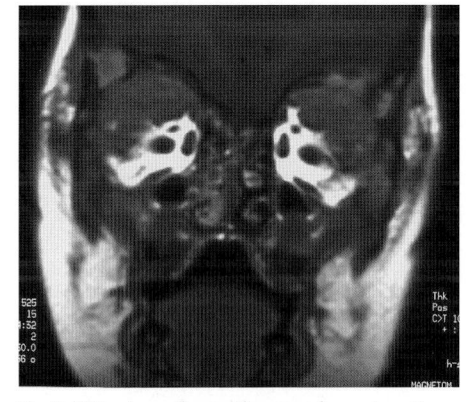

Fig. 2.213 Juvenile xanthogranuloma in a 3-year-old girl. Coronal enhanced T1W MR scan shows a marked infiltrative process involving both orbits, compatible with biopsy-proven xanthogranuloma.

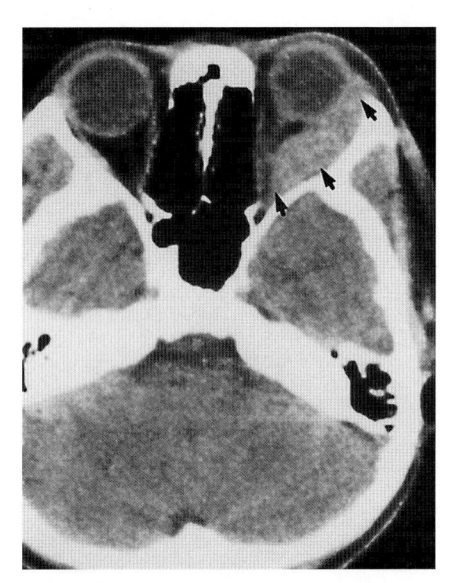

Fig. 2.214 Pseudorheumatoid nodule. Axial CT scan in a child shows an infiltrative process involving the left lateral rectus muscle, lateral orbital fat, and lacrimal gland (arrows).

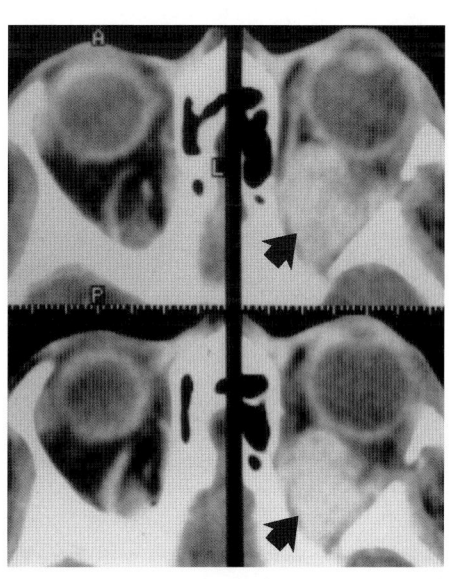

Fig. 2.215 Necrobiotic xanthogranuloma. Axial enhanced CT scans show an infiltrative process, involving the retrobulbar space of the left orbit (arrow), compatible with biopsy-proven necrobiotic xanthogranuloma. Note defect of lateral orbital wall, the site of biopsy. The right orbit was also involved (not shown here).

countered a very unusual and challenging case in which the clinical and radiological findings were typical of LCH (Hand–Schüller–Christian disease). A 3-year-old girl had bilateral proptosis and diabetes insipidus, but the histopathology was more consistent with JXG (Fig. 2.213). Additionally, the histiocytes were negative for the immunological marker S-100 protein and no Birbeck granules were found when electron microscopy was performed.

Erdheim–Chester Disease

Erdheim–Chester disease is a peculiar form of systemic xanthogranulomatosis that occurs in adults.[122, 123] Most patients do not have orbital involvement. The first two cases were reported by Shields et al.[123] The disease is characterized by the infiltration of many organs, including lung, kidney, heart, bones, orbit, and retroperitoneal tissues. Orbital involvement tends to be bilateral. These patients present with progressive bilateral exophthalmos, which may lead to ophthalmoplegia, and visual loss secondary to compressive optic neuropathy.[91] CT and MRI may show extensive soft-tissue infiltration of the orbital fatty reticulum.[106, 124] There may be no enhancement following the administration of Gd-DTPA contrast material, though at times delayed enhancement may be observed.

Pseudorheumatoid Nodules

Pseudorheumatoid nodules usually occur as focal masses in the dermis of children. This disease may involve the anterior orbit and periorbital region (Fig. 2.214), simulating pseudotumor, LCH, and orbital tumors. The subcutaneous nodules consist of zonular granulomas surrounding necrobiotic collagen. These are thought to be more common in sites of previous trauma and are managed by simple excision.[3]

Necrobiotic Xanthogranuloma

Necrobiotic xanthogranuloma is a histocytic disease characterized by the occurrence of multiple indurated xanthomatous subcutaneous nodules in patients with paraproteinemia and proliferative disorders such as multiple myeloma and leukemia.[3, 106, 125] Histologically, the lesion is composed of granulomatous inflammatory infiltrate, with Touton giant cells and xanthoma cells. Ophthalmic manifestations are common and include xanthogranulomas involving the eyelid, orbit, conjunctiva, and orbital fatty reticulum (Fig. 2.215).

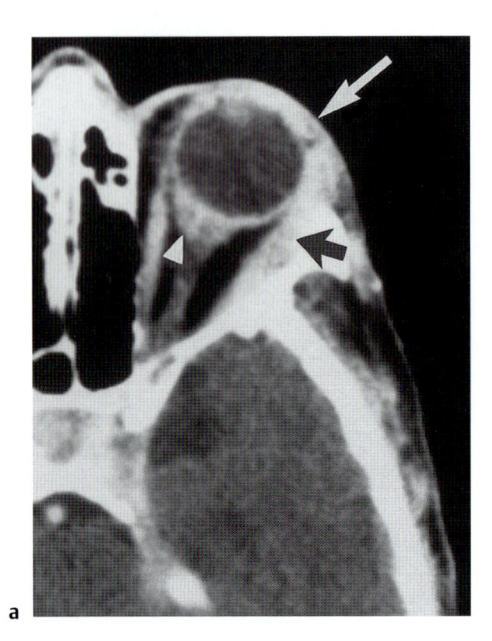

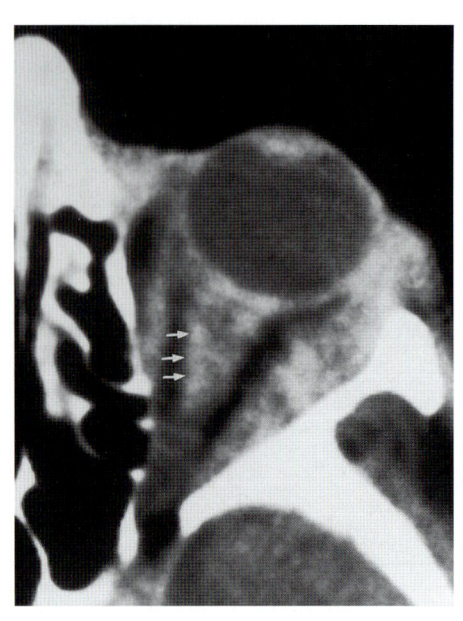

Fig. 2.**216** Lymphoma of the orbit.
a Axial enhanced CT scan shows moderate enlargement of lateral rectus muscle (black arrows), retrobulbar infiltrate (arrowhead), and thickening of the left eyelid (white arrow).
b Axial enhanced CT scan, obtained 10 months later, showing recurrence of lymphoma of the left orbit, associated with involvement of the left optic nerve (arrows).

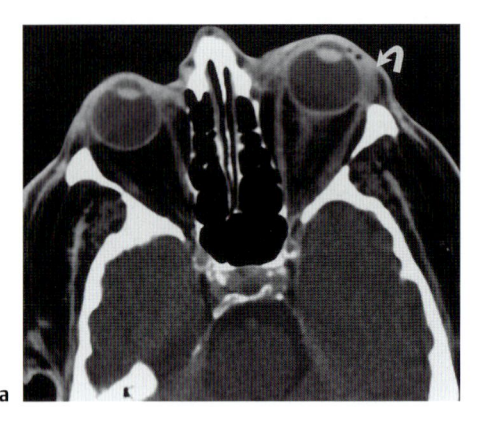

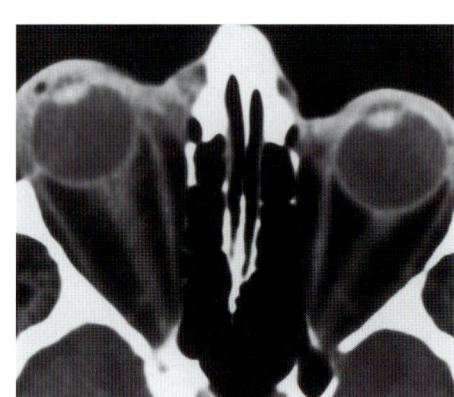

Fig. 2.**217** Lymphoma of the orbit.
a Axial enhanced CT scan shows proptosis of the left eye associated with slight enlargement of the left lateral rectus muscle as well as slight enlargement of the left lacrimal gland (arrow).
b Axial enhanced CT scan, taken five months later, showing proptosis of the right eye, associated with slight thickening of right optic nerve as well as thickening of right eyelid. The patient developed systemic lymphoma.

Tumors

Orbital Lymphoma

Orbital lymphomas are solid tumors of the immune system, which are primarily composed of (monoclonal) B cells. The extranodal presentation of non-Hodgkin lymphoma is common, with an incidence ranging from 21% to 64%, and with roughly 10% of non-Hodgkin lymphomas presenting in the head and neck region.[126] Lymphoid tumors account for 10–15% of orbital masses.[2,125]

Lymphoid neoplasms of the orbit span a large continuum of various classifications from the malignant lymphomas, to the benign pseudolymphomas or pseudotumors, to the reactive and atypical lymphoid hyperplasias.[2,126,127] There are no absolute imaging, clinical, or even laboratory tests that delineate all types of benign orbital lymphoid lesions from orbital lymphomas, or lesions that can simulate them.[2,16] A pleomorphic cellular infiltrate is correlated with more benign biological activity; the more uniform the cellular appearance, the greater the likelihood that a malignancy is present.[2] Of all patients with orbital lymphoma, 75% have or will have systemic lymphoma.[2,126] True lymphoid tissue in the orbit is found in the subconjunctival and lacrimal gland, and these two areas account for most of the lymphoreticuloses developing in the orbit.[2,128,129] Both benign and malignant lymphoid tumors of the orbit occur predominantly in adults and are extremely rare in children.[6,130] The two main types of lymphoid tumors that the ophthalmologists deal with are reactive lymphoid hyperplasia, a localized benign disease of unknown cause, and malignant lymphoma, which may arise in and be limited to the orbit or may arise in the sinonasal cavities, then extending into the orbit, or may be one focus of a systemic lymphoma.[6]

Diagnostic Imaging

Ultrasonography, CT, and MRI can be used to evaluate orbital lymphomas. CT and MRI have made it possible to make a strong presumptive diagnosis of orbital lymphoma, especially when CT and MRI features are examined in conjunction with the clinical signs and symptoms.[130] The CT and MRI findings are usually nonspecific, and it may be impossible to differentiate the lymphomas from orbital pseudotumors, benign lymphoid hyperplasia (Figs. 2.**216**–2.**220**), and lacrimal gland pseudotumor, and at times from primary epithelial lacrimal gland tumors (Fig. 2.**220**), optic nerve tumors, Graves orbitopathy, primary orbital tumors, or orbital cellulitis.[126–130] Orbital lymphomas are homogeneous masses of relatively high CT density and sharp or poor margins (Figs. 2.**221**, 2.**222**, 2.**223**), which are more often seen in the ante-

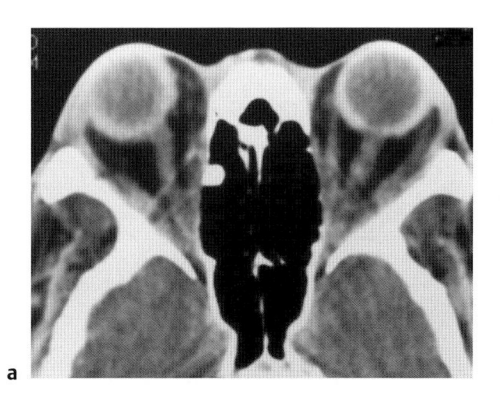

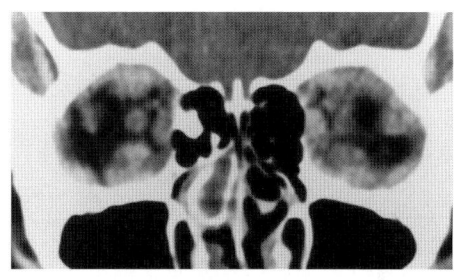

Fig. 2.218 Benign lymphoid hyperplasia.
a Axial enhanced CT scan shows moderate enlargement of the lateral and medial rectus muscles of both eyes, along with increased thickening of the scleral–Tenon coats.
b Coronal enhanced CT scan shows diffuse infiltrative process involving bilateral extraconal fat, associated with moderate enlargement of extraocular muscles.

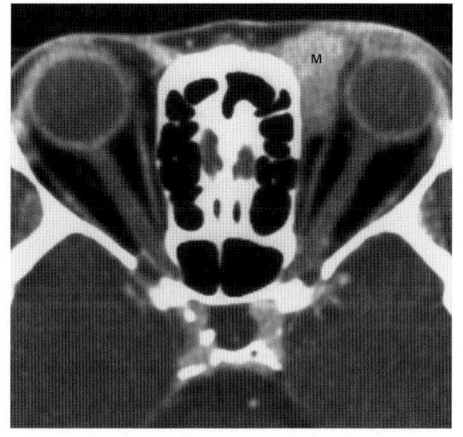

Fig. 2.219 Benign lymphoid hyperplasia. Axial enhanced CT scan in an elderly male shows a well-defined extraconal soft-tissue mass (M) compatible with benign lymphoid hyperplasia.

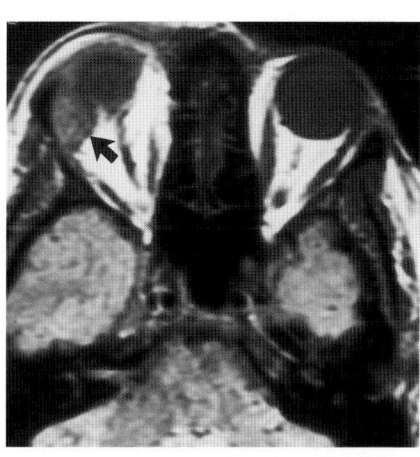

Fig. 2.220 Benign lymphoid hyperplasia of the lacrimal gland. a Axial T1W and b T2W MR scans showing enlargement of right lacrimal gland (arrow), compatible with benign lymphoid hyperplasia.

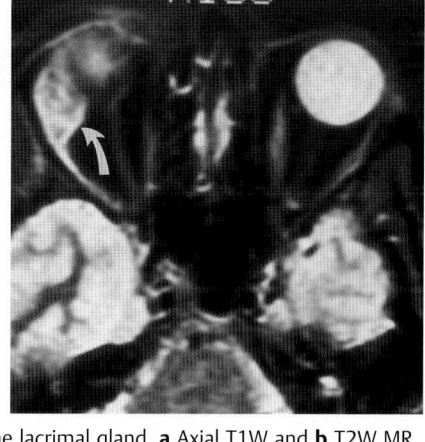

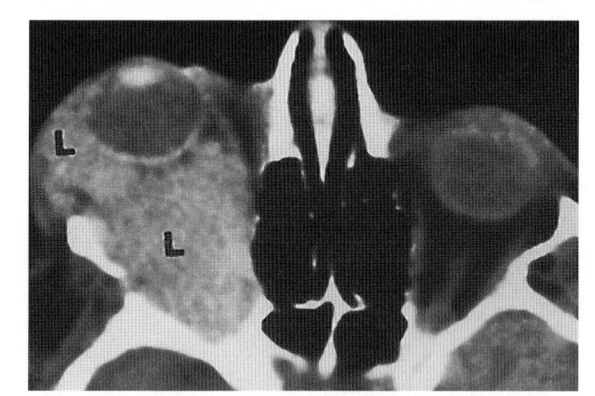

Fig. 2.221 Orbital lymphoma. Axial postcontrast CT scan shows a large orbital mass, proven to be lymphoma (L) involving the lacrimal gland and entire retrobulbar space. Note that the mass molds itself with the globe rather than invading it.

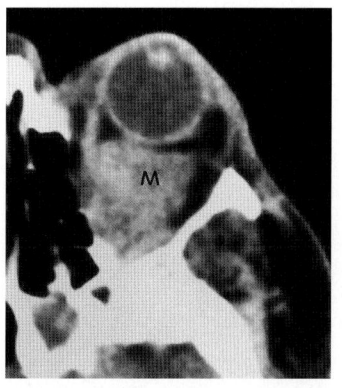

Fig. 2.222 Lymphoma. Axial enhanced CT scan shows a large mass (M), involving the retrobulbar space of the left orbit, compatible with lymphoma.

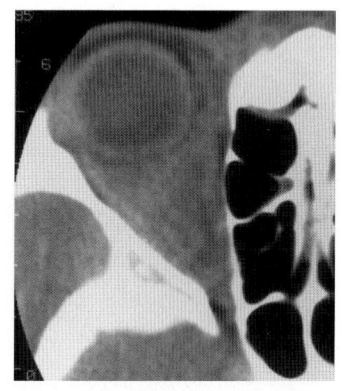

Fig. 2.223 Lymphoma. Axial CT scan shows a diffuse infiltrative process, involving the intraconal space of the right orbit, compatible with lymphoma.

rior portion of the orbit (Fig. 2.221), in the retrobulbar area (Figs. 2.222–2.224), within the muscle cone (Fig. 2.224), or in the superior or inferior orbital compartments (Figs. 2.225, 2.226). Mild to moderate enhancement is usually present (Figs. 2.225, 2.226).[126, 130] The shared feature of all orbital lymphoid tumors is their tendency to mold themselves around the orbital structures without producing bony erosion (Fig. 2.221).[129] Specifically, a bulky lesion in the region of the lacrimal fossa that does not produce bony erosion is most likely to be either inflammatory or lymphoid in character (Fig. 2.227).[16, 130] However, the aggressive malignant lymphomas can produce frank destruction of bone.[130] Lacrimal gland lymphoma displaces the globe medially and forward and appears as a moderately enhancing mass that diffusely involves the gland (Figs. 2.227, 2.228).[126]

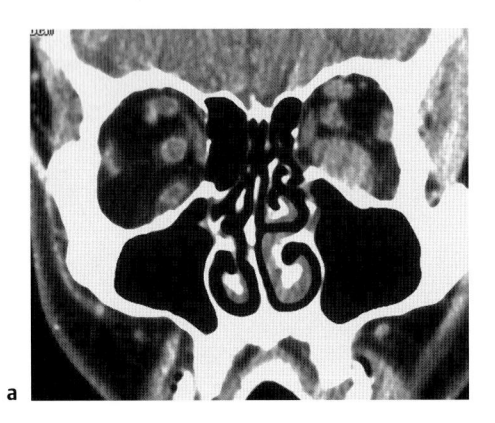

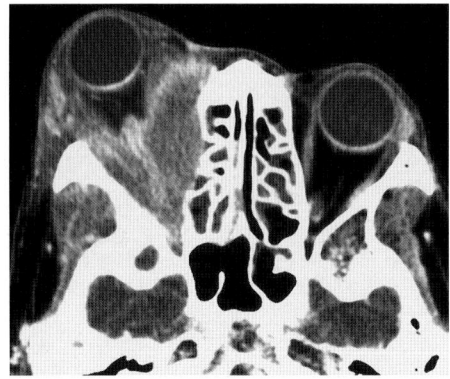

Fig. 2.224 Lymphoma.
a Coronal CT scan shows marked enlargement of the left inferior rectus muscle compatible with biopsy-proven lymphoma.
b Axial CT scan in another patient shows marked enlargement of the lateral and medial rectus muscles compatible with a presumed lymphoma.

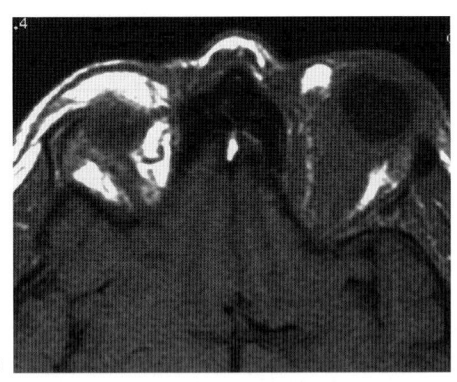

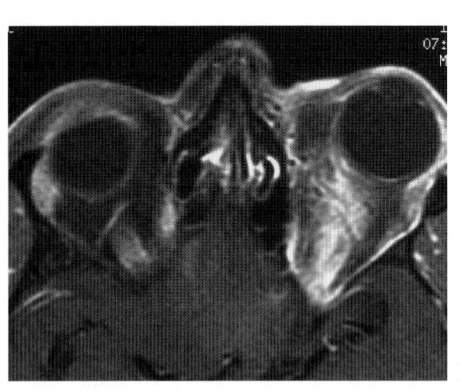

Fig. 2.225 Lymphoma. a Axial T1W and b axial enhanced fat-suppression MR scans showing orbital lymphoma involving the superior rectus and orbital fatty reticulum on the left eye.

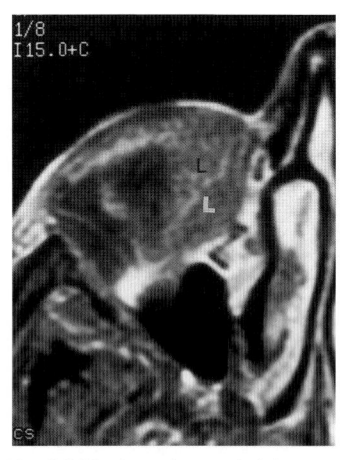

Fig. 2.226 Lymphoma. Axial enhanced fat-suppression T1W MR scan showing orbital lymphoma (L) involving the inferior aspect of the right orbit.

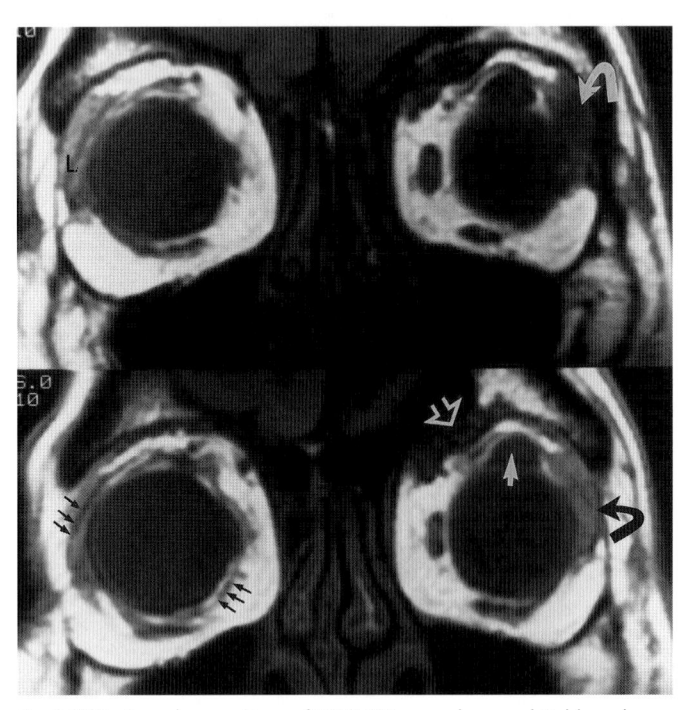

Fig. 2.227 Lymphoma. Coronal T1W MR scan shows orbital lymphoma involving the left lacrimal gland (curved arrows), superior rectus muscle (white arrow), and subperiosteal space (hollow arrow). Note the normal right lacrimal gland (L) and normal intermuscular fibrous sheath (black arrows).

MRI has proven to be as sensitive as CT for the diagnosis of orbital lymphoma and pseudotumors. Both pseudotumors and lymphoma may have intermediate or low signal intensity on T1-weighted and proton density images and appear isointense or less commonly hyperintense to fat in T2-weighted images (Figs. 2.227–2.229).[126] In children, orbital lymphoma may simulate orbital rhabdomyosarcoma (Fig. 2.229). At times lymphoma of the orbit may be associated with lymphoma of sinonasal cavities or systemic lymphoma (Figs. 2.230, 2.231).

Lymphoplasmacytic Tumors (Plasma Cell Tumor)

Tumors composed of pure plasma cells (plasmacytomas) and those composed of B lymphocytes and plasma cells (lymphoplasmacytoid tumors) are closely related to the various lymphomas.[2,3,106] The plasma cell is actually a B lymphocyte that has become modified to produce large quantities of immunoglobulin.[2,106] These so-called plasmacytoid lymphomas may secrete IgM paraprotein in sufficient quantities to cause a monoclonal peak in the serum; this is classically seen in Waldenström macroglobulinemia.[2,3] One of the important tumors of plasma cells is multiple myeloma (Fig. 2.232). There are also solitary forms of extramedullary plasmacytomas, which are not associated with systemic multiple myeloma. These plasma cell tumors, particularly as they affect the orbit and ocular structures, display the same spectrum of clinical involvement as seen in the lymphoproliferative disorders (Fig. 2.232).[2,3] Both isolated plasmacytoma and Waldenström macroglobulinemia can pro-

Pathology 251

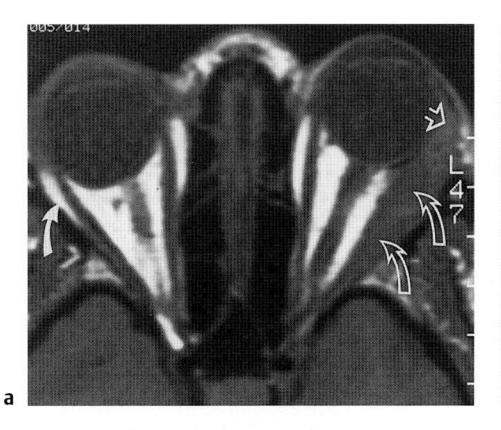

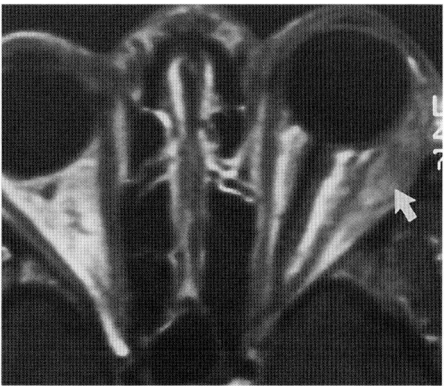

Fig. 2.**228** Orbital pseudotumor.
a Axial T1W MR scan shows an infiltrative process involving the lacrimal gland (short arrow) and extraconal space lateral to the left lateral rectus muscle (curved open arrows). Note the normal extraconal fat on the right side (solid curved arrow). The pseudotumor is isointense to the brain.
b Axial postcontrast T1W MR scan shows moderate enhancement of pseudotumor (arrow).

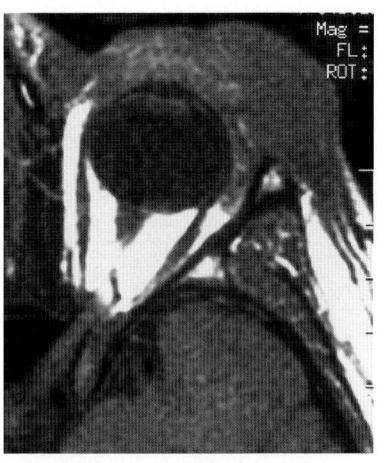

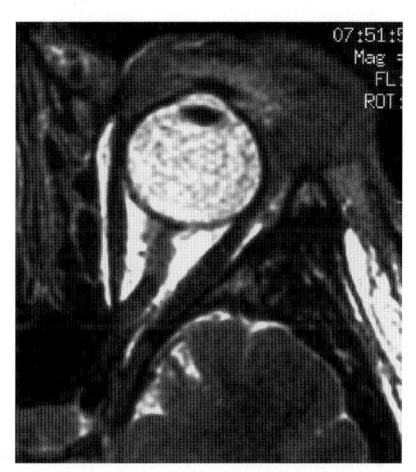

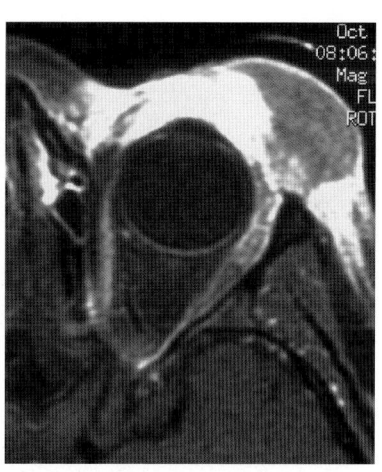

Fig. 2.**229** Lymphoma in a 16-year-old boy. **a** Axial T1W, **b** axial T2W, and **c** axial enhanced fat-suppression T1W MR scans showing large orbital lymphoma (Burkitt-like) involving the left eyelid.

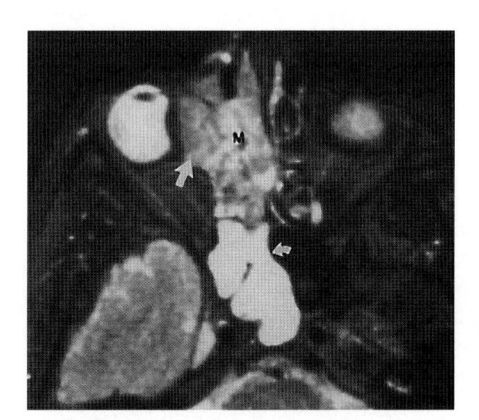

Fig. 2.**230** Sino-orbital lymphoma. Axial T2W MR scan shows a large ethmoid mass (M) involving the right orbit (arrow). As seen, this lymphoma is quite hyperintense. The hyperintensity of the right sphenoid sinus is due to retained secretion (curved arrow).

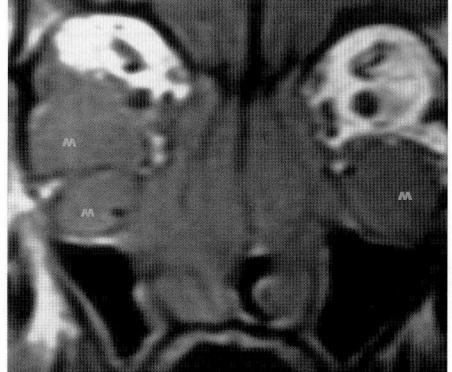

Fig. 2.**231** Presumed lymphoma of the orbits and sinonasal cavities. Coronal PW MR scan shows large subperiosteal masses (M), along with diffuse soft-tissue fullness in both nasal cavities and ethmoid air cells.

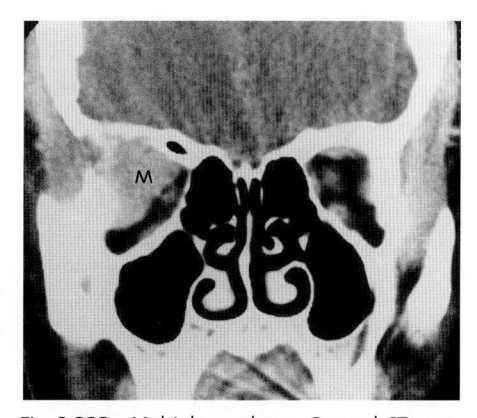

Fig. 2.**232** Multiple myeloma. Coronal CT scan showing a large mass (M), involving the superolateral aspect of the left orbit, associated with bone erosion.

duce a mass that can be visualized by both CT and MRI. The mass may be lobulated, densely enhancing, and well-defined, and can be present with or without bone erosion.[2, 16] In the case of systemic myelomatosis, a permeative or moth-eaten pattern of bone destruction or gross destruction may be present.[70]

Orbital Leukemia

Leukemia is one of the most common childhood cancers. It is estimated that of the approximately 7100 cancers in childhood in the United States each year, 35% are leukemia.[106, 125] Leukemic disorders in children fall mainly into the lymphoid and myeloid groups. About 75% of cases are acute lymphoblastic leukemia, 20% are acute myelogenous leukemia, and 5% are chronic myelogenous leukemia.[106] Chronic lymphocytic leukemia is a disease of

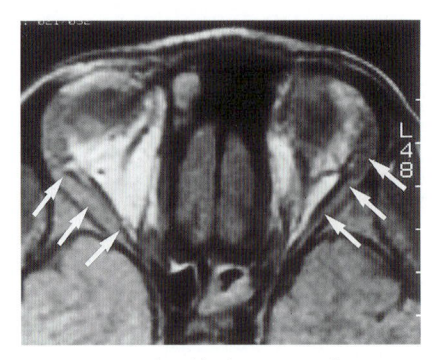

Fig. 2.233 Orbital leukemia. Axial PW MR scan shows bilateral subperiosteal leukemic infiltration (arrows).

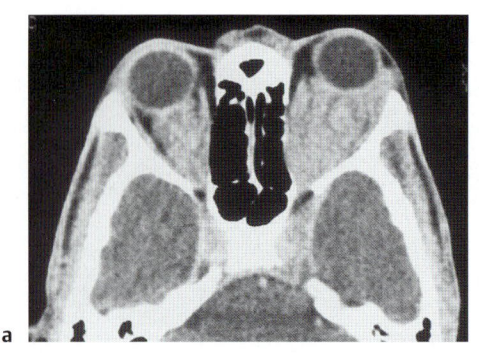

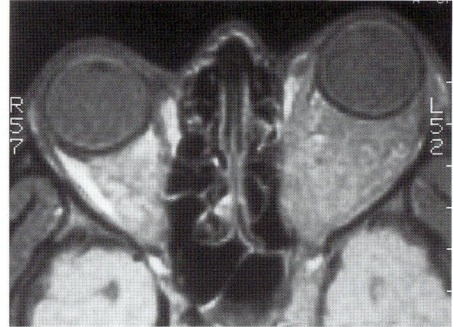

Fig. 2.234 Orbital leukemic infiltration. A 35-year-old man presented with bilateral proptosis.
a Axial enhanced CT scan shows a diffuse infiltrative process involving the retrobulbar spaces.
b In the PW MR scan, the retrobulbar infiltration appears isointense to muscles. The imaging diagnosis was pseudotumor vs. lymphoproliferative disorder. Further work-up revealed acute leukemia.

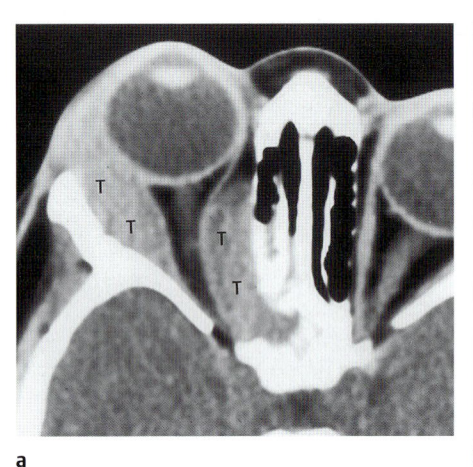

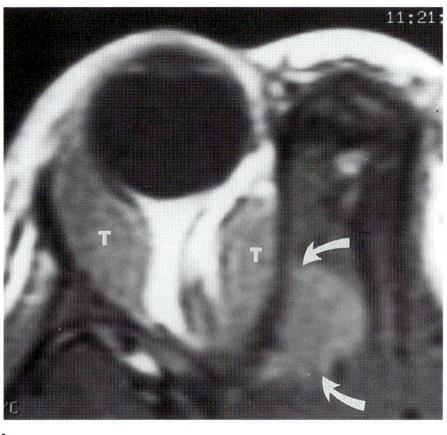

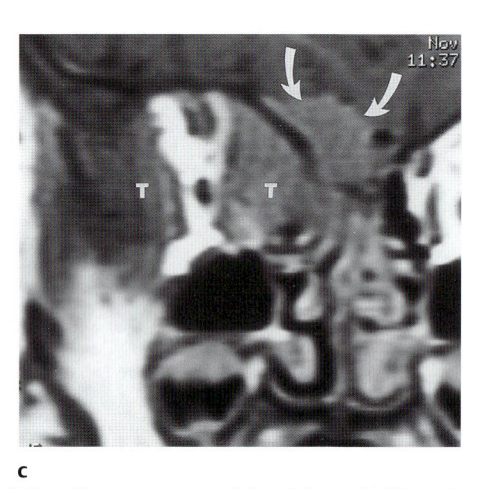

Fig. 2.235 Granulocytic sarcoma (leukemia). **a** Axial CT scan, **b** axial enhanced T1W MR scan and **c** coronal enhanced T1W MR scan in a 2-year-old child demonstrate extraconal (subperiosteal) soft-tissue tumor (T), involving both the medial and lateral aspects of the right orbit. There is involvement of the right posterior ethmoid air cells along with tumor involvement of the floor of the anterior cranial fossa (arrows in **b** and **c**).

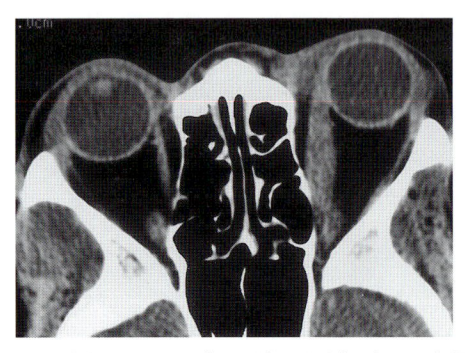

Fig. 2.236 Mycosis fungoides. Axial enhanced CT scan showing involvement of the left medial rectus muscle as well as thickening of the left eyelid.

adulthood and almost never affects children.[2] Involvement of the eye and adnexa is relatively common (Fig. 2.233). Orbital involvement with leukemia is the result of direct infiltration of orbital bone or soft tissue by leukemic cells (Fig. 2.233, 2.234).

In patients with acute myelogenous leukemia (AML), such infiltration most often occurs in the form of a granulocytic sarcoma (Fig. 2.235). A granulocytic sarcoma is commonly called a chloroma because the myeloperoxidase within the tumor imparts a green hue to it as seen on gross examination.[2,16,106] This may be the first manifestation of AML in many patients. The lesion typically involves the orbital subperiosteal space, usually the lateral wall of the orbit with extensions in the temporal fossa or the medial wall of the orbit with involvement of the ethmoid air cells, cribriform plate and anterior cranial fossa. There may be dural or leptomeningeal infiltration, demonstrating enhancement on enhanced CT and MRI (Fig. 2.235 b, c). The differential diagnosis of orbital leukemic infiltration includes rhabdomyosarcoma, Langerhans cell histiocytosis, subperiosteal abscess, subperiosteal hematoma, lymphoma, pseudotumor, metastasis (neuroblastoma, Ewing sarcoma, Wilms tumor), and mycosis fungoides (Fig. 2.236).

■ Orbital Vascular Conditions

Vascular lesions of the orbit represent an important group of orbital pathologies, particularly in infants and children. They also are the most controversial group of lesions because of confusion regarding their nature.[131] Debate continues about the classification of the various vascular malformations that may involve the orbit. In general, orbital vascular lesions include capillary hemangioma, cavernous hemangioma (cavernoma; a venous malformation), varices (venous malformation), lymphangioma, lymphangiovenous (venolymphatic) malformation, arteriovenous malformation (AVM), "sclerosing hemangioma," hemangiopericytoma, malignant hemangioendotheliomas (angiosarcomas), and hemangioblastoma (von Hippel–Lindau disease).

Pathology 253

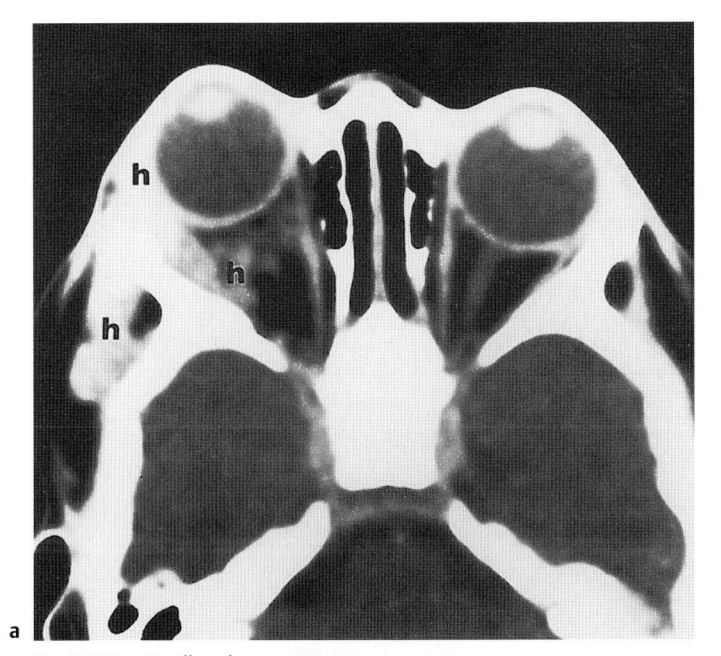

Fig. 2.**237** Capillary hemangioma.
a Axial postcontrast CT scan shows a diffuse intraorbital and extraorbital hemangioma (h).

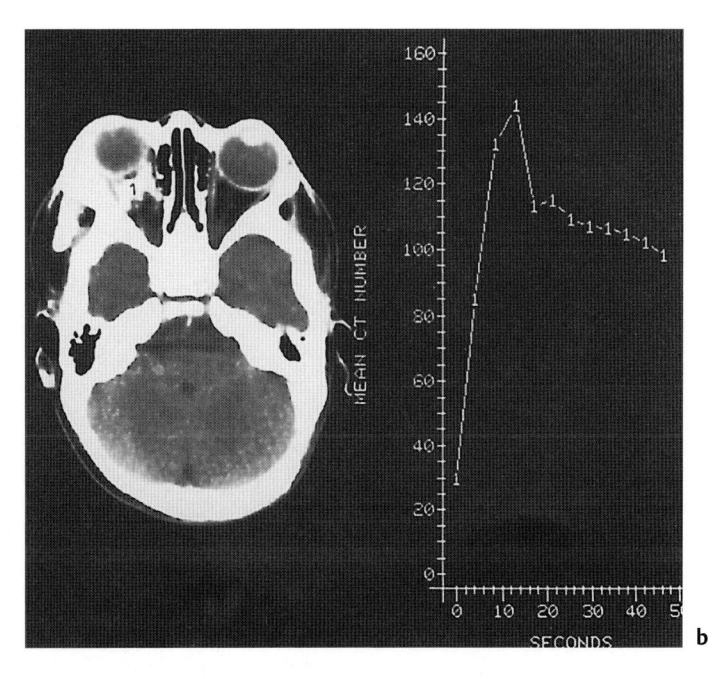

b Dynamic CT study shows the rapid wash-in phase, high peak, and rapid wash-out phase characteristic of highly vascular lesions.

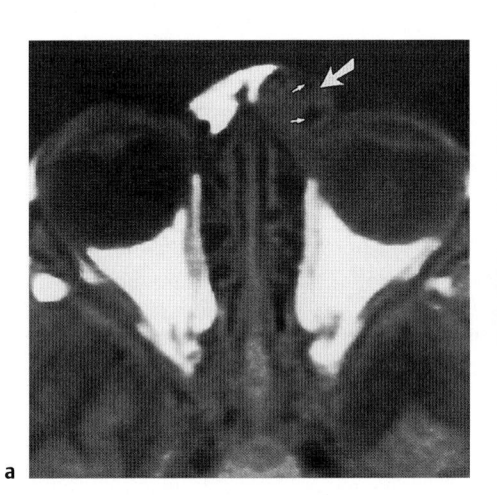

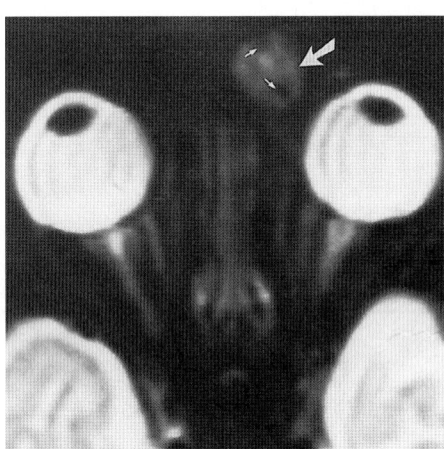

Fig. 2.**238** Capillary hemangioma. **a** Axial PW and **b** T2W MR scans show a mass in the right naso-orbital angle (large arrow). Note signal void due to prominent vessels (small arrows).

Capillary Hemangioma (Benign Hemangioendothelioma)

Capillary hemangiomas are tumors that occur primarily in infants during the first year of life. The tumor often increases in size for 6–10 months and then gradually involutes.[2,8,16,131,132] The tumor most commonly occurs in the superior nasal quadrant (Figs 2.**237**, 2.**238**). Microscopically the tumor is composed of endothelial and capillary vessel proliferation with benign endothelial cells surrounding small, capillary-sized vascular spaces.[8,16,131] Capillary hemangiomas in and around the orbit may have an arterial supply from either the external carotid or internal carotid arteries, and these tumors are capable of bleeding profusely.[8,131,132] These hemangiomas may extend intracranially through the superior orbital fissure, optic canal, and orbital roof. On CT or MRI, these lesions are seen as fairly well-marginated (Fig. 2.**238**) to poorly marginated, irregular, enhancing lesions. Most are extraconal, although some of these lesions may be seen in the intraconal space (Fig. 2.**239**). On dynamic CT or CT angiography, capillary hemangiomas characteristically show an intense, homogeneous enhancement (Fig. 2.**237b**). On MRI, capillary hemangiomas appear as hypointense or slightly hyperintense to brain on T1-weighted images and hyperintense to brain on proton density and T2-weighted images (Figs. 2.**238**, 2.**239**). They show intense enhancement following intravenous injection of Gd-DTPA contrast material. The vascularity of these lesions may not be appreciated on MR angiography (MRA). At the present time, therefore, one should not rely only on MRA for the diagnosis of these capillary hemangiomas.

Cavernous Hemangiomas

Cavernous hemangioma of the orbit, the most common orbital vascular tumor in adults, has distinctive clinical and histopathological features.[2,16,131] It tends to occur in the second to fourth decades of life. These tumors show a slowly progressive enlargement distinct from capillary hemangiomas, which gradually diminish in size. In contrast to capillary hemangiomas, a prominent arterial supply is absent.[8] Cavernous hemangiomas possess

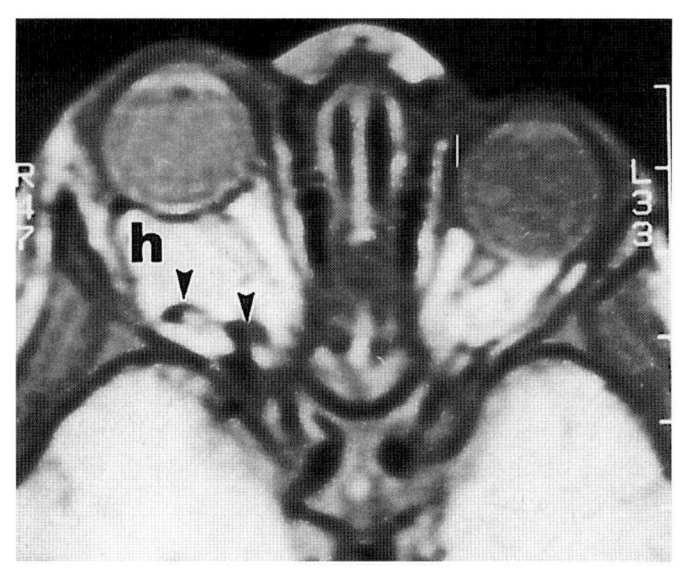

Fig. 2.**239** Intraconal capillary hemangioma. Axial PW MR scan in a 5-month-old girl shows a large retrobulbar mass compatible with a capillary hemangioma (h). Note signal voids due to prominent vessels (arrowheads).

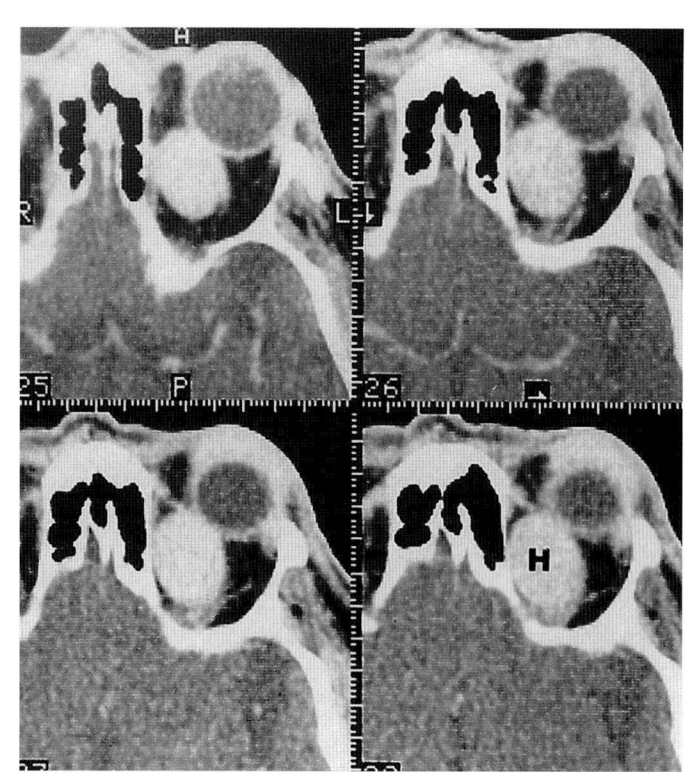

Fig. 2.**240** Cavernous hemangioma. Serial axial postcontrast CT scans show a well-defined intraconal enhancing mass compatible with a cavernous hemangioma (H).

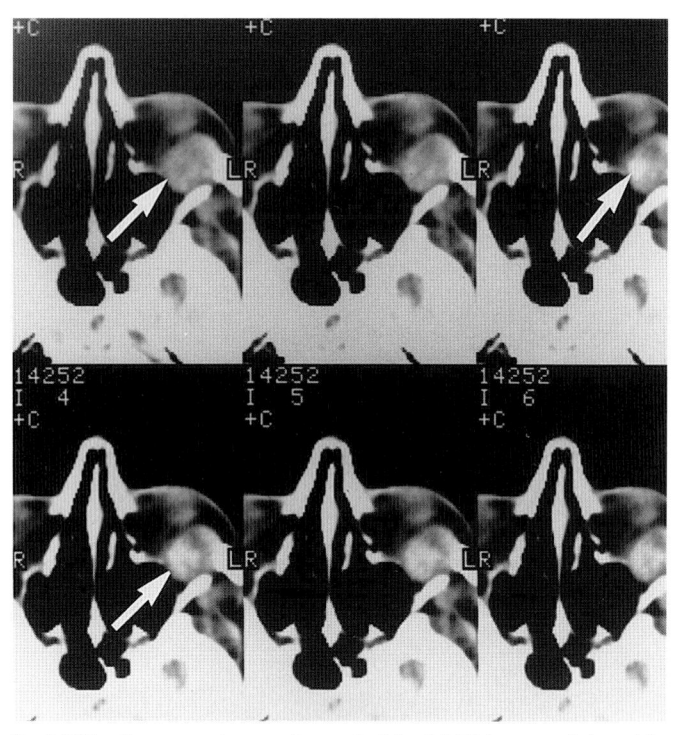

Fig. 2.**241** Cavernous hemangioma. Serial axial CT images of the orbit, taken following rapid intravenous injection of iodinated contrast material. Note gradual pooling of contrast (arrows) within this cavernous hemangioma.

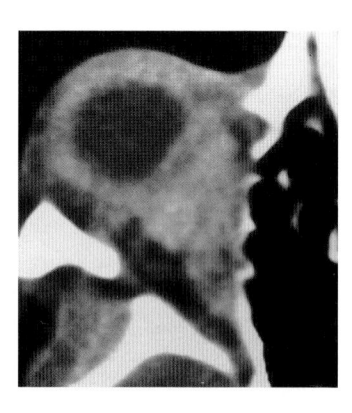

Fig. 2.**242** Cavernous hemangioma. Axial enhanced CT scan shows an irregular, ill-defined mass (arrows) within the right intraconal space. This is compatible with a partially resected cavernous hemangioma and reactive soft-tissue changes. Note surgical defect of lateral orbital wall.

a distinct fibrous pseudocapsule and therefore on CT and MRI appear as well-defined masses (Fig. 2.**140**). This observation, in addition to the fact that they are usually independent of the general circulation, enables excision of the entire lesion without fragmentation.[8] These hemangiomas may be located anywhere in the orbit, but frequently (83%) occur within the retrobulbar muscle cone (Figs. 2.**240**–2.**244**).

On CT, cavernous hemangiomas appear as well-defined, smoothly marginated, homogeneous, rounded, ovoid, or lobulated soft-tissue masses of increased density and variable contrast enhancement (Figs. 2.**240**, 2.**241**). Unless they are ruptured or surgically violated, cavernous hemangiomas always respect the contour of the globe and of surrounding structures (Fig. 2.**242**). The MRI characteristics of hemangiomas are shown in Figs. 2.**243**, 2.**244**. Histologically, cavernous hemangiomas are composed of large, dilated vascular channels (sinusoid-like spaces) lined by thin, attenuated endothelial cells.[8, 16, 131] These sinusoidal vascular spaces may demonstrate delayed increased enhancement on CT (Fig. 2.**241**) or MRI scans (Fig. 2.**245**). Cavernous hemangioma may be located in the extraconal space or have both intraconal and extraconal components (Fig. 2.**246**). At times, intraconal cavernous hemangiomas may be difficult to differentiate from other intraconal lesions such as meningiomas, hemangiopericytomas, and schwannomas (Fig. 2.**227**).[8, 16, 131] Uncommonly, an intramuscular hemangioma may occur. Orbital bone remodeling is not uncommon in cavernous hemangiomas and, rarely, calcification may be seen in these lesions. The so-called "sclerosing hemangioma" is another less well defined terminology, used to describe hemangiomas that show prominent sclerosis. These lesions often show foci of calcification (Fig. 2.**248**). Some hemangiomas may be associated with marked proptosis and orbital remodeling (Figs. 2.**249**, 2.**250**).

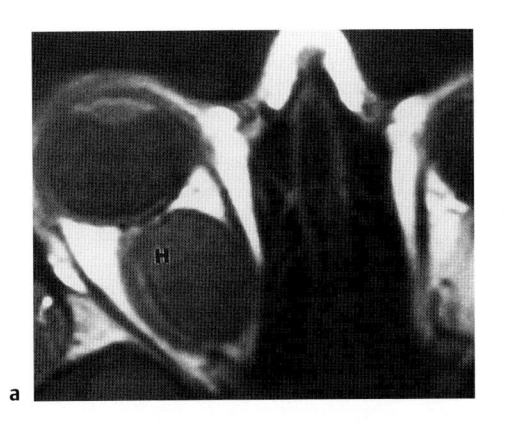

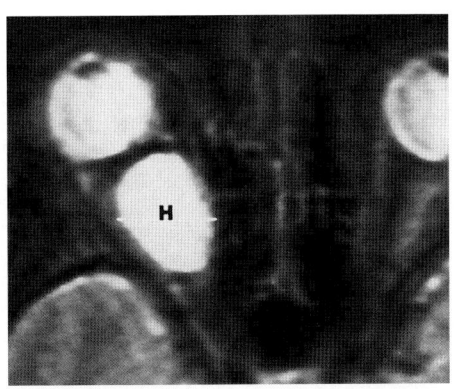

Fig. 2.**243** Cavernous hemangioma. **a** Axial T1W and **b** T2W MR scans show a well-defined intraconal mass compatible with cavernous hemangioma (H).

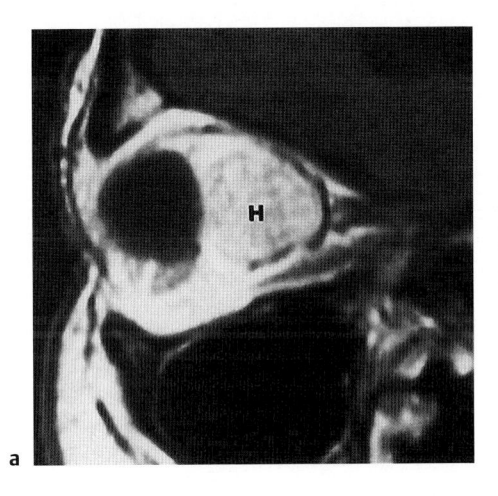

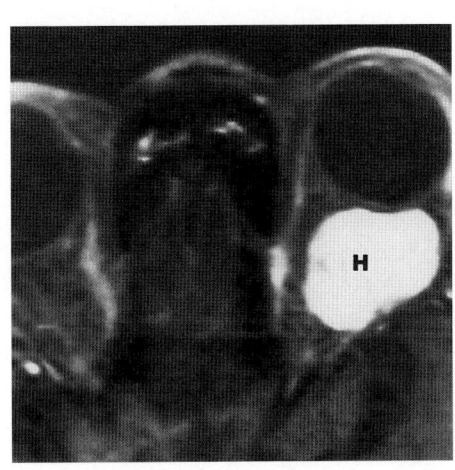

Fig. 2.**244** Cavernous hemangioma. **a** Sagittal postcontrast T1W and **b** axial postcontrast fat-suppression T1W MR scans show a well-defined intraconal mass compatible with cavernous hemangioma (H). The lesion is better outlined with fat-suppression technique.

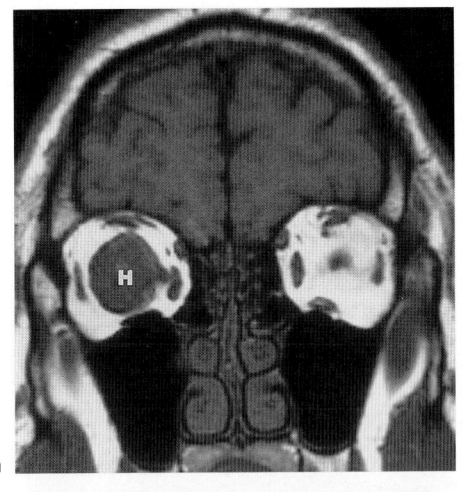

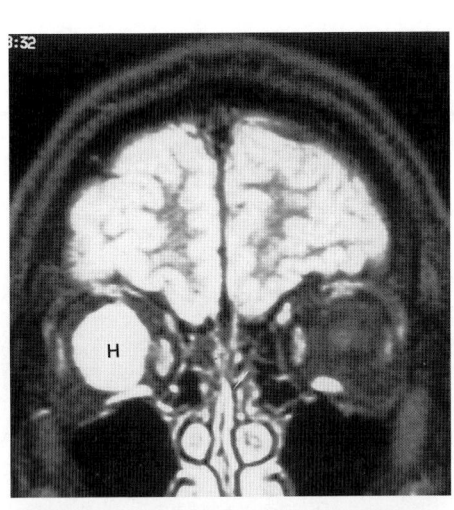

Fig. 2.**245** Cavernous hemangioma.
a Coronal unenhanced T1W, **b** coronal T2W, **c** axial enhanced T1W, and **d** coronal enhanced T1W MR scans, showing a cavernous hemangioma within the right intraconal space (H). Note heterogeneous enhancement in **c** and more diffuse enhancement in **d**. The coronal enhanced T1W MR image (**d**) was obtained several minutes after the axial enhanced T1W MR scan (**c**). Enhancement of cavernous hemangiomas becomes more homogeneous on delayed T1W MR images (see also Fig. 2.**241**).
Unlike in cavernous hemangiomas, hemangiopericytomas demonstrate intense homogeneous enhancement on early or late T1W MR pulse sequences.

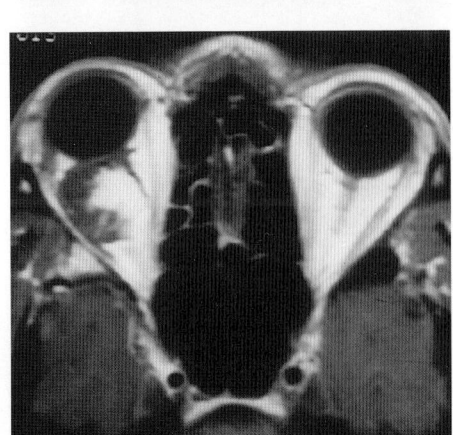

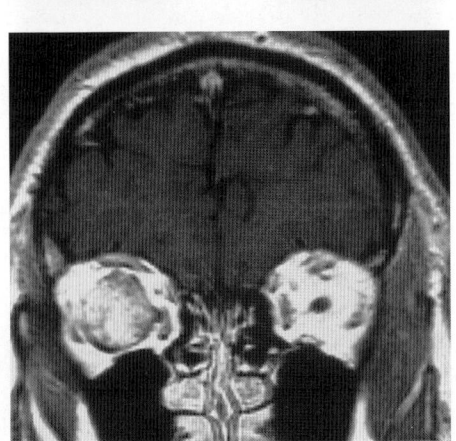

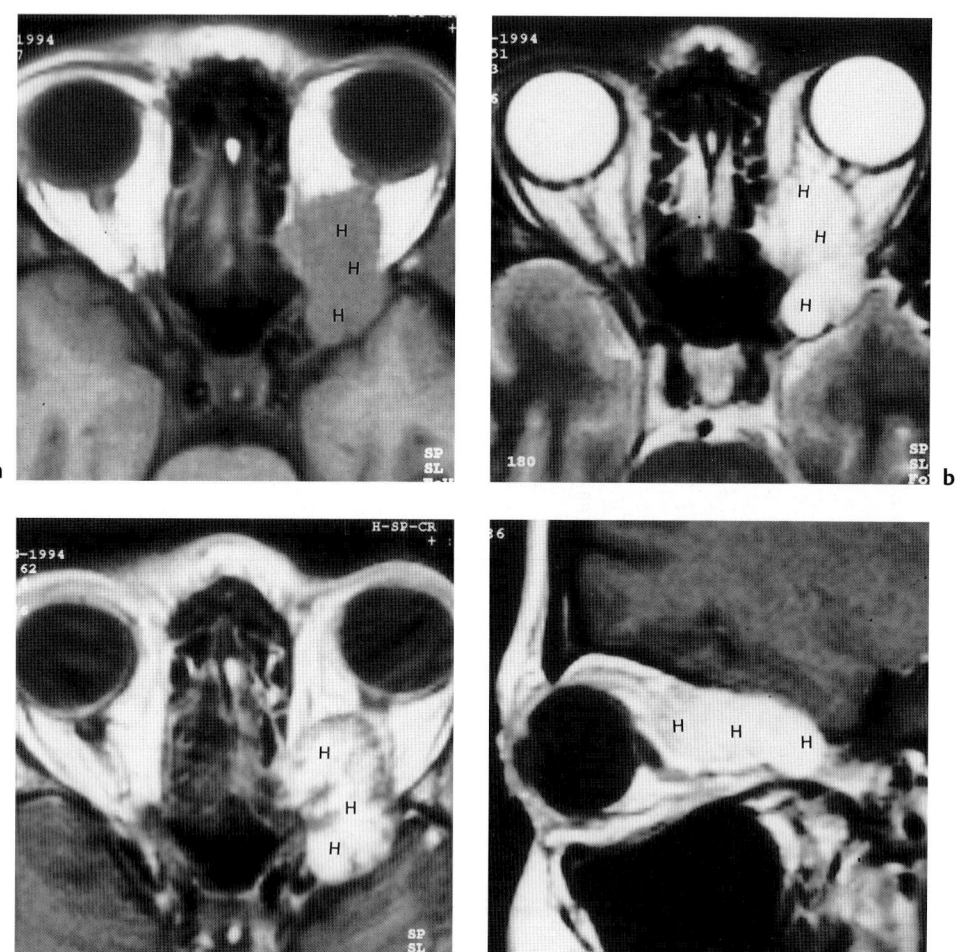

Fig. 2.**246** Cavernous hemangioma. **a** Axial T1W, **b** axial T2W, **c** axial enhanced T1W, and **d** sagittal enhanced T1W MR scans, showing a large cavernous hemangioma (H). Note extraconal extension, associated with remodeling of the posterior orbital wall of the left orbit. Courtesy of Richard Hewlett, MD, Christian Barnard Memorial Hospital, South Africa.

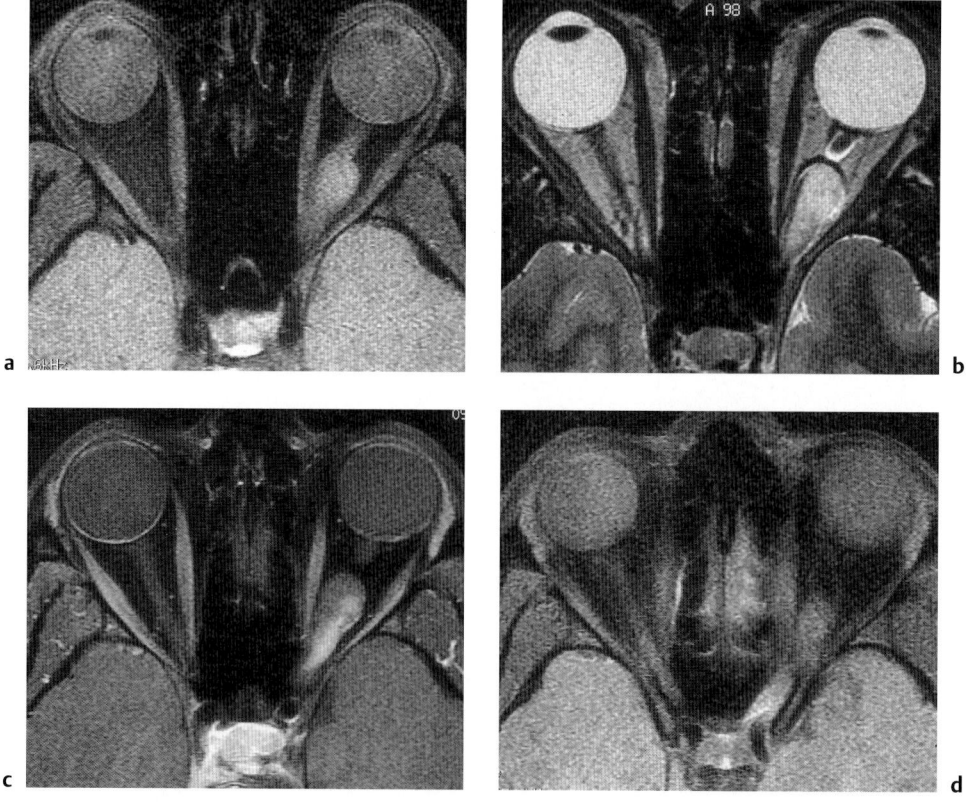

Fig. 2.**247** Presumed cavernous hemangioma (cavernoma). **a** Axial unenhanced fat-suppression T1W, **b** axial T2W, and **c** and **d** axial enhanced fat-suppression T1W MR scans. There is a smoothly marginated enhancing mass along the course of left optic nerve, including its intracanalicular portion (**d**). This is presumed to be a cavernous hemangioma. The mass did not change its shape in images taken with Valsalva maneuver. The lesion remained unchanged on follow-up a year later. All images were obtained on a 3 T MR scanner, using head coil.

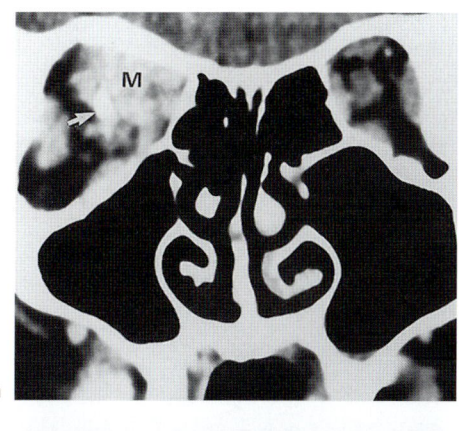

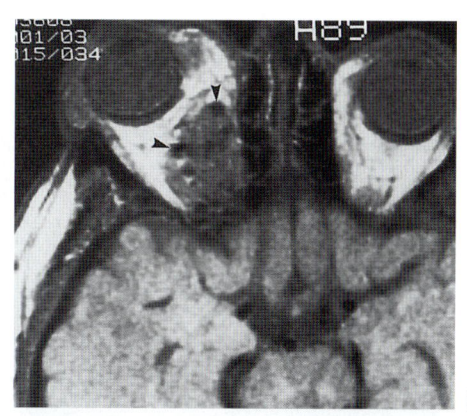

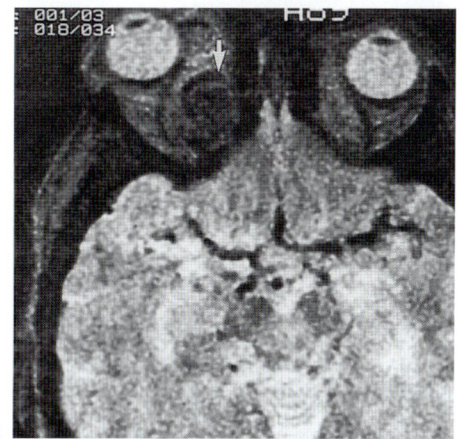

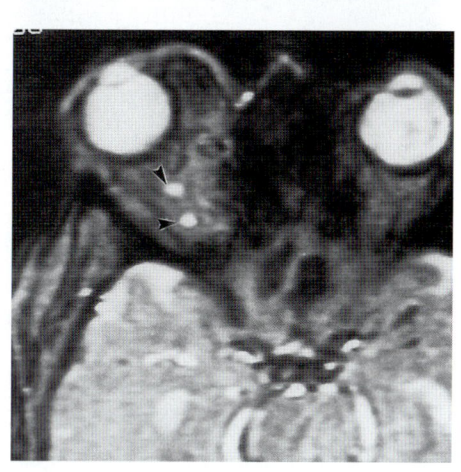

Fig. 2.248 "Sclerosing hemangioma."
a Coronal postcontrast CT scan shows an irregular enhancing mass (M). Note a prominent round calcification (arrow).
b Axial PW MR scan. The hemangioma is isointense to brain. Note several low-intensity images (arrowheads) due to calcifications.
c Axial T2W MR scan. The hemangioma appears hypointense to brain. This was due to increased interstitial sclerosis (dense fibrous tissue). Note the prominent vessel (arrow).
d Gradient-echo MR scan shows prominent vessels (arrowheads) within this "sclerosing hemangioma." An AVM with sclerosis may have similar imaging appearance.

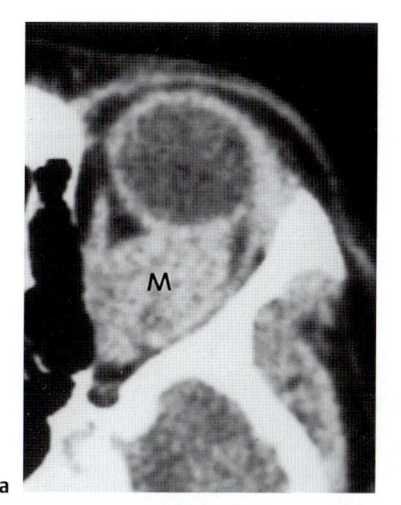

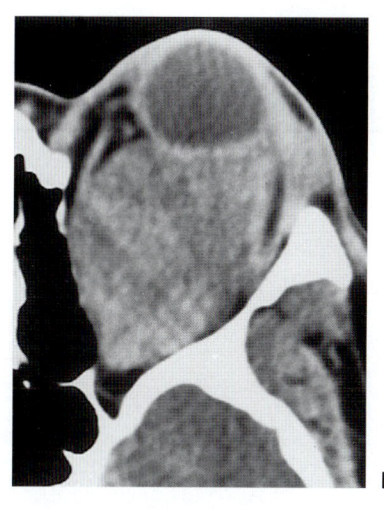

Fig. 2.249 Hemangioma.
a Axial enhanced CT scan in an 8-year-old girl shows an enhancing left retrobulbar mass (M).
b Axial enhanced CT scan, obtained eight years later, shows enlargement of the mass, which was proven to be consistent with a "sclerosing hemangioma."

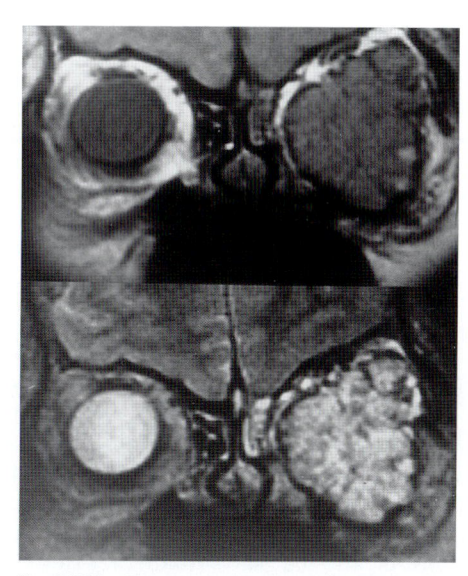

Fig. 2.250 Hemangioma. Coronal T1W (top) and T2W (bottom) MR scans in a 65-year-old woman, showing a large left orbital hemangioma.

Lymphangiomas

The origin of lymphangioma remains controversial, but the lesion is an unencapsulated mass consisting mostly of bloodless vascular and lymph channels.[72] Connective tissue between the channels may contain foci of lymphoid cells that proliferate in viral infections, resulting in the clinical finding of worsening proptosis when the child has an upper respiratory tract infection.[72] Orbital lymphangiomas occur in children and young adults. In contrast to the rapid, self-limited growth of infantile capillary hemangiomas, lymphangiomas gradually and progressively enlarge during the first two decades of life.[8, 131] Cavernous lymphangiomas are composed of delicate, endothelium-lined, lymph-filled sinuses (filled with clear fluid or chocolate-colored, unclotted fluid), which invade the surrounding connective-tissue

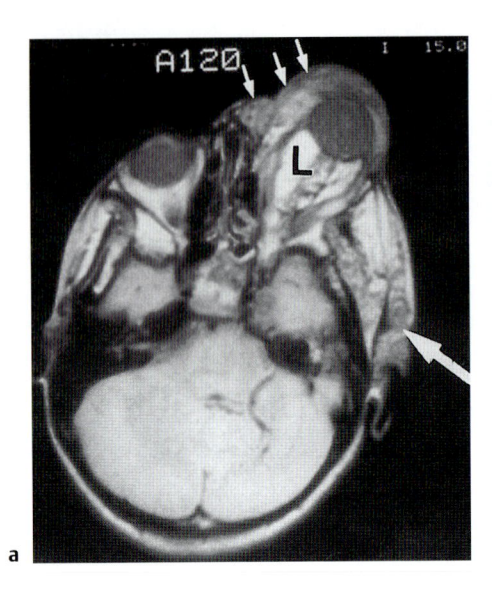

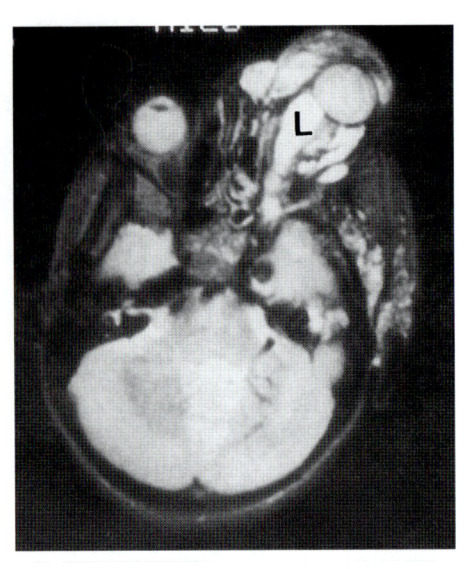

Fig. 2.251 Lymphangioma in a 10-year-old girl.
a Axial PW MR scan shows a large lymphangioma involving the eyelid (short arrows), intraconal space (L), and temporal fossa (arrow).
b Axial T2W MR scan. Lymphangioma (L) appears hyperintense.

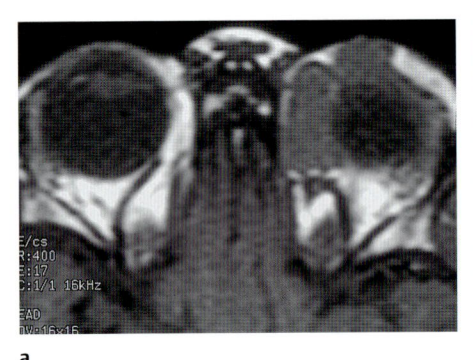

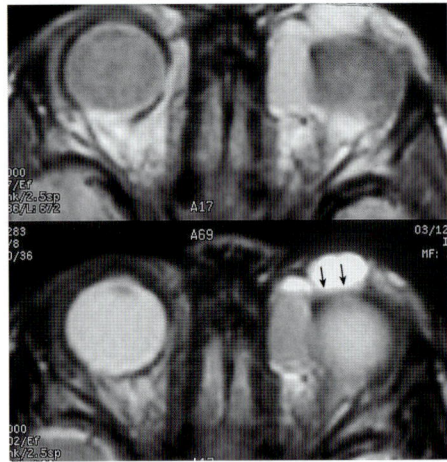

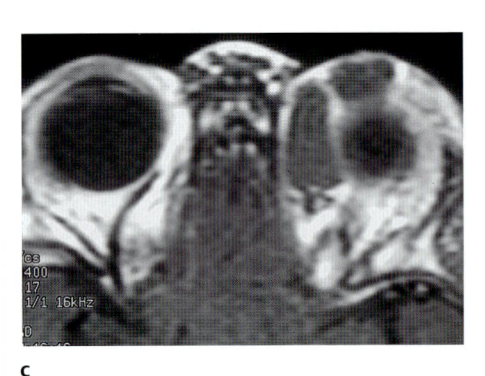

Fig. 2.252 Lymphangioma in a 3-year-old boy with proptosis of the left eye.
a Axial unenhanced T1W MR scan shows a lymphangioma involving the left orbit.
b PW (top) and T2W (bottom) MR scans. Note fluid–fluid level (arrows) which is due to hemorrhage.
c Axial enhanced T1W MR scan. Note lack of significant contrast enhancement.

stroma.[8,72,131] The interstitial tissue often shows lymphoid follicles and lymphocytic infiltration. Spontaneous (or after minor trauma) hemorrhage within the lesion is common, resulting in chocolate cyst.[8,16] Lymphangiomas may have distinct borders but are typically diffuse and not well-encapsulated (Figs. 2.251–2.253), with portions of the lesion infiltrating within normal tissues of the lid and orbit. They are usually multilobular (Fig. 2.252) and, because complete surgical excision is seldom accomplished, recurrence is common. They are more common in the extraconal space.[8,131]

On CT, these lymphangiomas appear as poorly circumscribed, often heterogeneous masses of increased density in the extraconal or intraconal space. Bony remodeling may be present, calcification is rare, and minimal to marked contrast enhancement may be present. On MRI, lymphangiomas are seen as relatively hypointense or hyperintense to brain on T1-weighted and usually very hyperintense on T2-weighted images (Figs. 2.251–2.253). Fluid–fluid level related to hemorrhages of varied ages is characteristic of lymphangioma. The MRI characteristics of lymphangiomas should help differentiate them from pseudotumors and hemangiomas (Figs. 2.251–2.253).[8]

Orbital Varix

Primary orbital varices are congenital venous malformations characterized by proliferation of venous elements and massive dilation of one or more orbital veins, presumably associated with congenital weakness in the venous wall.[8,16,72,133] A varix may include a single smooth-contoured dilated vein, a single vessel with segmental dilatation, or a tangled mass of venous channels.[72] Varices within the orbit may appear to have both cystic (chocolate) and solid components.[72] Orbital varices are the most common cause of spontaneous orbital hemorrhage.[134] Clinically, proptosis or globe displacement increases during a Valsalva maneuver, reflecting the varix's connection to the venous system.[8,72,125]

The CT appearance of orbital varix may be normal in axial sections (Fig. 2.254a) but, because of increased venous pressure, is quite abnormal in axial and particularly coronal sections, obtained in a prone position (Fig. 2.254b). Because the varix may be completely collapsed or barely visible when the patient is lying quietly supine, any time an orbital varix is suspected it is recommended that additional CT sections be taken during a Valsalva

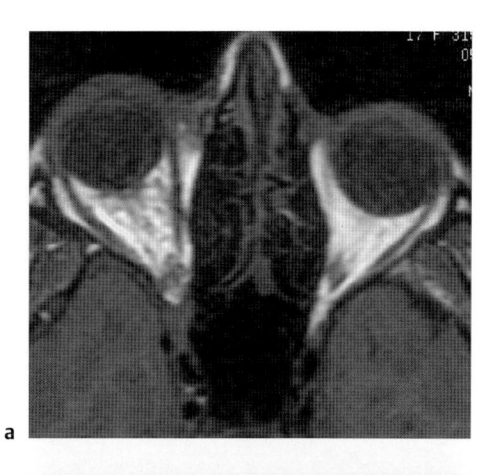

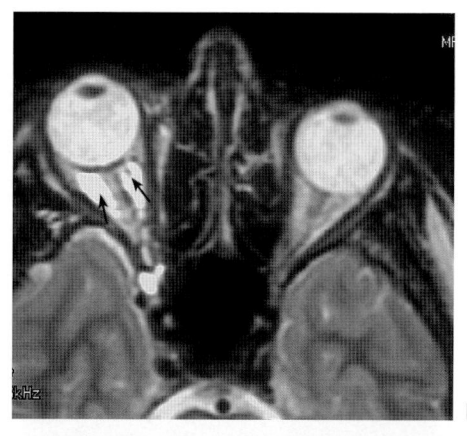

Fig. 2.**253** Lymphangioma. **a** Axial T1W, **b** axial T2W, **c** axial T2W, and **d** axial enhanced fat-suppression T1W MR scans, showing a poorly delineated intraconal lymphangioma. Note intense hyperintensity in T2W image (arrow) and hemorrhagic cyst ("chocolate cyst") (c) in the superior intraconal space. Note contrast enhancement of this lymphangioma (Fig. 2.**253 d**) as compared with unenhanced lymphangioma in Fig. 2.**252 c**.

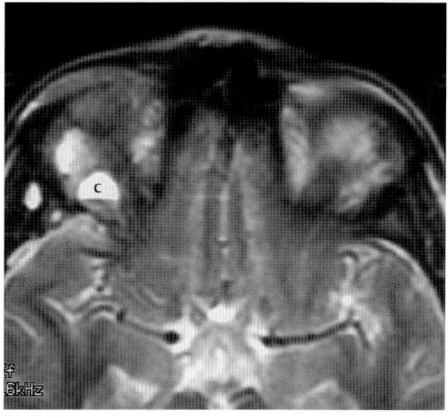

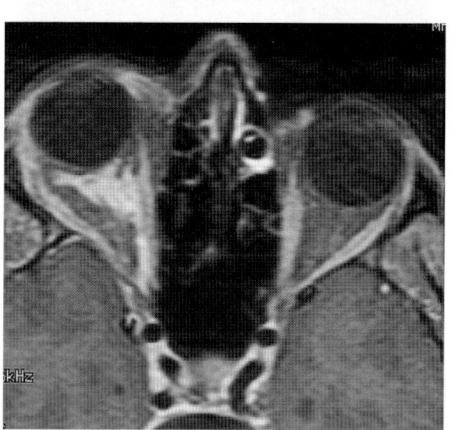

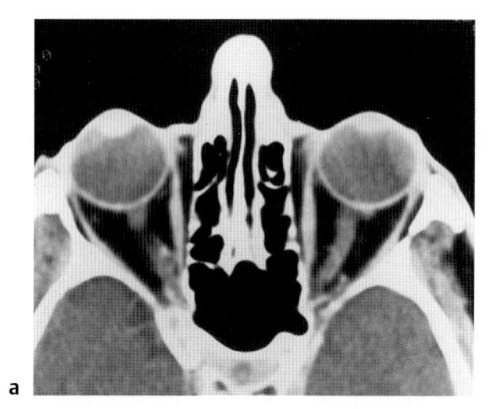

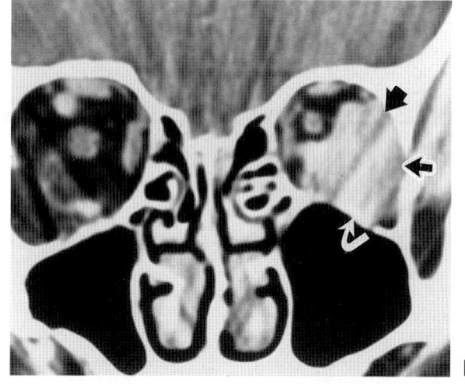

Fig. 2.**254** Orbital varix.
a Axial enhanced CT scan shows no obvious orbital lesion.
b Coronal CT scan, taken with patient in prone position, showing a large mass compatible with varix. The lesion is seen in coronal CT because of increased intravenous pressure, due to the patient's position. From Mafee MF, Putterman A, Valvassori GE, et al. Orbital space-occupying lesions: role of CT and MRI, an analysis of 145 cases. Radiol Clin North Am 1987; 25: 529–559. With permission.

maneuver. In a patient suspected of having an orbital varix, MRI also should be performed with the patient in the prone position. Some varices may have such small communication with the systemic venous system that they are undistensible. Because they have stagnant blood flow, they manifest themselves by thrombosis and hemorrhage.[131] Orbital varices may also be secondary to intracranial vascular malformation, particularly arteriovenous shunts.[2, 132] It is important to realize that some orbital varices may have the same CT appearance as cavernous hemangioma (Fig. 2.**255**).

MRI of orbital varices usually shows a varix to be hyperintense on T1-weighted, proton density, and T2-weighted images (Fig. 2.**256**). At times an orbital varix may have the same MRI characteristics as a cavernous hemangioma or other orbital masses, being hypointense on T1-weighted and hyperintense on T2-weighted MR images, and enhancing on postcontrast T1-weighted MR images (Fig. 2.**256**).

An orbital varix may be seen as several round or tubular structures with associated calcifications (phleboliths) (Fig. 2.**257**).[8] Venous anomalies of the orbit including varices may be associated with contiguous or noncontiguous intracranial or extracranial venous anomalies (Figs. 2.**258**, 2.**259**).[131]

Carotid Cavernous Fistulas and AVM

Carotid cavernous fistulas produce proptosis, chemosis, venous engorgement, pulsating exophthalmos, and an auscultable bruit. Ischemic ocular necrosis resulting from carotid–cavernous fistula has been reported.[16, 135] A carotid–cavernous fistula may result from trauma or surgery, or it may occur spontaneously. Spon-

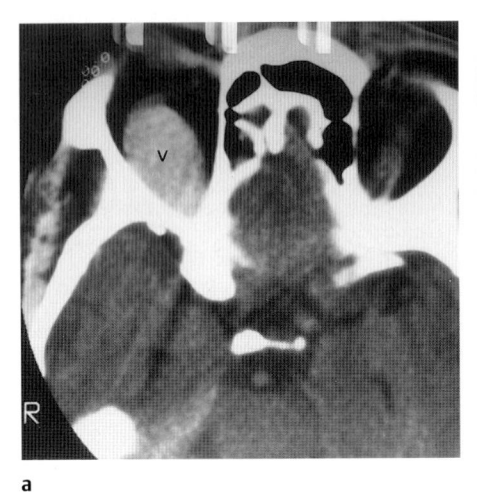

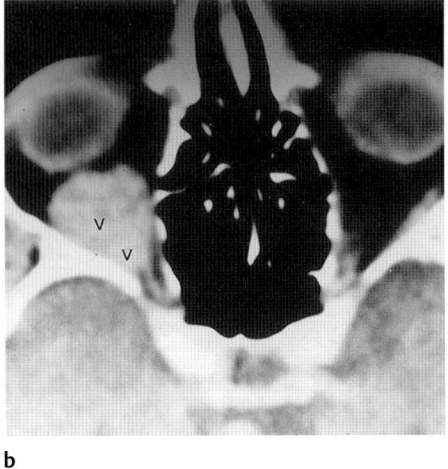

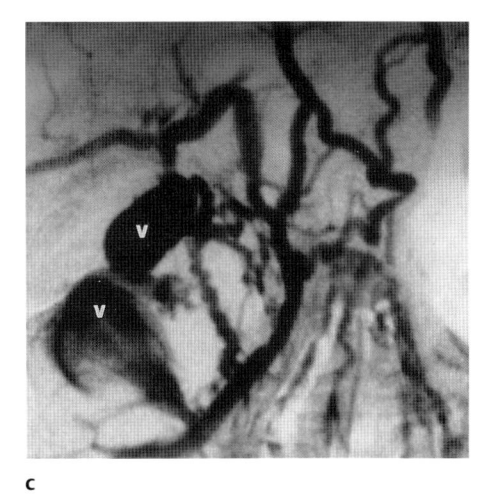

Fig. 2.**255** Orbital varix.
a Axial enhanced CT scan shows a large orbital varix (V), appearing to arise from the superior ophthalmic vein.
b Axial enhanced CT scan in another patient shows an orbital varix (V), appearing to arise from the inferior ophthalmic vein.
c Orbital venogram in another patient, showing massive dilatation of orbital veins compatible with varix (V). Case courtesy of John D. Bullock, MD, Dayton, OH, USA.

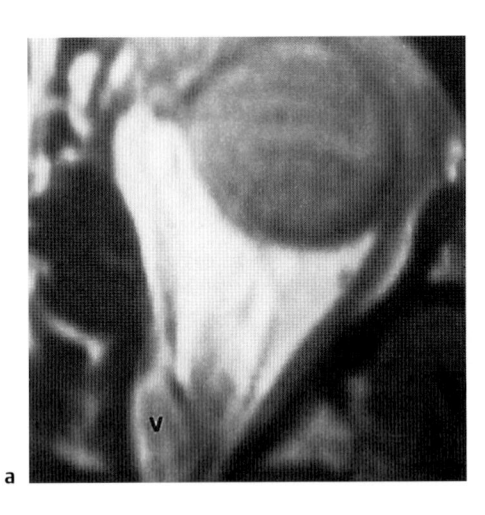

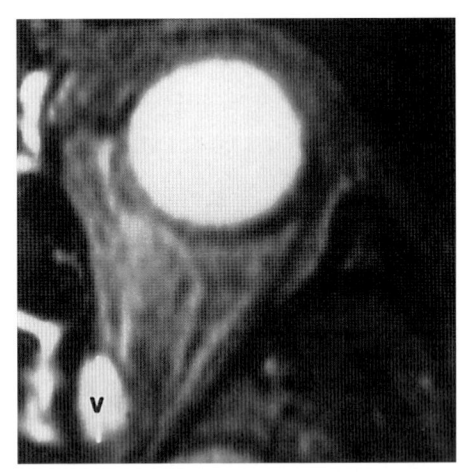

Fig. 2.**256** Orbital varix. **a** Axial PW and **b** T2W MR scans show a well-defined orbital mass compatible with orbital varix (V). This cannot be differentiated from a cavernous hemangioma. Engorgement of the mass following Valsalva maneuver on repeat MR or CT scans supports the diagnosis of varix.

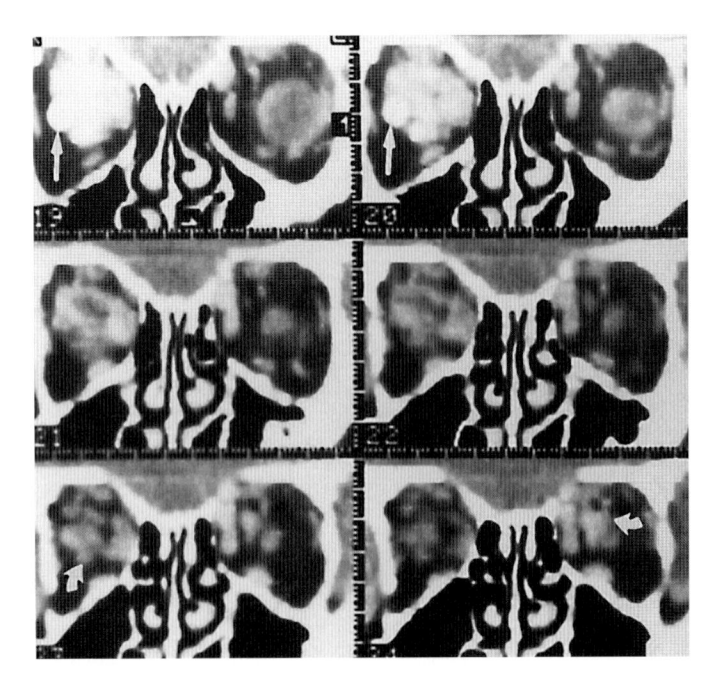

taneous carotid–cavernous fistula has been reported in patients with osteogenesis imperfecta, Ehlers–Danlos syndrome, and pseudoxanthoma elasticum. In these cases the fistula probably resulted from weakness of the vessel walls related to the connective-tissue disease.[135] CT and MRI demonstrate protopsis, with engorgement of the superior ophthalmic vein and infrequently the inferior ophthalmic vein and frequent enlargement of the ipsilateral extraocular muscles (Fig. 2.**260**). There may be CT or MRI evidence of venous thrombosis in the lumen of the superior ophthalmic vein or cavernous sinus. Arteriovenous shunts within the orbit itself are rare.[131] At times, anomalous intracranial venous malformations, and dural vascular malformations and fistulas may mimic the imaging appearance of carotid cavernous fistulas (Fig. 2.**261**).[135] Angiographic demonstration of the exact location of the carotid–cavernous fistula is essential for planning definitive therapy.

Fig. 2.**257** Orbital varix. Serial reformatted postcontrast CT scans show multiple bilateral enhancing masses (arrows). Note the round calcifications (straight arrows).

Pathology   261

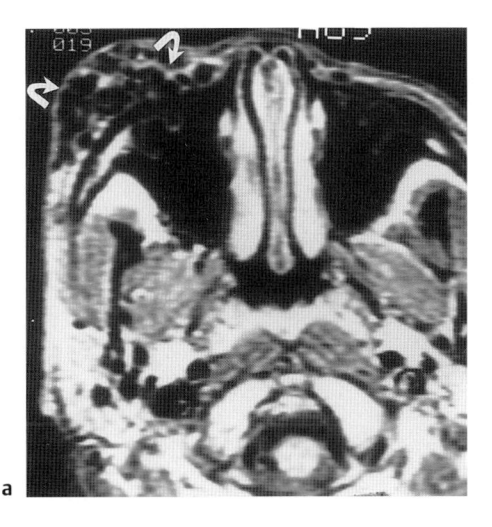

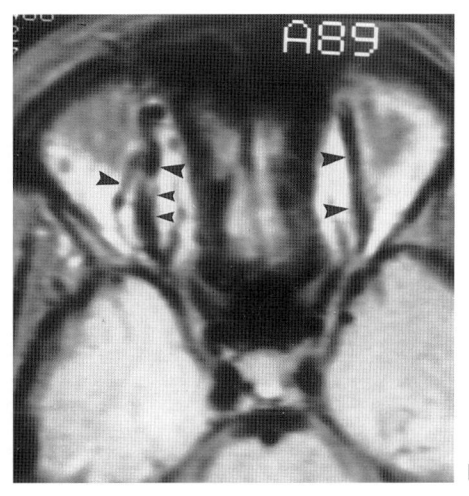

Fig. 2.**258** Orbitofacial vascular malformation.
a Axial PW MR scan shows multiple dilated vessels involving the right cheek region (arrows).
b Axial PW MR scan, taken superior to **a**, shows dilated right superior ophthalmic vein and its branches (arrows). The left superior ophthalmic vein (double arrows) appears normal.

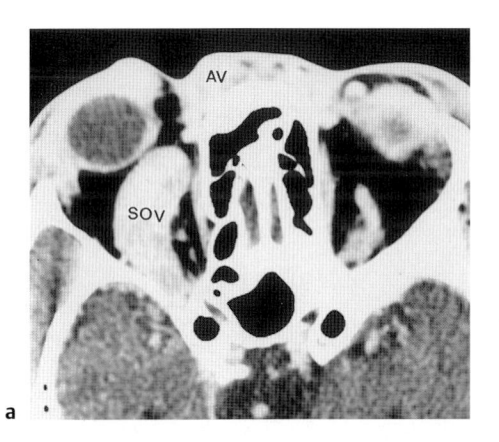

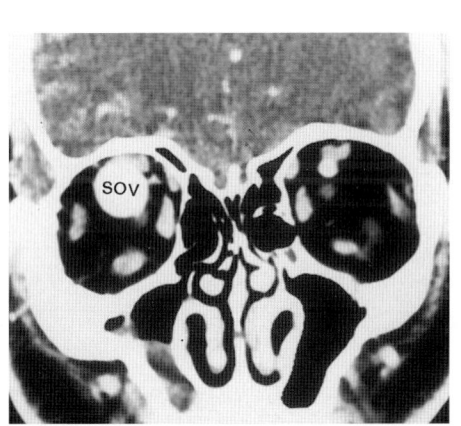

Fig. 2.**259** Dural vascular malformation.
a Axial enhanced CT scan shows marked dilatation of the right angular vein (AV) and superior ophthalmic vein (SOV). The left angular vein and superior ophthalmic vein also appear enlarged.
b Coronal enhanced CT scan shows marked dilatation of superior ophthalmic vein (SOV). Note increased vascularity of the right temporal lobe.

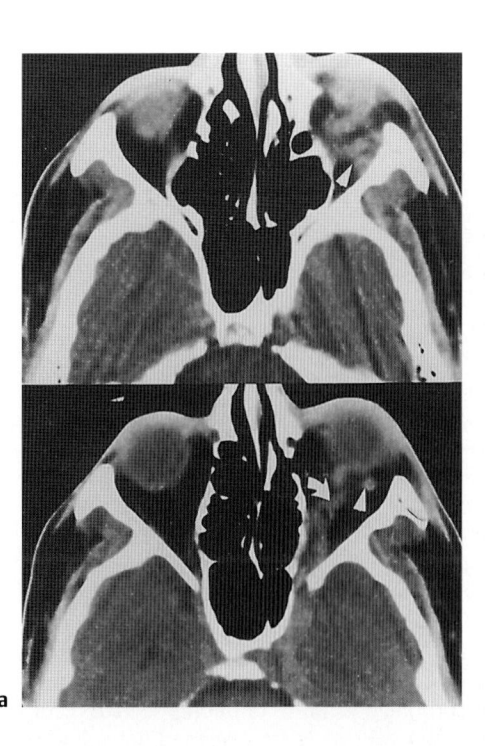

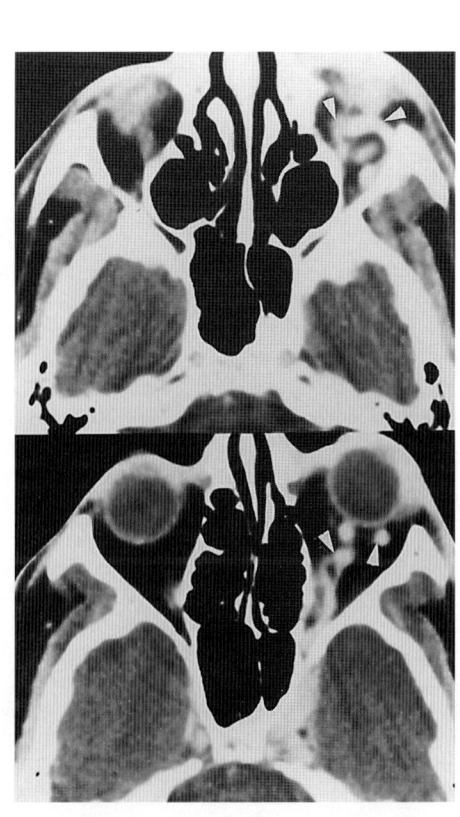

Fig. 2.**260** Carotid cavernous fistula. **a** Axial precontrast and **b** axial postcontrast CT scans show marked engorgement of orbital veins (arrowheads). Note increased contrast enhancement of both inferior and superior ophthalmic veins and collateral veins.

Fig. 2.**261** Dural vascular malformation mimicking carotid cavernous fistula. Sagittal PW MR scan shows marked dilatation of the superior ophthalmic vein (SOV). Note dilated vessels adjacent to the cavernous sinus (arrows) and engorged intracranial vessels (arrowheads).

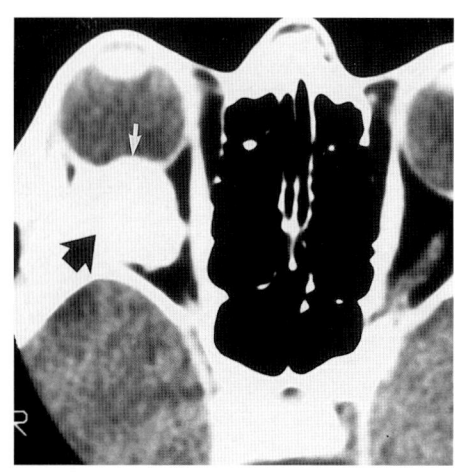

Fig. 2.**262** Hemangiopericytoma. Axial enhanced CT scan shows a large mass (arrows) with intense enhancement, compatible with a hemangiopericytoma. Note invasion of the globe (white arrow).

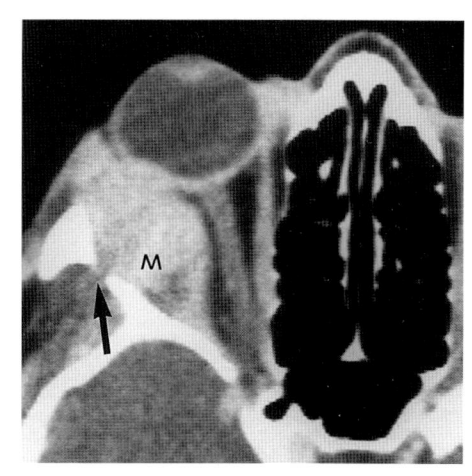

Fig. 2.**263** Hemangiopericytoma. Axial enhanced CT scan shows a large enhancing mass (M) compatible with hemangiopericytoma. Note focal bone erosion (arrow). Note that enhancement in this case is not as intense as seen in Fig. 2.**262**.

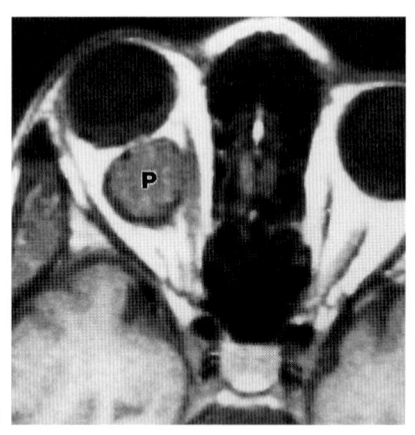

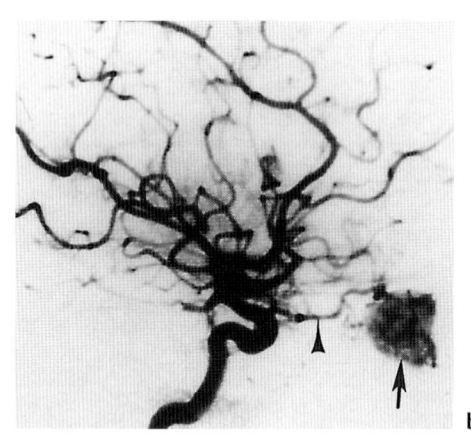

Fig. 2.**264** Hemangiopericytoma.
a T1W MR scan shows an intraconal hemangiopericytoma (P). Note focal invasion of adjacent medial rectus muscle.
b Angiogram shows a prominent ophthalmic artery (arrowhead), feeding hypervascular hemangiopericytoma (arrow).

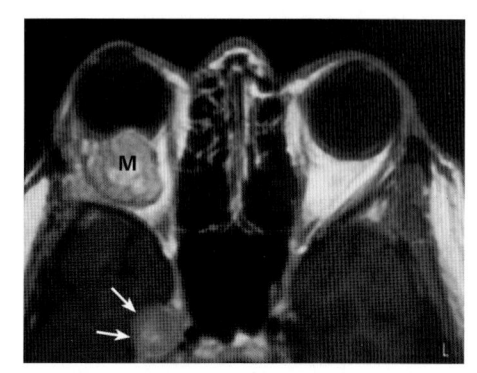

Fig. 2.**265** Recurrent hemangiopericytoma with perineural extension into the cavernous sinus. Axial enhanced T1W MR scan shows a large mass (M) compatible with recurrent hemangiopericytoma. Note perineural extension into the right cavernous sinus (arrows).

Hemangiopericytomas

Hemangiopericytomas are rare, slow-growing vascular neoplasms that arise from unique cells called pericytes of Zimmermann, which normally envelop capillaries and postcapillary venules of practically all types of tissues.[8, 136–138] Histologically these tumors are composed of scattered, capillary-like spaces surrounded by proliferating pericytes.[2, 8] Hemangiopericytomas may be divided into lobules by fibrovascular septa.[8, 136] About 50 % of the cases are malignant; distant metastases, although uncommon, occur via the vascular and lymphatic routes.[8, 139] Most such metastases go to the lungs.[8, 136, 138] If hemangioblastomas are not excised completely, they will recur. Wide surgical excision is the treatment of choice.

On CT the margins of an orbital hemangiopericytoma, in contrast to a cavernous hemangioma, may be slightly less distinct owing to its tendency to invade the adjacent tissues (Fig. 2.**262**).[8, 16] Erosion of the orbital bone may be present (Fig. 2.**263**), and marked contrast enhancement and hypervascularity are characteristic of hemangiopericytoma (Figs. 2.**262**, 2.**264**). Follow-up CT or MRI is extremely important to diagnose recurrence (Fig. 2.**265**). MRI and CT scanning may not differentiate these tumors from cavernous hemangiomas, neurogenic tumors, meningiomas, and other lesions (Figs. 2.**264**–2.**266**). Angiography may differentiate the tumors from cavernous hemangioma, meningiomas, and schwannomas.[8] Hemangiopericytomas usually have an early florid blush (Figs. 2.**264b**, 2.**266c**), and cavernous hemangiomas show a late minor pooling of contrast, or often appear as avascular masses.[8, 133, 140] Meningiomas may show multiple tumor vessels and a late blush, and schwannomas may show no tumor blush.[8, 16, 139, 140] Hemangiopericytomas may be difficult to differentiate from other rare vasculogenic tumors such as angioleiomyomas, malignant hemangioendotheliomas (angiosarcomas), and fibrous histiocytomas.[8] Hemangiopericytomas may originate from the sinonasal cavities and then invade the orbit (Fig. 2.**267**). Calcification is not a feature of hemangiopericytoma. It is more commonly seen in recurrent hemangiopericytoma following surgery and/or radiation therapy (Fig. 2.**267a**).

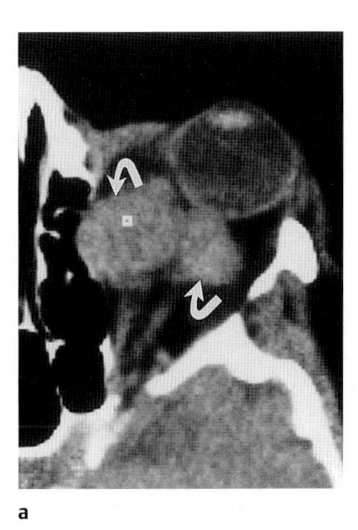

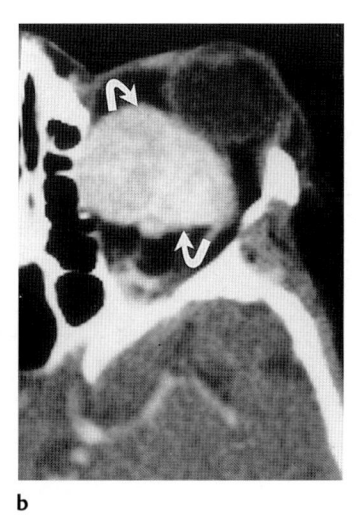

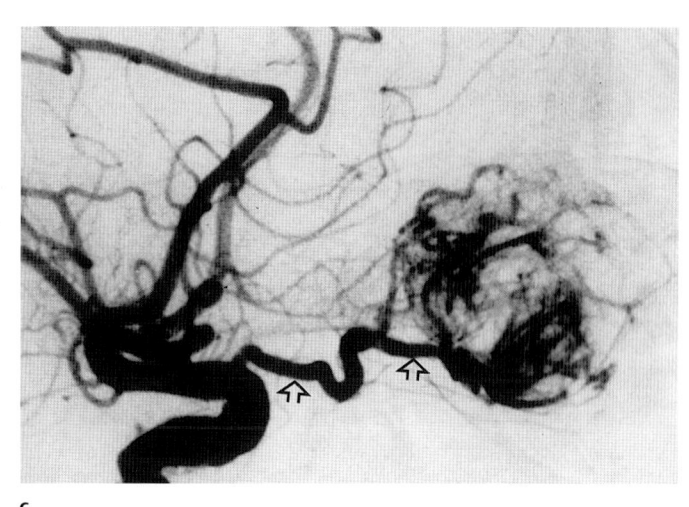

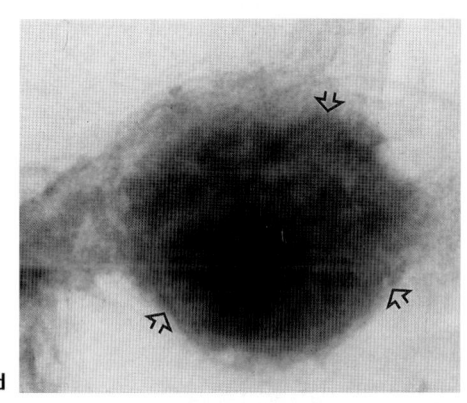

Fig. 2.**266** Hemangiopericytoma. **a** Axial unenhanced and **b** enhanced CT scans showing a large hemangiopericytoma (arrows). A cavernous hemangioma, exophytic optic nerve sheath meningioma, neurofibroma, fibrous histiocytoma, and orbital lymphoma may simulate this lesion. **c** Angiogram shows marked enlargement of ophthalmic artery (arrows) and intense vascularity of the hemangiopericytoma. **d** Angiogram (delayed capillary phase) shows marked tumor blush (arrows), characteristic of hemangiopericytoma.

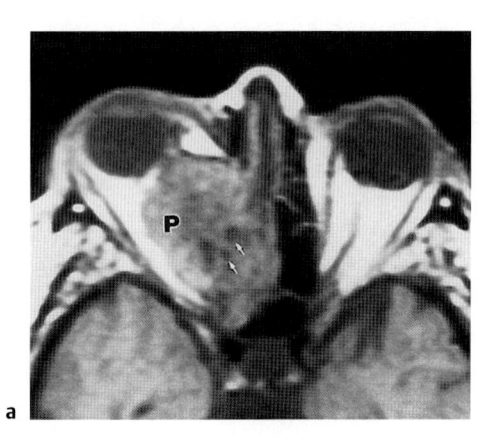

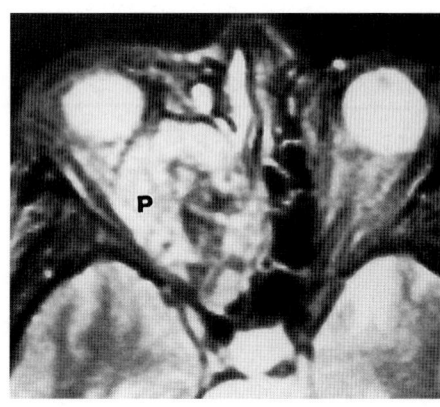

Fig. 2.**267** Hemangiopericytoma of the sinonasal cavity with secondary orbital involvement.
a Axial T1W MR scan shows a large hemangiopericytoma (P) invading the adjacent ethmoid. The hypointense areas (arrows) were due to calcifications, seen on CT but not shown here.
b Axial T2W MR scan shows the hemangiopericytoma (P).

Neural Lesions

Orbital Schwannomas

The orbit is host to many peripheral nerves. Approximately 4% of all orbital neoplasms are peripheral nerve tumors and primarily consist of neurofibromas and neurilemomas or Schwannomas. Of these, 2% of the lesions are plexiform neurofibromatosis; 1% isolated neurofibromas; and 1% Schwannoma (Figs. 2.**268**–2.**276**).[141]

Schwannomas are benign, slow-growing nerve sheath tumors that may arise anywhere within the orbit, although they are most common in the intraconal space.[8, 105, 106, 141] The malignant counterpart, the malignant schwannoma (malignant neurilemoma, neurogenic sarcoma, neurofibrosarcoma, and fibrosarcoma of the nerve sheath), is exceedingly rare in the orbit.[2, 8, 141] The optic nerve has no Schwann cells; orbital schwannomas must therefore arise from peripheral nerve fibers of the III, IV, V, VI, VII and autonomic nerves. Schwannomas and neurofibromas commonly involve the sensory nerves and are primarily differentiated on histopathology. Schwannomas are well-encapsulated by the perineurium of the nerve of origin and in contrast to neurofibromas, schwannomas do display clear-cut evidence of Schwann cell origin.[2, 16] Histologically they are surrounded by a thin, fibrous capsule that is formed by compression of perineural tissue. The tumor is composed of compactly arranged, spindle-shaped cells that interlace in cords and whorls, frequently oriented with their long axis parallel to one another. This cellular pattern is referred to as Antoni type A.[2, 8, 106, 141] Commonly, the Antoni type B part of the tumor has a less cellular pattern, which is characterized by haphazardly distributed cells in a collagenous matrix.[2, 6, 16, 106, 141] On CT and MRI orbital schwannomas appear as sharply marginated, oval or fusiform, intraconal or extraconal

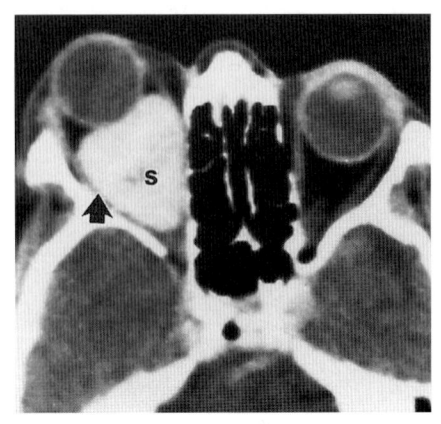

Fig. 2.268 Orbital schwannoma. Axial postcontrast CT scan shows a well-defined enhancing intraconal mass compatible with a schwannoma. (S). The mass abuts the lateral rectus (arrow) without involving it. The differential diagnosis should include cavernous hemangioma, hemangiopericytoma, optic nerve sheath meningioma, neurofibroma, and fibrous histiocytoma.

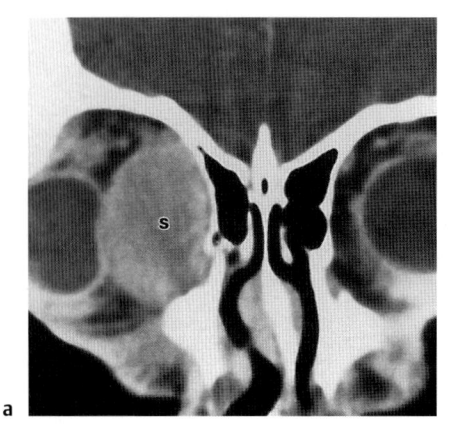

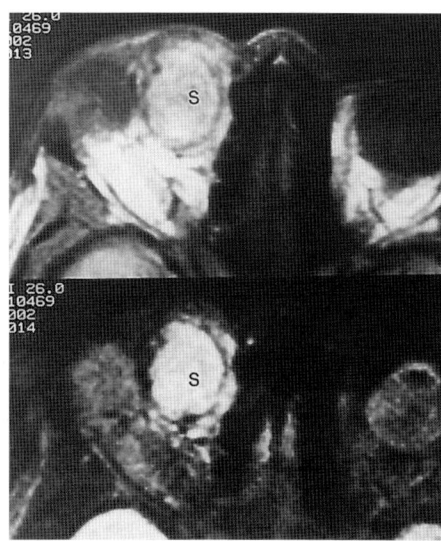

Fig. 2.269 Extraconal orbital schwannoma.
a Coronal postcontrast CT scan shows a well-defined (capsulated) enhancing mass compatible with a schwannoma (S). The extraconal nature of the lesion is better appreciated in the axial sections in **b**.
b Axial PW (top) and T2W (bottom) MR scans show the schwannoma (S). The medial rectus muscle was displaced laterally on lower sections not shown here. The differential diagnosis should include fibrous histiocytoma, hemangiopericytoma, neurofibroma, lymphoma, and rhabdomyosarcoma (rare in adult).

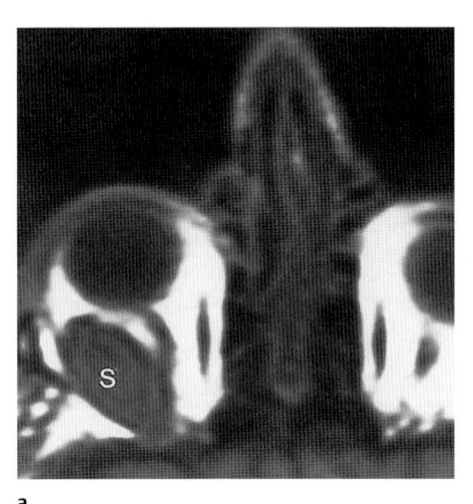

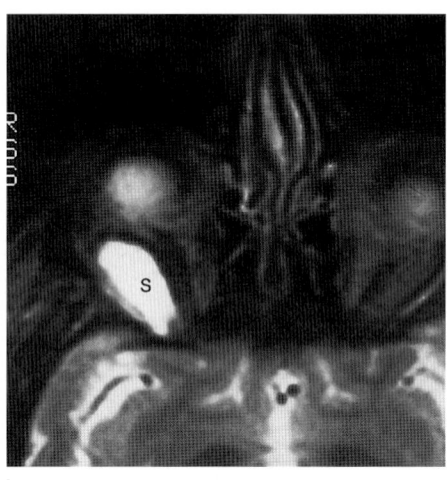

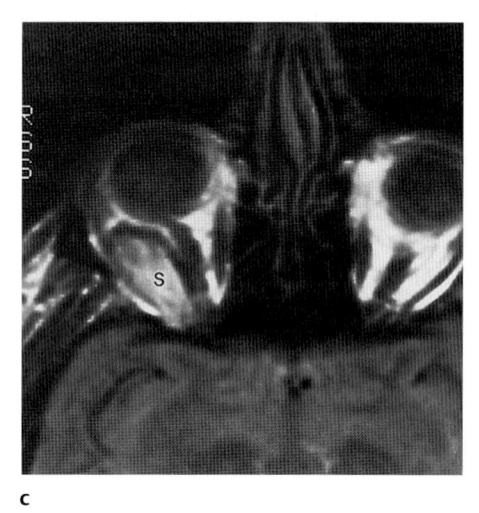

Fig. 2.270 Orbital schwannoma. **a** Axial T1W, **b** T2W and **c** axial postcontrast T1W MR scans show an orbital schwannoma (S). The differential diagnosis should include cavernous hemangioma, hemangiopericytoma, and fibrous histiocytoma.

masses, which demonstrate moderate to marked enhancement (Figs. 2.**268**–2.**272**). The optic nerve is always displaced and may be engulfed by the tumor (Fig. 2.**268**). Both schwannoma and neurofibroma may show areas of marked enhancement as well as areas of minimal or no enhancement (Fig. 2.**271 b**). On T2-weighted MR images, the myxoid regions of the tumor with its greater water content shows a greater signal intensity, as compared with the more cellular regions of the tumor (Figs. 2.**271 e**).

Neurofibroma

Neurofibromas may occur in one of four patterns: (1) plexiform, (2) diffuse, (3) localized or circumscribed, and (4) postamputation neuromas.[2, 141] When most of the fascicles in a segment of peripheral nerve are involved, cylindrical enlargement of the entire nerve segment is observed. This clinical and gross pathological configuration is referred to as plexiform neurofibroma.[6, 16, 141] Plexiform neurofibromas present in infancy or childhood and most commonly involve the eyelids (see Fig. 2.**216 a**). The tumor consists of cords and nodules giving rise to a "bag of worms" on palpation. Plexiform neurofibroma involvement of the eyelid is considered to be virtually pathognomonic for neurofibromatosis (von Recklinghausen disease).[141] Diffuse neurofibromas have an appearance similar to plexiform neurofibromatosis, with infiltration of orbital fat and extraocular muscles, but those lesions are less likely to be associated with von Recklinghausen disease.[2, 141] Circumscribed or localized neurofibromas often present as a slow-growing tumor that exerts a mass effect with displacement of the globe (Fig. 2.**273**). The tumor may occur along any sensory nerve but is more common in the superior quadrants (Figs. 2.**274**, 2.**275**). When arising from the lacrimal nerve, it may have the clinical appearance of a lacrimal gland tumor.

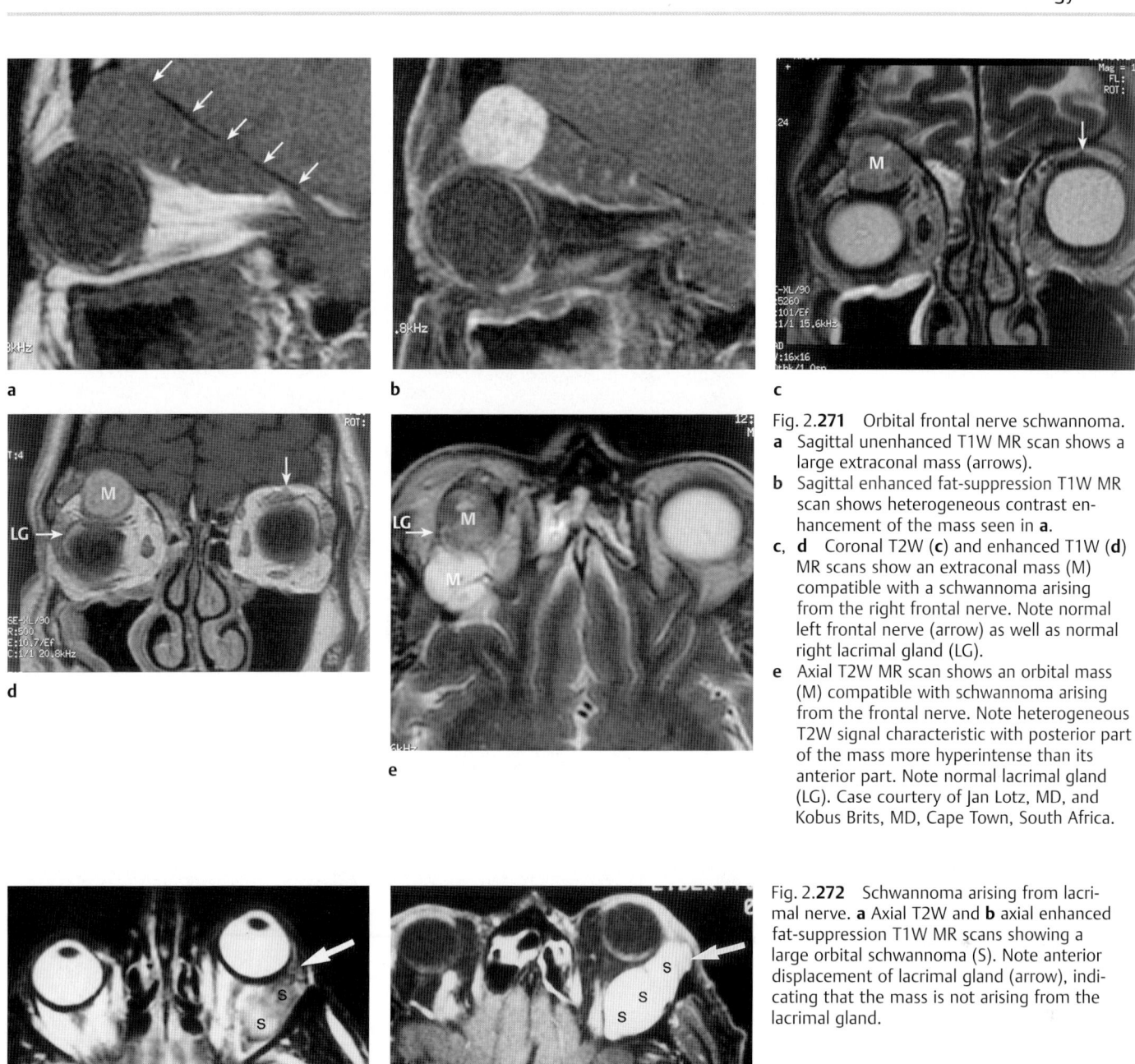

Pathology 265

Fig. 2.**271** Orbital frontal nerve schwannoma.
a Sagittal unenhanced T1W MR scan shows a large extraconal mass (arrows).
b Sagittal enhanced fat-suppression T1W MR scan shows heterogeneous contrast enhancement of the mass seen in **a**.
c, d Coronal T2W (**c**) and enhanced T1W (**d**) MR scans show an extraconal mass (M) compatible with a schwannoma arising from the right frontal nerve. Note normal left frontal nerve (arrow) as well as normal right lacrimal gland (LG).
e Axial T2W MR scan shows an orbital mass (M) compatible with schwannoma arising from the frontal nerve. Note heterogeneous T2W signal characteristic with posterior part of the mass more hyperintense than its anterior part. Note normal lacrimal gland (LG). Case courtesy of Jan Lotz, MD, and Kobus Brits, MD, Cape Town, South Africa.

Fig. 2.**272** Schwannoma arising from lacrimal nerve. **a** Axial T2W and **b** axial enhanced fat-suppression T1W MR scans showing a large orbital schwannoma (S). Note anterior displacement of lacrimal gland (arrow), indicating that the mass is not arising from the lacrimal gland.

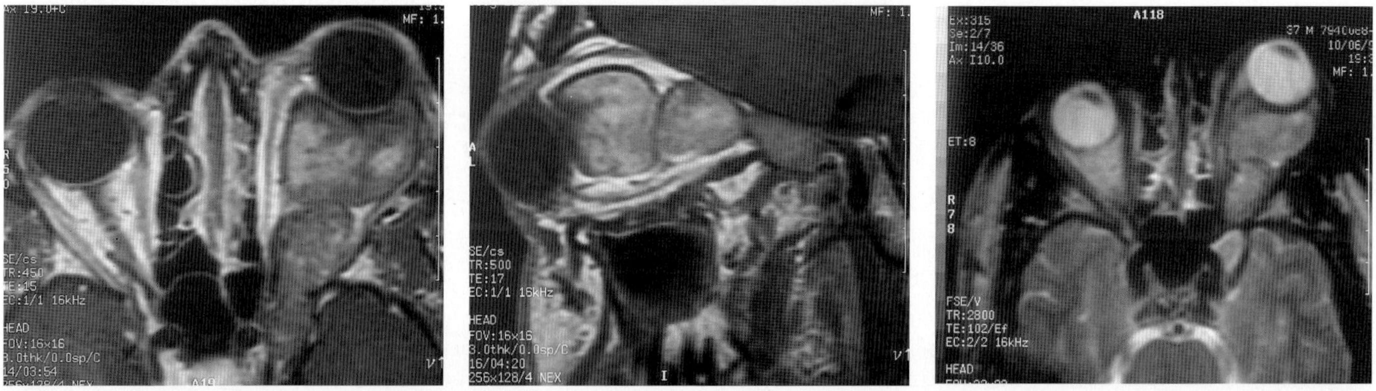

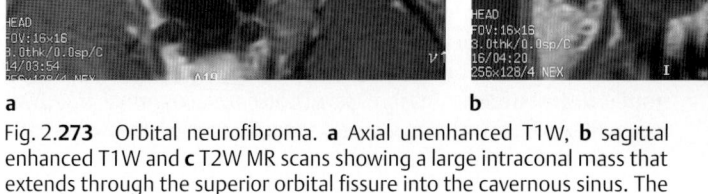

Fig. 2.**273** Orbital neurofibroma. **a** Axial unenhanced T1W, **b** sagittal enhanced T1W and **c** T2W MR scans showing a large intraconal mass that extends through the superior orbital fissure into the cavernous sinus. The extension into the cavernous sinus indicates that the lesion is not arising from the optic nerve, making the diagnosis of neurofibroma most likely.

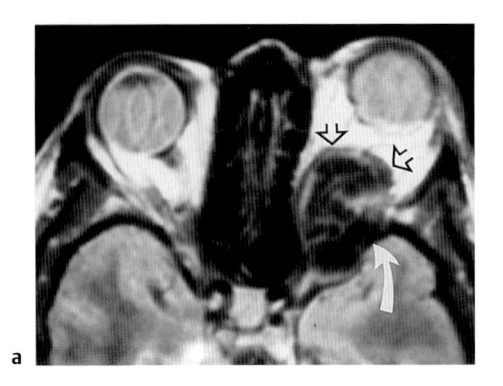

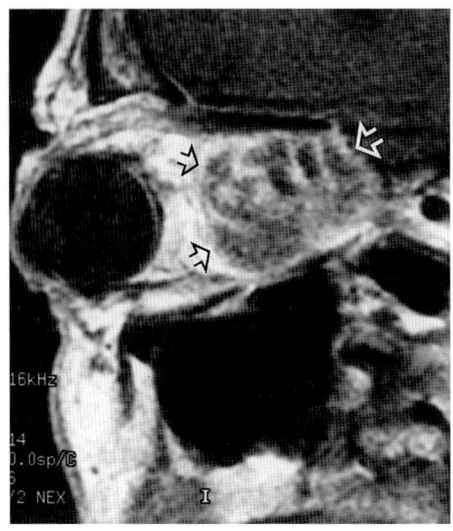

Fig. 2.274 Orbital neurofibroma. **a** Axial T2W and **b** sagittal enhanced T1W MR scans showing a neurofibroma (arrows). The mass shows hypointensity in the T2W MR image (**a**), related to dense fibrous stroma. Compare this case with the cases in Figs. 2.**269** and 2.**270**.

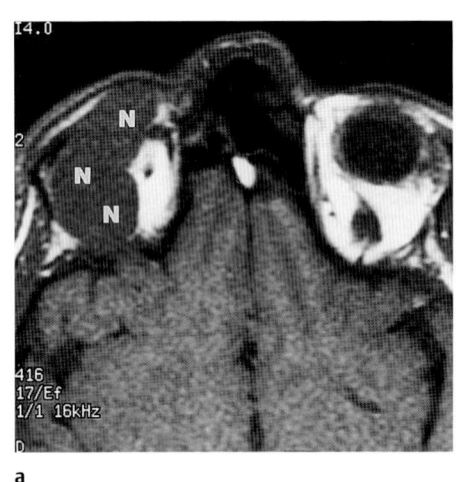

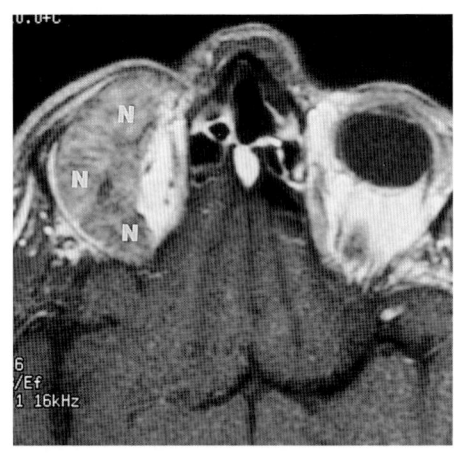

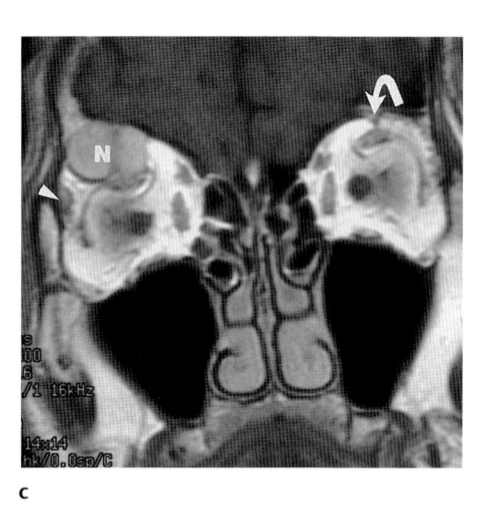

Fig. 2.275 Orbital frontal nerve neurofibroma. **a** Axial unenhanced T1W, **b** axial enhanced T1W, and **c** coronal enhanced T1W MR scans showing a large mass compatible with a neurofibroma (N) arising from the right frontal nerve. Note normal left frontal nerve (curved arrow). The tumor is separated from the lacrimal gland (arrowhead).

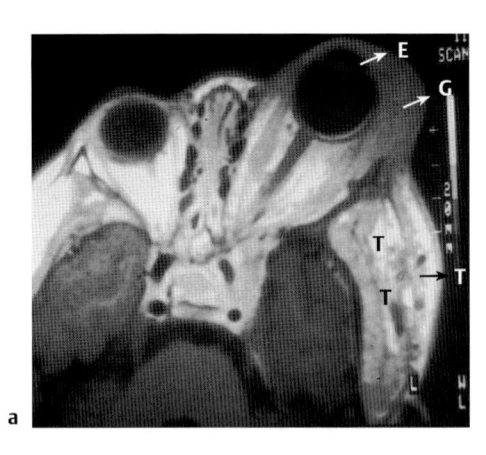

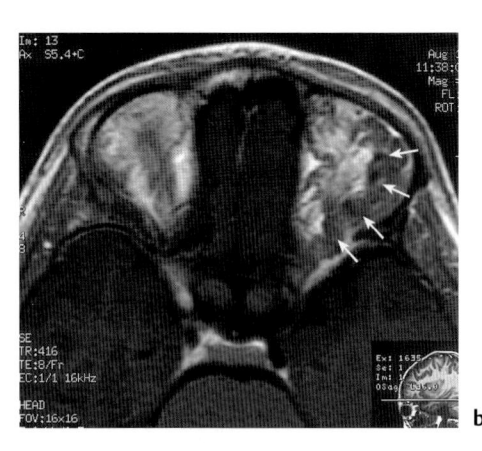

Fig. 2.276 a Plexiform neurofibromatosis. Axial enhanced T1W MR scan shows diffuse neurofibroma involving the left eyelid (E), lacrimal gland (G) lateral and medial rectus muscles, and neurofibroma involving the left temporal fossa (T). The left globe is enlarged and the entire uveal tract shows increased enhancement. The enhancement of the uveal tract was due to neurofibroma involving the choroid. Case courtesy of Ahmed A. Hidayat, MD, AFIP, Washington, DC, USA.
  b Plexiform neurofibromatosis. Axial enhanced MR scan in another patient with NF1 shows plexiform neurofibroma involving the superior left orbit (arrows).
  Fig. 2.**276 c** ▷

Orbital plexiform and diffuse neurofibromas appear as an ill-defined mass with extension into surrounding tissues and at times through the inferior and superior orbital fissures (Figs. 2.**276 a,b**). The CT and MRI appearance of malignant nerve sheath tumors is similar to nonmalignant tumors with the exception of bone destruction. Bilateral frontal nerve neurofibroma (Fig. 2.**276 c**) and intramuscular neurofibroma, resulting in enlargement of extraocular muscles, may be seen in patients with neurofibromatosis. The differential diagnoses of orbital schwannoma and neurofibroma are cavernous hemangioma, meningioma, fibrous histiocytoma, neurofibroma, fibrocystoma, hemangiopericytoma, and metastasis.

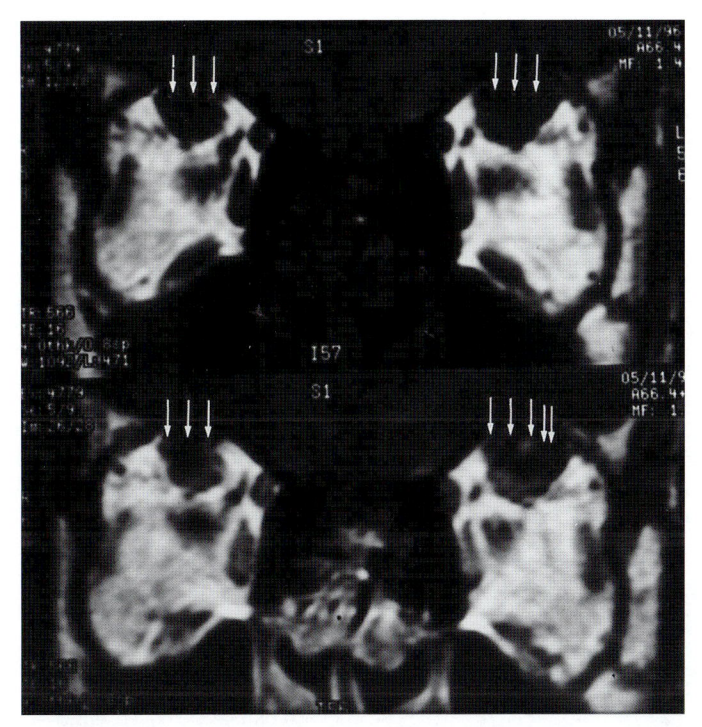

Fig. 2.**276c** Bilateral frontal nerve neurofibroma. Coronal T1W MR scan in another patient with NF1 shows bilateral frontal nerve neurofibromas (arrows).

■ Nontumoral and Tumoral Enlargement of the Optic Nerve Sheath

Optic Neuritis

This condition is an acute inflammatory process involving the optic nerve that may present as optic nerve enlargement.[2, 16] Multiple sclerosis is the most common cause of optic neuritis. Visual loss is typically unilateral in patients with optic neuritis, but it may be bilateral.[142] Radiation optic neuropathy is another cause of optic neuritis. Optic neuritis in children differs from that in adults, including a greater incidence of disk swelling and a tendency for bilateral simultaneous involvement.[142] Optic neuritis is often an early manifestation of multiple sclerosis, and on CT and MRI there may be some enlargement of the optic nerve, usually with some degree of contrast enhancement (Figs. 2.**277**–2.**281**). On MRI the optic nerve may appear thickened and hyperintense on T2-weighted images (Fig. 2.**280**).[15] In cases of optic neuritis, the MRI visualization of multiple sclerosis plaques may be accentuated by inversion recovery (STIR) technique.[2, 16] Postcontrast, fat-suppression T1-weighted MR images may be the best technique to demonstrate optic neuritis. Localized or diffuse areas of enhancement are seen within the nerve (Figs. 2.**280**, 2.**281**). In general, in patients with optic neuritis contrast enhancement on

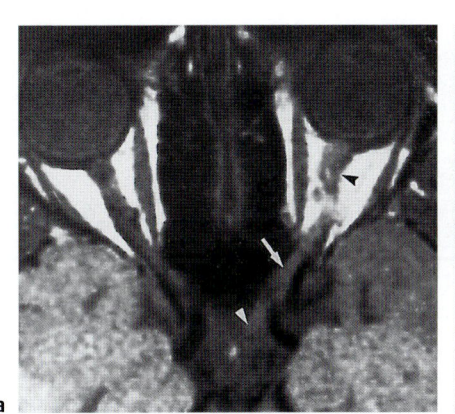

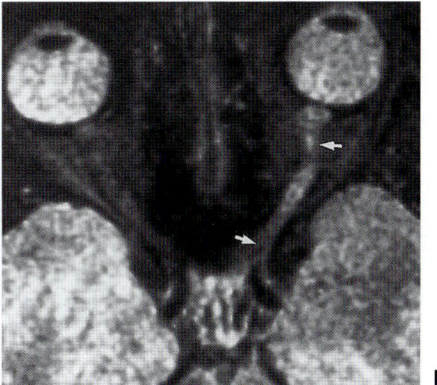

Fig. 2.**277** Optic neuritis. **a** Axial PW and **b** T2W MR scans show diffuse enlargement of the left optic nerve (arrows) in this 14-year-old girl with optic neuritis. The left optic nerve appears slightly more hyperintense compared to the uninvolved right optic nerve.

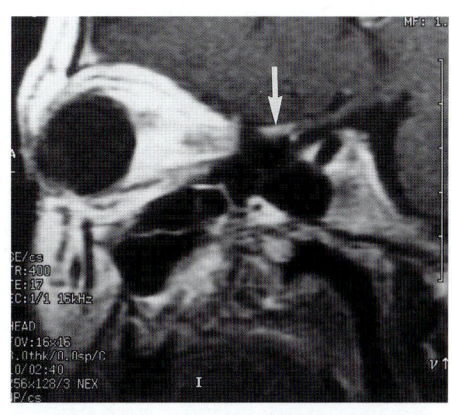

Fig. 2.**278** Optic neuritis. Sagittal enhanced T1W MR scan shows focal increased enhancement of the optic nerve (arrow), compatible with optic neuritis.

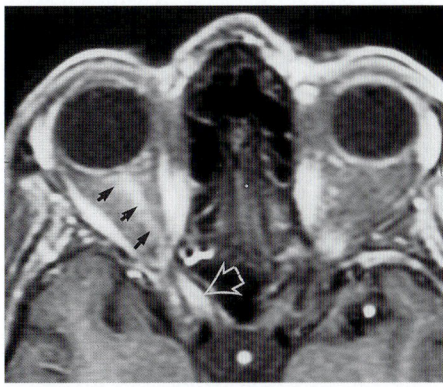

Fig. 2.**279** Optic neuritis. Axial enhanced fat-suppression T1W MR scans, showing diffuse enhancement of right optic nerve (arrows), including its intracanalicular segment (hollow arrow), compatible with demyelinating optic neuritis. Sarcoidosis may have a similar MR appearance.

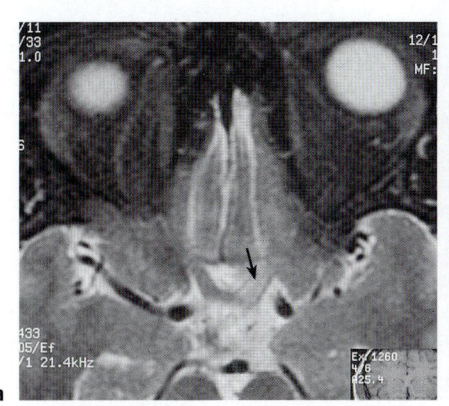

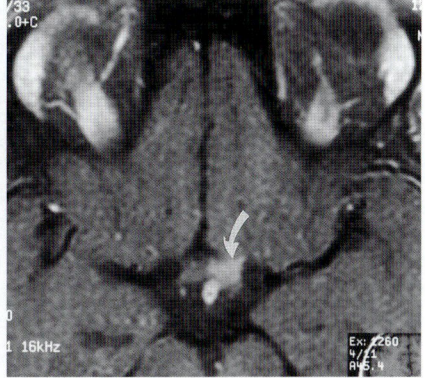

Fig. 2.**280** Optic neuritis localized to its intracranial segment. **a** Axial T2W and **b** axial enhanced fat-suppression T1W MR scans showing optic nerve involvement due to a demyelinating process limited to the intracranial segment of the left optic nerve. The lesion appears hyperintense in T2W and shows moderate enhancement (arrow).

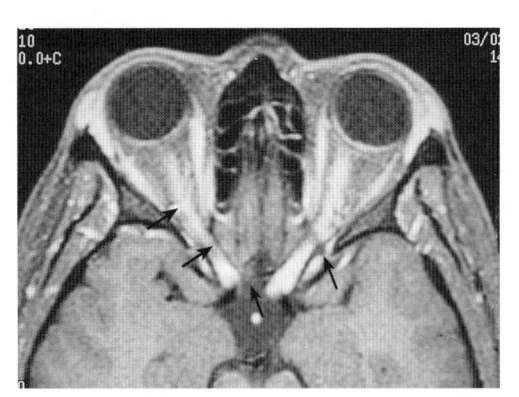

Fig. 2.281 Bilateral optic neuritis. Axial enhanced T1W MR scan shows increased enhancement of the optic nerves (arrows) in a patient with bilateral optic neuritis due to biopsy-proven demyelinating disease.

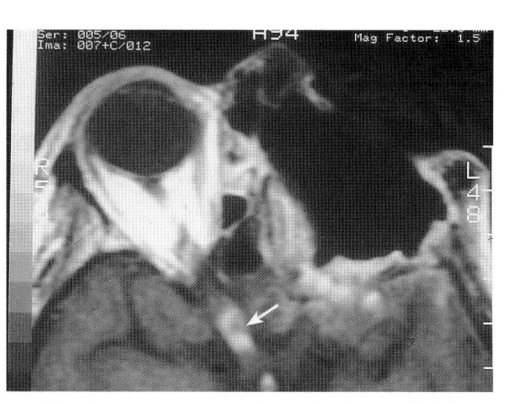

Fig. 2.282 Optic neuritis due to radiation therapy. Axial enhanced fat-suppression T1W MR scan shows enhancement of the right optic nerve (arrow) due to radiation optic neuritis. Note the postsurgical appearance of the left orbit following exenteration for an advanced carcinoma of the sinonasal cavities.

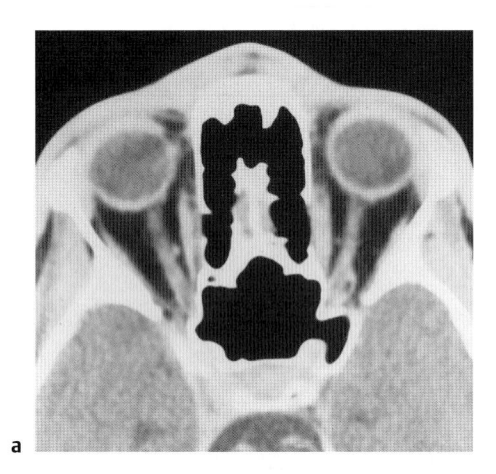

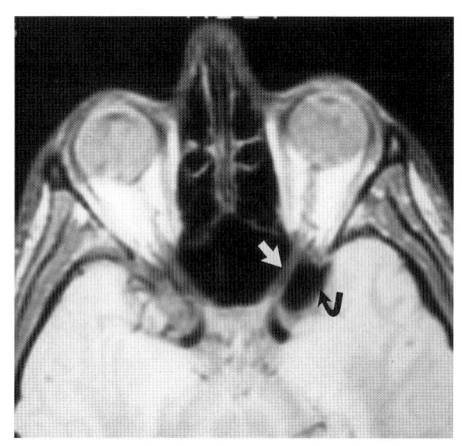

Fig. 2.283 Pneumosinus dilatans. **a** Axial CT scan and **b** axial PW MR scan showing pneumatization of the left anterior clinoid (black arrow). Note the intracanalicular segment of the left optic nerve (white arrow). The cortical bony outline of the left optic canal adjacent to the optic nerve is thinned out.

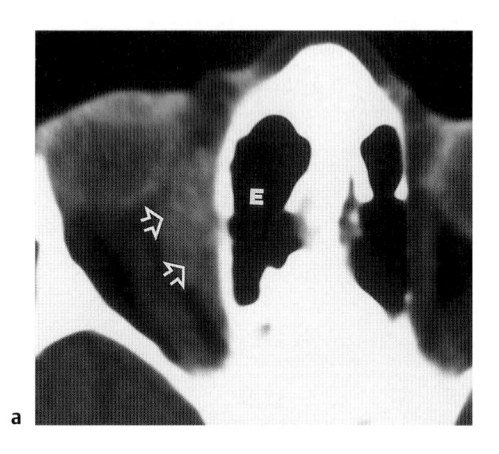

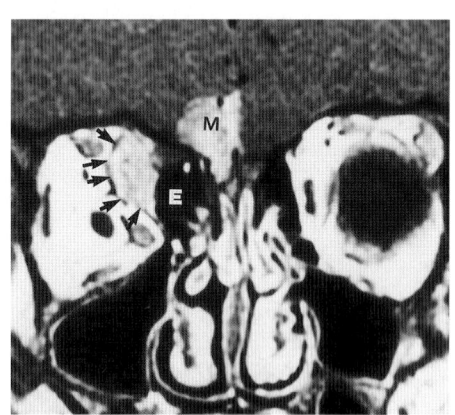

Fig. 2.284 Pneumosinus dilatans associated with meningioma.
a Axial CT scan shows a soft-tissue mass (arrows) involving the right orbit. Note dilatation of the right ethmoid sinus (E).
b Coronal enhanced T1W MR scan shows a meningioma (M) and its extension into the right orbit (arrows). Note dilatation of right ethmoid sinus (E). Case courtesy of Dr. E.L. Tajudine, Saudi Arabia.

CT and MRI is often subtle or present in a short segment of the optic nerve, particularly the intracanalicular portion of it (Figs. 2.**278**, 2.**280**, 2.**282**).

Pneumosinus Dilatans and Optic Neuropathy

Pneumosinus dilatans is a rare condition in which there is hyperpneumatization of paranasal sinuses lined with normal mucosa. In this condition, excessive pneumatization can lead to thinning and gross dehiscence of the bony wall. The frontal sinus is the most commonly affected, but the sphenoid sinus is the most important for visual loss because of its intimate relation with the optic canal (Fig. 2.**283**).[143] Sphenoidal or sphenoethmoidal pneumosinus dilatans may be associated with visual symptoms.[143] Pneumosinus dilatans has been associated with meningioma and fibro-osseous lesions (Fig. 2.**284**).[143] Pneumosinus dilatans without an associated pathological process rarely causes visual loss (Fig. 2.**283**). We have reported three cases of pneumosinus dilatans of the sphenoid sinus associated with visual loss.[143] The mechanism leading to optic neuropathy is uncertain. With direct communication between the sinus and the optic canal, one could postulate a direct compressive effect

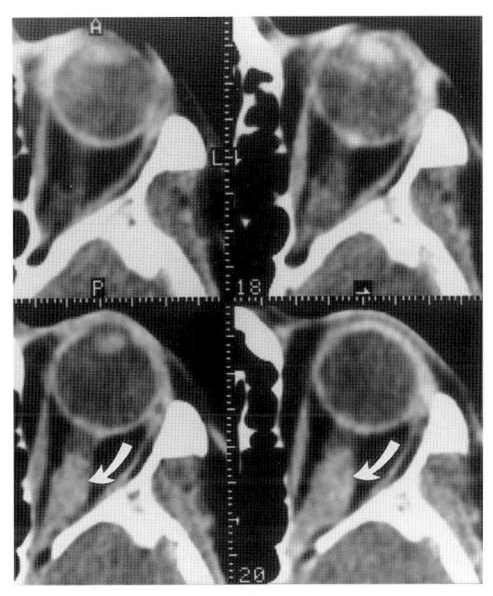

Fig. 2.**285** Optic nerve sheath meningioma. Axial enhanced CT scans showing tubular enlargement of the left optic nerve (arrows), compatible with optic nerve sheath meningioma.

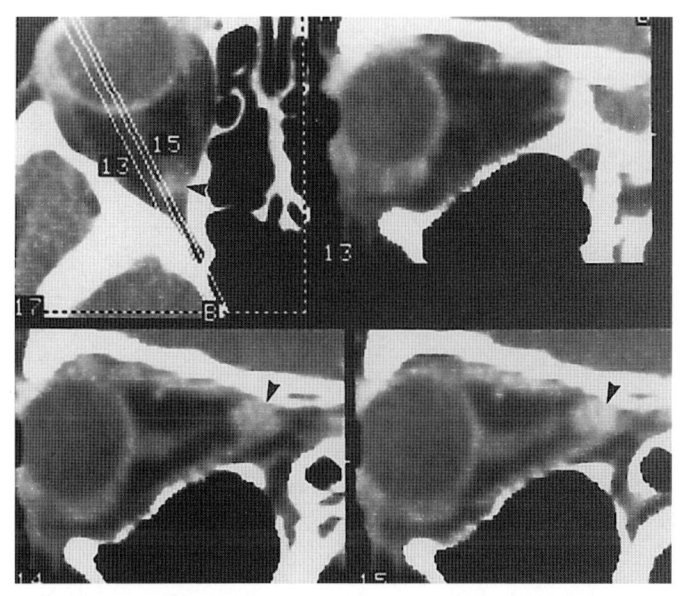

Fig. 2.**286** Optic nerve sheath meningioma. Serial reformatted sagittal CT scans showing a meningioma involving the apical segment of the optic nerve (arrowheads).

by mucosa or air leading to ischemic damage.[143] It has been suggested that sudden elevation of the intrasinus pressure, as with sneezing or with altitude change, may cause direct damage to an exposed optic nerve.[143]

Optic Nerve Sheath Meningioma

Optic nerve meningioma arises either from the arachnoid cells (meningothelial) covering the optic nerve or from an extension into the orbit (optic canal) of an intracranial meningioma. Another rare group of meningiomas consists of tumors that arise from ectopic arachnoid cells within the orbital cavity, either in the muscle cone or in the walls of the orbit. These ectopic intraorbital "extradural" meningiomas do not appear to have any connection to the optic nerve sheath or the optic canal and do not appear to originate intracranially. Their origin is uncertain, but they probably arise from congenitally displaced nests of meningothelial cells along the orbital walls or within the muscle cone. They are frequently associated with characteristic, localized expansion of adjacent ethmoid air cells, which is termed "blistering" (Fig. 2.**284**). Meningiomas are usually seen in middle-aged women. Childhood optic nerve meningioma is rare, but the disease is much more aggressive than the adult form. Bilateral optic nerve meningiomas may occur in patients with or without neurofibromatosis. Bilateral optic nerve gliomas, however, always occur in patients with neurofibromatosis (NF1).

CT is an excellent imaging study for evaluating optic nerve meningiomas. CT is best performed with and without infusion of iodinated contrast medium. Thin sections, 1.5–3 mm, are essential to visualize the actual extent of the tumor. Since optic nerve meningioma is confined to the dura mater, it appears as a well-defined tubular thickening in 64% of the cases (Fig. 2.**285**).[2, 16, 142] Optic nerve sheath meningiomas are commonly seen as localized eccentric expansion, often at the orbital apex (Figs. 2.**286**, 2.**287**). Following intravenous administration of contrast media, meningiomas often show homogeneous and well-defined enhancement. The "tram-track" sign originally described with optic nerve meningioma, where enhanced CT shows lucency in the center of an enlarged optic nerve sheath complex with peripheral enhancement, is not a specific finding in optic nerve meningioma.[16, 142] This pattern of enhancement may be seen in pseudotumors and optic neuritis.[16] On CT images, linear or granular calcifications within an optic nerve mass are almost always an indication of optic nerve sheath meningioma (Fig. 2.**288**).[16]

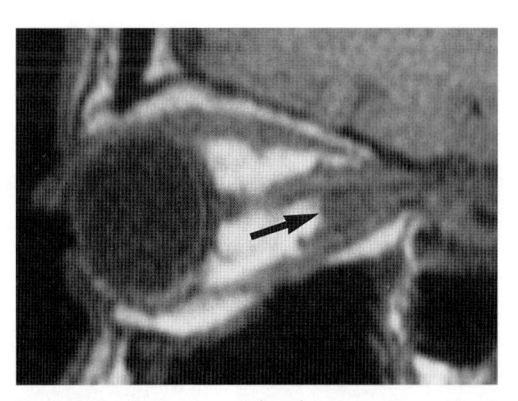

Fig. 2.**287** Optic nerve sheath meningioma. Sagittal T1W MR scan shows a localized eccentric enlargement of the optic nerve, compatible with surgically proven meningioma (arrow).

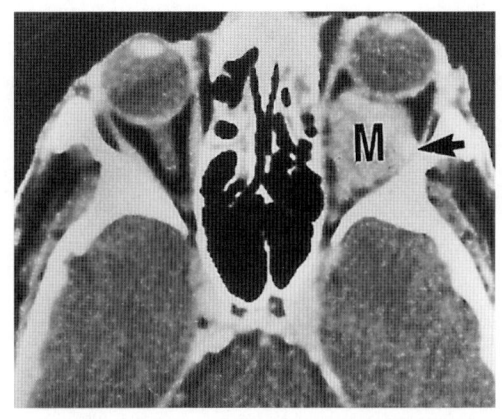

Fig. 2.**288** Optic nerve sheath meningioma. Axial postcontrast CT scan shows an enhancing mass (M) growing around the left optic nerve. Note the small calcifications (arrow), characteristic of meningiomas.

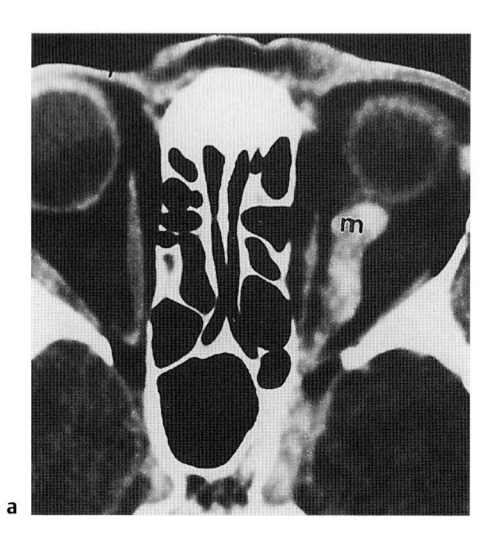

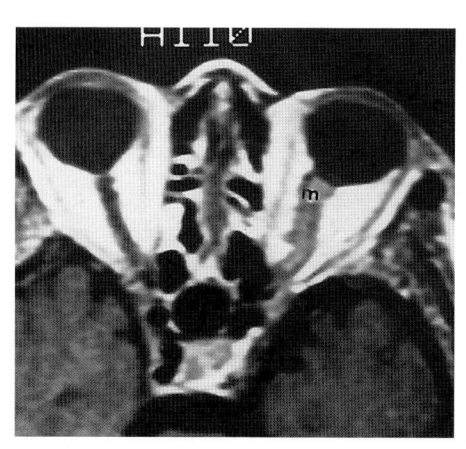

Fig. 2.**289** Optic nerve sheath meningioma.
a Axial postcontrast CT scan shows an enhancing mass (m) along the left optic nerve.
b Axial postcontrast T1W MR scan shows moderate enhancement of the meningioma (m).

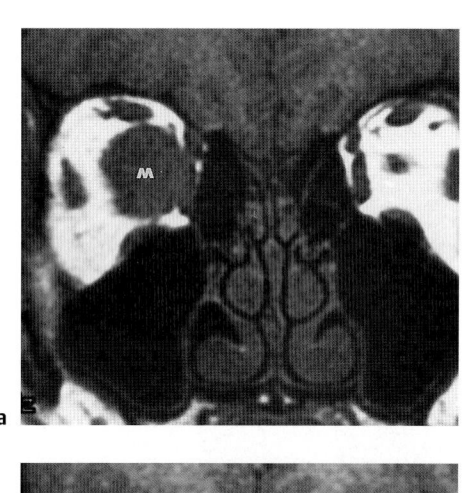

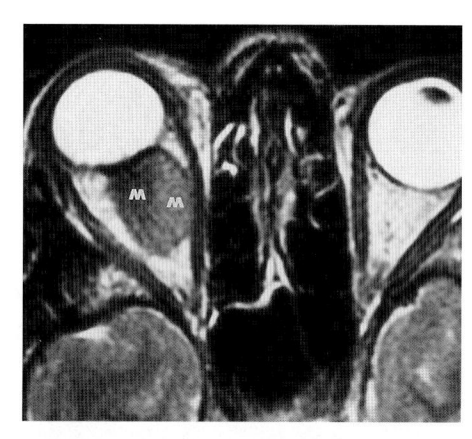

Fig. 2.**290** Optic nerve sheath meningioma. **a** Coronal unenhanced T1W, **b** axial T2W, **c** coronal enhanced fat-suppression T1W, and **d** axial enhanced fat-suppression T1W MR scans, showing a large optic nerve sheath meningioma (M). Note constricted optic nerve (arrows).

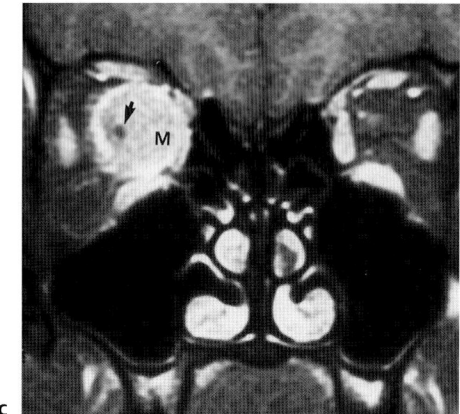

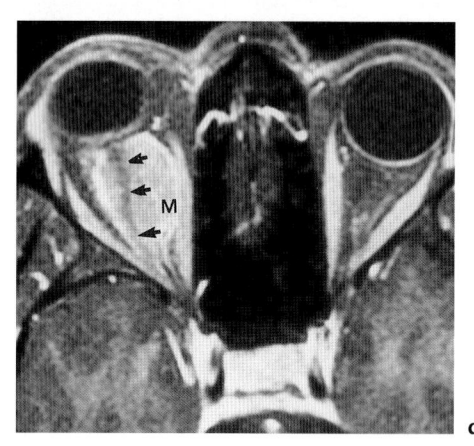

MRI can make significant contributions to the imaging evaluation of optic nerve sheath meningiomas. On MR images, meningioma can be seen as a uniform or round enlargement of the optic nerve (Figs. 2.**289**, 2.**290**). Meningiomas usually retain an isointense appearance to the normal fellow optic nerve and brain tissue on most MRI pulse sequences. Meningiomas may be hypointense in T1-weighted and proton-weighted MR images, and hyperintense in T2-weighted MR images.[2,16,142] Intravenous injection of paramagnetic gadolinium-based contrast medium usually shows marked enhancement of meningiomas. When contrast is used, an additional T1-weighted fat suppression pulse sequence may prove extremely valuable for enhancing meningioma (Fig. 2.**291**). At times, small meningioma may not be detected by MRI (Fig. 2.**292**); however, focal optic nerve calcification may be detected by CT (Fig. 2.**292b**). It should be noted that occasionally focal dural calcification may be detected as an incidental finding in individual with no visual disturbance (Fig. 2.**293**). Because benign dural calcification of the optic nerve sheath is very uncommon, those detected as an incidental finding, and with no symptom, need follow-up examination.

Intraorbital extension of an intracranial meningioma (Fig. 2.**294**) or intracranial extension of an orbital optic nerve meningioma can easily be demonstrated by CT and MRI (Fig. 2.**294**). En plaque meningiomas may produce marked hyperostotic changes, at times with no significant soft-tissue component (Fig. 2.**295**).

Pathology

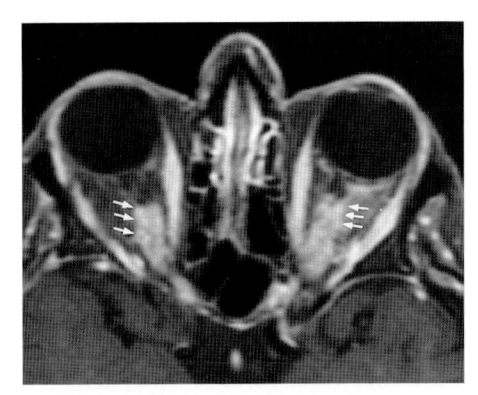

Fig. 2.**291** Bilateral optic nerve sheath meningioma. Axial enhanced fat-suppression T1W MR scan shows enhancement of bilateral "en plaque" optic nerve sheath meningiomas (arrows).

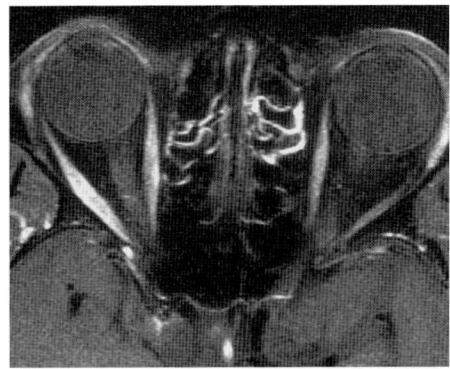

Fig. 2.**292** Small optic nerve sheath meningioma.
a Axial enhanced fat-suppression T1W MR scan, taken with a 3 T MR unit, showing no obvious lesion.
b Axial unenhanced CT scan showing diffuse small calcifications of a presumed right optic nerve sheath meningioma.

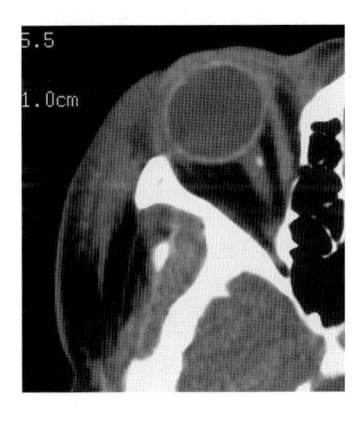

Fig 2.**293** Optic nerve sheath dural calcification. Axial CT scan showing a focal calcification in a 26-year-old woman with no visual disturbance.

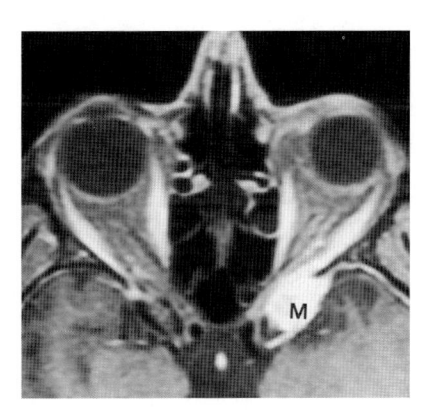

Fig. 2.**294** Paraclinoid meningioma extending into the optic canal. Axial enhanced fat-suppression T1W MR scan shows a meningioma (M) with extension into the left optic canal.

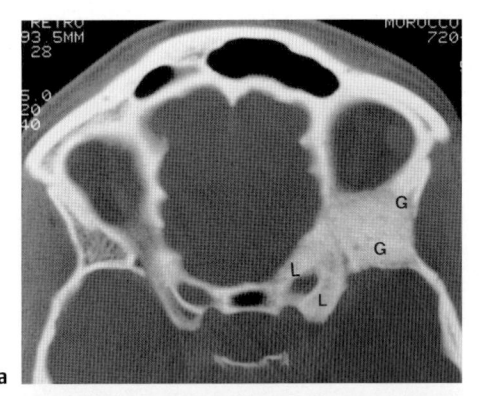

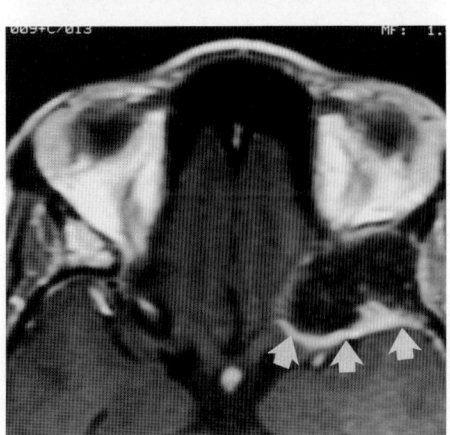

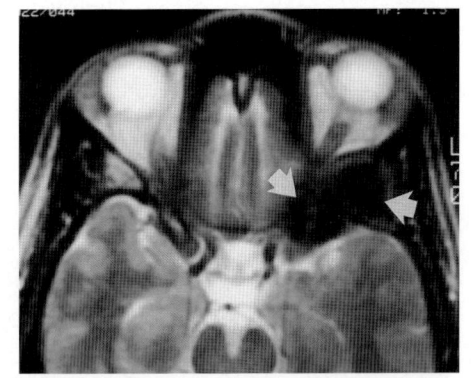

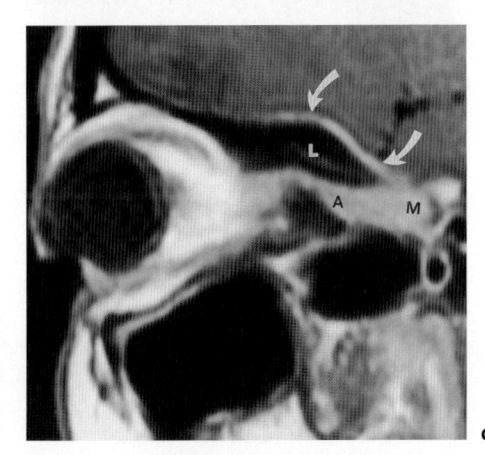

Fig. 2.**295** En plaque meningioma.
a Axial CT scan shows increased thickening and sclerosis of the lesser (L) and greater (G) wings of left sphenoid bone. This is related to extensive hyperostotic changes, characteristic of en plaque meningioma. This CT appearance may be mistaken for fibrous dysplasia.
b Axial T2W MR scan shows hypointensity of hyperostotic bone (arrows).
c Axial enhanced T1W MR scan. The abnormal enhancement (arrows) represents en plaque meningioma. This is the key to the diagnosis, as in a benign fibro-osseous lesion there will be no such enhancement around the sclerotic bone. In a benign fibro-osseous lesion, there will be heterogeneous enhancement within the sclerotic bone.
d Sagittal enhanced T1W MR scan showing extension of en plaque meningioma (M) along the superior orbital fissure into the orbital apex (A). Note the hyperostotic lesser wing (L) and en plaque meningioma over the lesser wing (arrows).

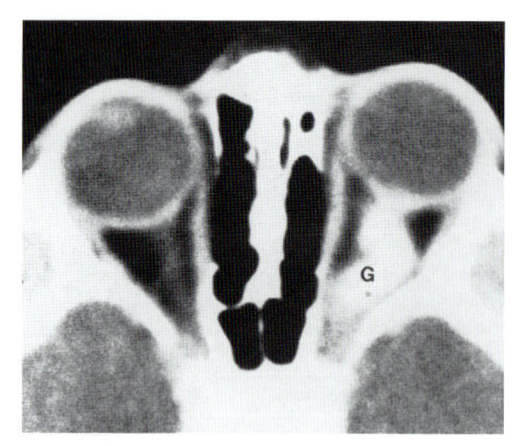

Fig. 2.296 Optic nerve glioma. Axial postcontrast CT scan shows marked enhancement of an optic nerve glioma (G) in this 5-year-old boy with no history of neurofibromatosis. Note the kinking and tortuosity of the tumor, characteristic of juvenile pilocytic glioma.

Optic Nerve Glioma

Optic nerve glioma is a tumor arising from the neuroglia.[2, 16] Although it is usually a tumor of childhood (2–6 years), it can be seen at birth and in adults. Nine out of ten cases show symptoms in the first two decades. Optic nerve glioma in children is a benign, well-differentiated, and slow-growing tumor (juvenile pilocytic glioma). Bilateral optic nerve gliomas are characteristic of neurofibromatosis type 1 (NF1). The natural history of childhood optic glioma does not involve malignant transformation or systemic metastasis.[2, 16] Local invasion into the extrocular muscles rarely occurs. Thickening of perineural tissue (arachnoid hyperplasia) seems to be responsible for the fusiform shape of optic nerve glioma.[2, 16] The primary sequela of this tumor is atrophy that results from damage to the optic nerve fibers and the optic nerve nutrient arteries.[16] Malignant optic glioma is primarily seen in adults. It is a rare, fatal disease (glioblastoma multiformis) that usually extends from intracranial glioma. It often begins with unilateral loss of vision and rapidly progresses to bilateral blindness and death within one or two years.[2, 16] Diffuse, tortuous enlargement of the optic nerve with a characteristic kinking and buckling (sinusoid) appearance is a characteristic feature of the childhood form of optic glioma (Fig. 2.296). Calcification is rare in optic nerve gliomas. Following intravenous contrast administration they may show homogeneous or nonhomogeneous enhancement. The inhomogeneity is the result of tumor infarction secondary to obliteration of the small nutrient arteries of the optic nerve.[2, 16]

MRI readily demonstrates an enlarged fusiform and kinked optic nerve (Fig. 2.297). On T1-weighted and proton-weighted MR images, the optic glioma will appear isointense or slightly hypointense compared to the white matter (Figs. 2.298a, 2.299). On T2-weighted images, the lesion may show greater variability in intensity; however, it may appear hyperintense compared to the white matter (Fig. 2.298b). The use of paramagnetic Gd-DTPA contrast media results in moderate to marked enhancement of gliomas (Figs. 2.297c, 2.298c). At times, there may be moderate to marked arachnoid hyperplasia, surrounding the optic glioma. On postcontrast CT and MRI, arachnoid hyperplasia demonstrates moderate to marked enhancement around the optic glioma. This feature of optic nerve glioma may simulate an optic nerve meningioma. Optic nerve meningioma, however, is quite rare in children and in addition results in an irregular outline of the enlarged optic nerve, related to focal invasion of surrounding dural sheath of the optic nerve. Low-grade optic nerve glioma in an adult with no history of neurofibromatosis is very uncommon (Fig. 2.300). Malignant optic nerve gliomas are extremely rare and behave very aggressively (Fig. 2.301). Another rare tumor of optic nerve is hemangioblastoma, seen in patients with von Hippel–Lindau disease (Fig. 2.302).

■ Fibrous Tissue Tumors of the Orbit

Fibrous tumors of the orbit are a group of lesions that present a confusing clinical, histological, and imaging spectrum of disease. These include fibroma, fibrous histiocytoma, fibrocystoma, aggressive fibromatosis, nodular fasciitis and fibrosarcoma. Fibrohistiocytic tumors are more common than fibroblastic (fibroma, fibromatosis) tumors.[144]

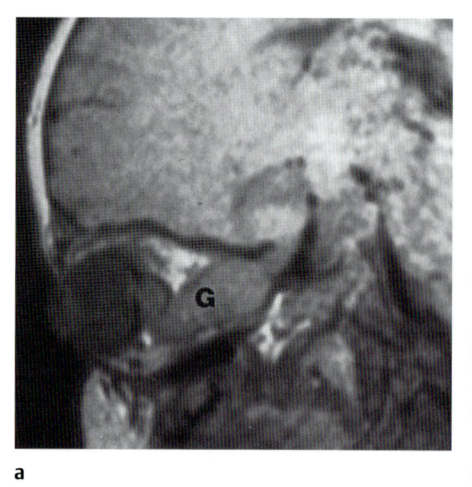

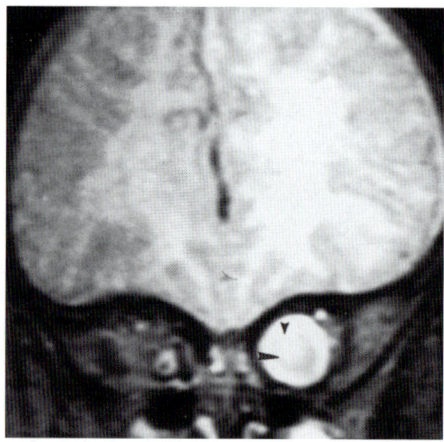

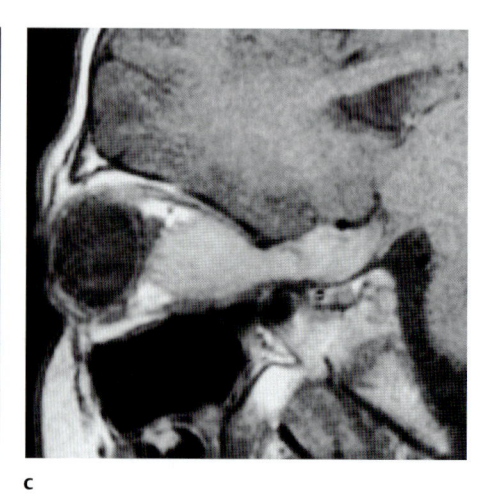

Fig. 2.297 Optic nerve juvenile pilocytic glioma.
a Sagittal PW MR scan shows a large optic nerve glioma (G).
b Coronal T2W MR scan shows the glioma (arrows) surrounded by hyperintense CSF.
c Sagittal enhanced T1W MR scan in another child, an 8-year-old boy, showing marked enhancement of a large left low-grade (pilocytic) optic nerve glioma.

Pathology 273

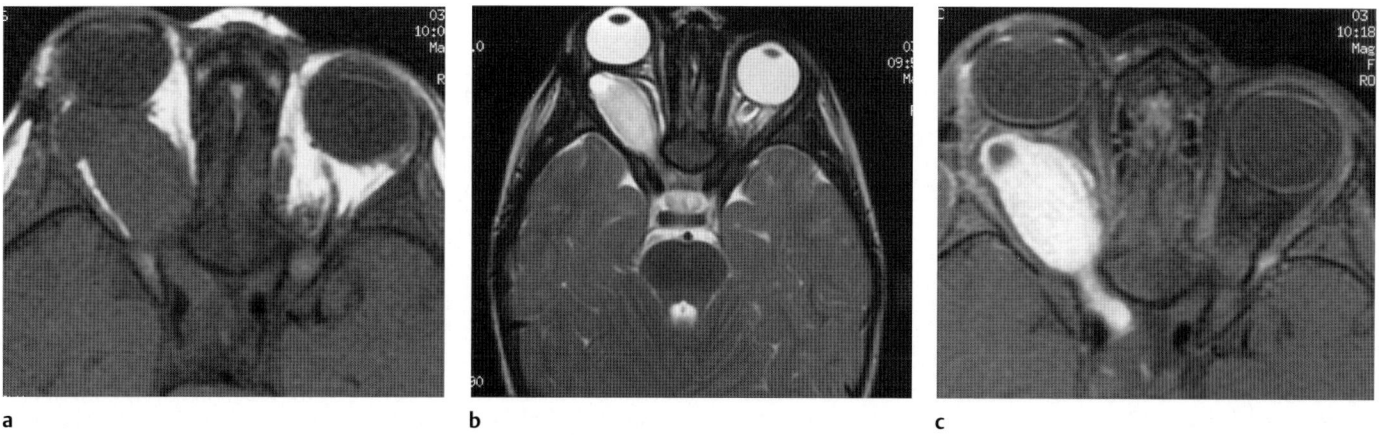

Fig. 2.**298** Low-grade optic nerve glioma in a 17-month-old boy. **a** Axial unenhanced T1W, **b** axial T2W, and **c** axial enhanced fat-suppression T1W MR scans, showing a large optic nerve glioma involving the right optic nerve.

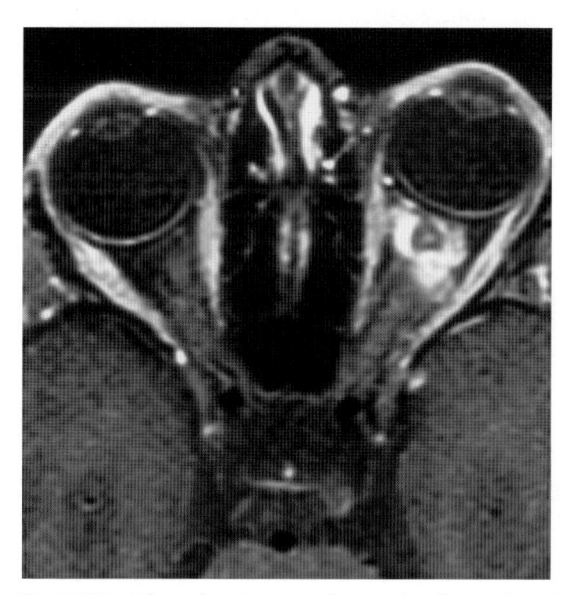

Fig. 2.**299** Bilateral optic nerve low-grade gliomas in a 4-year-old girl. Axial enhanced fat-suppression T1W MR scan showing bilateral optic nerve glioma, characteristic of NF1.

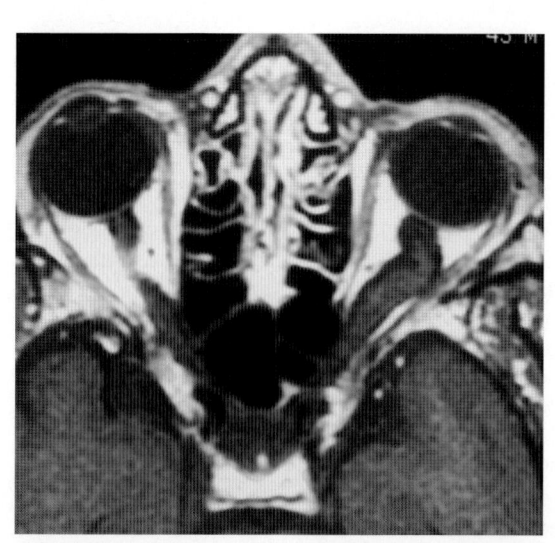

Fig. 2.**300** Low-grade optic nerve glioma in a 43-year-old man. Axial enhanced T1W MR scan shows moderate diffuse enlargement of the left optic nerve.

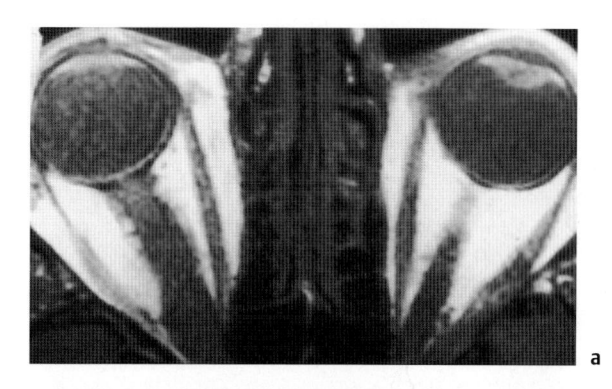

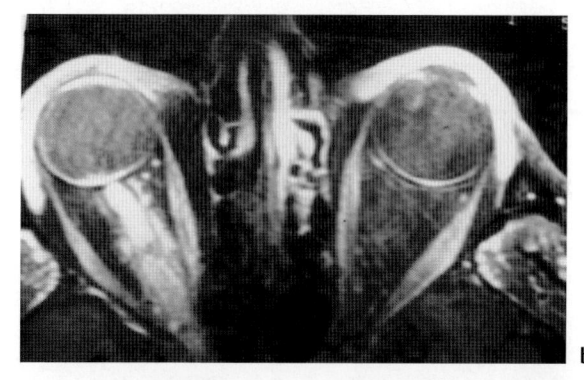

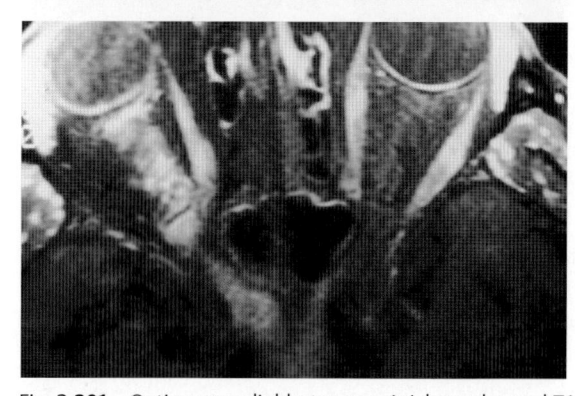

Fig. 2.**301** Optic nerve glioblastoma. **a** Axial unenhanced T1W MR scan and **b**, **c** axial enhanced fat-suppression T1W MR scans. There is marked enlargement of the right optic nerve with marked contrast enhancement. Note the irregular outline of the tumor. There is infiltration into the retrobulbar fat (**b**) and extension into the cranial segment of the left optic nerve (**c**). Case courtesy of Adam Flander, MD, Thomas Jefferson Hospital, Philadelphia, PA, USA.

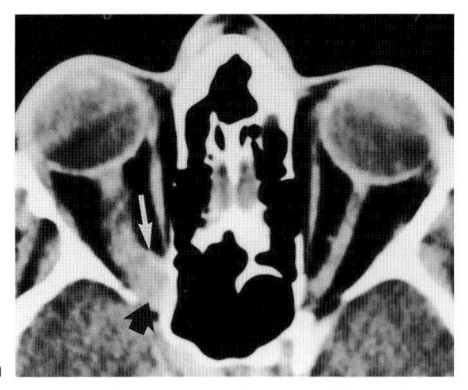

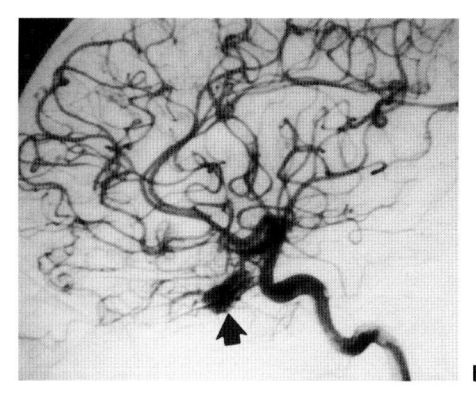

Fig. 2.302 Optic nerve hemangioblastoma. **a** Axial enhanced CT scan and **b** lateral angiogram demonstrating an optic nerve hemangioblastoma (arrows). Courtesy of the Armed Forces Institute of Pathology, Washington, DC, USA.

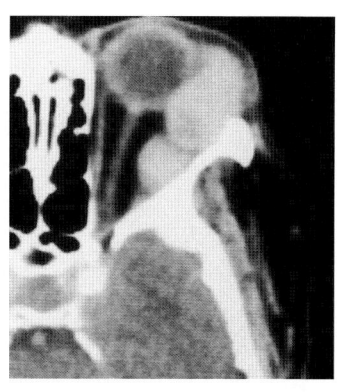

Fig. 2.303 Fibrous histiocytoma. Axial enhanced CT scan shows a bilobed enhancing mass (M) compatible with fibrous histiocytoma.

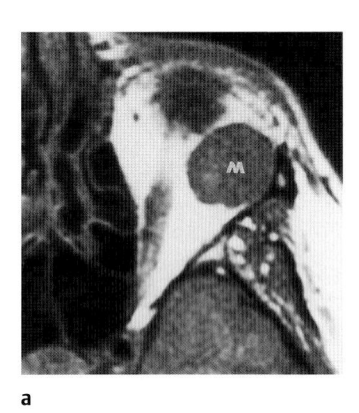

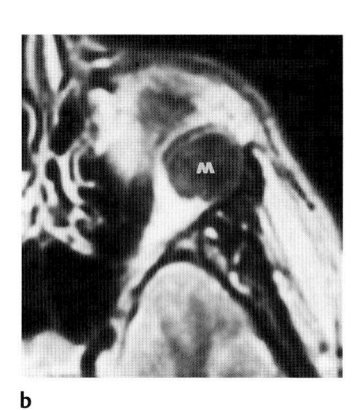

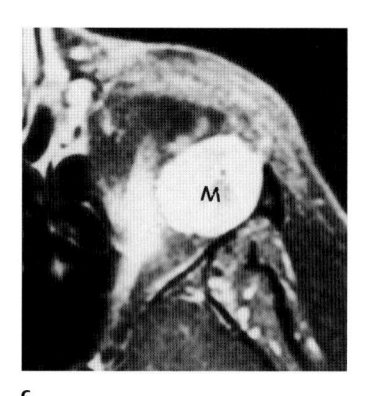

Fig. 2.304 Presumed fibrous histiocytoma. **a** Axial unenhanced T1W, **b** axial T2W, and **c** axial enhanced fat-suppression T1W MR scans showing a mass (M), presumed to be a fibrous histiocytoma.

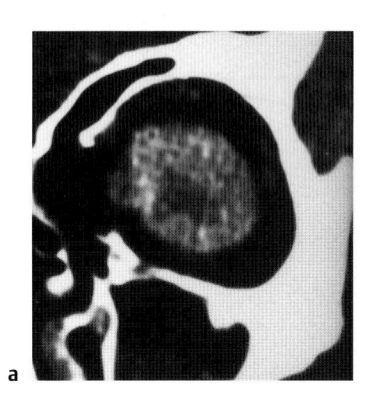

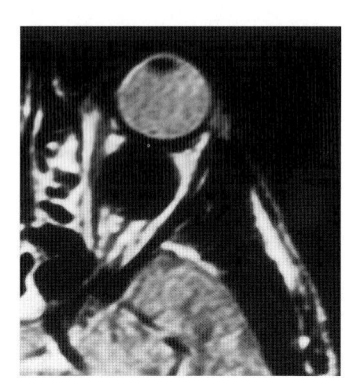

Fig. 2.305 Fibrocytoma.
a Coronal enhanced CT scan shows a mass (M) with moderate enhancement, compatible with surgically proven fibrocytoma.
b Axial T2W MR scan. The mass appears very hypointense owing to dense fibrous tissue.

Fibrous Histiocytoma

Fibrous histiocytoma is a mesenchymal tumor that involves the fascia, muscle, and soft tissues of the body.[3, 144–147] It is considered by some authors to be the most common mesenchymal tumor of the orbit.[145] The neoplasm is made up of fibroblasts, myofibroblasts, undifferentiated mesenchymal cells and fibrous-appearing histiocytic cells that tend to form a characteristic cartwheel or storiform pattern.[2, 3, 147] Fibrous histiocytoma probably arises from a fibroblast precursor. It bears no relationship to the systemic reticuloendothelioses or malignant histiocytoses. The tumor may be benign or malignant.[145, 146] Fibrous histiocytomas are seen on CT and MRI as well-circumscribed masses that may be intraconal or extraconal and demonstrate moderate to marked contrast enhancement (Figs. 2.**303**, 2.**304**).[144] Some of the tumors may be bilobed. Some of the densely cellular fibrous histiocytomas may appear moderately to markedly hypointense on T2-weighted MR scans. These T2-weighted hypointense lesions may not be differentiated on imaging from some of the neurofibromas (see Fig. 2.**274**), fibrocystomas (Fig. 2.**305**), and orbital meningioma (Fig. 2.**306**). The differential diagnosis should include cavernous hemangioma, hemangiopericytoma, schwannoma, meningioma, neurofibroma, fibrocystoma, leiomyoma (vasculogenic), lymphoma, and metastasis. Malignant fibrous histiocytomas may be seen following radiation to the orbit for retinoblastoma.[16] Malignant fibrous histiocytomas produce bone erosion (Fig. 2.**307**).[2, 8]

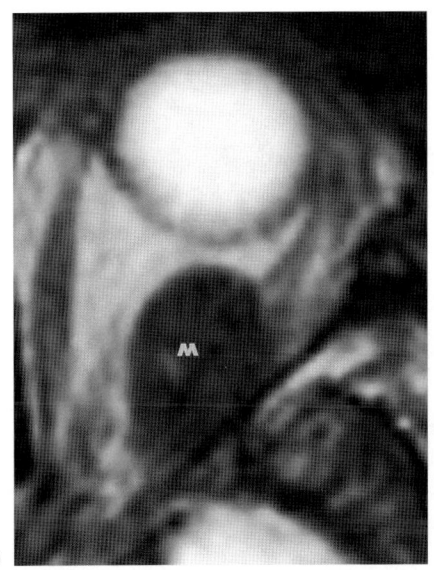

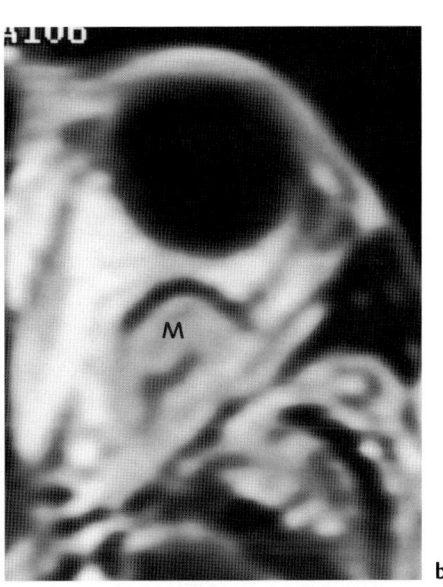

Fig. 2.**306** Orbital meningioma. **a** Axial T2W MR scan showing a hypointense mass (M). **b** Axial enhanced T1W MR scan shows moderate to marked enhancement of the tumor. This orbital meningioma is believed to have arisen from ectopic arachnoid tissue within the orbit. The hypointensity on T2W MR image is due to compact fibrous tissue and dense tumor.

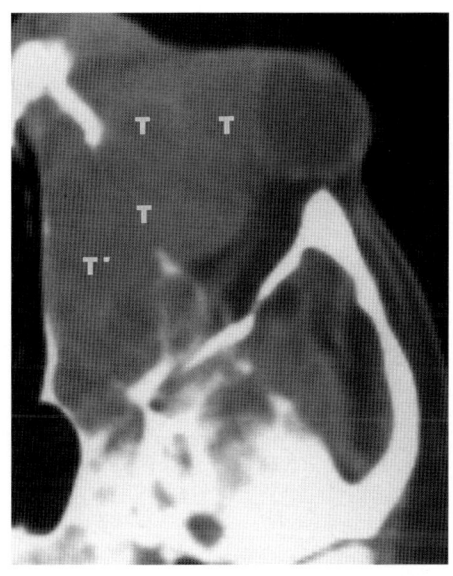

Fig. 2.**307** Malignant fibrous histiocytoma. Axial CT scan shows a large destructive tumor mass (T) involving the left orbit and adjacent sinonasal cavities.

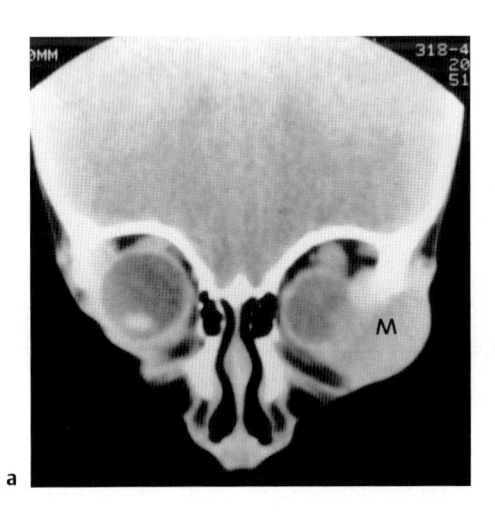

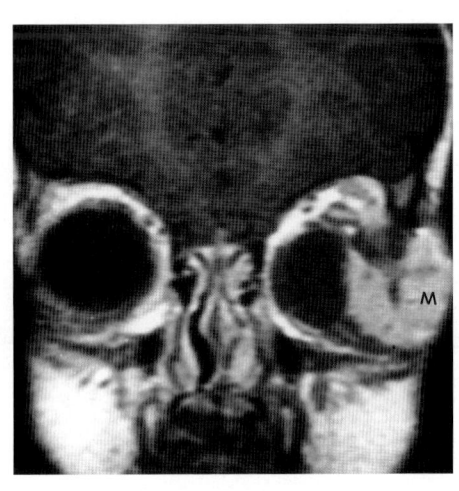

Fig. 2.**308** Aggressive fibromatosis in a 3-year-old girl. **a** Coronal enhanced CT scan and **b** coronal enhanced T1W MR scan showing a large mass (M) with moderate to marked enhancement, compatible with histologically proven aggressive fibromatosis. This cannot be differentiated from orbital rhabdomyosarcoma.

Fibroma and Fibrosarcoma

Fibroma is the least common fibrous tumor of the orbit, and most fibromas are found in young adults.[144] It is usually encapsulated and has slow growth spanning years. It arises from the fascia of the extraocular muscles or Tenon's capsule in the orbit. Fibrosarcoma is also rare in the orbit. Congenital, infantile, juvenile, and adult forms of fibrosarcoma are recognized.[144] Aggressive fibromatosis is a benign but locally invasive fibroblastic lesion lying clinically and pathologically in the spectrum between fibrosis and low-grade fibrosarcoma. CT and MR imaging of aggressive fibromatosis may show a lesion with benign-appearing or invasive characteristics (Fig. 2.**308**).

Rhadomyosarcoma of the Orbit

Although rhabdomyosarcoma (RMS) is a rare tumor, it is still the most common primary orbital malignancy in children and the most common soft-tissue malignancy of childhood. Soft-tissue sarcomas account for 6% of all childhood cancers.[148–152] RMS occurs primarily in patients from ages 2 to 5 years, but the tumor may occur at any age from birth to adulthood. In most cases the average age at diagnosis is 7–8 years, with 90% of patients presenting before age 16 years. Orbital RMS is invariably unilateral and, although the tumor may involve any part of the orbit and adnexa, it tends to involve more the superior portion of the orbit. The most characteristic presenting features of orbital RMS are a fairly rapid onset and progression with proptosis and displacement of the globe. RMS originates from embryonic tissue, either from immature prospective muscle fibers or from pluripotential embryonic mesenchymal tissue with a potential for aberrant differentiation into muscle fibers.[153]

Any rapidly developing proptosis in childhood must presumptively be diagnosed as RMS. The differential diagnosis also includes leukemic and metastatic deposits (neuroblastoma), lymphoma, Langerhans cell histiocytosis, aggressive fibromatosis, plexiform neurofibromatosis, ruptured dermoid/epidermoid cyst, subperiosteal hematoma after trauma, and a chocolate cyst related to hemorrhage in a lymphangioma. Rhabdomyosarcomas are pleomorphic tumors, and the cells may be anaplastic. On the basis of the histopathological characteristics, RMS is classified into one of three histological types: (1) embryonal, (2) differen-

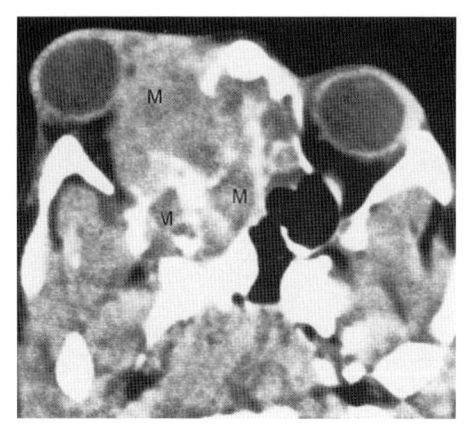

Fig. 2.**309** Rhabdomyosarcoma in a 17-year-old female. Axial postcontrast CT scan shows a large destructive mass (M) involving the right orbit and extending into the ethmoid.

tiated, and (3) alveolar. Orbital RMS generally presents painlessly with rapidly progressive unilateral exophthalmos, or less commonly with superficial swelling with palpable mass and proptosis. Patients may even present with a confusing or misleading history, such as recent trauma. Most tumors are retrobulbar, resulting in proptosis, but can arise extraconally, especially superiorly or supranasally. RMS may arise intraocularly from the ciliary body.[148] Tumors arising in the paranasal sinuses, nasal cavity, pterygopalatine fossa, nasopharynx, and parapharyngeal space may secondarily invade the orbit, and RMS arising elsewhere can metastasize to the orbit.[148]

Diagnostic Imaging

CT and MRI play an important role in the preoperative evaluation and staging of RMS. Imaging should include CT and MRI scans of primary and metastatic sites (i.e., lung, liver, brain, and so forth). CT and MRI are also important in evaluating recurrent and residual diseases. A baseline CT or MRI study, to be taken 8–10 weeks after completion of treatment, is essential. Without a baseline CT or MR scan, the follow-up studies may not be specific for tumor recurrence. Because of the dramatic improvement in survival of patients treated promptly with appropriate chemotherapy and radiation therapy, these tumors must be diagnosed as soon as possible. On CT images, rhabdomyosarcomas are isodense in relation to normal muscles and appear as homogeneous, well-defined, soft-tissue masses without bone destruction. Larger tumors appear as less well-defined soft-tissue masses with bone destruction or invasion of surrounding structures (Fig. 2.**309**). Tumors that have focal hemorrhage appear heterogeneous on CT scans. All tumors demonstrate moderate to marked contrast enhancement.[148] On T1-weighted MR images, rhabdomyosarcomas are isointense or slightly hypointense compared with brain (Figs. 2.**310 a**, 2.**311 a**). On T2-weighted MR images, the tumors will appear to be of slightly to moderately increased signal intensity compared with brain (Fig. 2.**311 b**).

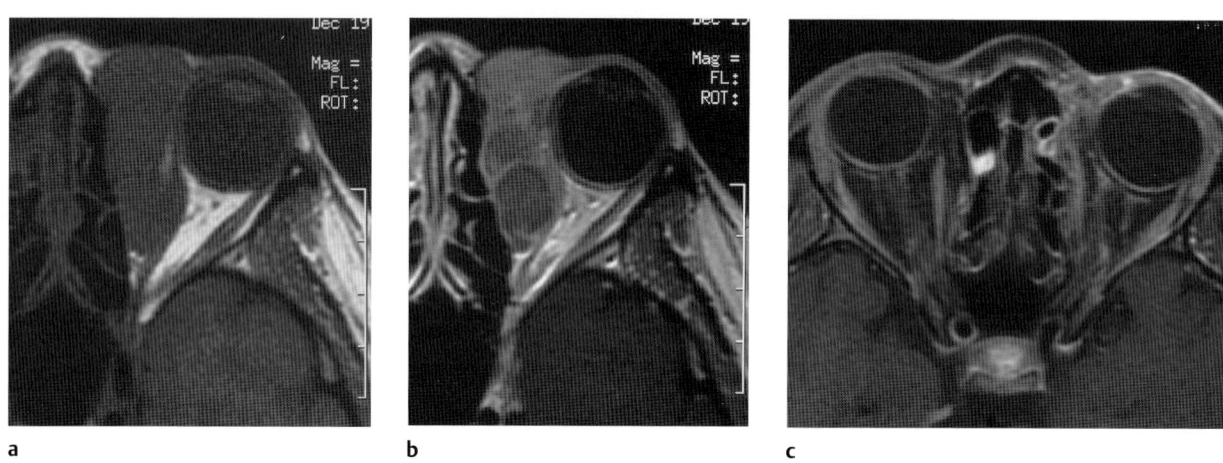

a b c

Fig. 2.**310** Rhabdomyosarcoma. **a** Axial unenhanced T1W and **b** axial enhanced T1W MR scans show a large mass compatible with rhabdomyosarcoma. **c** Axial enhanced fat-suppression T1W MR scan, taken following chemotherapy and radiation therapy, shows complete resolution of the tumor.

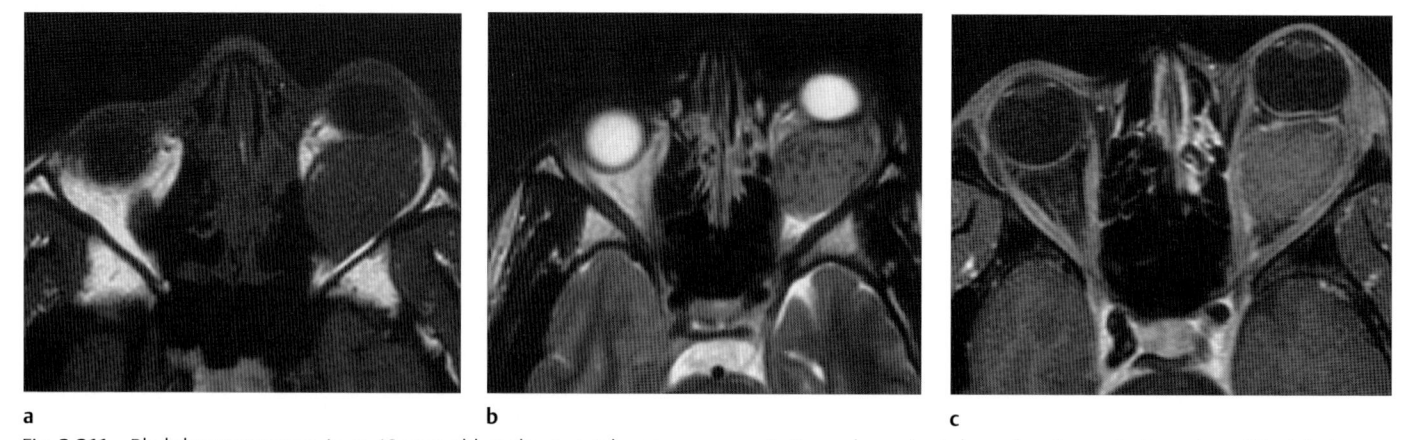

a b c

Fig. 2.**311** Rhabdomyosarcoma in a 19-year-old male. **a** Axial unenhanced T1W, **b** axial T2W, and **c** axial enhanced fat-suppression T1W MR scans. There is a well-defined intraconal mass that shows mild enhancement. Coronal scan (not shown here) revealed invasion of the inferior rectus muscle. Histological diagnosis was consistent with a rhabdomyosarcoma.

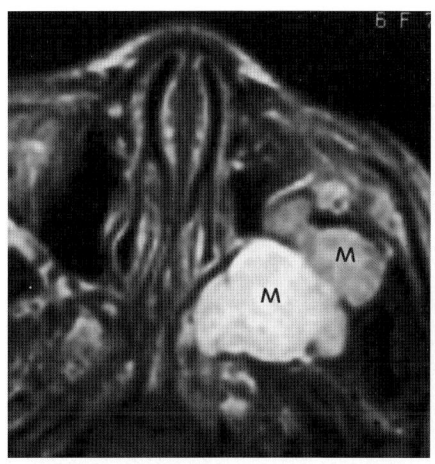

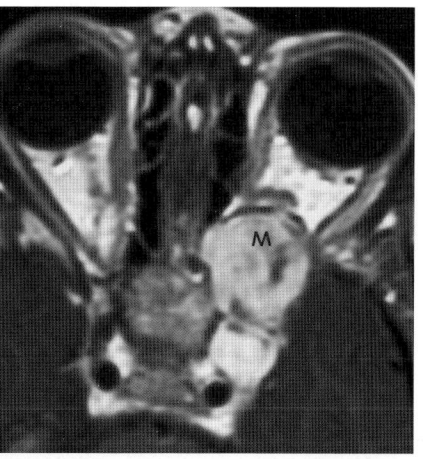

Fig. 2.312 Rhabdomyosarcoma in a 6-year-old female. **a** Axial T2W and **b** axial enhanced T1W MR scans showing a large mass (M), compatible with rhabdomyosarcoma, arising in the infratemporal fossa (**a**) with extension into the left orbit (**b**).

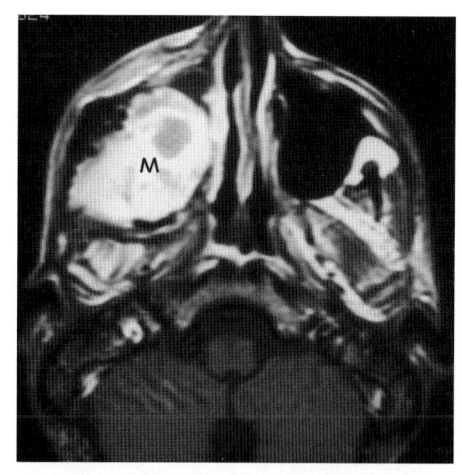

Fig. 2.313 Rhabdomyosarcoma. Axial enhanced T1W MR scan shows a right infratemporal mass (M) with marked enhancement, compatible with rhabdomyosarcoma.

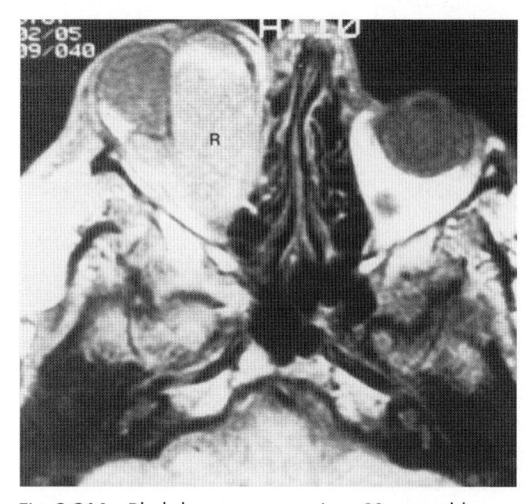

Fig. 2.314 Rhabdomyosarcoma in a 60-year-old patient. Axial PW MR scan shows a large orbital mass compatible with rhabdomyosarcoma (R). The "senile" rhabdomyosarcoma is very rare. The differential diagnosis should include lymphoma, primary orbital melanoma (see Fig. 2.317), malignant histiocytoma, hemangiopericytoma, and metastasis.

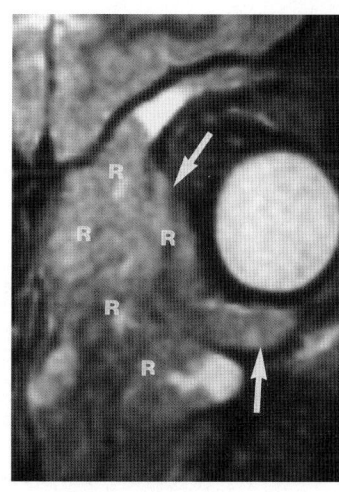

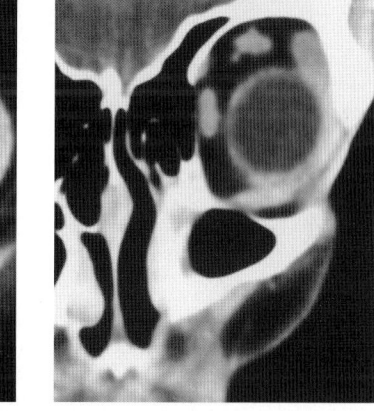

Fig. 2.315 Rhabdomyosarcoma.
a Coronal T2W MR scan shows a large rhabdomyosarcoma (R) of the left sinonasal cavities, extending into the orbit (arrows).
b Coronal enhanced CT scan following treatment shows complete resolution of tumor.

Tumors that have chronic or subacute areas of hemorrhage demonstrate focal areas of increased signal on T1-weighted and T2-weighted MR images.[151] RMS demonstrates moderate to marked enhancement on enhanced CT and enhanced T1W MRI scans (Figs. 2.**310b**, 2.**311c**).

RMS may arise in the infratemporal fossa and then extend into the orbit (Figs. 2.**312**, 2.**313**). When the diagnosis is suspected, sectional imaging with primarily CT or MRI is performed to confirm the presence of an infiltrative mass and evaluate the extent of involvement of adjacent structures, including the brain. Although the two techniques may be equivalent in detecting the mass and determining its origin, MRI better delineates the full extent of involvement owing to its superior soft-tissue contrast and multiplanar capability. Although RMS of the orbit is most often seen in children and adults under 20 years of age, at times it affects older patients (Fig. 2.**313**, 2.**314**). MRI and CT scan are both very useful to demonstrate the effectiveness of treatment (Fig. 2.**315**) as well as recurrence of tumor (Fig. 2.**316**).

Nevertheless, many common and less common orbital and head and neck lesions, such as hemangiomas, lymphangiomas, lymphoma, leukemic infiltration, plexiform neurofibromatosis, aggressive fibromatosis, Langerhans cell histiocytosis, pseudorheumatoid nodule, pseudotumor, subperiosteal abscess, subperiosteal hematoma, Ewing sarcoma, and metastasis (neuroblastoma) can appear similar to RMS with similar CT and MR characteristics. Thus, the findings are nonspecific in many cases, necessitating a tissue diagnosis. Subperiosteal hematoma in children may simulate RMS. MRI in these cases may be extremely valuable to make the correct diagnosis. Orbital pseudotumors in children may simulate orbital RMS (Figs. 2.**186**, 2.**187**). Aggressive fibromatosis in children (Fig. 2.**308**) and capillary hemangiomas and other vasculogenic lesions, including vascular malformations, may also simulate RMS. Dynamic CT study is sometimes very helpful in the diagnosis of capillary hemangiomas. At times RMS may present with a clinical picture and imaging features of an orbital subperiosteal abscess.[154] In adults, lymphoma and primary and secondary orbital tumors should be included in the differential diagnosis (Fig. 2.**317**).

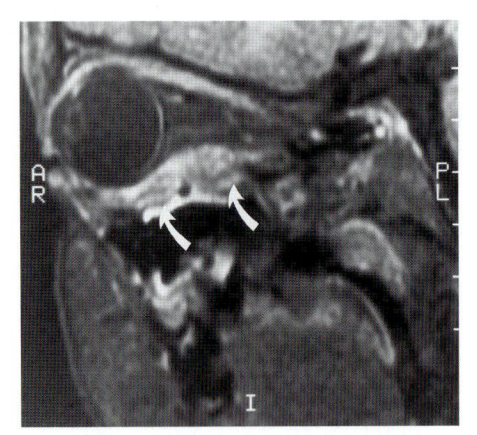

Fig. 2.316 Recurrent rhabdomyosarcoma. Sagittal enhanced fat-suppression T1W MR scan shows recurrent rhabdomyosarcoma (arrows).

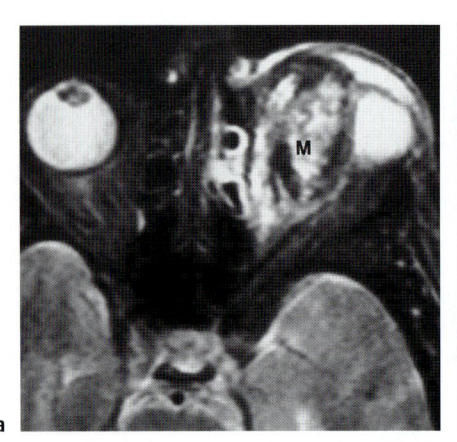

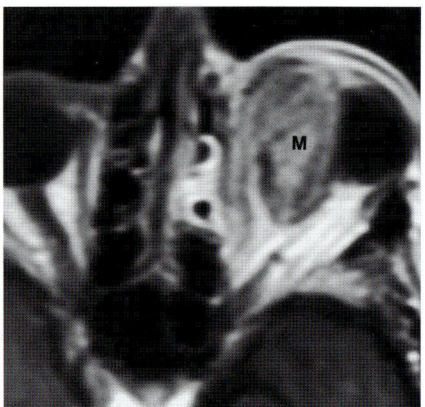

Fig. 2.317 Primary malignant melanoma of the orbit in a 69-year-old man. **a** Axial T2W and **b** axial enhanced T1W MR scans showing a large mass (M) compatible with primary uveal melanoma. Differential diagnosis include lymphoma and metastasis.

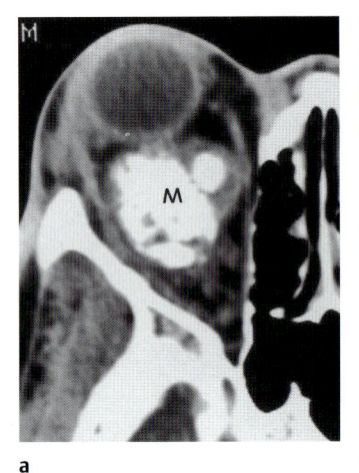

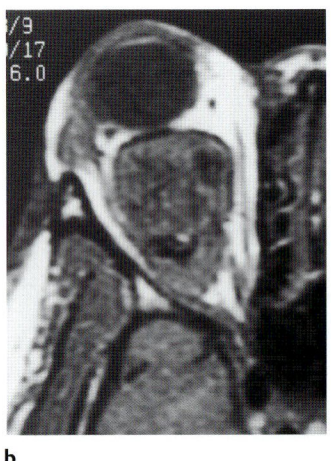

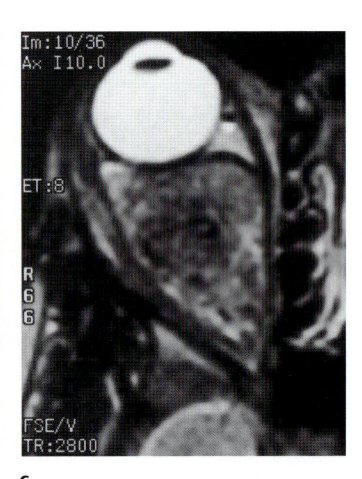

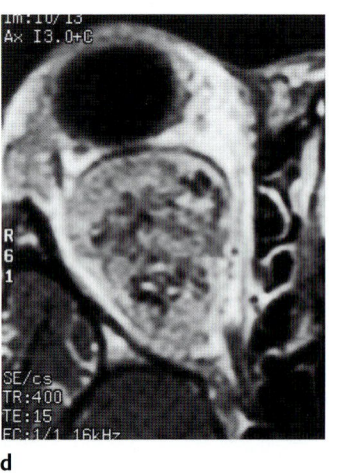

Fig. 2.318 Mesenchymal chondrosarcoma of the orbit. **a** Axial CT scan shows an intraconal mass (M) associated with marked calcifications. **b** Axial unenhanced T1W, **c** axial T2W, and **d** axial enhanced T1W MR scans. The mass appears hypointense on T2W MR image (**c**) and shows moderate contrast enhancement (**d**).

Mesenchymal Chondrosarcoma of the Orbit

Extraskeletal malignant cartilaginous tumors are subdivided into two major categories: mesenchymal and myxoid chondrosarcoma. Mesenchymal chondrosarcomas commonly occur within the bones. Extraskeletal locations include the head and neck, cranial and spinal dura mater, and, less frequently, the leg, especially the thigh.[155, 156] Orbital mesenchymal chondrosarcoma (OMC) remains an extremely rare entity occurring more frequently in young women.[2, 155, 156] The most common presenting symptom of OMC is proptosis, with orbital pain, diplopia, and headache. Histologically, OMC is relatively distinct, containing islands of chondroid tissue. The cartilaginous areas have the appearance of mature cartilage. Most of them contain amorphic calcification and foci of ossification of the cartilaginous matrix.[155] Other areas of undifferentiated mesenchymal tissue are seen with a predominance of spindle-shaped cells. Mitoses are not frequent.

CT imaging characteristics include a relatively well-defined soft-tissue mass with areas of mottled coarse calcification (Fig. 2.318); moderate, delayed contrast enhancement is noted. MRI characteristics include signal intensity lower than or equal to brain on T1-weighted MR scans and isointense to brain on T2-weighted MR scans, with moderate enhancement after iv administration of gadolinium-DTPA contrast medium (Figs. 2.318 b–d).

The calcified component of the tumor shows low signal on both T1-weighted and T2-weighted MR scans (Figs. 2.318 b, c). On enhanced T1-weighted MR scans, however, mild enhancement is seen even within the calcified component.[155] Differential diagnosis for an intraorbital calcified mass includes meningioma, sclerosing hemangioma, hemangiopericytoma, vascular malformation, varix, and orbital amyloidosis.[2, 8, 155] Calcification in cavernous hemangioma, fibrous histiocytoma, fibrocystoma, schwannoma, neurofibroma, and optic glioma is extremely rare. Orbital amyloidosis demonstrates a soft-tissue mass with coarse, streaky, amorphous calcification diffusely scattered throughout the lesion (Fig. 2.207). In addition, certain areas that appear to be calcific density actually represent amyloid.[155]

■ Lacrimal Gland and Fossa Lesions

The lacrimal gland is about the size and shape of an almond and is located in the superolateral extraconal orbital fat in the lacrimal fossa, adjacent to the tendons of the superior and lateral rectus muscles. The more anterior palpebral lobe is separated from the deeper orbital lobe by the lateral horn of the levator muscle aponeurosis.[23, 125] The lacrimal gland can be involved by acute and chronic inflammatory disease (dacryoadenitis) including abscess formation (Fig. 2.319), as well as by a wide spectrum of orbital pathology, and meticulous clinical and preoperative imaging of these patients is imperative so that an inappropriate incisional biopsy is avoided. This situation is especially true when a benign mixed tumor of the lacrimal gland is suspected. This tumor requires en bloc excision through a lateral orbitotomy to ensure complete extirpation and prevent late recurrences.[23, 157, 158] If an incisional biopsy of a benign mixed tumor is performed, there is an increased likelihood of operative tumor spillage and thus late recurrences.[23, 159, 160] The excellent prognosis of benign mixed tumor, provided it is completely removed at first surgery, is now widely accepted.

In general, epithelial tumors represent about 50% of the masses involving the lacrimal gland. The remaining 50% of lacrimal gland masses are either lymphoid or inflammatory in nature.[23, 159] Metastasis to the parenchyma of the lacrimal gland is rare.[23] Dermoid cysts are not true lacrimal gland tumors, but rather they arise from epithelial rests located in the orbit, particularly in the superolateral quadrant. Epithelial cysts, on the other hand, are intrinsic lesions that result from dilation of the lacrimal gland ducts.[23, 159] Inflammatory diseases of the lacrimal gland can be divided into two categories, acute and chronic. Acute dacryoadenitis (bacterial or viral) is more commonly seen in children and in younger people.[23, 155, 162] It may be related to trauma and clinically is associated with local tenderness, erythema, lid swelling, conjunctival chemosis, discharge or suppuration, enlarged preauricular and cervical nodes, and systemic findings.[23, 155] Acute dacryoadenitis is usually unilateral and tends to respond very rapidly to therapy.[23, 155] Acute dacryoadenitis may be part of the spectrum of idiopathic inflammatory orbital pseudotumor, and this diagnosis is made often on the basis of clinical presentation, CT or MRI findings, and the prompt and favorable response to the administration of systemic corticosteroids.[23, 155, 162, 163]

Chronic dacryoadenitis may follow acute infection or be caused by sarcoidosis (see Fig. 2.**182**), thyroid ophthalmopathy, Mikulicz syndrome, "sclerosing pseudotumors," and Wegener's granulomatosis. In sarcoid there is usually bilateral disease, with either symmetric or asymmetric lacrimal gland enlargement (see Figs. 2.**194**, 2.**195**). Mikulicz syndrome is a nonspecific swelling of the lacrimal gland and salivary glands associated with conditions such as leukemia, lymphoma, pseudotumor, tuberculosis, syphilis, and sarcoidosis. In Sjögren syndrome, there is enlargement and lymphocytic infiltration of the lacrimal glands. Half of these patients have a connective-tissue disease such as rheumatoid arthritis, systemic lupus erythematosus, scleroderma, or polymyositis. Inflammatory pseudotumor in the region of the lacrimal gland accounts for about 15% of all orbital pseudotumors (see Fig. 2.**183**).[155, 163]

Ocular involvement in Wegener granuloma is common, affecting 40% of patients with generalized disease.[2, 23, 81] Involvement of the lacrimal gland is not uncommon (see Figs. 2.**204**, 2.**205**). Histological examination of involved lacrimal glands shows infiltration with histiocytes, plasma cells, lymphocytes, polymorphs, and eosinophils, with giant cell formation.[23, 163] Massive enlargement of lacrimal glands may be present and has been demonstrated on CT.[23, 163, 164] Lymphomatous lesions of the lacrimal gland include a broad spectrum from reactive lymphoid hyperplasia to malignant lymphomas of various types (see Figs. 2.**220**, 2.**227**). Shield et al., in a review of 645 space-occupying orbital lesions that underwent biopsy, found 71 cases of lymphocytic and plasmacytic lesions.[165] Of these, 12 were located in the lacrimal gland. Benign mixed lacrimal gland tumors tend to occur in patients in the third to sixth decade of life. The tumors present with slowly progressive, painless upper lid swelling, proptosis, or both, without inflammatory symptoms or signs (Figs. 2.**320**–2.**322**).

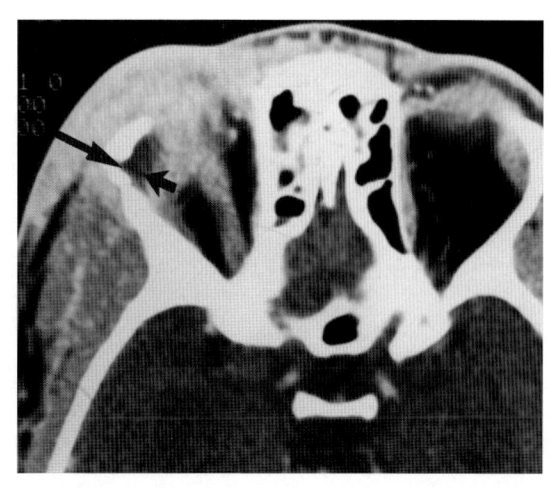

Fig. 2.**319** Acute dacryoadenitis. Axial enhanced CT scan shows diffuse enlargement of the right lacrimal gland and adjacent orbital soft tissue, including the temporal fossa, due to inflammation. Note bone erosion due to osteomyelitis (large arrow) and abscess formation (short arrow).

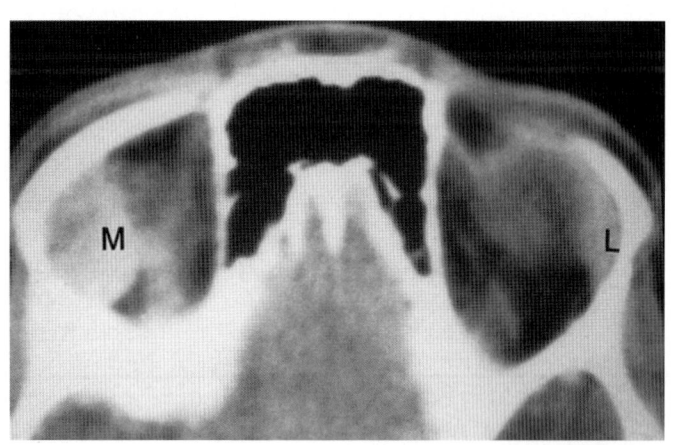

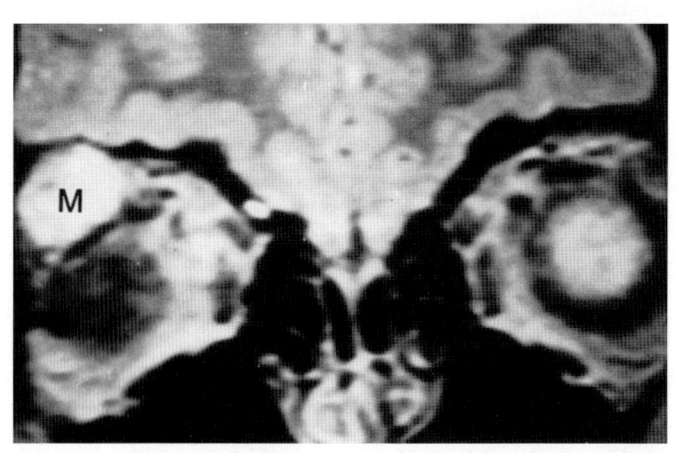

Fig. 2.**320** Benign lacrimal gland tumor.
a Axial postcontrast CT scan shows a well-defined right lacrimal gland mass (M) compatible with benign mixed tumor. Note the normal left lacrimal gland (L).
b T2W MR scan shows the lacrimal mass (M) compatible with a surgically proven benign mixed tumor.

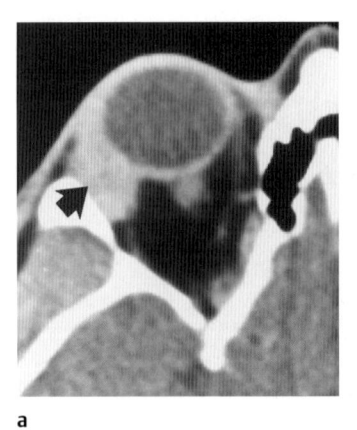

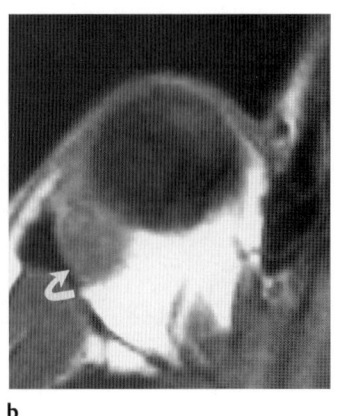

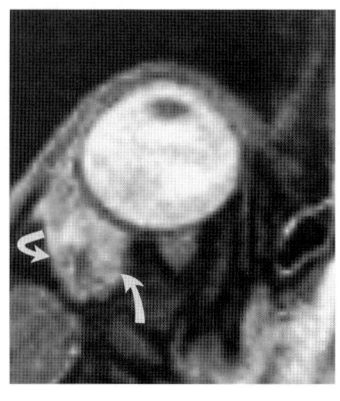

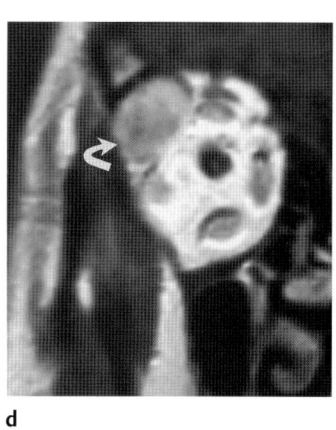

Fig. 2.**321** Benign mixed tumor of the lacrimal gland. **a** Axial enhanced CT scan, **b** axial unenhanced T1W MR scan, **c** axial T2W MR scan, and **d** coronal enhanced T1W MR scan, showing a right lacrimal gland mass (arrows) compatible with surgically proven benign mixed tumor.

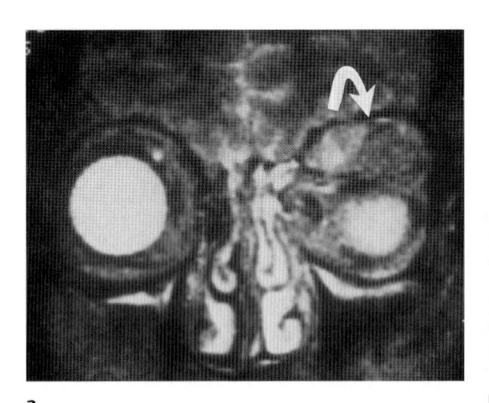

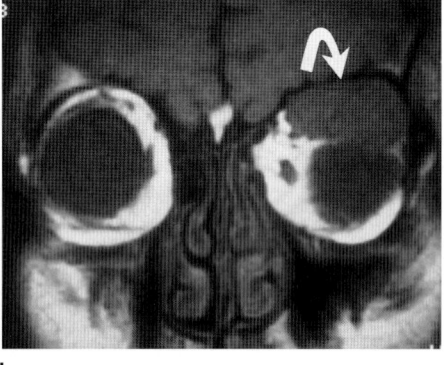

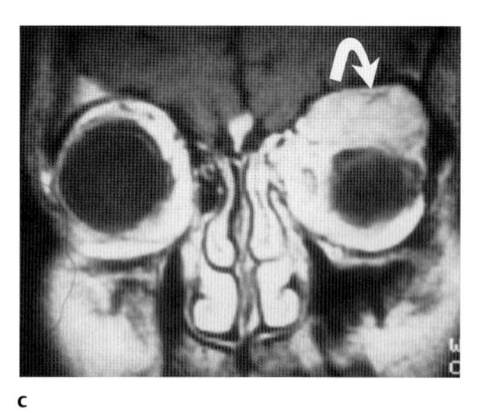

Fig. 2.**322** Benign mixed tumor of the lacrimal gland.
a Coronal T2W MR scan shows a large heterogeneous lacrimal gland mixed tumor (arrows).

b, c Coronal unenhanced T1W (**b**) and enhanced T1W (**c**) MR scans. The mass (arrows) appears homogeneous on T1W MR images and demonstrates marked enhancement. Case courtesy of August F. Mark, MD, München, Germany.

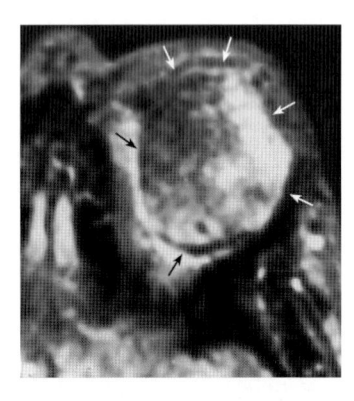

Fig. 2.**323** Benign mixed tumor of the lacrimal gland. Axial T2W MR scans shows a large benign mixed tumor of the lacrimal gland (arrows).

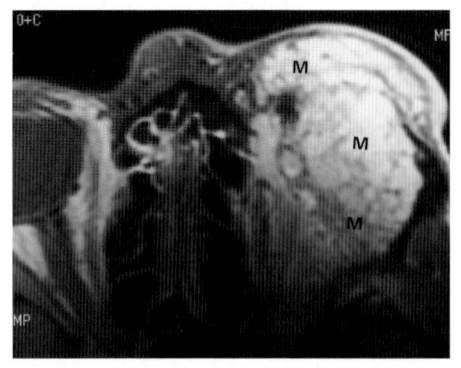

Fig. 2.**324** Large benign mixed tumor of lacrimal gland. Axial enhanced T1W MR scan shows a large enhancing lacrimal gland mass (M) compatible with surgically proven benign mixed tumor.

CT and MRI

Inflammatory lesions of the lacrimal gland show diffuse enlargement of the gland. Contrast enhancement may be marked, and there may be associated acute lateral rectus muscle myositis. There may be associated scleritis with fluid in Tenon's space and a ring of uveoscleral enhancement. In chronic dacryoadenitis, the gland also shows diffuse oblong enlargement (see Figs. 2.**195**, 2.**197**). The glands may be massively enlarged in cases of sarcoidosis (see Fig. 2.**194**) or in other conditions such as Mikulicz syndrome, pseudotumor (see Figs. 2.**197**, 2.**198**), and Wegener granulomatosis.[23, 81, 163] Benign and malignant lymphoid tumors situated in the lacrimal gland also display diffuse enlargement with oblong contouring of the gland (see Fig. 2.**182**).[23, 163] However, these lesions are usually bulky (see Fig. 2.**197**), frequently have anterior and posterior extension, and mold and drape themselves on the globe. In general, inflammatory processes and lymphomas tend to involve all aspects of the lacrimal gland, often including its palpebral lobe (see Figs. 2.**221**, 2.**227**). By comparison, neoplastic lesions rarely originate in the palpebral lobe of the gland, and therefore there is often only posterior extension of the mass rather than anterior growth beyond the orbital rim (Figs. 2.**320**, 2.**321**). Some of the mixed tumor may appear heterogeneous on T2-weighted MR images (Fig. 2.**322**). Some of the tumors may be large and associated with fossa formation in the superior temporal bony orbit (Figs. 2.**323**, 2.**324**).

Because the lacrimal gland is histologically similar to a salivary gland, the diseases that affect these glands are similar.

Epithelial tumors represent 50% of the masses involving the lacrimal gland.[23, 159, 163] Half of these tumors are pleomorphic (benign mixed) adenomas, and the other half are malignant lesions. Of the malignant tumors, adenocystic carcinoma is the most common, followed by pleomorphic tumor (malignant mixed tumor), mucoepidermoid carcinoma, adenocarcinoma (Figs. 2.325, 2.326), squamous cell carcinoma, and undifferentiated (anaplastic) carcinoma. A significant number of these tumors arise within pleomorphic adenomas.[23, 158] Benign mixed tumors may undergo spontaneous malignant degeneration, and are increasingly likely to undergo such malignant degeneration the longer the patient has the tumor.[158–160, 164] In such a malignant mixed tumor, the malignant cell clone develops from the preexisting benign mixed tumor, and the malignancy is often a poorly differentiated adenocarcinoma, or an adenoid cystic carcinoma.[23, 162] In general, patients with these carcinomas have a poor prognosis.[23, 157]

Bony changes in the lacrimal gland fossa may be produced by both benign or malignant epithelial tumors.[23] However, bone changes also can be produced by lacrimal gland cysts (Fig. 2.327) and other orbital lesions such as schwannoma, neurofibroma, fibrous histiocytoma, and lesions originating within the subperiosteal space or bone such as a benign orbital cyst, hematic cyst (cholesterol granuloma) (see Fig. 2.160), or Langerhans cell histiocytosis; and in particular eosinophilic granuloma, dermoid cyst, epidermoid cyst, or metastatic carcinoma.[160] Lymphoid and inflammatory processes rarely produce bone changes.[23]

Miscellaneous Lacrimal Gland Lesions

Amyloid Tumor of the Lacrimal Gland

Infiltration of the lacrimal gland with amyloid is a very uncommon disorder.[163] Amyloidosis of the lacrimal gland and orbit is usually associated with the primary, localized variant of the disorder, although it can be seen as a secondary form of the disease due to degeneration and amyloid depositions.[163] Isolated lacrimal gland involvement is rare and may mimic inflammatory and infiltrative lesions and even neoplasms of the lacrimal gland. The CT and MRI findings of lacrimal gland amyloidosis consist of an enlarged lacrimal gland with or without calcification. A castlike amorphous calcification of the lacrimal gland should raise the possibility of lacrimal amyloidosis (see Fig. 2.207). Calcifications may be multiple, resembling pheboliths.[163]

Kimura Disease

Kimura disease is a chronic self-limited inflammatory condition of unknown etiology and a rare cause of tumorlike masses in the head and neck. Kimura et al[166] reported this entity in 1948. Kimura disease was long regarded to be synonymous with angiolymphoid hyperplasia with eosinophilia; however, it is now clear that they are separate entities despite some similar histological features. The patients typically present with painless tumorlike nodules in the head and neck region, often associated with regional lymphadenopathy. Peripheral blood eosinophilia and an elevated serum level of IgE are almost always present. Histologically, Kimura disease is characterized by a mixed lymphoeosinophilic infiltration, reactive lymphoid follicles, ill-defined fibrosis, and capillary proliferation. Major salivary glands as well as the lacrimal gland may be involved in Kimura disease. The CT appearance of Kimura disease is shown in Figure 2.328. The differential diagnosis of Kimura disease of the lacrimal gland includes dacryoadenitis, sarcoidosis, pseudotumor, lymphoma, and lacrimal gland and fossa tumors.[163]

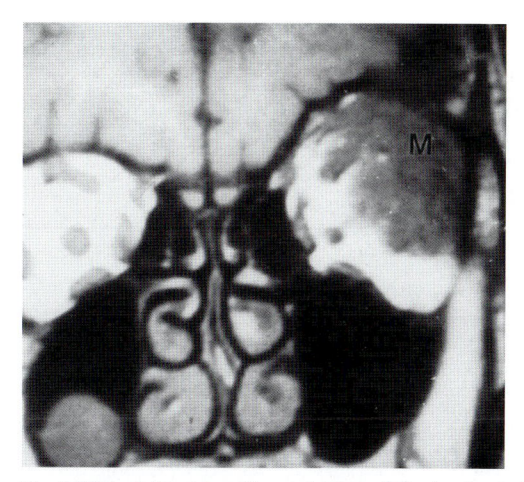

Fig. 2.325 Adenoid cystic carcinoma of the lacrimal gland. Coronal MR scan shows an irregular infiltrative mass (M) invading the adjacent superior and lateral rectus muscles, as well as the extracoronal and intraconal fatty reticulum.

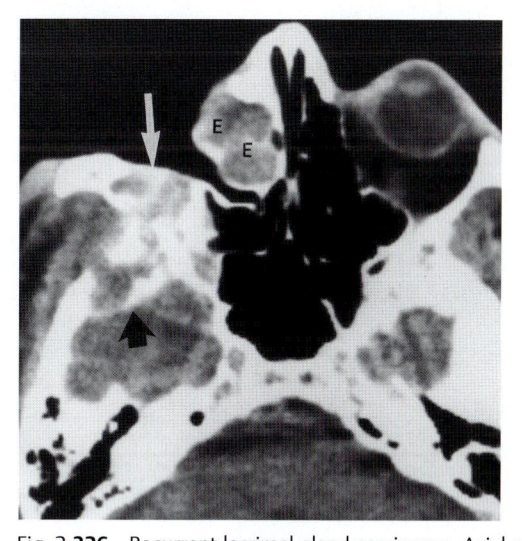

Fig. 2.326 Recurrent lacrimal gland carcinoma. Axial enhanced CT scan shows the postsurgical appearance of a right orbital exenteration. There is tumor recurrence in the right ethmoid (E) and at the surgical bed (arrows).

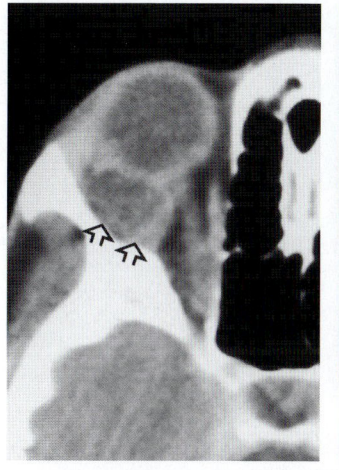

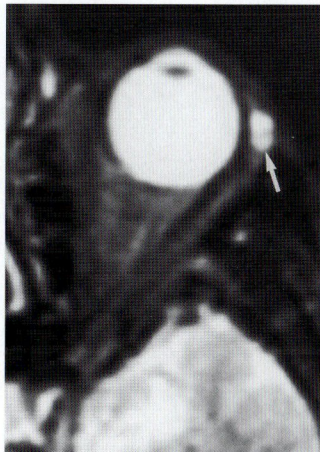

Fig. 2.327 Lacrimal gland duct cyst.
a Axial enhanced CT scan shows a large lacrimal gland cyst (arrows). Note smooth remodeling of the lateral bony orbit adjacent to the cyst.
b Axial T2W MR scan in another patient shows a small lacrimal gland duct cyst (arrow).

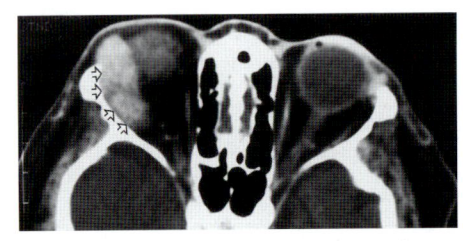

Fig. 2.328 Kimura disease of the lacrimal gland. Axial enhanced CT scan shows diffuse enlargement of the right lacrimal gland with marked contrast enhancement (arrows), consistent with Kimura disease. Case courtesy of Robert A. Weiss, MD, Chicago, IL, USA.

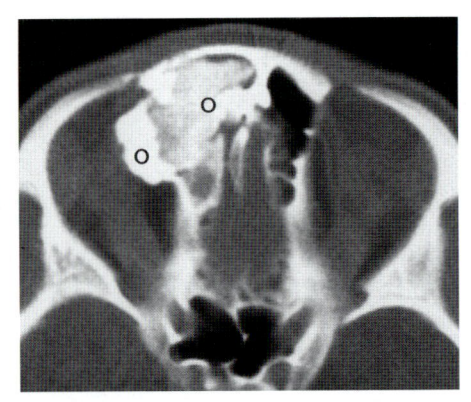

Fig. 2.329 Osteoma. Axial CT scan shows a fronto-ethmoid osteoma (O) extending into the left orbit.

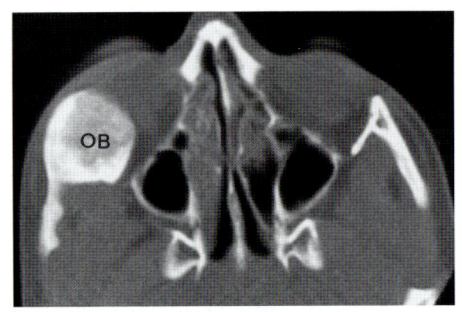

Fig. 2.330 Osteoblastoma. Axial CT scan shows an osteoblastoma (OB) involving the lateral wall of the right orbit.

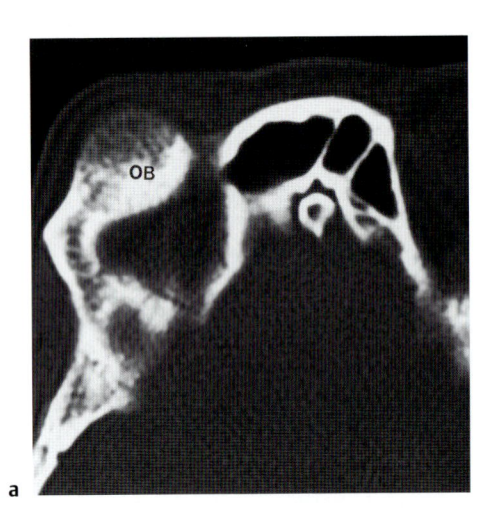

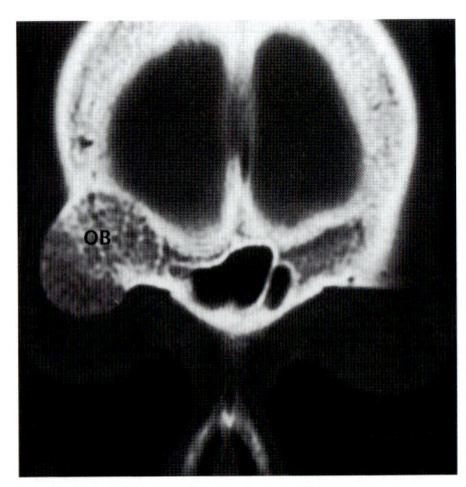

Fig. 2.331 Osteoblastoma. Axial (a) and coronal (b) CT scans showing a presumed osteoblastoma of the frontal bone (OB). Case courtesy of Robert A. Weiss, MD, Chicago, IL, USA.

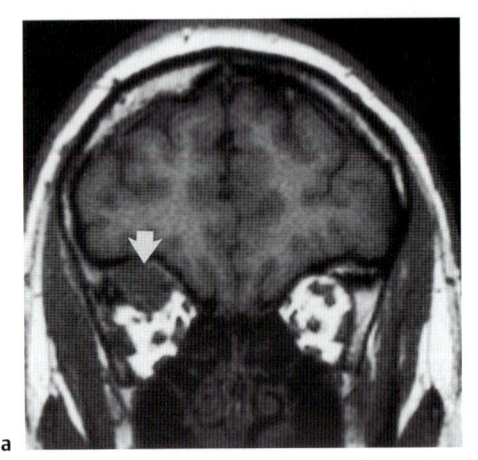

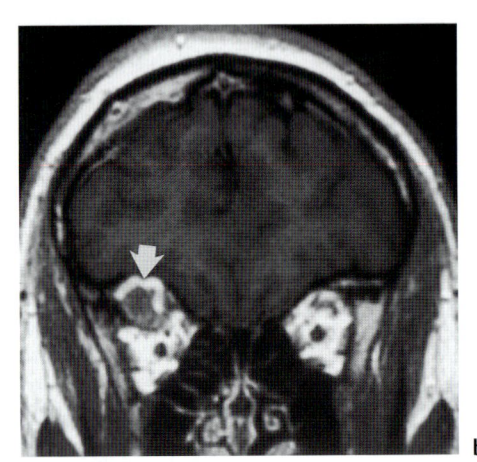

Fig. 2.332 Osteoblastoma. a Coronal unenhanced T1W and b coronal enhanced T1W MR scans showing a presumed osteoblastoma (arrows). The CT scan (not shown here) showed a well-defined sclerotic lesion.

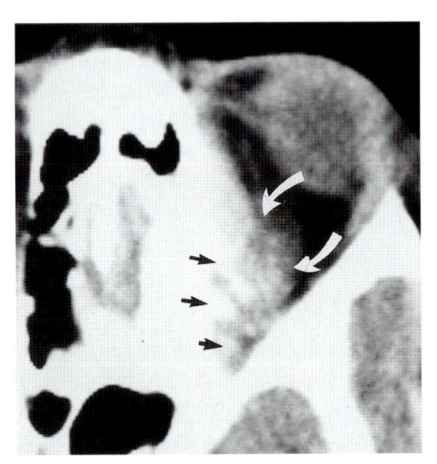

Fig. 2.333 Osteogenic sarcoma of the ethmoid invading the orbit. Axial enhanced CT scan shows irregular mass (white arrows) involving the left orbit. Note tumor bone formation (black arrows).

Fibro-Osseous Lesions of the Orbit

Fibro-osseous, osseous, and cartilaginous lesions of the orbit and paraorbital regions are relatively uncommon. These lesions may share overlapping clinical, radiological, and pathological features, causing potential difficulties in diagnosis.[2, 125] The specific entities that are shown in this chapter include osteoma (Fig. 2.329), osteoblastoma (Figs. 2.330–2.332), and osteosarcoma (Figs. 2.333, 2.334). Fibro-osseous lesions are described in more detail in Chapter 4.

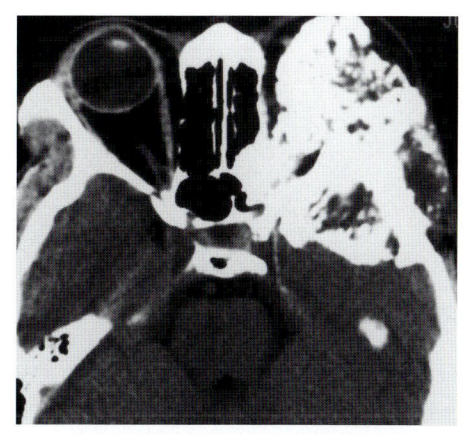

Fig. 2.334 Osteogenic sarcoma. Axial CT scan shows a destructive mass involving the left orbit. Note marked tumor bone formation.

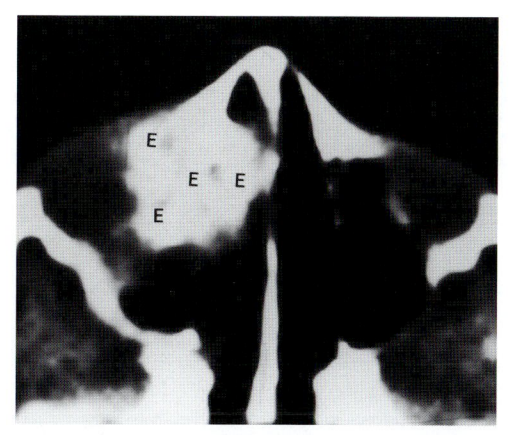

Fig. 2.335 Calcified esthesioneuroblastoma. CT scan shows a calcified esthesioneuroblastoma (E) invading the right orbit. This can be mistaken for a benign fibro-osseous lesion.

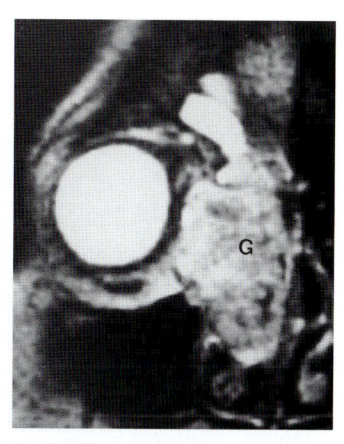

Fig. 2.336 Giant cell tumor in a 20-year-old woman. Coronal T2W MR scan showing a giant cell tumor (G) of the sinonasal cavities invading the right orbit.

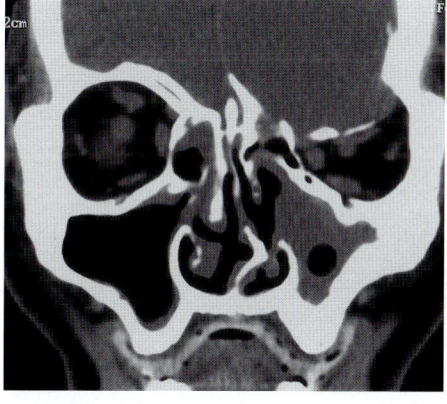

Fig. 2.337 Mucocele invading orbit. a Coronal CT scan showing a large frontal mucocele extending into the left orbit. Note erosion and downward desplacement of the roof of the left orbit. b Axial T2W and c coronal enhanced T1W MR scans. The mucocele is hyperintense on T1W and T2W MR images. The appearance of mucocele was the same on unenhanced T1W scans (not shown here).

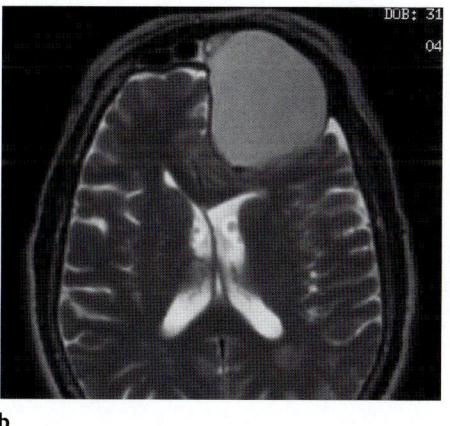

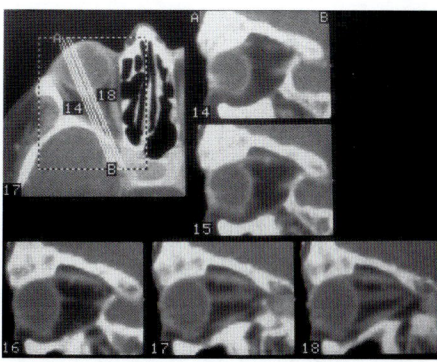

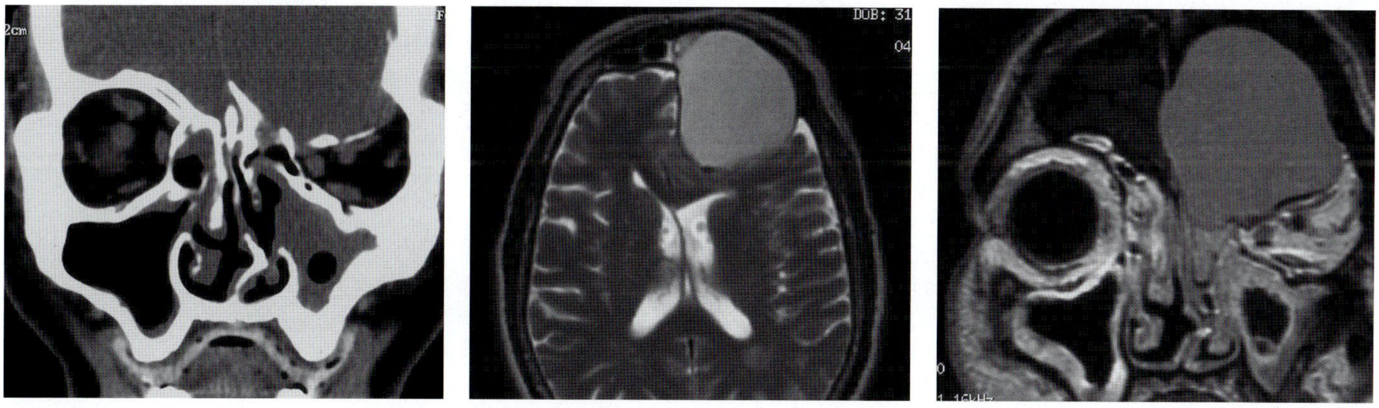

Fig. 2.338 Intraosseous hemangioma.
a Serial reformatted sagittal CT scans, showing a frontal bone hemangioma encroaching on the superior orbit. This may be mistaken for a benign fibro-osseous lesion such as fibrous dysplasia.

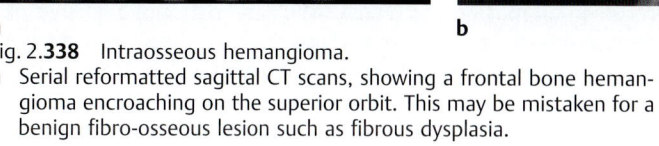

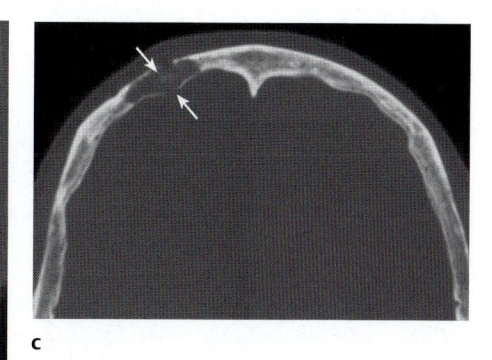

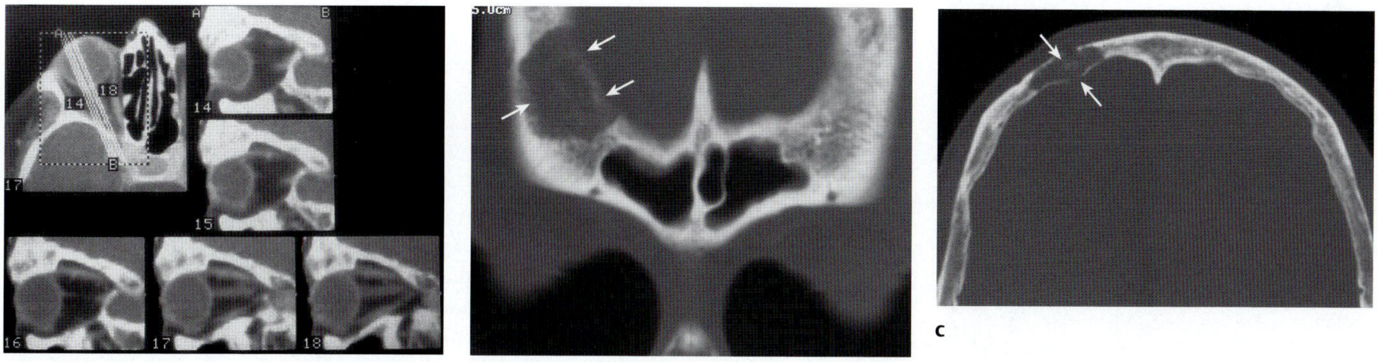

b, c Coronal (b) and axial (c) CT scans in another patient, showing a histologically proven hemangioma of the right frontal bone (arrows).

Secondary Orbital Tumors

Malignant and benign tumors, including cysts, of the sinonasal cavities may invade the orbit directly (Figs. 2.335–2.338). Tumors of the skin of the face such as basal cell and squamous cell carcinomas and malignant melanoma can invade the orbit (Fig. 2.339). The inferior orbital fissure is a pathway for tumors arising from or extending into the pterygopalatine or infratemporal fossae. Adenoid cystic tumors of the oral cavity and sinonasal cavities, as well as squamous cell carcinoma, melanoma, and lymphoma of the sinonasal and oral cavities, can extend

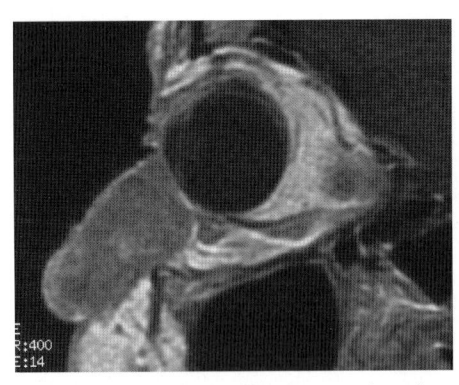

Fig. 2.**339** Malignant melanoma invading the orbit. Sagittal enhanced T1W MR scan showing a large cutaneous melanoma invading the left orbit.

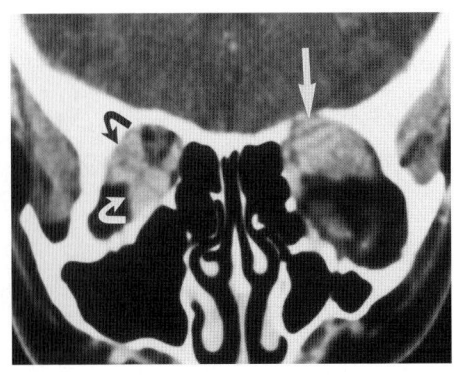

Fig. 2.**340** Metastasis. Coronal enhanced CT scan shows bilateral metastases (arrow) from primary breast carcinoma.

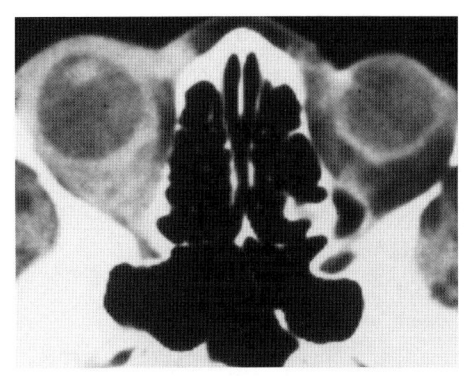

Fig. 2.**341** Metastasis. Axial CT scan shows a diffuse infiltrative process compatible with metastasis from a scirrhous carcinoma of the breast. Patients with orbital metastatic scirrhous carcinoma usually present with enophthalmia due to retraction of the globe.

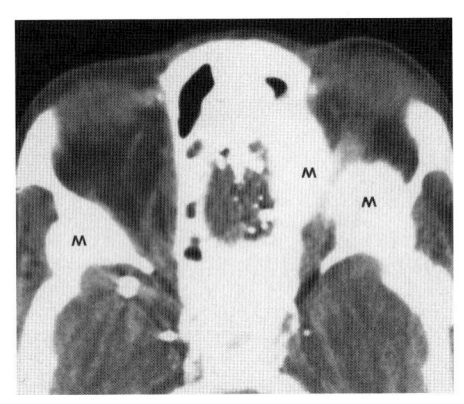

Fig. 2.**342** Metastasis. Axial CT scan shows multiple hyperostotic metastases (M) from prostate carcinoma.

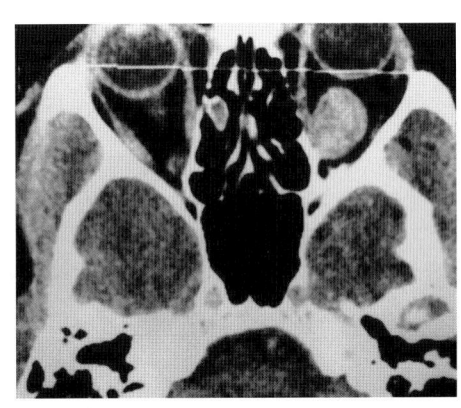

Fig. 2.**343** Metastasis. Axial enhanced CT scan shows a metastasis (arrow) from carcinoid tumor. Case courtesy of Debra J. Sheltar, MD, Houston, TX, USA.

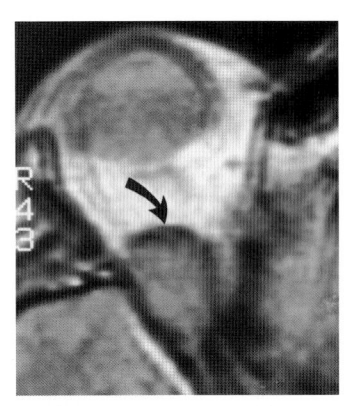

Fig. 2.**344** Metastasis. Axial PW MR scan shows a metastasis (arrow) from a primary leiomyosarcoma.

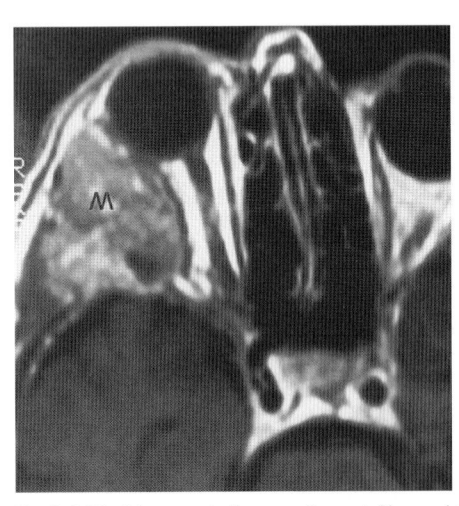

Fig. 2.**345** Metastasis from malignant fibrous histiocytoma. Axial post-contrast T1W MR scan shows a large destructive, markedly enhancing mass (M) compatible with metastasis to the greater wing of the sphenoid.

along the perineural–perivascular pathways into the pterygopalatine fossa and then into the orbit (see Chapters 4 and 9). Intracranial lesions such as meningioma may extend through the posterolateral wall of the orbit, the optic canal, or the sphenoid fissures, or ethmoidal foramina, or less resistant bony walls such as the lamina papyracea and orbital roof. Metastases to the orbit are most commonly the result of breast carcinoma in women (Figs. 2.**340**, 3.**341**) and carcinoma of the lung, kidney, or prostate in men (Fig. 2.**342**). Metastases can simulate primary orbital tumors, myositis, or diffuse orbital pseudotumor (breast carcinoma). Multiplicity of lesions can be helpful in suggesting the diagnosis of metastatic disease. Metastatic lesions may occur in any of the orbital compartments.[167] At times, metastatic deposit may be single and well-defined, simulating benign orbital tumor. This appearance in our experience has been seen in patients with known or unknown primary breast, prostate, malignant melanoma, and carcinoid tumor (Fig. 2.**343**). Sclerosing orbital metastases (desmoplastic fibrosis) from scirrhous carcinoma of the stomach (linitis plastica) or scirrhous carcinoma of the breast result in enophthalmos (Fig. 2.**341**). Sarcomas can also give rise to metastasis to the orbit (Figs. 2.**344**, 2.**345**). In children, metastases are usually from neuroblastoma (Fig. 2.**346**), Ewing sarcoma and Wilms tumor. At times optic nerve metastasis and seeding may simulate optic neuritis (Fig. 2.**347**). In patients that have undergone enucleation for malignant uveal melanoma, retinoblastoma, and ocular medulloepithelioma, any unexplained tumor mass within the surgical bed should highly be considered for recurrence.

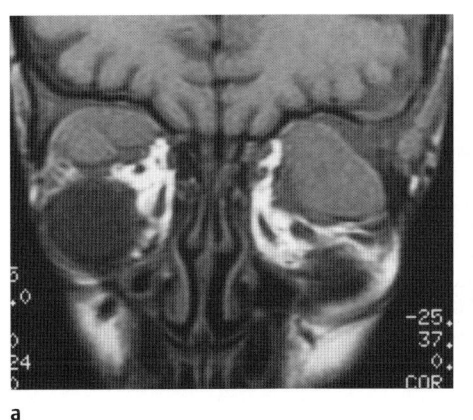

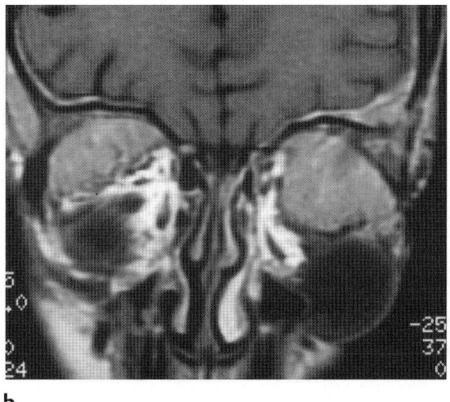

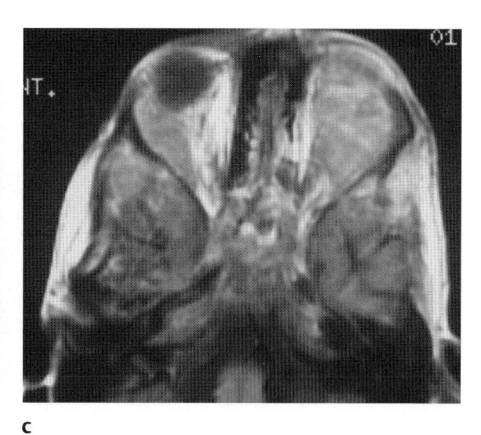

Fig. 2.**346** Metastasis in a 9-year-old girl with neuroblastoma. **a** Unenhanced coronal, **b** enhanced coronal and **c** enhanced axial MR scans, showing bilateral subperiosteal metastatic neuroblastoma. Case courtesy of Ayman A. El Sayad, MD, Saudi Arabia.

Ocular Motility Disorders

Ocular muscle disturbances (strabismus) are relatively common in the population, occurring at a rate of approximately 2–4%.[14] While the onset is usually in infancy or early childhood, acquired forms may occur at any age. If the object being viewed does not fall on the macula of both eyes, strabismus exists and the position of the nonaligned eye determines the description of the type of deviation (esotropia = inward deviation, exotropia = outward turning; vertical imbalance is described as hypertropia or hypotropia).[14]

Acquired Ocular Motility Disturbances Associated with Orbital Pathology

Many patients with classic hyperthyroidism show no ocular muscle involvement; conversely, patients manifesting severe eye muscle restriction often have normal thyroid function but are considered to have a form of euthyroid myopathy. Patients with orbital myositis or other conditions may present with an onset of limitation of ductions (monocular movement in test fields of gaze) in one or both eyes, with variable signs of inflammation and proptosis. In patients with cavernous sinus fistula, orbital venous congestion occurs with subsequent swelling of EOM and mechanical interference with movement.

Brown Superior Oblique Tendon Sheath Syndrome

In 1950, Brown described a clinical syndrome (superior oblique tendon sheath or Brown syndrome) characterized by an impaired ability to raise the eye in adduction. Typically, the patient may have straight eyes or a hypotropia (one eye lower in the primary position). Brown further classified this condition into true and simulated syndromes.[168] True (congenital) Brown syndrome includes only those patients with a congenitally short or taut superior oblique tendon sheath complex. Patients with simulated (acquired) Brown syndrome acquire the clinical features of the syndrome secondary to a variety of etiologies. Most authors, including Brown, have postulated that acquired Brown syndrome is primarily a disease of the tendon sheath–trochlear complex of the superior oblique muscle secondary to an inflammatory process of the adjacent tissues. Normal ocular movement of the superior oblique muscle requires a loose sheath and free movement of the tendon in the sheath. When the eye is adducted, the primary action of the inferior oblique muscle is elevation. When the eye is elevated in the adducted position, the superior oblique muscle normally relaxes, causing its tendon to lengthen and slide freely through the trochlea. If the superior oblique muscle cannot relax or its tendon cannot lengthen, the eye cannot be elevated while adducted. This limitation of elevation in adduction simulates an inferior oblique palsy, although the pathological process is postulated to be located primarily in the superior oblique complex. This restriction in the physiological passage of the tendon through the trochlea may be permanent or occur on an intermittent basis in the acquired form.

In acquired Brown syndrome, the symptom and findings often are intermittent. Affected patients usually complain of intermittent double vision (diplopia) on upward gaze and sometimes a "clicking" sensation in the area of the trochlea when attempting to look up (Figs. 2.**348**, 2.**349**). CT and MRI may show abnormalities in the area of the trochlea in acquired Brown syndrome (Figs. 2.**348**–2.**350**). One patient who had a history of head trauma showed significant thickening of the reflected portion of the superior oblique tendon in the involved eye, which was confirmed at the time of surgery.[169] The association of acquired Brown syndrome and rheumatoid arthritis has been well documented in the literature and may disappear spontaneously.

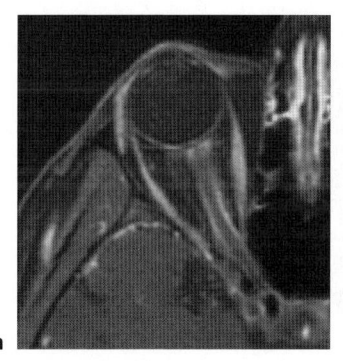

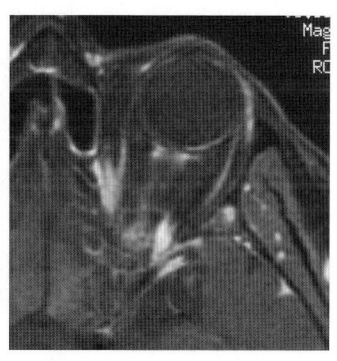

Fig. 2.**347** Optic nerve metastasis. **a**, **b** Axial enhanced fat-suppression T1W MR scans show bilateral optic nerve enhancement compatible with diffuse subarachnoid seeding from a primary breast carcinoma.

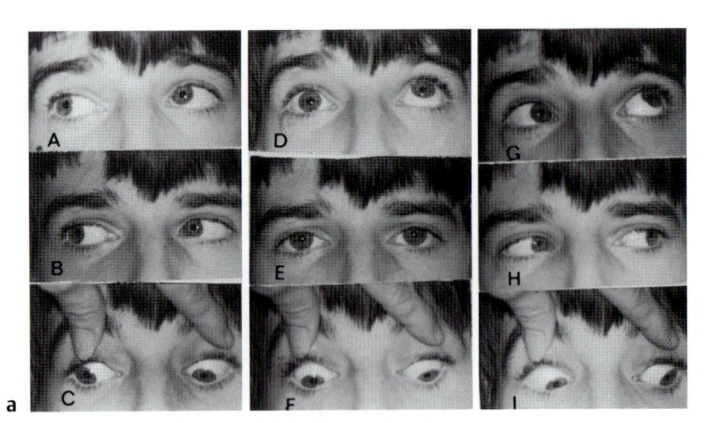

Fig. 2.348 Left acquired Brown syndrome.
a The eyes are shown in various gazing positions. The eyes are normal in the primary (phoria) (E), right lateral (B), left lateral (H), down and right (C), downward midline (F), and down and left positions (I). However, in the upward midline (D) and up and left positions (adduction of right eye) (G), elevation of the right eye is lacking. As the eye is abducted, the level of elevation remains the same until the midline is reached (D, G), at which point full elevation is usually possible (A). When the eye is adducted nasally (G) from the primary gaze (E), the primary action of the inferior oblique muscle is elevation. Thus, lack of elevation of the right eye during adduction (G), as in this patient, simulates paralysis of the right inferior oblique muscle, which is the hallmark of Brown syndrome. This actually represents "pseudoparalysis" because the cause is not dysfunction of the right inferior oblique muscle but rather inadequate relaxation of its antagonist, the right superior oblique muscle.

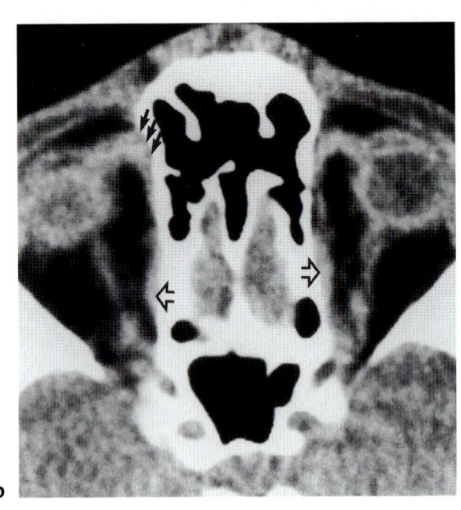

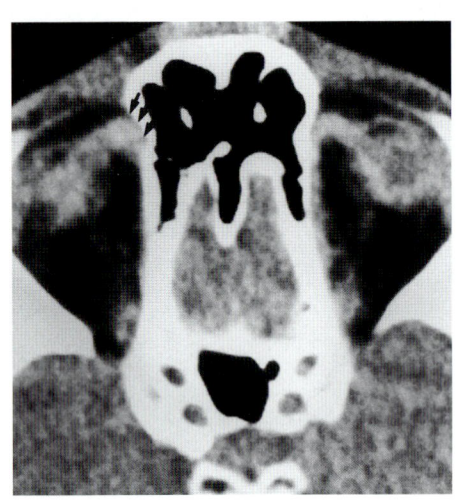

Fig. 2.**348 b** and **c** Axial CT scans show superior oblique muscles (hollow arrows) and thickening of the reflected portion of the right superior oblique tendon (solid arrows). Reproduced from Mafee et al. CT in the evaluation of Brown syndrome of the superior oblique tendon sheath. Radiology 1985; 154: 691–695. With permission.

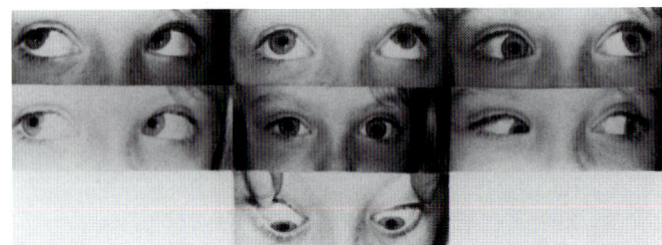

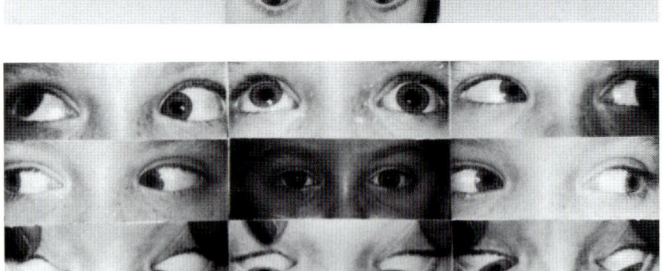

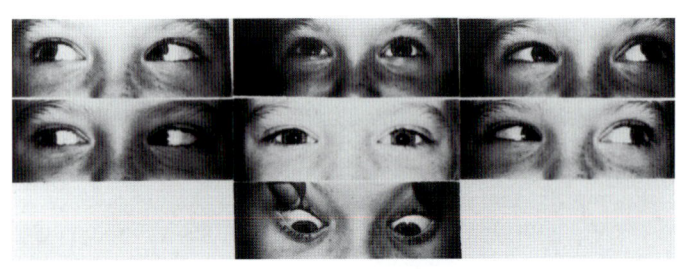

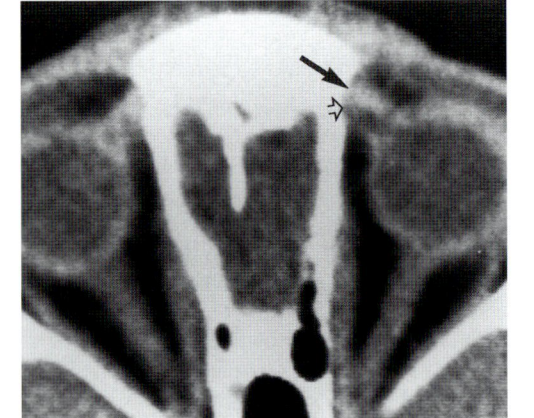

Fig. 2.**349 a** Congenital Brown syndrome, showing the eyes in various gazing positions. Note the markedly limited elevation of the right eye in the upward midline position (top middle), which is even more pronounced on adduction of the right eye (top right).
b Eleven months after tenotomy of the right superior oblique muscle, elevation is markedly improved on both adduction and abduction.
c Acquired Brown syndrome developed on the opposite side following trauma. Note the limited elevation of the left eye in the straight up position (top midline) and during the adduction (top right).
d Axial CT scan demonstrates slight thickening of the reflected tendon of the left superior oblique muscle (arrow). The open arrow points to area of edema. Reproduced from Mafee et al. CT in the evaluation of Brown syndrome of the superior oblique tendon sheath. Radiology 1985; 154: 691–695. With permission.

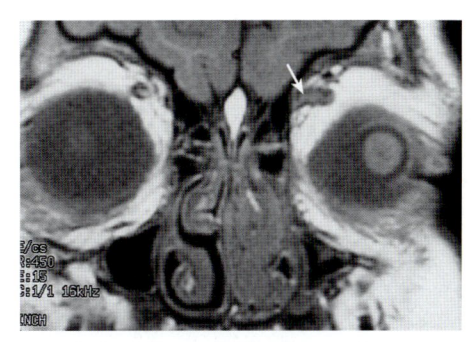

Fig. 2.**350** Left acquired Brown syndrome. Coronal T1W MR scan showing thickening of the reflected portion of the left superior oblique muscle (arrow).

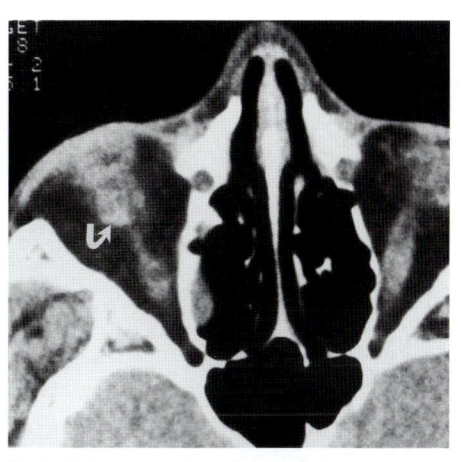

Fig. 2.**351** Laceration of the inferior rectus muscle. Axial CT scan shows deformity of the right inferior rectus (arrow) due to knife injury.

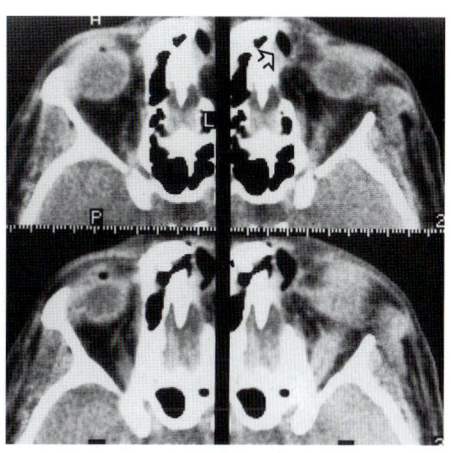

Fig. 2.**352** Deformity of trochlea following frontal sinus surgery. Axial CT scans show postsurgical deformity of the left trochlear region (arrow). The patient developed dysfunction of the left superior oblique muscle.

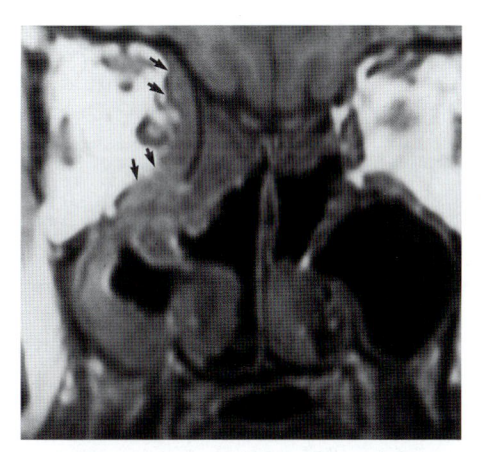

Fig. 2.**353** Deformity of the right medial rectus muscle following endoscopic sinus surgery. Coronal T1W MR scan shows subperiosteal soft-tissue (hematoma) along the medial wall of the right orbit (arrows).

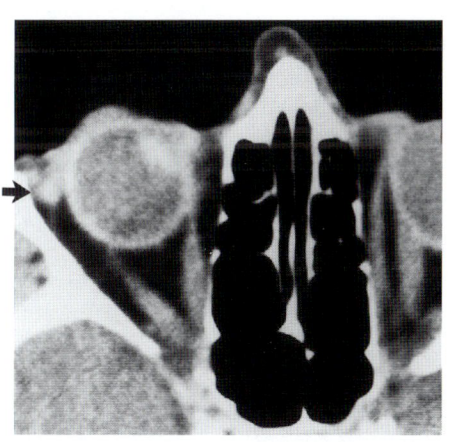

Fig. 2.**354** Pseudo-lost muscle. Axial CT scan in left lateral gaze, showing nonvisualization of the right lateral rectus. There is posttraumatic scar formation (arrows), causing limitation of function of the right lateral rectus. At surgery, the lateral rectus was found to be present.

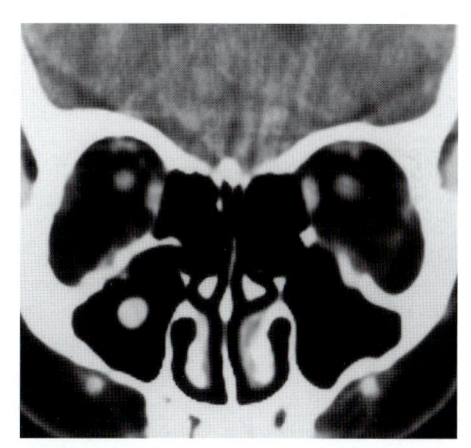

Fig. 2.**355** Nonvisualization of superior oblique muscles. Coronal CT scan shows absent superior oblique muscles.

■ Traumatic Injury of Ocular Muscles

Orbital tissues are frequently incarcerated in an orbital floor fracture. Ocular motility disturbances may be due to entrapment of the inferior rectus or inferior oblique or both (Fig. 2.**351**), or may be related to damage to their tendons (Fig. 2.**352**) or due to hematoma and scar formation (Figs. 2.**353**, 2.**354**). The medial rectus muscle is frequently damaged in orbital medial wall fracture. Early positive forced duction tests do not necessarily prove entrapment, and these disturbances may be the result of hematoma or inflammation. Soft-tissue damage may play a significant role in causing the typical findings of a "blowout fracture."

■ Congenital Anomalies of the Extraocular Muscles

Congenital Syndromes

Ocular motility disturbances frequently occur in craniosynostosis syndromes, and the observed patterns of abnormal movement are characteristically predictable. This is particularly true for the craniosynostosis syndromes of Apert and Crouzon. The type of abnormal movement noted in these two groups may be affected by mechanical factors induced by abnormal anatomy but may also show abnormalities in size of muscles and location of insertion. In rare conditions, the superior oblique muscles may be absent on imaging (Fig. 2.**355**).

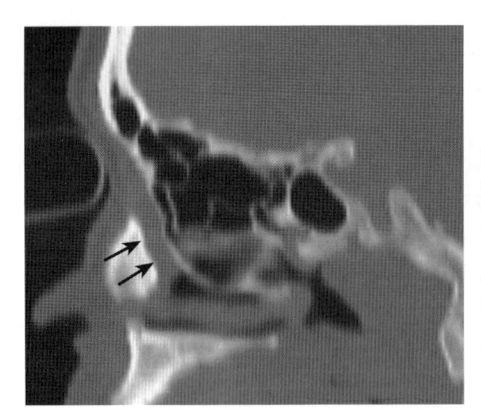

Fig. 2.**356** Sagittal reformatted CT scan shows the normal nasolacrimal canal (arrow).

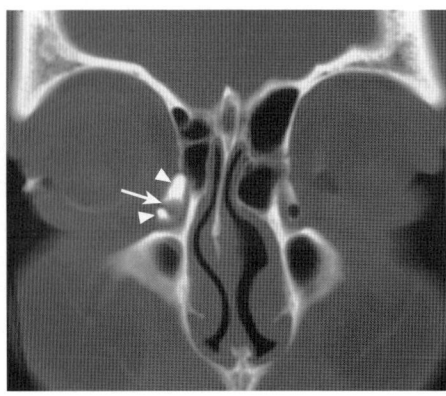

Fig. 2.**357** Dacryolith. CT dacryocystography shows a filling defect (arrow) in the right lacrimal sac, compatible with a dacryolith. Contrast material is seen outlining the lacrimal sac (arrowheads).

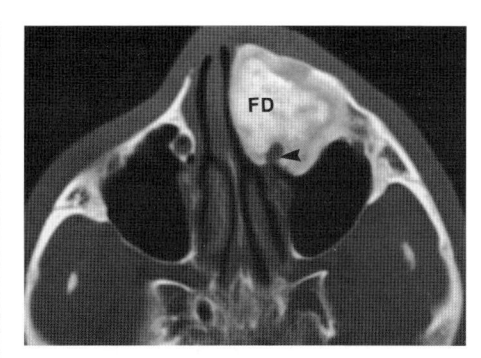

Fig. 2.**358** Constriction of nasolacrimal duct. Axial CT scan shows typical appearance of fibrous dysplasia (FD). Note narrowing of the left nasolacrimal duct (arrowhead).

Lacrimal Apparatus

Abnormalities of the lacrimal sac, superior and inferior lacrimal canaliculus, and nasolacrimal duct may cause many symptoms. The majority of these patients, however, present with increased tearing (epiphora). The cause of patients' symptoms may be intrinsic or extrinsic to the lacrimal drainage system. The nasolacrimal sac groove/fossa and nasolacrimal duct can be readily visualized by CT scan (Fig. 2.**356**). The lacrimal canaliculi, common canaliculus, lacrimal sac, and nasolacrimal duct can be visualized by dacryocystography.[170] The dacryocystographic technique has changed very little since Ewing's description in 1909.[171] Modern advances in digital subtraction and scintigraphy are useful adjuncts to standard dacryocystography. Current standard dacryocystographic technique includes injection of a water-soluble iodinated contrast agent into the lacrimal drainage system.[170] Following topical anesthesia, the lower punctum is dilated and a lacrimal cannula is inserted. While the upper punctum is occluded with a cotton-tipped applicator, 2–3 ml of contrast such as Sinografin is injected. Caldwell and lateral views are taken before and immediately after injection of contrast at 5, 15, and 30 minutes.[170] Late films (60 minutes) are obtained to evaluate dye retention. The normal dacryocystogram shows filling of superior and inferior canaliculi, the common duct, the lacrimal sac, and the nasolacrimal duct. Delayed film should show complete clearing of the dye within the lacrimal drainage system. CT dacryocystography allows better assessment of the lacrimal drainage system (Fig. 2.**357**) and the extent of adjacent tissue involvement.

Canalicular Obstructions

These obstructions are present proximal to the common canaliculus. Trauma is the most common cause for these obstructions. Canaliculitis and canalicular papillomas are other causes of obstruction. The common canalicular obstructions are usually due to chronic dacryocystitis or a ball-valve effect of dacryoliths. Dacryocystography shows contrast in ascending and descending canaliculi, up to or including the common canaliculus (sinus of Maier); the lacrimal sac does not fill. Lack of patency of the common lacrimal canaliculus usually requires conjunctivodacryocystorhinostomy and insertion of a Jones tube or microdissection of the common canaliculus with dacryocystorhinostomy.[170]

High Nasolacrimal Duct Obstruction

The typical location of high nasolacrimal duct obstructions is at the bony entrance to the nasolacrimal duct. These are the most common abnormalities found on dacryocystograms.[170] The constriction is usually a lesion of the membranous duct, although deformity of the osseous duct due to bony pathology or trauma is not uncommon (Fig. 2.**358**). The typical dilatation of the lacrimal sac, forming a lacrimal sac mucocele or abscess, should be noted. Chronic dacryocystitis is the most common etiology for constriction of the membranous duct.[170] Dacryoliths, secondary to chronic dacryocystitis, can also lodge in the nasolacrimal duct, resulting in complete or incomplete obstruction. Fibro-osseous lesions may cause constriction of the nasolacrimal duct, resulting in incomplete obstruction of the lacrimal drainage system (Fig. 2.**358**).

Dacryocele

A dacryocele (lacrimal sac mucocele) is a cystic expansion of the lacrimal sac or a diverticulum of the sac. The expansion is caused by a proximal or distal block of the nasolacrimal duct.[172] Dacryoceles are considered a congenital anomaly of the lacrimal drainage system and are usually apparent in the first few days of life. On CT scans and MR images, dacryoceles appear as well-circumscribed, rounded lesions centered in the nasolacrimal sac region (Fig. 2.**359**).[172] On CT scan, the density of the lesion is homogeneous when it is uninfected. On MR images, dacryocele appears hypointense on T1-weighted and hyperintense on T2-weighted images (Fig. 2.**360**). If the lesion is infected, there may be a rim of contrast enhancement.

Lacrimal Sac Tumors

Lacrimal sac tumors are rare and include epithelial and nonepithelial tumors. Benign epithelial tumors include papilloma, oncocytoma, and benign mixed tumors. Malignant epithelial tumors include squamous carcinoma (Fig. 2.**361**), adenocarcinoma (Fig. 2.**362**), mucoepidermoid carcinoma (Fig. 2.**363**), oncocytic adenocarcinoma, adenoid cystic carcinoma, acinic cell carcinoma (Fig. 2.**364**), and poorly differentiated carcinoma. Other tumors of the lacrimal sac include malignant melanoma (Fig. 2.**365**), lymphoma (Fig. 2.**366**), neurogenic tumors, fibrous histiocytoma, and other rare tumors.

Pathology 289

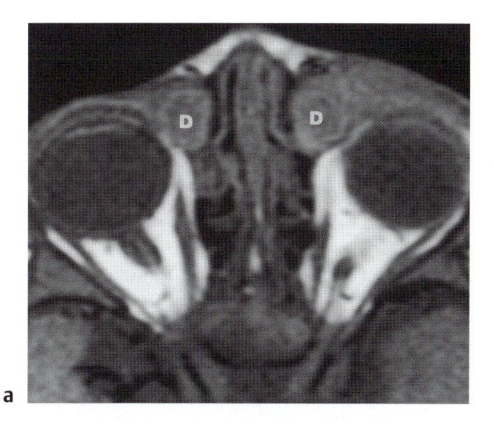

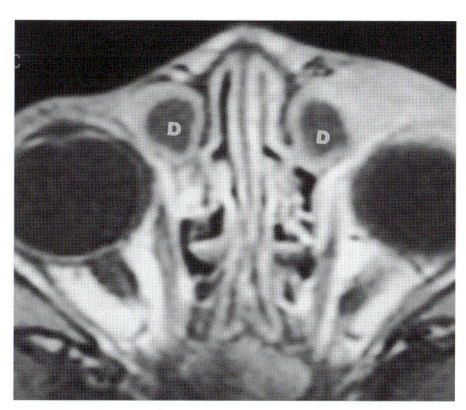

Fig. 2.**359** Dacryocele. **a** Axial unenhanced T1W and **b** axial enhanced T1W MR scans showing bilateral lacrimal sac mucocele (dacryocele) (D).

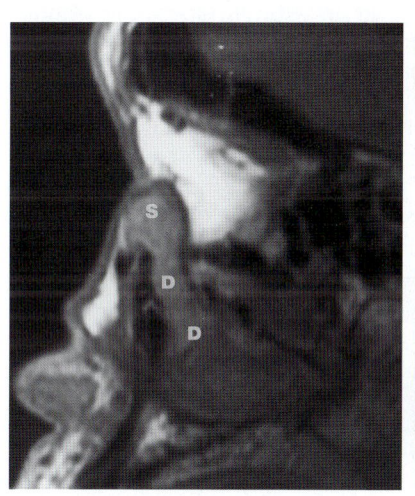

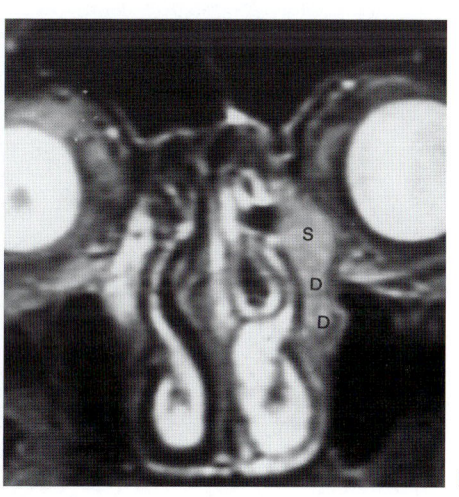

Fig. 2.**360** Dilated lacrimal drainage system. **a** Sagittal T1W and **b** coronal T2W MRI scans show marked dilatation of the left nasolacrimal duct (D) and sac (S) due to distal blockage of the nasolacrimal duct.

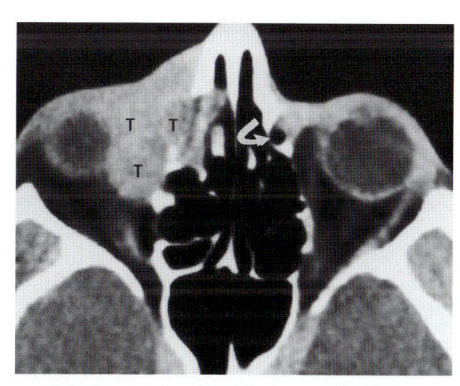

Fig. 2.**361** Squamous cell carcinoma of the lacrimal sac. Axial enhanced CT scan shows a right lacrimal sac tumor (T). Note normal left nasolacrimal duct (arrow).

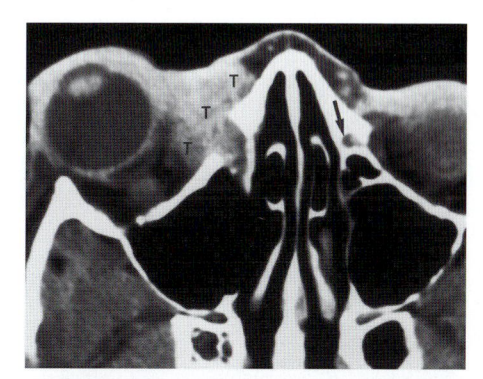

Fig. 2.**362** Adenocarcinoma of lacrimal sac. Axial enhanced CT scan shows a right lacrimal sac tumor (T) compatible with an adenocarcinoma. Note normal left nasolacrimal duct (arrow).

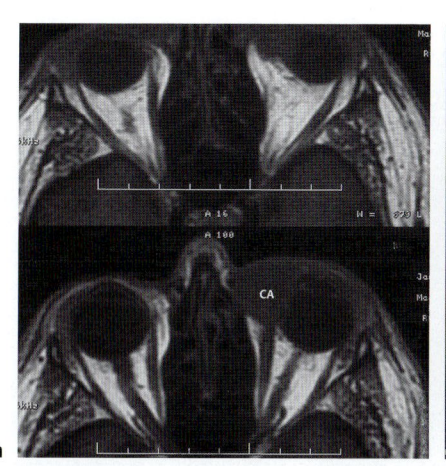

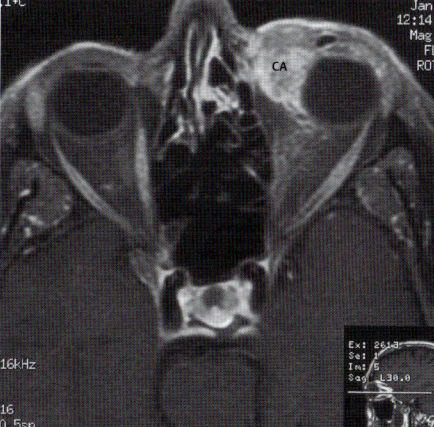

Fig. 2.**363** Mucoepidermoid carcinoma of the lacrimal sac region. **a** Axial T1W and **b** axial enhanced fat-suppression T1W MR scans, showing a mucoepidermoid carcinoma (CA) of the left lacrimal sac region.

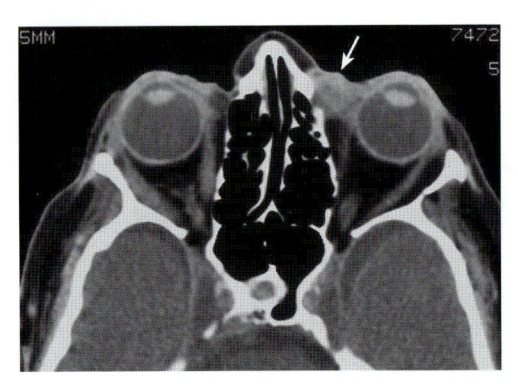

Fig. 2.364 Acinic cell carcinoma of the lacrimal sac. Axial CT scan, showing a left lacrimal sac acinic cell carcinoma (arrow).

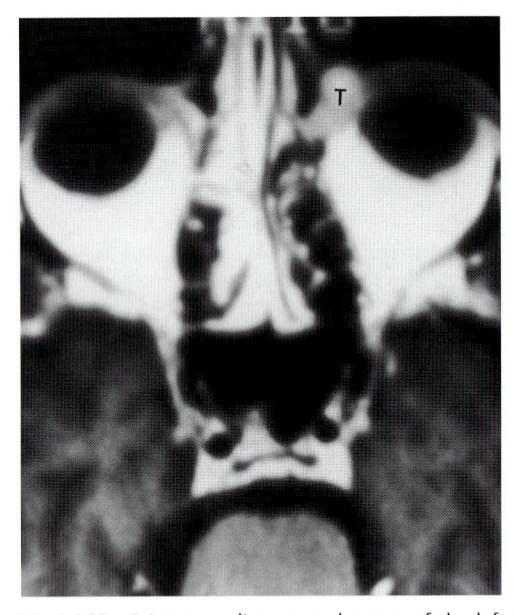

Fig. 2.365 Primary malignant melanoma of the left lacrimal sac. Axial enhanced T1W MR scan shows a left lacrimal sac tumor (T) compatible with primary malignant melanoma of the lacrimal sac.

Orbital Trauma

Orbital trauma includes: fractures of the floor; medial wall fractures; lateral wall fractures; roof fractures; combined fractures, such as tripod fractures, nasal-ethmoidal-orbital fractures, Le Fort fractures; and penetrating injuries to the orbit and globe, including foreign bodies.[172, 173]

The classic blow-out fracture involves the floor of the orbit, usually sparing the orbital rim. Frequently, orbital tissues are incarcerated in the fracture site (Figs. 2.367–2.369). CT better delineates the soft tissue along with the bony deformity of the orbit.[172] This imaging technique allows visualization of the position of the inferior rectus muscle (e.g., free, hooked, or entrapped) and better identification of soft-tissue changes, such as hematoma and herniation of fat into the fracture site. Blow-in fractures involve the displacement of orbital floor fragments toward the orbit, resulting in decrease in the orbital volume. Orbital floor fractures commonly involve the medial wall of the orbit. Isolated fracture of the medial orbital wall may also occur. Orbital emphysema (pneumo-orbitus) is commonly associated with medial orbital wall fractures. Coronal scans are best to demonstrate these fractures as well as to evaluate the possible damage to the medial rectus muscle at the fractured site.

Orbital roof fractures may be the result of penetrating or nonpenetrating injuries. These fractures may be associated with pneumocephalus, CSF leak, and intracranial complications. Associated frontal sinus fractures may be present. CT and MR imaging are both indicated to evaluate the fracture and possible intracranial complications.

Fractures of the optic canal, superior orbital fissure, and orbital apex may be associated with optic nerve damage. CT scan is best to localize the fracture, and MR imaging is necessary to evaluate damage to the optic nerve. Compression of the optic nerve may develop when bony fragments impinge on the nerve within the optic canal. Optic nerve compression may also occur due to hemorrhage within the optic nerve sheath or be related to subperiosteal hemorrhage or retrobulbar hemorrhage. Rapid diagnosis and surgical treatment of treatable causes, such as optic nerve compression by bony fragments, or acute retrobulbar and subperiosteal hemorrhages that compress the optic nerve, may result in significant visual recovery.[173]

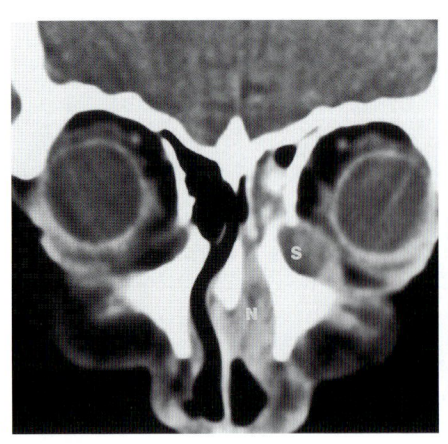

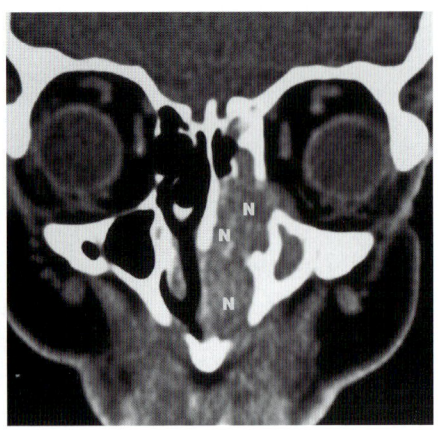

Fig. 2.366 Lymphoma involving the lacrimal sac. a, b Coronal enhanced CT scans showing lymphoma involving the left nasal cavity (N) and left lacrimal sac (S).

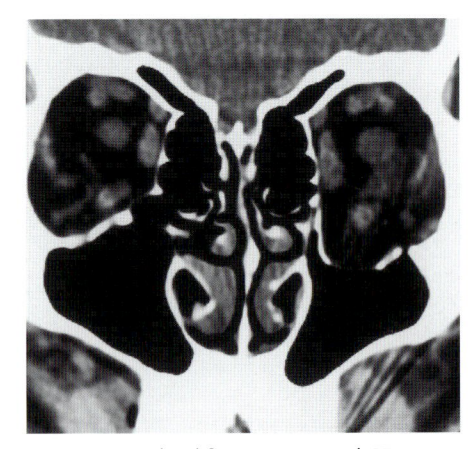

Fig. 2.367 Orbital fracture. Coronal CT scan shows blow-out fracture of the floor of the left orbit, associated with herniation of orbital fat into the left maxillary sinus.

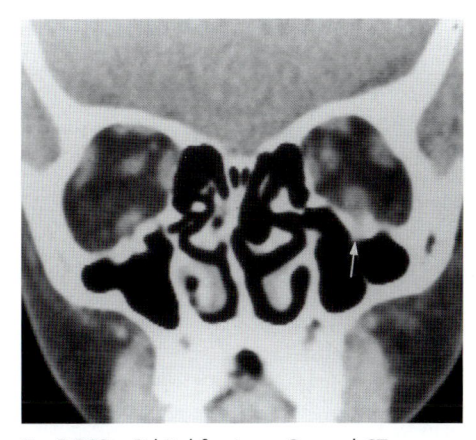

Fig. 2.**368** Orbital fracture. Coronal CT scan shows deformity of the left inferior rectus with entrapment (arrow) due to minimally displaced blow-out fracture of the left orbital floor.

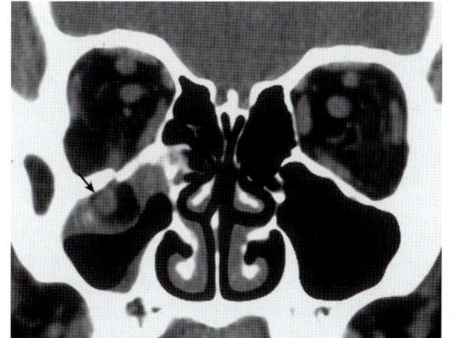

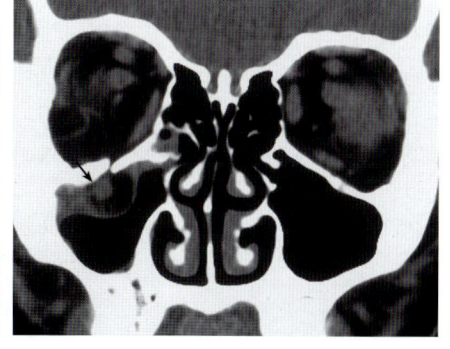

Fig. 2.**369** Orbital fracture.
a Coronal CT scan shows herniation of the orbital fat, and inferior rectus (arrow) into the right maxillary antrum.
b Coronal CT scan shows entrapment of the right inferior rectus at the site of minimally displaced fracture of the floor of the right orbit. At this level, the entire inferior rectus muscle is within the maxillary antrum (arrow).

Lateral orbital wall fractures are often associated with tripod or complex Le Fort III fractures. These fractures are discussed in Chapter 4.

CT scan is the study of choice for the evaluation of complications associated with orbital fractures as well as for the evaluation of postsurgical orbit (Fig. 2.**370**).

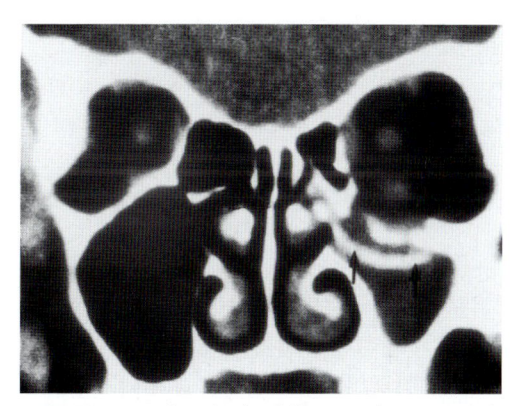

Fig. 2.**370** Displaced orbital floor implant. Coronal CT scan shows displacement of a left orbital floor implant (arrow) into the left maxillary antrum.

References

1. Warwick R, Williams PL, eds. Gray's Anatomy. 35th British edition. Philadelphia: W.B. Saunders; 1973.
2. Mafee MF. The eye, orbit: embryology, anatomy, and pathology. In: Som PM, Curtin HD, eds. Head and Neck Imaging. St. Louis: Mosby; 2003: 441–654.
3. Rootman J, ed. Diseases of the Orbit. Philadelphia: J.B. Lippincott; 1988.
4. Reeh MJ, Wobij JL, Wirtschafter JD. Ophthalmic Anatomy: A Manual with Some Clinical Applications. San Francisco: American Academy of Ophthalmology; 1981: 11–54.
5. Smith MF. Orbit, eyelids, and lacrimal system. Basic and Clinical Science Course. San Francisco: American Academy of Ophthalmology; 1987–1988.
6. Wilson FM. Fundamentals and principles of ophthalmology. Basic and Clinical Science Course. San Francisco: American Academy of Ophthalmology; 1991–1992.
7. Daniels DL, Yu S, Pech P, et al. Computed tomography and magnetic resonance imaging of the orbital apex. Radiol Clin North Am 1987; 25: 803–817.
8. Mafee MF, Putterman A, Valvassori GE, et al. Orbital space-occupying lesions: role of CT and MRI, an analysis of 145 cases. Radiol Clin North Am 1987; 25: 529–559.
9. Duhamel HL. Sur le development et la crue des os des animax. Mem Acad R Sci 1742; 55: 354–370.
10. Mafee MF, Miller MT. Computed tomography scanning in the evaluation of ocular motility disorders. In: Gonzalez CF, Becker MH, Flanagan JC, eds. Diagnostic Imaging in Ophthalmology. New York: Springer-Verlag; 1985: 39–54.
11. Dale RT, ed. Fundamentals of Ocular Motility and Strabismus. New York: Grune and Stratton; 1982.
12. Helveston EM, Merriam WW, Ellis FD, et al. The trochlea: a study of the anatomy and pathology. Ophthalmology 1982; 89: 124–133.
13. Fink WH. The anatomy of the extrinsic muscles of the eye. In: Allen JH, ed. Strabismus Ophthalmic Symposium. St. Louis: Mosby; 1950: 17–62.
14. Miller TM, Mafee MF. Computed tomography scanning in the evaluation of ocular motility disorders. Radiol Clin North Am 1987; 25: 733–752.
15. Snell RS, Lemp MA, eds. Clinical Anatomy of the Eye. Boston, MA: Blackwell Scientific; 1989.
16. Mafee MF. Imaging of the orbit. In: Valvassori GE, Mafee MF, Carter B, eds. Imaging of the Head and Neck. Stuttgart: Georg Thieme Verlag; 1995: 248–327.
17. Zonneveld FW, Koorneef L, Hillen B, et al. Direct Multiplanar, High Resolution, Thin-Section CT of the Orbit. Eindhoven, NL: Philips Medical Systems; 1986.
18. Mafee MF, Pruzansky S, Corrales MM, et al. CT in the evaluation of the orbit and the bony interorbital distance. AJNR 1986; 7: 265–269.
19. Mafee MF, Kumar A, Tahmoressi CN, et al. Direct sagittal CT in the evaluation of temporal bone disease. AJNR 1988; 9: 371–378.
20. Barakow JA, Dillon WP, Chew WM. Orbit, skull base and pharynx: contrast-enhanced fat suppression MR imaging. Radiology 1991; 179: 191–198.
21. Tien RD, Hesselink JR, Szumowski J. MR fat suppression combined with Gd-DTPA enhancement in optic neuritis and perineuritis. J Comput Assist Tomogr 1991; 15: 223–227.
22. Tien RD, Chu PK, Hesselink JR, et al. Intra- and paraorbital lesions: value of fat-suppression MR imaging with paramagnetic contrast enhancement. AJNR 1992; 12: 245–253.
23. Mafee MF, Haik BG. Lacrimal gland and fossa lesions: role of computed tomography. Radiol Clin North Am 1987; 25: 767–779.
24. Langer BG, Mafee MF, Pollack S, et al. MRI of the normal orbit and optic pathway. Radiol Clin North Am 1987; 25: 429–446.
25. Zonneveld FW, Koornneef L, Hiller B, et al. Normal direct multiplanar CT anatomy of the orbit with correlative anatomic cryosections. Radiol Clin North Am 1987; 25: 381–407.
26. Ettl A, Salomonowitz E, Koorneef L, Zonneveld FW. High resolution MR imaging anatomy of the orbit. Correlation with comparative cryosectional anatomy. Radiol Clin North Am 1998; 36: 1021–1045.

27. Currario G, Silverman FN. Orbital hypotelorism, arhinencephaly, and trigoncephaly. Radiology 1960; 74: 206–216.
28. Gerald BE, Silverman FN. Normal and abnormal interorbital distances with special reference to mongolism. AJR 1956; 95: 154–161.
29. Morin J, Hiu J, Anderson J, et al. A study of growth in the interorbital region. Am J Ophthalmol 1936; 56: 895–901.
30. Cameron J. Interorbital width: new cranial dimension, its significance in modern and fossil man and in lower mammals. Am J Phys Anthropol 1931; 15: 509–515.
31. Hansman CF. Growth of interorbital distance and skull thickness as observed in roentgenographic measurements. Radiology 1966; 86: 87–96.
32. Linder B, Campos M, Schafer M. CT and MRI of orbital abnormalities in neurofibromatosis and selected craniofacial anomalies. Radiol Clin North Am 1987; 25: 787–802.
33. Converse JM, McCarthy JG. Orbital hypertelorism. Scand J Plast Reconstr Surg 1985; 15: 265–276.
34. DeMyer WM. Neurologic evaluation associated forebrain maldevelopment and orbital hypotelorism. In: Symposium on Diagnosis and Treatment of Craniofacial Anomalies, Vol. 20. St. Louis: Mosby; 1979: 153–163.
35. Becker MH, McCarthy JG. Congenital abnormalities. In: Gonzalez CF, Becker MH, Flanagan JC, eds. Diagnostic Imaging in Ophthalmology. New York: Springer-Verlag; 1985: 115–187.
36. Gorlin RJ, Pindberg JJ, Cohen MM Jr. Syndromes of the Head and Neck, 2 d ed. New York: McGraw Hill; 1976.
37. Smith DW. Recognizable Patterns of Human Malformation. Philadelphia: W.B. Saunders; 1970.
38. Taybi H. Radiology of Syndromes and Metabolic Disorders. 2 d ed. St. Louis: Mosby; 1983.
39. Mafee MF, Jampol LM, Langer BG, et al. Computed tomography of optic nerve colobomas: morning glory anomaly, and colobomatous cyst. Radiol Clin North Am 1987; 25: 693–699.
40. Mann I. Developmental Abnormalities of the Eye, 2 d ed. Philadelphia: J.B. Lippincott; 1957: 74–78.
41. Mann I. The Development of the Human Eye. New York: Grune and Stratton; 1969.
42. Brown G, Tasman W, eds. Congenital anomalies of the optic disc. New York: Grune and Stratton; 1983: 97–191.
43. Arey LB. Developmental Anatomy, 6 th ed. Philadelphia: W.B. Saunders; 1970.
44. Duke-Elder S, Wybar KC. System of ophthalmology: the anatomy of the visual system, Vol. 2. St. Louis: Mosby; 1961.
45. Hamilton WJ, Boyd JD, Mossman HW, eds. Human Embryology: Development of Form and Function, 3 d ed. Baltimore, MD: Williams and Wilkins; 1962.
46. Tessier P. The definitive plastic surgical treatment of the severe facial deformities of craniofacial dysostosis: Crouzon's and Apert's diseases. Plast Reconstr Surg 1971; 48: 419–442.
47. Campbell JA. Craniofacial anomalies. In: Newton TH, Potts DG, eds. Radiology of the Skull and Brain, Vol. 1, Book 2. St. Louis: Mosby; 1971: 571–633.
48. Pruzansky S. Time: the fourth dimension in syndrome analysis applied to craniofacial malformations. Birth Defects 1977; 13: 3–28.
49. Mafee MF, Valvassori GE. Radiology of the craniofacial anomalies. Otolaryngol Clin North Am 1981; 14: 939–988.
50. Harwood-Nash DC. Coronal synostosis. In: Rogers LF, ed. Disorders of the Head and Neck Syllabus, Second Series. Reston, VA: American College of Radiology. 1977.
51. Anderson FM, Geiger L. Craniosynostosis: a survey of 204 cases. J Neurosurg 1965; 22: 229–240.
52. Shillito J Jr., Matson DD. Craniosynostosis: a review of 519 surgical patients. Pediatrics 1968; 41: 829–853.
53. Crouzon O. Dysostose cranio-faciale hereditaire. Bull Mem Soc Med Hop, Paris; 1912: 33: 545–555.
54. Lombardi G. Radiology in Neuro-ophthalmology. Baltimore, MD: Williams and Wilkins; 1967.
55. Saethre H. Ein beitrag zum turnschadel problem (pathogenese, erblickeit und symptomatologie). Deutsch Z Nervenh 1931; 119: 533–555.
56. Chotzen F. Eine eigenartige familiare entwicklungsstorung (akrocephalo- syndaktylie), dysostosis craniofacialis und hypertelorisms). Mschr Kinder 1932; 55: 97–122.
57. Bartsocas CS, Weber AL, Crawford JD. Acrocephalosyndactyly type 3: Chotzen's syndrome. J Pediatr 1970; 77: 267–272.
58. Lewis A, Gerson P, Axelson K, et al. Von Recklinghausen neurofibromatosis II. Incidence of optic glioma. Ophthalmology 1984; 91: 929–935.
59. Zimmerman RA, Bilaniuk LT, Mezger RA, et al. Computed tomography of orbitofacial neurofibromatosis. Radiology 1983; 146: 113–116.
60. Kobrin JL, Block FC, Wiengiest TA. Ocular and orbital manifestations of neurofibromatosis. Surv Ophthalmol 1979; 24: 45–51.
61. Jacoby CG, Go RT, Beren RA. Cranial CT of neurofibromatosis. AJR 1980; 135: 553–557.
62. Berry GA. Note on a congenital defect (? Coloboma) of the lower lid. Royal London Ophthalmologic Hospital Reports 1889; 12: 225.
63. Treacher-Collins E. Case with symmetrical congenital notches in the outer part of each lower lid and defective development of the malar bones. Trans Ophthal Soc 1900; 20: 190–191.
64. Pires deLima JA, Monteior HB. Aparello branquiale suas pertur-bacoes evolutivas. Arch Anat Anthrop (Lisboa) 1923; 8: 185.
65. Francheschetti A, Klein D. The mandibulo-facial dysostosis, a new hereditary syndrome. Acta Ophthalmol 1949; 27: 141–224.
66. Gorlin RJ, Pindberg JJ, Cohen MM Jr. Syndromes of the Head and Neck, 2nd ed. New York: McGraw-Hill; 1976.
67. Poswillo D. The pathogenesis of the Treacher Collins syndrome (mandibulofacial dysostosis). Br J Oral Surg 1975; 13: 1–26.
68. Herring SW, Rowlatt UF, Pruzansky S. Anatomical abnormalities in mandibulofacial dysostosis. Am J Med Genet 1979; 3: 225–259.
69. Henderson JW. Orbital Tumors. Philadelphia: W.B. Saunders; 1973: 116–123.
70. Mafee MF, Dobben GD, Valvassori GE. Computed tomography assessment of paraorbital pathology. In: Gonzalez CA, Becker MH, Flanagan JC, eds. Diagnostic Imaging in Ophthalmology. New York: Springer-Verlag; 1985: 281–302.
71. Grove AS. Giant dermoid cysts of the orbit. Ophthalmology 1979; 86: 1513–1520.
72. Kaufman LM, Villablanca JP, Mafee MR. Diagnostic imaging of cystic lesions in the child's orbit. Radiol Clin North Am 1998; 36: 1149–1163.
73. Rubenstein J. Disorders of the conjunctiva and limbus. In: Yanoff M, Duker JS, eds. Ophthalmology. St. Louis: Mosby; 1999: 1.1–1.21.
74. Dutton J. Orbital diseases. In: Yanoff M, Duker JS, eds. Ophthalmology. St. Louis: Mosby; 1999: 14.1–14.7.
75. Chang DF, Dallow RL, Walton DS. Congenital orbital teratoma: Report of a case with visual preservation. J. Pediatr Ophthalmol Strabismus 1980; 17: 88.
76. Garrity JA, Trautmann JC, Bartley GB, et al. Optic nerve sheath meningoceles: clinical and radiographic features in 13 cases with a review of the literature. Ophthalmology 1990; 97: 1519.
77. Laventer DB, Merriman JC, Defendini R, et al. Enterogenous cysts of the orbital apex and superior orbital fissure. Ophthalmology 1994; 101: 1614.
78. Dobben GD, Philip B, Mafee MF, et al. Orbital subperiosteal hematoma, cholesterol granuloma, and infection. Evaluation with MR imaging and CT. Radiol Clin North Am 1998; 36: 1185–1200.
79. Polito E, Leccisotti A. Diagnosis and treatment of orbital hemorrhagic lesions. Ann Ophthalmol 1994; 26: 85–93.
80. Gomez-Morales A, Croxatto JO, Croxatto L, et al. Hydatid cysts of the orbit: a review of 35 cases. Ophthalmology 1988; 95: 1027.
81. Mafee MF, Atlas SW, Galetta SL. In: Atlas SW, ed. Magnetic Resonance Imaging of the Brain and Spine, 3 d ed. Philadelphia: Lippincott Williams and Wilkins; 2002: 1433–1524.
82. Weber AL, Mikulis DK. Inflammatory disorders of the paraorbital sinuses and their complications. Radiol Clin North Am 1987; 25: 615–630.
83. Hawkins DD, Clark RW. Orbital involvement in acute sinusitis. Clin Pediatr 1977; 16(5): 464–471.
84. Eustis HS, Mafee MF, Walton C, Mondonca J. MR imaging and CT of orbital infections and complication in acute rhinosinusitis. Radiol Clin North Am 1998; 36: 1165–1183.
85. Chandler JR, Langenbrunner DJ, Stevens ER. The pathogenesis of orbital complications in acute sinusitis. Laryngoscope 80: 1414; 1970.
86. Dolan RW, Choudhury K. Diagnosis and treatment of intracranial complications of paranasal sinus infection. J Oral Maxillofac Surg 53: 1080; 1995.
87. Igarishi H, Igarishi S, Fujio N, et al. Magnetic resonance imaging in the early diagnosis of cavernous sinus thrombosis. Ophthalmologica 209: 292; 1995.
88. Saah D, Schwartz A. Diagnosis of cavernous sinus thrombosis by magnetic resonance imaging using flow parameters. Ann Otol Rhinol Laryngol 103: 487; 1994.

89 Centeno RS, Bentson RJ, Mancuso AA. CT scanning in rhinocerebral mucormycosis and aspergillosis. Radiology 1981; 140: 383–389.
90 Courey WR, New PFJ, Price DL. Angiographic manifestations of craniofacial phycomycosis: report of three cases. Radiology 1972; 103: 329–334.
91 Weber AL, Vitale Romo L, Sabates NR. Pseudotumor of the orbit. Clinical, pathologic, and radiologic evaluation. Radiol Clin North Am 1999; 37: 151–168.
92 Blodi FC, Gass JDM. Inflammatory pseudotumor of the orbit. Br J Ophthalmol 1968; 52: 79–93.
93 Flanders AE, Mafee MF, Rao VM, et al. CT characteristics of orbital pseudotumors and other orbital inflammatory processes. J Comput Assist Tomogr 1989; 13(1): 40–47.
94 Birch-Hirschfield A. Zur diagnostik and pathologie der orbitaltumoren. Deutsche Ophth Ges 1905; 32: 127–135.
95 Motto-Lippa L, Jakobiec FA, Smith M. Idiopathic inflammatory orbital pseudotumor in childhood. II. Results of diagnostic tests and biopsies. Ophthalmology 1981; 88: 565–574.
96 Trokel SL, Hilal SK. Recognition and differential diagnosis of enlarged extraocular muscles in computed tomography. Am J Ophthalmol 1979; 87: 503–512.
97 Tolosa E. Periartritic lesions of the carotid siphon with the clinical features of a carotid infraclinoid aneurysm. J Neurol Neurosurg Psychiatry 1954; 17: 300–302.
98 Hunt WE, Meagher JN, LeFever HE, et al. Painful ophthalmoplegia. Neurology 1961; 11 (Suppl):56–62.
99 Smith JL, Taxdal DSR. Painful ophthalmoplegia: the Tolosa-Hunt syndrome. Am J Ophthalmol 1966; 61: 1466–1472.
100 Sondheimer FK, Knapp J. Angiographic findings in the Tolosa-Hunt syndrome: painful ophthalmoplagia. Radiology 1973; 106: 105–112.
101 Hurwitz CA, Faquin WC. Case record 5-2002. N. Engl J Med 2002; 346(7): 513–520.
102 Rubin RM, Sadun AA. Ocular myopathies. In Yanoff M, Duker JS, eds. Ophthalmology. St. Louis: Mosby; 1999: 11.18.1–11.18.8.
103 Kendler DL, Lippa J, Rootman J. The initial clinical characteristics of Graves' orbitopathy vary with age and sex. Arch Ophthalmol. 111: 197–201; 1993.
104 Mafee MF, Dorodi S, Pai E. Sarcoidosis of the eye, orbit, and central nervous system: role of MR imaging. Radiol Clin North Am 1999; 37: 73–87.
105 Mafee MF. Case 25: Optic nerve sheath meningioma. In: Head and Neck Disorders (Fourth Series) Test and Syllabus. Reston VA: American College of Radiology; 1992: 552–595.
106 Shields JA, ed. Diagnosis and Management of Orbital Tumors. Philadelphia: W.B. Saunders; 1989.
107 Dykhuizen RS, Smith C, Kennedy MM, et al. Necrotizing sarcoid granulomatosis with extrapulmonary involvement. Eur Respir J. 1997; 10: 245–247.
108 Raskin Em, McCormick SA, Maher EA, et al. Granulomatous idiopathic orbital inflammation. Ophthal/Plast Reconstr Surg 1995; 11: 131–135.
109 Monfort-Gouraud M, Chokre R, Dubiez M, et al. Inflammatory pseudotumor of the orbit and suspected sarcoidosis. Arch Pediatr 1996; 3: 697–700.
110 Mombaerts I, Schlingemann RO, Goldschmeding R, Koornep L. Idiopathic granulomatous orbital inflammation. Ophthalmology 1996; 103: 2135–2141.
111 Carmody RF, Mafee MF, Goodwin JA, et al. Orbital and optic pathway sarcoidosis: MR findings. AJNR 1994; 15: 775–783.
112 Ing EB, Garrity JA, Gross SA, Ebersold MJ. Sarcoid masquerading as optic nerve sheath meningioma. Mayo Clinic Proc 1997; 72: 38–43.
113 Beardsley TL, Brown SV, Sydner CF, et al. Eleven cases of sarcoidosis of the optic nerve. Am J Ophthalmol 1984; 97: 67–77.
114 Vidal RW, Devaney K, Ferlito A, et al. Sinonasal malignant lymphomas: a distinct clinicopathological category. Ann Otol Rhino Laryngol 1999; 108: 411–419.
115 Lichtenstein L. Histiocytosis X: Integration of eosinophilic granuloma of bone, "Letterer-Siwe disease" and "Hand Schüller-Christian disease" as related manifestations of a single nosologic entity. Arch Pathol 1953; 56; 84–102.
116 Nezelof C, Barbey S. Histiocytosis: Nosology and pathobiology. Pediatr Pathol 1985; 3: 1–41.
117 Hidayat AA, Mafee MF, Laver NV, Noujaim S. Langerhans' histiocytosis and juvenile xanthogranuloma of the orbit. Clinicopathologic, CT, and MR imaging features. Radiol Clin North Am 1998; 36: 1229–1240.
118 Stanley SS: Taking the X out of histiocytosis X. Radiology 1997; 204: 322–324.
119 Nezelof C, Basset F. Langerhans cell histiocytosis research: post, present, and future. Hematol Oncol Clin North Am 1998; 12: 385–406.
120 Zimmerman LE. Ocular lesions of juvenile xanthogranuloma. Nevoxanthoendothelioma. Trans Am Acad Ophthalmal Otolaryngol 1965; 69: 412–442.
121 Jakobiac FA, Mills MD, Hidayat AA, et al. Periocular xanthogranulomas associated with severe adult-onset asthma. Trans Am Opthalmol Soc 1993; 91: 99–129.
122 Alper MG, Zimmerman LE, LaPiana FG. Orbital manifestations of Erdheim-Chester disease. Trans Am Ophthalmal Soc. 1983; 8: 64.
123 Shields AK, Karcioglu ZA, Shields C, et al. Orbital and eyelid involvement with Erdheim-Chester disease: A report of two cases. Arch Ophthalmol 1991; 109: 850–854.
124 Tien RD, Brasch RC, Jackson DE, et al. Cerebral Erdheim-Chester disease: persistent enhancement with Gd-DTPA on MR images. Radiology 1989; 172: 791–792.
125 Mafee MF. Eye and orbit. In: Som PM, Curtin HD, eds. Head and Neck Imaging. St. Louis: Mosby-Yearbook; 1996: 1009–1128.
126 Flanders AE, Espinosa GA, Markie- wicz DA, et al. Orbital lymphoma. Radiol Clin North Am 1987; 25: 601–612.
127 Peyster RG, Hoover ED. Computerized Tomography in Orbital Disease and Neuro-ophthalmology. Chicago: Mosby; 1984: 21–56.
128 Fitzpatrick PJ, Macko S. Lymphoreticular tumors of the orbit. Int J Radiat Oncol Biol Phys 1984; 10: 333–340.
129 Yeo JH, Jakobiec FA, Abbott GF, et al. Combined clinical and computed tomographic diagnosis of orbital lymphoid tumors. Am J Ophthalmol 1982; 94: 235–245.
130 Valvassori Ge, Sabnis SS, Mafee RF, et al. Imaging of orbital lymphoproliferative disorders. Radiol Clin North Am 1999; 37: 135–150.
131 Bilaniuk LT. Orbital vascular lesions: Role of imaging. Radiol Clin North Am 1999; 37: 169–183.
132 Mafee MF, Miller MT, Tan WS, et al. Dynamic computed tomography and its application to ophthalmology. Radiol Clin North Am 1987; 25: 715–731.
133 Ruchman MC, Stefanyszn MA, Flanagan JC, et al. Orbital tumors. In: Gonzalez CA, Becjer MH, Flanagan JC, eds. Diagnostic Imaging in Ophthalmology. New York: Springer-Verlag; 1985: 201–238.
134 Krohel GB, Wright JE. Orbital hemorrhage. Am J Ophthalmol 1979; 88: 254–258.
135 Tan WS, Wilbur AC, Mafee MF. The role of the neuroradiologist in vascular disorders involving the orbit. Radiol Clin North Am 1987; 25: 849–861.
136 Panda A, Dayal Y, Singhal V, et al. Hemangiopericytoma. Br J Ophthalmol 1984; 68: 124–127.
137 Stout AP. Tumors featuring pericytes, glomus tumor and hemangioperibytoma. Lab Invest 1956; 5: 217–223.
138 Stout AP, Murray MR. Hemangiopericytoma. Ann Surg 1972; 116: 26–32.
139 Bockwinkel KD, Diddams JA. Haemangiopericytoma: report of care and comprehensive review of literature. Cancer 1970; 25: 896–901.
140 Rootman J, Goldberg C, Robertson W. Primary orbital schwannomas. Br J Ophthalmol 1982; 66: 194–204.
141 Carroll GS, Haik BG, Fleming JC, et al. Peripheral nerve tumors of the orbit. Radiol Clin North Am 1999; 37: 195–202.
142 Mafee MF, Goodwin J, Dorodi S. Optic nerve sheath meningiomas: Role of MR imaging. Radiol Clin North Am 1999; 37: 37–58.
143 Skolnick CA, Mafee MF, Goodwin JA. Pneumosinus dilatans of the sphenoid sinus presenting with visual loss. J Neuroophthalmol 2000; 20(4): 259–263.
144 Dalley R. Fibrous histiocytoma and fibrous tissue tumors of the orbit. Radiol Clin North Am 1999; 37: 185–194.
145 Font RL, Hidayat AA. Fibrous histiocytoma of the orbit: a clinicopathologic study of 150 cases. Hum Pathol 1982; 13: 199.
146 Ros PR, Kursunoglu S, Batle JF, et al. Malignant fibrous histiocytoma of the orbit. J Clin Neuroophthalmol 1985; 5: 116.
147 Jacomb-Hood J, Moseley IF. Orbital fibrous histiocytoma: Computed tomography in 10 cases and a review of radiological findings. Clin Radiol 1991; 43: 117–120.
148 Mafee MF, Pai E, Philip B. Rhabdomyosarcoma of the orbit. Evaluation with MR imaging and CT. Radiol Clin North Am 1998; 36: 1215–1227.
149 Vade A, Armstrong D. Orbital rhabdomyosarcoma in childhood. Radiol Clin North Am 1987; 25: 701–714.
150 Mafee MF. Case 10: Myositic orbital pseudotumor. In: Head and Neck Disorders (Fourth Series) Tested Syllabus. Reston VA: Am Coll of Radiology; 1992: 213–259.

151 Mafee MF. The orbit proper. In: Som PM, Bergeron RT, eds. Head and Neck Imaging. St. Louis: Mosby-Yearbook; 1991: 747–813.
152 Mafee MF. Orbital and intraocular lesions. In: Edelman RR, Hesselink JR, Zlatkin MC, eds. Clinical Magnetic Resonance Imaging. Philadelphia: W.B. Saunders; 1995: 985–1020.
153 Rao BN, Santana VM, Fleming et al. Management and prognosis of head and neck sarcomas. Am J Surg, 158: 373–377; 1989.
154 Seedat RY, Hammlton PD, deJager LP, et al. Orbital rhabdomyosarcoma presenting as an apparent orbital subperiosteal abscess. Int J Pediatr Otorhinolaryngol 2000; 52: 177–181.
155 Shinaver CN, Mafee MF, Choi KH. MRI of mesenchymal chondrosarcoma of the orbit: case report and review of the literature. Neuroradiology 1997; 39: 296–301.
156 Koeller KK. Mesenchymal chondrosarcoma and simulating lesions of the orbit. Radiol Clin North Am 1999; 37: 203–217.
157 Stewart WB, Krohel GB, Wright JE. Lacrimal gland and fossa lesions: an approach to diagnosis and management. Ophthalmology 1979; 86: 886–895.
158 Wright JE. Factors affecting the survival of patients with lacrimal gland tumors. Can J Ophthalmol 1982; 17: 3–9.
159 Zimmerman LE, Sanders LE, Ackerman IV. Epithelial tumors of the lacrimal gland: prognostic and therapeutic significance of histologic types. Int Ophthalmol Clin 1962; 2: 337–367.
160 Jakobiec FA, Yeo JH, Trokel SL, et al. Combined clinical and computed tomographic diagnosis for primary lacrimal fossa lesions. Am J Ophthalmol 1982; 94: 785–807.
161 Hesselink J, Davis K, Dallow R, et al. Computed tomography of masses in the lacrimal gland region. Radiology 1979; 131: 143–147.
162 Jones BR. Clinical features and etiology of dacryoadenitis. Transophthalmol Soc UK 1955; 75: 435–452.
163 Mafee MF, Edward DP, Koeller KK, Dorodi S. Lacrimal gland tumors and simulating lesions. Clinicopathologic and MR imaging features. Radiol Clin North Am 1999; 37: 219–239.
164 Hoffman GS, Kerr GS, Leavitt RY, et al. Wegener granulomatosis: an analysis of 158 patients. Ann Intern Med 1992; 116: 488.
165 Shield SJA, Bakewell B, Augsburger JJ, et al. Classification and incidence of space-occupying lesions of the orbit: a survey of 645 biopsies. Arch Ophthalmol 1984; 102: 1606–1611.
166 Kimura T, Yoshimura S, Ishikawa E. Eosinophilic granuloma with proliferation of lymphoid tissue. Trans Soc Pathol Jpn 1948; 37: 179.
167 Char DH, Unsöld R. Computed tomography: Ocular and orbital pathology In: Newton TH, Bilaniuk LT, eds. Radiology of the Eye and Orbit. New York: Raven Press; 1990: 9.1–9.64.
168 Brown HW. True and simulated superior oblique tendon sheath syndromes. Doc Ophthalmol 1973; 34: 123, 134.
169 Mafee MF, Folk ER, Langer BG, et al. CT in the evaluation of Brown syndrome of the superior oblique tendon sheath. Radiology 1985; 154: 691–695.
170 Millman AL, Liebeskind A, Putterman AM. Dacryocystography: The technique and its role in the practice of ophthalmology. Radiologic Clin North Am.; 1987: 25: 781–786.
171 Ewing AE. Roentgen ray demonstration of the lacrimal abscess cavity. Am J Ophthalmol; 1909: 241: 1–4.
172 Mafee MF, Mafee RF, Malik M, Pierce J. Medical imaging in pediatric ophthalmology. Pediatr Clin North Am.; 2003: 50: 259–286.
173 Mauriello JA, Lee HL, Nguyen L. CT of soft tissue injury and orbital fractures. Radiol Clin North Am 1999; 37: 241–252.

3 Base of the Skull

Mahmood F. Mafee

Embryology

The mesenchyme that surrounds the developing brain condenses and makes the skull bones. Like other parts of the skeleton, the cranial bones pass through blastemal and cartilaginous stages before they reach the osseous stage. Desmocranium (blastemal skull) is a term applied to the skull in which ossification follows immediately after the blastemal stage, with the chondrification stage being omitted (membranous bone formation). Chondrocranium is a term applied to the parts of the skull that pass through, and at times remain in, a cartilaginous stage (chondrification and cartilaginous bone formation).[1] Certain craniofacial bones are derived from the branchial or visceral arches (viscerocranium). The base of the skull, except for the orbital plate of the frontal bone and lateral parts of the greater sphenoidal wings, is preformed in cartilage, while the whole of the vault is ossified directly in mesenchyme (Table 3.1).[1] The desmocranium begins to form around the developing brain by the end of the first month of embryogenesis. The occipital plate is the first to appear and eventually forms the basiocciput. Ossification commences before the chondrocranium has fully developed.[1] However, parts of it still exist at birth, and therefore small regions remain cartilaginous in the adult skull.[1] At birth, unossified chondrocranium presents at the following sites: (1) the nasal alae and septum; (2) the sphenoid bone; (3) the spheno-occipital and sphenopetrous junctions; (4) the petrous apices (foramen lacerum); and (5) the occipital bone.[1]

Anatomy

The cranial cavity contains the brain, its meninges, and their blood vessels. Its walls are lined with a fibrous membrane, the so-called endocranium (inner periosteum), which is the outer zone (endosteal layer) or periosteal layer of the dura mater. It passes through the various foramina that lead to the exterior, and becomes continuous with the periosteum on the outer surface of the skull, the pericranium (outer periosteum). Both of these fibrous membranes are continuous with the sutural ligaments, which extend the narrow interosseous intervals at the sutures.[1] Most of the cranial bones display outer and inner tables, formed by compact bone and separated from each other by the diploë (diploic space), cancellous bone containing red bone marrow in its interstices.[1]

The vertebrate skull is adapted to support and protect its contents: the brain and its membranes, and special senses. When the inner surface of the base of the skull is exposed, it shows a natural and clearly defined subdivision into three regions, the anterior, middle, and posterior cranial fossae (Fig. 3.1).[1] The anterior cranial fossa forms less than the anterior third of the skull base and is limited behind by a sharp edge (posterior margin of the lesser wing) on each side of the median plane. The floor of the anterior cranial fossa constitutes the orbital roof on each side, and the roof of the nasal cavity and ethmoid labyrinths (fovea ethmoidalis) in the median area (Fig. 3.2). The cribriform plate (including its lateral lamella) of the ethmoid bone is located between the orbital roofs. The crista galli is a crestlike elevation attached to the most anterior part of the cribriform plate (Fig. 3.2). The posterior part of the floor of the anterior cranial fossa is formed by the sphenoid bone (Fig. 3.2). On each side, the lesser wing of the sphenoid projects laterally from the body and meets the posterior margin of the orbital plate of the frontal bone. The sharp posterior margin of the lesser wing of the sphenoid bone forms the posterior limit of the floor of the anterior cranial fossa on each side.

The middle cranial fossa is immediately behind the anterior fossa. Its median portion is formed by the body of the sphenoid, the upper surface of which is the sella turcica (Figs. 3.1, 3.2). The floor of the lateral part of the fossa is formed by the greater wing of the sphenoid in front, and by the petrous part of the temporal bone

Table 3.1 Endochondral and dermal (membrane) elements of the cranium

A. Chondrocranium (endochondral bone)	B. Desmocranium (membranous bone)
1. Nasal capsule	1. Frontal bone
2. Orbitosphenoid	2. Nasal bone
3. Presphenoid	3. Squama of temporal bone
4. Postsphenoid	4. Squama of occipital bone (interparietal)
4. Basiocciptal	5. Parietal bone
5. Otic capsule	6. Tympanic bone
6. Exoccipital	7. Medial pterygoid bone
7. Supraoccipital	8. Vomer bone
8. Alisphenoid	9. Palatine bone
10. Meckel's mandibular cartilage	10. Lacrimal bone
11. Cartilage of malleus	11. Zygomatic bone
12. Styloid cartilage	12. Maxilla
13. Hyoid cartilage	13. Mandible

Modified from reference 1.

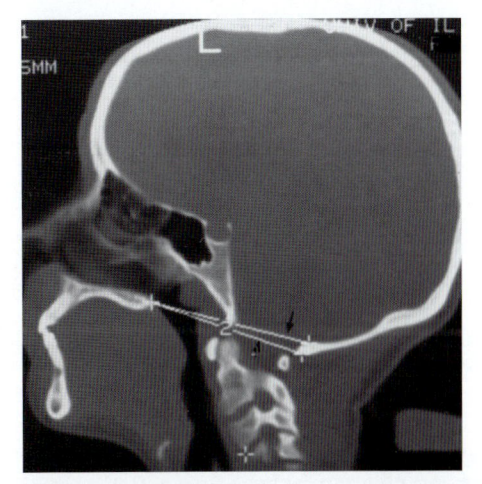

Fig. 3.1 Sagittal CT scan of midline cranio-cervical region, showing the midline structures of the floor of the calvaria. Note Chamberlain (arrow) and McGregor (arrowhead) lines and the exquisite midline anatomy of the cranio-cervico-facial regions.

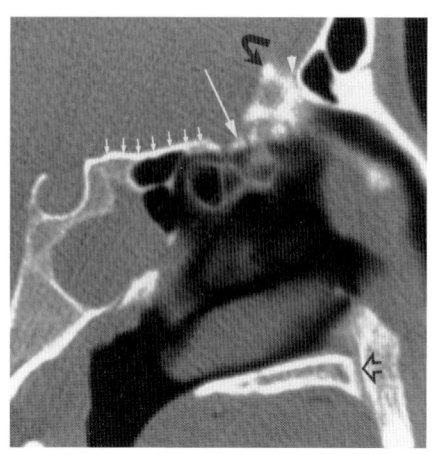

Fig. 3.2 Sagittal CT scan shows incisor foramina (hollow arrow), foramen caecum (arrowhead), crista galli (curved black arrow), cribriform plate (white arrow), jugum sphenoidale (short arrows), sella, and the clivus. Note postsurgical changes of sphenoidotomy.

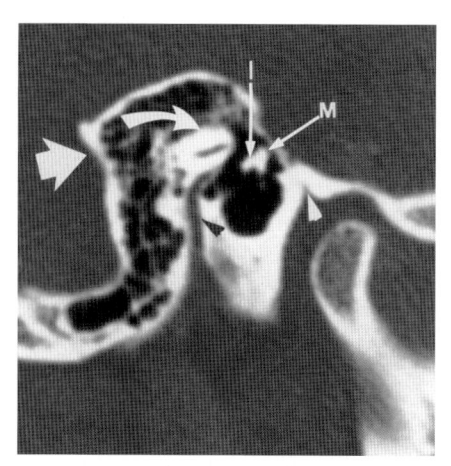

Fig. 3.3 Sagittal CT scan of the skull base, showing the floor of the middle and posterior cranial fossa. The posterior petrous bone (large arrow) in this section contributes to the lateral wall of the posterior fossa. The superior border of it separates the posterior cranial fossa from the middle cranial fossa. Note squamotympanic fissure (white arrowhead), malleus (M), incus (I), lateral semicircular canal (curved arrow) and facial nerve canal (black arrowhead). Note tegmen tympani, a thin bony lamella forming the roof of the tympanic cavity.

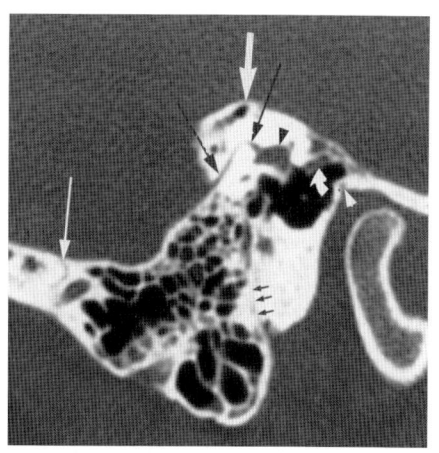

Fig. 3.4 Sagittal CT scan of the skull base, showing petrosquamous fissure (white arrowhead), canal for tensor tympani (curved arrow), vestibule (black arrowhead), vestibular aqueduct (black arrows), arcuate eminence (short white arrow), the mastoid-occipital suture (long white arrow), and the tympanomastoid suture (short black arrows).

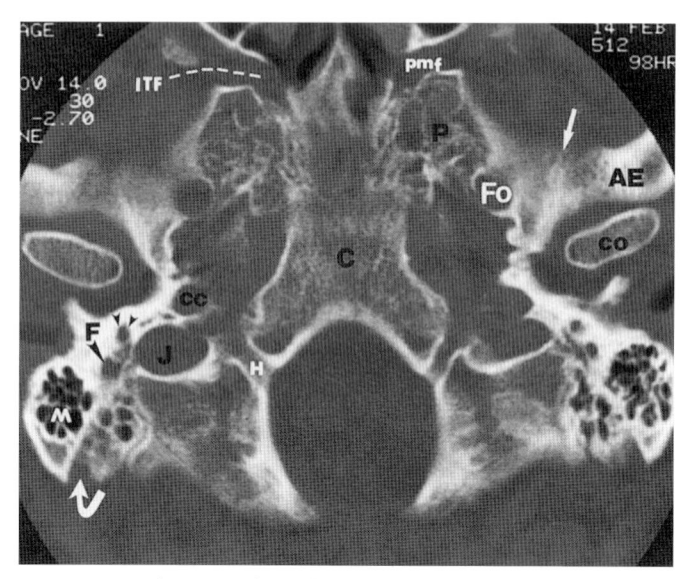

Fig. 3.5a Axial CT scan shows the digastric notch (curved arrow), mastoid process (M), facial nerve canal (F) and anterior to that bone marrow of the root of the styloid process (double arrowheads), jugular fossa (J), carotoid canal (cc), hypoglossal canal (H), clivus (C), madibular condyle (co), articular eminence (AE), sphenotemporal suture (straight arrow), foramen ovale (Fo), base of the pterygoid plate (P), and pterygomaxillary fissure (pmf), entering into the infratemporal fossa (ITF, dashed line).

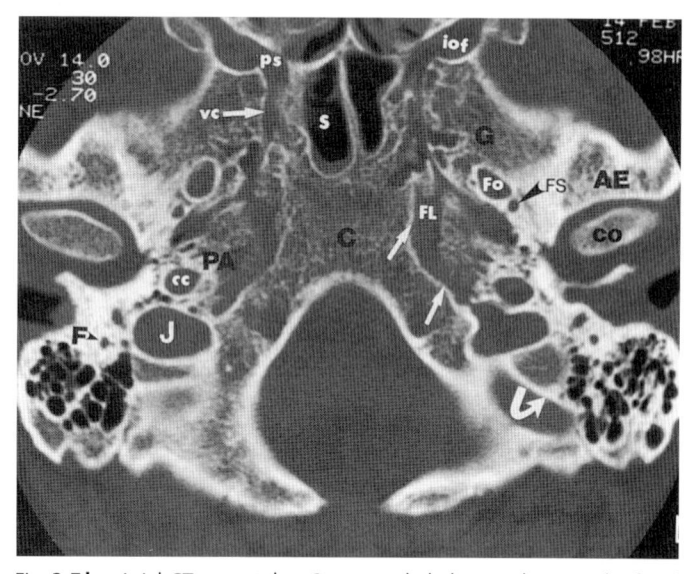

Fig. 3.5b Axial CT scan, taken 3 mm cephalad to a, showing the facial nerve canal (F), jugular fossa (J), carotid canal (cc), petrous apex (PA), clivus (C), vidian canal (vc), pterygopalatine fossa (ps), sphenoid sinus (s), inferior orbital fissure (iof), greater wing of the sphenoid (G), foramen ovale (Fo), foramen lacerum (FL), foramen spinosum (FS), articular eminence (AE), mandibular condyle (co), petrooccipital fissure (straight arrows), and sigmoid sinus plate (curved arrow). The inferior petrosal vein runs along the petro-occipital fissure to join the jugular bulb.

Fig. 3.5 c–f ▷

behind (Fig. 3.3).[1] Posteriorly, the floor of the middle cranial fossa is formed by the anterior surface of the petrous bone (Figs. 3.3, 3.4). The greater wing of the sphenoid bone extends laterally from the side of the body and curves upward in the side of the skull to join the squamous portion of the temporal bone and the anteroinferior part of the parietal bone to complete the fossa (Fig. 3.5).

The posterior cranial fossa, which lies behind the petromastoid plate of the temporal bone on each side, occupies roughly two-fifths of the base of the skull (Figs. 3.4, 3.5).[1] It is formed for the most part by the occipital bone. The anterior part of the fossa is the basiocciput (basilar part of the occipital bone), which is fused in front with the basisphenoid to form the clivus. On each side, the lateral wall of the posterior fossa is formed by the posterior surface of the petrous bone above and by the lateral or the so-called condylar part of the occipital bone below. The mastoid segment of the temporal bone joins the squamous part of the occipital bone at the occipital–mastoid suture to complete the formation of the posterior fossa.

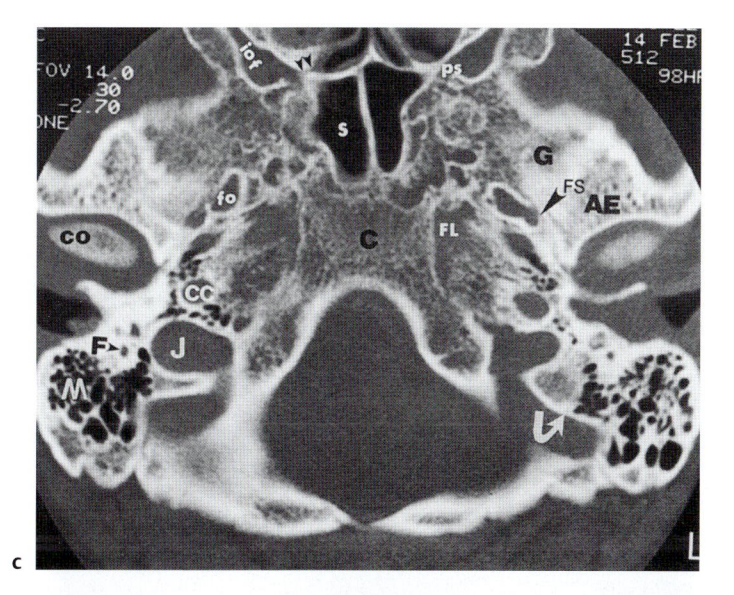

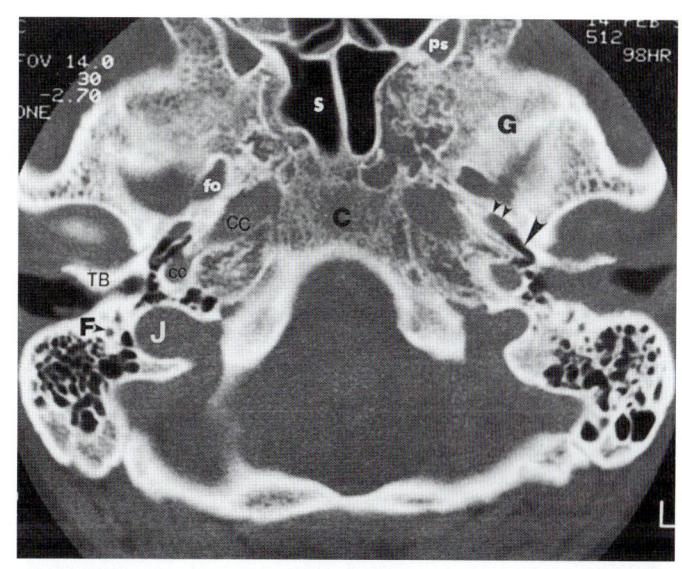

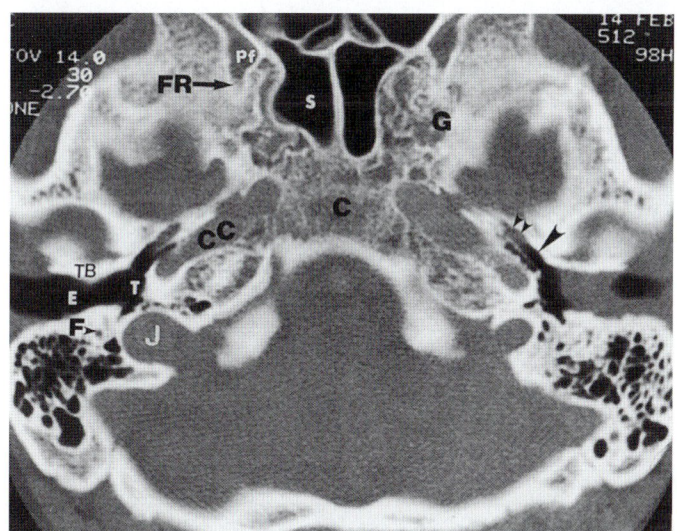

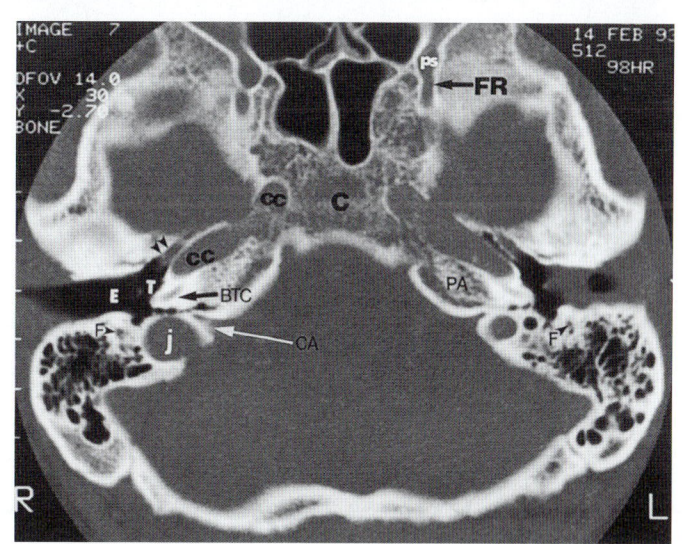

Fig. 3.5

c Axial CT scan, taken 3 mm cephalad to **b**, showing mastoid process (M), facial nerve canal (F), jugular fossa (J), carotid canal (CC), condyle (co), foramen ovale (fo), sphenoid sinus (s), inferior orbital fissure (iof), sphenopalatine foramen (arrowheads), pterygopalatine fossa (ps), greater wing of sphenoid (G), foramen spinosum (FS), foramen lacerum (FL), articular eminence (AE), sigmoid sinus plate (curved arrow), and clivus (C). Note squamotympanic fissure running laterally and posteriorly towards the floor of the mandibular fossa.

d Axial CT scan, taken 1.5 mm cephalad to **c**, showing the facial nerve canal (F), jugular fossa (J), tympanic bone (TB), carotid canal (cc), clivus (C), foramen ovale (fo), sphenoid sinus (s), pterygopalatine fossa (ps), greater wing of the sphenoid (G), tensor tympani muscle (short arrowheads), and eustachian tube (large arrowhead).

e Axial CT scan, taken 1.5 mm cephalad to **d**, showing the facial nerve canal (F), jugular fossa (J), external auditory canal (E), tympanic cavity (T), tympanic bone (TB), carotid canal (CC), clivus (C), sphenoid sinus (s), foramen rotundum (FR), pterygopalatine fossa (pf), greater wing of the sphenoid (G), tensor tympani muscle (short arrowheads), and eustachian tube (large arrowhead).

f Axial CT scan, Taken 1.5 mm cephalad to **e**, showing the facial nerve canal (F), jugular fossa (j), cochlear aqueduct (CA), basal turn of the cochlea (BTC), tympanic cavity (T), external auditory canal (E), tensor tympani muscle (arrowheads), carotid canal (cc), clivus (C), pterygopalatine fossa (ps), foramen rotundum (FR), and bone marrow of the petrous apex (PA).

The foramen magnum lies in the floor of the fossa. Through it the brainstem becomes continuous with the spinal cord. The foramen transmits certain neural and vascular structures. These are summarized in Table 3.2.

■ The External Surface of the Cranial Base

The inferior surface of the skull base is very irregular and is connected anteriorly to the skeleton of the face. Multiple channels (fissures) and foramina perforate the skull base and transmit neural and vascular structures, summarized in Table 3.2. The incisor canals are located in the anterior aspect of bony palate and each leads upward into the corresponding half of the nasal cavity and through it pass the terminal branch of the greater palatine artery and the nasopalatine nerve (Fig. 3.2) (Table 3.2).[1] Occasionally there are two additional apertures in the median plane: the anterior and posterior incisive foramina.

The greater palatine foramen, which is the lower orifice of the greater palatine canal, opens close to the lateral border of the palate immediately behind the palatomaxillary suture (Figs. 3.6, 3.7).[1] The lesser palatine foramina, usually two on each side, are situated behind the greater palatine foramina and are best seen on axial CT scan. The greater palatine foramen transmits the greater palatine nerves and vessels. The lesser palatine foramina contain the lesser palatine nerves and vessels (Table 3.2).

Table 3.2 Contents of cranial basal foramina, canals and fissures

Name	Location	Contents
Foramen caecum	Floor of anterior cranial fossa between crista galli and internal crest of frontal bone	Ends blindly, but rarely is patent, transmits a vein from nasal cavity to superior sigittal sinus
Anterior ethmoid canal	Frontal and ethmoid	Anterior ethmoid artery and nerve
Posterior ethmoid canal	Frontal and ethmoid	Posterior ethmoid artery and nerve
Optic canal	Lesser wing of sphenoid	Optic nerve, ophthalmic artery, sympathetic fibers
Superior orbital fissure	Lesser and greater wing of sphenoid	Motor III, IV, VI, sensory V1 (frontal, lacrimal and nasociliary) Sympathetic fibers Superior ophthalmic vein Anastomosis of recurrent lacrimal and middle meningeal artery
Inferior orbital fissure	Greater wing of sphenoid, palatine, zygomatic, and maxillary bones	V2 (infraorbital and zygomatic), parasympathetic branches from pterygopalatine ganglion
Foramen rotundum	Greater wing of sphenoid	Maxillary nerve, venous plexus of foramen rotundum
Foramen ovale	Greater wing of sphenoid	Mandibular nerve, lesser petrosal nerve, venous plexus (emissary veins) of foramen ovale unites the caverous sinus with pterygoid plexus, accessory meningeal artery
Foramen spinosum	Greater wing of sphenoid	Middle meningeal artery and veins Meningeal branch of the mandibular nerve
Foramen of Vesalius (Sphenoidal emissary foramen)	Greater wing of sphenoid, inconstant small opening anterior to foramen ovale	Emissary vein
Foramen lacerum	Petrous apex, body of sphenoid bone and posterior border of greater wing	Internal carotid artery and its accompanying sympathetic and venous plexuses. Meningeal branches of the ascending pharyngeal artery and emissary vein to the cavernous sinus Vidian nerve. Two or three small emissary veins, connecting the cavernous sinus with the pharyngeal veins and pterygoid plexus
Carotid canal	Petrous temporal bone	Internal carotid artery. The internal carotid nervous plexus and venous plexus.
Jugular foramen	Petrous and occipital bones	Internal jugular vein, (inferior petrosal sinus), 9th, 10th, 11th cranial nerves.
Internal auditory canal	Petrous bone	VII and VIII cranial nerves. Labyrinthine vessels.
Hypoglossal canal	Occipital bone	Hypoglossal nerve, the venous plexus of the hypoglossal canal, or occasionally a single vein, meningeal branch of ascending pharyngeal artery
Condylar canal (inconsistent)	Occipital bone	Posterior condylar emissary vein unites the lower end of sigmoid sinus with the veins in the suboccipital triangle
Mastoid canal (Foramen)	Mastoid temporal bone	Emissary vein from the upper end of sigmoid sinus with posterior auricular or occipital vein. Meningeal branch from occipital artery.
Foramen magnum	Occipital bone	Medulla oblongata, meninges, roots of accessory nerve, vertebral arteries, spinal arteries.
Stylomastoid foramen	Styloid and mastoid	Facial nerve, stylomastoid branch of posterior auricular artery.
Pterygoid canal (Vidian canal)	Sphenoid bone	(Vidian) Pterygoid nerve and vessels
Greater palatine foramen	Palatine bone	Greater palatine nerves and vessels
Lesser palatine foramina	Palatine bone	Lesser palatine nerves and vessels
Incisor canal	Maxilla	Terminal branches of the greater palatine artery and the nasopalatine nerve
Petrotympanic fissure	Temporal bone	Chorda tympani, anterior tympanic branch of the maxillary artery.
Mastoid canaliculus, a minute canal	Petrous temporal bone (floor of jugular fossa)	Auricular branch of the vagus nerve (Arnold's nerve)
Tympanic canaliculus (Jacobson's canal)	Petrous temporal bone (near the ridge between jugular fossa and the orifice of carotid canal)	Tympanic branch of glossopharyngeal nerve (Jacobson's nerve)

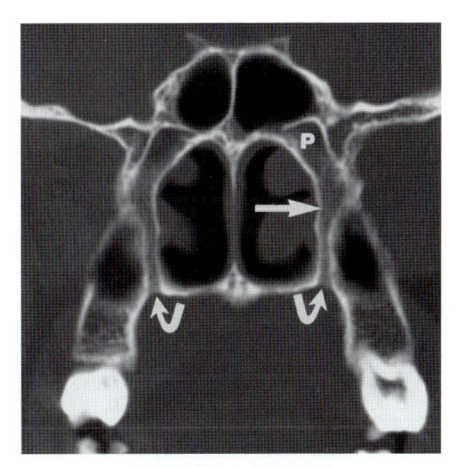

Fig. 3.6 Coronal CT scan showing the pterygopalatine fossa (P), greater palatine canal (straight arrow), and greater palatine foramina (curved arrows).

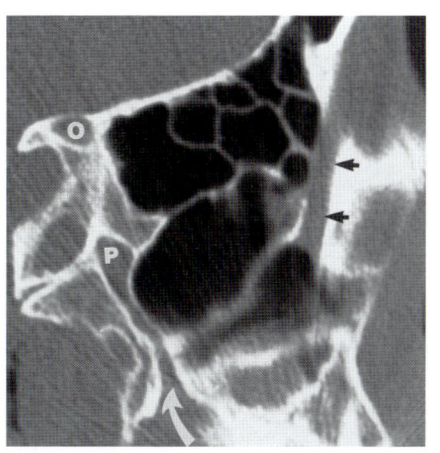

Fig. 3.7 Direct sagittal CT scan showing optic canal (O), pterygopalatine fossa (P), greater palatine foramen (curved arrow), which is the lower orifice of the greater palatine canal. Note nasolacrimal duct (black arrows).

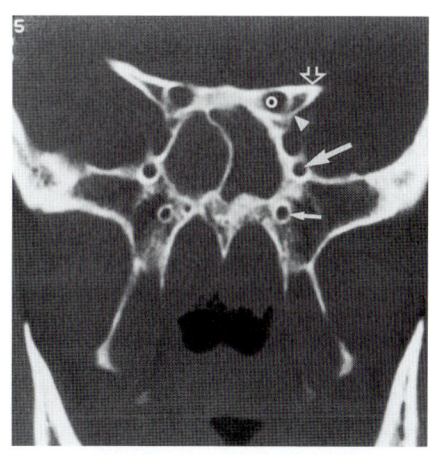

Fig. 3.8 Direct coronal CT scan showing the lesser wing of the sphenoid (hollow arrow), optic canal (o), optic strut (arrowhead), foramen rotundum (large arrow), and vidian canal (short arrow). Note the opacification of the sphenoid sinuses.

■ The Pterygoid Processes, Pterygoid Plates, Scaphoid Fossa, Spine of the Sphenoid Bone, Foramen Ovale, and Foramen Spinosum

Each pterygoid process descends behind the maxillary from the junction of the greater wing and body of the sphenoid bone (Figs. 3.7–3.10). It has two laminae, the medial and lateral pterygoid plates, separated from each other by an interval termed the pterygoid fossa.[1] The medial surface of medial pterygoid plate in life is covered with mucous membrane and takes part in the formation of the lateral boundary of the posterior nasal aperture (choana) and part of the lateral wall of the nasopharynx.[1] The posterior border of the medial pterygoid plate at its upper end divides to enclose a shallow fossa, the so-called scaphoid fossa. The anterior fibers of the tensor veli palatini muscle originate from the scaphoid fossa.[1] The lateral pterygoid plate projects backward and laterally and its lateral surface forms the medial wall of the infratemporal fossa.[1] The ovale and spinosum foramina are important openings on the infratemporal surface of the greater wing of the sphenoid (Figs. 3.5, 3.8–3.10). The foramen ovale passes through the greater wing, posterior to the foramen rotundum. It transmits the mandibular division of the trigeminal nerve (Table 3.2).

In addition to the mandibular nerve, the foramen ovale transmits the accessory meningeal artery and, sometimes, the lesser petrosal nerve (Table 3.2).[1] In the interval between the foramen ovale and the scaphoid fossa the bone sometimes presents a small foramen, the sphenoidal emissary foramen (foramen Vesalius), which transmits an emissary vein to the cavernous sinus (Table 3.2).[1] Posterior and slightly lateral to the foramen ovale, the foramen spinosum pierces the greater wing and transmits the middle meningeal artery, its accompanying veins, and the meningeal branch of the mandibular nerve (Fig. 3.5) (Table 3.2).[1] Immediately posterolateral to the foramen spinosum, this surface of the greater wing has an irregular downward projection, named the spine of the sphenoid bone.[1] The medial surface of the sphenoid spine with the adjoining part of the posterior border of the greater wing forms the anterolateral border of a groove, which is completed posteromedially by the petrous part of the temporal bone. This groove contains the cartilaginous part of the eustachian tube (Fig. 3.5).[1] Behind and medial to the groove for the tube, the inferior surface of the petrous bone occupies the interval between the greater wing and the basilar part of the occipital bone.

■ The Foramen Lacerum

Posteromedial to the foramen ovale is the foramen lacerum. It is bounded behind by the petrous apex and in front by the body of sphenoid bone and the posterior border of the greater wing (Fig. 3.5). The foramen contains the internal carotid artery and its accompanying sympathetic and venous plexuses (Table 3.2).[1] The inferior surface of the petrous bone in this region is rough and uneven. Behind this rough area, a large circular foramen leads upward into the bone, the inferior opening of the carotid canal (Fig. 3.5). The canal turns forward and medially and opens on the posterior wall of the foramen lacerum (Fig. 3.6). The lower part of the foramen lacerum is occupied by fibrocartilage, and no large structure enters or leaves the skull through this opening. The foramen lacerum is also traversed by minute meningeal branches from the ascending pharyngeal artery and emissary veins from the cavernous sinus pass right through the foramen (Table 3.2). The greater petrosal nerve turns downward through the foramen lacerum on the lateral side of the internal carotid artery and is joined by the deep petrosal nerve to form the nerve of the pterygoid canal (vidian canal) (Figs. 3.5, 3.6, 3.10) (Table 3.2).

■ Pterygoid (Vidian) Canal

Pterygoid canal, or vidian canal, lies in the line of fusion of the pterygoid process and greater wing with the body of the sphenoid bone (Figs. 3.5, 3.8). The vidian canal opens on the anterior wall of the foramen lacerum and leads forward to open on the posterior wall of the pterygopalatine fossa (Figs. 3.5b, 3.8, 3.10). It transmits the nerve and vessels of the pterygoid (vidian) canal (Table 3.2).[1]

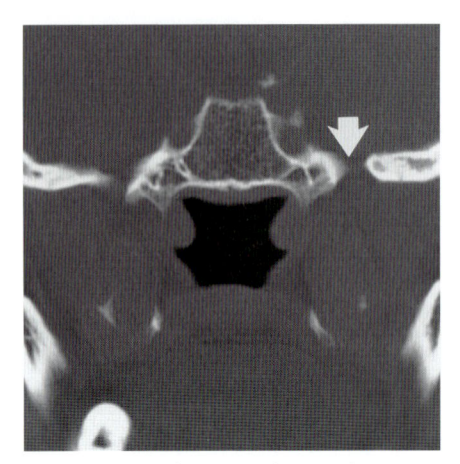

Fig. 3.9 Coronal CT scan showing foramen ovale on each side (arrow).

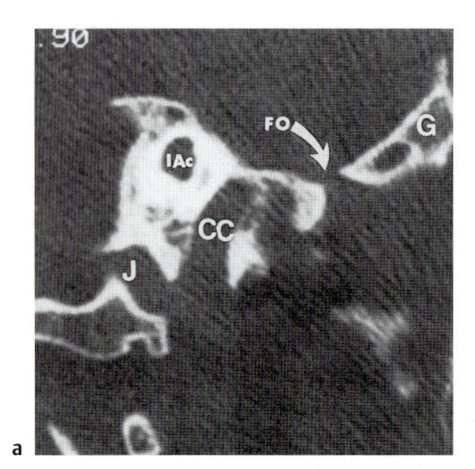

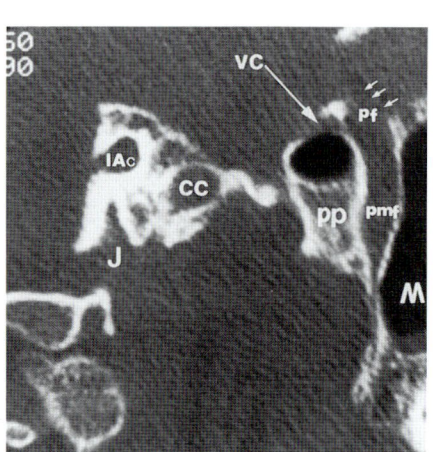

Fig. 3.10 a Direct semisagittal CT scan showing the greater wing of the sphenoid (G), foramen ovale (FO), carotid canal (CC), internal auditory canal (IAc), and jugular fossa (J).
b Direct semisagittal CT scan, taken medial to a, showing the maxillary sinus (M), pterygomaxillary fissure (pmf), pterygopalatine fossa (pf), vidian canal (VC), pterygoid process (pp), carotid canal (cc), internal auditory canal (IAc), and jugular fossa (J). Note the relationship of the inferior orbital fissure (arrows) to the pterygopalatine fossa.

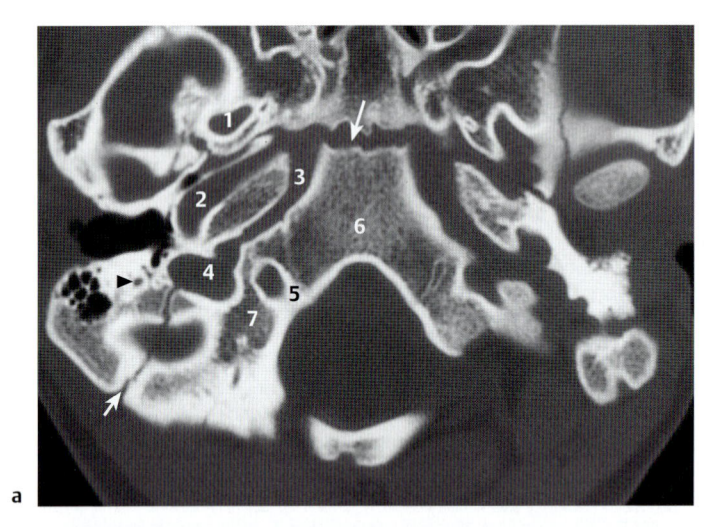

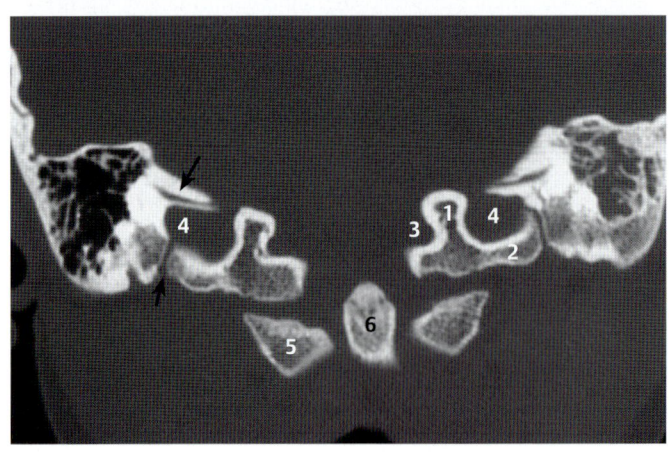

Fig. 3.11
a Axial CT scan of the base of the skull of a 6-year-old boy showing: **1** foramen ovale; **2** carotid canal; **3** petro-occipital fissure; **4** jugular fossa; **5** hypoglossal canal; **6** basiocciput; **7** jugular process of occipital bone; arrowhead = descending portion of facial nerve canal; long arrow = spheno-occipital synchondrosis; short arrow = occipital-mastoid suture.
b Coronal CT scan of the same subject as in a, showing: **1** occipital condyle; **2** jugular process of occipital bone; **3** hypoglossal canal; **4** jugular fossa; **5** superior articular facet of atlas; **6** odontoid process; short arrow = occipital-mastoid suture; long arrow = vestibular aqueduct. Note opacification of the left mastoid air cells.

■ The Squamotympanic Fissure

From the base of the sphenoid spine, the squamotympanic fissure runs laterally and slightly posteriorly between the upper part of the tympanic plate of the temporal bone and the floor of the mandibular fossa (Fig. 3.5 c,d).[1] A thin edge of bone may be visible in the depth of the medial end of the squamotympanic fissure (Figs. 3.3, 3.4). It is the lower border of the down-turned lateral portion of the tegmen tympani and therefore a part of the petrous temporal (Figs. 3.3, 3.4). It divides the upper part of the squamotympanic fissure into petrotympanic and petrosquamous fissures (Figs. 3.3, 3.4). Through the petrotympanic fissure the chorda tympani travels in the anterior canaliculus as it passes downward and forward from the tympanic cavity. The anterior tympanic branch of the maxillary artery also traverses the petrotympanic fissure (Table 3.2).[1]

■ Foramen Magnum and Hypoglossal Canal

The median region of the posterior part of the external surface of skull base features anteriorly the foramen magnum (Fig. 3.5). The foramen transmits the lower end of the medulla oblongata and the meninges. In the subarachnoid space the spinal roots of the spinal accessory nerves and the vertebral arteries, with their sympathetic plexuses, ascend into the cranium, and the posterior spinal arteries descend, one on each posterolateral aspect of the brainstem, as does the anterior spinal artery on the front of the brainstem in the median plane (Table 3.2).[1] In addition, the lower part of the cerebellar tonsils may project into the foramen on each side of the medulla oblongata. Anteriorly, the margin of the foramen magnum is overlapped slightly on each side by the occipital condyle, which projects downward to articulate with the superior articular facet on the lateral mass of the atlas (Fig. 3.11). The anterior part of the occipital condyle in its upper aspect is pierced by the hypoglossal (anterior condylar) canal (Figs. 3.5 a, 3.11). The hypoglossal canal contains the hypoglossal nerve, a meningeal branch of the ascending pharyngeal artery, and a small emissary vein from the basilar plexus (Table 3.2).[1] Not uncommonly the canal is divided into two by a spicule of bone.[1] A depression of variable depth occurs behind the condyle.

This is the condylar fossa; it may be pierced by the condylar canal, which, when present, transmits an emissary vein from the sigmoid sinus.[1] Lateral to the condyle the jugular process of the occipital bone articulates with the petrous temporal. The anterior border of the process is free and forms the posterior boundary of the jugular foramen (Figs. 3.5a, 3.11).

■ The Jugular Foramen

The jugular foramen is a large, irregular hiatus between the jugular process of the occipital bone and the jugular fossa of the petrous temporal, and is set at the posterior end of the petro-occipital suture (fissure) (Figs. 3.5a, 3.10, 3.11). In front, it is separated from the lower orifice of the carotid canal by a raised ridge of bone (Fig. 3.10). Medially, it is separated from the hypoglossal canal by a thin bar of bone (Figs. 3.5a, 3.11). Laterally, it is related to the medial aspect of the sheath of the styloid process.[1] The anterior part of the foramen transmits the inferior petrosal sinus (Table 3.2); its intermediate part transmits the glossopharyngeal, vagus, and spinal accessory nerves; its posterior part transmits the internal jugular vein (bulb) (Table 3.2). The floor of the jugular fossa separates the jugular bulb from the tympanic cavity, and its lateral wall is pierced by a minute canal, the mastoid canaliculus, which transmits the auricular branch (Arnold's nerve) of the vagus nerve (Table 3.2). Passing laterally through the bone, this nerve is very near to the facial canal, and finally emerges in the tympanomastoid suture (Fig. 3.4).[1] It is extracranial at birth but becomes surrounded by bone as the tympanic plate and the mastoid process develop.[1] On or near the ridge between the jugular fossa and the orifice of the carotid canal, the canaliculus for the tympanic nerve pierces the bone to transmit to the middle ear the tympanic branch (Jacobson's nerve) from the glossopharyngeal nerve (Table 3.2). On the upper boundary of the jugular foramen, near its medial end, there is a small notch, more easily identified on the internal surface, which contains the inferior ganglion of the glossopharyngeal nerve (Fig. 3.5f). The orifice of the cochlear aqueduct lies at the apex of the notch (Fig. 3.5f). The aqueduct contains the perilymphatic duct.[1]

■ Stylomastoid Foramen

Posterior to the root of the styloid process, the stylomastoid foramen transmits the facial nerve. The stylomastoid foramen lies at the anterior end of the mastoid notch (digastric notch) (Fig. 3.5a), from which the posterior belly of the digastric muscle takes origin. As the facial nerve emerges from the foramen it is close to the posterior belly of the digastric, which it supplies before entering the parotid gland.[1] In addition to the facial nerve, the foramen carries the stylomastoid branch of the posterior auricular artery (Table 3.2).[1]

■ The Internal Surface of the Cranial Base

The internal surface of the cranial base, unlike its external surface, shows a natural division into anterior, middle, and posterior cranial fossae (Fig. 3.1). The anterior cranial fossa is limited in front and on each side by the frontal bone. Its floor is formed by the orbital parts (horizontal plate) of the frontal bone, the cribriform plate of the ethmoid, and the lesser wings and anterior part of the sphenoid bone. The sphenoid bone completes the posterior region of the floor of the fossa. Centrally is the anterior part of the upper surface of its body, termed the jugum sphenoidale (Fig. 3.2). The jugum articulates with the posterior margin of the cribriform plate (Fig. 3.2).[1] Posteriorly, the jugum is limited by the anterior border of a groove, termed the chiasmatic sulcus, which crosses the body of the sphenoid in the forepart of the middle cranial fossa and leads from one optic canal to the other.[1] The foramina of the anterior skull base include optic canals/foramina (Fig. 3.7), anterior and posterior ethmoid canals, and the foramen cecum (Fig. 3.2). The foramen cecum usually ends blindly, but on rare occasions it is patent and accommodates a vein from the nasal cavity to the superior sagittal sinus (Table 3.2). The optic canal contains the optic nerve, ophthalmic artery, and meninges (Table 3.2). The anterior ethmoidal canal opens on the line of the suture between the orbital part of the frontal bone and cribriform plate. It is placed behind the crista galli and is difficult to identify because it is overlapped above the medial edge of the orbital plate.[1] It transmits the anterior ethmoid nerve, artery, and veins, which run forward under the dura mater and gain access to the nasal cavity at the side of crista galli (Table 3.2). The posterior ethmoidal canal opens at the posterolateral corner of the cribriform plate and is overhung by the anterior border of the sphenoid bone. It transmits the posterior ethmoid vessels (Table 3.2).[1]

■ Superior Orbital Fissure, Foramen Rotundum, Tegmen Tympani, and Tegmen Antri

The middle cranial fossa is more extensive on each side than in the midline. It is bounded in front by the posterior borders of the lesser wings, the anterior clinoid processes, and the anterior margin of the sulcus chiasmatis; bounded behind by the superior borders of the petrous bones and the dorsum sellae of the sphenoid bone; and bounded laterally by the temporal squamae, the frontal angles of the parietal bones, and the greater wings of the sphenoid (Figs. 3.3, 3.4, 3.5f, 3.8).[1] Centrally, the floor is formed by the body of the sphenoid, including the sella turcica, tuberculum sellae, dorsum sellae, and posterior clinoid processes. Laterally, the middle cranial fossa is deep. It is formed in front by the cerebral surface of the greater wing and behind by the anterior surface of the petrous bone, and laterally by the cerebral surface of the temporal squamosa. Anteriorly, it communicates with the orbit through the superior orbital fissure. The fissure transmits the terminal branches of the ophthalmic nerve, the superior ophthalmic vein, the oculomotor, trochlear and abducent nerves, and some smaller vessels (Table 3.2).[1] The foramen rotundum pierces the greater wing immediately below and a little behind the medial end of the superior orbital fissure (Figs. 3.5f, 3.8). It contains the maxillary nerve and leads forward into the pterygopalatine fossa (Table 3.2). The foramen ovale passes through the greater wing posterior to the foramen rotundum. It transmits the mandibular nerve (Figs. 3.5b, c, d, 3.9) (Table 3.2). Posteromedial to the foramen ovale is the foramen lacerum (Fig. 3.5b, c, d). Behind the foramen lacerum the anterior surface of the petrous apex presents a shallow depression, the trigeminal impression, occupied by the trigeminal ganglion (see Fig. 3.13d). The arcuate eminence is posterolateral to the trigeminal impression. The eminence is produced by the superior semicircular canal, which is closely related here to the floor of the middle cranial fossa (Fig. 3.4).[1] Anterolateral to the arcuate eminence, the anterior surface of the petrous bone is formed by the tegmen tympani, a thin osseous lamella which forms the roof of the tympanic cavity (Fig. 3.4). Lateral to the arcuate eminence, the posterior part of the tegmen tympani forms the roof of the mastoid antrum, the tegmen antri. The superior border of the petrous bone separates the middle cranial fossa from the posterior cranial fossa (Figs. 3.**3**, 3.**4**). Behind the trigeminal impression, the superior border of the petrous bone is grooved by the superior petrosal sinus, which connects the posterior end of the cavernous sinus to the upper end of the sigmoid sinus.

Cavernous Sinus

On each side of the body of the sphenoid, the cavernous sinus extends from the medial end of the superior orbital fissure to the apex of the petrous bone. In addition to the internal carotid artery and its plexus of sympathetic nerves, the sinus contains the oculomotor, trochlear, abducent, and ophthalmic nerves, but these structures are not in contact with bone (Fig. 3.**12**). An anterior intercavernous sinus, which crosses the tuberculum sellae, and a posterior intercavernous sinus, which crosses the front of the dorsum sellae, connect the two cavernous sinuses to each other.[1] Numerous trabeculae cross the interior of the cavernous sinuses, giving them a spongy appearance (hence the name). The third and fourth cranial nerves and the ophthalmic and maxillary divisions of the trigeminal nerve run forward in the lateral wall of the cavernous sinus (Fig. 3.**12**). They lie between the endothelial lining and the dura mater. The abducent nerve passes through the sinus. The tributaries are the superior and inferior ophthalmic veins, the cerebral veins, the sphenoparietal sinus, and the central vein of the retina. The sinus drains posteriorly into the superior and inferior petrosal sinuses, and inferiorly into the pterygoid venous plexus. The superior and inferior petrosal sinuses are small sinuses situated on the superior and inferior borders of the petrous bone on each side. The superior petrosal sinus drains the cavernous sinus into the transverse sinus, and the inferior petrosal sinus drains the cavernous sinus into the internal jugular vein. The anterior surface of the petrous bone has two grooves for nerves; the larger, medial groove is for the greater petrosal nerve, a branch of the facial nerve; the smaller, lateral groove is for the lesser petrosal nerve, a branch of the tympanic plexus. The greater petrosal nerve enters the foramen lacerum deep to the trigeminal ganglion and joins the deep petrosal nerve (sympathetic fibers from around the internal carotid artery), to form the pterygoid or vidian nerve which runs into the pterygoid (vidian) canal. The lesser petrosal nerve passes forward to the foramen ovale.

Trigeminal Cavity (Meckel's Cave), Trigeminal Cistern, and Ganglion

The trigeminal cavity (cave), or Meckel's cave, occupies the shallow depression (trigeminal impression) of the petrous apex. Meckel's cave is formed by the evagination of the meningeal layer of the dura from the posterior cranial fossa near the tip of the petrous bone downward and medially beneath the dura (Fig. 3.**12 c–e**) of the middle cranial fossa (Fig. 3.**12 c–e**). It encloses the roots of the trigeminal nerve and the trigeminal ganglion. The trigeminal (gasserian or semilunar) ganglion is a flattened sensory ganglion of the trigeminal nerve (Fig. 3.**12 c–e**), lying in close relation to the cavernous sinus along the medial part of the middle cranial fossa (Fig. 3.**12 c–e**). The fibers of the sensory divisions of the fifth cranial nerve arise from the cells of the trigeminal ganglion. This ganglion occupies a recess (trigeminal or Meckel's cave) in the dura mater covering the trigeminal impressions near the petrous apex. Extension of arachnoid mater into the trigeminal cavity, the so-called trigeminal (gasserian, Meckel's) cistern, can easily be visualized on MR images (Fig. 3.**12 c–e**).

The Posterior Cranial Fossa

The posterior cranial fossa is the largest and deepest of the three cranial fossae, occupying roughly two-fifths of the base of the skull. It houses the cerebellum, pons, and medulla oblongata. The fossa is bounded anteriorly by the superior border of the petrous bone (Figs. 3.**3**–3.**5**) and posteriorly by the internal surface of the squamous part of the occipital bone (Fig. 3.**5**). The floor is formed by the basilar, condylar, and squamous parts of the occipital bone and the mastoid part of the temporal bone (Fig. 3.**5 b**); the occipital bone forms much of the back and base of the cranium. It encloses the foramen magnum and has an expanded plate, termed the squamous part, above and behind this foramen; the thick somewhat quadrilateral piece in front of it is the basilar part (Fig. 3.**5**); on each side of the foramen is a lateral part. The lateral (condylar) parts of the occipital bone are situated at the sides of foramen magnum (Figs. 3.**5 a**, **b**, 3.**11**); on their inferior surfaces are the occipital condyles, two processes for articulation with the superior facets of the atlas (Fig. 3.**11 b**).[1] Above the anterior part of each condyle the bone presents the hypoglossal canal (Fig. 3.**11**). The canal transmits the hypoglossal nerve and a meningeal branch of the ascending pharyngeal artery.[1] The condylar fossa lies behind the condyle. The floor of this fossa is sometimes perforated by the condylar canal, through which an emissary vein passes from the sigmoid sinus (Table 3.**2**).

The jugular process extends laterally from the posterior half of the condyle (Fig. 3.**11**). It is a quadrilateral plate of bone, indented in front by the jugular notch, which forms the posterior part of the jugular foramen.[1] The jugular notch is sometimes partly divided into two by a bony spicule named the intrajugular process, which projects forward and laterally.[1] From the undersurface of the jugular process an eminence, the paramastoid

Fig. 3.**12** Cavernous sinus, trigeminal cavity and ganglion ▷
- **a** Coronal T1W (top) and Gd-enhanced T1W (bottom) MR scans, taken with a 1.5 T MR imager, through the middle cranial fossa, showing the cavernous sinuses. Note enhancement of the endothelium-lined interior of the cavernous sinuses, signal void of the internal carotid artery, oculomotor nerve (straight white arrow), ophthalmic nerve (arrowhead), maxillary nerve (black arrow), and abducent nerve (curved arrow). The trochlear nerve is small and, when visualized, it is seen just below the oculomotor nerve.
- **b** Coronal Gd-enhanced T1W MR scan, taken with a 3 T MR imager, through the middle cranial fossa, showing cavernous sinuses. Note oculomotor nerve (straight white arrow), trochlear nerve (small black arrow), ophthalmic nerve (hollow black arrow), maxillary nerve (large black arrow), abducent nerve (curved white arrow), and mandibular nerve in foramen ovale (arrowhead).
- **c** Axial T2W MR scan, obtained with 3 T MR imager, shows cochlea (1), cochlear nerve (2), vestibule (3), inferior vestibular nerve (4), posterior semicircular canal/common crus, (5) and endolymphatic duct (6).
- **d** Axial T2W MR scan, taken 2 mm superior to **c**, shows cochlea (1), facial nerve (2), vestibule (3), superior vestibular nerve (4), horizontal semicircular canal (5), posterior semicircular canal (6), endolymphatic duct (7), bone marrow of petrous apex (8), and gasserian cistern and ganglion (9).
- **e** Axial T2W MR scan of another subject, taken with 3 T MR imager, shows the cisternal portion of the trigeminal nerve (curved arrow) and the trigeminal (gasserian) cisterns (straight arrows). The trigeminal (gasserian) ganglion, or semilunar ganglion, is a flattened sensory ganglion of the fifth cranial nerve. It is seen on the right side lying in close relation to the petrous apex. The trigeminal nerve branches are seen within the gasserian cisterns. Arrowheads = superior semicircular canal.
- **f** Sagittal T2W (4117/84, TR/TE, 512×264/4.00 NEX, 12×12 FOV) MR scan, obtained with 3 T MR imager. Note chiasmatic (1), infundibular (2) recesses of the third ventricle, lamina terminalis (arrow), and exquisite anatomy of the midline intracranial structures.

Anatomy 303

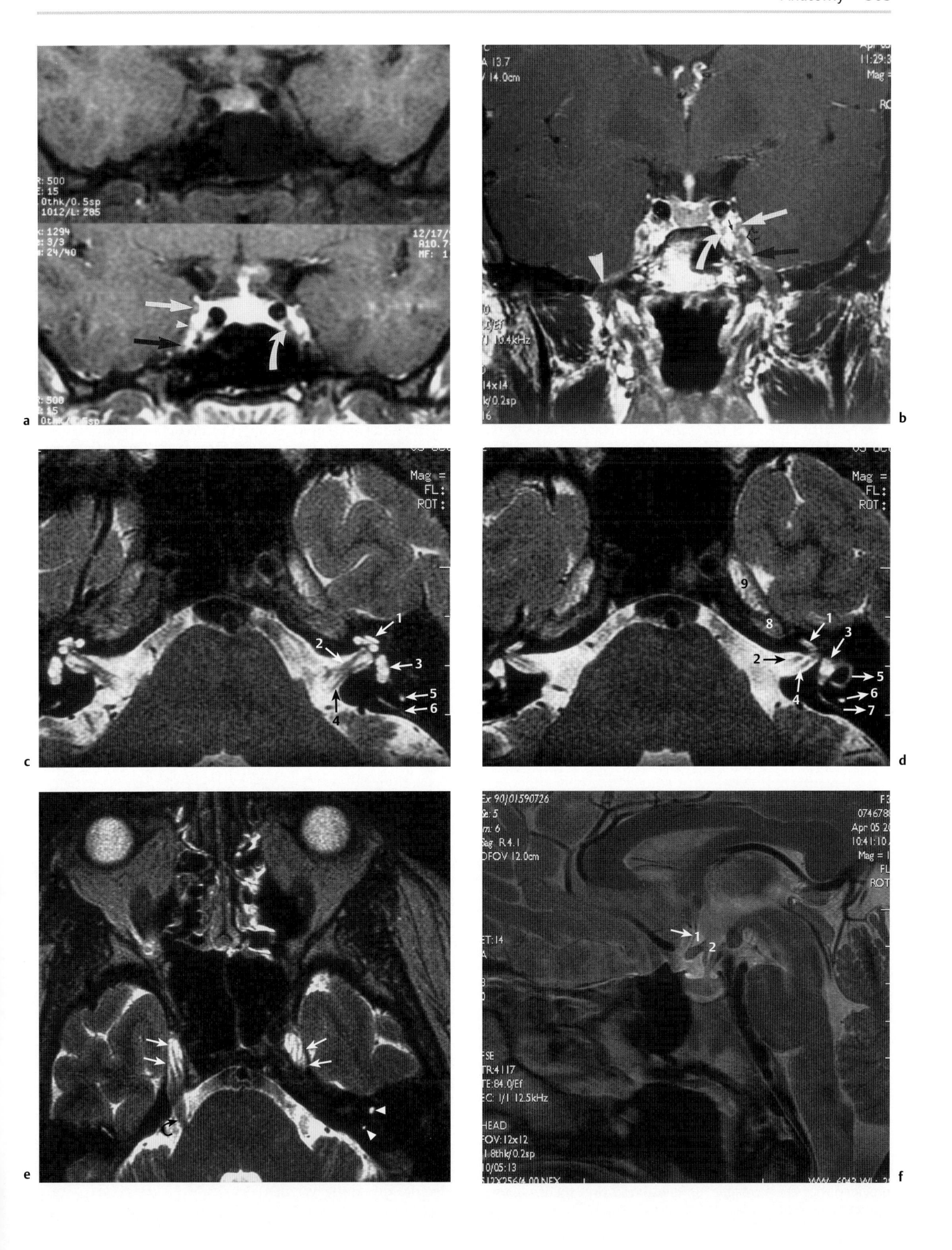

process, sometimes projects downward, and may be of sufficient length to articulate with the transverse process of the atlas.[1] Laterally the jugular process presents a rough quadrilateral or triangular area that is joined to the jugular surface of the temporal bone by a growth plate of cartilage; at about the age of 25 years this plate begins to ossify (Figs. 3.**5a**, 3.**11**).[1] In front of the foramen magnum are the basilar part (basiocciput) of the occipital bone, the basilar part of the sphenoid bone (basisphenoid), and the dorsum sellae form the clivus (Fig. 3.**1**). On each side this area is separated from the petrous bone by the petro-occipital fissure, occupied in life by a thin plate of cartilage (Fig. 3.**5b**).[1] This fissure is limited behind by the jugular foramen, and its margins are grooved by the inferior petrosal sinus.[1] The posterior part of the jugular foramen contains the internal jugular bulb. In front of the vein the accessory, vagus and glossopharyngeal nerves, in that order from behind forward, traverse the foramen.[1] Medial to the lower border of the jugular foramen, a rounded elevation, termed the jugular tubercle, lies above and somewhat in front of the inner opening of the hypoglossal canal (Fig. 3.**11**), which contains the hypoglossal nerve and a meningeal branch of the ascending pharyngeal artery.[1] The posterior surface of the petrous bone forms a large portion of the lateral (anterolateral) wall of the posterior fossa. The internal auditory canal (IAC) runs in a lateral direction, containing the acoustic nerve, facial nerve, nervus intermedius, labyrinthine vessels, meninges, and subarachnoid space (Fig. 3.**12c–e**). Behind the petrous bone the lateral wall of the posterior cranial fossa is formed by the mastoid part of the temporal bone. It bears a wide groove, which runs forward and downward, then downward and medially, and finally forward to the posterior limit of the jugular foramen. This groove contains the sigmoid sinus and is termed the sigmoid sulcus. In this part of its course the mastoid foramen opens near its posterior margin and transmits an emissary vein from the sinus.[1] In addition to an emissary vein, the mastoid foramen transmits a meningeal branch of the occipital artery (Table 3.**2**). The condylar canal which is inconsistent, transmits an emissary vein from the lower end of the sigmoid sinus.[1] The anterior wall of the posterior fossa (the clivus) is related to the plexus of basilar venous sinuses that connects the two inferior petrosal sinuses and communicates below with the internal vertebral venous plexus.[1]

Role of Diagnostic Imaging in Skull Base Pathology and Surgery

The base of the skull, a site crowded with functionally important structures, is an anatomical region where a variety of congenital, inflammatory, benign and malignant neoplastic, and traumatic lesions may develop. CT and MRI are the most sensitive methods of detecting various lesions of the skull base.[2–9] Recent advances in cranial base surgical techniques have improved access to and repair of this complex anatomical region.[10–14] The precise identification of the site of origin as well as the extension of craniofacial tumors is exceedingly important for clinical tumor classification, appropriate modes of treatment, and determining the prognosis. Nodal and distant metastases of malignant sinonasal tumors are uncommon. Therefore, if extension of sinonasal tumors into the base of the skull can be precisely determined, provided they are accessible for radical resection, there will be a chance to cure the patient.[10–12]

CT has proved invaluable in detecting the bone involvement and soft-tissue component of lesions of the skull base.[2–9] MRI proved superior to CT in the evaluation of the soft tissue component.[6,7,15] In one series, all features of tumor extension that were used in classification of malignant ethmoid tumors to distinguish one stage from another could easily be assessed with clinical examination, CT scan, and MRI.[16] Staging can be done clinically and by means of CT and MRI scanning, which accurately reveal tumor extension and involvement of those anatomical structures that determine a change of stage.[16] Anterior craniofacial resection is now recognized as the treatment of choice for ethmoid tumors involving the cribriform plate with or without invasion of the anterior cranial fossa.[16]

The difficulty of gaining access to the central skull base has led to the development of many surgical approaches to this area during the past decade.[10,12–14,17] Numerous techniques, including the following, have been described to safely access the central base. (1) Transnasal approach via anterior facial degloving. (2) Transpalatal approach, which provides direct access to the sphenoid rostrum and proximal clivus. This requires the removal of part of the hard palate and the splitting of the soft palate.[17] (3) The transoral route provides direct access to the lower clivus and upper cervical spine, but the nasopharynx is still inaccessible unless the surgeon divides the soft palate, which might cause postoperative fistulae and velopharyngeal incompetence.[17] (4) The transmandibular or mandibular swing approach to the nasopharynx and clivus. (5) Transmaxillary and (6) Le Fort-I approaches to the central skull base.[10,17] Despite the remarkable advances in skull base surgery, operating on the skull base still poses a technical challenge. Radical surgical treatment of skull base lesions has been limited by the inaccessibility of the area and the close proximity of many significant vascular and neural structures.

Imaging Techniques

Computed tomography (CT) is the study of choice for assessment of the bony structures, foramina, fissures, carotid canal, jugular fossa, facial nerve canal, and craniocervical junction (Figs. 3.**1**–3.**11**). The examination should be carried out with axial and direct coronal 2–5 mm sections with a bone and soft-tissue algorithm. A reformatted sagittal view is very helpful in many cases. The study should be performed with and without contrast. MRI examination is performed in the axial, coronal, and sagittal planes with two 3–5 mm sections (Fig. 3.**12**).[7] Gadolinium contrast MRI study with and without fat suppression is mandatory for defining intracranial extension. Gradient echo pulse sequences and MR angiography (MRA) and MR venography (MRV) may define the vascularity of the lesions and the vascular anatomy in relation to tumors and cysts such as glomus tumor, meningioma, neurogenic tumors, epidermoid cyst, and cholesterol granuloma.[7,15] FLAIR as well as diffusion-weighted imaging (DWI) pulse sequences are invaluable for differentiating epidermoid cyst (cholesteatoma) from simulating lesions.[18] Epidermoid cysts appear hyperintense on both FLAIR and DWI pulse sequences. Epidermoid cysts that have calcification or "desiccated keratomas" may not be homogeneously hyperintense on FLAIR and DWI pulse sequences. Most of the MR images presented in this chapter were obtained with a 1.5 T MR imager. A few images were obtained, using a 3 T MR imager (General Electric, Milwaukee, WI, USA).

Angiography and Embolization

Tumors that involve the skull base may develop a rich vascular supply from branches of the external and internal carotid and vertebral arteries.[19] MRI and CT imaging are excellent for diagnosing the presence of these tumors and determinning the extent and boundaries of the tumors. MR angiography can be performed to demonstrate the vascularity and arterial supply of the lesions as well as to supply evidence of displacement or encasement.[19] True evaluation of arterial supply, however, cannot be performed by MR angiography.[19]

Angiography should be performed before the embolization of skull base tumors. Endovascular embolization of tumors is performed to decrease the blood supply to the tumor before surgical excision.[19] Surgery should be performed within 1–5 days after embolization.[19] Revascularization and recruitment of extensive blood supply from other vessels has been shown to occur if surgery is not performed within this period.[19] In cases where there is an anticipation of internal carotid artery sacrifice, angiography with balloon test occlusion should be performed to evaluate the outcome of such sacrifice. If cross filling from the other carotid is not present, an external carotid–middle cerebral artery bypass should be performed before surgery.[19] Surgery should be avoided for 8 weeks following permanent balloon occlusion to allow organization of thrombus and prevention of embolization of blood clot during manipulation of the distal internal carotid artery.[19]

Imaging Anatomy of the Skull Base

The base of the skull is an anatomical region that can be evaluated best using CT. The combination of CT and MRI provides maximum information concerning hard-tissue and soft-tissue structures (Figs. 3.1–3.12). Part of the anatomy of the base of the skull has been reviewed in Chapter 1. Most of the important structures of the skull base, as well as a number of base of skull foramina, are illustrated in Figs. 3.1–3.12.

Anatomical Variations

Preoperative CT, MRI, and angiography make surgery technically less difficult and may facilitate the opportunity for complete resection of tumors. The preoperative knowledge of anatomical variations is of utmost importance to otological, ophthalmic, maxillofacial, and skull base surgeons and to neurosurgeons. Anatomical variations and anomalies, at times, may contribute to increased morbidity and even mortality associated with surgery. Some of the important anatomical variations include dehiscence of the optic canal (Fig. 3.13), dehiscence or abnormal course of the internal carotid artery canal (Figs. 3.14, 3.15), high jugular fossa (Fig. 3.16), dehiscence of jugular fossa with protruding internal jugular vein into the hypotympanum (Fig. 3.17), forward-lying sigmoid sinus plate (Fig. 3.18), prominent emissary vein (Fig. 3.18), dehiscence of facial nerve canal, low-lying tegmen tympani and tegmen antri, and low-lying cribriform plate. Some anatomical variation/anomaly may result in symptoms such as limitation of motion in cases such as elongated coronoid process (Fig. 3.19). Aberrant internal carotid artery with or without per-

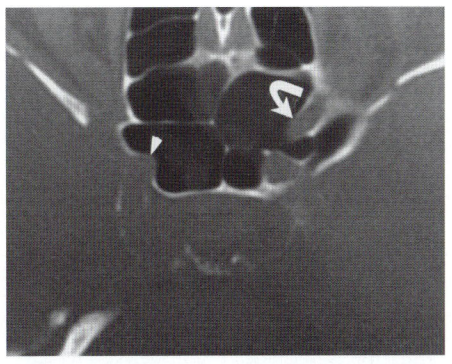

Fig. 3.13 Dehiscent optic and internal carotid artery canals. CT scan shows dehiscence of the internal carotid artery canal (arrowhead), protruding on both sides into the sphenoid sinuses, as well as dehiscent optic canal (curved arrow).

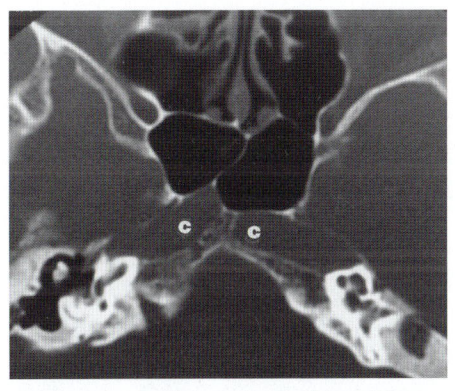

Fig. 3.14 Retrosphenoid internal carotid artery canal. CT scan shows retrosphenoid course of internal carotid artery canals (C).

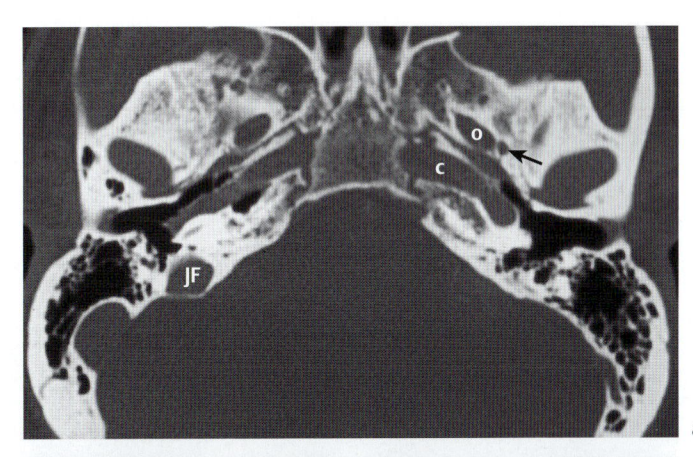

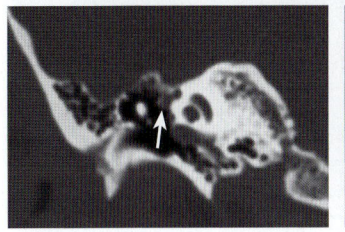

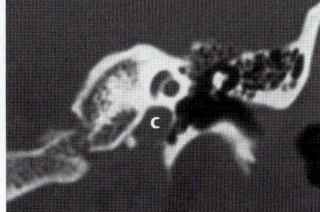

Fig. 3.15 Aberrant internal carotid atery.
a Axial CT scan shows normal left internal carotid artery canal (C) and aberrant course of right internal carotid artery. Note absence of right and normal left foramen spinosum (arrow). JF = jugular fossa. O = foramen ovale.
b Coronal CT scan shows slight enlargement of the right facial canal (arrow). This finding should raise the possibility of persistent stapedial artery, which is seen as a tiny dot over the aberrant internal carotid in Fig. 3.15a.
c Coronal CT scan shows normal left facial canal for comparison. Case courtesy of S. Noujaim, MD, Royal Oak, Michigan, USA.

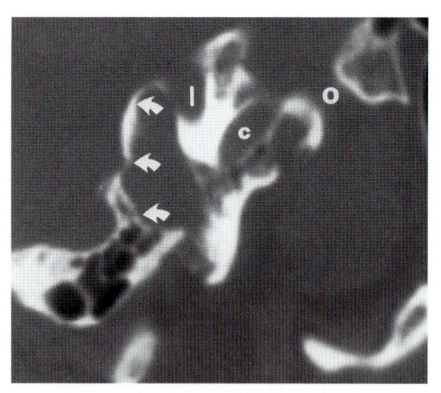

Fig. 3.16 High jugular fossa. Direct semisagittal CT scan, showing high jugular fossa (arrows), internal auditory canal (I), carotid canal (C), and foramen ovale (O).

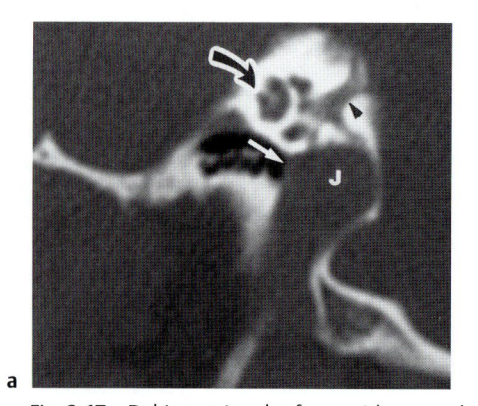

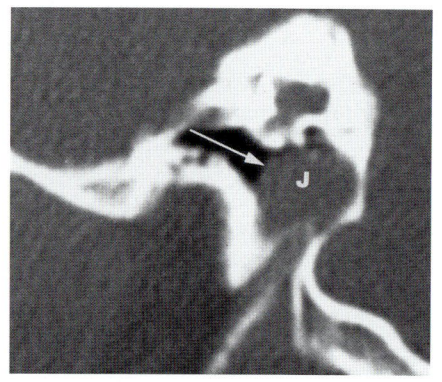

Fig. 3.17 Dehiscent jugular fossa with protruding jugular bulb into the hypotympanum.
a Direct semisagittal CT scan, showing a high jugular fossa (J), with focal bony dehiscence (straight arrow). Note cochlea (curved arrow) and common crus (arrowhead).
b Direct semisagittal CT scan, showing high jugular fossa/bulb (J), bone dehiscence, and protruding jugular vein (arrow).

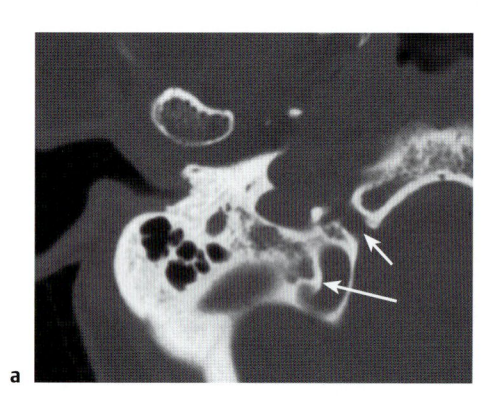

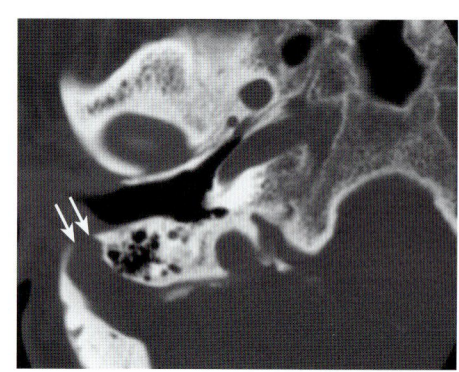

Fig. 3.18 a CT scan shows a large emissary canal (long arrow) adjacent to hypoglossal canal (short arrow).
b CT scan in the same subject as in a shows a markedly anterior and laterally located sigmoid sinus plate with focal area of bony dehiscence (arrows).

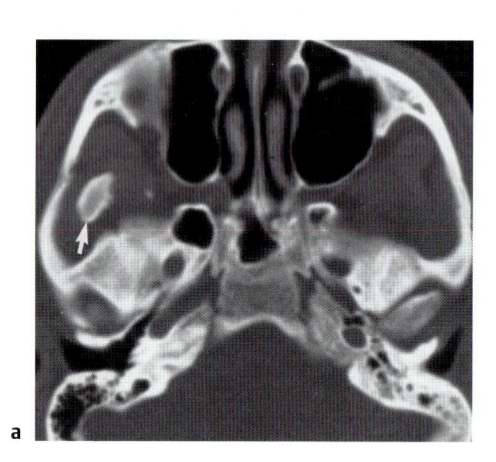

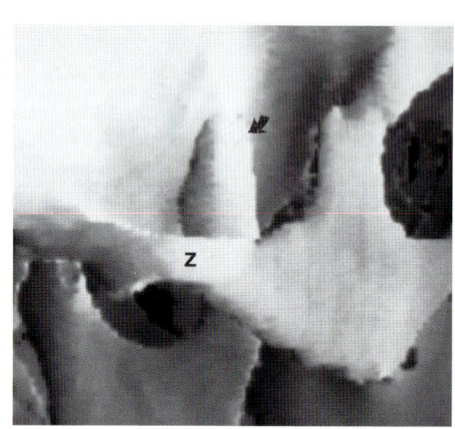

Fig. 3.19 Elongated coronary process.
a Axial CT scan and b reformatted 3D view, showing an elongated coronary process (arrow) of the mandible. Z = zygomatic arch.

sistent stapedial artery (Fig. 3.15) as well as a protruding internal jugular bulb into the hypotympanum (Fig. 3.17) may result in pulsatile tinnitus. Other anatomical variation such as sphenoid pneumosinus dilatans, associated with extensive pneumatization of the anterior clinoid, and dehiscent optic canal may rarely cause visual field defects (see Chapter 2).

Skull Base Pathology

In general, skull base lesions can be divided into three categories: (1) intracranial lesions that involve the skull base; (2) primary or secondary fibro-chondro-osseous lesions, as well as fractures; and (3) extracranial lesions that involve the skull base (Tables 3.3–3.5). The intracranial lesions that affect the skull base may result from congenital anomalies such as meningoencephalocele (Figs. 3.20–3.25), developmental inclusion cysts (epidermoid, dermoid, craniopharyngiomas, and neurenteric cysts) (Figs. 3.26–3.44), neoplasms such as meningiomas, chordomas, ag-

Table 3.3 Anterior skull base lesions

- Meningoencephalocele
- Developmental cysts (epidermoid, dermoid)
- Teratoma
- Neurenteric cyst
- Infections (epidural abscess) and invasive mycotic infection and granulomas (sarcoid)
- Mucoceles (frontoethmoid)
- Cholesterol granuloma (orbit)
- Hemangioma
- Lymphangioma
- Inverted papilloma (extension of sinonasal papilloma)
- Polyps (extension of sinonasal polyps)
- Carcinomas (extension of sinonasal cancers)
- Esthesioneuroblastoma
- Hemangiopericytoma (primary meningeal or extension of sinonasal and orbital tumor)
- Schwannoma/neurofibroma (extension of sinonasal tumor)
- Lymphoma
- Plasmacytoma
- Melanoma (extension of intranasal melanoma)
- Wegener granuloma
- Malignant fibrous histiocytomas
- Rhabdomyosarcoma (children)
- Fibro-osseous lesion (fibrous dysplasia, ossifying fibroma, osteoblastoma)
- Osteopetrosis
- Paget disease
- Giant cell tumor
- Langerhans cell histiocytosis
- Meningioma
- Metastases (breast, lung, kidney, prostate, thyroid, neuroblastoma, etc.)

Table 3.4 Central skull base lesions

- Meningoencephalocele
- Epidermoid cyst
- Dermoid cyst
- Teratoma
- Neurenteric cyst
- Craniopharyngioma
- Arachnoid cyst
- Cholesterol granuloma cyst (extension of orbital or petrous apex cyst)
- Mucocele of petrous apex (rare)
- Infections (epidural abscess) and invasive mycotic infection
- Mucocele (sphenoid sinus)
- Hemangioma
- Invasive pituitary adenoma
- Schwannoma/neurofibroma
- Meningioma
- Giant aneurysm of internal carotid artery
- Carotid cavernous fistula, dural arteriovenous fistula
- Carcinoma of nasopharynx invading skull bone
- Perineural extension of head and neck tumor
- Lymphoma
- Plasmacytoma
- Rhabdomyosarcoma (children)
- Fibrous histiocytoma
- Aggressive fibromatosis
- Giant-cell tumor
- Langerhans cell histiocytosis
- Chordoma
- Chondro-osteogenic tumor
- Chondromyxoid tumor
- Fibro-osseous lesion (fibrous dysplasia, ossifying fibroma, and osteoblastoma)
- Osteopetrosis
- Paget disease
- Metastases (breast, lung, kidney, prostate, thyroid, neuroblastoma, GI tract, etc.)

gressive pituitary adenomas, neuromas, lymphomas including plasmacytoma, teratoma, and vascular lesions such as aneurysms. Intra-axial lesions of the brain rarely affect the skull base. In our experience involvement of the base of skull is seen more with ependymomas.

Developmental Cysts of the Skull Base

Epidermoid and Dermoid Cysts

Epidermoid cyst or congenital cholesteatoma may be intradural, extradural, or intraosseous. The cyst develops from epithelial rest that becomes pinched-off along the suture lines or diploë in the course of embryonic development. Epidermoid cysts are lined by epidermis only, are filled with keratin, and do not contain the dermal appendages. Dermoid cysts are lined by keratinizing epithelium with dermal appendages in the walls, such as hair follicles, sebaceous gland and may contain fat. Both epidermoid and dermoid cysts may involve the base of the skull (Figs. 3.**26**–3.**31**). On CT scans, epidermoid cysts appear as low-density, unenhanced mass. Intraosseous epidermoids are bone-expanding and bone-destructive lesions (Figs. 3.**26**–3.**29**). In rare cases, calcifications may be seen in epidermoid cysts, either within or at the periphery of the cyst (Fig. 3.**31**). Dermoid cysts that contain true fatty tissue (well-differentiated teratoma) show characteristics of fat on CT and MRI (Fig. 3.**27**). Dermoid cysts that do not contain true fatty tissue cannot be differentiated from epidermoid cysts on CT and MRI scans. On MRI, epidermoid cysts appear hypointense on T1-weighted and hyperintense on T2-weighted, FLAIR

Table 3.5 Posterior skull base lesions

- Epidermoid–dermoid cyst
- Neurenteric cyst (intraclival, preclival)
- Cholesterol granuloma
- Mucocele of petrous apex (rare)
- Infections (epidural abscess), osteomyelitis of skull base (necrotizing otitis externa) and invasive mycotic infection
- Rheumatoid arthritis (atlanto-odontoid joint)
- Synovial cyst
- Meningioma
- Glomus jugular tumor
- Schwannoma (5, 7, 8, 9, 10, 11, 12)
- Neurofibroma
- Chondrosarcoma/chondroma
- Chordoma
- Internal carotid aneurysm (petrous portion)
- Dural arteriovenous fistula (transverse sinus)
- Osteogenic sarcoma
- Langerhans cell histiocytosis
- Lymphoma
- Plasmacytoma
- Chondromyxoid tumor
- Extension of carcinoma of temporal bone and parotid gland
- Endolymphatic sac tumor (low-grade papillary adenocarcinoma)
- Fibro-osseous lesion (osteochondroma, chondroblastoma, fibrous dysplasia, etc.)
- Metastases

308 3 Base of the Skull

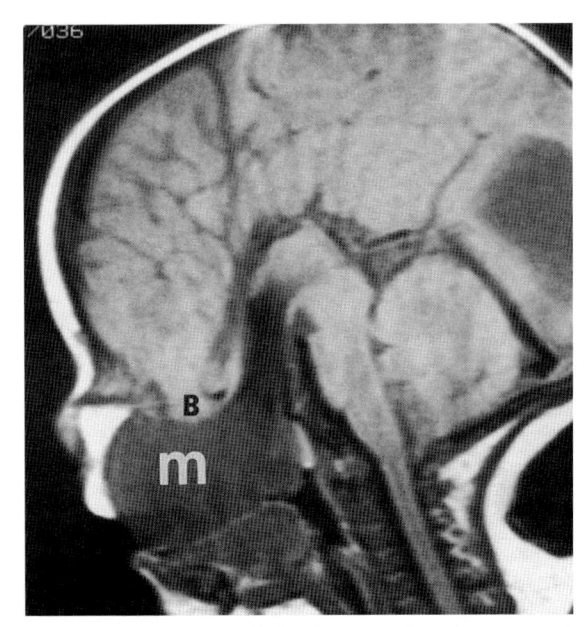

Fig. 3.**20** Menincoencephalocele. Sagittal T1W MR scan shows a large defect in the floor of the anterior cranial fossa with part of the brain (B) and meninges (m) extending into the nasal–ethmoid complex. As seen, the large CSF-filled component (meningocele) has significantly compromised the airway.

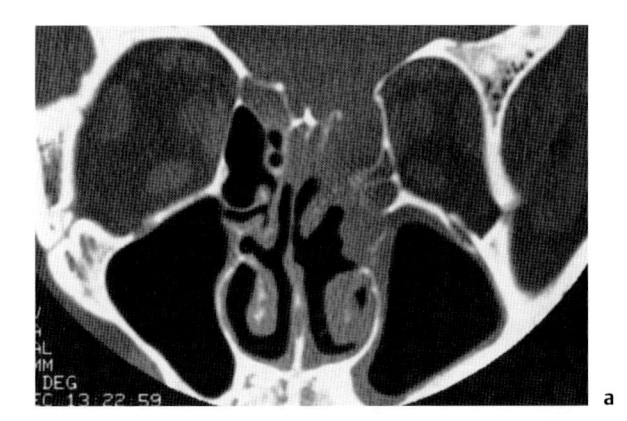

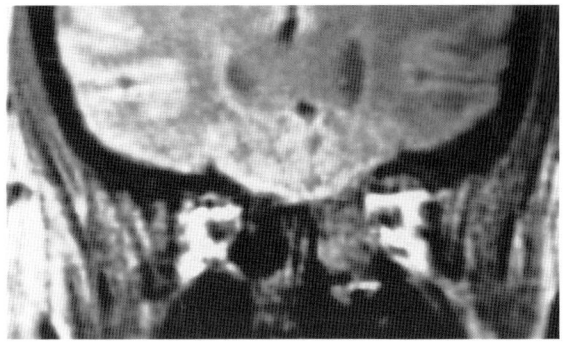

Fig. 3.**21** Meningoencephalocele. **a** Coronal CT and **b** PD (PW) MR scans showing a bony defect of the floor of the anterior cranial fossa on the left side, associated with brain herniation into the ethmoid labyrinth.

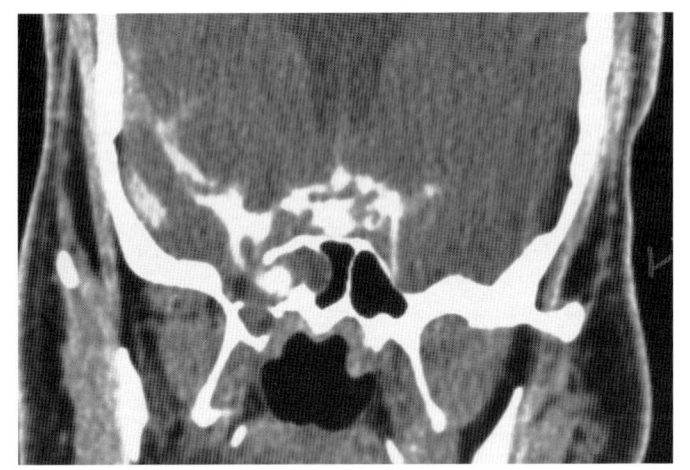

Fig. 3.**22** Meningoencephalocele. Cisternogram. Coronal CT scan showing a large defect of the floor of the middle cranial fossa on the right side, associated with brain herniation into the right sphenoid sinus.

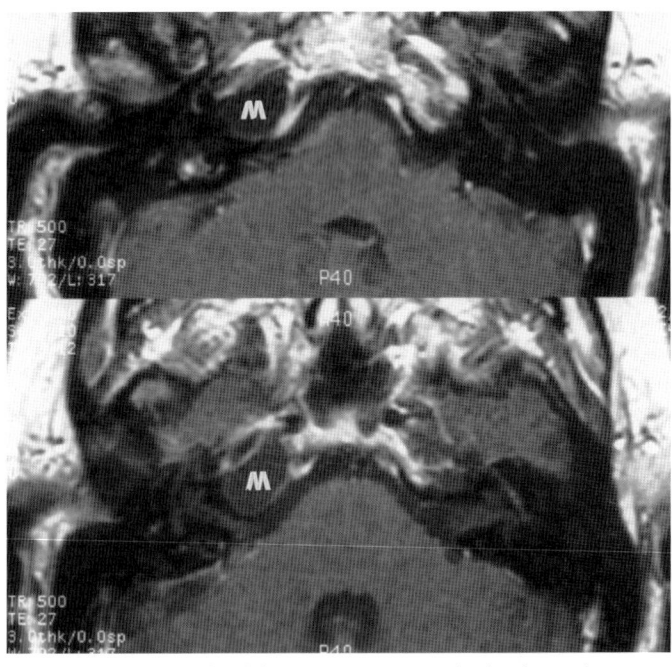

Fig. 3.**23** Meningocele of the petrous apex. Axial Gd-enhanced T1W MR scans showing a meningocele (M) at the right petrous apex. This cannot be differentiated from an arachnoid cyst or an epidermoid cyst in this region. However, epidermoid cyst, unlike meningocele and arachnoid cyst, will appear hyperintense on FLAIR and DWI scans.

Skull Base Pathology 309

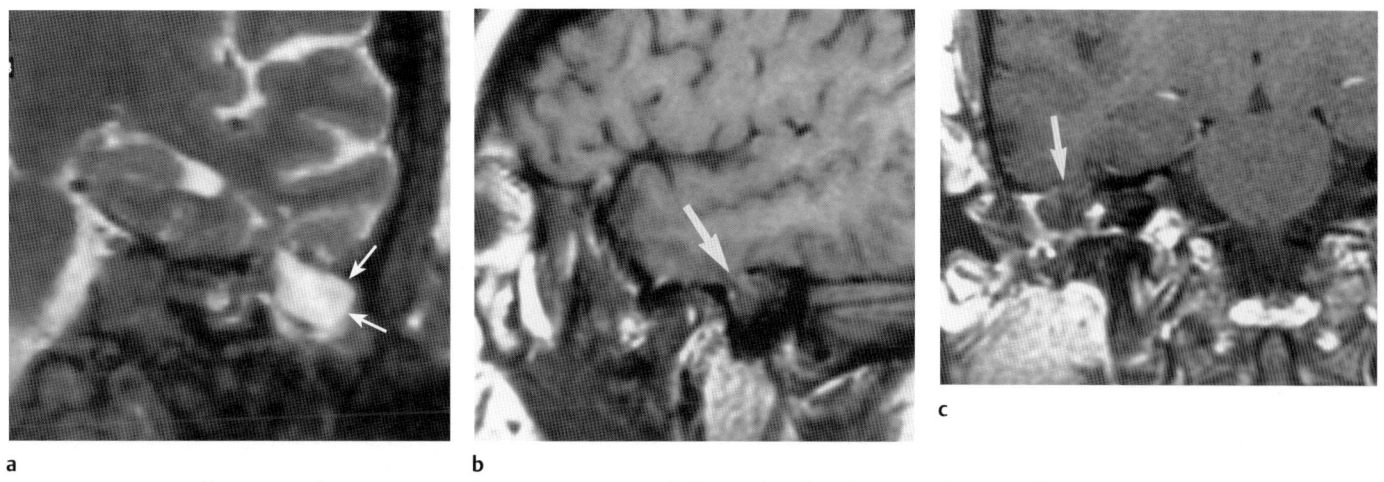

Fig. 3.24 Meningocele. **a** Coronal T2W MR scan showing a meningocele (arrows) within the mastoid antrum. **b** Sagittal T1W and **c** coronal Gd-enhanced T1W MR images in another patient showing an encephalocele within the mastoid (arrows).

Fig. 3.25 Meningocele. Coronal CT cisternogram in a patient with no history of trauma, showing CSF in the middle ear (white arrows). Note the CSF collection in the sublabyrinthine air cells (black arrow) and an air bubble in the CPA cistern (white curved arrow). At surgery, CSF was found in this region. It is possible that ectopic aggressive arachnoid tissue in the sublabyrinthine region has caused this CSF communication. Case courtesy of Dr. R. Devasthali, Chicago, USA.

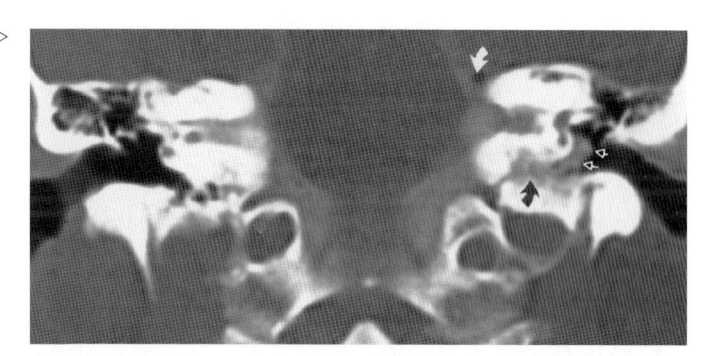

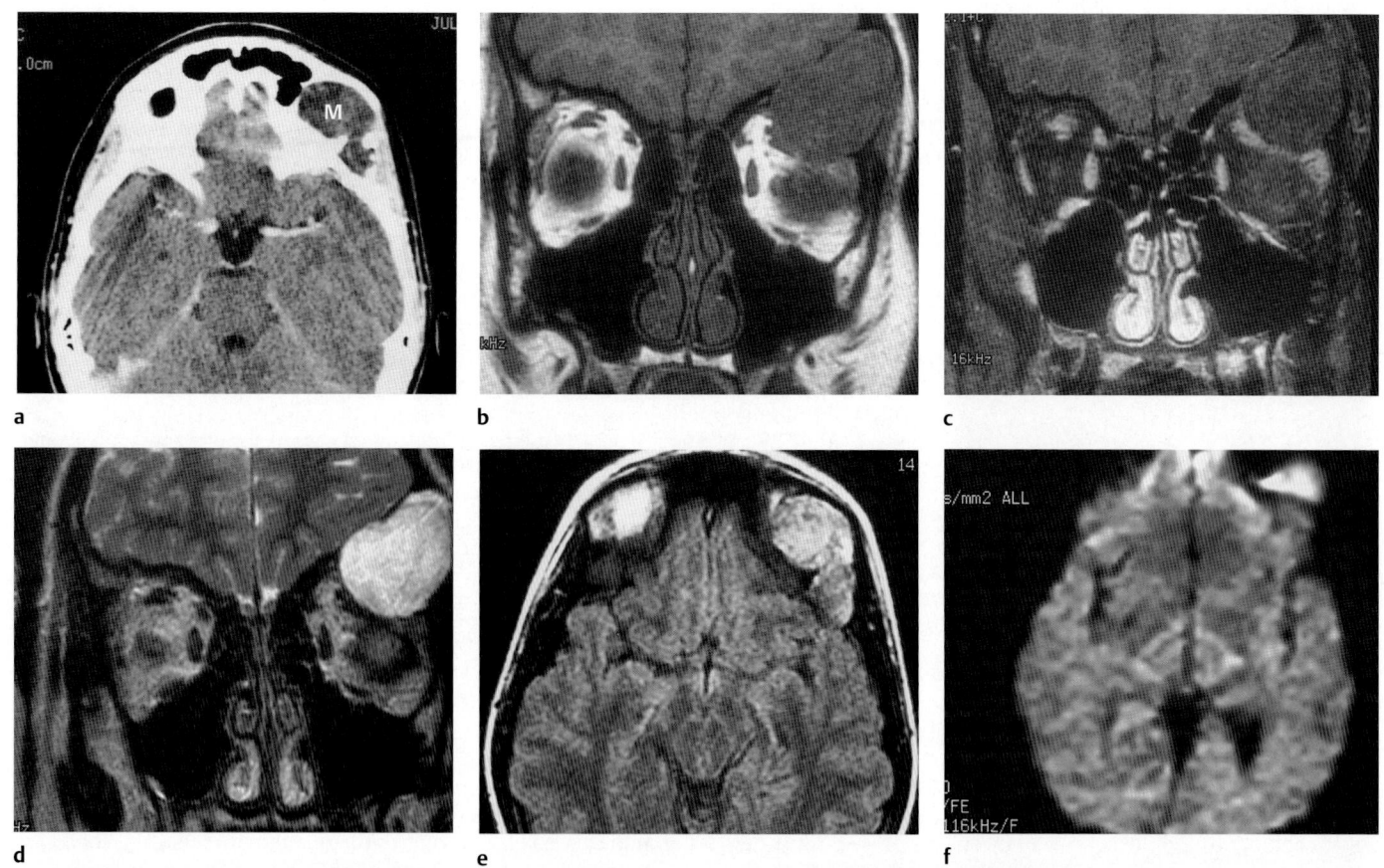

Fig. 3.26 Edipermoid cyst of anterior cranial fossa; 14-year-old boy. **a** Enhanced CT scan, showing a nonenhancing mass (M), involving the roof of the left orbit. **b** Coronal T1W MR scan, showing a large hypointense mass in the superior-temporal region of the left orbit. **c** Coronal fat-suppression Gd-enhanced T1W MR scan. **d** Coronal T2W MR scan. **e** Axal FLAIR MR scan. **f** Axial DWI MR scan. The epidermoid remains hyperintense on FLAIR, DWI, and demonstrates no contrast enhancement. Case courtesy of Yoon S. Hahn, MD, Chicago, IL, USA.

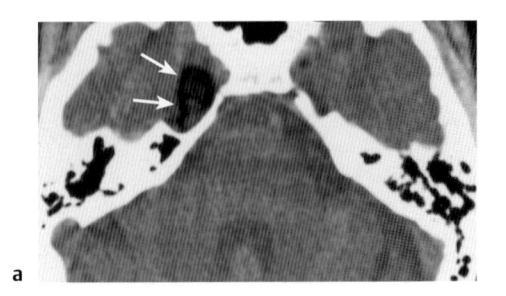

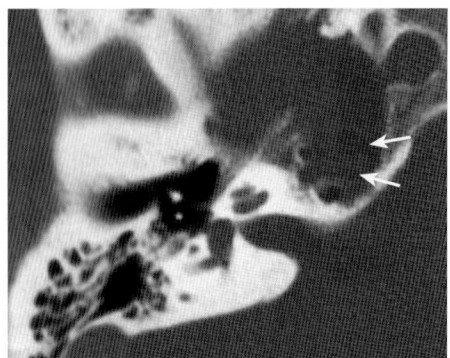

Fig. 3.27 Dermoid in the trigeminal cistern. **a** Axial CT scan shows a fat-containing mass in the right trigeminal cistern (arrows). **b** Axial CT scan shows expansion of the trigeminal impression of the petrous apex (arrows). Case courtesy of Keith Schaible, MD, Chicago, IL, USA.

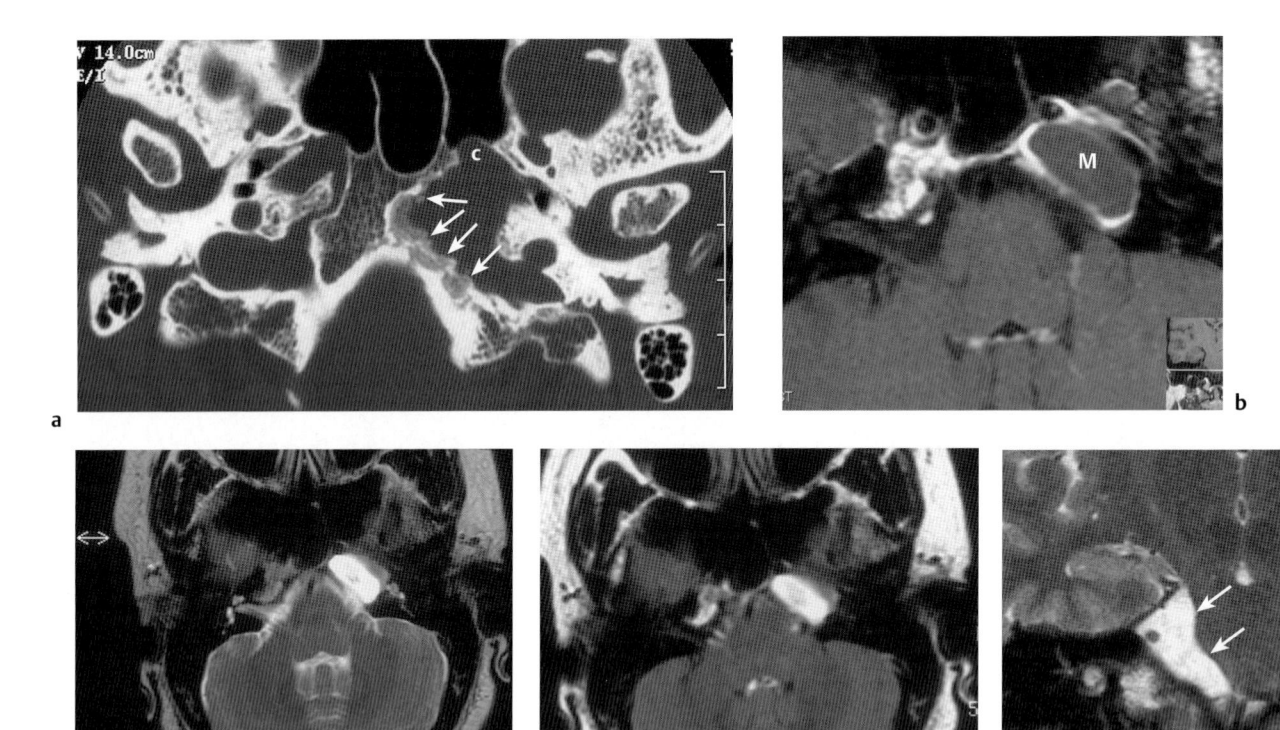

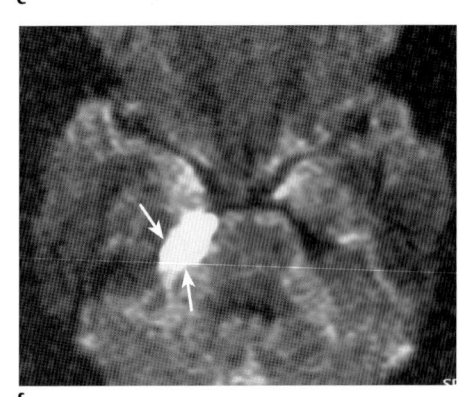

Fig. 3.28 Epidermoid cyst of the petrous bone. **a** CT scan shows an expansile mass involving the left petrous apex. Note erosion of the medial aspect of the carotid canal (c) and scalloping as well as sclerosis of the left side of the clivus (arrows). **b** Axial Gd-enhanced T1W MR scan, showing minimal enhancement at the peripheral (capsule) portion of the mass (M) replacing the petrous apex. **c** Axial T2W and **d** axial FLAIR MR scans. The epidermoid appears hyperintense on T2W and FLAIR MR images. **e** Coronal T2W and **f** axial DWI MR scans in another patient, showing a right intradural CPA epidermoid cyst (arrows). The epidermoid appears hyperintense on DWI scans.

and diffusion-weighted images (DWI) (Figs. 3.26, 3.27, 3.28). On Gd-enhanced T1-weighted MR images, there will be a thin line of enhancement around the capsule of these lesions (Fig. 3.28). Calcification is rare in epidermoids and more common in dermoids and teratomas. Some epidermoid cysts that contain compacted squamous debris (keratin) may appear somewhat heterogeneous on various MR pulse sequences. Epidermoid cyst should be differentiated from cholesterol granuloma and mucoceles. In contrast to epidermoid and dermoid cysts, cholesterol granuloma has a different etiology and pathogenesis. These are secondary lesions that are formed due to posttraumatic, postsurgical, or postinflammatory events and are referred to as cholesterol cysts or cholesterol granulomas.[4–6, 15–20] Cholesterol granulomas are bone-pushing and bone-destructive lesions

Skull Base Pathology 311

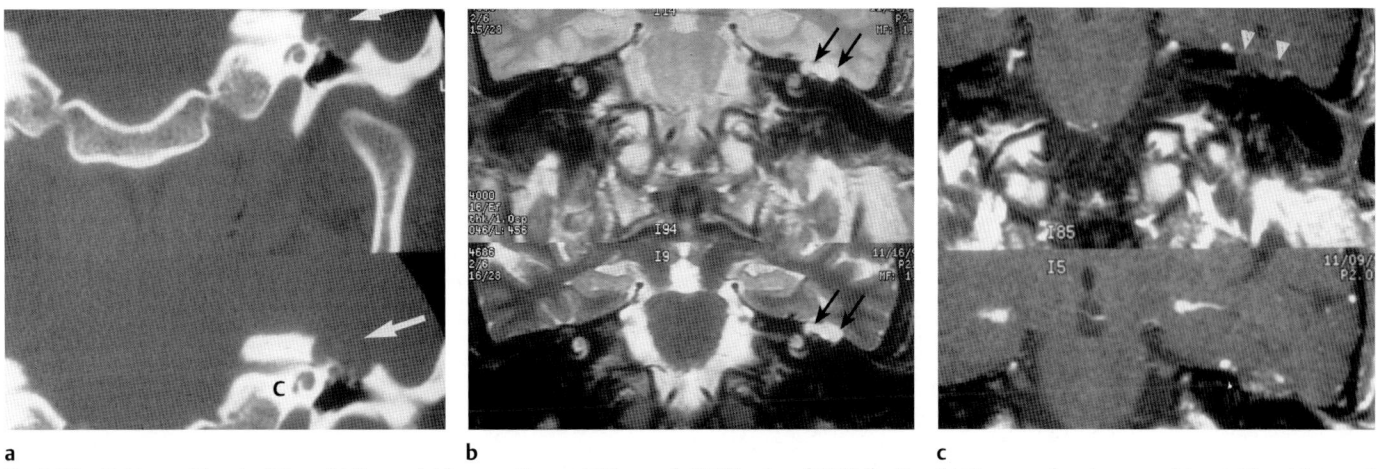

Fig. 3.**29** Epidermoid cyst of the middle cranial fossa. **a** Coronal CT scan, **b** PW (top) and T2W (bottom) MR scans, showing an epidermoid cyst (arrows) in the left middle cranial fossa adjacent to the geniculate portion of the facial canal. C = cochlea. The epidermoid appears hyperintense on T2W (Fig. 3.**29 b**) and demonstrates no contrast enhancement (Fig. 3.**29 c**).

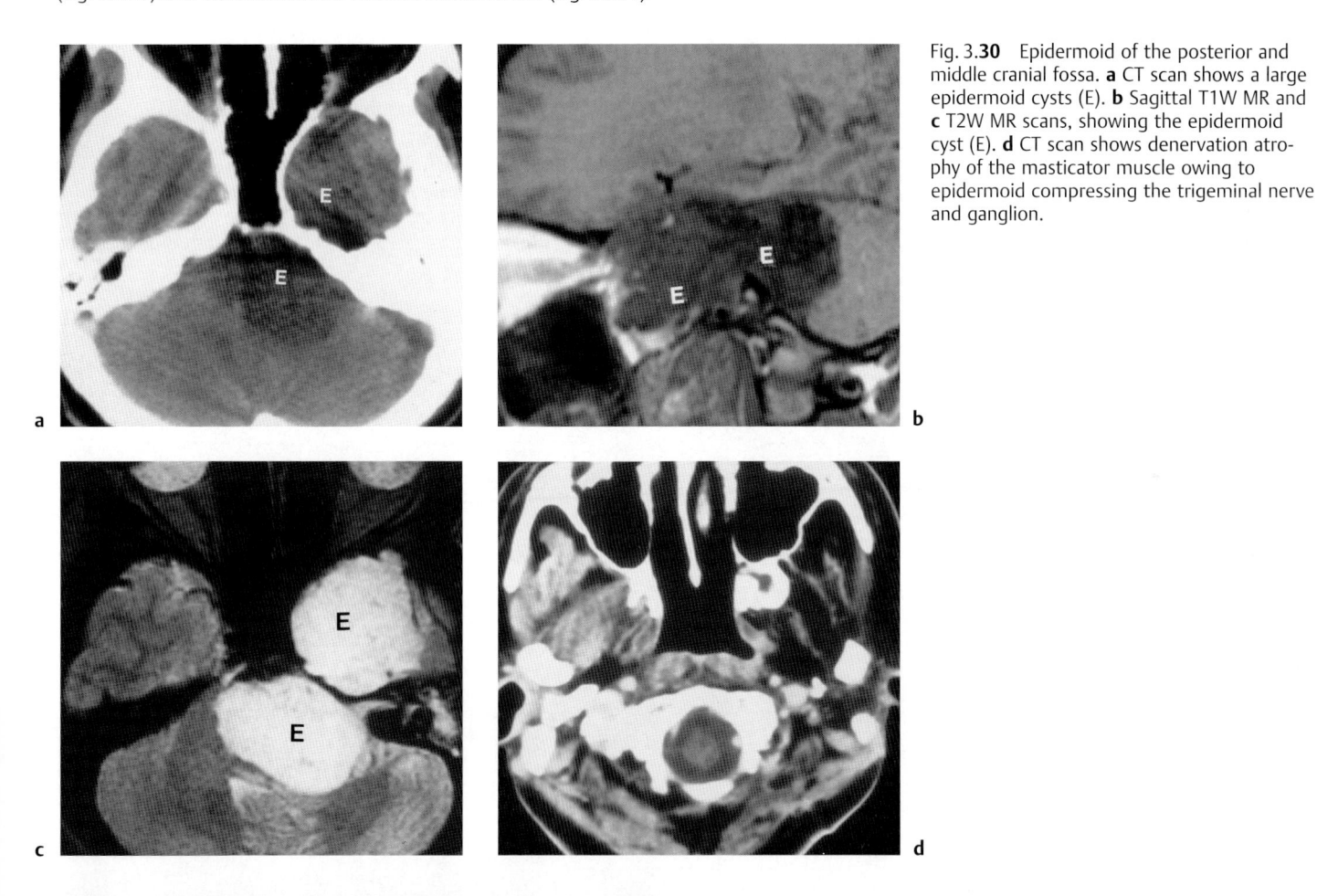

Fig. 3.**30** Epidermoid of the posterior and middle cranial fossa. **a** CT scan shows a large epidermoid cysts (E). **b** Sagittal T1W MR and **c** T2W MR scans, showing the epidermoid cyst (E). **d** CT scan shows denervation atrophy of the masticator muscle owing to epidermoid compressing the trigeminal nerve and ganglion.

Fig. 3.**31** Epidermoid cyst. CT scan shows an intradural CPA epidermoid cyst. On rare occasions epidermoid like this may show calcification.

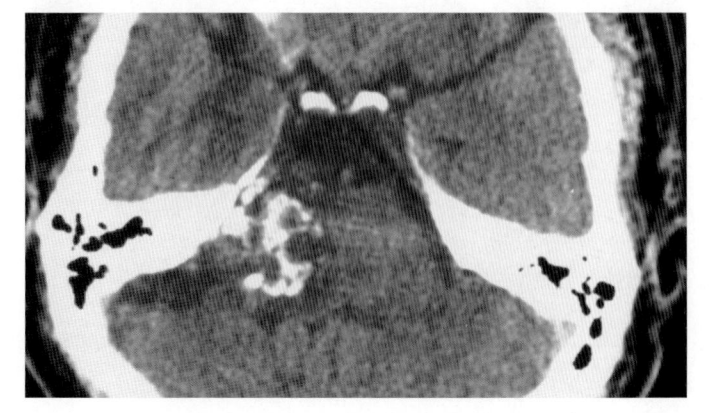

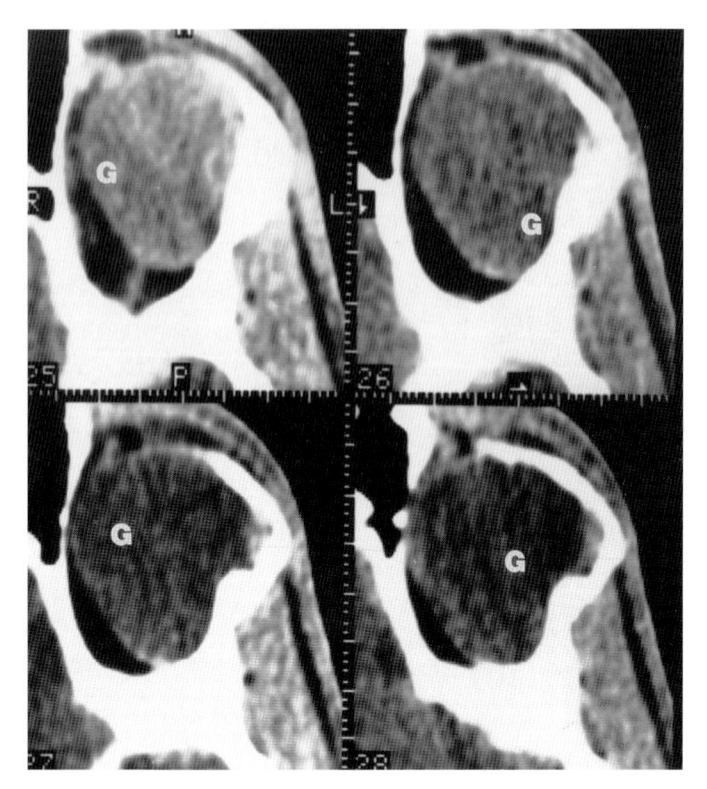

Fig. 3.32 Cholesterol granuloma. Axial CT scans showing a large cholesterol granuloma cyst (G) involving superior aspect of the left orbit.

(Figs. 3.32, 3.33). CT scan shows unenhanced expansile lytic lesions (Figs. 3.32, 3.33b). Cholesterol granulomas give rise to high signal on T1-weighted and T2-weighted MR images, characteristic of chronic hemorrhage (Fig. 3.33).[20] Some of the cholesterol granulomas may have heterogeneous signal characteristics (Fig. 3.34). At times cholesterol granuloma may be bilateral (Fig. 3.35). Epidermoid cyst and cholesterol granuloma cyst are described in more detail in Chapter 2 on the orbit and Chapter 1 on the temporal bone.

Mucoceles of the paranasal sinuses are cystic lesions, lined by a respiratory epithelium, that occur as a result of obstruction of the main ostium of the individual paranasal sinuses. Mucoceles are most commonly seen in the frontal and ethmoid sinuses. Expansion, erosion, and destruction of the sinus walls are characteristics of mucoceles (Fig. 3.36). Mucoceles are described in detail in Chapter 4 on the paranasal sinuses.

Craniopharyngioma

Craniopharyngioma is an epithelial tumor that resembles the adamantinoma (ameloblastoma) of the jaw. Most craniopharyngiomas occur during the first and second decades of life, although a second peak occurs in the 5th decade. The tumor constitutes 2–5% of all primary intracranial tumors. It usually arises in the suprasellar area but can be intrasellar (Figs. 3.37, 3.38). Craniopharyngioma arises from nests of squamous epithelial cells that are believed to be remnants of Rathke's pouch, lying between the anterior and posterior lobes of pituitary gland. About

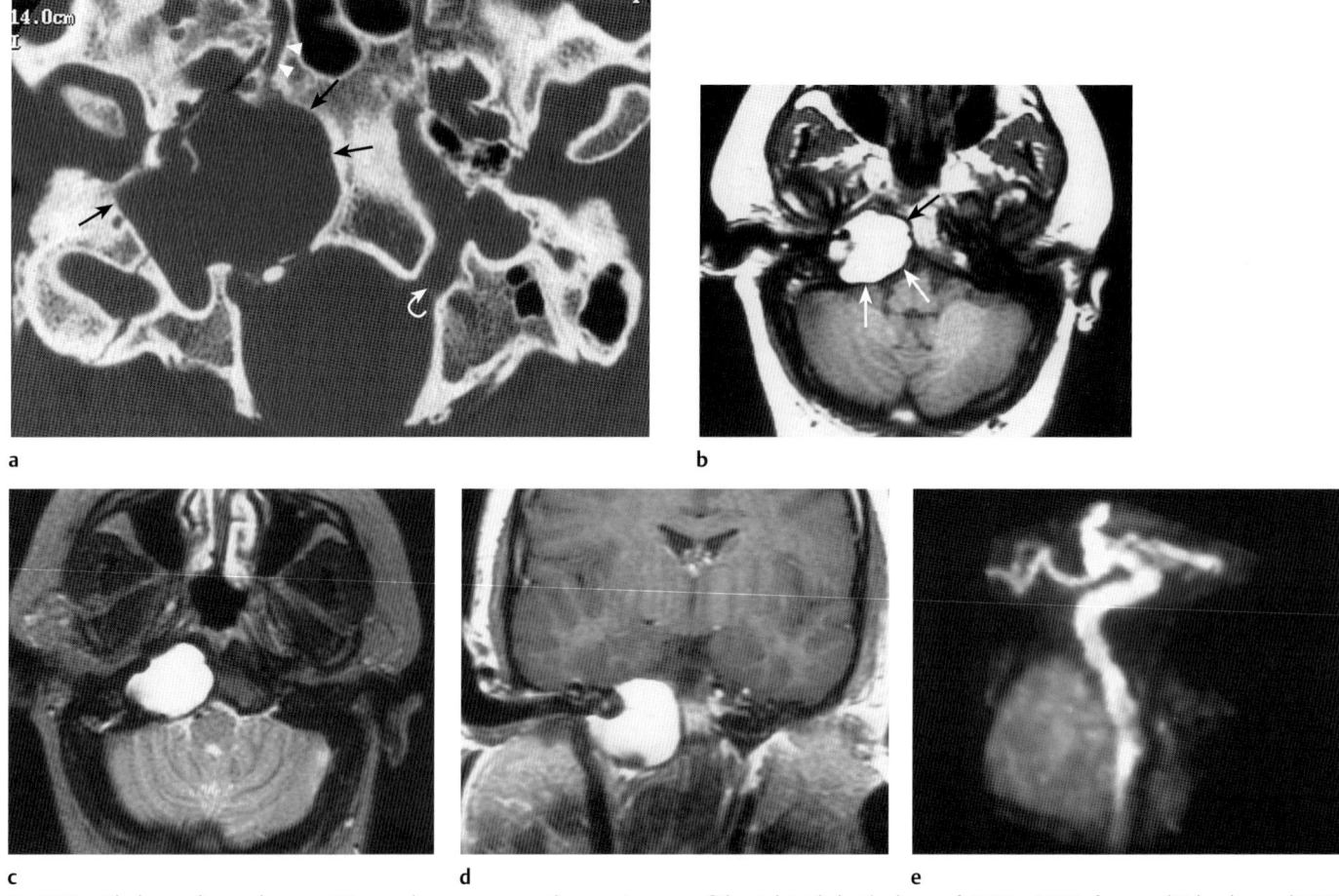

Fig. 3.33 Cholesterol granuloma. a CT scan shows an expansile mass involving the right petrous apex (arrows); arrowheads = vidian canal. Note normal hypoglossal canal on the left side (curved arrow) and involvement of the right side by the lesion. b T1W, c T2W, d coronal Gd-enhanced T1W, and e MRA images, showing hyperintensity of this cholesterol granuloma on T1W (arrows), as well as on T2W and MRA pulse sequences.

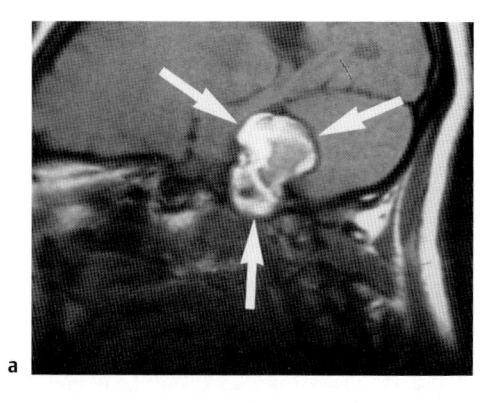

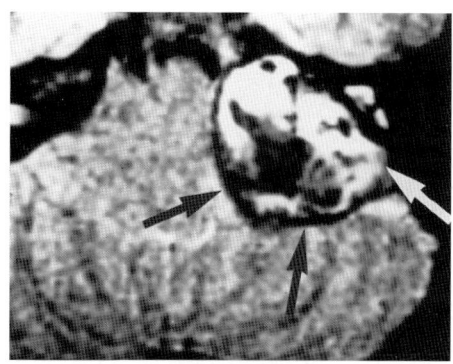

Fig. 3.34 Cholesterol granuloma. **a** Sagittal T1W and **b** axial T2W MR scans showing a large cholesterol granuloma of the left petrous apex (arrows).

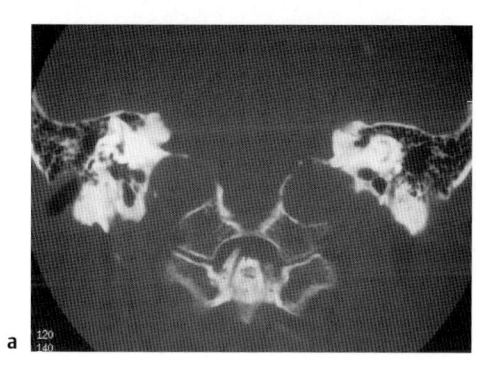

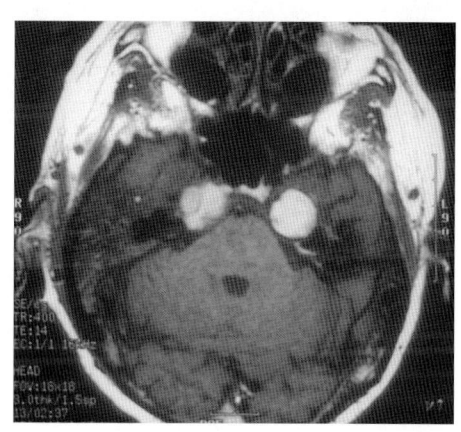

Fig. 3.35 Bilateral cholesterol granuloma. **a** Coronal CT scan and **b** axial T1W MR scan showing bilateral petrous apex cholesterol granulomas.

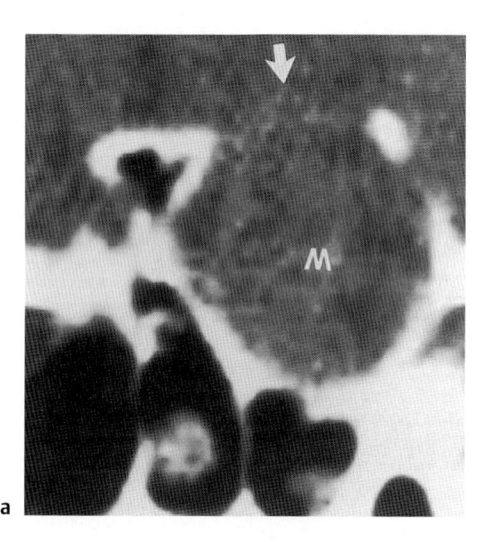

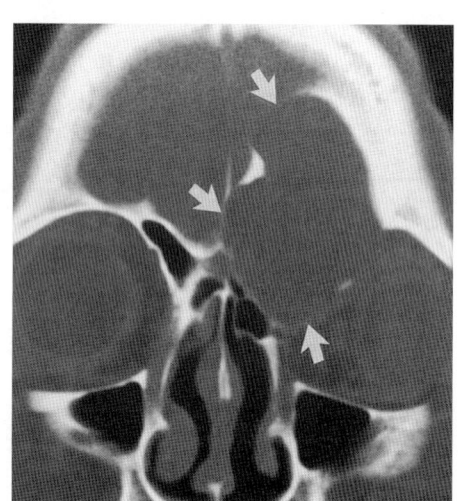

Fig. 3.36
a Sphenoid sinus mucocele. Coronal CT scan shows marked expansion of the sphenoid sinuses, representing a large mucocele (M), extending into the suprasellar middle cranial fossa region (arrow).
b Frontal sinus mucocele. Coronal CT scan shows marked expansion of the left frontal sinus representing a large mucocele (arrows), extending into the anterior cranial fossa and left orbit.

80% of craniopharyngiomas are suprasellar and 20% are intrasellar. We have seen intraventricular (third ventricle) and extracranial (within the sphenoid sinus and base of the skull) craniopharyngiomas (Fig. 3.39). The resemblance to the adamantinoma (ameloblastoma) of the jaw is striking and there are cases of craniopharyngioma with tooth formation that suggest a common cell of origin. Craniopharyngiomas vary greatly in size and composition. The CT and MR imaging characteristics reflect this heterogeneous internal architecture. On CT scans, they usually have a combination of cystic (80%), solid, and calcified components (Fig. 3.38).[21] Calcifications are frequently ringlike or nodular and are seen in about 80% of cases.[21] Rarely, cystic craniopharyngiomas may be homogeneously isodense or even hyperdense on CT scans.[21] The high density is related to high protein content. The solid component of craniopharyngioma usually enhances homogeneously on CT scans. On MR scans, calcification in craniopharyngioma often has a low signal intensity on all pulse sequences. Cystic areas are isointense to brain on T1-weighted and hyperintense on T2-weighted MR images.[21] About half of craniopharyngiomas contain focal or diffuse regions of bright hyperintensity on T1-weighted MR images.[21] These areas correspond to cysts containing aqueous proteinaceous materials, cholesterol, or methemoglobin.[21] If the protein content is very high, however, they may appear hypointense on T2-weighted MR images.[21] The solid component of tumor shows both long T1 and long T2 characteristics with marked enhancement after intravenous administration of Gd-DTPA contrast material (DTPA = diethylenetriamine pentaacetic acid). Craniopharyngioma may

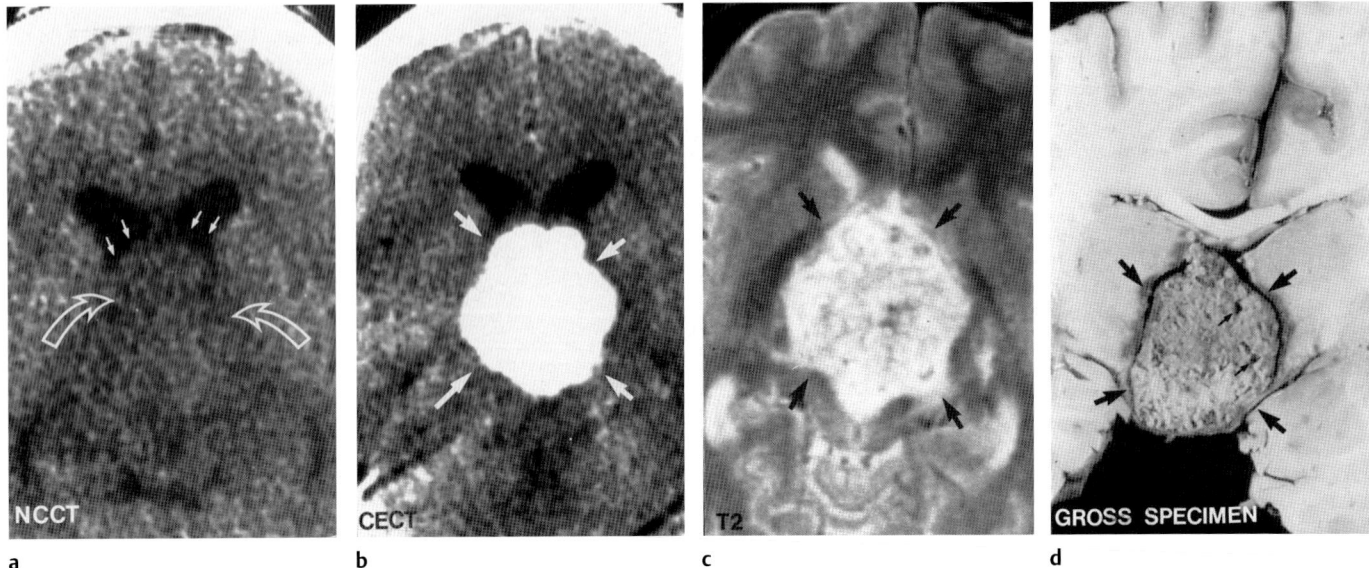

Fig. 3.37 Craniopharyngioma. a Noncontrast CT (NCCT) scan shows a suprasellar mass (arrows). **b** Contrast-enhanced CT (CECT) scan shows marked enhancement of this noncystic craniopharyngioma (arrows). **c** T2W MR scan shows hyperintensity of the craniopharyngioma (arrows). **d** Gross specimen shows suprasellar solid craniopharyngioma (arrows).

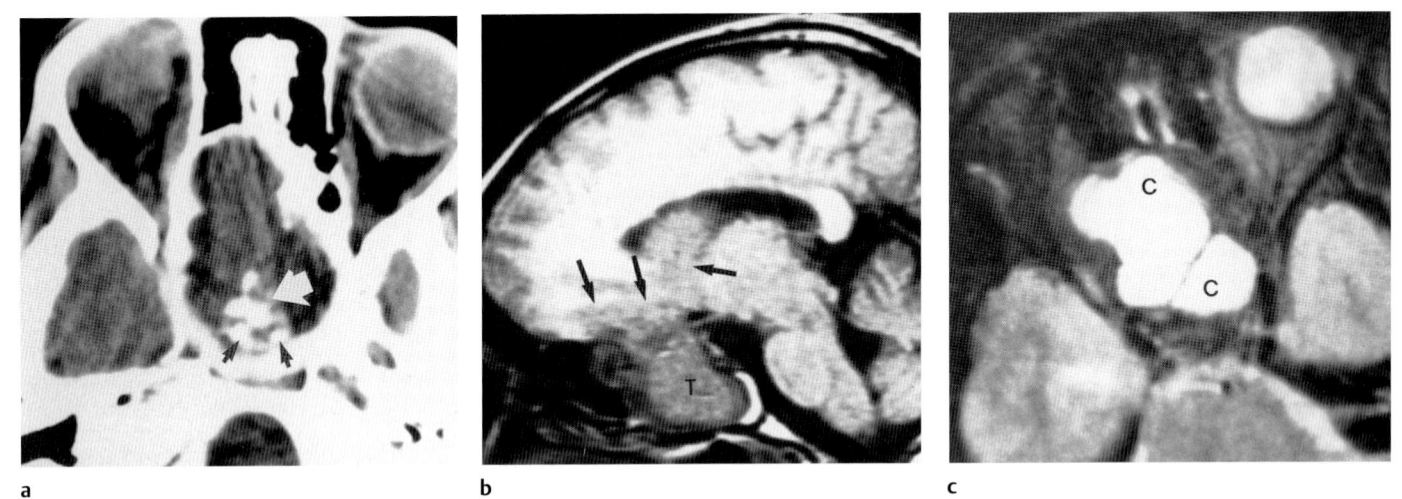

Fig. 3.38 Craniopharyngioma. a CT scan shows a large cystic mass involving the floor of the anterior cranial fossa as well as sellar middle cranial fossa. Note calcifications (arrows). **b** T1W MR scan shows an intrasellar tumor (T) with large suprasellar component (arrows) with extension into the floor of the anterior cranial fossa. **c** T2W MR scan shows extension of craniopharyngioma (c) into the anterior cranial fossa.

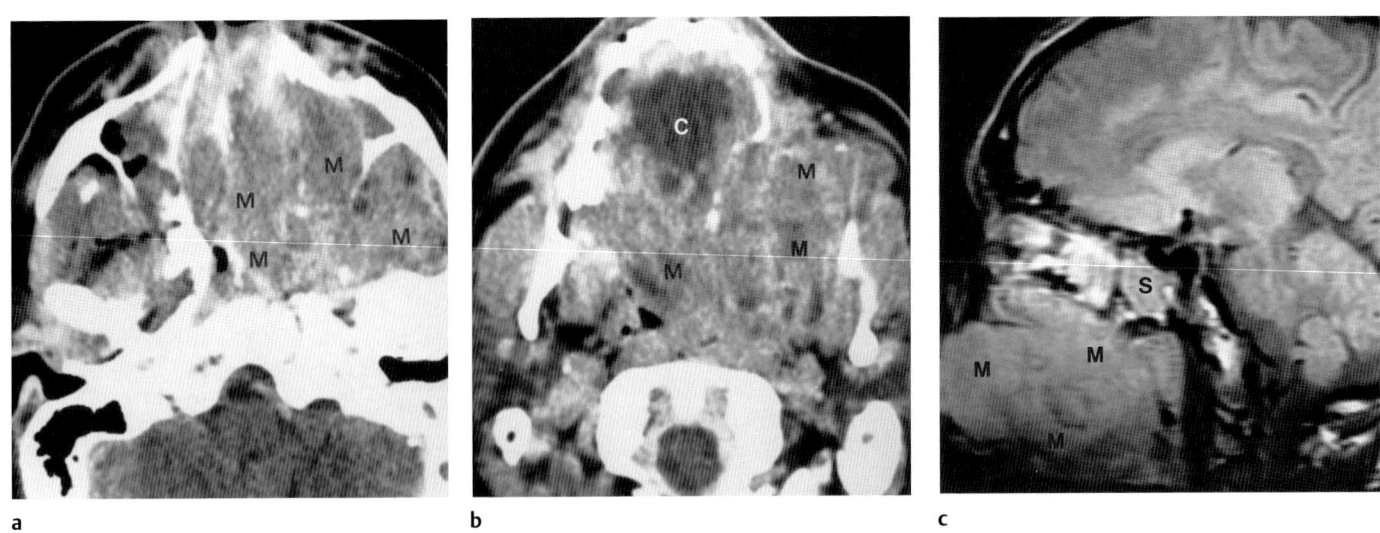

Fig. 3.39 Extracranial craniopharyngioma. a CT scan shows an extensive mass (M) involving the nasopharynx, nasal cavities, with extension into the left maxillary sinus and left infratemporal fossa. **b** CT scan shows extension of the mass (M) into the oropharynx and left buccal space, with total replacement of the hard palate by tumor. Part of the tumor appears cystic (c). **c** Sagittal PW MR scan showing extensive craniopharyngioma within the sphenoid sinus (S), oropharynx and oral cavity (M). There was no intrasellar or supraseller mass present in this case.

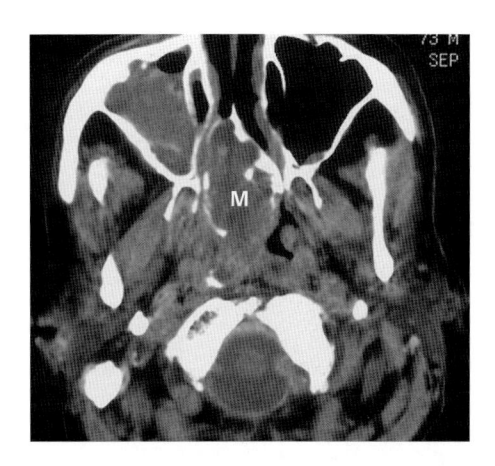

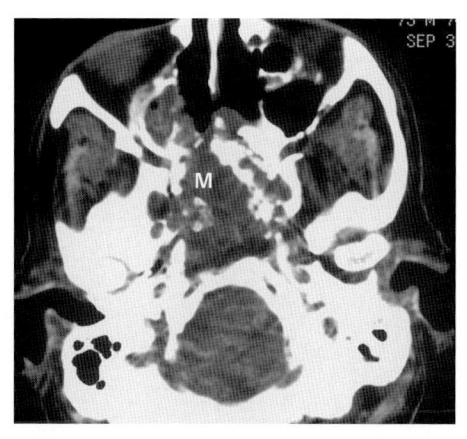

Fig. 3.40 Ameloblastoma. **a** Unenhanced CT scan shows a mass (M) in the nasopharynx. **b** Unenhanced CT scan shows a destructive mass (M) in the central skull base compatible with an ameloblastoma. Differential diagnosis should include chordoma, chondrosarcoma, invasive pituitary adenoma, craniopharyngioma, giant-cell tumor, esthesioneuroblastoma, carcinoma of the sphenoid sinus, and metastasis.

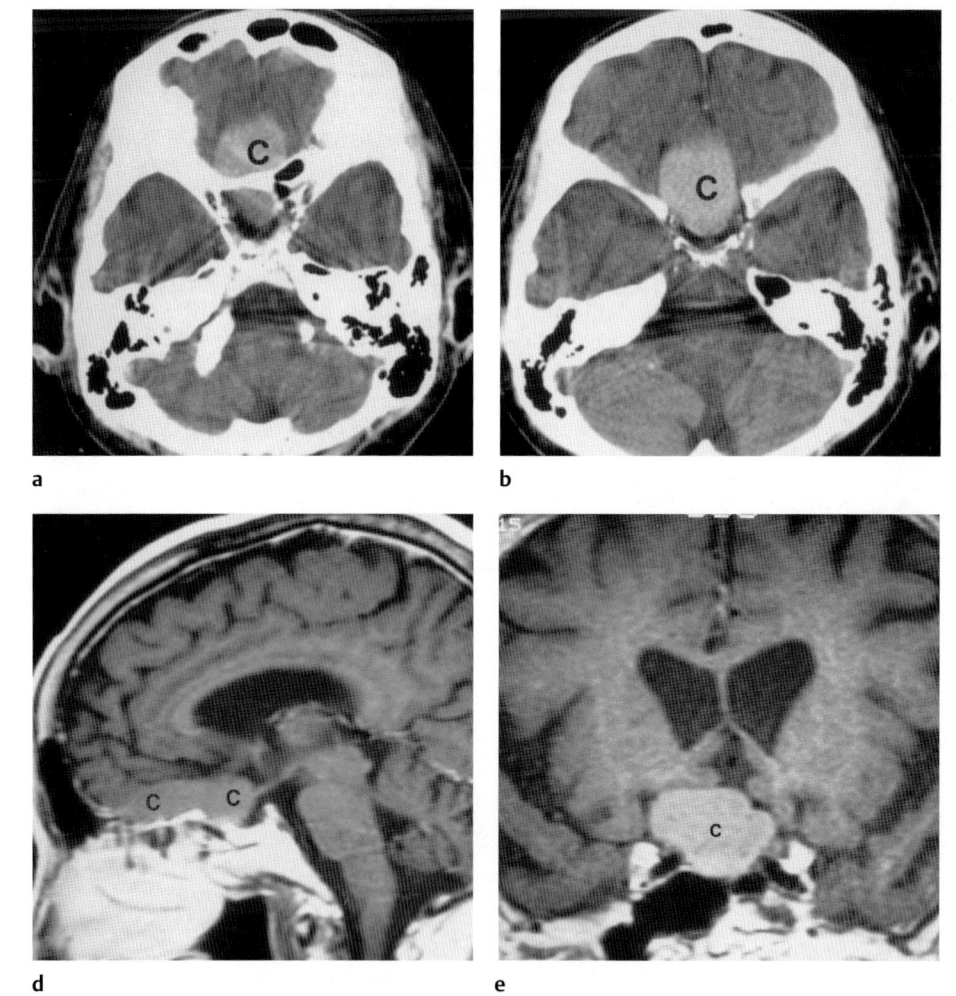

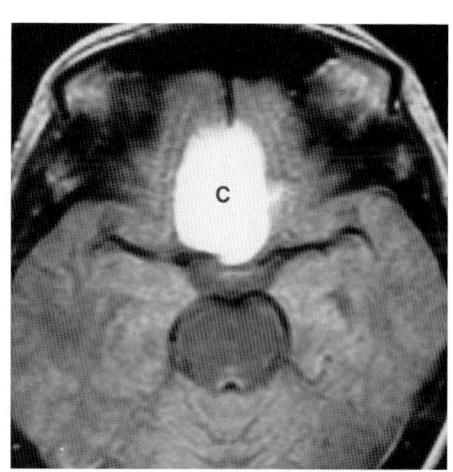

Fig. 3.41 Neurenteric cyst of the anterior cranial fossa. **a, b** CT scans show a hyperdense anterior cranial mass compatible with a neurenteric cyst (c). **c** PW, **d** sagittal Gd-enhanced T1W, and **e** coronal Gd-enhanced MR scans, showing the cyst (c). The mass also appeared hyperintense on unenhanced T1W MR images.

be extensive, with extension into the skull base, clivus, and sphenoid and ethmoid sinuses (Fig. 3.**39**). Sphenoid sinus and base of the skull ameloblastoma is a rare entity that can simulate extracranial craniopharyngioma with extensive involvement of the base of the skull and sinonasal cavities (Fig. 3.**40**).

Rathke's Cleft Cyst

Rathke's cleft cyst is histologically similar to craniopharyngioma.[21] Like craniopharyngioma, the Rathke's cyst is derived from remnants of Rathke's pouch; however, it is smaller, exclusively intrasellar, and has thin walls lined by a single layer of columnar or cuboidal epithelium.[21] Craniopharyngiomas have a thicker wall, composed of squamous or basal cells.[21]

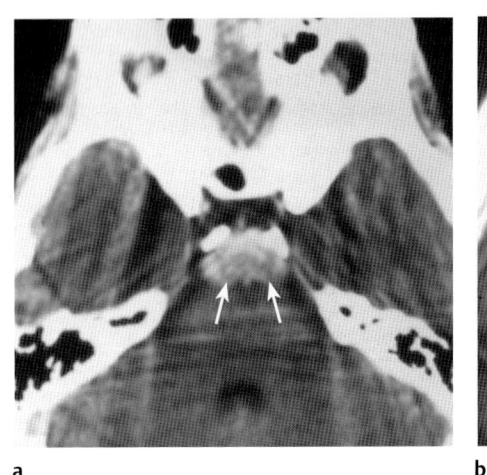

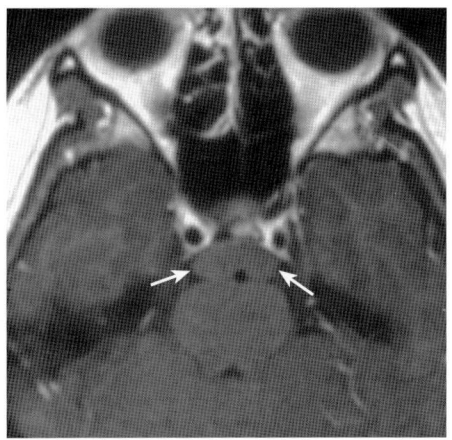

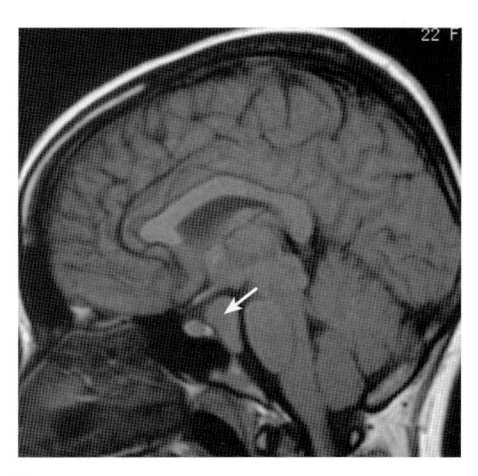

Fig. 3.42 Presumed neurenteric cyst of the posterior cranial fossa. **a** CT scan shows a hyperdense mass in the prepontine region (arrows). **b** Gd-enhanced axial T1W MR scan shows the mass (arrows) in front of the basilar artery. **c** Sagittal unenhanced T1W MR scan showing the mass (arrow), just behind the clivus and dorsum sella, with extension into the posterior aspect of the suprasellar region. Case courtesy of James Ausman, MD, Chicago, IL, USA.

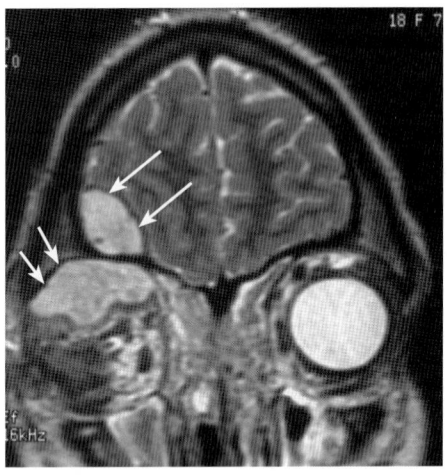

Fig. 3.43 Sinogenic epidural abscess of the anterior cranial fossa. Coronal T2W MR scan showing opacification of ethmoid sinuses, subperiosteal orbital abscess (small arrows), and an epidural abscess (long arrows).

Neurenteric Cyst

Neurenteric cysts are developmental cysts that are believed to be related to dysgenesis of the notochord and/or neurenteric canal during early embryogenesis. Neurenteric cysts arise secondary to the persistence of the neurenteric canal, which is the temporary connection between the amniotic cavity and yolk sac during the third week of embryogenesis.[22] Intracranial neurenteric cysts have been described in the anterior cranial fossa (Fig. 3.41),[23] posterior cranial fossa including cerebellopontine and prepontine cisterns, suprasellar cistern, preclival (Fig. 3.42), and within the clivus.[24] Neurenteric cysts are believed to arise from the developing endodermal and notochordal tissues and represent persistence of the transient neurenteric canal.[25] The desmocranium (blastemal skull) starts to form around the developing brain with condensation of the mesenchyme by the end of the first month of embryogenesis.[24] The occipital plate is first to appear, and eventually forms the basiocciput. At the same time, the notochord obliquely traverses the occipital plate, where it comes close to the epithelium of the dorsal wall of the developing pharynx.[24,25] Transiently, it fuses with the dorsal wall of the pharynx and then reenters the cranial base and courses ventrally to end just caudal to the hypophysis.[25] Hence, the notochord could conceivably carry some of the endodermal elements of the neurenteric canal with it as it invaginates into the clivus (Fig. 3.42). Neurenteric cysts, colloid cysts, and Rathke's cleft cysts are similar on histological and immunochemical analysis, and their locations are important distinguishing features.[25] A Rathke's cleft cyst is sellar or rarely suprasellar; a neurenteric cyst is usually in the posterior fossa (Fig. 3.42), and rarely in the anterior cranial fossa (Fig. 3.41);[23] and a colloid cyst is typically in the region of the foramen of Monro along the anterior superior wall of the third ventricle. Intraspinal neurenteric cysts are more common in the cervical region, typically anterior to the spinal cord and without associated spinal defects.[25] Intraspinal neurenteric cyst may be seen at the level of the conus, posterior to the cord or roots; intraspinal neurenteric cysts are frequently associated with spinal defects.[23,24,25] Persistent endoectodermal adhesions or a persistent adhesion between notochord and the endoderm may produce a notochordal dysgenesis such as diastematomyelia, and a neurenteric cyst may result.[23,25]

The histological appearance of neurenteric cysts includes a lining epithelium that ranges from nonciliated to ciliated, cuboidal to columnar (and occasionally stratified columnar epithelium), with a variable number of admixed goblet cells.[23,24,25] These mucinous features permit overall comparison with the normal respiratory or gastrointestinal tract lining.[25] On CT scans, neurenteric cysts that contain thick proteinaceous fluid appear hyperdense on unenhanced scans. These lesions appear hyperintense on T1-weighted and T2-weighted MR images (Figs. 3.41, 3.42). A case of extra-axial cerebellopontine neurenteric cyst has been reported, associated with a small solid component.[22] The solid component was composed of foamy histiocytes, chronic inflammatory cells, giant cells, and cholesterol clefts.[22] At times lesions may appear isointense to hypointense to CSF on T2-weighted MR images. We have seen cervical spinal neurenteric cyst that had similar signal characteristics to arachnoid cyst. The location, position anterior to the cervical spinal cord, and lack of enhancement of such an intradural mass should favor the diagnosis of spinal neurenteric cyst.

Inflammatory Conditions

Inflammatory lesions of the sinonasal cavities, orbit, temporomandibular joint, and temporal bone (necrotizing otitis externa) may spread intracranially through the skull base (Figs. 3.43–

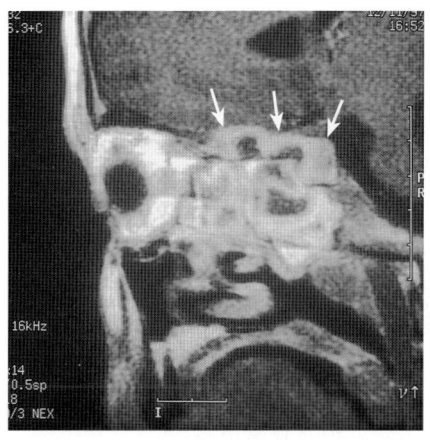

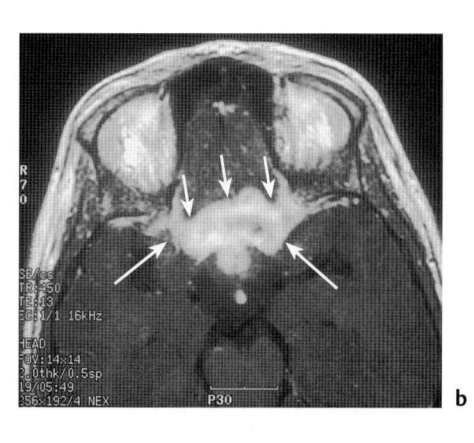

Fig. 3.44 Sinogenic epidural abscess. **a** Gd-enhanced sagittal and **b** axial MR scans showing inflammatory mucosal enhancement within the sphenoid sinus, as well as a large epidural abscess (arrows) in the anterior cranial fossa.

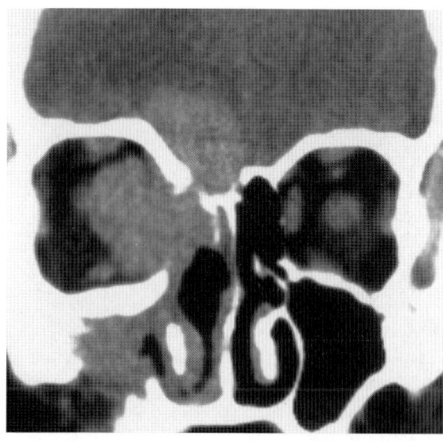

Fig. 3.45 Mucormycosis involving anterior cranial fossa. Coronal enhanced CT scan shows postsurgical changes of the sinonasal cavity on the right side and extensive mucormycosis infection involving the right orbit and anterior cranial fossa. Case courtesy of Dr. H. Sherif, Cairo, Egypt.

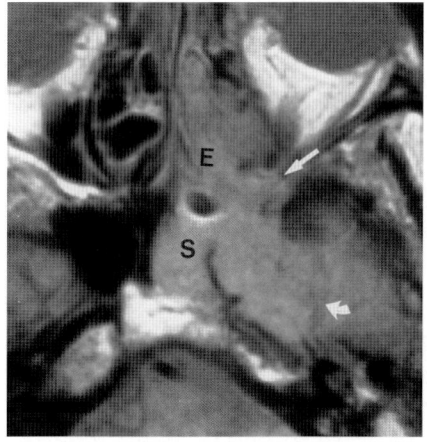

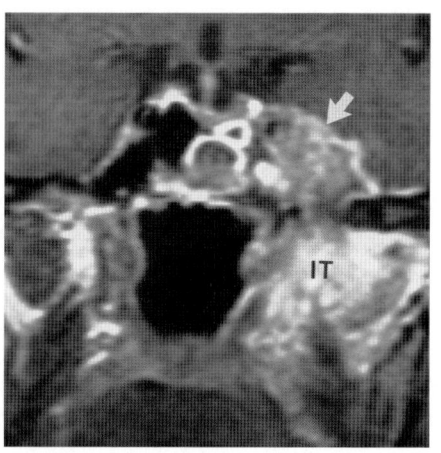

Fig. 3.46 Aspergillosis involving middle cranial fossa. **a** PD (PW) MR scan shows inflammatory opacification of the sphenoid (S) and ethmoid (E) sinuses. Note extension of the inflammation beyond the periosteum, into the middle cranial fossa (arrows). **b** Gd-enhanced coronal T1W MR scan shows inflammatory involvement of the cavernous sinus (arrow) as well as involvement of the skull base and infratemporal fossa (IT).

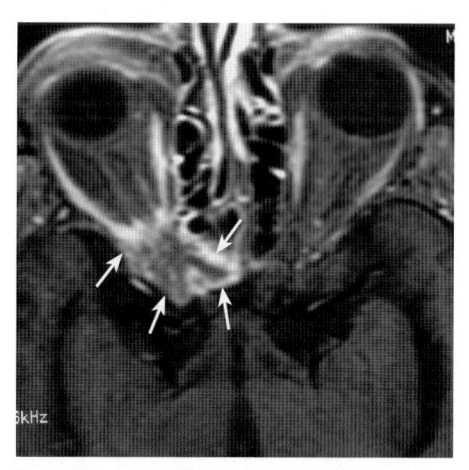

Fig. 3.47 Aspergillosis of the middle cranial fossa. Axial fat-suppression, Gd-enhanced T1W MR scan shows an infiltrative process in the right superior orbital fissure (arrows) compatible with surgically proven invasive aspergillosis in this 78-year-old woman who presented with Tolosa–Hunt syndrome. This patient had no known immunocompromising condition.

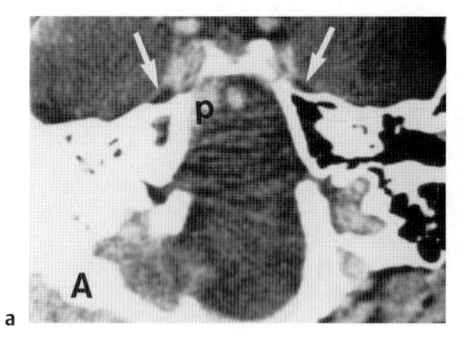

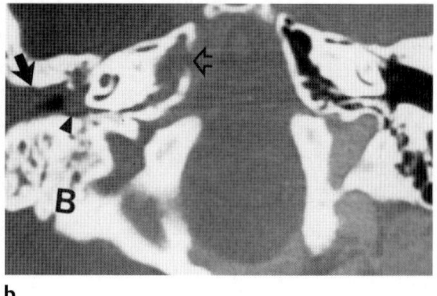

Fig. 3.48 Petrous apicitis. **a** Axial enhanced CT scan shows opacification of right mastoid air cells and abnormal enhancement adjacent to the right petrous apex (P). Note gasserian cisterns (arrows). **b** Axial CT scan shows focal erosion of the petrous apex (hollow arrow), opacified right mastoid air cells, and inflammatory changes in the right middle ear (arrowhead) and external auditory canal (solid black arrows). Patient presented with Gradenigo syndrome following surgical drainage for an external canal abscess.

3.52). In patients with diabetes and those who are immunocompromised, opportunistic fungal infections, such as mucormycosis and aspergillosis, may involve the sinonasal cavities and rapidly invade the skull base (Figs. 3.45–3.47). Invasive necrotizing fungal osteomyelitis of the base of the skull is a rare and frequently misdiagnosed clinical entity. It frequently involves an immunocompromised host, prior long-term antibiotic therapy, and steroid therapy (Figs. 3.46, 3.47).[11] At times the disease may be seen in an immunocompetent host (Fig. 3.48).[11] In contrast to bacterial skull base osteomyelitis, fungal osteomyelitis of the skull base in the region of the temporal bone (necrotizing otitis externa) has not been associated with diabetes mellitus. However, involvement of the anterior and middle cranial fossa by mucormycosis in patient with diabetes, and aggressive aspergil-

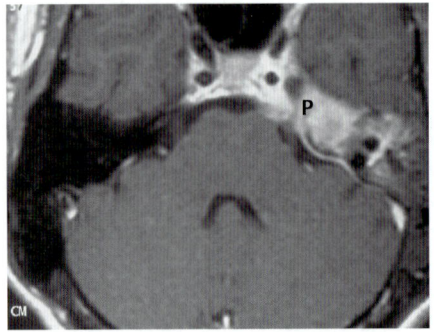

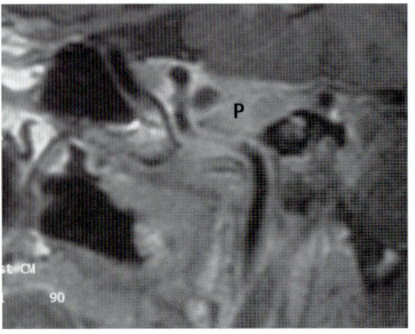

Fig. 3.49 Petrous apicitis. **a** Axial Gd-enhanced T1W MR scan, showing increased inflammatory enhancement in the left petrous apex (P). **b** Sagittal Gd-enhanced T1W MR scan, showing inflammatory enhancement of the petrous apex (P). Note abnormal enhancement around the internal carotid artery, if severe enough, may cause Horner syndrome. Case courtesy of Kamel Ayadi, MD, Saudi Arabia.

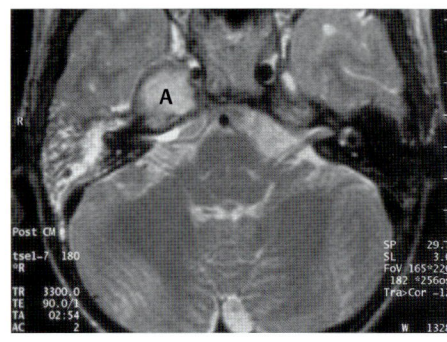

Fig. 3.50 Otogenic petrous apex abscess. Axial T2W MR scan, showing a petrous apex intradural (Meckel's cave) abscess (A). Case courtesy of Kamel Ayadi, MD.

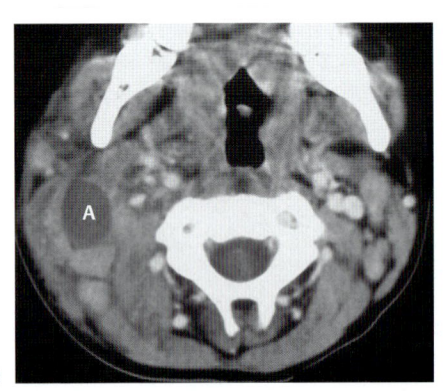

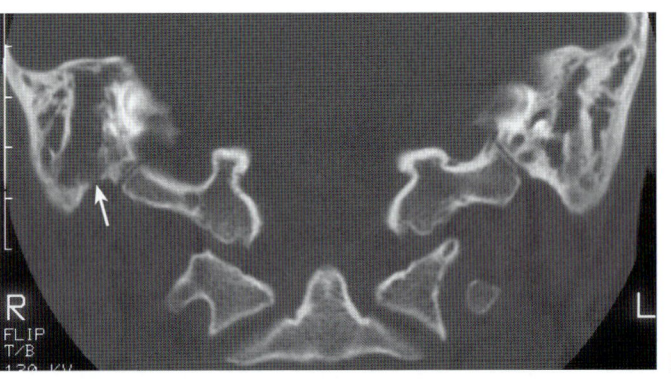

Fig. 3.51 Bezold abscess. **a** Enhanced CT scan shows a neck abscess (A), under the right sternocleidomastoid muscle. **b** Coronal CT scan shows opacification of the right mastoid with cortical break (arrow), the site of extension of mastoid abscess into the deep facial neck structures.

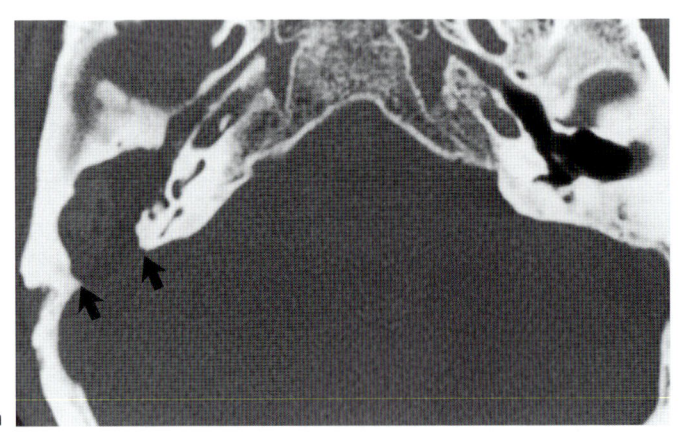

Fig. 3.52 Acquired cholesteatoma. **a** Axial CT scan shows marked expansion of the mastoid antrum, which is filled with cholesteatomatous debris. Note erosion of petromastoid plate (arrows). **b** Coronal CT scan shows erosion of tegmen (solid arrows) and fistula of lateral semicircular canal (hollow arrow) by this acquired cholesteatoma.

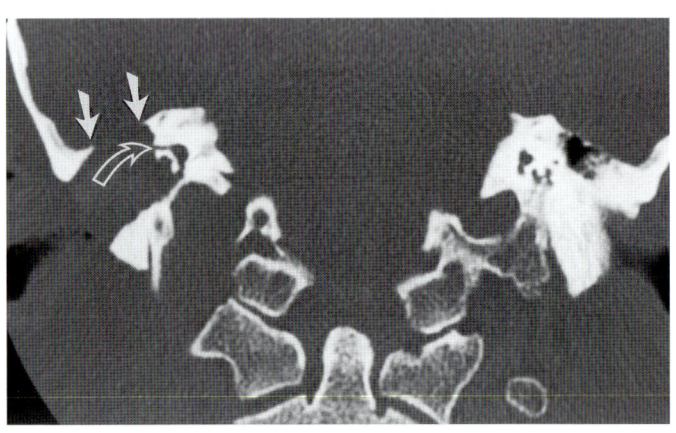

losis in immunocompromised patients have been reported. Chronic inflammatory conditions of the sinonasal cavities and temporal bone may be associated with formation of mucocele and cholesterol granuloma cyst and, in the case of chronic otomastoiditis, an acquired cholesteatoma may develop. Acquired cholesteatomas like primary cholesteatomas (epidermoid cysts) may result in erosion of the skull base (Fig. 3.52).

■ Tumors

The extracranial tumors commonly affecting the skull base include tumors of the paranasal sinuses, carcinoma of the nasopharynx, juvenile angiofibroma, Langerhans cell histiocytosis (Fig. 3.53), multiple myeloma, lymphoma, rhabdomyosarcoma, temporal bone tumors, neurogenic tumors, perineural extension

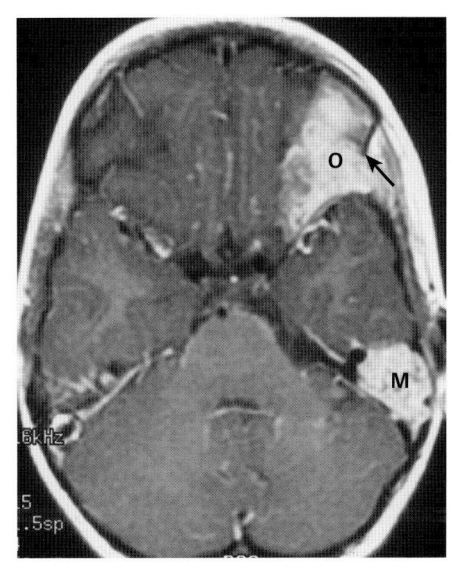

Fig. 3.53 Langerhans cell histiocytosis. Enhanced CT scan shows orbital (o) and mastoid (M) involvement by Langerhans cell histiocytosis. Note erosion of the lateral wall of the left orbit (arrow) as well as marked contrast enhancement of the involved sites. Case courtesy of Robert Schamschula, MD, Australia.

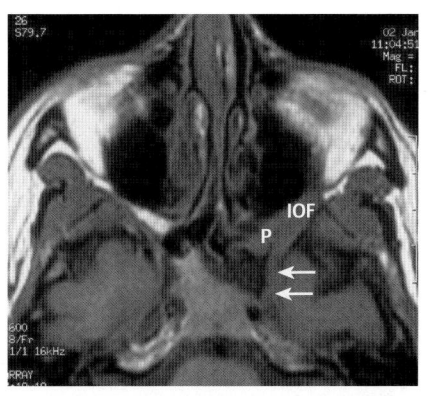

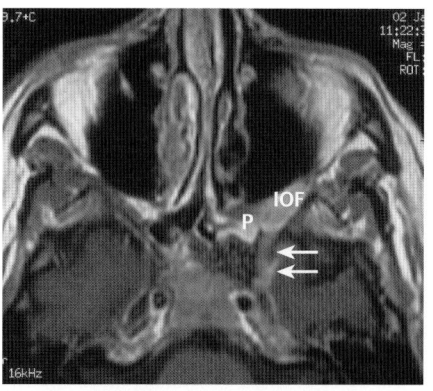

Fig. 3.54 Perineural extension of adenoid cystic carcinoma of the hard palate. a Unenhanced axial T1W MR scan shows tumor in the left pterygopalatine fossa (P), extending along the maxillary nerve in the foramen rotundum (arrows) and inferior orbital fissure (IOF). b Gd-enhanced axial T1W MR scan shows tumor enhancement in the same regions as in a.

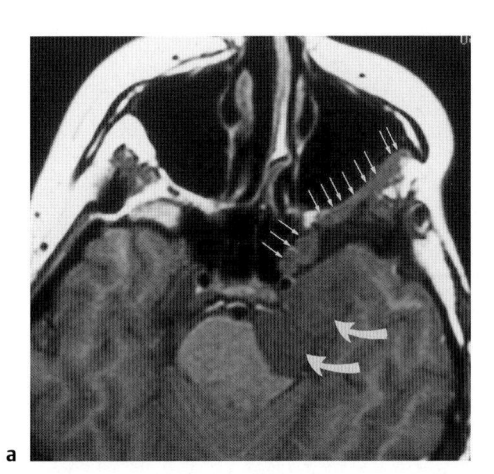

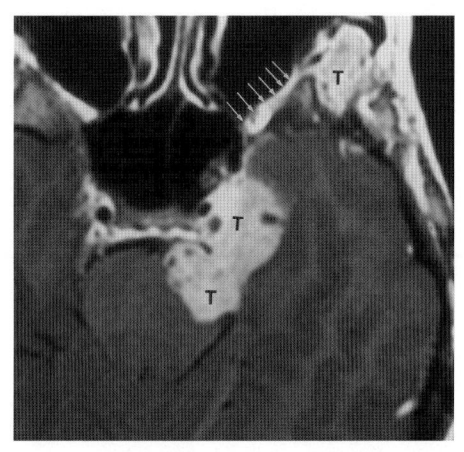

Fig. 3.55 Perineural extension of adenoid cystic carcinoma of the left parotid, years following total parotidectomy. a Unenhanced axial T1W MR scan shows tumor along the left infratemporal fossa, inferior orbital fissure, and pterygopalatine fossa (small arrows). Note tumor along the fifth cranal nerve (large curved arrows). b Gd-enhanced T1W MR scan shows marked enhancement of tumor (T) in the left temporal fossa, along the inferior orbital fissure (arrows) and along the fifth cranial nerve.

of adenoid cystic carcinoma or other tumors (Figs. 3.54, 3.55), and metastatic retropharyngeal and skull base nodal or soft-tissue deposits as well as bony metastases. These lesions will be described in more detail in other sections of this chapter. Intracranial tumors that commonly involve the skull base are invasive pituitary adenoma and meningioma and neurogenic tumors.

Invasive Pituitary Adenomas

The pituitary gland, a combined epithelial and neuroectodermal gland, lies in the sella turcica of the sphenoid bone. The gland is composed of a glandular anterior lobe, the adenohypophysis, and a neural posterior lobe, the neurohypophysis.[21] The most common primary neoplasm of the pituitary gland is pituitary adenoma.[21] The incidence of pituitary adenomas approaches 10% of intracranial neoplasms.[21] This high incidence is related to the more ready detection of microadenomas by improved radioimmunoassay and imaging techniques.[26] Less than one-half of operated pituitary hormone-secreting pituitary tumors are prolactinoma. In young productive females, many prolactinomas are microadenoma. In males, virtually all are macroadenomas and many are invasive. Some pituitary adenomas, despite histology, will demonstrate invasive characteristics and infiltrate cavernous sinuses, sphenoid sinus, nasopharynx, base of the skull, and adjacent brain parenchyma (Fig. 3.56). Tumor may extend from the nasopharynx into the nasal cavity and present itself clinically as a polyp. Rarely an ectopic pituitary adenoma may be seen in the nasopharynx. Tumor can erode the clivus and extend along dural planes into the petrous apex (Fig. 3.56). Aneurysm of the internal carotid artery may simulate a small or large pituitary tumor (Fig. 3.57).

Meningiomas

Meningiomas constitute between 13% and 18% of all primary intracranial neoplasms. They originate from meningothelial cells of the arachnoid membrane (arachnoidal cap cells), which are most abundant in the arachnoid granulations but are also found in small clusters in intracranial and intraspinal arachnoid membrane, as well as in the choroid plexus, where they give rise to in-

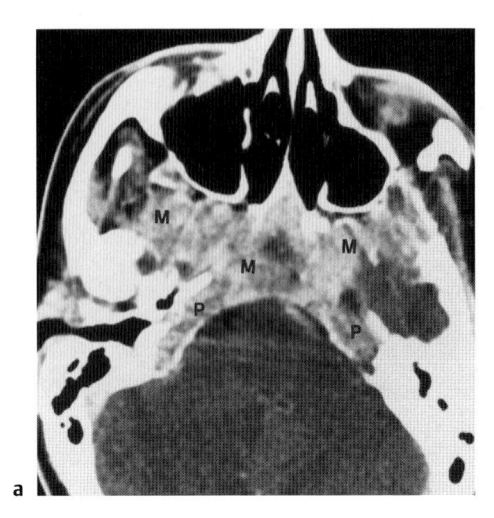

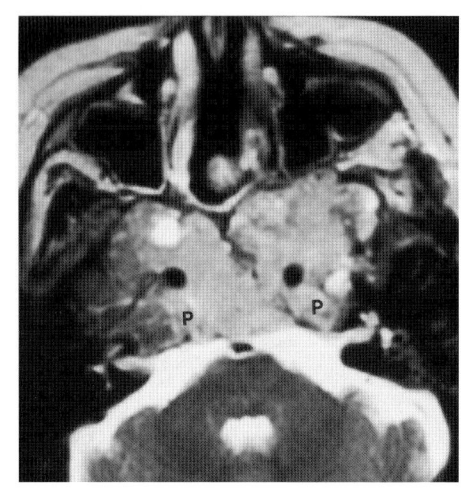

Fig. 3.56 Invasive pituitary adenoma. **a** CT scan shows destructive mass (M) of the base of skull, involving the sphenoid body and its lateral recesses as well as extension into the petrous apices (P), related to an invasive prolactin adenoma. **b** Axial T2W MR scan in another patient with invasive pituitary adenoma, showing a large midline mass, with extension into the cavernous sinuses, lateral recesses of sphenoid sinus, and petrous apices (P).

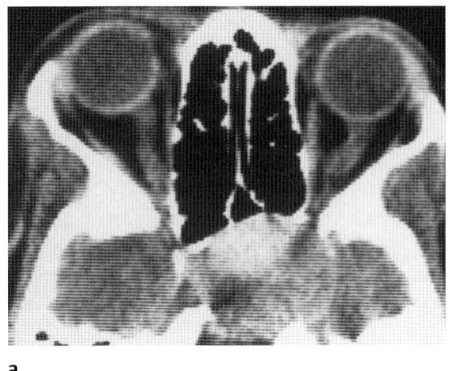

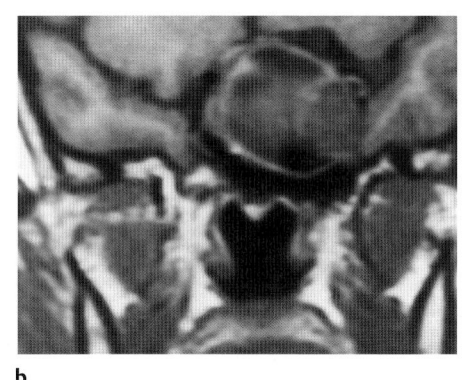

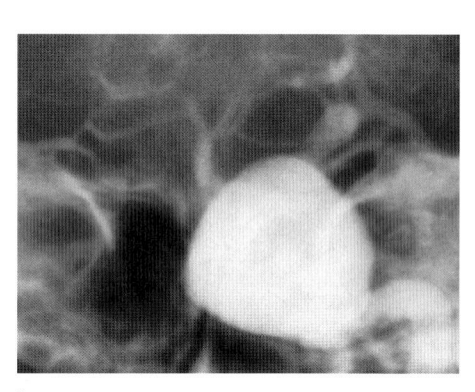

Fig. 3.57 Giant aneurysm of internal carotid artery. **a** Enhanced CT scan, **b** coronal T1W MR scan and **c** angiogram showing a partially thrombosed internal carotid artery aneurysm.

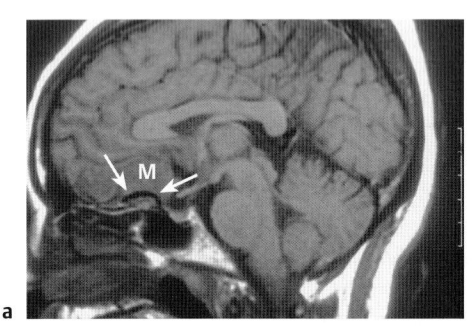

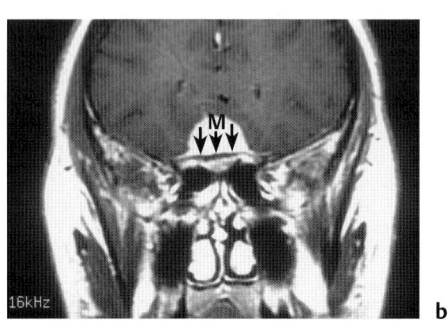

Fig. 3.58 Skull base meningioma. **a** Sagittal T1W and **b** coronal Gd-enhanced T1W MR scans, showing a meningioma (M) in the region of the jugum sphenoidale. Arrows point to hyperostotic changes.

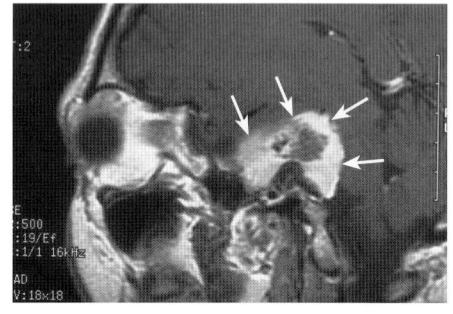

Fig. 3.59 Skull base meningioma. Sagittal Gd-enhanced T1W MR scan, showing a clivus meningioma (arrows) extending into the middle cranial fossa.

traventricular meningiomas.[21] Arachnoidal cap cells have a tendency to form psammoma bodies, features that are common in meningiomas. Meningiomas usually grow as bulky masses (Figs. 3.58–3.61); however, especially at the sphenoid ridge, or less commonly at the superior or posterior surfaces of petrous bone, the neoplasm grows as a flattened plate or sheet and is referred to as en plaque meningioma (Figs. 3.62, 3.63).[27] Intracranial meningiomas can extend into the extracranial space via the natural pathways (skull base foramina and fissures) (Figs. 3.64, 3.65). At times extracranial meningiomas may be seen within the sinonasal cavity (Figs. 3.64, 3.65) or tympanic cavity (Fig. 3.66) and jugular fossa (Fig. 3.67), arising from ectopic arachnoid tissue (Figs. 3.66, 3.67). We have seen primary meningioma arising from the inferior nasal turbinate, clinically simulating a papilloma. The lesion was removed but recurred at the same site, which required further surgery. Meningiomas have slight to moderately high attenuation values on CT scans. This is related to psammomatous calcification as well as dense connective tissue.[21] The majority of meningiomas show homogeneous enhancement on enhanced CT scans (Fig. 3.68).[21] On T1-weighted MR images, most meningiomas are isointense to brain (Fig. 3.58); less commonly they are hypointense. They become isointense

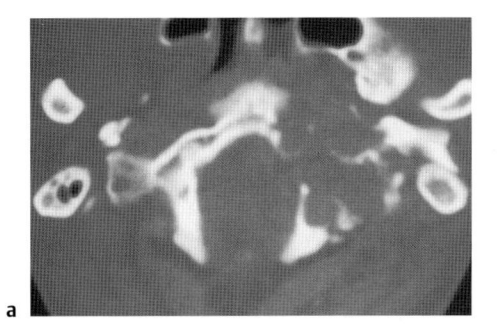

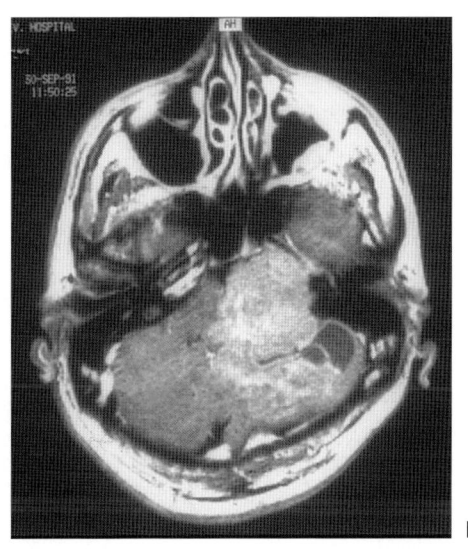

Fig. 3.**60** Meningioma. **a** Axial CT scan shows erosion of the lateral mass of the occipital bone on the left side. **b** Gd-enhanced T1W MR scan shows large meningioma involving the left CPA region. Case courtesy of Dr. Y. Inoui, Osaka, Japan.

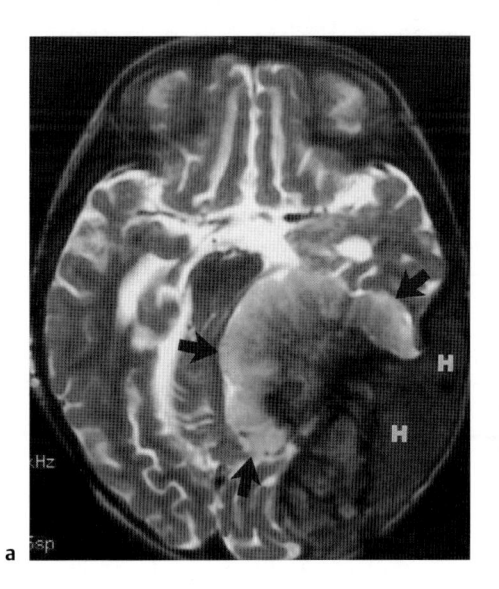

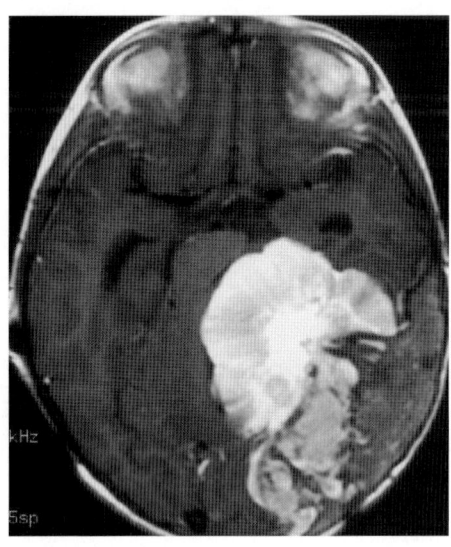

Fig. 3.**61** Meningioma. **a** Axial T2W MR scans in this 6-year-old girl show marked hyperostotic changes (H) and a large meningioma (arrows). **b** Gd-enhanced T1W MR scan shows marked tumor enhancement.

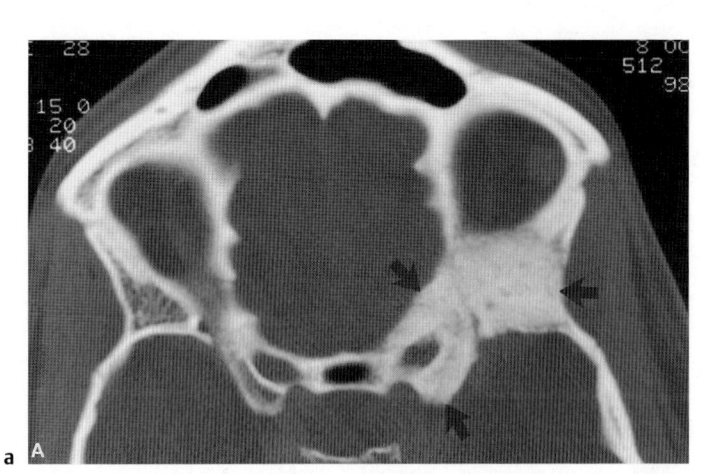

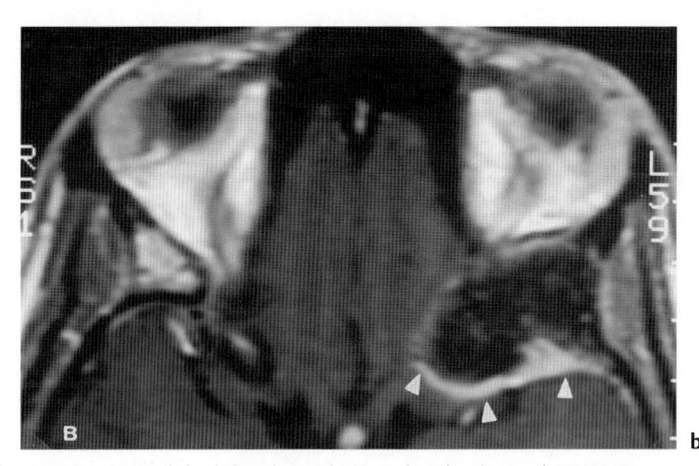

Fig. 3.**62** En plaque meningioma. **a** CT scan shows marked hyperostotic changes (arrows) of the left sphenoid wings. **b** Gd-enhanced T1W MR scan shows a rim of enhancement (arrowheads) compatible with an en plaque meningioma.

322   3 Base of the Skull

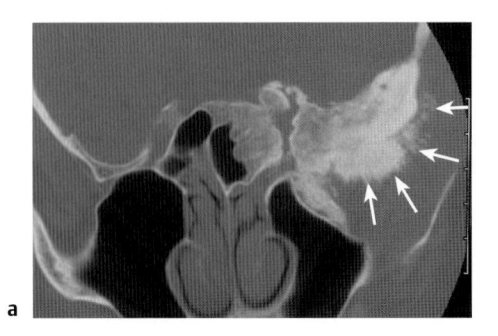

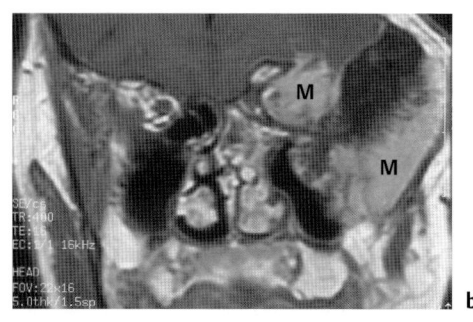

Fig. 3.63 Aggressive meningioma. **a** Coronal CT scan shows marked hyperostotic changes of the left sphenoid bone. Note irregular spicules of calcification, mimicking tumor bone formation of osteogenic sarcoma. **b** Coronal Gd-enhanced T1W MR scan shows enhancement of the meningioma (M) involving the intracranial as well as extracranial structures.

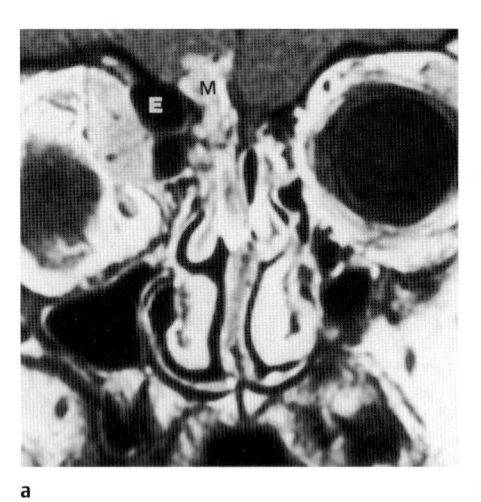

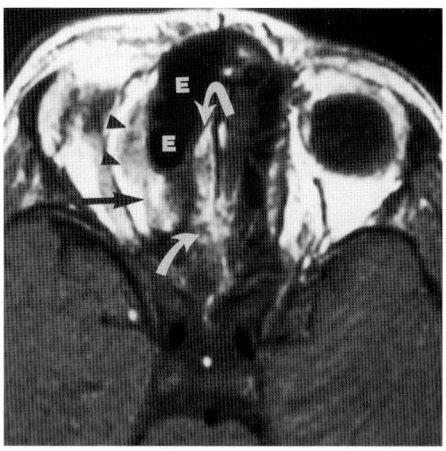

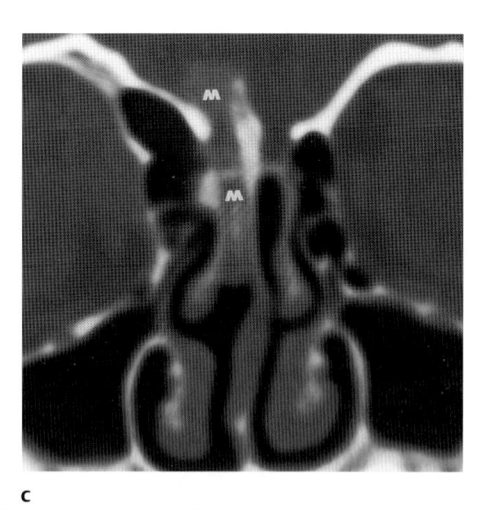

Fig. 3.64 Meningioma. Ten-year-old boy with neurofibromatosis. **a** Gd-enhanced coronal MR scan shows an antrior cranial fossa meningioma (M). Note expansion of the adjacent ethmoid air cell (E). **b** Gd-enhanced axial MR scan shows anterior cranial fossa meningioma (arrows). Note tumor extension into the right orbit (arrowheads) and expansion of adjacent ethmoid air cells (E). **c** Coronal CT scan shows meningioma (M) in the anterior cranial fossa and superior nasal cavity. Case courtesy of Dr. E.L. Tajudine, Saudi Arabia.

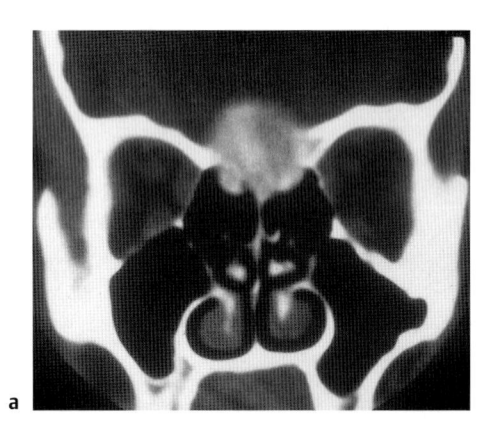

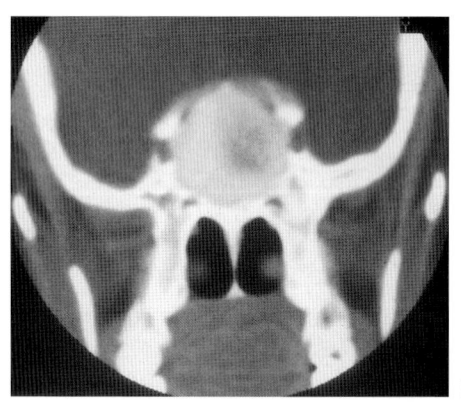

Fig. 3.65 Meningioma. **a** and **b** CT scans, showing a hyperdense mass on the floor of the anterior cranial fossa and within the sphenoid sinus, compatible with a meningioma.

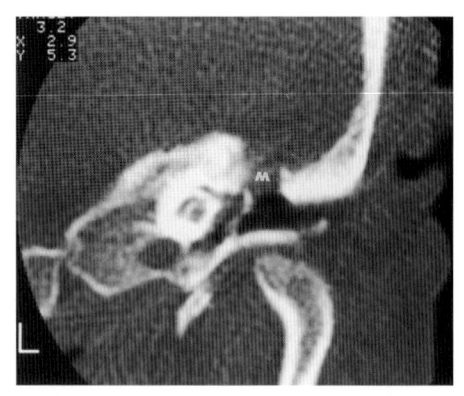

Fig. 3.66 Intratympanic meningioma. Coronal CT scan shows a mass (M) in the attic, simulating an attic cholesteatoma. Note absent tegmen. This meningioma could have been developed either from ectopic arachnoid tissue in the attic or from herniated brain into the attic.

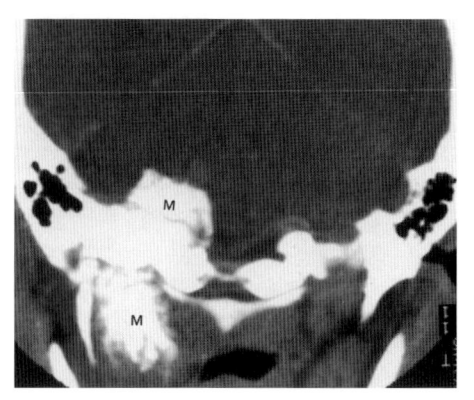

Fig. 3.67 Calcified meningioma. Coronal CT scan shows a large meningioma (M) with marked calcification in the base of the posterior cranial fossa, associated with marked extracranial extension into the right parapharyngeal space.

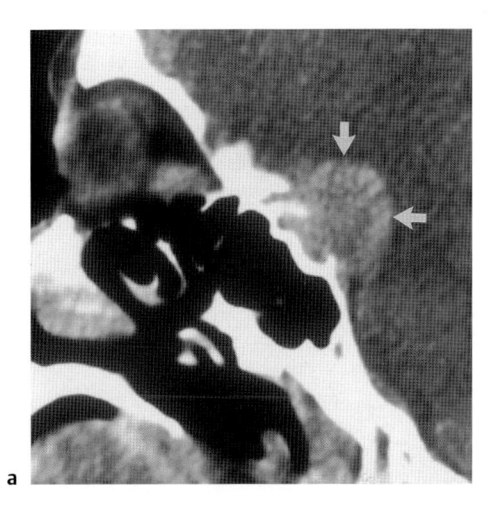

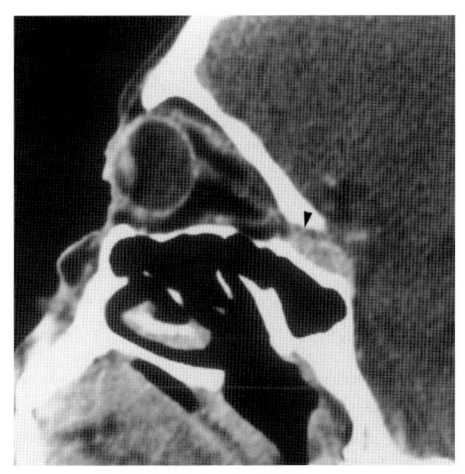

Fig. 3.**68** Meningioma. Enhanced parasagittal CT scan shows a parasellar meningioma (arrows). **b** CT scan, taken slightly medial to **a**, shows extension of parasellar meningioma into the optic canal (arrowhead).

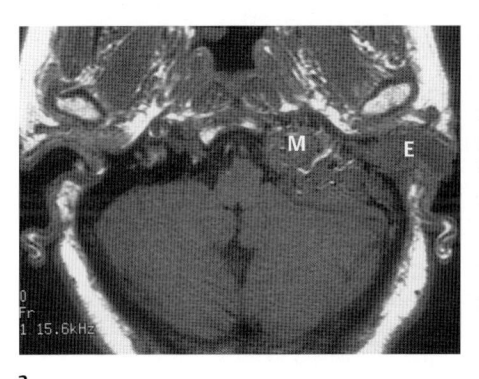

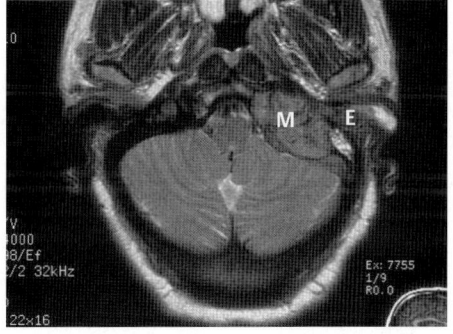

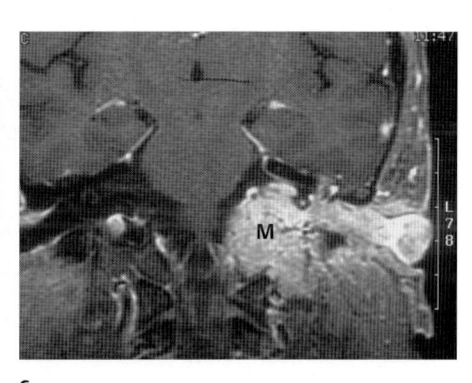

Fig. 3.**69** Glomus jugulare. **a** Axial T1W and **b** T2W MR scans, showing a mass (M), involving the left petrous bone, with extension into the external auditory canal (E). **c** Coronal fat-suppression Gd-enhanced T1W MR scan shows marked enhancement of the mass (M), involving the petrous bone with extension into the middle ear and external canal.

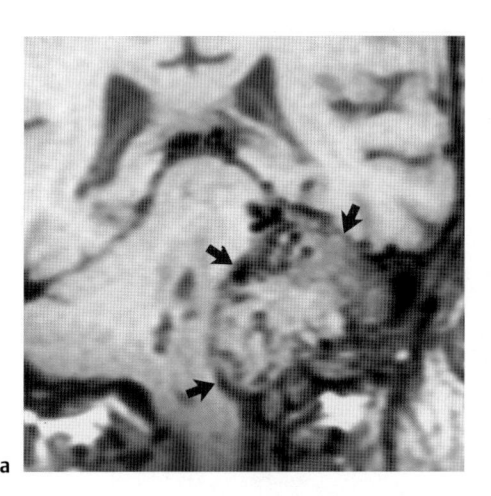

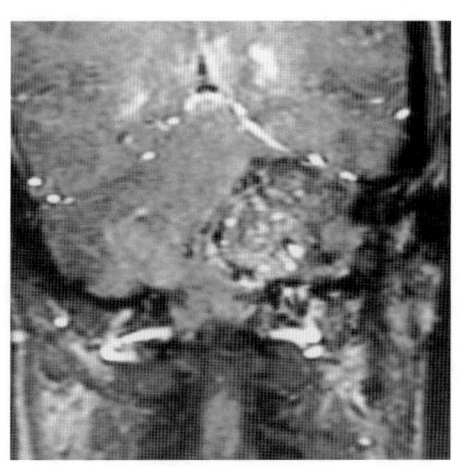

Fig. 3.**70** Glomus jugulare. **a** Coronal T1W and **b** gradient-echo (GRE/60°, 24/14, TR/TE) MR scans showing a large hypervascular CPA mass, related to extension of a glomus jugulare (arrows).

(50%) or hyperintense (40%) on T2-weighted MR images (Fig. 3.**61**).[21] They frequently show intense and homogeneous enhancement with gadolinium-DTPA contrast (Figs. 3.**58**–3.**61**).[21] Enhancement of thickened adjacent dura, the so-called dural tail, is commonly seen in meningiomas.

Paragangliomas, Schwannomas, and Neurofibromas of Skull Base

Paragangliomas, schwannomas, and neurofibromas of the head and neck have been reviewed in the chapters on the temporal bone (Chapter 1) and parapharyngeal spaces (Chapter 8). These lesions can involve the base of the skull.[28, 29] Paragangliomas, or glomus tumors, often involve the skull base, arising within the jugular fossa (glomus jugulare); tympanic cavity (glomus tympanicum), inferior nodosum of the vagus nerve (glomus vagale), or, rarely, along the facial nerve (glomus faciale).[28, 29] Paragangliomas are hypervascular and locally more invasive than schwannomas. On MRI, signal voids are often seen within these lesions, reflecting their hypervascularity (Figs. 3.**69**, 3.**70**). There will be intense enhancement on enhanced CT and MRI scans (Figs. 3.**71**, 3.**72**).[28, 29] On rare occasions, chemodectoma may arise in the sellar/parasellar region (Fig. 3.**73**). Schwannomas have long T1 and T2 characteristics. Large schwannomas often

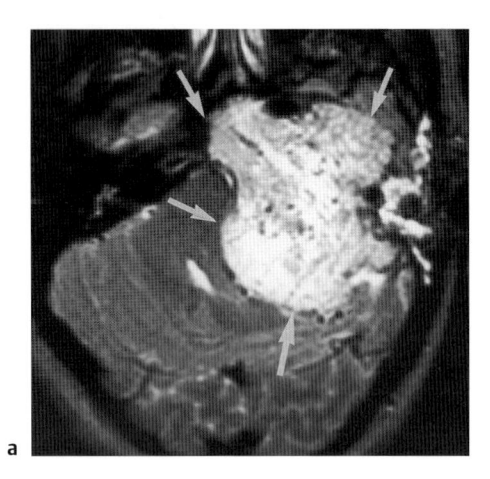

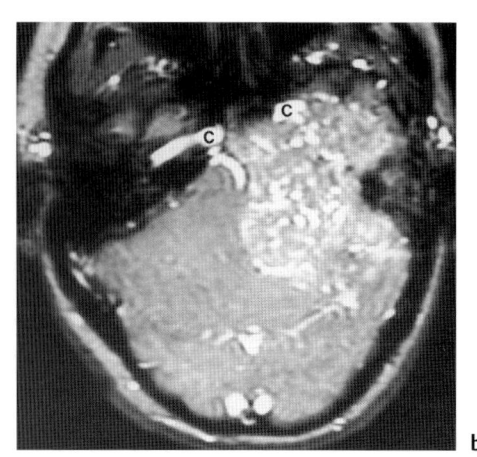

Fig. 3.71 Glomus jugulare. **a** Gd-enhanced MR scan shows an extensive tumor with marked contrast enhancement involving the posterior and middle cranial fossa (arrows). **b** Gradient-echo (GRE/60°, 24/14, TR/TE) MR scan shows marked vascularity of this mass. C = internal carotid artery.

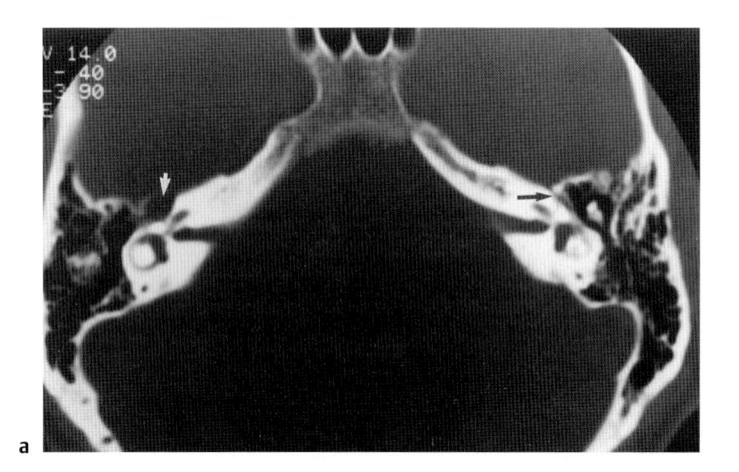

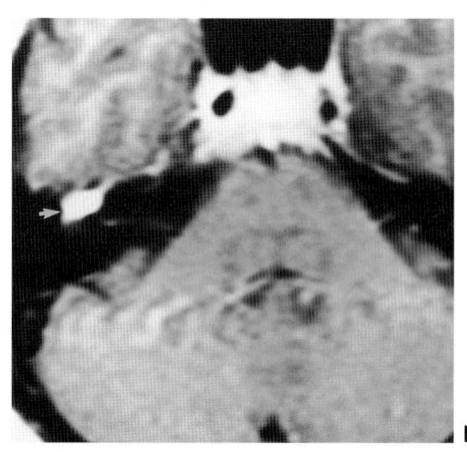

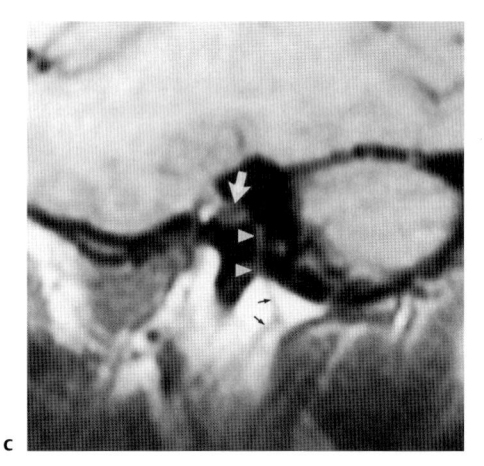

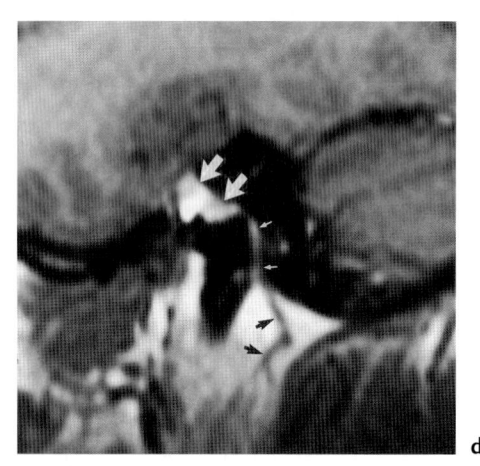

Fig. 3.72 Glomus faciale. **a** CT scan shows expansion as well as erosion of the geniculate portion of the right facial canal (white arrow). Note normal left facial canal (black arrow). **b** Gd-enhanced T1W MR scan shows a mass (arrow) with marked enhancement at the geniculate portion of the right facial nerve. **c** Sagittal unenhanced T1W MR scan shows a mass at the geniculate portion of the facial nerve (large arrow) and normal mastoid and parotid segments of the facial nerve (arrowheads and small arrows). **d** Sagittal Gd-enhanced T1W MR scan shows marked enhancement of glomus faciale (large arrows). Note normal mastoid segment and parotid segment of facial nerve (small arrows).

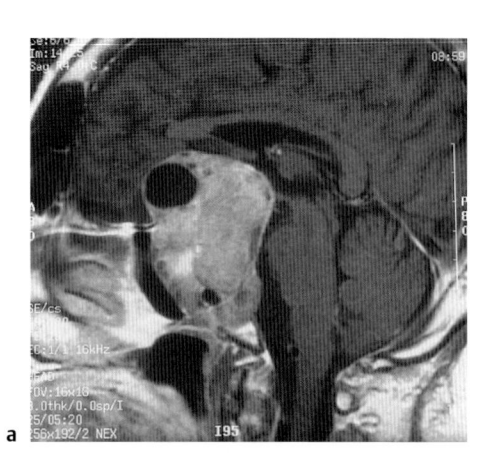

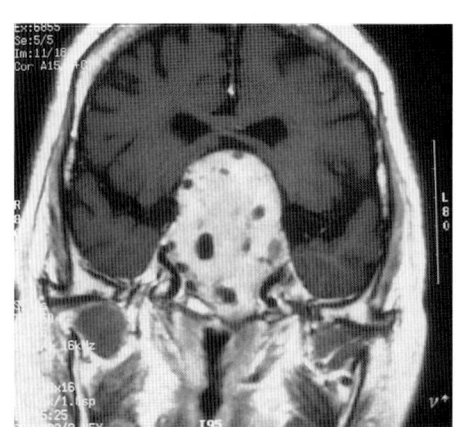

Fig. 3.73 Chemodectoma of the sellar region. **a** Gd-enhanced sagittal and **b** coronal T1W MR images, showing a large sellar mass with marked contrast enhancement. Note marked increased vascularity, as demonstrated by several signal-void images within the tumor.

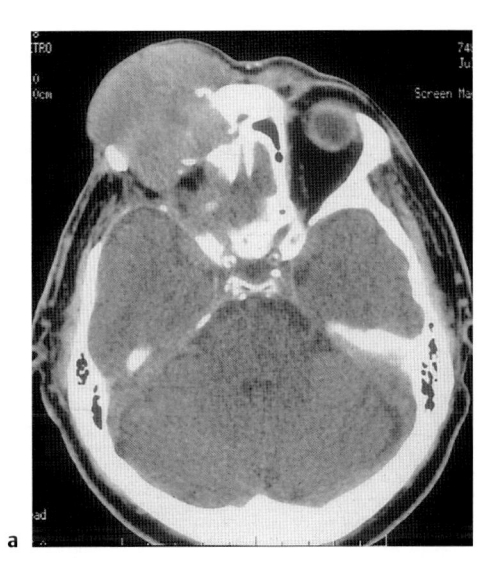

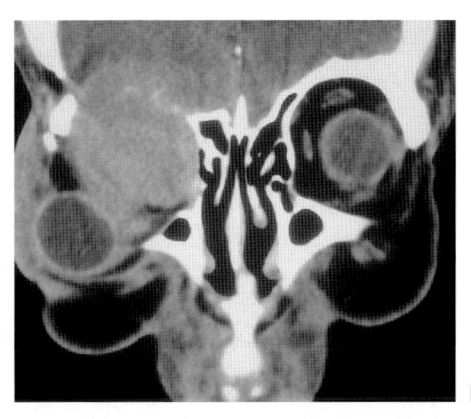

Fig. 3.**74** Neurofibroma of the anterior cranial fossa. **a** Axial and **b** coronal CT scans, showing a large destructive mass involving the roof of the right orbit, compatible with presumed aggressive neurofibroma in this patient with neurofibromatosis type 1. Malignant transformation in this case cannot be excluded on the basis of CT findings.

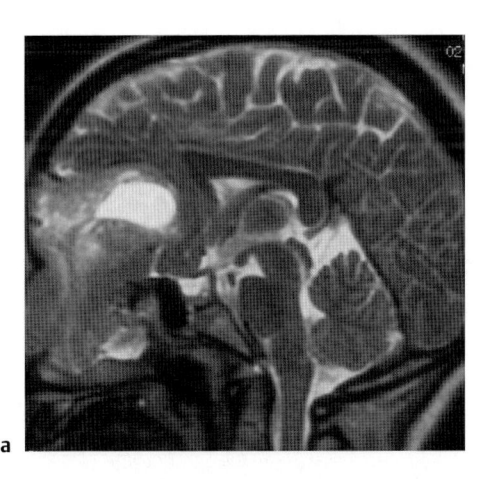

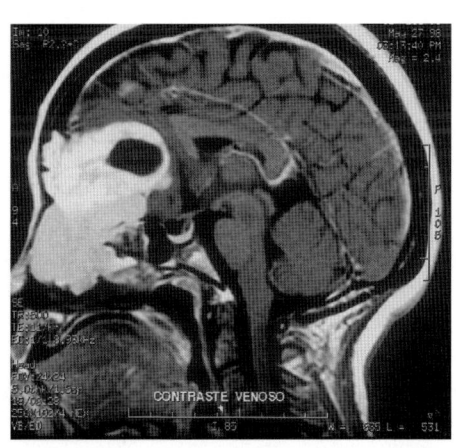

Fig. 3.**75** Neurofibroma of the anterior cranial fossa. **a** Sagittal T2W and **b** Gd-enhanced T1W MR scans, showing a large nasal–ethmoidal mass with extension into the anterior cranial fossa in this patient with type 1 neurofibromatosis. Case courtesy of Heraldo Belmont, MD, Rio de Janeiro, Brazil.

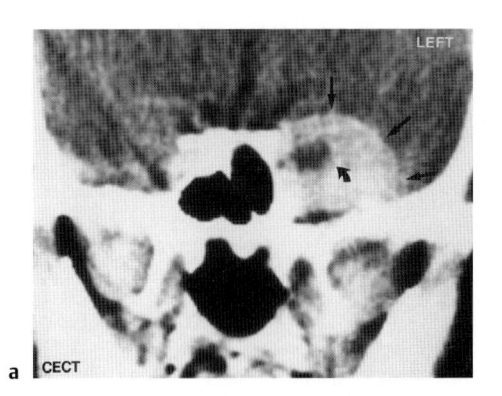

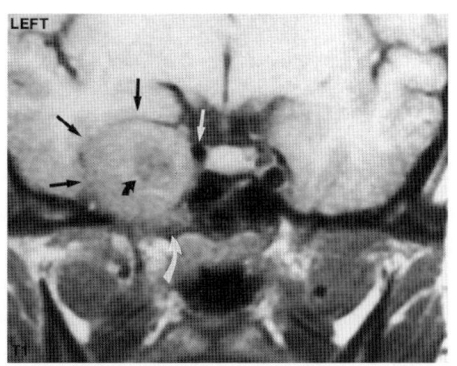

Fig. 3.**76** Isolated neurofibroma of the fifth cranial nerve. **a** Coronal contrast-enhanced CT (CECT) shows a mass arising from the maxillary nerve within the left cavernous sinus (arrows). **b** Coronal T1W MR scan showing the mass (arrows). Note a small cystic component (black curved arrow). Note displacement of the internal carotid artery (white straight arrow) and tumor extension along the foramen rotundum (white curved arrow).

appear heterogeneous, associated with intense enhancement in one part and no enhancement in another portion of tumor (Figs. 3.**74**–3.**83**). Schwannomas and neurofibromas result in smooth expansion of the jugular fossa and foramina and fissures of the base of skull (Figs. 3.**80**–3.**82**). Aggressive patterns of bone destruction and invasion of adjacent tissues should raise the question of malignant schwannoma and neurofibrosarcoma. A rare case of pigmented schwannoma of the jugular fossa is presented in Figure 3.**84**. The differential diagnosis of tumors of the jugular fossa is outlined in Table 3.**6**.

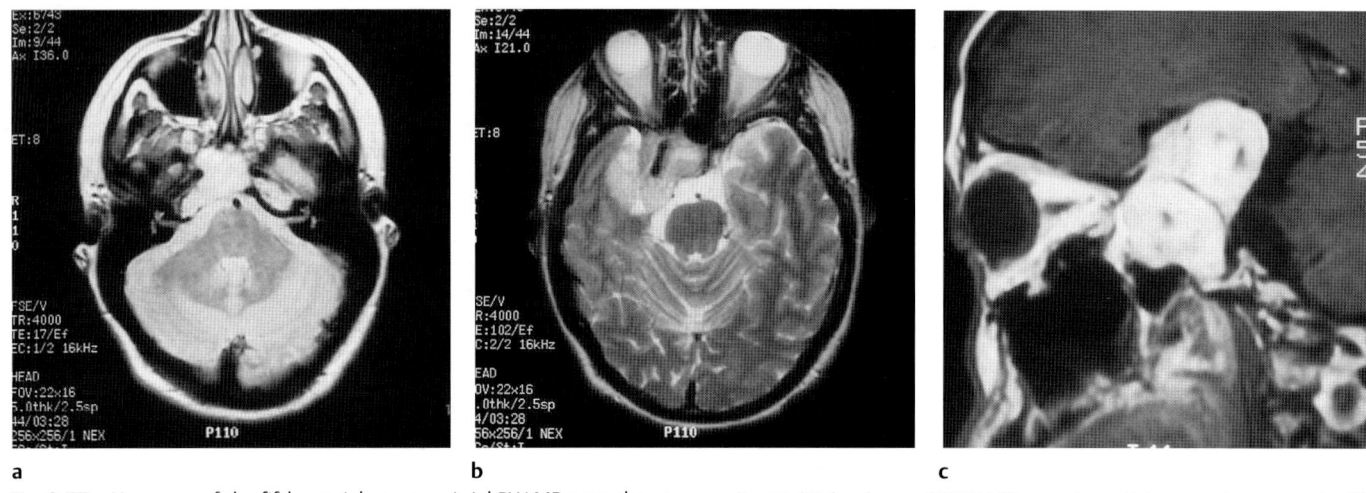

Fig. 3.77 Neuroma of the fifth cranial nerve. **a** Axial PW MR scan shows a mass adjacent to the right petrous apex, extending into the cavernous sinus. **b** Axial T2W MR scan shows a mass in the right cavernous sinus. **c** Sagittal Gd-enhanced T1W MR scan shows intense enhancement of the mass with large parasellar and base of the skull extension.

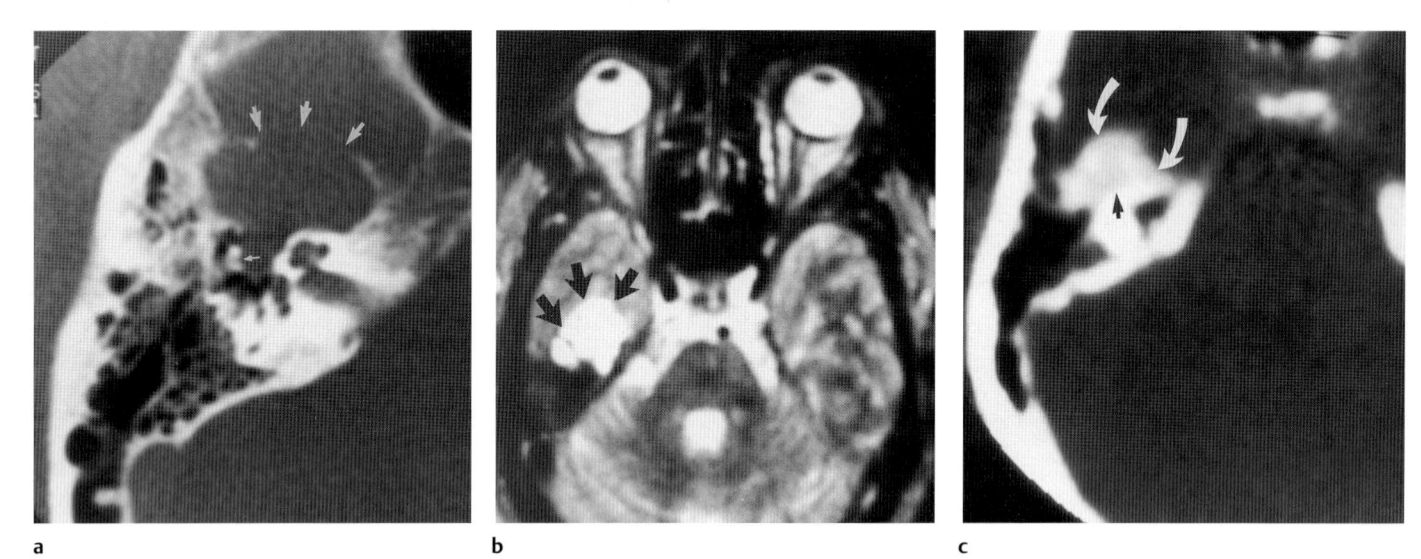

Fig. 3.78 Facial neuroma. **a** Axial CT scan shows marked expansion of the geniculate portion of the facial canal (arrows). Note tumor adjacent to the middle ear ossicles (small arrow). **b** T2W MR scan shows hyperintense facial neuroma (arrows). **c** Axial CT scan of a patient with calcified "sclerosing hemangioma" of the facial nerve for comparison.

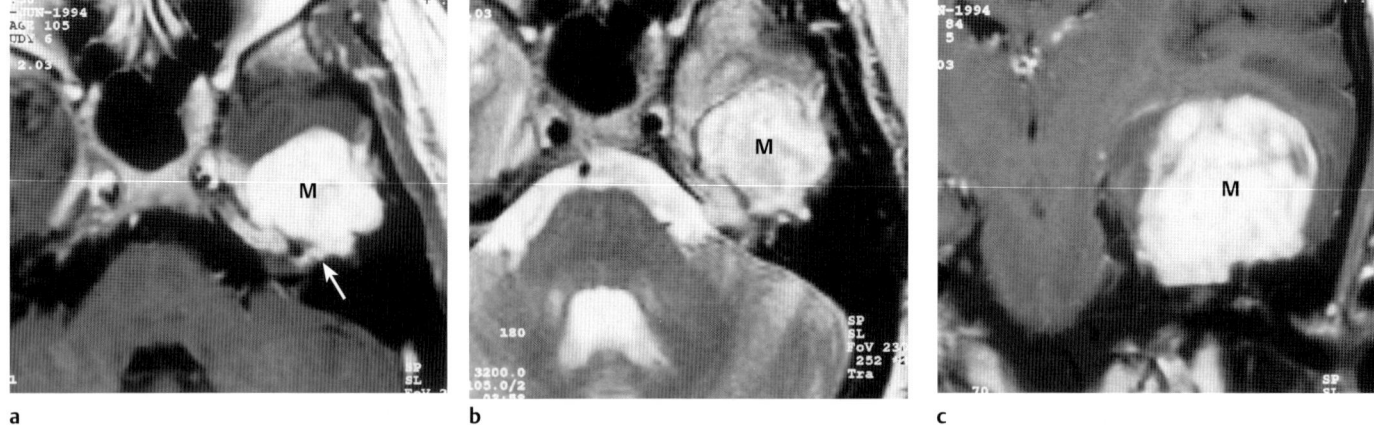

Fig. 3.79 Facial neuroma. **a** Gd-enhanced T1W MR scan shows a large enhancing mass (M) with tumor extending along the facial nerve (arrow). **b** Axial T2W MR scan shows hyperintense facial neuroma (M). **c** Gd-enhanced coronal T1W MR scan showing enhanced facial neuroma. This tumor is thought to have arisen from the greater superficial petrosal nerve. Case courtesy of Richard Hewlett, MD, University of Stellenbosch, South Africa.

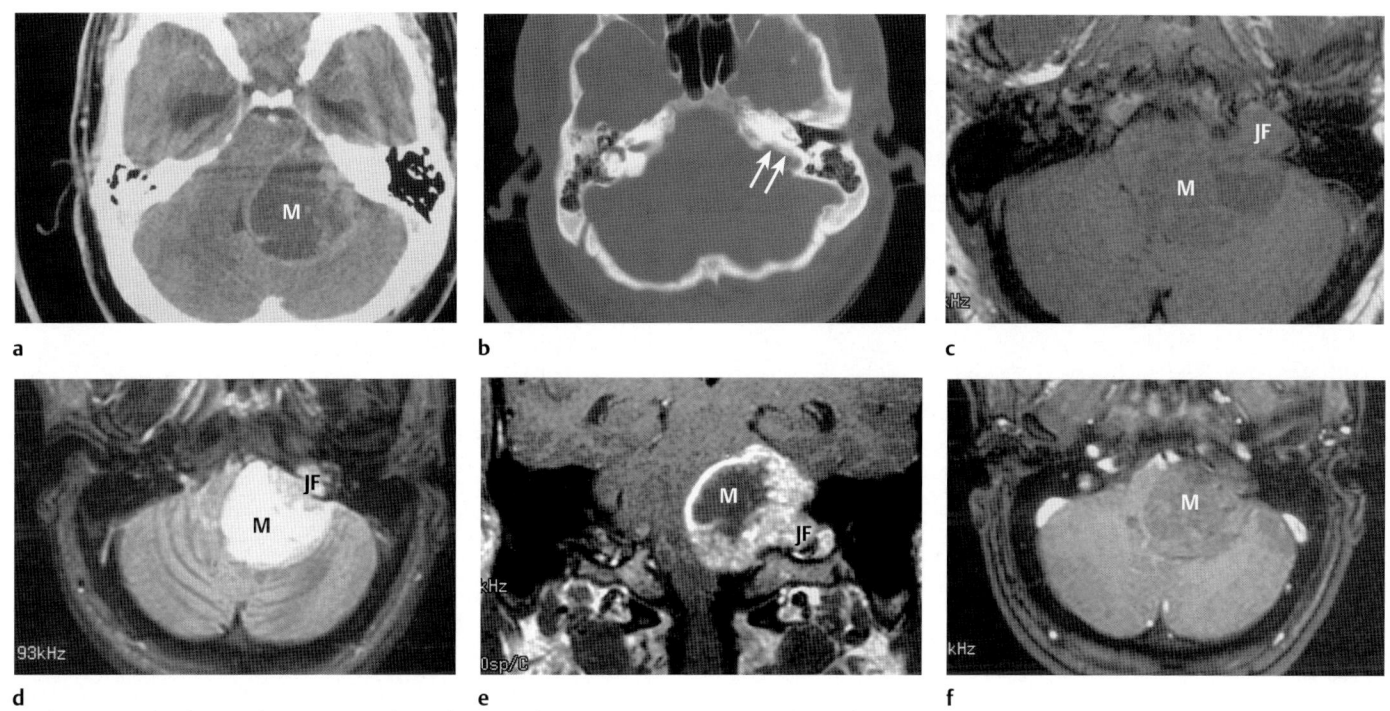

Fig. 3.**80** Jugular fossa schwannoma (glossopharyngeal nerve). **a** Enhanced CT scan shows a partially enhancing left CPA mass (M). **b** CT scan shows erosion of jugular fossa (arrows). **c** Axial T1W and **d** axial T2W scans show a mass in the jugular fossa (JF), extending into the posterior fossa (M). **e** Gd-enhanced coronal T1W MR scan shows jugular fossa tumor (JF) and its extension (M) into the posterior fossa with compression of the left middle cerebellar peduncle. **f** Gradient-echo (GRE/50, 100/7 ms, TR/TE) shows the mass (M). Note that, unlike chemodectoma, there is no hypervascularity present in this pulse sequences. Compare this with Fig. 3.**71**.

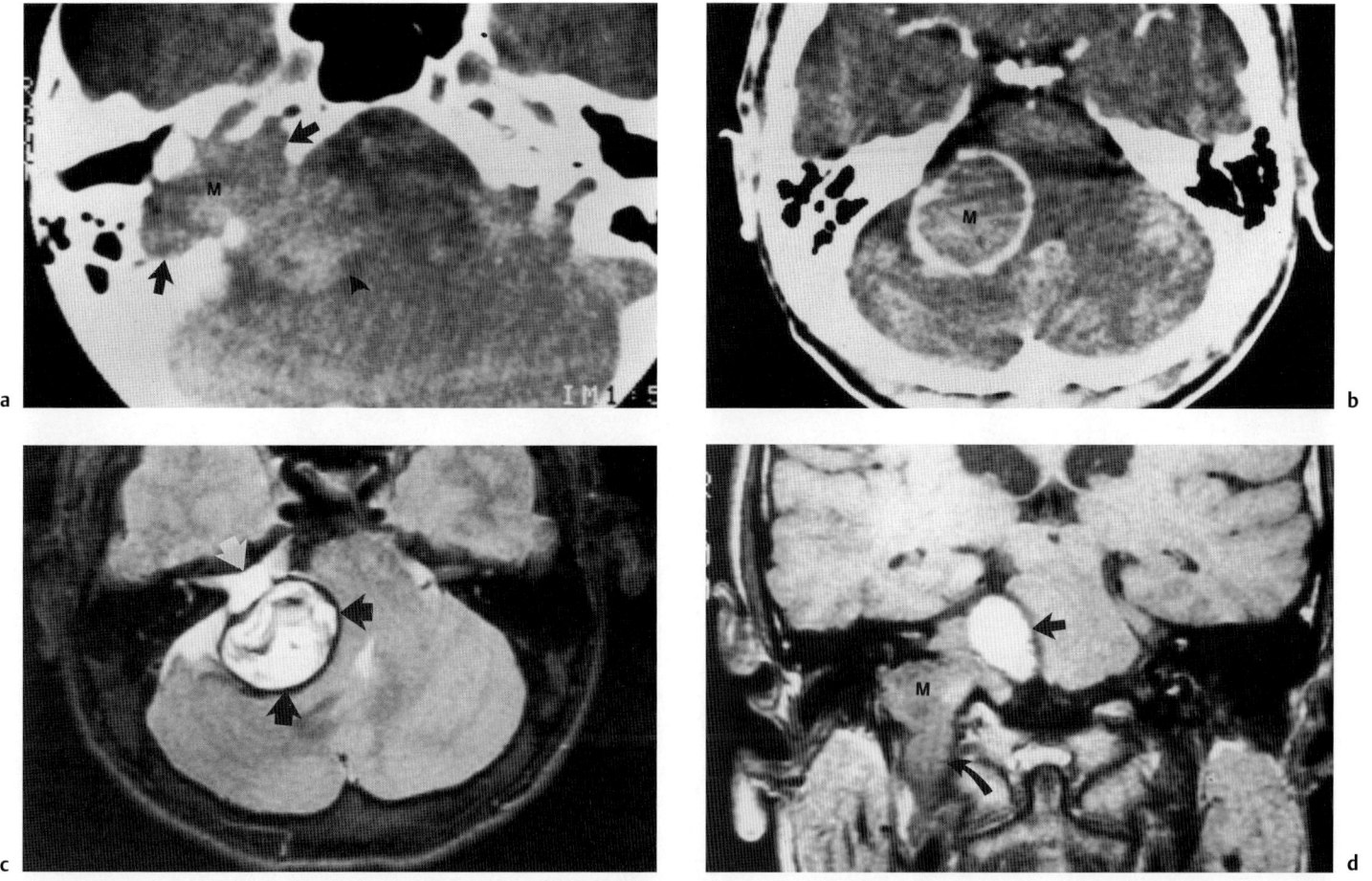

Fig. 3.**81** Schwannoma of the vagus nerve. **a** Enhanced CT scan shows a soft-tissue mass (M) in the enlarged jugular fossa (arrows). Note extension of tumor in the CPA region (arrowhead). **b** Enhanced CT scan shows extension of the tumor (M) in the CPA region with more enhancement along its peripheral portion. **c** T2W MR scan shows extension of this jugular schwannoma in the CPA region (arrows). **d** Coronal unenhanced T1W MR scan shows schwannoma in the jugular fossa (M), extending into the CPA region (straight arrow) and upper neck (curved arrow).

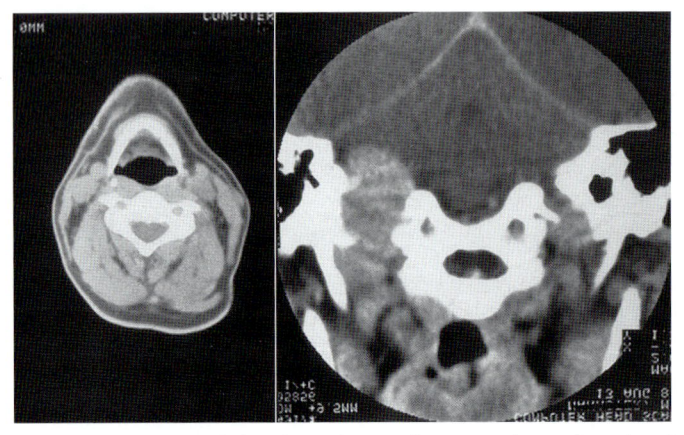

Fig. 3.82 Neuroma of the eleventh cranial nerve. Enhanced axial and coronal CT scans, showing a mass in the right jugular fossa. Note denervation atrophy of the right trapezoid and sternocleidomastoid muscles.

Table 3.6 Differential diagnosis of tumors of the jugular fossa

- Glomus jugulare (most common)
- Extension of glomus tympanicum
- Jugular fossa schwannoma (9, 10, 11) (second most common)
- Extension of facial nerve schwannoma
- Extension of hypoglossal nerve schwannoma
- Meningiomas*
- Extension of endolymphatic sac adenocarcinoma*
- Chondrosarcoma*
- Chordoma*
- Osteosarcoma*
- Chondroblastoma*
- Chondromyxoid tumor*
- Lymphoma
- Plasmacytoma (multiple myeloma)
- Metastases (lung, breast, thyroid, kidney)

* Calcification may be present

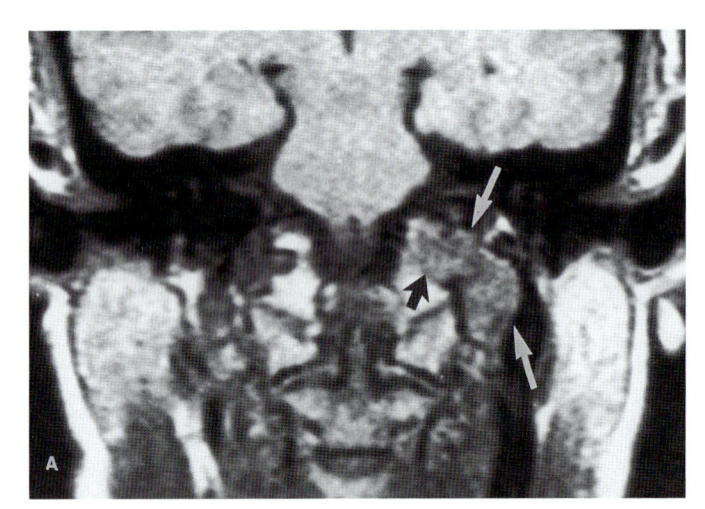

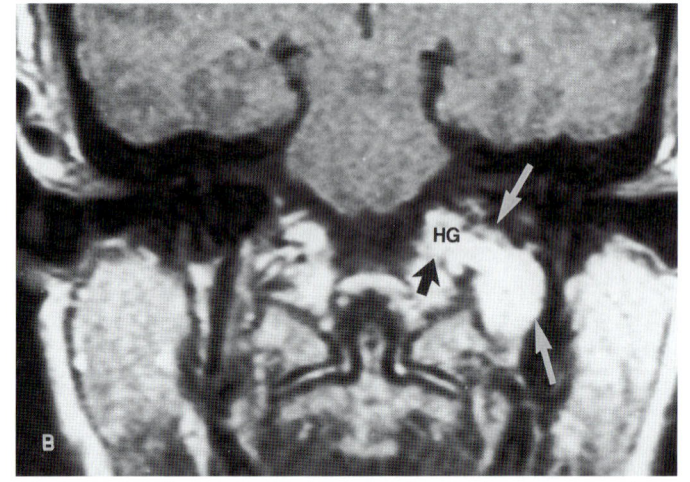

Fig. 3.83 Hypoglossal neuroma. **a** Coronal T1W MR scan shows a mass along the base of skull (arrows). **b** Gd-enhanced coronal T1W MR scan shows marked enhancement of this hypoglossal neuroma within the enlarged hypoglossal canal (HG) and its extension in the upper neck (arrows).

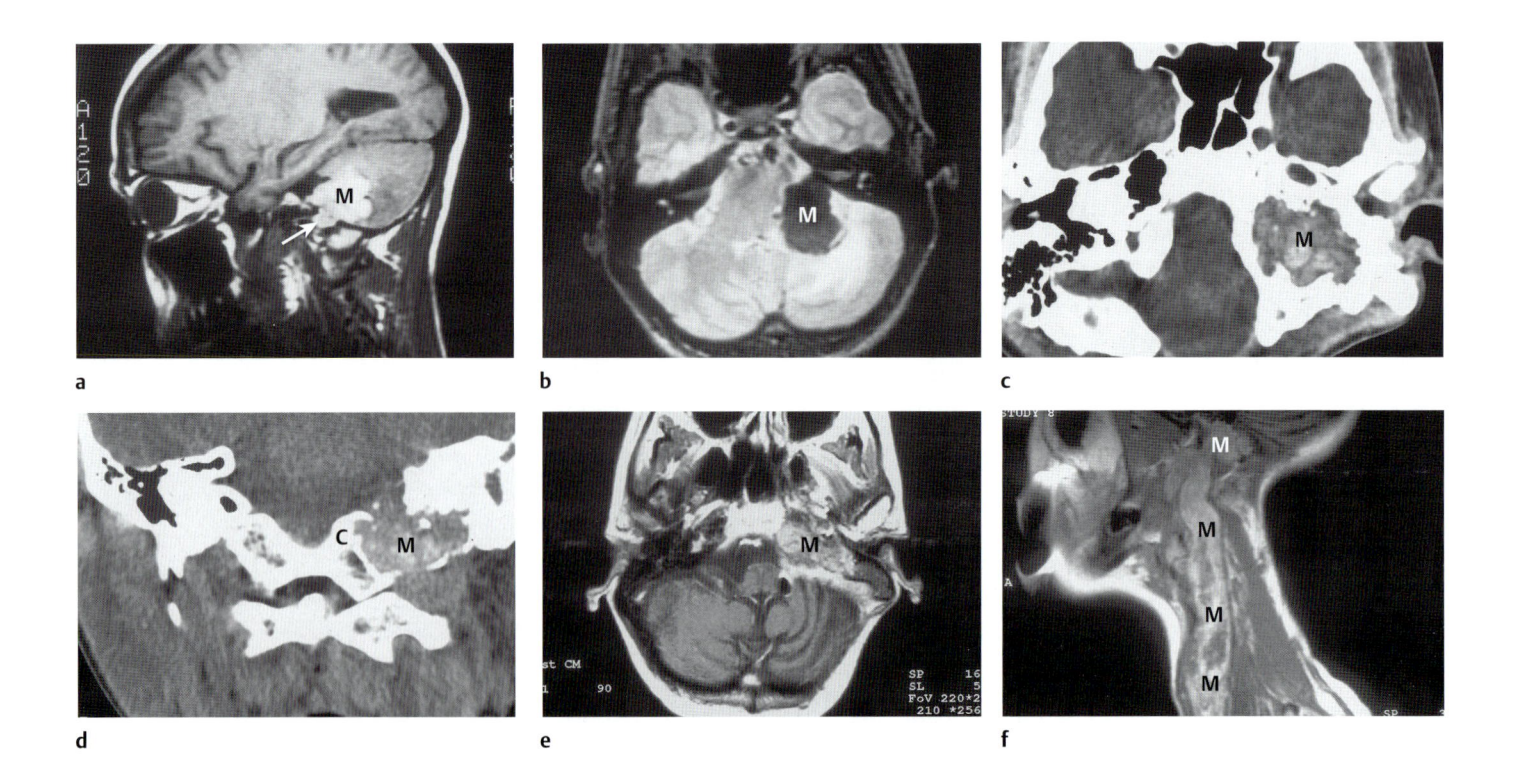

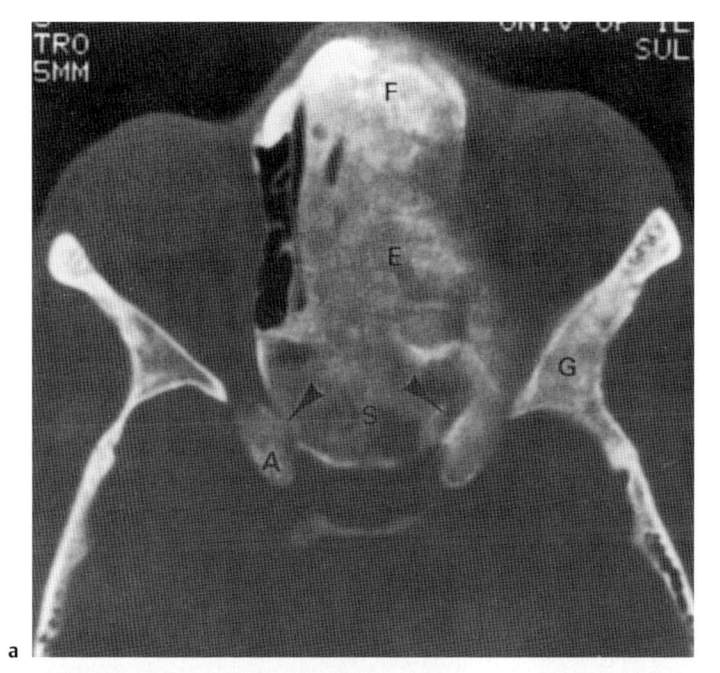

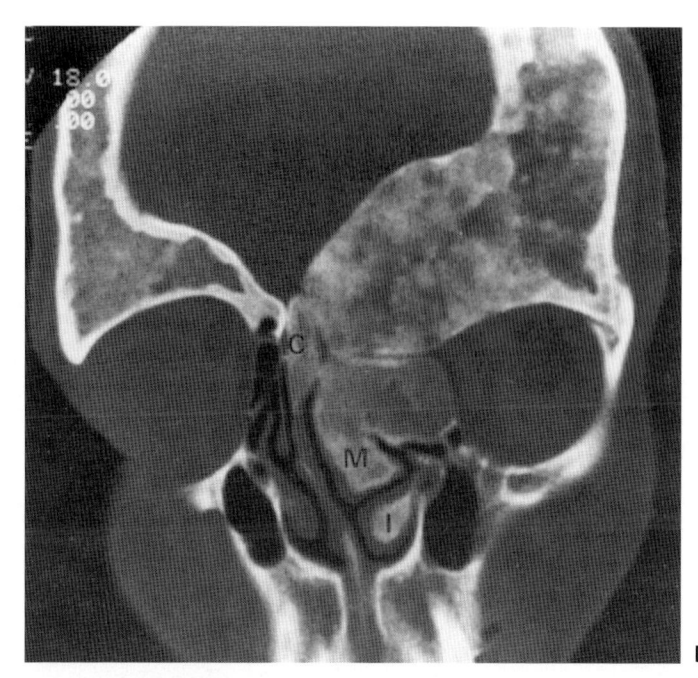

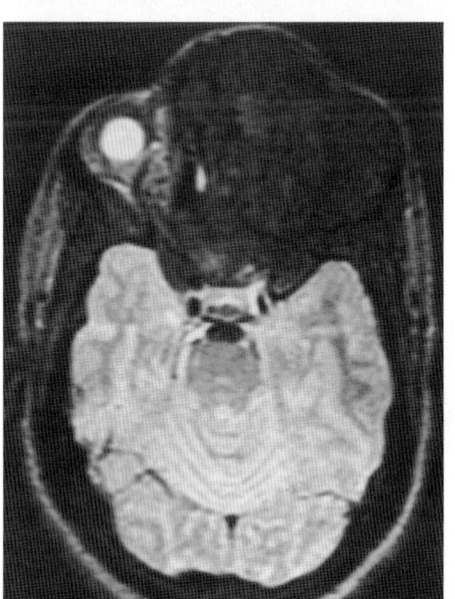

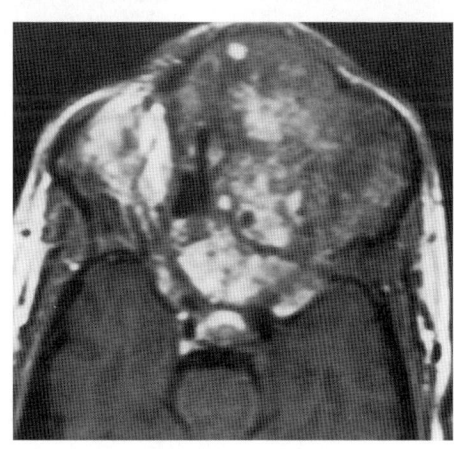

Fig. 3.**85** Fibrous dysplasia.
a Axial CT scan shows characteristic changes indicative of fibrous dysplasia involving the frontal (F), ethmoidal (E), and sphenoidal (S) bones. Note the involvement of the greater wing (G) and anterior clinoid (A) of the sphenoid bones. The optic canals are markedly constricted (arrows).
b Coronal CT scan shows marked involvement of the frontal bone. Note the involvement of crista galli (C), middle concha (M) and inferior concha (I). Involvement of the inferior concha is less common.
c Axial T2W MR scan. Note the hypointensity of the involved bones, seen in **a**.
d Postcontrast axial T1W MR scan. Note the heterogeneous enhancement of the involved bone. On precontrast T1W images (not shown here) the involved areas appeared almost isointense to brain.

◁ Fig. 3.**84** Pigmented schwannoma of the jugular fossa. **a** Unenhanced sagittal T1W MR scan shows a hyperintense mass (M). **b** T2W MR scan shows a hypointense mass (M). The tumor was removed and pathology was considered as primary leptomeningeal melanoma. **c** Unenhanced CT scan, obtained six years following resection of tumor, reveals mass (M) in the enlarged jugular fossa. **d** Unenhanced coronal CT scan shows jugular fossa mass (M) and partial erosion of the occipital condyle (C). **e** Gd-enhanced T1W MR scan shows recurrent tumor in the jugular fossa (M). **f** Gd-enhanced sagittal T1W MR scan shows tumor along the entire course of the jugular vein (M). The tumor was excised and the pathology was considered to be a pigmented schwannoma rather than primary leptomeningeal malignant melanoma.

Fibro-Osseous Lesions of the Skull Base

Fibro-osseous lesions of the skull base include fibrous dysplasia (Figs. 3.**85**, 3.**86**), ossifying fibroma (Fig. 3.**87**), intraosseous hemangioma (Fig. 3.**88**), osteoma, osteoblastoma, osteoclastoma (giant-cell tumor) (Figs. 3.**89**, 3.**90**), chondroblastoma (Figs. 3.**91**, 3.**92**), chondromyxoid tumors (Figs. 3.**93**, 3.**94**), hemangiopericytoma (Fig. 3.**95**), chondroma, chondrosarcoma (Figs. 3.**96**–3.**98**), osteogenic sarcoma (Figs. 3.**99**–3.**100**), chordoma (Figs. 3.**101**–3.**106**), fibrous histiocytoma, and aggressive fibromatosis. Other pathologies that may involve the skull base include rhabdomyosarcoma (Figs. 3.**107**–3.**110**), adenocarcinoma of the temporal bone (Figs. 3.**111**–3.**113**), aggressive fibromatosis (Fig. 3.**114**), lymphoma (Figs. 3.**115**–3.**117**), Langerhans cell histiocytosis (Figs. 3.**118**, 3.**119**), leukemic infiltration (Fig. 3.**120**), and metastasis. Metastatic lesions are most commonly from primary tumors of the lung, breast, prostate, thyroid, and kidney. In children, leukemia, neuroblastoma, Wilms' tumor, and Ewing's tumor are the most common primary sites.

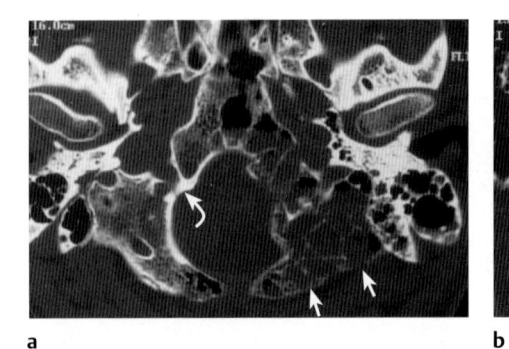

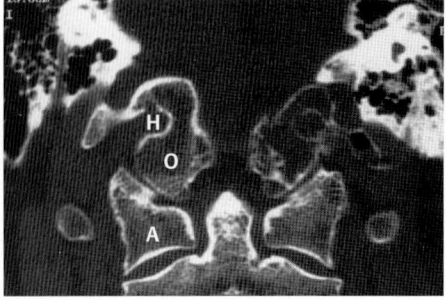

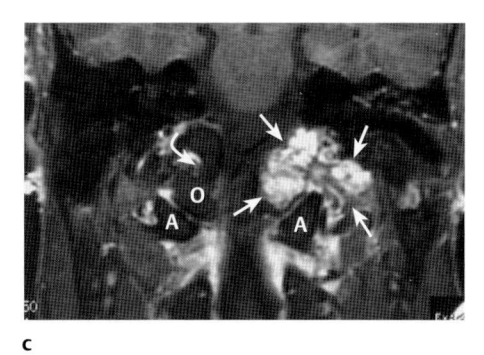

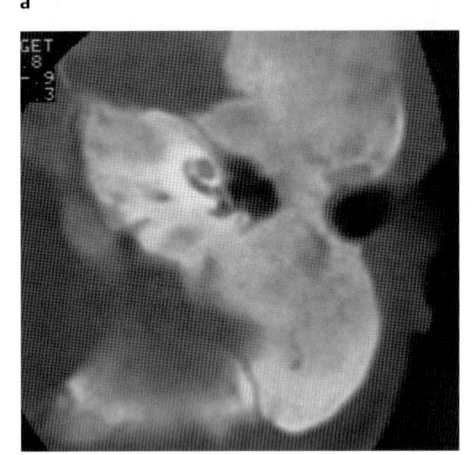

Fig. 3.86 Fibrous dysplasia. **a** CT scan shows expansion of occipital bone on the left side (arrows), related to histologically proven benign fibro-osseous process. Note involvement of the basi-occiput on the left side along with pneumatization of the occipital bone. Note normal right hypoglossal canal (arrow) and irregularity of cortical outline of left hypoglossal canal. **b** Coronal CT scan shows pathological fracture of the left occipital condyle due to involvement by fibro-osseous process and likely related to loss of hard-tissue support of the craniocervical junction. CT scan following treatment, not shown here, revealed complete healing with marked increased bony trabeculae. A = lateral mass of atlas, O = occipital condyle, H = hypoglossal canal. **c** Gd-enhanced coronal fat-suppression T1W MR scan shows marked enhancement of fibro-osseous process involving the left occipital condyle (arrows). A = superior articular facet of atlas; O = occipital condyle; curved arrow = hypoglossal canal. **d** CT scan in another patient shows fibrous dysplasia involving the entire temporal bone except the optic capsule.

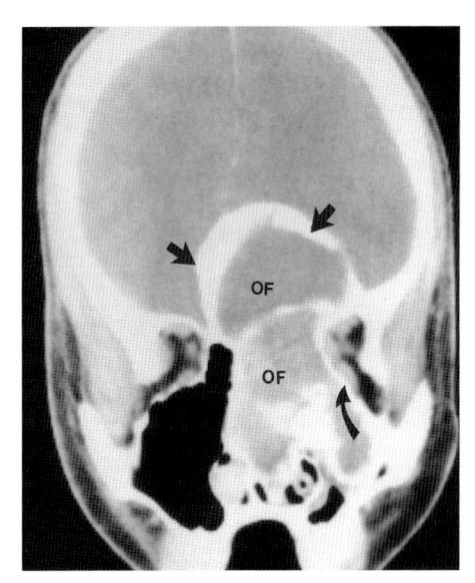

Fig. 3.87 Ossifying fibroma. Coronal CT scan shows a large fibro-osseous lesion compatible with ossifying fibroma (OF). Note thick surrounding rim (arrows). The floor of the left orbit is slightly thickened without evidence for periosteal reaction (curved arrow).

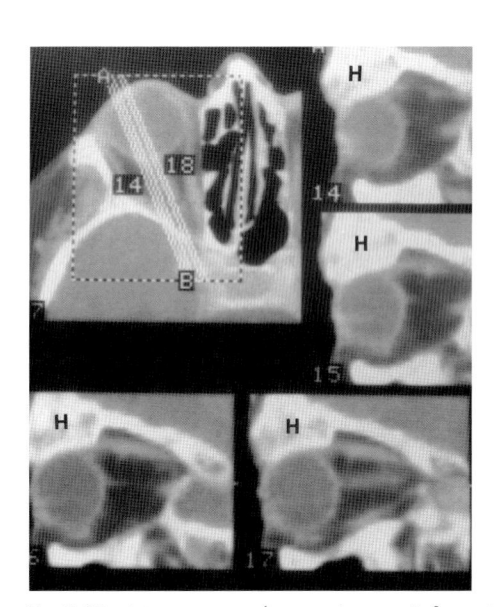

Fig. 3.88 Intraosseous hemangioma. Reformatted parasagittal CT scans, showing an intraosseous hemangioma (H) involving the orbital plate of the frontal bone. Differential diagnoses: osteoblastoma, osteoma, localized fibrous dysplasia, and hemangiopericytoma.

Skull Base Pathology

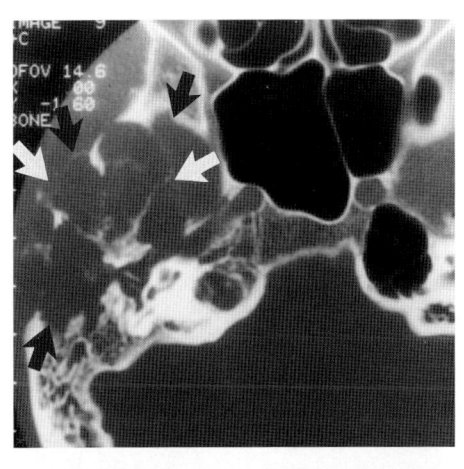

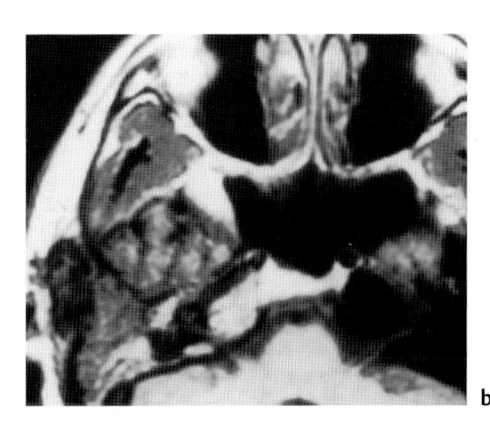

Fig. 3.**89** Giant-cell tumor of the temporal bone. **a** Axial CT scan, **b** T1W, **c** T2W, and **d** Gd-enhanced T1W MRI scans, showing an expansile, bone-destructive mass, involving the squamous temporal bone with extension into the middle ear and anterior portion of the mastoid bone (arrows in Fig 3.**89a**). The mass is heterogeneous in signal (**b**, **c**) and demonstrates marked enhancement (**d**). Differential diagnosis includes chondromyxoid fibroma, chondroblastoma, aggressive fibromatosis, metastasis, etc.

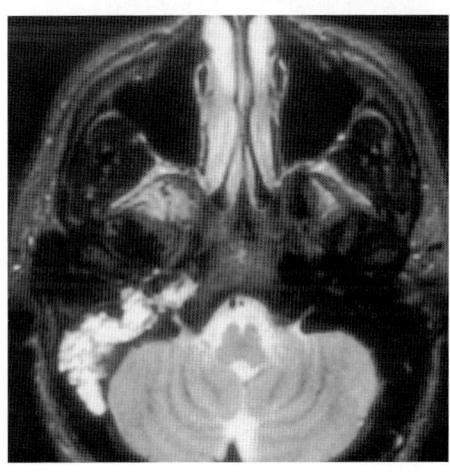

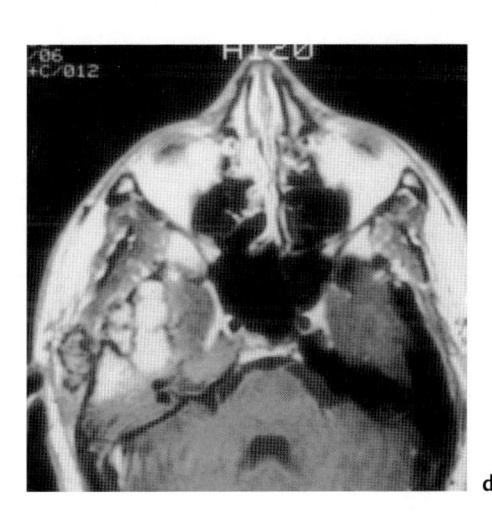

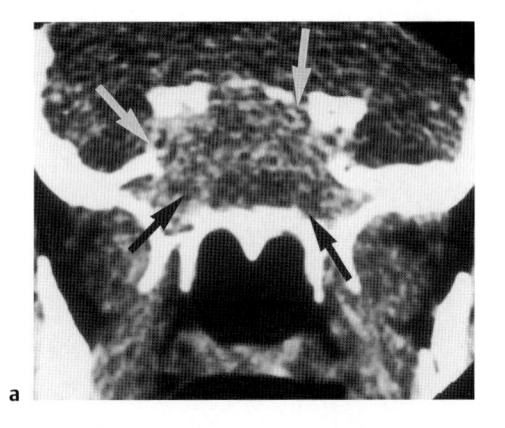

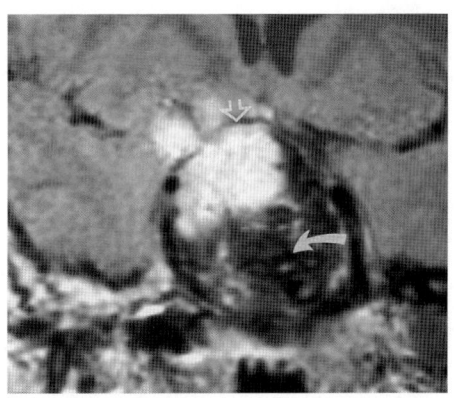

Fig. 3.**90** Recurrent giant-cell tumor of the sphenoid bone. **a** Coronal CT scan shows an expansile mass (arrows) in the sphenoid sinus. Tumor was removed and the site was filled with bone chips. **b** Gd-enhanced coronal T1W MRI scan, obtained a few years later, showing recurrence of the giant-cell tumor (hollow arrow). The bone chips and scar tissue appear hypointense (curved arrow).

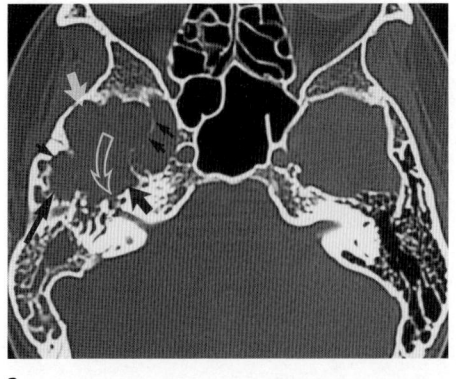

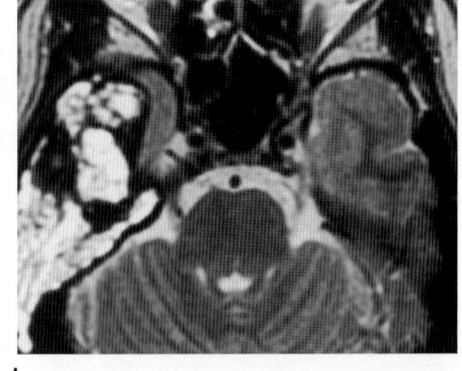

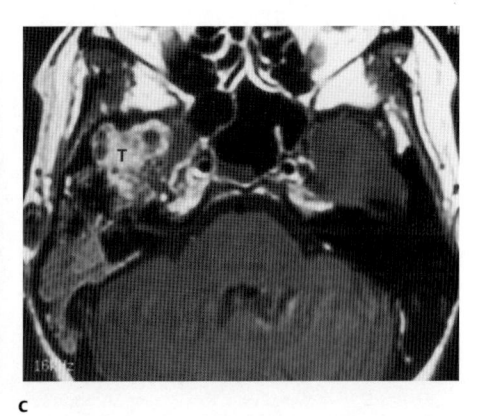

Fig. 3.**91** Chondroblastoma of the squamous temporal bone. **a** CT scan shows an expansile bone-destructive mass (arrows), involving the squamous temporal bone. There is extension into the middle ear with erosion of the cochlear capsule as well (hollow white arrow). **b** T2W MR scan shows that the mass is heterogeneous but primarily hyperintense. Note hyperintensity of inflammatory changes of the mastoid air cells. **c** Gd-enhanced T1W MR scan shows marked enhancement of the tumor (T). Case courtesy Tony Peduto, MD, Westmead, Australia.

Fig. 3.**92** Chondroblastoma of the petrous temporal bone. **a** Axial and **b** coronal CT scans showing a destructive mass involving the petrous apex (arrows). Note increased calcified matrix and invasion of the internal auditory canal. **c** T1W and **d** Gd-enhanced T1W MR scans showing the mass at the petrous apex (arrows) and extension of tumor into the internal auditory canal (arrowheads). Case courtesy Dr. G. Lee, Kansas City, MO, USA.

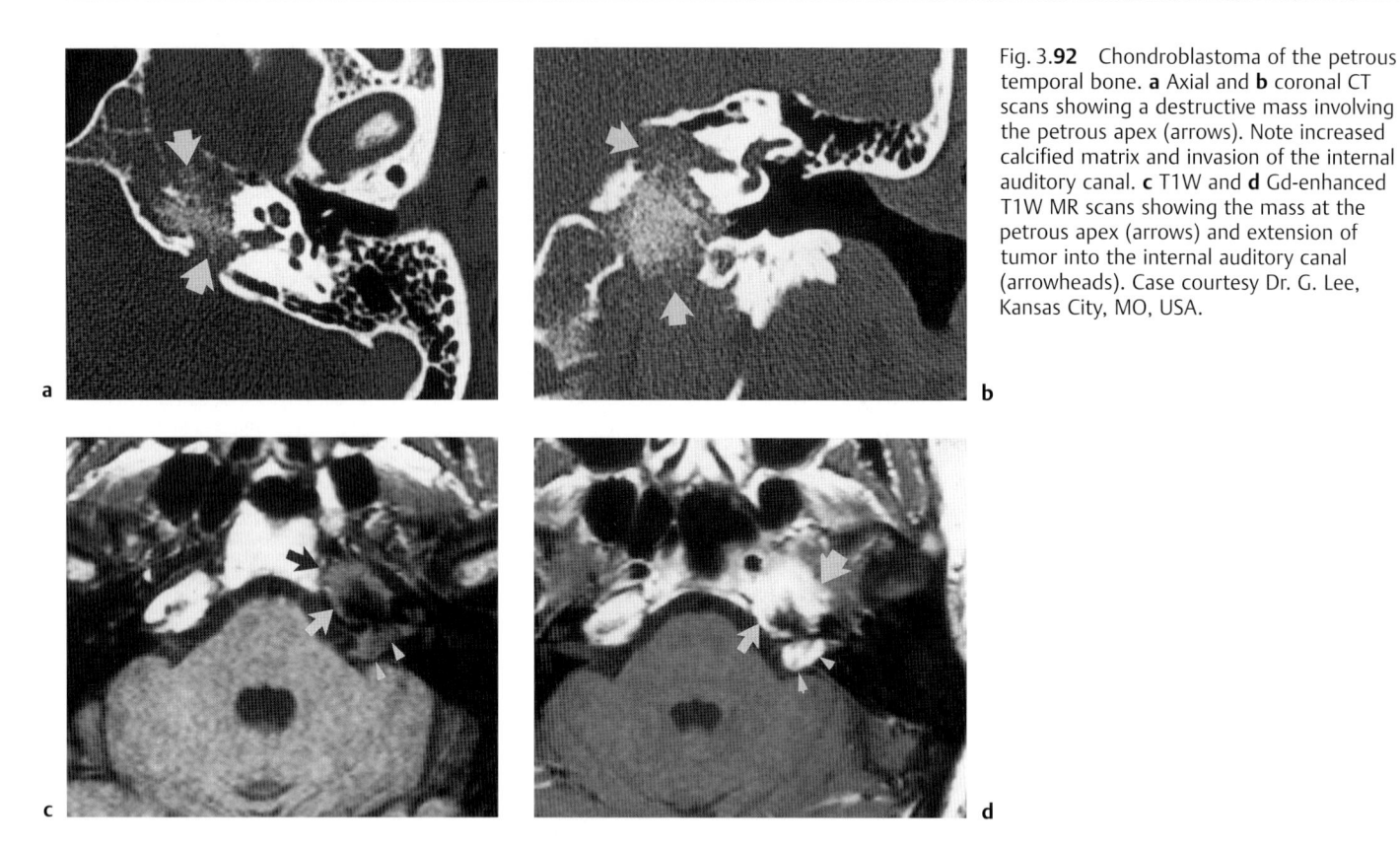

Fig. 3.**93** Fibromyxoma of the temporal bone. CT scan shows a destructive mass, involving the petrous apex (M), extending into the middle ear and external auditory canal.

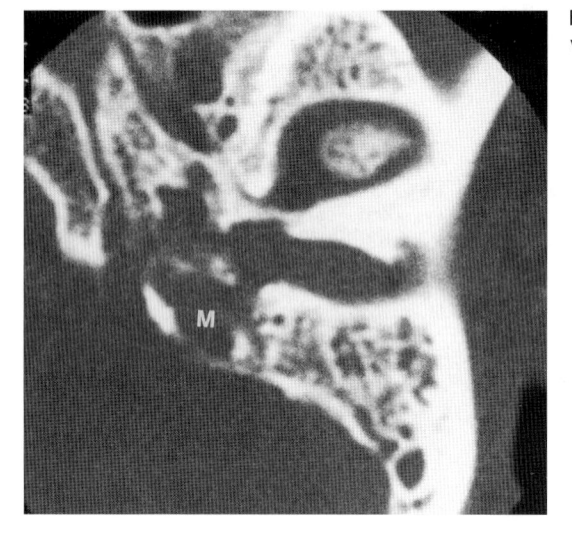

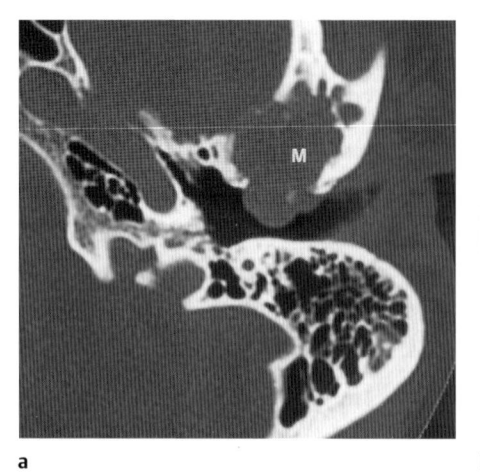

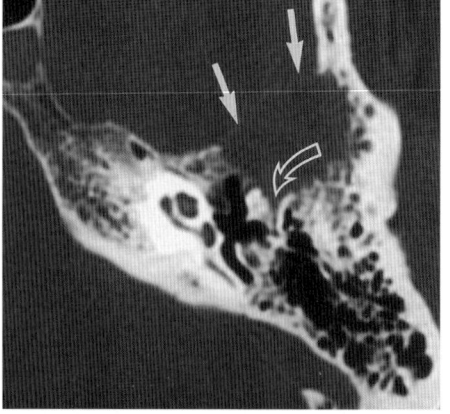

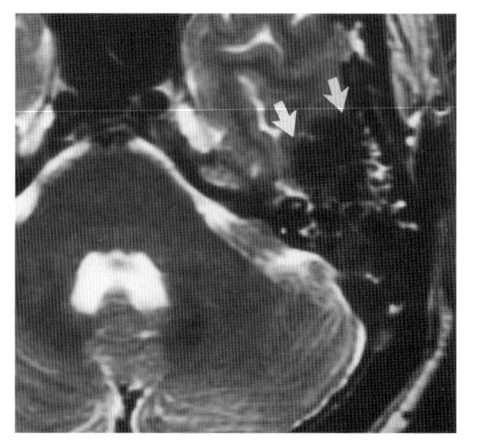

Fig. 3.**94** Chondromyxoid fibroma. **a** CT scan shows an expansile mass (M), involving the squamous temporal bone, extending into the external auditory canal. **b** CT scan, taken superior to **a**, shows extension of the mass into the middle cranial fossa (arrows) as well as into the attic (curved arrow). **c** Axial T2W MR scan shows the tumor to be mainly hypointense in appearance, representing a predominantly compact fibrous component. Case courtesy Dr. G. Lee, Kansas City, MO, USA.

Skull Base Pathology 333

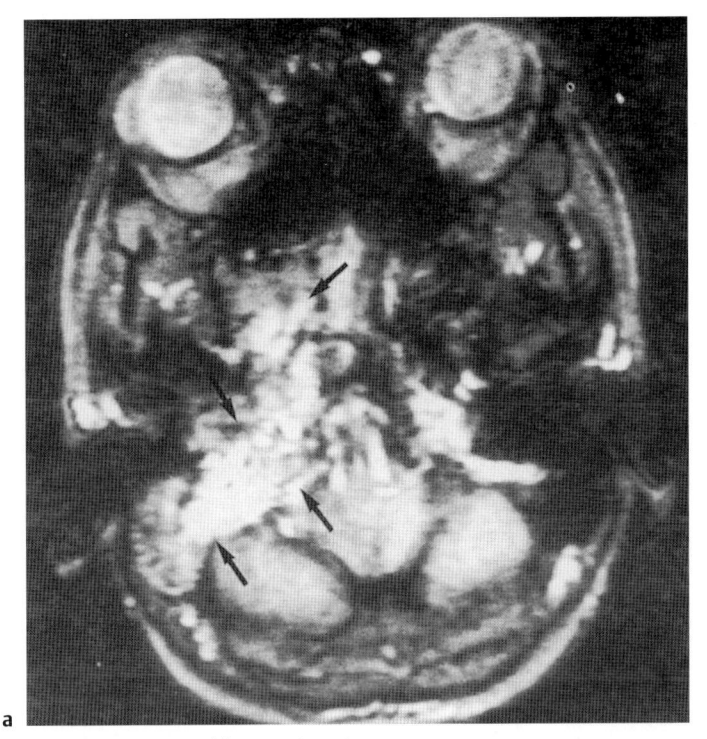

Fig. 3.**95** Presumed hemangiopericytoma.
a Axial gradient-echo MR scan shows a hypervascular mass (arrows), involving the posterior cranial fossa and extending into the middle cranial fossa.

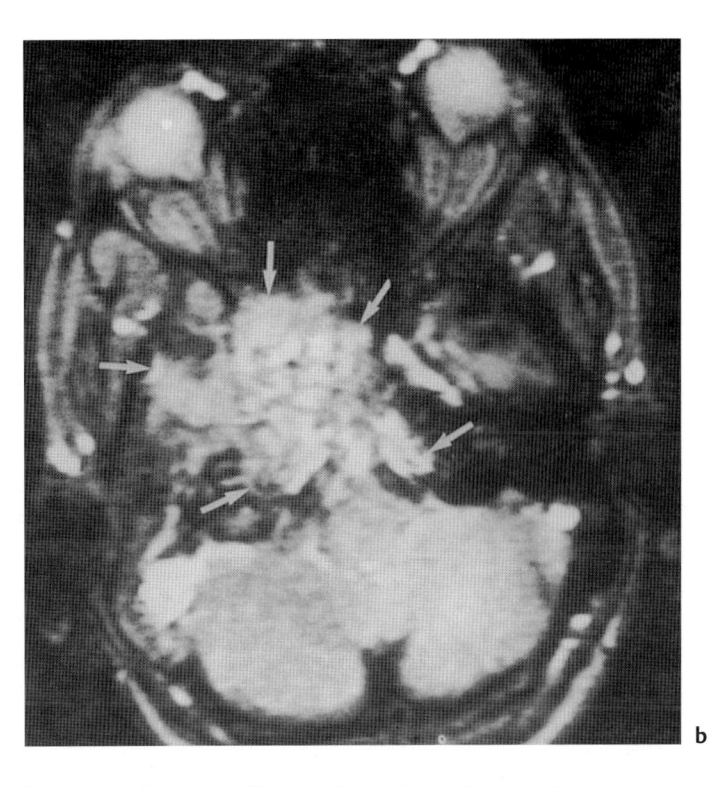

b Axial gradient-echo MR scan, obtained cephalad to **a**, shows massive involvement of the clivus and sphenoid bone (arrows).

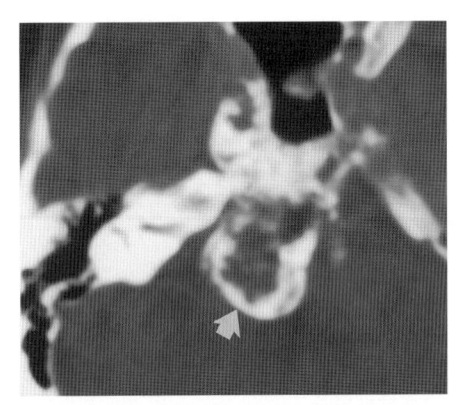

Fig. 3.**96** Chondrosarcoma of skull base. CT scan shows a large partially calcified (tumor calcification) mass (arrow), centered at the clivus with extension into the posterior cavernous sinus. The site of the origin of this tumor is likely to be the spheno-occipital and spheno-petrosal synchondrosis. Case courtesy of Marina Grisoli, MD. Italy.

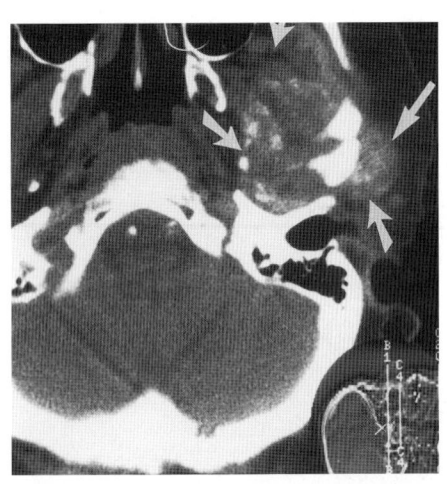

Fig. 3.**97** Chondrosarcoma of the TMJ. CT scan shows a large mass (arrows) in the left TMJ region. Note tumor calcifications and irregularity of the left condyle.

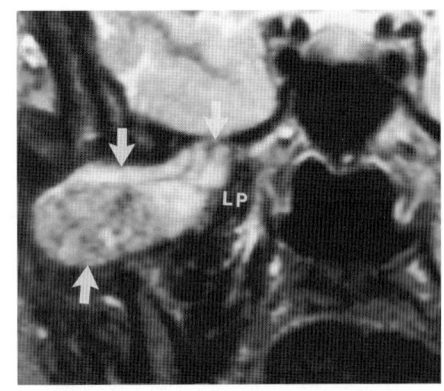

Fig. 3.**98** Chondrosarcoma of the TMJ. Coronal T2W MR scan shows a large heterogeneous mass (arrows), involving the right TMJ region. Note displaced lateral pterygoid muscle (LP).

Chondrosarcoma of the Skull Base

Sarcomas of the skull base are rare but potentially lethal tumors and invariably challenging for otolaryngologists and oromaxillofacial surgeons and neurosurgeons. Prognosis is considered poor; local recurrence and distant metastases are common.[31] Chondrosarcomas account for 0.1 % of all head and neck tumors.[32] The most common skull base sites include temporo-occipital junction (petro-occipital fissure) (Fig. 3.**96**), middle cranial fossa (foramen lacerum), sphenoethmoid complex, clivus, anterior cranial fossa, and temperomandibular joint (Figs. 3.**97**, 3.**98**).[31] The spheno-occipital synchondrosis, the spheno-petrosal synchondrosis, and a large part of petrous portion of the temporal bone are sites in the mature skull that undergo endochondral ossification. It is hypothesized that islands of residual endochondral cartilage may be present in these areas and that chondroid tumors develop from these chondrocytes.[31] Some authors have suggested that these tumors may arise from pleuripotential mesenchymal cells or they may be arising from metaplasia of mature fibroblasts.[31–33] Although most chondrosarcomas arise

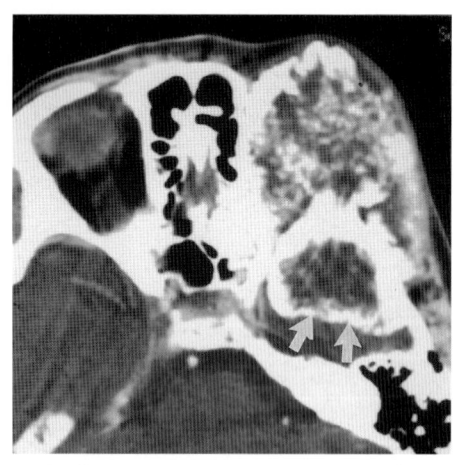

Fig. 3.**99** Osteogenic sarcoma. CT scan shows an extensive destructive tumor involving the left orbit with extension into the left middle cranial fossa (arrows). There are numerous foci of tumor bone formation.

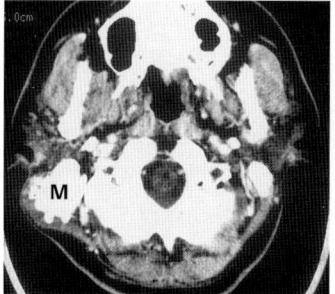

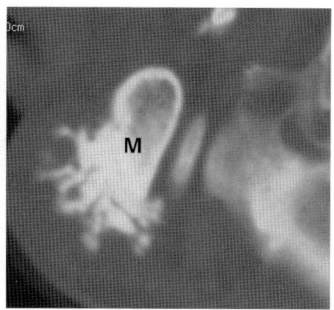

Fig. 3.**100** Parosteal osteogenic sarcoma of the mastoid. **a** CT scan shows increased size of the right mastoid (M), with irregular cortical outline as well as soft-tissue thickening of the mastoid region. **b** CT scan, obtained to show bony detail, showing sclerosis of the mastoid (M), associated with multiple bone islands related to tumor bone formation. Note a cleft between the mastoid and tumor invading the mastoid region. Case courtesy of Dr. Paterson, Seattle, WA, USA.

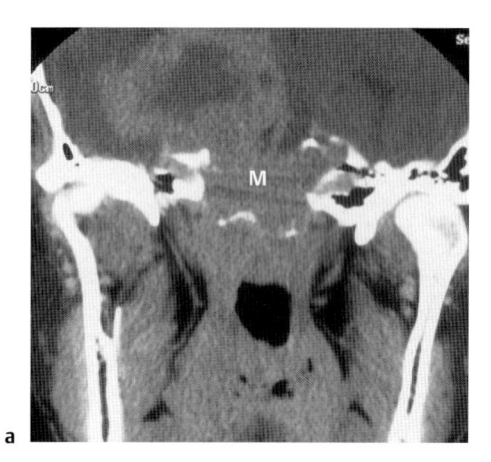

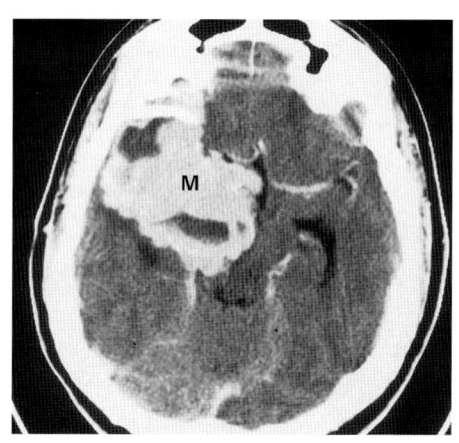

Fig. 3.**101** Presumed chordoma. **a** Coronal CT scan in a 24-year-old man shows a destructive mass (M) involving the clivus and extending into the right temporal lobe. **b** Axial enhanced CT scan shows marked enhancement of the intradural component of the mass (M). Courtesy of Dr. S. Raju, Chicago, IL, USA.

from cartilagenous or bony structures, they may also develop in soft tissues, in which cartilage is normally not found (see Chapter 2).[33,34] It is not clear whether these soft-tissue chondrosarcomas develop from mesenchymal differentiation or ectopic chondroid precursor cells.[34] Several subtypes of chondrosarcoma have been proposed. The conventional subtype consists of hyaline or myxoid areas or a combination of two. Chondrosarcomas are classified into three categories based on varying cellularity and nuclear atypia.[35] Rosenberg et al[35] reviewed 200 cases of skull base chondrosarcoma and found that 50.5% of tumors were grade I (well differentiated), 21% were grade II (moderately differentiated), 28.5% were mixed grade I and II, and 0% were grade III (poorly differntiated) tumors. The differential diagnosis for chondrosarcoma includes chordoma, chondroid chordoma, chondroma, osteochondroma, osteogenic sarcoma (Figs. 3.**99**, 3.**100**), meningioma, schwannoma, chondroblastoma, enchondroma, osteoblastoma, fibro-osseous lesion, glomus tumor, brown tumor, and metastases.[36,37] At times, adenoid cystic tumor of oral and sinonasal cavities may produce calcifications and reactive periosteal bone formation simulating chondro-osteogenic tumors. (See Chapter 4.)

Imaging Diagnosis

CT and MRI play an important role in the diagnosis of chondrosarcoma and other lesions of the base of the skull. CT scan is most helpful in chondrosarcoma and osteogenic sarcoma because it shows bone destruction and tumor calcification (Figs. 3.**96**–3.**100**). At the early stage, chondrosarcoma may be well-defined, expansile and bone-pushing. A rim of calcification may be present. At times, tumor may be limited to the sphenoid sinus, simulating a benign lesion. MRI helps to evaluate tumor involvement of intracranial as well as extracranial structures.[36] Chondrosarcomas appear as low to intermediate signal intensity on T1W and hight signal intensity on T2W MR images, with marked enhancement on enhanced T1W MR images (Fig. 3.**98**). This is similar to signal characteristics of chordoma (see Figs. 3.**103**–3.**106**).

Chordomas

Chordomas are malignant neoplasms arising from the embryonic remnants of the notochord. They represent approximately 1% of all malignant bone tumors.[38] The notochord, which functions as a primitive axial skeleton in humans, develops in the third to fourth week of gestation.[38] It extends from the sphenoid (cartilaginous) bone at the junction of the occipital bone to the coccyx. It exits the sphenoid bony confine to run in close apposition to the primitive pharynx, reenters the bone in the basiocciput, and then courses via the apical odontoid ligament through the center of the vertebral bodies to end at the coccyx.[38] Accordingly, chordomas are identified in the sacrococcygeal region, the bones of the skull (Figs. 3.**101**, 3.**102**), and the vertebra (cervical, lumbar, and thoracic in order of increasing frequency).[38] Craniocervical chordomas are frequently identified in the dorsum sella (Fig. 3.**103**), clivus (Fig. 3.**101**), sphenoid sinus (Fig. 3.**104**), and nasopharynx, and less frequently they may be identified anterior to the jugular foramen (Fig. 3.**105**), petrous apex (Fig. 3.**102**), and middle cranial fossa. Pathologically, chordomas are well-demarcated or encapsulated, soft, mucoid, or gelatinous masses with solid and cystic components. The cells are epithelioid with abundant vacuolated cytoplasms and vesicular nuclei.[38] The cells are associated with a copious extracellular mucinous matrix. Vacuolization of the cytoplasm represents glycogen or mucus and, when extensive, can appear with a "soap bubble" appearance, compressing the nucleus and creating the characteristic physaliphorous cells seen in chordomas.[38] Immunohistochemically, chordomas are cytokeratin, epithelial membrane antigen, and S-100 protein positive.[38] A variant of the chordoma, called chondroid chordoma (Fig. 3.**105**), is identified and is noted for being more common in women and younger patients than nonchondroid chordoma, its virtually exclusive occurrence at the skull base, the presence of a benign or malignant cartilaginous component, and S-100 protein immunoreactivity but absence of cytokeratin immunoreactivity, and its better prognosis.[38]

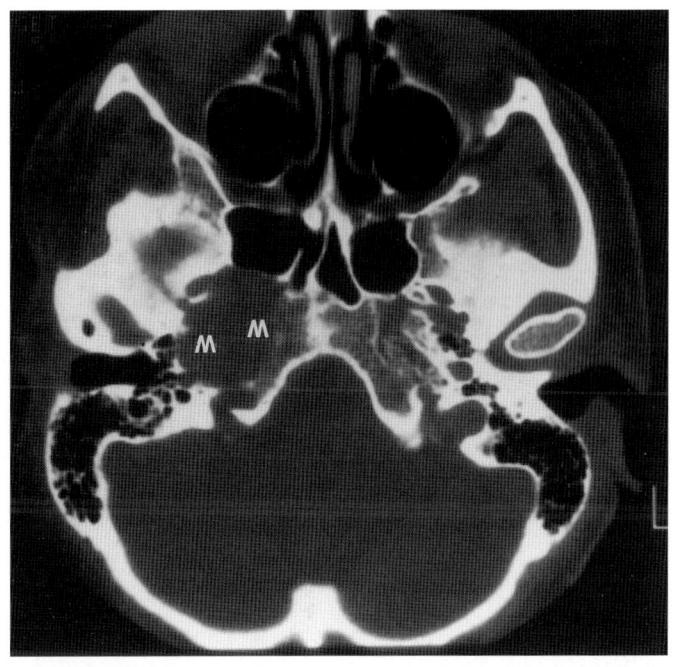

Fig. 3.**102** Chordoma. CT scan shows a mass (M) centered at the right petro-occipital region, associated with erosion of petrous apex and adjacent clivus.

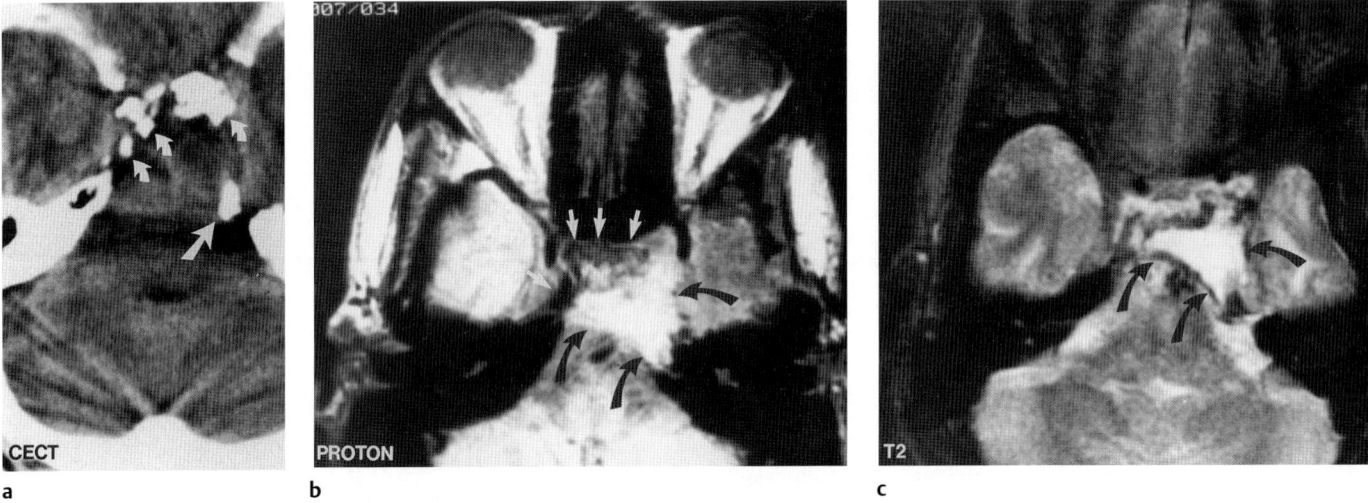

Fig. 3.**103** Chordoma. **a** Contrast-enhanced CT (CECT) scan shows a large mass adjacent to the dorsum sella. Note lack of significant contrast enhancement and associated multiple coarse calcifications (arrows). **b** Proton-weighted and **c** T2W MR scans showing hyperintense chordoma (arrows).

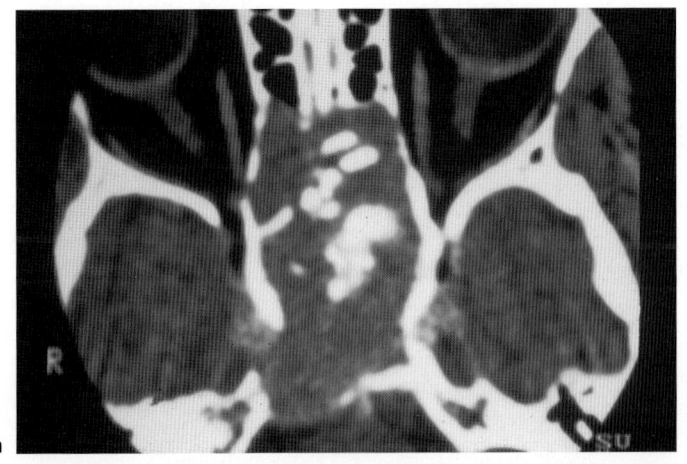

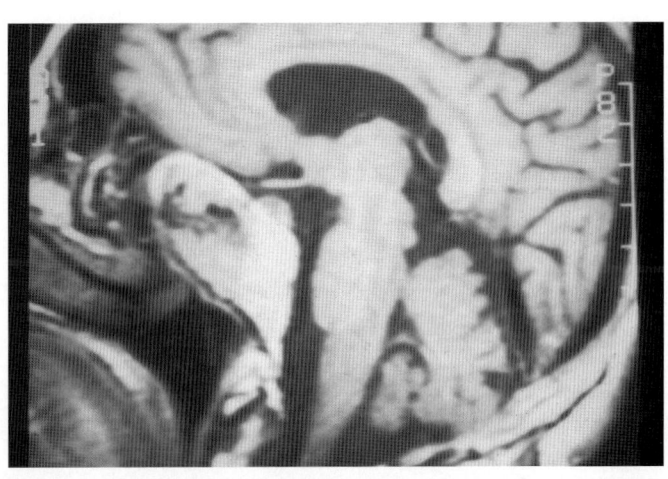

Fig. 3.**104** Chordoma. **a** CT scan shows a mass involving the sphenoid sinus and the clivus. Note coarse calcifications. **b** T1W MR scan shows chordoma within the entire sphenoid sinus.

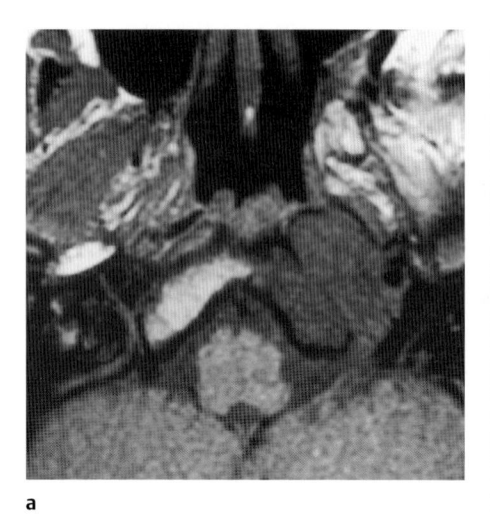

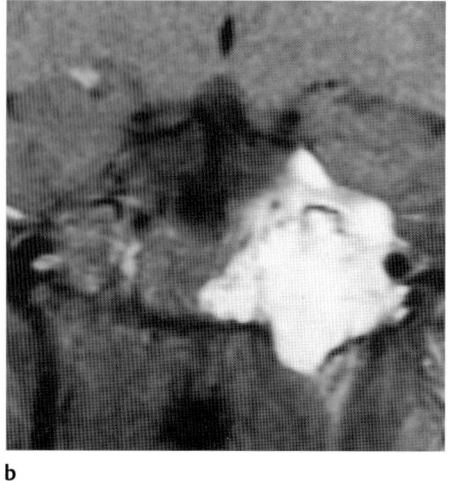

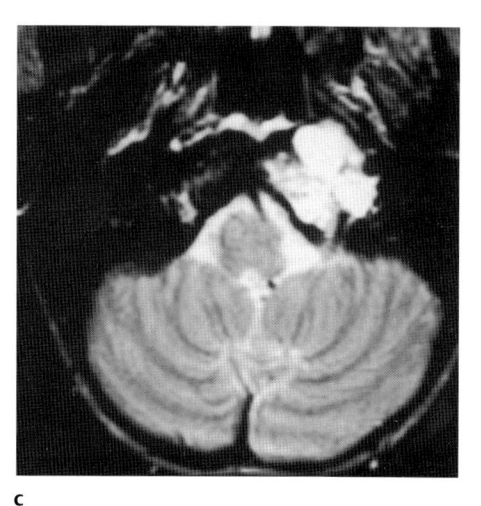

Fig. 3.**105** Chondroid chordoma. **a** Axial T1W MR scan shows a hypointense mass in the left inferior petrous apex region. **b** Coronal enhanced T1W MR scan shows marked enhancement of this chordoma. **c** Axial T2W MR scan shows characteristic intense hyperintensity of this chordoma.

Differential diagnosis: chondroma, chondrosarcoma, and metastic hypernephroma and thyroid carcinoma. Case courtesy of B.D. Doust, MD, Chicago, IL, USA.

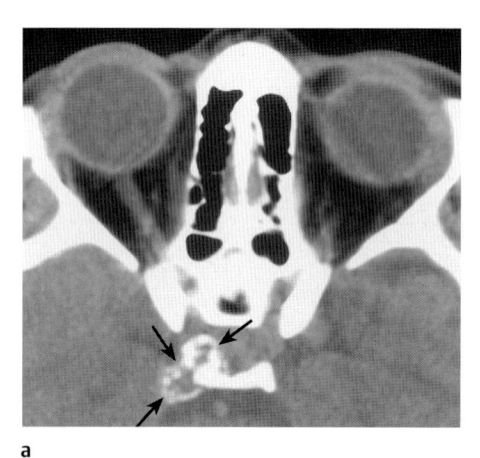

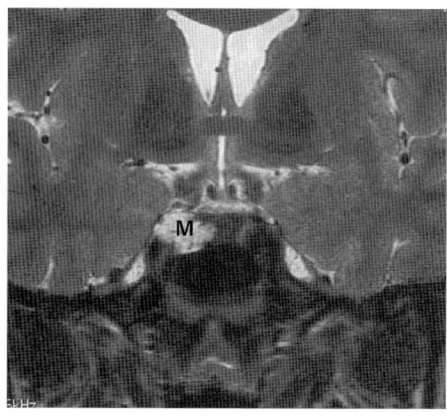

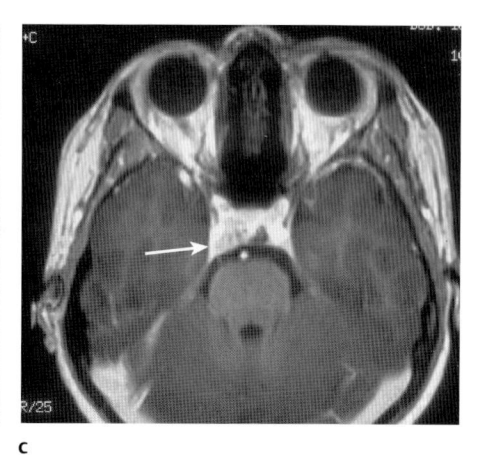

Fig. 3.**106** Chordoma. **a** CT scan shows a calcified mass (arrows) in the right parasellar region. **b** Coronal T2W MR scan, obtained with a 3 T MR imager. The mass (M) appears moderately hyperintense in appearance. **c** Gd-enhanced T1W MR scan shows mild enhancement of this chordoma (arrow).

Chordoma, chondroid chordoma, and chondrosarcoma are difficult to differentiate reliably by CT and MRI (Figs. 3.**96**, 3.**103**–3.**106**. The histological diagnosis of these lesions is also often difficult.[31] Chordomas contain an abundance of cells with bubbly eosinophilic cytoplasm, called physaliphorous cells. Chondroid chordoma contains features of both chondrosarcoma and chordoma. Chondroid chordoma contain neoplastic chondrocytes along with physaliphorous cells that are present but are much rarer than in chondromas.[31] Chordomas stain positive for cytokeratin, epithelial membrane antigen (EME), S-100 protein, and vimentin. Conversely, chondrosarcomas stain positive for vimentin and S-100 and negative for cytokeratin and EME.[31] Differentiation of chordomas may occur and includes transformation to fibrosarcoma, malignant fibrous histiocytoma, osteosarcoma, and chondrosarcoma.[38]

Imaging Diagnosis

On CT scans, the typical appearance of a chordoma is of a midline expansile and destructive lesion involving the clivus (Figs. 3.**101**–3.**104**). The tumor mass often contains multiple calcifications or bony fragments of the adjacent destroyed bone. As the tumor enlarges, it involves the nasopharynx, sella, cavernous sinus, petrous apex, sphenoid sinus, and posteriorly the brainstem and basilar artery. The T1W MR images show a mass of low signal intensity that may contain foci of high signal due to old bleeding or proteinaceous fluid. Calcifications appear hypointense on T1W, T2W, and gradient echo MR images. In the T2W MR images, chordoma has typical high-signal intensity (Figs. 3.**103c**, 3.**106b**). Following the i.v. injection of a gadolinium-based contrast medium, the tumor undergoes a homogeneous or nonhomogeneous enhancement (Fig. 3.**105b**).

Chordomas may have a very high signal intensity on T2-weighted MR images (Fig. 3.**103**). Contrast enhancement in chordoma is variable and at times may be minimal (Fig. 3.**106**). Tumors that have matrix calcification may appear heterogeneous on MR images. There will usually be a marked enhancement with gadolinium contrast (Fig. 3.**105**).[36] At present, total resection of chordomas followed by radiation therapy (ideally proton beam) appears to offer the best chance for cure.[31] The differential diagnosis of tumor of the base of skull, centered at the petro-occipital fissure, includes chordoma, chondrosarcoma, jugular fossa schwannoma, glomus jugulare, meningioma, chondroblastoma, chondromyxoid tumor, lymphoma, rhabdomyosarcoma, Langerhans cell histiocytosis, endolymphatic sac tumor, extension of nasopharyngeal carcinoma, and metastasis. Schwannomas are generally smooth in margin and relatively hypovascular. They do not show significant enhancement on a dynamic CT study, nor do they demonstrate increased vascularity on flow-sensitive MR pulse sequences such as gradient echo sequence. Schwannomas and neurofibromas, however, demonstrate intense contrast enhancement on routine postcontrast CT and MR scans (Figs. 3.**80**, 3.**83**). Glomus jugular tumors (paragangliomas) are locally destructive as well as infiltrative, causing irregular enlargement of the jugular fossa. These lesions are hypervascular, demonstrating signal flow voids on T1-weighted and T2-weighted MR images (Figs. 3.**69**, 3.**70**, 3.**71**). Paragangliomas show intense enhancement on dynamic CT scans and marked vascularity on flow-sensitive MR pulse sequences (Figs. 3.**70 b**, 3.**71 b**). Meningioma is seen as a dural-based mass, demonstrating intense enhancement as well as enhancement of adjacent thickened dura (dural tail) (Figs. 3.**60**, 3.**61**). Chordoma is typically a destructive tumor of the clivus, expanding the clivus and extending into the soft tissue of the posterior nasopharynx. Calcifications are common in chondrosarcoma, chordoma, and meningioma. Calcification is very rare in schwannoma. We have seen marked calcification in a fifth cranial and tenth cranial nerve schwannoma.

Rhabdomyosarcoma

Although, rhabdomyosarcoma (RMS) is a rare disease in adults, it is the most common primary orbital malignancy in children and the most common head and neck sarcoma in children (Figs. 3.**107**, 3.**108**).[37,39] There are three types of RMS: embryonal, differentiated, and alveolar.[37] The malignant alveolar type in the adult is the most aggressive.[39] The acute and subacute symptoms of orbital RMS may be mistaken for symptoms of orbital inflammation.[40] RMS, Ewing sarcoma and other soft-tissue sarcomas occur in the head and neck of children and less commonly in young adults. The soft-tissue sarcomas include fibrosarcoma, angiosarcoma, malignant fibrous histiocytoma, malignant schwannoma, liposarcoma, hemangiopericytoma, synovial sarcoma, and other less common sarcomas.[37] RMS may be adjacent to or involve the temporal bone (Figs. 3.**109**, 3.**110**). Radiation therapy with the addition of chemotherapy has significantly improved the survival rate of patients with RMS. Recent studies in gene therapy have been directed at targeting tumor suppression for the treatment of RMS.[39]

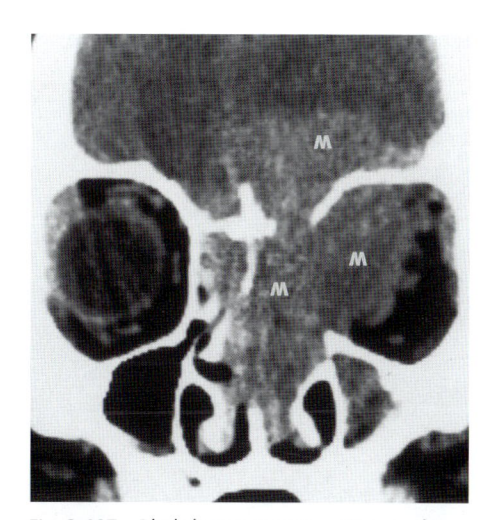

Fig. 3.**107** Rhabdomyosarcoma. CT scan shows a sino-orbital mass (M), involving the anterior cranial fossa. Case courtesy of Hafez Sharif, MD, Cairo, Egypt.

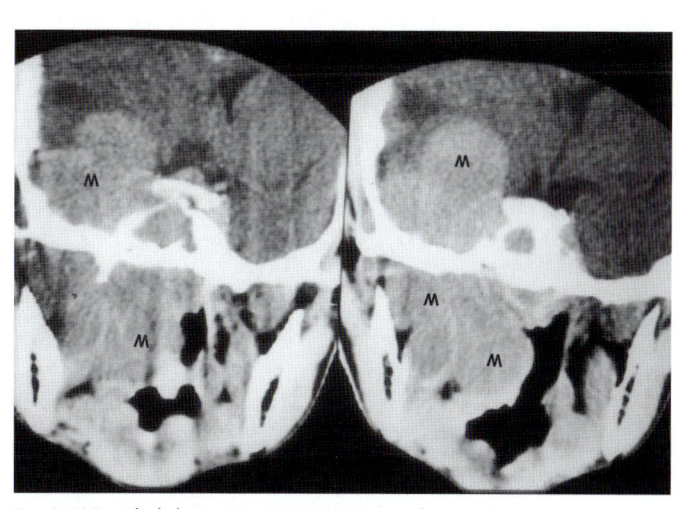

Fig. 3.**108** Rhabdomyosarcoma. CT scans shows a large extra- and intracranial mass (M) compatible with advanced rhabdomyosarcoma. Case courtesy of Hafiz Sharif, MD, Cairo, Egypt.

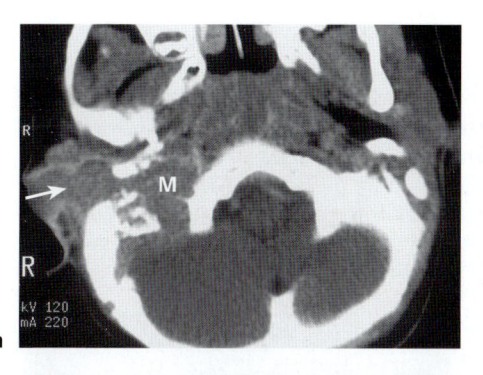

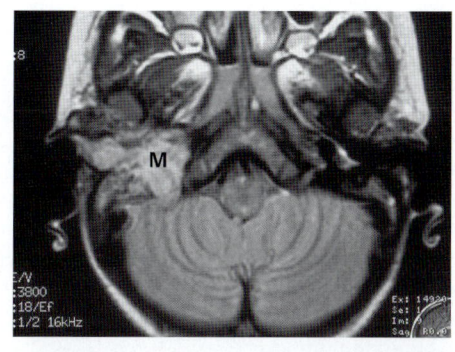

Fig. 3.**109 a** Rhabdomyosarcoma. Enhanced CT scan shows a mass (M), involving the skull base with erosion of petromastoid plate and tumor extension into the middle ear and external auditory canal (arrow). **b** PW MR scan showing the mass (M). **c** Gd-enhanced T1W MR scan shows marked tumor (M) enhancement. **d** Gd-enhanced coronal T1W MR scan shows enhancement of the skull base mass (M).

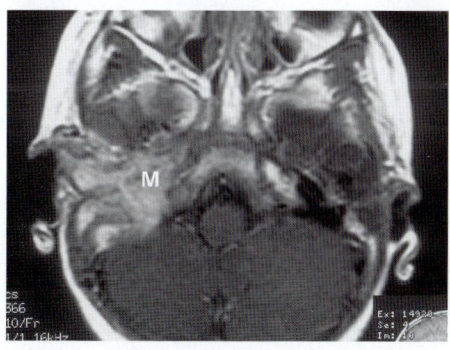

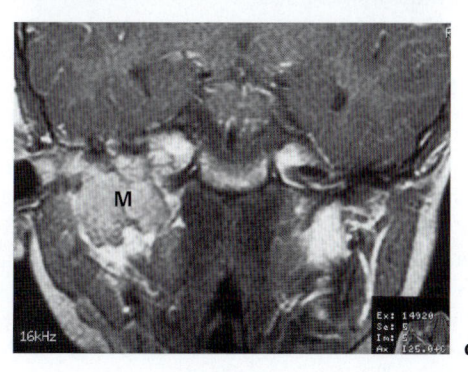

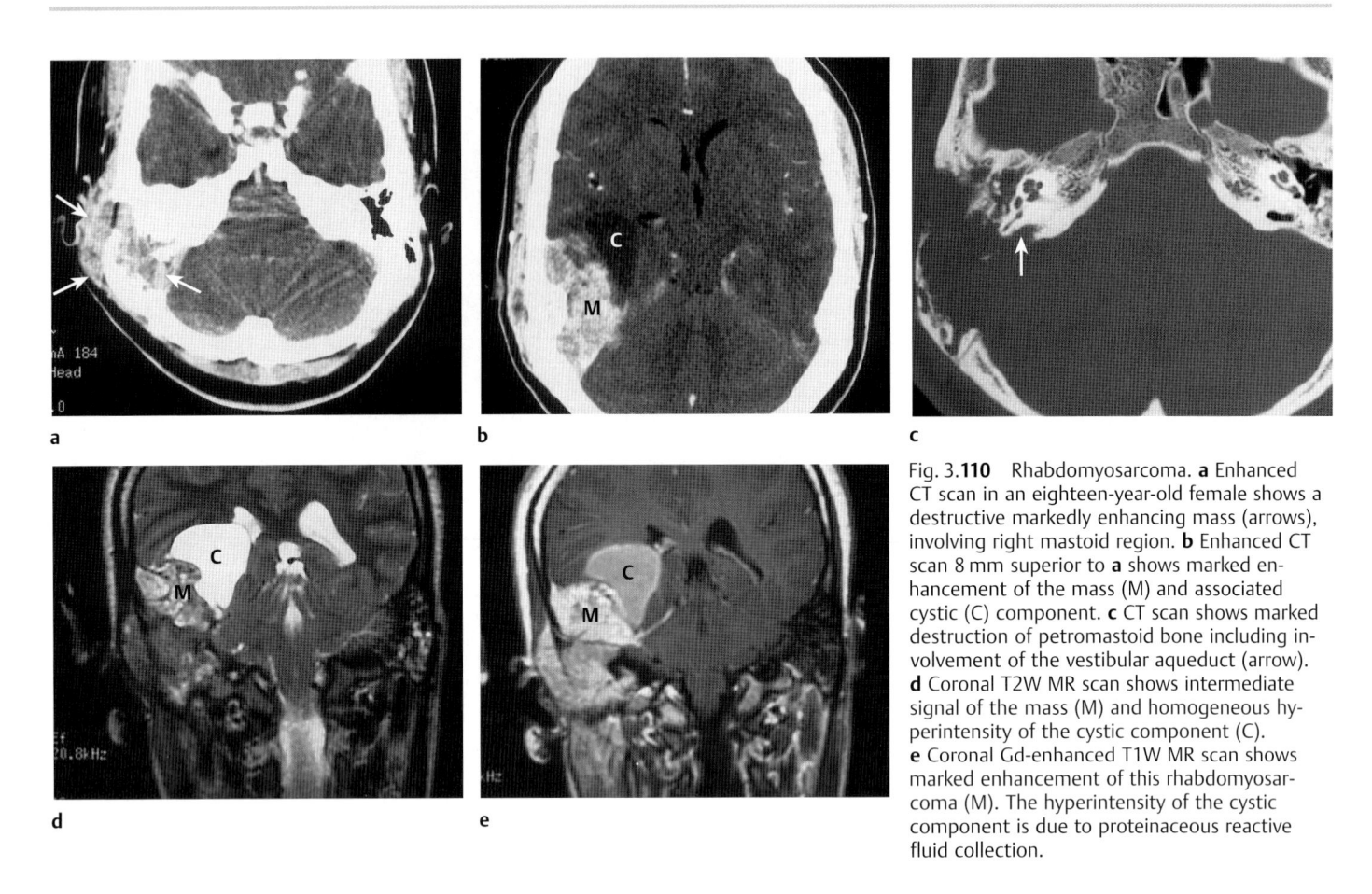

Fig. 3.**110** Rhabdomyosarcoma. **a** Enhanced CT scan in an eighteen-year-old female shows a destructive markedly enhancing mass (arrows), involving right mastoid region. **b** Enhanced CT scan 8 mm superior to **a** shows marked enhancement of the mass (M) and associated cystic (C) component. **c** CT scan shows marked destruction of petromastoid bone including involvement of the vestibular aqueduct (arrow). **d** Coronal T2W MR scan shows intermediate signal of the mass (M) and homogeneous hyperintensity of the cystic component (C). **e** Coronal Gd-enhanced T1W MR scan shows marked enhancement of this rhabdomyosarcoma (M). The hyperintensity of the cystic component is due to proteinaceous reactive fluid collection.

Low-grade Adenocarcinoma of Endolymphatic Sac Origin

Primary adenocarcinomatous lesions of the temporal bone are distinctly unusual, rare tumors. Even today controversy remains with regard to their cell of origin. In 1989, Heffner[41] described 20 cases of a type of papillary cystic temporal bone neoplasm in which the neoplasm destroyed a large portion of the posterior temporal bone and included a prominent extension into the posterior cranial fossa. Patient histories indicated a slow growth rate of the lesions. There were resemblances of the normal distal endolymphatic sac tissue to some portions of many of the neoplasms. Tissue submitted to the Armed Forces Institute of Pathology from a rare case of papillary adenomatous neoplasm of endolymphatic sac origin, reported by Hassard et al[42] had a strong similarity to the larger, destructive neoplasms. Heffner concluded that tumors in his series grew slowly, but the neoplasms manifested a destructive, infiltrating growth into the temporal bone. Heffner preferred to diagnose them as low-grade adenocarcinomas. Because the neoplasms were epithelial and manifested a destructive growth along the posterior-medial face of the temporal bone, Heffner inferred that the endolymphatic sac seems an ideal location to give rise to these tumors with their combined intrabony and posterior fossa components. These tumors characteristically cause destruction of the vestibular aqueduct and at times marked erosion of the petromastoid plate (Fig. 3.**111**). There may be fine or coarse calcifications present within the tumor. The neoplasm may be solid or a combination of solid and cystic components. There will be moderate to marked contrast enhancement on CT and MRI scans (Fig. 3.**111**). Some of these tumors may originate from sublabyrinthine mastoid air cells with intact endolymphatic sac (Fig. 3.**112**).[43a] Bilateral tumors have been reported in patients with Von Hippel–Lindau disease.[43] Other rare tumors of the temporal bone such as mucoepidermoid carcinoma may have similar CT and MR findings to low-grade papillary adenocarcinoma (Fig. 3.**113**). These tumors should be included in the differential diagnosis of destructive or nondestuctive tumors about the posteromedial face of the petrous bone as well as extra-axial cerebellopontine tumors.

Fibromatosis

Fibromatosis is an infiltrating and aggressive fibroblastic proliferation. Other names for this entity include aggressive fibromatosis, desmoid tumor, tumefactive fibroinflammatory tumor, and inflammatory pseudotumor.[38] The disease lacks features of either an inflammatory process or a neoplasm.[38] It is identified in the head and neck in 10–15% of the cases. In children this area of the body may be affected in up to 30% of cases.[38] Excluding the neck, the common sites of occurrence are nasal cavity, paranasal sinuses, nasopharynx, tongue, and oral cavity. The disease may involve the parapharyngeal space, orbit, and mastoid temporal

Fig. 3.**112** Low-grade papillary adenocarcinoma of the temporal bone of non-endolymphatic sac origin. **a** Axial T2W MR scan shows several foci of abnormal high signal in the right retrolabyrinthine region (arrow). **b** Sagittal T2W MR scans showing abnormal high signal in the sublabyrinthine region (large arrow). Note normal endolymphatic duct and sac (small arrows). **c** Sagittal T2W MR scan in another patient with large endolymphatic duct and sac, for comparison with **b**. **d** Sagittal T2W MR scan shows a hyperintense mass in the sublabyrinthine region (arrow) with extension superiorly in the juxtaendolymphatic duct region (arrowhead).

Skull Base Pathology

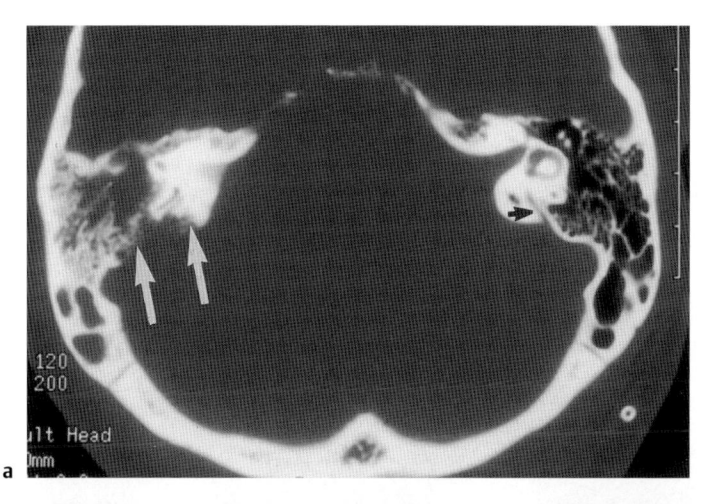

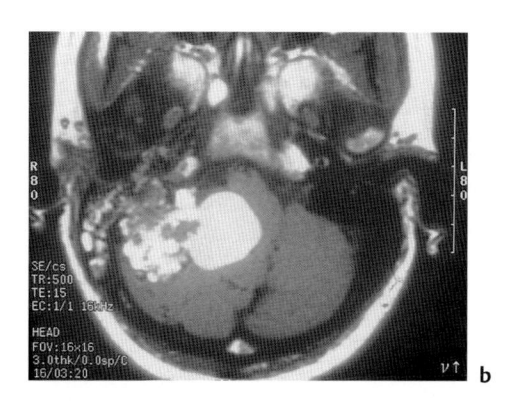

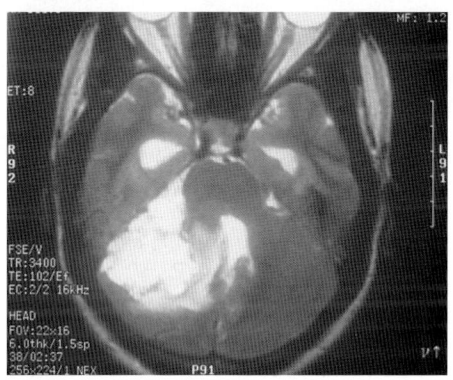

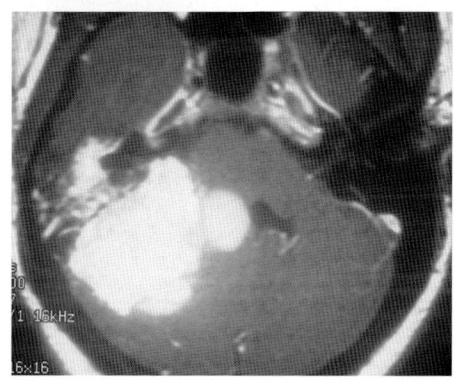

Fig. 3.111 Endolymphatic sac low-grade papillary adenocarcinoma. **a** CT scan shows focal bony destruction of the petromastoid plate (white arrows), in the expected location of the vestibular aqueduct. Note normal left vestibular aqueduct (black arrow). **b** Unenhanced T1W MR scan shows a large posterior fossa mass. **c** T2W and **d** enhanced T1W MR scans, showing large mass with cystic and enhancing solid components.

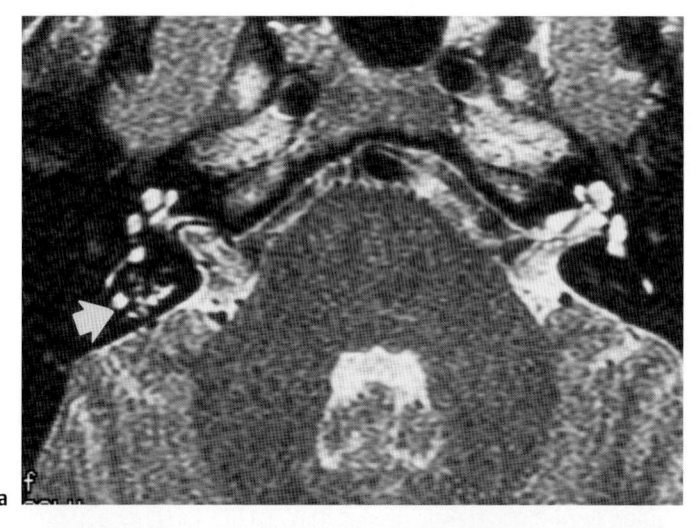

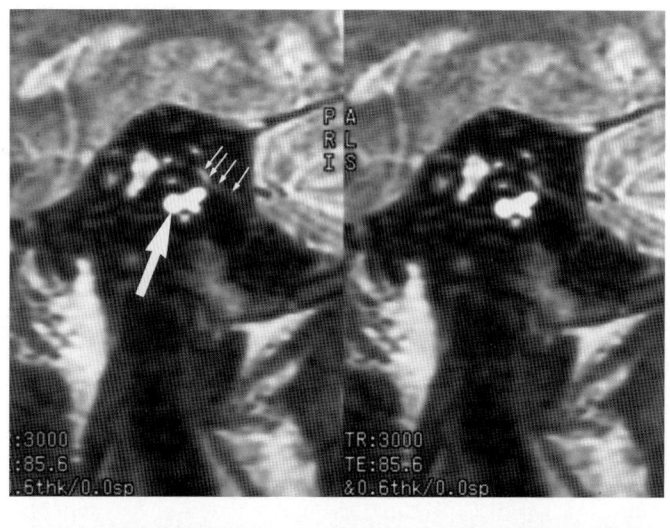

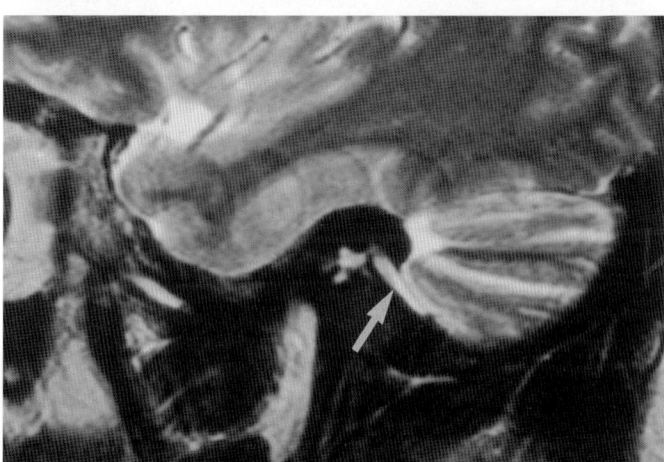

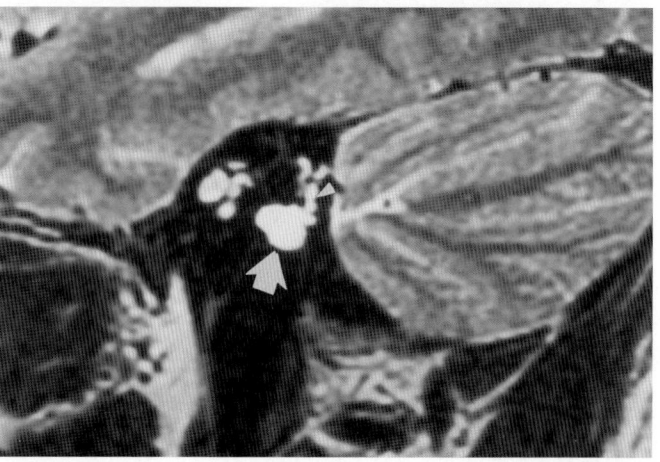

Fig. 3.112 e and f ▷

340   3 Base of the Skull

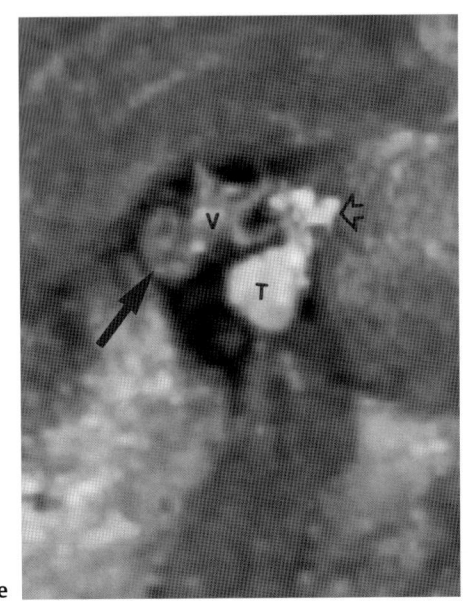

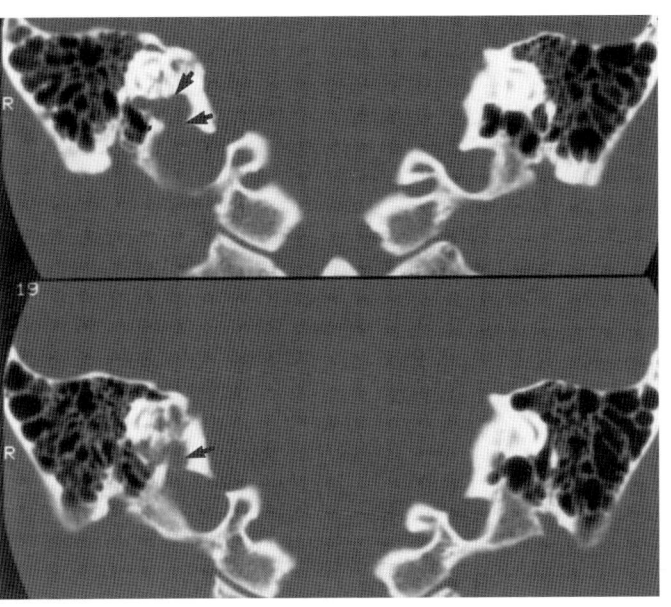

Fig. 3.**112 e**   3D MRI, using MIP technique, showing the tumor (T) and its superior infiltration around and adjacent to the endolymphatic duct (hollow arrow). Note cochlea (solid arrow) and vestibule (v). **f** Coronal CT scans showing enlargement of the superior aspect of the jugular fossa in the region of the tumor (arrows). At surgery the endolymphatic sac and duct were normal. This tumor is believed to arise from the mucosal gland of sublabyrinthine mastoid air cells.

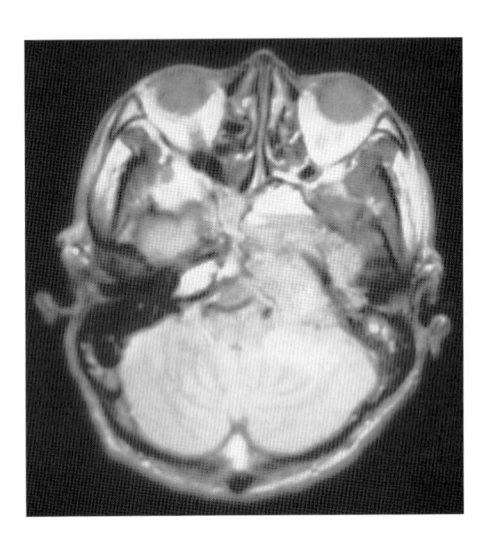

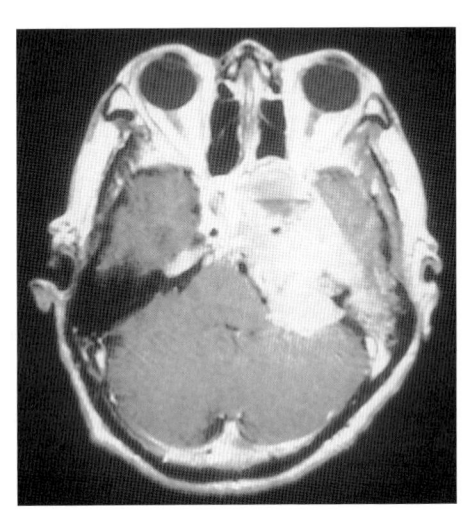

Fig. 3.**113**   Mucoepidermoid carcinoma of the temporal bone. **a** Precontrast and **b** postcontrast axial MR scans showing a mass with marked enhancement, replacing the entire left petrous apex.

bone (Fig. 3.**114**). Differential diagnosis based on CT and MRI findings should include rhabdomyosarcoma, nerve sheath tumor, myxoma, soft-tissue sarcoma, fibro-osseous lesion, Langerhans cell histocytosis, lymphoma, and metastases.

Lymphoproliferative Disorders

Lymphoma, plasmacytoma, histiocytoses, and leukemia may involve the skull base.[44–48] Malignant lymphomas are divided into non-Hodgkin lymphomas (NHL) and Hodgkin disease. NHL are comprised of polymorphous cellular infiltrate which includes B and T lymphocytes, histiocytes, and plasma cells. The predominant cell type determines the pathological classification. Meningeal infiltration is the most common lesion in secondary NHL (Fig. 3.**115**). Involvement of bony structures of the skull base including the craniocervical region, clivus, petrous bone, and sphenoethmoid complex may be present as an initial presentation or during a systemic disease (Fig. 3.**116**). In some patients, lymphoma may extend along the adjacent nerve or primarily involve the intracranial/extracranial nerves (Fig. 3.**116**). Primary central nervous system NHL were formerly rare neoplasms, but more recently the yearly incidence has been increasing. This is due to organ transplantation and AIDS.[44] Hodgkin disease is often localized to groups, or a single group, of lymph nodes and extranodal involvement is very rare. Histologically it is characterized by the presence of the neoplastic Reed–Sternberg cell or its variants intermixed with an inflammatory infiltrate composed variably of lymphocytes, neutrophils, histiocytes, plasma cells, and eosinophils. A few subgroups are identified: (1) lymphocyte predominance, (2) mixed cellularity, (3) lymphocyte depletion, and (4) nodular sclerosis. The meninges and the structures of the skull base may be involved in Hodgkin disease. Parenchymal involvement of the brain is rare.[45, 46]

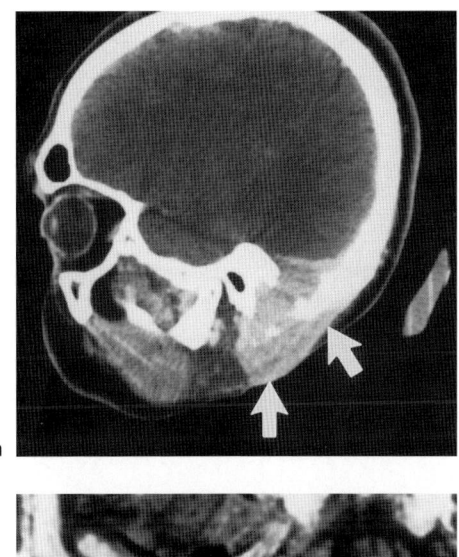

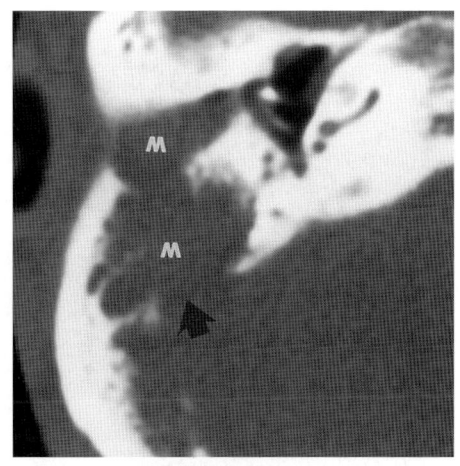

Fig. 3.**114** Aggressive fibromatosis. **a** Enhanced sagittal CT scan shows destructive mass with marked enhancement involving the mastoid region (arrows). **b** CT scan shows mass (M) in the mastoid and external canal. Note erosion of petromastoid plate (arrow). **c** T1W MR scan shows the mass (M), erosion of petromastoid plate (arrow), and tumor infiltration adjacent to the facial nerve (arrowheads). **d** Sagittal T1W MR scan shows the mass (M) extending into endolymphatic sac (S) region. Note endolymphatic duct (small arrows), vestibule (V) and common crus (curved arrow).

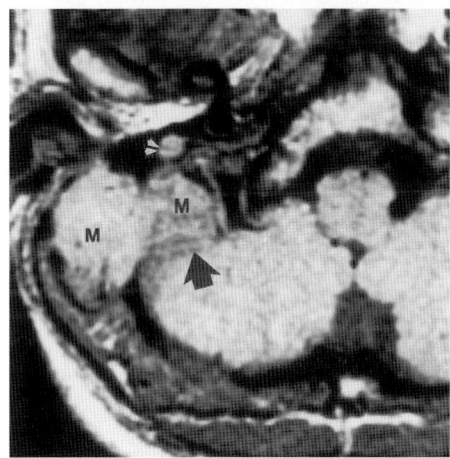

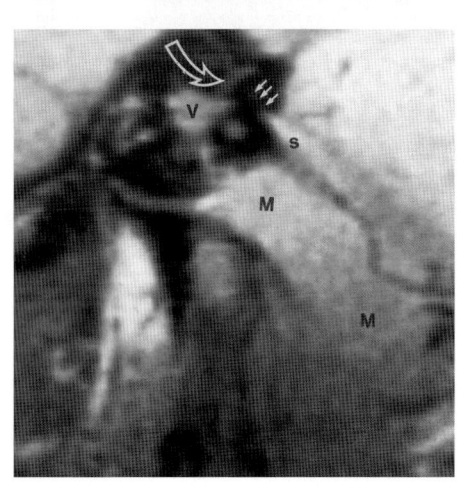

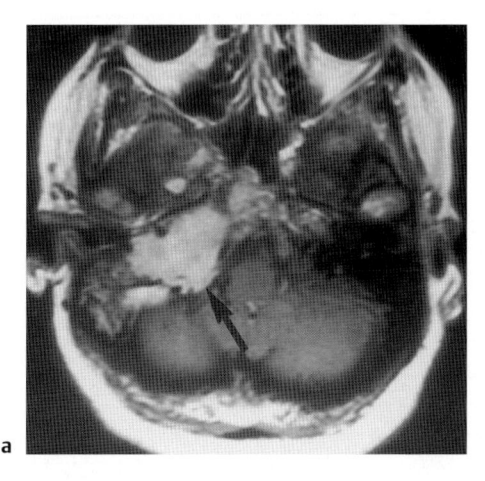

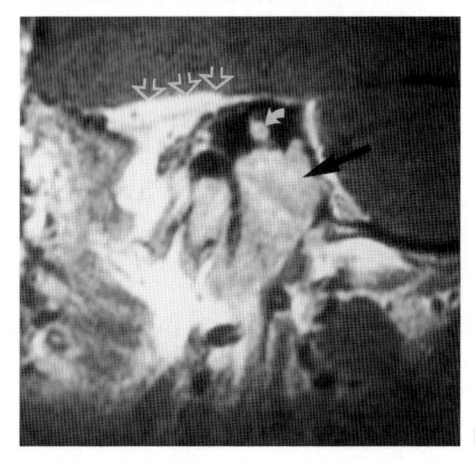

Fig. 3.**115** Lymphoma. **a** Axial Gd-enhanced T1W MR scan shows an enhancing mass involving the region of petrous apex (arrow). **b** Sagittal Gd-enhanced T1W MR scan shows tumor in the jugular fossa (black arrow), within the internal auditory canal (curved arrow) and the floor of the middle cranial fossa (hollow arrows).

Plasmacytoma (Multiple Myeloma)

Plasmacytomas are characterized by the proliferation of monoclonal plasma cells that secrete a single immunoglobulin or its fragments. In the blood the immunoglobulin is identified as the M (myeloma) component, and it could be IgA, IgD, IgG, IgE, or IgM. The neoplastic proliferation of the plasma cells may be confined to multiple bones (multiple myeloma) or to a single bone (solitary myeloma).[47] The disease, which starts within the bone marrow, is characterized by mature and immature plasma cells with nuclear atypia and mitotic activity. Russell bodies, which correspond to packed immunoglobulin, are usually present. Primary intracranial solitary plasmacytoma involving the meninges or cerebrum and lesions localized to the bones of skull base have been reported (Fig. 3.**117**).

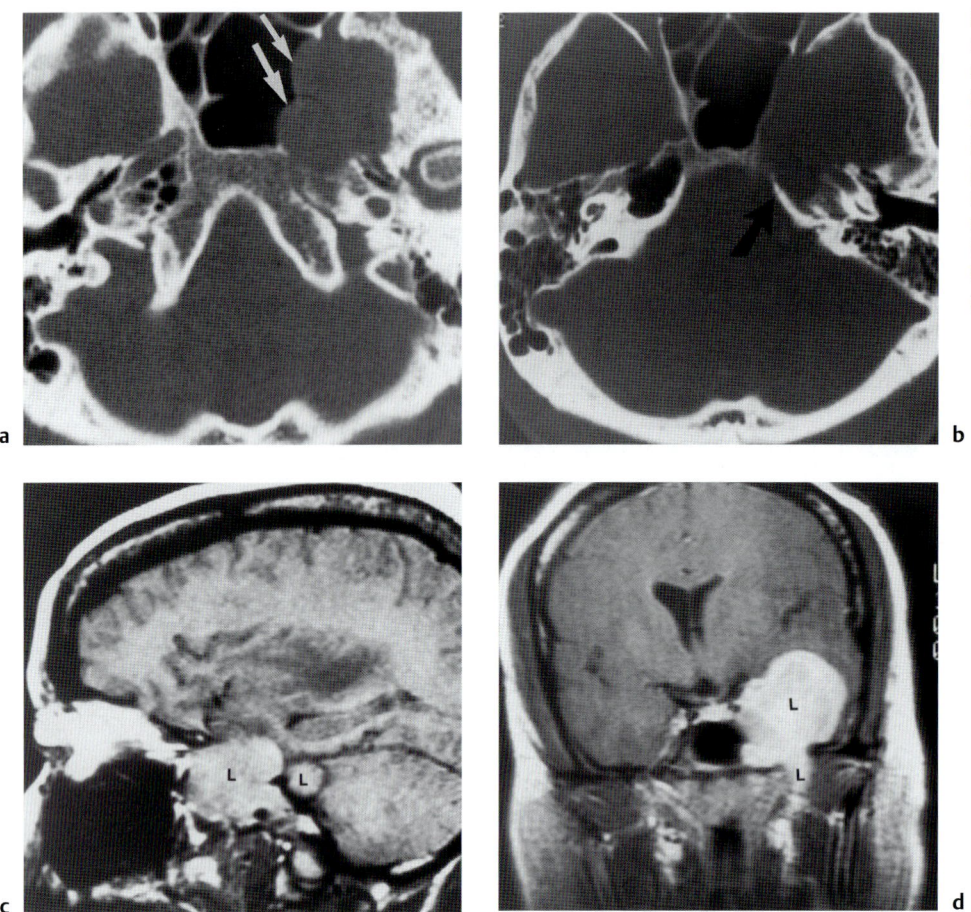

Fig. 3.**116** Plasmacytoma. **a** CT scan shows a mass (arrows) adjacent to the petrosphenoid region. **b** CT scan taken superior to **a** shows partial erosion of left petrous apex (arrow). **c** Sagittal T1W MR scan shows a lesion (L) involving the base of skull at the expected position of trigeminal nerve. **d** Coronal Gd-enhanced MR scan shows marked enhancement of lesion (L) that extends along the trigeminal nerve into the foramen ovale. Histological evaluation was consistent with plasmacytoma.

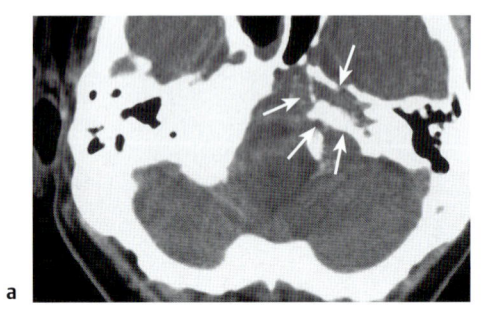

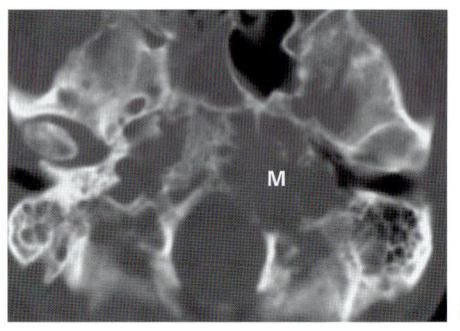

Fig. 3.**117** Multiple myeloma. **a** Unenhanced CT scan shows a destructive mass (arrows) involving the left petrous apex. **b** CT scan shows a mass (M) with bone erosion in the region of the left jugular fossa and adjacent clivus.

■ Histiocytoses

The histiocytoses comprise a group of heterogeneous disorders characterized by proliferation of histiocytic cells that belong either to the monocyte-macrophage system or to the dendritic cell system (Langerhans cell and dendritic reticulum cell).[38,48] The histiocytoses include Langerhans cell histiocytosis; histiocytoses of mononuclear phagocytes other than Langerhans cells, such as juvenile xanthogranuloma, sinus histiocytosis associated with massive lymphadenopathy (Rosai–Dorfman disease), reticulohistiocytoma; and other less common entities. Malignant histocytic disorders include monocytic leukemia, malignant histiocytosis, and histiocytic lymphoma. Unifocal Langerhans cell histiocytosis (eosinophilic granuloma) is a benign disorder that affects children and young adults. Skull bones, particularly petromastoid, orbit, and sphenoidal regions, are the sites of involvement (Figs. 3.**118**, 3.**119**). Multifocal Langerhans cell histiocytosis involves the lymph nodes, liver, spleen, bones, and other organs. In the cranial cavity, the lesions tend to present in multiple bones, the orbit, and the pituitary hypothalamic region. The classical triad of Hand–Schuller–Christian disease includes lytic bone lesions of sphenoid, exophthalmus, and diabetes insipidus.

■ Leukemia

Craniospinal complications of leukemias include diffuse or focal infiltrate, solid neoplastic masses (chloroma) (Fig. 3.**120**), and intraparenchymal and extraparenchymal hemorrhages. Leptomeningeal and dural infiltration is the most common and can be

Skull Base Pathology

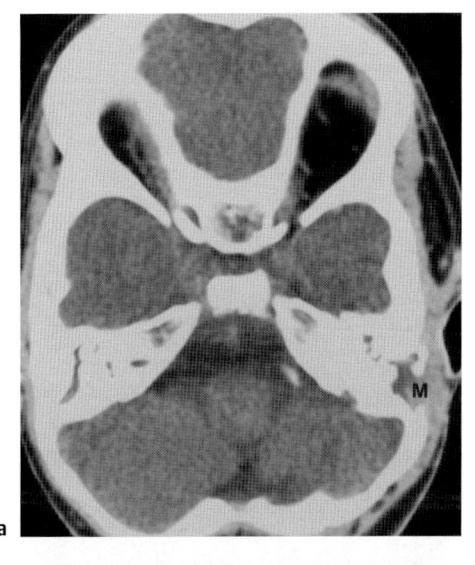

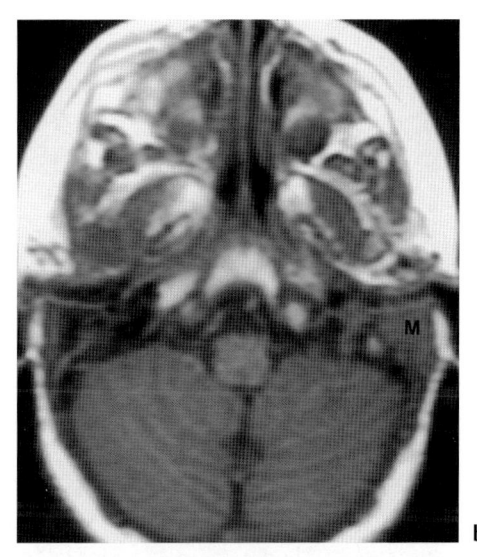

Fig. 3.**118** Langerhans cell histiocytosis of both mastoid temporal bones. **a** CT scan shows a mass (M) involving the left mastoid region. **b** T1W MR scan shows that the mass (M) is hypointense. **c** Coronal CT shows a destructive mass (M) involving the left mastoid. **d** Coronal CT scan shows a mass (M) with cortical bone erosion, involving the right mastoid as well. Note multiple lytic lesions, involving the mandible. This child also had bilateral pneumothorax.

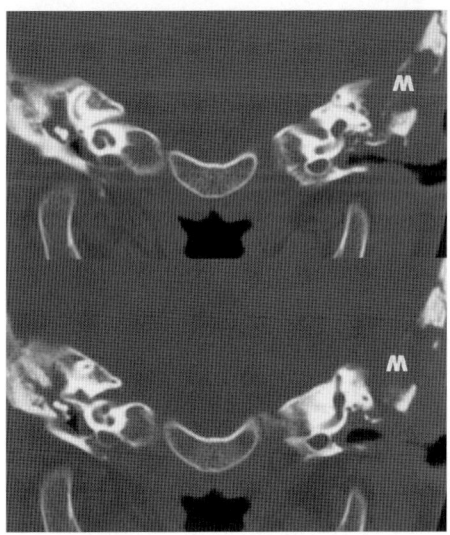

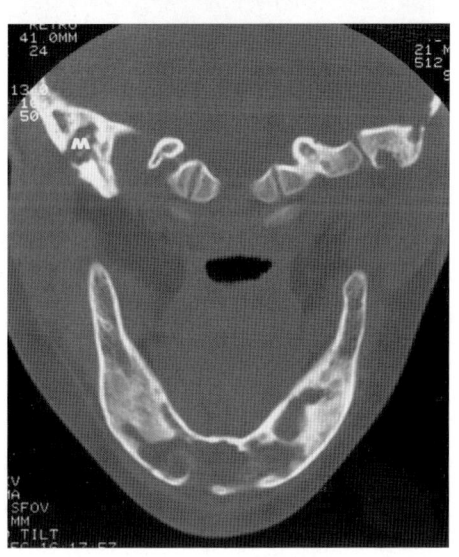

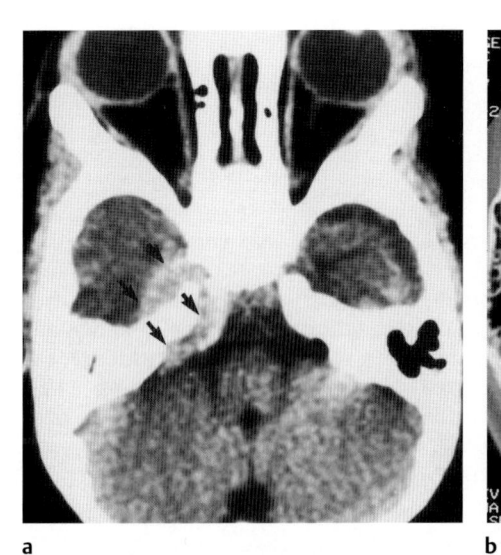

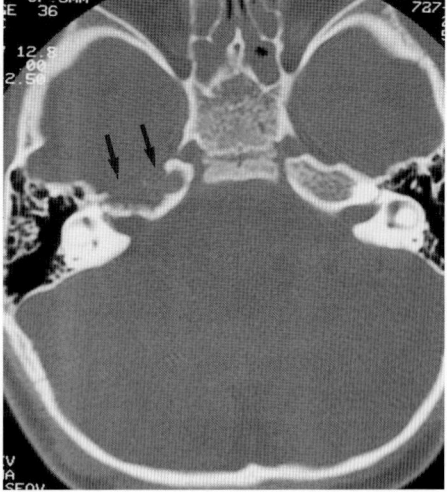

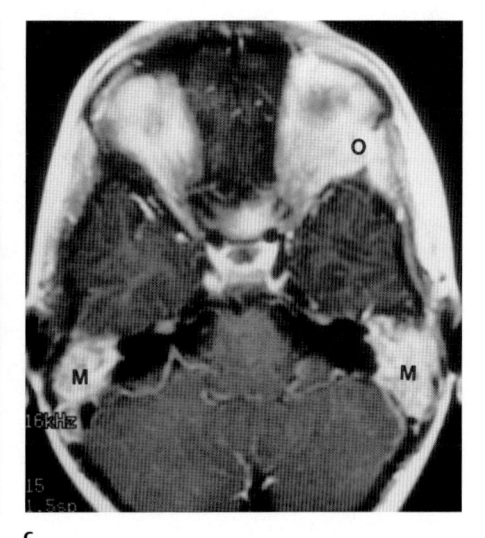

Fig. 3.**119** Langerhans histiocytosis. **a** Enhanced CT scan shows an infiltrative process with marked enhancement involving the right petrous apex (arrows). **b** CT scan shows cortical erosion of the petrous apex (arrows). **c** Gd-enhanced T1W MR scan in another patient shows bilateral mastoid (M) and left orbital (O) involvement with Langerhans cell histiocytosis. Figure **c** courtesy of Robert Schamschula, MD, Australia.

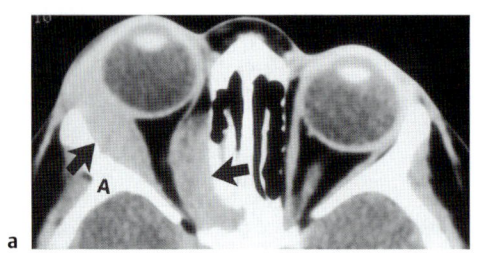

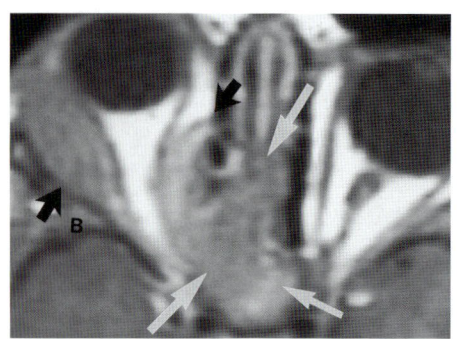

Fig. 3.**120** Chloroma. **a** Enhanced CT scan and **b** Gd-enhanced T1W MR scans, showing subperiosteal leukemic infiltration (arrows) involving the right orbit and the floor of the anterior cranial fossa (white arrows).

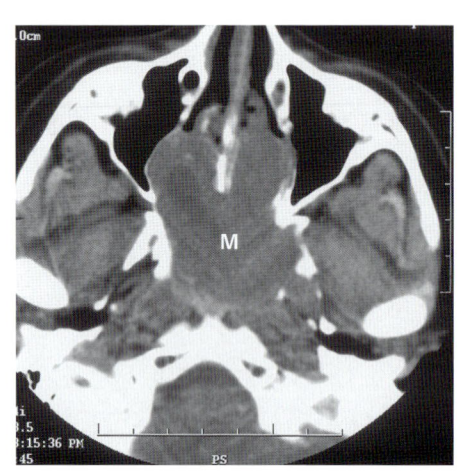

Fig. 3.**121** Angiofibroma. Axial unenhanced CT scan, showing a large nasopharyngeal mass (M) extending into the nasal cavities.

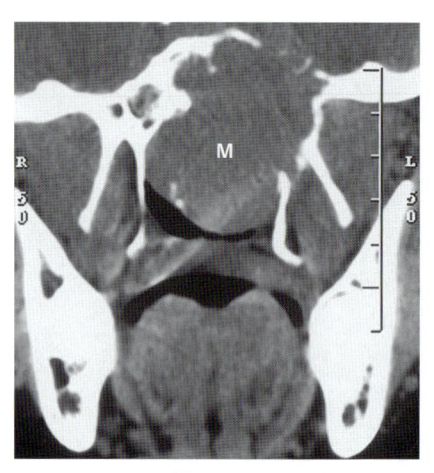

Fig. 3.**122** Angiofibroma. Coronal unenhanced CT scan, showing extension of a nasopharyngeal mass (M) into the sphenoid sinus. Note erosion of the pterygoid base with tumor reaching the left cavernous sinus.

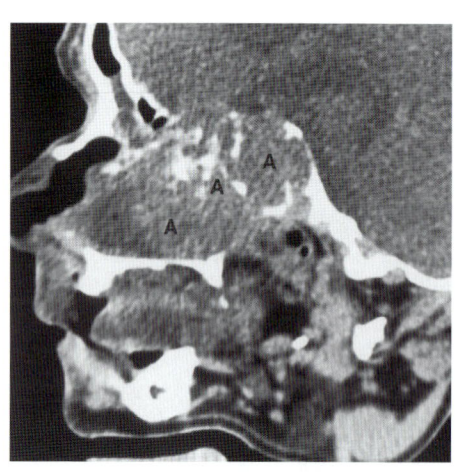

Fig. 3.**123** Adenocarcinoma of ethmoid invading the anterior cranial fossa. Sagittal CT scan shows adenocarcinoma (A) involving the naso-ethmoid complex, extending into the sphenoid sinus and eroding the floor of the anterior cranial fossa.

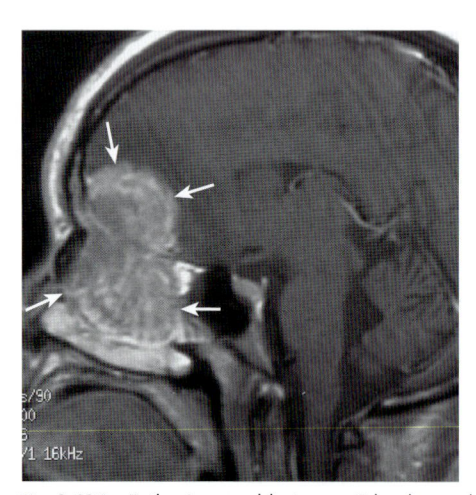

Fig. 3.**124** Esthesioneuroblastoma. Gd-enhanced sagittal T1W MR scan shows marked enhancement of this esthesioneuroblastoma with marked extension into the anterior cranial fossa (arrows).

associated with extension into cranial nerves and spinal nerve roots. Chloroma (granulocytic sarcoma) is related to the formation of solid tumor masses by leukemic infiltrates in bones and soft tissues (Fig. 3.**120**). The characteristic green color of the lesions is due to the myeloperoxidase content of the neoplastic cells.

■ Extracranial Lesions Affecting the Skull Base

The extracranial lesions commonly affecting the skull base include juvenile angiofibroma (Fig. 3.**121**, 3.**122**); carcinoma of the nasopharynx; tumors (Figs. 3.**123**–3.**125**)[49–52] and infections of the paranasal sinuses (Figs. 3.**43**–3.**47**)[53] and temporal bone (necrotizing otitis externa) (Figs. 3.**48**–3.**51**); glomus complex tumors (Figs. 3.**69**–3.**72**); hemangiopericytoma; aggressive fibromatosis (Fig. 3.**114**); neurogenic tumors (Figs. 3.**80**–3.**84**); and metastatic retropharyngeal and skull base nodal or soft-tissue deposits.

Tumors and inflammatory lesions of the paranasal sinuses may spread intracranially through the base of the skull. Lesions of the paranasal sinuses, orbits, or nasal cavities, which may involve the skull base, include mucoceles (Fig. 3.**36a,b**); carcinomas (Fig. 3.**123**); esthesioneuroblastoma (Figs. 3.**124**, 3.**125**); lacrimal gland tumors (adenoid cystic carcinoma, adenocarcinoma); parotid gland tumors (Fig. 3.**126**); rhabdomyosarcoma; lymphoma; and Langerhans cell histiocytosis. In adults, the most common lesion of the sinuses that invades the skull base is squamous cell carcinoma and esthesioneuroblastoma. Esthesioneuroblastoma arises from neuroepithelial cells of the olfactory region.[50–52] The sense of smell is located in a specialized sensory neuroepithelium that covers the superior nasal turbinates and the upper portion of the nasal septum. Since the superior turbinates, the cribriform plate, and the upper portion of the

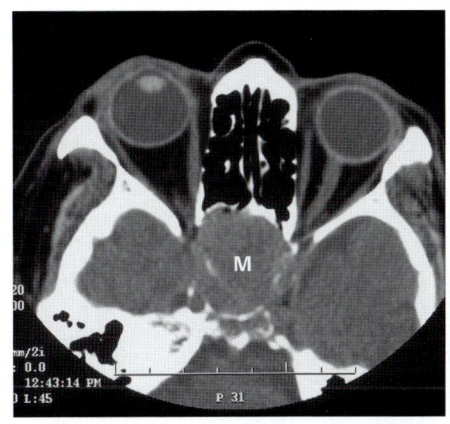

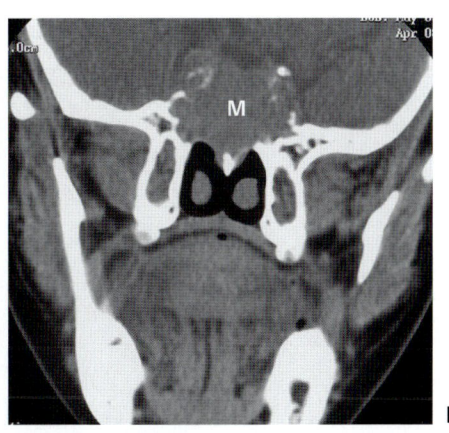

Fig. 3.**125** Esthesioneuroblastoma, originating in the sphenoid sinus and invading the skull base. **a** Unenhanced axial and **b** coronal CT scans, showing a mass (M) in the sphenoid sinus invading the pterygoid processes and floor of the sphenoid sinus.

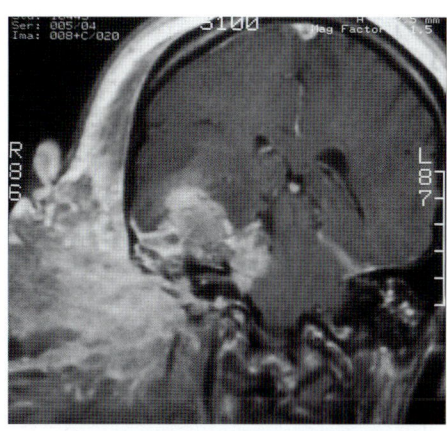

Fig. 3.**126** Undifferentiated carcinoma of the right parotid in a 25-year-old woman, with extension into the intracranial space. Gd-enhanced coronal T1W MR scan showing massive tumor involving the right parotid gland region with intracranial extension.

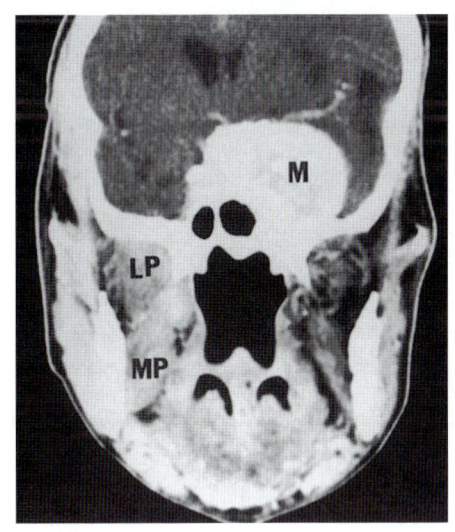

Fig. 3.**127** Denervation atrophy of masticator muscles. Postcontrast coronal CT scan shows a presumed parasellar meningeoma (M). Note the marked atrophy of the lateral and medial pterygoid muscles, as well as right masseter and temporalis muscles. Note the normal lateral (LP) and medial (MP) pterygoid muscles on the opposite side.

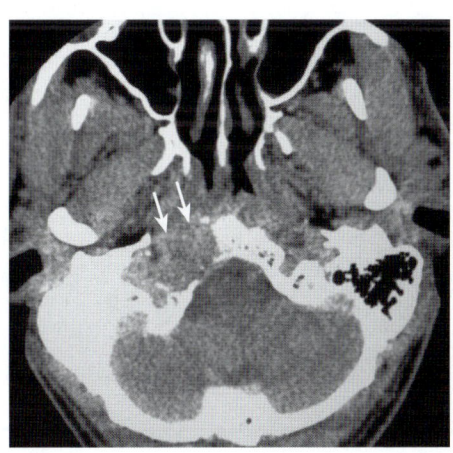

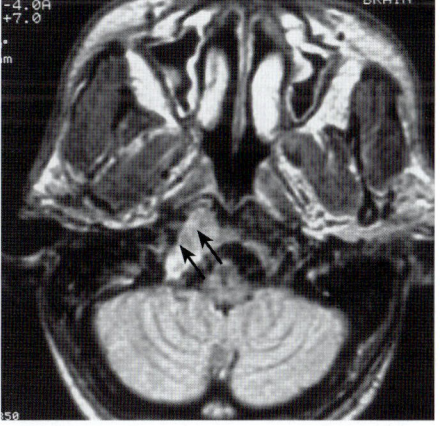

Fig. 3.**128** Base of skull metastasis from small-cell carcinoma of the lung. **a** CT scan shows a soft-tissue mass (arrows) with bony erosion of the right side of the clivus as well as the right hypoglossal canal. **b** PW MR scan shows replacement of the bone marrow in the same area as seen in **a** by a hyperintense pathological process.

nasal septum belong to the ethmoid, and because this tumor spreads very rapidly to the ethmoid sinus, it seems appropriate to include esthesioneuroblastomas in the classification of ethmoid tumors. In younger age groups, juvenile angiofibroma and lymphoma are more common. Lymphomas may be expansile or destructive. Although juvenile nasopharyngeal angiofibroma (JNA) is a benign neoplasm, it is an aggressive and extremely vascular one that is capable of bone destruction and intracranial extension (Fig. 3.**121**, 3.**122**).[49] Maxillary removal and reinsertion is a technique developed by Schuller and colleagues[14] as a method to gain wide surgical access to the anterior cranial base for resection of a tumor such as JNA, while preserving adjacent critical structures. Finally, atrophy of the muscles in the infratemporal fossa should call to mind possible abnormalities of the skull base, affecting cranial nerve V (Fig. 3.**127**).[7] Any abnormality involving the fifth cranial nerve may cause atrophy of the muscles of mastication (see Fig. 3.**30**). Any abnormality involving the tenth cranial nerve may involve the muscles of deglutition, namely, the pharyngeal and palatal muscles. Pseudoenlargement of the pterygoid muscles may occur after hemimandibulectomy. After hemimandibulectomy, the pterygoid and masseter muscles may pull the remnant of the ramus anteriorly and superiorly, effectively shortening the lateral pterygoid muscle and making it appear to be larger than the contralateral muscle. This should not be mistaken for tumor.

■ Metastasis

Metastatic lesions of the skull base are common in advanced cancers. They may be lytic (breast, kidney, thyroid, lung, plasmacytoma) or sclerotic (prostate) or mixed (prostate,

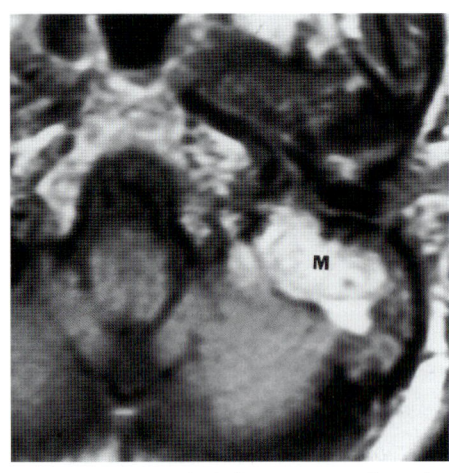

Fig. 3.**129** Base of skull metastasis from breast carcinoma. Gd-enhanced MR scan shows a markedly enhancing mass (M), involving the left petromastoid region.

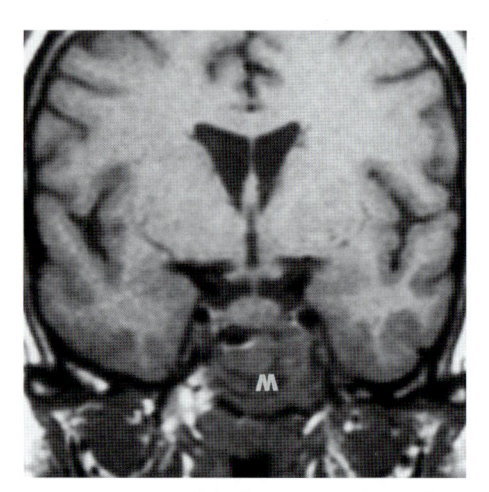

Fig. 3.**130** Base of skull metastasis from adenocarcinoma of the colon. Unenhanced T1W coronal MR scan shows a mass (M) involving the sphenoid bone.

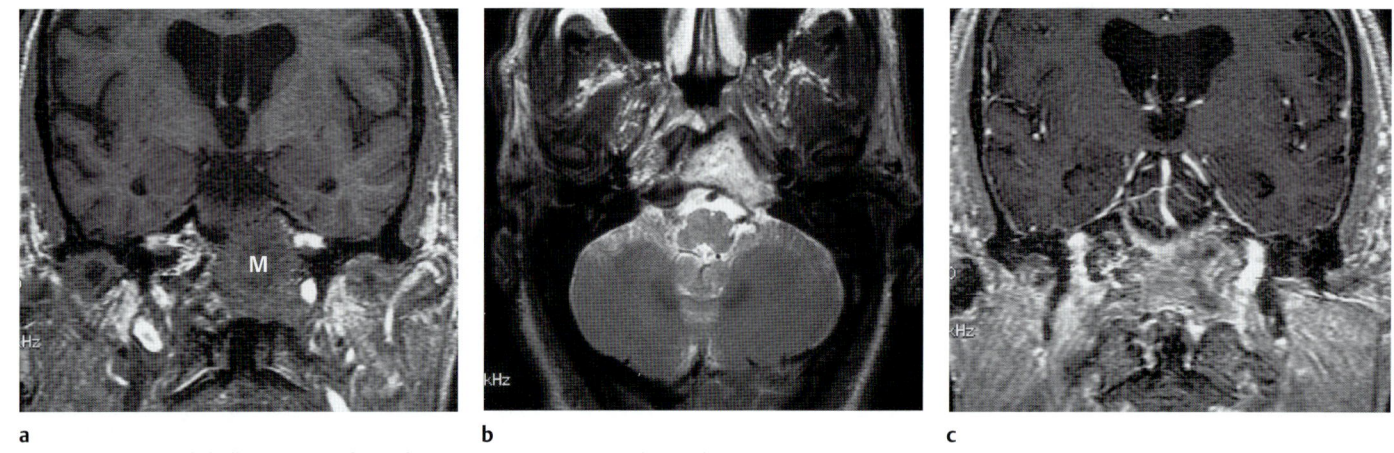

Fig. 3.**131** Base of skull metastasis from thyroid carcinoma. **a** Unenhanced coronal T1W, **b** axial T2W, and **c** Gd-enhanced coronal T1W MR scans obtained with a 3 T MRI unit, showing a metastatic lesion (M) involving the skull base.

breast). CT is the preferred method to demonstrate these bony lesions (Fig. 3.**128**).[7] MRI may be used to evaluate the soft-tissue component, bone marrow replacement, and the intracranial extension of the metastatic skull base deposits (Figs. 3.**129**–3.**131**).

■ Trauma

CT is the modality of choice for fracture of the base of the skull (Figs. 3.**132**–**137**). The site of the leak in CSF rhinorrhea and otorrhea can be detected most accurately using CT water-soluble iodinated contrast cisternography (Figs. 3.**138**, 3.**139**).[8,9] MRI is most valuable for showing soft-tissue contusion (Fig. 3.**140**) and extracerebral and intracerebral hemorrhages. Further discussions on skull-base trauma are presented in Chapters 1, 2, and 4.

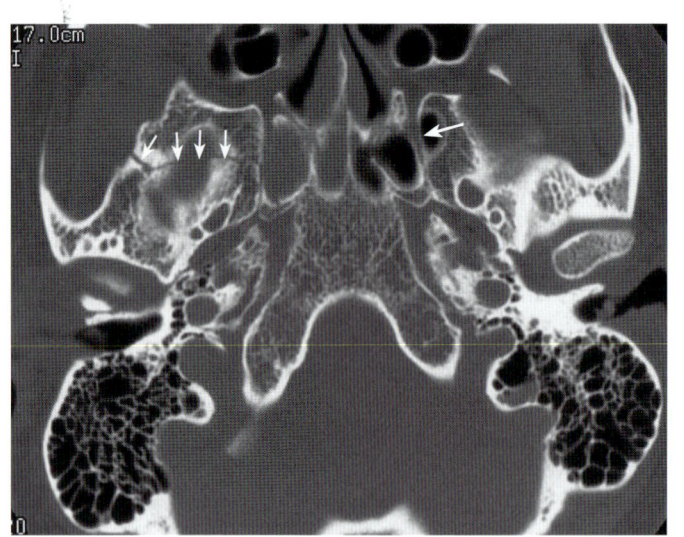

Fig. 3.**132** Base of skull fracture. Axial CT scan shows fracture involving the greater wing of sphenoid (small arrows), extending to involve the vidian canal. Note normal left vidian canal (long arrow). Opacification of right sphenoid sinus is due to hematoma.

Skull Base Pathology 347

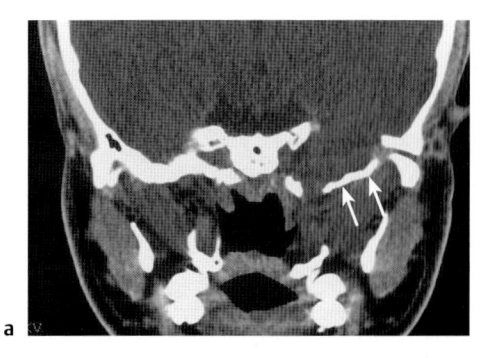

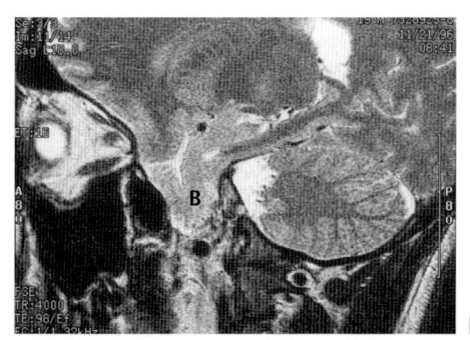

Fig. 3.**133** Depressed fracture of skull base with brain herniation. **a** Coronal CT scan shows depressed fracture of the left middle cranial fossa (arrows). **b** T2W sagittal MRI scan shows brain herniation (B).

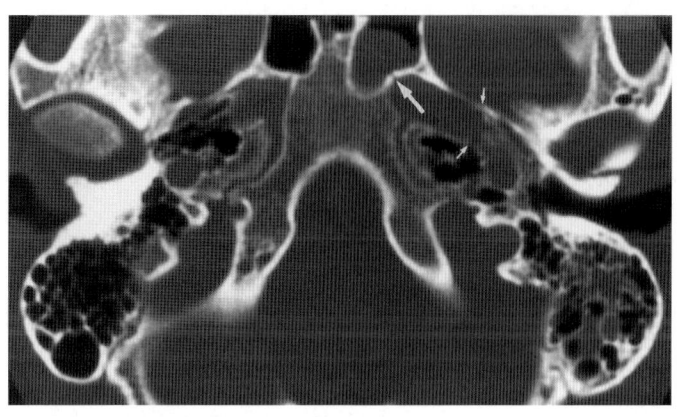

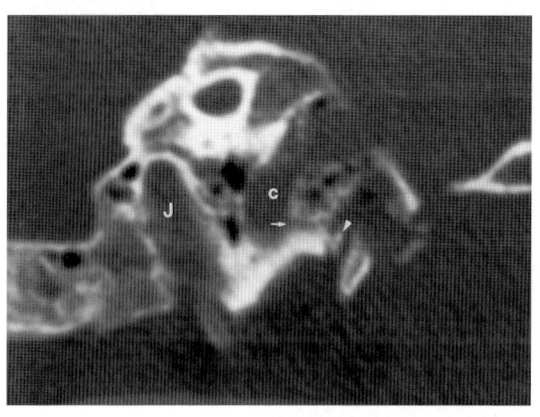

Fig. 3.**134** Fracture of carotid canal. **a** Axial CT scan shows fractures involving the left carotid canal (small arrows) and left sphenoid sinus (large arrow). **b** Sagittal CT shows normal jugular fossa (J) and fracture (arrow) of the carotid canal (C). Note bone fragment (arrowhead).

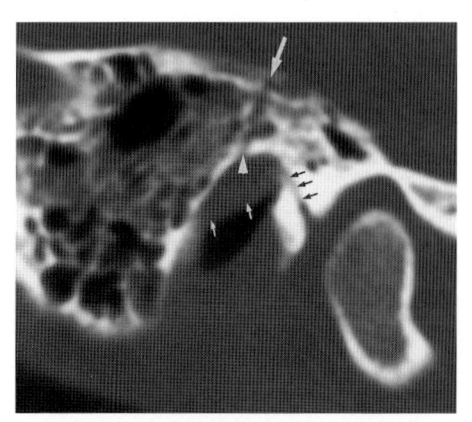

Fig. 3.**135** Base of skull fracture. Sagittal CT scan shows a fracture involving the floor of the middle cranial fossa (long arrow), extending to involve the superior wall of the external auditory canal (arrowhead). Note separation of the squamotympanic suture (black arrows) and soft-tissue, related to hematoma within external auditory canal (small white arrows).

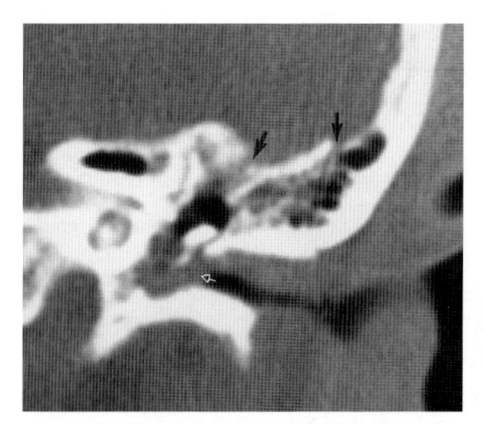

Fig. 3.**136** Depressed fracture of the floor of the middle cranial fossa, associated with CSF leak. Coronal CT scan shows fracture involving the floor of the middle cranial fossa (black arrows), including tegmen tympani. Note the thickened tympanic membrane (white arrow). The increased density in the middle ear is due to CSF and hemotympanum.

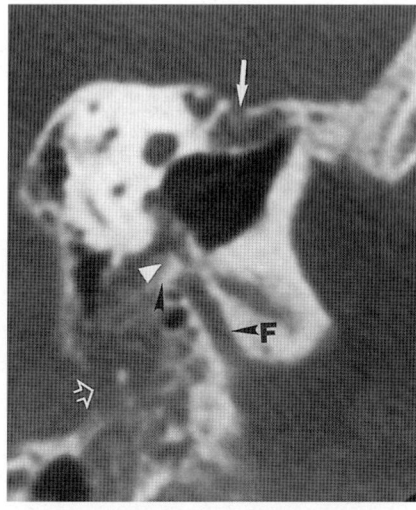

Fig. 3.**137** Fracture of the temporal bone. Direct semisagittal CT scan shows fracture of the mastoid involving the sigmoid sinus plate (hollow arrow), fracture of the facial canal with a bony fragment (arrowheads), extending into the facial canal (F), and a fracture involving the floor of the middle cranial fossa (solid arrow).

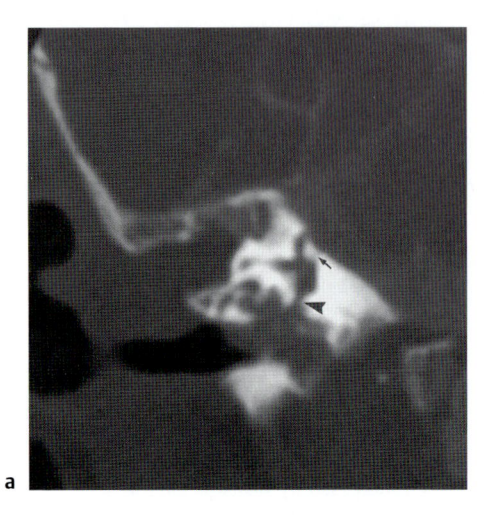

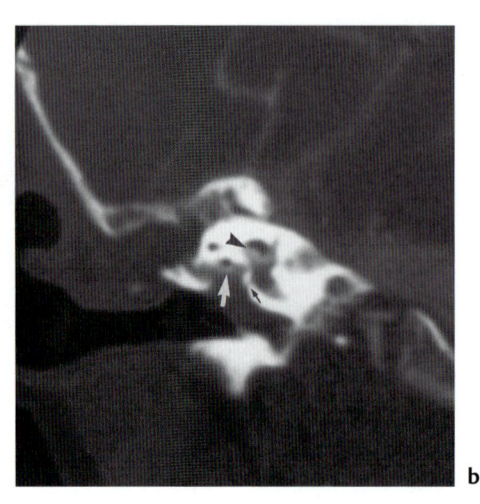

Fig. 3.**138** CSF otorrhea due to skull base fracture. **a** Coronal CT scan obtained following intrathecal injection of iodinated contrast material shows fracture along the basal turn of the cochlea (arrowhead), extending into the vestibule (arrow). Note soft-tissue changes in the middle ear and mastoid, related to prior mastoidectomy. **b** Coronal CT cisternogram shows CSF leaking into the vestibule (arrowhead) and middle ear cavity (white arrow). Note fracture of the basal turn of the cochlea (black arrow). This patient had mastoidectomy with soft-tissue obliteration of the mastoid cavity which did not resolve the CSF leak. Repair of the otic capsule fracture resolved the leak.

Fig. 3.**139** CSF leak. Direct coronal CT cisternogram shows the presence of CSF mixed with contrast within the ethmoid sinus (E). Note the defect of the cribiform plate. This patient had intranasal surgery for CSF leak, which did not solve the problem.

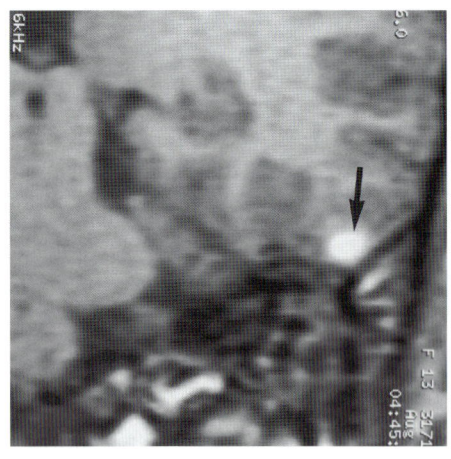

Fig. 3.**140** Skull base fracture. Coronal unenhanced T1W MR scan shows focal hematoma (arrow) at the site where a tegmental fracture was seen on CT scan.

References

1. Warwick R, Williams PL, eds. Gray's Anatomy, 35th British ed. Philadelphia: W.B. Saunders; 1973.
2. Noyek AM, Kassel EE, et al. Clinically directed CT in occult disease of the skull base involving foramen ovale. Laryngoscope 1982; 92: 1021–1027.
3. Som PM, Shugar JM, et al. A clinical radiographic classification of skull base lesions. Laryngoscope 1979; 89: 1066–1076.
4. Mafee MF, Aimi K, et al. CT in the diagnosis of primary tumors of the petrous bone. Laryngoscope 1984; 94: 1423–1430.
5. Mafee MF, Valvassori GE, et al. The role of radiology in surgery of the ear and skull base. Otolaryngol Clin North Am 1982; 15: 723–723.
6. Kumar A, Valvassori GE, et al. Skull base lesions: a classification and surgical approach. Laryngoscope 1986; 96: 252–263.
7. Weber AL. Imaging of the skull base. Eur J Radiol 1996; 22: 68–81.
8. Mafee MF, Valvassori GE " et al. Tumors and tumor-like conditions of the middle ear and mastoid: role of CT and MRI: an analysis of 100 cases. Otolaryngol Clin North Am 1988; 21: 349–375.
9. Mafee MF, Valvassori GE, Dobben GD. The role of radiology in surgery of the ear and skull base. Otolaryngol Clin North Am, 1982; 15(4): 723–753.
10. Lewark TM, Allen GC, Chowdhury K, et al. LeFort I osteotomy and skull base tumors. Arch Otolaryngol Head Neck Surg 2000; 126: 1004–1008.
11. Shelton JC, Antonelli PJ, Hackett R. Skull base fungal osteomyelitis in an immunocompetent host. Otolaryngol Head Neck Surg 2002; 126: 76–78.
12. Schuller DE, Hart MC, Goodman JH. The surgery of benign and malignant neoplasms adjacent to or involving the skull base. Am J Otolaryngol 1989; 1: 305–313.
13. Powell DM, Shah N, Carr A, et al. Maxillary removal and reinsertion in pediatric patients. Arch Otolaryngol Head Neck Surg 2002; 128: 29–34.
14. Schuller DE, Goodman JH, Brown BL, et al. Maxillary removal and re-insertion for improved access to anterior cranial base tumors. Laryngoscope 1992; 102: 203–212.
15. Pisneski M, Mafee MF, Samii M. Applications of MR angiography in head and neck pathology. Otolaryngol Clin North Am 1995; 28(3): 543–561.
16. Cantu G, Solero CL, Mariani L, et al. A new classification for malignant tumors involving the anterior skull base. Arch Otolaryngol Head Neck Surg 1999; 125: 1252–1257.
17. Colreavy MP, Baker T, Campbell M, et al. The safety and effectiveness of the LeFort I approach to removing central skull base lesions. ENT Ear Nose Throat J 2001; 80: 315–320.
18. Fitzek C, Mewes T, Fitzek S, et al. Diffusion-weighted MRI of cholesteatoma of the petrous bone. J Magn Reson Imaging 2002; 15: 636–641.
19. Thorton J, Bachir Q, Aletich VA, et al. Role of MRI and diagnostic and interventional angiography in vascular and neoplastic diseases of the skull base associated with vestibulocochlear symptoms. Topics Magn Reson Imaging 2000; 11(2): 123–137.
20. Dobben GD, Philip B, Mafee MF, et al. Orbital subperiosteal hematoma, cholesterol granuloma, and infection: evaluation with MR imaging and CT. Radiol Clin North Am 1998; 36: 1185–1200.

21 Mafee MF, Smirniotopoulos JG, Goodwin J. Imaging of chiasmal and juxtasellar regions. Ophthalmol Clin North Am 1994; 7: 347–366.
22 Shin JH, Byun BJ, Kim DW, Choi DL. Neurenteric cyst in the cerebellopontine angle with xanthogranulomatous changes: serial MR findings with pathological correlation. AJNR 2002; 23: 663–665.
23 Bevetta S, El-Shunnar K, Hamlyn PJ. Neurenteric cyst of the anterior cranial fossa. Br J Neurosurg 1996; 10: 225–227.
24 Kapoor V, Douglas R, Melanie J, et al. Neuroradiological-pathological correlation in a neurenteric cyst of the clivus. AJNR 2002; 23: 476–479.
25 Brooks BS, Duvall ER, Gammal TE, et al. Neuroimaging features of neurenteric cysts: analysis of nine cases and review of the literature. AJNR 1993; 14: 735–746.
26 Randall RV, Scheithauer BW, Laws ER, et al. Pituitary adenomas associated with hyperprolactinemia: a clinical and immunohistochemical study of 97 patients operated on transsphenoidally. Mayo Clin Proc 1985; 60: 753–762.
27 Charbel FT, Hyun H, Misra M, et al. Juxtaorbital en plaque meningiomas; report of four cases and review of literature. Radiol Clin North Am 1999; 37: 89–100.
28 Mafee MF, Valvassori GE, Shugar MA, et al. High resolution and dynamic sequential computed tomography: use in the evaluation of glomus complex tumors. Arch Otolarynol 1983; 109: 691–696.
29 Mafee MF, Raofi B, Kumar A, Muscato C. Glomus faciale, glomus jugulare, glomus tympanicum, glomus vagale, carotid body tumors, and simulating lesions. Radiol Clin North Am 2000; 38: 1059–1076.
30 Wenig BM, Mafee MF, Ghosh L. Fibro-osseous, osseous, and cartilaginous lesions of the orbit and paraorbital lesion: correlative clinicopathological and radiographic features, including the diagnostic role of CT and MR imaging. Radiol Clin North Am 1998; 36: 1241–1259.
31 Neff B, Sataloff RT, Storey L, et al. Chondrosarcoma of the skull base. Laryngoscope, 2002; 112: 134–139.
32 Koch BB, Karnell LH, Hoffman HT, et al. National cancer database report on chondrosarcoma of the head and neck. Head Neck 2000; 22: 408–425.
33 Shinaver CN, Mafee MF, Choi KH. MRI of mesenchymal chondrosarcoma of the orbit: case report and review of the literature. Neuroradiology 1997; 39: 296–301.
34 Chen CC, Hsu L, Hecht JL, Janecka I. Bimaxillary chondrosarcomas: clinical, radiological, and histologtic correlation. AJNR 2002; 23: 667–670.
35 Rosenberg AE, Nielson GP, Kiel SB, et al. Chondrosarcoma of the base of the skull: a clinical pathological study of 200 cases with emphasis in its distinction from chardoma. Am J Surg Pathol 1999; 23: 1370–1378.
36 Brown E, Hug EB, Weber AL. Chondrosarcoma of the skull base. Neuroimaging Clin North Am 1994; 14: 429–541.
37 Mafee MF, Pai E, Philip B. Rhabdomyosarcoma of the orbit: evaluation with MR imaging and CT. Radiol Clin North Am 1998; 36: 1215–1227.
38 Wenig B, ed. Atlas of Head and Neck Pathology. Philadelphia: W.B. Saunders; 1993.
39 Amato MM, Esmaeli B, Shore JW. Orbital rhabdomyosarcoma metastatic to contralateral orbit. Ophthalmology 2002; 109: 753–756.
40 Seedat R, et al. Rhabdomyosarcoma. Int J Pediatr Otorhinolaryngol 2000; 52: 177–181.
41 Heffner DK. Low grade papillary adenocarcinoma of endolymphatic sac. Cancer 1989; 64: 2292–2302.
42 Hassard AD, Boudreau SF, Cron CE. Adenoma of the endolymphatic sac. J. Otolaryngol 1984; 13: 213–216.
43 Mafee MF, Wee R Lee, Mafee RF. Imaging of vestibular aqueduct, endolymphatic duct and sac and adenocarcinoma of probable endolymphatic sac origin. Rivista Neuroradiol 1995; 8: 951–961.
43a Mafee MF, Shah H. Endolymphatic sac tumors and papillary adenocarcinoma of the temporal bone. Role of MRI and CT. Iranian J Radiol, in press.
44 De Angelis LM. Primary central nervous system lymphoma: a new clinical challenge. Neurology 1991; 41: 619.
45 Sapozink MD, Kaplan HS: Intracranial Hodgkin disease: a report of 12 cases and review of the literature. Cancer 1983; 52: 1301.
46 Ashby MA, Barber PC, Holmes AE, et al. Primary intracranial Hodgkin's disease: a case report and discussion. Am J Surg Pathol 1988; 12: 294.
47 Mancardi GL, Mandybur TI. Solitary intracranial plasmacytoma. Cancer 1983; 51: 2226.
48 Hydayat AA, Mafee MF, Laver NV, Noujaim S. Langerhans cell histiocytosis and juvenile xanthogranuloma of the orbit. Clinicopathological, CT, and MR imaging features. Radiol Clin North Am 1998; 36: 1229–1240.
49 Gullane PJ, Davidson J, O'Dwyer T, Forte V. Juvenile angiofibroma: a review of the literature and case series report. Laryngoscope 1992; 102: 928–933.
50 Kadish S, Goodman M, Wang CC. Olfactory neuroblastoma: a clinical analysis of 17 cases. Cancer 1976; 37: 1571–1576.
51 Austin JR, Cebrun H, Kershisnik MM, et al. Olfactory neuroblastoma and neuroendocrine carcinoma of the anterior skull base: treatment results at the M.D. Anderson Cancer Center. Skull Base Surg 1996; 6: 1–8.
52 Dulguerov P, Calcaterra T. Esthesioneuroblastoma: the UCLA experience 1970–1990. Laryngoscope 1992; 102: 843–849.
53 Som PM, Brandwein M. Sinonasal cavities: Inflammatory diseases, tumors, fractures and postoperative findings. In: Som PM, Curtin HD, eds. Head and Neck Imaging, Vol 1. St. Louis: Mosby-Yearbook Inc; 1996: 126–315.

Section III Nasal Cavity and Paranasal Sinuses

Chapter 4 **Imaging of the Nasal Cavity and Paranasal Sinuses**

Nasal Cavity: Embryology and Development 353

Paranasal Sinuses: Embryology and Development 353

Anatomy of the Nasal Cavity 355

Anatomy of the Paranasal Sinuses 358

Pterygomaxillary Fissure, Pterygopalatine (Sphenopalatine) Fossa, and Palatine Bone 371

Imaging Techniques 379

Sinonasal Pathology 386

4 Imaging of the Nasal Cavity and Paranasal Sinuses

M. F. Mafee

Nasal Cavity: Embryology and Development

The branchial apparatus (i.e., branchial arches, branchial grooves, pharyngeal pouches, and branchial membranes) plays an important role in the formation of the face, nasal cavity, oral cavity, and neck, as it also does in the formation of the pharynx and larynx.[1] The first branchial arches are usually referred to as the mandibular and the second as the hyoid arches. Each branchial arch consists of an ectodermal exterior, a mesenchymal core, and an endodermal interior. The mesenchyme produces a skeletal element, which subsequently chondrifies either wholly or in part.[1] Most of the remainder of the core of mesenchyme (paraxial and prechordal) becomes striated muscle. Most of the facial mesenchymes are provided by the neural crest cells. The human mandibular arch grows ventromedially in the floor of the primitive pharynx to meet its fellow in the midline. The hyoid arch similarly grows ventrally to meet and fuse in the midline. While the mandibular prominence (process) is invading the floor of the primitive pharynx, the mesenchyme between the central aspect of the forebrain and the epithelial roof of the primitive mouth proliferates and bulges under the ectoderm to form the frontonasal elevation (prominence) or process. The facial prominences (frontonasal, maxillary, and mandibular) appear around the fourth week of gestation and give rise to the boundaries and structures of the face (Fig. 4.1).[2] The paired mandibular and maxillary prominences give rise to the lateral facial structures; the frontonasal prominence gives rise to the structures of the midface. During the fifth week a thickened plaque of ectoderm develops on each side ventrolaterally to the frontonasal elevation, dividing this into medial (nasomedial) and lateral (nasolateral) nasal elevations (swelling) or folds (Fig. 4.1). These thickenings are the olfactory or nasal placodes. They are at first widely separated and, as the elevations develop, they soon become depressed to form the olfactory pits (nasal pits).[1] Extensions of mesenchyme from the nasomedial elevation into the roof of the primitive mouth (stomatodeum) proliferate to form the premaxillary or the globular fields: the globular processes of His.[1]

The growth of the mesenchyme surrounding the olfactory pit (nasal pit) leads to a deepening of the pit to become a primitive nasal cavity, or nasal sac, the forerunner of the nasal cavities. The paired maxillary prominences, like the frontal prominence, consist of proliferating mesenchyme covered by ectoderm. The maxillary prominence grows in a ventral direction and becomes fused with the lateral nasal prominence (fold), the two being at first separated by the nasomaxillary groove. The ectoderm along the boundary between the nasolateral and maxillary elevations gives rise to the solid cellular rod, which becomes canalized to form the nasolacrimal duct. During the next weeks, the internal aspects of the maxillary processes produce palatine processes, which grow toward the midline. The palatine bone is ossified in a membrane of connective tissue from one center, which appears during the eighth week of fetal life in its perpendicular plate.[1] The nasal capsule is well-developed by the end of the third month.[1] The free caudal border of each of its lateral parts becomes incurved to form the

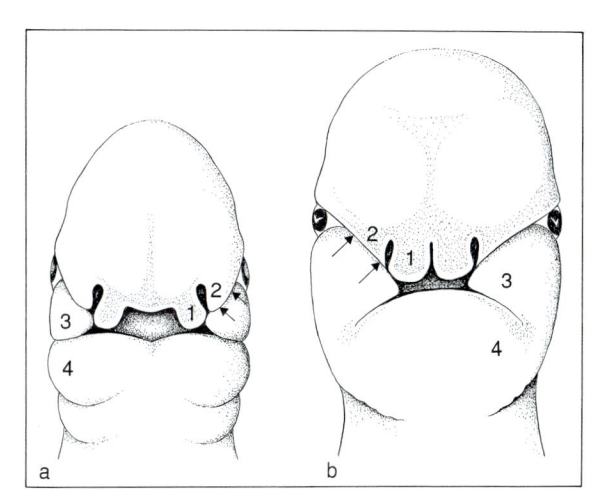

Fig. 4.1 Frontal views of the fetal face at **a** 5 weeks and **b** 6–7 weeks of gestation. 1 = Nasomedial process; 2 = nasolateral process; 3 = maxillary process; 4 = mandibular process; arrows indicate nasolacrimal grooves. Modified from Castillo M. Congenital abnormalities of the nose: CT and MR findings. AJR 1994; 162: 1211–1217, with permission.

inferior nasal concha, which ossifies (membranous bone) during the fifth fetal month and becomes a separate bone.[1] Posteriorly, the lateral portion of the nasal capsule becomes ossified as the ethmoidal bone, bearing on its medial surface ridges that become the middle, superior, and supreme chonchae. Part of the rest of the nasal capsule remains cartilaginous as the septal and alar cartilages of the nose; part is replaced by the mesenchymal vomer and nasal bones.[1] The anterior portion of the nasal cavity is called the vestibule, the epithelium of which is ectodermally derived and represents the internal extension of the integument of the external nose; similarly, the epithelium lining the nasal cavities proper (schneiderian membrane) is of ectodermal origin.[2] The olfactory epithelia develop in the superoposterior portion of each nasal cavity and differentiate from cells in the ectodermally derived nasal cavity epithelium.[2]

Paranasal Sinuses: Embryology and Development

■ Maxillary Sinuses

The paranasal sinuses develop as outgrowths of the walls of the developing nasal cavities in the regions of the nasal meatuses.[2,3] Maxillary and ethmoid sinuses develop during fetal life. Although the frontal and sphenoid sinuses originate during fetal life, they are not large enough to be present at birth but develop during the early years of life.[2,3] The maxillary sinuses begin as a bud in the lateral wall of the ethmoid portion of the nasal capsule in the third fetal month.[3] The size of the sinus at birth is estimated at 6–8 mm.[3] By 4–5 months after birth, the maxillary sinus can be readily identified, particularly on CT scans (Fig. 4.2). After birth, growth of the maxillary sinus continues rapidly until

354 4 Imaging of the Nasal Cavity and Paranasal Sinuses

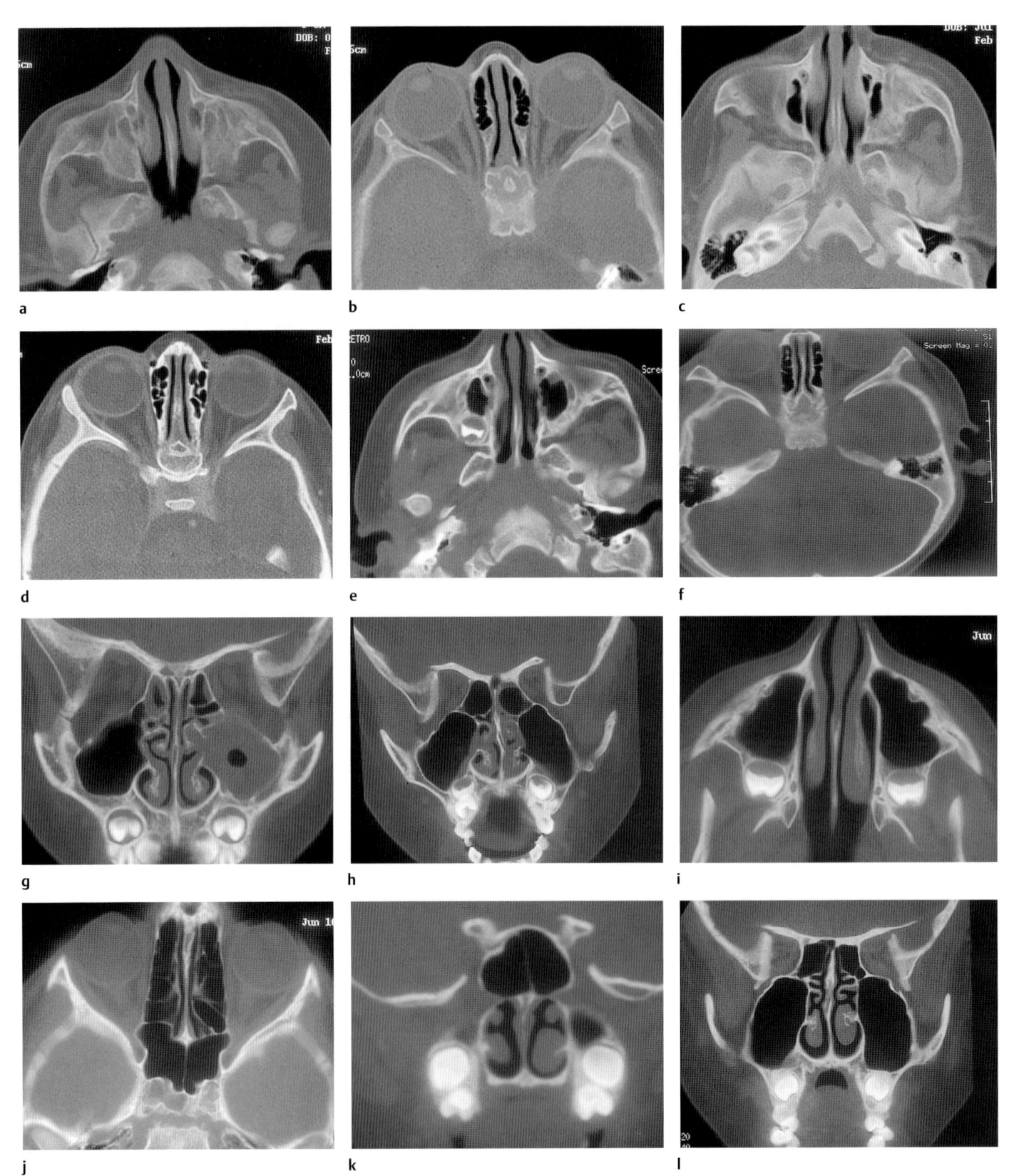

Fig. 4.2 Development (longitudinal) of paranasal sinuses. **a, b** CT scans of a 3-month-old infant. Note that the maxillary sinuses are small and not yet pneumatized. In some infants, air may be present within maxillary sinuses in the first few days or weeks of life. The ethmoid air cells are well pneumatized (**b**). **c** Axial and **d** CT scans of a 7-month-old infant showing normal pneumatization of maxillary sinuses and ethmoid air cells. **e, f** CT scans of a 2-year-old child. **g** CT scans of a 3-year-old child, **h** a 5-year-old child, **i, j, k** a 6-year-old child, and **l** a 10-year-old child, showing normal longitudinal development of paranasal sinuses except in **g**, which shows left maxillary sinusitis in a 3-year-old child.

about 3 years of age (Fig. 4.2 c, e, g), and then slowly progresses until the seventh year (Fig. 4.2 h).[3] At this time another acceleration in growth occurs until the age of 12 years. Following the eruption of the secondary dentition, further growth occurs related to invasion of the alveolar process of the maxilla.[3]

■ Ethmoid Sinuses

The anterior and middle ethmoid air cells begin as evaginations of the lateral wall of the developing nasal cavity, in the region of the future mucosa of the middle meatus, approximately in the third month of fetal life.[3] Shortly afterward, posterior ethmoid cells begin to evaginate the nasal mucosa in the superior meatus. At birth the anterior group is approximately 5 mm in height, 2 mm in length, and 2 mm in width, and the posterior group is 5 mm in height, 4 mm in length, and 2 mm in width.[3] After birth or a few months later, the ethmoid air cells can be readily identified on CT scans (Fig. 4.2 b, d). By the age of 12 years, the ethmoids have almost reached their adult size (Fig. 4.2 h) (24 mm in height, 23 mm in length, and 11 mm in width for the anterior group; and 21 mm in height, 21 mm in length, and 12 mm in width for the posterior group).[3]

■ Frontal Sinuses

Each frontal sinus develops in the ethmoid portion of the nasal capsule in the region of the frontal recess. At birth it is indistinguishable from the anterior ethmoid air cells.[3] Postnatal growth is slow, and at one year the sinus is barely perceptible anatomically. At about the fourth year, the frontal sinus begins to invade the vertical plate of the frontal bone. The sinus increases progressively in size until the late teens.[3]

■ Sphenoid Sinuses

The sphenoid sinuses develop in the third month of fetal life as an extension (evagination) of the developing nasal cavities. Although the sphenoid sinus can be identified as a tiny cavity in sections of the fetus at 4 months, the sinus remains small at birth and is little more than an evagination of the sphenoethmoid recess.[3] After the fifth year, development of the sphenoid sinuses is more rapid, and by the age of 7 years the sinuses have extended posteriorly to the level of the sella turcica (Fig. 4.2 k).[3] Further growth occurs until 12 years. After the twelfth year, the growth may extend to include the basisphenoid and pterygoid processes (lateral processes) of the sphenoid bone.

Anatomy: The Nasal Cavity

The nasal cavity, the first of the upper airway passages, extends from the roof of the mouth upward to the base of the skull (Fig. 4.3 a). It is divided by the nasal septum into two halves that open on the face via the external nares or nostrils, and communicates behind with the nasopharynx via the posterior nasal apertures, the choanae (Fig. 4.3 b, c). The framework of the external nose is composed of bones and hyaline cartilages. Its bony framework consists of the nasal bones, the frontal (nasal) processes of the maxillae, and the nasal part of the frontal bone. The cartilaginous framework consists of septal, lateral, and major and minor alar nasal cartilages. These are connected with one another and with the bones by the continuity of the perichondrium and the periosteum.[1]

The septal cartilage forms almost the whole of the nasal septum in the anterior part of the nasal cavity. Its posterosuperior border is attached to the perpendicular plate of the ethmoid bone and its posteroinferior border is attached to the vomer and the nasal crest of the maxillae and the anterior nasal spine (Fig. 4.3 a, c). The vomer is a thin trapezoidal bone that forms the posteroinferior part of the bony nasal septum. It has two surfaces and four borders. Its superior border is the thickest and presents a deep furrow, bounded on each side by a projecting ala. The furrow fits over the rostrum of the sphenoid bone.[1] The alae articulate with the sphenoidal conchae, the sphenoidal processes of the palatine bones, and the vaginal process of the medial pterygoid plates.[1] The inferior border articulates with the nasal crest, formed by the maxilla and palatine bones. Its anterior border is the longest; its upper half articulates with the perpendicular plate of the ethmoid, and its lower half is cleft to receive the inferior margin of the cartilage of the nasal septum. The posterior border is free and separates the posterior nasal apertures (choanae). The anterior end of the vomer articulates with the posterior margin of the incisor crest of the maxillae and projects downward between the incisive canals. The posterior nasal apertures or choanae are two oval openings, each measuring about 2.5 cm in the vertical and 1.25 cm in the transverse dimension. Each half of the nasal cavity can be described as having a roof, a floor, a medial (septal) wall and a lateral wall. It consists of three regions: vestibular, respiratory, and olfactory. The nasal vestibule is a slight dilatation just inside the aperture of the nostril. It is lined with skin, coarse hairs, and sebaceous and sweat glands. The vestibule is limited above and behind by a curved elevation, named the limen nasi (mucocutaneous junction), which corresponds to the upper margin of the lower nasal cartilage and along which the skin of the vestibule is continuous with the mucous membrane of the nasal cavity.[1] The respiratory region is the largest region of the nasal cavity and is located between the vestibule and the olfactory region. The olfactory region is limited to the superior nasal concha, the upper part of the nasal septum, and the intervening roof.[1]

The roof of the nasal cavity is narrow from side to side and may be divided into frontonasal, ethmoidal, and sphenoidal parts, corresponding to the bones that contribute to its formation. Its anterior, the frontonasal part, is formed by the nasal spine of the frontal bone and the nasal bones. The ethmoidal (horizontal) part is formed by the cribriform plate of the ethmoid bone and separates the nasal cavity from the medial part of the floor of the anterior cranial fossa (Fig. 4.3 a, c). It contains numerous small openings for the passage of the olfactory nerves. The sphenoidal part is formed by a portion of the body of the sphenoid bone.

The floor of the nasal cavity is concave from side to side. Its anterior three-fourths is formed by the palatine process of the maxilla, its posterior one-fourth by the horizontal part of the palatine bone (Figs. 4.3, 4.4). In its anterior part, there is a small tunnel-shaped opening that leads into the incisor (incisive) canals (Fig. 4.3 c).

The medial wall is formed by the bony nasal septum and the septal cartilage, and is often deviated from the median plane. The bony nasal septum is formed almost entirely by the vomer and the perpendicular plate of the ethmoid (Fig. 4.3 a).

The lateral wall of the nasal cavity is very irregular owing to the presence of three bony projections: the superior, middle, and inferior nasal conchae (Fig. 4.3). Its bony portion is formed, for the most part, below and in front by the nasal surface of the maxilla (Fig. 4.3 a), posteriorly by the perpendicular plate of the palatine bone, and above by the nasal surface of the ethmoidal labyrinth, which intervenes between the nasal cavity and the

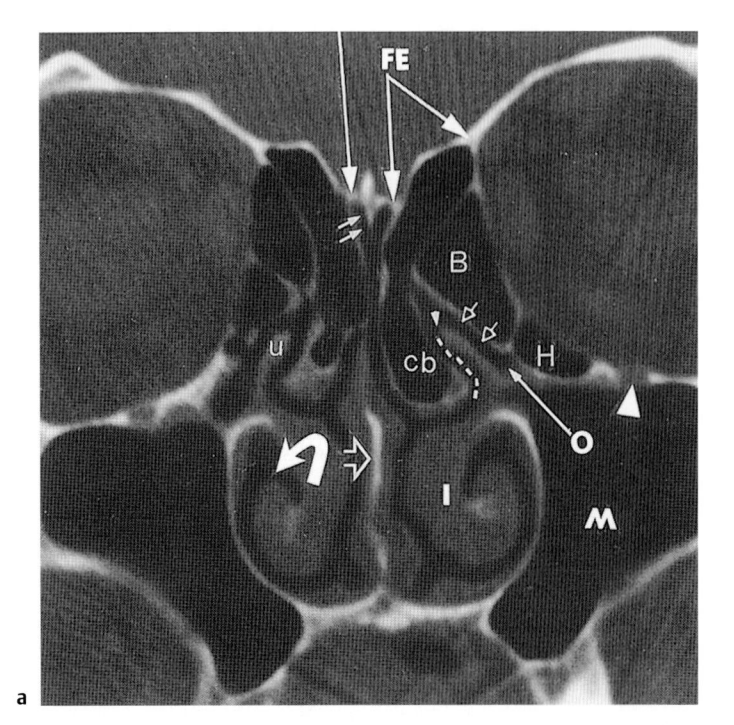

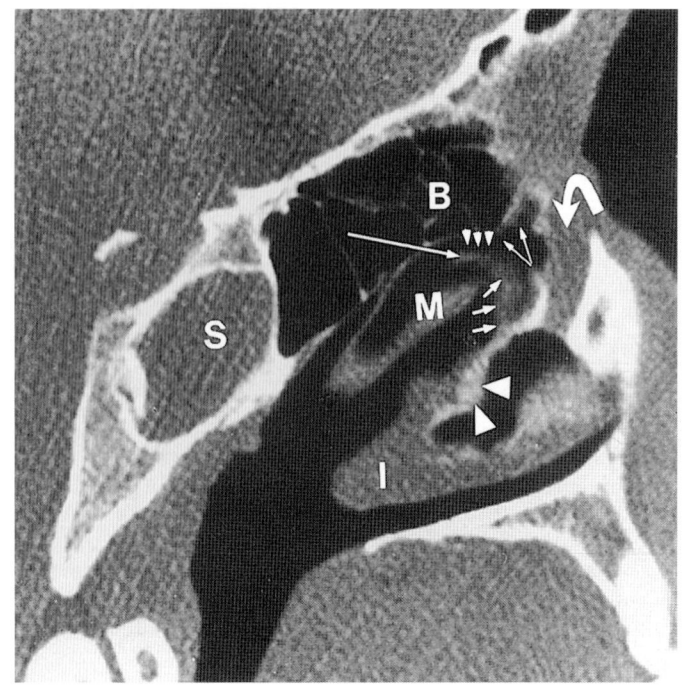

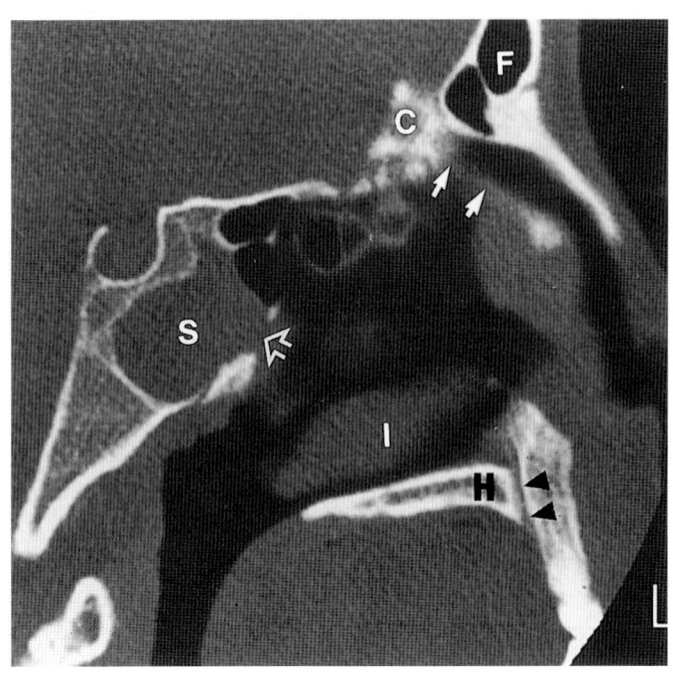

Fig. 4.3
a Coronal CT scan showing the inferior turbinate (I), nasal septum (hollow arrow), inferior meatus (curved arrow), uncinate process (u), superior nasal cavity (small double arrows), cribriform plate (long arrow), fovea ethmoidalis (FE), bulla ethmoidalis (B), infundibulum (double hollow arrows), pneumatized middle turbinate, so-called concha bullosa (cb), maxillary sinus ostium (o), infraorbital canal (large arrowhead), and maxillary sinuses (M). The small arrowhead points to the region of the hiatus semilunaris, which allows communication of the middle meatus (dashed line) with the infundibulum.
b Direct semisagittal CT scan showing the nasolacrimal canal (curved arrow), inferior turbinate (I), middle turbinate (M), bulla ethmoidalis (B), and opacified sphenoid sinus (S). Note the partially volumed uncinate process (three small arrows) and its attachment to the ethmoidal process of inferior nasal concha (double arrowheads). The infundibulum is between the bulla ethmoidalis and uncinate process (three arrowheads). The anterior ethmoid air cells (crossed arrows), including the bulla ethmoidalis, drain into the infundibulum. The long arrow points to the posterior portion of the uncinate process.
c Direct semisagittal CT scan showing the frontal sinus (F), crista galli (C), opacified sphenoid sinus (S), posterior ethmoid cells, partially volumed nasal septum and perpendicular plate of ethmoid bone (double arrows), inferior turbinate (I), hard palate (H), and incisor canal (arrowheads). Note the sella turcica, tuberculum sella, planum sphenoidale, and cribriform plate with multiple small holes for the passage of olfactory nerve fibers. The hollow arrow points to the surgical defect of the anterior wall of the sphenoid sinus.

orbit (Fig. 4.3a).[1,4,5] The nasal conchae project downward and slightly medially, each forming the roof of a passage or meatus (inferior, middle, and superior), which communicates freely with the nasal cavity (Fig. 4.3a). The inferior concha is an independent thin bone that articulates with the nasal surface of the maxilla and the perpendicular plate of the palatine bone (Fig. 4.3).[4,5] The inferior meatus is under the inferior concha and extends downward to the floor of the nasal cavity. It is the largest of the three meati and extends almost the entire length of the lateral wall of the nose. The inferior meatus receives the orifice of the nasolacrimal canal (Fig. 4.3b).

The middle and superior conchae are bony projections from the medial surface of the ethmoidal labyrinth (Fig. 4.3). The middle concha extends backward to articulate with the perpendicular plate of the palatine bone.[2,4,5] The middle meatus receives the opening of anterior and middle ethmoid air cells, and maxillary and frontal sinuses (Fig. 4.4). The superior concha is a small, curved lamina that lies above and behind the middle concha. The superior meatus receives the opening of the posterior ethmoidal air cells (Fig. 4.4). A narrow interval, the sphenoethmoidal recess (Fig. 4.4), separates the superior concha from the anterior surface of the body of the sphenoid, through which the sphenoidal sinus opens into the nasal cavity.[4–6] A fourth concha (concha suprema) is often present on the medial surface of the ethmoidal labyrinth above and behind the posterior end of the superior concha. Immediately behind the superior meatus, the sphenopalatine foramen (Fig. 4.4), which opens into the pterygopalatine fossa, pierces the lateral wall of the nasal cavity.[4–6] It transmits the sphenopalatine artery and the nasopalatine and superior nasal nerves from the pterygopalatine fossa.[1]

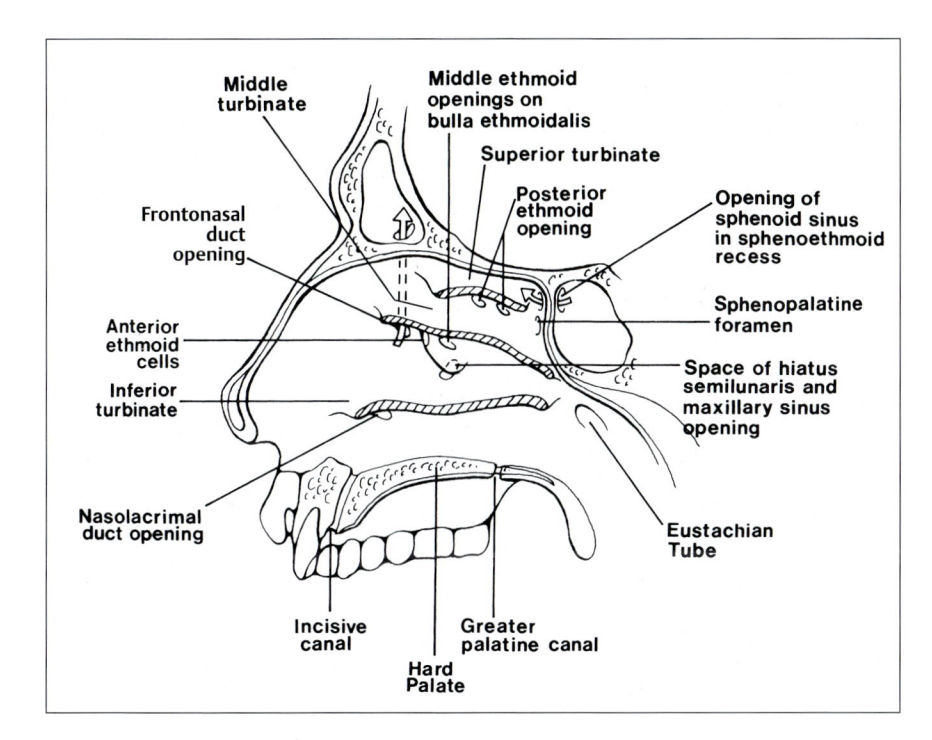

Fig. 4.4 Schematic drawing of the nasal cavity showing relative positions of the ostia of the sinuses. The frontal sinus ostium opens into the frontonasal duct and this in turn drains into the anterior part of the middle meatus. Modified from Davies J. Embryology and anatomy of the head, neck, face, palate, nose and paranasal sinuses. In: Paparella MM, Shurrick DA, eds., Otolaryngology, Vol 1. Philadelphia: W.B. Saunders, 1980; and Som PM. The paranasal sinuses. In: Bergeron RT, Osborn AG, Som PM, eds., Head and Neck Imaging. St. Louis: Mosby, 1984.

The Nasal Mucous Membrane

The nasal mucous membrane lines the nasal cavities with the exception of the vestibules, and is intimately adherent to the periosteum or perichondrium. The nasal vestibule is a cutaneous structure composed of keratinizing squamous epithelium and underlying subcutaneous tissue with cutaneous adnexal structures (hair follicles, sebaceous glands, and sweat glands).[2] The nasal mucosa is thickest and most vascular over the nasal conchae, especially at their extremities. It is also thick over the nasal septum, but very thin in the meati, on the floor of the nasal cavity, and in the opening of the paranasal sinuses. The nonsensory epithelium of the nasal cavity is composed of ciliated pseudostratified columnar epithelium interspersed with goblet cells, collectively termed the respiratory epithelium. Beneath the basal lamina are groups of serous and mucous (modified minor salivary) glands, opening by branched ducts on the epithelial surface. The vascular cavernous tissue lying beneath the respiratory mucosa is extensive. The endothelium of these cavernous sinuses demonstrates "fenestration." Immediately under the basal membrane, there is a fibrous layer infiltrated with lymphocytes, forming in many parts a diffuse lymphoid tissue; under this is a nearly continuous layer of mucous and serous glands, the ducts of which pass through the lymphoid layer before opening upon the surface. The mucus secreted by the glands and goblet cells makes a mucous film covering the membrane, which is moved by ciliary action downward and backward.[4–9]

The olfactory epithelium is considerably thicker than the surrounding nonsensory epithelium of the nasal cavity. It is composed of three chief cell types: olfactory receptor cells, supporting (sustentacular) cells, and basal cells.[1] The receptor cells are the primary sensory olfactory neurons. The cells are bipolar, spindle-shaped neurons, positioned vertically in the olfactory epithelium, composed of myelinated axons that penetrate the basal lamina to protrude from the mucosal surface and nonmlyelinated proximal processes that traverse the cribriform plate.[1,2] The supporting cells are irregular columnar elements that separate and partially enwrap the receptors. The basal cells are irregular or polygonal in shape and are confined to the regions abutting the basal lamina of the epithelium. The nonmyelinated axons of the receptor cells run in small bundles within the epithelium among the processes of the supporting and basal cells and finally penetrate the basal lamina, where each bundle becomes ensheathed by Schwann cells.[1] The ensheathed bundles (fila olfactoria) join with others to form the fasciculi of the olfactory nerve.[1] These fibers eventually enter the olfactory bulb, where they synapse with the second-order sensory neurons.[1]

Nasal Cycle

The nasal cycle is a physiological phenomenon in which the nasal mucosa undergoes alternating cycles of left- and right-sided mucosal swelling. The cycle varies from 20 minutes to 6 hours.

Innervation

The nerves of the nasal cavity include branches of the trigeminal and olfactory cranial nerves.

Innervation of the mucous membranes of the nose is supplied by the ophthalmic (anterior ethmoidal branch of the nasociliary nerve) and maxillary branches of trigeminal nerve as well as branches from the nerve of the pterygoid canal via the pterygopalatine (sphenopalatine) ganglion.[1,2] Accompanying the sensory fibers in these nerves are postganglionic vasomotor sympathetic fibers to the nasal blood vessels, while running with the branches from the pterygopalatine ganglion are postganglionic parasympathetic fibers, the latter being secretomotor to the nasal glands.[1] The olfactory mucous membranes contain the cells of origin of olfactory nerve fibers, which collect into bundles that traverse the cribriform plate and end in the olfactory bulb.[2]

■ Blood Supply and Lymphatic Drainage

The nasal cavities receive their blood supply from several sources, including the sphenopalatine artery, the facial artery, and the anterior and posterior ethmoidal arteries, branches of the ophthalmic artery (a branch of the internal carotid artery). The sphenopalatine artery is the end artery of the internal maxillary artery (a branch of the external carotid artery), located in the sphenopalatine foramen. It supplies the mucosa of the nasal septum; fontanelle (membranous portion of the medial wall of the maxillary sinus); superior, middle, and inferior turbinates; and the lateral nasal wall. The veins of the nose parallel the arteries, with drainage via the sphenopalatine foramen into the pterygoid venous plexus and then into the internal jugular vein, via the ophthalmic veins into the cavernous sinuses and then into the dural venous sigmoid sinuses/jugular bulbs, and also via the facial vein into either the internal or external jugular vein.[2]

■ Lymphatics

The anterior portion of the nose drains to the lymphatics, draining the skin covering the external nose, and passes to the submandibular nodes. The majority of the lymphatics of the nasal cavity drain via the retropharyngeal lymph nodes to the deep cervical lymph nodes.[2]

Anatomy of the Paranasal Sinuses

The paranasal sinuses are air-filled cavities and include the frontal, ethmoidal, maxillary, and sphenoidal sinuses. They vary in size and form in different individuals and are lined with upper respiratory mucosa, continuous with that of the nasal cavity. The mucous membrane, compared to the nasal mucosa, is thinner, less vascular, and more loosely adherent to the bony walls of the sinuses.[1] The sinuses lighten the skull and add resonance to the voice.

■ The Frontal Sinuses

The frontal sinuses are two irregular cavities that extend posteriorly, superiorly, and laterally for a variable distance between the laminae (tables) of the frontal bone (Fig. 4.5). Developmentally, each frontal sinus begins during the fourth month of fetal life in the regions of the frontal recess.[10] At birth, they are indistinguishable from the anterior ethmoid cells. Postnatal growth is slow. They are visible after the first or second year of life and are well-developed by 7–8 years but reach their full size only after puberty.[1,5,10] They are larger in males. The sinuses undergo a primary expansion with the eruption of the first deciduous molars and a secondary expansion when the permanent molars begin to appear in the sixth year.[1] With advancing age, absorption of bone from the inner walls of the sinuses may occur as an atrophic change leading to further enlargement. Their average measurements are height 3.2 cm, breadth 2.6 cm, depth 1.8 cm.[1] Each sinus extends backward into the medial part of the roof of the orbit (Fig. 4.5). The part of the sinus extending upward in the frontal bone may be small and the orbital part large, or vice versa (Fig. 4.6). Each frontal sinus opens into the anterior part of the corresponding middle meatus of the nose through the frontonasal duct (frontonasal recess), which traverses adjacent to the anterior part of the labyrinth of the ethmoid (Fig. 4.5d).[1,4–6]

Innervation

Innervation of the frontal sinuses is provided by the supraorbital and supratrochlear branches of the frontal nerve, a derivative of the ophthalmic division of the fifth (trigeminal) cranial nerve.[2]

Blood Supply and Lymphatic Drainage

The arterial blood supply of the frontal sinuses comes from the supraorbital and supratrochlear arteries of the anterior ethmoidal arteries; venous drainage is into the anastomotic vein in the supraorbital notch connecting the supraorbital and superior ophthalmic veins and then into the cavernous sinus.[1,2] The lymphatic drainage of the frontal sinuses is to the submandibular lymph nodes.[2]

■ The Ethmoidal Sinuses and Surgical Anatomy of the Ethmoid Bone

The advent of minimally invasive surgical techniques (MIST), using powered instruments with real-time suction, has further enhanced knowledge of the surgical anatomy of the paranasal sinuses. The ethmoid bone is a delicate and complex structure. It articulates with 13 other bones: the frontal, sphenoid, nasals, maxillae, lacrimals, palatines, inferior nasal conchae, and vomer.[1,6] The ethmoid bone consists of four parts: a horizontal lamina, called the cribriform plate; a perpendicular plate; and two lateral masses, called the labyrinths (Fig. 4.7). Ethmoid cells begin to develop around the third to fourth months of fetal life, and there may be a few cells (four or five) present at birth (Fig. 4.2b).[10] By the age of 12 years, the ethmoid air cells have almost reached their adult size (Figs. 4.2j, l).[3,10] Each ethmoidal labyrinth consists of thin-walled highly variable air cells arranged in three groups: anterior, middle, and posterior clusters (Fig. 4.8). The anterior and middle groups are usually referred to as anterior air cells (2–8 cells), separated from the posterior compartment by the vertical portion of the basal lamella of the middle concha. Fundamentally, anterior ethmoid cells are defined as those whose ostia open into the infundibulum and via the hiatus semilunaris superior into the middle meatus.[3,11,12] Bullar ethmoid cells are those opening above, or on, or under the bulla.[3] Posterior ethmoid cells have their ostia in the superior meatus. The anterior ethmoidal air cells include frontal recess air cells, infundibular (suprainfundibular) air cells, agger nasi air cells, terminal cells, ethmoid bulla, and concha bullosa (pneumatized anterior middle turbinate).[3] Although the limit of the ethmoid labyrinth is thought to be the ethmoid bone, ethmoid cells may encroach on any of the adjacent bones: the nasal and lacrimal bones anteriorly, the sphenoid bone posteriorly, the maxilla inferiorly, and the orbital plate of the frontal bone superiorly.[3] Some air cells are not entirely enclosed by the ethmoid bone (extramural cells); instead, the ethmoid bone may be perforated so that the air-cell mucosa extends upward against the ethmoidal notch of the frontal bone, anteriorly against the lacrimal and maxillary bones, and posteriorly against the sphenoid and palatine bones. The most anterior intramural ethmoidal air cells are the frontal recess air cells (cells developed in relation to and adjacent to frontal recess), which extend toward the frontal bone anterosuperiorly (Fig. 4.9a). The frontal sinus arises from these cells, as do the supraorbital ethmoidal air cells.[4,11] The next most

Anatomy of the Paranasal Sinuses 359

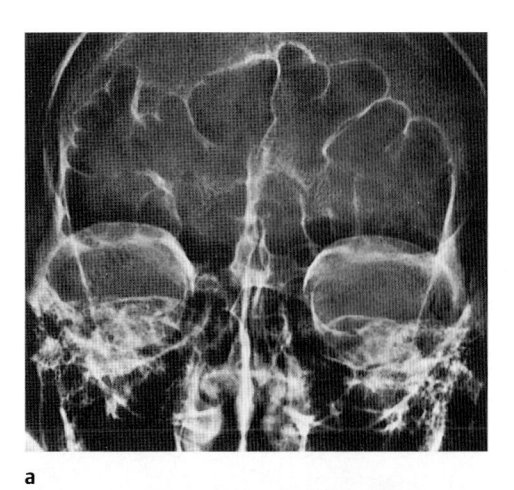

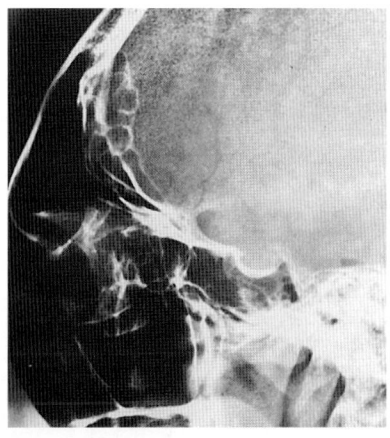

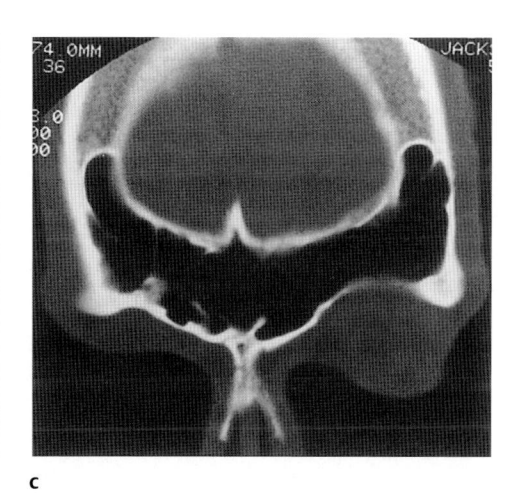

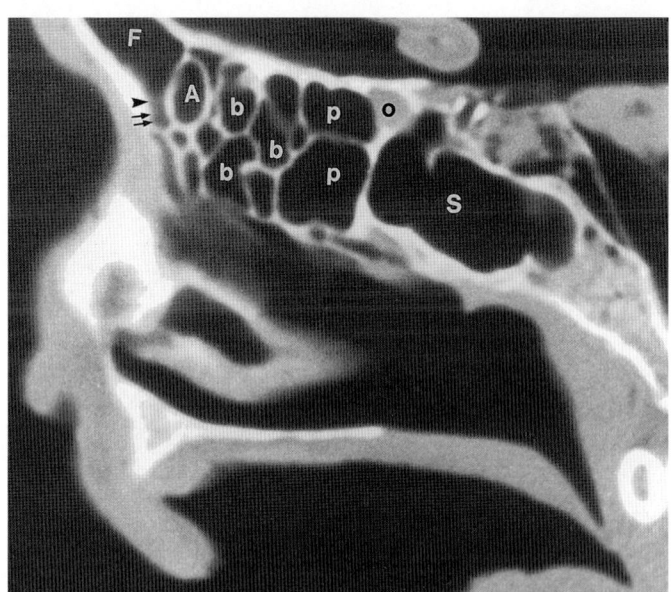

Fig. 4.5 a, b Large frontal sinuses depicted in the Caldwell (**a**) and lateral (**b**) projections.
c Coronal CT scan shows extensive pneumatization of the frontal sinuses.
d Sagittal CT scan of a cadaveric head, showing frontal sinus (F), frontal ostium (arrowhead), frontal (frontonasal) recess (arrows), anterior ethmoid (suprainfundibular cell) (A), bullar cells (b), posterior ethmoid cells (p), optic nerve and optic canal (o), and sphenoid sinus (S).

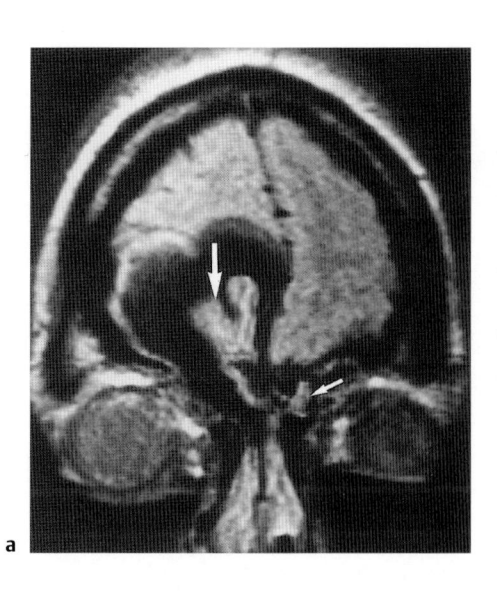

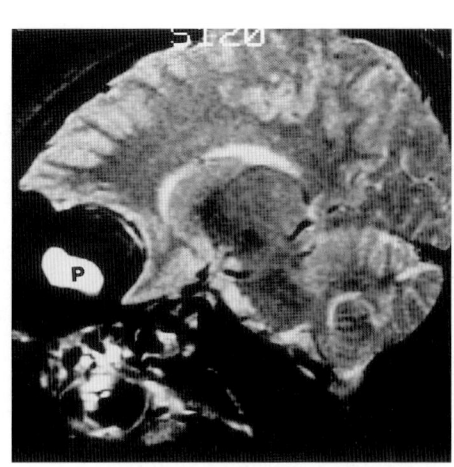

Fig. 4.6 Asymmetry of the frontal sinuses.
a Coronal proton-weighted MR scan shows marked enlargement of the right frontal sinus. Note the polyps (arrows), which were removed at surgery.
b Sagittal T2W MR scan, same patient as in Fig. 4.6a, showing a giant frontal sinus with a polyp (P) within it.

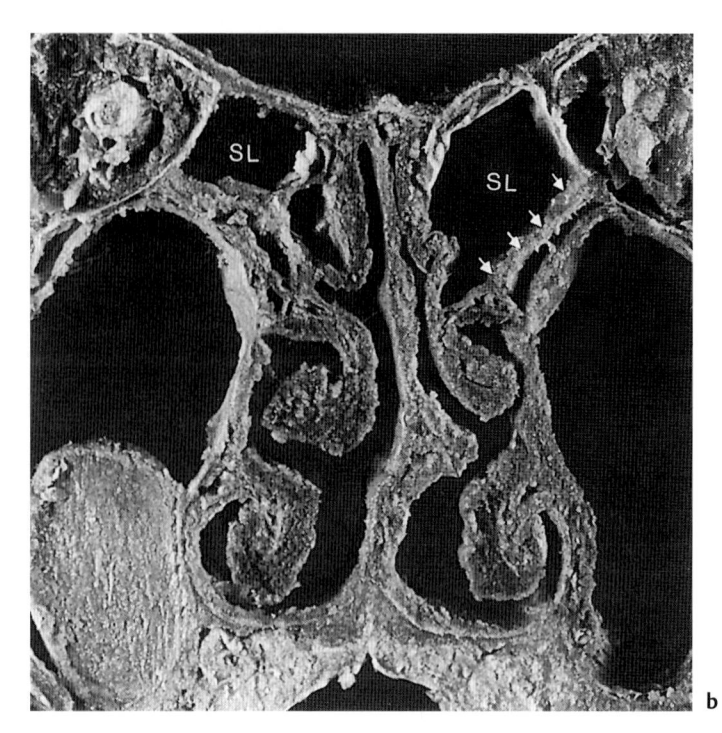

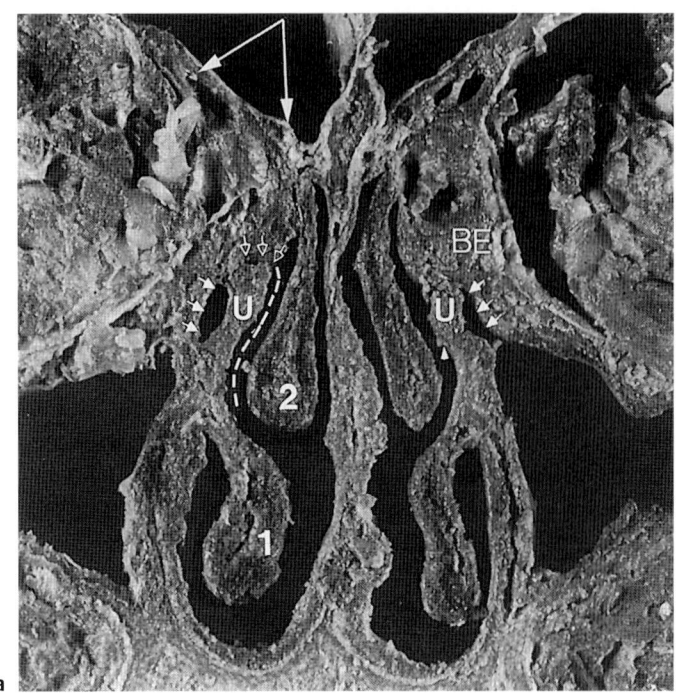

360   4 Imaging of the Nasal Cavity and Paranasal Sinuses

Fig. 4.7

a Coronal section through the ostiomeatal complex of a cadaveric head shows the inferior turbinate (1), middle turbinate (2), uncinate process (U), and bulla ethmoidalis (BE). Note the attachment of the uncinate process (arrowhead) to the ethmoidal process of the inferior concha. The infundibulum (three solid arrows) is a passage between the uncinate process and the inferior border of the bulla. The three open arrows indicate communication of the middle meatus (dashed line) with the infundibulum through the semilunar hiatus. As seen, the hiatus (three open arrows) is a passage between the inferior aspect of the bulla and the superior aspect of the uncinate process. The long arrows at the top of the photograph indicate the fovea ethmoidalis (roof of the lateral masses of the ethmoid bone). Note the attachment of the middle turbinate to the junction of the fovea ethmoidalis and cribiform plate.

b Coronal section posterior to **a**, taken just posterior to the bulla ethmoidalis. Note the lateral attachment of the middle turbinate, the so-called basal or ground lamella (arrows). The basal lamella separates the posterior ethmoidal air cells from bullar air cells. The sinus lateralis (SL) in this section is superior to the basal lamella. The sinus lateralis, if it is present, is above the bulla and anterior to the basal lamella. Note retention cyst along the floor of the right maxillary sinus. Reproduced from Mafee MF. Endoscopic sinus surgery: role of the radiologist. AJNR 1991; 12: 855–860, with permission.

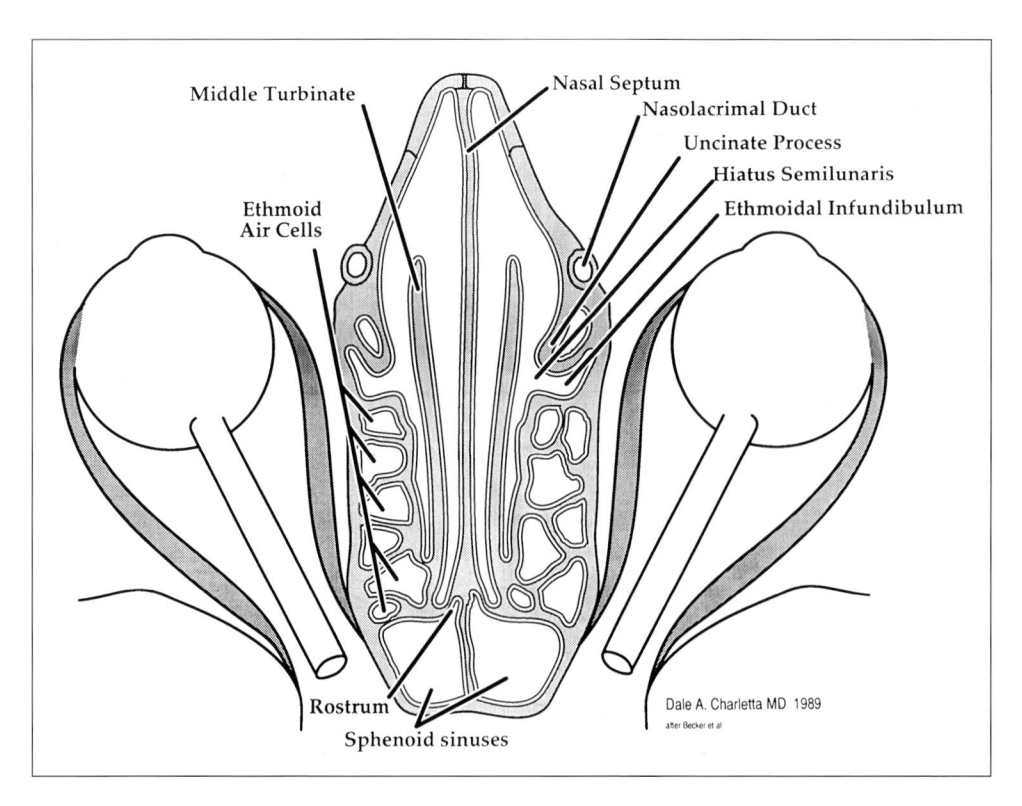

Fig. 4.8a Schematic drawing of the ethmoid, sphenoid, and nasal cavities, demonstrating the anatomy of the ostiomeatal complex.

Fig. 4.8b ▷

Anatomy of the Paranasal Sinuses

anterior group is the infundibular cells. From these arise the most anterior extramural cells, the agger nasi cells, which pneumatize the lacrimal bone and the adjacent frontal process of the maxilla (Fig. 4.9b).[3,4,5,11,12] The agger nasi cells are located on the lateral nasal wall immediately anterior to the anterior end of the middle turbinate (Fig. 4.10).[13,14] These cells drain into the ethmoid infundibulum (Figs. 4.8, 4.9b). The agger nasi cells are notable because they occur in about 80% of individuals.[9] The agger nasi cells occupy the lateral nasal wall anterosuperiorly to the hiatus semilunaris (Figs. 4.9a, 4.9b) and form an elevated area of bone (rudimentary concha) in the anterior part of the middle meatus (Fig. 4.9b).[9] The ostia of these cells open into the superior part of the infundibulum.[9]

The medial surface of the ethmoidal labyrinth forms a part of the lateral wall of the corresponding half of the nasal cavity. Within the nasal cavity, scrolls of bone on the lateral walls, the conchae, project medially to divide the passageway into meati, or channels for air (Fig. 4.7).[1,6] The superior and middle conchae are parts of the ethmoid bone, but the inferior nasal conchae (a turbinate is a concha plus a soft-tissue complex) are a separate pair of bones. The superior, middle, and inferior meati (air channels), which are formed under the respective conchae, have increased contact with the nasal surfaces to permit more effective warming and moistening of inspired air (air conditioning).[6] The posterior ethmoidal air cells drain into the superior meatus (Fig. 4.4). The middle meatus connects via various ostia and air passages with the anterior and middle ethmoidal air cells and the frontal and maxillary sinuses. The frontal sinuses communicate with the middle meatus of the corresponding half of the nasal cavity by means of a passage called the frontonasal canal (duct) or recess (Fig. 4.5d, 4.9b). This communication between frontal sinus and nasal cavity is not strictly a duct[15,16] but rather an internal channel positioned between the frontal sinus ostium and the anterior middle meatus and referred to as the frontal recess (Fig. 4.5d, 4.9b). Just anterior to the anterior superior attachment of the middle turbinate and anterior to the frontal recess are the agger (ridge) nasi and agger nasi cells (Fig. 4.9b).[3,4,5,11] This prominence on the lateral nasal wall represents the most anterior of the anterior ethmoidal cells (Fig. 4.10). These cells (agger nasi cells) can invade the lacrimal bone or the ascending process of the maxilla. Because of their closeness to the frontal recess, they are excellent surgical landmarks. Opening

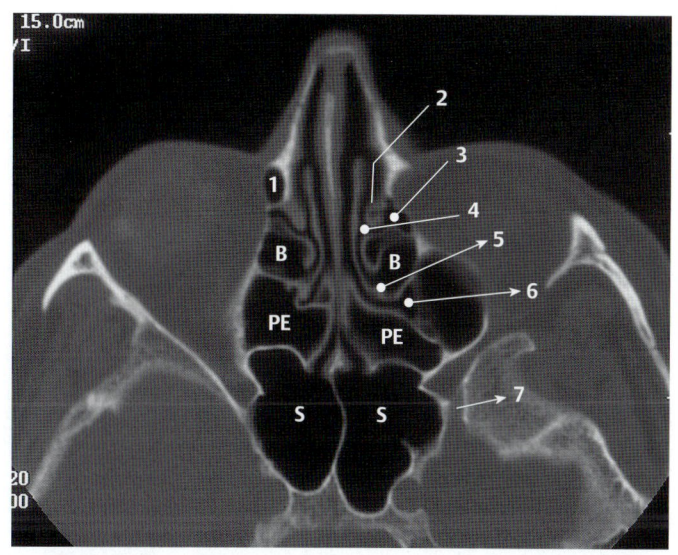

Fig. 4.8b Infundibulum, hiatus semilunaris, basal lamella, and sinus lateralis. Axial CT scan shows nasolacrimal canal (1), uncinate process (2), infundibulum (3), hiatus semilunaris (4), basal lamella of the middle turbinate (5), sinus lateralis (6), foramen rotundum (7), bulla ethmoidalis (B), posterior ethmoid cells (PE), and sphenoid sinus (S). Note: There is no space (cleft) between the basal lamella and posterior ethmoid cells on the right side; therefore, there is no sinus lateralis on this side.

these agger nasi cells during external ethmoidectomy provides a good view of the nasofrontal duct (Figs. 4.9b, 4.10). Obstruction of the frontonasal canal (frontal recess) results in mucocele formation of the frontal sinus. On the other hand, complete obliteration of the frontonasal canal is necessary to perform complete frontal sinus obliteration (Fig. 4.9c).

Just posterior and inferior to the agger nasi cells lies the ethmoidal uncinate process (Figs. 4.10b, 4.11–4.13), the starting point in anterior-to-posterior endoscopic sinus surgical procedures. The uncinate process is a thin, curved bar of bone from the lateral side of the ethmoidal labyrinth that forms a portion of the lateral nasal wall (Figs. 4.10b, 4.11–4.13). It projects downward and backward and is subject to considerable variation in size. It ranges in height from 2 to 4 mm and is 14–22 mm

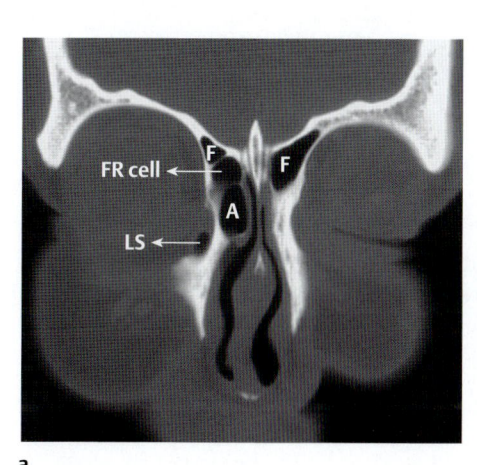

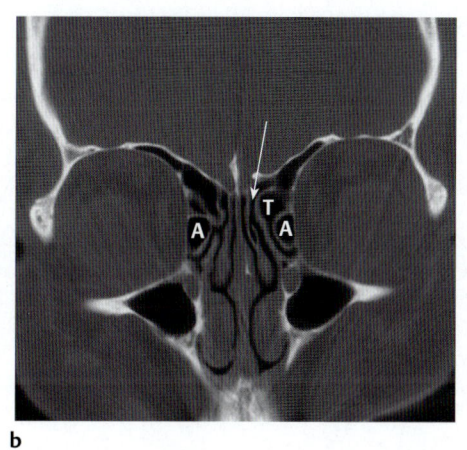

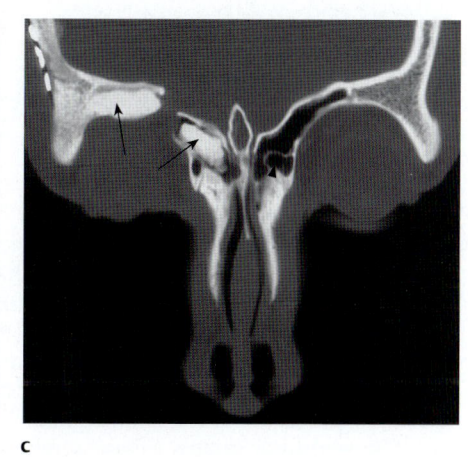

Fig. 4.9
a Coronal CT scan showing frontal sinus (F), frontal recess anterior ethmoid cell (FR cell), agger nasi cell (A), and air within right lacrimal sac (LS).
b Coronal CT scan showing agger nasi cells (A) and nasofrontal recess (arrow). Note: The anterior attachment of the uncinate process on the left to an anterior ethmoid air cell, creating the so-called terminal cell (T). In this individual, the left nasofrontal recess (arrow) drains into the middle meatus, medial to the uncinate process. The right nasofrontal recess drains into the right infundibulum.
c Frontal sinus obliteration, using hydroxyapatite cement. Coronal CT scan shows hydroxapatite cement (arrows) in the right frontal sinus, including nasofrontal recess. Arrowhead = frontal recess air cell.

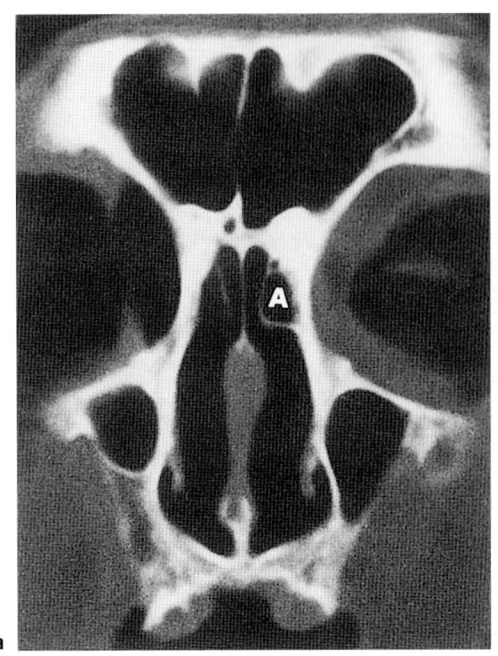

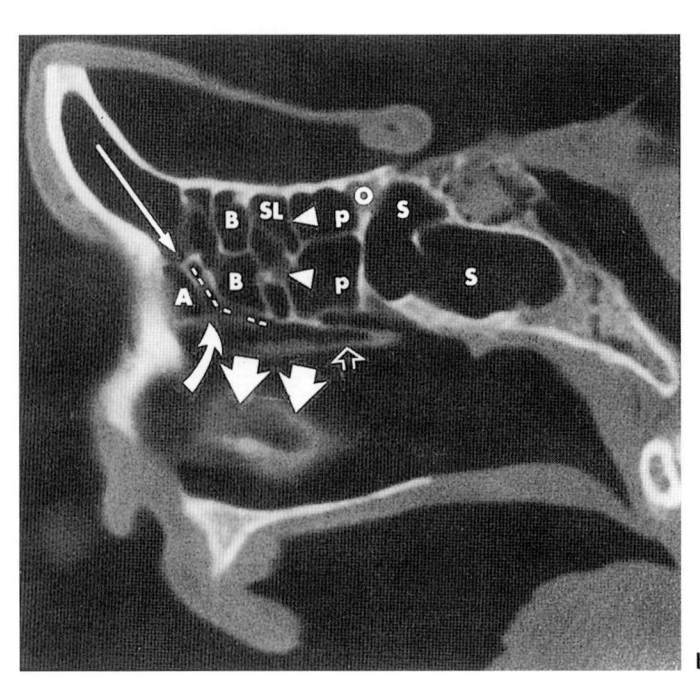

Fig. 4.**10a** CT scan of cadaveric head shows agger nasi cell (A).
b Paramidline sagittal CT scan of a cadaveric head shows agger nasi cell (A), ethmoidal bulla (B), sinus lateralis (SL), posterior ethmoidal cells (p), optic nerve (O), and sphenoid sinus (S). Note the middle turbinate (open arrow), uncinate process (curved arrow), and partially volumed inferior turbinate (double arrows). The infundibulum (broken line) is a curved passage below the bulla and above the uncinate process. Note the frontonasal duct or frontal recess (long straight arrow). The ostium of the frontal sinus opens into the frontonasal duct and this in return drains into the middle meatus. Note the posterior attachment of the middle turbinate to the cribriform plate (arrow heads). This is called the basal lamella of the middle turbinate. The basal lamella is L-shaped and is also attached to the medial wall of the orbit.

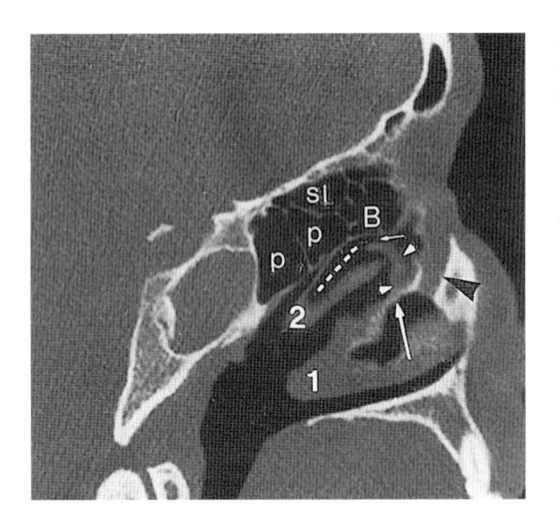

Fig. 4.**11** Direct parasagittal CT scan showing the inferior turbinate (1), middle turbinate (2), bulla ethmoidalis (B), sinus lateralis (sl), and posterior ethmoidal air cells (p). The basal lamella is the bony partition between bulla ethmoidalis and posterior ethmoidal air cells. The basal lamella is also between the sinus lateralis and bulla ethmoidalis. A partially volumed uncinate process (white arrowheads) is seen in this section. Note its anterior attachment (long arrow) to the ethmoidal process of the inferior concha. Just superior and anterior to the uncinate process are the agger nasi cells. The infundibulum is a curved passage (short white arrow) below the bulla and above the uncinate process. The area between the posterosuperior border of the uncinate process and the anteroinferior border of the bulla ethmoidalis is the semilunar hiatus (dashed line), which courses around the inferoposterior border of bulla to connect the infundibulum with the middle meatus. Note opacification of the sphenoid sinus by a surgically proven mucous retention cyst. This image clearly explains why the nasolacrimal duct (black arrowhead) or sac is injured during endoscopic anterior ethmoidectomy. Reproduced from Mafee MF. Endoscopic sinus surgery: role of the radiologist. AJNR 1991; 12: 855–860, with permission.

long.[13] Anteriorly it articulates with the lacrimal bone and ethmoidal process of the inferior nasal concha (Figs. 4.**7**, 4.**8**, 4.**11**, 4.**12**). The superior edge of this process is free and forms the medial boundary of the hiatus semilunaris (Figs. 4.**8**, 4.**12**) in the middle meatus of the nose.[1] As it progresses posteroinferiorly, it forms the inferior border of the semilunar hiatus (Figs. 4.**7**, 4.**12**) and the medial wall of the infundibulum (Fig. 4.**8**).

The semilunar hiatus (hiatus semilunaris) is a curvilinear opening of the lateral nasal wall that lies above the uncinate process and below the bulla ethmoidalis (Figs. 4.**8**, 4.**9**, 4.**11**, 4.**12**). The opening separates the uncinate process from the ethmoidal bulla and serves as a connection between the infundibulum and the middle meatus (Fig. 4.**8**). The middle ethmoidal air cells produce a rounded swelling, called the bulla ethmoidalis, on the lateral wall of the middle meatus (Figs. 4.**8a**, 4.**11**–4.**13**, 4.**14b**), whose lateral border forms a portion of the medial orbital wall. These cells open into the ethmoid infundibulum or onto the medial wall of the bulla into the middle meatus.[4]

The ethmoidal infundibulum is a trough-shaped cleft (deep curved passage) that is below the bulla and above and lateral to the uncinate process (Figs. 4.**8**, 4.**9**, 4.**11**, 4.**12**, 4.**14b**). It potentially receives drainage from the anterior and middle ethmoidal air cells and the frontal and maxillary sinuses.[14] In more than 50% of crania, the infundibulum continues superiorly as the frontonasal duct into the frontal sinus.[1] Kasper,[15] however, found that in 62% of cases, the ethmoidal infundibulum and nasofrontal connections were anatomically discontinuous channels.

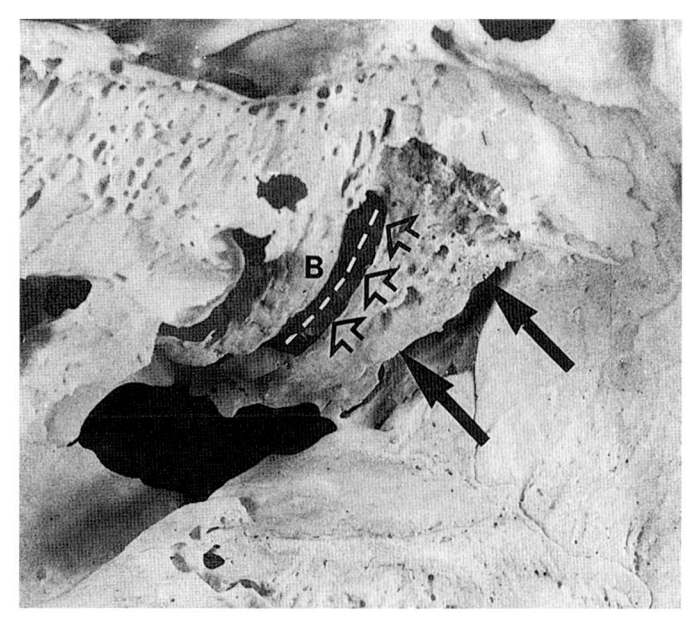

Anatomy of the Paranasal Sinuses 363

Fig. 4.12 Anatomy of the lateral nasal wall. The middle concha in this dry skull has been removed, allowing visualization of left nasal wall. Note the anteroinferior (large arrows) and posterosuperior (open arrows) borders of uncinate process; B = bulla ethmoidalis. The passage (dashed line) between the posterosuperior border of the uncinate process and the anteroinferior border of the bulla is the semilunar hiatus (hiatus semilunaris). The hiatus courses around the outer anteroinferioposterior border of the bulla to reach the middle meatus. Reproduced from Mafee MF. Endoscopic sinus surgery: role of the radiologist. AJNR 1991; 12: 855–860, with permission.

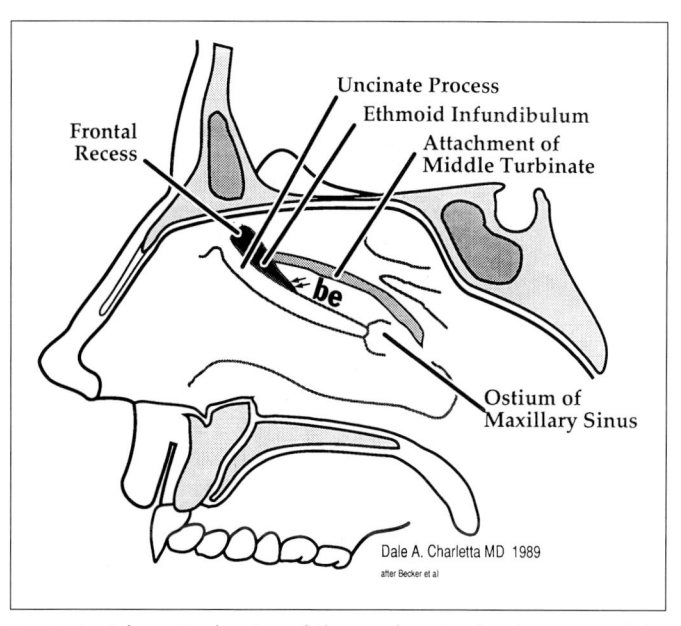

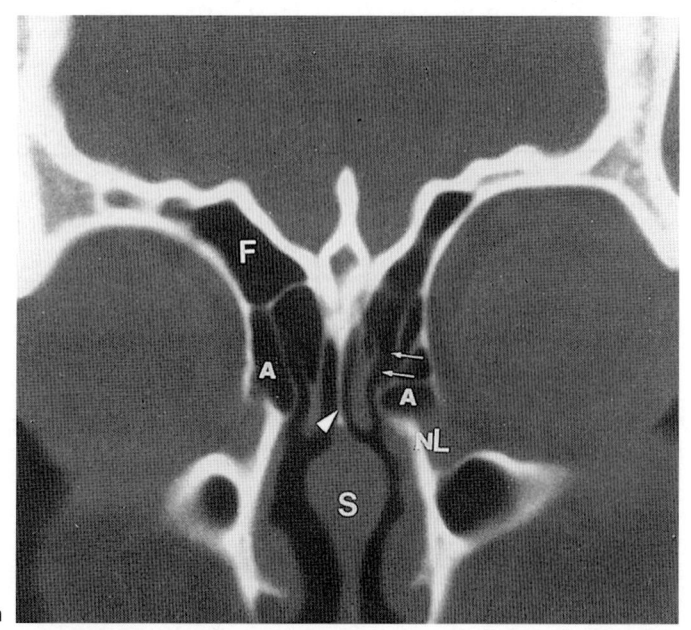

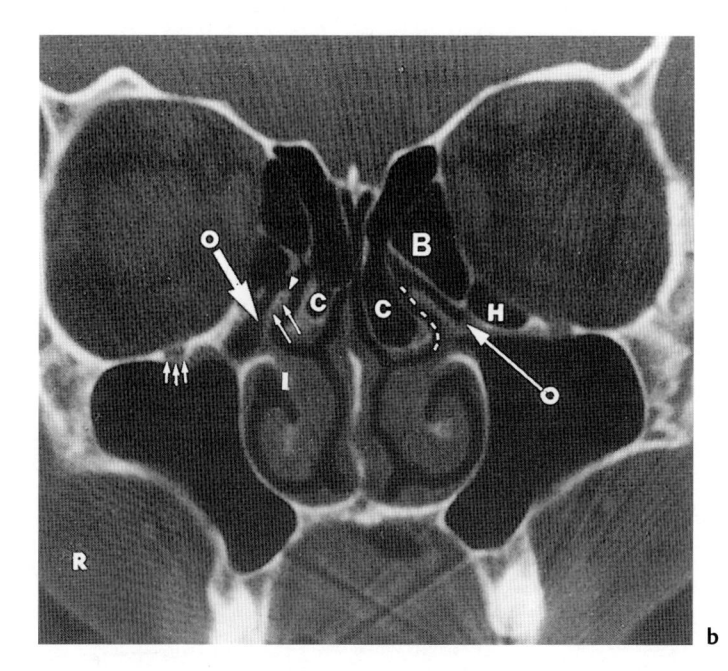

Fig. 4.13 Schematic drawing of the nasal cavity showing some of the anatomical landmarks of the ostiomeatal complex. be = bulla ethmoidalis. Note that the ostium of the maxillary sinus is close to the more posterior portion of the uncinate process.

Fig. 4.14
a Coronal CT scan shows agger nasi cells (A), frontal recess (arrows), frontal sinus (F), lacrimal sac fossa and nasolacrimal canal (NL), perpendicular plate of ethmoid bone (arrowhead), and nasal septum (S).
b Coronal CT scan showing the ethmoid bulla (B), uncinate process (double arrows), concha bullosa (c), Haller cell (H), inferior turbinate (I), and infraorbital canal (triple arrows). The infundibulum is the passage between the uncinate process and the bulla. The hiatus semilunaris (arrowhead) is the communication passage between the middle meatus (dashed line) and infundibulum; o = orifice of maxillary sinus.

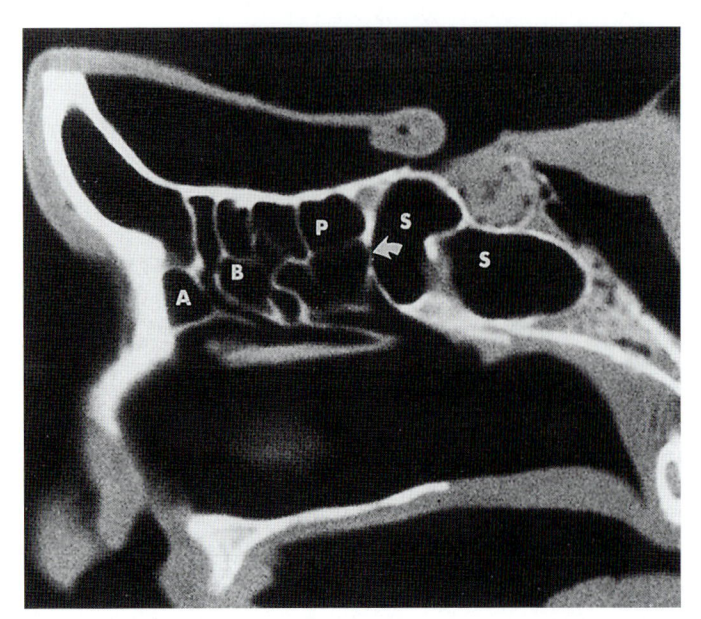

4 Imaging of the Nasal Cavity and Paranasal Sinuses

Fig. 4.15 Midline sagittal CT scan of cadaveric head shows the sphenoid sinus (S) with its ostium opening (curved arrow) into the sphenoethmoidal recess. (This section was taken along the lateral, rather than central margin of the ostium.) Note agger nasi cell (A), bulla (B), posterior ethmoidal cells (P), and basal lamella between the bulla and posterior ethmoidal cells.

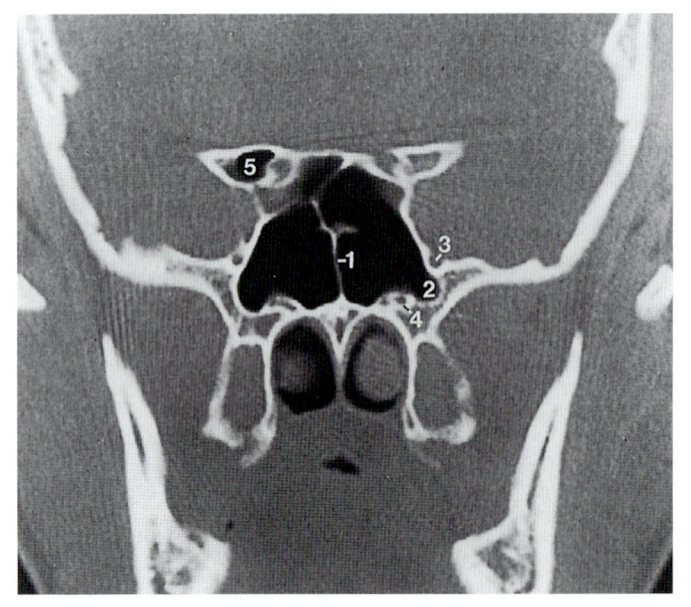

Fig. 4.16 Normal sphenoid sinus; CT scan, coronal plane. A septum (1) separates the right and left sphenoid sinuses. A small lateral recess (2) projects out between the foramen rotundum (3) and pterygoid (vidian) canal (4). Also note pneumatization of the right anterior clinoid (5).

The exact drainage system of the frontal sinus depends on its embryological development. The drainage may occur by way of rudimentary ethmoidal cells into the frontal recess[15] or directly into the frontal recess.[4, 5, 11, 13, 14] Medial to the bulla ethmoidalis and the uncinate process is the middle turbinate (Fig. 4.7). Anteriorly, it attaches to the medial wall of the agger nasi and the superoanterior edge of the uncinate process (Figs. 4.9, 4.10).[16] Superiorly, it attaches to the cribriform plate. The attachment of the middle turbinate changes direction at its most posterior extent. Instead of running in an anteroposterior direction, it curves laterally, and the final lateral attachment of the middle turbinate is oriented in the frontal plane and is called the basal or ground lamella (Figs. 4.7b, 4.8b, 4.11).[11, 14, 16] The posterior ethmoidal air cells are between the basal lamella and the sphenoidal sinus. The basal lamella is an excellent landmark for separating the anterior and middle ethmoidal air cells from the posterior ethmoidal air cells.[4–6, 11]

Sinus Lateralis (Retrobullar, Suprabullar Recesses)

An air space (cleft) is usually found between the ground lamella and the bulla ethmoidalis, which may extend superiorly to the bulla (suprabullar recess). This is called the sinus lateralis (Figs. 4.7b, 4.8b). This sinus lateralis, unlike the anterior ethmoidal air cells that open into the infundibulum, may communicate with the frontal recess[4, 5, 16] or open directly and independently into the middle meatus. Bolger et al[17] found that a separate and discrete retrobullar recess was present in 93.8% of human cadavers they dissected by both gross and endoscopic techniques. A single, discrete, well-developed suprabullar recess was present in 70.9%. They found that the suprabullar recess did not communicate with the frontal recess. They recommended that the sinus lateralis is more correctly called the retrobullar and suprabullar recesses.[17]

Innervation

Innervation for ethmoid sinuses is provided by the branches of the ophthalmic and maxillary division of the trigeminal nerve, including the nasociliary, anterior ethmoid, and posterior ethmoid nerves and the orbital branches of the pterygopalatine (sphenopalatine) ganglion.[2]

Blood Supply and Lymphatic Drainage

The ethmoid sinuses receive their blood supply from both the internal and external carotid arteries via the branches of the ophthalmic (anterior and posterior ethmoidal) arteries and the nasal branch of the sphenopalatine artery, the terminal branch of the artery of the internal maxillary artery, a branch of the external carotid artery. Venous drainage of the ethmoid sinuses occurs by two routes: (1) into the nose via the nasal veins, which flow to the maxillary vein, and then into the retromandibular vein and ultimately into the external jugular vein;[2] (2) via the ethmoid veins into the ophthalmic veins to the cavernous sinuses.[2] The lymphatic drainage of the ethmoid sinuses is to the submandibular lymph nodes (from the anterior and middle ethmoid air cells) and the retropharyngeal lymph nodes (from the posterior air cells).[2]

■ Sphenoidal Sinuses

The sphenoidal sinuses are contained within the body of the sphenoid bone. They originate during the third fetal month as evaginations of the mucosa of the nasal cavity. At birth, the sinus remains very small and is little more than an evagination of the sphenoethmoid recess.[3, 9, 10] After the fifth year, invasion of the sphenoid bone is more rapid, and by the age of 7 years the sinus extends posteriorly to the level of the sella turcica. Further enlargement occurs after puberty. The sphenoid sinuses are related above to the pituitary gland (Figs. 4.10, 4.11, 4.15) and the optic nerves and chiasm, and on each side to the internal carotid artery and the cavernous sinuses. The sphenoid sinuses, like frontal sinuses, can vary considerably in size and shape. The main intersphenoid septum is often deflected to one side; they are therefore rarely symmetrical (Figs. 4.16–4.18). The average measurements of the sphenoid sinus are vertical height 2 cm, transverse breadth 1.8 cm, anteroposterior depth 2.1 cm.[1] At times there may be lateral expansion (lateral recess) into the roots of the pterygoid processes or greater wings of the sphenoid (Fig. 4.17), and it may invade the lesser wing (Fig. 4.16) and the basilar part of the sphenoid bone. There are sometimes gaps in the bony walls, and the mucous membrane may lie directly against the dura mater. Bony bridges, produced by the internal carotid artery and the pterygoid (vidian) canal, may project into the sinuses from the lateral wall and floor, respectively.[1, 14] A posterior ethmoidal sinus may extend into the body of the sphenoid and largely replace a sphenoidal sinus.[1] Each sphenoid sinus drains into the nasal cavity via the sphenoethmoidal recess by an aperture in the upper part of its anterior wall (Fig. 4.15). The sphenoid ostium is well above the floor of the sinus and always drains medial to the superior turbinate. On average, the ostium measures 2 mm × 3 mm and lies 10 mm above the floor of the sinus.[3] Blood supply is from the posterior ethmoidal arteries, and lymph drainage is to the retropharyngeal nodes. Their nerve supply is from the posterior ethmoidal nerves and the orbital branches of the pterygopalatine ganglion.[1]

■ The Maxillary Sinuses

The maxillary sinuses are first to develop, around the 65 th day of gestation.[3] The size of the sinus at birth is about 6–8 mm³. They can be seen on plain radiography and particularly on CT scans (Fig. 4.2a) at 4–5 months of age or earlier. Rapid expansion occurs from 7 to 18 years, related to eruption of permanent teeth. Ethmoid and maxillary sinuses are the only sinuses that are large enough at birth to be clinically significant in rhinosinusitis (see Fig. 4.56).[3] The maxillary sinuses are pyramidal cavities within the bodies of the maxillae and are the largest accessory air sinuses of the nose (Figs. 4.14, 4.19, 4.20). The base of the pyramid is formed by the lateral wall of the nasal cavity; the apex extends into the zygomatic process of the maxilla and may reach the zygomatic bone itself. Its base faces medially and is the lateral wall of the nasal cavity and presents the maxillary hiatus in the disarticulated bone (Fig. 4.12). In the articulated skull, this aperture hiatus is much reduced in size by the uncinate process of the ethmoid above, the maxillary process of the inferior nasal concha below, and the perpendicular plate of the palatine bone behind (Figs. 4.19, 4.20). The roof of the maxillary sinus is the orbital floor, which is ridged by the infraorbital canal which usually projects into the sinus (Figs. 4.19, 4.20). The floor is formed by the alveolar process of the maxilla. Several conical projections corresponding with the roots of the first and second molar teeth project into the floor. The floor is sometimes perforated by one or more of these roots. Occasionally the roots of the first and second premolars, of the third molar, and at times of the canine may also project into the sinus. The size of the maxillary sinuses varies in different individuals, and even on the two sides of the same individual. The average measurements of an average-sized maxillary sinus are vertical height opposite the first molar tooth 3.5 cm, transverse breadth 2.5 cm, and anteroposterior depth 3.2 cm.[1] The maxillary sinus communicates with the middle meatus of the nasal cavity, generally by two small apertures, one of which is usually closed by the mucous membrane in life (fontanelle). The natural ostium of the maxillary sinus is located in the superior portion of its medial wall, usually posterior to the midpoint of the bulla ethmoidalis (Figs. 4.4, 4.13, 4.14b).[4, 5] The posterior extent of the uncinate process points to the position of the ostium and is an excellent imaging and endoscopic landmark for its localization (Figs. 4.12, 4.14b). Accessory ostia are present in 10–30% of cases, usually in the membranous medial aspect of the maxillary sinus, where a double layer of mucosa with no in-

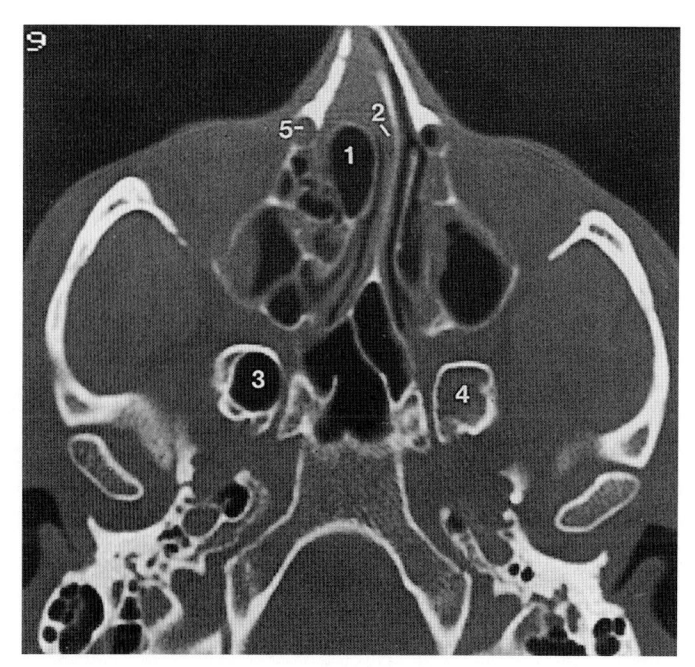

Fig. 4.17 Axial CT scan, normal variant. Note the pneumatized middle turbinate (1) as part of the right ethmoid air cells. The nasal septum (2) is deviated to the left. A right lateral recess (3) of the sphenoid sinus extends into the pterygoid bone, whereas the left pterygoid bone is solid (4). Also note the nasolacrimal duct (5) containing air on the left and fluid and soft tissue on the right, both normal. Note the vidian canals, which run through the base of the pterygoid processes. From Reference 17 a.

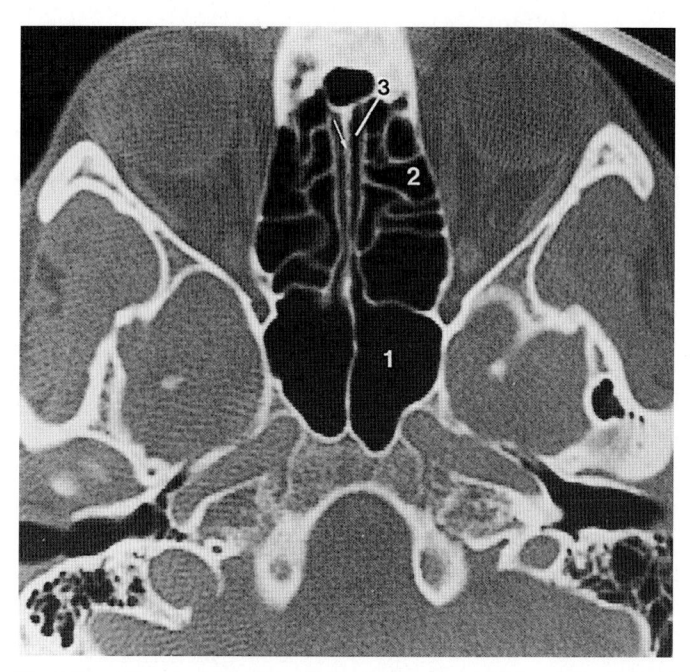

Fig. 4.18 CT scan, axial plane, through the sphenoid sinus (1), ethmoid sinuses (2), and top of the nasal cavity (3) with the nasal septum (arrow). From Reference 17 a.

tervening bone forms the nasoantral wall inferior to the uncinate process. The natural opening of the maxillary sinus is above the floor and is poorly placed for natural drainage. The middle meatus is of such a form that pus running down from the frontal and anterior ethmoidal sinuses is directed by the hiatus semilunaris into the opening of the maxillary sinus, which may, in some cases, act as a secondary reservoir for pus discharged from these sinuses.

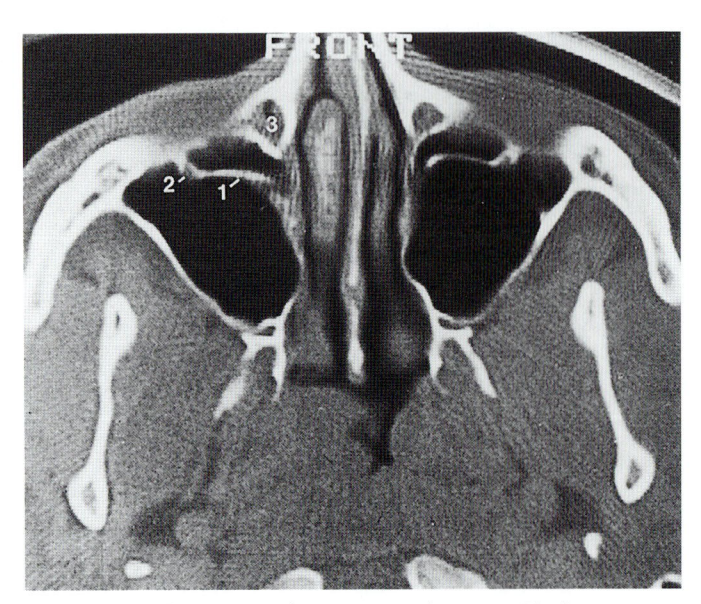

Fig. 4.**19** Maxillary sinus with septum; axial CT scan. The bony septum (1) extends from the infraorbital nerve canal (2) to the medial wall of the maxillary sinus, partially separating the anterior compartment from the main chamber of the maxillary sinus. The nasolacrimal duct (3) is located anteriorly.

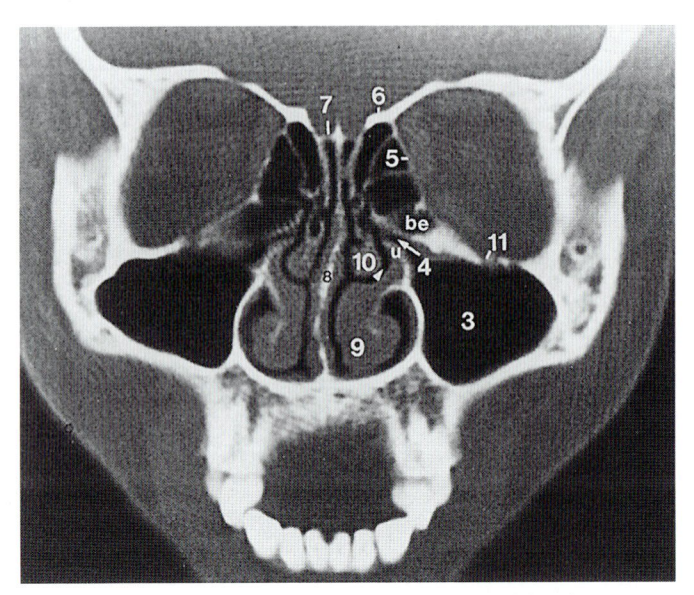

Fig. 4.**20** Coronal CT scan shows the maxillary sinus (3) with its ostium (4), opening into the infundibulum (arrow). The infundibulum is located between the bulla ethmoidalis (be) and the uncinate process (u). Note the lamina papyracea (5), fovea ethmoidalis (6), cribriform plate (7), nasal septum (8), and inferior (9) and middle turbinates (10). The lateral lamella of cribriform plate is between 6 and 7.

Innervation

Innervation of the maxillary sinuses is supplied by the branches of the maxillary division of the trigeminal nerve, including the anterior, middle, and posterior superior alveolar nerves and the infraorbital nerve.[1,2]

Blood Supply and Lymphatic Drainage

The blood supply of the maxillary sinus is by means of the facial, infraorbital, and greater palatine vessels; major blood comes from branches of the maxillary artery (infraorbital, greater palatine, posterosuperior and anterosuperior alveolar arteries, and sphenopalatine artery),[2] with a smaller contribution from the facial artery; both maxillary and facial arteries are branches of the external carotid artery. Venous drainage occurs anteriorly via the anterior facial vein to the jugular vein and posteriorly via the maxillary vein to the jugular system by way of the retromandibular vein, and additionally in the region of the infratemporal fossa. The maxillary vein communicates with the pterygoid plexus, which anastomoses with the dural sinuses (cavernous sinuses) through the base of the skull.[2] The maxillary sinuses lymphatics drain into the submandibular nodes.[2]

■ Functional Endoscopic Sinus Surgery and the Role of the Radiologist

Endoscopic sinus surgery has become an increasingly popular procedure since Messerklinger[18] and Wigand et al.[19] described the advantages of the intranasal endoscope and its surgical application. The concept of "functional endoscopic sinus surgery"[20] evolved from the work of Hilding,[21,22] Proctor,[23,24] and Messerklinger[25–27] on mucociliary clearance and air flow in the paranasal sinuses and on the importance of establishing drainage and preserving the mucosa of the sinuses. Functional endoscopic sinus surgery is based on the hypothesis that the ostiomeatal complex (maxillary sinus ostium, anterior and middle ethmoid ostia, frontal recess, infundibulum, and middle meatal complex) is the key area in the pathogenesis of chronic sinus diseases.[11,13,25–31] Minor pathological changes in the nasal mucosa in the vicinity of the ostiomeatal complex (OMC) may interfere with mucociliary clearance or with the ventilation of the maxillary, ethmoidal, and frontal sinuses. The underlying principle of functional endoscopic sinus surgery is that the sinus mucosa will return to normal if adequate drainage can be established.[4,5,6,14] No attempt is made to remove the sinus mucosa; rather, it is allowed to return to normal and to resume its normal function. Obstruction of the OMC is believed to be a critical step in the development of chronic rhinosinusitis. Much of the endoscopic treatment of chronic rhinosinusitis is mainly directed at addressing disease involving the OMC.[25] In the functional concept, surgical relief of obstruction at the OMC region is a critical element in the ventilation of the paranasal sinuses. Sinonasal mucociliary clearance is a fundamental function, required to maintain the health and defense of the nose.[8] Ultrastructural changes of the respiratory mucosa can result from acute and chronic infections.[9] Mucociliary transport plays an important role in the defense mechanism of the respiratory tract.[7] Mucociliary transport depends to a large extent on the activity of cilia and the properties of the mucus layer.[7] Measuring ciliary beat frequency with a photoelectric device is a direct method for assessing ciliary activity.[7]

Knowledge of the anatomy of the ethmoid bone, nasal cavity, ostiomeatal complex and natural ostium of the maxillary sinus, and the exact drainage system of the frontal sinus, is of considerable importance in this operative technique. A successful outcome of endoscopic sinus surgery is based on a clearly defined diagnostic evaluation of the disease in the ostiomeatal complex in patients with chronic sinusitis.[4,14,20,31] This evaluation includes a good medical history; careful physical examination, including intranasal endoscopy; and, after medical therapy, a CT scan to examine the ostiomeatal complex.[14,15,31] Familiarity with the anatomy of the paranasal sinuses, particularly the ethmoidal sinuses, is critical for interpreting imaging studies of the paranasal sinuses. In the endoscopic approach, the most important landmarks are the agger nasi cells, frontal recess, middle turbinate, middle meatus, uncinate process, ethmoid infundibulum, hiatus semilunaris, bulla ethmoidalis, natural ostium of the maxillary sinus, basal lamella, superior meatus, and sphenoethmoidal recess (Figs. 4.7–4.14).

Ostiomeatal Complex

The ostiomeatal complex or unit has been referred to as the maxillary sinus ostium and infundibulum[4,5,14,20] and also as the normally aerated channels, providing air flow and mucociliary clearance for the maxillary sinus and the anterior and middle ethmoidal, and frontal sinuses (Tables 4.1, 4.2).[16] However, the term "ostiomeatal complex" is often used to refer to the maxillary sinus ostium, anterior and middle ethmoidal air cells ostia, frontonasal duct (frontal recess) (Figs. 4.11, 4.12, 4.14), infundibulum, and middle meatal complex (Table 4.1).[1] Also, in many otolaryngological communications, the anterior and middle ethmoidal air cells are collectively referred to as anterior ethmoidal air cells. Recognition of the importance of the ostiomeatal complex has given the radiologist an important role in the examination of patients who are scheduled for functional endoscopic sinus surgery. Radiologists should be familiar with the basic structures and spaces of the sinonasal cavities, in particular with the more subtle and complex ethmoid anatomical features. Some of the recesses, such as the frontal recess, sinus lateralis (retrobullar, suprabullar recesses)[17] and sphenoethmoid recess, are rather vague, elusive, and rather difficult to understand. Radiologists should also be familiar with the principles of endonasal endoscopic operation, and make a careful evaluation of the paranasal sinuses, in particular the ethmoid bone, the middle meatus region, and the lateral wall of the nasal cavity.

Anatomical Variations

Certainly, individual structural differences in the ethmoidal complex, ostiomeatal units, and other paranasal sinuses are to be expected, and the reader should not be discouraged if certain illustrations in the literature are not identical with the images he or she will review for any individual patient. Certain anatomical variations are occasionally observed and should be included in the imaging report. These are as follow.

Drainage of the Ethmoid Bulla

On the basis of the configuration of the bulla, three classes of ethmoid bulla development have been described.[32] (1) The simple bulla is a single, usually large, cavity with one medial opening. The drainage from the ethmoid simple bulla, the largest and most constant anterior ethmoid air cell, opens into the middle meatus. The ostium of the simple ethmoid bulla is often found in the hiatus semilunaris superior (HSS); however, it can also be found in the anterior or lateral bullar wall, the ethmoid infundibulum, the hiatus semilunaris inferior, and the retrobullar recess.[33] (2) The compound ethmoid bulla has two or three separate compartments, each of which opens medially and communicates to the HSS.[32] (3) The complex ethmoid bulla has two or three compartments, one of which communicates with the HSS. The other components will communicate with the ethmoid infundibulum.[32] As in the compound bulla, no communication between the components has been found.[32]

Table 4.1 Ostiomeatal unit (complex) and its regional anatomy

- Middle meatus
- Infundibulum
- Hiatus semilunaris
- Frontal recess (nasofrontal duct)
- Frontal sinus ostium
- Bullar cell ostia
- Other anterior ethmoid air cell ostia
- Primary ostium of maxillary sinus
- Regional anatomy; middle turbinate, uncinate process, bulla ethmoidalis, maxillary sinus and frontal sinus

Table 4.2 Sphenoethmoidal recess and its regional anatomy

- Superior meatus
- Primary ostium of sphenoid sinus
- Posterior ethmoid cell ostia
- Regional anatomy; superior turbinate, sphenoid, and posterior ethmoid sinuses

Concha Bullosa, a Pneumatized Middle Turbinate

The base of the middle turbinate can be invaded by ethmoid air cells, which can enlarge the turbinate; an enlarged, pneumatized turbinate is known as a concha bullosa. This anatomical variant is relatively common. The otolaryngologist is interested in knowing whether the concha bullosa has compromised the middle meatus or even the ethmoid infundibulum (Fig. 4.14 b).

Low Position of Fovea Ethmoidalis (Roof of the Ethmoid Labyrinth)

A low position of the cribriform plate and fovea ethmoidalis and lateral lamella of the cribriform plate (thin bone between the cribriform plate proper and fovea ethmoidalis) is a potentially dangerous anatomical variation, which can be penetrated easily unless the surgeon is aware of the finding (Fig. 4.20). The attachment of the middle turbinate to the cribriform plate is at the junction of the cribriform plate and its lateral lamella (Figs. 4.14, 4.20). The anterior ethmoid artery canal is at the junction of the fovea ethmoidalis with the lateral lamella of the cribriform plate (Fig. 4.21 h). The fovea ethmoidalis (roof of ethmoid) is part of the frontal bone. It is thicker than the cribriform plate and its lateral lamella, which are part of the ethmoid bone.

Variation of the Uncinate Process

The uncinate process may be symmetrically or asymmetrically short and stubby. Rarely, uncinate process may be atelectatic (Fig. 4.22) or be pneumatized ("uncinate bulla") (Fig. 4.23). The superior edge of the uncinate process may deviate medially to obstruct the middle meatus or, more importantly, may deviate laterally to obstruct the infundibulum (Fig. 4.22). Marked lateral deviation or even fusion of the uncinate process to the medial orbital wall may endanger the orbit and, hence, the optic nerve, while uncinectomy is performed during anterior endoscopic sinus surgery.

Haller Cells

These are ethmoidal air cells extending along the medial floor of the orbit (infraorbital ethmoid air cells) (Figs. 4.14 b, 4.21 j), which may cause narrowing of the infundibulum.

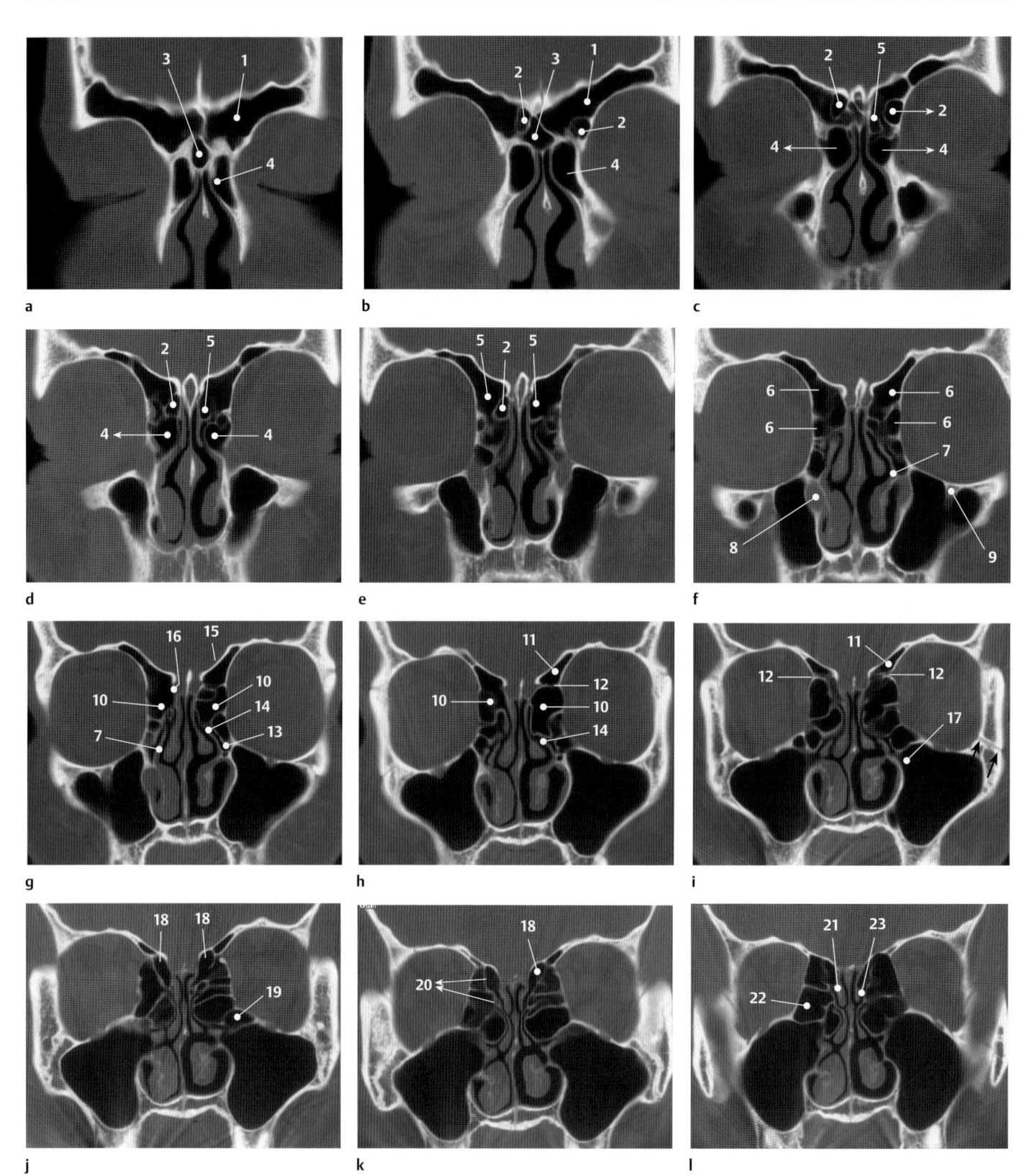

Fig. 4.21 a–l Imaging anatomy of paranasal sinuses and ostiomeatal complex. All images are from the same individual. 1 = frontal sinus; 2 = frontal recess anterior ethmoid air cell; 3 = frontal bulla; 4 = agger nasi cell; 5 = frontal (frontonasal) recess; 6 = anterior ethmoid cells; 7 = uncinate process; 8 = nasolacrimal canal; 9 = infraorbital canal and nerve; 10 = bulla ethmoidalis; 11 = suprabullar cell; 12 = anterior ethmoid artery canal; 13 = infundibulum; 14 = hiatus semilunaris, where the infundibulum opens into the middle meatus; 15 = fovea ethmoidalis; 16 = lateral lamella of cribriform plate proper; 17 = maxillary sinus ostium; 18 = sinus lateralis; 19 = Haller cell; 20 = basal lamella; 21 = superior turbinate; 22 = posterior ethmoid cells; 23 = superior meatus; arrows = zygomatic canal in malar bone. The inferior meatus and middle meatus are air spaces, lateral and inferior to the inferior and middle turbinates, respectively.

Anatomy of the Paranasal Sinuses 369

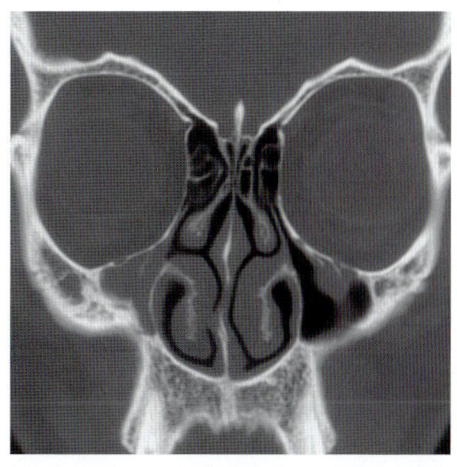

Fig. 4.**22** Anatomical variations of the uncinate process. Coronal CT scan showing lateral attachment of the right uncinate process to the medial wall of the orbit ("atelectatic uncinate process"). Note opacified right maxillary sinus due to obstruction of the infundibulum.

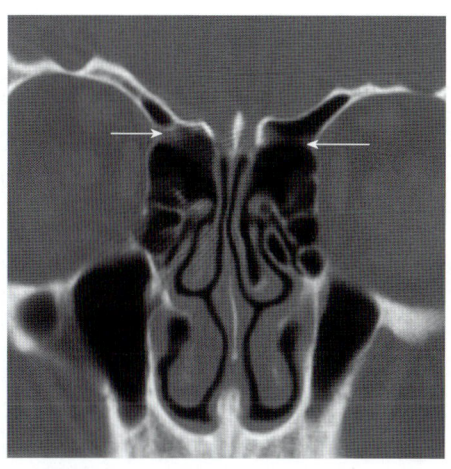

Fig. 4.**23** Pneumatized uncinate process. Coronal CT scan shows pneumatized left uncinate process. Note the anterior ethmoid artery canal (arrows).

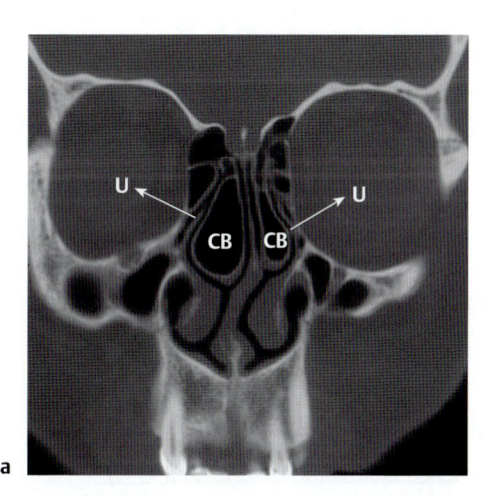

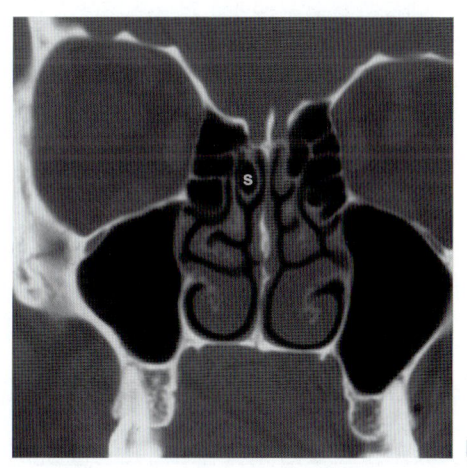

Fig. 4.**24** Bilateral concha bullosa, and pneumatized superior turbinate. **a** Coronal CT scan, showing bilateral concha bullosa (CB). u = uncinate process. **b** Coronal CT scan shows pneumatized superior turbinate (S).

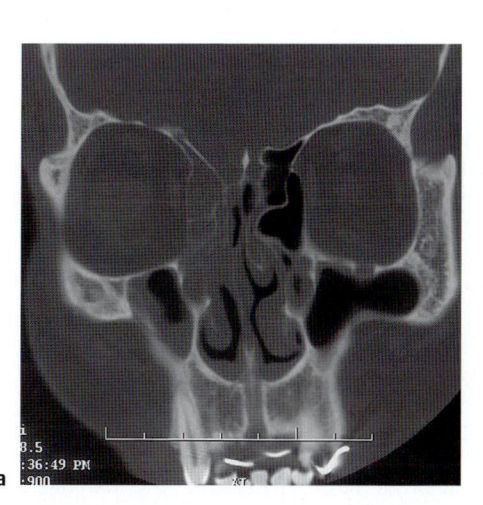

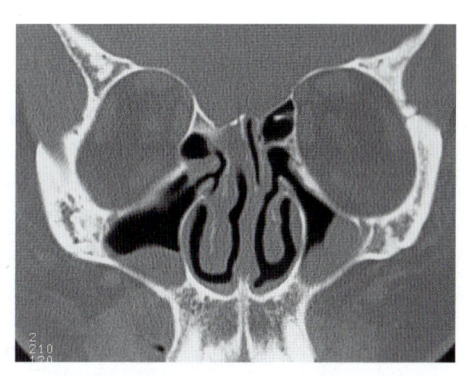

Fig. 4.**25** Low-lying fovea ethmoidalis. **a** Coronal CT scan shows low position of right fovea ethmoidalis. Note opacified right anterior ethmoid cells. **b** Coronal CT scan in another patient showing inferior displacement as well as bony defect of the right fovea ethmoidalis. The partly opacified right ethmoid cells and the superior nasal mass were found to be due to brain herniation.

Pneumatized Superior Concha

The superior turbinate can be invaded by posterior ethmoid air cells, which can enlarge the turbinate (Fig. 4.**24 b**).

Bulging of the Optic Canal into the Posterior Ethmoidal Complex

An important observation is extensive lateral pneumatization of the posterior ethmoidal air cells, which can increase the vulnerability of the optic nerve (Figs. 4.**15**, 4.**16**). In rare instances, the internal carotid artery may be exposed in the posterior ethmoidal and sphenoid sinuses. In addition, identification of an asym-

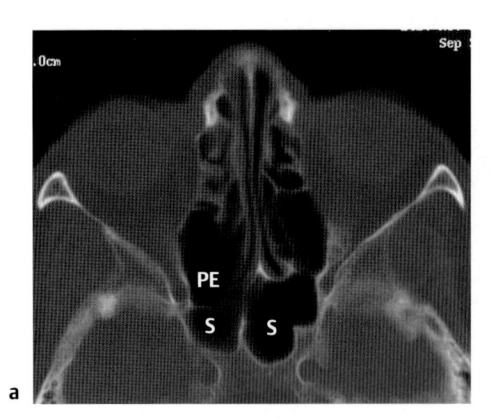

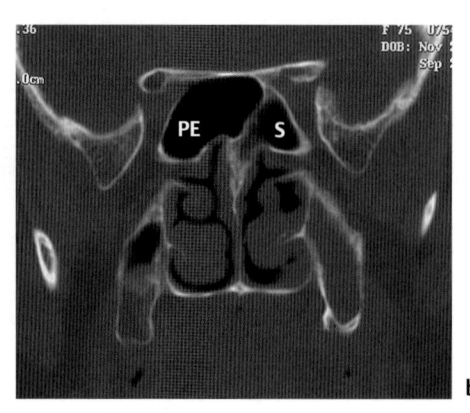

Fig. 4.26 Onodi cell. **a** Axial and **b** coronal CT scans, showing extension of the right posterior ethmoid cell (PE), the "Onodi cell", into the right sphenoid sinus (S). At surgery this Onodi cell may be mistaken for the sphenoid sinus as seen in Fig. 4.26b.

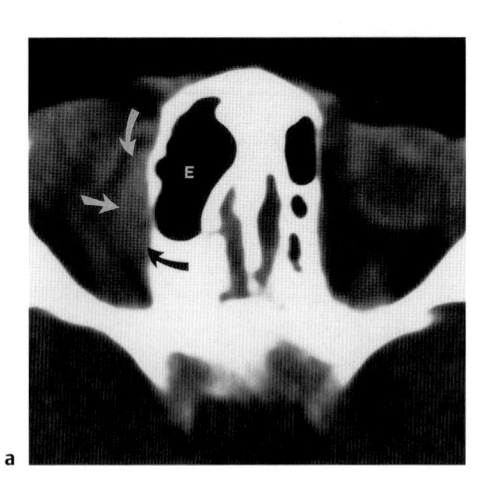

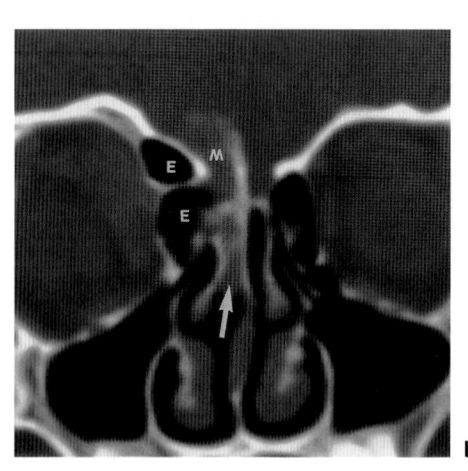

Fig. 4.27 Meningioma and associated penumosinus dilatans. **a** Axial CT scan shows extension of an anterior cranial fossa meningioma into the right orbit (arrows). Note enlargement of right ethmoid cells (E).
b Coronal CT scan shows meningioma (M) in the anterior cranial fossa and its extension into the right nasal cavity (arrow). Note enlargement of right anterior ethmoid air cells (E). Case courtesy of Dr. E.L. Tajudine, Saudi Arabia.

metric intersphenoid septum is important because the posterior extension of this partition usually marks the location of the internal carotid artery.

Onodi Cell

This is a posterior ethmoid air cell encroaching into the anterior aspect of the sphenoid sinus. Adolf Onodi,[33] a professor of laryngology at the University of Budapest in Hungary, first described the sphenoethmoid ("Onodi") cell. He reported that the posterior ethmoid cell could pneumatize laterally or superolaterally to the sphenoid sinus, resulting in an anatomical variation in which the sphenoid sinus could be inferior and medial to the posterior ethmoid cell. In 1995, an attempt was made to standardize the definition of the Onodi cell. The Anatomic Terminology Group[35] defined the Onodi cell as the most posterior ethmoid cell that pneumatizes laterally and superiorly to the sphenoid sinus and is intimately associated with the optic nerve (Fig. 4.26).[35] Given this definition, the incidence of the Onodi cell has been estimated to range from 8% to 14% in the population.[34] Extensive pneumatization of the sphenoid sinus may result in pneumatization of the medial aspect of the lesser wing, including the anterior clinoid. This has been called "pneumosinus dilatans."[34] The surgical significance of the presence of the Onodi cell makes its identification of paramount significance.[34] The presence of the Onodi cell can increase the risk of orbital complications of endoscopic and other surgical approaches to the sphenoid and posterior ethmoid sinuses. During endoscopic sinus surgery, the Onodi cell may be mistaken for the sphenoid sinus, causing a distorted spatial perception for the surgeon.[34] The presence of the Onodi cell and pneumatized anterior clinoid may contribute to an increase in the risk of injury to the optic nerve and to the internal carotid artery.

Pneumosinus Dilatans of the Paranasal Sinuses

Pneumosinus dilatans (PD) is a rare condition that is characterized by an unusual dilation of the paranasal sinus by air, which can lead to marked thinning of bony boundaries.[36-39] Involvement of the sphenoid sinus can cause compression of the optic nerve, leading to visual loss.[36] The dehiscence of the roof of the sphenoid sinus may lead to cerebrospinal fluid (CSF) leaks.[40-45] The pathogenesis of PD remains unclear, but five possible mechanism have been postulated: congenital, developmental, neoplastic, fibro-osseous, and obstructive.[38] Congenital agenesis of a cerebral hemisphere or cerebral atrophy can cause frontal sinus overdevelopment. Anophthalmos can cause overdevelopment of the ethmoid sinuses.[38] Developmental anomalies in bone growth and remodeling resulting from alteration in osteoblasts and osteoclast function may cause a generalized overdevelopment of all paranasal sinus.[38] Local meningiomas can cause hyperostosis of surrounding bone and dilation of the adjacent sinus (Fig. 4.27). Fibro-osseous lesions, such as fibrous dysplasia or ossifying fibroma, have also been reported to cause sinus overgrowth.[39] Obstruction of the ostiomeatal complex can also cause an abnormal one-way valve between the nasal cavity and the paranasal sinuses, leading to chronic air trapping and increased intrasinus pressure.[38] Finally, PD may be an anatomical variation and be detected as an incidental finding on imaging studies. PD of the sphenoid sinus is important in patients exposed to barotrauma, such as in diving and flying and forced Valsalva maneuver. Extensive pneumatization of the sphenoid sinus may result in a relatively thin roof as well as the floor of the middle cranial fossa. This may be an important factor in predisposing certain individuals to developing spontaneous CSF leaks (Fig. 4.28).[40-44]

Other anatomical variations include deviation of the nasal septum, paradoxical middle turbinate, horizontal orientation of the uncinate process, vertical orientation of the lateral lamella of the cribriform plate, hypoplastic maxillary sinus (which endangers the orbit during uncinectomy), and posttraumatic or congenital deformity of the medial wall or floor of the orbit. CT scanning and endoscopy are complementary in the diagnosis and treatment of disorders of the nasal cavity and paranasal sinuses.[4–6] Endoscopic nasal sinus surgery, like traditional sinus surgery, is associated with serious risks. Complications such as blindness, ocular motility dysfunction, orbital hematoma, CSF leak, anterior cranial fossa brain and/or vascular damage, brain abscess, pneumocephalus, carotid–cavernous sinus fistula, and death have been reported.[45–49] Buus et al[48] reported bilateral blindness in a 39-year-old woman following endoscopic ethmoidectomy. Pathological specimens from both sides revealed optic nerve tissues. As an entire generation of otolaryngologists learns these new techniques, complications will continue to evolve. Prevention begins with proper preoperative endoscopic and CT evaluation and surgical preparation.[46, 48, 49]

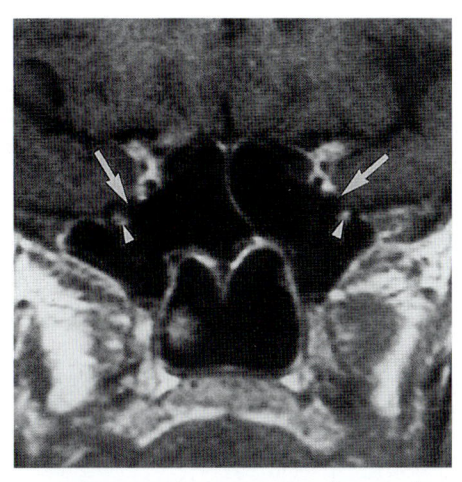

Fig. 4.**28** Coronal T1W MR scan showing the sphenoid sinuses and intersphenoid septum. Note lateral extension into the base of the pterygoid processes. Note the thinning of the middle cranial fossa bone, with the dura lying directly against the mucous membrane of the sphenoid sinuses (arrows). The maxillary nerves project through the foramen rotundum (arrowheads).

Pterygomaxillary Fissure, Pterygopalatine (Sphenopalatine) Fossa, and Palatine Bone

The infratemporal fossa lies below the infratemporal crest on the greater wing of the sphenoid, which is at a level with the upper border of the zygomatic arch[1]. The pterygomaxillary fissure (PMF), the lateral opening of the pterygopalatine fossa (PPF), is a triangular interval that lies within the medial portion of the infratemporal fossa, formed by the divergence of the maxilla from the pterygoid process of the sphenoid bone (Figs. 4.**29**–4.**30**).[1] The PMF has a well-defined posterior margin formed superiorly by the lateral margin of the anterior surface of the base of the pterygoid process and inferiorly by the fused pterygoid plates, and a less well-defined anterior margin, owing to the curving contour of the posterior wall of the maxillary sinus (Fig. 4.**30**). The pterygopalatine fossa (PPF) is a small space, in continuity with the superior aspect of the PMF, and behind and below the orbital apex (Figs. 4.**29**–4.**31**). This relatively small inverted triangular space is bounded posteriorly by the fused pterygoid plates and the base (root) of the sphenoid bone, medially and more superiorly anteromedially by the vertical plate of palatine bone, and anteriorly by the posterior wall of the maxillary bone (Figs. 4.**29**–4.**31**).[1, 50] The fossa is a major crossroad between the nasal cavity (via the sphenopalatine foramen) (Figs. 4.**29 d**, 4.**31**), orbit (via the inferior orbital fissure) (Figs. 4.**30**, 4.**31**), infratemporal fossa (via the PMF), cranial cavity (via the foramen rotundum and vidian canal) (Fig. 4.**29**), nasopharynx (via the palatovaginal canal), and oral cavity (via the palatine canal) (Fig. 4.**31**) (see Table 4.**3**).[50, 51] When viewed laterally, the PPF appears as a narrow and inferiorly tapering space contiguous with the more anteriorly positioned inferior orbital fissure and formed by a gap between the curving margins of the maxillary and sphenoid bones (Figs. 4.**29**–4.**31**). The gap is bridged inferiorly and medially by the palatine bone, which has a unique configuration.[50]

The palatine bone has an L-shaped appearance in a frontal view owing to its horizontal and perpendicular plates (Figs. 4.**33**, 4.**34**). The horizontal plates of each palatine bone unite to form the posterior part of the hard palate that fuses to the palatine processes of the maxillary bones. At the upper part of the perpendicular plate, processes are present that fuse with the maxillary and sphenoid bones. The orbital process extends superolaterally to attach to the posterior margin of the orbital surface of the maxillary bone and partly to the inferior surface of the body of the sphenoid bone. The sphenoidal process extends superomedially to attach to the base of the medial pterygoid plate.[50] The perpendicular plate fuses anteriorly with the rough posterior surface of the medial wall of the maxillary bone, thus covering part of the maxillary hiatus of the maxillary sinus (Fig. 4.**32**).[50] Posteriorly, the perpendicular plate is variably contoured and fuses with the medial surface of the medial pterygoid plate (Fig. 4.**34**). The perpendicular plate has complex medial and

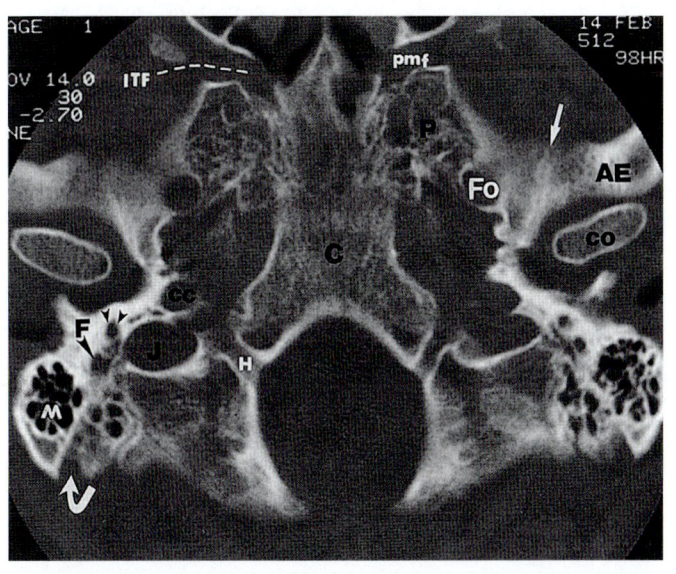

Fig. 4.**29 a** Normal anatomy of the base of the skull. Axial CT scan shows the digastric notch (curved arrow), mastoid process (M), facial nerve canal (F) and anterior to that bone marrow of the root of the styloid process (double arrowheads), jugular fossa (J), carotid canal (cc), hypoglossal canal (H), clivus (C), mandibular condyle (co), articular eminence (AE), sphenotemporal suture (straight arrow), foramen ovale (Fo), base of the pterygoid plate (P), and pterygomaxillary fissure (pmf), entering into the infratemporal fossa (ITF, dashed line).

Fig. 4.**29 b–e** ▷

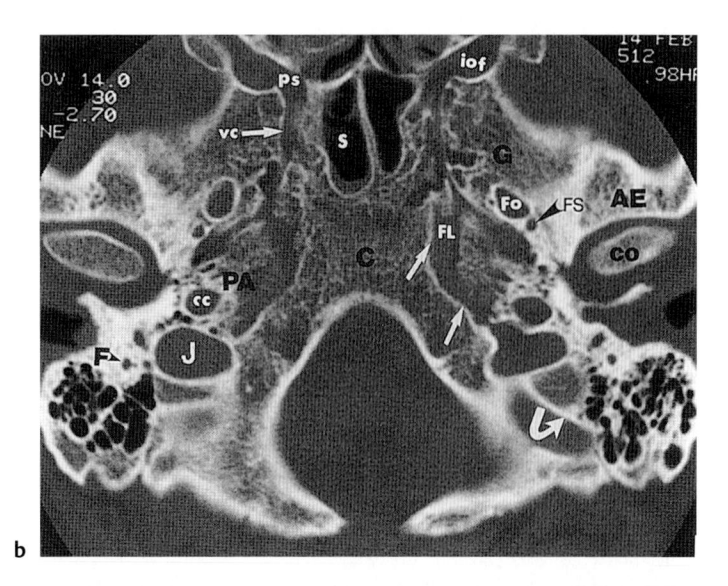

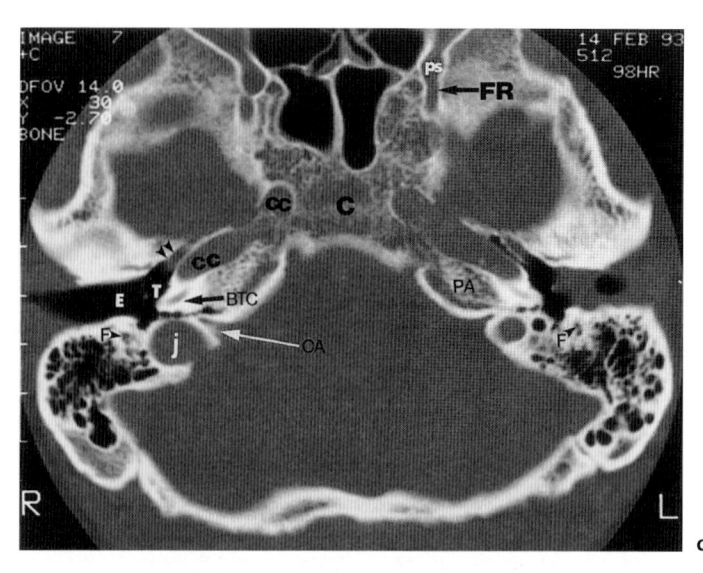

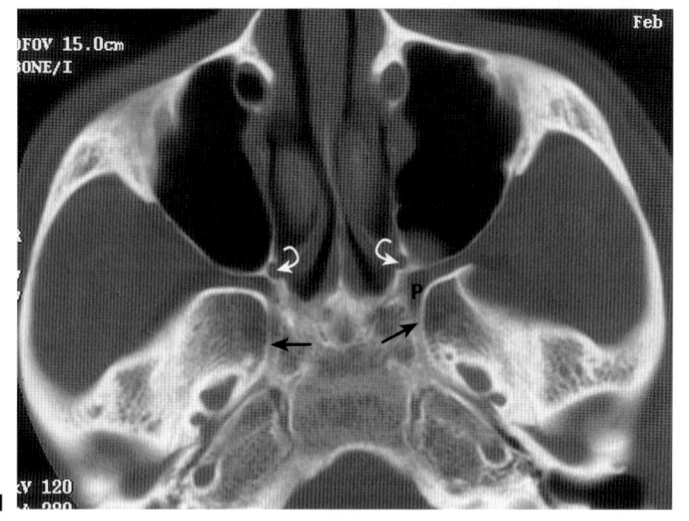

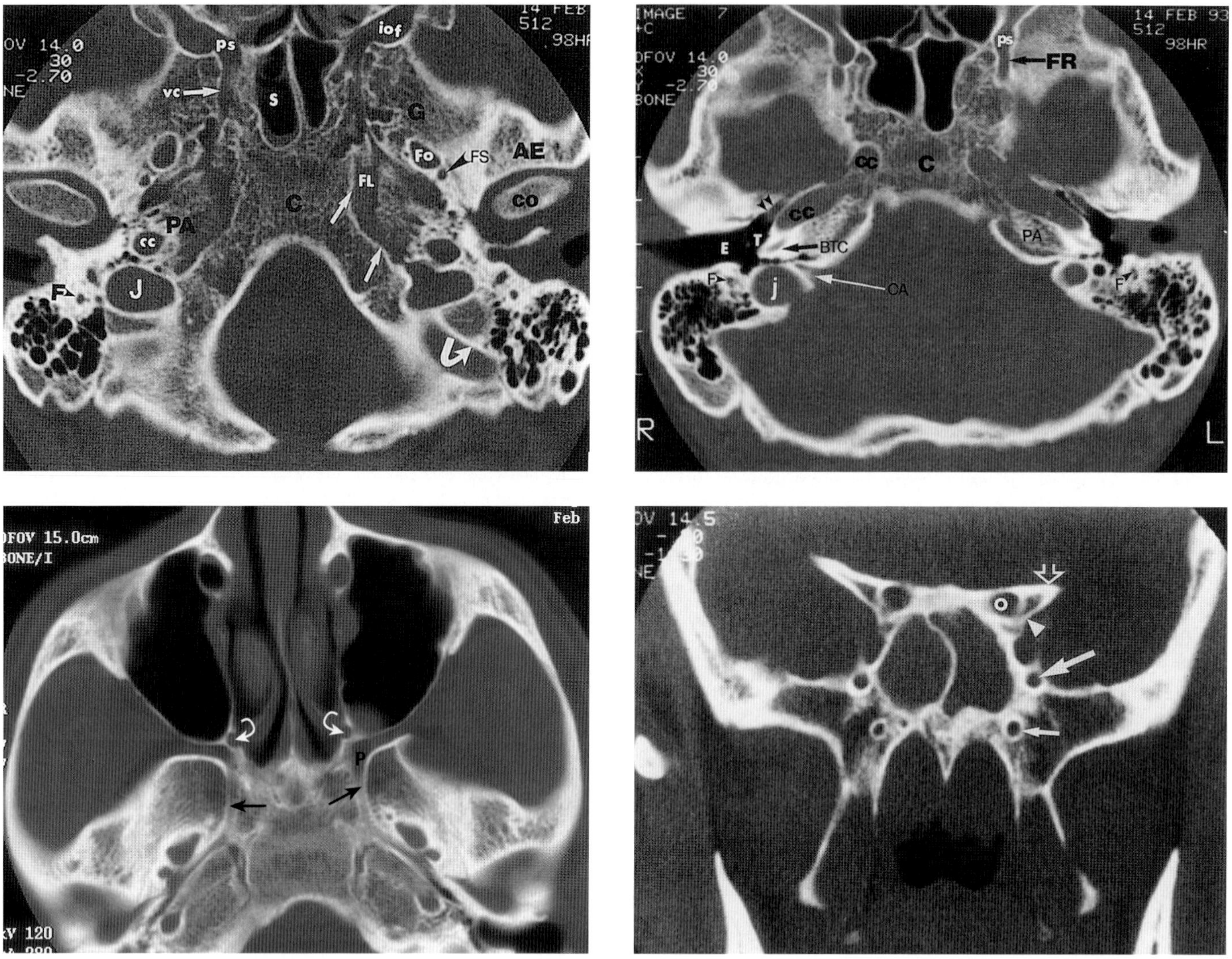

Fig. 4.29
b Axial CT scan, taken 3 mm cephalad to **a**, showing the facial nerve canal (F), jugluar fossa (J), carotid canal (cc), petrous apex (PA), clivus (C), vidian canal (vc), pterygopalatine fossa (ps), sphenoid sinus (s), inferior orbital fissure (iof), greater wing of the sphenoid (G), foramen ovale (Fo), foramen lacerum (FL), foramen spinosum (FS), articular eminence (AE), mandibular condyle (co), petro-occipital fissure (straight arrows), and sigmoid sinus plate (curved arrow). The inferior petrosal vein runs along the petro-ocipital fissure to join the jugular bulb.

c Axial CT scan showing the facial nerve canal (F), jugular fossa (j), cochlear aqueduct (CA), basal turn of the cochlea (BTC), tympanic cavity (T), external auditory canal (E), tensor tympani muscle (arrowheads), carotid canal (cc), clivus (C), pterygopalatine fossa (ps), foramen rotundum (FR), and bone marrow of the petrous apex (PA).

d Axial CT scan showing sphenopalatine canal (curved arrows), vidian canal (straight arrow), and pterygopalatine fossa (P).

e Direct coronal CT scan showing the lesser wing of the sphenoid (hollow arrow), optic canal (o), optic strut (arrowhead), foramen rotundum (large arrow), and vidian canal (short arrow). Note the opacification of the sphenoid sinuses. With advancing age, absorption of bone from the inner walls of the skull bone may occur as an atrophic change. This may result in thinning of the middle cranial fossa with the dura and subarachnoid space directly against the mucous membrane of the sphenoid sinuses (see Fig. 4.28). This thinning may result in spontaneous CSF rhinorrhea.

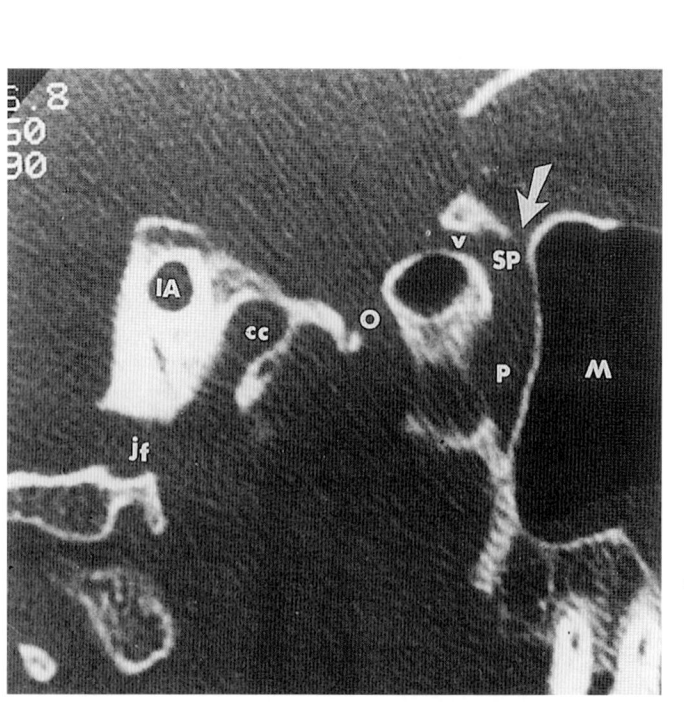

Fig. 4.30 Sphenopalatine fossa. Semisagittal CT scan showing the maxillary sinus (M), pterygomaxillary fissure (P), sphenopalatine fossa (SP), inferior orbital fissure (arrow), foramen ovale (O), pterygoid (vidian) canal (v), internal carotid canal (cc), jugular fossa (jf), and internal auditory canal (IA).

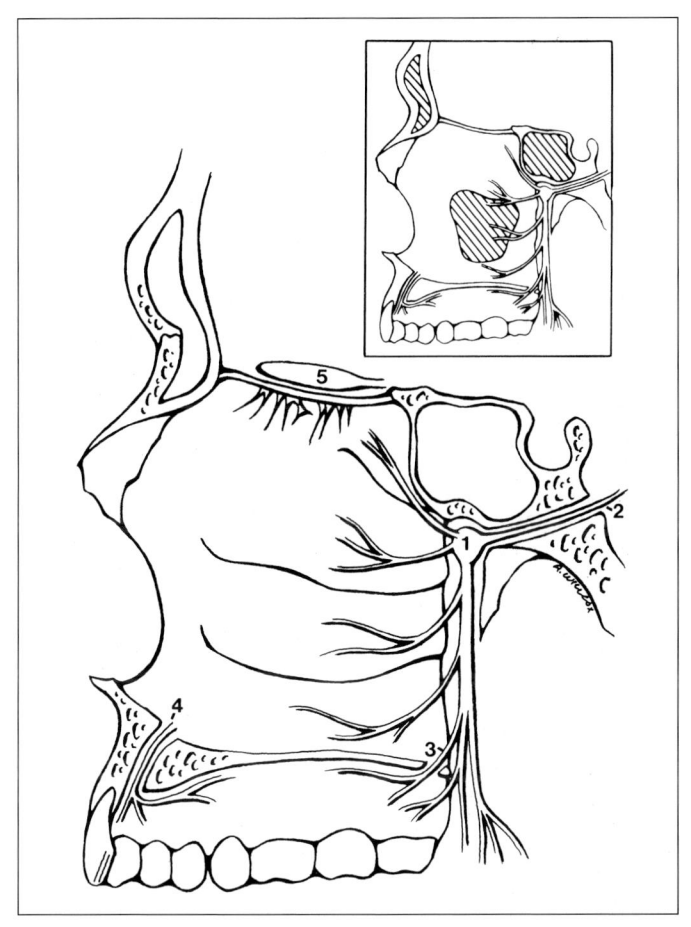

Fig. 4.31 Schematic drawing of the sphenopalatine ganglion and its branches, with insert showing the sinuses. Note the sphenopalatine ganglion (1), vidian nerve within the pterygoid canal (2), greater palatine nerve (3), nasopalatine nerve (4), and olfactory bulb (5). Modified from Warwick R, Williams PL, eds. Gray's Anatomy, 35th British ed. Philadelphia: W.B. Saunders, 1973.

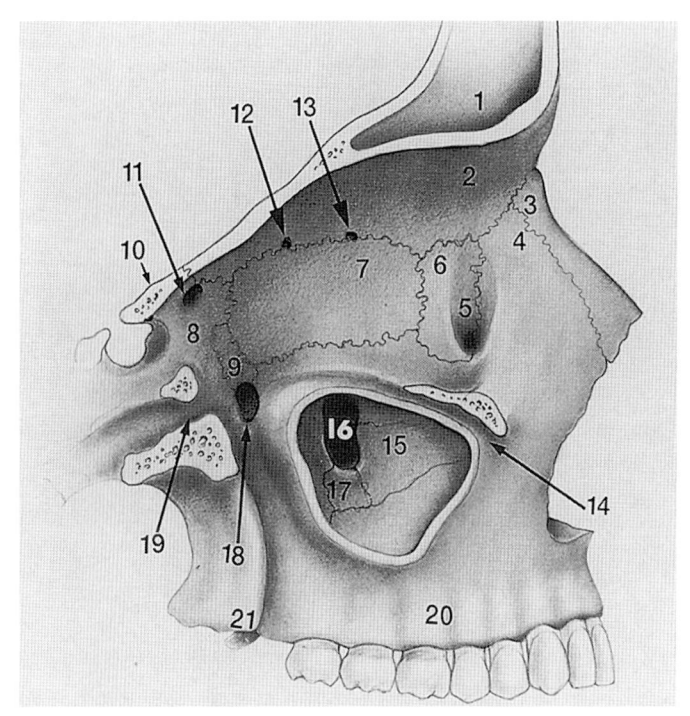

Fig. 4.32 Schematic drawing of the orbital maxillary region.
1 = frontal sinus
2 = orbital plate of frontal bone
3 = nasal bone
4 = frontal process of maxilla
5 = lacrimal groove
6 = lacrimal bone
7 = lamina papyracea
8 = sphenoid bone
9 = palatine bone
10 = lesser wing of the sphenoid
11 = optic canal
12 = posterior ethmoid foramen
13 = anterior ethmoid foramen
14 = infraorbital canal (foramen)
15 = inferior concha
16 = maxillary hiatus
17 = palatine bone
18 = sphenopalatine foramen opening into pterygopalatine fossa
19 = vidian canal, opening into pterygopalatine fossa
20 = alveolar process of maxilla
21 = pterygoid plate

lateral surfaces (Fig. 4.34). The lateral surface from anteriorly to posteriorly consists of a smooth part that covers part of the maxillary hiatus of the maxillary sinus; a rough part attaching to the rough posterior surface of the medial wall of the maxillary bone; a somewhat V-shaped part that superiorly attaches to the orbital and sphenoidal processes of the palatine bone which together form the anterior-medial wall of the PPF (Fig. 4.34); next a curving ridge that attaches to the anteriorly fused pterygoid plates and anterior edge of the superior part of the medial pterygoid plate; and most posteriorly a variably contoured bony plate that fuses with the anterior part of the medial surface of the medial pterygoid plate.[50] The medial surface forming part of the lateral wall of the nasal fossa has an ethmoidal crest contiguous with the middle turbinate and also a conchal crest contiguous with the inferior turbinate. The upper part of the perpendicular plate, and the orbital and sphenoidal processes and the sphenopalatine groove between the processes, form an acute angle with the anterior surface of the sphenoid bone, while the inferior part of the perpendicular plate is nearly parasagittally oriented.[50]

Important attachments are also made by the orbital, sphenoidal, and pyramidal processes of the palatine bone. The orbital process extends superolaterally to attach to the posterior margin of the orbital surface of the maxillary bone and partly to the inferior surface of the body of the sphenoid bone. The sphenoidal process extends superomedially to attach to the base of the medial pterygoid plate. Both orbital and sphenoidal processes form part of the walls of the PPF and nasal fossa (Figs. 4.33, 4.34).[50,51] The pyramidal process arising from the junction of the horizontal and perpendicular plates attaches to the maxillary bone and extends posterolaterally to attach to the angled inferior margins of the pterygoid plates. In addition to the palatine bone, the anatomy of the pterygoid processes of the sphenoid bone is also complex. The pterygoid process positioned inferiorly to the body and greater wing of the sphenoid bone consists of the base and medial and lateral pterygoid plates (Fig. 4.34). The anterior surface of the base forms a shallow recess slightly deeper medially following the curve of the medial pterygoid plate and bounded by the greater wing and body of the sphenoid bone, inferior margin of the superior orbital fissure, fused pterygoid plates, and superior part of the medial pterygoid plate. This recess, containing the anterior openings of the foramen rotundum superiorly and vidian (pterygoid) canal inferomedially, forms most of the posterior wall of the PPF (Figs. 4.29b, c, 4.30); its lateral edge forms most of the posterior margin of the pterygomaxillary fissure with the small inferior part formed by the pterygoid plates. More inferiorly, the separated pterygoid plates attach to the pyramidal process of palatine bone. The pterygomaxillary fissure, superiorly the lateral opening of the PPF, has a well-defined posterior margin formed superiorly by the lateral margin of the base of the pterygoid processes and inferiorly by fused pterygoid plates and an anterior margin formed by the curving contour of the medial aspect of the posterior wall of the maxillary sinus (Fig. 4.30). The

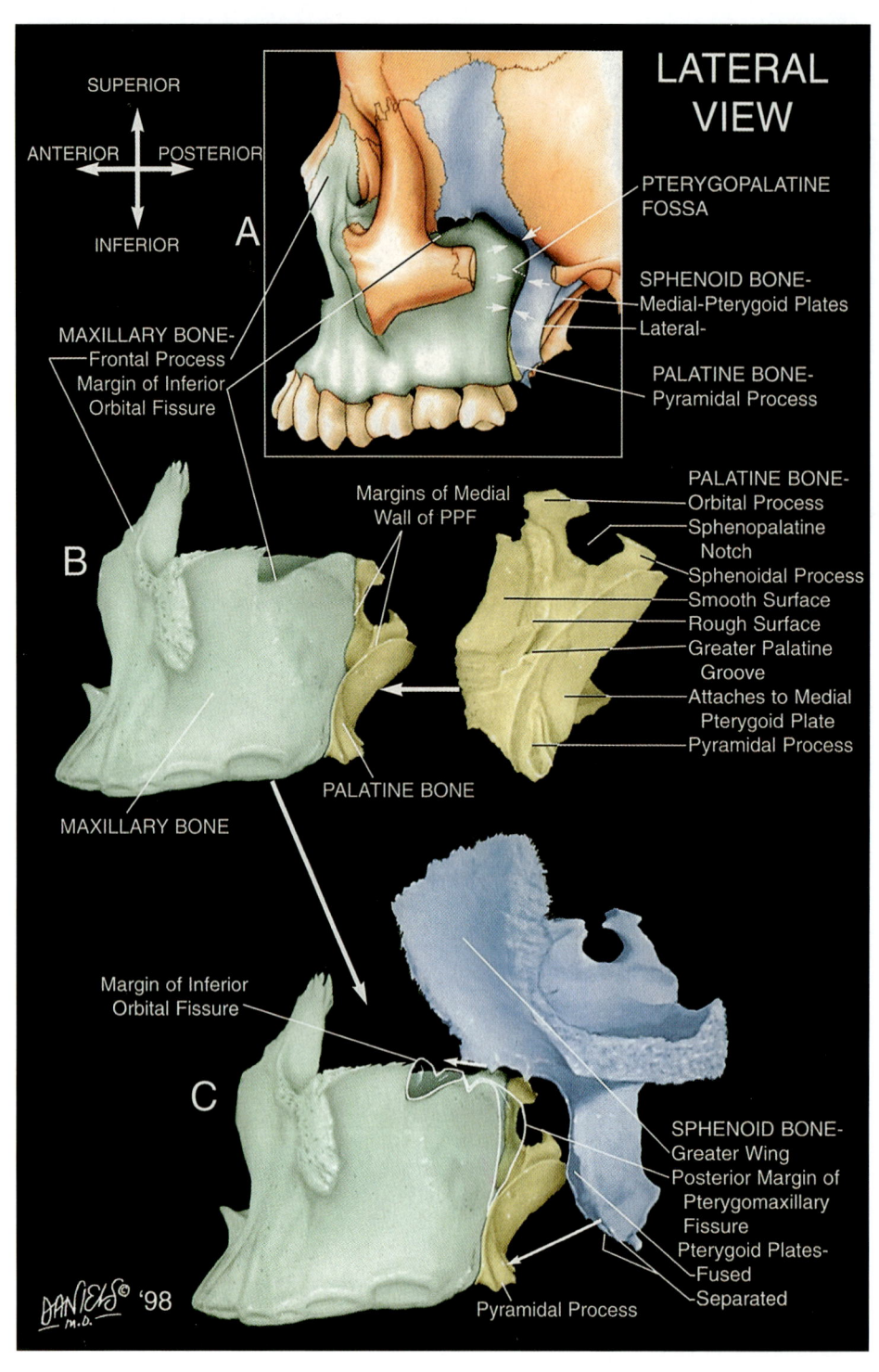

Fig. 4.33 Lateral views of the sphenoid, palatine, and maxillary bones.

A Shown in the intact skull is the curving gap between the sphenoid and maxillary bones, consisting of the pterygopalatine fossa (PPF) and its lateral opening, the pterygomaxillary fissure (arrows), and the more anteriorly positioned inferior orbital fissure.

B To form the anterior margin of the medial wall of the PPF, the rough surface of the palatine bone is shown attaching to the posteromedial surface of the maxillary bone. More inferiorly, the anterior surface of the pyramidal process of the palatine bone attaches to the maxillary bone. The medial wall of the PPF tapers inferiorly.

C Completing the PPF, the medial surface of the medial pterygoid plate attaches to the most posterior part of the perpendicular plate of the palatine bone. More inferiorly, the pyramidal process fuses with the angled inferior margins of the pterygoid plates. The pterygomaxillary fissure is formed anteriorly by the maxillary bone, posteriorly by the lateral edge of the base of the pterygoid process, and inferiorly by the fused pterygoid plates. The margins of the pterygomaxillary and inferior orbital fissures are shown in white. From Daniels D, et al. Osseous anatomy of pterygopalatine fossa. AJNR 1998; 19: 1425, with permission.

greater anterior palatine canal(s) (Fig. 4.35) formed by the junction of an obliquely descending groove at the posterior-inferior aspect of the medial wall of the maxillary bone and the greater palatine groove, deep to lateral surface of the perpendicular plate of the palatine bone, opens inferiorly at the greater palatine foramen located at the lateral margin of the horizontal plate. The lesser palatine canal(s) extends through the pyramidal process to open at the lesser palatine foramen at the anterior aspect of the inferior surface of the pyramidal process (Fig. 4.36).

The palatine nerves (Fig. 4.31) are distributed to the roof of the mouth, the soft palate, the tonsil, and the lining membrane of the nasal cavity.[1] The greater (anterior) palatine nerve descends through the greater palatine canal and emerges upon the hard palate through the greater palatine foramen (Figs. 4.31, 4.35, 4.36).[1] It supplies the gums, and the mucous membrane and glands of the hard palate. While in the greater palatine canal (Fig. 4.31), it gives off nasal branches, which emerge through openings in the perpendicular plate of the palatine bone and ramify over the inferior nasal concha and the walls of the middle and inferior meati; at its exit from the canal, palatine branches are distributed on the soft palate. The lesser (middle and posterior) palatine nerves descend through the greater palatine canal, emerge through the lesser palatine foramina, and supply branches to the uvula, tonsil, and soft palate.

Pterygomaxillary Fissure, Pterygopalatine (Sphenopalatine) Fossa, and Palatine Bone 375

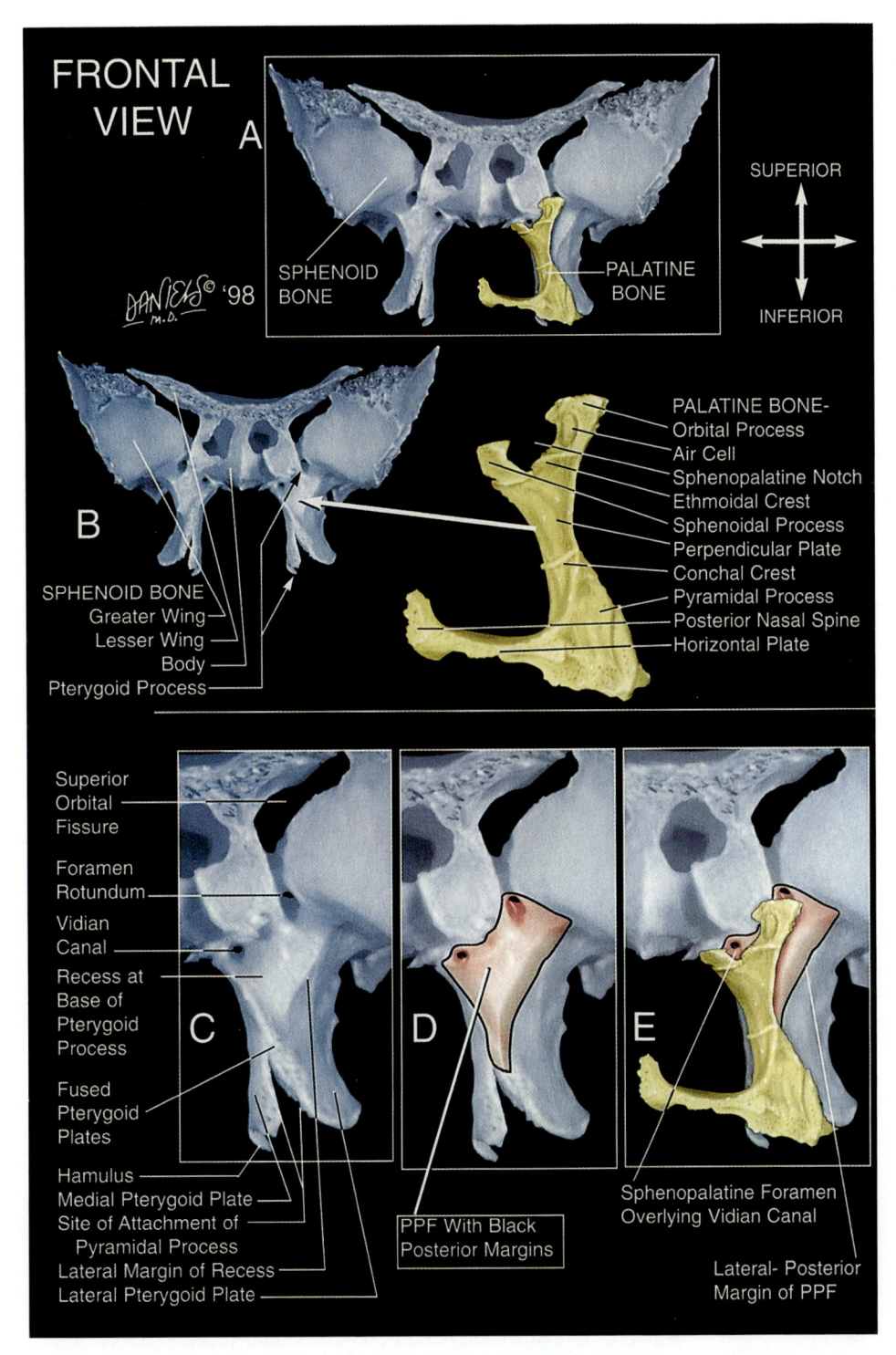

Fig. 4.34 Frontal views of the sphenoid and palatine bones.
A Overview of the palatine bone attached to the pterygoid process and inferior aspect of the body of the sphenoid bone.
B The palatine bone is shaped like a right angle owing to its horizontal and perpendicular plates. The pyramidal process arises at the junction of these plates and extends posterolaterally between the inferior margins of the pterygoid plates.
C Magnified view of the pterygoid process shows the shallow recess at the base of the sphenoid bone. It is deeper medially, forms most of the posterior wall of the PPF, and contains the openings of the foramen rotundum and the more inferomedially positioned vidian canal.
D The posterior margins of the PPF correspond to the margins of the recess at the base of the sphenoid bone and taper inferiorly.
E With the palatine bone in place, note the angled configuration of the upper part of the perpendicular plate, the orbital and sphenoidal processes, and the sphenopalatine foramen. The sphenopalatine foramen is shown overlying the vidian canal, a relationship that can be seen on axial CT scans (see Fig. 4.29d). The PPF extends lateral to the upper part of the perpendicular plate of the palatine bone. From Daniels D, et al. Osseous anatomy of the pterygopalatine fossa. AJNR 1998; 19: 1425, with permission.

■ The Pterygopalatine (Sphenopalatine) Ganglion

The pterygopalatine ganglion (PPG) (Fig. 4.31) is the largest of the peripheral ganglia of the parasympathetic system. It is deeply placed in the pterygopalatine fossa (PPF), in front of the pterygoid (vidian) canal (Figs. 4.29b, 4.31, 4.32).[1] It is situated just below the maxillary nerve as it crosses the fossa. The motor or parasympathetic root is formed by the nerve of the pterygoid canal, the so-called vidian nerve. The greater petrosal nerve arises from the genicular ganglion of the facial nerve and consists chiefly of taste fibers that are distributed to the mucous membrane of the palate; but it also contains preganglionic parasympathetic fibers that are destined for the PPG. It passes forward and reaches the foramen lacerum. In this foramen it is joined by the deep petrosal nerve from the sympathetic plexus on the internal carotid artery, and forms the nerve of the pterygoid (vidian) canal, which passes forward through the vidian canal and ends in the PPG. The sympathetic root of the PPG is also incorporated into the nerve of the pterygoid canal. Its fibers, which are postganglionic, arise in the superior cervical ganglion and travel into the internal carotid plexus and the deep petrosal nerve.[1] The branches that appear to arise from the pterygopalatine ganglion are, for the most part, derived from the maxillary nerve through its ganglionic branches and, though intimately related to the

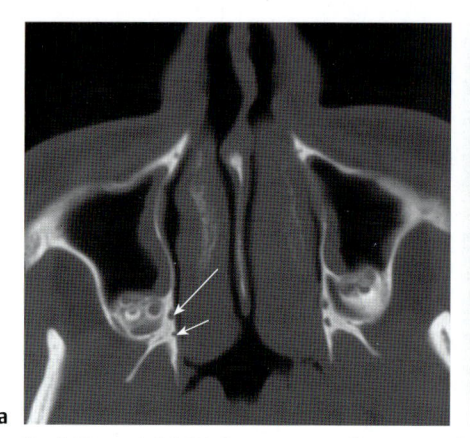

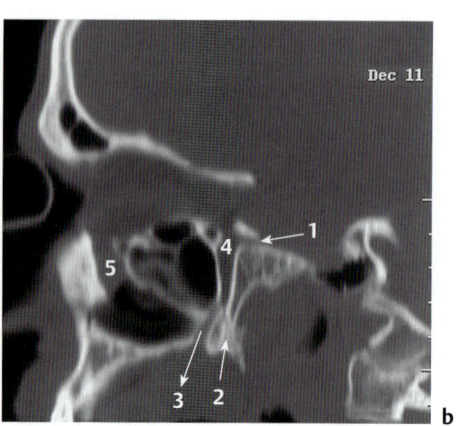

Fig 4.35 a Axial CT shows greater (large arrow) and lesser (short arrow) palatine foramina. b Reformatted sagittal CT scan, showing vidian canal (1), lesser palatine canal (2), greater palatine canal (3), pterygopalatine fossa (4) and nasolacrimal canal (5).

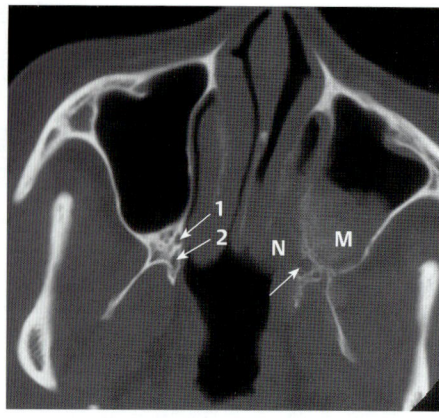

Fig. 4.36 Palatine foramina. Axial CT scan, showing greater (1) and lesser (2) palatine foramina. Note enlargement of the left greater palatine (arrow) due to perineural extension of an adenoid cystic carcinoma in the left maxillary sinus (M) and nasal cavity (N).

ganglion, do not establish any synaptic connection with its cells.[1] They include orbital, palatine, nasal and pharyngeal branches. The orbital branches enter the orbit by the inferior orbital fissure and are distributed to the periosteum and the orbitalis muscles.[1] Some twigs pass through posterior ethmoid foramen to the ethmoid and sphenoidal sinuses. The palatine nerves are distributed to the roof of the mouth, the soft palate, the tonsil, and the lining membrane of the nasal cavity.[1] The nasal branches enter the nasal cavity through the sphenopalatine foramen (Fig. 4.29d). The pharyngeal nerve, a small branch, arises from the posterior aspect of the PPG, passes through the palatovaginal canal with the pharyngeal branch of the maxillary artery (see Table 4.3), and is distributed to the mucous membrane of the nasal part of the pharynx, behind the auditory tube.[1] The palatovaginal canal is formed by the inferior surface of the vaginal process of the ala of the vomer bone and by the upper surface of the sphenoidal process of the palatine bone.[1] The canal opens anteriorly through the posterior wall of the PPF.

The fossa communicates laterally with the infratemporal fossa through the pterygomaxillary fissure (Fig. 4.29a, 4.3b), medially with the nasal cavity through the sphenopalatine foramen (Fig. 4.29d), anteriorly with the orbit through the inferior orbital fissure (Fig. 4.29d, 4.30), and superiorly with the cranial fossa through the foramen rotundum (Fig. 4.29c) and pterygoid (vidian) canal (Fig. 4.29d, 4.30, 4.31). The sphenopalatine foramen through the vertical portion of the palatine bone transmits the sphenopalatine vessels and the superior nasal and nasopalatine nerves. The foramen serves as a communication medially between the pterygopalatine fossa and the superior meatus of the nasal cavity.

■ Applied Anatomy

The various communications of the PPF provide a means of spread of infection and tumor among the nasal cavity, orbit, infratemporal fossa, cranial cavity, nasopharynx, oral cavity, and oropharynx (Table 4.3). Tumor and infection can extend through the PPF via the orbital apex, the inferior orbital fissure, the foramen rotundum (which allows access to the cavernous sinus), the vidian canal (leading to the foramen lacerum and petrous apex), the vidian nerve (leading to the geniculate ganglion of the facial nerve), the sphenopalatine foramen (providing access to the posterosuperior part of the nasal cavity), the greater and lesser palatine canals (leading to the palatine foramina and hence the oral cavity) (Figs. 4.35, 4.37, 4.38), the pterygomaxillary fissure (which communicates with the masticator space), and the palatovaginal (pharyngeal) canal (which communicates with the nasopharynx). The palatovaginal canal, which transmits the pharyngeal nerve and artery from the PPF to the roof of the pharynx, is a potential communication between the nasopharynx and the PPF. The canal opens anteriorly through the posterior wall of the PPF. It transmits the pharyngeal branch of the pterygopalatine ganglion and a pharyngeal branch of maxillary artery. Inferiorly at the narrow inferior portion of the pterygomaxillary fissure, the pterygopalatine (palatine) canal (Fig. 4.31) transmits the palatine vessels and nerves, serving as a potential communication with the oral cavity.

The sphenopalatine artery, a major blood vessel of the nasal mucosa, exits from the sphenopalatine foramen and supplies the nasal turbinates, the fontanelle, and the nasal septum.[52] The sphenopalatine artery is the end artery of the internal maxillary artery located in the sphenopalatine (pterygopalatine) or vidian canal.[52] Posterior epistaxis develops from injury to various branches of the sphenopalatine artery.[52] In cases of massive bleeding unresponsive to conservative treatment such as nasal packing or electrocautery, the bleeder is identified and ligated. Damage to the sphenopalatine artery (SPA) during nasal surgery causes severe bleeding.[52] The sphenopalatine foramen is bounded superiorly by the body of the sphenoid, anteriorly by the orbital process of the palatine bone, and posteriorly by the sphenoidal process of the palatine bone (Fig. 4.29d).[52–54] The sphenopalatine foramen is located between the posterior end of the horizontal lamella of the middle turbinate and the posterior end of the horizontal lamella of the superior turbinate (Fig. 4.29d).[52] On CT scans, the sphenopalatine foramen can be recognized by its angled contour and location just anterior to the vidian canal (Fig. 4.29b, d). Also, on CT scan and during surgery, it is helpful to assume that the sphenopalatine foramen is located above the posterior end of the horizontal lamella of the middle turbinate (Fig. 4.29d).[52] In most cases, the sphenopalatine foramen is located posterior to the ethmoidal crest in the perpendicular plate of the palatine bone. Therefore, during the intranasal surgical approach, the ethmoidal crest that is exposed after removing the mucosa may be used as a landmark in searching for the sphenopalatine foramen.[52] The important surgical technique for maxillary sinusitis is middle meatal antrostomy. When removing the fontanelle to perform antrostomy by removing only

Table 4.3 Canals, foramina, and fissures communicating with the pterygopalatine fossa (PPF) and pathways of spread of malignancy and infection of the head and neck via the PPF

Name	Location	Contents	Pathway of spread via PPF
Foramen rotundum	Greater wing of sphenoid	Maxillary nerve, and venous plexus	From PPF to cavernous sinus
Pterygoid canal (vidian canal)	Sphenoid bone	(Vidian) Pterygoid nerve and vessels	From PPF to foramen lacerum
Inferior orbital fissure	Greater wing of sphenoid, palatine, zygomatic, and maxillary bones	V2 infraorbital, and zygomatic parasympathetic branches from pterygopalatine ganglion	From PPF to orbital apex
Sphenopalatine foramen	Body of sphenoid, sphenoidal process, and orbital process of palatine bone	Nasopalatine nerve and accompanying vessels	Nasal cavity to PPF and vice versa
Greater palatine canal	Maxilla and palatine bone	Anterior, middle, and posterior palatine nerves and the greater and lesser palatine vessels that emerge through foramina on the bony palate	From oral cavity to PPF and vice versa
Palatovaginal canal	Vaginal process of vomer bone and palatine bone	Pharyngeal branch of the pterygopalatine ganglion and a minute pharyngeal branch of the maxillary artery	From the roof of pharynx (nasopharynx) to PPF and vice versa
Petrygomaxillary fissure	Maxilla and pterygoid process of sphenoid bone	Terminal branches of the maxillary artery, maxillary nerve	From PPF to infratemporal fossa and vice versa

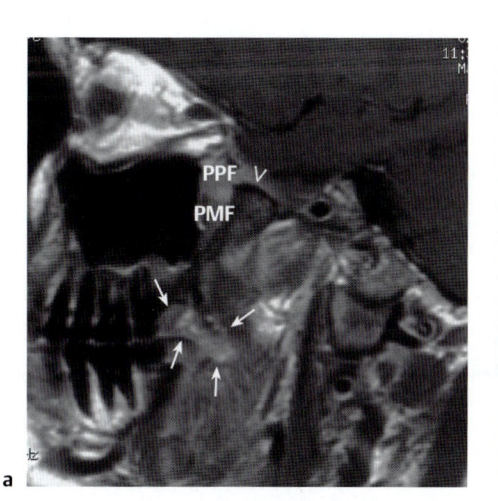

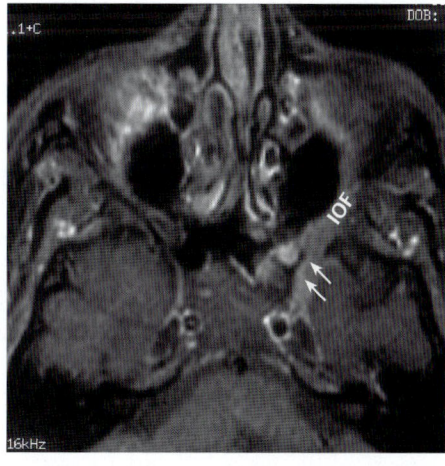

Fig. 4.37 Perineural extension of adenoid cystic carcinoma. **a** Enhanced sagittal T1W MR scan, showing an adenoid cystic carcinoma of the hard palate (arrows). Note extension of tumor along pterygomaxillary fissure (PMF), pterygopalatine fossa (PPF), and vidian canal (V). **b** Axial enhanced fat-suppression T1W MR scan, showing tumor extension along the left maxillary nerve (arrows) and along the inferior orbital fissure (IOF).

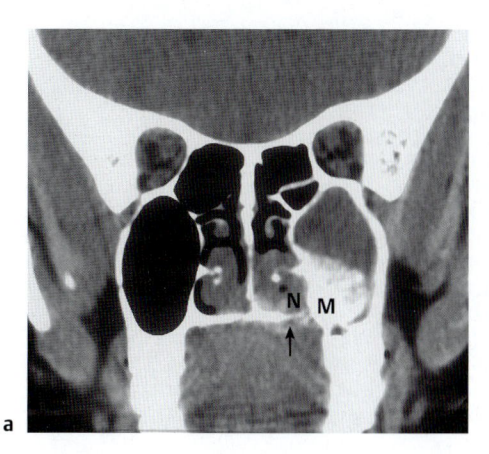

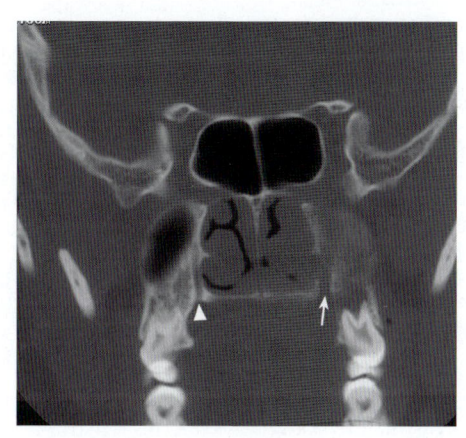

Fig. 4.38 Perineural extension of adenoid cystic carcinoma. **a** Coronal CT scan shows a calcified mass (M) in the left maxillary sinus, with extension into the nasal cavity (N) and hard palate (arrow). **b** Coronal CT scan shows enlargement of left greater palatine foramen (arrow) and palatine canal. Note normal right palatine foramen and canal (arrowhead).

the fontanelle area, arterial bleeding is occasionally encountered. When removing the perpendicular plate of the palatine bone to create a large middle meatal antrostomy opening, the main branch of the posterior lateral nasal artery, a branch of SPA, may be injured.[52] During conchotomy, massive arterial bleeding does not usually occur when removing the anterior and inferior half of the inferior turbinate, but it can be expected when removing the posterior and superior portion.[52]

References

1. Warwick R, Williams PL, eds. Gray's Anatomy, 35th British ed., Philadelphia: W.B. Saunders; 1973.
2. Wenig BM. Atlas of Head and Neck Pathology. Philadelphia: W.B. Saunders; 1993.
3. Graney DO, Rice DH. Paranasal sinuses—anatomy. In: Cummings CW, Fredrickson JM, Harker LA, Krause CJ, Schuller DE, eds. Otolaryngology Head and Neck Surgery. St. Louis: Mosby-Year Book; 1993: 901–906.
4. Mafee MF. Endoscopic sinus surgery: role of the radiologist. AJNR 1991; 12: 855–860.
5. Mafee MF, Chow JM, Meyers R. Functional endoscopic sinus surgery: Anatomy, CT Screening, indications, and complications. AJR 1993; 160: 735–744.
6. Mafee MF. Preoperative imaging anatomy of nasal-ethmoid complex for functional endoscopic sinus surgery. Radiol Clin North Am 1993; 31(1): 1–20.
7. Boek W, Graamans K, Natzijl H, et al. Nasal mucociliary transport: New evidence for a key role of ciliary beat frequency. Laryngoscope 2002; 112: 570–573.
8. Jang YJ, Myong NH, Park KH, et al. Mucociliary transport and histologic characteristics of the mucosa of deviated nasal septum. Arch Otolaryngol Head Neck Surg 2002; 128: 421–424.
9. Rautiainen M, Nuutinen J, Kiukaanniemi H, Collan Y. Ultrastructural changes in human nasal cilia caused by the common cold and recovery of ciliated epithelium. Ann Otal Rhinol Laryngol 1992; 101: 982–987.
10. Mafee MF. Imaging of the nasal cavities, paranasal sinuses, nasopharynx, orbits, infratemporal fossa, pterygomaxillary fissure, parapharyngeal space, and base of skull. In: Ballenger JJ, Snow JD, eds. Ballenger's Otorhinolaryngology Head and Neck Surgery, 16th ed. Ontario: BC Decker; 2002.
11. Becker SP. Anatomy for endoscopic sinus surgery. Otolaryngol Clin North Am 1989; 22: 677–682.
12. Van Ayela OE. Ethmoid labyrinth: anatomic study with consideration of the clinical significance of its structural characteristics. Arch Otolaryngol 1939; 39: 881–902.
13. Rice DH. Endoscopic sinus surgery: anterior approach. Oper Tech Otolaryngol Head Neck Surg 1990; 1: 99–103.
14. Zinreich SJ, Kenney DW, Rosenbaum AE, Gayer BW, Kumar AJ, Stammberger H. Paranasal sinuses: CT imaging requirements for endoscopic surgery. Radiology 1987; 163: 709–775.
15. Kasper KA. Nasofrontal connections: a study based on one hundred consecutive dissections. Arch Otolaryngol 1936; 23: 322–343.
16. Zinreich SJ, Abidin M, Kennedy DW. Sectional imaging of the nasal cavity and paranasal sinuses. Oper Tech Otolaryngol Head Neck Surg 1990; 194–98.
17. Bogler WE, Mawn CB. Analysis of the suprabullar and retrobullar recesses for endoscopic sinus surgery. Ann Otol Rhinol Pharyngol Suppl 2002; 186: 3–14.
17a. Carter BL. Paranasal sinuses, nasal cavity, pterygoid fossa, nasopharynx, and infratemporal fossa. In: Valvassori GE. Buckingham RA, Carter BL, Hanafee WN, Mafee MF, eds. Head and Neck Imaging. Stuttgart: Georg Thieme Verlag; 1988: 173–250.
18. Messerklinger W. Endoscopy of the Nose. Baltimore: Urban and Schwarzenberg; 1978.
19. Wigand ME, Steiner W, Jaumann MP. Endonasal sinus surgery with endoscopical control: from radical operation to rehabilitation of the mucosa. Endoscopy 1978; 10: 255–260.
20. Kennedy DW, Zenrich J, Rosenbaum AE, Johns ME. Functional endoscopic sinus surgery: theory and diagnostic evaluation. Arch Otolaryngol 1985; 111: 576–582.
21. Hilding AC. The physiology of drainage of nasal mucus. IV Drainage of the accesory sinuses in man. Otolaryngol Rhinol Laryngol 1944; 53: 34–41.
22. Hilding AC. Physiological basis of nasal operations. Calif Med 1950; 72: 103–107.
23. Procter DF. The nose, paranasal sinuses and pharynx. In: Waters W, ed. Lewis-Walters Practice of Surgery, Vol. 4. Haerstown, MD: Prior; 1966: 1–37.
24. Proctor DF. The mucociliary system. In: Proctor DF, Anderson IHP, eds. The Nose: Upper Airway Physiology and Atmospheric Environment. New York: Elsevier; 1982.
25. Messerklinger W. On the drainage of the normal frontal sinus of man. Acta Otolaryngol 1967; 673: 176–181.
26. Messerklinger W. Uber die Drainage der menschlichen Nasennebenhohlen unter normalen and pathologischen Bedingungen. II. Mitteilung: Die Stirnhohle und ihr Ausfuhrungssystem. Monatsschr Ohrenheilkd 1967; 101: 313.
27. Messerlinger W. Endoscopy of the Nose. Baltimore: Urban and Schwarzenberg; 1978.
28. Winther B, Gross CW. Introduction and indications for functional endonasal (endoscopic) sinus surgery. Oper Tech Otolaryngol Head Neck Surg 1990; 1: 92–93.
29. Schaefer SD. Endoscopic sinus surgery: posterior approach. Oper Tech Otolaryngol Head Neck Surg 1990; 1: 104–107.
30. Stammberger H. Endoscopic endonasal surgery: concepts in treatment of recurring rhinosinusitis. Part I. Anatomic and pathologic considerations. Otolaryngol Head Neck Surg 1986; 94: 143–147.
31. Chow JM, Mafee MF. Radiologic assessment preoperative to endoscopic sinus surgery. Otolaryngol Clin North Am 1989; 22: 691–701.
32. Setliff RC, Catalano PJ, Catalano LA, Francis C. An anatomic classification of the ethmoidal bulba. Otolaryngol Head Neck Surg 2001; 125: 598–602.
33. Onodi A. The Optic Nerve and the Accessory Sinuses of the Nose. New York: William Wood & Co.; 1910.
34. Allmond L, Murr AH. Opacified Onodi cell. Arch Otolaryngol Head and Neck Surg 2002; 128: 598–599.
35. Stammberger HR, Kennedy DW. Paranasal sinuses: anatomic terminology and nomenclature. The Anatomic Terminology Group. Ann Otol Rhinol Laryngol Suppl 1995; 167: 7–16.
36. Skolnick CA, Mafee MF, Goodwin J. Pneumasinus dilatans of the sphenoid sinus presenting with visual loss. J Neuroophthalmol 2000; 20: 259–263.
37. Benjamins LE. Pneumosinus frontalis dilatans. Acta Otolaryngol 1981; 1: 412–423.
38. Ganly I, McGuiness R. Pneumosinus dilatans of the maxillary, ethmoid, and sphenoid sinuses. Arch Otolaryngol Head Neck Surg 2002; 128: 1428–1430.
39. Lloyd GA. Orbital pneumosinus dilatans. Clin Radiol 1985; 36: 381–386.
40. Davis S, Kaye AH. A dynamic pressure study of spontaneous CSF rhinorrhea in the empty sella syndrome. J Neurosurg 1980; 52: 103–105.
41. Clark D, Bullock P, Hui T, Firth J. Benign intracranial hypertension: a cause of CSF rhinorrhea. J. Neurol Neurosurg Psychiatry 1994; 57: 847–849.
42. Kaufman B, Nusen FE, Weiss MH, et al. Acquired spontaneous, nontraumatic normal pressure cerebrospinal fluid fistulas originating from the middle fossa. Radiology 1977; 122: 379–387.
43. Gassner HG, Ponikau JU, Sherris DA, Kern EB. CSF rhinorrhea: 95 consecutive surgical cases with long-term follow-up at the Mayo Clinic. Am J Rhinol 1999; 13: 439–447.
44. Shetty PG, Shroff MM, Fatterpeckar GM, et al. A retrospective analysis of spontaneous sphenoid sinus fistula: MR and CT findings. Am J Neuroradiol 2000; 21: 337–342.
45. Stankiewicz JA. Blindness and intranasal endoscopic ethmoidectomy. Laryngoscope 1987; 97: 1270–1273.
46. Stankiewicz JA. Complications of endoscopic sinus surgery. Otolaryngol Clin North Am 1989; 22: 749–758.
47. Maniglia AJ. Fatal and major complications secondary to nasal and sinus surgery. Laryngoscope 1989; 99–276.
48. Buus DR, Tse DT, Farris BK. Ophthalmic complications of sinus surgery. Ophthalmology 1990; 97: 612–619.
49. Neuhaus RW. Orbital complications secondary to endoscopic sinus surgery. Ophthalmology 1990; 97: 1512–1518.
50. Daniels DL, Mark LP, Ulmer JL, et al. Osseous anatomy of the pterygopalatine fossa.
51. Daniels DL, Mark LP, Mafee MF, Massaro B, et al. Osseous anatomy of the orbital apex. AJNR 1995; 16: 1929–1935.
52. Lee HY, Kim HU, Kim SS, et al. Surgical anatomy of the sphenopalatine artery in lateral nasal wall. Laryngoscope 2002; 112: 1813–1818.
53. El-Guindy A. Endoscopic transseptal sphenopalatine artery ligation for intractable posterior epistaxis. Ann Otol Rhinol Laryngol 1998; 107: 1033–1037.
54. Bolger WE, Bargie RC, Melder P. The role of the crista ethmoidalis in endoscopic sphenopalatine artery ligation. Am J Rhinol 1999; 13: 81–86.

Imaging Techniques

■ General Considerations

The sinonasal cavities are an important component of the upper respiratory tract. A variety of inflammatory and allergic conditions, benign and malignant tumors, and tumorlike lesions can occur in this region. Conventional plain film radiography may be used as a screening method for various pathological conditions of the sinonasal cavities.[1] This will provide orientation and direction to further examinations that are indicated such as CT and MRI.[1] Developmental malformations, such as palatomaxillary cleft, congenital anomalies and inflammatory disorders of the nose and paranasal sinuses, as well as fractures and fibro-osseous lesions, and the detailed bony structures of the paranasal sinuses and base of the skull, are best evaluated by CT scan.[2–4] MRI, on the other hand, provides more information concerning soft-tissue structures of the sinonasal cavities, face, and base of the skull. The intracranial connections of lesions such as nasal dermoids, nasal gliomas, and intracranial extensions of sinonasal tumors and infections are best evaluated using MRI.[1–4]

Although a plain film sinus series can be of much value in acute sinusitis and for the initial evaluation of subacute or chronic sinusitis and other sinonasal diseases, significant discrepancies are sometimes noted between a sinus series and a CT scan.[1–5] Chronic sinusitis associated with inspissated mucus has a characteristic CT appearance (Fig. 4.**39**). This characteristic CT finding may be very hard to appreciate on plain film and could be totally missed or misinterpreted on MRI (see Fig. 4.**77b**).[6,7]

Although CT scan can be more specific in the diagnosis of osteogenic and chondrogenic lesions, MRI is more sensitive in showing the extent of their soft-tissue components as well as the presence of subtle or obvious intracranial spread.[3] MRI is superior to CT in differentiating inflammatory conditions from neoplastic processes.[1–4,7,8] Most inflammatory lesions are quite hyperintense on T2-weighted (T2W) MR scans as opposed to most malignant tumors, lymphoreticular proliferative, myeloproliferative, and chronic granulomatous disorders.[3,7] Most tumors of the sinonasal cavities are not as hyperintense as the surrounding inflammation and retained secretions; therefore, MRI plays an important role in the mapping and staging of these tumors. Sinogenic intracranial complications are best evaluated using MRI. The intracranial and intraorbital complications of sinus surgery are also often best evaluated using MRI. CT has proved to afford the best preoperative and postoperative evaluation for endoscopic sinus surgery.[5,6,8,10–13]

■ Computed Tomography

CT scan is an excellent imaging modality to evaluate the sinonasal cavities. It provides an accurate assessment of the paranasal sinuses and craniofacial bones as well as the extent of pneumatization of the paranasal sinuses. Five-millimeter sections are often adequate for the evaluation of most sinonasal and skull base structures. The axial sections are taken parallel to the orbitomeatal line or parallel to the hard palate. The coronal sections are obtained with the patient supine or prone, the head hyperextended, and the gantry tilted to a plane as close to 90° to the canthomeatal line as possible. Dental artifacts may be minimized by adjustment of the gantry tilt. The degree of angulation of the gantry should be determined by adjusting the angle of the beam on the lateral digital scout view. Thinner sections (3 mm) are used to identify small lesions and evaluate the ostiomeatal unit. In terms of filming, some authors recommend an intermediate window width/level (W/L) technique (2500/250, W/L).[7,19]

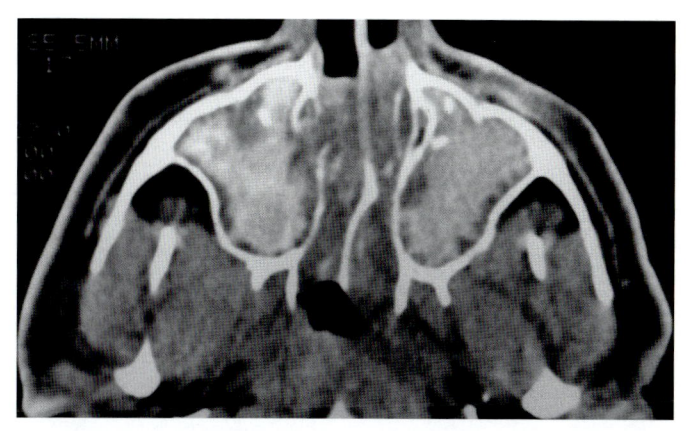

Fig. 4.**39** Chronic sinusitis. CT scan shows bilateral nasal polyps and increased density of maxillary sinuses, related to inspissated retained secretion. Note marked thickened mucosa of both maxillary sinuses.

We prefer CT images to be viewed or filmed with extended window width–window level bone technique (4000/700–800 W/L). If the study is interpreted on hard-copy films, we recommend that the technicians provide an additional set, using soft-tissue window technique. The soft-tissue technique allows better evaluation of inspissated mucosal secretions and microcalcifications. The quality of reformatted images obtained on new ultrafast spiral CT scanners is excellent.

Optimal imaging protocols for preoperative CT scanning of the paranasal sinuses, including preparation of the patient, CT technique, and data display (filming), have been reported by many authors.[4,7,9,11,19] In chronic as well as allergic sinusitis, treatment with appropriate medical therapy and adequate preparation of patients enable the best CT assessment of mucosal disease of the sinonasal cavities.[2,4,19] Three-millimeter section direct coronal CT scanning, with the patient preferably in the prone position and the head hyperextended, currently affords the best preoperative evaluation for endoscopic sinus surgery.[1,2,4,5,7,9,10] A complete CT study of the paranasal sinuses should include axial and coronal views;[2,3,5] however, a single coronal series in most cases provides the maximum amount of information one needs for evaluating the ostiomeatal complex.[4] Coronal scanning should extend from the frontal sinus anteriorly to the sphenoidal sinus posteriorly. However, the combination of coronal and axial CT scans allows the surgeon more easily to assess the three-dimensional aspects of the ostiomeatal complex.[5]

Axial CT scanning should be included whenever coronal CT scans show a mass or mucosal disease associated with expansion of the sinuses.[5] Erosion of the posterior table of the frontal sinus, the sphenoethmoidal bony plates, basal lamella, pterygomaxillary fissure, and pterygopalatine fossa are best evaluated in axial and direct or reformatted sagittal CT scans (Fig. 4.**40**).[21,22] The introduction of spiral and helical CT scanning has had a great impact in sectional imaging. The speed with which studies can be carried out allows much faster patient throughput. With spiral CT technique, the quality of reformatted images has improved significantly (Fig. 4.**41**). For children and agitated patients, spiral CT is extremely useful in providing acceptable diagnostic information in a matter of a few minutes. Contrast-enhanced CT should not be part of preoperative CT for endoscopic sinus surgery. Contrast material is used only when the preliminary evaluation of CT scans suggests a mass. In addition, contrast

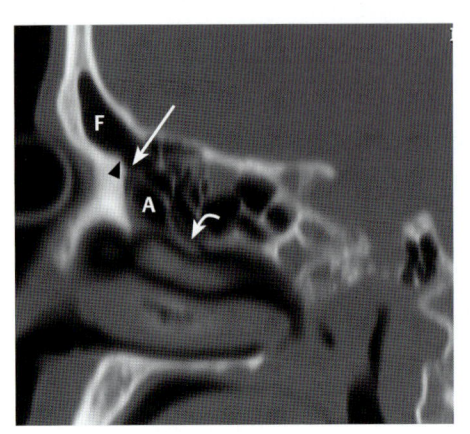

Fig. 4.40 Sagittal reformatted CT scan, showing frontal sinus (F), frontal sinus ostium (arrowhead), frontal (frontonasal) recess (arrow), agger nasi cell (A), and uncinate process (curved arrow).

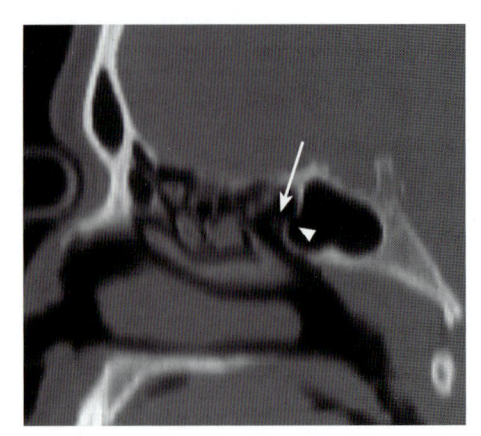

Fig. 4.41 Sagittal reformatted CT scan, showing the ostium of the sphenoid sinus (arrowhead) and sphenoethmoid recess (arrow).

material should be given whenever extracranial (orbital) and intracranial complications of sinonasal infections or tumors are suspected. Three-dimensional reconstruction CT imaging has been most useful for studying facial deformity and for planning surgery.[23,24] For sinonasal tumors, the combination of CT and MRI provides the maximum diagnostic imaging information. Our protocol for MRI of sinonasal disease, using a head coil, includes 5 mm thick sections, sagittal T1-weighted (T1W) localization, axial T1-weighted and T2-weighted and coronal T1-weighted sections. Following intravenous administration of gadolinium contrast material, postcontrast T1-weighted axial, coronal, and sagittal views are obtained. We prefer to obtain only one of the postcontrast T1-weighted pulse sequences with fat suppression. The magnetic susceptibility artifacts as well as those related to dental fillings are more pronounced on fat-suppression pulse sequences.

Image-Guided Endoscopic Surgery

Image guidance systems are available that can provide otolaryngologists with precise anatomical localization during head and neck surgery.[25–27] The use of both the optically based and electromagnetically based image guidance systems has proved valuable to provide anatomical localization with an accuracy of 2 mm or better at the start of surgery.[27] Our CT protocol for image-guided endoscopic surgery includes 2.5 mm axial sections and reformatted sagittal and coronal views (Figs. **4.40**, **4.41**). The video display from the optically based image guidance system during surgery will demonstrate the tip of the surgical instrument and the corresponding position on axial, coronal, and sagittal and three-dimensional images of the patient's preoperative CT scan. The use of the image guidance system was found to increase the mean total operating time by 17.4 minutes per case.[27]

■ Standard Film Radiography

Radiographic anatomy of the paranasal sinuses and nasal cavities can be well recognized in the four standard sinus projections: Waters, Caldwell, lateral, and submentovertical (Figs. **4.42–4.47**).

Waters view. This view is obtained with the chin raised and placed on the x-ray cassette with the nose 1–1.5 cm off the plate, and with the central ray perpendicular to the cassette plate. A number of anatomical structures, including the maxillary sinuses, frontal sinuses, anterior ethmoidal air cells, and the anterior orbital rim, can be seen in this projection as outlined in Fig. **4.42**. The maxillary sinuses are best visualized in this view. This view is not appropriate for more posterior ethmoidal air cells. The frontal sinuses are well shown, and the main cavity of the sphenoid sinus is often poorly demonstrated within the outline of the nasal or oral cavities. Other structures that can be evaluated in this projection include the floor of the orbit, orbital rim, infraorbital foramen, superior orbital fissure, foramen rotundum, and temporal line (Fig. **4.42**). Fluid level in the maxillary and frontal sinuses can easily be identified in this projection taken in the upright position. A questionable fluid level may be confirmed by repeating the Waters view with the head tilted to the side (Fig. **4.43**).

Caldwell view. This posteroanterior view is obtained by placing the nose and forehead against the x-ray cassette with the canthomeatal line (external auditory canal and outer canthus of the eye) perpendicular to the cassette. The central x-ray beam is tilted caudally 15–25° so that the petrous ridges are projected at or below the floor of the orbits (Fig. **4.44**). The anatomical structures that are visible in this view are demonstrated in Fig. **4.44**. This view is most appropriate for evaluating the frontal and ethmoid sinuses. The lamina papyracea, superior orbital fissure, foramen rotundum, superior orbital rim, frontozygomatic suture, innominate line, and some other structures can also be seen well in this view (Fig. **4.44**). The sphenoid sinus and sella are superimposed on the ethmoidal air cells and nasal cavities. Although the maxillary sinuses are superimposed over the petrous bone, they can often be evaluated in this projection. In this regard the Caldwell view is complementary to the Waters view for the evaluation of maxillary sinus disease.

Lateral view. This view is usually obtained with the patient seated in front of a vertical cassette holder so that the patient's head can be adjusted in a true lateral position. The x-ray beam is perpendicular to the center of the film. Certain anatomical structures, as seen in Fig. **4.45**, are visualized in this projection. The sphenoid sinuses and sella turcica are shown to the best advantage in this view. The frontal, ethmoid, and maxillary sinuses are superimposed on each other. The anterior and posterior tables of the frontal sinuses can be evaluated in this view. Other structures that can be assessed with this view include the pterygomaxillary fissure, pterygopalatine fossa, nasopharynx, hard and soft palates, and mandible. The zygoma may appear as a triangular bone superimposed on the maxillary sinuses (Fig. **4.45 a, c**). The orbital walls and rims are superimposed on each other. The clivus can be seen extending from the dorsum sella down to the anterior mar-

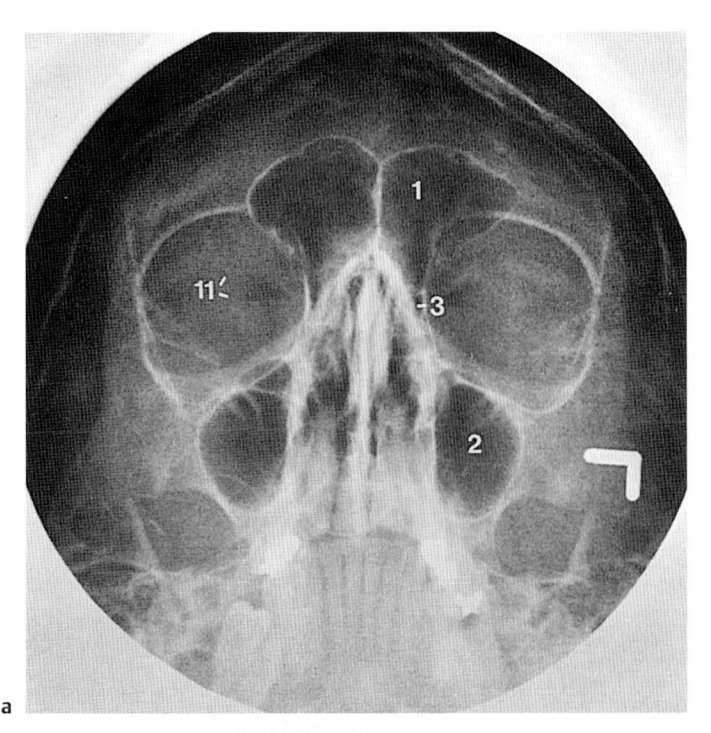

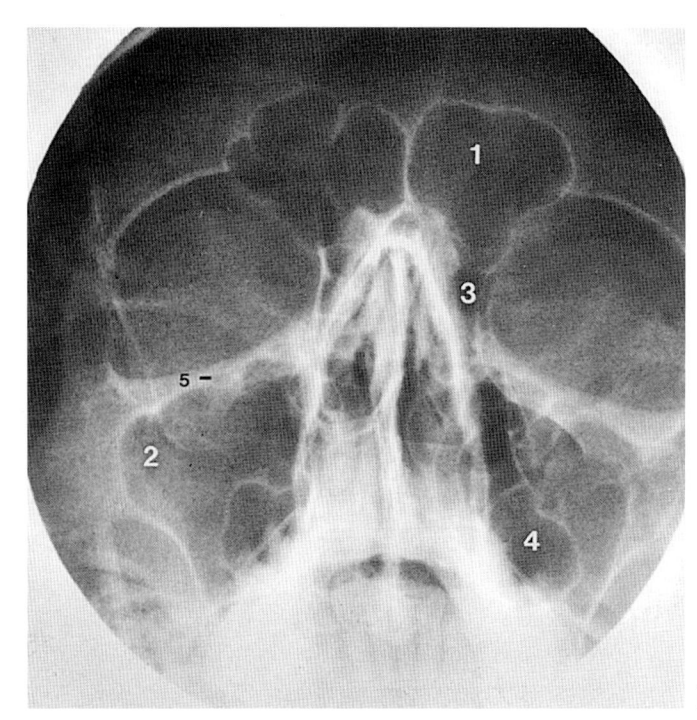

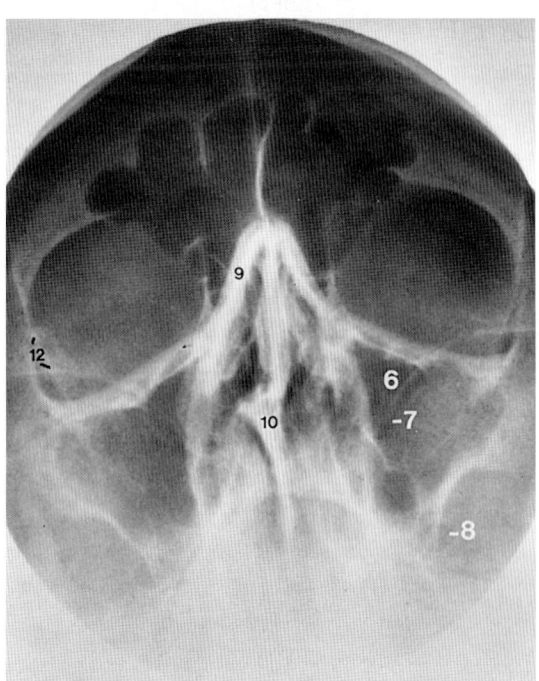

Fig. 4.**42 a–c** Normal Waters projection. Three different patients to show variations in the sinuses and the normal landmarks. The frontal (1) and maxillary (2) sinuses are seen together with the anterior ethmoid air cells (3). The sinuses are fairly symmetrical. Lateral recesses of the sphenoid sinuses (4) are projected through the maxillary sinuses in **b** and **c**. The infraorbital nerve canal (5) is seen in the anterior inferior rim of the orbit. The lesser wing of the sphenoid (6), best seen in **c**, is separated medially from the greater wing by the superior orbital fissure (7). Since the latter structure is located posteriorly at the apex of the orbit, it is projected inferiorly with the elevated chin in the Waters projection. Note the foramen ovale (8), occasionally seen projected behind the floor of the maxillary sinus. The nasal bone (9) and nasal septum (10) are clearly seen. Soft-tissue structures such as the palpebral fissure (11) are more subtle. The innominate line (12) of the greater wing of the sphenoid is also evident, but better evaluated on the Caldwell projection. In this view, the floor of the orbit is projected inferior to the inferior orbital rim. From Reference 20.

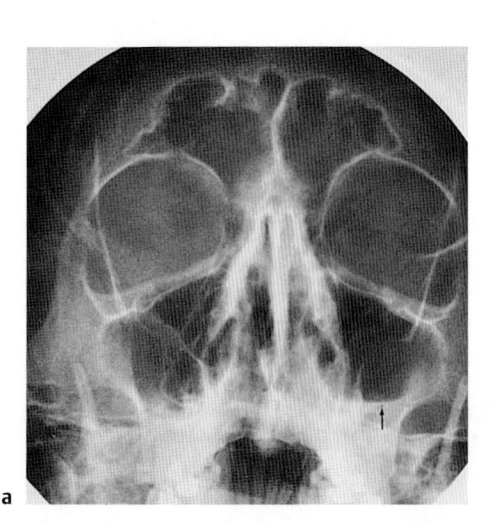

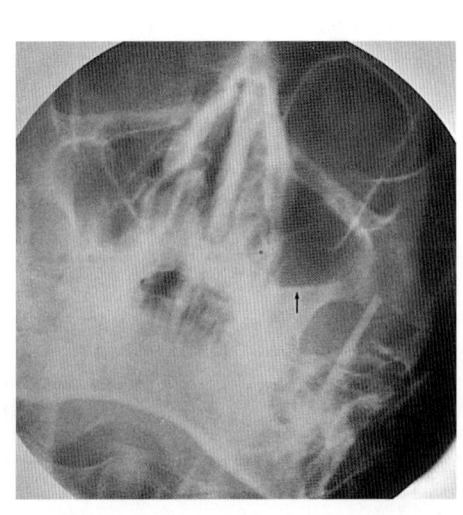

Fig. 4.**43** Waters projection to show fluid level. A standard Waters projection seen in **a** shows the fluid level (arrow), which shifts as shown in **b** on tilting the head to the side. From Reference 20.

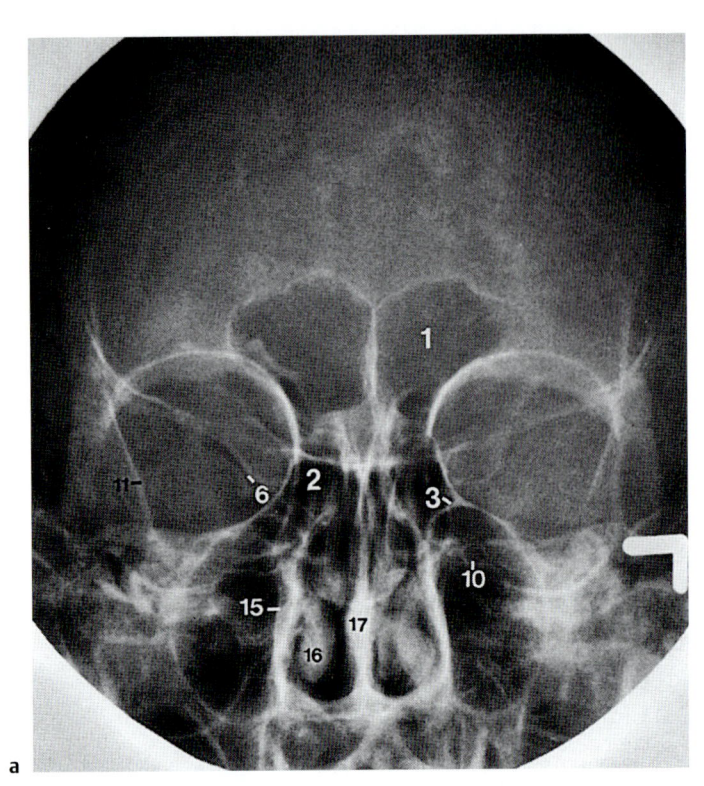

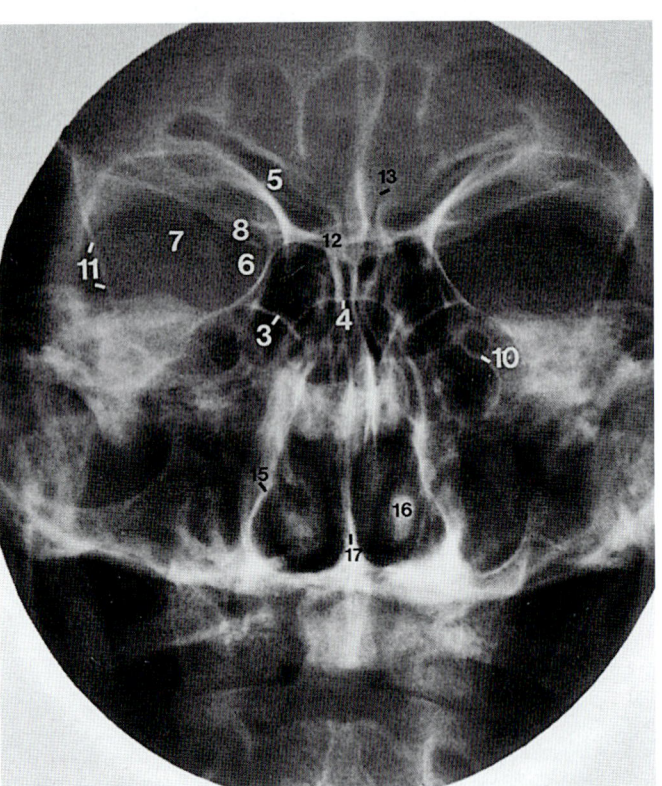

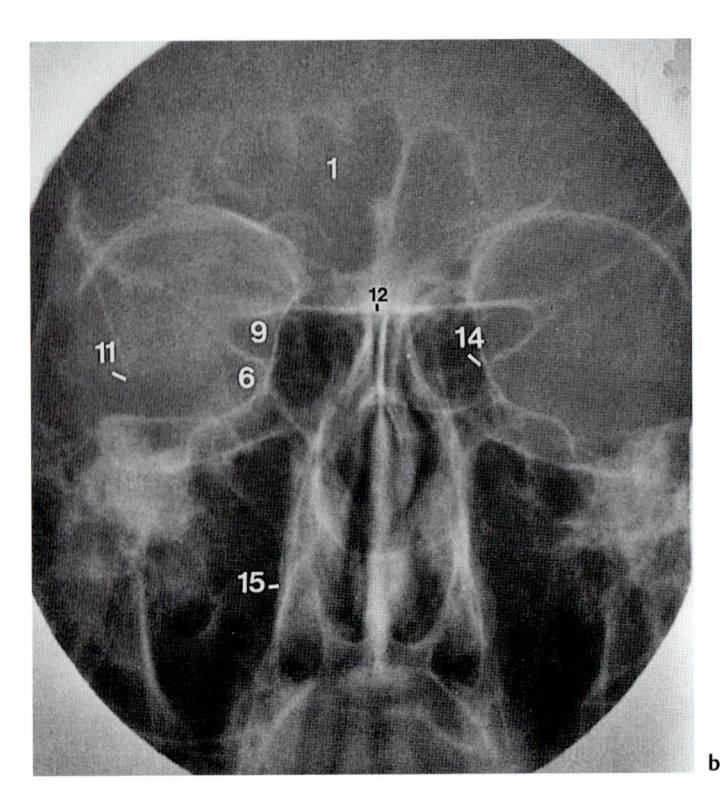

4 Imaging of the Nasal Cavity and Paranasal Sinuses

Fig. 4.**44 a–c** Caldwell projection. The frontal (1) and ethmoid (2) sinuses are seen to good advantage, but the maxillary sinuses are superimposed over the petrous portion of the temporal bone. The ethmomaxillary plate (3) and the floor of the sella (4) are best seen in **c**. Supraorbital cells (5) are an extension of the ethmoid cells over the roof of the orbit. The superior orbital fissure (6) between the greater (7) and lesser (8) wings of the sphenoid is at the apex of the orbit. The anterior clinoids (9) are pneumatized in **b** and are projected through the upper portion of the superior orbital fissure. The foramen rotundum (10) is located below the superior orbital fissure. Note the innominate line (11) of the greater wing of the sphenoid, the planum sphenoidale (12), and the crista galli (13) in **c**. The lamina papyracea (14) forms the medial wall of the orbit. The medial wall of the maxillary sinus (15), inferior turbinates (16), nasal septum (17), and floor of the nasal cavity, or hard palate, are also evident. From Reference 20.

gin of the foramen magnum. This view is important for seeing air–fluid levels in the sphenoid, frontal, and maxillary sinuses. In skull base fracture or in patients with CSF rhinorrhea, the air–fluid level in the sphenoid sinus may be the only sign seen in standard radiography.

Submentovertical base view. This base or basal view is obtained by passing the central x-ray beam at an angle through the base of the skull. In this projection, the vertex is placed on the cassette, and the canthomeatal line is perpendicular to the central x-ray beam. This projection provides the visualization of certain bones and foramina of the base of the skull, which are depicted in Fig. 4.46. The sphenoid sinuses are shown best in this view. The so-called "lateral three lines" as seen in Fig. 4.46 are: (1) an S-shaped line formed by the lateral wall of the maxillary antrum (antral or sinus line), (2) a straight line formed by the lateral wall of the orbit (orbital line), and (3) a curved line formed by the anterior wall of the middle cranial fossa (middle cranial

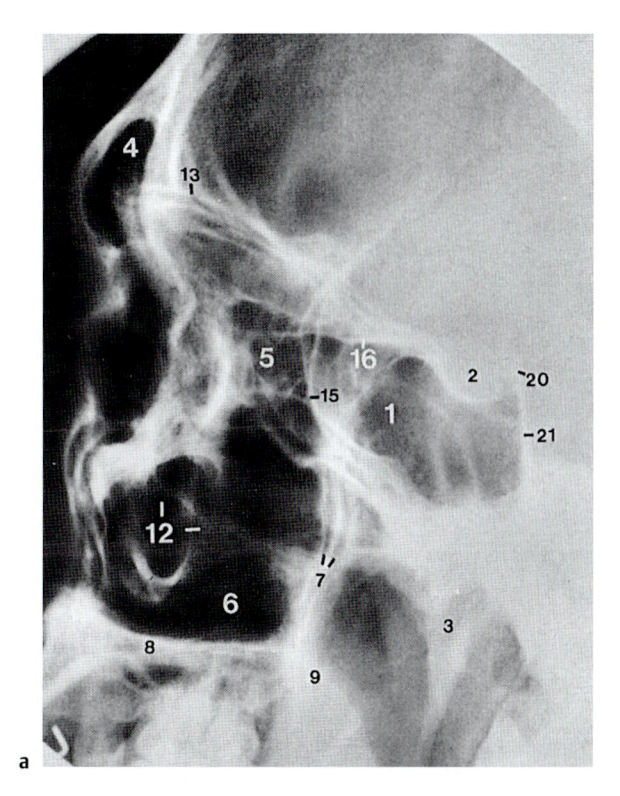

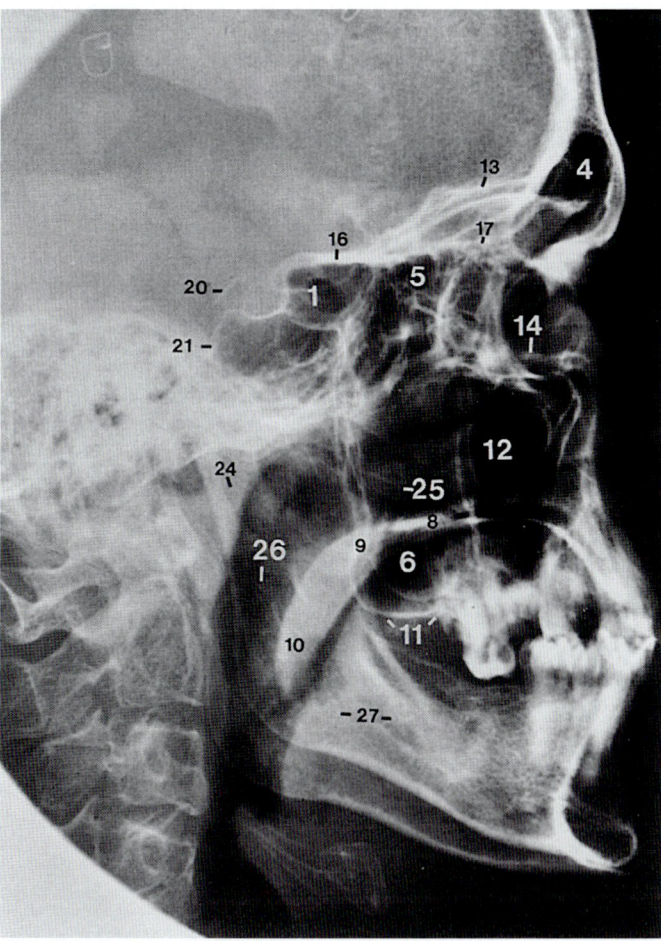

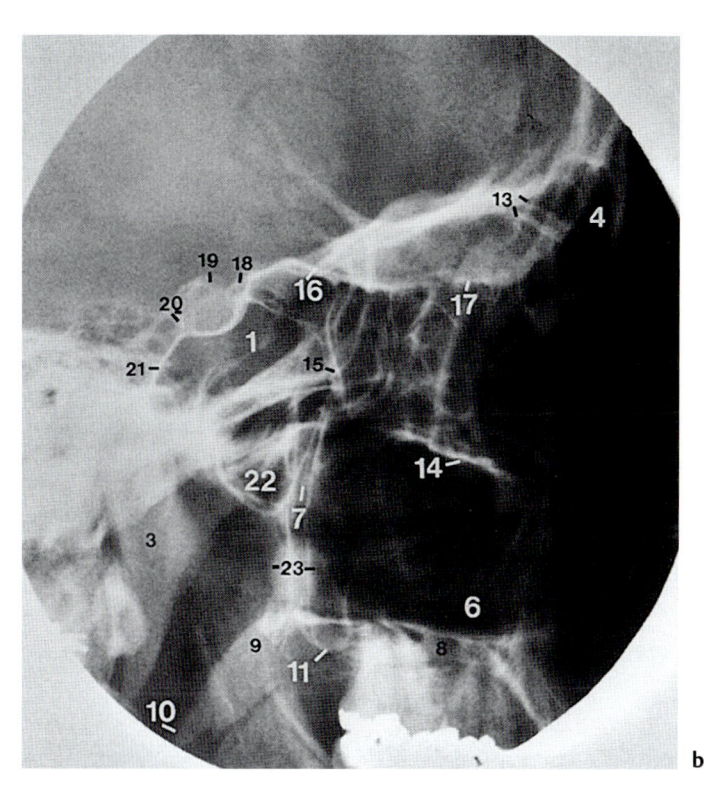

Fig. 4.**45 a–c** Lateral projection. The sphenoid sinus (1), sella (2), and soft tissues of the nasopharynx (3) are seen to best advantage. The two frontal sinuses (4), ethmoid sinuses (5), and maxillary sinuses (6) are superimposed. The pterygomaxillary fissure (7) between the posterior wall of the maxillary sinus and the pterygoid process is a long inverted triangle. Note the hard palate (8) and soft palate (9) with the uvula (10). The floor of the maxillary sinus (11) is located at the level of the hard palate (**b**) or below it (**c**) when the sinus is large and extending into the alveolar process. The zygoma (12) contains the lateral portion of the maxillary sinus to varying degrees. Also note the roof (13) and floor (14) of the orbit, the floor (15) of the middle cranial fossa formed by the greater wing of the sphenoid, the planum sphenoidale (16), the roof of the ethmoid air cells (17), the anterior (18) and posterior (19) clinoids, the dorsum sella (20) and the clivus (21). The lateral recess of the sphenoid sinus (22) extends inferiorly into the pterygoid behind the pterygomaxillary fissure. The inferior turbinate (23) is best seen in **b**. The condylar neck (24), coronoid process (25), ramus (26), and body (27) of the mandible are best seen in **c**. From Reference 20.

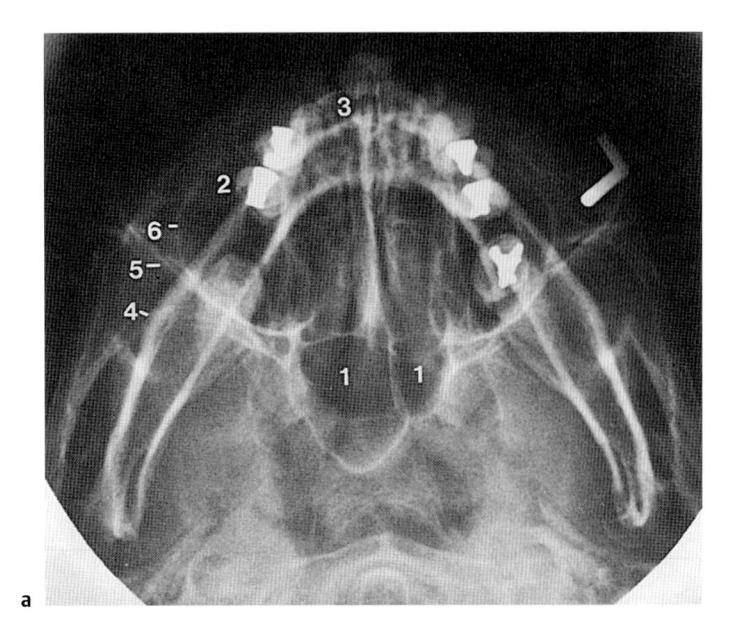

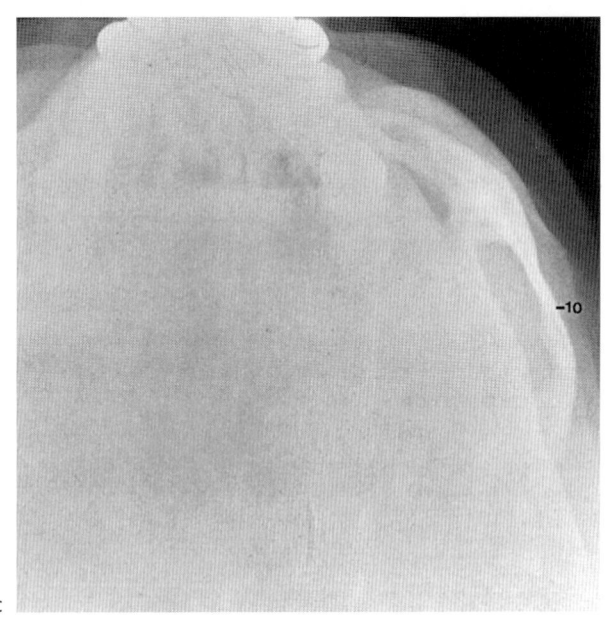

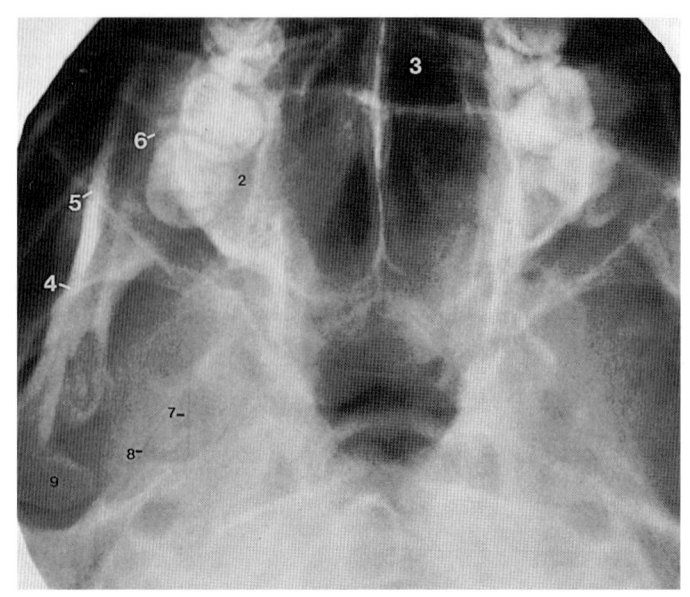

Fig 4.**46a–c** Base projection. The sphenoid sinuses (1) are often asymmetrical as in **a** and are more difficult to see with the hyperextended projection as in **b**. The maxillary sinuses (2) are best seen in **a**, whereas the frontal sinuses (3) are better seen with the hyperextended base view as in **b**. Three lines forming landmarks in the base projection are the greater wing of the sphenoid, representing the anterior wall of the middle cranial fossa (4), the straight line of the orbit (5), and the more curved line of the maxillary sinus (6). The lines 4 and 5 join each other because they are both part of the greater wing of the sphenoid bone. The foramen ovale (7) and spinosum (8) can also be seen. The mandibular condyle (9) is located within the condylar fossa. **c** An underexposed film taken for visualization of the zygomatic arch (10) is called the "bucket handle" view. From Reference 20.

fossa line or sphenoid line). The orbital line and middle cranial fossa line are part of the greater wing of the sphenoid; therefore, when they are followed medially, they are seen to meet each other. Several modifications of the base projection are used, depending on the area of interest. The usual projection is taken with the mandible superimposed on the frontal sinus (Fig. 4.**46**). The sphenoid sinuses, posterolateral wall of the maxillary sinuses, the floor of the middle cranial fossa containing the foramen ovale and foramen spinosum, the temporomandibular joint, and the petrous apices are seen in this projection.[1,20] The ethmoidal air cells are superimposed on the nasal cavities. The hyperextended base projection is taken with the mandible projected anterior to the frontal sinuses, allowing visualization of the anterior and posterior walls of the frontal sinuses. Another modification of the base view, taken with the mandible projected behind the frontal bone or halfway between the Waters and base views, is used primarily for evaluating more posterior structures, such as the jugular fossa.[20] An underexposed film may be used for visualization of the zygomatic arch (Fig. 4.**46c**).

Oblique view. The oblique view may be obtained to separate anterior and posterior ethmoidal air cells and to study the optic nerve canal and the walls of the orbit.

Chamberlain–Town view. This projection is obtained with the chin down and the x-ray beam angled caudally, passing through the inferior orbital fissure, separating the posterior wall of the maxillary sinus from the sphenoid bone. This projection may occasionally be used in trauma patients to assess the posterior wall of the maxillary sinus and the sphenoid bone and mandibular condyles.[20]

Nasal bone views. The lateral projection coned down to the nasal bones and premaxilla best depicts the nasal bone and the anterior nasal spine (Fig. 4.**47**). The frontonasal and maxillonasal sutures are seen in this projection. The vascular and neural grooves run parallel to the maxillonasal suture line and should not be mistaken for fractures. Occlusal film (Fig. 4.**47b**) may occasionally be used to identify medial and lateral displacement of nasal bone fracture fragments.

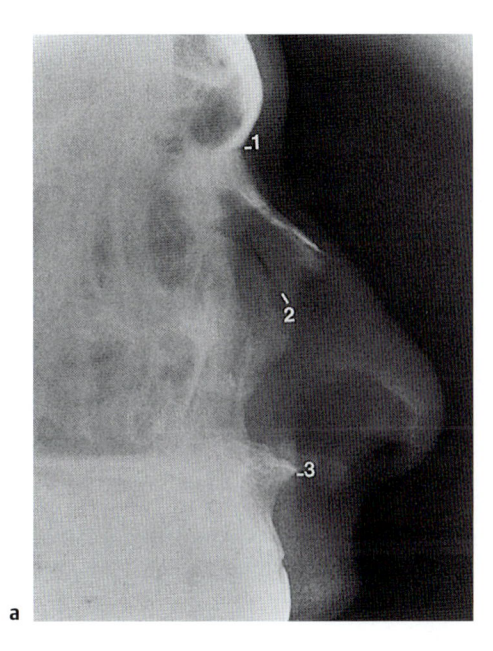

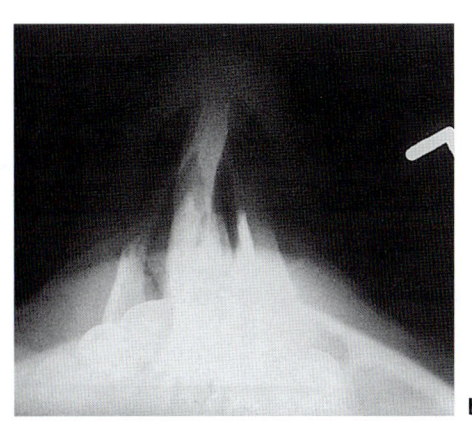

Fig. 4.**47** Nasal bones. Coned down lateral (**a**) and occlusal (**b**) films show the nasal bones. They are separated at the nasion (1) from the frontal bone. Vascular and neural grooves are parallel to the suture line (2) between the nasal bone and nasal process of the maxilla. The spinous process (anterior nasal spine) (3) of the maxilla is also evident. The occlusal view **b** may be used for identification of any displacement of the nasal bones. From Reference 20.

■ Magnetic Resonance Imaging

An opinion one frequently hears with regard to sinonasal imaging is that MRI is often not very helpful compared with CT scanning. This may be true for few specific entities such as fibro-osseous lesions; however, for benign and malignant tumors, MRI is superior to CT scans in differentiating tumor from surrounding associated inflammatory disease and retained secretions. The marked hyperintensity of the inflammatory mucosal disease on T2-weighted MR images as well as marked enhancement of inflammatory mucosal thickening on enhanced T1-weighted MR images often allow the radiologist to differentiate tumors from surrounding inflammatory disease. Intracranial tumor extension and intracranial complications of sinonasal infections are better evaluated by MRI than CT scanning. In general, the combination of MR and CT imaging in most cases will allow for better evaluation of the disease and at times for making a more specific diagnosis. The radiologist should always be consulted in determining the most appropriate imaging study (or studies) for each individual case. In the evaluation of suspected sinonasal disease processes, a typical MRI protocol consists of short TR/TE sagittal localization, unenhanced short TR, short TE and long TR long TE axial sequences, followed by contrast-enhanced short TR short TE axial, coronal, and sagittal pulse sequences.

Other pulse sequences may provide additional information. A long TR long TE coronal sequence can be particularly helpful. This protocol also permits the evaluation of intracranial extension of sinonasal pathology. In our institution, the MRI images are routinely obtained with a slice thickness of 5 mm, an image acquisition matrix of 256×256 or 256×128, and one or two signal averages, using the head coil as the receiving coil. Gadolinium-DTPA (0.1 mmol/kg) contrast is used when tumor or infiltrative processes or complications of sinonasal inflammatory processes are suspected. In some cases, postcontrast fat-suppression short TR short TE sequences are obtained to increase the contrast between normal and abnormal tissues and in particular to evaluate intraorbital extension of sinonasal diseases.

■ Risk of Radiation from Sinus Imaging

The biological side-effects of ionizing radiation have always been a matter of concern.[4, 14, 15] In general, absorbed doses from most diagnostic studies are quite low.[16] There are no exposure limits for medical radiation as long as the study is clinically indicated.[14] On the average, diagnostic radiology is second to background radiation as a source of exposure for the population in industrialized countries.[15, 17, 18] Natural background radiation may vary by three orders of magnitude throughout the world.[15] It has been postulated that only 1–2% of all genetically determined diseases are attributable to natural background radiation.[3, 15] The dose required to double human mutation rates lies between 2 and 2.5 sievert (Sv).[18] The incidence of radiation-induced cataract depends on the dose time and age.[15] The cornea demonstrates few effects until fractionated doses are in the range of 50 gray (Gy) (5000 rads). Currently the SI unit of radiation dose equivalent is the sievert;[19] the former unit was the rem. For diagnostic x-rays, 1 Gy = 1 Sv and 1 Sv = 100 rem.[19]

The risk of radiation from the sinus series or screening sinus CT is small.[14] Approximately 0.3 cGy is given for each film view obtained during plain x-ray sinus series.[3, 14] The organs most likely to be affected by a cumulative radiation dose are the lens, the thyroid gland, and the gonads. The dose to the lens of the eye is small if Waters and Caldwell views are obtained posterior-inferior as they should be.[14] With the combination of high-speed film and a posterior-inferior projection, the dose to the eye in a sinus series should be on the order of 0.0001 Gy (0.01 cGy) to 0.0005 Gy (0.05 cGy).[3, 14] The radiation dose to the lens of the eye from a CT examination of the head may range from 3 to 6 cGy.[2, 3] The radiation dose is dependent on the kilovolt peak (kVp) and mAs.[19] For sinus CT scan, the relative radiation dose, utilizing 125 kVp and 160 mAs will be 1.76–1.92 cSv (1.76–1.92 rem). The radiation from a CT scan of the sinuses to the lens, cornea, and other organs included in the CT sections can be significantly reduced by decreasing mAs (80–125 mAs), without significantly sacrificing details. The imaging plane also can be chosen to avoid scanning directly through the lens of the eye.

References

1. Mafee M F. Imaging of the nasal cavities, paranasal sinuses, nasopharynx, orbits, infratemporal fossa, pterygomaxillary fissure, parapharyngeal space " and base of skull. In: Ballenger JJ, Snow JB, eds. Ballenger's Otorhinolaryngology Head and Neck Surgery, 16th ed. Ontario: BC Decker; 2002.
2. Mafee MF. Imaging of paranasal sinuses and nasal cavity. In English GM, ed. Diseases of the Nose and Sinuses. Vol. 2. Philadelphia: Lippincott-Raven; 1995: 1–42.
3. Mafee MF. Modern imaging of paranasal sinuses a role of limited sinus CT scanning consideration of time, cost and radiation. Ear Nose Throat J 13: 532–546.
4. Mafee MF. Imaging methods for sinusitis. JAMA 1993; 269(20): 2808.
5. Chow J M, Mafee M F. Radiologic assessment preoperative to endoscopic sinus surgery. Otolaryngol Clin North Am 1989; 22: 691–701.
6. Mafee M F, Chow J M, Meyers R: Functional endoscopic sinus surgery: Anatomy, CT screening, indications, and complications. AJR 1993; 160: 735–744.
7. Som P M, Curtin H D. Chronic inflammatory sinonasal diseases including fungal infections; the role of imaging, Radiol Clin North Am 1993; 31: 33–34.
8. Mafee MF. Nonepithelial tumors of the paranasal sinuses and nasal cavity: Role of CT and MR imaging. Radiol Clin North Am 1993; 31: 75–90.
9. Zinreich S J, Kennedy DW, Rosenbaum AE, et al. Paranasal sinuses: CT imaging requirements for endoscopic survey. Radiology 1987; 31: 709–775.
10. Kennedy DW, Zinrich J, Rosenbaum AE, et al. Functional endoscopic sinus surgery: Theory and diagnostic evaluation. Arc Otolaryngol 1985; 111: 576–582.
11. Mafee M E Endoscopic sinus surgery: Role of the radiologist. AJNR 1991; 12: 855–860.
12. Mafee ME Preoperative imaging anatomy of nasal-ethmoid complex for functional endoscopic sinus surgery. Radiol Clin North Am 1993; 31: 1–20.
13. Rice DH. Basic surgical techniques and variations of endoscopic sinus surgery. Otolaryngol Clin North Am 1989; 22: 713–726.
14. Poznanski AK. Do sinus roentgenograms in children pose a radiation risk? JAMA 1989; 262: 3058.
15. Mettler FA, Moseley RD. Medical Effects of Ionizing Radiation. Orlando: Grune and Stratton; 1985.
16. Wagner L K. Absorbed dose in imaging. Why measure it? Radiology 1991; 178: 622–623.
17. Upton AC. The biological effects of low-level ionizing radiation. Sci Am 1982; 246: 41–49.
18. Exposure of the U.S. Population from Diagnostic Medical Radiation. Bethesda, MD: National Council on Radiation Protection and Measurement; 1989
19. Zinreich SJ, Albayram S, Benson ML, Oliverio PJ. The ostiomeatal complex and functional endoscopic surgery. In: Som PM, Curtin HD, eds. Head and Neck Imaging, Vol. I, 3rd ed. St. Louis: Mosby; 2003: 149–173.
20. Carter BL. Paranasal sinuses, nasal cavity, pterygoid fossa, nasopharynx, and infratemporal fossa. In: Valvassori GE, Buckingham RA, Carter BL, Hanafee WN, Mafee MF, eds. Head and Neck Imaging. Stuttgart: Georg Thieme Verlag; 1988: 173–250.
21. Mafee MF, Kumar A, Tahmoressi CN, et al. Direct saggital CT in the evaluation of temporal bone disease. AJNR 1988; 9: 371–378.
22. Ball JB, Towbin RB, Staton RE, Cowdrey K. Direct sagittal computed tomography of the head. Radiology 1985; 155: 822.
23. Friedmann M, Mafee M, Ray C, et al. Three-dimensional imaging for evaluation of head and neck tumors. Arch Gynecol Head Neck Surg 1993; 119: 601–607.
24. Ray CE, Mafee MF, Friedmann M, Tahmoressi CN. Applications of three-dimensional CT imaging in head and neck pathology. Radiol Clin North Am 1993; 31: 181–194.
25. Zinreich SJ, Tebos, Long DL, et al. Frameless stereotaxic integration of CT imaging data accuracy and initial applications. Radiology 1993; 188: 735–742.
26. Fried MP, Kleefield J, Gopal H, et al. Image-guided endoscopic surgery: results of accuracy and performance in a multicenter clinical study using an electromagnetic tracking system. Laryngoscope 1997 107: 594–601.
27. Metson R, Coseza M, Gliklich RE, Montgomery WW. The role of image-guidance systems for head and neck surgery. Arch Otolaryngol Head Neck Surg 1999; 125: 1100–1104.

Sinonasal Pathology

Congenital Anomalies of the Nose and Paranasal Sinuses

Congenital anomalies of the face may occur as an isolated malformation or may be coupled with malformations in other regions of the body as part of various craniofacial syndromes.[1–4] Congenital abnormalities of the nose can occur with or without respiratory obstruction. Nasal obstruction is usually detected in the neonatal period.[3] Cleft lip and cleft palate are the most frequent anomalies, but other less common defects are important considerations in the differential diagnosis of mass lesions of the facial area.[1,2] In more complex cases, evaluation of the face may require both CT and MR imaging. All congenital abnormalities of the face are due to failures in the embryological development of the face.[1–5] The arrested development may be associated with disturbances in embryonic nutrition during the second and third months of gestation.[4]

Embryology

During the four weeks of gestation when the anterior neuropore closes in the vicinity of the optic recess, mesodermal tissue begins to form bone, cartilage, and connective tissue. At this time, several swellings appear on the fetal face. The rostrally situated frontal prominence is bounded inferolaterally by the maxillary processes (see Fig. 4.**1**). Superior and medial to the maxillary processes lie the nasal medial and lateral processes (see Fig. 4.**1**). The frontal and maxillary processes merge and become involved in the formation of the lateral two-thirds of the upper lip, superior alveolar ridge, and palatal shelves. The nasal medial processes merge with the maxillary processes to form the philtrum and columella.[3,4] The nasal medial processes also merge with the frontal prominence to form the frontonasal process, which eventually gives origin to nasal bones, nasal cartilages, central incisors, hard palate, and ethmoid bones (see Fig. 4.**1**). The nasolacrimal sacs and ducts develop from the nasolacrimal groove and are situated between the maxillary process and the orbits (see Fig. 4.**1**). Failure of both nasal medial processes to fuse and failure of the frontonasal process to form result in midline facial clefting.[3,4] The fetal ectoderm may become entrapped with the overgrowth of the frontonasal process, a postulated explanation for ectopic gliomas, epidermoids, dermoids, and sinus tracts. If the neuropore fails to close, an encephalocele through the frontonasal, frontoethmoidal, or frontosphenoidal complexes may result, producing an external, intranasal, or nasopharyngeal encephalocele or meningocele.[3,4]

Cleft Palate

Congenital malformations consequent upon arrest of development and failure of fusion of components in the formation of the face and palate are not uncommon. At the simplest, one maxillary process may fail completely to fuse with the corresponding premaxillary region (globular process), leading to a persistent fissure between the philtrum and lateral part of the upper lip on that side (Fig. 4.**48**)—so called cleft lip or "hare" lip. Failure of fusion between a maxillary process and the lateral nasal process (elevation) results in facial cleft, in which the nasolacrimal duct is an open furrow, a condition usually associated with a cleft lip on the same side (see Fig. 4.**1**).[4] Many varieties of cleft palate have been observed; the commonest type is unilateral, only one side of the nasal cavity being in communication with the mouth,

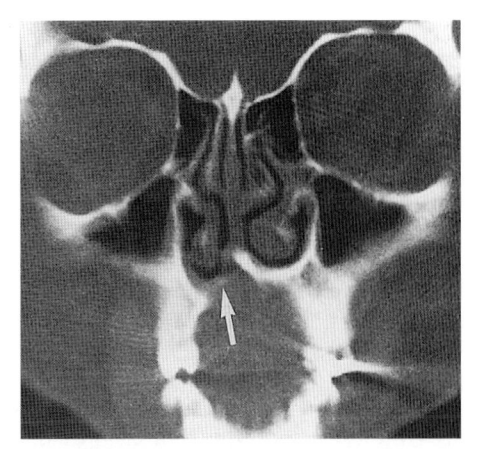

Fig. 4.48 Coronal CT scan shows a palatomaxillary cleft (arrow).

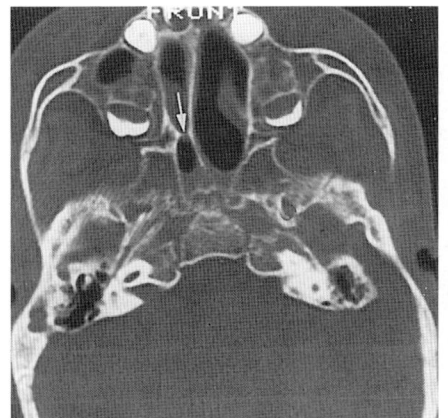

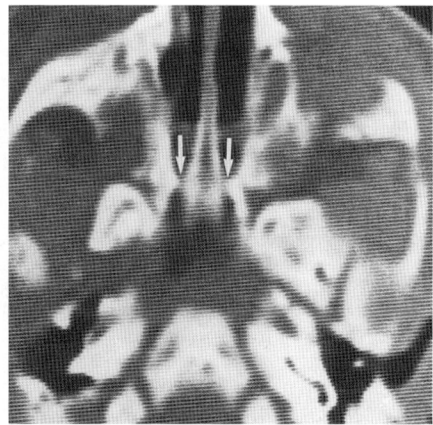

Fig. 4.49 Choanal atresia. **a** Unilateral, **b** bilateral. Axial CT scans showing bony atresia (arrows) on the right side (**a**) and bilaterally (**b**). Note the hypoplasia of the nasal cavity on the side of the choanal atresia, and abnormally thick vomer bone, seen in Fig. 4.49 b. From B.L. Carter, MD. Thieme 1988

the extent of cleft being variable (Fig. 4.48). In the mildest forms, only the soft palate is cleft, or even merely the uvula.[4]

Choanal Atresia (Choanal Obliteration)

The stomatodeum (primitive mouth) is separated from the end of the pharyngeal gut by the buccopharyngeal membrane. The ectoderm forming the cranium and brain is separated inferiorly from the stomatodeum by a mesenchymal plate. Failure of resorption of this mesodermal plate produces bony choanal atresia. Membranous choanal atresia results from failure of perforation of the buccopharyngeal membrane. Choanal atresia may be unilateral or bilateral as an isolated congenital anomaly, but 75 % are reported to be associated with other defects.[3] The atresia occurs in one of every 7000 to 8000 live births and is more frequent in girls than in boys.[6] Forty-five percent of cases are bilateral; although most atresias are partly or completely bony, 5–10 % are membranous. Some are incomplete and manifest as a stenosis rather than an atresia.[6] The anomaly may be associated with hypoplasia of the nasal structures, the palatine process of the maxilla, an outgrowth of the palatal bone, a broad vomer, or an abnormality of the perpendicular plate of the palatine bone.[2,6,7] Bilateral choanal atresia results in severe respiratory difficulty in early neonatal life. The newborn infant is a nasal breather. Mouth breathing is a learned reflex that takes the infant from hours to days to acquire. Choanal atresia is suspected clinically when there is respiratory distress in the neonate and is confirmed when a catheter does not pass from the nose to the oropharynx. Further confirmation of the diagnosis and delineation of the area is made by CT scan after suctioning the nasal passage and applying decongestant nose drops. The definition of choanal atresia and the structure of the atretic plate are not clear in the literature.[6] "Choanal obliteration" is a more descriptive term than "choanal atresia" because the abnormally thick vomer bone and the medial pterygoid plate are usually more contributive in the problem than the atretic plate itself.[6] In many cases the obstruction of the posterior nasal opening (choana) is made by meeting of both medial and lateral nasal walls posteriorly with or without thin soft tissue or a small bony plate between.[7] The CT scan is the imaging study of choice to evaluate patients suggestive of choanal atresia (Fig. 4.49). Axial sections are taken with the gantry angled 5° cephalad to a line perpendicular to the hard palate; 1.5–3 mm sections should be taken and processed for soft-tissue and high-resolution bone algorithm. Normal choanal orifices measure more than 0.37 cm in children younger than 2 years. In patients younger than 8 years, the width of the posterior and inferior parts of the vomer is normally less than 0.34 cm.[8] A thickened vomer is usually the underlying cause of bony atresia.[2,6,7] Membranous atresia is usually treated using endoscopic perforation, and bony atresia requires transpalatine resection of the vomer.[6]

Congenital Nasal Piriform Aperture Stenosis

Premature fusion and overgrowth of the nasal medial processes (see Fig. 4.1) causes narrowing of the piriform aperture (anterior nasal opening). In 75 % of the cases, the central upper incisors are fused as a single central megaincisor.[3] Some of these patients may also have holoprosencephaly and abnormalities of the pituitary–adrenal axis.

Congenital Dacrocystocele and Mucocele of the Lacrimal Sac and Duct (Submucosal Nasal Mass)

Embryologically, the nasolacrimal drainage system develops from surface ectoderm located between the maxillary and frontonasal processes (see Fig. 4.1).[3,4] Canalization of the nasolacrimal duct occurs in the third fetal month and is completed by the sixth month or with respiration at birth.[3,9] The most frequent site of incomplete canalization is at the junction of the nasolacrimal duct and the nasal mucosa, the valve of Hasner. The next site is at the junction of the common lacrimal canaliculus and the lacrimal sac, the valve of Rosenmüller.[9] A congenital dacryocystocele (CD) is believed to result from obstruction at these two sites. This causes accumulation of mucosal fluid in the drainage system and distension of the lacrimal sac. The term mucocele also has been used, describing glandular tissue within the sac which produces mucus. Dacryocystocele is the preferable term as it is more anatomically accurate and makes no reference to the source of the fluid in the lacrimal sac.[9] An uninfected dacryocystocele presents as a blue mass in the medial canthal region. CD differs from the more common classic neonatal nasolacrimal duct obstruction by the absence of a mass in the medial canthal region and the free flow of pus or tears onto the surface of the eye and eyelids.[9] In simple neonatal nasolacrimal duct obstruction, the system is blocked at a single point, the valve of Hasner. In CD, the system is blocked both distally and proximally, with resultant distension of the lacrimal sac.[9] The differential diagnosis of a medial canthal mass in infants includes CD, capillary hemangioma, lymphangioma, solid dermoid, dermoid cyst, encephalocele, meningoencephalocele, nasal glioma, and heterotopic brain.[9] In children, inflammatory conditions, rhabdomyosarcoma, and other tumors of the sinonasal cavities should be considered (Table 4.4).

4 Imaging of the Nasal Cavity and Paranasal Sinuses

Although the formation of the nasolacrimal system occurs early in life, canalization of the nasolacrimal duct occurs either in late intrauterine life or with respiration at birth. Failure of canalization of the proximal nasolacrimal duct, along with obstruction of the common lacrimal canaliculus, produces lacrimal sac mucocele. Failure of canalization of the distal nasolacrimal duct (at the valve of Hasner), along with obstruction of the Rosenmüller valve, produces nasolacrimal duct mucocele. The problem may be bilateral or unilateral. CT and MRI show a cystic medial canthus mass, dilatation of the nasolacrimal duct, and a submucosal intranasal mass (Fig. 4.50). There may be expansion of the fossa for the lacrimal sac. The nasolacrimal duct mucocele appears as a soft-tissue mass, along with dilated nasolacrimal duct under the respective inferior turbinate. The mucoceles are seen on CT scans as a fluid density and on MRI as fluid intensity in the lower naso-orbital angle (mucocele of lacrimal sac) or within the nasal cavity (Fig. 4.50) If infected, there will be some enhancement of the lesion (pyocele) on enhanced CT or MR scans. Complete resection or marsupialization generally results in cure.[9]

Midline Facial Clefting

Midline facial clefting results from failure of both nasal medial processes to fuse and failure of the frontonasal process to form (see Fig. 4.1). The rare median cleft syndrome is always associated with hypertelorism and may be divided into low and high groups. In the low group, the cleft involves the upper lip, hard palate, and occasionally the nose.[2,3] Basal encephaloceles, anomalies of the corpus callosum (agenesis), intracranial lipomas, and optic nerve dysplasia (colobomas) are accompanying anomalies.[2] In the high group, the cleft involves the nose and forehead and, less commonly, the upper lip and hard palate.[2] Associated anomalies include intraorbital cephaloceles, frontoethmoidal and nasal encephaloceles (Fig. 4.51), cranium bifidum occultum, microphthalmos, anophthalmos, intracranial lipomas and, less commonly, callosal anomalies.[2,10]

Anomalies of Closure of the Prenasal Space: Encephaloceles, Nasal Gliomas, Epidermoids, and Dermoids

An encephalocele is the protrusion of intracranial contents, including meninges and brain matter, through a defect in the cranium or skull base.[11] Encephalocele may be congenital or due to spontaneous or traumatic causes.[11,12] Most encephaloceles involve the herniation of frontal lobe tissue through an anterior cranial fossa defect into the nasal or ethmoid cavity (Fig. 4.51).[11] Intrasphenoid and intratemporal (petrous apex, mastoid) encephaloceles are rare subsets of this disease process (Fig. 4.52).[11,12] In early life, the frontal bone is separated from the nasal bones by the fonticulus frontalis (anterior fontanelle, bregmatic fontanelle).[2,3] The prenasal space separates the nasal

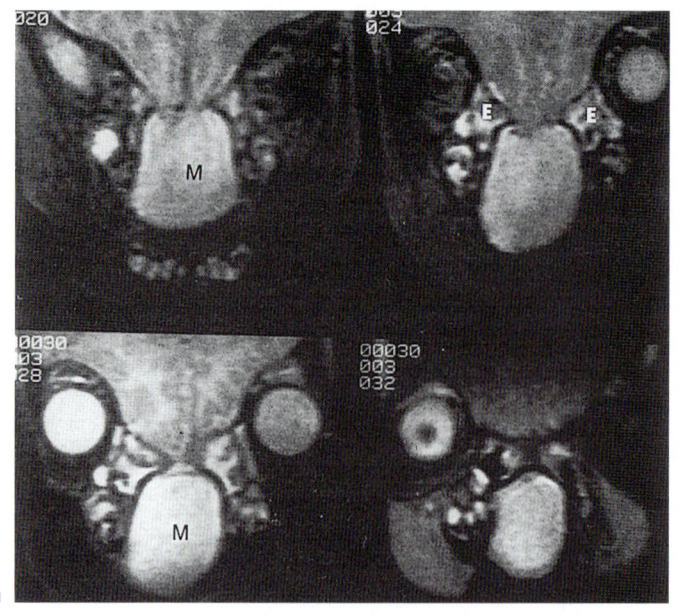

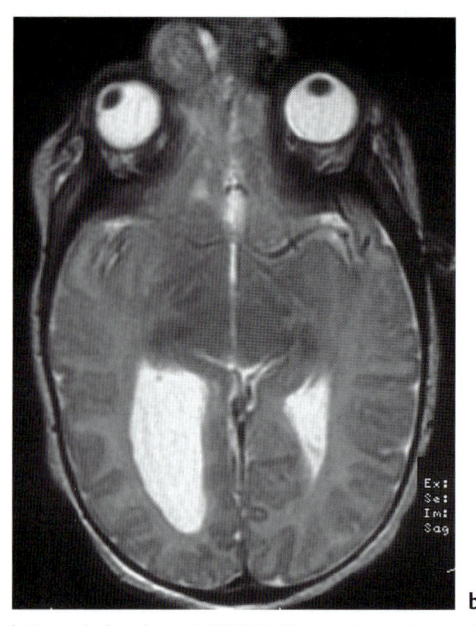

Table 4.4 Differential diagnosis of a medial canthal mass in an infant

- Congenital dacryocystocele (mucocele)
- Capillary hemangioma
- Dermoid/epidermoid cyst
- Encephalocele
- Meningoencephalocele
- Heterotopic brain tissue
- Rhabdomyosarcoma
- Inflammatory conditions (dacryocystitis)

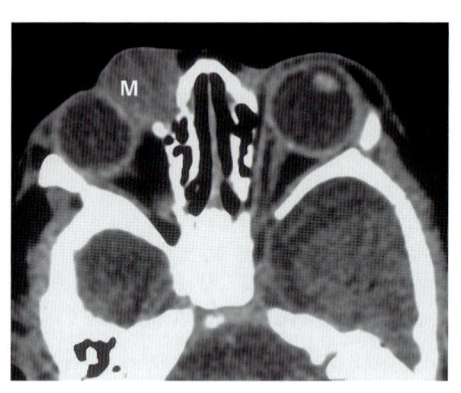

Fig. 4.50 Congenital dacryocele. Axial CT scan shows a right naso-orbital mass (M), compatible with a congenital dacryocele (mucocele).

Fig. 4.51 **a** Meningoencephalocele. Coronal T2W MR images showing marked hypertelorism, herniation of the brain between the ethmoid labyrinths (E), and a large CSF intensity mass (M) representing a meningocele.

b Encephalocele. Axial T2W MR scan, in another patient, showing marked hypertelorism and displacement of the brain between the orbits.

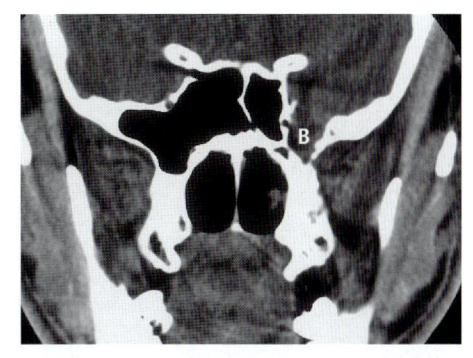

Fig. 4.52 Intrasphenoid sinus encephalocele. Coronal CT scan, showing brain tissue (B) in the lateral recess of the left sphenoid sinus.

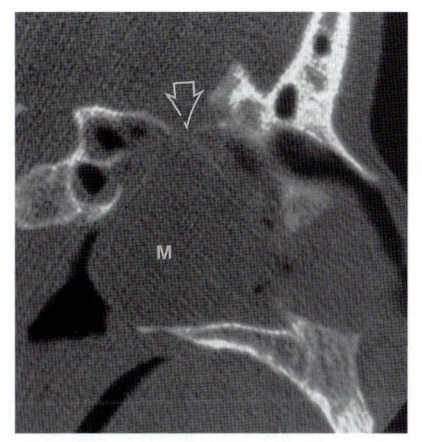

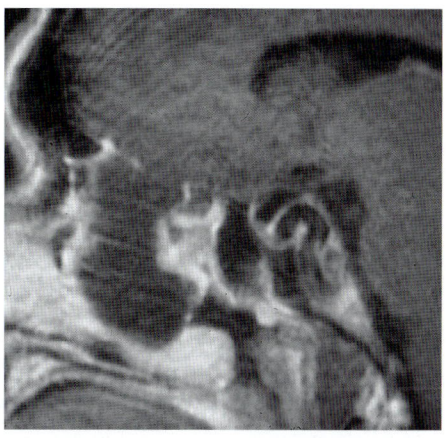

Fig. 4.53 a Nasal glioma. Direct sagittal CT scan shows a large nasal mass (M). This was clinically considered to be a polyp. Note inferior displacement of the cribriform plate (arrow). CSF leak developed after surgery. b Enhanced T1W sagittal MR scan in another patient, an adult, shows a large intranasal meningocele. This was clinically considered to be a polyp.

bones from the underlying cartilaginous nasal capsule. The prenasal space contains a dural diverticulum,[2,10] which gradually regresses, leaving behind the foramen cecum, located just anterior to the base of the crista galli.[11] Protrusion of brain through the fonticulus frontalis results in a nasofrontal encephalocele (40–60% of sincipital cephaloceles).[2,3] The sinciput is the anterior part of the head just above and including the forehead. If the brain protrudes into the prenasal space, nasoethmoidal encephaloceles result (30% of sincipital cephaloceles) (Fig. 4.51). Nasal gliomas result from sequestration of brain in the distal part of the dural diverticulum (Fig. 4.53a). These extracranial rests of neuroglial tissue (astrocytes and gliosis) grow slowly and have no malignant potential. Approximately 15% of nasal gliomas are reported to have a fibrous connection to the subarachnoid space, but no CSF connection. However, a CSF leak may develop following surgery (Fig. 4.53). Intranasal gliomas as well as meningocele or meningoencephalocele may present later in life as nasal masses (Fig. 4.53).

Encephaloceles within the sphenoid sinus are subdivided by their location into a medial, perisellar type and a lateral, sphenoid recess type. Those of the lateral sphenoid recess type are found lateral to the foramen rotundum in a pneumatized portion of the pterygoid process and greater wing of the sphenoid and evolve from the herniation of temporal lobe tissue through a middle cranial fossa defect.[12] Extensive lateral pneumatization of sphenoid sinus into the pterygoid process may result in a relatively thin floor of the middle cranial fossa and may predispose certain individuals to develop spontaneous encephalocele or CSF leak.[12] Any fluid level or soft-tissue mass in the lateral recess of sphenoid sinus, detected on CT scan or MRI, in an otherwise well-aerated sphenoid sinus in the presence of thinning or defect of the sphenoid sinus roof should be considered strongly suspicious for CSF leak/meningoencephalocele (Fig. 4.52). CT in patients who have had surgery for encephalocele resection with repair of the skull base defect will demonstrate osteoneogenesis adjacent to the defect or around the entire peripheral sphenoid lateral recess.[12] The multiple layers of fascia or other soft tissue in place result in obliteration of the lateral sphenoid recess.

Dermoid, Epidermoid, and Dermal Sinus

If the dural diverticulum of the prenasal space reaches the skin of the nose, it may drag ectoderm with it as it regresses, resulting in a dermal sinus (50%), or a dermoid or epidermoid cyst (50%) may develop.[3,11,13,14] Neuroectodermal tissue has been found extending through the foramen cecum from the falx to the nasal septum. The distal opening of a dermal sinus may be found anywhere from the glabella (a smooth elevation medial to supraorbital/supraciliary arches of the frontal squama) to the columella (a skin–cartilage septum between the nares). Epidermoids are more common at the tip of the nose or slightly lateral to the nose; dermoids are usually midline and often seen at the upper nasal dorsum (Figs. 4.54, 4.55). Intracranial communication is found in some of these cases.[2,3,11,13,14] Although a nasal dermoid or nasal pit (dimple) may be limited to the nose, the possibility of a sinus tract communicating with the intracranial cavity should be considered in the presence of an enlarged foramen cecum, a bifid crista galli, or a bifid or broadened nasal septum (Fig. 4.55b), or whenever there is a history of recurrent meningitis and/or anterior cranial fossa abscesses.[2,3] The bony defect is best evaluated and identified with thin-section (1.5–3 mm) CT scan. In our institution, we obtain thin sections of the frontonasal region in children who present with a nasal pit, dermoid, epidermoid, or lipoma at or near the base of the nose. If a sinus tract or intracranial communication is shown or suspected, additional MRI of the brain will be performed. The intracranial component may lie within the falx at its attachment to the crista galli,[2] or may be seen as a moderate to large mass embedded within the subfrontal region.

■ References

1. Mafee MF, Valvassori GE. Radiology of craniofacial anomalies. Otolaryngol Clin North Am 1981; 14: 939–988.
2. Naidich TP, Blaser SI, Bauer BS, Armstrong DC, McLone DG, Zimmerman RA. Embryology and congenital lesions of the midface. In: Som PM, Curtin HD, eds. Head and Neck Imaging, 4th ed. St. Louis: Mosby; 2003; 3–86.
3. Castillo M. Congenital abnormalities of the nose: CT and MR findings. AJR 1994; 162: 1211–1217.
4. Warwick R, Williams PL, eds. Gray's Anatomy, 35th British ed., Philadelphia: W.B. Saunders, 1973: 116–119.
5. Carter BL. Paranasal sinuses, nasal cavity, pterygoid fossa, nasopharynx, and infratemporal fossa. In: Valvassori GE, Buckingham RA, Carter BL, Hanafee WN, Mafee M F, eds. Head and Neck Imaging. Stuttgart: Georg Thieme Verlag, 1988: 192–250.
6. Khafagy YW. Endoscopic repair of bilateral congenital choanal atresia. Laryngoscope 2002; 112: 316–319.
7. Harner SG, McDonald TJ, Reese DF. The anatomy of congenital choanal atresia. Otolaryngol Head Neck Surg 1981; 89: 7–9.
8. Chinwuba C, William J, Strand R. Nasal airway obstruction. CT assessment. Radiology 1986; 159: 503–506.

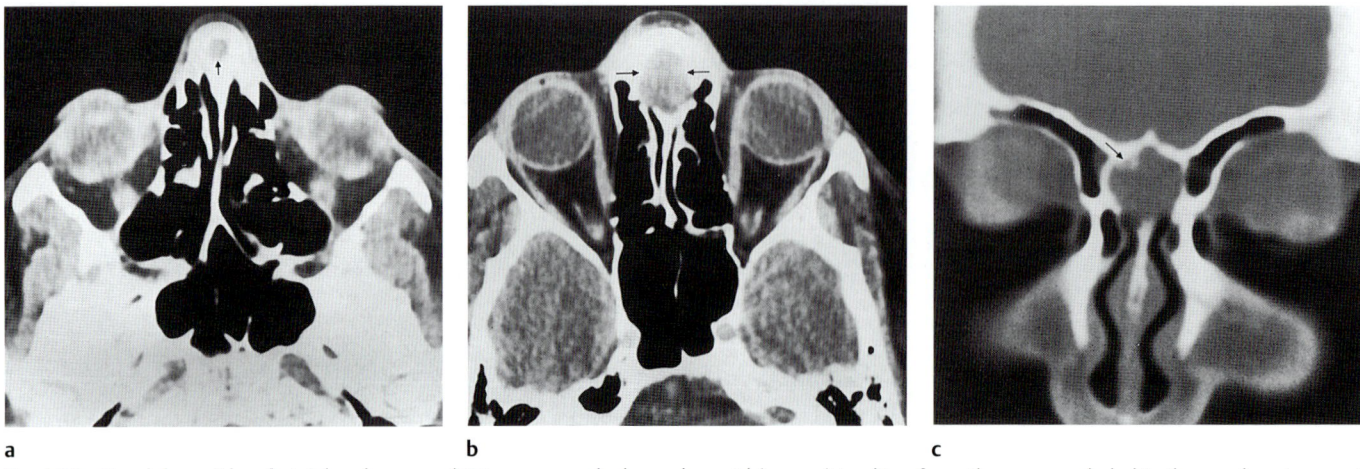

Fig. 4.54 Nasal dermoid. **a, b** Axial and **c** coronal CT scans reveal a large dermoid (arrows) tracking from the nose cephalad in the nasal septum up to the foramen cecum. No intracranial communication was found at surgery. Courtesy of Bertram Giulian, MD and Daniel Hottenstein, MD, Harrisburg, PA, USA.

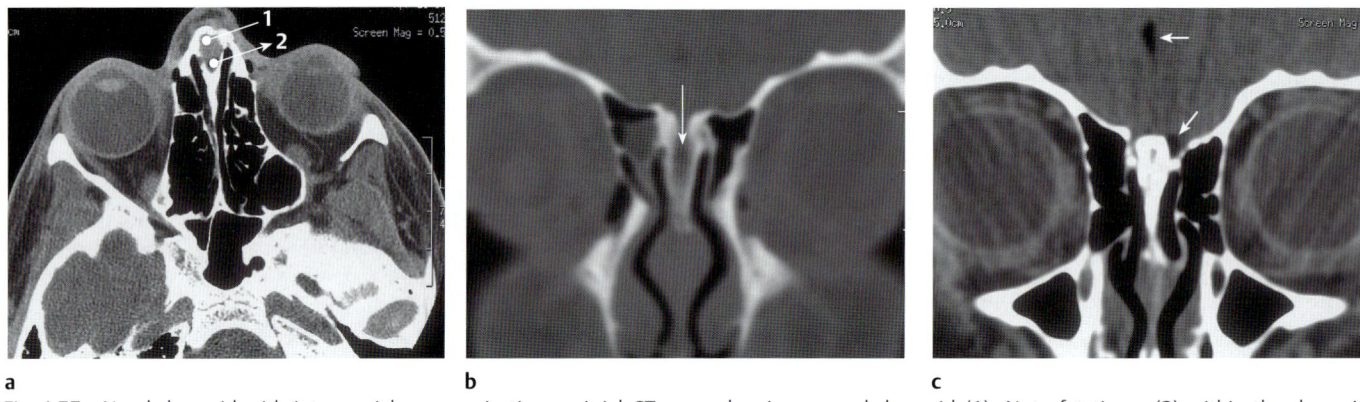

Fig. 4.55 Nasal dermoid with intracranial communication. **a** Axial CT scan, showing a nasal dermoid (1). Note fat tissue (2) within the dermoid. **b** Coronal CT scan showing a bifid nasal septum (arrow). **c** Coronal CT scan, showing tracking of nasal dermoid fat in the anterior cranial region (arrows).

9 Shashy RG, Durairaj V, Holmes JM, et al. Congenital dacryocystocele associated with intranasal cysts: diagnosis and management. Laryngoscope 2003; 113: 37–40.
10 Simpson DA, David DJ, White J. Cephaloceles: Treatment, outcome, and antenatal diagnosis. Neurosurgery 1984; 15: 14–21.
11 Barkovich A J, Vandermarck P, Edwards MSB, Cohen PH. Congenital nasal masses: CT and MR imaging lectures in 16 cases. AJNR 1991; 12: 105–116.
12 Lai Sy, Kennedy DW, Bolger WE. Sphenoid encephaloceles: disease management and identification of lesions within the lateral recess of the sphenoid sinus. Laryngoscope 2002; 112: 1800–1805.
13 Sessions RB. Nasal dermal sinuses: new concepts and explanations. Laryngoscope 1982; 92: 1–25.
14 Clark WD, Bailey BJ, Stiernberg CM. Nasal dermoid with intracranial involvement. Otolaryngol Head Neck Surg 1985; 93(l): 102–104.

■ Inflammatory Diseases

Acute Sinusitis

The diagnosis of sinusitis is not only or necessarily an imaging diagnosis. The radiologist should always require some information, positive or negative, about symptoms or signs that might suggest sinusitis, such as nasal discharge or congestion, fever, sinus pain and tenderness, and prior history of sinus draining, irrigation, or surgical procedures. It is important to realize that the ethmoid and maxillary sinuses are the only sinuses that are large enough at birth to be clinically significant in rhinosinusitis (Fig. 4.**56**). Mucosal thickening, the most common finding on imaging studies, usually indicates the presence of chronic sinusitis, but it may certainly be related to an episode of acute sinusitis as well. Postoperative scarring, and periosteal reaction after sinus surgery such as Caldwell–Luc operation, may result in loss of normal aeration of the sinuses. These changes may be permanent, even in the absence of any sinus disease.[1] Although the lack of sclerosis and periosteal reaction speaks against chronic sinusitis, it does not at all rule out a chronic infection. Bilaterality and absence of erosion weigh in favor of an inflammatory rather than a neoplastic process. Diffuse thickening of the mucosa and submucosa lining the paranasal sinuses is a common finding on plain films, CT, and MR scans. Indeed, 20–40% of patients undergoing MRI of the head are found to have edematous tissue of the paranasal sinuses as an incidental finding. Sinusitis may accompany a viral infection or systemic disease but it is also seen in patients with allergies. An acutely infected sinus that is producing symptoms may show thickening of the mucosa, an air–fluid level, or both. The most common cause for acute sinusitis is a viral upper respiratory tract infection. A secondary acute bacterial infection is often caused by *Streptococcus pneumoniae*. Other prevalent pathogens include *Haemophilus influenzae* and *Moraxella*

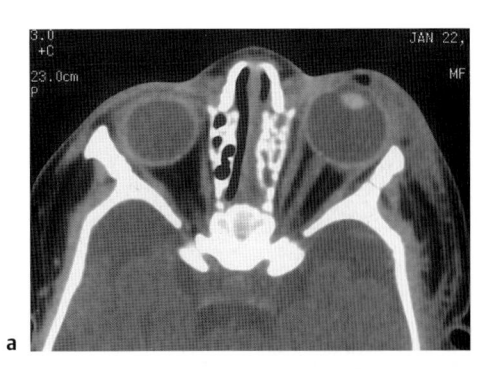

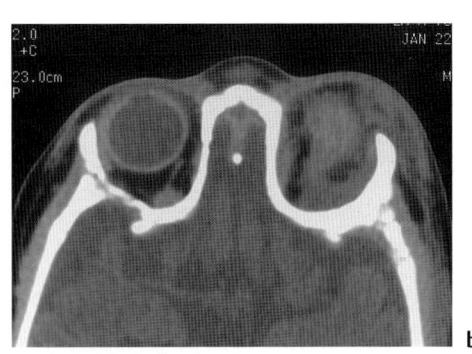

Fig. 4.**56** Acute sinusitis with orbital cellulitis in an 8-week-old infant. **a** Axial CT scan shows opacification of left ethmoid air cells. **b** Axial CT scan shows extension of preseptal orbital inflammation along the postseptal superolateral left orbit.

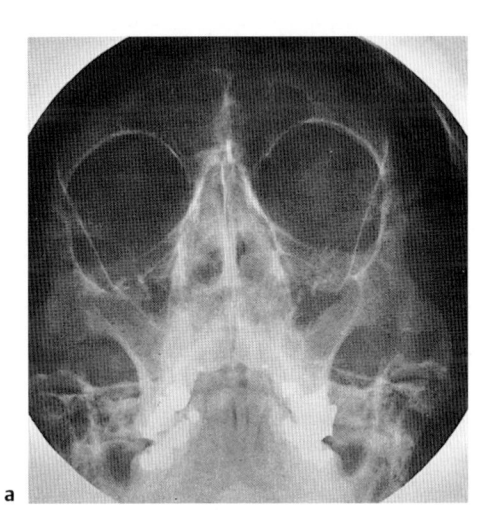

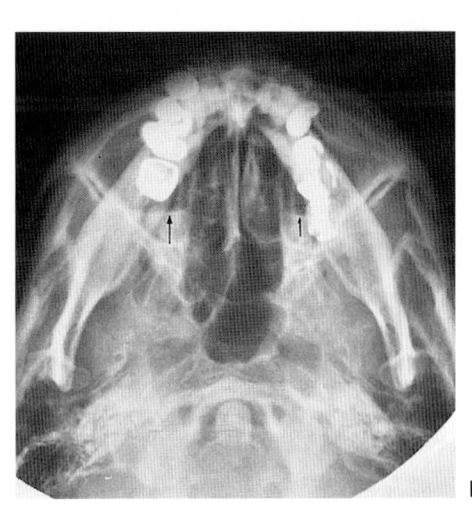

Fig. 4.**57 a** Allergic sinusitis. Waters projection. Diffuse opacification of the paranasal sinuses is commonly seen with allergic type sinusitis. **b** Acute sinusitis with air–fluid level. Base projection shows a fluid level (arrows) in both maxillary antra.

catarrhalis.[2] Isolated infections of the maxillary sinus may be due to dental caries in about 20% of cases. More severe types of sinusitis occur in patients with diabetes and in patients who are immunosuppressed by various drugs, toxins, and systemic disease. These patients are more prone to aggressive types of fungal infections, such as mucormycosis and aspergillosis, which tend to invade the local blood vessels, causing extensive destruction, osteomyelitis, and even cerebral infarction.[3–7] Treatment of fungal sinusitis consists of surgical debridement and administration of amphotericin B. Thus, the type of infection needs to be diagnosed as early as possible and treated appropriately. Biopsy and special cultures may be required to establish the diagnosis of fungal infection.[6]

Radiological Diagnosis

It should be noted that an air–fluid level does not necessarily indicate the presence of acute sinusitis. Knowledge of the history and physical findings is necessary to differentiate other causes of an air–fluid level, such as a previous antral lavage, recent trauma, a recent surgical procedure, barotrauma, or hemorrhage caused by a coagulopathy disorder.[1] Acute sinusitis is usually evident on clinical examination, confirmed by plain film studies (Fig. 4.**57**) and followed by CT study as needed. Complications of sinusitis are an indication for CT and/or MRI.[1, 8–10] CT scanning is preferable for identifying bone destruction and osteomyelitis. MRI shows the orbital and intracranial sinogenic complications to better advantage.[11]

Sinus Infections and Their Complications

Conventional radiography is adequate for the diagnosis of clinically uncomplicated acute sinusitis. Although antibiotics have cut down the incidence of complicated sinusitis with orbital involvement, it still occurs and orbital involvement may even be the first sign of sinus infection in children.[1, 12] Infection may spread from sinuses to the orbit by direct extension. It may also spread by way of numerous valveless communicating veins between the sinuses and the orbit.[12] In sinusitis associated with complications, CT is the best method for demonstrating the nature and the source of the problem. The orbital involvement from sinusitis includes inflammatory edema (Fig. 4.**58**), orbital periostitis, subperiosteal induration (phlegmon) (Fig. 4.**59**), subperiosteal abscess (Fig. 4.**60**), orbital and facial cellulitis (Fig. 4.**61**), and orbital abscess (Fig. 4.**62**). Should the infection spread from the sinuses into the cranial cavity, one or more of the following complications may ensue: cavernous sinus thrombosis (Fig. 4.**63**), meningitis (Fig. 4.**64**), and epidural (Fig. 4.**65**), subdural (Fig. 4.**66**), and brain abscesses (Fig. 4.**67**). Periostitis and osteomyelitis of the frontal sinus severe enough to involve the orbit may also extend through the posterior plate of the frontal sinus to involve the anterior cranial fossa (Fig. 4.**68**).

Osteomyelitis of the frontal bone may be accompanied by doughy edema overlapping the affected sinus and/or a subgaleal abscess, causing a mass effect termed a "Pott's puffy tumor." (Fig. 4.**69**). Acute, subacute, or chronic sinusitis that has not responded to appropriate antibiotic and other medical treatments should be biopsied to rule out the presence of any underlying tumor, particularly if infection is limited to a single sinus. In the

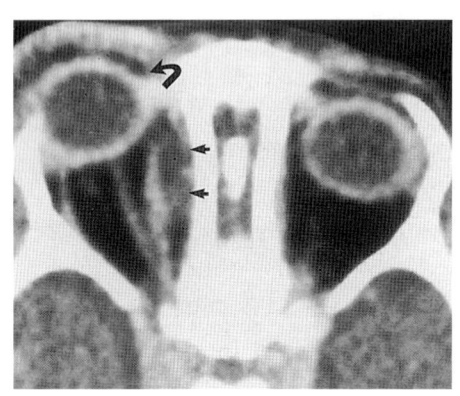

392   4 Imaging of the Nasal Cavity and Paranasal Sinuses

Fig. 4.**58** Inflammatory edema of the eyelid and subperiosteal space. Axial CT scan showing edema of the eyelid (curved arrow) and edema in the subperiosteal space (straight arrows).

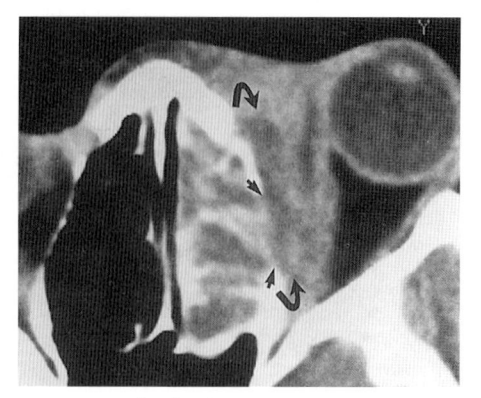

Fig. 4.**59** Orbital subperiosteal phlegmon. CT scan shows opacification of the left ethmoid air cells. Note erosion of the lamina papyracea (arrows) and a subperiosteal phlegmon (curved arrows).

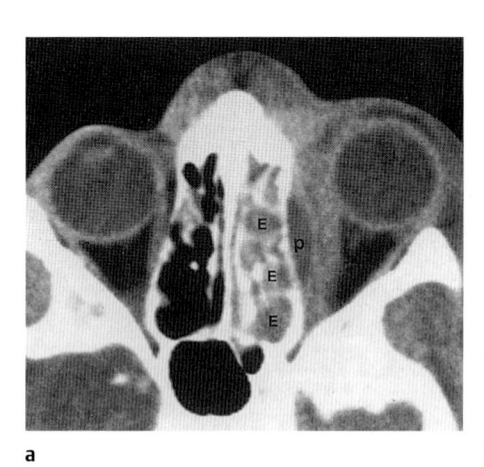

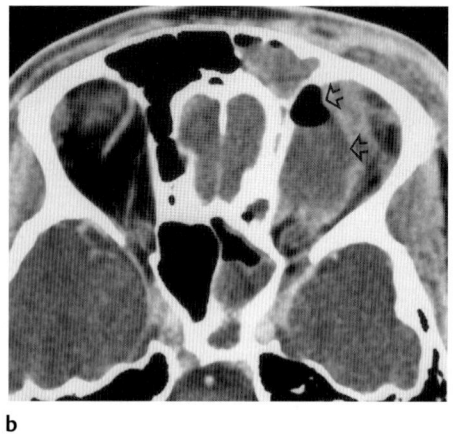

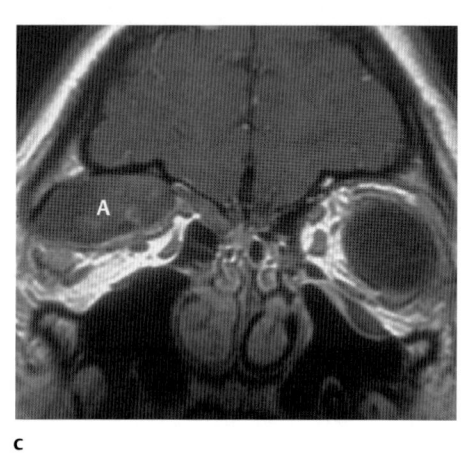

Fig. 4.**60**
a Orbital subperiosteal abscess. CT scan shows opacification of the left ethmoid air cells (E) and collection of fluid (pus) in the subperiosteal space (P).

b Subperiosteal abscess. CT scan shows opacified left frontal sinus and a large orbital subperiosteal abscess (arrows). Note mucosal thickening of the left sphenoid sinus.
c Subperiosteal abscess. Enhanced coronal T1W MR scan showing a large subperiosteal abscess (A).

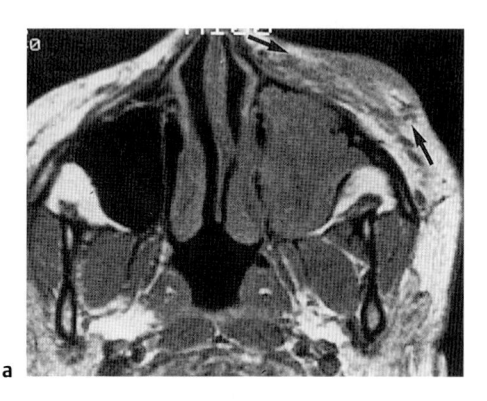

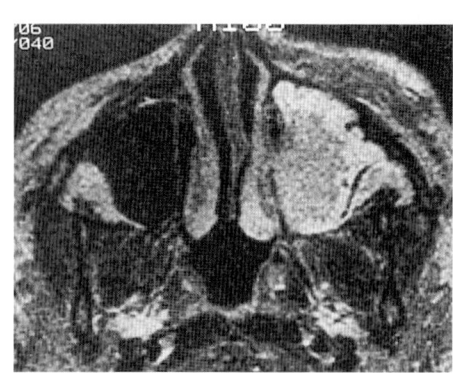

Fig. 4.**61** Facial cellulitis. **a** PW and **b** T2W axial scans show diffuse inflammatory edema of the left cheek (arrows) and opacification of the left maxillary sinus. This patient developed facial and orbital cellulitis following a dental procedure, resulting in an orbital abscess associated with some visual loss.

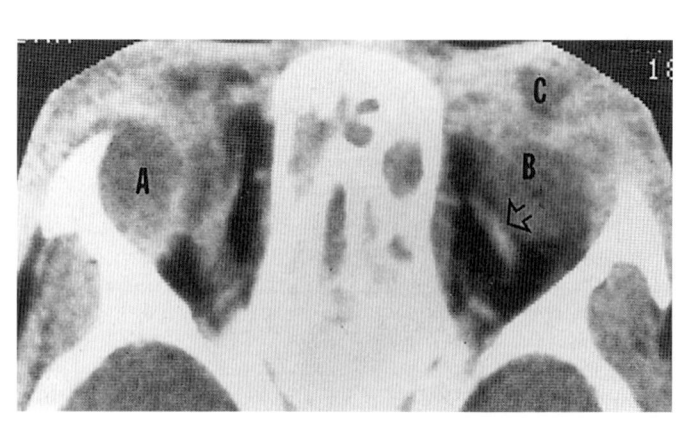

◁ Fig. 4.**62** Orbital abscesses. CT scan shows orbital (A and B) and eyelid (C) abscesses. Note the moderate engorgement of the superior ophthalmic vein (arrow).

Sinonasal Pathology

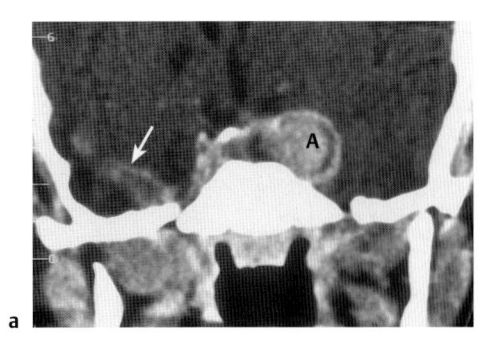

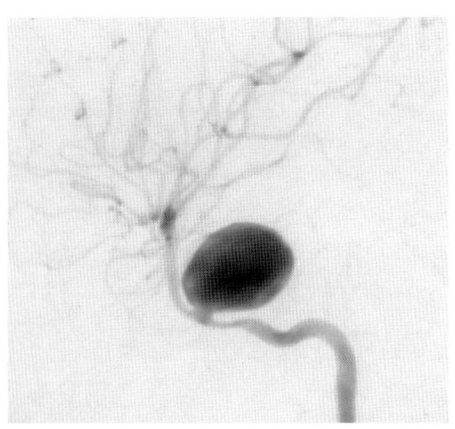

Fig. 4.63 Sinogenic mycotic aneurysm. **a** Enhanced coronal CT scan, showing a mycotic aneurysm of the left internal carotid artery (A). Note temporal lobe abscess (arrow). **b** Angiogram shows mycotic aneurysm. Case Courtesy of Jose Mondoncca, MD, Brazil.

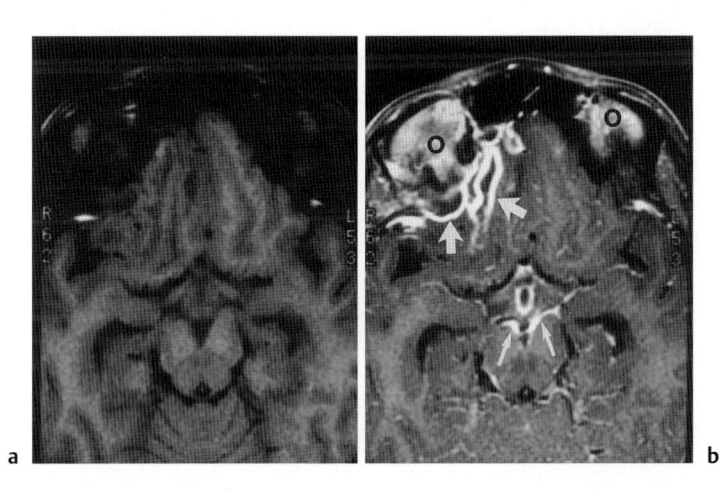

Fig. 4.64 Sinogenic orbital cellulitis and meningitis. Precontrast fat-suppression (**a**) and postcontrast fat-suppression (**b**) T1W MR scans, showing enhancement of superior orbital fatty-reticulum (O) and leptomeningeal enhancement (arrows). Case Courtesy of Hamid Mohazab, MD, Chicago, IL, USA.

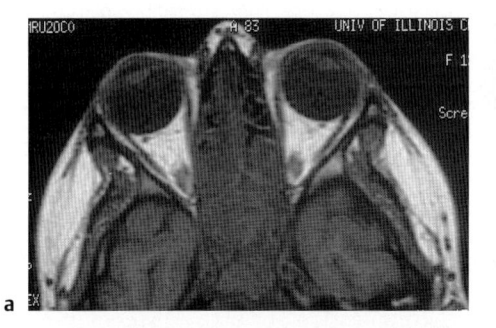

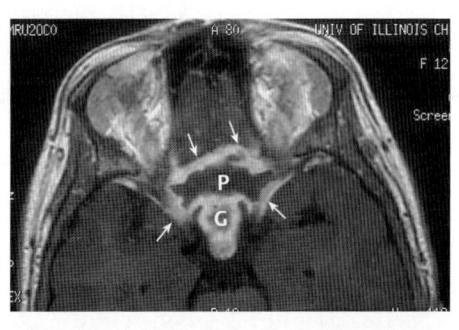

Fig. 4.65 Sinogenic epidural abscess. **a** T1W MR scan in a 12-year-old girl shows opacified sphenoid and ethmoid sinuses. **b** Enhanced T1W MR scan shows pus (P) and granulation tissue (G) in the epidural space. Note granulation along the planum sphenoidale (arrow).

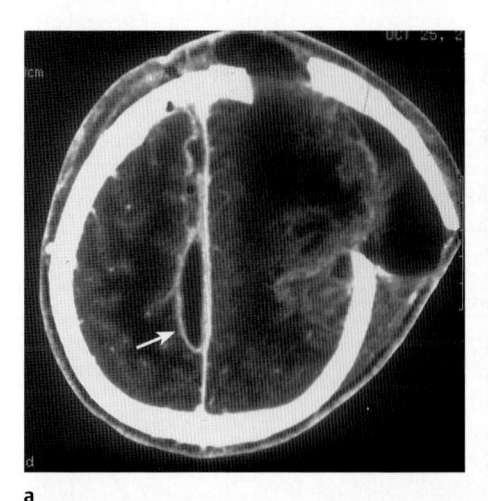

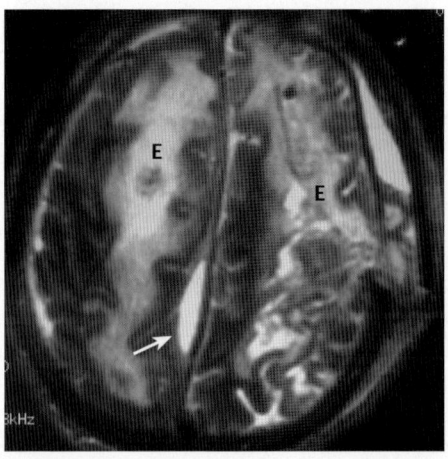

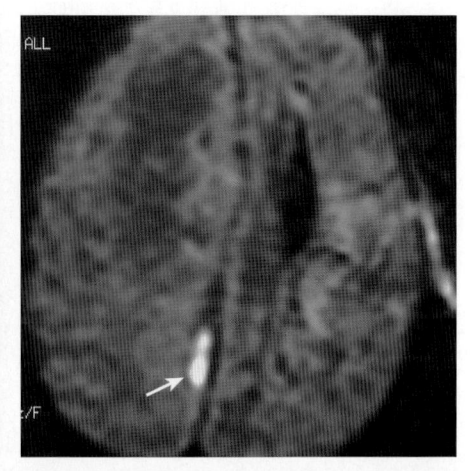

Fig. 4.66 Sinogenic subdural abscess and encephalitis. **a** Enhanced CT scan shows subdural abscess along the falx (arrow). Note postoperative changes, related to drainage of a sinogenic subdural abscess, and marked edema of left frontal lobe due to encephalitis. **b** T2W MR scan shows subdural abscess (arrow) and marked bilateral white-matter cerebral edema (E). **c** DW MR image shows subdural abscess (arrow).

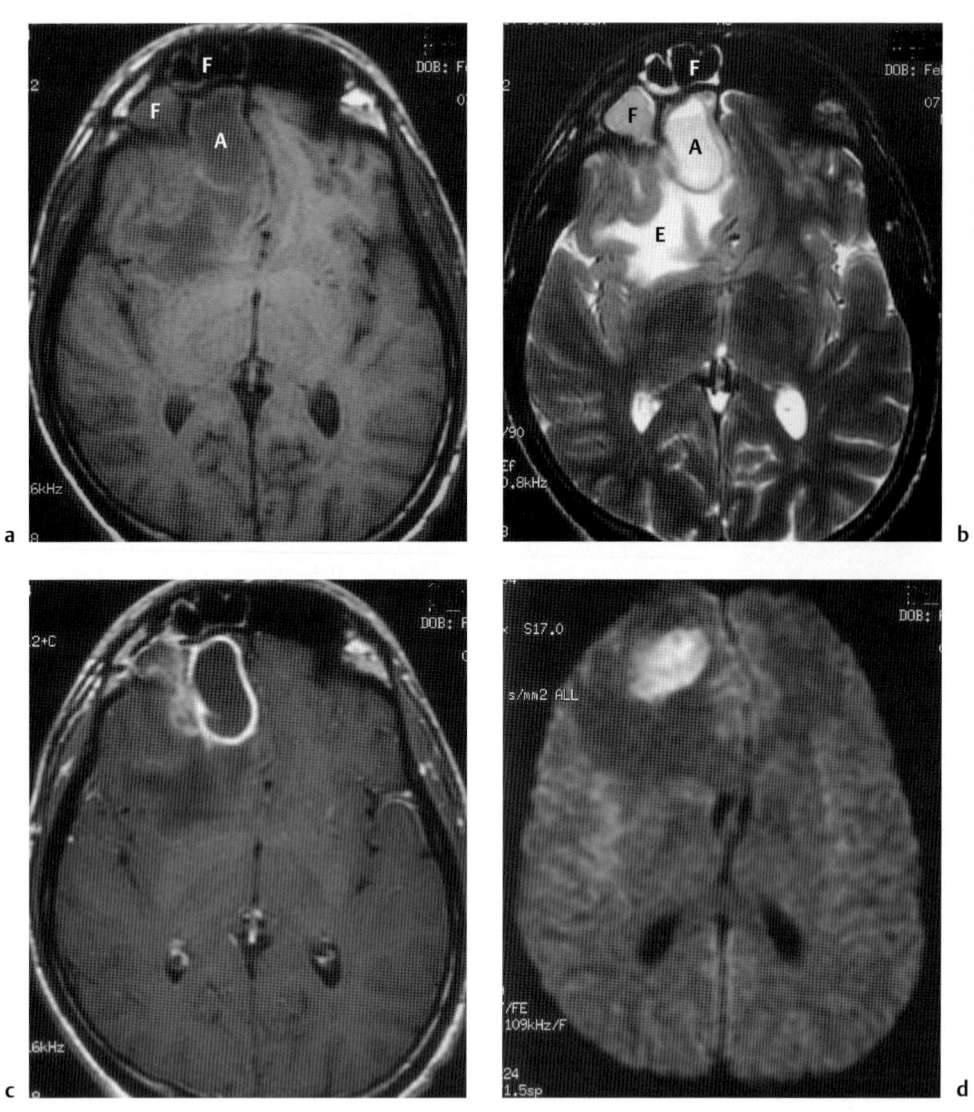

Fig. 4.**67 a–d** Sinogenic brain abscess in a patient with right frontal sinusitis. **a** T1W and **b** T2W MR scans, showing inflammatory changes in the right frontal sinus (F), frontal lobe abscess (A) and edema (E). **c** Enhanced T1W and **d** DW MR scans, showing the frontal lobe abscess. The abscess appears hyperintense in the DW MR scan (**d**). This patient responded well to treatment.

case of maxillary sinus, an underlying dental cause should be excluded. A persistent air–fluid level following dental extraction may indicate an oral–antral fistula.[1] Orbital complications resulting from acute or chronic sinusitis can be best evaluated with CT and MRI (Figs. 4.**58**–4.**60**, 4.**62**). The most common complications of rhinosinusitis in children occur in the orbit. These complications include the following in order of increasing severity: orbital edema, orbital cellulitis, subperiosteal orbital abscess, intraorbital abscess, thrombosis of the superior ophthalmic vein, and cavernous sinuses. Inflammatory orbital edema due to sinusitis is edema of the eyelid, which is the first stage; it is often misdiagnosed as orbital or periorbital cellulitis. The infection in this early stage is actually still confined to the sinus.[12] A CT or MR scan at this stage will demonstrate the edema of the eyelids and conjunctivae and inflammatory changes of the infected sinus or sinuses. As the reaction of the orbital periosteum begins and gradually advances, the edema of the eyelids and conjunctivae becomes more generalized, and the eye begins to protrude. Inflammatory tissue collects beneath the periosteum to form a subperiosteal edema (Fig. 4.**58**) or phlegmon (Fig. 4.**69**); subsequently, pus may form to represent a subperiosteal abscess (Fig. 4.**60**). As the disease progresses, bacteria may infiltrate the periorbital and retro-orbital fat, giving rise to true orbital cellulitis and abscess (Fig. 4.**62**). These two conditions frequently coexist. At this stage, extraocular mobility is progressively impaired. With severe involvement, visual disturbances can result from optic neuritis, ischemia (compression), or both. Abscess formation in the orbit may result from extension of a subperiosteal abscess through the periosteum or from localization of orbital and facial cellulitis (Fig. 4.**61**).[12] Ethmoid sinus infection is frequently responsible for orbital swelling, subperiosteal abscess, and orbital cellulitis, which extends from the ethmoid through the lamina papyracea. CT is an excellent method for evaluating an acute sinusitis. The information obtained from the CT scan and MRI, together with clinical findings (proptosis, limitation of extraocular muscle movement, and decreased visual acuity), may be the best guideline for treatment.[9]

Intracranial Complications of Sinusitis

Although intracranial complications of sinusitis are relatively rare, prompt recognition of these disease states is important to prevent permanent neurological deficit or fatality.[8, 12, 13] Intracranial complications of sinus infection derive either from indirect extension, via retrograde thrombophlebitis of valveless emissary veins, or directly, through bony contiguity associated with septic erosion, trauma, or structural abnormality.[12] These complications include osteomyelitis, epidural empyema, subdural empyema, meningitis, cerebritis, brain abscess, sinodural

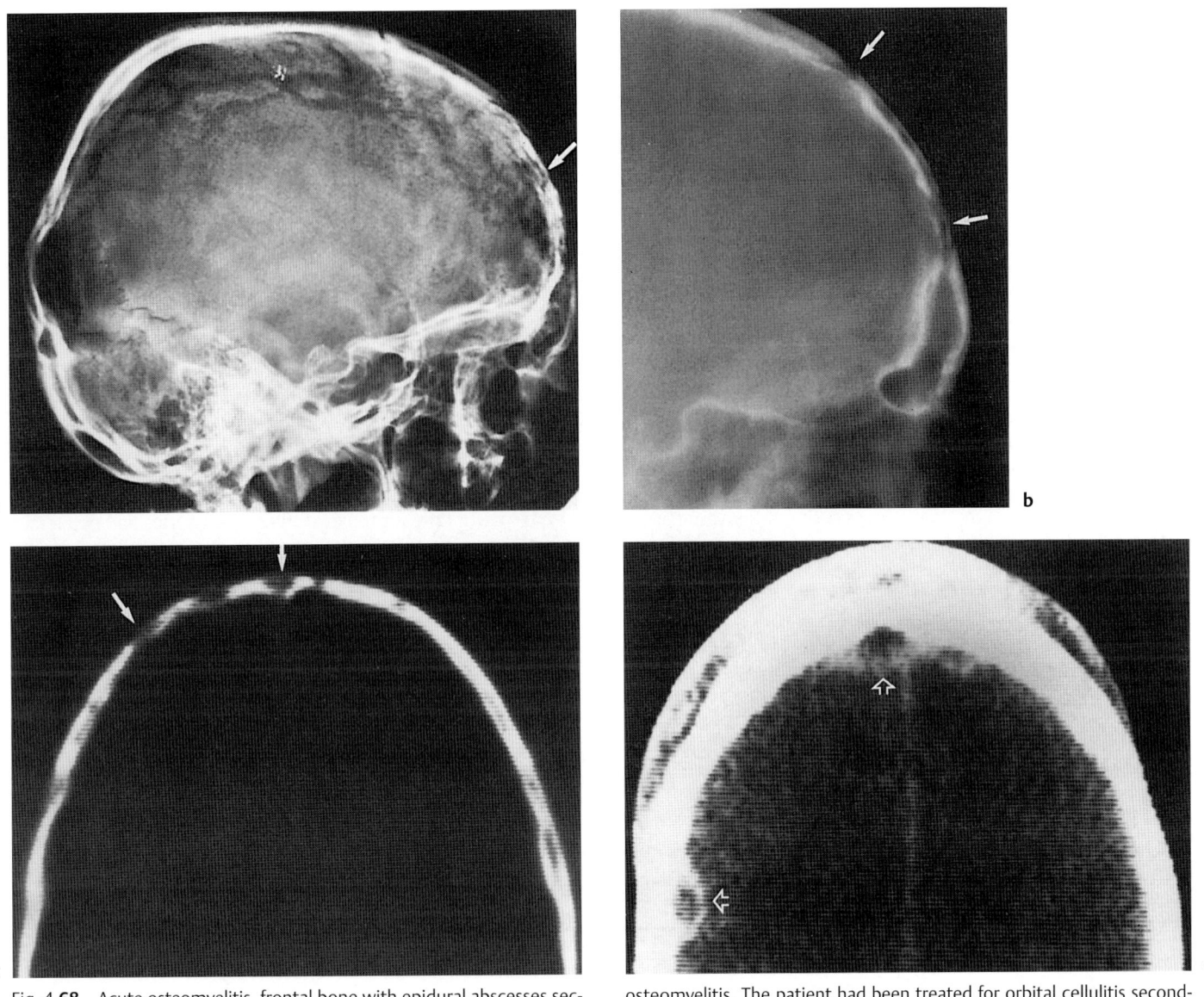

Fig. 4.**68** Acute osteomyelitis, frontal bone with epidural abscesses secondary to sinusitis. **a** Lateral projection, **b** lateral tomogram, **c** and **d** axial CT scans. Destruction of the frontal bone due to osteomyelitis (arrows) is evident on the plain film, lateral tomogram, and CT scan in **a**, **b**, and **c**, respectively. The epidural abscesses noted in **d** (open arrows) are due to the osteomyelitis. The patient had been treated for orbital cellulitis secondary to sinusitis, but the acute osteomyelitis was unsuspected. Reproduced from Carter BL, Bankoff MS, Fisk JD. Computed tomographic detection of sinusitis responsible for intracranial and etracranial infections. Radiology 1983; 147: 739–742, with permission.

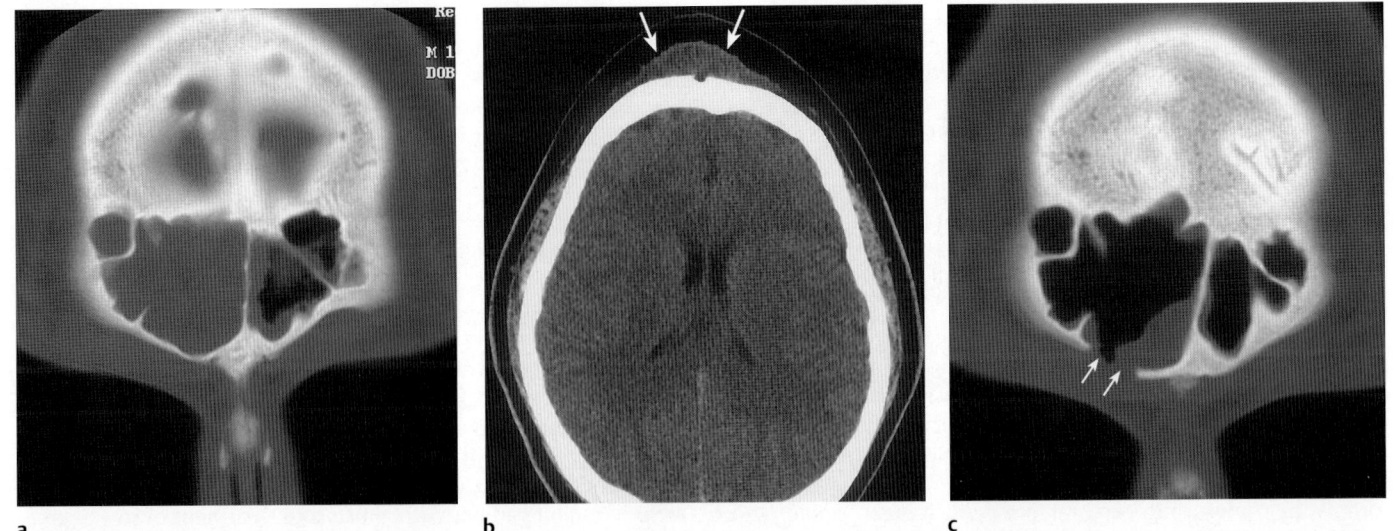

Fig. 4.**69** Subgaleal abscess ("Pott's puffy tumor") in a 15-year-old boy. **a** Coronal CT scan shows opacification of right frontal sinus as well as mucosal thickening of the left frontal sinus. **b** Axial CT scan shows a subgaleal phlegmon over the external table of the frontal bone (arrows). **c** Coronal CT following trephination of right frontal sinus, showing the trephinized frontal sinus (arrows) with marked improvement of frontal sinusitis.

thrombosis (cavernous sinus thrombosis),[8,9] infarct, and tension pneumocephalus related to ruptured intracranial abscess into the ventricles while in continuity with the sinonasal cavities.

Subdural empyema (SDE) is thought to be the most common complication of the sinus infection.[8,11] With timely intervention, mortality rates associated with SDE range from 10% to 20% but may be as high as 70% under certain circumstances.[8] SDE is the most common intracranial complication of sinusitis, and the most common cause of SDE is sinusitis.[11] SDE is a neurosurgical emergency that requires drainage to avert a rapidly evolving and fulminant clinical course. Inoculation of the subdural space most often occurs indirectly via thrombophlebitis of valveless emissary veins.[8] The triad of fever, sinusitis, and neurological deficits is suggestive of intracranial spread of infection. In SDE, the infection lies adjacent to the leptomeninges; therefore, patients with SDE may present with meningeal signs, hemiparesis, seizure, or mental status changes. CT with contrast is usually sufficiently sensitive to detect SDE, which is appreciated on the scan as a low-density extra-axial fluid collection in the setting of marked cortical swelling.[9] There may be increased vascular enhancement related to generalized increased permeability of the vasculature caused by the inflammatory response. Small interhemispheric subdural collection may be difficult to detect by CT scanning (Fig. 4.**66**). MRI is superior to CT scanning for detection of subdural collection and pyogenic lesions. SDE is a very serious sequela of sinusitis that is seen commonly in young men and is frequently associated with *Streptococcus anginosus*.[8] Changes of mental status in a patient with sinusitis should be treated aggressively, and the diagnosis of SDE should be pursued with MRI including contrast study. Small SDE may not be detected by CT scan including contrast enhancement.[8] MRI is the imaging study of choice for the diagnosis of SDE as well as other sinogenic intracranial complications.[8,11] Early recognition and treatment are essential to reduce any subsequent morbidity or mortality.[11] It is prudent to perform MRI of the sinuses, orbits, and brain whenever extensive or multiple complications of sinusitis are suspected.[13]

Acute Mycotic Sinonasal Diseases

Mucormycosis

Mycotic infection of the nasal and paranasal sinuses and craniofacial structures is a serious disease that requires prompt surgery and medical therapy to reduce its high morbidity rate.[1,10,12] This is usually seen in individuals such as AIDS patients or patients who have undergone therapy with immunosuppressive drugs and antimetabolites.[1,12,14,15] Rhino-orbito-cerebral mucormycosis is typically seen in debilitated patients, patients with diabetic ketoacidosis, and patients who are severely immunocompromised. Leukemia and dialysis have also been reported to predispose patients to this infection.[3] Recently, cases of rhino-orbito-cerebral mucormycosis have been described in patients with iron overload.[4,5] Rhinocerebral mycotic infection may be caused by the members of the family Mucoraceae (mucormycosis), which belongs to the class of Phycomycetes, and *Aspergillus* (aspergillosis).[10] The fungi responsible for mucormycosis are ubiquitous and normally saprophytic in humans: they rarely produce severe disease, except in those with predisposing conditions.[2,3,6,10] There are five major clinical subtypes of mucormycosis: rhino-orbito-cerebral, pulmonary, gastrointestinal, disseminated, and cutaneous forms.[10,14,15] The most common form is the rhino-orbito-cerebral form, which is associated with the highest mortality rate. The infection usually begins in the nose and spreads to the paranasal sinuses; it then extends into the orbit and cavernous sinuses.[1,2,10,14] Orbital involvement results in such orbital signs as ophthalmoplegia, proptosis, loss of vision, and orbital cellulitis. At times orbital cellulitis may be associated with rapid and sudden loss of vision due to occlusion of central retinal artery or vein.[3] When one encounters a patient with rapid development of ocular arterial disease, giant-cell arteritis (also called temporal arteritis) or rhino-orbito-cerebral mucormycosis and aspergillosis enter the differential diagnosis.[3] The orbital vessels are very resistant to compression by surrounding abnormal tissue. Malignant orbital tumors as well as pseudotumors are less likely to cause occlusion of orbital vessels.[3] The inflammatory process soon extends along the intracranial and infraorbital routes and into the infratemporal fossa (Figs. 4.**70**, 4.**71**). Black necrosis of a turbinate is a diagnostic clinical sign in mucormycosis, but it may not be present until late in the course of the disease.[10] The pathological landmark of mucormycosis is invasion of the walls of the vessels, particularly the arteries.[1,2] The organism presumably enters the nasal cavity and paranasal sinuses in inhaled dust particles.[10] It sporulates in tissues that have lost their internal resistance to the fungus. Hyphae are produced, and blood vessels are invaded.[10] The organism proliferates within the muscular walls of the arteries and to a lesser extent the veins and lymphatics, thus producing purulent arteritis, thrombophlebitis, and consequent infarction.[10] The nasal and sinus wall are invaded via these vessels, with subsequent invasion of the meninges, brain, cavernous sinuses, cranial nerves, and carotid arteries. Fungal arteritis may result in an aneurysm, thrombosis, or cerebral infarction.[10]

The radiographic findings of mucormycosis of the sinuses were first described by Green et al.,[14] who noted three signs: nodular mucosal thickening, absence of fluid levels, and spotty destruction of bony walls. None of these signs can be considered typical for the diagnosis of fungal sinusitis; however, a CT scan or MRI study may be very helpful and sometimes characteristic for the diagnosis of mucormycosis.[10,12] The main contribution of CT or MR scanning to the diagnosis of mucormycosis is its clear demonstration of the relationship between nasal, sinus, and orbital disease, a relationship so typical of mucormycosis that, in appropriate clinical setting, this diagnosis should be considered whenever combined nasal, sinus, and orbital diseases are encountered. Invasion of the medial orbit by the infecting organism results in phlegmon of the periorbital and, therefore, elevation of the medial rectus, which later becomes involved via direct invasion by hyphae (Fig. 4.**70**). Effacement and edema of the facial planes outside the involved sinus, bone destruction of the sinus walls, and, in particular, periosteal irregularity and cortical bony rarefaction indicative of periostitis and osteitis are common. In an appropriate clinical setting, CT and MR scans usually help to differentiate the overall picture from that of a sinonasal malignant process. Amphotericin B with aggressive debridement remains the mainstay of treatment of rhino-orbito-cerebral mucormycosis.[15]

Aspergillosis

Aspergillus is a ubiquitous mold found primarily in agricultural dust. It may produce rhinocerebral infection and orbital involvement similar to mucormycosis, although hematogenous spread from the lungs to the brain is more common.[10,14] This fungus also has a well-known propensity for invading blood vessels, including the internal carotid artery. The combination of orbital sinus involvement is not pathognomonic of rhinocerebral mucormycosis or aspergillosis; however, awareness of its possibility, particularly when any of the predisposing factors are present, would help in making an early diagnosis and treatment of this aggressive and fatal disease. In our practice, CT and MR scanning have been the most effective imaging modalities for making the correct diagnosis (Fig. 4.**71**). It is important to include the nasal cav-

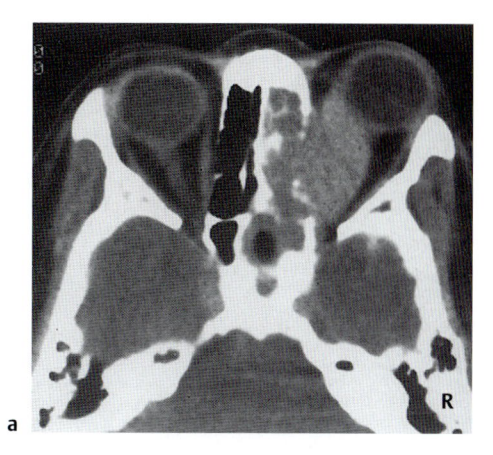

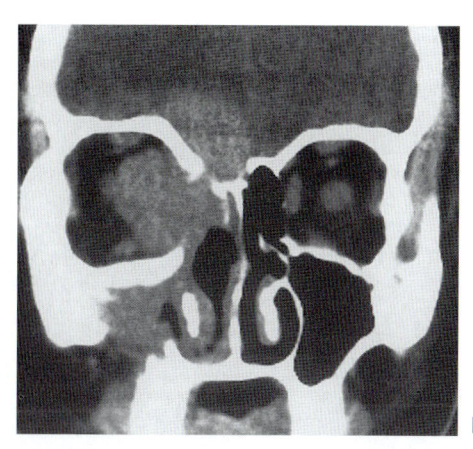

Fig. 4.70 Mucormycosis. **a** Axial and **b** coronal CT scans show soft-tissue changes in the right ethmoid with marked infiltration into the right orbit and intracranial space. Note the postoperative changes of the right maxillary and ethmoid sinuses. R = right side. Case courtesy of Dr. H. Sherif, Cairo, Egypt.

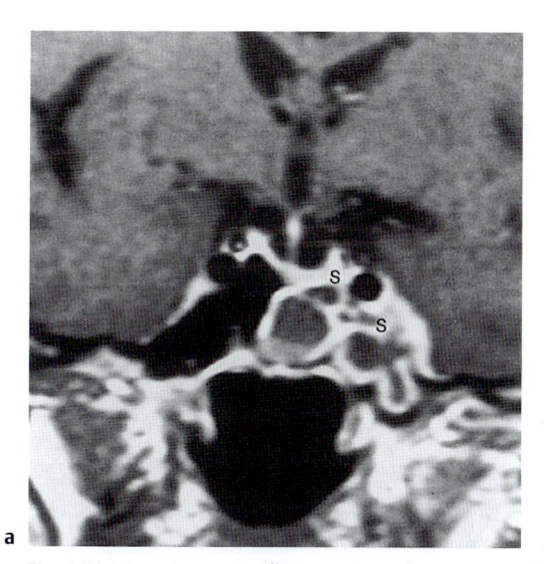

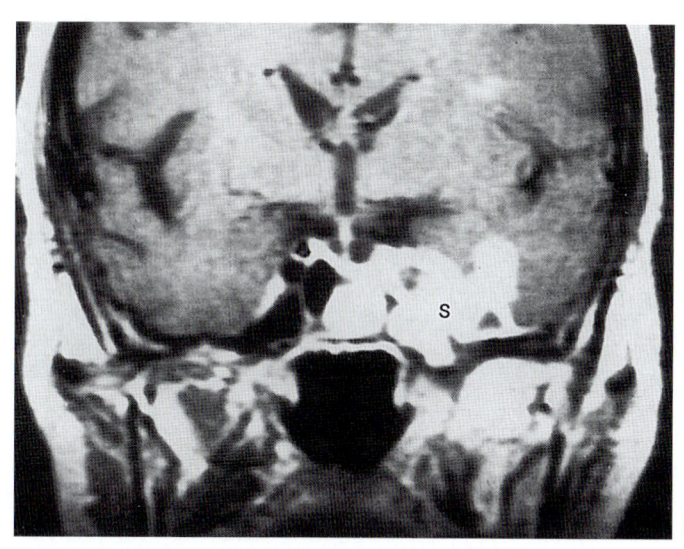

Fig. 4.71 Invasive aspergillosis. **a** Post-Gd-DTPA coronal T1W MR scan and **b** a follow-up study about five months later. Note the marked enhancement of the left sphenoid sinus (S) and invasion of the carotid artery, cavernous sinus, and temporal lobe on follow-up study **b**.

ity, the nasopharynx, and the base of the skull and the brain when performing CT or MRI in a patient with a potential or tentative diagnosis of mucormycosis or aspergillosis or other opportunistic infections of the sinonasal tracts.

Chronic Sinusitis

Chronic sinusitis is an extremely common disease that each year affects more than 31 million people in the United States alone.[16] It is defined as inflammation that endures for more than three months despite treatment.[16] Chronic sinusitis is often a complication of bacterial infection, a chronic allergic problem, or in patients with cystic fibrosis (CF).[1] The inflammatory-cell types and cytokine profiles of chronic sinusitis are well documented in the literature. Eosinophils, T lymphocytes, and cells expressing T_H2-like cytokines such as interleukin (IL)-4, IL-5, and IL-13 are found in higher numbers in mucosal specimens of atopic patients with chronic sinusitis than in controls.[17,18] CF is a heterogeneous recessive genetic disorder with pathological features that reflect mutations in the cystic fibrosis transmembrane conductance regulator (CFTR) gene.[17] The classic CF reflects two loss-of-function mutations in the CFTR gene and is characterized by chronic bacterial infection of the airways and sinuses, fat maldigestion due to pancreatic exocrine insufficiency, infertility in males due to obstructive azoospermia, and elevated concentrations of chloride in sweat.[17] Most patients with cystic fibrosis develop chronic sinusitis. The paranasal sinuses in patients with CF are often hypoplastic, with 90–100% of patients older than 8 months demonstrating radiological evidence of sinusitis.[18] Sinus disease in patients with CF presents different inflammatory-cell and cytokine profiles from that seen in other patients with chronic sinusitis.[17,18] There are a higher number of neutrophils, macrophages, and cells expressing messenger RNA for interferon δ and IL-δ in patients with CF.[18] Chronic rhinosinusitis is a clinical diagnosis, confirmed and staged with the CT scan of sinonasal cavities.[19,20] Often, the CT scan is used to plan the extent of surgery for disease that fails to respond to medical management. Chronic inflammatory disease is often associated with mucosal thickening and sclerosis of the bone, particularly within the sinuses (Figs. 4.72, 4.73). Acute infections cause demineralization (rarefaction) of the wall of the sinus and subsequently, when the process becomes chronic, results in reactive sclerosis of the sinus walls (Fig. 4.73). These changes in the wall of the sinus often indicate the presence of osteitis, which requires a prolonged course of antibiotics.[1]

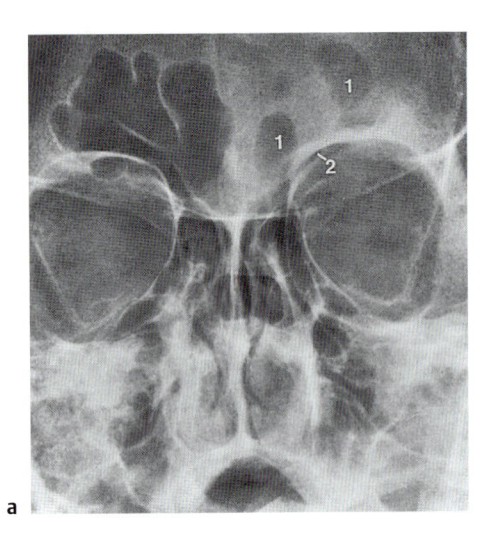

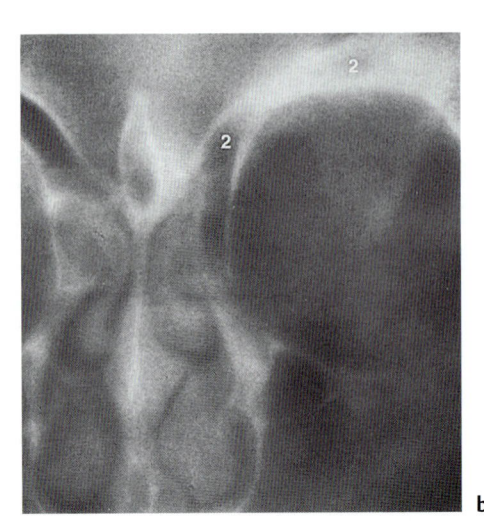

Fig. 4.72 Chronic sinusitis. **a** Caldwell projection; **b** AP tomogram. The partial obliteration of the left front sinus (1) is due to a previous episode of sinusitis 15 years previously. Recent symptoms are due to an infection of the left supraorbital cell (2), which is also chronic, as demonstrated by some associated reactive sclerosis. From Reference 20a.

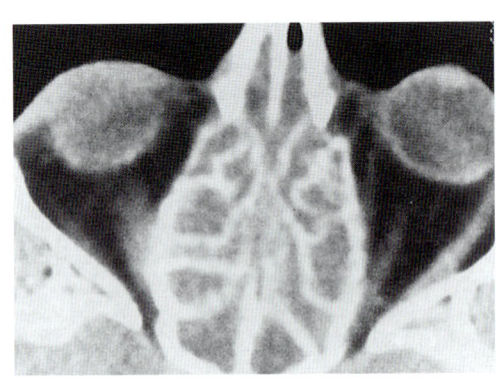

Fig. 4.73 Chronic ethmoid sinusitis. Note opacified ethmoid air cells and associated sclerosis of the trabeculae. The sphenoid sinuses are small, as well as opacified.

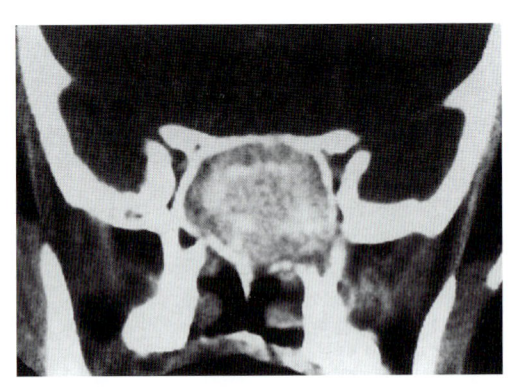

Fig. 4.74 Chronic noninvasive aspergillosis. Coronal unenhanced CT scan shows opacification and slight expansion of the sphenoid sinuses. Note multiple areas of marked increased density related to calcifications and inspissated mucus.

Chronic Fungal (Mycotic) Sinusitis and Chronic Allergic Fungal Rhinosinusitis (AFS)

Fungal sinus disease is often diagnosed because an apparently routine infection fails to respond to a commonly used antibiotic regimen.[10] In immunocompetent patients, fungal sinus disease may first be recognized as a slowly progressing extramucosal fungus ball, a slowly noninvasive disease.[21] In immunocompromised patients, however, fungal mucosal sinus diseases of the sinonasal cavities have more typically been attributed to fulminant mucormycosis and aspergillosis. The benign extramucosal fungal disease has been attributed to *Aspergillus* species.[21] However, appraisal of the aggressiveness of the fungal disease on the basis of the organism alone may not always be valid.[22-27] Extramucosal fungal sinusitis develops as a saprophytic growth in retained secretions in a sinus cavity. This disorder is usually benign and is rarely associated with mucosal invasion (Figs. 4.74, 4.75). The treatment of extramucosal fungal disease entails removing the fungal ball and restoring mucociliary drainage and sinus ventilation (Fig. 4.75). A biopsy should be obtained from the mucosa to rule out mucosal invasion.[28] Saferstein[29] was the first to report the combination of nasal polyposis, crust formation, and sinus cultures yielding *Aspergillus*. Subsequently, other reports supported the existence of this observation as a distinct clinical entity.[30-32] The constellation of allergic mucin, sinonasal polyposis, and the presence of extramucosal fungi has been called allergic fungal rhinosinusitis (AFS) for its similarity to "allergic bronchopulmonary aspergillosis[29, 33] (Fig. 4.76). Although the disease has been the subject of numerous reports and studies, its exact pathophysiology, criteria for diagnosis, and ultimate treatment regimens remain controversial.[33] Most investigators agree that surgical marsupialization of the affected sinuses and removal of allergic mucin is the initial step, but surgery alone cannot be considered to be curative.[33] Even after adequate surgical treatment, fungal hyphae and spores remain in the involved sinuses.[34] Systemic steroids help to reduce the rate of recurrence. However, once the steroids are reduced or discontinued, disease will return.[34] Some investigators recommend the use of topical antifungal therapy as well as postoperative immunotherapy with relevant fungal antigens.

Allergic fungal sinusitis, by definition, demonstrates central areas of allergic mucin composed clinically of a pasty, brownish green, dense material and histologically comprising sheets of degenerated inflammatory cells with fungal fragments (usually aspergillus) visible under fungal stain and with Charcot–Leyden crystals visible under hematoxylin–eosin stain.[35] The highly proteinaceous central mucin creates areas of high attenuation on CT images (Fig. 4.76) and corresponding low signal on both T1-weighted and T2-weighted MR images.[35] Allergic fungal rhinosinusitis (AFS) is thought to be an allergic reaction to aerosolized, environmental fungi, usually of the dematiaceous species. In an immunocompetent host, AFS is a noninvasive form characterized by the presence of allergic mucin, which is composed of eosinophils and Charcot–Leyden crystals alternating with layers of mucus, creating a lamellar, inspissated pattern.[33] Fungal hyphae are scattered throughout the allergic mucin but there is no

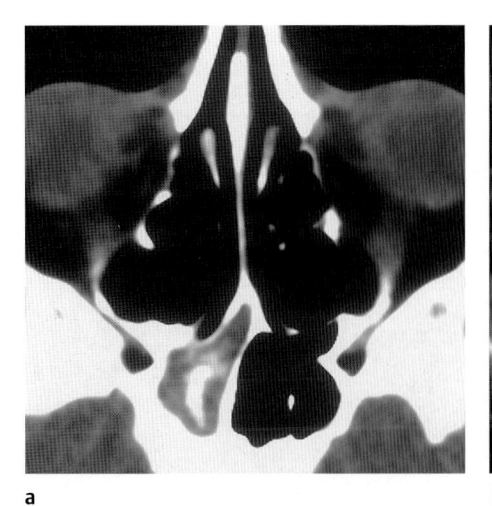

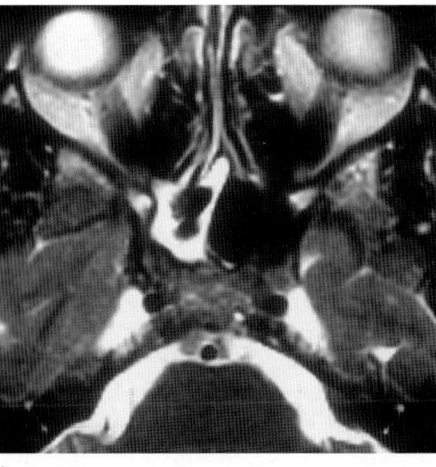

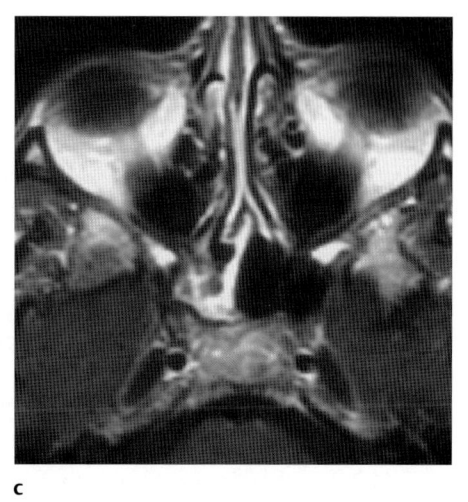

Fig. 4.**75** Chronic noninvasive sphenoid sinus aspergillosis. **a** Axial unenhanced CT scan showing an opacified right sphenoid sinus, associated with a central calcification. **b** T2W and **c** enhanced T1W MR scans, showing inflammatory changes of the right sphenoid sinus. Note hypointense central area, related to calcification seen on CT scan.

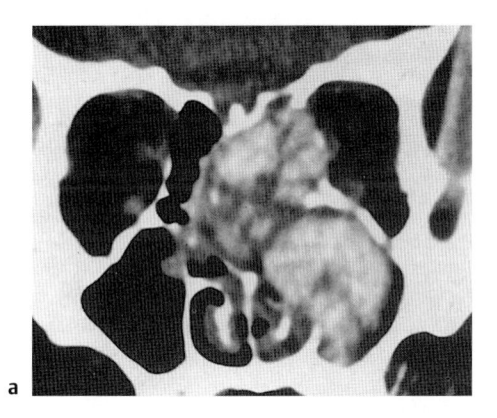

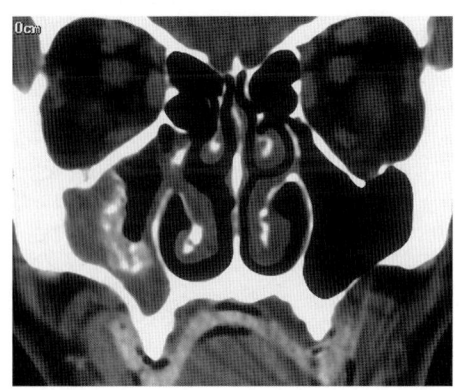

Fig. 4.**76** **a** Chronic allergic sinusitis. Coronal CT scan shows masses of increased density within the maxillary, nasal, and ethmoid sinuses on the left side. At surgery, polyps and marked inspissated retained secretions were removed. **b** Chronic noninvasive aspergillosis. Coronal CT scan, showing an opacified right maxillary sinus, associated with a central calcification ("fungus ball").

evidence of invasion into the host tissue.[34] A fungal ball is also a noninvasive form of the disease in which fungus forms a mass of intertwined hyphae without host invasion.[34] Presentation in pediatric patients with AFS is different from that in adults, with children having obvious abnormalities of their facial skeleton (facial dysmorphism, proptosis), unilateral sinus disease, and asymmetrical disease more often.[36] The types of fungus cultured in the sinus cavities were similar in both groups with the exception of *Aspergillus*, which was seen only in adults.[36]

Imaging Diagnosis of Chronic Mycotic Sinusitis

The imaging manifestations of mycotic sinusitis may be nonspecific or highly suggestive of the presence of fungal infection. The sinuses most often involved are the maxillary, ethmoid, and sphenoid sinuses. The findings on plain radiography may vary from those of nonspecific mucosal disease without any bone involvement to an opacified sinus with a polypoid mass with a central or peripheral hyperdense (calcified) mass (fungal ball, mycetoma).[10, 21, 28] The fungal balls or mycetomas may appear either as a homogeneous soft-tissue mass or in some cases as a well-defined density similar to that seen with calcium or bone (Fig. 4.**76**).[21] The increased density within the polypoid sinus mass in cases of chronic mycotic sinusitis is believed to be due to calcium phosphate and calcium sulfate deposits within necrotic areas of the mycelium.[28, 37] CT is superior to plain radiography and complex motion tomography in detecting fungal concretions. Zinreich et al.[21] reported 25 patients with fungal sinusitis. Of these, 22 had foci of increased attenuation on CT scans. Areas of focal hyperattenuation varied in size. The smallest area measured 4 mm in diameter; the largest almost formed a cast of the maxillary sinus. It has been suggested that the focal increased densities seen within the sinuses represent calcium phosphate and calcium sulfate deposits within necrotic areas of the mycelium.[28, 37] The presence of areas of increased densities in the paranasal sinuses correlated well with fungal sinusitis in the study of Zinreich et al.[21] However, since pus, desiccated mucosal secretions, dystrophic calcifications (concretions, antrolith), and acute hemorrhage are also dense on CT scans, CT findings alone are not conclusive within a partially or totally opacified sinus. The finding should therefore serve as a high index of suspicion for chronic noninvasive or chronic indolent fungal sinusitis, especially aspergillosis. The increased central density, with or without calcifications, reflects the extra mucosal saprophytic growth of fungi in retained desiccated secretions. The presence of highly proteinaceous inspissated mucus creates areas, often with lamellar pattern of very high attenuation values on CT images.[38] The presence of diffuse increased attenuation within the paranasal sinuses and nasal cavity should be considered as chronic allergic hypersensitivity fungal sinusitis, usually due to aspergillosis (chronic noninvasive aspergillosis) (Fig. 4.**76**) or chronic hyperplastic sinusitis and polyposis associated with desiccated retained mucosal secretions (concretions) (Fig. 4.**77**). As these materials accumulate within the sinus, bony demineralization of the sinus walls ensues secondary to the release of inflammatory mediators and pressure, resulting in expansion of the sinus and mucocele formation.[38] The MRI characteristics of

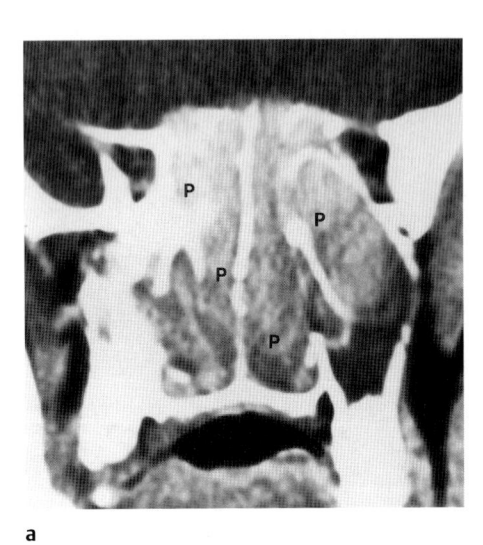

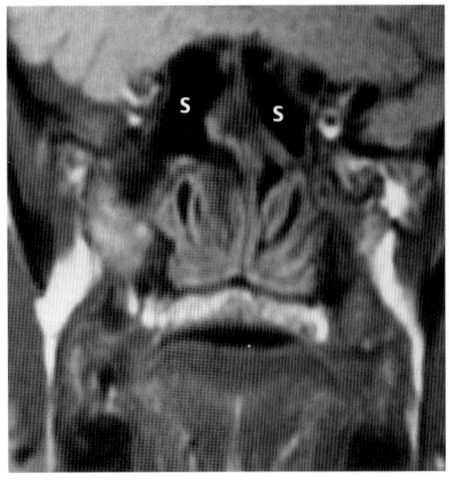

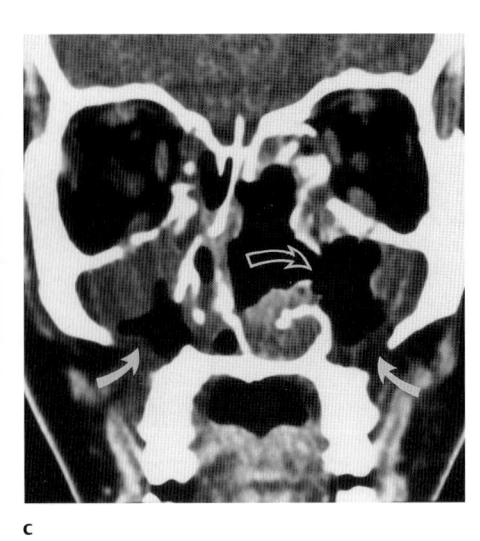

Fig. 4.77 Chronic hyperplastic sinusitis and polyposis, associated with desciccated retained mucosal secretion (concretion). **a** Coronal CT, **b** PW coronal MR, and **c** postsurgical CT scan images, showing sinonasal polyps (P). Note postsurgical changes of bilateral Caldwell–Luc procedures (solid arrows) and middle meatal antrostomy (hollow arrow) in **c**. Note that the concretions in the sphenoid sinuses (S) on MRI cannot be appreciated. Note characteristic lamellar pattern of inspissated mucus in preoperative CT (**a**).

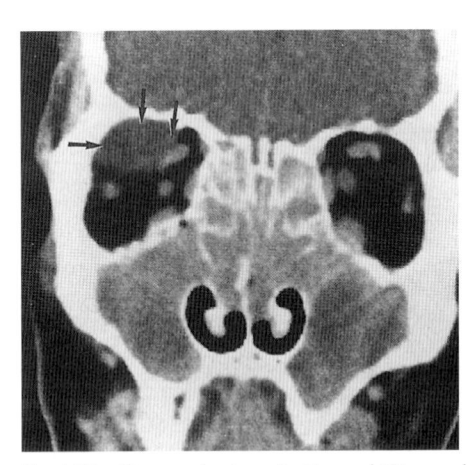

Fig. 4.78 Sinonasal polyposis. Coronal CT scan shows soft-tissue masses within the maxillary sinuses, nasal cavities, and ethmoid sinuses in this patient with a long-standing history of nasal polyposis. The soft tissue in the right superior orbit (arrows) is due to a frontal sinus polyp eroding into the orbit.

fungal sinusitis depend on the stage of the disease. In acute invasive fungal sinusitis, regardless of the offending organism, there will be significant inflammatory edema and cellular infiltrate, resulting in marked hyperintensity in PW and particularly in T2-weighted MR images. The process appears relatively hypointense in T1-weighted MR images. In chronic noninvasive or indolent fungal sinusitis, the presence of concretions and desiccated mucosal secretions results in low signal on T1-weighted and marked hypointensity on T2-weighted MR images (Fig. 4.77). The reactive granulations or associated subacute or acute sinusitis will demonstrate hyperintense signal on T2-weighted MR images. There will be enhancement only of mucosal rim on enhanced MR images. All of the fungal concretions in the study of Zinreich et al.[17] stained positively for calcium. Decreased signal intensity on T1-weighted and very decreased signal intensity on T2-weighted MR images were thought by Zinreich et al.[21] to be due to calcium as well as iron and manganese found in fungal sinusitis. Iron, magnesium, and manganese are known to be essential in fungal amino acid metabolism.[39] Zinreich et al.[21] examined specimens of fungal concretions from two patients, as well as specimens obtained from four patients with bacterial sinusitis, for the presence of iron, magnesium, and manganese. They found that iron and manganese, both paramagnetic elements, were present in two patients with proven aspergillus sinusitis in larger quantities than in four patients with bacterial sinusitis. They concluded that increased concentrations of iron and manganese, as well as the presence of calcium in the fungal concretions, may explain the hypointensity on T2-weighted MR images. It is now known, however, that the presence of inspissated mucosal secretions within the sinus cavity or along the crevices of polyps result in a markedly hypointense T2-weighted signal.[12,38] In fact, it seems that in practice the majority of sinus cases with hypointense T2-weighted signal are related to desiccated retained mucosal secretion without the presence of fungal organisms. Chronic noninvasive aspergillus sinusitis and chronic allergic hypersensitivity aspergillus sinusitis may have the same MR appearance as chronic hyperplastic sinonasal polyposis with inspissation of the retained mucosal secretion.

Allergy

Allergic reactions of the upper respiratory tract may result in characteristic change in the nasal cavity and paranasal sinuses. These vary from mild thickening of the mucosa to complete opacification of the sinus. Hypertrophy of the nasal turbinates is common, occasionally accompanied by the presence of nasal polyps. Approximately 10% of the population has this manifestation of allergy, which is most commonly seasonal, due to a ragweed allergy, although spores from molds are also important antigens.[1] Extensive, bilateral opacification of the sinuses and diffuse polyposis (Fig. 4.78) are far more common in allergic disease than in bacterial sinusitis (Fig. 4.79). Pregnancy rhinitis is a well-recognized clinical entity that is believed to be due to elevated estrogen level. Pregnancy rhinitis is defined as nasal congestion present in the last six or more weeks of pregnancy without other signs of respiratory tract infection and with no known allergic cause, disappearing completely within two weeks after delivery.[40]

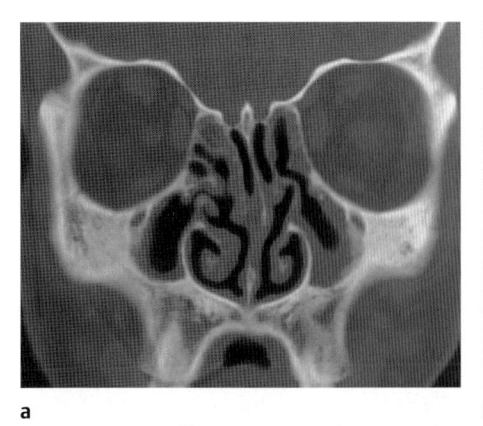

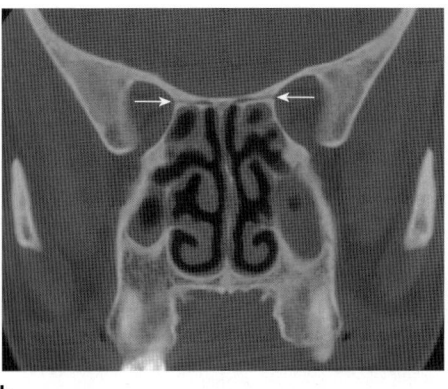

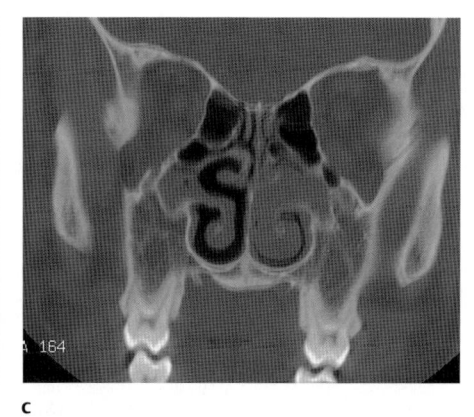

Fig. 4.79 Cystic fibrosis. **a** Coronal CT scan showing hypoplastic paranasal sinuses, along with mucosal thickening. Note posterior ethmoid canals (arrows) in **b**. **c** Kartagener syndrome. Coronal CT scan in a patient with Kartagener syndrome shows hypoplastic and opacified maxillary sinuses.

Vasomotor Rhinitis (Rhinitis Medicamentosa)

The pronounced nasal vasoconstriction effect of topical nasal decongestants may at times be followed by rebound vasodilatation and nasal stuffiness.[41] This is especially likely after long-term use of these nasal decongestants. The stuffiness is relieved by additional doses of the vasocontrictor. Eventually the patient becomes increasingly dependent on the topical decongestant and a vicious circle is established with long-term daily overdose.[41] This phenomenon is termed rhinitis medicamentosa.

Chronic Sinonasal Inflammation Secondary to Nasal Cocaine Abuse

Intranasal cocaine abuse can cause a variety of otolaryngological complications from a combination of its potent vasoconstriction and direct irritation of the nasal mucosa.[42] Repeated intranasal "snorting" or "sniffing" of cocaine can lead to ischemia and necrosis of the nasal septum, resulting in septal perforation, synechia, and chronic sinusitis.[42] Other complications of cocaine abuse include osteolytic sinusitis, nasolacrimal duct obstruction, hypertensive crisis, vasculitis, ventricular arrhythmia, cardiopulmonary arrest, clonic-tonic seizures, and hyperpyrexia.[42]

Silent Sinus Syndrome

Common symptoms associated with chronic sinusitis include congestion, rhinorrhea, pressure, or facial pain. There are a few patients who present with orbital structural changes such as enophthalmos and at times diplopia on upward gaze.[43–45] Silent sinus syndrome has been described as spontaneous enophthalmos with chronic maxillary sinusitis, associated with maxillary sinus atelectasis. Nasal endoscopy will commonly show retraction of the uncinate shelf ("atelectatic uncinate") and obliteration of the infundibulum (Fig. 4.**80**).[44] There are three theories regarding the pathogenesis of silent sinus syndrome. The most popular theory involves obstruction of the outflow tract of the maxillary sinus, resulting in hypoventilation of the sinus, negative antral pressure, and subsequent atelectasis of sinus walls. The second theory suggests that inflammatory disease induces erosion of the floor of the orbit, and the third describes sinusitis in a hypoplastic sinus.[43] Radiological findings include obstruction of the ostiomeatal complex at the maxillary component of the infundibulum, atelectatic uncinate process, contracted maxillary antrum, opacification of the maxillary sinus, inferior bowing of the antral roof (floor of orbit), lateral bowing of the medial wall, and anterior bowing of the posterior maxillary sinus. The maxillary walls may be thickened (chronic osteitis), thinned, or partially dehiscent (Fig. 4.**80**).

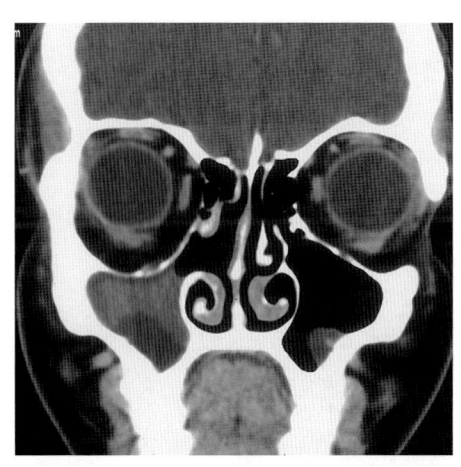

Fig. 4.**80** Silent sinus disease. Coronal CT scan in a 31-year-old woman with no prior history of surgery or trauma, showing opacified right maxillary sinus and nonvisualization of the right uncinate process ("atelectatic uncinate").

Rhinolith

Foreign bodies within the nose and paranasal sinuses tend to become encrusted and calcified when retained for a long period and are thus known as rhinoliths and sinoliths, respectively. These calcareous bodies may be endogenous or exogenous in origin. Teeth, sequestra, and dried blood clots are considered endogenous.[46] Exogenous material includes fruit seeds, beads, buttons, pieces of dirt and pebbles, and the remains of gauze tampons.[46] A nidus of purulent exudate, deposits of blood products, cellular debris, and mineral salts such as calcium phosphate and carbonate may form a rough surface. Rhinoliths may produce nasal obstruction, a malodorous nasal discharge with local pain, and epistaxis. They may even project into the maxillary sinus by pressure necrosis of the nasoantral wall. Foreign bodies within the nose may be self-induced or due to dental root canal fillings, bullets, shrapnel, or buckshot. A calcified nasal mass (Fig. 4.**81**) on CT scan is characteristic of a rhinolith. The calcification appears as a cast surrounded by soft tissue related to inflammatory reaction associated with rhinolithiasis. A sinolith appears similar to a rhinolith, and is most commonly seen in the maxillary antrum.

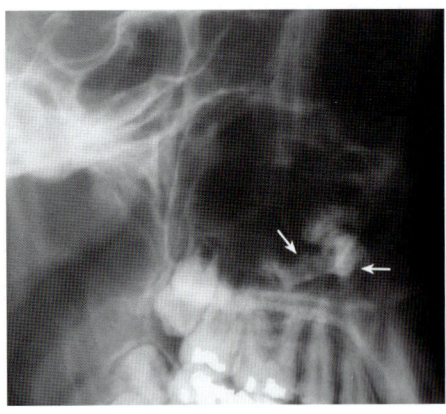

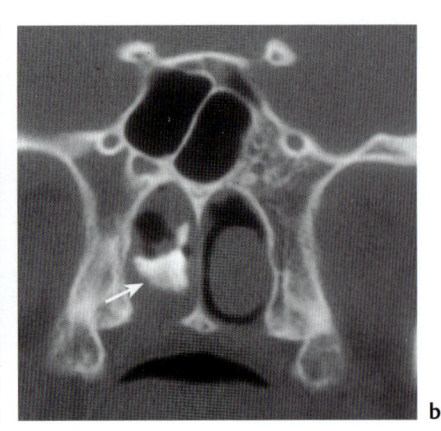

Fig. 4.81 Rhinolith. **a** Lateral projection of the head and face shows a calcified mass (arrows) in the nasal cavity. **b** CT scan shows a calcified mass (arrow) in the posterior right nasal cavity, compatible with a rhinolith.

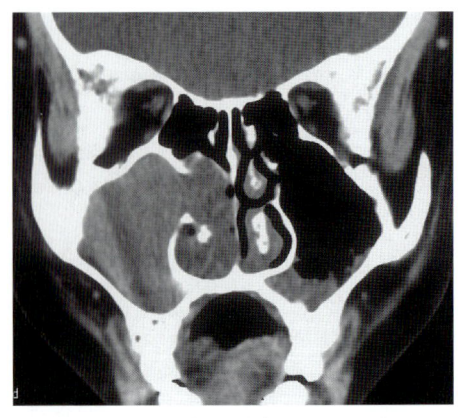

Fig. 4.82 Sinonasal sarcoidosis. Coronal CT scan showing soft-tissue mass in the right maxillary sinus and right nasal cavity compatible with sarcoidosis. This cannot be differentiated from an antronasal polyp or an inverted papilloma.

Table 4.5 Differential diagnosis of granulomatous lesions of sinonasal cavities

- Fungal infections
- Sarcoidosis
- Tuberculosis
- Leprosy
- Syphilis
- Rhinoscleroma
- Allergic granuloma and hypersensitivity angiitis
- Polyarteritis nodosa and systemic lupus
- Granuloma gravidarum
- Angiitis (Churg–Straus syndrome)
- Foreign-body granuloma (lipogranuloma, paraffinoma)
- Cholesterol granuloma
- Pyogenic granuloma
- Idiopathic granuloma (destructive or nondestructive)
- Nonspecific granuloma in nasal polyps
- Wegener granuloma
- Lymphomatoid granuloma (T-cell lymphoma, formerly referred to as pseudotumor or midline reticulosis)

Atrophic Rhinitis

The presence of a dry nasal mucosa may indicate a variety of problems. Primary atrophic rhinitis or ozena affects females in their early teens or early adulthood and usually is associated with crusting and a foul odor. Examination shows widening of the nasal cavities and a thin mucosa. Secondary atrophic rhinitis may follow repeated episodes of infection, multiple intranasal surgical procedures, or cocaine abuse.[1] Addiction to decongestant nose drops may also dry the nasal mucosa. An end stage of prolonged infection may result in atrophic rhinitis, an uncommon condition in the United States.[1] Progressive chronic inflammatory changes, atrophy, and fibrosis are seen with crusting and atrophic changes of the respiratory endothelium with islands of squamous metaplasia. These patients often have foul mucous discharge, not appreciated by the patient, who has lost the sense of smell.

Granulomatous Diseases of Sinonasal Cavities

There are many causes for granulomatous processes of the upper respiratory tract.[47–63] Sinonasal granulomas have an extensive differential diagnosis (Table 4.5). The list includes sarcoidosis (Fig. 4.82), fungal infections, tuberculosis, syphilis, leprosy, rhinoscleroma, Wegener granulomatosis, allergic granulomatosis and angiitis (Churg–Strauss syndrome), lymphoplasmatoid granuloma (pseudotumor), cholesterol granulomas, foreign body granulomas such as lipogranuloma due to oil drops, injected corticosteroids, and paraffin, and unknown causes. The finding of isolated granulomas in nasal tissue is nonspecific, having been reported to occur in 1% of nasal polyps.[48] In one study, granulomas in nasal polyps were found to be idiopathic in 6 of 19 cases.[48] In the past, the term midline granuloma referred to a group of disorders that produce destructive lesions of the midline of the head and face. A review of the literature reveals a lack of general consensus on the individual disorders.[47, 63] The entities often referred to as "midline granuloma" or lethal midline granulomas, polymorphic reticulosis, lymphomatoid granulomatosis, and others,[47, 63] are no longer described by these terms. Advances in immunocytochemical phenotyping and molecular genetics have revealed that the majority of the sinonasal destructive lesions referred to as midline destructive lesions can be classified into two distinct pathological groups: Wegener granulomatosis and non-Hodgkin T-cell lymphoma. Terms used to refer to such lesions include lethal midline granuloma, nonhealing midline granuloma (Stewart syndrome), idiopathic midline destructive disease, polymorphic reticulosis, lymphomatoid granuloma, pseudolymphoma, and others. It has now clearly been established that polymorphic reticulosis is a non-Hodgkin lymphoma[64] and midline destructive granuloma is linked to T-cell lymphoma (Fig. 4.83).[47] Sinonasal lymphoma is one of the rarest forms of extranodal lymphoma in western populations.[47] This contrasts with the prevalence in some Asian countries, in which sinonasal lymphoma is the second most common type of extranodal lymphoma.[47] In this geographic group, over 90% of cases have T-cell markers, and Epstein–Barr virus has been consistently demonstrated in the cell genome.[47] Wegener granulomatosis and lymphoma are not the main causes of destructive lesions of the sinonasal tract. There are other more common etiologies that should be excluded (Table 4.6).

Rhinoscleroma

Rhinoscleroma (hard nose) is a tumorlike expansion of the nose and upper lip, seen more commonly in Africa (especially Egypt), Central and South America, and Eastern Europe. It is caused by *Klebsiella rhinoscleromatis*, a Gram-negative encapsulated bac-

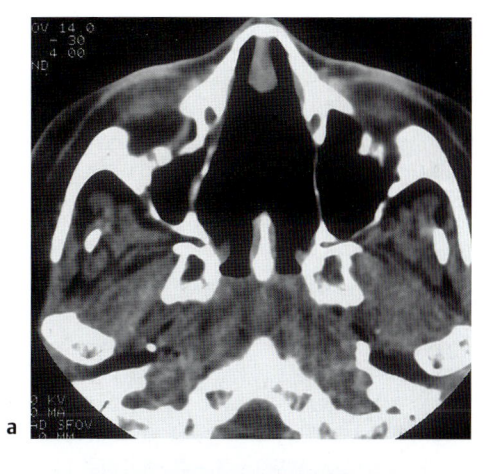

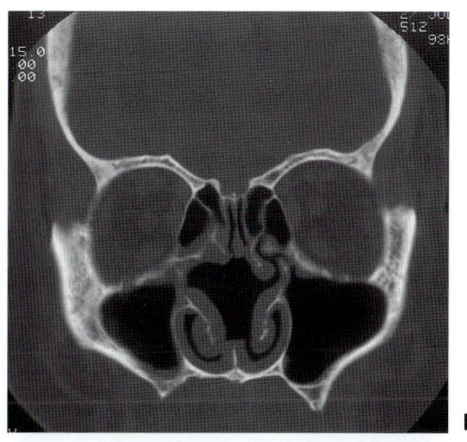

Fig. 4.83 a, b Wegener granulomatosis.
a Axial and **b** coronal CT scans, showing large perforation of nasal septum, along with mucosal thickening of nasal cavities. **c, d** "Idiopathic midline granuloma." **c** Coronal CT and **d** PW MR scans in another patient, showing destructive tumor (T) in the sinonasal cavities. This entity, which is most likely a T-cell lymphoma, can be mistaken for Wegener granulomatosis.

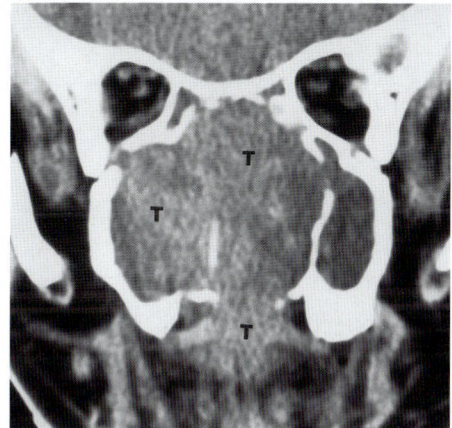

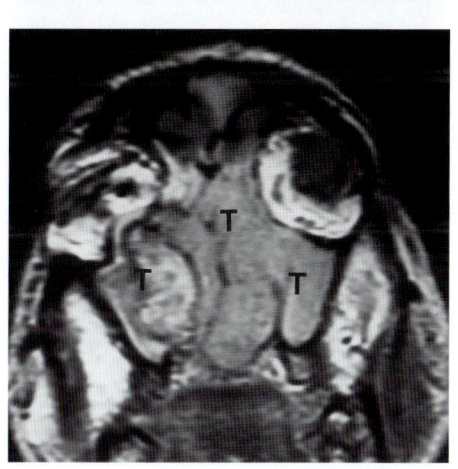

terium of low virulence.[1] The disease process usually involves the nasal cavity and the nasopharynx, but it can also involve the larynx, trachea, bronchi, middle ear, and orbit.[52]

Rhinosporidiosis

Rhinosporidiosis is an infective condition caused by the organism *Rhinosporidium seeberi*.[53] The organism is classified as fungus. It is endemic in South India and Sri Lanka and commonly affects nasal and conjunctival mucosa.[53] The lesion may be very large and simulate a pedunculated nasal polyp or papilloma. A diagnostic feature of the masses is the presence of whitish spots on the masses, which are actually the rhinosporidium itself.[53] The mass is painless and bleeds easily. Differential diagnosis includes coccidioidomycosis and other fungal infections.

Myospherulosis

Myospherulosis is an innocuous, iatrogenically induced pseudomycotic disease, resulting from the interaction of red blood cells and petrolatum-based ointment.[54] Histological examination reveals pseudocysts embedded within fibrotic tissue, with an associated chronic inflammatory infiltrate composed of lymphocytes, histiocytes, giant cells, and plasma cells. Pseudocysts contain round, saclike structures called "parent bodies"; these parent bodies in turn contain numerous spherules or endobodies. The origin of the myospherules are from red blood cells that react with petrolatum or lanolin found in ointment used in "packing."

Table 4.6 Differential diagnosis of destructive lesions of the sinonasal cavities

1 **Trauma**
   - Accidental
   - Iatrogenic (postsurgical)
   - Self-induced (rhinosillexomania)
2 **Infection**
   - Bacterial: Mycobacteria, syphilis, rhinoscleroma, leprosy, actinomycosis
   - Fungal: Aspergillosis, mucormycosis, other mycotic rhinosinusitis
3 **Toxic**
   - Cocaine abuse
   - Chromium salts
4 **Inflammatory**
   - Sarcoidosis
   - Foreign-body granuloma
   - Wegener granulomatosis
   - Polyarteritis nodosa
   - Systemic lupus
   - Allergic hypersensitivity angiitis
5 **Neoplastic**
   - Basal cell carcinoma
   - Squamous cell carcinoma
   - Adenocarcinoma
   - Hemangiopericytoma
   - Esthesioneuroblastoma
   - Lymphoma
   - Melanoma
   - Rhabdomyosarcoma, fibrosarcoma
   - Kaposi sarcoma
   - Posttransplantation lymphoproliferative disease (PTLD)
   - Osteochondrogenic sarcoma
   - Metastasis

Modified from Borges A, Fink J, Villablanca P, et al. Midline destructive lesions of the sinonasal tract: simplified terminology based on histopathologic criteria. AJNR 2000; 21: 331–336.

Nasal Granuloma Gravidarum

Granuloma gravidarum (GG) is an uncommon benign vascular proliferation that usually occurs in the mucous membranes of the mouth and gums, and rarely in the nose, during pregnancy.[49] This is a lobular capillary hemangioma that occurs in the gravid state and regresses after parturition. The term granuloma is a misnomer because this lesion is not granulomatous. Physical examination reveals a reddish brown mass that bleeds readily on probing and whose surface is usually ulcerated.[49] It may arise from nasal septum, turbinates, or floor of the nose and may be sessile or pedunculated. Differential diagnoses include antrochoanal polyp, inverted papilloma, schwannoma, angiomatous polyp, mucosal melanoma, lymphoma, Kaposi sarcoma and metastasis. The etiology of GG remains unknown. Its occurrence during pregnancy and its tendency to regress spontaneously after delivery indicate a clear dependency on the hormonal stimulation of pregnancy.

Sarcoidosis

Sarcoidosis of the paranasal sinuses usually presents with nasal obstruction and chronic sinusitis.[50] The reported incidence of nasal sarcoidosis varies from 1–2% to 18% of all cases of sarcoidosis. At the Mayo Clinic, 2319 cases of sarcoidosis were seen between 1950 and 1981.[51] Nine percent had head and neck involvement. The nose was involved in 13 percent of the cases. Nasal sarcoidosis commonly affects the mucosa of the septum and turbinates, in particular, the inferior turbinates.[1]

Imaging Findings

The CT and MRI findings of sinonasal sarcoidosis are nonspecific. Mucosal thickening may be present, which usually indicates the presence of chronic mucosal disease (Fig. 4.**82**). The sinusitis in sarcoidosis is due either to nasal disease interfering with proper sinus drainage, resulting in infection, or to invasion by the sarcoidosis. At times imaging studies may show a nasal mass with bony destruction of sinonasal structures. Nasal involvement in sarcoidosis may be external. Nasal cutaneous sarcoidosis is called lupus pernio[50] and can be seen as soft-tissue thickening of the nose and face, including eyelids, on CT and MR images.

Wegener Granulomatosis

Wegener granulomatosis (WG) is a severe, noninfectious systemic necrotizing granulomatous vasculitis that characteristically involves the respiratory tract and the kidneys (focal necrotizing glomerulonephritis).[54,55] The etiology of WG is unknown. It is somehow related to an autoimmune reaction to an unknown allergen that eventually affects a number of organs. The sedimentation rate is elevated and an antineutrophil cytoplasmic autoantibodies (ANCA) assay is usually positive. Because WG may mimic other inflammatory and neoplastic conditions, biopsies of affected tissues in conjunction with measurement of serum ANCA are used to make the diagnosis. ANCA were first reported by Davies and co-workers in 1982 in the serum of patients with necrotizing glomerulonephritis and systemic vasculitis.[56] These antibodies to the components of an autoantigen were subsequently shown to be present in patients with various forms of systemic vasculitis, including Wegener granulomatosis, polyarteritis nodosa, and idiopathic crescentic glomerulonephritis.[57] With ANCA-associated disease there may be vasculitis or granulomatous lesions in the lungs, kidneys, and elsewhere.[58–60] Wegener granulomatosis typically produces slowly progressive ulceration and destruction of the nose and paranasal sinuses. Septal perforation and friable nasal mucosa and thick crusts are seen on clinical examination. Neurological involvement has been reported in up to 54% of cases. Reversible meningeal and cerebral involvement has been reported in the absence of nasal or renal disease and with a negative ANCA test.[61,62] Aggressive therapeutic regimens using cyclophosphamide, azathioprine, and corticosteroids have significantly improved survival of patients with WG.

Imaging Findings

The radiographic and MRI findings of early Wegener granulomatosis may be nonspecific, revealing mucosal thickening suggestive of inflammatory sinonasal disease. Extensive soft-tissue tumor and associated bone destruction (Figs. 4.**83a, b**) are the hallmarks of the late stage of the disease but are still not characteristic of the disease (Fig. 4.**83**), eliciting a long differential diagnosis (Table 4.**6**) (Fig. 4.**83**). The lesion may be well-defined, simulating nasal polyp, or diffuse and nodular in appearance with or without bone destruction. The distinction from sinonasal lymphoma and other granulomatous and neoplastic lesions cannot be confidently made on the basis of CT and MRI characteristics.

Allergic Granulomatosis and Angiitis (Churg–Strauss Syndrome)

Allergic granulomatosis and angiitis were initially described by Churg and Strauss as a triad of bronchial asthma, eosinophilia, and vasculitis.[65] At the Mayo Clinic, 32 cases were seen between 1950 and 1978; patients' ages ranged from 11 to 70 years.[1] Nasal involvement is quite common and nasal manifestations are similar to Wegener granulomatosis and polymorphic reticulosis,[1] namely, obstruction, pain, purulent or bloody discharge, anosmia, polyps, crusting, and granular and friable mucosa. The systemic manifestations are prominent and may include fever, night sweats, malaise, weight loss, myalgia, anemia, leukocytosis, and a high sedimentation rate.[1]

Imaging Findings

CT and MRI may show nonspecific mucosal thickening of the nasal cavities associated with changes indicative of sinusitis. There may be pansinusitis with nodular and polypoid thickening of the mucosa.

Foreign-Body Granuloma (Paraffinoma and Cholesterol Granuloma)

Paraffin is a mineral oil that consists of straight-chain saturated hydocarbons.[66] The injection of paraffin into tissues may cause a paraffinoma, characterized as a granulomatous foreign-body reaction. Paraffinoma has been reported as a complication of nasal packing and sinus packing with petrolatum-impregnated gauze.[66] Cholesterol granuloma (CG) is another chronic foreign-body granuloma related to reaction to hemorrhage. In the head and neck region, it most frequently occurs in the petrous apex, middle ear, and mastoid, but it has been reported in the orbit, frontal bone, and paranasal sinuses.[67] Irrespective of its location, the histology of CG is the same. Typical needle-shaped cholesterol clefts are surrounded by foreign body giant cells. The tissue also contains histiocytes with foamy cytoplasm, hemosiderin, and chronic inflammatory reaction.[67] Cholesterol granulomas are characterized by high signal intensity on both T1-weighted and T2-weighted MR images. Some CG may show hypointense areas on T2-weighted MR images.

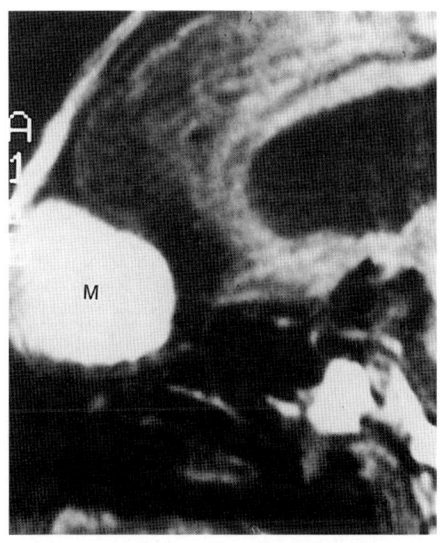

Fig. 4.84 Frontal sinus mucocele. Sagittal unenhanced T1W MR scan shows a hyperintense expansile mass (M) compatible with a mucocele.

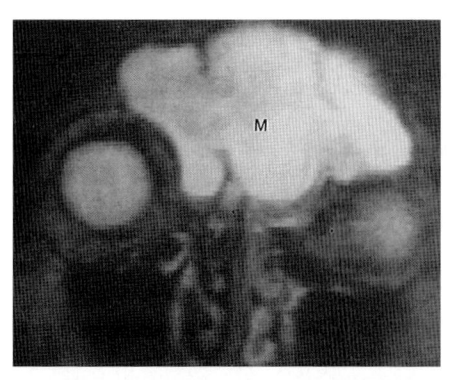

Fig. 4.85 Frontal sinus mucocele. Coronal T2W MR scan shows a hyperintense expansile mass (M), compatible with a mucocele.

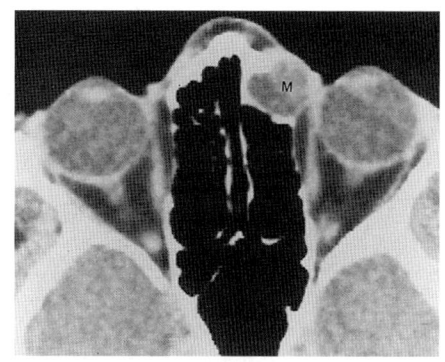

Fig. 4.86 Ethmoidal mucocele. Axial CT scan shows an expansile mass (M) compatible with an anterior ethmoidal sinus mucocele.

Mucoceles in Paranasal Sinuses

The etiology of mucocele (collection of mucus) is debatable. Most otorhinolaryngologists believe that mucoceles are secondary to obstruction of the main ostium of the sinus.[68,69] This obstruction may be the result of inflammation, trauma, osteoma, fibrous dysplasia, or repeated surgery in and around the nasal cavity.[1,10,12] A minority of investigators believe that mucoceles arise as small cysts within the mucous membrane and, by continued growth, finally obstruct the ostium of the sinus. Similarly, inflammation, trauma, and surgery may contribute to the initial cyst, or it may arise de novo.[10,12] Isolated noninvasive fungal sinusitis particularly of the sphenoid sinus is a rare but well-documented phenomenon.[68] *Aspergillus* is the organism most commonly involved in those cases, with the formation of a fungal ball being the predominant pathological process as opposed to the other types of fungal rhinosinusitis, i.e. allergic, chronic diffuse noninvasive, and acute fulminant.[68] Chronic noninvasive fungal sinusitis may result in the formation of sinus mucoceles.[68] Mucoceles are the cystlike lesions that most commonly produce bone destruction within the paranasal sinuses.[10,12] They are expanding cystic lesions covered by mucous membrane, which result from the continued accumulation of secretion and desquamation within an obstructed sinus cavity.[1,12] Bilateral mucoceles are rare. Their secretion is usually clear, thick (mucoid), and tenacious unless the mucocele has been converted to a pyocele by the invasion of bacteria.[10] In pyoceles, the cyst contains a thick, viscid green or yellow material.

Mucoceles are frequently discussed from the standpoint of sinus of origin. There is a definite predilection for the frontal and ethmoidal sinuses, presumably because of the dependent position of their ostia. Approximately two-thirds of all mucoceles involve the frontal sinuses (Figs. 4.84, 4.85); the majority of the remainder involve the ethmoidal labyrinth (Figs. 4.86, 4.87). Maxillary and sphenoid mucoceles (Figs. 4.88, 4.89) are rare. The sinus of origin, of course, is most important for treatment planning. The persistent expansion of the mucocele causes erosion of surrounding bone, with frequent exit into the adjacent orbit (Figs. 4.87, 4.90). Proptosis (displacement of the eye), puffiness of the upper eyelid, a mild ophthalmoplegia, some degree of visual disturbance, and a palpable mass are clinical features encountered with a supraorbital mucocele. The mucocele usually enters the more anterior portion of the orbital cavity (usually from the frontal and ethmoid sinuses) in the upper nasal quadrant (Fig. 4.87); this results in a peculiar droopy appearance, and the puffy soft tissue of the upper eyelid and a mass will be palpable beneath and slightly behind the superior orbital rim. In a large frontal sinus mucocele, if bone erosion occurs along the orbital roof, it may imitate signs of other tumors of the posterior orbit and sphenoid. The sphenoidal mucocele may cause serious neurological symptoms by intracranial extension. There may be destructions of the floor of the sella and encroachment of the pituitary gland. An orbital apex syndrome with loss of vision or constriction of the visual field may occur (Fig. 4.89). A mucocele of the maxillary sinus, although infrequent, may result in upward displacement of the orbital contents and exophthalmos caused by elevation of the roof of the antrum (Fig. 4.90).

Imaging Diagnosis of Mucocele

CT and MRI should be considered the diagnostic methods of choice for the diagnosis and management of mucocele. The radiographic characteristics of mucoceles have been well described.[10,12] A large mucocele produces a classic radiographic appearance of an enlarged, distorted sinus with a large bony defect representing a breakthrough into the adjacent structures (Figs. 4.84–4.91). Not all mucoceles are so classic, and there are many with subtle bone erosion. The gradual pressure atrophy and erosion of the bone by the enlarging soft-tissue mass of mucocele produces the expansile appearance on CT scanning (Figs. 4.84–4.90), with no enhancement after contrast infusion (except around the inflamed capsule and peripheral induration), and occasional peripheral calcification. Occasionally, a large frontal sinus inflammatory polyp, if bone erosion occurs along the orbital roof, may imitate the CT scan appearance of a mucocele (Fig. 4.78) or other tumors of the orbit. Mucoceles are typically seen on MRI as hypointense or less frequently as hyperintense images on T1-weighted and hyperintense on T2-weighted MR scans (Figs. 4.84, 4.85, 4.91). Because of variable protein content within long-standing mucoceles, signal intensity can be highly variable on both T1-weighted and T2-weighted MR sequences.

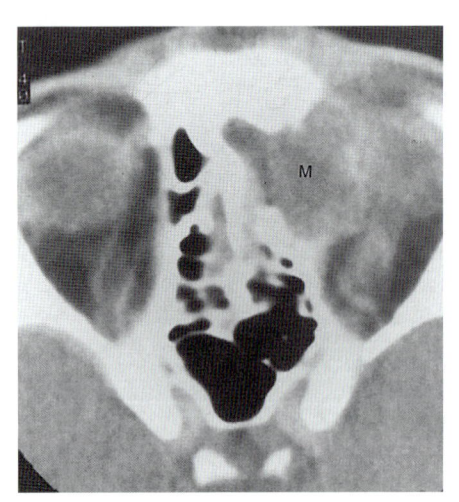

Fig 4.87 Ethmoidal mucocele. Axial CT scan shows an ethmoidal mucocele (M), extending into the orbit.

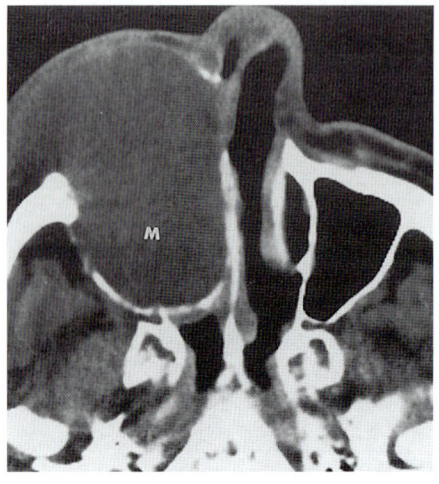

Fig. 4.88 Maxillary sinus mucocele. Axial CT scan shows a large expansile mass (M), compatible with a maxillary mucocele.

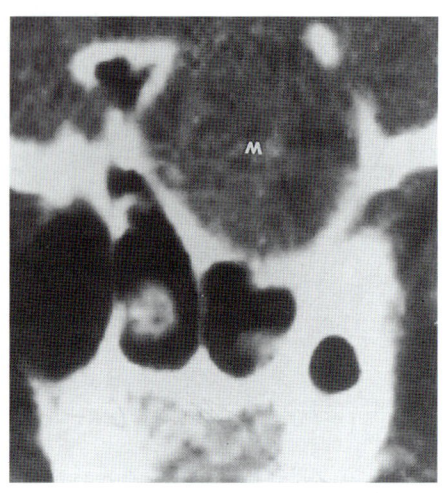

Fig. 4.89 Sphenoid sinus mucocele. Coronal CT scan shows a large sphenoidal mucocele (M). This was caused by nasoethmoidal fibrous dysplasia, obstructing the left sphenoid sinus ostium.

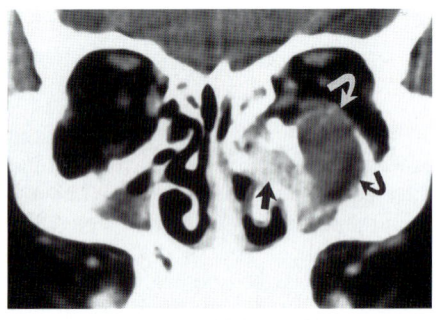

Fig. 4.90 Mucocele of left maxillary sinus secondary to nasal cancer. Enhanced CT scan shows a nasal carcinoma (straight arrow), resulting in obstruction of the maxillary ostium and mucocele formation (curved arrows). Courtesy Hatef Sherif, MD, Cairo, Egypt.

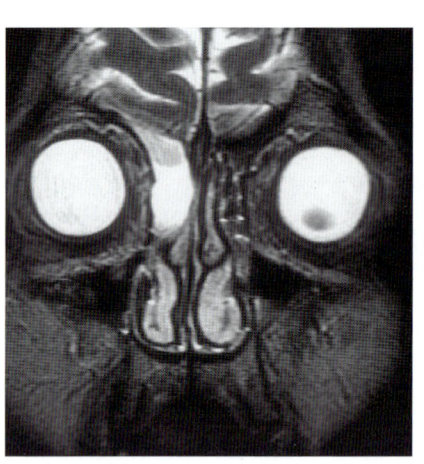

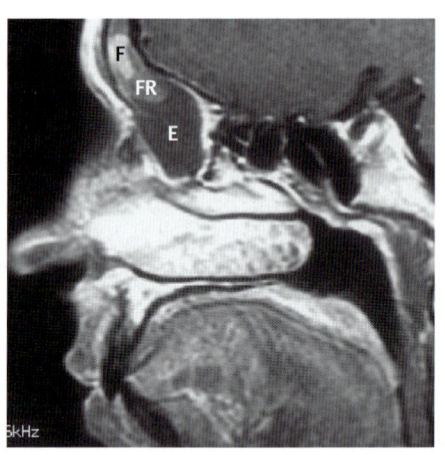

Fig. 4.91 Mucocele of the ethmoid sinus. **a** Coronal T2W MR scan, showing the hyperintense ethmoidal mucocele. The retained secretion in the right frontal sinus is less hyperintense. **b** Enhanced sagittal T1W MR scan showing the anterior ethmoidal mucocele (E). Note a ring of enhancement along the peripheral portion of the mucocele. Note retained secretion in frontal sinus (F) and frontal recess (FR).

Some mucoceles which contain thick mucus and inspissated mucosal retained secretions may be hypointense on T2-weighted MR scans. The increased signal intensity of mucocele on T1-weighted MR images is related to the proteinaceous content of mucosal secretions. Therefore, depending on the protein content, a mucocele may be slightly or markedly hyperintense on T1-weighted MR images (Figs. 4.84, 4.91b). Chronic fungal rhinosinusitis (both fungal balls and allergic fungal rhinosinusitis) and fungal mucoceles demonstrate a low or intermediate signal intensity on both T1-weighted and T2-weighted MR images,[68] with expansion of affected sinuses as well as peripheral rim enhancement on enhanced MR images. CT and MRI may also demonstrate neoplastic or inflammatory disease obstructing the sinus ostium, the cause of mucocele formation. The traditional teaching has emphasized the need for complete removal of the mucocele lining to achieve a cure.[69] However, simple drainage and marsupialization of mucoceles has been performed with good long-term results.[69]

■ Retention Cysts

Intramural maxillary sinus cysts, defined by Lindsay as nonsecreting cysts,[70] are a common incidental finding in plain radiography, CT and MRI of the sinuses. They are estimated to be present in about 10% of the healthy adult populations.[71] These cysts result from the obstruction of the ducts of mucosal serous and/or mucinous glands, and the cysts are usually small; rarely, however, they can enlarge sufficiently to fill a sinus cavity (Fig. 4.92). The maxillary sinuses are the largest of the paranasal sinuses and they are the most commonly found to harbor intramural retention cysts.[19] The sphenoid sinuses are the second most commonly to harbor retention cysts. These retention cysts are usually asymptomatic but may become clinically important when they cause obstruction of the maxillary sinus outflow tract, when they occur in the setting of symptoms compatible with chronic rhinosinusitis.[19] These retention cysts originate from the mucosa of the sinuses owing to obstruction of the drainage sites of submucosal glands. These cysts make up one of the most common incidental findings within the paranasal sinuses on CT or MR scans.[72] The incidence may range from 4.3% to 12.4%.[19] The

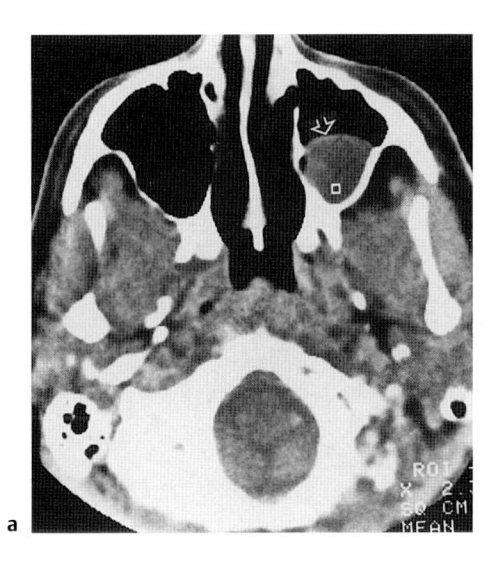

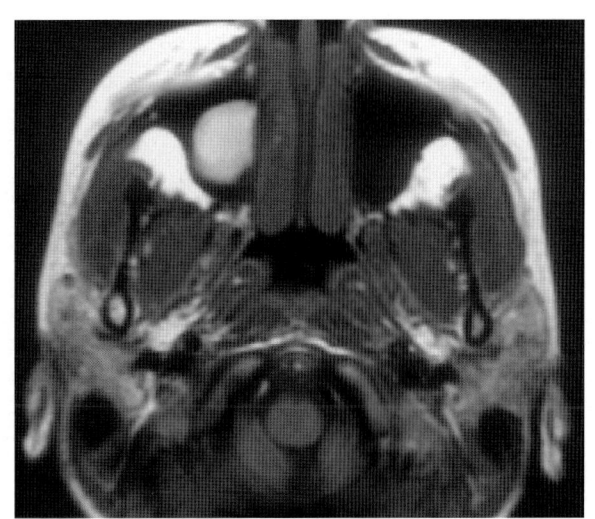

Fig. 4.**92 a** Retention cyst. Axial CT scan shows a well-defined soft-tissue mass of water density in an otherwise normal maxillary sinus (arrow). **b** Axial T1W MR scan shows a mucous retention cyst in the right maxillary sinus. The increased intensity is due to proteinaceous fluid content. The cyst was hypointense on T2W and FLAIR pulse sequences owing to increased protein content.

pathogenesis of maxillary retention cyst remains unclear. Some studies propose a postobstructive or allergic cause.[73] Other reports have included barotrauma in the formation of these cysts.[74] It is likely that the initial event leading to the formation of a sinus retention cyst is an inflammatory process as well as inflammatory obstruction of the ostiomeatal complex. In general, it is important to realize that maxillary sinus retention cysts are not related to anatomical variations of the ostiomeatal complex and do not reflect persistent obstruction of the maxillary outflow tract.[19] Consideration also should be given to not scoring maxillary sinus retention cysts as positive radiographic disease in the Lund scoring system.[20] Of course, in the setting of large and in particular medially located maxillary retention cysts and those associated with bony changes, diagnostic and therapeutic intervention may be indicated.[75] Berg et al.[76] suggested that these cysts, a frequent finding in the healthy population, seem to be the origin of choanal polyps. They argued that an expanding intramural cyst, when totally occupying the antrum, will emerge through the ostium into the nasal cavity, resulting in a choanal polyp or, better, a "choanal cyst." The macroarchitecture and microarchitecture of the antral part of the polyps, as well as the protein distribution in the cyst fluids, was identical to the structure and the protein distribution in the intramural cysts.[76] These cysts are seen as a smoothly marginated, convex configuration (dome shaped) of water or soft-tissue density on CT scans.[77] The MRI appearance of retention cysts reflects an image with long T1 and long T2 characteristics. These are seen as low signal intensity on T1-weighted MR images. Mucous retention types, as opposed to serous types, may show slightly higher signal intensity on T1-weighted MR images, related to their increased protein content. Retention cysts do not show contrast enhancement on enhanced CT and MR scans.

■ Nasal Polyps

Nasal polyps (NPs) are the most common mass lesion in the nose.[78] They are benign mucosal protrusions into the nasal cavity of multifactorial origin and characterized by chronic mucosal inflammation. The suggested pathological mechanisms comprise several factors including cytokines, immunoglobulin E (IgE), interleukins (IL), IL-4, IL-5, IL-6, and IL-8, and transforming growth factor-β1 (TGF-β1) in the pathogenesis of nasal polyposis.[79] IL-5 plays a key role in eosinophil recruitment and activation.[79] Ming et al.[78] reported that the pathogenesis of NP involves nasal polyp fibroblasts (NPFs) through synthesizing IL-6 to modulate the activation of immune responses (plasma cell formation) and synthesis of stroma. Cyclooxygenase also contributes to NP development by promoting vasodilatation. Interleukin 6 is a multifunctional cytokine that is involved in a variety of inflammatory conditions. One of its primary roles is the modulation of host immunity such as differentiation of B-cells into antibody-producing plasma cells and stimulating T-cell proliferation with the subsequent leukocytosis.[78] Interleukin 6 also stimulates fibroblast proliferation, increases collagen deposition, and decreases collagen breakdown.[78] Cyclooxygenase (COX) is an enzyme responsible for the conversion of arachidonic acid to prostaglandins (PGs).[78] Two isoforms of COX have been identified: COX-1 maintains tissue homeostasis, whereas inducible cyclooxygenase (COX-2) is responsible for the excessive PG synthesis of the PG family. PGE_2 increases vascular permeability and thereby facilitates cell migration to inflammatory areas.[78] The important role of COX-2 and IL-6 in the pathogenesis of nasal polyps was detected by Ming et al.[78] The role of bacterial infection and/or allergy is still debated but seems to be secondary as follows.[79]

Chronic sinus inflammation most commonly results from repeated episodes of acute or subacute inflammatory diseases of the sinonasal cavities. The sinus mucosa reflects these pathological alterations as a combination of areas of hypertrophic, polypoid, atrophic, and fibrotic changes intermixed with regions of acute or chronic inflammation and edema that are of either an infectious or an allergic origin. Chronic infections and allergies have both been regarded as probable causes in the formation of nasal polyps. Many different explanations for the formation of sinonasal polyps have been proposed. Some authors suggested that recurrent infections lead to chronic vascular changes. Tos and Mogensen[80] suggested that a rupture of the epithelium initiates formation of granulation tissue. Previously, however, it has not been possible to explain what initiates the growth of polyps.[81] In 1988, Petruson et al.[81] reported that insulin-like growth factor 1 (IGF-1) is a possible pathogenic mechanism in the formation of nasal polyps.[81,82] They presented findings of high local concentrations of a trophic growth peptide, IGF-1, in the epithelial and vascular cells, as well as in the activated macrophages and in nasal polyps. The authors argued that if these cells are enclosed in the mucosa of blocked inflamed paranasal sinuses, there may be an excessive increase in the concentration of IGF-1, exerting its growth-stimulating effect over long periods and therefore resulting in abnormal proliferation and eventually, in the formation of nasal polyps. Nasal polyps have been histologically classified as edematous (60%), glandular–cystic (27%), and fibrous types (13%) types, which exhibit intact epithelium on the surface[83] with massive edema/fluid and pseudocyst formation in the deeper layers.[79,83] Polyp tissue seems to be significantly denervated, and the open endothelial junctions of venules might be responsible for the vascular leakage,[78] and therefore for contrast enhancement on CT and MRI. Accumulation of eosinophils, neutrophils, plasma and mast cells, macrophages, and lymphocytes is a frequent finding.[78] Proliferation of connective-tissue and epithelial cells, basal membrane thickening, and fibrosis have also been described. It is difficult to estimate the growth rate of nasal polyps, but many patients have observed that growth accelerates when they develop infections.[81,82] The basal cells in the polyps from which the epithelial cells are developed show variable mitotic activity ranging from almost every cell to no cells at all being mitotically active.[82] Petruson et al.[81,82] demonstrated that the mitotic activity in the nasal mucosa was usually higher than in the nasal polyps and, concomitantly, the activity of the growth factor was lower. This observation suggested that increased growth factor activity is more important for the formation of nasal polyps than is increased mitotic activity. In the nasal mucosa, the epithelial cells are desquamated after some weeks.[81,82] During an infection, this rate increases[84] and, sometimes, large areas showing no epithelial cells may be seen. Petruson et al.[81,82] found that the lifetime of an epithelial cell on a nasal polyp was longer than in the nasal mucosa. They also noted that in most of the nasal polyps it was possible to observe IGF-1 immunoreactivity in endothelial cells and in vessel wall cells. Petruson et al[81,82] hypothesized that when macrophages, seen both in allergies and in infections, are enclosed in the paranasal sinuses, they release growth factors and, owing to reduced drainage, high concentrations accumulate and as a result stimulate the growth of both epithelium and blood vessels in the sinuses; the polyps start to bulge out through the ostia of the sinuses into the nasal cavity. It is known that steroids inhibit the activity of IGF-1 and treatment with local steroids slows down the growth of nasal polyps.[85]

Aspirin-sensitive Nasal Polyp[1]

The approximate number of asthmatic patients in the United States exceeds 10 million: within this group, approximately 500 000 patients differ clinically from those who have bronchial asthma alone.[86] In these patients, nasal polyps develop, followed by bronchial asthma and, subsequently, an extraordinary sensitivity to aspirin and other nonsteroidal anti-inflammatory drugs (NSAIDs) such as ibuprofen.[86-89] Patients with this syndrome, known as aspirin-sensitive asthma, often have severe rhinosinusitis and nasal polyposis. This clinical triad was first described by Dr. Max Samter and hence was given the name of Samter's triad.[89] The significance of this disorder is that it tends to worsen over time and can result in a fatal asthmatic attack.[86] The cause of the triad of nasal polyp, bronchial asthma, and aspirin sensitivity is unknown. A fundamental defect in aspirin sensitivity is excessive production of cysteinyl leukotrienes, both at baseline and after aspirin challenge.[87,88] These mediators are derived from arachidonic acid by the actions of 5-lipoxygenase C_4 synthase.[88] Enhanced activity of key synthetic enzymes, perhaps genetically determined, has been implicated as the cause of the elevated production of cysteinyl leukotrienes in patients with aspirin-sensitive asthma.[88] The common feature of drugs that provoke asthma attacks in aspirin-intolerant persons is that they inhibit cyclooxygenase-1 (COX-1).[88] Receptors for the cysteinyl leukotrienes have been characterized at molecular level.[88] The

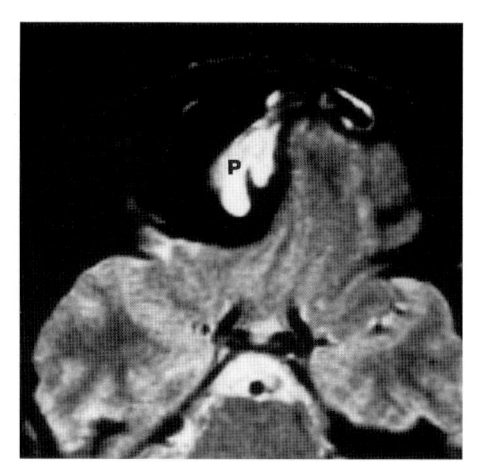

Fig. 4.**93** Frontal sinus polyp. Axial T2W MR scan shows a frontal sinus polyp (P).

two receptors have been designated $CysLT_1$ and $CysLT_2$. The $CysLT_1$ receptor is prominent in the airways. Sousa and colleagues[87] have reported that aspirin-sensitive persons with rhinosinusitis have increased expression of the $CysLT_1$ receptor on leukocytes infiltrating the nasal mucosa. The interrelationship between aspirin intolerance and bronchial asthma may be secondary to the release of inflammatory mediators such as leukotrienes, which result in the symptoms of bronchial asthma.

Imaging Studies of Sinonasal Polyps

A solitary polyp may not be distinguished from a retention cyst on unenhanced CT and MRI (Fig. 4.**93**). Unlike cysts, polyps demonstrate moderate to marked contrast enhancement (Figs. 4.**94**, 4.**95**). When multiple polyps are present, sinus secretions become entrapped within the crevices between the polyps, as well as on the surfaces of the polyps. On CT scans, polyps show soft-tissue attenuation values; however, depending on the concentration of the entrapped mucosal secretions, the CT attenuation values rises, and the chronic sinonasal polyposis may show mixed CT attenuation values with areas of increased density, simulating focal or diffuse dystrophic calcifications (Fig. 4.**96**). One important observation on CT or MRI of nasal polyps is the smooth expansion of nasal fossae (see Fig. 4.**78**) and pressure atrophy of the adjacent bony wall of the sinonasal cavities. Bone erosion is not common with polyps. However, in aggressive, long-standing polyposis, there may be significant expansion of the sinuses as well as bone erosion (see Fig. 4.**78**). Polyps tend to have various signal intensities on MR pulse sequences. The MRI characteristics of polyps reflect the various stages of polyps (edematous, glandular, cystic, and fibrous), as well as various stages of desiccation of the entrapped mucosal secretions within the crevices between the polyps and on the surfaces of the polyps. This appearance distinguishes them from tumors that usually do not have variable signal intensities in each MRI sequence. Polyps may coexist with mucoceles. At times it may be impossible to distinguish between mucoceles and multiple polyps.[90]

Choanal Polyp

The choanal polyp develops from an expanding intramural cyst/polyp that protrudes through the maxillary antrum ostium and into the nasal cavity.[76] The close relationship between choanal polyps and the maxillary sinus was first described by Killian in 1906[91] when he traced the polyps from the nasopharynx to the

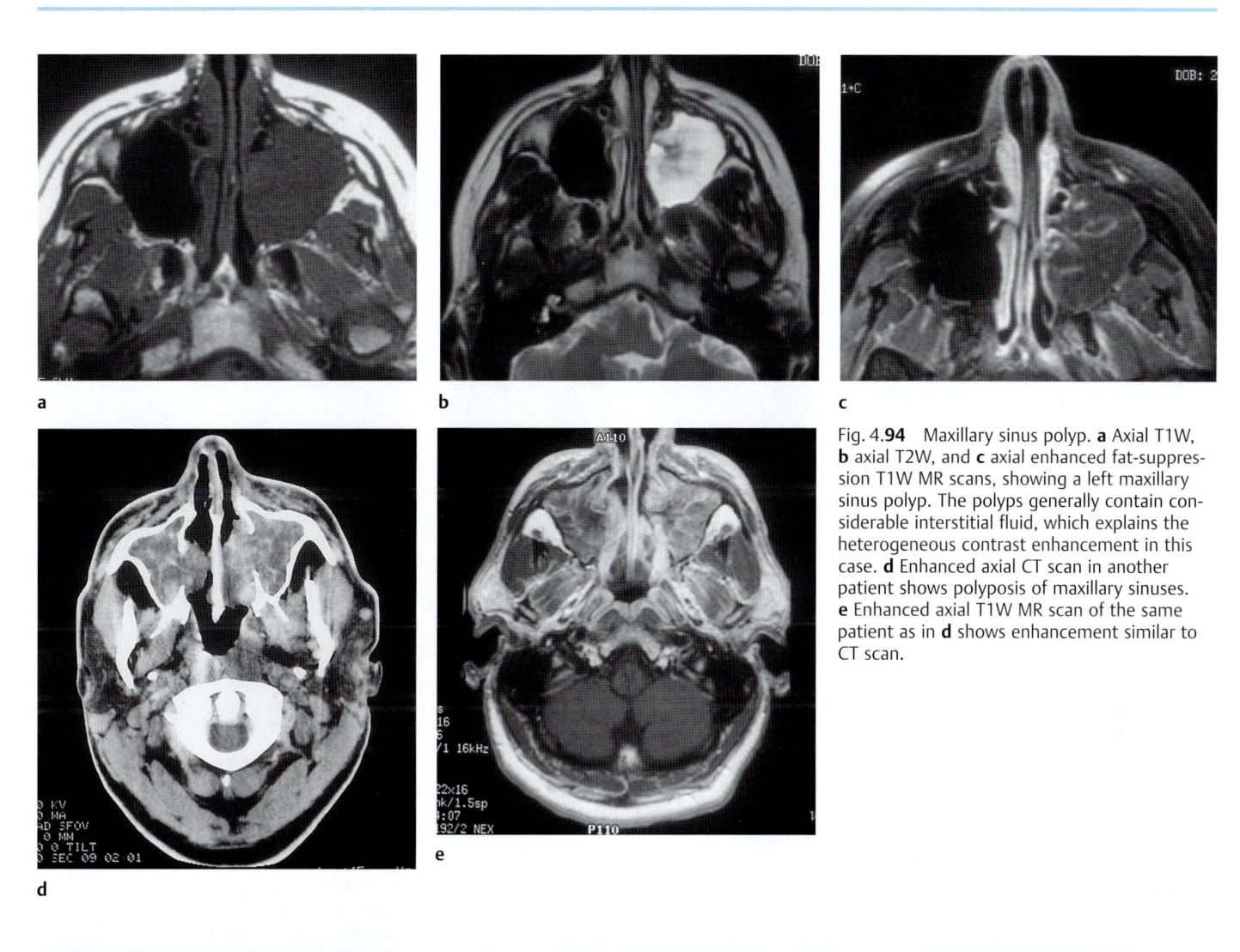

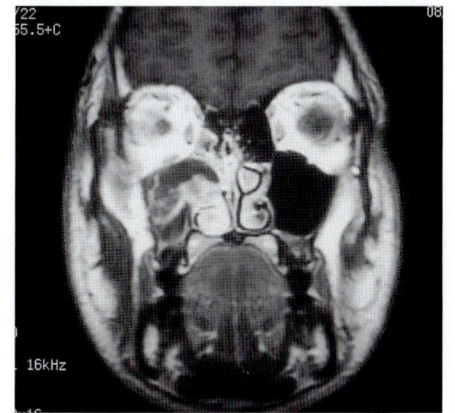

Fig. 4.**94** Maxillary sinus polyp. **a** Axial T1W, **b** axial T2W, and **c** axial enhanced fat-suppression T1W MR scans, showing a left maxillary sinus polyp. The polyps generally contain considerable interstitial fluid, which explains the heterogeneous contrast enhancement in this case. **d** Enhanced axial CT scan in another patient shows polyposis of maxillary sinuses. **e** Enhanced axial T1W MR scan of the same patient as in **d** shows enhancement similar to CT scan.

Fig. 4.**95** "Angiomatous polyp." Coronal enhanced MR scan shows an angiomatous polyp in the right nasal cavity and right maxillary sinus. A component of polyp shows intense enhancement.

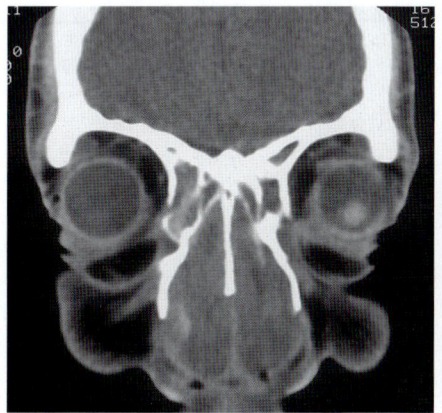

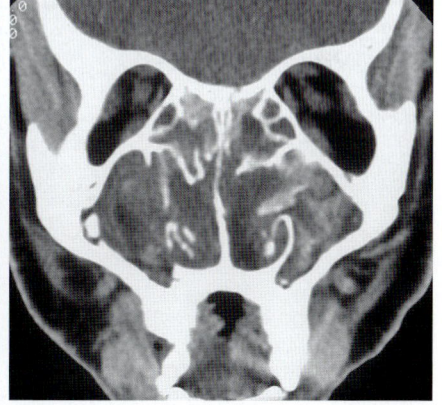

Fig. 4.**96** Massive sinonasal polyposis in a 28-year-old man with a history of nasal polyposis and several surgical procedures for removal of polyps. **a, b** Coronal CT scans showing bilateral nasal polyps and polyposis of maxillary and ethmoid sinuses. The increased linear densities within the maxillary sinuses are due to desciccated mucus.

region of the ostium of the maxillary sinus, but not into the maxillary sinus cavity. Other authors found choanal polyps to be attached to the lateral wall of the maxillary sinus with a fibrous or polypoid pedicle.[92] Mills[93] suggested that the antrochoanal polyps arise from blocked and ruptured mucous glands during the healing process of bacterial sinusitis. Berg et al.[76] using the preservative technique used in surgical antral exploration, were able to show the intrasinusoidal choanal polyps. An antral part of the polyps was recognized without exception. The polyps continued into the maxillary sinus with a thin-walled cyst that, in most cases, completely filled the cavity (Fig. 4.**97**). The cyst wall was separated from the regular sinus mucosa. The histopathological picture of the nasal part of the choanal polyps shows a central cavity surrounded by monomorphic edematous stroma in which

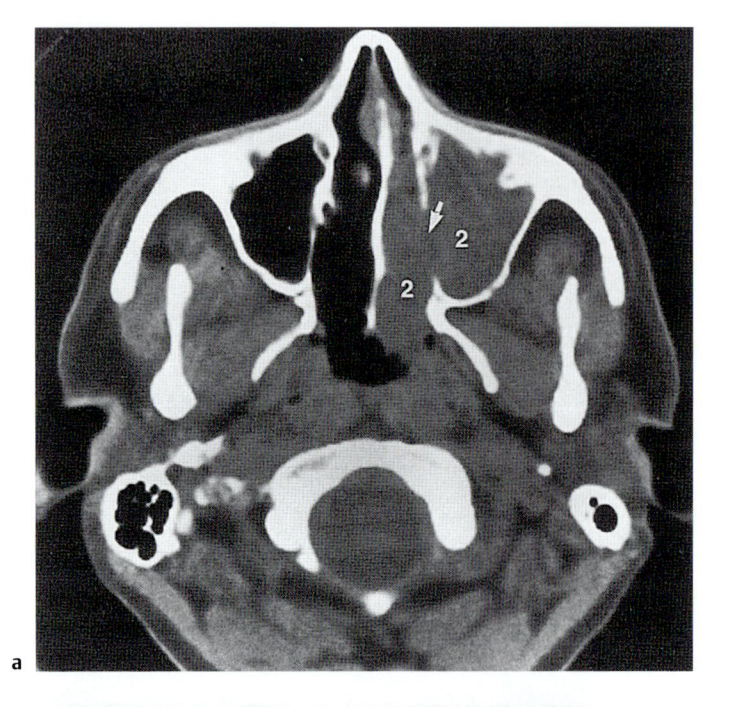

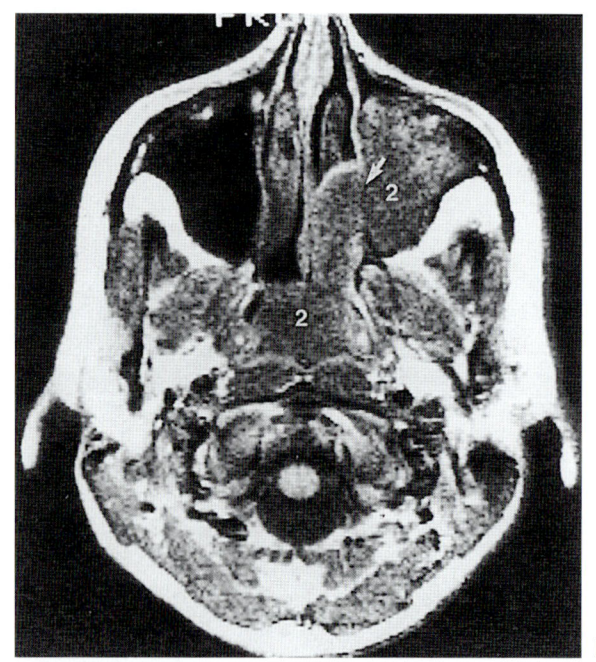

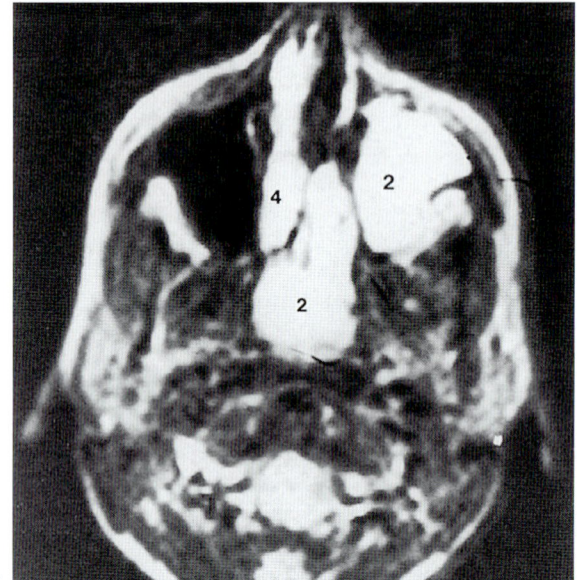

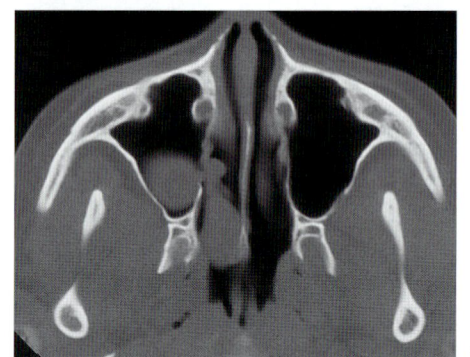

Fig. 4.**97 a–c** Antrochoanal polyp. An axial CT scan (**a**) reveals the polyp (2) extending from the left maxillary sinus through a wide ostium (arrow) into the nasal cavity and nasopharynx. The entire polyp (2) is seen by MRI in the axial plane on a T1W image (**b**) and on a T2W image (**c**). Edematous changes are apparent with the low signal on the T1W image **b** and the high signal on the T2W image **c**. The right turbinate (4) also has a normal high signal on the T2W image due to the mucosal secretions. **d** Antrochoanal polyp. CT scan in another patient, shows an antrochoanal polyp within the right antrum and nasal cavity.

only a few cells are seen.[76] The external surface is covered by normal respiratory epithelium; the antral part of the choanal polyps demonstrates the same histological appearances, but the cyst wall may be thinner and less organized. Berg et al.[76] were not able to distinguish microscopically any portion of the choanal polyps from the structures observed in the intramural cysts. The cyst fluid aspirated from the choanal polyps revealed a similar distribution and concentration of proteins to that found in intramural cysts.[76]

■ References

1. Salmon SD, Graeme-Cook F. Case records of the Massachusetts General Hospital. N Engl J Med 1990; 322: 116–123.
2. Ferguson BJ, Amon J, Poole MD et al. Short treatment durations for acute bacterial rhinosinusitis: Five days of gemifloxacin versus 7 days of gemifloxacin. Otolaryngol Head Neck Surg 2002; 127: 1–6.
3. Mafee MF. Imaging of paranasal sinuses and nasal cavity. In: English GM, ed. Otolaryngology, Vol. 2. Philadelphia: Lippincott-Raven;1996: 11–44.
4. Bienfang DC, Karluk D. Mucormycosis, rhino-orbital. Case records of the Massachusetts General Hospital. N Engl J Med 2002; 346: 924–929.
5. Abe F, Inaba H, Katoh T, Hotchi M. Effects of iron and desferrioxamine on *Rhizopus* infection. Mycopathologica 1990; 107: 782–783.
6. Mora-Duarte J, Betts R, Rotsstein C, et al. Comparison of Caspofungin and Amphotericin B for invasive candidiasis. N Engl J Med 2002; 347: 2020–2029.
7. Stammberger H, Jakse R, Beaufort F. Aspergillosis of the paranasal sinuses. X-ray diagnosis, histopathology, and clinical aspects. Ann Otol Rhinol Laryngol 1984; 93: 251–256.
8. Hutchin ME, Shores CG, Bauer MS, Yarbrough WG. Sinogenic subdural empyema and streptococcus anginosus. Arch Otolaryngol Head Neck Surg 1999; 125: 1262–1266.
9. Eustis HS, Mafee MF, Walton C, Mondonca J. MR imaging and CT of orbital infections and complications in acute rhinosinusitis. Radiol Clin North Am 1998; 36: 1165–1183.

10. Mafee MF. Orbital and intraocular lesions. In: Edelman RR, Hesselink JR, Zlatkin MG, eds. Clinical Magnetic Resonance Imaging. Philadelphia: W.B. Saunders; 1996: 985.
11. Jones NS, Walker JL, Bassi S, et al. The intracranial complications of rhinosinusitis: Can they be prevented? Laryngoscope 2002; 112: 59–63.
12. Mafee MF. Eye and orbit. In: Som PM, Curtin HD, eds. Head and Neck Imaging. St. Louis: Mosby; 2003: 441–654.
13. Younis RT, Anand VK, Davidson B. The role of computed tomography and magnetic resonance imaging in patients with sinusitis with complications. Laryngoscope 2002;112: 224–229.
14. Green WH, Goldberg HI, Wohl GT. Mucormycosis infection of the craniofacial structures. AJR 1967; 101: 802–806.
15. Talmi YP, Reouven AG, Bakon M, et al. Rhino-orbital and rhino-oribito-cerebral mucormycosis. Otolaryngol Head Neck Surg 2002; 127: 22–31.
16. Berger G, Kattan A, Bernheim J, Ophir D. Polypoid mucosa with eosinophilia and glandular hyperplasia in chronic sinusitis: A histopathological and immunohistochemical study. Laryngoscope 2002; 112: 738–745.
17. Knowles MR, Durie PR. What is cystic fibrosis? N Engl J Med 2002; 347: 439–442.
18. Sobol SE, Christodoulopoulos P, Manoukian JJ, et al. Cytokine profile of chronic sinusitis in patients with cystic fibrosis. Arch Otolaryngol Head and Neck Surg 2002; 128: 1295–1298.
19. Bhattacharyya N. Do maxillary sinus retention cysts reflect obstructive sinus phenomena? Arch Otolaryngol Head Neck Surg 2002; 126: 1369–1371.
20. Lund VJ, Kennedy DW. Staging for rhinosinusitis. Otolaryngol Head Neck Surg 1997; 117(Suppl): 35–40.
20a. Carter BL. Paranasal sinuses, nasal cavity, pterygoid fossa, nasopharynx, and infratemporal fossa. In: Valvassori GE, Buckingham RA, Carter BL, Hanafee WN, Mafee MF, eds. Head and Neck Imaging. Stuttgart: Georg Thieme Verlag; 1988: 173–250.
21. Zinreich SJ, Kennedy DW, Malat J, et al. Fungal sinusitis: diagnosis with CT and MR imaging. Radiology 1988; 169: 439–444.
22. Pillsbury HC, Fischer ND. Rhinocerebral mucormycosis. Arch Otolaryngol 1977; 103: 600–604.
23. Young RC, Bennett JE, Vogel CL, et al. Aspergillosis: the spectrum of disease in 98 patients. Medicine 1970; 49: 147–173.
24. Meikle D, Yarington CT Jr., Winterbauer R H. Aspergillosis of the maxillary sinuses in other healthy patients. Laryngoscope 1985; 95: 776–779.
25. McGill T J, Simpson G, Nealy G B. Fulminant aspergillosis of nose and paranasal sinuses: a new clinical entity. Laryngoscope 1980; 90: 748–754.
26. Beck-Mannagetta J, Necek K, Grasserbauer M. Solitary aspergillosis of maxillary sinus: A complication of dental treatment. Lancet 1983; 2: 1260.
27. Terry D. Blastomycosis of the paranasal sinuses. Presented at the American Rhinologic Society, April 17–18, 1993; Los Angeles, California.
28. Stammberger H. Endoscopic surgery for mycotic and chronic recurrent sinusitis. Ann Otorhinolaryngol 1985; 94(Suppl) 119: 3–10.
29. Saferstein B. Allergic bronchopulmonary aspergillosis with obstruction of the upper respiratory tract. Chest 1976; 70: 788–790.
30. Katzenstein AL, Sale SR, Greenberger PA. Allergic aspergillus sinusitis: a newly recognized form of sinusitis. J Allergy Clin Immunol 1983; 72: 89–93.
31. Marple B, Newcomer M, Schwade N, Mabry R. Natural history of allergic fungal rhinosinusitis. A 4- to 10-year follow-up. Otolaryngol Head Neck Surg 2002; 127: 361–366.
32. Beamis JF, Mark EJ. Case records of the Massachusetts General Hospital. N Engl J Med 2001; 345: 443–449.
33. Bassichis BA, Marple BF, Mabry R, Newcomer MT. Use of immunotherapy in previously treated patients with allergic fungal sinusitis. Otolaryngol-Head Neck Surg 2001; 125: 487–490.
34. Schell WA. Histopathology of fungal rhinosinusitis. Otolaryngol Clin North Am 2000; 33: 251–276.
35. Manning SC, Wash S. Diagnosis of allergic fungal sinusitis vs a mucocele. Arch Otolaryngol Head Neck Surg 1999; 125: 1169.
36. McClay JE, Marple B, Kapadia L, et al. Clinical presentation of allergic fungal sinusitis in children. Laryngoscope 2002; 112: 565–569.
37. Kopp W, Fotter R, Steiner H, et al. Aspergillosis of the paranasal sinuses. Radiology 1985; 156: 715–716.
38. Mukherji SK, Figueroa RE, Ginsberg LE, et al. Allergic fungal sinusitis: CT findings. Radiology 1998; 207: 417–422.
39. Kubicek C P, Rohr M. Metabolic effects of managenese deficiency in *Aspergillus niger*: evidence of increased protein degradation. Arch Microbiol 1985; 141: 266–268.
40. Ellegard E, Karlsson G. IgE-mediated reactions and hyperreactivityin pregnancy rhinitis. Arch Otolaryngol Head Neck Surg 1999; 125: 1121–1125.
41. Graf P, Enerdal J, Hallen H. Ten days' use of oxymetazoline nasal spray with or without benzalkonium chloride in patients with vasomotor rhinitis. Arch Otolaryngol Head Neck Surg 1999; 125: 1128–1132.
42. Ayala C, Watkins L, Deschler DG. Tension orbital pneumocele secondary to nasal obstruction from cocaine abuse: a case report. Otolaryngol Head Neck Surg2002; 127: 572–574.
43. Kim SA, Mathog RH. Radiology quiz case 2; Silent sinus syndrome: maxillary sinus atelectasis with enophthalmos. Arch Otolaryngol Head Neck Surg 2002; 128: 81–83.
44. Boyd JH, Yaffee K, Holds J. Maxillary sinus atelectasis with enophthalmos. Ann Otol Rhinol Laryngol 1998; 107: 34–39.
45. Gillman GS, Schaitkin BM, May M. Asymptomatic enophthalmos: the silent sinus syndrome. Am J Rhinol 1999; 13: 459–462.
46. Hadi U, Ghossaini S, Zaytoun G. Rhinolithiasis: a forgotten entity. Otolaryngol Head Neck Surg 2002; 126: 48–51.
47. Borges A, Fink J, Villablanca P, et al. Midline destructive lesions of the sinonasal tract: Simplified terminology based on histopathologic criteria. AJNR 2000; 21: 331–336.
48. Coup AJ, Hooper IP. Granulomatous lesions in nasal biopsies. Histopathology 1980; 4: 293–308.
49. Krishna I, Balakrishnan K, Kumar N. Quiz case 4; Nasal granuloma gravidum. Arch Otolaryngol Head Neck Surg 2000; 126: 1156–1160.
50. Neville E, Mills RG, James DG. Sarcoidosis of the upper respiratory tract and its relation to lupus pernio. Ann NY Acad Sci 1976; 278: 416–426.
51. McCaffrey TV, McDonald TJ. Sarcoidosis of the nose and paranasal sinuses. Laryngoscope 1983; 93: 1281–1294.
52. Thompson LDR. Rhinoscleroma. ENT Ear Nose Throat J 2002; 81: 506.
53. Loh KS, Chong SM, Pang YT, Soh K. Rhinosporidiasis: Differential diagnosis of a large nasal mass. Otolaryngol Head Neck Surg 2001; 124: 121–122.
54. Wenig BM, ed. Atlas of Head and Neck Pathology. Philadelphia: W.B. Saunders; 1993.
55. Hoffman GS, Kerr GS, Leavitt RY, et al. Wegener's granulomatosis: an analysis of 158 patients. Ann Intern Med 1992; 116: 458–498.
56. Davies DJ, Moran JE, Neall JF, Ryan GB. Segmental necrotizing glomerulonephritis with antineutrophil antibody: possible arbovirus aetiology? BMJ 1982; 285: 606.
57. Jennette JC, Charles LA, Falk RJ. Antineutrophil cytoplasmic autoantibodies: disease associations, molecular biology, and pathophysiology. Int Rev Exp Pathol 1991; 32: 193–221.
58. Fanburg BL, Niles JL, Mark BJ. Case records of the Massachusetts General Hospital. N Engl J Med 1993; 329: 2019–2026.
59. van der Woude FJ, Rasmussen N, Lobatto S, et al. Autoantibodies against neutrophils and monocytes: Tool for diagnosis and marker of disease activity in Wegener's granulomatosis. Lancet 1985; 1: 425–429.
60. Jayne DRW, Marshall PD, Jones SJ, Lockwood CM. Autoantibodies to GBM and neutrophil cytoplasm in rapidly progressive glomerulonephritis. Kidney Int 1990; 37: 965–970.
61. Weinberger LM, Cohen ML, Remler BF, Naheedy MH, Leigh RJ. Intracranial Wegener's granulomatosis. Neurology 1993; 43: 1831–1834.
62. Marsot-Dupuch K, Clement DeGivry S, Quayoun M. Wegener granulomatosis involving the pterygopalatine fossa: An unusual case of trigeminal neuropathy. AJNR. 2002; 23: 312–315.
63. McDonald TJ, Deremee RA, Harrison EG Jr., Facer GW, Devine KD. The protein clinical features of polymorphic reticulosis (lethal midline granulomatosis). Laryngoscope 1976; 86: 936–945.
64. Weymuller EA, Rice DH. Surgical management of infections and inflammatory diseases. In: Cummings CW, Fredrickson JM, Harker LA, Krause EJ, Schuller DE, eds. Otolaryngology Head and Neck Surgery. 2nd ed. Vol. 1. St. Louis: Mosby-Year Book; 1993: 955–964.
65. Churg J, Strauss L. Allergic granulomatosis, allergic angiitis, and periarteritis nodosa. Am J Pathol 1951; 27: 277–301.
66. Keefe MA, Bloom DC, Keefe KS, Killian PJ. Orbital paraffinoma as a complication of endoscopic sinus surgery. Otolaryngol Head Neck Surg 2002; 127: 575–577.
67. Aferzon M, Millman B, O'Donell T, Gilroy PA. Cholesterol granuloma of the frontal bone. Otolaryngol Head Neck Surg 2002; 127: 578–581.
68. Lee JT, Bhuta S, Lufkin R, Calcaterra TC. Fungal mucoceles of the sphenoid sinus. Laryngoscope 2002; 112: 779–783.
69. Har-El G. Endoscopic management of 108 sinus mucoceles. Laryngoscope 2001; 111: 2131–2134.
70. Lindsay JR. Nonsecreting cysts of the maxillary sinus mucosa. Laryngoscope 1942; 52: 84–100.

71. Hanna HH. Asymptomatic sinus disease in air-crew members. Clin Aviation Aerospace Med 1974; 45: 77–81.
72. Cooke LD, Hadley DM. MRI of the paranasal sinuses: Incidental abnormalities and their relationship to symptoms. J Laryngol Otol 1991; 105: 278–281.
73. Berg O, Carenfelt C, Sobin A. On the diagnosis and pathogenesis of intramural maxillary cysts. Acta Otolaryngol 1989; 108: 464–468.
74. Garges LM. Maxillary sinus barotrauma. Aviat Space Environ Med 1985; 56: 796–802.
75. Fisher EW, Whittet HB, Croft CB. Symptomatic mucosal cysts of the maxillary sinus: antroscopic treatment. J Laryngol Otol 1989; 103: 1184–1186.
76. Berg O, Carenfelt C, Silfversward C, Sobin A. Origin of the choanal polyp. Arch Otolaryngol Head Neck Surg 1988; 114: 1270–1271.
77. Mafee MF. Imaging of the head and neck: computed tomography, magnetic resonance. In: Ballenger JJ, Snow JB, eds. Otorhinolaryngology Head and Neck Surgery. 15th ed. Baltimore: Williams and Wilkins; 1996; 699.
78. Ming CM, Hong CY, Shun CT, et al. Inducible cyclooxygenase and interleukin 6 gene expressions in nasal polyp fibroblasts. Arch Otolaryngol Head and Neck Surg 2002; 128: 945–951.
79. Hirschberg A, Darvas AJZ, Almay K, et al. The pathogenesis of nasal polyposis by immunoglobulin E and interleukin-5 is completed by transforming growth factor β1. Laryngoscope 2003; 113: 120–124.
80. Tos M, Mogensen C Pathogenesis of nasal polyps. Rhinology 1977; 15: 87–95.
81. Petruson B, Hansson HA, Petruson K. Insulin-like growth factor I immunoreactivity in nasal polyps. Arch Otolaryngol Head Neck Surg 1988; 114: 1272–1275.
82. Petruson B, Hansson HA, Petruson K. Insulin-like growth factor I is a possible pathogenetic mechanism in nasal polyps. Acta Otolaryngol 1988; 106: 156–160.
83. Kakoi H, Hiraide E. A histological study of formation and growth of nasal polyps. Acta Otolaryngol 1987; 103: 137–144.
84. Winther B, Brofeldt S, Christensen B, et al. Light and scanning electron microscopy of nasal biopsy material from patients with naturally acquired common colds. Acta Otolaryngol 1984; 97: 309–318.
85. Karlsson G, Runderantz H. A randomized trial of intranasal biclomethasone dipropionate after polypectomy. Rhinology 1982; 20: 144–148.
86. Ziroli NE, Na H, Chow JM, et al. Aspirin-sensitive versus non-aspirin-sensitive nasal polyp patients: analysis of leukotrienes/FaS and FaS-ligand expression. Otolaryngol Head Neck Surg 2002; 126: 141–146.
87. Sousa AR, Parikh A, Scadding G, et al. Leukotriene-receptor expression on nasal mucosal inflammatory cells in aspirin-sensitive rhinosinusitis. N Engl J Med 2002; 347: 1493–1499.
88. Arm JP, Austre KP. Leukotriene receptors and aspirin sensitivity. N Engl J Med 2002; 347: 1524–1526.
89. Samter M, Beers RF. Intolerance to aspirin: clinical studies and consideration of its pathogenesis. Ann Intern Med 1968; 68: 975–983.
90. Som PM, Dillon WP, Sze G, et al. Benign and malignant sinonasal lesions with intracranial extension: their MR differentiation. Radiology 1989; 172: 763–766.
91. Killian G. The origin of choanal polypi. Lancet 1906; 2: 81–82.
92. Van Alyea OE. Management of non-malignant growths in the maxillary sinus. Ann Otolaryngol 1951; 65: 714–722.
93. Mills CE. Secretory cysts of the maxillary antrum and their relation to the development of antrochoanal polypi. J Laryngol Otol 1959; 73: 324–3344.

Tumor and Tumorlike Lesions of the Paranasal Sinuses and Nasal Cavity

Introduction

Malignant tumors of the nasal cavity and paranasal sinuses account for only 0.2–0.8% of all malignant neoplasms and just 3% of all tumors occurring in the head and neck.[1–4] Approximately 50–65% of malignant sinonasal tumors arise within the maxillary sinuses, 10–25% in the ethmoid sinuses, and 15–30% in the nasal cavity.[2,5–8]

Tumors and tumorlike lesions of the sinonasal tract may be classified (1) as benign or malignant; (2) as carcinoma, sarcoma, or lymphoma; (3) according to the tissue of origin (e.g., epithelial, bone, lymphoid, mesenchymal, etc.); or (4) as a combination of the above. The World Health Organization prefers to classify the tumors according to the tissue of origin and subdivide them into benign or malignant. Some of the more common tumors and tumorlike lesions of the sinonasal tract are shown in Tables 4.**7** and 4.**8**.

Because many sinonasal tumors are accompanied by underlying or superimposed chronic inflammatory or allergic disease, tumors may be easily overlooked.[4] Although it is possible to distinguish tumor from associated inflammatory disease on CT, the differentiation may be difficult. In this type of situation, CT has some deficiency with regard to the location of the actual tumor margin.[9,10] As imaging technology improved and MRI became available for clinical application, superior tumor mapping became possible. Today, with MRI, it is possible in most sinonasal tumors to differentiate inflammatory reactions and retained secretions from the bulk of the tumor, because the high water content of inflammatory conditions results in markedly increased signal on T2-weighted MR scans.[9] In contrast, the overwhelming majority of sinonasal tumors are highly cellular[2,3] and therefore have an intermediate signal intensity on T2-weighted MR images.[5,9] It is important to realize, however, that the more benign tumors and glandular-type tumors, such as polyps, papillomas, minor salivary gland tumors, and schwannomas, usually have sufficient water content to produce hyperintensity on T2-weighted MR scans.[5]

Conventional plain films, although infrequently used, may still be used as the screening study in various pathological conditions of the nasal cavity and paranasal sinuses to give orientation and direction to further indicated examinations such as CT and MRI. In the appropriate clinical setting, the CT and MR appearances, location, expansion, and type of bone destruction will allow the radiologist to provide a preferred list of differential diagnoses. For example, chronic inflammatory disease is often associated with mucoperiosteal thickening and, at times, marked sclerosis of the bone.[10–12] Chronic sinusitis associated with inspissated mucus has a characteristic hyperdense CT appearance. Polyposis of the nasal cavity and paranasal sinuses, mucocele, chronic noninvasive fungal infections (*Aspergillus*), and benign tumors tend to expand the area of origin by virtue of their slow growth or mass effect as well as bone demineralization. The gradual pressure atrophy and erosion of the bone by the enlarging soft-tissue mass, such as polyp or mucocele, can be readily seen on CT scans. Malignant tumors, on the other hand, usually destroy bone and invade the adjacent hard-and soft-tissue structures. Extension into the orbit, pterygopalatine fossa, infratem-

Table 4.**7** Benign neoplasms of sinonasal cavities

1	Osteoma
2	Hemangioma, lymphangioma
3	Sinonasal or schneiderian papilloma
4	Angiofibroma
5	Schwannoma
6	Lobular capillary hemangioma (pyogenic granuloma)
7	Sinonasal hemangiopericytoma
8	Benign fibrous histiocytoma*
9	Fibromatosis*

10	Benign fibro-osseous and osseous lesions
	  a Fibrous dysplasia
	  b Ossifying fibroma
	  c Juvenile active ossifying fibroma

11	Sinonasal myxoma and fibromyxoma
12	Ameloblastoma*
13	Giant-cell tumor*

Modified from Wenig BM. Atlas of Head and Neck Pathology. Philadelphia, W.B. Saunders, 1993. * = potentially malignant.

poral fossa, and cranial cavity can be demonstrated by contrast-enhanced CT scans and in particular by MR scans. Osteogenic or chondrogenic sarcomas of the paranasal sinuses demonstrate irregular periosteal reaction, cortical break, and islands of tumor bone formation, as well as marked bone destruction.[10–12] Most inflammatory lesions are quite hyperintense on T2-weighted MR images as opposed to malignant tumors, lymphoreticular proliferative disorders, and chronic granulomatous diseases, all of which appear relatively less hyperintense on T2-weighted MR images.[5, 10–12] Most tumors of the nasal cavity and paranasal sinuses are not as hyperintense as the surrounding inflammation and retained secretions on T2-weighted MR images. On enhanced MRI, most tumors demonstrate less enhancement than inflammatory reaction; therefore, MRI plays an important role in mapping and staging these tumors.

Benign Tumors

Benign tumors of the nose are rare in comparison with malignant tumors. In decreasing order of frequency, the benign tumors are osteoma, hemangioma, papilloma, angiofibroma, benign mixed tumor, schwannoma, and other less common tumors (Table 4.7).

Osteoma

An osteoma is seen primarily in the frontal and ethmoid sinuses and can consist of very dense, compact bone, or of lamellar bone with intertrabecular fibrous tissue (Fig. 4.98). A fibrous osteoma appears less dense on plain film studies and thus may be confused with a cyst.[12] Intraosseous hemangioma can mimic an osteoma on plain film and CT.[13] More information with regard to the clinical, histological, and CT scan and MRI features of osteomas can be found in the section describing the fibro-osseous lesions of the sinonasal cavity (p. 442).

Sinonasal or Schneiderian Papillomas

The mucosa of the nasal cavity and paranasal sinuses (Schneiderian mucosa) is composed of pseudociliated columnar epithelium and gives rise to three distinct histological papillomas, which include fungiform (septal, squamous, or exophytic papilloma), 50%; inverted (endophytic papilloma) (Figs. 4.99, 4.100), 47%; and cylindrical cell papilloma (oncocytic schneiderian), 3% (Fig. 4.101). These are collectively referred to as schneiderian papillomas (Table 4.8).[3, 5, 9, 14–16] These are benign neoplasms composed of squamous or columnar epithelial proliferation with associated mucous cells or pools, and a myxomatous stroma.[3] Biological behavior is essentially the same for all types, but clinical findings may differ.[3] Fungiform papillomas arise on the nasal septum and have a verrucous appearance. They are not considered to be premalignant.[5] Inverted papillomas characteristically arise from the lateral nasal wall in the vicinity of the middle turbinate and extend into the ethmoid and maxillary sinuses (Fig. 4.99). They are almost always unilateral and are notorious for recurrence after partial resection. The fungiform type is almost invariably limited to the nasal septum. The inverted and cylindrical cell papillomas occur along the lateral nasal wall (middle meatus, middle turbinate), and less frequently in the paranasal sinuses (Figs. 4.99–4.102).[3] The cylindrical cell papilloma is characterized by a multilayered proliferation of columnar or cylindrical cells with minimal squamous cell components. The cylindrical cell papilloma may exhibit inverting and exophytic components, and its anatomical distribution and clinical behavior parallel those of the inverted type.[14–16] In general, papillomas are unilateral, but bilateral papillomas occur infrequently.[3]

Table 4.8 Classification of tumors and tumorlike lesions of the sinonasal cavities

Origin	Type
Epithelial	Schneiderian papillomas Fungiform (septal, squamous, or exophytic papilloma) (50%) Inverted (endophytic papilloma) (47%) Oncocytic schneiderian (cylindric cell papilloma) (3%) Squamous cell carcinoma Adenocarcinoma Undifferentiated carcinoma
Salivary gland	Pleomorphic adenoma Adenoid cystic carcinoma (cylindroma) Acinic cell carcinoma Mucoepidermoid carcinoma
Neuroectodermal–neural	Schwannoma Neurofibroma Ectopic meningioma Invasive (aggressive) pituitary adenoma Olfactory neuroblastoma Malignant schwannoma Neuroendocrine carcinoma
Soft tissue	Hemangioma Angiofibroma Fibroma Lymphangioma Hemangiopericytoma Hemangiosarcoma Rhabdomyosarcoma Malignant and benign fibrous histiocytoma
Bone, cartilaginous, and odontogenic tissue	Osteoma, osteoblastoma, osteoclastoma (giant-cell tumor) Cemento-ossifying fibroma Myxoma Chondroma Chordoma Chondrosarcoma Osteosarcoma Ewing sarcoma Odontogenic keratocyst Ameloblastoma Fibrous dysplasia Paget disease
Hematopoietic	Plasmacytoma Lymphoma Langerhans cell histiocytosis Thalassemia Polymorphic reticulosis (lymphomatoid granulomatosis) = non-Hodgkin lymphoma
Developmental	Nasal glioma-encephalocele Hamartoma Dermoid/Epidermoid Teratoma Malignant teratoma
Metastatic	Kidney Lung Breast GI tract Others
Miscellaneous	Inflammatory polyps Fungal infections Wegener granulomatosis Granular cell tumor Merkel cell tumor Retention cyst Mucocele

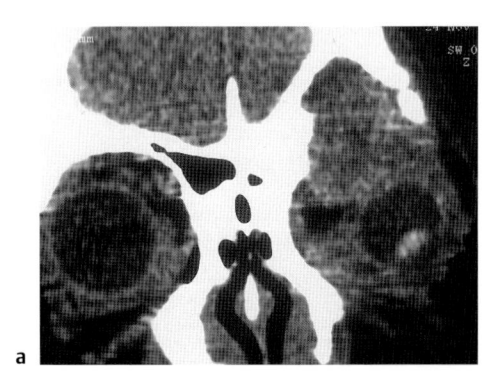

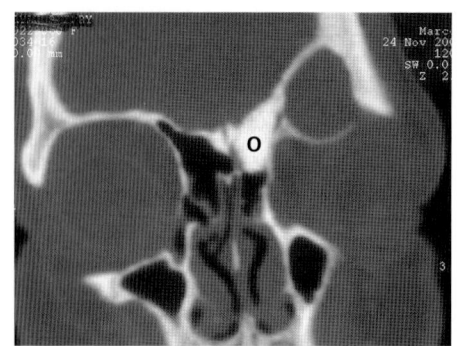

Fig. 4.98 Osteoma causing secondary mucocele. **a** Coronal CT scan shows expansion of the left frontal sinus, compatible with a large mucocele, secondary to an osteoma. **b** Coronal CT scan shows osteoma (o), obstructing the left frontal recess. Note the supraorbital extent of the left frontal mucocele. Case courtesy of Michael Friedman, MD, Chicago, IL, USA.

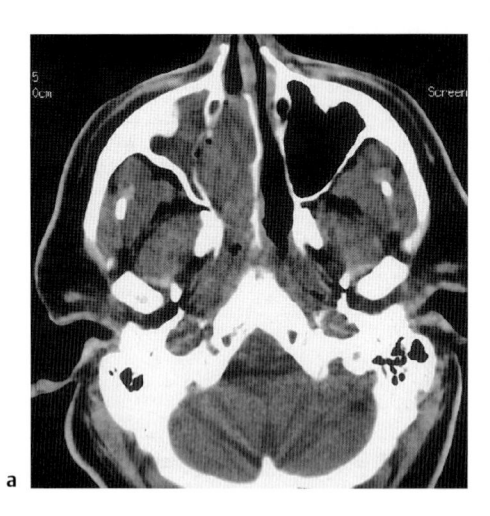

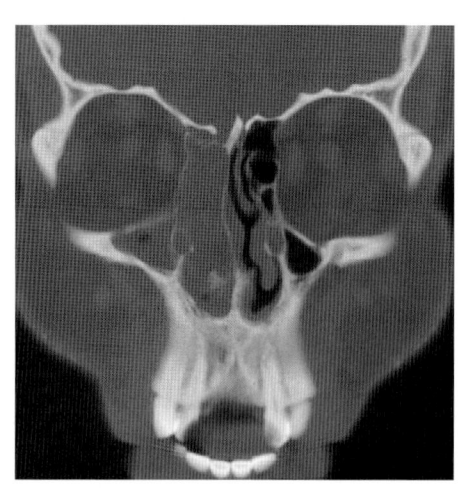

Fig. 4.99 Inverted papilloma. **a**, **b** Axial and coronal CT scans, showing a right nasal mass, compatible with surgically proven inverted papilloma, extending into the right side of the nasopharynx.

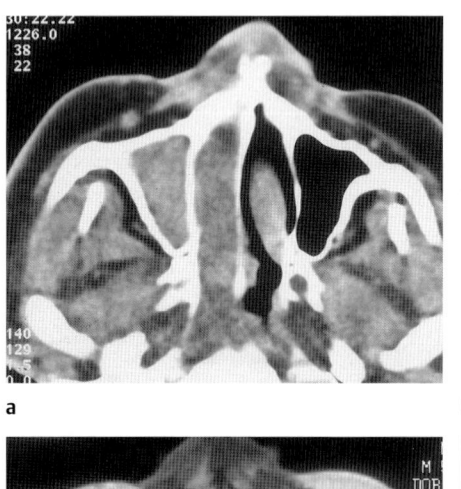

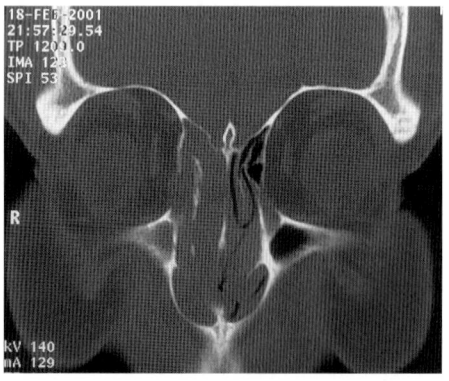

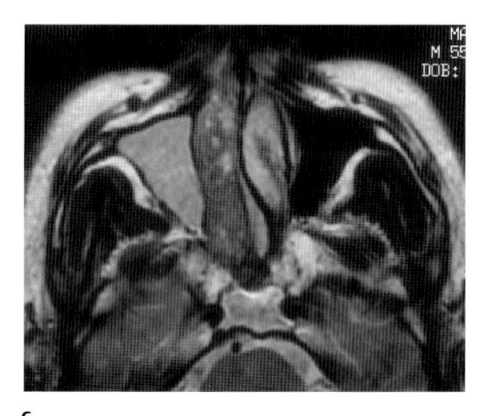

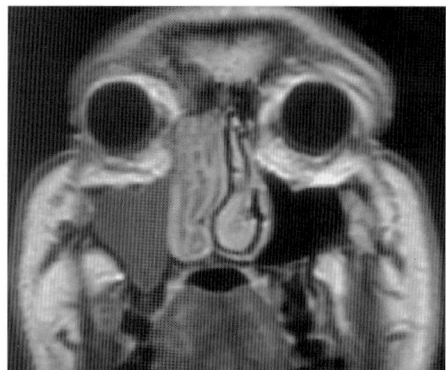

Fig. 4.**100 a–e** Inverted papilloma. **a** Enhanced axial and **b** coronal CT scans, showing a large right nasal mass compatible with an inverted papilloma. Note that the right maxillary sinus opacification may be due either to tumor extension or to an obstructive inflammatory process. **c** Axial T2W, **d** axial postcontrast T1W, and **e** coronal postcontrast T1W MR scans, showing inverted papilloma. The opacification of the right maxillary sinus is due to obstructive sinus disease, which could not be distinguished from tumor extension on CT scans.

Fig. 4.**100 f, g** ▷

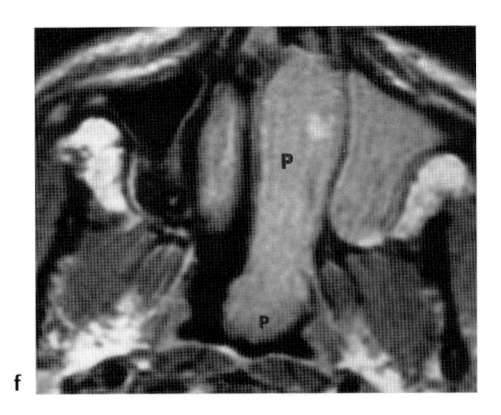

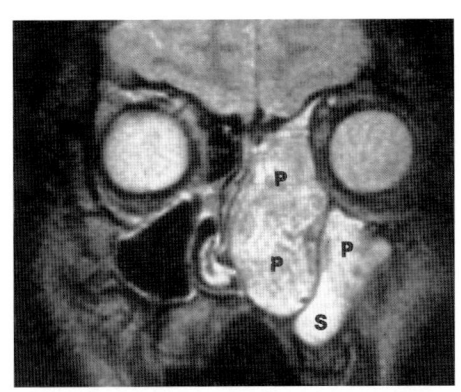

Fig. 4.**100f, g** Inverted papilloma. **f** Axial PW and **g** coronal T2W MR scans in another patient, showing a large inverted papilloma (P), extending into the left maxillary sinus and nasopharynx. Note the hyperintense retained secretion along the floor of the maxillary sinus (S).

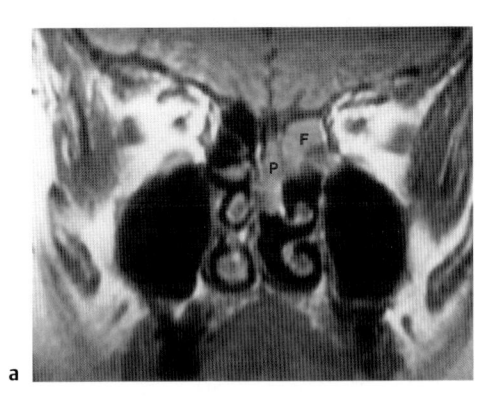

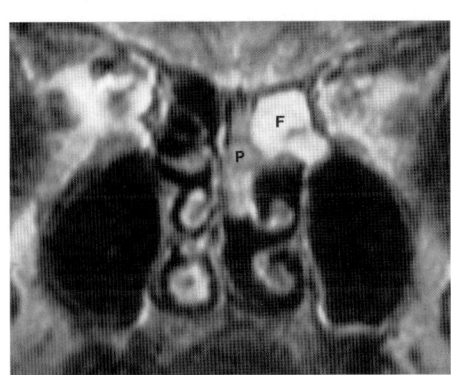

Fig. 4.**101** Cylindrical papilloma. **a** Axial PW and **b** T2W MR scans, showing an intranasal papilloma (P). Note retained fluid in the posterior ethmoid (F).

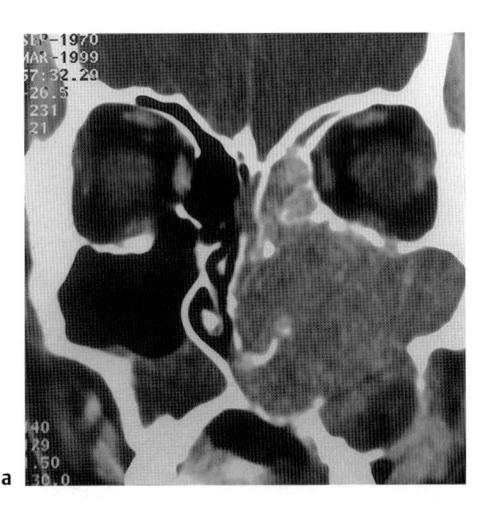

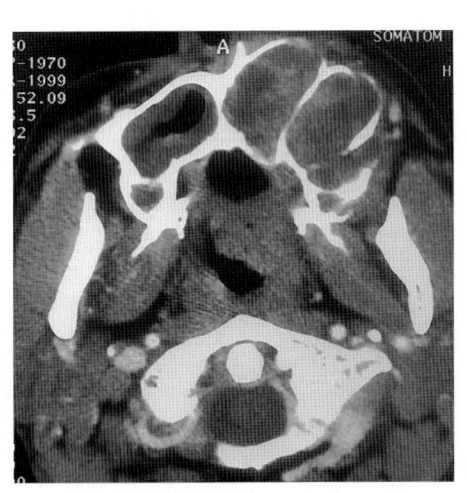

Fig. 4.**102** Exophytic and inverting papilloma. **a** Enhanced coronal and **b** axial CT scans, showing a large nasal papilloma extending into the left maxillary sinus, resulting in marked expansion of the lower aspect of the maxillary sinus. On histological examination this was interpreted as a papilloma with mainly exophytic as well as inverting components.

The etiology of papillomas remains unproven, though human papilloma virus (HPV) types 6/11 have been identified in sinonasal papillomas.[3] Papillomas may occur simultaneously with nasal inflammatory polyps.[3] Sinonasal papillomas are not associated with an increased risk or with the development of additional papillomas elsewhere in the upper respiratory tract.[3] The consistent identification of microscopic mucous cysts interspersed throughout the neoplastic epithelium is one histological characteristic that differentiates papillomas of the sinonasal cavities from those arising from stratified squamous epithelium elsewhere in the body.[16] Inverted papillomas (IP), although benign, are locally invasive, exhibiting a characteristic endophytic growth pattern with inversion of the surface epithelium into the underlying stroma. Most cases involve the nasal cavity and the paranasal sinuses; only 5% of cases demonstrate exclusive sinus involvement.[17] IP have been found to have an associated malignancy rate of 7–15%, with squamous cells being the most common pathological type.[17] Schneiderian papilloma of the middle ear may arise in association with a sinonasal papilloma or rarely may develop in the middle ear with no evidence of tumor in the sinonasal cavity.[15, 16] It is hypothesized that during embryogenesis there may be an ectopic migration of the ectodermally derived schneiderian membrane that lines the sinonasal cavities to the endodermally derived mucosa of the other part of the upper aerodigestive tract, including the tubotympanic recess.[16]

The most common clinical presentation of IP is unilateral nasal obstruction and epistaxis. The characteristic imaging ap-

Fig. 4.**103** Pleomorphic adenoma of hard palate. **a** Sagittal T1W and **b** coronal T2W MR scans, showing a hard palate mass (M), compatible with a pleomorphic adenoma.

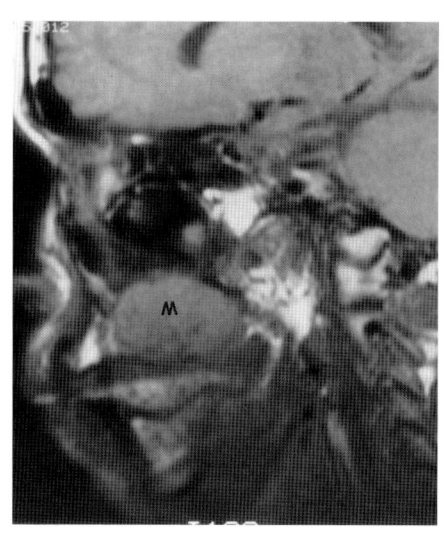

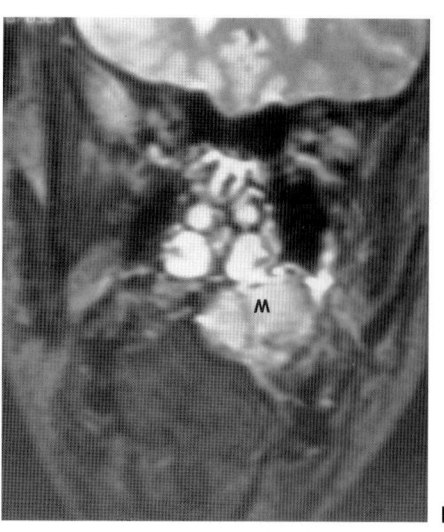

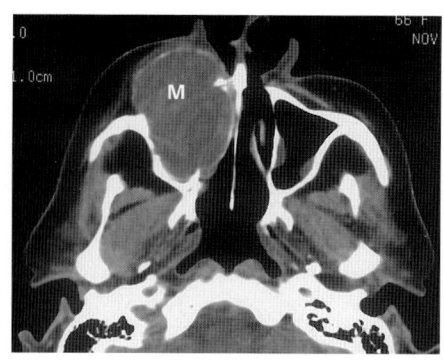

Fig. 4.**104** Pleomorphic adenoma of maxillary sinus. Axial CT scan shows a well-defined mass (M) involving the right maxillary antrum and extending into the adjacent soft tissue of the right cheek.

pearance of IP is a unilateral polypoid mass occupying the lateral nasal wall and paranasal sinus (Figs. 4.**99**–4.**101**). Seventy percent of cases have been found to show evidence of bony erosion (pressure erosion) on CT scan.[17] However, this finding is usually secondary to bony remodeling and pressure atrophy rather than true bone erosion. Papillomas demonstrate more signal intensity on T2-weighted MR images than malignant tumors of the nasal cavities. Experience with sinonasal papillomas has proved that recurrence is related to inadequate excision.[16] Transnasal excision, Caldwell–Luc procedure, and lateral rhinotomy with medial maxillectomy have all been used with recurrence rates of 58–71%, 35%, and 13%, respectively. Therefore, the latter procedure has been considered to be the best treatment by multiple centers.[17] It is therefore important to have a baseline CT scan 8–10 weeks after surgery for comparison purposes when the patient will have follow-up CT scanning years later. Associated squamous cell carcinoma has been noted in 5–13% of sinonasal papillomas of the inverted and cylindrical types.[16] Hyams[14] reported that a transition line from benign papilloma to the malignant lesion could be demonstrated in some instances.

Adenoma

Adenomas occur wherever there are glandular elements in the epithelium, such as the nose, paranasal sinuses, and nasopharynx. These may simulate a nasal polyp but are locally invasive and again show local recurrence if not completely excised. The pleomorphic adenoma arising from minor salivary glands can arise from the palate or from ectopic glands in the nares, or very rarely in a paranasal sinus (Figs. 4.**103**, 4.**104**). Malignant mixed tumors are much more common in the minor salivary glands than in the major glands (Fig. 4.**105**).[1, 3, 12]

Hemangiomas

Hemangiomas must always be considered wherever blood vessels are present.[12] They may be capillary or cavernous, an isolated finding or part of a syndrome, such as the Osler–Weber–Rendu (AV fistula) syndrome. Cavernous hemangiomas occur less frequently in the upper respiratory tract, as compared with the capillary hemangiomas.[3] Cavernous hemangiomas are more often identified on the turbinates rather than on the septum.[3] The lobular polypoid form of capillary hemangioma is a form of hemangioma occurring on skin and mucous membranes. The lesion has been synonymously referred to as pyogenic granuloma.

However, the term is a misnomer in that the lesion is neither an infectious process nor granulomatous.[3] The lesion is most often identified in the anterior portion of the nasal septum referred to as Little's area or Kisselbach's triangle.[3] The next most common site is the tip of the turbinates. The etiology remains unclear but is associated with prior trauma and with pregnancy ("pregnancy" tumor). Histologically, the vascular component are arranged in lobules or clusters composed of central capillaries that give off smaller ramifying tributaries.[3] The vascular component is surrounded by granulation tissue and chronic inflammatory cell infiltrate.[3] The "pregnancy" tumor is a lobular capillary hemangioma that occurs in the gravid state and that regresses after parturition.[3] Hemangioma of the cartilaginous septum is the most aggressive, and tends to recur if not completely excised.[12] Intraosseous hemangiomas are uncommon tumors; the most frequent sites are the calvaria and the vertebral column. Involvement of the facial bones is rare, and occurs most commonly in the maxilla, mandible, nasal bone, zygoma and frontal bone.

Hemangiomas are now thought to be hamartomas with an anomalous proliferation of endothelial-lined vascular channels.[13] Intraosseous hemangiomas have a characteristic sharply marginated expansile lesion with intact cortical outline and sunburst pattern of radiating trabeculae. Hemangiomas are hypointense on T1-weighted and hyperintense on T2-weighted MR images. The trabeculae typically show low signal intensity. There will be intense enhancement on dynamic CT scans as well as on post-gadolinium MR images. The CT and MRI characteristics of intraosseous hemangioma may be similar to hemangiopericytoma (Fig. 4.**106**, see also Fig. 4.**149**).

Angiofibroma

Angiofibroma is a benign, highly vascular, nonencapsulated neoplasm that occurs almost exclusively in adolescent males, with intracranial involvement in 20–36% of patients.[1, 12, 18–20] The lesion is histologically benign but locally aggressive. Angiofibromas almost always have a nasopharyngeal origin near the pterygopalatine fossa. The tumor then spreads into the nasopharynx, nasal cavity, maxillary sinus, sphenoid sinus, ethmoid sinus (Fig. 4.**107**), and infratemporal fossa, into the orbit through the inferior orbital fissure, and intracranially through the foramen rotundum, pterygoid canal, and superior orbital fissure. In the clinical setting, CT scans, MR images, and angiographic findings are diagnostic. Angiofibromas demonstrate marked enhance-

Sinonasal Pathology   417

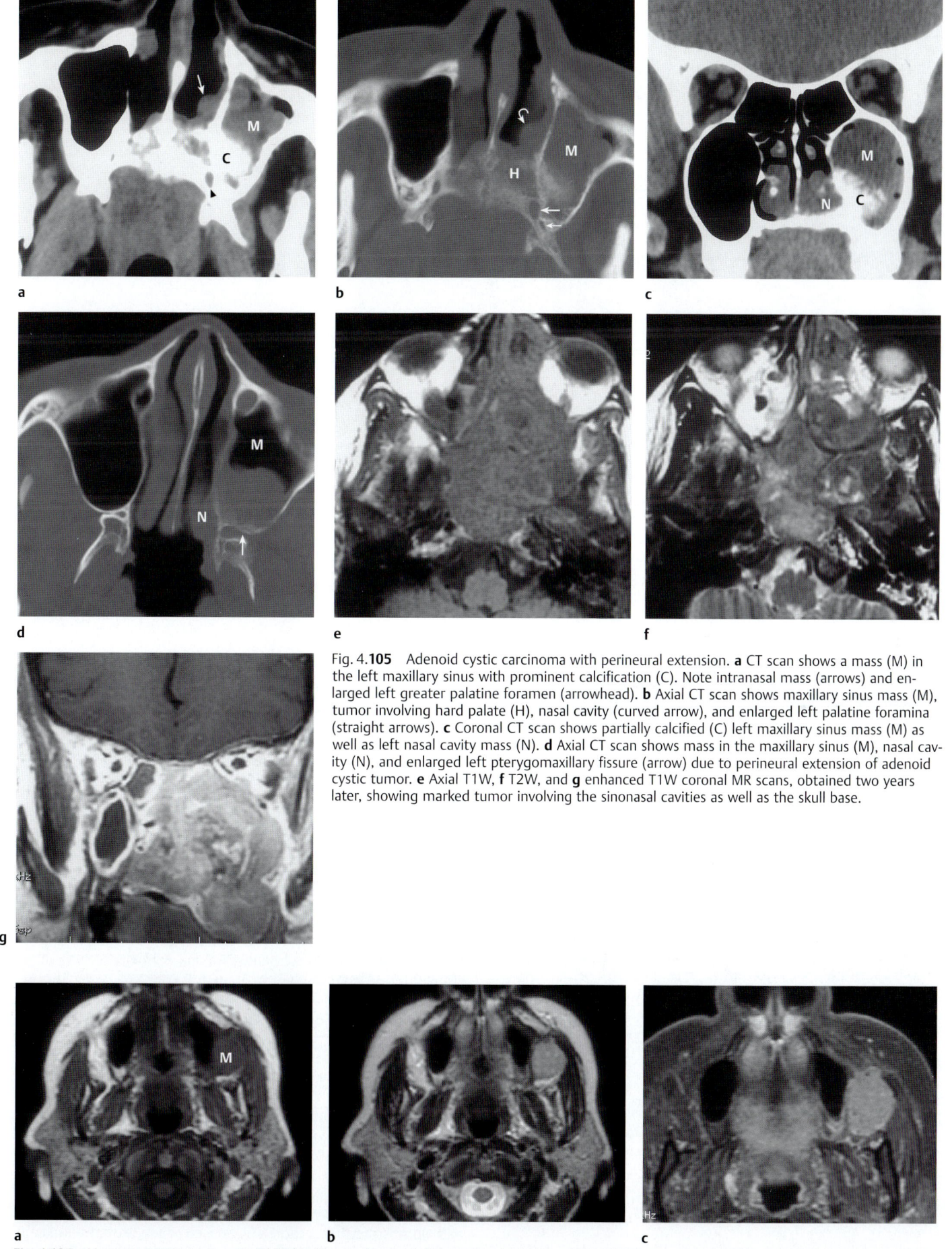

Fig. 4.**105** Adenoid cystic carcinoma with perineural extension. **a** CT scan shows a mass (M) in the left maxillary sinus with prominent calcification (C). Note intranasal mass (arrows) and enlarged left greater palatine foramen (arrowhead). **b** Axial CT scan shows maxillary sinus mass (M), tumor involving hard palate (H), nasal cavity (curved arrow), and enlarged left palatine foramina (straight arrows). **c** Coronal CT scan shows partially calcified (C) left maxillary sinus mass (M) as well as left nasal cavity mass (N). **d** Axial CT scan shows mass in the maxillary sinus (M), nasal cavity (N), and enlarged left pterygomaxillary fissure (arrow) due to perineural extension of adenoid cystic tumor. **e** Axial T1W, **f** T2W, and **g** enhanced T1W coronal MR scans, obtained two years later, showing marked tumor involving the sinonasal cavities as well as the skull base.

Fig. 4.**106** Hemanigopericytoma. **a** Axial T1W MR scan shows a left buccal mass (M). **b** Axial T2W MR scan. **c** Axial enhanced fat-suppression T1W MR scan. The tumor is hyperintense on T2W (**b**) and demonstrates marked enhancement (**c**).

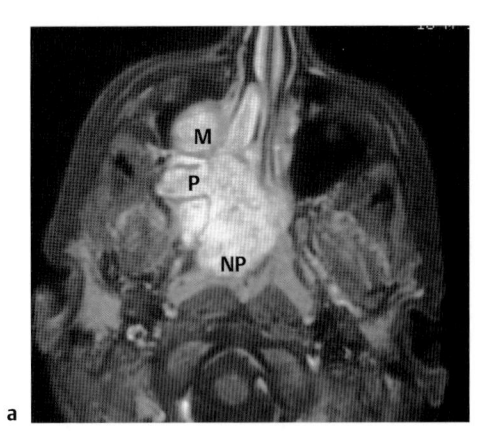

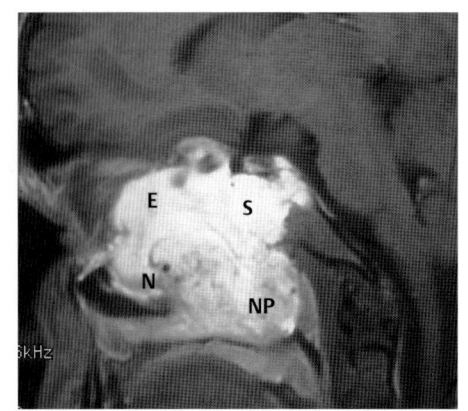

Fig. 4.**107** Juvenile angiofibroma in 13-year-old boy. **a** Axial enhanced T1W fat-suppression MR scan shows a large tumor with intense enhancement within the nasopharynx (NP), pterygomaxillary fissure (P), and maxillary sinus (M). **b** Sagittal enhanced T1W fat-suppression MR scan shows tumor in the nasopharynx (NP), nasal cavity (N), ethmoid (E), and sphenoid (S) sinuses.

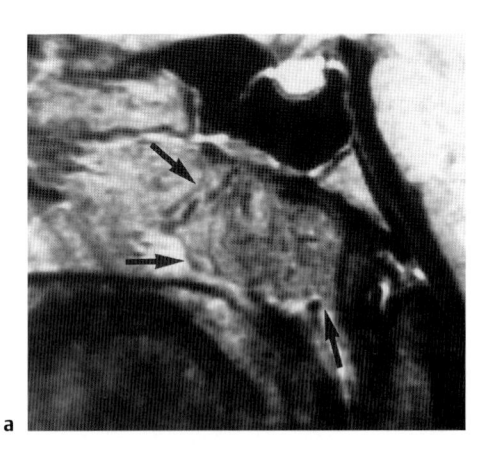

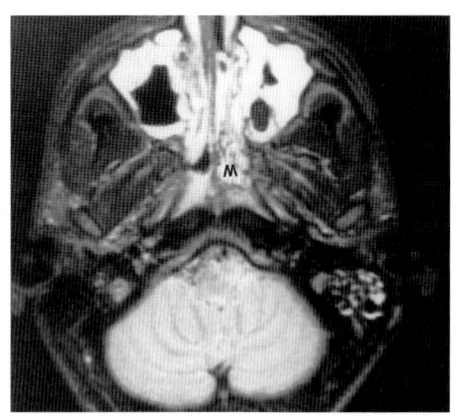

Fig. 4.**108** Recurrent juvenile angiofibroma in a 19-year-old man. **a** Sagittal PW MR scan shows a posterior nasal cavity mass (arrows) extending into the nasopharynx. Note several signal flow voids, indicative of increased vascularity. **b** Axial T2W MR scan shows nasal and nasopharyngeal mass (M). Note inflammatory changes in the maxillary sinuses.

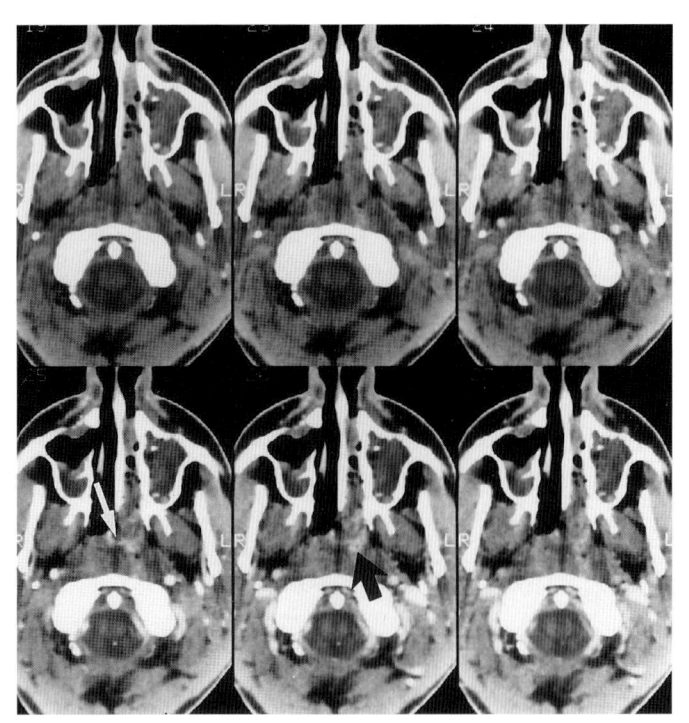

Fig. 4.**108 c** Serial dynamic CT scans, obtained following rapid injection of intavenous contrast material, showing rapid enhancement of angiofibroma (arrows).

ment on CT scans (Fig. 4.**107**). On dynamic CT scans they reveal intense early enhancement characteristic of highly vascular lesions.[19] On MR images, these lesions appear as a mass of low-to-intermediate signal intensity on T1-weighted and proton-density-weighted images and of intermediate-to-high signal intensity on T2-weighted MR scans (Fig. 4.**108**). There may be multiple flow-void channels, which represent increased vascularity. This increased vascularity can be confirmed by performing gradient-echo MR pulse sequences. Angiofibromas reveal marked enhancement on Gd-DTPA enhanced T1W MR images (Fig. 4.**108**).

Neurogenic Tumors

Nasal Glioma

Nasal gliomas are attributed to glial cell rests and can occur as nodules at the base of the nose, simulating a dermoid, or as an intranasal mass simulating polyp (see Fig. 4.**53 a**). As with other congenital anomalies in this area, a connection with the intracranial cavity should be excluded prior to any attempted removal of the tumor.[1, 12]

Schwannoma

Peripheral nerve sheath tumors are divided into schwannomas, neurofibromas, and neurogenic sarcomas. Most of these tumors arise from sensory nerves; motor nerves are infrequent sites of these tumors. In the sinonasal cavities, neurogenic tumors arise from the first and second divisions of the trigeminal nerve and from the autonomic nerves. The olfactory nerve, like the optic nerve, has no Schwann cells and therefore cannot be the site of these tumors. Schwannomas are often solitary and encapsulated and do not recur if completely excised. They are infrequent in sinonasal cavities. Those that have been reported were found in the nasal fossa and maxillary, ethmoidal, and sphenoid sinuses.

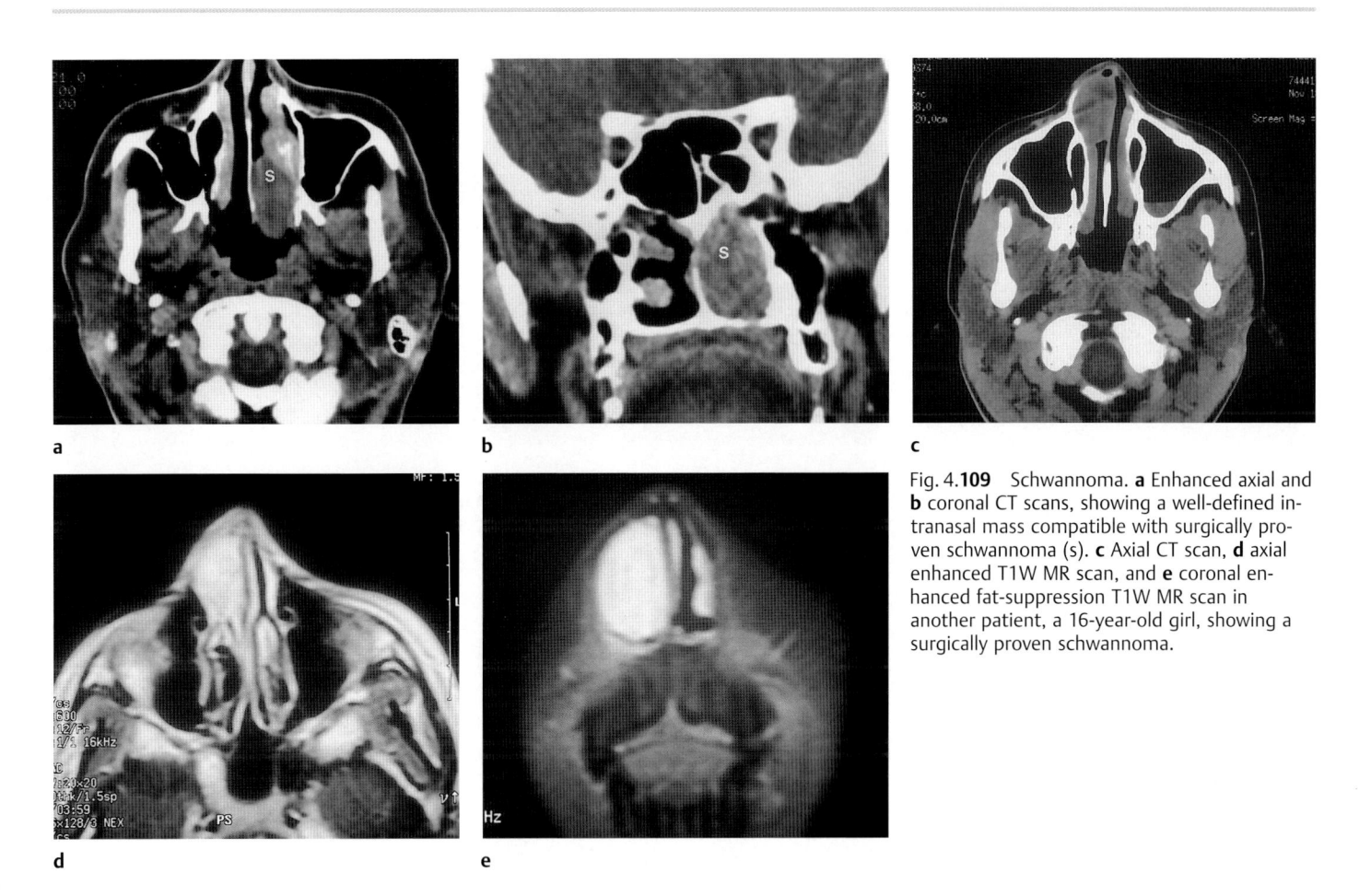

Fig. 4.**109** Schwannoma. **a** Enhanced axial and **b** coronal CT scans, showing a well-defined intranasal mass compatible with surgically proven schwannoma (s). **c** Axial CT scan, **d** axial enhanced T1W MR scan, and **e** coronal enhanced fat-suppression T1W MR scan in another patient, a 16-year-old girl, showing a surgically proven schwannoma.

On CT scans, schwannomas appear as well-defined, homogeneous masses, and reveal moderate enhancement after intravenous injection of contrast material (Fig. 4.**109**). Schwannomas, however, may be inhomogeneous as well as cystic. Malignant schwannomas are destructive. On MR images, schwannomas reveal low to intermediate signal intensity on T1-weighted and hyperintensity on T2-weighted images (Figs. 4.**109**, 4.**110**). They demonstrate moderate to marked enhancement after intravenous administration of Gd-DTPA (Figs. 4.**110c, d**). Schwannomas may have varied signal characteristics depending upon their histological patterns (Antoni type A and B) and the presence or absence of cystic as well as cholesterol degeneration. Schwannomas are bone-pushing and remodeling lesions (Fig. 4.**110**), and the presence of aggressive bone destruction should be considered an indication of malignant degeneration. Some of the sinonasal schwannomas may be extensive without evidence for malignancy (see Chapter 3). Hemangiopericytomas may simulate a sinonasal schwannoma (Fig. 4.**111**).

Meningioma

Meningiomas may extend into the sinonasal cavities (Figs. 4.**112**, 4.**113**). In rare situations, a meningioma may be found in the sinonasal cavities, arising from ectopic arachnoid tissue (Fig. 4.**114**). Intrasinus meningioma may be completely calcified, simulating an osteoma or fibrous dysplasia.

Epithelial Odontogenic Cysts Involving the Sinonasal Cavities

Many odontogenic cysts and tumors arise in the maxilla and mandible.[12] These include dentigerous cysts, which are epithelialized sacs that develop from the enamel organ of an unerupted tooth (Fig. 4.**115**). Dentigerous cysts tend to be expansile and well-circumscribed, and may grow at varying rates. A definite diagnosis of dentigerous cyst and other odontogenic cysts such as odontogenic keratocyst (OKC)[21] can only be made histopathologically.[21] OKC was first reported by Philipsen[22] in 1956. It is classically described as an intraosseous lesion of the jaw that is notorious for its destructive, aggressive nature and high propensity for recurrence.[21] The OKC is believed to arise from the cell rests of the enamel dental lamina, the oral epithelial lining of the developing tooth follicle before dental hard tissues are formed. Another theory is that the OKC develops owing to extension of cells from the basal layer of oral epithelium into the mandible or maxilla.[21] OKC may appear as a simple or multiloculated cyst. It is aggressive and may involve significant portion of the mandible or maxilla (Fig. 4.**116**). Multiple odontogenic cysts, especially the keratocyst, occur in the first and second decades as part of the basal cell nevus (Gorlin–Goltz syndrome),[12] inherited in an autosomal dominant manner (Fig. 4.**117**). These patients also have developmental anomalies of the skeleton. OKC appears on CT as an expansile cystic mass. The mandibular lesions are often scalloped and may occasionally demonstrate high attenuation values related to high protein concentrations. At times, calcifications may be seen in the peripheral or central portions of the cyst.[21] The lesion may be extensive, involving half of the mandible or maxilla, associated with cortical break and displacement or of, extension into, the adjacent soft tissues (Figs. 4.**118**, 4.**119**). Those involving the maxilla would appear as an expansile or nonexpansile cystic mass arising from the alveolar ridge and extending into the maxillary sinus (Figs. 4.**116**, 4.**117**). There may be a calcified rim, separating the cyst from the mucoperiosteal outline of the maxillary sinus (Fig. 4.**115b**). On MRI, the OKC has low to intermediate signal intensity on T1-weighted and high signal intensity on T2-weighted MR images (Figs. 4.**118b**, 4.**119**). There will be no contrast enhancement on CT and MR scans. At times, inho-

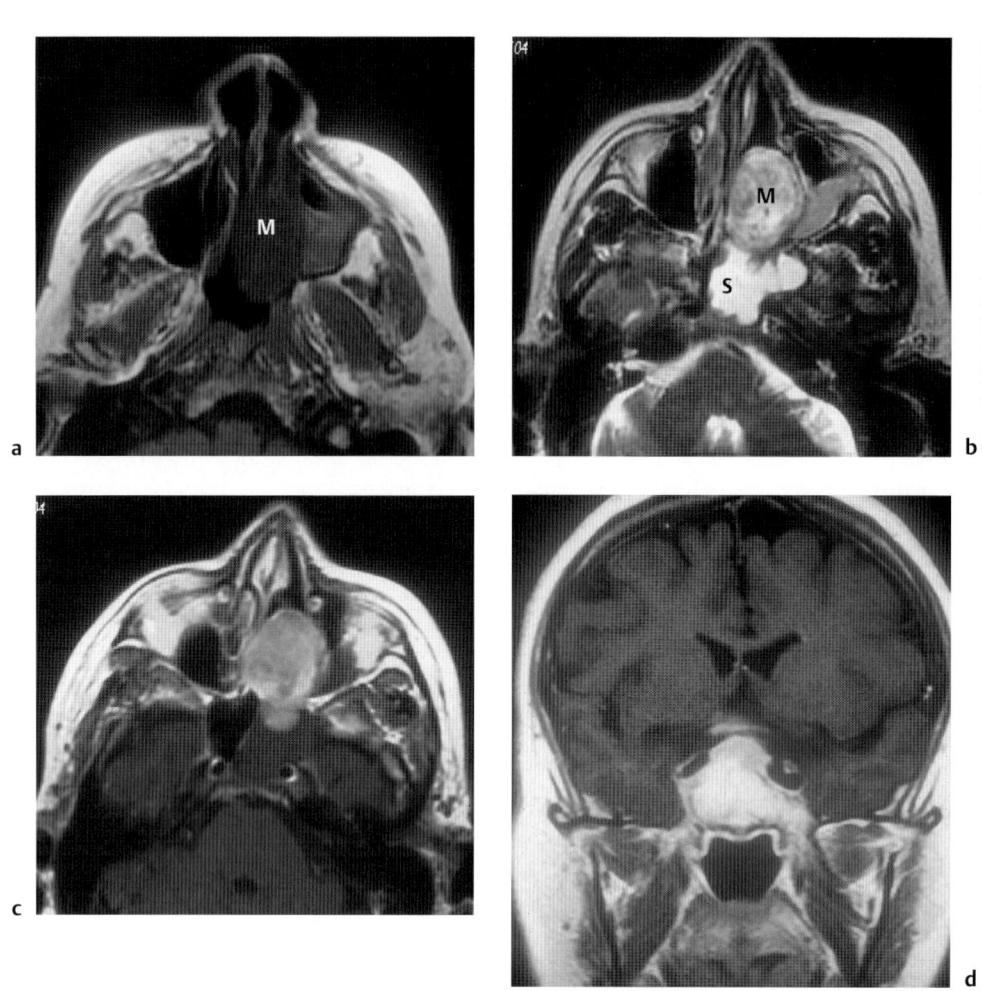

420   4 Imaging of the Nasal Cavity and Paranasal Sinuses

Fig. 4.**110** Schwannoma. **a** Axial T1W MR scan shows a mass (M) in the left nasal cavity, compatible with a schwannoma. **b** Axial T2W MR scan reveals a heterogeneous, predominantly hyperintense mass (M), compatible with schwannoma. Note retained secretion in the sphenoid sinus (S). **c** Enhanced axial T1W MR scan reveals homogeneous enhancement of tumor. Note extension into the sphenoid sinus and the resultant retained secretion within left sphenoid sinus. **d** Enhanced coronal T1W MR scan in another patient shows an enhanced mass within the sphenoid sinus, compatible with a schwannoma. Fig. **d** courtesy of Harish Shownkeen, MD, Chicago, IL, USA.

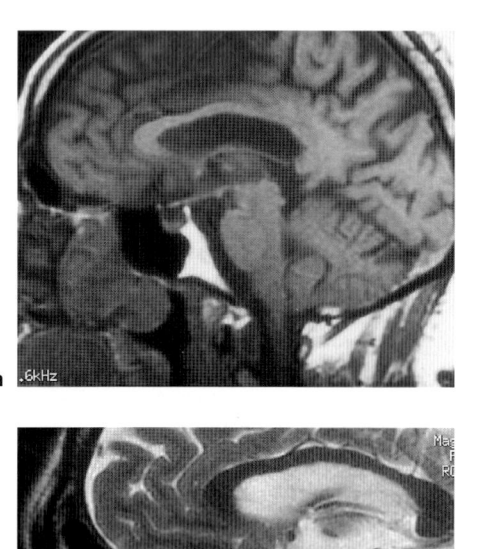

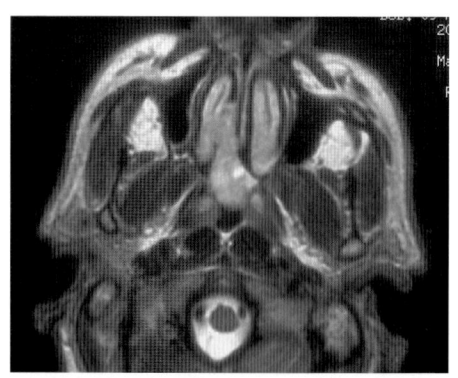

Fig. 4.**111** Nasal mass. **a** Sagittal T1W, **b** axial T2W, **c** sagittal T2W, and **d** coronal enhanced T1W MR scans showing a well-defined intranasal mass medial to the right middle turbinate. Differential diagnoses include papilloma, schwannoma, pleomorphic adenoma, hemangiopericytoma, ethesioneuroblastoma and nasal polyp. The tumor was very vascular at surgery. Histological evaluation was consistent with hemangiopericytoma.

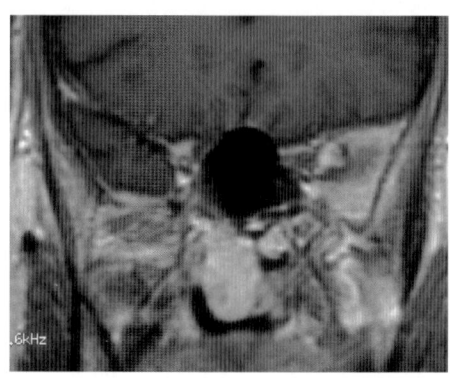

Sinonasal Pathology 421

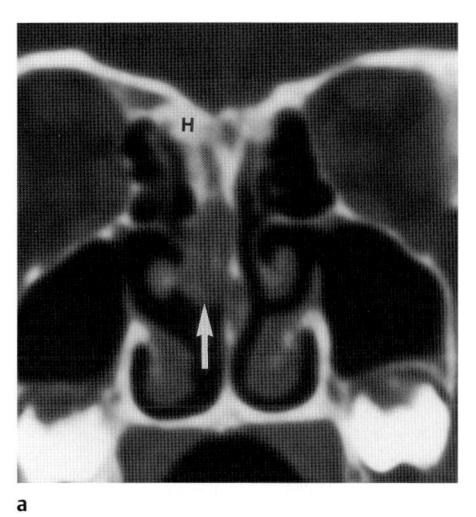

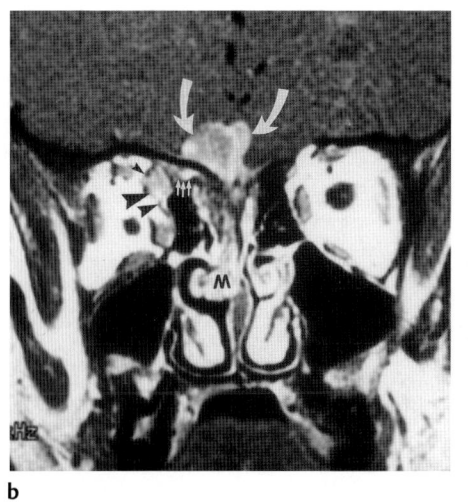

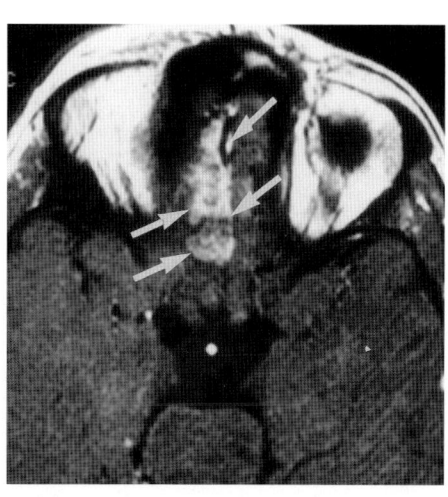

Fig. 4.112 Olfactory meningioma extending into the nasal cavity. a Coronal CT scan shows a nasal mass (arrow) compatible with extension of a meningioma into the nasal cavity. Note hyperostotic changes (H). b Coronal enhanced T1W MR scan shows olfactory plate meningioma (large arrows). Note extension of tumor along the ethmoid canal (triple white arrows) into the orbit (arrowheads). Note also tumor extension into the nasal cavity (M). c Axial enhanced T1W MR scan shows olfactory plate meningioma (arrows). Case Courtesy of Dr. E.L. Tajudine, Saudi Arabia

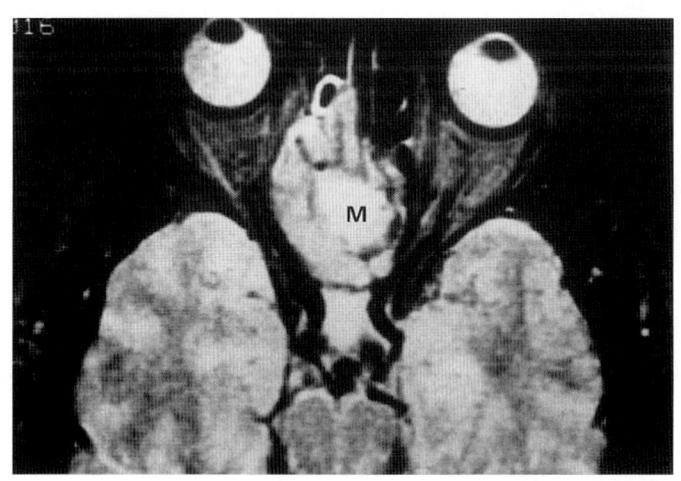

Fig. 4.113 Meningioma. T2W MR scan shows a large mass (M) involving the sphenoidal and right ethmoidal sinuses. This was due to extension of an intracranial meningioma. Primary intrasinus or intranasal meningioma may occur, arising from ectopic arachnoid tissue (see Fig. 4.114).

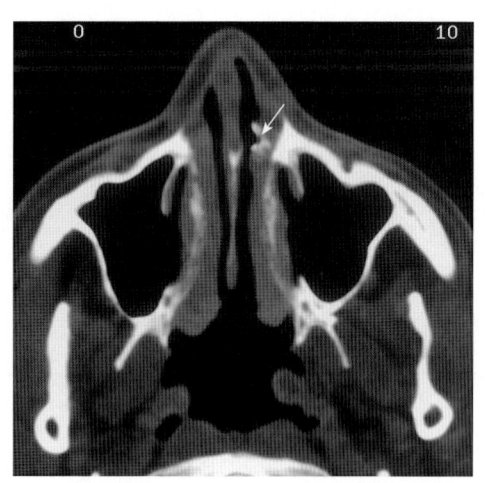

Fig. 4.114 Meningioma of the nasal cavity, arising from ectopic arachnoid granulation. Axial CT scan shows small calcification along the anterior aspect of the left inferior turbinate (arrow). This is related to a recurrence of intranasal meningioma. Clinically, it was thought that the patient had a small papilloma. The lesion was biopsied twice and pathology was consistent with meningioma.

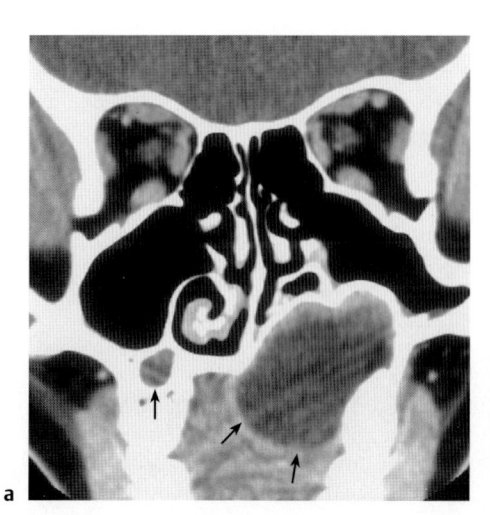

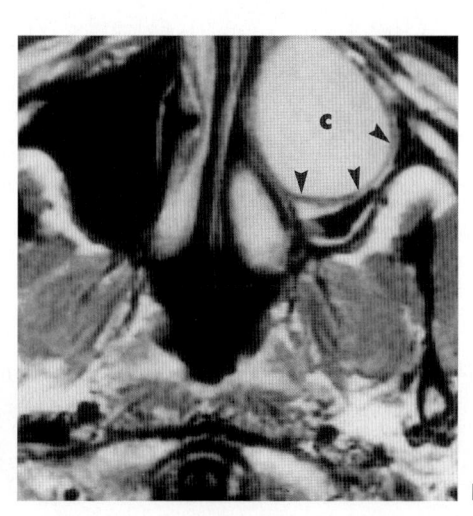

Fig. 4.115 Odontogenic cyst. a Coronal CT scan shows a large left maxillary and a small right maxillary odontogenic cysts (arrows). b Axial PW MR scan in another patient shows a hyperintense keratogenic cyst (C) protruding into the left maxillary sinus. Note the characteristic cyst capsule (arrows), separated by air from the sinus mucosal lining.

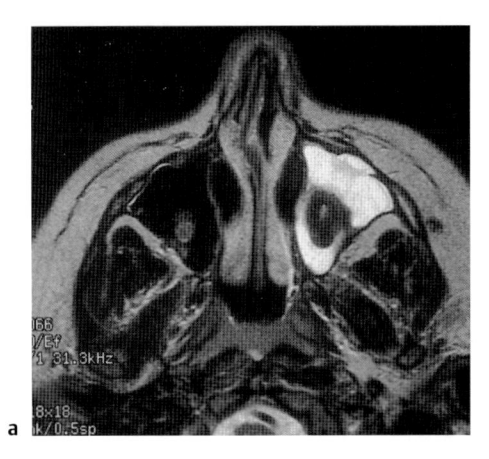

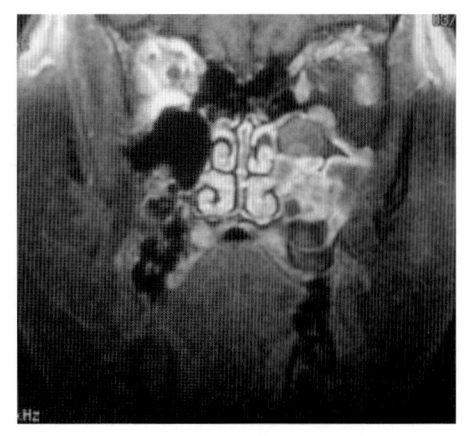

Fig. 4.116 Multiple odontogenic cyst. **a** Axial T2W MR scan shows a large left maxillary odontogenic cyst. Note a hypointense molar tooth within it. There are small cysts within the right maxillary antrum. **b** Enhanced fat-suppression coronal T1W MR scan, showing moderate enhancement within the cysts. Enhancing component within an odontogenic cyst should be carefully examined for possible malignant transformation.

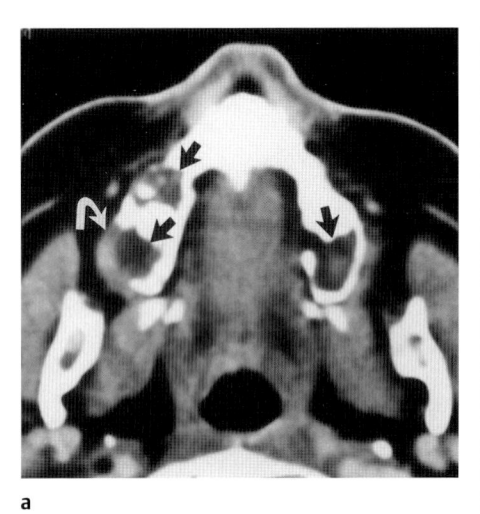

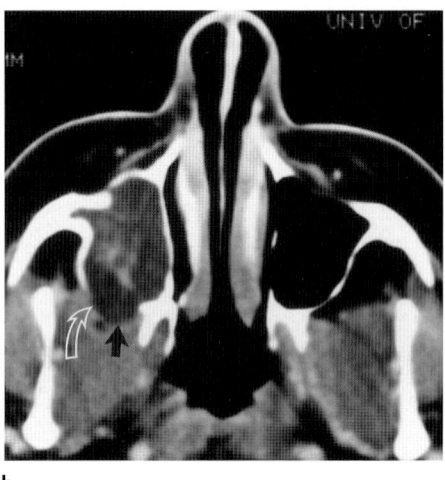

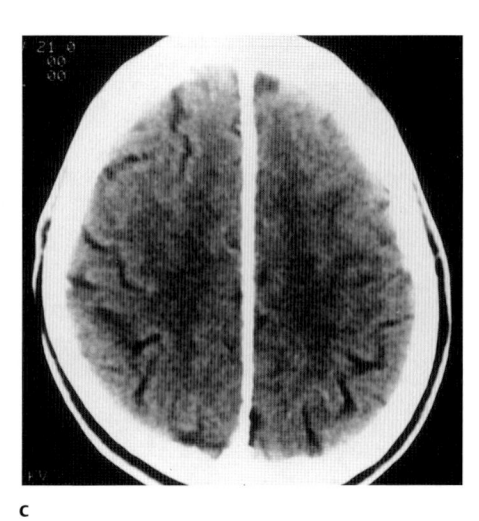

Fig. 4.117 Multiple keratogenic cysts (= basal cell nevus syndrome). **a** Enhanced CT scan shows multiple cysts (arrows) involving the alveolar process of the maxilla. **b** Scan at a higher level to that of **a** shows extension of cyst within the right maxillary antrum. Note some enhancement within the lesion. Some of this cyst may not show any enhancement. **c** CT scan shows marked calcification of the falx.

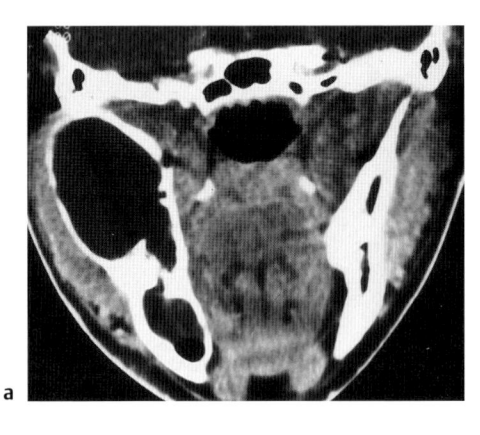

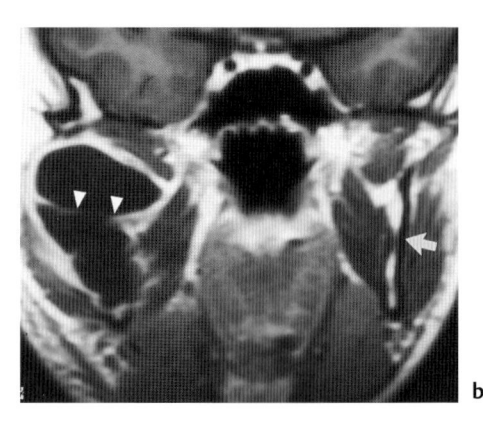

Fig. 4.118 Large odontogenic keratogenic cyst. **a** Coronal CT scan and **b** coronal contrast-enhanced T1W MR scan showing cystic expansion of the right mandible. The MR scan (**b**) shows the fluid-filled cyst, with air–fluid level from recent biopsy (arrowheads). The walls/septae of the cyst demonstrate contrast enhancement (**b**), but no soft-tissue component is seen. Arrow = normal left mandibular ramus.

mogeneous contrast enhancement may be present (Figs. 4.**116b**, 4.**118b**, 4.**119d**). Radicular cysts of the periodontal membrane occur at the root of a carious tooth. These cysts tend to be destructive and may tend to develop an oral–antral fistula after tooth extraction. Ameloblastomas may occur in the maxilla and mandible, and are often multicystic and honeycombed in appearance (Figs. 4.**120**–4.**122**). They may undergo malignant degeneration and thus must be completely excised. The mesodermal type of odontic tumor arising from the mesenchyme of the tooth bud may also be seen, such as the myxoma, odontogenic fibroma, and cementoblastoma. The mixed types of tumor consisting of ectodermal and mesodermal components include the odontoma, the complex composite odontoma, and the compound composite odontoma (Figs. 4.**123**, 4.**124**).

Nonodontogenic Cysts

Nonodontogenic cysts are named according to their location. The median or fissural cyst is frequently found in the maxilla and is usually lined with squamous epithelium. The nasopalatine duct cyst (NDC) (Fig. 4.**125**) or cyst of the incisive canal is the most

Sinonasal Pathology 423

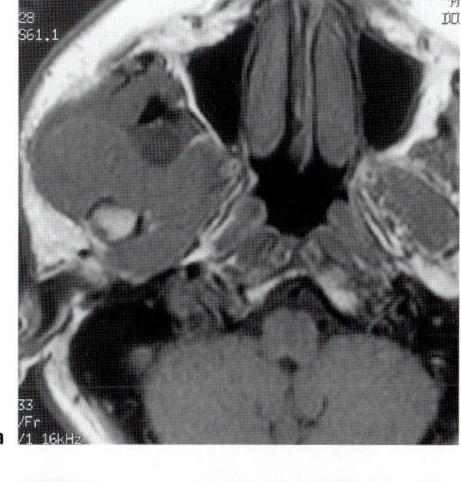

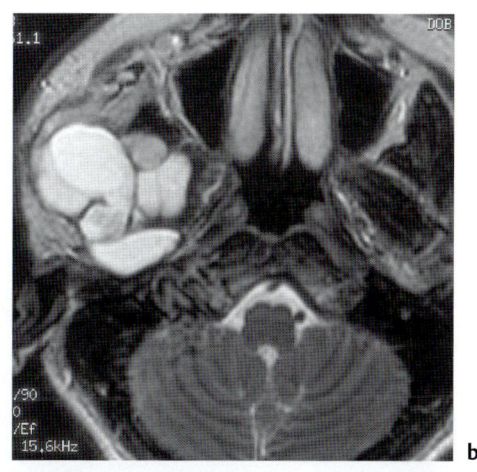

Fig. 4.**119** Large keratogenic cyst extending into the infratemporal fossa. **a** T1W MR scan shows a large mass in the right infratemporal fossa. **b** T2W MR scan shows multicystic hyperintense lesion in the right infratemporal fossa. **c** Enhanced T1W and **d** fat-suppression enhanced T1W MR scans showing no significant enhancement within the cystic lesion. However, note deformity as well as increased enhancment of the right masseter muscle. The enhancement is a reactive response to invasion of the cyst into the masseter muscle (M) confirmed at surgery.

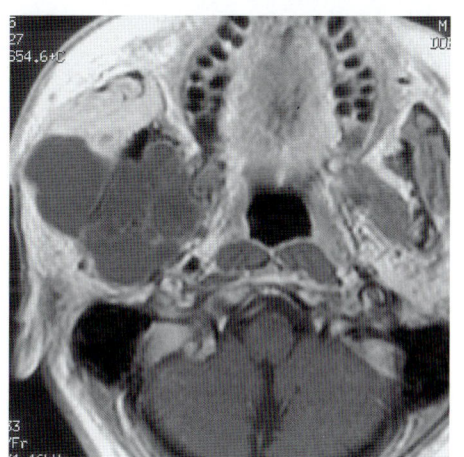

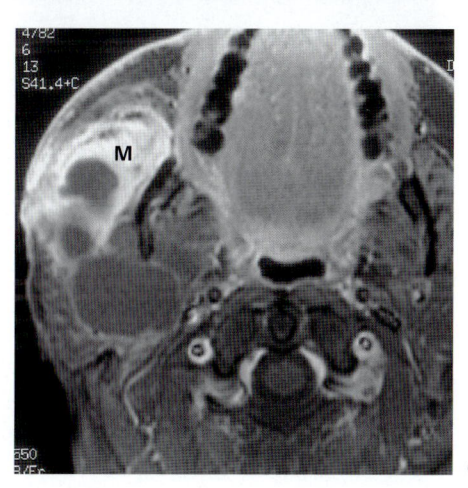

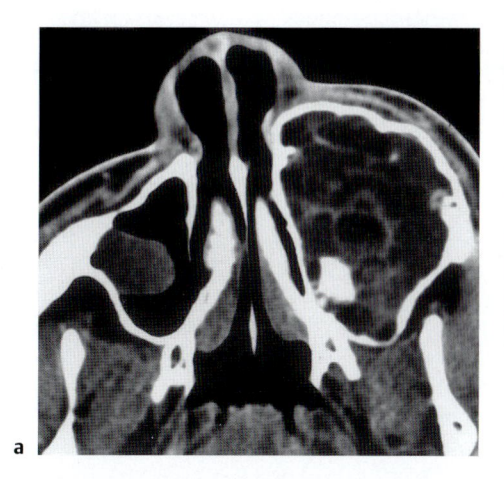

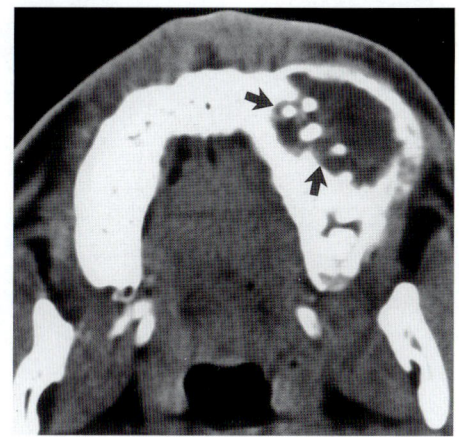

Fig. 4.**120** Ameloblastoma. **a**, **b** Axial CT scans show an expansile heterogeneous mass involving the maxillary alveolar process (arrows) and maxillary antrum on the left side. Case Courtesy of Hatem Sherif, MD, Cairo, Egypt.

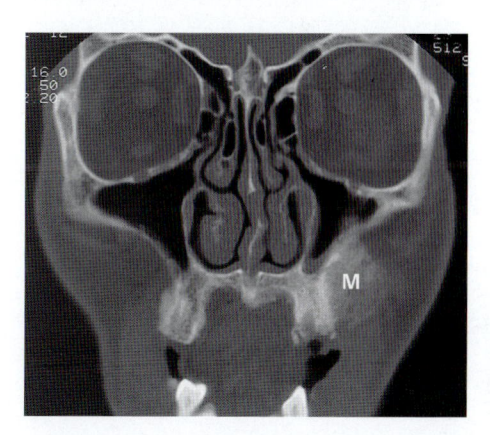

Fig. 4.**121** Ameloblastoma. Coronal CT scan shows an expansile partially calcified mass (M), involving the alveolar process of the maxilla.

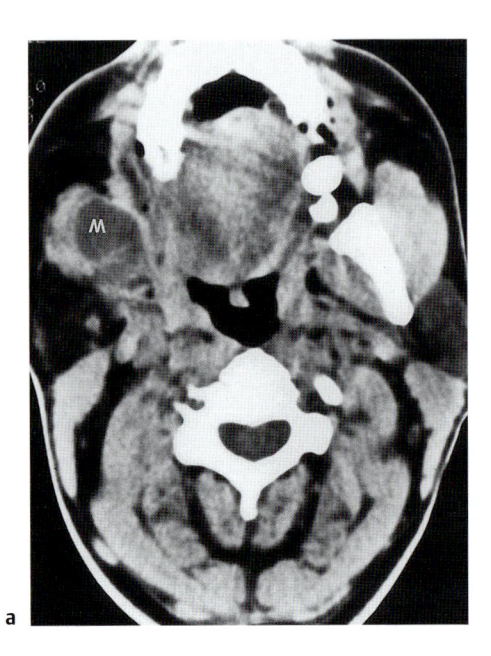

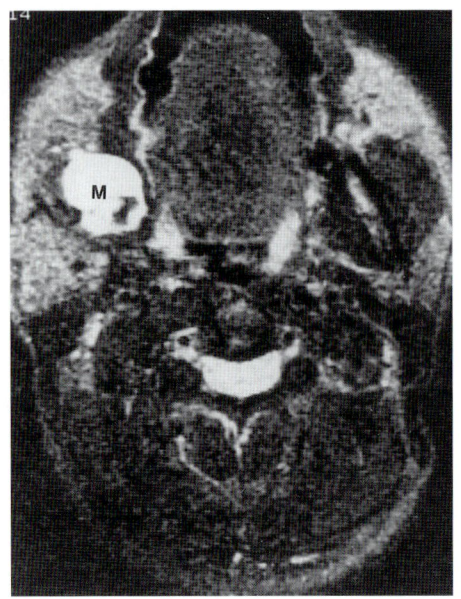

Fig. 4.**122** Recurrent ameloblastoma. **a** CT scan shows a large buccal mass (M) compatible with recurrent ameloblastoma. Note surgical absence of right mandibular ramus. **b** Axial T2W MR scan showing a hyperintense buccal mass (M) compatible with recurrent ameloblastoma.

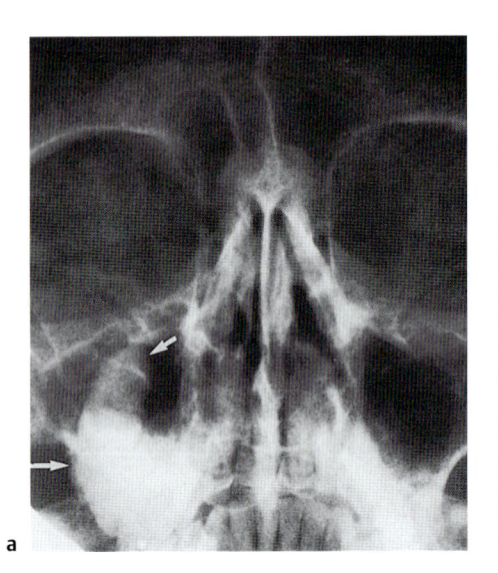

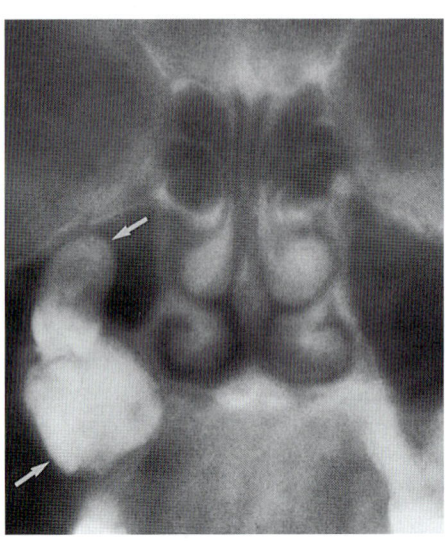

Fig. 4.**123** Compound composite ondontoma, right. **a** Waters projection; **b** AP tomogram. A well-defined tooth and a dense mass in the alveolar process are part of the compound composite ondontoma (arrows). From Reference 12.

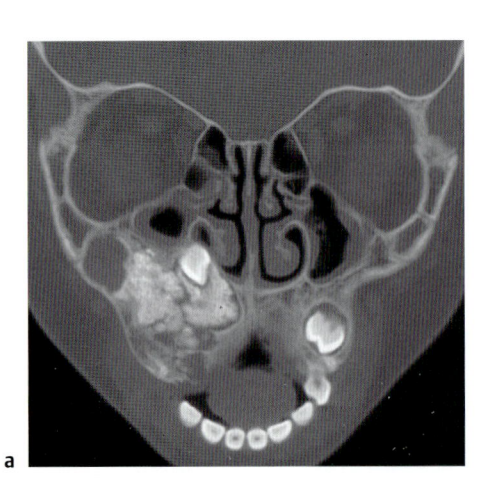

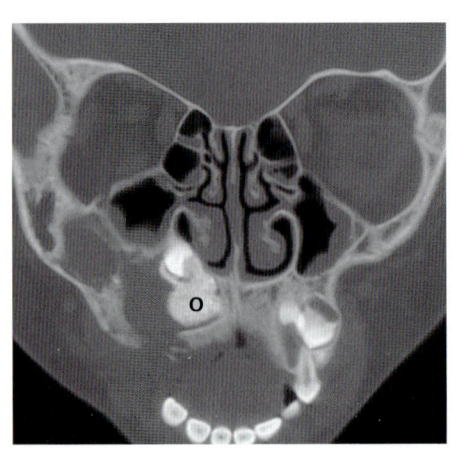

Fig. 4.**124** Compound composite odontoma in a 7-year-old girl. **a** Coronal CT scan shows a dense mass and a tooth in the alveolar process of the right maxilla compatible with odontoma. **b** Postoperative coronal CT scan shows residual odontoma (O).

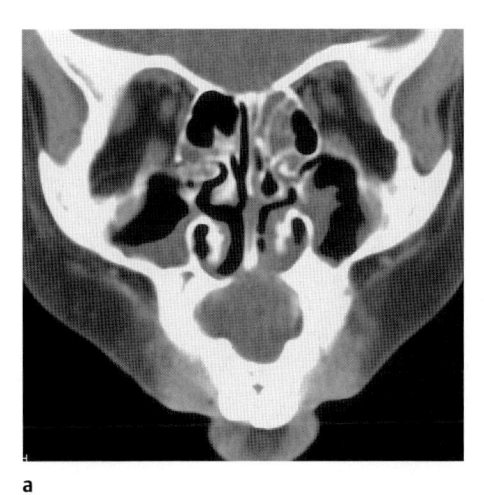

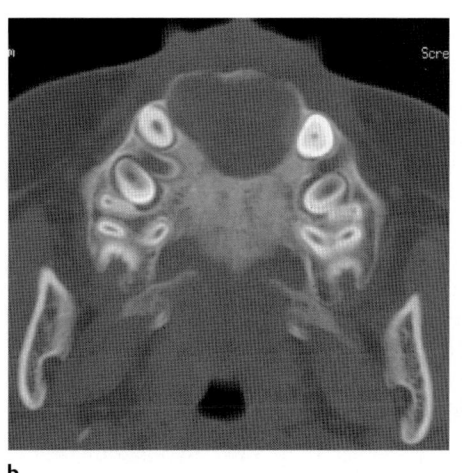

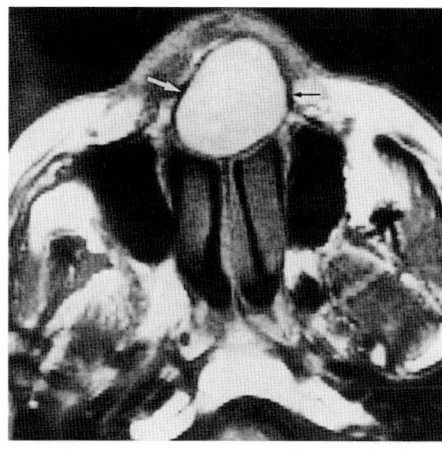

Fig. 4.**125 a**, **b** Nasopalatine duct cyst ("incisural cyst"). **a** Coronal and **b** axial CT scans showing a nasopalatine duct cyst ("incisural cyst") involving the premaxilla. **c** Incisive canal cyst; T1W MR image. The cyst (arrows) is seen to be enlarging the incisive canal. Fig. 4.**125 c** from B.L. Carter, MD, Thieme 1988.

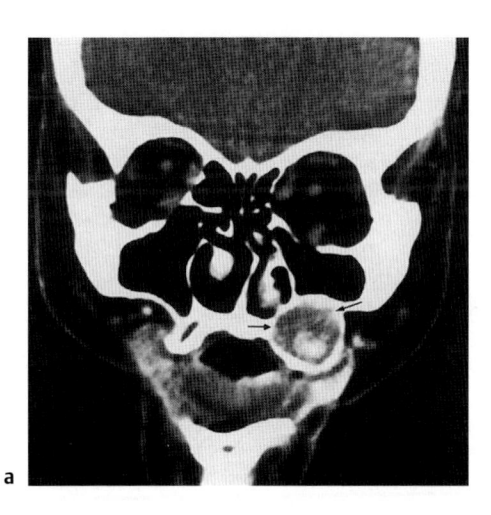

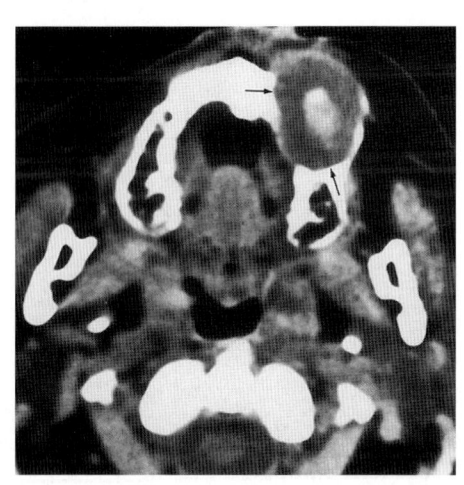

Fig. 4.**126 a**, **b** Globulomaxillary cyst, left maxilla. **a** Coronal CT, **b** axial CT. The cyst (arrows) has expanded bone and contains proteinacious material with some calcification. From Reference 12.

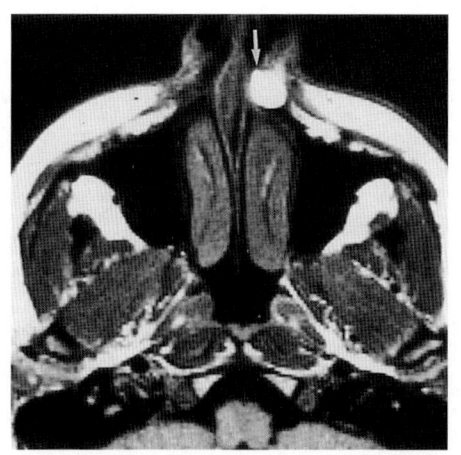

Fig. 4.**127** Nasoalveolar cyst. T1W MR scan. The cyst (arrow) is displacing the nasal process of the maxilla and has a high protein content with a strong signal. From Reference 12.

common cyst of nonodontogenic origin in the maxilla. The NPD cyst was previously thought, like all fissural cysts, to originate from epithelium that was trapped during the fusion of the embryonic process. This concept has since been discarded, and it is now believed that the NDC develops from epithelial remnants of the oronasal ducts present within the incisive canals.[12,23] These cysts may become secondarily infected or activated by trauma. Other cysts in the area are the globulomaxillary cyst (Fig. 4.**126**), located between the lateral incisor and canine teeth, the nasoalveolar cyst (Fig. 4.**127**) in the lateral nasal floor, radicular cyst, and the "aneurysmal bone cyst."[12,23] The midline location of nasoalveolar cyst and vitality of underlying incisors reduces the possibility of radicular cyst, and the precise midline location generally eliminates the possibility of ameloblastoma.[23] The cysts are prone to infection and may become enlarged, resulting in facial deformity; they should be excised.[12,21] Globulomaxillary cyst is a historical term used to describe a cyst that is located between the lateral incisor and cuspid, originating from epithelial rests between the medial nasal and maxillary processes during embryonic fusion. Nasoalveolar cysts are found between the ala and the maxilla and do not invade or separate bone (Fig. 4.**127**).

Extracranial Craniopharyngioma

Craniopharyngioma is an epithelial tumor that resembles the ameloblastoma of the jaw. It arises from rests of squamous epithelial cells that are believed to be remnants of Rathke's pouch. It usually arises in the suprasellar region but can be in-

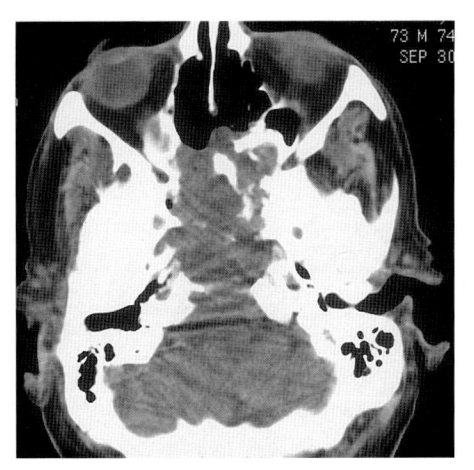

Fig. 4.**128** Ameloblastoma of the sphenoid sinus. Axial CT scan shows a destructive midline mass, replacing the sphenoid sinus and extending into the posterior ethmoid cells. The lesion was highly hyperintense on T2W MR images, simulating a mucocele.

trasellar. Although rarely, similarly to ameloblastoma it can arise within the sphenoid sinus and base of the skull (Figs. 4.**128**, 4.**129**). Extracranial craniopharyngioma may be extensive. Intrasphenoid ameloblastoma and craniopharyngioma have similar CT and MR appearance of sphenoid sinus mucocele. Extracranial craniopharyngioma may appear as a destructive mass with both soft-tissue and cystic components (Fig. 4.**129**). This subject is discussed further in Chapter 3.

Epithelial Odontogenic Tumors

Odontogenic tumors include ameloblastoma, calcifying epithelial odontogenic tumor (Pindborg tumor) and clear cell odontogenic carcinoma[24–27]. Ameloblastoma is the most common benign, but aggressive, epithelial odontogenic tumor. More than 80% involve the mandible. Maxillary ameloblastomas primarily occur in the molar region (Figs. 4.**120**–4.**122**). The tumor may arise in or extend into the soft tissue adjacent to retromolar region (Fig. 4.**130**). Ameloblastoma is discussed in more detail in Chapter 6. Calcifying epithelial odontogenic tumor (CEOT) is a benign neoplasm characterized by solid epithelial layers or islands, an acellular hyalinized stromal bridge interspersed with foci of an amyloid-like substance, and variable amounts of round, conglomerate, or concentric laminar (Liesegang ring) calcifications.[24] Two-thirds of the CEOTs arise in the mandible, whereas one-third arise in the maxilla. The maxillary tumor appears on CT scan as an expansile partially calcified mass. The lesion may contain an unerupted tooth within it. On T1-weighted and T2-weighted MR images the tumor appears heterogeneous in signal characteristics. The noncalcified component of tumor shows moderate to marked enhancement on enhanced T1-weighted pulse sequences.[24]

Granular Cell Tumor

Granular cell tumor (granular cell myoblastoma) is an uncommon benign lesion affecting the mucous membranes of the upper aerodigestive tract.[28] The most common site is the anterior third of the tongue. In the palate, the tumor may simulate a mixed tumor (pleomorphic adenoma) or an adenoid cystic tumor. Perineural extension has been reported.[28] Most are benign, but approximately 10% have malignant behavior with metastasis to the regional lymph nodes as well as distant metastasis.[28] This tumor was thought to arise from myoblasts, but recent investigations, including immunohistochemical analysis, have suggested a neurogenic origin on the basis of the close association of the tumor with the nerves and ultrastructural findings of neurofilaments in the granular tumor cells.[3, 28] This has been supported by the fact that S-100 protein has been found in granular cell tumor. The S-100 protein is found in neurons and in Schwann cells in the late phase of cell development.[28] It is not found in myoblasts.[28] The use of S-100 protein and neuron-specific enolase stains has confirmed the neurogenic origin of this tumor. The presence of myelinated and nonmyelinated axonlike structures is evidence that granular cell tumors are of Schwann cell origin. The tumor typically appears as a solid mass, although multifocal tumors have been reported.

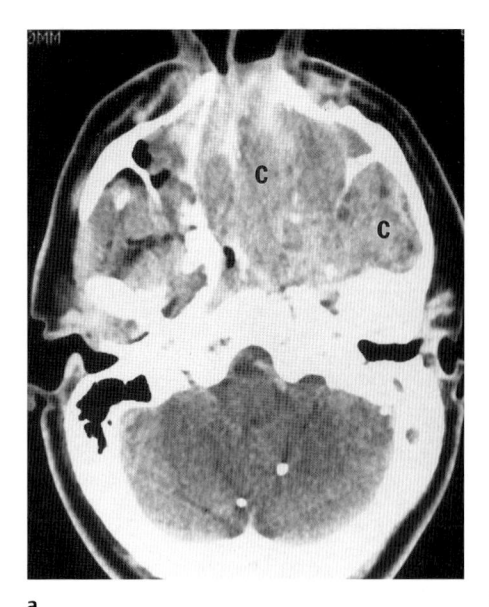

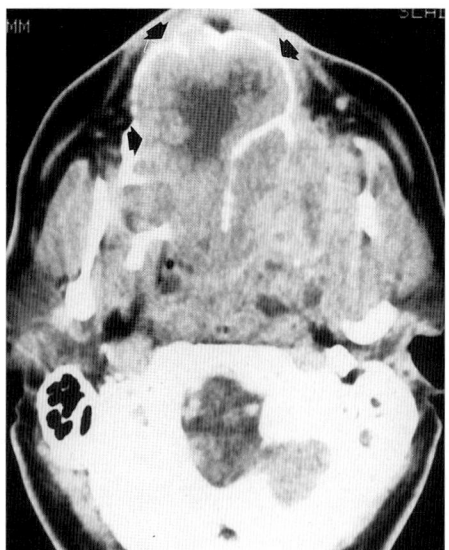

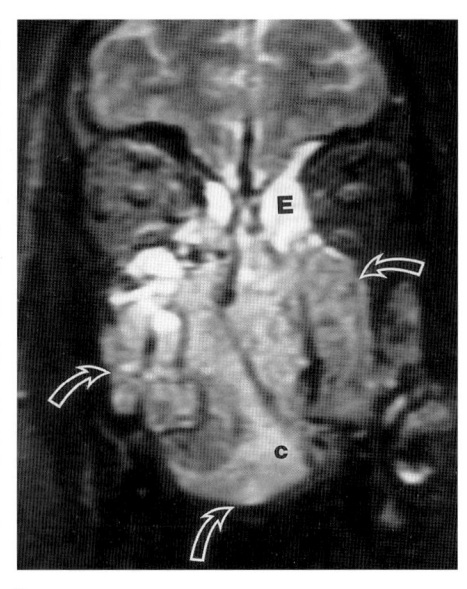

Fig. 4.**129** Extracranial craniopharyngioma. **a** Enhanced CT scan shows soft-tissue infiltration in the nasopharynx, nasal cavities, maxillary sinuses, and left infratemporal fossa, related to a large extracranial craniopharyngioma (C). **b** Enhanced CT scan shows further extension into the hard palate (arrows). **c** Coronal T2W MR scan shows extensive tumor in the sinonasal cavities (arrows). Note fluid collection in the hard palate component (C) and retained mucosal secretion in the ethmoid (E).

Malignant Odontogenic Tumors

Clear Cell Odontogenic Carcinoma

Clear cell odontogenic carcinoma (CCOC) is a rare neoplasm that has been described within the past two decades.[25] It is an indolent, locally aggressive tumor with a propensity for multiple local recurrences. Waldron et al.[26] and Hansen et al.[27] described the first five patients. Since then, more than 30 different cases have been reported. The mandible is the most commonly affected. The differential diagnosis of intraosseous clear cell tumors of the jaws includes metastatic carcinoma, particularly renal cell carcinoma, central (primary osseous) salivary gland tumors (which may undergo clear cell change such as mucoepidermoid carcinoma, clear cell carcinoma, acinic cell carcinoma, or epithelial–myoepithelial carcinoma),[27] and odontogenic tumors (which may have a clear cell component, such as calcifying epithelial odontogenic tumor and ameloblastoma with clear cell change).[27]

Epithelial Tumors of the Sinonasal Cavities

Malignant epithelial tumors of the nasal cavity and paranasal sinuses account for a small percentage of the number of cancer cases in the United States, with the incidence estimated to be less than 0.4% of all new cancers.[1] Most nasal cavity and paranasal sinus malignancies, however, are epithelial tumors (Table 4.**9**).

These tumors can be subdivided into tumors of epithelial origin or of salivary gland origin. Tumors of epithelial origin can be further divided into papillomas, squamous cell carcinomas, adenocarcinomas, and anaplastic cacinomas.[5, 9, 10, 11, 20, 29, 30, 31] Tumors of salivary gland origin include pleomorphic adenomas, adenoid cystic carcinomas, acinic cell carcinomas, and mucoepidermoid carcinomas.[5, 9, 10, 11, 20] In general, malignant tumors of the nasal cavity are rare. The differential diagnosis of cancer in the nasal cavity includes squamous cell carcinoma, adenocarcinoma, undifferentiated carcinoma, melanoma, lymphoma, adenoid cystic carcinoma, and rarely mucoepidermoid carcinoma.

Malignant neoplasms arising from the paranasal sinuses are rare. These cancers represent less than 5% of all head and neck malignancies.[1, 32] Myers and co-workers[32] reported their 18-year single-institution experience at the University of Michigan from 1980 to 1997. Their cancer registry identified 170 patients treated for a paranasal sinus malignancy; 141 of them had complete data. There were 87 male and 54 female patients. The pathologies and distribution of affected sites in their series are summarized in Table 4.**10**.

Most of the patients presented with advanced-stage disease regardless of histopathological type. Only 6 of 141 patients (4.3%) presented with regional metastasis. Even with aggressive primary treatment, 71 patients developed a recurrence with a median time to recurrence of 336 days.[32] The 5- and 10-year disease-specific survival rates in their series were 52% and 35%, respectively.

Squamous Cell Carcinomas

Squamous cell carcinomas of the paranasal sinuses are twice as common in men as in women and most commonly occur in the sixth and seventh decades of life. Dull unilateral pain and unilateral purulent nasal secretion may be relatively early signs of a nasal cavity or paranasal sinus carcinoma. In one study, the most common presenting symptom was facial pain (42% of patients). Nasal obstruction was the second most common symptom, occurring in 29% of patients, followed by facial swelling, which occurred in 26% of patients.[32] The presence of lymph node metastases at the time of the initial evaluation was uncommon and was reported to be approximately 10%.[32] Within the maxillary sinus, squamous cell carcinoma frequently presents as a swelling or distortion of surrounding structures, such as the

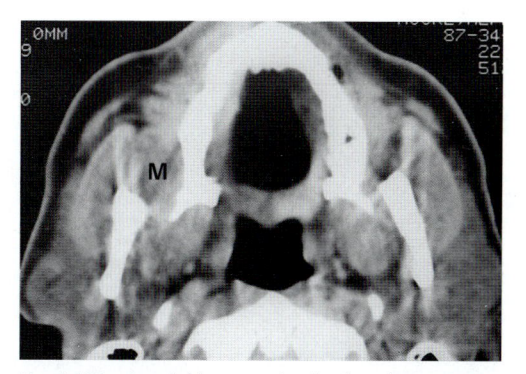

Fig. 4.**130** Ameloblastoma in the bucal space. CT scan shows a right buccal mass (M) compatible with histologically proven ameloblastoma.

Table 4.**9** Classification of nasal cavity and paranasal sinus malignant neoplasms

1	Epithelial
	• Squamous cell carcinoma
	• Respiratory carcinoma
	• Adenocarcinoma (mucosal)
	• Minor salivary gland neoplasms
2	Mesenchymal/neuroectodermal/hematopoietic
	• Malignant melanoma
	• Olfactory (esthesio)neuroblastoma
	• Midline malignant reticulosis = non-Hodgkin-lymphoma
	• Malignant lymphoma
	• Malignant fibrous histiocytoma
	• Fibrosarcoma
	• Malignant schwannoma
	• Leiomyosarcoma
	• Angiosarcoma
	• Osteosarcoma
	• Chondrosarcoma
	• Tetracarcinoma
	• Others

Table 4.**10** Pathologies and distribution of affected sites in 141 malignancies of paranasal sinuses

Histology	Affected sinus				
	Maxillary	Ethmoid	Frontal	Sphenoid	Total
Squamous cell carcinoma	61	8	1	3	73
Adenoid cystic carcinoma	12	5	0	0	17
Adenocarcinoma	7	9	0	0	16
Lymphoma	9	0	0	1	10
Olfactory neuroblastoma	0	9	0	0	9
Osteosarcoma	4	0	0	0	4
Fibrosarcoma	2	1	0	0	3
Sinonasal undifferentiated carcinoma	0	2	0	0	2
Plasmacytoma	1	1	0	0	2
Anaplastic sarcoma	1	0	0	0	1
Hemangiopericytoma	0	1	0	0	1
Melanoma	0	1	0	0	1
Ewing sarcoma	0	0	0	1	1
Malignant schwannoma	1	0	0	0	1
Total	98	37	1	5	141

From Myers LL, Nussenbaum B, Bradford CR, et al. Paranasal sinus malignancies: an 18-year single institution experience. Laryngoscope 2002; 112: 1964–1969.

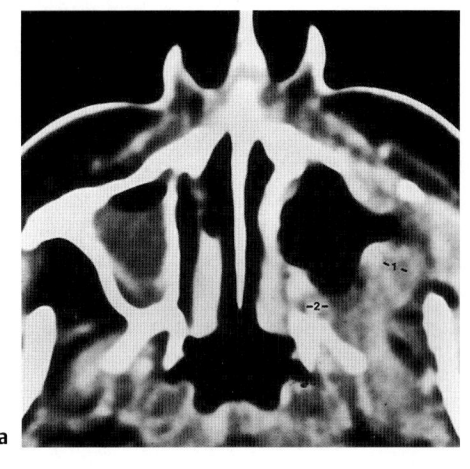

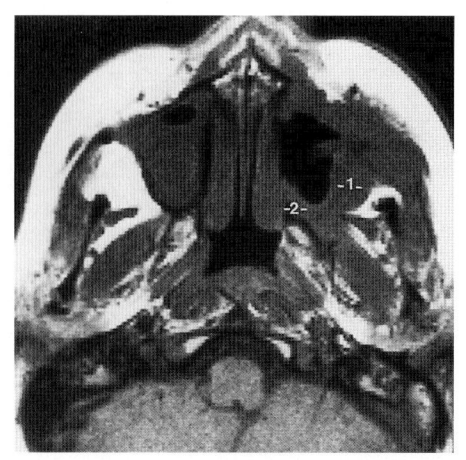

Fig. 4.**131** Carcinoma, left maxillary sinus. **a** Axial CT scan and **b** axial T1W, **c** axial T2W, and **d** coronal T1W MR scans all show extensive destruction including the posterolateral wall of the sinus, with the extension laterally to the infratemporal fossa (1) and posteriorly to the pterygopalatine fossa (2). The coronal image (**d**) also reveals extension inferiorly into the alveolar ridge (3) and hard palate. The medial wall (4) of the sinus is also destroyed, and tumor is extending into the left ethmoidal cells (5). Inflammatory changes in the right maxillary sinus (6) with an air–fluid level (**c**) show a bright signal on the T2W image (**c**), whereas tumor (1 and 2) in the left sinus has a moderate signal. From Reference 12.

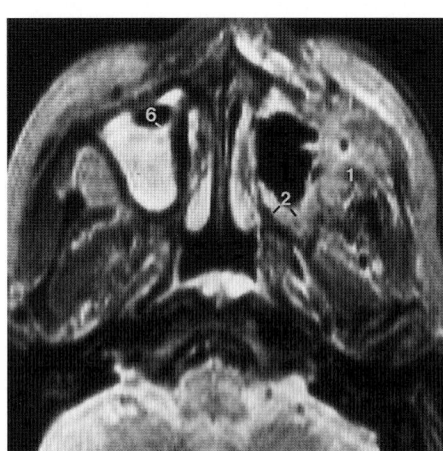

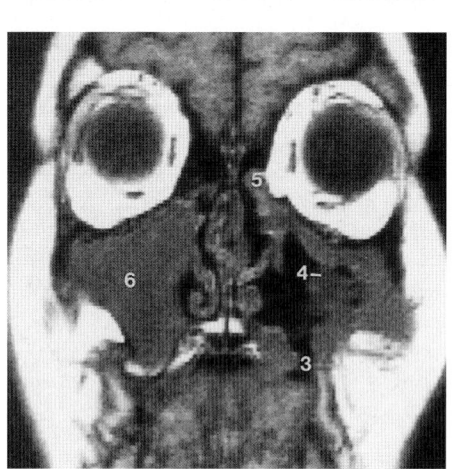

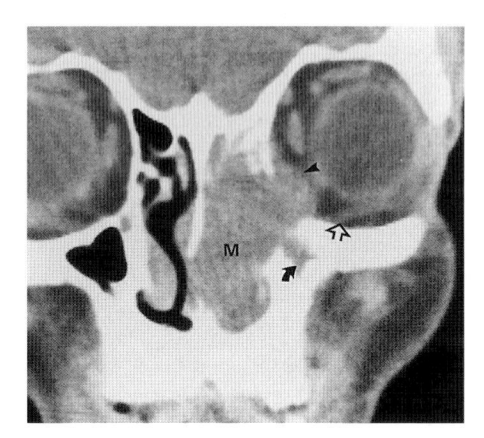

Fig. 4.**132** Squamous cell carcinoma. Coronal CT scan shows a large mass (M) involving the left nasal cavity and left ethmoidal cells. Note the bone erosion (curved arrow) and extension into the orbital subperiosteal space (arrowhead); normal inferior oblique muscle (hollow arrow).

cheek, gingivobuccal sulcus, nose, or eye. These symptoms tend to be present in 40–60% of patients at the time a diagnosis is made. Other studies have determined facial pain, nasal obstruction, and epistaxis also to be frequent presenting symptoms.[2,5] Facial pain or hypoesthesia may be related to perineural extension of sinonasal cancers or other head and neck cancers.[33–36] In sphenoid sinus carcinoma, cranial neuropathies may be the initial presenting symptoms, with the abducent nerve being the most commonly involved.[37] Maxillary sinus carcinomas have a propensity for extension into the orbit, ethmoid sinus, pterygopalatine fossa, or infratemporal fossa (Fig. 4.**131**). Extension of the tumor posteriorly into the pterygopalatine fossa may allow extension of tumor into the orbit through the inferior orbital fissure. Very few data are available regarding squamous cell carcinoma of the ethmoid sinus, with most carcinomas of the ethmoid sinus being adenocarcinomas.[38,39]

Ethmoid sinus carcinomas also have a propensity for spread into the orbit (Fig. 4.**132**). The location of ethmoid sinus carcinomas, however, allows spread through the fovea ethmoidalis or medially through the cribriform plate into the anterior cranial fossa. Extension of the tumor into the middle cranial fossa can occur from a posterior ethmoidal carcinoma extending through the superior orbital fissure.[9] A mean 5-year cure rate of approximately 35% is frequently reported after a combination of surgery and radiation therapy.[2,40,41] Orbital involvement indicates a poor prognosis, with pterygoid fossa involvement and cervical lymph node metastases being ominous findings.[2] The initial evaluation of patients who have epithelial tumors of the nasal cavity or paranasal sinuses, after the detailed history and physical examination, consists of obtaining imaging studies. These studies are necessary to delineate the full extent of the tumor, which is frequently underestimated by clinical evaluation.

Imaging Diagnosis

The radiological evaluation of patients includes a CT and/or MR scan (Figs. 4.**131**–4.**136**). MR imaging delineates the tumor from surrounding soft tissue, inflammatory edema, and retained secretions, whereas CT allows evaluation of fine bony detail and osseous involvement (Figs. 4.**132**, 4.**133**).

Critical areas to be assessed include the bony orbital walls (Figs. 4.**132**, 4.**137**), the cribriform plate, the fovea ethmoidalis, the posterior wall of the maxillary sinus, the pterygopalatine

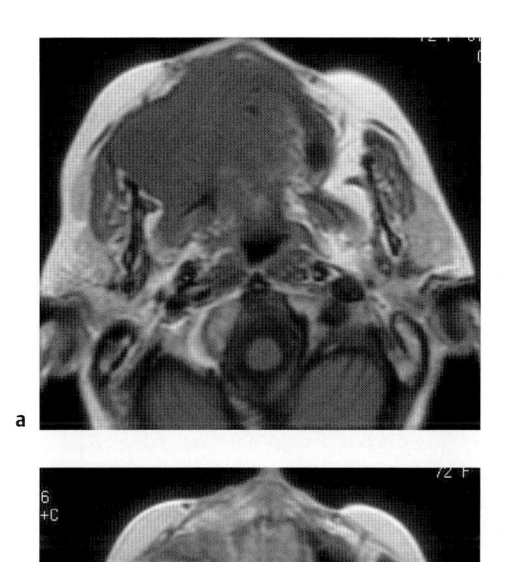

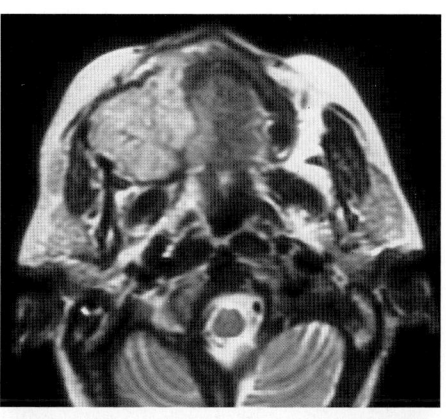

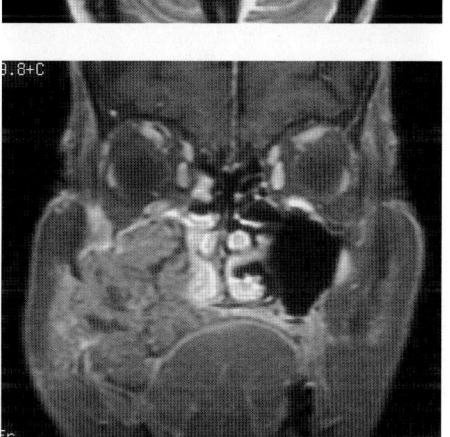

Fig. 4.**133** Squamous cell carcinoma of the maxillary sinus in a 72-year-old woman. **a** Axial T1W MR scan shows a large hypointense mass, replacing the alveolar process of right maxilla with large buccal extension. **b** Axial T2W MR scan shows a hyperintense tumor. **c** Axial enhanced T1W MR scan shows moderate tumor enhancement. **d** Coronal enhanced fat-suppression T1W MR scan shows massive tumor in the right maxillary sinus and buccal space. Differential diagnoses include adenocarcinoma and lymphoma.

fossa, the confines of the sphenoid sinus, and the posterior wall of the frontal sinus. Erosion of bone in these areas indicates spread of the tumor beyond the confines of the nasal cavity and paranasal sinuses. Administration of contrast medium is usually not helpful in evaluating squamous cell carcinomas of the sinonasal cavities, because of the somewhat similar CT densities of tumor and inflammatory as well as scar and granulation tissues. Nevertheless, contrast administration may be beneficial in several instances, for example:

1. The use of contrast may help to delineate intracranial spread of tumor, involved meninges, and brain parenchyma, resulting from breakdown of the blood–brain barrier.
2. Contrast study can differentiate fluid from solid tissue and areas of necrosis.

Despite the significant amount of information that can be garnered from a CT scan, there are several limitations of CT scanning:

1. It cannot always determine whether the tumor has invaded or just approached the periorbita.
2. Upon examination of the CT scan, it is difficult to differentiate tumor from soft-tissue swelling. Consequently, it is difficult to determine the degree of actual tissue invasion.
3. It is difficult to determine the extent of tumor infiltration into obstructed sinuses because of similar soft-tissue attenuation values of tumor and retained secretions.

Although difficulty may also at times be encountered in differentiating *encroachment* of the periorbita by tumor from *invasion* of the periorbita by tumor through the use of MR imaging, the latter two limitations of CT are areas in which MR imaging excels. MR imaging provides excellent delineation of tumor from surrounding soft tissue, inflammatory tissue, and retained secretions within the sinuses (Figs. 4.**134**, 4.**137**). This characteristic, in combination with multiplanar capability and lack of radiation exposure, gives MR a distinct advantage over CT. The ability of MR imaging to differentiate tumor from benign processes such as surrounding soft tissues, inflammatory tissue, and retained secretions is based on differences in proton mobility. It might be anticipated that the typical appearance of edema or retained secretions within the sinuses on MR images would be of low intensity on T1-weighted images and high intensity on T2-weighted images (Figs. 4.**134**, 4.**135**), reflecting the high water content associated with the excessive interstitial fluid or retained secretions. However, because of the frequently chronic nature of these benign processes in patients who have a nasal cavity or paranasal sinus tumor, especially in those patients in whom an advanced tumor has been diagnosed, sufficient time has elapsed to allow for the concentration of high water affinity mucoproteins and the absorption of free water. This leads to various degrees of shortening of both the T1 and T2 relaxation times. The areas of almost complete desiccation can have low signal, which can be seen adjacent to areas that are still predominantly composed of water. This can produce a wide variety of signal intensities on both T1-weighted and T2-weighted MR images.[9,29]

Carcinomas of the nasal cavity and paranasal sinuses share similar gross and microscopic pathological characteristics:

1. They are highly cellular tumors with little free water and, as such, are represented by a homogeneous MR appearance, with low to intermediate signal intensity on T1-weighted and T2-weighted MR images (Fig. 4.**135**).
2. There may be focal, well-defined areas of intermediate to high signal intensities on T1-weighted and T2-weighted MR images that represent subacute or chronic hemorrhage.
3. There may be areas of low to intermediate signal intensity on T1-weighted MR images and areas of high intensity on T2-weighted MR images that represent fluid-filled sites of necrosis.

430   4 Imaging of the Nasal Cavity and Paranasal Sinuses

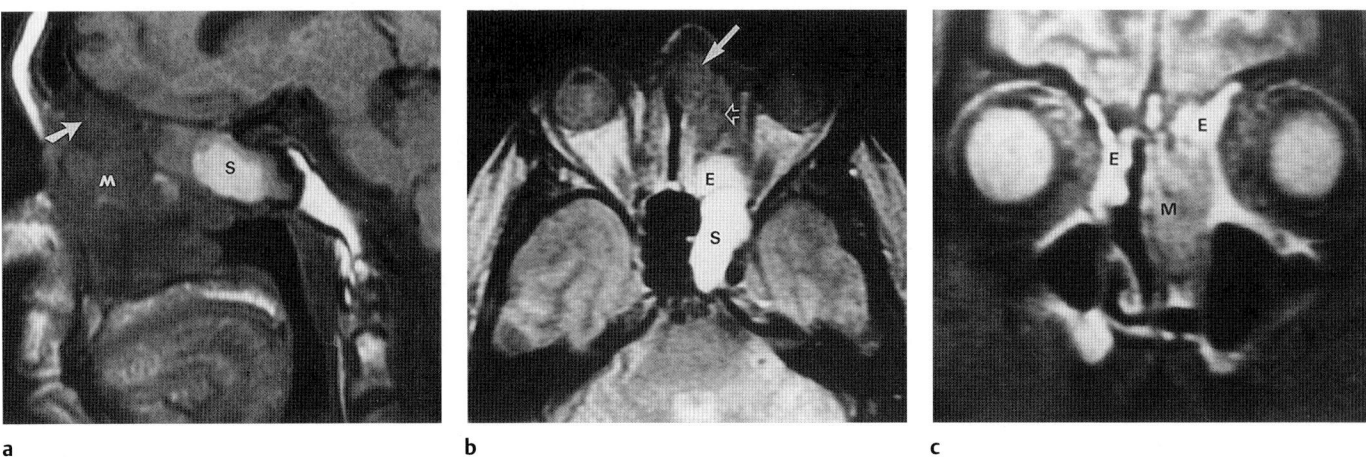

Fig. 4.**134** Squamous cell carcinoma
a Sagittal T1W MR scan shows a mass (M) involving the nasal cavity and ethmoidal sinus (arrow). The retained secretion in the sphenoid sinus (S) appears hyperintense.
b Axial proton-density-weighted (PW) MR scan shows tumor in the nasal cavity (solid arrow) and ethmoid (hollow arrow). Note the hyperintense retained mucosal secretion in the posterior ethmoid (E) and left sphenoid sinus (S).
c Coronal T2W MR scan shows tumor mass (M) and hyperintense mucosal secretions in the ethmoidal cells (E).

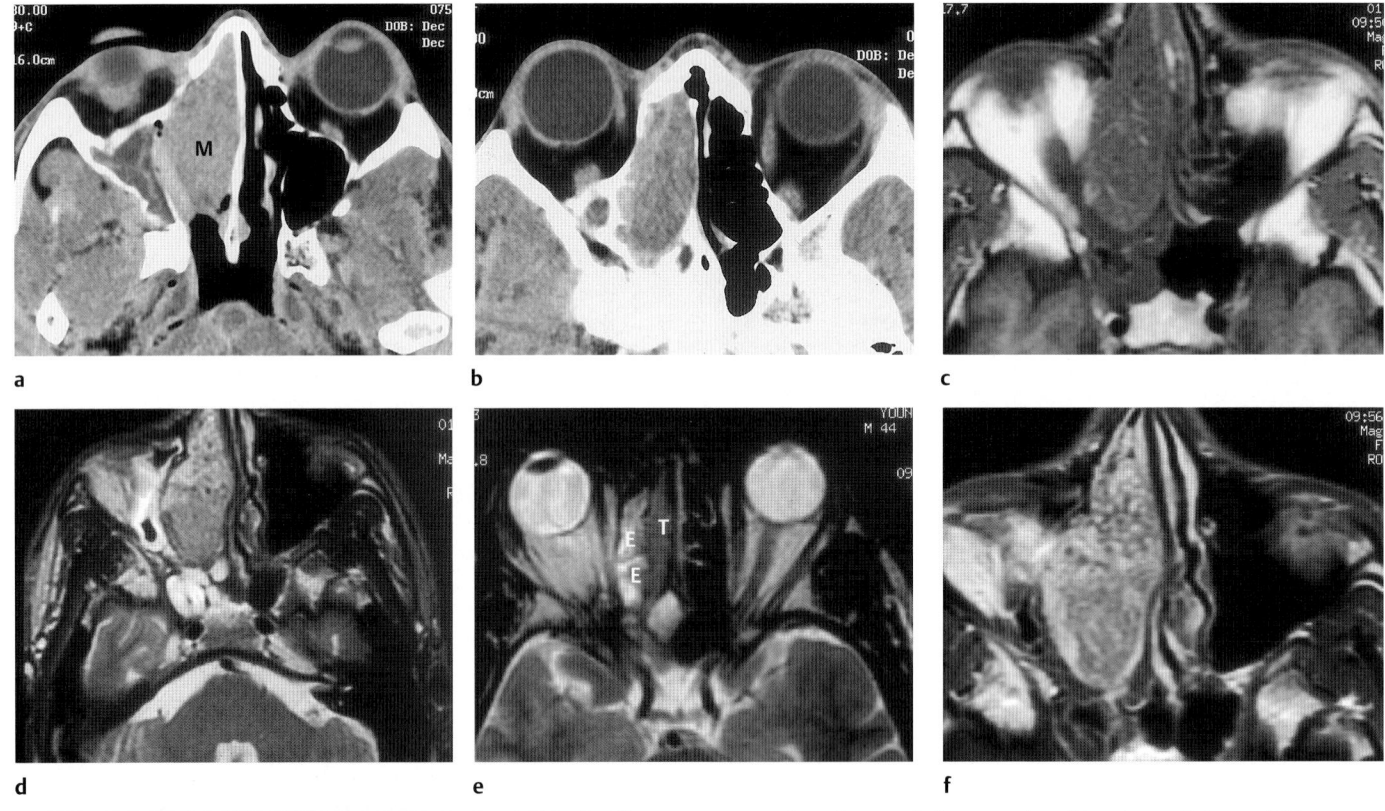

Fig. 4.**135** Papillary squamous cell carcinoma of the nasoethmoid region. **a** Enhanced CT scan shows a moderately enhancing mass (M). **b** Enhanced CT scan shows involvement of entire right ethmoid air cells. **c** T1W and **d** T2W MR scans show that the mass is isointense to brain. **e** T2W MR scan shows that the tumor (T) is hypointense with regard to inflammatory mucosal changes in the ethmoid cells (E). **f** and **g** Enhanced T1W MR scans showing tumor enhancement. Note that tumor (T) enhances less than inflammatory mucosal thickening of ethmoid cells (E).

Fig. 4.**135 h–n** ▷

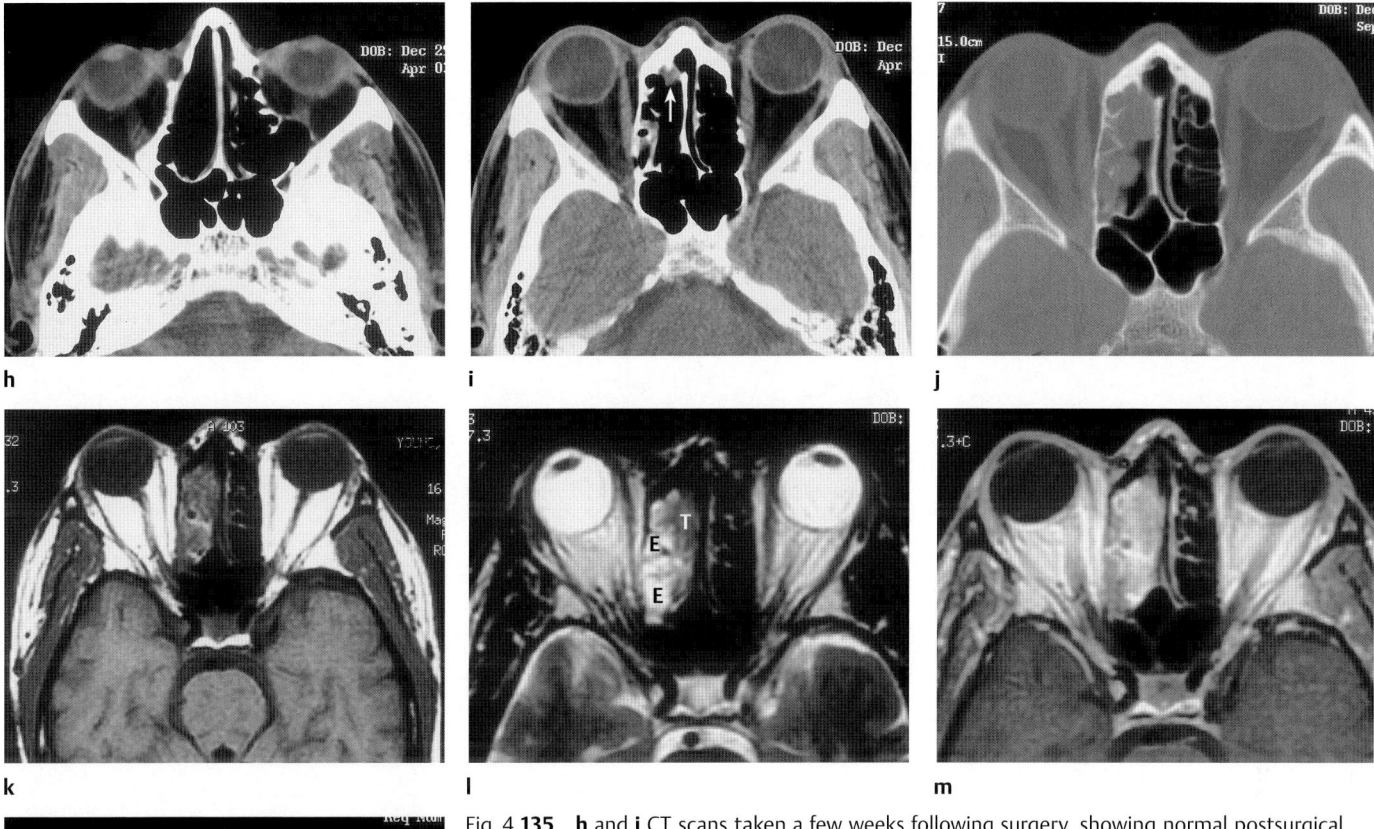

Sinonasal Pathology   431

Fig. 4.**135**   **h** and **i** CT scans taken a few weeks following surgery, showing normal postsurgical appearance. Note a small focus of increased density (arrow in Fig. 4.**135i**). **j** CT scan taken five months following surgery, showing marked opacification of the ethmoid in the surgical bed. The appearance is nodular and therefore highly suggestive of recurrence. **k** T1W, **l** T2W, and **m** enhanced T1W MR scans, showing abnormal signal intensity in the right ethmoid. Note that the recurrent tumor (T), as in the original MRI (**d**, **e**), is hypointense to inflammatory changes of the ethmoid cells (E). **n** Enhanced CT scan, taken several months later, showing marked tumor recurrence. The appearance of recurrence is now similar to the initial CT image (**b**).

4 Benign processes within the nasal cavity and paranasal sinuses, such as polyps and papillomas (Figs. 4.**94**, 4.**97**) can often be differentiated from malignant lesions by their morphological appearance (contour) and signal intensities on T1-weighted and T2-weighted MR images. Extension of benign processes intracranially is seen as a polypoid intracranial mass.[29]

Gd-DTPA-enhanced MR study may offer additional information. In most instances, enhancement of the tumor is less intense than enhancement of the thickened mucosa (Fig. 4.**135g**). The extent of tumor enhancement with Gd-DTPA appears to correlate with the vascularity of the tumor, with the more vascular tumors having the greater amount of enhancement.[29] Mucosal enhancement, however, may help differentiate an obstructed sinus from tumor.

Glandular Tumors of Sinonasal Cavities

Adenoid Cystic Carcinoma

Tumors of minor salivary gland origin and other glandular neoplasms constitute between 4% and 10% of malignant neoplasms of the sinonasal cavities.[5,42] The minor salivary gland tumors can occur anywhere within the sinonasal cavities; however, they frequently arise from minor salivary glands within the palate and then extend into the nasal cavity or paranasal sinuses (Fig. 4.**138**). These tumors include adenoid cystic carcinomas (Figs. 4.**138**–4.**141**), mucoepidermoid carcinomas (Figs. 4.**136**, 4.**142**), acinic cell carcinomas, and mixed tumors (pleomorphic adenomas). Several authors have remarked on the prevalence of adenoid cystic carcinomas,[5,42] which typically both destroy and remodel bone. Adenoid cystic tumors have the ability to extend through submucosal and fibrous tissue planes around the primary site, as well as a propensity for invasion along the nerve sheath and perivascular structures (Figs. 4.**140**, 4.**141**).[33] Perineural spread is also common in squamous cell carcinoma of the head and neck, including cutaneous type.[33–35] Perineural spread can be seen in other head and neck tumors such as lymphoma (including post-transplantation lymphoproliferative disorder), Wegener granulomatosis, malignant melanoma, as well as granular cell tumor.[28] Adenoid cystic carcinoma (ACC) accounts for fewer than 1% of all head and neck malignancies and 10% of all salivary gland neoplasms.[33] It occurs more often in minor salivary glands than in the major ones. The palate and paranasal sinuses are the most com-

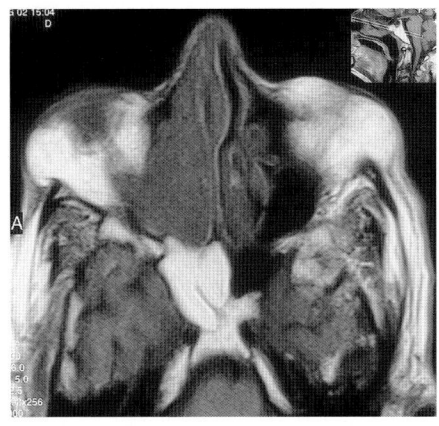

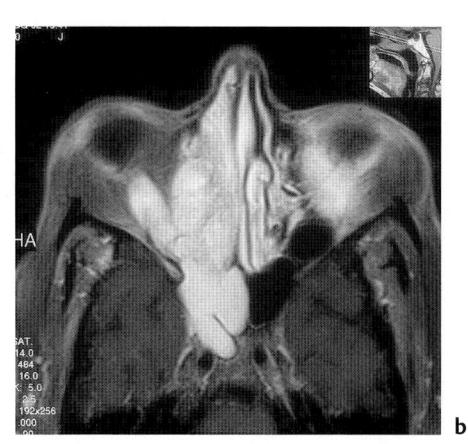

Fig. 4.**136** Mucoepidermoid carcinoma of the nasal cavity. **a** Axial T1W MR scan shows a hypointense mass in the right nasal cavity. The retained secretion in the sphenoid sinus is hyperintense. **b** Axial enhanced fat-suppression T1W MR scan shows intense enhancement of tumor. Final histological diagnosis was mucoepidermoid carcinoma.

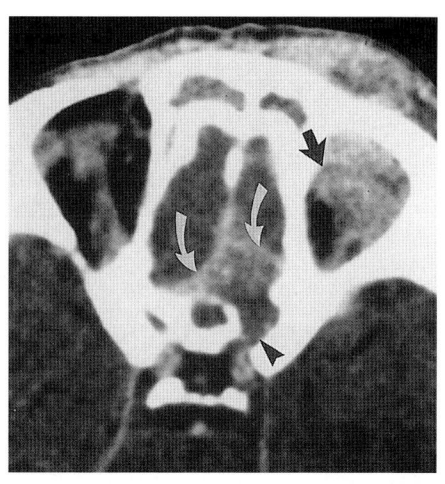

Fig. 4.**137** Axial enhanced CT scan shows extension of ethmoid carcinoma into the anterior cranial fossa (white arrows), optic canal (arrowhead), and superior orbit (black arrow).

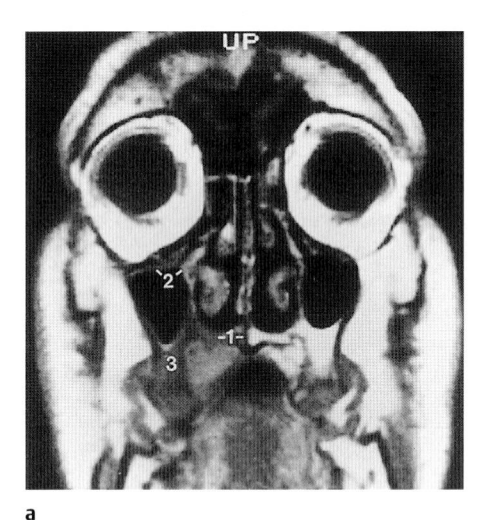

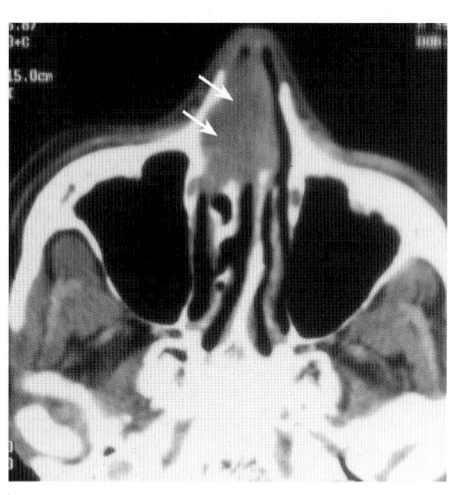

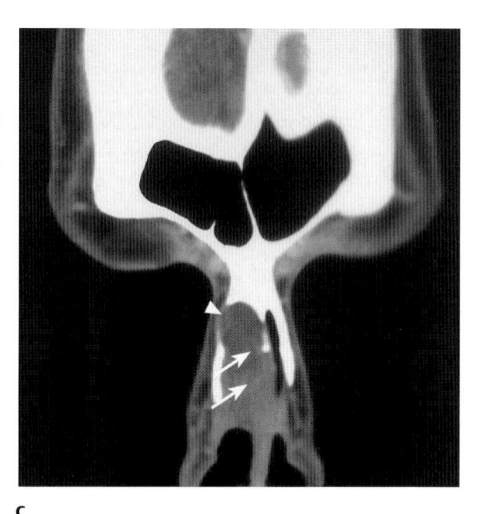

Fig. 4.**138** **a** Adenoid cystic carcinoma of the hard palate and right alveolar ridge. Coronal T1W MR. Note soft-tissue change of the maxillary sinus (2). Involvement of the palate (1) with the underlying soft tissues and hypointensity of the alveolar ridge (3) can be seen. **b** Axial and **c** coronal CT scans in another patient showing an adenoid cystic tumor of the nasal cavity (arrows). Note erosion of the nasal bone (arrowhead) in **c**. Histological study revealed perineural involvement.

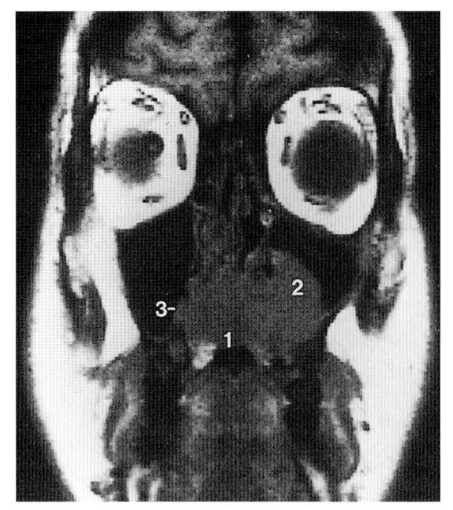

Fig. 4.**139** Adenoid cystic carcinoma of the palate. Coronal T1W MR image. A large tumor involving the palate (1) and left maxillary sinus (2) also barely extends to the right maxillary sinus (3).

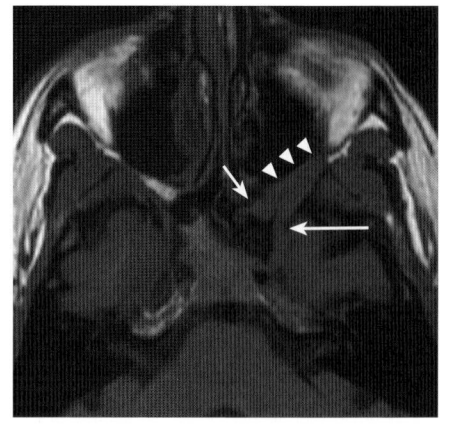

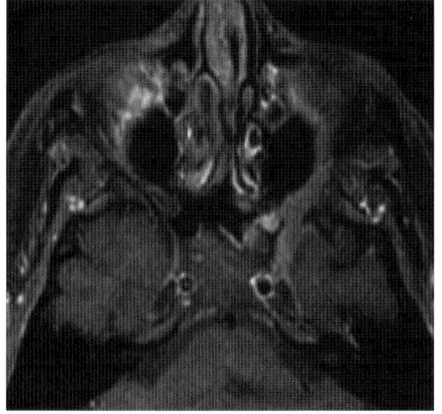

Fig. 4.**140** Adenoid cystic tumor with perineural extension. **a** Axial T1W MR scan shows perineural extension of an adenoid cystic carcinoma of the hard palate, not shown here, into the sphenopalatine fossa (short arrow), along the inferior orbital fissure (arrowheads) and along the maxillary nerve (long arrow). **b** Enhanced fat-suppression T1W MR scan shows moderate contrast enhancement of involved structures.

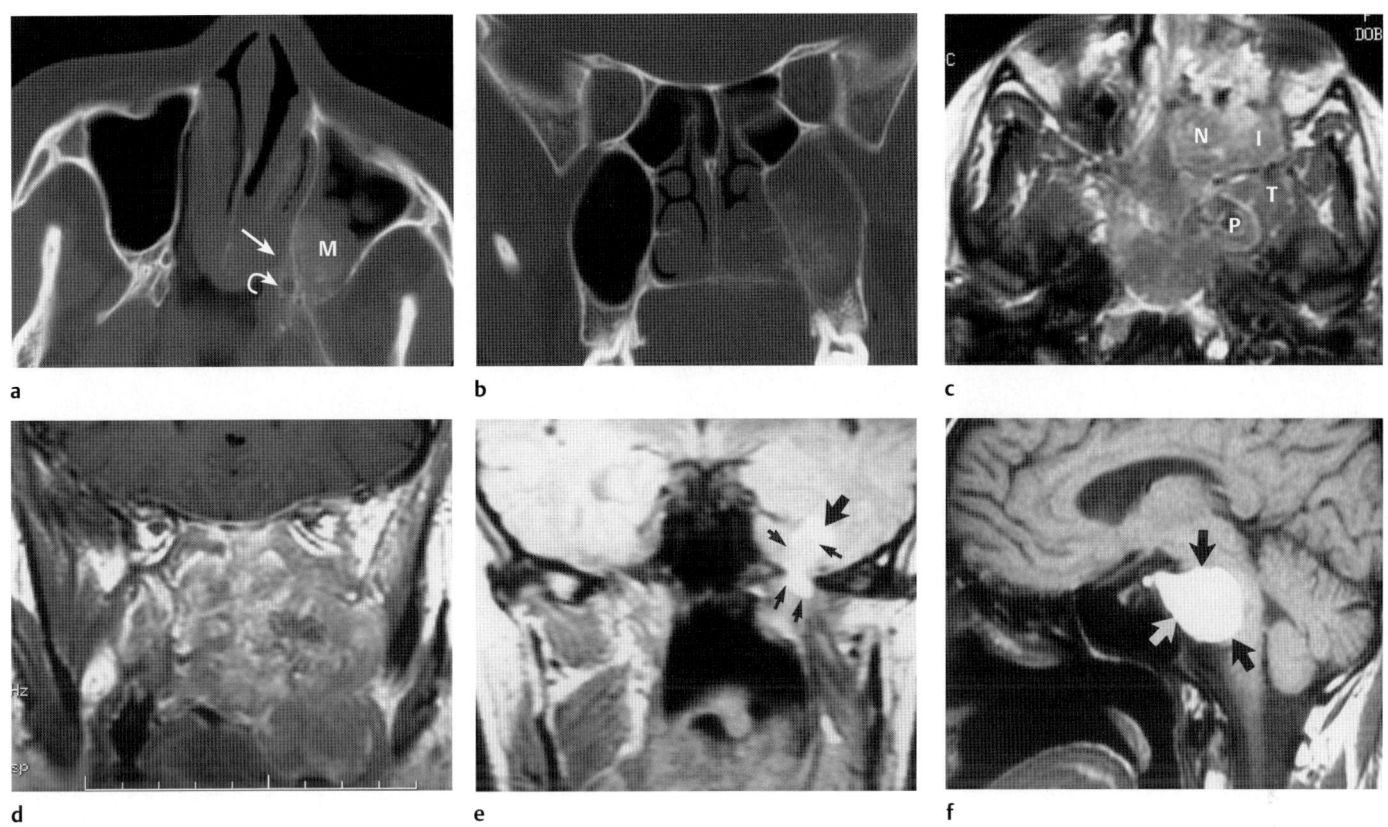

Fig. 4.141 Adenoid cystic carcinoma tumor with perineural extension. **a** CT scan shows a partially calcified mass in the left maxillary sinus (M). Note extension of tumor in the nasal cavity (straight arrow). The left greater palatine foramen (curved arrow) is enlarged owing to perineural extension of this tumor. **b** Coronal CT scan shows partially calcified mass in the left maxillary sinus. Note tumor involvement of the adjacent left nasal cavity and hard palate. There is demineralization of the left side of the hard palate. **c** Axial enhanced T1W MR scan, taken two years later, shows marked tumor, involving nasal cavity (N), inferior orbital fissure (I), pterygopalatine fossa (P), and infratemporal fossa (T). **d** Coronal enhanced T1W MR scan shows extensive tumor in the left nasal cavity, left maxillary sinus, and left hard palate. **e** Coronal PW MR scan in another patient who had an adenoid cystic tumor of the hard palate removed almost 20 years previously, showing a mass at the base of the skull (arrows), with enlarged foramen ovale. **f** Sagittal T1W MR scan, taken 10 months later, showing extension of tumor along the trigeminal nerve with a large hyperintense mass (arrows) in the prepontine region. This was removed and the pathology was adenoid cystic carcinoma, identical to primary tumor.

mon site of minor salivary gland involvement. Of all malignant paranasal sinus tumors, 5–15% are ACC.[34] ACC is a slowly progressive and relentless tumor that has a tendency to recur locally and to metastasize distantly.[33] Recurrence and metastasis can occur even decades after treatment of the primary tumor (Fig. 4.**141 f**).[35] Of all patients with ACC of the head and neck, those whose disease originates in the paranasal sinuses or nasal cavity have the poorest prognosis.[33] Most of the surgical patients studied by Wiseman et al.[33] had positive microscopic margins despite aggressive surgery, including maxillectomy, orbital exenteration, and craniofacial resection. Their data suggest that, despite the difficulty of achieving negative margins, doing so does appear to confer some benefit.[33] ACC is considered to be a radiosensitive but not radiocurable tumor. Postoperative irradiation most likely delays rather than prevents local recurrence. Unlike other head and neck cancer patients, patients with ACC of the sinonasal tract often survive for long periods with distant metastatic disease.[33] Therefore, the presence of distant metastases is not a contraindication to surgical treatment of the primary tumor in order to achieve local control. Cervical lymph node metastasis of ACC is rare and no patients in Wiseman and colleagues' series of 35 cases presented with such metastasis.[33]

Mucoepidermoid Carcinoma

Mucoepidermoid carcinoma (MEC) occurs most often in the major salivary glands, the minor salivary glands of the oral cavity and pharynx, and the lacrimal glands.[44,45] Only rarely does it arise in the respiratory tract (i.e., the larynx, trachea, and bronchi) or the sinonasal cavities (Figs. 4.**136**, 4.**142**).[44,45] When these tumors do occur in the sinonasal tract, the most common site is the maxillary antrum; other sites, in order of decreasing incidence, include the nasal cavity, nasopharynx, and ethmoid sinus.[45] The CT and MRI appearances of mucoepidermoid carcinoma of the sinonasal cavities cannot be used to reliably distinguish this tumor from other malignant lesions of the sinonasal tract (Figs. 4.**136**, 4.**142**).

Adenocarcinoma

Primary adenocarcinomas are rare and most often occur in the ethmoid region (Fig. 4.**143**).[9,42] Adenocarcinomas, in general, constitute a heterogeneous group of neoplasms that can be subclassified into several morphological subgroups, including papillary, tubular, mucinous, nonmucinous, clear cell, colonic, and solid tumors.[6] In general, a malignant neoplasm of the sinonasal cavity that does not fit the classic features of salivary gland tumors is usually classified as an adenocarcinoma.[6] These tumors may expand the bony margins and at any time may appear on CT and MR images as relatively benign lesions.[9] The high-grade adenocarcinomas often exhibit invasive, destructive margins (Fig. 4.**143**) in contrast to the pushing margins of low-grade tumors. High-grade adenocarcinomas are arranged in a predominantly solid pattern with ill-defined glandular formations that have severe nuclear pleomorphism and an increased mitotic ratio.[6] This may explain their intermediate-intensity signal on

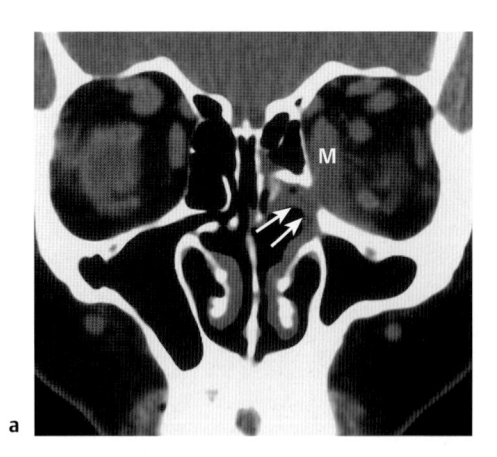

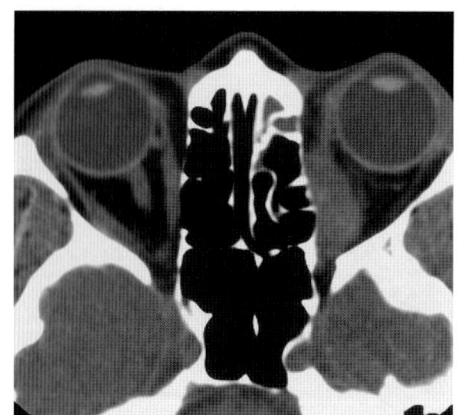

Fig. 4.**142** Low-grade mucoepidermoid carcinoma of the ethmoid sinus. **a** Coronal CT scan shows irregular soft tissue (arrows), where a nasal–ethmoid tumor had recently been resected. Note an orbital mass (M), related to tumor extension. **b** CT scan shows tumor extension along the medial wall of the left orbit.

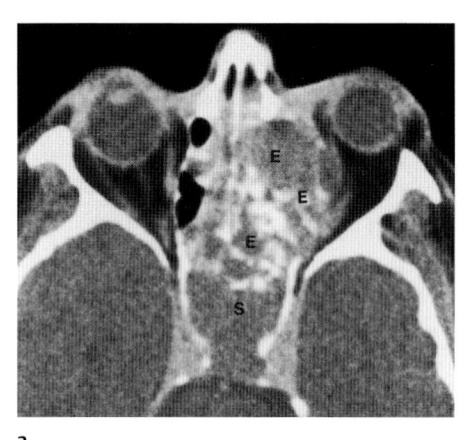

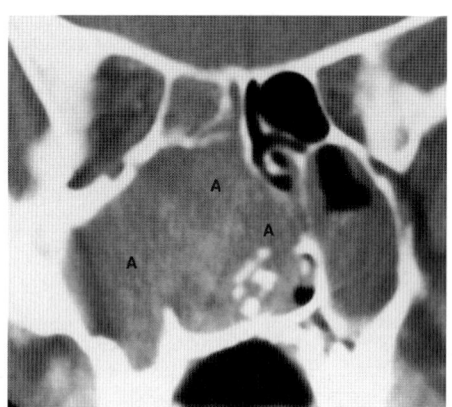

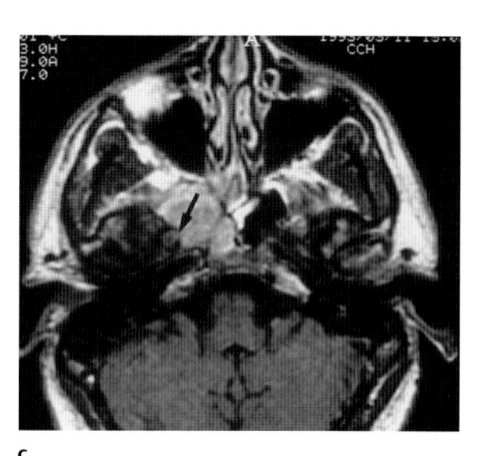

Fig. 4.**143** Adenocarcinoma of the ethmoid sinus and nasal cavity. **a** Axial CT scan shows a large tumor involving the ethmoid (E) air cells. The opacified sphenoid sinus (S) was due to retained mucous secretion. Note several dystrophic calcifications. **b** Coronal CT in another patient, showing adenocarcinoma (A), involving the nasal cavity and right maxillary sinus. Note dystrophic calcifications. **c** Axial enhanced T1W MR scan in another patient showing a markedly enhancing mass (arrow), involving the right sphenoid sinus, extending into the posterior ethmoid. Histological diagnosis was undifferentiated carcinoma. Case **c** courtesy of Calvin Flowers, MD, Chicago, IL, USA.

T2-weighted MR images. The majority of low-grade tumors consist of small uniform glands in which cystic and papillary formations with psammoma bodies (calcifications) are often present (Fig. 4.**143**). The cells are uniform without substantial nuclear pleomorphism, and mitoses are rare.[7,43] In contrast to high-grade tumors, this structural configuration produces higher T2-weighted signal intensities. Intraneural and perineural spread is more common in adenoid cystic carcinomas (Figs. 4.**140**, 4.**141**).[9] The mainstay of treatment for adenoid cystic carcinomas and adenocardinomas remains surgical resection, with or without preoperative or postoperative radiation therapy.

Sinonasal Neuroendocrine Carcinoma and Undifferrentiated Carcinoma

Neuroendocrine carcinoma is a malignant neoplasm with divergent differentiation along both epithelial and neuroendocrine cell lines.[3] It is an uncommon class of neoplasms that may be identified in virtually all sites of the head and neck, including sinonasal cavity, salivary glands, larynx, and middle ear.[3] Sinonasal undifferentiated (anaplastic) carcinoma is a highly aggressive and invasive tumor typically affecting adults and identified in the nasal cavity and/or multiple paranasal sinuses (see Fig. 4.**200**).[3] Absence of any histological differentiating features (squamous, glandular, neurofibrillary material, or rosettes) is the feature of this lesion. It may be very difficult to differentiate it from higher-grade olfactory neuroblastomas (Fig. 4.**143c**).[3,47]

Olfactory Neuroblastoma (Olfactory Neuroepithelioma/Esthesioneuroblastoma)

Olfactory neuroblastoma, known as esthesioneuroblastoma, is a rare malignant neoplasm of neuroectodermal origin that arises from the olfactory epithelium in the cribriform region, the upper third of the nasal septum, and along the superior and supreme nasal turbinates.[47] It accounts for 6% of sinonasal cancers and 0.3% of the upper aerodigestive tract malignancies.[48] The incidence peaks once in the 11- to 20-year-old group and again in the 50- to 60-year old age group. A simple staging system was introduced by Kadish et al.,[49] according to which disease stage is classified as stage A, which denotes tumor confined in the nasal cavity; stage B, having tumor extension outside the nasal cavity but confined in paranasal sinuses; and stage C, having extension beyond the sinuses.[49] The microscopic appearance of the tumor is varied, and thus the tumor may be mistaken for lymphoma, melanoma, undifferentiated carcinoma, extramedullary plasmacytoma, Ewing sarcoma, and embryonal rhabdomyosarcoma.[5,47] Electron microscopy and immunohistochemical analysis are done essentially to differentiate between these lesions. Grossly, the tumors usually have a broad-based or pedunculated attachment in the region of the cribriform plate. The primary cell type ranges from an immature neuroblast to a benign-appearing neurocyte. Pathological studies have shown a tendency of these tumors to spread submucosally and intracranially without obvious involvement of the anterior cranial fossa dura.

Sinonasal Pathology 435

The most common presenting symptoms of these tumors are epistaxis and nasal obstruction. Local recurrence has been reported in up to 57% of patients.[47] In one of our patient local recurrence occurred 23 years following treatment. A metastatic rate of 20–62% has been reported in the literature,[3,47] with the most common site being the cervical lymph nodes. Other sites include the parotid glands, skin, lung, bone, liver, eye, and spinal cord and canal. Because of the tendency for tumor to spread in a submucosal manner, the surgical excision must be wide,[47] and a frozen-section examination of the biopsy specimen should be performed at the time of excision. The preoperative assessment of these lesions must include CT scanning, MR imaging, or both (Figs. 4.**144**, 4.**145**), including the use of contrast enhancement, to evaluate dural or frontal lobe involvement (Figs. 4.**144**, 4.**145**). For tumor removal, the craniofacial approach, with an en bloc excision of the cribriform region (anterior craniotomy and rhinotomy) should be used in all cases of dural or frontal lobe involvement.[47] The 5-year survival rate is 58–75%.[2,10]

Although insidious and capable of intracranial involvement, these tumors usually expand within the nasal cavity and ethmoid sinus (Figs. 4.**144**, 4.**145**). CT and MR scanning generally demonstrate a homogeneous mass with moderate to marked enhancement. These tumors are hypointense to brain on T1-weighted and appear rather hypointense to brain on T2-weighted MR images (Fig. 4.**146**). At times, the tumor may be inhomogeneous, with areas of cystic degeneration. These tumors may show calcifications (Fig. 4.**147**). In one patient in our series, the tumor was completely calcified, simulating an ossifying fi-

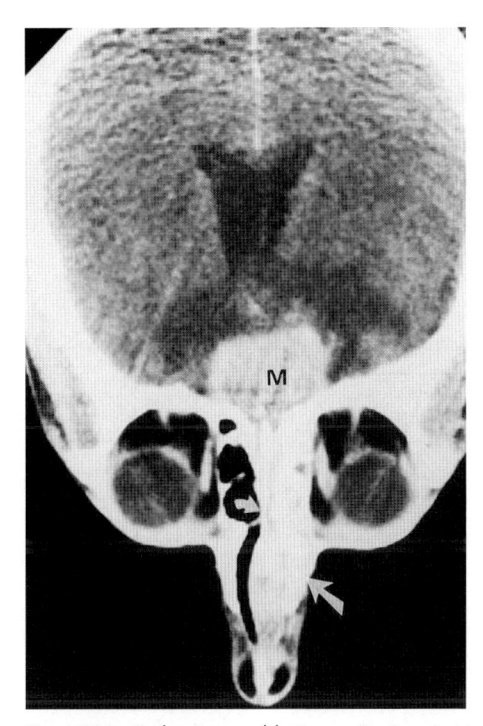

Fig. 4.**144** Esthesioneurablastoma. Postcontrast coronal CT scan shows a mass in the nasal cavity (straight arrow) and left ethmoid (curved arrow). Marked involvement of the anterior cranial fossa and frontal lobes is evident as an enhancing mass (M) and peripheral brain edema.

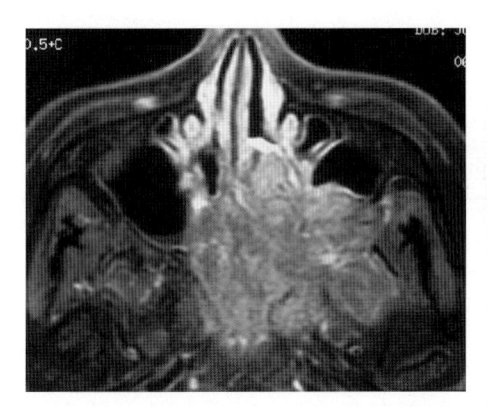

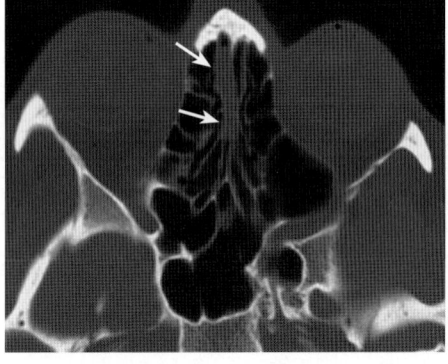

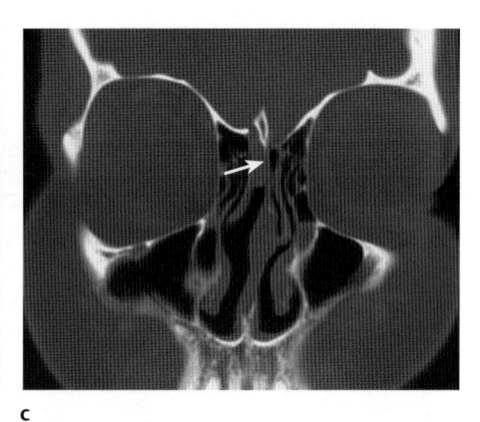

Fig. 4.**145 a, b** Esthesioneuroblastoma in a 56-year-old woman. **a** Axial enhanced fat-suppression T1W MR scan shows marked tumor enhancement, involving both nasal cavities, nasopharynx, and left maxillary sinus, with extension into the left infratemporal fossa. **b, c** Esthesioneuroblastoma in a 31-year-old woman. **b** Axial and **c** coronal CT scans showing a small esthesioneuroblastoma (arrows). A slightly larger mass had been resected a few weeks prior to this examination. The lesion was enhanced intensely on enhanced MR images. This residual tumor was resected.

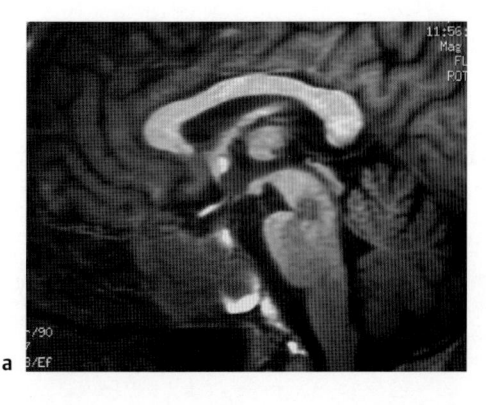

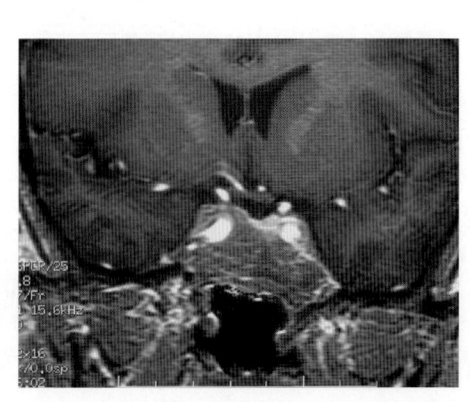

Fig. 4.**146** Esthesioneuroblastoma within the sphenoid sinus in a 67-year-old woman.
a Sagittal T1W and **b** coronal enhanced T1W MR scans, performed on a 3 T MR unit, shows a mass within the sphenoid sinus, compatible with histiologically proven esthesioneuroblastoma.

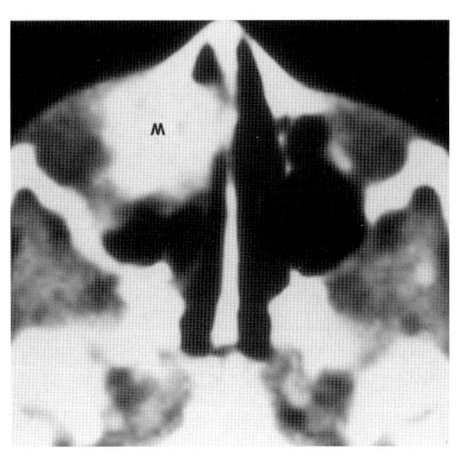

Fig. 4.**147** Calcified esthesioneuroblastoma. Axial CT scan shows a calcified mass (M), compatible with an esthesioneuroblastoma.

broma (Fig. 4.**147**). Although rare, it can arise within sphenoid sinus (Fig. 4.**146**). Primary intracranial esthesioneuroblastomas have been reported. Bone is the most common metastatic site.[48] The neck lymph nodes are also common sites of metastases. Other potential sites of metastatic involvement include liver, pancreas, lung, mediastinal lymph node, skin, and leptomenigeal and epidural spaces. Esthesioneuroblastoma is usually manged by craniofacial resection followed by postoperative radiation therapy.[48, 49]

Ganglioneuroma

Neuroblastic tumors of the maxillofacial region are rare entities, constituting only 6% of tumors in the pediatric age group.[50] Tumors originate from neural crest that normally migrates into the medulla and sympathetic ganglia.[50, 51] These tumors typically occur within the first months of life as an indolent mass in the cervical region. The tumor may involve the cranial nerves, the carotid sheath and the skull base.[50] Pathologically, neuroblastic tumors have different degrees of maturation. Neuroblastoma is the most primitive type of tumor, and it has the highest potential for metastasis. Ganglioneuromas represent the most differentiated (mature) variant and have no metastatic potential.[51] The differential diagnosis of a head and neck mass in pediatric age group should include infectious processes, developmental anomalies (cystic hygroma, branchial cleft cyst), and malignancies such as rhabdomyosarcoma, non-Hodgkin lymphoma, Ewing sarcoma, and variants of neuroblastic tumors, including infantile melanotic neuroectodermal tumors.[50, 51]

Melanotic Neuroectodermal Tumor of Infancy

Melanotic neuroectodermal tumor of infancy (MNTI) is a very rare primitive neuroectodermal tumor, originating from neural crest cells, containing large melanin-containing cells around nests of neuroblastic cells.[52, 53] More than 90 percent of MNTI tumors arise in the head and neck.[53] The tumor cells contain abundant intracytoplasmic melanin.[53] The tumors always occur within the first year of life as a rapidly growing, painless, expansile, pigmented soft-tissue mass in the mandibulo-maxillofacial region. The anterior portion of the maxilla is the most common (70%) site of involvement.[53] The tumor may be located in the orbit as well as in the brain and intracranial dura.[53] There have been occasional reports of an increase in the level of vanillylmandelic acid, which returned to normal values after removal of the tumor, as is the case after the excision of other tumors of neural crest origin, such as neuroblastomas, ganglioneuroblastomas, and pheochromocytomas. The CT and MRI studies show a destructive, osteolytic lesion, displacing the adjacent bone and tooth buds.[53] There may be sclerosis of the adjacent expanded bone as well as intratumoral calcification. The treatment of choice is surgical excision.[52, 53] Overall the local recurrence rate is 10–15%.[53] Metastases occur in less than 5% of cases.[53] It is impossible to predict clinically or pathologically which tumors will have a malignant component. In rare cases it has been reported that a malignant component acquired the features of neuroblastoma.[52, 53]

Ewing Sarcoma

Ewing sarcoma (ES) is a highly malignant small, round cell (blue cell) tumor of children, adolescents, and young adults that accounts for 5–10% of all malignant primary bone tumors.[5] Only 1–4% of all Ewing sarcomas occur in the head and neck, most commonly the mandible, followed by the maxillae, calvaria, and cervical vertebrae.[54] Pathologically, ES appears as a malignant primitive type of "small blue round cells." Primary ES of sinonasal cavities is extremely rare. We have seen one case in an 18-year-old man. The tumor originated in the anterior ethmoid. The CT scan revealed a small but destructive lesion of the ethmoid bone, associated with soft tissue at the left naso-orbital angle. Ewing sarcoma and primitive neuroectodermal tumor of bone are closely related.[54a] The standard chemotherapy protocol for Ewing sarcoma has been based on four drugs: doxorubicin, cyclophosphamide, vincristine, and dactinomycin.[54a] A new drug combination, ifosfamide and etoposide has been found to be highly effective in patients with Ewing sarcoma or primitive neuroectodermal tumor of bone who have had a relapse after standard therapy.[54a]

Extracranial Primitive Neuroectodermal Tumor (PNET)

The peripheral primitive neuroectodermal tumors (PNETs) are unusual, often highly aggressive, malignant neoplasms, rarely presenting in the head and neck.[55–57] PNETs occur most commonly as a soft-tissue tumor of the trunk or lower extremity. In soft tissues, tumors arise from the nonautonomic nervous system and display neuronal differentiation.[55] They share certain features and characteristics with classic neuroblastoma and with some CNS tumors.[56] Although there is some uncertainty regarding their histopathological classification, the development of special stains and immunohistochemistry has resulted in better characterization and recognition of this tumor as a distinct entity among other small, round cell tumors such as Ewing sarcoma, rhabdomyosarcoma, lymphoma, and classic neuroblastoma.[56] The category of PNETs includes central neuroectodermal tumors that involve the brain and spinal cord, and peripheral neuroectodermal tumors (Fig. 4.**148**). By definition, a peripheral neuroepithelioma is a PNET arising from peripehral, nonautonomic neural tissue.[55] PNETs are considered to have originated from the neural crest.[56] Both PNET and Ewing sarcoma have been reported following radiation therapy in patients with retinoblastoma.[58]

Merkel Cell Carcinoma

Merkel cell carcinoma is a rare aggressive tumor. The origin of the Merkel cells is controversial. There is evidence supporting their origin from the neural crest as well as from transitional cells in the basal layer of the epidermis (Merkel cell). Although the majority of the Merkel cell tumors are found on sun-exposed sites, there have been reports of these tumors involving nasal, palatal and other parts of the head and neck.[59, 60] One recent report described a highly vascular nasal mass.[60] The mass appeared expansile with bone destruction on CT and demonstrated long T1 and T2 characteristics on MR images, along with marked enhancement on enhanced T1-weighted MR images.

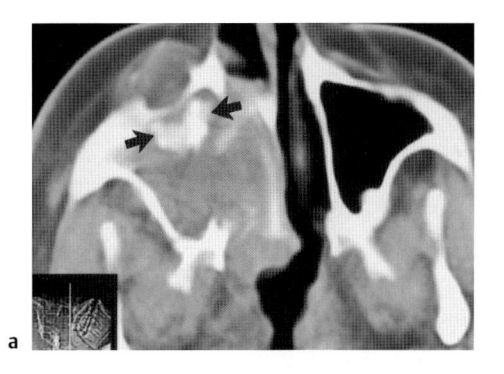

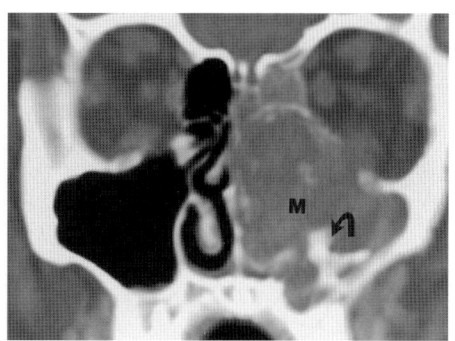

Fig. 4.**148** Primitive neuroectodermal tumor (PNET). **a** Axial CT scan shows a right destructive mass, involving the maxillary sinus, nasal cavity, and cheek on the right side. Note clumps of calcification (arrows), commonly found in these lesions. **b** Coronal CT scan shows maxillary sinus mass (M) and calcification (arrow). Note invasion of the floor of the left orbit.

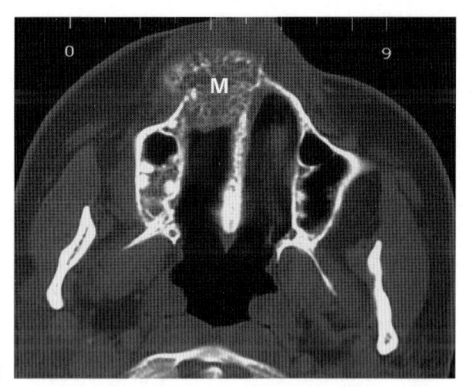

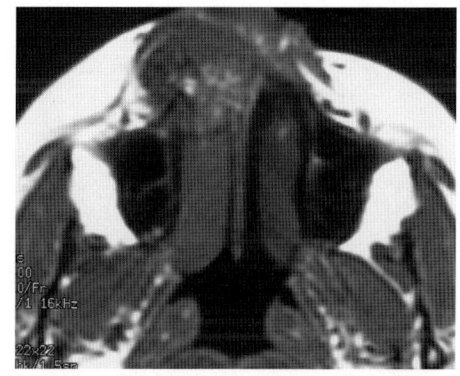

Fig. 4.**149** Hemangiopericytoma. **a** Axial CT scan shows a mass (M) with increased mineralized trabeculae involving the premaxilla. **b** Axial T1W, **c** axial T2W, and **d** axial enhanced T1W MR scans. The mass has mixed signal intensity in T1W (**b**), is hyperintense in T2W (**c**) and shows marked enhancement in **d**.

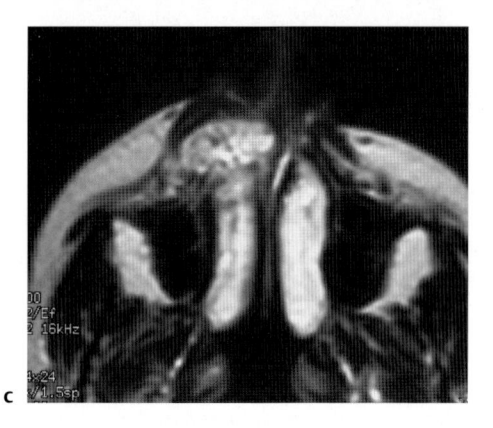

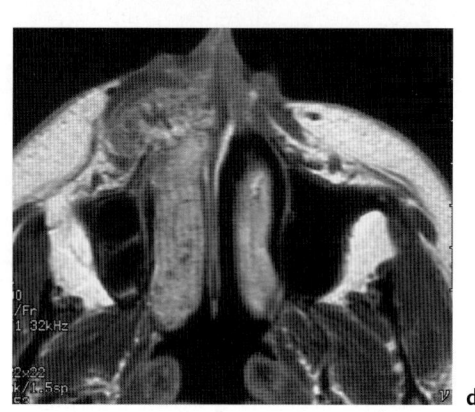

Hemangiopericytoma of Sinonasal Cavities

Sinonasal hemangiopericytomas are rare lesions that usually present with obstruction of nasal passage and epistaxis. The term pericyte was first introduced by Zimmerman in 1923[61,62] and refers to a specific cell type lying external to the reticulin sheath of capillaries. They are small, round, or spindle-shaped cells with bracing cytoplasmic processes that envelop capillaries. They are external to the endothelial cells, surrounded by the basement membrane, and are thought to regulate the size of capillary lumina through contractile properties and to synthesize collagen.[62,63] Nasal hemangiopericytomas represent 1% of all vasoformative tumors, most of which occur in the lower extremity, retroperitoneum, and pelvis. However, 15–20% occur in the head and neck region.[64] In the latter, the nose and paranasal sinuses are the most common sites of occurrence, followed by the orbital region, parotids, and neck.[65] These hemangiopericytomas appear on CT scans as moderate to markedly enhancing masses. They may show some calcification (Fig. 4.**149**), particularly in recurrent tumor following surgical resection or radiation therapy. The tumors may be large and associated with bone erosion. On MR images they appear as low to intermediate signal intensity on T1-weighted and intermediate to hyperintensity on T2-weighted images (Figs. 4.**111**, 4.**149**). They disclose moderate to marked enhancement following injection of Gd-DTPA contrast material (Fig. 4.**149**). Treatment of sinonasal hemangiopericytoma is generally surgical, with wide local excision.

Rhabdomyosarcoma of Sinonasal Cavities

Rhabdomyosarcoma is the most common soft-tissue sarcoma in infants and children.[66] It ranks seventh among the common malignancies of childhood, accounting for 5–15% of all neoplasms in children.[67,68] The peak incidence is in the 2- to 5-year-old age group, with a second peak occurring between 15 and 19 years of age.[69] The head and neck are the most common sites of origin, followed by the genitourinary tract, the extremities, trunk, and retroperitoneum.[66] Rhabdomyosarcomas are pleomorphic tumors, and the cells may be anaplastic. On the basis of their histopathological characteristics, rhabdomyosarcomas are classified into one of three histological types: embryonal, differentiated, or alveolar.[69] Differentiated rhabdomyosarcoma is the

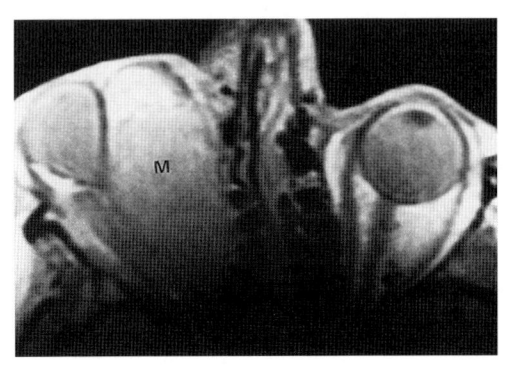

Fig. 4.**150** Rhabdomyosarcoma. Axial CT scan shows a large orbital mass (M) compatible with rhabdomyosarcoma in this elderly patient.

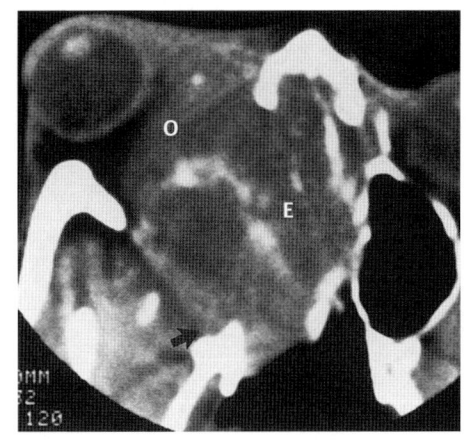

Fig. 4.**151** Rhabdomyosarcoma. Axial CT scan shows a large mass, involving the ethmoid (E) and orbit (O), and with extension into the sphenopalatine region (arrow), in this 17-year-old girl.

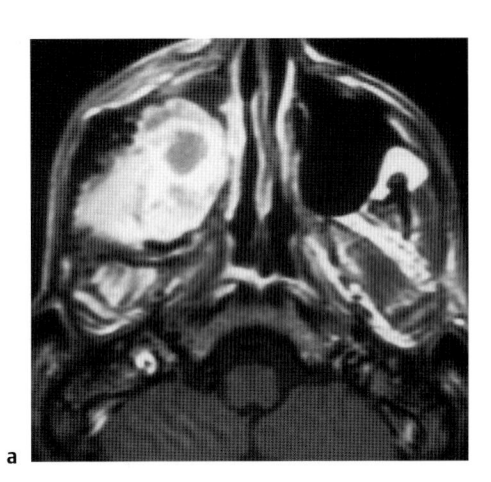

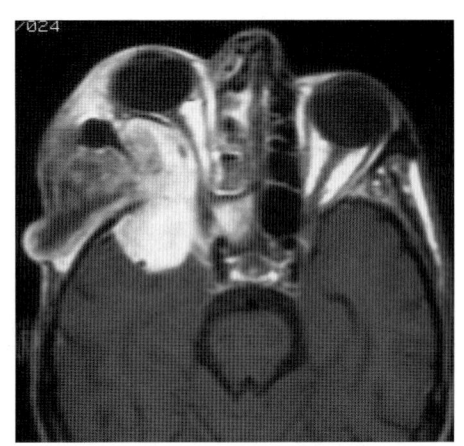

Fig. 4.**152** Recurrent rhabdomyosarcoma in a 28-year-old man. **a** Axial enhanced T1W MR scan shows massive tumor, showing intense contrast enhancement in the right infratemporal fossa, and extending into the right maxillary sinus. **b** Axial enhanced T1W MR scan shows tumor in the right temporal fossa, orbit, and anterior aspect of the right middle cranial fossa.

least frequent type and is rarely misdiagnosed because cells with eosinophilic cytoplasmic fibrils that are usually cross-striated are used to identify the tumor. Embryonal rhabdomyosarcoma, the most common histological subtype, is believed to arise from the primitive muscle cell, as would be found in a fetus at 7–10 weeks of gestation.[67] The histological diagnosis of embryonal and alveolar type rhabdomyosarcoma may be difficult; it has been estimated that up to 50% of the proven cases of rhabdomyosarcoma are incorrectly diagnosed on initial biopsy.[67]

Rhabdomyosarcoma of the sinonasal tract and orbit often presents as a relatively innocuous problem (e.g., recurrent sinusitis, proptosis, or a small naso-orbital mass). Secondary sinonasal tumors may arise from adjacent orbital spread from orbital rhabdomyosarcoma or pharyngeal rhabdomyosarcoma (Figs. 4.**150**–4.**152**). Rhabdomyosarcomas are aggressive bone-destroying and bone-pushing lesions. CT and MR studies should be performed with or without contrast enhancement, paying particular attention to detecting bone erosion at the skull base and intracranial extension of the tumor (Figs. 4.**150**–4.**152**).[66,69] The initial surgical procedure should include an adequate biopsy for confirmation and complete excision of tumor if feasible without causing excessive morbidity.[66,69] Chemotherapy has been very successful in treating primary tumors and controlling metastatic disease.[70] Radiation therapy is used primarily for local control.[59] In general, chemotherapy and radiation therapy are the primary treatment modalities for patients with rhabdomyosarcomas. Since the introduction of combination therapy (surgical, chemotherapy, and radiation), there has been a significant, continuing improvement in the survival rate of children with head and neck rhabdomyosarcomas.[66]

Lymphoma of Sinonasal Cavities

Lymphomas are commonly classified into Hodgkin disease and non-Hodgkin lymphomas. In general, Hodgkin disease develops within lymph nodes and spreads by involving adjacent nodal groups. Non-Hodgkin lymphomas may originate within a lymph node group, but in 40% of the cases they originate in extralymphatic organs or tissue.[71] Non-Hodgkin lymphomas have the capacity to differentiate into lymphocytic leukemia.[72] The majority of extranodal lymphomas are B-cell lymphomas, with T-cell lymphomas accounting for fewer than 1% of them.[73] Sinonasal lymphoma of the natural killer (NK)/T-cell type is a rare clinical presentation of extranodal lymphoma in the United States; it occurs more frequently in Asia.[73–76] In a series of 113 patients with nasal lymphoma, Cheung et al.[77] reported the following distribution: 45.1% of the patients had NK/T-cell lymphoma; 21.3% had pure T-cell lymphoma; and 33.6% had B-cell lymphoma. Thus, in Asia, NK/T-cell lymphoma is the most common variant of non-Hodgkin lymphoma that presents in the nose and nasopharynx.[76,77] Angiocentricity is a common finding in NK/T-cell lymphoma.[74] Extranodal lymphomas of NK/T cell type can occur in other sites, including the GI tract, skin, nervous system, and eyes although the nasal cavity is the most common site.[73] Although the nasopharyngeal region, as a portion of the Waldeyer's ring area, is a potential site of lymphoma, in the United States actual involvement of the nose and paranasal sinuses is rare.[71] Lym-

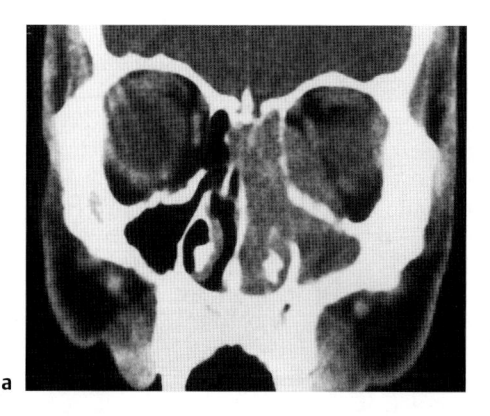

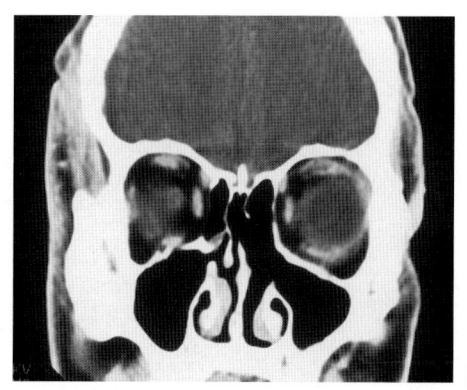

Fig. 4.**153** Lymphoma. **a** Enhanced coronal CT scan shows lymphoma, involving the left nasal cavity and ethmoid air cells. Note extension along the left medial orbital wall. **b** Coronal CT scan following treatment shows complete resolution of tumor.

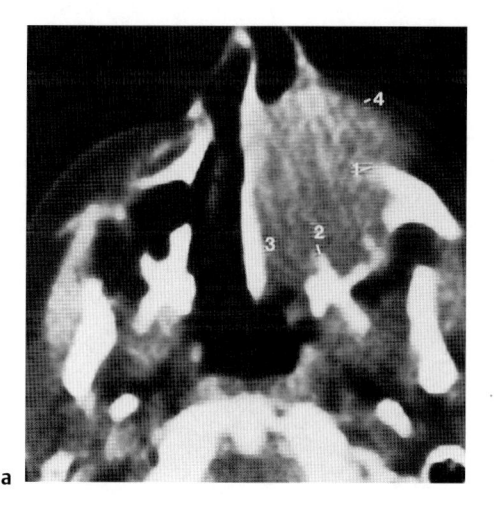

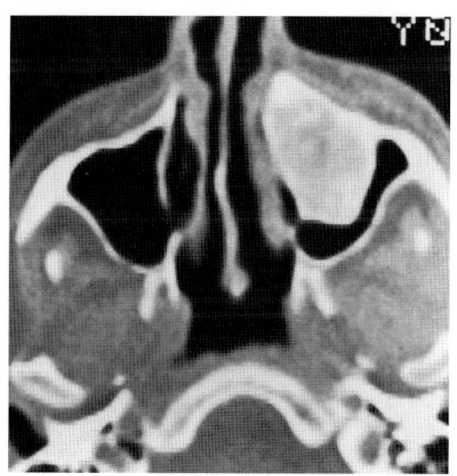

Fig. 4.**154** Lymphoma, left maxillary sinus. **a** Axial CT scan shows a large mass with destruction of the anterior (1) and medial walls (2) of the sinus, and extension into the nasal cavity (3) and subcutaneous area anterior to the sinus (4). This was treated with radiotherapy. **b** A scan taken several years later shows replacement of tumor by dense calcification.

phomas arising in the nose and paranasal sinuses are of the non-Hodgkin type and are frequently observed in patients who have disseminated lymphoma or AIDS. In a series of 1467 patients with lymphoma, Freeman et al.[78] found 37 lymphomas in the nasopharynx and 33 in the nasal cavity and paranasal sinuses. Lymphomas may be unicentric at an extralymphatic site when diagnosed early.[71] The clinical appearance of lymphomas in this area may be easily confused with that of an infection or granulomatous or nonlymphomatous neoplastic process.[67] The entity known previously as polymorphic reticulosis, lymphomatoid granulomatosis, midline granuloma syndrome, nonhealing midline granuloma, necrosis with atypical cellular exudate, or idiopathic midline destructive disease is now clearly defined as a T-cell lymphoma. The majority of nasal lymphomas manifest markers of T-cell lineage. In the New World Health Organization's Classification of Tumors,[76] these tumors are classified as extranodal/natural killer NK/T-cell lymphoma, nasal type. Extranodal NK/T-cell lymphoma occurs mainly in Asian men, with a mean age of 50 years at the time of diagnosis.[73] The disease is strongly associated with Epstein–Barr virus.[75,76] The distinction between lymphoma and Wegener granulomatosis is important because the treatment of lymphoma is radiation and that of Wegener granulomatosis is cyclophosphamide and steroids in cases of fulminant disease. On CT and MR studies, lymphomas of the nose and paranasal sinuses may mimic the much more common entities of sinusitis, polyposis, granulomatous processes, and benign and malignant neoplasms (Figs. 4.**153**–4.**160**). They are often seen as bulky masses, and there may be changes to indicate expansion, erosion, or infiltration (Figs. 4.**155**, 4.**158**, **159**). Chemotherapy and radiation therapy remain the methods of choice for treating lymphomas.

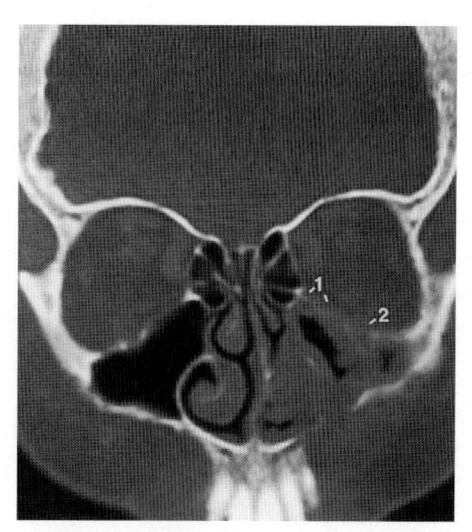

Fig. 4.**155** Lymphoma, left maxillary sinus. Coronal CT scan. A soft-tissue mass within the sinus with considerable bone destruction had at first been considered to be carcinoma but was later proven to be lymphoma. Note destruction of the floor of the orbit (1) and bone destruction in the region of the infraorbital nerve canal (2). From Reference 12.

Plasmacytoma of Sinonasal Cavities

Plasma cell neoplasms are designated as multiple myeloma, solitary medullary plasmacytoma of bone, and extramedullary plasmacytoma. Multiple myeloma and plasmacytoma are part of a continuum of B-cell lymphoproliferative disorders.[18] Extramedullary plasmacytoma (EMP) is characterized by monoclonal proliferation of plasma cells, a neoplasm of B-lymphocyte populations. EMP accounts for 4% of all nonepithelial tumors of the nasal cavity, paranasal sinuses, and nasopharynx and for 0.4% of all head and neck malignancies.[79] It accounts for about 20% of plasma cell neoplasms and occurs frequently (75–80%)[79] in the upper airways. The nasal cavity, nasal septum, and nasopharynx are the most common locations. It is confined to the soft tissues; there is no generalized bone involvement or systemic manifestations. The tumor may arise in the sinonasal cavity and nasopharynx and has been reported in the tonsil, oropharynx, larynx, orbit, thyroid glands, parotid gland, soft tissues of anterior cervical spine, mandible, TMJ, hyoid bone, sphenoid sinus,[18] petrous bone, base of the skull, and clivus, and within the cranium alone.[18] However, approximately 30% of patients with extramedullary plasmacytoma develop systemic manifestations of multiple myeloma after 20 years or more.

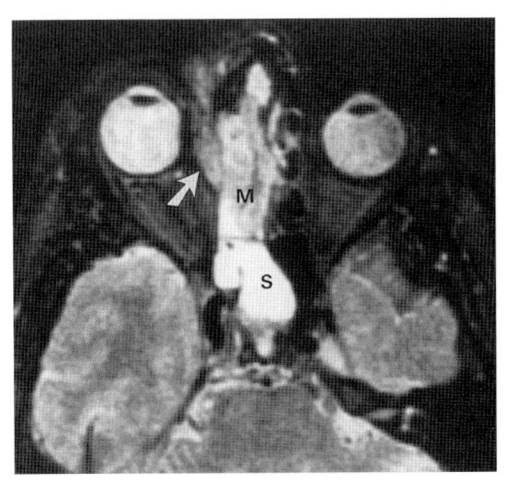

Fig. 4.**156** Large cell lymphoma. Axial T2W MR scan. The tumor mass (M) appears less hyperintense than the retained fluid in the sphenoid sinus (S). Note the involvement of the orbit with elevation of the periosteum (arrow).

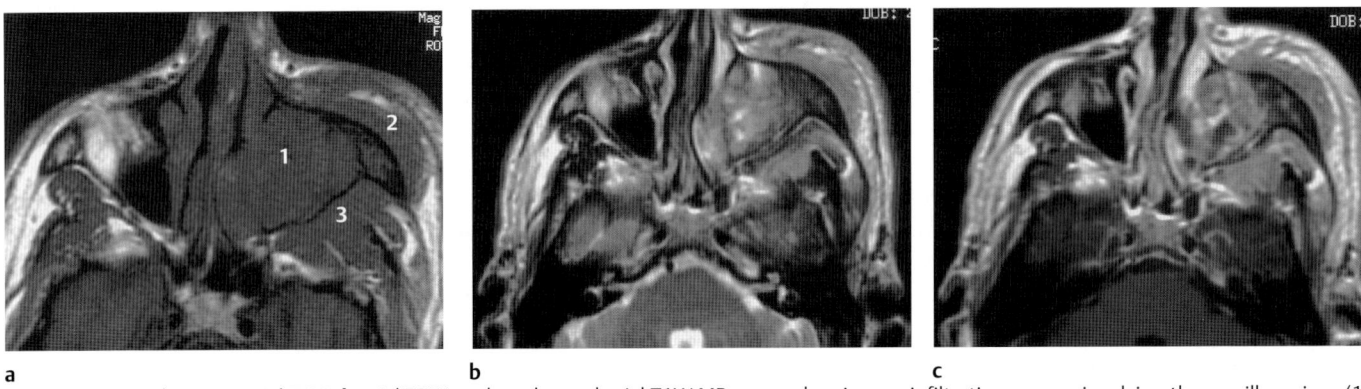

Fig. 4.**157** Lymphoma. **a** Axial T1W, **b** axial T2W, and **c** enhanced axial T1W MR scans, showing, an infiltrative process involving the maxillary sinus (1), cheek (2), infratemporal fossa (3), and nasal cavity on the left side.

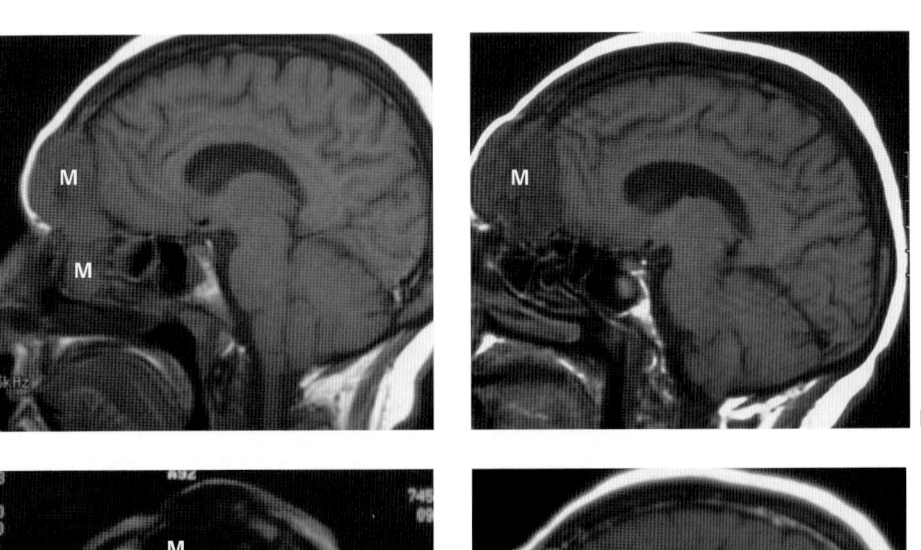

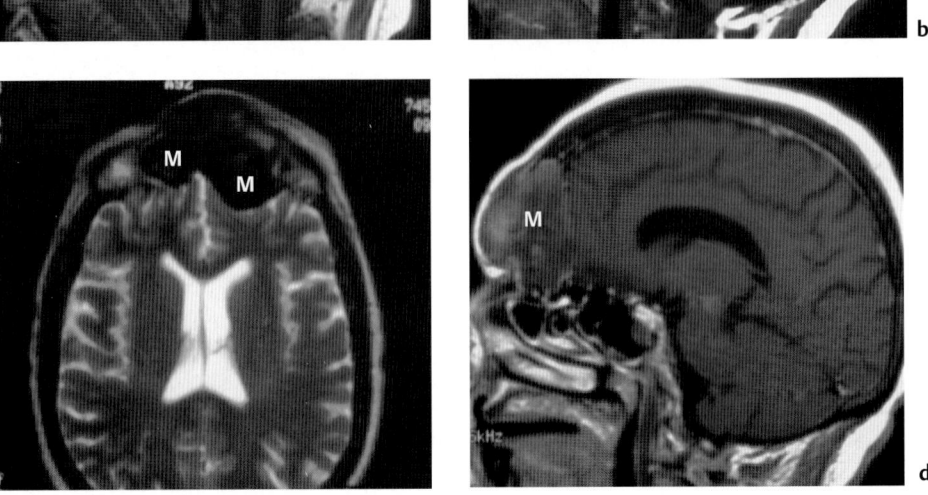

Fig. 4.**158** Lymphoma, frontal sinus. **a** Sagittal T1W MR scan shows a mass (M) in the frontal sinus and frontal recess. **b** Sagittal T1W MR scan, obtained seven months later, shows marked expansion of the frontal sinus due to tumor growth. **c** Axial T2W MR scan shows hypointense mass within the frontal sinuses. **d** Enhanced sagittal T1W MR scan shows moderate contrast enhancement of frontal sinus lymphoma.

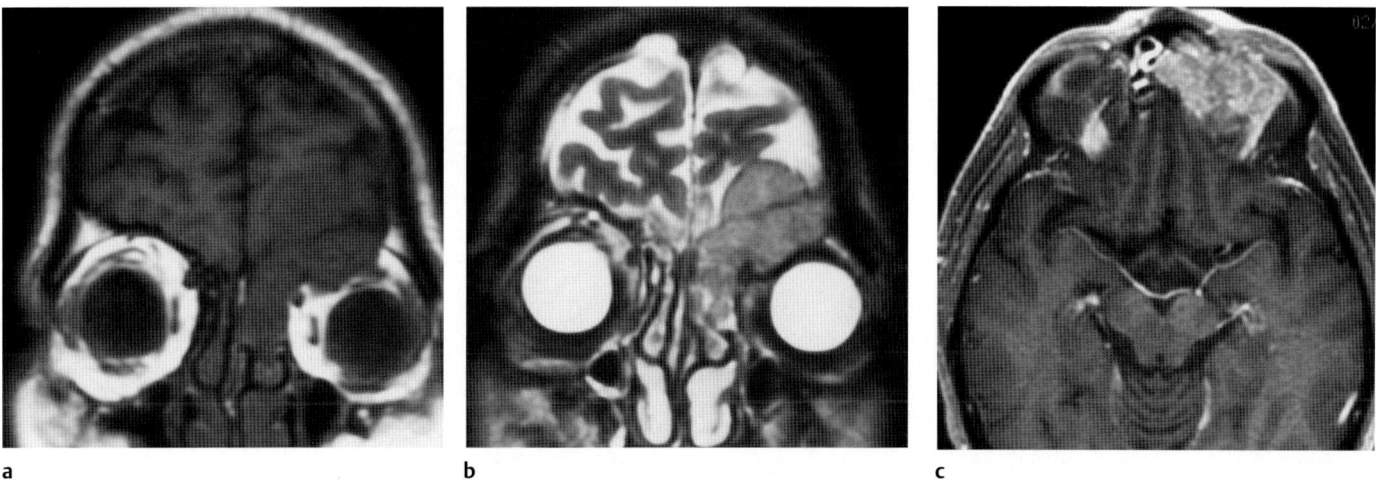

Fig. 4.159 Frontal sinus lymphoma. **a** Coronal T1W MR scan shows a mass in the left frontal sinus and frontonasal recess. **b** Coronal T2W MR scan shows the mass to be hypointense to brain. **c** Axial enhanced T1W MR scan shows marked enhancement of frontal sinus lymphoma. Case courtesy of Harish Shownkeen, MD, Chicago, IL, USA.

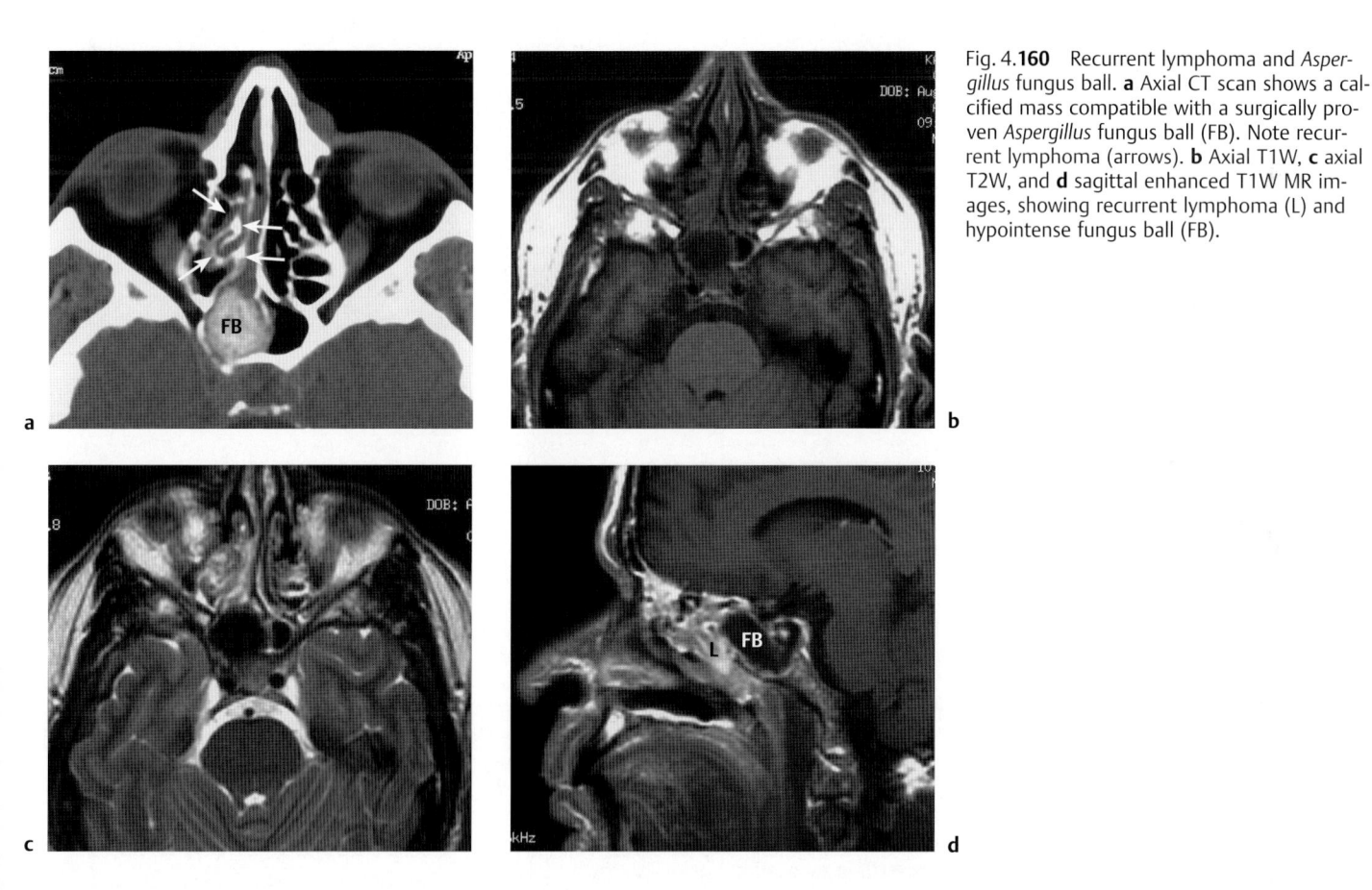

Fig. 4.160 Recurrent lymphoma and *Aspergillus* fungus ball. **a** Axial CT scan shows a calcified mass compatible with a surgically proven *Aspergillus* fungus ball (FB). Note recurrent lymphoma (arrows). **b** Axial T1W, **c** axial T2W, and **d** sagittal enhanced T1W MR images, showing recurrent lymphoma (L) and hypointense fungus ball (FB).

Plasmacytoma of the sinonasal tract appears on CT scans as a fairly well-defined mass, which often has expansile characteristics and is associated with bone remodeling, as well as bone erosion (Fig. 4.**161**). There will be moderate to marked enhancement after intravenous infusion of contrast material. On MR images, plasmacytoma appears as a mass of low signal intensity on T1-weighted and intermediate to high signal intensity on T2-weighted images (Fig. 4.**161**). It may disclose moderate to marked enhancement following intravenous administration of gadolinium-based contrast material. Imaging alone cannot be used to reliably distinguish this tumor from other malignancies of the sinonasal tract.[80]

Posttransplantation Lymphoproliferative Disorders (PTLD)

The chronic use of immunosuppressive agents has been associated with an increase in the incidence of lymphoproliferative disorders. The process has a strong predilection for extranodal sites, most frequently involving the gastrointestinal tract, the CNS, and the allografted organ.[81,82] Involvement of the sinonasal cavities and other parts of the head and neck is relatively rare, presenting as focal submucosal masses involving Waldeyer's ring or as cervical lymphadenopathy.[81,82] Gordon et al.[82] reported a case of a patient who presented with multiple cranial nerve palsies due to PTLD that arose in the paranasal sinuses and spread to the skull base, mimicking invasive fungal infection on CT and MRI scans.[82]

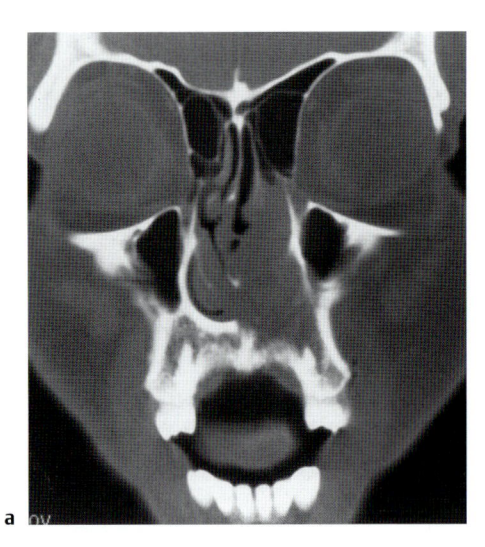

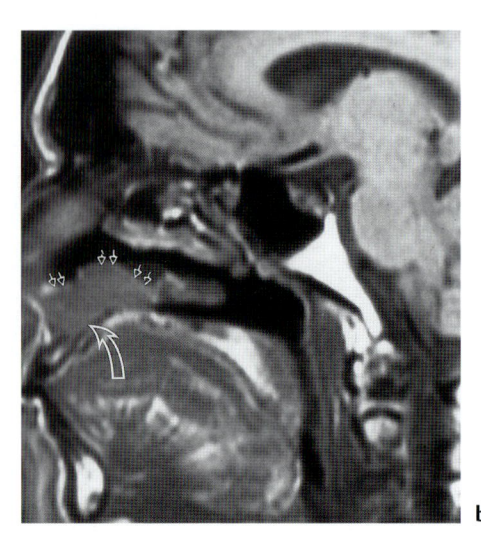

Fig. 4.**161** Plasmacytoma. **a** CT scan shows a left nasal cavity mass, along with erosion of the floor of the left nasal cavity. **b** Sagittal T1W MR scan shows a hypointense mass (arrows).

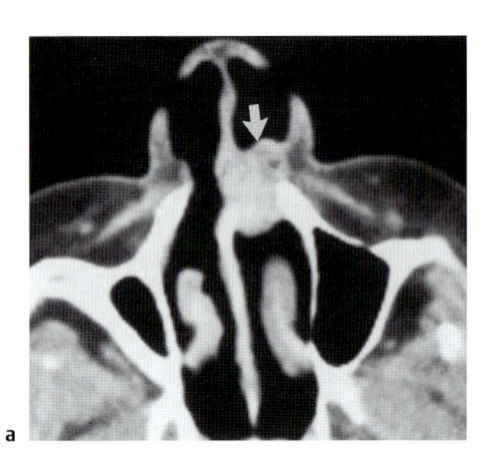

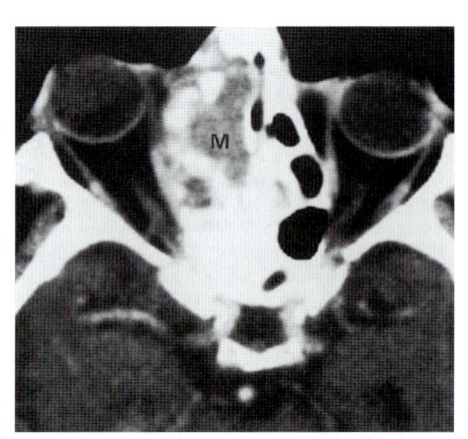

Fig. 4.**162** **a** Malignant melanoma. Axial CT scan shows a well-defined mass in the anterior left nasal cavity (arrow). **b** Malignant melanoma. Postcontrast axial CT scan in another patient shows a large mass (M) involving the right nasal cavity and right ethmoid air cells, and with extension into the right orbit.

Leukemic Manifestation in the Paranasal Sinuses

Chronic lymphocytic leukemia (CLL) is the most common leukemia of adults. It is an indolent disease most prevalent in older patients; 90% of patients are more than 50 years old.[83] Head and neck manifestations of CLL are commonly associated with cervical lymphadenopathy. Expression of CLL in the paranasal sinuses is very rare; there are only three cases reported in the literature. CT findings are similar to chronic inflammatory polypoid mucosal thickening. Granulocytic sarcoma is a rare extramedullary collection of immature cells with myelogenous differentiation. It is also known as chloroma because the tumor has a greenish hue. Secondary to the presence of intracellular myeloperoxidase, the occurrence of chloroma usually heralds acute myelogenous leukemia or the onset of the blastic phase of chronic myelogenous leukemia. It occurs commonly in soft tissue, skin, periosteum, and lymph nodes, although it can occur anywhere throughout the body. Involvement of the sino-orbital region has been shown in Chapter 8.

Malignant Melanoma of Sinonasal Cavities

Malignant melanoma involving the nasal and paranasal sinus mucosa is rare and difficult to treat; it has a poor prognosis, which is generally even worse than that of cutaneous malignant melanoma.[84] Approximately 20% of all malignant melanomas occur in the head and neck region,[84] of which less than 10% affect the mucous membranes of the oral cavity or upper respiratory tract.[84–86] Less than 1% of all malignant melanomas arise in the nasal cavity or adjacent sinuses.[84] The majority of lesions originate in the nasal cavity (Figs. 4.**162**, 4.**163**), and less than 25% begin in the maxillary sinus.[84] Local recurrence and distant metastases may occur many years after initial therapy.[84] The 5-year survival is 10–25%.[5, 84] Melanotic tumors may have a characteristic MR appearance, namely, hyperintense on T1-weighted and hypointense on T2-weighted MR images, although this MR appearance may often not be present (Fig. 4.**163**).

■ Benign Fibro-osseous, Osseous, and Cartilaginous Lesions of the Sinonasal Region

Fibro-osseous, osseous, and cartilaginous lesions of the facial region, including the sinonasal cavities and orbital region, are relatively uncommon.[87–90] These lesions may share overlapping clinical, radiological, and pathological features causing potential difficulties in diagnosis. Included within this spectrum of sinonasal and other craniofacial fibro-osseous and cartilaginous lesions are both nonneoplastic proliferation and neoplasms.

Included under the category of benign fibro-osseous lesions are fibrous dysplasia and ossifying fibroma. In a perfect world, fibrous dysplasia (FD) and ossifying fibroma (OF) would be readily differentiated on the basis of radiographic and his-

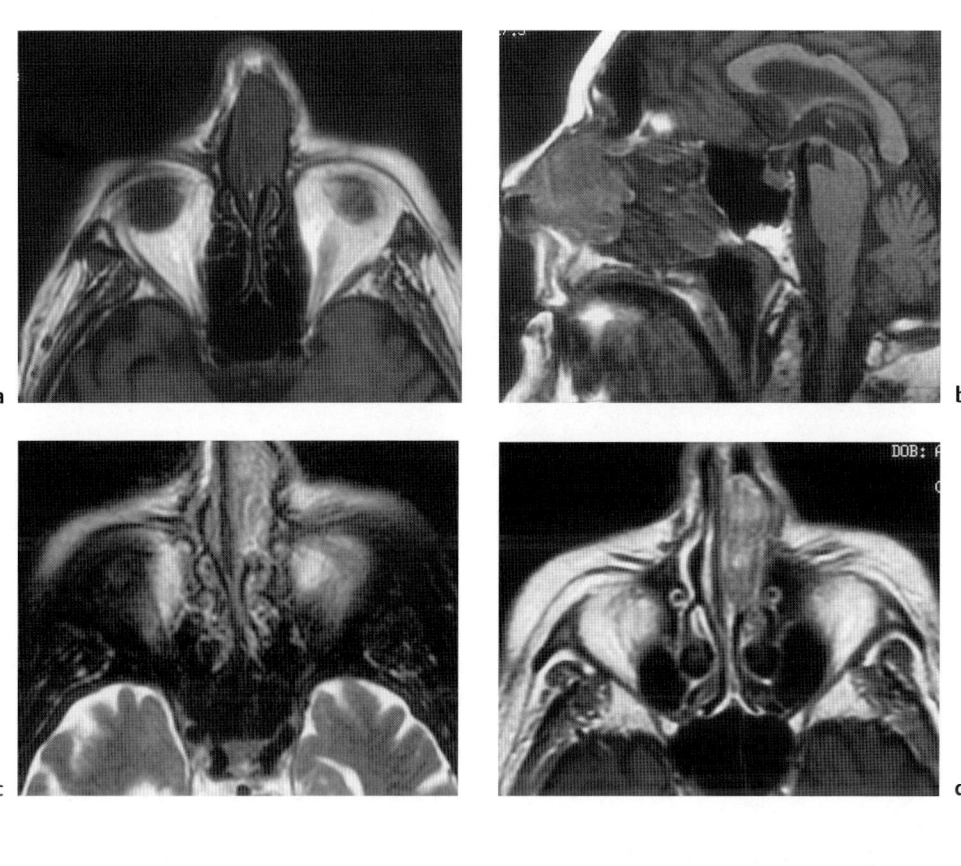

Fig. 4.**163** Nasal malignant melanoma. **a** Axial T1W MR scan shows a mass in the left nasal cavity. **b** Sagittal T1W MR scan shows the nasal mass, which appears slightly hyperintense to brain. **c** T2W axial MR scan. The mass is hyperintense to brain. **d** Axial enhanced T1W MR scan shows marked tumor enhancement.

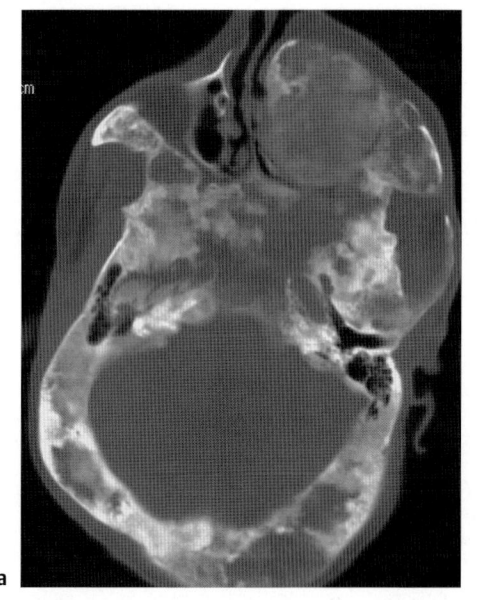

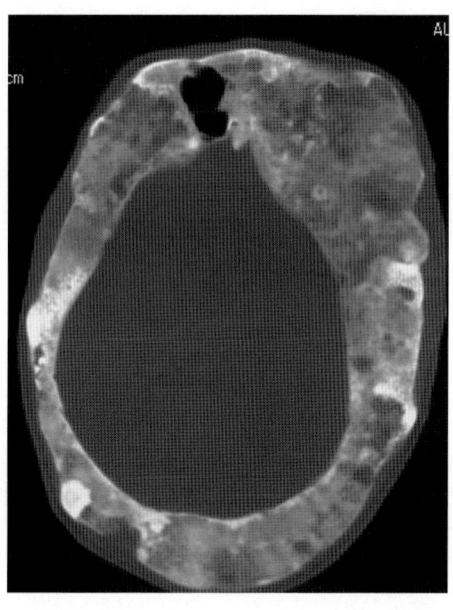

Fig. 4.**164** McCune–Albright syndrome. **a, b** CT scans show diffuse form of fibrous dysplasia involving the craniofacial bones.

topathological features. Craniofacial benign fibro-osseous lesions, however, may not be separable by histopathological evaluation. FD may show histological features normally attributable to OF (e.g., lamellar bone and osteoblastic rimming). OF may show features normally attributable to FD (e.g., woven bone with absent osteoblastic rimming). In the absence of radiographic correlation, such lesions are designated by pathologists as benign fibro-osseous lesion, not further specified.[90]

Fibrous Dysplasia

Fibrous dysplasia (FD) is an idiopathic nonheritable benign bone disease in which normal medullary bone is replaced by structurally weak fibrous and osseous tissue.[90,91] Three general subtypes of disease are recognized: monostotic (70% of cases), polyostotic (27% of cases), and McCune–Albright syndrome (3% of cases). The monostotic form is the mildest form. The most severe form of the disease, McCune–Albright syndrome, is more commonly found in females, is associated with short stature, and is associated with endocrine abnormalities and pigmented cutaneous lesions (Fig. 4.**164**).[92,93] The monostotic form is not believed to be a precursor to the polyostotic form.[90] Congenital fibrous dysplasia, also known as cherubism, is an autosomal dominant disease characterized by bilateral swelling of gnathic bones, usually the mandible (Fig. 4.**165**).[90] Expansion of the maxilla with involvement of the maxillary sinuses and infraorbital rim of the maxilla produces upward bulging of the orbital floor resulting in lifting of the eye, exposure of the lower portion of the sclera, and tightening

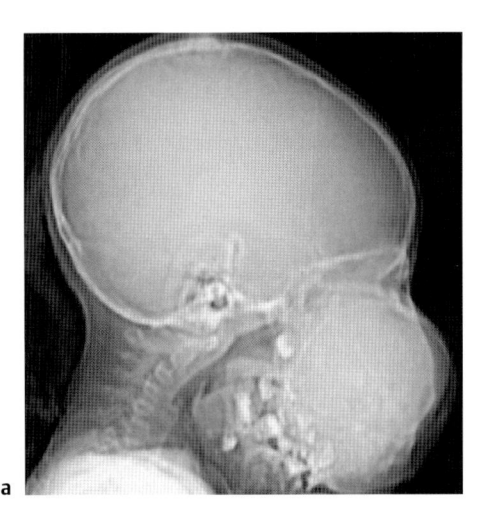

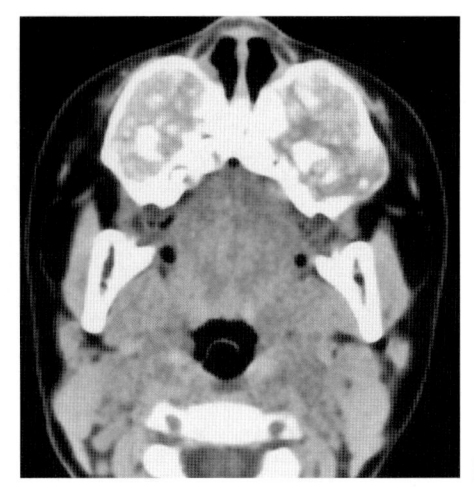

Fig. 4.**165** Cherubism. **a** Lateral scanogram and **b** CT scan show bilateral involvement of maxilla by fibrous dysplasia. Note expansion of the maxilla and involvement of maxillary sinuses.

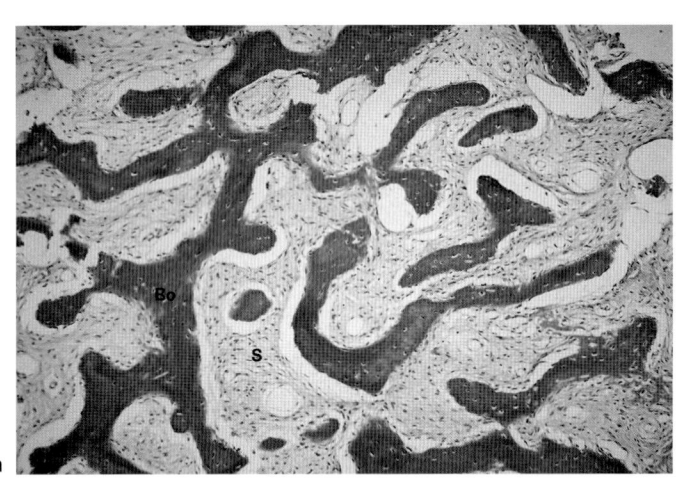

Fig. 4.**166** Fibrous dysplasia. **a** Low-power and **b** high-power photomicrographs. This fibro-osseous lesion is characterized by irregularly shaped, immature (woven) bone (Bo) that typically lacks osteoblastic rimming. The trabeculae of bone are not lamellar bone but coarse immature woven bone. The stroma (S) is moderately cellular. The fibrous tissue component is similar to that of ossifying fibroma (see Fig. 4.**171**); it includes nondescript, fibrous tissue without pattern and can be of variable cellularity. Case courtesy of Bruce Wenig, MD, Washington D.C., USA.

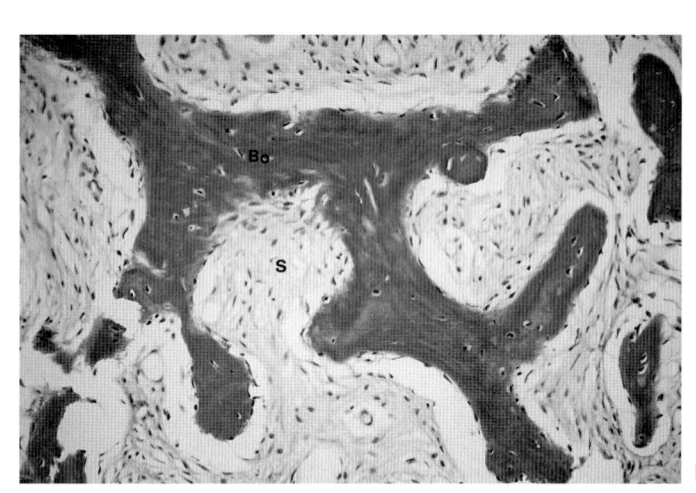

of the overlying facial skin with retraction of the lower eyelids. The overall result is the cherubic appearance as depicted in Renaissance art with upward gaze toward heaven.[90]

The precise etiology of FD is unknown. Lee and co-workers[94] proposed that abnormal intracellular regulation of cyclic adenosine monophosphate or protein kinase A is a possible etiological factor in the development of FD. Several other researchers[91, 95] have identified mutations in the $G_s\alpha$ gene, resulting in altered activity of intrinsic GTPase activity or the G_s protein signal transduction pathway as a cause of FD. It is now believed that FD is caused by a postzygotic, somatic mutation of the protein transcript of the *GNAS-1* gene, which encodes the alpha (α) subunit of the stimulatory G protein.[96, 97] Mutations at position 201 of $G_s\alpha$ in which arginine is replaced by cysteine or by histidine were found first in endocrine organs in patients with McCune–Albright syndrome,[96, 97] and then in monostotic and polyostotic FD. The natural progression of FD includes two phases: an active phase which persists until puberty and a subsequent quiescent phase.[98] The majority of patients affected by FD are under 30 years of age and are usually in the first two decades of life.[99] A significant number of cases may not be present until adulthood.[99]

The histopathological appearance of FD is overgrowth of the fibrous stroma surrounding disorganized trabeculae (Fig. 4.**166**). The fibrous tissue component is nondescript, without pattern, and is of variable cellularity. The osseous component includes irregularly shaped trabeculae of osteoid and immature (woven) bone arising metaplastically from the fibrous stroma; it is poorly oriented with misshapen bony trabeculae, increased cellularity, and irregular margins, and forms odd geometric patterns including C-shaped or S-shaped configurations (so-called Chinese characters). The trabeculae typically lack osteoblastic rimming (Fig. 4.**166**).[90] Multinucleated giant cells, macrophages, increased vascularity, and calcification may be seen.[90] FD and ossifying fibroma may be histologically indistinguishable. FD may be complicated by aneurysmal bone cyst formation because of the vascularity of the lesion. Aneurysmal bone cyst is a radiographic term and not a clinical entity. Anatomically the most commonly involved area of the skull is the ethmoid bone, followed by the sphenoid, frontal, and maxillary bones.[91]

The appropriate management of FD around the optic nerve within the optic canal in patients with normal vision is controversial. In a study by Lee et al.,[99] statistically significant narrow-

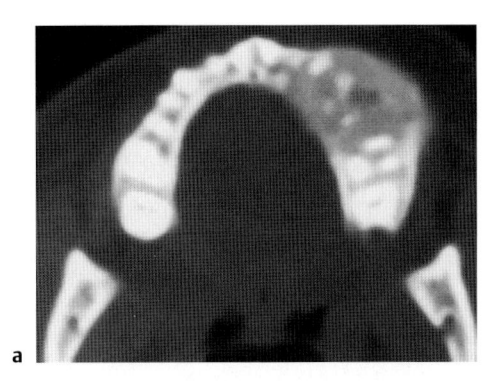

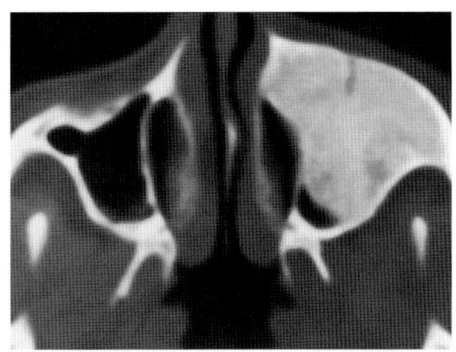

Fig. 4.**167** Fibrous dysplasia. **a**, **b** CT scans show local expansion of the alveolar process of the left maxilla. Note absence of periosteal reaction/elevation or penetration of adjacent soft tissues. Section through the maxillary sinuses (**b**) demonstrates typical ground-glass appearance with imperceptible blending into normal cortical bone.

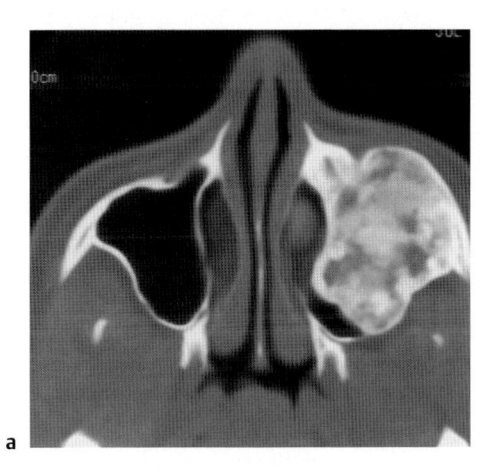

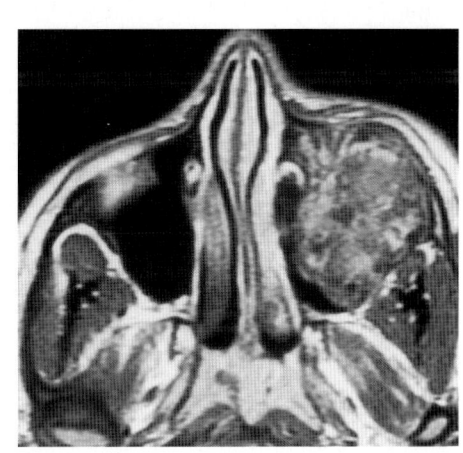

Fig. 4.**168** Fibrous dysplasia. **a** CT scan and **b** enhanced T1W MR scan showing fibrous dysplasia of the left maxillarly antrum. Note heterogeneous, marked contrast enhancement in **b**.

ing of the encased optic canal was observed in patients with FD, as compared with normal controls. However, despite the optic canal constriction, 95% of the patients had normal vision. The authors concluded that prophylactic decompression of the optic nerve cannot be recommended on the basis of diagnostic imaging alone. The cause of both the acute and gradual loss of vision associated with FD remains unclear.[99] Possible causes include optic nerve compression, optic nerve traction, trauma, pathological fracture, and cystic masses such as aneurysmal bone cyst associated with some cases of FD.[99] There are some pharmacological agents available that may have limited effects in patients with FD. These include bisphosphonates, which inhibit osteoclastic bone resorption, aromatase inhibitors, and tamoxifen citrate, which have proved successful in the treatment of precocious puberty in patients with McCune–Albright syndrome.[91] In the absence of curative medication for FD, surgery remains the mainstay of therapy.[91] Lesions discovered incidentally on CT or MRI scans that are asymptomatic should be followed by imaging. Radiation therapy is ineffective and is contraindicated because of the possibility of malignant transformation.[91]

Diagnostic Imaging

The radiological features of fibrous dysplasia depend on the stage of development and amount of bony matrix within the lesion. Radiographic changes range from lucent zones to diffuse areas of sclerosis (Figs. 4.**164**, 4.**167**). Periosteal reaction or cortical break are not a feature of benign fibro-osseous lesions. Facial bones and the base of the skull are preferentially involved by the sclerotic form of fibrous dysplasia. The lytic form is often seen in cranial bones. Expansion of involved bone with a heterogeneous pattern of CT densities, along with intact thin cortex, is characteristic of fibrous dysplasia (Fig. 4.**167**). In ossifying fibroma, often there is a moderately thick peripheral rim of bone density present (see Fig. 4.**172**). Fibrous dysplasia has an intermediate signal intensity on T1-weighted MR images and heterogeneous hypointense signal intensity on T2-weighted MR images (Figs. 4.**168**–4.**170**). There may be areas of T2-weighted hyperintensity, particularly in early stages of the disease. Following intravenous administration of Gd-DTPA contrast material, there is often moderate to marked contrast enhancement (Figs. 4.**168**–4.**170**). Fibrous dysplasia or ossifying fibroma, particularly of sphenoid bone, may be mistaken for meningioma on MR scans.

Ossifying Fibroma

Ossifying fibromas have a predilection for women and tend to occur in older age groups, most frequently seen in the third and fourth decades of life, although any age may be affected.[90] A predilection for African-American women has been reported.[90] Orbital and paraorbital involvement is generally asymptomatic, unassociated with pain or swelling, and is often diagnosed incidentally following radiographic examination. Symptomatic tumors manifest by displacement of teeth or as an expansile unilateral swelling that may eventually result in facial asymmetry. Ossifying fibroma has been suggested as arising from the mesenchyme of the periodontal ligament and, as such, is related to the cementifying fibroma and cemento-ossifying fibroma.[90]

Ossifying fibromas appear as tan-gray to white, gritty, and firm, varying in size from 0.5 to 10 cm. Histologically, ossifying fibromas are composed of randomly distributed mature (lamellar) bone spicules rimmed by osteoblasts admixed within a fibrous stroma (Fig. 4.**171**). Although the osseous component is generally

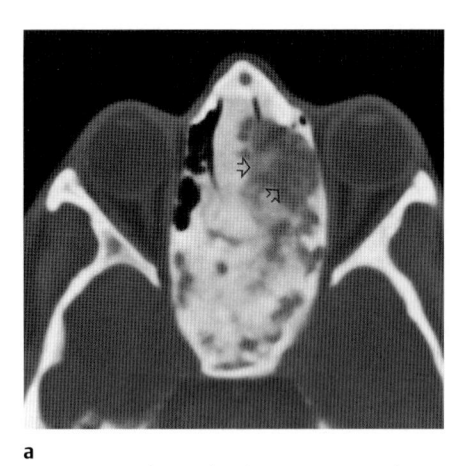

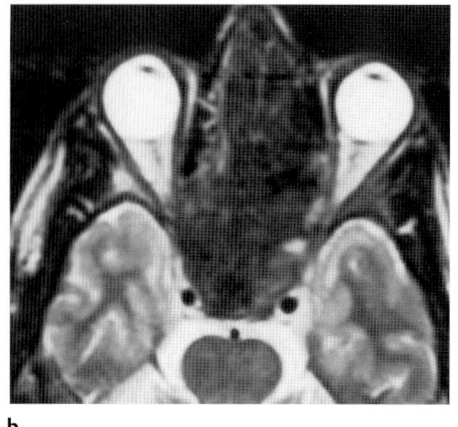

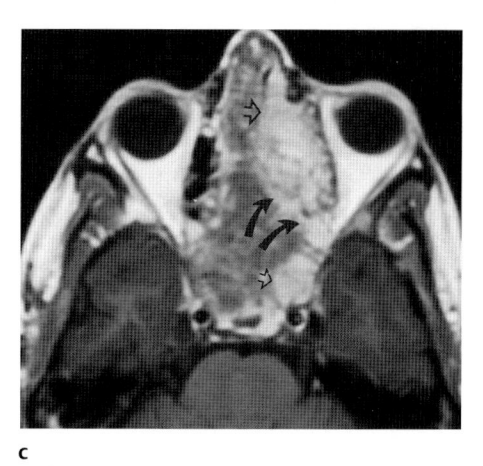

Fig. 4.**169** Fibrous dysplasia. **a** CT scan, **b** T2W MR scan, and **c** enhanced T1W MR scan showing fibrous dysplasia of the ethmoid and sphenoid bones. Note that the less-mineralized portion (arrows in **a**) appears to show more contrast enhancement on contrast-enhanced MRI (arrows in **c**).

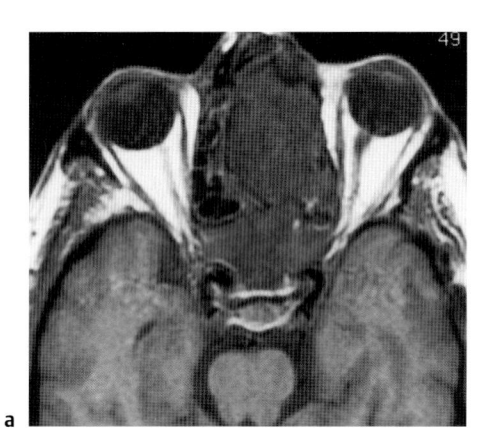

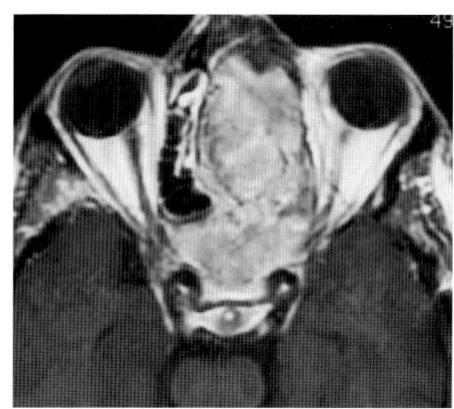

Fig. 4.**170** Fibrous dysplasia. **a** T1W and **b** enhanced T1W MR scans, showing fibrous dysplasia of the ethmoid and sphenoid bones. Note intense homogeneous enhancement.

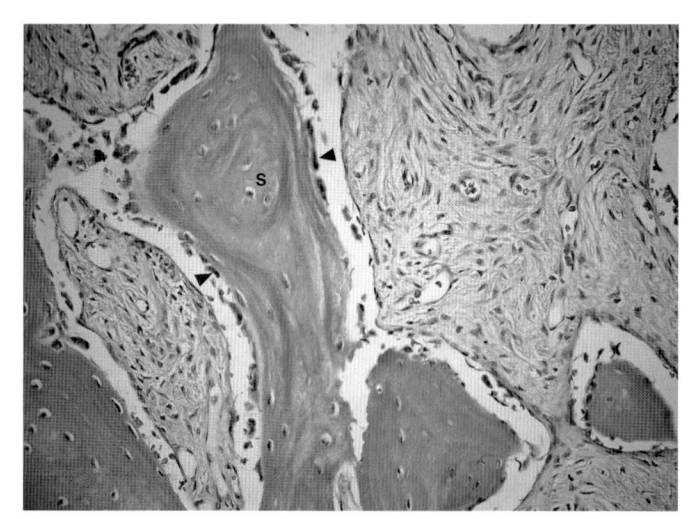

Fig. 4.**171** Ossifying fibroma (photomicrograph). This fibro-osseous lesion is characterized by the presence of mature (lamellar) bony spicules (S), rimmed by osteoblasts (arrowheads), and mixed with a fibrous stroma. Courtesy of Bruce Wenig, MD, Washington D.C., USA.

described as mature, the central portions may be woven bone with lamellar bone at the periphery. Complete bone maturation is seldom seen. A fibrous stroma may be densely cellular; mitotic figures are rare to absent.[90] Secondary changes, including hemorrhage, inflammation, and giant cells, may be seen. The differential diagnosis of ossifying fibroma is primarily from fibrous dysplasia. For ossifying fibromas, surgical excision is the treatment of choice. The prognosis is excellent following complete excision. Recurrences rarely occur.[90]

Radiological features depend on the stage of development and amount of mineralized matrix present. The lesion is seen as a well-circumscribed or sharply demarcated mass with smooth contours (Fig. 4.**172**). In its early stage, the lesion may appear as a solitary cystlike or solid soft tissue with minimal or no mineralized (calcified) components. At a later stage, the lesions become radiopaque. On CT scans, ossifying fibromas appear as an expansile mass, surrounded by a thick or thin radiodense rimming. There may be islands of bone formation within the lesion (Figs. 4.**173**, 4.**174**). On MR imaging scans, ossifying fibromas appear heterogeneous and usually have low to intermediate signal intensity on T1-weighted and hypointense signal intensity on T2-weighted MR images. There is moderate contrast enhancement on postgadolinium T1-weighted MRI scans.

Variants of Ossifying Fibroma

Included within the spectrum of ossifying fibroma are its variants, which are essentially the same lesion but perhaps differ in the nature of the calcified material that is present (cementum versus bone); in the location of the lesion in question (oral versus paranasal sinus or orbital); or in other morphological variations (presence of psammomatoid concretions) and overall biological

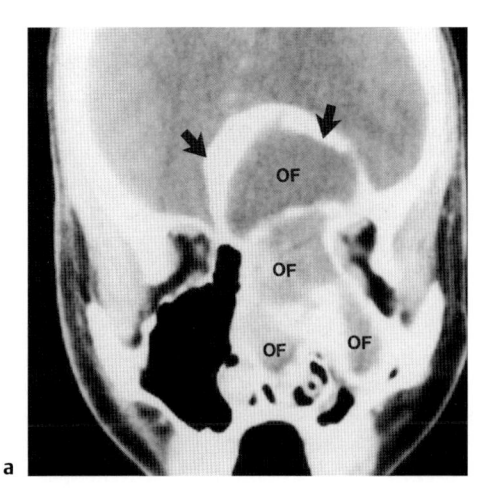

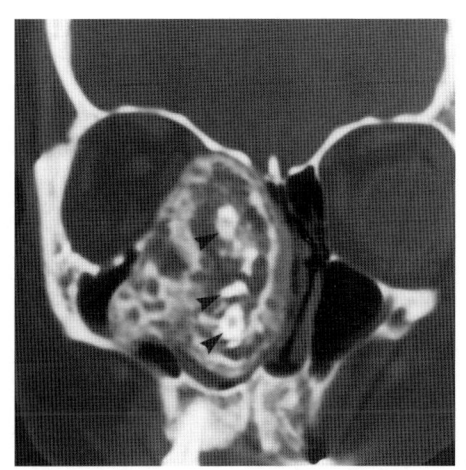

Fig. 4.**172** Ossifying fibroma. **a** CT scan shows a large ethmoid ossifying fibroma (OF), demonstrating an expansile lesion involving the floor of the anterior cranial fossa (arrows). Note extension into the left nasal cavity and maxillary sinus. **b** Coronal CT scan in another patient shows an ossifying fibroma involving the nasoethmoid complex, demonstrating multiple islands of mineralized bodies (mature bone) (arrows) Note a shell-like appearance of the lesion without CT evidence for invasion of adjacent orbit.

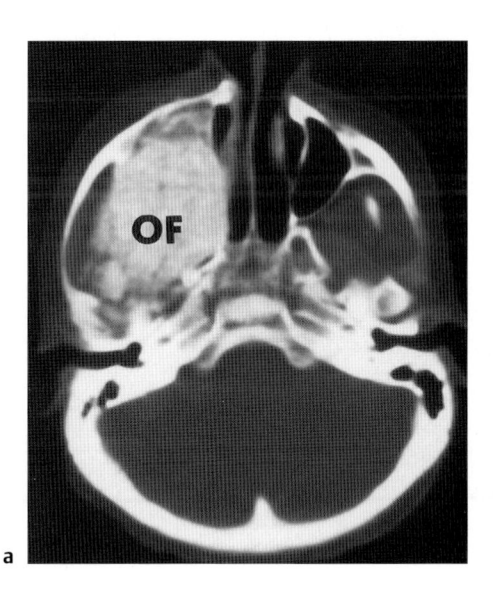

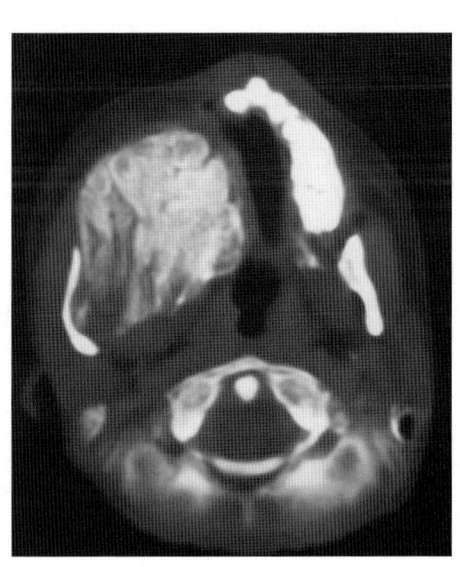

Fig. 4.**173** Ossifying fibroma. **a**, **b** Axial CT scans in a child, showing a presumed ossifying fibroma (OF).

behavior (aggressive versus static). Gnathic lesions likely originate from periodontal ligament. The cells of the periodontal ligament are capable of producing cementum, bone, or fibrous tissue.[90] Such lesions, depending on the presence of cementum or bone, are designated as cementifying fibromas or ossifying fibromas. Those lesions with an admixture of both matrix materials are called cemento-ossifying fibroma. The histogenesis for similar-appearing lesions that occur in areas not associated with the periodontal ligament (e.g., paranasal sinuses, orbit) is not entirely known. It is possible that these lesions originate from displaced periodontal ligamentous tissue in embryogenesis. Alternatively, they originate from other cells capable of producing cementum, bone, and fibrous tissue. In the orbital and paraorbital regions, these usually lack cementum; may have oval-to-round calcified concretions with concentric laminations (psammomatoid concretion); and may behave in a locally aggressive manner with extension into adjacent anatomical compartments and destruction of bony confines. These lesions have been designated by a variety of names, including aggressive psammomatoid ossifying fibromas and juvenile active ossifying fibroma.[90, 95]

Psammomatoid Active Ossifying Fibroma

The psammomatoid active ossifying fibroma, also called the juvenile aggressive psammomatoid ossifying fibroma, is a variant of conventional ossifying fibroma that typically occurs in the sinonasal tract and potentially may behave aggressively with locally invasive and destructive capabilities.[90, 95] There is no gender predilection. These lesions occur in younger age groups (first and second decades) resulting in their designation as juvenile psammomatoid ossifying fibroma. Their designation as juvenile, however, is not always accurate because they occur over a wide age range, including older-aged individuals.[90, 95] Presenting symptoms include facial swelling, nasal obstruction, pain, sinusitis, headache, and proptosis. These lesions may occur in any area of the sinonasal tract but show predilection for the ethmoid sinus, nasal, and supraorbital frontal region.[90, 95] There may be involvement of a single site or multiple sinuses, and the orbit may be involved.

Histologically, the most distinctive component of ossifying fibroma is the presence of mineralized or calcified psammomatoid bodies or ossicles. These ossicles vary from a few in number to a dense population of innumerable spherical bodies. The ossicles vary from small with a round-to-oval shape to a larger irregularly shaped ossicle pattern, and are present within the bony trabeculae as well as within the adjacent cellular stroma (Fig. 4.**174**). Osteoclasts are present within the ossicles and osteoblasts can be seen along their peripheral aspects. The bony trabeculae vary in appearance and include odd shapes with a curvilinear pattern to coarse bone trabeculae. The trabeculae are composed of lamellar bone with associated osteoclasts and osteoblastic rimming. Transition zones between the spherical ossicles and bony trabeculae can be seen. The nonosseous component includes a cellular stroma with a fascicular-to-storiform growth composed of round-to-polyhedral spindle-shaped cells with prominent basophilic nuclei and apparent cytoplasmic borders. Mitotic figures can be seen, but mitotic activity is not prominent and atypical mitoses are not present.

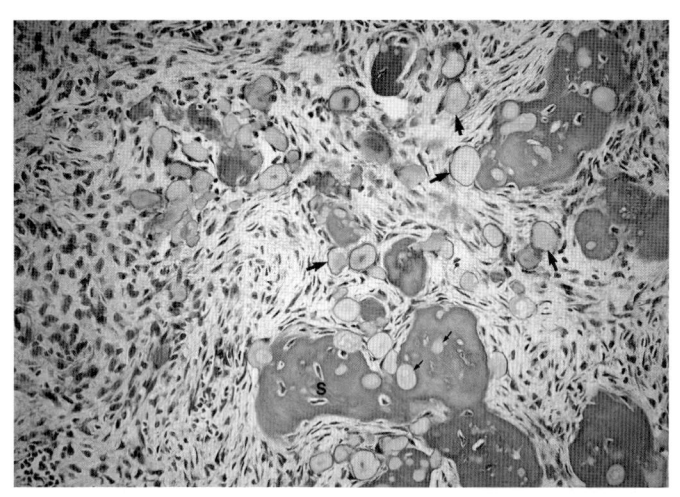

Fig. 4.**174** Aggressive psammomatoid ossifying fibroma (photomicrograph). The most distinctive component of this variant of ossifying fibroma is the mineralized or calcified psammomatoid bodies or ossicles (arrows). The ossicles vary from small, with a round to oval shape, to a larger, irregularly shaped ossicle pattern, and are present within the bony trabeculae (smaller arrows) as well as within the adjacent cellular stroma. Note spicules of woven bone (S) dispersed within a cellular fibrous stroma. In this histological variant of ossifying fibroma, trabeculae of newly formed bone are very small, suggesting cementicles or psammoma bodies (arrows). Courtesy of Bruce Wenig, MD, Washington D.C., USA.

Radiological features are similar to ossifying fibroma with admixture of both soft-tissue and bone density pattern. The lesion has an aggressive appearance with marked expansion of bone with or without apparent cortical break (Fig. 4.**175**). Periosteal reaction and new bone formation, seen in osteochondrogenic sarcomas, is not a feature of ossifying fibroma or psammomatoid active ossifying fibroma. The lesion may extend into surrounding tissue by virtue of expansion but not invasion (Figs. 4.**175 b, c**). On CT and MR images there may be areas of soft-tissue fluid-like levels. The most characteristic feature is the presence of numerous round or oval calcified bodies of varied sizes, representing the psammomatoid (cementicle) bodies (Fig. 4.**175**). The MR imaging appearance of psammomatoid active ossifying fibroma is also similar to ossifying fibroma, including moderate to marked enhancement on postgadolinium MRI scans. On T2-weighted MR images, there may be areas of hyperintensity signal simulating cysts or soft-tissue fluid levels. Complete surgical excision is the treatment of choice. The prognosis is good following complete excision, but recurrences may occur and the tumors may behave in an aggressive manner with local destruction and potential invasion into vital structures.[90, 95]

Extramedullary Hematopoiesis of Paranasal Sinuses

Extramedullary hematopoiesis of the paranasal sinuses (EHPS) may simulate the radiographic appearance of fibrous dysplasia.[100] It is uncommon, but it needs to be included in the differential diagnosis of fibro-osseous lesions, and when the cause of apparent soft-tissue masses or opacifications of the sinuses is being investigated in patients with hyperactive hematopoietic disorders.[100] This is particularly true in patients who suffer from thalassemia, sickle cell anemia, or myeloproliferative disorders. Radiographic features of EHPS may include hypertrophy of the sinuses, obliteration of the sinuses, and expansion of the sinuses. On CT scans there will be linear and fine increased densities within the opacified sinuses, resembling islands of calcification, seen in benign fibro-osseous lesions and those of low-grade chondrosarcoma. On MRI, the lesions appear hypointense on T1-weighted and T2-weighted MR images and demonstrate

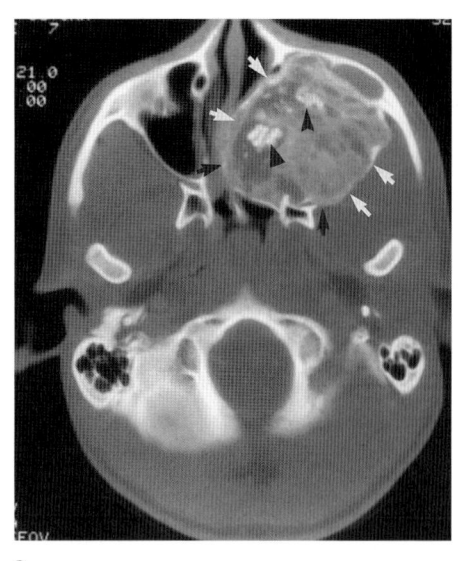

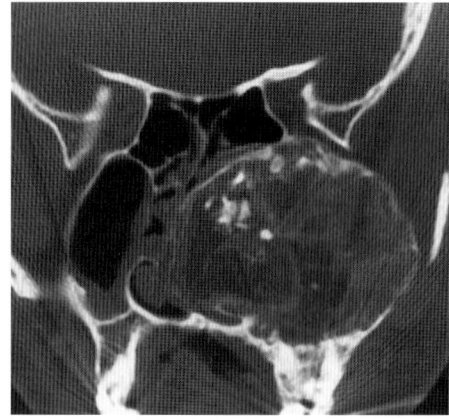

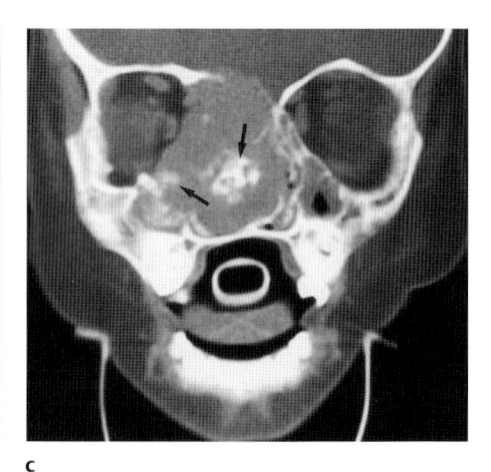

Fig. 4.**175** Aggressive psammomatoid ossifying fibroma. **a** Axial CT scan shows a large expansile mass of mixed density. Note several small mineralized foci, psammomatoid bodies (arrowheads). Note expansion of the posterior and medial walls of the maxillary antrum (arrows). **b** Coronal CT scan shows a pathologically proven psammomatoid ossifying fibroma in this patient. **c** CT scan in an 18-month-old child shows a soft-tissue mass, with involvement of medial wall of the orbit as well as the roof of the ethmoid bone. Note intralesional islands of mineralization (arrows). Case in Fig. 4.**175 c** courtesy of Tony Pedulo, MD, Westmead, Australia.

Paget Disease of Bone (Osteitis Deformans)

Paget disease of bone represents a common disorder affecting 3–4% of the population over the age of 40 years.[101] The cause of Paget disease remains uncertain. A probable viral origin has been proposed because intranuclear inclusion bodies (resembling those of a paramyxovirus variety) are found in the osteoclasts in histological specimens of Paget disease.[101] Paget disease is characterized by excessive and abnormal remodeling of bone, with both active and quiescent phases. In the lytic phase (incipient-active), osteoclasts predominate. In the mixed phase (active), osteoblasts begin to appear superimposed on osteoclastic activity and eventually predominate. Finally, the blastic phase (late-inactive) appears in which osteoclastic activity gradually declines.[101] Paget disease of differing phases may be seen in the same patient. Paget disease is predominantly located in the axial skeleton, with the most commonly affected site being the pelvis. The spine and skull are the next most common sites of involvement. Bone enlargement as well as trabecular and cortical thickening can be depicted on CT and MR images (Fig. 4.**176**). On MRI, the bone marrow frequently maintains its yellow marrow signal characteristic. The increased blood flow seen pathologically in Paget disease is reflected as increased enhancement, following intravenous administration of gadolinium contrast material.[101] Sarcomatous transformation which occurs in 1% of patients with Paget disease is heralded by findings of masslike replacement of the marrow space, cortical destruction, and an associated enhancing soft-tissue mass on CT or MR images.[101]

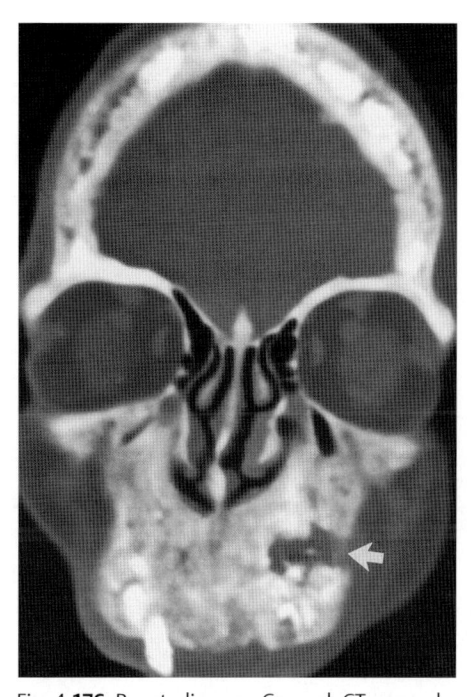

Fig. 4.**176** Paget disease. Coronal CT scan shows involvement of the craniofacial bones by Paget disease. Note typical bone enlargement and mixed excessive bone formation as well as loss of bone density. The bone defect (arrow) is the site of biopsy. Case courtesy of Calvin Flowers, MD, Chicago, IL, USA.

Osteopetrosis

Osteopetrosis is believed to result from more than one genetic or biochemical defect, with at least five types of the disease having been described.[102] The osteopetroses are a heterogeneous group of genetic conditions characterized by increased bone density due to impaired bone resorption by osteoclasts.[103, 104] The two most commonly seen forms are autosomal recessive (malignant) osteopetrosis (AROP) and autosomal dominant (benign) osteopetrosis (ADOP). The different forms can easily be differentiated by mode of inheritance, clinical and radiological findings, and prognosis.[103] In humans, currently, only three genes have been associated with osteopetrosis.[104] The precocious type of osteopetrosis is an autosomal recessive form that presents at birth or early in life and causes death, usually in early childhood, due to severe anemia and major infections.[103] Nerve palsies, related to bone thickening, can cause complications such as deafness and blindness, and reduced marrow space results in extramedullary hematopoiesis and hepatosplenomegaly. Treatment of these patients currently involves mostly bone marrow transplantation or the administration of recombinant human interferon.[103] Radiographically, a generalized increased bone density (osteosclerosis) is seen. Osteopetrosis with renal tubular acidosis and cerebral calcifications is an autosomal recessive type of osteopetrosis that manifests in early childhood with pathological fractures, failure to thrive, short stature, and in most cases mental retardation.[103] The radiographic findings are similar to the other types of osteopetrosis but there seems to be a spontaneous regression of the osteosclerosis in later childhood.[103] All patients show intracranial calcifications in the basal ganglia and in the cortex.[103] The intermediate type of osteopetrosis is an autosomal recessive type characterized by a much milder clinical picture than the precocious type (malignant type). This type is very rare and radiographically there is a diffuse osteosclerosis.

The delayed type of osteopetrosis is an autosomal dominant form, also known as the benign or adult type. This is much milder than the previously described types. Most patients are asymptomatic and are at times incidentally detected by radiological examination.[103] Depending on the distribution of sclerosis, two basic phenotypes are distinguished within this adult group. These two types also show some clinical differences.[102–104] The autosomal dominant osteopetrosis type I (ADOP I) usually presents without symptoms.[103] Radiologically, a generalized, uniform osteosclerosis is present (Fig. 4.**177**). The disease-causing gene is assigned to chromosome 11q12–13.[104] ADOP I is the only type of osteopetrosis not associated with an increased fracture rate.[103, 104] Autosomal dominant osteopetrosis type II (ADOP II), the form originally described by Albers-Schönberg,[104] is characterized by a sandwich-like appearance of the spine because of the thickened vertebral end plates. The gene carrying ADOP II is assigned to chromosome 1p21.[103] The distribution of bone sclerosis in ADOP I is generalized and mainly at the skull, the spine, and the long bones.[103] Unlike ADOP I, the distribution of bone sclerosis in ADOP II is a more focal hyperostosis pattern, resulting in endobones ("bones-within-bones"), a sandwich-like ("rugger-jersey spine") appearance of the spine, and the predominant sclerosis of the skull base.[103, 104] The CT appearance of ADOP types I and II includes increased sclerosis, bone thickening, and obliteration of the marrow space (Fig. 4.**177**). Bone thickening is associated with stenosis of the optic canal, superior and inferior orbital fissures, petrous carotid canal, vertebral transverse foramina (vertebral artery), and other skull base foramina. Optic canal stenosis and optic nerve atrophy are mainly seen in ADOP II and the autosomal recessive (malignant) osteopetrosis.[102] The MRI appearance of osteopetrotic bones includes marked hypointense signal on all pulse sequences.[102] The involved craniofacial bones appear thickened and the hypointensity on MRI includes the marrow space as well. The involved bones do not reveal contrast enhancement on enhanced T1-weighted MR im-

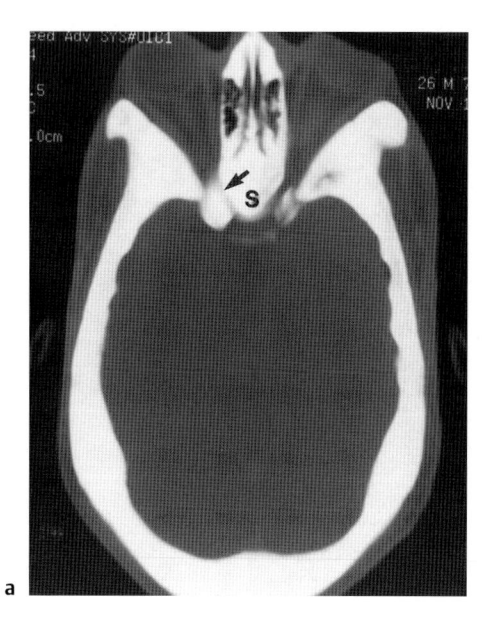

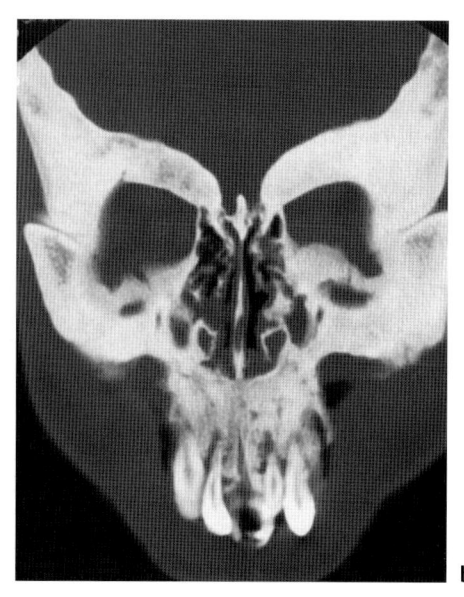

Fig. 4.177 Osteopetrosis in a 26-year-old man. **a** CT scan shows marked sclerosis and bone thickening of the craniofacial bones. Note constriction of the right optic canal (arrow). Note small size of ethmoid air cells and nondeveloped sphenoid sinus (S). **b** Coronal CT scan shows marked sclerosis and bone thickening of the craniofacial bones with obliteration of the marrow spaces. Note hypoplastic maxillary and ethmoid sinuses.

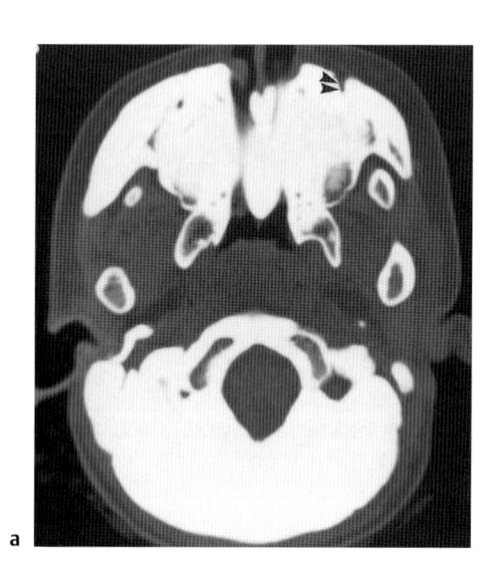

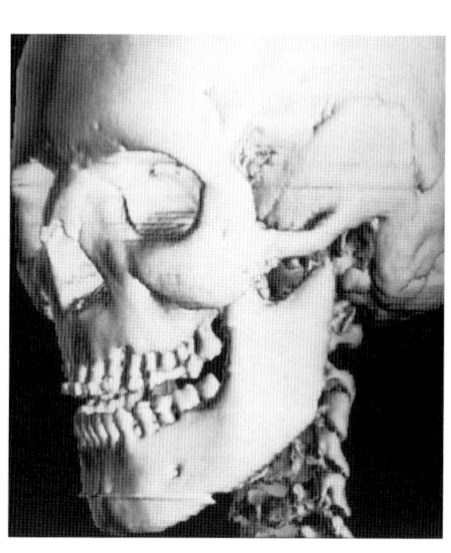

Fig. 4.178 Presumed Camurati–Englemann disease. **a** CT scan and **b** 3D reconstruction image showing sclerosis and bone thickening of the craniofacial bones. Note constriction of the inferior orbital canal (arrows in **a**). Courtesy James Goodwin, MD, Chicago, IL, USA.

ages. However, if there is associated extramedullary hematopoiesis, there will be moderate enhancement following intravenous administration of gadolinium contrast material.

Camurati–Engelmann Disease

Camurati–Engelmann disease is a rare sclerosing bone dysplasia, inherited as an autosomal dominant disorder.[103] The facial and cranial bones may be involved. The patients present in childhood with muscle weakness and pain, gait disturbances, hearing loss, and exophthalmos.[103] Radiographically, it consists of a craniotubular hyperostosis (Fig. 4.178). The distribution of the disease is usually symmetrical and bilateral.

Osteoma

Osteomas are benign bone-forming tumors that are almost exclusively identified in the craniofacial skeleton. In the craniofacial region, osteomas may be found in all sites but are most common in the frontal and ethmoid sinuses (Fig. 4.179).[12,90] These tumors are usually asymptomatic and are found by radiographic studies. Symptoms associated with paraorbital osteomas include headaches, facial swelling or deformity, and ocular disturbances.[12] Although usually asymptomatic, osteomas may obstruct the ostium of the sinus and result in a secondary infection or mucocele formation (see Fig. 4.98), or they may grow and encroach on adjacent structures, such as the orbit. They may also account for the severe sinus pain that some individuals experience during airplane flights. At times, a large osteoma of the frontal sinus may erode into the posterior table, resulting in marked pneumocephalus, and if there is underlying infection of the frontal sinus, there will be associated intracranial inflammation and abscess formation. Paraorbital osteomas usually occur as a single lesion but may be associated with Gardner syndrome, an inherited autosomal dominant trait characterized by intestinal (colorectal) polyposis; soft-tissue lesions (fibromatosis), cutaneous epidermoid cysts, lipomas, leiomyomas); and multiple craniofacial osteomas.[90] Histologically, osteomas are well-circumscribed and composed of dense, mature, predominantly lamellar bone sometimes rimmed by osteoblasts. Interosseous

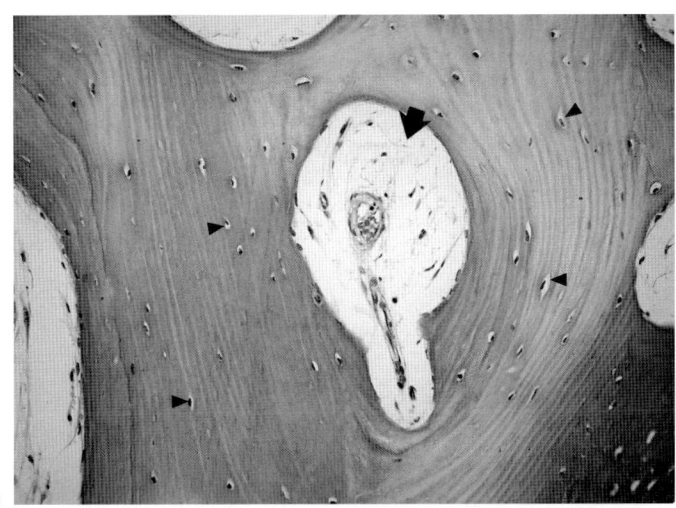

Fig. 4.**179** **a** Osteoma (photomicrograph). This ivory osteoma is composed of dense, mature, lamellar bone. Note osteocytes (arrowheads), haversian canal (arrow), and lack of fibrous stroma. In fibrous osteoma, the interosseous spaces include fibrous, fibrovascular, and fatty tissue. **b** Osteoma. CT scan shows an osteoma of the right anterior ethmoid sinus.

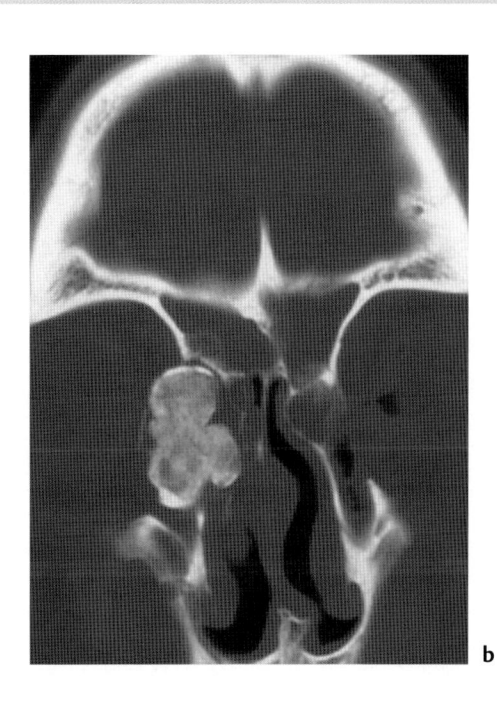

spaces may be composed of fibrous, fibrovascular, or fatty tissue, and hematopoietic elements may be present. Osteomas usually require no treatment but surgical excision may be required for symptomatic osteomas or for cosmetic reasons. Complete surgical excision is curative.

Diagnostic Imaging

The radiographic appearance is that of a sharply delineated radiopaque lesion arising in and confined to bone or protruding into a sinus (Fig. 4.**179b**). At times the border may be irregular. Dense (ivory) osteomas appear hypointense on T1-weighted and T2-weighted MR images. Cancellous osteomas appear as intermediate signal intensity on T1-weighted and T2-weighted MR images and demonstrate moderate enhancement on gadolinium-enhanced T1-weighted MR scans. Even those osteomas that appear uniformly dense on CT will demonstrate some degree of enhancement on MRI.

Osteoblastoma

Osteoblastoma is a benign osteoblastic neoplasm sharing histological appearance with osteoid osteoma but of larger size. Osteoblastomas are uncommon osseous neoplasms accounting for about 3% of all benign osseous neoplasms.[90] Osteoblastomas occur in the vertebrae; in long bones, particularly the femur and tibia; and in small bones of the hands and feet. Head and neck sites of involvement include the mandible (most common site); maxilla; temporal bone; orbit; and paranasal sinuses.[90] Osteoblastomas occur more often in men and, although these tumors can occur at any age, the majority of patients (70–90%) are under 30 years of age.[90] Signs and symptoms associated with head and neck involvement include pain, facial swelling and asymmetry, loosening of teeth, and eating problems. In contrast with osteoid osteoma, the pain associated with osteoblastoma is less often nocturnal and less responsive to aspirin. There are no known causative factors.

Histologically, osteoblastomas are hypercellular with haphazardly arranged interlacing trabeculae of osteoid associated with a loose fibrovascular connective tissue.[90] The osseous trabeculae are composed of woven bone, vary in thickness, and are lined by uniform-appearing osteoblasts. Multinucleated giant cells are variably present and in any given lesion may be prominently seen. The cellular component in osteoblastoma appears loose with intervening, fibrovascular stroma. The stroma contains prominent dilated capillaries, extravasated blood, and fibrous tissue.[90]

Diagnostic Imaging

On CT scans, osteoblastoma appears as a well-defined round expansile lesion with prominent calcified rim. The central portion may have a similar appearance as ossifying fibroma (Fig. 4.**180**). On MR imaging, osteoblastomas appear to have similar MR imaging characteristics to ossifying fibroma. The central portion may be hyperintense on T2-weighted MR images. Osteoblastoma may show moderate to marked enhancement on T1-weighted Gd-DTPA-enhanced MR images (see Fig. 5.**35b–d** and Chapters 3 and 5). Conservative surgery, including curettage or local excision, is the treatment of choice and is curative. Incompletely excised lesions may recur, although partially resected or incompletely curetted tumor may regress.[90]

Chondroma

Chondromas of the paraorbital region, including the sinonasal tract and nasopharynx, are rare. The most frequent sites of occurrence include the nasal cavity (septum); the ethmoid sinus; and the nasopharynx.[105, 106, 107] There is equal gender predilection and most patients are less than 50 years of age.[106] Symptomatic patients may present with nasal obstruction, enlarging painless mass, proptosis, and headaches. Craniofacial chondromas may appear as a polypoid, firm, smooth-surfaced nodule measuring from 0.5 to 2 cm and rarely greater than 3 cm. Histologically, these are lobulated tumors composed of chondrocytes recapitulating the normal histology of cartilage. Cellular pleomorphism, binucleate chondrocytes, or increased mitotic activity are not present. Craniofacial chondromas should be viewed with some suspicion. Chaudhry et al.[106] found that approximately 20% of craniofacial chondrosarcomas are initially misdiagnosed as chondromas. The differentiation of a chondroma from a well-differentiated chondrosarcoma may at times be difficult if not

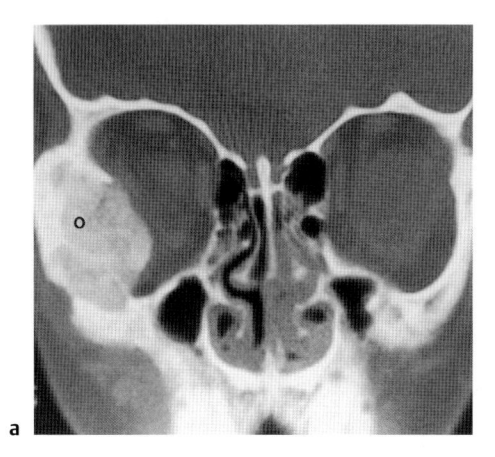

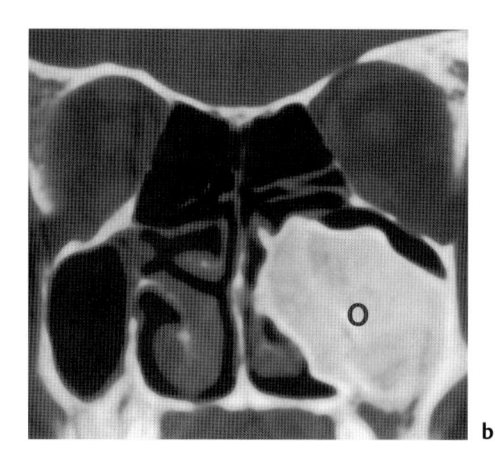

Fig. 4.**180** Osteoblastoma. **a** Coronal CT scan shows an osteoblastoma (O) involving the lateral wall of the right orbit. **b** Coronal CT scan shows an osteoblastoma (O) of the left maxilla. A calcified brown tumor of the maxilla may simulate this maxillary osteoblastoma as well as a post-radiation calcified lymphoma (see Fig. 4.**154**).
Fig. **b** courtesy of Randall Weingarten, MD, Chicago, IL, USA.

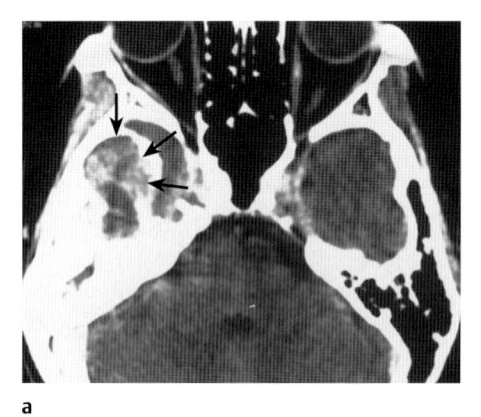

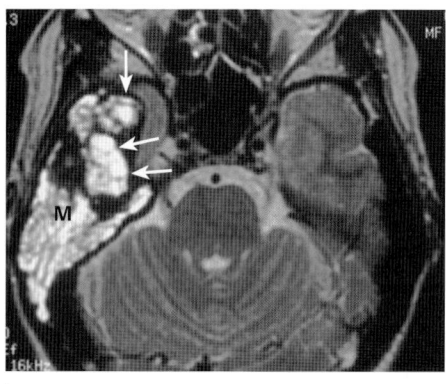

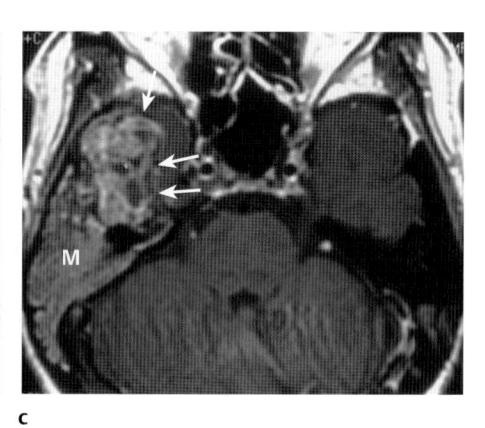

Fig. 4.**181** Chondroblastoma of temporal bone. **a** Axial CT scan shows an expansile mass in the right middle cranial fossa. Note mineralized medial border (arrows). **b** Axial T2W MR scan shows hyperintense mass (arrows) as well as hyperintensity of mastoid air cells (M), secondary to retained secretion as a result of invasion by the tumor. **c** Axial enhanced T1W MR scan shows marked tumor enhancement (arrows) as well as moderate enhancement of mastoid inflammatory mucosal thickening. Case courtesy of Tony Pedulo, MD, Westmead, Australia.

impossible. For this reason, conservative but complete surgical excision of all craniofacial chondrogenic tumors is the treatment of choice. Recurrences of chondromas are uncommon. Tumor recurrence may be indicative of a very well-differentiated chondrosarcoma missed earlier at the time of first diagnosis.

Chondroblastoma

Chondroblastoma is a benign cartilaginous neoplasm predominantly composed of immature chondrocytes (chondroblasts). Chondroblastomas are uncommon, representing less than 1% of osseous neoplasms.[108] Less than 2% of chondroblastomas occur in the head and neck region.[106] The most common head and neck site of involvement is the temporal bone (Fig. 4.**181**); less often, chondroblastomas occur in other sites, including other craniofacial bones.

Histologically, chondroblastomas are hypercellular tumors composed of mononuclear cells (chondroblasts), randomly distributed multinucleated giant cells, chondroid areas, and calcification. Mitotic figures are present but generally are limited in number and without atypical forms.[90]

Curettage with or without bone grafting is the treatment of choice and is curative in greater than 90% of cases.[106, 108] Local tumor recurrence occurs within three years of surgery and is successfully treated by the repeat curettage and resection. Although Huvos and Marcove[108] found the presence of a coexisting aneurysmal bone cyst component in chondroblastomas to impact adversely on tumor recurrence, Bloem and Mulder[109] found no such correlation. Aggressive behavior in the form of local invasion or distant metastasis (so-called *metastasizing chondroblastomas*) may rarely occur.[106, 107] Treatment for these lesions should include complete resection.

Giant-cell Tumor (Osteoclastoma)

Giant-cell tumors (GCTs) are benign but locally aggressive neoplasms characterized by the presence of osteoclast-like giant cells admixed with epithelioid and spindle-shaped mononuclear cells.[90, 110] GCT of bone was first described by Sir Astley Cooper in 1818.[110] Historically, the lesion has been referred to by numerous terms, including myeloid sarcoma, osteoblastoma, and osteoclastoma.[110] GCT is a relatively common skeletal tumor, accounting for 4–9.5% of all primary osseous neoplasms and 18–23% of benign bone neoplasms.[110] Giant-cell tumors are also referred to as *osteoclastoma* because of the resemblance of the giant cells to osteoclasts. This tumor is most often found in the metaphyses of long bones of adults. The vast majority of GCTs affect skeletally mature patients, between 20 and 50 years of age. Giant-cell tumors of the head and neck are uncommon.[2, 29, 90] The most common sites of occurrence include the sphenoid (most common), temporal, and ethmoid bones. Symptoms include headache, diplopia, decreased vision, and proptosis.[90] Multicentric tumors are uncommon but when present may be associated with a more aggressive clinical course,[90] or may be due to an unrecognized parathyroid gland adenoma, hyperplasia, or adenocarcinoma (see Fig. 4.187).

Pathological Features

Histologically, true giant-cell tumors are characterized by the presence of a large number of multinucleated giant cells in a diffuse distribution in a background of mononuclear cells. The giant cells are evenly distributed throughout the lesion and include numerous nuclei that tend to cluster in more central portions of the cell (Fig. 4.182). The multinucleated giant cells are thought to originate from fusion of the mononuclear cells.[90] Giant-cell tumors lack matrix production, but in the presence of a pathological fracture, osteoid (reactive new bone) may be present. The presence of chondroid matrix is unusual and, if present, likely represents evidence that the lesion in question is not a giant-cell tumor. In addition, thin-walled vascular spaces, hemorrhage, and hemosiderin-laden macrophages (foam cells) can be seen. Aneurysmal bone cyst (ABC) components in GCTs are relatively common. GCT is the most common lesion associated with secondary ABC. The identification of solid component of GCT allows differentiation from primary ABC, which contains only hemorrhagic cystic regions.[110] The pathological differential diagnosis of GCT is extensive, including but not limited to giant-cell reparative granuloma, brown tumor of hyperparathyroidism, osteoblastoma, chondroblastoma, ABC, nonossifying fibroma, foreign-body reaction, fibrous dysplasia associated with cystic hemorrhagic changes, and osteosarcoma with abundant giant cells.[110]

Diagnostic Imaging

Giant-cell tumors of the sinonasal cavities cause local expansion and destruction (Figs. 4.183, 4.184). On CT scans, the solid components of tumor demonstrate attenuation values similar to that of muscle. The ABC regions may show a fluid–fluid level on CT and MRI and appear as low attenuation on CT. On MR scans, the solid component of GCT frequency reveals low to intermediate signal intensity on T1-weighted and T2-weighted MR images. The cause of this MR appearance has been reported as hemosiderin deposition, increased vascularity, increased cellularity, or high collagen content. The ABC regions may show high or low signal intensity on T1-weighted and markedly increased signal intensity on T2-weighted MR images. The solid components of GCTs enhance diffusely on enhanced T1-weighted MR images, reflecting the hypervascular tissue seen on pathological analysis. Enhanced T1-weighted MR images are most valuable in detecting recurrent tumor (Fig. 4.184 d). The differential diagnosis of giant-cell tumor of the sinonasal cavities should include rhabdomyosarcoma, lymphoma, epithelial tumors, brown tumor of hyperparathyroidism, giant-cell reparative granuloma, chondroblastoma (Fig. 4.181), and metastasis. The treatment for giant-cell tumors is surgical excision, with the extent of surgery dependent on the size and extent of the tumor. Up to 60 % of giant-cell tumors recur if treated by simple curettage alone.[90] Radiotherapy has been used in the treatment of giant-cell tumors but is usually reserved for lesions that are not amenable to surgical resection and cryotherapy.[90]

Giant-cell Reparative Granuloma

In 1953 Jaffe[111] coined the term "giant-cell reparative granuloma" to represent that variety of giant-cell tumor found exclusively in the maxilla and mandible, where areas of osteoid deposition are seen alongside areas of bone destruction, giving the appearance of attempted repair.[111, 112] Giant-cell reparative granuloma is an uncommon benign nonneoplastic reactive lesion of bone usually

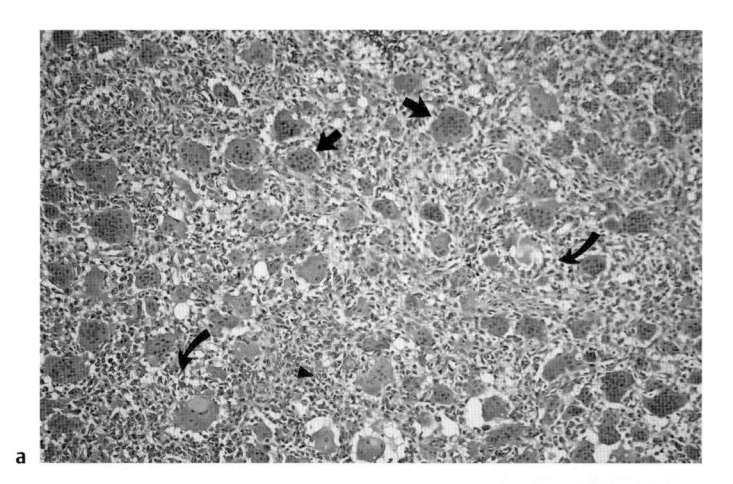

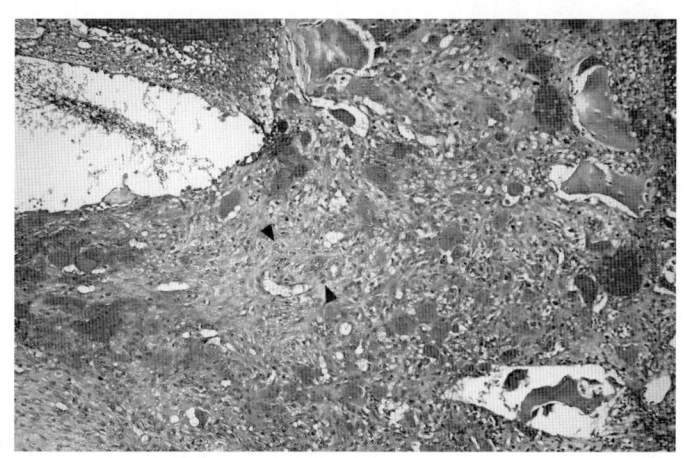

Fig. 4.182 Giant-cell tumor (photomicrographs) showing multinucleated giant cells (arrows) that are uniformly dispersed within a cellular stroma (**a**). Stroma consists of primitive mesenchymal cells, differentiating into histiocytes (arrowheads) and fibroblasts (curved arrows). Note cystic changes in **b**. Courtesy Bruce Wenig, MD, Washington D.C., USA.

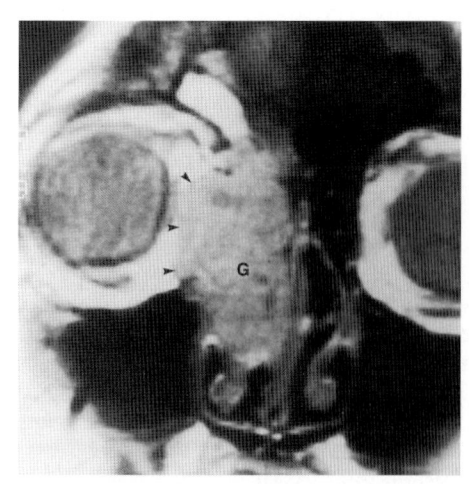

Fig. 4.183 Giant-cell tumor. 19-year-old man. Coronal PW MR scan shows a large mass compatible with giant cell tumor (G), involving the right nasal cavity and right ethmoid air cells and extending into the orbit (arrows).

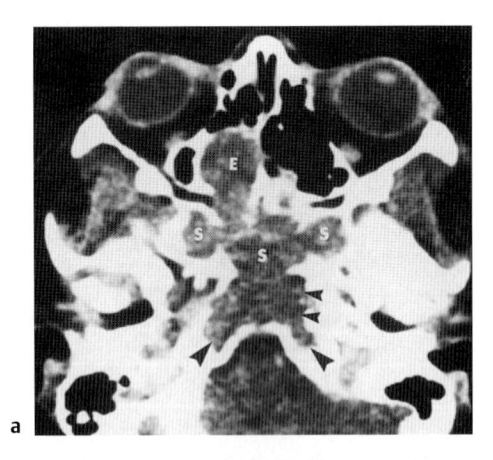

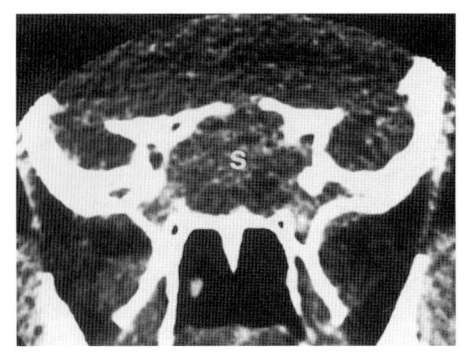

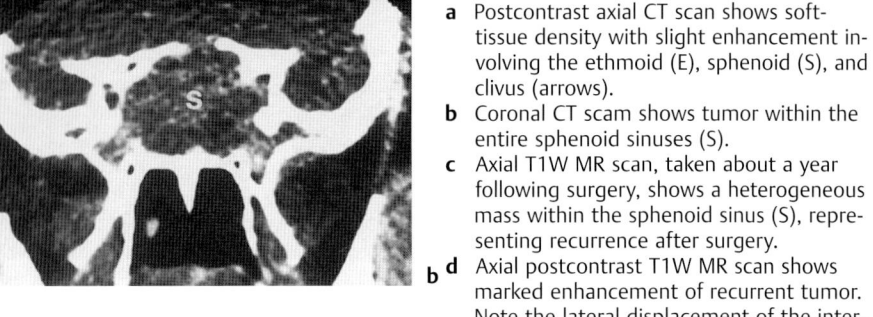

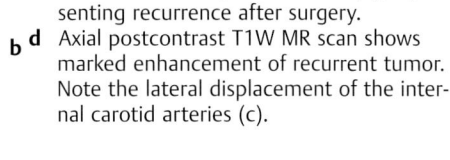

Fig. 4.184 Giant cell tumor (osteoclastoma). 25-year-old woman.
a Postcontrast axial CT scan shows soft-tissue density with slight enhancement involving the ethmoid (E), sphenoid (S), and clivus (arrows).
b Coronal CT scam shows tumor within the entire sphenoid sinuses (S).
c Axial T1W MR scan, taken about a year following surgery, shows a heterogeneous mass within the sphenoid sinus (S), representing recurrence after surgery.
d Axial postcontrast T1W MR scan shows marked enhancement of recurrent tumor. Note the lateral displacement of the internal carotid arteries (c).

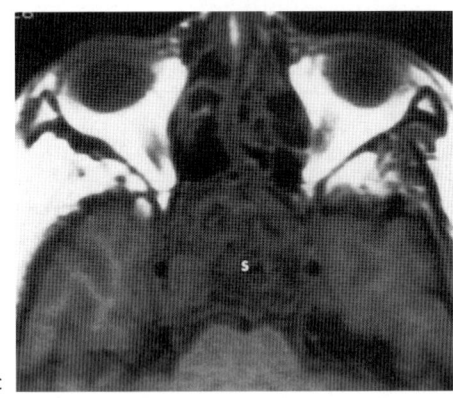

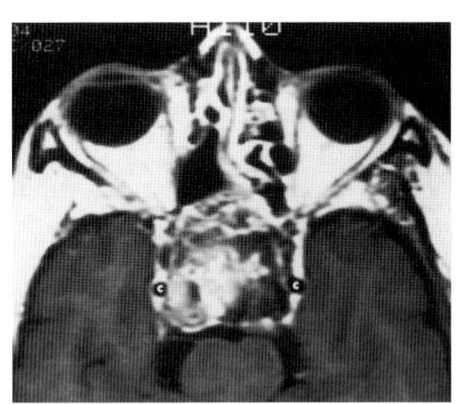

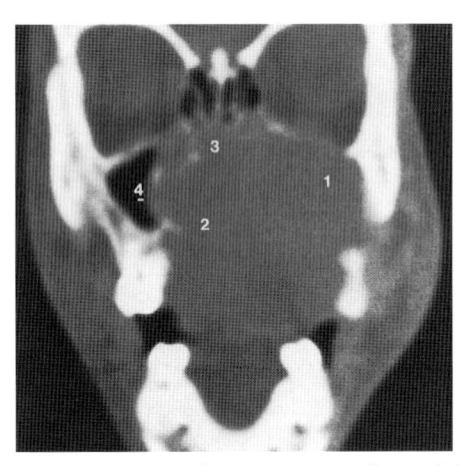

Fig. 4.**185** Giant cell reparative granuloma of the maxilla in an 8-year-old patient. Coronal CT scan. A large, expansile soft tissue mass arising from the left maxilla and palate is occupying the entire left maxillary sinus (1), the palate (2), and encroaching on the nasal cavity (3) and the right maxillary sinus (4). The mass was resected and the patient was given radiotherapy. From Reference 12.

occurring in the mandible and is seen predominantly in children and young adults.[112] Giant-cell reparative granulomas (GCRGs) share many features with true giant-cell tumor, brown tumor, and aneurysmal bone cysts, and in many regards these lesions may be indistinguishable.[90, 111, 112] In the head and neck area, the maxilla and mandible are the most common sites of occurrence (Figs. 4.**185**, 4.**186**). GCRGs have been described affecting other organs of the head and neck, including the paranasal sinuses, nasal septum, temporal bone, other skull bones, as well as cricoid cartilage and hyoid bone.[113] Orbital, paraorbital, or nasopharyngeal involvement is less common. Those lesions that are predominantly confined to intraosseous sites (e.g., jaws) are referred to as *central giant-cell reparative granulomas* (Fig. 4.**185**, 4.**186**) and those primarily involving soft tissues (e.g., paraorbital, sinonasal, or oral) are termed *peripheral giant-cell reparative granulomas*.[90] Paraorbital involvement is associated with pain and swelling.

The central and peripheral giant-cell reparative granulomas are histologically identical, composed of a cellular fibroblastic stroma that includes multinucleated giant cells. The giant cells are unevenly distributed but tend to be clustered in limited areas of the lesion. The giant cells often aggregate in and around foci of hemorrhage or are seen in vascular spaces. Less often, the giant cells are diffusely distributed in the fibroblastic stroma. The giant cells are smaller, with fewer nuclei, than those seen in true giant-cell tumors. The stroma includes spindle-shaped to oval-appearing fibroblasts. Mitotic figures are seen in the fibroblasts but not the giant cells; in general, the mitotic activity is less than in true giant-cell tumors. Both the giant cells and stromal fibroblasts lack cytological atypia. Cyst formation and reactive bone may be present. The latter may or may not include osteoblastic rimming. A stromal inflammatory cell infiltrate, including lymphocytes and plasma cells, is present.

Brown Tumor and Renal Osteodystrophy

In 1934 Albright and colleagues[114] described a variety of giant-cell tumors secondary to hyperparathyroidism, which they called "brown tumor" because of its naked-eye appearance. Primary hyperparathyroidism results in the direct release of parathyroid hormone from an adenoma or, less commonly, glandular hyperplasia or parathyroid adenocarcinoma. Secondary hyperparathy-

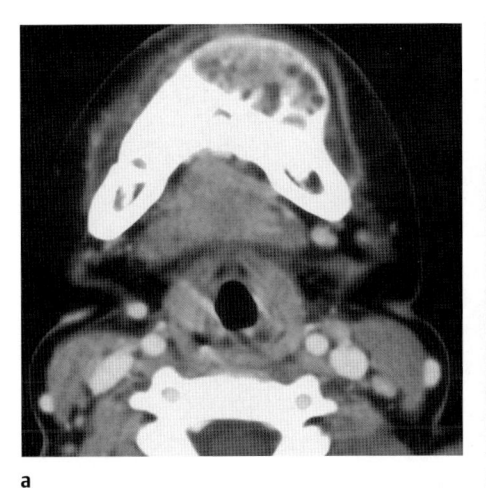

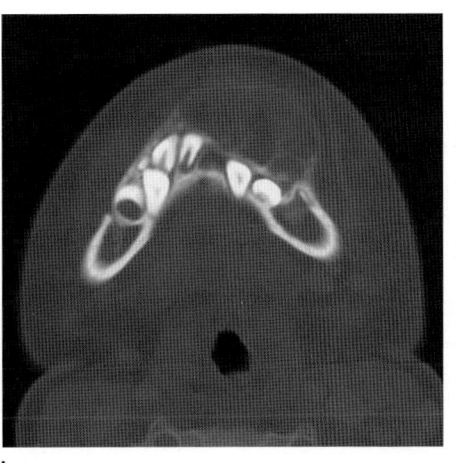

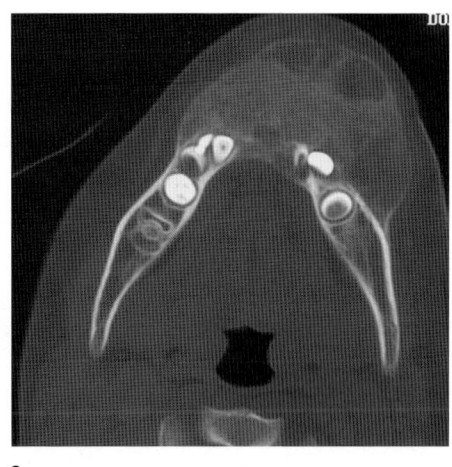

Fig. 4.**186** Giant-cell reparative granuloma of the mandible in a 5-year-old girl. **a** Enhanced axial CT scan shows an expansile mass with moderate enhancement involving the anterior mandible. **b** High-resolution axial CT scan shows marked thinning of the mandibular cortex. Note intralesional fine mineralized septae. **c** CT scan taken six months later following treatment with bone chips, showing increased mineralization (repair) within the lesion.

roidism is caused by an imbalance of calcium and phosphorus metabolism. Osteitis fibrosa, bone cyst, and brown tumor are rare clinical entities in the Western world, but are commonly seen in other parts of the world.[115] Osteitis fibrosa cystica as a manifestation of primary hyperparathyroidism was first described by Von Recklinghausen in 1891.[115] It results from the direct effect of parathyroid hormone on bone, causing the conversion of potentially osteogenic cells from osteoblasts to osteoclasts. An imbalance of osteoclastic activity causes bone resorption with fibrous replacement of the marrow and thinning of cortex. Cysts may also develop as a result of intraosseous bleeding within a vascular fibroblastic tissue. Clusters of hemosiderin-laden macrophages, giant cells, and proliferating plump fibroblasts fill the cystic lesions.[115] Increased vascularity, hemorrhage, and deposits of hemosiderin impart the characteristic brown hue to the lesion, hence the name "brown tumor." Brown tumor, therefore, is not a neoplastic lesion and represents a reactive and reparative cellular process. Grossly, a brown tumor appears as a mass with partly cystic and partly solid areas.[115] Clinically, brown tumors are slow-growing lesions that can be locally destructive. Although initially associated with primary hyperparathyroidism, they are being seen with greater frequency in secondary hyperparathyroidism, as a result of longer survival rates in the latter group. Brown tumors most commonly involve the ribs, clavicles, pelvic girdle, and mandible. Brown tumors of the maxilla and hard palate are uncommon (Fig. 4.**187**). Orbital involvement has been reported.

Histopathology

Histologically, brown tumors are rich in giant cells and are indistinguishable from true giant-cell tumor and giant-cell reparative granuloma. The differentiation between brown tumor, true giant-cell tumor, giant-cell reparative granuloma, and other bone tumor variants containing giant cells requires a synthesis of the information obtained from the clinical course of the disease, the radiographic imaging including CT, MRI, and radioisotope scan, the laboratory tests, and histological examination of biopsy material because no single feature can be claimed to be characteristic of any of these lesions.[115] This differentiation is essential as all these lesions are treated differently. While both true giant-cell tumor and giant-cell reparative granuloma are treated surgically, brown tumor is known to regress spontaneously after removal or treatment of the underlying cause (Fig. 4.**187**). Therefore, brown tumor should always be excluded by simple routine biochemical serum analysis in case of an expansile bone lesion, especially in the facial region.

Diagnostic Imaging

Brown tumors present as expansile, lytic lesions of the bone, causing thinning of the cortex, bone remodeling, and bone destruction.[116] The radiological picture can be complicated by pathological fractures. Occasionally faint osteoid matrix can be seen within the lesion since these lesions elaborate osteoid material in their stroma. On routine bone scans these lesions show increased uptake of radiopharmaceuticals, indicating their vascular nature. Technetium-99m sestamibi scan is commonly used for localization of parathyroid adenoma or hyperplasia; metabolically active brown tumor may demonstrate uptake of ^{99m}Tc. On CT, brown tumors are seen as expansile, with marked thinning of the cortex and break in the cortex with soft-tissue extension (Fig. 4.**187**). The CT attenuation values of lesions are typically in the range of blood and fibrous tissue (Fig. 4.**187a**). On intravenous administration of iodinated contrast material, moderate to marked enhancement is seen, reflecting the vascular nature of the lesion. The MRI appearance of brown tumor is variable. These lesions show generally low to intermediate signal intensity on both T1-weighted and T2-weighted MR images (Figs. 4.**187**, 4.**188**). Areas of very low signal intensity can be seen in the lesions, owing to presence of hemorrhage and hemosiderin. Fluid–fluid levels may be present, suggestive of the hemorrhagic nature of the lesion and secondary ABC formation. On intravenous administration of gadolinium contrast material, marked enhancement of the solid component of the lesion is seen on enhanced T1-weighted MR images.

The cornerstone of treatment of brown tumor is reversal of the hypercalcemia, which is achieved by parathyroidectomy.[115] Following treatment of underlying metabolic disorder, brown tumors frequently become sclerotic and show regression (Fig. 4.**187i**).[115] Based on the imaging features alone, brown tumors have to be differentiated from other expansile and destructive lesions of the facial and cranial bones, viz., true giant-cell tumor, giant-cell reparative granuloma, plasmacytoma, "aneurysmal bone cyst," odontogenic and nonodontogenic tumors, fibro-osseous lesions, and metastases.

Other than giant-cell tumor, the differential diagnosis of giant-cell reparative granuloma (GCRG) includes the brown tumor of hyperparathyroidism (Figs. 4.**187**, 4.**188**). In fact, the

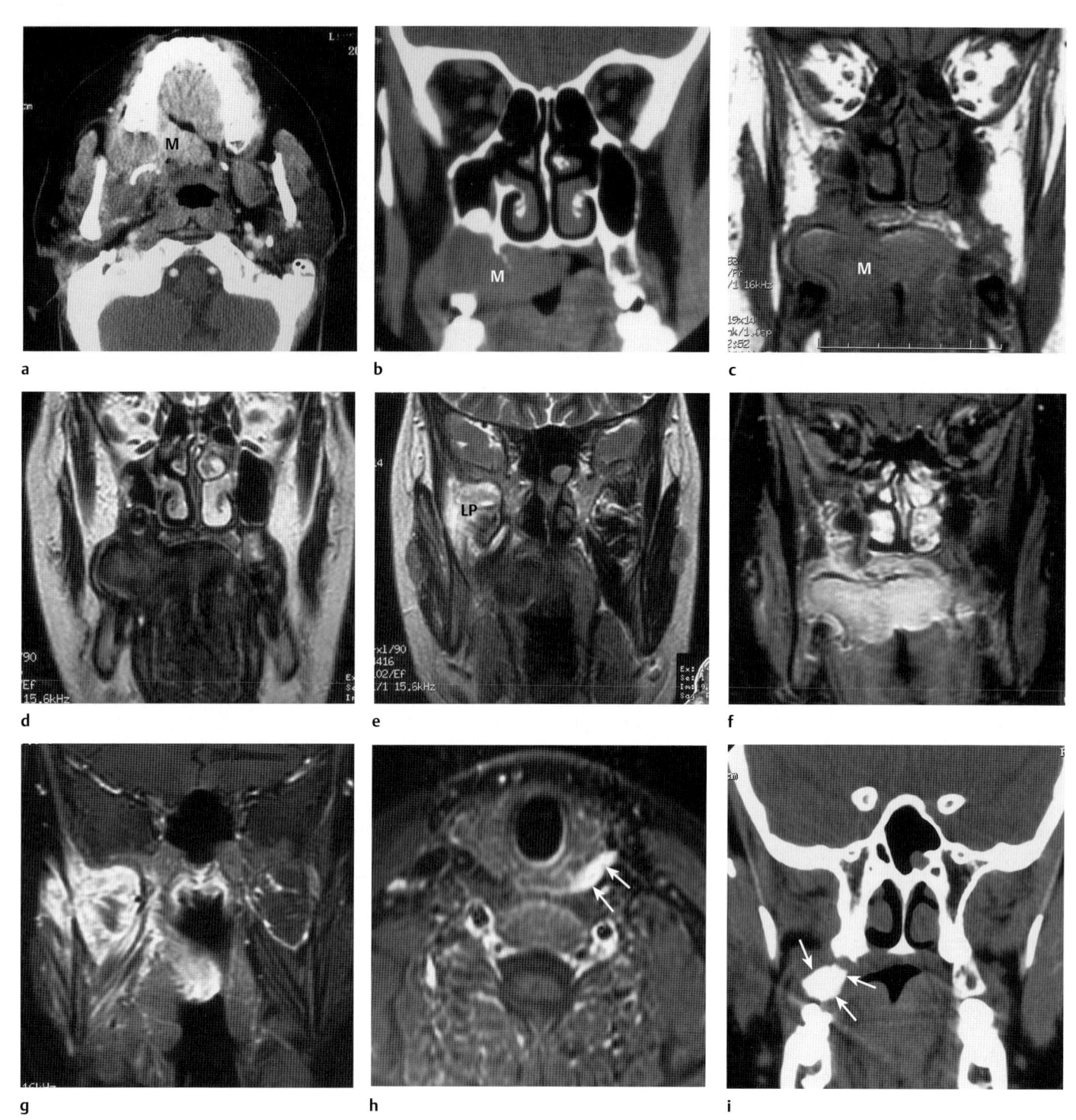

Fig. 4.**187** Brown tumor. 19-year-old woman. **a** Enhanced axial CT scan shows a large palatalomaxillary mass (M). **b** Coronal CT scan shows the mass (M) along with erosion of ipsilateral maxillary tuberosity. **c** Coronal T1W MR scan shows a hypointense right palatomaxillary mass (M). **d** The lesion appears hypointense on coronal T2W MR scan. **e** Enhanced coronal T1W MR scan shows abnormal enhancement of right lateral pterygoid muscle (LP). **f**, **g** Enhanced fat-suppression coronal T1W MR scans showing marked enhancement of the palatomaxillary mass as well as abnormal enhancement of the right lateral pterygoid muscle. **h** Enhanced fat-suppression MR scan shows a large left parathyroid adenoma (arrows). **i** Coronal CT scan following removal of parathyroid adenoma shows almost complete resolution of the right palatomaxillary mass. Note dystrophic calcification (arrows) at the site of brown tumor. Histological diagnosis of hard palate mass was consistent with Brown tumor. After removal of the parathyroid adenoma, the palatal mass decreased in size and became calcified. The abnormal enhancement of the pterygoid muscle also resolved. The CT and MRI diagnosis in another institution was rhabdomyosarcoma. The biopsy diagnosis was malignant giant cell tumor. The radiologist's diagnosis in our institution was brown tumor. An MRI of the parathyroid gland established the diagnosis (Fig. 4.**187h**). Maxillofacial surgery was cancelled, and instead a parathyroid adenoma (26 mm) was removed. This resulted in almost total resolution of the oral mass (Fig. 4.**187i**), and resolution of reactive changes of right lateral pterygoid muscle.

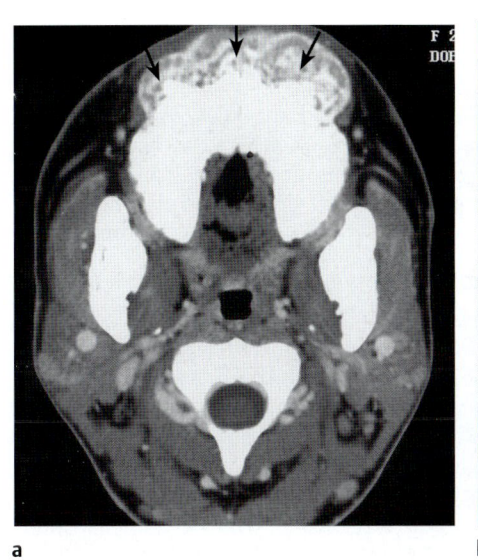

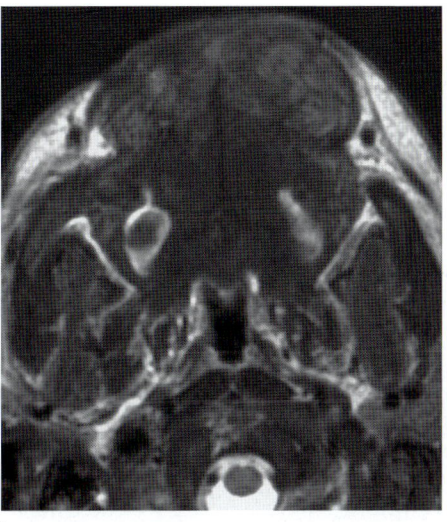

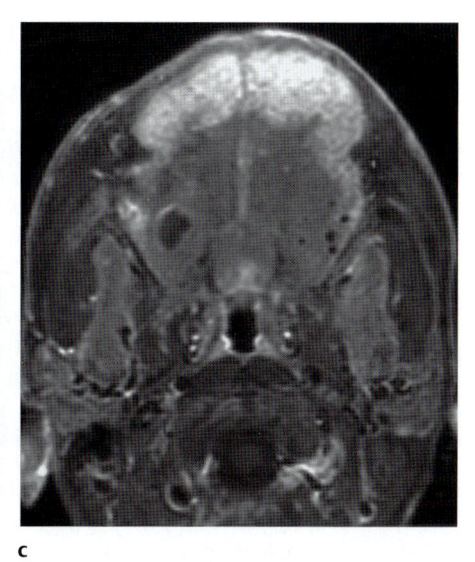

Fig. 4.188 Brown tumor and renal osteodystrophy. **a** Axial CT scan shows increased thickening of the alveolar process of the maxilla as well as rami of the mandible, related to renal osteodystrophy. Note extensive soft-tissue infiltration of the upper gum (arrows). **b** Axial T2W and **c** enhanced fat-suppression T1W MR scans showing soft-tissue infiltration of the upper gum. Note marked enhancement in **c**. Pathological diagnosis of gum lesion was compatible with brown tumor.

histology of these two lesions is identical.[90] Accordingly, all patients suspected of having a giant-cell reparative granuloma should be evaluated for hyperparathyroidism with laboratory determination of serum calcium, parathyroid hormone, phosphate, and alkaline phosphate levels. Surgical curettage is the treatment of choice for GCRG. Up to 15% of gnathic lesions recur,[90] but sinonasal tract lesions are less likely to recur following curettage.

Renal Osteodystrophy

Renal osteodystrophy (RO) is a term used to describe the skeletal complications of end-stage renal failure (ESRF) (Fig. 4.**188**). RO is a multifactorial disorder of bone remodeling. Factors such as parathyroid hormone (PTH), tumor necrosis factor α (TNF-α) and interleukin 1 (IL-1) activate the remodeling cycle through actions on the existing osteoblasts.[117] Existing osteoclasts are attracted to the site and activated by matrix-dissolution products.

Renal osteodystrophy is classified as osteitis fibrosa, osteomalacia, or mixed or adynamic disease, according to histological features.[116] Bone disease in patients with chronic renal disease (CRD) is caused by both hyperparathyroidism and other factors.[118] Some patients with CRD have hyperparathyroid uremic bone disease, which is characterized by an activation of osteoclasts and osteoblasts with excess bone resorption. Other patients have an adynamic bone disease or osteomalacia. Adynamic bone disease is characterized by low activity of the bone cells, no excess accumulation of matrix, and little parathyroid hypersecretion.[118]

The parathyroid glands, through the secretion of parathyroid hormone (PTH), regulate serum calcium concentrations and bone metabolism. In turn, serum calcium concentrations regulate PTH secretion. Low or falling calcium concentrations act within seconds to stimulate PTH secretion, initiated by means of a calcium-sensing receptor on the surface of the parathyroid cells.[118] Hypocalcemia from any cause stimulates parathyroid hormone secretion, and chronic hypocalcemia also stimulates the growth of the parathyroid glands. This secondary hyperparathyroidism usually resolves with the treatment of the underlying cause of hypocalcemia. However, in patients with chronic renal failure, secondary hyperparathyroidism often lasts longer and is more severe than in patients with other hypocalcemic disorders, such as deficiency or malabsorption of vitamin D.[118] Eventually, either before or, more often, after renal transplantation, secondary hyperparathyroidism can develop into a disorder of oversecretion of parathyroid hormone with hypercalcemia (tertiary hyperparathyroidism).[118] The classic histological form of renal osteodystrophy is osteitis fibrosa cystica (OFC), which is caused by secondary hyperparathyroidism with contributions from locally derived cytokines and a deficiency of 1α,25-dihydroxycholecalciferol. A hallmark of osteitis fibrosa is marrow fibrosis, caused by the activation of marrow mesenchymal cells, which differentiate into fibroblast-like cells secreting the fibrous tissue occupying peritrabecular spaces.[117] Another feature of this disorder is the increased frequency of bone remodeling, leading to increased resorption of bone. The increased resorption is caused by an increase in both the number and the activity of osteoclasts. Bone formation is also increased, as reflected by increased amounts of osteoid and nonlamellar bone, which are hallmarks of a high rate of bone turnover.[117]

In OFC, the focus of abnormal remodeling activity is often in the cortical osteons of long bones, leading to increased cortical porosity as a result of resorption and remodeling.[117] OFC may become filled with fibrous tissue. When this highly vascularized fibrous tissue develops, microhemorrhages, microfractures, and blood by-products will accumulate. Deposits of intracellular and extracellular hemosiderin will accumulate and impart a reddish-brown hue and hence the name "brown tumor" (Figs. 4.**185**, 4.**187**).

■ Malignant Osseous and Cartilaginous Tumors of Sinonasal Cavities

Osteosarcoma (Osteogenic Sarcoma)

Up to about 10% of conventional osteosarcomas occur in the head and neck region.[90] Craniofacial osteosarcomas (excluding those arising in the setting of Paget disease) have an equal gender predilection and occur in patients who are generally a decade or two older than those with extrafacial osteosarcomas. The jaws are most commonly affected, with the mandible more often involved than the maxilla. Osteosarcomas may occur in other head and neck sites, including the paranasal sinuses, the orbital region, and the skull.[10,11,90] The most common clinical complaints include painful swelling of the face, dentition problems, nasal obstruction, and epistaxis. Elevated serum alkaline phosphatase represents the sole laboratory value of clinical importance in osteosarcoma, and an abrupt elevation in patients with preexisting benign bone lesions may be indicative of malignant transformation.

Most osteosarcomas occur de novo without an identifiable preexisting condition, but osteosarcomas may develop secondary to a preexisting bone disease, including Paget disease, fibrous dysplasia, osteoblastoma, osteochondromas, giant-cell tumors, chronic osteomyelitis, osteogenesis imperfecta, and bone infarct.[90] Ionizing radiation is also implicated in the development of osteosarcoma.[10,11] Osteogenic sarcoma may be familial.[90] Patients with the heritable form of retinoblastoma are at risk (approximately 10% by age 25 years) of developing osteosarcoma.[2]

The gross appearance of osteosarcoma is dependent on the extent of mineralization versus the extent of the stromal component. As such, osteosarcomas vary from firm, hard, and gritty to fleshy and fibrous. The histopathological features of osteosarcoma include a sarcomatous stroma intimately admixed and giving rise to osteoid. Osteoid, the unmineralized precursor of bone, appears as eosinophilic, hyaline-like material with irregular contours, and is surrounded by a rim of osteoblasts. Stromal cells display variable anaplasia and are spindled to polygonal, containing hyperchromatic nuclei with or without nucleoli. Necrosis, invasive growth, and mitotic activity, including typical and atypical (bizarre) mitoses are commonly present. Tumor vascularity varies from relatively inconspicuous to dominant.

Diagnostic Imaging

Radiographically, osteosarcomas are destructive, poorly delineated osteolytic, osteosclerotic, or mixed lesions (Figs. 4.**189**–4.**192**). There may be minimal or massive tumor bone formation within the tumor proper and invading surrounding tissue (Figs. 4.**189**, 4.**190**). On MR imaging, the tumor appears heterogeneous and demonstrates intermediate signal on T1-weighted and mixed signal intensity (hyperintense and hypointense zones) on T2-weighted MR images (Fig. 4.**191c**). Osteosarcomas demonstrate heterogeneous enhancement on Gd-DTPA-enhanced T1-weighted MR images (Fig. 4.**190**).

Chondrosarcoma

Chondrosarcomas account for only 10–20% of primary bone tumors.[105] The incidence of chondrosarcoma of head and neck sites varies from 5% to 12%.[90] In the head and neck, chondrosarcomas are slightly more common in men that in women and primarily occur in the fourth to seventh decades of life. Approximately 2% of chondrosarcomas occur in patient less than 20 years of age.[90,119] The most common site of occurrence in the head and neck is the larynx; however, chondrosarcomas occur in virtually all other sites in which cartilage is found but primarily occur in the craniofacial area, including the mandible, maxilla, and maxillofacial skeleton (nose and paranasal sinuses), as well as the base of the skull and the nasopharynx (see Chapter 3).[6,119] Lesions arising from the nasal septum have been reported, but they are rare and only 50 cases have been reported to date. Symptoms vary according to the site of origin. Craniofacial chondrosarcomas may cause nasal obstruction; epistaxis; changes in dentition (loosening or eruption of teeth); proptosis; visual disturbances; and an expanding mass associated with pain, trismus, headaches, and neural deficits.

Histologically, chondrosarcomas are lobulated, hypercellular tumors composed of cells with hyperchromatic, pleomorphic

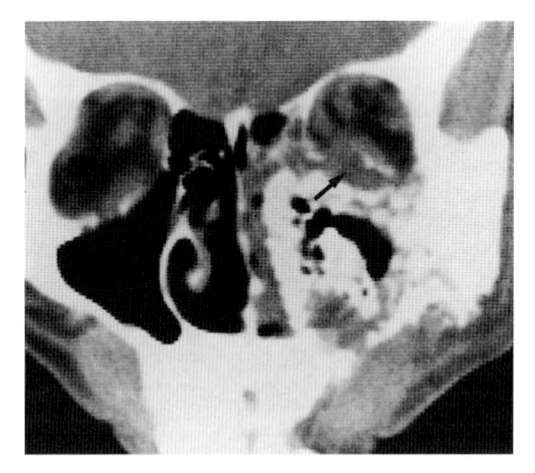

Fig. 4.**189** Osteogenic sarcoma. Coronal CT scan shows a destructive lesion with marked tumor bone formation involving the left maxilla. Note the involvement of the inferior rectus muscle (arrow).

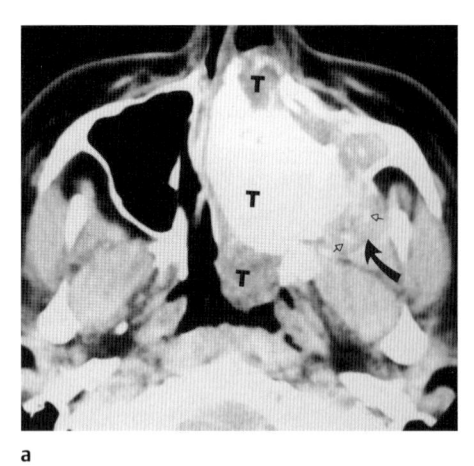

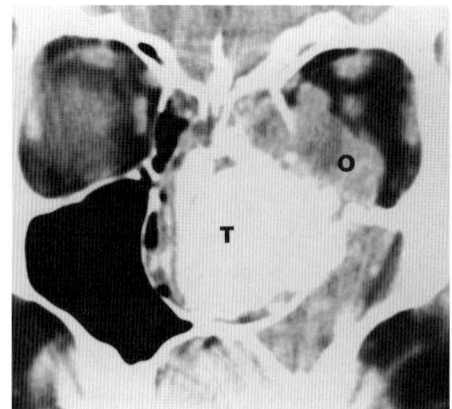

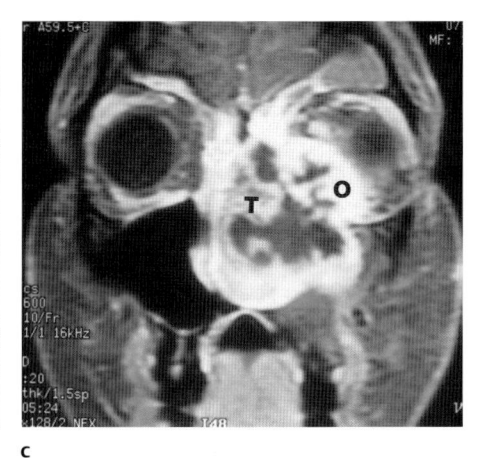

Fig. 4.**190** Osteogenic sarcoma of the ethmoid bone. **a** Axial CT scan shows a large destructive tumor (T) involving the nasal cavity and left maxillary sinus. Note extension into the left infratemporal fossa (curved arrow). Note tumor bone formation in the nasal cavity as well as within the infratemporal component of the tumor (small arrows). **b** Enhanced coronal CT scan shows intranasal tumor (T). Note invasion of the orbit (O). **c** Coronal fat-suppression enhanced T1W MR scan showing necrotic tumor (T). Note significant orbital invasion (O).

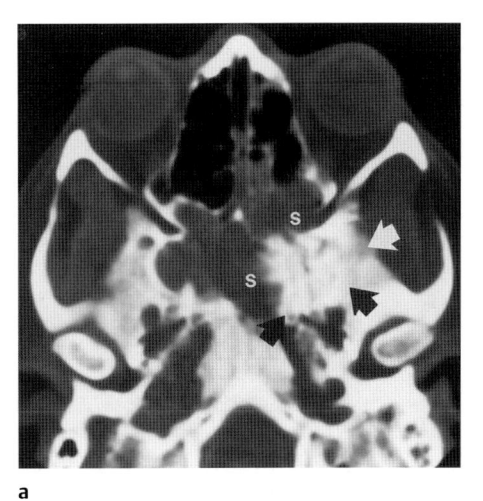

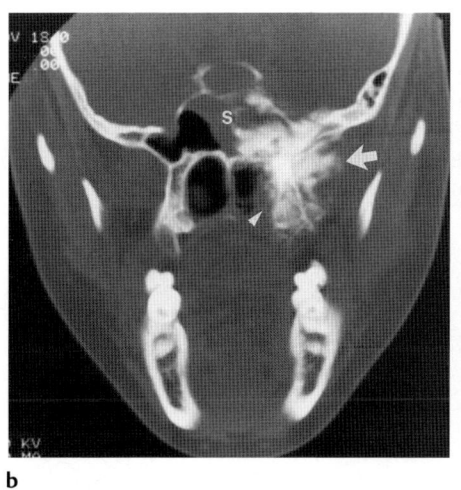

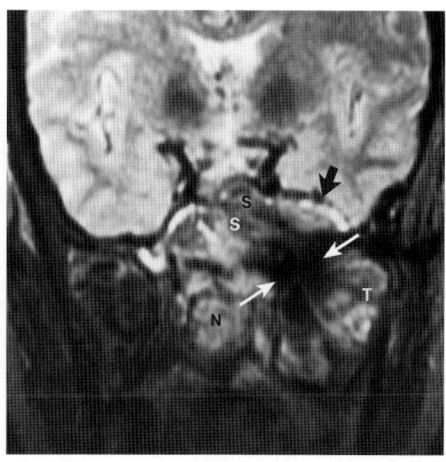

Fig. 4.191 Osteogenic sarcoma of the sphenoid bone. **a** Axial CT scan shows an osteosarcoma of the base of the sphenoid. Note marked tumor bone formation (arrows). The remainder of the tumor within the sphenoid sinus (S) shows no evidence of mineralization. **b** Coronal CT scan shows tumor within the sphenoid sinus (S). Note marked irregular tumor bone formation (arrow) and periosteal reaction (arrowhead). **c** PW coronal MR scan shows tumor in the nasopharynx (N), sphenoid sinus (S), and infratemporal fossa (T). Note hypointense tumor bone formation (white arrows) and elevation of dura (black arrow) due to involvement of the epidural space.

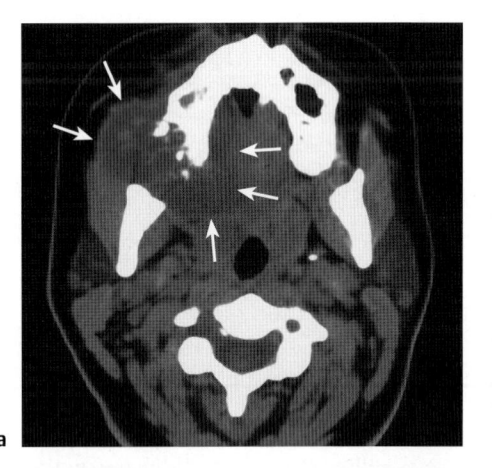

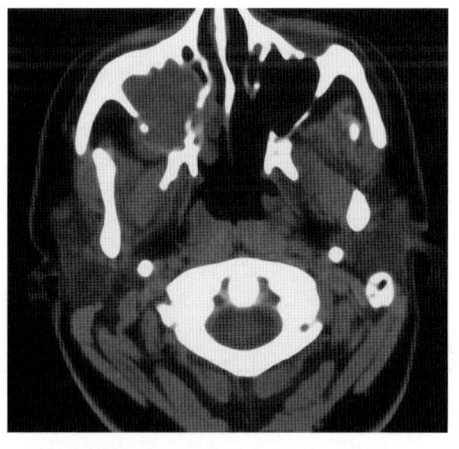

Fig. 4.192 Osteogenic sarcoma of the maxillary alveolar ridge. **a** Axial CT scan shows a large intraoral mass (arrows) involving the alveolar process of the maxilla and extending into the right buccal space. Note small foci of mineralization. **b** Axial CT scan shows tumor within the right maxillary sinus. Note erosion of the posterior wall of the maxillary sinus. **c** Axial and **d** coronal CT scans, taken two months later, demonstrate marked irregular tumor bone formation characteristic of osteogenic sarcoma.

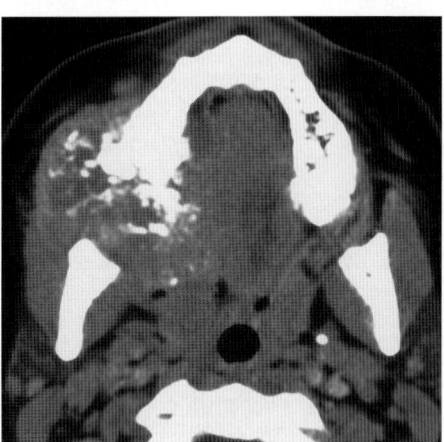

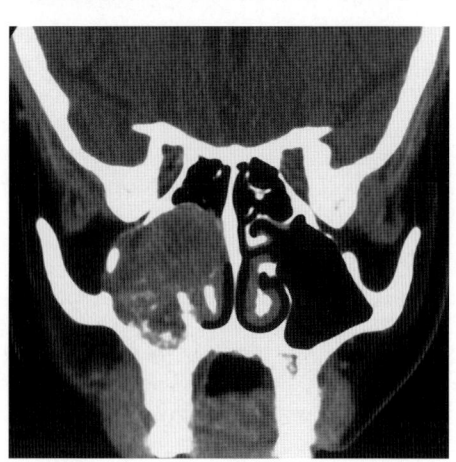

nuclei; are binucleated or multinucleated; have prominent nucleoli; and have increased mitotic activity. Histological variants of chondrosarcoma, including dedifferentiated chondrosarcoma, mesenchymal chondrosarcoma, and clear cell chondrosarcoma, are rare in the sinonasal tract and nasopharynx.[105] Chondrosarcomas are divided histologically into three grades on the basis of the degree of cellularity, nuclear size and atypia, and mitotic activity.

Grade 1 tumors have an abundant chondroid matrix with clusters of chondrocytes with normal or slightly irregular nuclei, rare nucleoli, and absent mitoses. Grade 2 tumors exhibit more cellularity, less matrix, enlarged nuclei, increased mitoses, and higher number of binucleate cells. Grade 3 tumors demonstrate high cellularity, prominent nuclear pleomorphism, prominent mitotic figures, and irregular and satellite-shaped chondrocytes.[105]

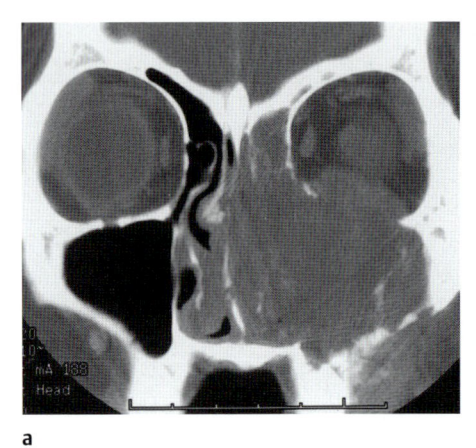

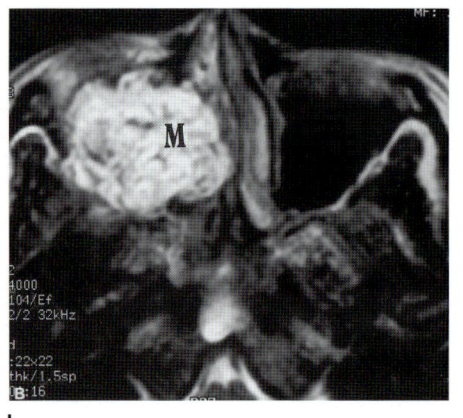

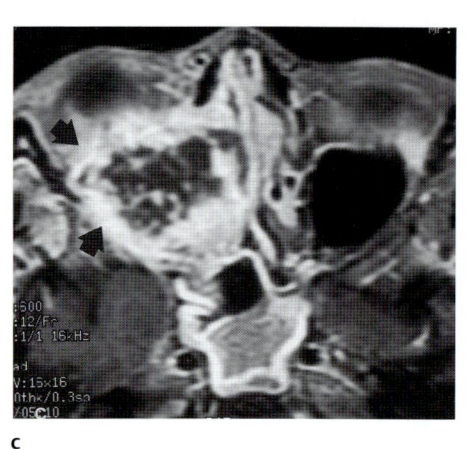

Fig. 4.**193** Chondrosarcoma? **a** Coronal CT scan shows a destructive mass of the left maxilla with invasion of the floor of the orbit. **b** Axial T2W MR scan shows a hyperintesne mass (M), involving the maxillary antrum and extending into the right nasal cavity. **c** Enhanced fat-suppression T1W MR scan shows marked enhancement of a partially necrotic tumor (arrows). Initial diagnosis was chondrosarcoma but final pathology was considered to be chondrogenic osteosarcoma.

Diagnostic Imaging

The radiological appearance of craniofacial chondrosarcomas is that of a destructive, rather expansile lesion of soft-tissue matrix with scattered, ring-forming calcifications. There may be multiple fine calcifications or a combination of small and coarse calcifications (Fig. 4.**193**). The radiographic appearance may correlate with histological grade.[105] Low-grade chondrosarcomas are uniformly calcified and there is a well-defined demarcation between the tumor and the nonneoplastic bone. In high-grade chondrosarcomas, there are larger portions of the tumor that are not calcified, the calcification that is present tends to be faint and amorphous, and the tumor has an irregular growth and is not well defined from the nonneoplastic host bone.

Chondrosarcomas may be seen as a nondestructive, fairly well-delineated or destructive, poorly delineated osteolytic or mixed lesion. On MR imaging, they appear hypointense on T1-weighted MR images and moderately to markedly hyperintense on T2-weighted MR images (Fig. 4.**193**). There may be moderate to significant enhancement on Gd-DTPA-enhanced T1-weighted MR scans. For maxillofacial chondrosarcomas, radical resection with adequate margins is indicated.[90, 120] In these sites, chondrosarcoma is a slow-growing but persistent tumor characterized by multiple recurrences.

■ Miscellaneous Tumors of Sinonasal Cavities

Sinonasal Myxoma and Fibromyxoma

Myxomas/fibromyxomas of the craniofacial bones are rare. In 1958, Zimmerman and Dahlin[121] reviewed 2276 cases of primary bone neoplasms and found only 26 myxomatous jaw tumors. In 1973, Ghosh et al.[122] found 10 odontogenic myxomas among 8723 primary bone neoplasms. Myxomas can occur at any age but most arise between the ages of 25 and 35 years.[123] In general, myxoma/fibromyxoma is a tumor of the jaw bones and is uncommon in extragnathic locations; the mandible (posterior and condylar regions) is affected more often than the maxilla (zygomatic process and alveolar base).[3] Extragnathic involvement includes paranasal sinuses, primarily the maxillary sinus (antrum), often associated with extension into the nasal cavity.[3] Localization to the jaw bones has led to the belief that these tumors take origin from the primordial odontogenic mesenchyme or from osteogenic embryonic connective tissue.[3] Although myxomas of the mandible and maxilla are benign, slow-growing, expansible tumors, they can be locally aggressive.[123] Maxillary tumor most commonly presents as a palatal or facial swelling.

Histologically, myxomas are composed of small, benign-appearing, stellate cells lying in a myxoid stroma rich in polysaccharides. Given the large amount of myxoid stroma, the tumor appears very hypocellular. This histological appearance of myxoid stroma is responsible for relative hyperintensity on T1-weighted and heightened hyperintensity on T2-weighted MR images.

The histological appearance of craniofacial myxomas resembles that of other tumors. Lesions that can be mistaken for myxomas on the basis of myxoid areas include inflammatory polyp, mucocele, pleomorphic adenoma, myxoid neurofibroma, chondromyxoid fibroma, myxolipoma, fibrous histiocytoma, chondrosarcoma, chordoma, inverted papilloma, fibrosarcoma, leimyosarcoma, and rhadbomyosarcoma.[124] Rhabdomyosarcomas are positive for desmin and myxomas are not. Metastases from a presumptive myxoma/fibromyxoma should place that diagnosis seriously in doubt.[3] In fact, the lesion may represent a myxoid variant of a sarcoma (liposarcoma, malignant fibrous histiocytoma, or rhabdomyosarcoma).[3]

Radiographically, the lesion appears as expansible unilocular or multilocular radiolucences with a "honeycomb" or "soap bubble" appearance similar to the radiographic appearance of ameloblastoma (Fig. 4.**194**). On CT scans, myxoma has a soft-tissue density with moderate contrast enhancement on enhanced CT scans. Maxillary myxomas often demonstrate expansion, thinning, and even frank destruction of the bone cortex.[123]

The differential diagnosis of an expansile lesion in the maxillary sinus is listed in Table 4.**11**. The mucocele is the most common expansile mass in the maxillary and other paranasal sinuses. On CT images, a mucocele is usually a unilocular collection that centrifugally expands the sinus walls. Expansile cystic lesions associated with impacted and unerupted teeth are likely to be odontogenic cysts.[125, 126] Ameloblastomas, the most common odontogenic tumors, are benign yet invasive neoplasms that usually originate in the molar and premolar areas of the mandible. The CT appearance of ameloblastoma consists of a multilocular or unilocular cystic-appearing lesion. There may be a soft-tissue component that shows moderate contrast enhancement. The Pindborg tumor (calcifying epithelial odontogenic tumor) is also a benign noninvasive tumor that, similarly to ameloblastoma, invades and destroys bone.[123] Pindborg tumor is a benign neoplasm of unknown cause related to the odontogenic structures.¹²³ Most tumors occur in the mandible. The tumor comprises solid epithelial layers with variable amounts of round, conglomerate, or concentric laminar calcifications.¹²³ Association with adenomatoid odontogenic tumor and dentigerous cyst has been reported. Pindborg tumor may therefore be present as a mandibular or maxillary expansile mass with amorphous calcifications, associated with or without a central tooth. Odontoma may be mistaken for Pindborg tumor or ossifying fibroma. In contrast to Pindborg tumor, odontoma will appear as a lesion with amorphous opacity with innumerable toothlike densities (denticles).[123]

Aspiration prior to excision of cystic-appearing lesions of the maxillary sinus may provide important information. Straw-colored fluid denotes a cystic lesion; pus indicates an inflammatory or infectious mass; and white keratin-containing fluid strongly suggests an odontogenic keratocyst. Bloody aspirates could represent a vascular malformation. MRI is superior to CT for the differentiation of various expansile lesions of paranasal sinuses.

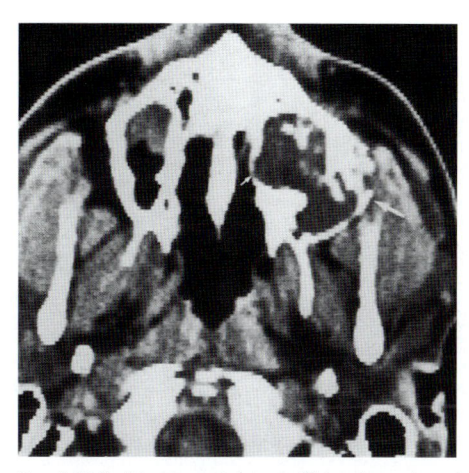

Fig. 4.**194** Myxoma, right maxillary sinus. An axial CT scan reveals an expansile lesion of the left maxillary sinus (arrows). It contains some areas of calcification. From Reference 12.

Chondromyxoid Fibroma

A separate and distinct benign tumor of cartilaginous origin that may involve the craniofacial bones, including paranasal sinuses, is the chondromyxoid fibroma.[3] The tumor may involve temporal bone. With time, the myxoid component may become fibrotic; the presence of cartilage, though, varies but never exceeds 75 % of the total tumor volume.[3] Osteoclastic giant cells and numerous calcifications may be seen. Surgery (en bloc resection) is the treatment of choice. Recurrence may occur if the tumor is incompletely excised.

Table 4.**11** Differential diagnosis of expansile lesion in the maxillary sinus

- Fibrous dysplasia
- Ossifying fibroma
- Dentigerous cyst (keratogenic cyst)
- Ameloblastoma
- Adenoid adamentinoma
- Pindborg tumor
- Cystic odontoma
- Myxoma
- Pleomorphic adenoma
- Neurofibroma
- Inverted papilloma
- Chondromyxoid fibroma
- Osteoblastoma
- Adenoid cystic tumor
- Extramedullary hematopoiesis
- Thalassemia
- Giant-cell tumor

Fibromatosis

Aggressive fibromatosis (Desmond tumor) is an infiltrating fibroblastic proliferation lacking histological features of either an inflammatory process or a neoplasm.[3] The head and neck is affected in 10–30 % of cases. Excluding the neck, the common sites of occurrence are nasal cavity and paranasal sinuses, nasopharynx, tongue, oral cavity, and orbit.[3, 127] It may involve the mastoid and external ear canal areas. The disease usually presents as a painless enlarging mass. The sinonasal fibromatosis causes facial deformity, nasal obstruction, epistaxis, and proptosis. Histologically, the lesion is composed of uniform-appearing spindle-shaped cells with sharply defined, pale-staining nuclei associated with and separated by abundant collagen production. There is mild pleomorphism and there are rare mitotic figures.[3]

Histologically, nodular fasciitis (NF), a nonneoplastic (reactive) proliferation of fibroblasts may be mistaken for aggressive fibromatosis.[3] In the head and neck, the most common site of NF is the neck. It may arise in the mastoid and external ear canal. Sinonasal involvement is extremely rare. On imaging, sinonasal fibromatosis appears as a soft-tissue mass, often with ill-defined margins with infiltration into surrounding structures, and associated with bone destruction (Fig. 4.**195**). The treatment of choice is complete surgical excision. Typically, the lesion is difficult to manage because it insinuates into adjacent structures.[3] In rare cases, transformation to an overt fibrosarcoma may occur.[3]

Fibrosarcoma

Fibrosarcoma is a malignant tumor of fibroblasts. Approximately 10–15 % of fibrosarcomas occur in the head and neck region.[3] Common head and neck sites are the nasal cavity and paranasal sinuses, followed by the larynx and neck. Grossly, the lesion may appear polypoid or sessile. Sinonasal fibrosarcomas are often associated with bone erosion or destruction. Histologically, fibrosarcoma is divided into low-grade and high-grade based on cellularity, cellular maturity, and the amount of collagen production.[3] On imaging, sinonasal fibrosarcoma appears as a soft-tissue mass, associated with bone erosion or destruction (Fig. 4.**196**). Differential diagnosis includes fibromatosis, fibrous histiocytoma, malignant schwannoma, sinonasal carcinoma, malignant melanoma, and lymphoma.

Benign Fibrous Histiocytoma

Benign fibrous histiocytoma (BFH) is a neoplasm composed of an admixture of fibroblastic and histiocytic cells.[3] BFH is an uncommon neoplasm in the head and neck, accounting for less than 5 % of all fibrous histiocytomas. Excluding cutaneous sites, the most common locations in the head and neck are the nasal cavity, paranasal sinuses, and orbit.[127] The CT and MRI appearances of BFH cannot be differentiated from sinonasal schwannoma, papilloma, and early stages of carcinoma.

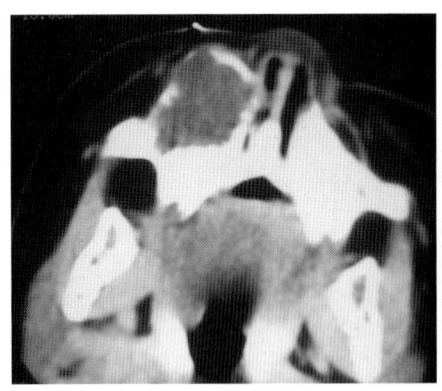

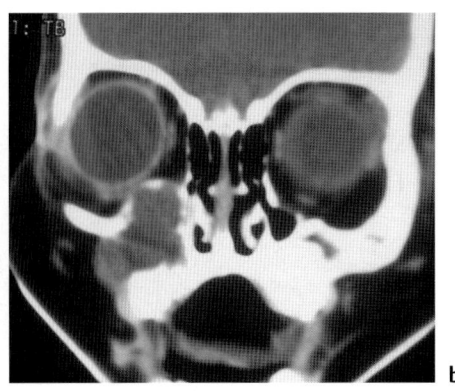

Fig. 4.**195** Aggressive fibromatosis. 16-year-old boy. **a** Axial CT scan shows a soft-tissue mass involving the right cheek region. **b** Coronal CT scan shows involvement of the underlying right maxilla. Courtesy of Ahmad Monajati, MD, New York, USA.

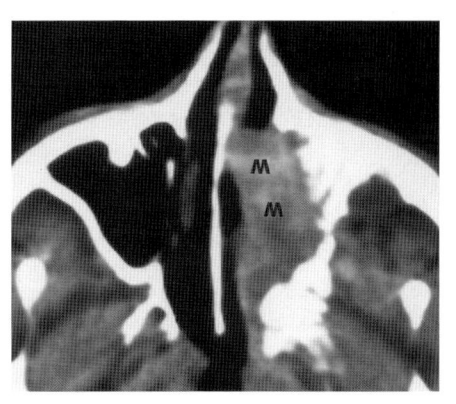

Fig. 4.**196** Recurrent fibrosarcoma. Axial CT scan shows a soft-tissue mass (M) in the nasal cavity, compatible with recurrent fibrosarcoma. Note reactive bony changes of the left maxillary antrum and pterygoid plates. Courtesy of Hatef Sharif, MD, Cairo, Egypt.

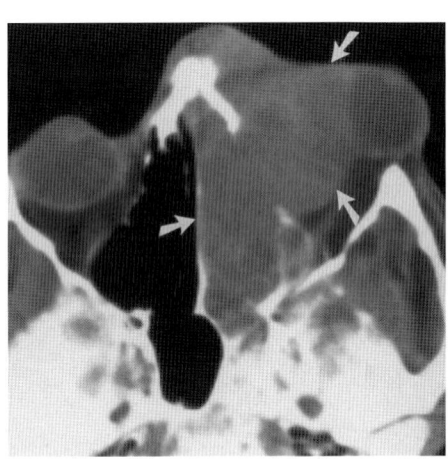

Fig. 4.**197** Malignant fibrous histiocytoma. CT scan shows a large soft-tissue mass (arrows) involving the nasoethmoid and orbital regions. Courtesy of Hatef Sharif, MD, Cairo, Egypt.

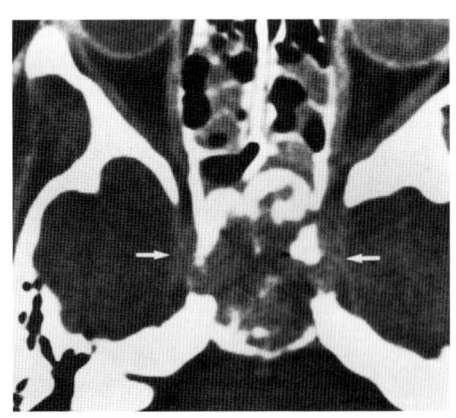

Fig. 4.**198** Langerhans cell histiocytoma. Axial enhanced CT scan shows an enhancing soft tissue mass (arrows) replacing parts of the clivus, compatible with eosinophilic granuloma. From Reference 12.

Malignant Fibrous Histiocytoma

Malignant fibrous histiocytoma (MFH) is a neoplasm consisting of an admixture of fibroblastic and histiocytic cells with features of malignant nature.[3] MFH is the most common soft-tissue sarcoma of late adult life, primarily affecting the soft tissues of the lower extremities. The most common noncutaneous locations in the head and neck are the sinonasal cavity, orbit,[127] and neck. Symptoms vary and include a mass with or without associated pain, nasal obstruction, epistaxis, facial deformity, and proptosis. The neoplasm consists of spindle-shaped cells admixed with histiocytic cells and marked by prominent pleomorphism and increased mitotic activity.[3] The CT and MRI appearances of sinonasal MFH are similar to those of fibrosarcoma, rhabdomyosarcoma, lymphoma, and sinonasal carcinoma (Fig. 4.**197**). Some MFH may appear very hypointense on T2-weighted MR images, related to high cellularity and increased mitotic activity. The myxoid variant of MFH may show higher signal intensity on T2-weighted MR images. Lymph node metastases occur in 15 % of cases. Other sites of metastasis include lung, liver, and bone. The majority of MFHs occur de novo; however, cases that are radiation-induced are reported. Complete surgical excision is the treatment of choice.[3]

Langerhans Cell Histiocytosis

A granulomatous disease that occurs in children more often than sarcoidosis or Wegener granulomatosis is Langerhans cell histiocytosis (LCH). The term histiocytosis-X was coined to describe a group of histiocytic conditions, with the letter X indicating their unknown nature. It is now known that these histiocytic conditions result from the proliferation and infiltration of abnormal histiocytes within various tissues. These cells are morphologically and immunologically similar to Langerhans cells, hence the name Langerhans cell histiocytosis. The head and neck are frequently involved in LCH, usually the skull bones or the jaws. Sinonasal involvement is uncommon. Involvement of maxillary and sphenoid sinuses has been reported (Fig. 4.**198**).[127] LCH is discussed in more detail in Chapter 2 as well as in Chapter 3.

Pituitary Adenoma and Sellar Paraganglioma

Tumors of the pituitary gland, particularly prolactinoma (Fig. 4.**199**), and other intracranial or extracranial tumors, such as meningiomas, chordomas, carcinoma (Fig. 4.**200**) and paragangliomas (Fig. 4.**201**), as well as giant aneurysm of the internal carotid artery may erode the floor or lateral wall of the sella and present as a mass in the sphenoid sinus or nasopharynx. Aggressive pituitary adenomas may extend into the nasal cavity and maxillary sinuses and present clinically as a nasal polyp.

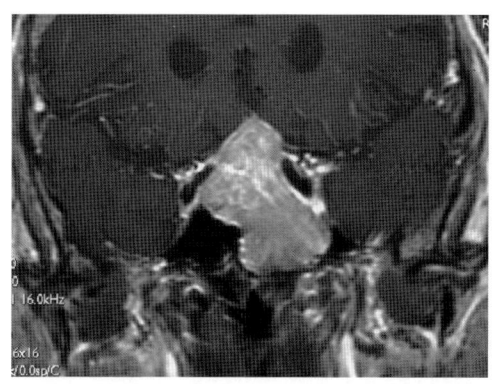

Fig. 4.**199** Pituitary adenoma. Coronal T1W MR image showing a large pituitary adenoma extending into the left sphenoid sinus.

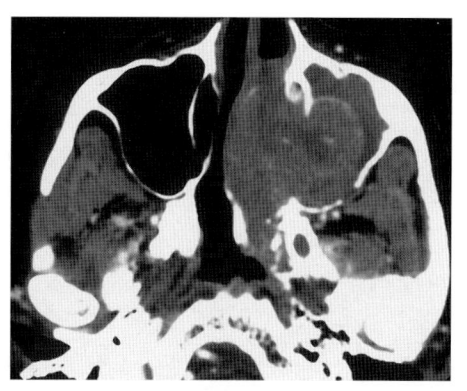

Fig. 4.**200** Undifferentiated carcinoma. Enhanced CT scan shows extension of an undifferentiated carcinoma of the sphenoid sinus (not shown here), into the nasal cavity and left maxillary sinus.

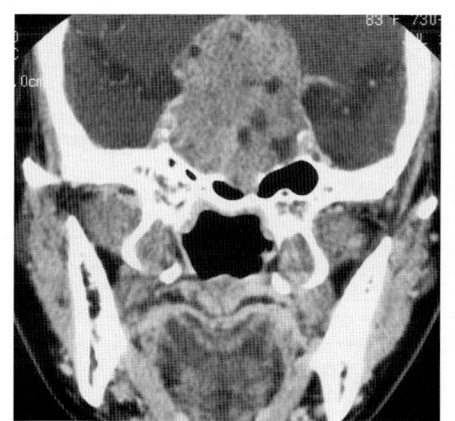

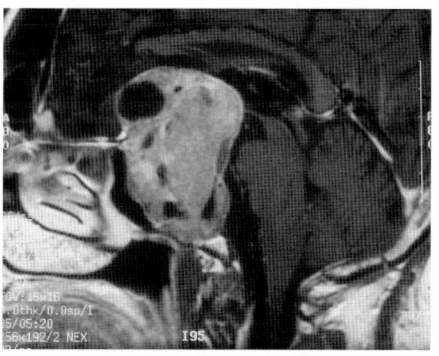

Fig. 4.**201** Paraganglioma of the sellar region. **a** Enhanced coronal CT scan showing a large intrasellar mass, demonstrating intense contrast enhancement. **b** Enhanced sagittal T1W MR scan shows extension of a parasellar paraganglioma into the sphenoid sinus.

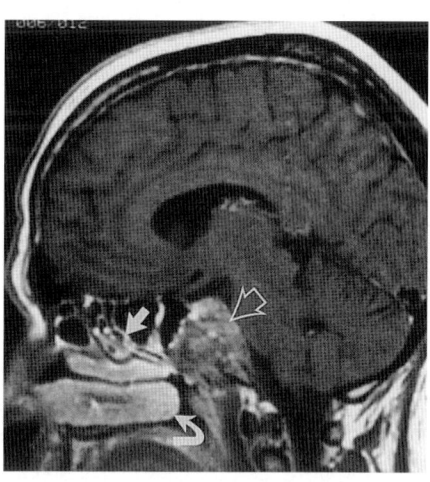

Fig. 4.**202** Metastasis. Postcontrast sagittal T1W MR scan shows enhancement of a metastatic adenocarcinoma of colon (open arrow). Note the normal mucosa of the turbinate (curved arrow) and ethmoid air cells (white arrow), which enhance more than the tumor.

Metastatic Tumors

The sinonasal tract can be host for the initial presentation of metastatic tumors. Some unusual sinonasal entities require a systemic work-up before they can be deemed "primary tumors." Among tumors metastasizing to the sinonasal cavities, renal cell carcinoma is the most common.[128] Next in frequency are tumors of the lung, breast, prostate, testis, and gastrointestinal tract. The majority of metastases to the paranasal sinuses are to the bone and are mainly hematogenic. A review of 98 paranasal sinus metastases showed that renal cell carcinoma constituted 54% of these tumors, most commonly affecting the maxilla (36%), followed by the ethmoidal sinus (25%), frontal sinus (17%), and nasal cavity (11%).[128] In more than 40% of the cases, a lesion of the base of the skull accounted for presenting manifestations that included headaches, facial pain, visual abnormalities, and, especially, oculomotor symptoms.[89] The prostate gland and lung were the most common primary sites of metastasis.[89] The clinical features were similar to those of a primary sphenoid malignant tumor. Metastatic tumors to the paranasal sinuses have a tendency to center their expansion around the margins of the sinus rather than a mucosal thickening. On CT scans, metastases from renal cell carcinomas and melanomas appear as markedly enhancing, soft-tissue masses that may remodel or destroy the walls of the sinonasal cavities. Prostatic metastatic lesions often result in sclerotic bone with abnormal irregular margins associated with small or large soft-tissue components. Metastases from lung, breast, bladder, distal genitourinary tract, and gastrointestinal tract are usually aggressive and bone-destroying. The MR characteristics of a sphenoid sinus metastasis from a colon carcinoma are shown in Fig. 4.**202**.

References

1 Boring CC, Squires TS, Tong T. Cancer statistics. CA Cancer J Clin 1992; 42: 19–38.
2 Mafee MF. Imaging of paranasal sinuses and nasal cavity. In: English GM, ed. Otolaryngology. Vol. 2. Philadelphia: Lippincott-Raven; 1996; 1–44.
3 Wenig BM. Atlas of Head and Neck Pathology. Philadelphia: W.B. Saunders; 1993.
4 Gadeberg CC, Hjelm-Hansen M, Sogaard H, et al. Malignant tumors of the paranasal sinuses and nasal cavity. A series of 180 patients. Acta Radiol 1984; 23: 181–187.
5 Som P. Tumors and tumor-like conditions of sinonasal cavity. In: Som P, Curtin H, eds. Head and Neck Imaging, 3d ed. St. Louis: Mosby-Year Book; 2003.
6 Goepfert M. Luna MA, Lindberg RD, et al. Malignant salivary gland tumors of the paranasal sinuses and nasal cavity. Arch Otolaryngol 1983; 10: 662–668.
7 Knegt PP, de Jong PC, van Andel JG, et al. Carcinoma of the paranasal sinuses: results of a prospective pilot study. Cancer 1985; 56: 57–62.
8 Konno A, Togawa K, Inous S. Analysis of the results of our combined therapy for maxillary cancer. Acta Otolaryngol Suppl (Stockh) 1980; 372: 1–16.
9 Chow JM, Leonetti JP, Mafee MF. Epithelial tumors of the paranasal sinuses and nasal cavity. Radiol Clin North Am 1993; 31: 61–73.
10 Mafee MF. Imaging of the head and neck: computed tomography, magnetic resonance imaging. In: Ballenger JJ, Snow JB, eds. Otolaryngology Head and Neck Surgery, 15th ed.. Baltimore: Williams and Wilkins; 1996: 699.
11 Mafee MF. Nonepithelial tumors of the paranasal sinuses and nasal cavity. Role of CT and MR imaging. Radiol Clin North Am 1993; 31: 75–90.
12 Carter BL. Tumors of the paranasal sinuses and nasal cavity. In: Valvassori GE, Buckingham RA, Carter BL, Hanafee WN, Mafee MR, eds. Head and Neck Imaging. Stuttgart: Thieme Verlag, 1988; 219–250.
13 Moore S, Chun JK, Mitre SA, Som PM. Intraosseous hemangioma of the zygoma: CT and MR findings. AJNR 2001; 22: 1383–1385.
14 Hyams VJ. Papillomas of the nasal cavity and paranasal sinus: a clinicopathological study of 315 cases. Ann Otol Rhinol Laryngol 1971; 80: 192–206.
15 Seshul MJ, Eby TL, Crowe DR, Peters GE. Nasal inverted papilloma with involvement of middle ear and mastoid. Arch Otolaryngol Head Neck Surg 1995; 121: 1045–1048.
16 Chherti DK, Gajjar NA, Bhuta S, Andrews JC. Quiz case 2. Schneiderian-type papilloma of the middle ear. Arch Otolaryngol Head Neck Surg 2001; 127: 79–80.
17 Lea JT, Bhuta S, Lufkin R, Castro DJ. Isolated inverting papilloma of the sphenoid sinus. Laryngoscope 2003; 113: 41–44.
18 Norris CM, Goodman ML. Case records of the Massachusetts General Hospital. N Engl J Med 1992; 326: 1417–1424.
19 Mafee MF. Dynamic CT and its application to otolaryngology and head and neck surgery. J Otolaryngol 1982; 77: 5.
20 Hill JH, Soboroff BJ, Appelbaum EL. Nonsquamous tumors of the nose and paranasal sinuses. Otolaryngol Clin North Am 1986; 19: 723–739.
21 Grafenberg MR, Kim S, Sorenson D. Pathology quiz case 2. Odontogenic keratocyst (OKC). Arch Otolaryngol Head Neck Surg 2002; 128: 1100–1102.
22 Philipsen HP. Om Keratocyster (Kolesteatom) 1 Kaeberbe. Tandelaegebladet 1956; 60: 963–980.
23 Albayram MS, Sciubba J, Zinreich JJ. Nasopalatine duct cyst. Arch Otolaryngol Head Neck Surg 2001; 127: 1283–1285.
24 Sik-Ching Ching A, Wai Pak M, Kew J, Metreweli C. CT and MR imaging appearances of an extraosseous calcifying epithelial odontogenic tumor (Pindborg Tumor). AJNR 2000; 21: 343–345.
25 Brandwein M, Said-Al-Naief N, Gordon R, Urken M. Clear cell odontogenic carcinoma: report of a case and analysis of the literature. Arch Otolaryngol Head Neck Surg 2002; 128: 1089–1095.
26 Waldron CA, Small IA, Silverman H. Clear cell ameloblastoma—an odontogenic carcinoma. J Oral Maxillofac Surg 1985; 43: 707–717.
27 Hansen LS, Eversole LR, Green TL, Powell NB. Clear cell odontogenic tumor—a new histologic variant with aggressive potential. Head Neck Surg 1985; 8: 115–123.
28 Boulos R, Marsot-Dupuch K, DeSaint-Maur P, et al. Granular cell tumor of the palate: a case report. AJNR 2002; 23: 850–854.
29 Som PM, Dillon WP, Sze G, et al. Benign and malignant sinonasal lesions with intracranial extension: differentiation with MR imaging. Radiology 1989; 172: 763–766.
30 Som PM, Brandwein M. Sinonasal cavities: Inflammatory disease, tumors, fractures, and postoperative findings. In: Som PM, Curtin HD, eds. Head and Neck Imaging, 3d ed. Vol. I.. St. Louis: Mosby; 1996.
31 Spiro JD, Soo KC, Spiro RH. Squamous carcinoma of the nasal cavity and paranasal sinuses. Am J Surg 1989; 158: 3328–3332.
32 Myers LL, Nussenbaum B, Bradford CR, et al. Paranasal sinus malignancies: An 18-year single institution experience. Laryngoscope 2002; 112: 1964–1969.
33 Schmalfuss IM, Tart RP, Mukerji S, Mancuso AA. Perineural tumor spread along the auriculotemporal nerve. AJNR 2002; 23: 303–311.
34 Wiseman SM, Popat SR, Rigual NR, et al. Adenoid cystic carcinoma of the paranasal sinuses and nasal cavity: a 40-year review of 35 cases. ENT Ear Nose Throat J 2002; 81: 510–517.
35 Kim GE, Park HC, Keum KC, et al. Adenoid cystic carcinoma of the maxillary antrum. Am J Otolaryngol 1999; 20: 77–84.
36 Fordice J, Kershaw C, El-Naggar A, Goepfert H. Adenoid cystic carcinoma of the head and neck. Predictors of morbidity and mortality. Arch Otolaryngol Head and Neck Surg 1999; 125: 149–152.
37 Moore GF, Massey JD, Yonkers AS. Abducens nerve paralysis: A potential presentation of sphenoid sinus cancer. Otolaryngol Head Neck Surg 1986; 94: 249–253.
38 Bridger MWM, Beale FA, Bryce DP. Carcinoma of the paranasal sinuses—ûa review of 158 cases. J Otolaryngol 1978; 7: 379–388.
39 Larson DL, Christ JE, Jesse RH. Preservation of the orbital contents in cancer of maxillary sinus. Arch Otolaryngol 1982; 108: 370–372.
40 Lund VS. Malignant tumors of the nasal cavity and paranasal sinuses. ORL 1983; 45: 1–12.
41 Sisson GA. Carcinoma of the paranasal sinuses and craniofacial resection. J Laryngol Otol 1976; 90: 59–68.
42 Batsakis JG. Tumors of the Head and Neck: Clinical and Pathological Considerations. 2d ed. Baltimore: Williams and Wilkins: 1979; 177–187.
43 Lund VS, Howard DJ, Lloyd GAS, et al. Magnetic resonance imaging of paranasal sinus tumor for craniofacial resection. Head Neck 1989; 11: 279–283.
44 Kaznelson DJ, Schindel J. Mucoepidermoid carcinoma of the air passages. Report of three cases. Laryngoscope 1979; 89: 115–121.
45 Thomas GR, Regolado JJ, McClinton M. A rare case of mucoepidermoid carcinoma of the nasal cavity. ENT Ear Nose Throat J 2002; 81: 519–521.
46 Skolnik EM, Massari FS, Tenta LT. Olfactory neuroepithelioma: reviews of the world literature and presentation of two cases. Arch Otolalryngol 1966; 84: 644–653.
47 Som PM, Lidov M, Brandwein M, et al. Sinonasal esthesioneuroblastoma with intracranial extensions: marginal tumor cysts as a diagnostic MR finding. AJNR 1994; 15: 1259–1262.
48 Argiris A, Dutra J, Tseke P, Haines K. Esthesioneuroblastoma: The Northwestern University Experience. Laryngoscope 2003; 113: 155–160.
49 Kadish S, Goodman M, Wang CC. Olfactory neuroblastoma: a clinical analysis of 17 cases. Cancer 1976; 37: 1571–1576.
50 Califano L, Zupi A, Mangone GM, et al. Cervical ganglioneuroma: Report of a case. Otolaryngol Head Neck Surg 2001; 124: 115–116.
51 Joshi VV, Cantor AB, Altshuler G, et al. Recommendations for modification of terminology of neuroblastic tumors and prognostic significance of Shimada Classification. A clinicopathologic study of 213 cases from the pediatric oncology group. Cancer 1992; 69: 2183–2196.
52 Kapadia S, Frisman D, Hitchcock C, et al. Melanotic neuroectodermal tumor of infancy. Clinicopathological, immmunohistochemical, and flow cytometric study. Am J Surg Pathol 1993; 17: 566–573.
53 Volk MS, Nielsen GP. Case records of the Massachusetts General Hospital. Case 7—2001. A male infant with a right maxillary mass. N Engl J Med 2001; 344: 750–757.
54 Howard D, Daniels H. Ewing's sarcoma of the nose. J Ear Nose Throat 1993; 72: 277–279.
54a Grier HE, Krailo MD, Tarbell NJ, et al. Addition of ifosfamide and etoposide to standard chemotherapy for Ewing's sarcoma and primitive neuroectodermal tumor of bone. N Engl J Med 2003; 348: 694–701.
55 Dehner LP. Peripheral and central primitive neuroectodermal tumors. Arch Pathol Lab Med 1986; 110: 997–1003.
56 Chowdhury K, Manoukian JJ, Rochon L, et al. Extracranial primitive neuroectodermal tumor of the head and neck. Arch Otolaryngol Head Neck Surg 1990; 116: 475–478.
57 Jurgens H, Bier V, Harms D, et al. Malignant peripheral neuroectodermal tumors: a retrospective analysis of 42 cases. Cancer 1988; 61: 349–357.

58 Klein E, Anzil A, Mezzacappa P, et al. Sinonasal primitive neuroectodermal tumor arising in a long-term survivor of heritable unilateral retinoblastoma. Cancer 1992; 70: 423–431.
59 Azizi L, Marsot-Dupuch K, Bigel P, et al. Merkel cell carcinoma: a rare cause of hypervascular nasal tumor. AJNR 2001; 22: 1389–1393.
60 Rice RD, Choukich GD, Thompson KS, Chase DR. Merkel cell tumor of the head and neck: five new cases with literature review. Arch Otolaryngeal Head Neck Surg 1993; 119: 782–786.
61 Chawla OP, Oswal VH. Hemangiopericytoma of the nose and paranasal sinuses. J Laryngol Otol 1987; 101: 729–737.
62 Stout AP, Murray MR. Hemangiopericytoma: a vascular tumor featuring Zimmerman's pericytes. Ann Surg 1942; 116: 26–33.
63 Rhodin JAG. Ultrastructure of mamalian venous capillaries, venules and small collecting veins. J Ultrastruct Res 1968; 25: 452–500.
64 Batsakis JG, Rice DH. The pathology of head and neck tumors: Vasoformative tumors. Part 9B. Head Neck 1981; 3: 326–339.
65 Batsakis JG, Jacobs JB, Templeton AC. Hemangiopericytoma of the nasal cavity: electron-optic study and clinical correlations. J Laryngol Otol 1983; 97: 361–368.
66 Anderson GJ, Tom LW, Womer RB, et al. Rhabdomyosarcoma of the head and neck in children. Arch Otolaryngol Head Neck Surg 1990; 116: 428–431.
67 Feldman BA. Rhabdomyosarcoma of the head and neck. Laryngoscope 1982; 92: 424–440.
68 Malogolowkin MH, Orega JA. Rhabdomyosarcoma of childhood. Pediatr Ann 1988; 17: 251–268.
69 Mafee MF, Pai E, Philip B. Rhabdomyosarcoma of the orbit: evaluation with MR imaging and CT. Radiol Clin North Am 1998; 36: 1215–1229.
70 Pinkel D, Pickren F. Rhabdomyosarcoma in children. JAMA 1961; 175: 293–298.
71 Wilder WH, Harner SG, Banks PM. Lymphoma of the nose and paranasal sinuses. Arch Otolaryngol 1983; 109: 310–312.
72 Aisenberg AC. Malignant lymphoma. N Engl J Med 1973; 288: 883–890.
73 Farhat F, Djokic M, Naclerio RM. Extranodal natural killer (NK)T-cell lymphoma (Epstein-Barr virus associated). Arch Otolaryngol Head Neck Surg 2002; 128: 1327–1329.
74 Jaffe ES, Chan JK, Sui J, et al. Report of the workshop on nasal and related extranodal angiocentric T/Natural killer cell lymphoma: definitions, differential diagnosis, and epidemiology. Am J Surg Pathol 1996; 20: 103–111.
75 Oai GC, Chim CS, Liang R, et al. Nasal T-cell/natural killer cell lymphoma: CT and MR imaging features of a new clinicopathologic entity. AJR 2000; 174: 1141–1145.
76 Khariwala SS, Litman DA, McQuone SJ, et al. Natural killer (NK) cell/peripheral T-cell lymphoma. Arch Otolaryngol Head Neck Surg 2000; 126: 1391–1393.
77 Cheung MMC, Chan JKC, Lau WH, et al. Primary non-Hodgkin's lymphoma of the nose and nasopharynx: clinical features, tumor immunophenotype, and treatment outcome in 113 patients. J Clin Oncol 1998; 16: 70–77.
78 Freeman C, Berg JW, Cutler SJ. Occurrence and prognosis of extranodal lymphomas. Cancer 1972; 29: 252–260.
79 Miller FR, Lavertu P, Wanamaker, et al. Plasmacytomas of the head and neck. Otolaryngol Head Neck Surg 1998; 19: 614–618.
80 Ching ASC, Khoo JBK, Chong VFH. CT and MR imaging of solitary extramedullary plasmacytoma of the nasal tract. AJNR 2002; 23: 1632–1636.
81 Loevner LA, Karpati RL, Kumar P, et al. Posttransplantation lymphoproliferative disorder of the head and neck: imaging features in seven adults. Radiology 2000; 81: 139–148.
82 Gordon AR, Loevner LA, Sonners AL, et al. Posttransplantation lymphoproliferative disorder of the paranasal sinuses mimicking invasive fungal sinusitis: Case report. AJNR 2002; 23: 855–857.
83 Johnston R, Altman KW, Gartenhaus RB. Chronic lymphocytic leukemia manifesting in the paranasal sinus. Otolaryngol Head Neck Surg 2002; 127: 582–584.
84 Conley J, Hamaker RC. Melanoma of the head and neck. Laryngoscope 1976; 29: 760–764.
85 Conley J, Pack GT. Melanoma of the mucous membranes of the head and neck. Arch Otolaryngol Head Neck Surg 1974; 99: 315–319.
86 Moore ES, Martin H. Melanoma of the upper respiratory tract and oral cavity. Cancer 1955; 8: 1167–1176.
87 Mafee MF, Langer B, Valvassori GE, et al. Radiologic diagnosis of nonsquamous tumors of the head and neck. Otolaryngol Clin North Am 1986; 19: 507–521.
88 Fu Y, Perzin AH. Nonepithelial tumors of the nasal cavity, paranasal sinuses and nasopharynx: a clinical pathologic study: II. Osseous and fibro-osseous lesions, including osteomas, fibrous dysplasia, ossifying fibroma, osteoblastoma, giant cell tumor, and osteosarcoma. Cancer 1974; 33: 1289–1305.
89 Mickel RA, Zimmerman MC. The sphenoid sinus: A site for metastasis. Otolaryngol Head Neck Surg 1990; 102–709–716.
90 Wenig BM, Mafee MF, Ghosh L. Fibro-osseous, osseous, and cartilaginous lesion of the orbit and paraorbital region: correlative clinicopathologic and radiographic features, including the diagnostic role of CT and MR imaging. Radiol Clin North Am 1998; 36: 1241–1259.
91 Lustig LR, Holliday MJ, McCarthy EF, Nager GT. Fibrous dysplasia involving the skull base and temporal bone. Arch Otolaryngol Head Neck Surg 2001; 127: 1239–1247.
92 Albright F, Butler M, Hamptom A, Smith P. Syndrome characterized by osteitis fibrosa disseminata, areas of pigmentation and endocrine dysfunction with precocious puberty in female. N Engl J Med 1937; 216: 727–746.
93 McCune D, Bruch H. Osteodystrophia fibrosa: report of a case in which the condition was combined with precocious puberty, multiple pigmentation of the skin and hyperthyroidism. Am J Dis Child 1937; 52: 745–748.
94 Lee P, Van Dop C, Migeon C. McCune-Albright syndrome: long term follow-up. JAMA, 1986; 256: 2980–2984.
95 Cohen M, Howell R. Etiology of fibrous dysplasia and McCune-Albright syndrome. Int J Oral Maxillofac Surg 1999; 28: 366–371.
96 Schwindinger WF, Francomano CA, Levine MA. Identification of a mutation in the gene encoding the alpha subunit of the stimulator G-protein of adenylyl cyclase in McCune–Albright syndrome. Proc Natl Acad Sci USA 1992; 29: 5152.
97 Weinstein LS, Shenker A, Gejman PV, et al. Activating mutations of the stimulatory G-protein in the McCune–Albright syndrome. N Engl J Med 1991; 325: 1688.
98 Tokano H, Sugimoto T, Noguchi Y, Kitamura K. Sequential tomography images demonstrating characteristic changes in fibrous dysplasia. J Laryngol Otol 2001; 115: 751.
99 Lee J, Fitzgibbon E, Butman JA. Normal vision despite narrowing of the optic canal in fibrous dysplasia. N Engl J Med 2002; 347: 1670.
100 Kearney PR, Nasser A. Pathology quiz case 2; extramedullary hematopoiesis of the paranasal sinuses. Arch Otolaryngol Head Neck Surg 2002; 128: 76–79.
101 Smith SE, Murphey MD, Motamedi K, et al. From the Archives of the AFIP Radiologic Spectrum of Paget disease of bone and its complications with pathologic correlation. Radiographics 2002; 22: 1191–1216.
102 Curé JK, Key LL, Goltra DD, Van Tassel P. Cranial MR imaging of osteopetrosis. AJNR 2000; 21: 1110–1115.
103 Hul WV, Vanhoenacker F, Balemans W, et al. Molecular and radiological diagnosis of sclerosing bone dysplasias. Eur J Radiol 2001; 40: 198–207.
104 Hul EV, Gram J, Bollerslev J, et al. Localization of the gene causing autosomal dominant osteopetrosis Type I to chromosome 11q12–13. J Bone Miner Res 2002; 7: 1111–1117.
105 Coppit GI, Eusterman VD, Bartels J, Downey TJ. Endoscopic resection of chondrosarcomas of the nasal septum: A report of 2 cases. Otolaryngol Head Neck Surg 2002; 127: 569–571.
106 Chaudhry AP, Robinovitch MR, Mitchell DR, et al. Chondrogenic tumors of the jaws. Am J Surg 1961; 102: 403.
107 Dahlin DC, Lenni RR. Bone Tumors: General Aspect and Data on 8,542 Cases, 4th ed. Springfield, IL: Charles C. Thomas; 1986.
108 Huvos AG, Marcove RC. Chondroblastoma of bone: A critical review. Clin Orthop 1973; 95: 300.
109 Bloem JL, Mulder JD. Chondroblastoma: a clinical and radiological study of 104 cases. Skeletal Radiol 1985; 14: 1.
110 Murphey MD, Nomikos GC, Glemming DJ, et al. From the archives of the AFIP. Imaging of giant cell tumor and giant cell reparative granuloma of bone: Radiologic–pathologic correlation. Radiographics 2001; 21: 1283–1209.
111 Jaffe HL. Giant cell reparative granuloma, traumatic bone cyst and fibrous (fibro-osseous) dysplasia of jawbones. Oral Surg 1953; 6: 159–175.
112 Quick CA, Anderson R, Stoal S. Giant cell tumors of the maxilla in children. Laryngoscope 1980; 90: 784–791.
113 Khademi B, Gandomi B. Giant cell reparative granuloma of the hyoid bone. Otolaryngol Head Neck Surg 2001; 124: 117–118.
114 Albright F, Aub J, Bauer W. Hyperparathyroidism: a common and pleomorphic condition as illustrated by 17 proved cases from one clinic. JAMA 1934; 102: 1276–1287.

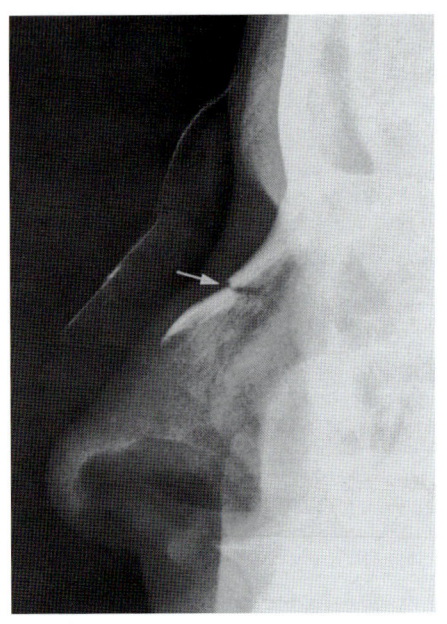

Fig. 4.**203** Nasal bone fracture, lateral projection. The fracture line (arrow) crosses the nasociliary groove and shows slight displacement of the fracture fragments.

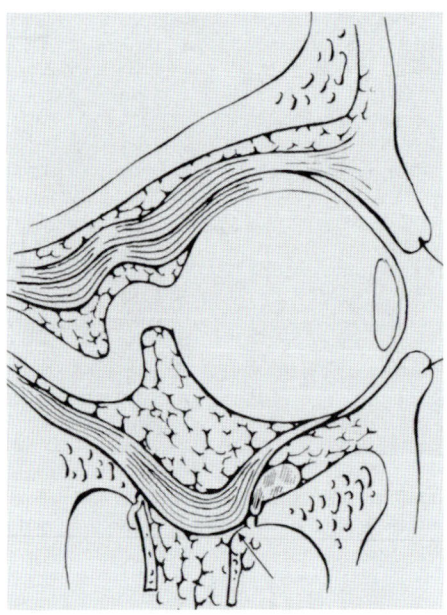

Fig. 4.**204** Schematic drawing of a blowout fracture. The inferior rectus muscle (arrow) is displaced inferiorly with orbital fat through the fracture defect. Modified from Zizmor J. Trans Am Acad Ophthalmol Otolaryngol 1957; 44: 733–739.

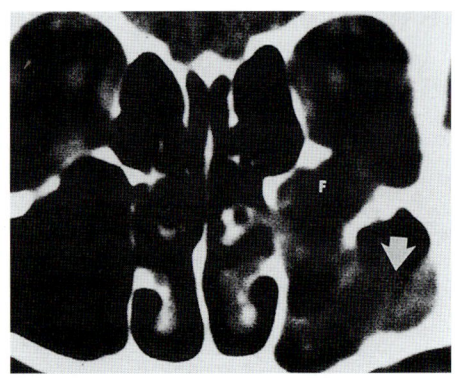

Fig. 4.**205** Blowout fracture. Coronal CT scan shows fracture of the left orbital floor, associated with herniation of orbital fat (F) and air–fluid level (arrow) in the maxillary sinus.

115 Kar DK, Gupta SK, Gupta SK, et al. Brown tumor of the palate and mandible in association with primary hyperparathyroidism. J Oral Maxillofac Surg 2001; 59: 1352–1354.
116 Mafee MF, Yang G, Tseng A, et al. Fibro-osseous and giant cell lesions including brown tumor of the mandible, maxilla and other craniofacial bones. Radiol Clin North Am 2003; 13: 525–540.
117 Hruska RA, Teitelbaum SL. Renal osteodystrophy. N Engl J Med 1995; 33: 166.
118 Marx SJ. Hyperparathyroidism and hypoparathyroid disorders. N Engl J Med 2000; 343: 1863–1875.
119 Burkey BB, Hoffman HT, Baker SR, et al. Chondrosarcoma of the head and neck. Laryngoscope 1990; 100: 1301.
120 Finn DG, Goeppert H, Batsakis JG. Chondrosarcoma of the head and neck. Laryngoscope 1984; 95: 1539.
121 Zimmermann DC, Dahlin DC. Myxomatous tumors of the jaws. Oral Surg 1958; 11: 1069–1080.
122 Ghosh BC, Huvos AG, Gerald FP, Miller TR. Myxoma of the jaw bones. Cancer, 1973; 31: 237–240.
123 Batti JS, Zahtz G, O, Reilly B. Quiz Case 4: Myxoma of the maxillary sinus. Arch Otolaryngol Head Neck Surg 2000; 126: 679–683.
124 Heffner DK. Sinonasal myxomas and fibromyxomas in children. ENT Ear Nose Throat J 1993; 72: 365–368.
125 Mabrie DC, Francis HW, Zinreich SJ, et al. Imaging quiz case 4: Dentigerous cyst. Arch Otolaryngol Head Neck Surg 2001; 126: 1269–1273.
126 Yonetsu K, Bianchi JG, Troulis MJ, Curtin HD. Unusual CT appearance in an odontogenic keratocyst of the mandible: case report. AJNR 2001; 22: 1887–89.
127 Mafee MF. Orbit: embryology, anatomy, and pathology. In: Som PM, Curtin HD, eds. Head and Neck Imaging. Vol. 1. St. Louis: Mosby; 2003: 529–654.
128 Berstein JM, Montgomery WW, Balgh K, Jr. Metastatic tumors to the maxilla, nose, and paranasal sinuses. Laryngoscope 1966; 76: 621–650.

Traumatic and Postoperative Findings

Trauma

Maxillofacial trauma occurs in significant number of severely injured patients. Motor vehicle accident (MVA) and assault remain the primary causes of maxillofacial fractures. Cerebral and pulmonary injuries are often associated with maxillofacial fractures in severely injured patients.[1] Orbital and maxillary fractures are the most common overall facial fractures, though other studies have indicated that the mandible is the most common facial bone involved in facial fractures.[1] Plain film studies, although less frequently used for patients with facial injury, can provide useful information.[1,2] Displaced fractures caused by direct blows to the nose may be disfiguring and obstruct normal breathing. The degree of deformity is usually apparent on the direct lateral and occlusal films (Fig. 4.**203**). CT scanning may be required to evaluate accompanying fractures of other bones of the face. In the nasal bone, fracture lines usually cross other vascular and neural grooves, which are parallel to the suture lines between the nasal bones and the nasal processes of the maxilla (Fig. 4.**203**). More severe injuries are often accompanied by fractures through the anterior spinous process of the maxilla (anterior nasal spine) and other bones. Fractures with severe deformity or with complications require further study with CT scanning. Facial fractures are often multiple, complex, and asymmetric, but they tend to fall into various categories, such as blowout fracture of the orbit, tripod injuries, and Le Fort injuries.[1,2] The blowout fracture (Figs. 4.**204**–4.**208**) most commonly involves the floor of the orbit, which is depressed inferiorly by the soft tissues of the orbit when displaced by a fist, ball or other blunt trauma to the globe. The anterior rim of the orbit remains intact. A depressed floor fracture may be associated with inferior herniation of orbital fat or with entrapment of the inferior rectus and/or inferior oblique muscles (Figs. 4.**204**, 4.**205**, 4.**206**). Contusion of the inferior rectus muscle is almost always present. This is seen as deformity of the muscle as compared with the normal side. Direct coronal and reformatted sagittal CT scans clearly demonstrate this type of injury. A medial blowout fracture involving the lamina papyracea is less common than the inferior type (Fig. 4.**207**). This is often associated with contusion or entrapment of the medial rectus muscle.

Facial trauma may be such that it can result in a blow-in fracture of the orbital floor as well as blowout or blow-in fractures of the orbital roof. The fracture may involve the orbital apex (Fig. 4.**208**).

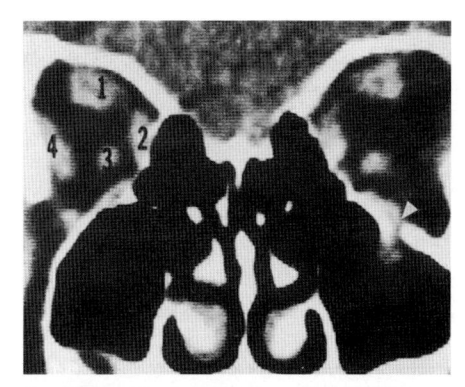

Fig. 4.**206** Blowout fracture. Coronal CT scan shows minimally displaced orbital floor fracture. Note the partially herniated inferior rectus (arrowhead) and soft tissue (hematoma) at the site of the fracture. 1 = superior rectus; 2 = medial rectus; 3 = inferior rectus; 4 = lateral rectus.

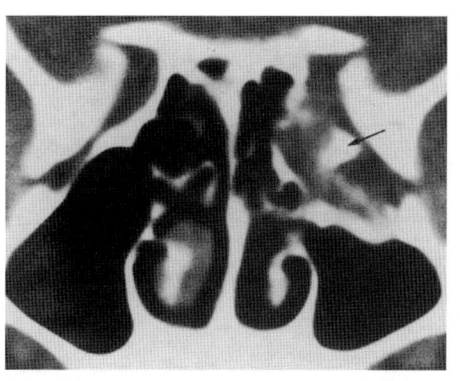

Fig. 4.**207** Blowout fracture. Coronal CT scan shows a fracture of the left orbital floor. Note a bony fragment (arrow) at the orbital apex.

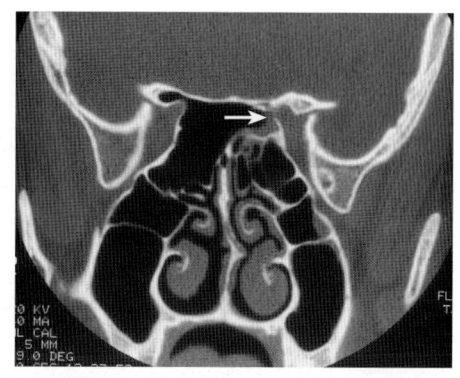

Fig. 4.**208** Optic canal fracture. Coronal CT scan shows a fracture (arrow) of the left orbital apex involving the optic canal.

Fig. 4.**209** Schematic drawing of a tripod fracture. The fracture extends through the frontozygomatic region (1), zygomatic arch (2), anterior rim of the orbit (3), and maxilla. Note also separation of the sphenozygomatic suture, between the greater sphenoid wing and zygoma. After Zizmor J, Noyek A. Orbital trauma. In: Newton T H, Potts D G, eds., Radiology of the Skull and Brain. St. Louis: Mosby, 1971.

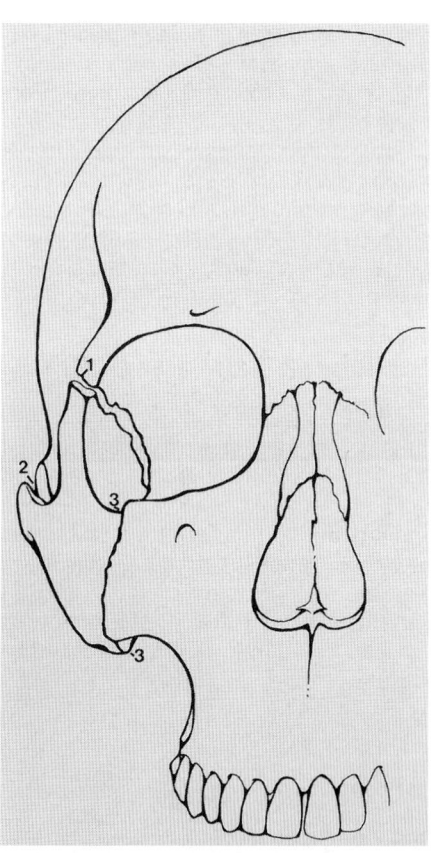

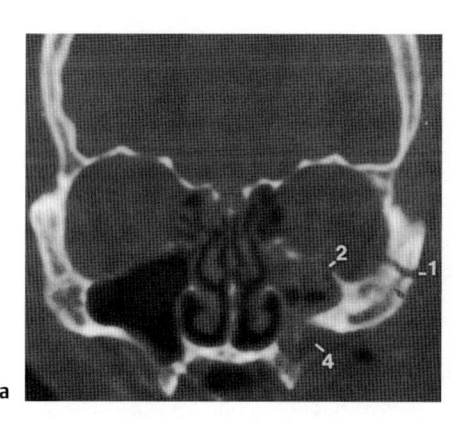

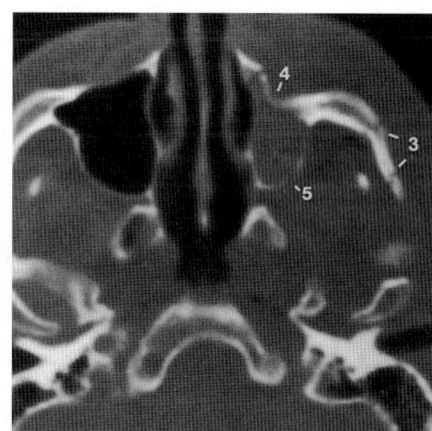

Fig. 4.**210** Tripod fracture. **a** Coronal and **b** axial CT scans. Fractures through the left frontozygomatic suture, anterior rim (2) to floor of the orbit, and the zygomatic arch (3) are clearly seen. In addition, the fracture line through the zygomatic/maxillary area involves the wall of the maxillary sinus anteriorly (4) and posterolaterally (5). Depression in the zygoma is visible in **b**. Note the fracture involving the frontal process of the zygoma (1), seen on coronal CT scan. Note normal right frontozygomatic suture, as compared with left irregular, deformed frontozygomatic suture. From Reference 2a.

Tripod Fracture

A tripod fracture (Figs. 4.**209**, 4.**210**) is the result of an oblique injury to the face with three main fracture sites; the frontozygomatic suture line, the zygomatic arch, and the maxilla (including the inferior rim of the orbit and the lateral wall of the maxillary sinus). The zygoma is often depressed in this type of injury, but the direction of rotation and displacement may vary depending on the direction and force of the blow (Fig. 4.**211**). Le Fort fractures are a result of direct anterior facial injuries. The classification as originally described by Le Fort in 1901 referred to symmetrical fractures of the facial bones, extending back to and involving the pterygoid plates (Fig. 4.**212**). Since the injuries are often asymmetric, they are usually designated as Le Fort-type fractures. The Le Fort I injury is a horizontal fracture extending across the floor of the maxillary sinuses above the dentition line

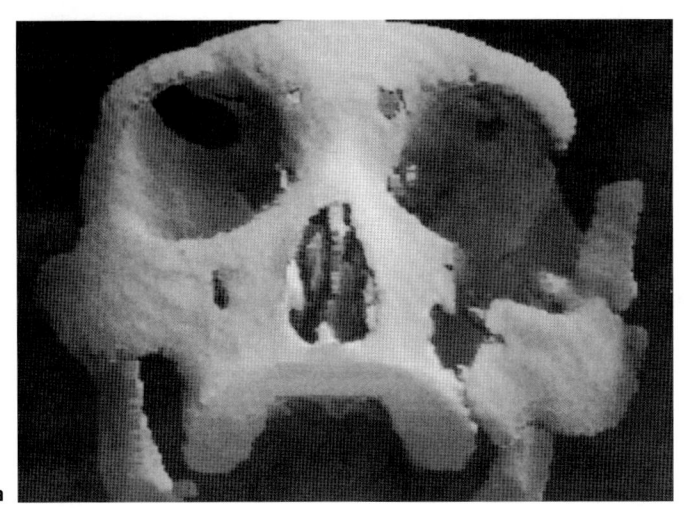

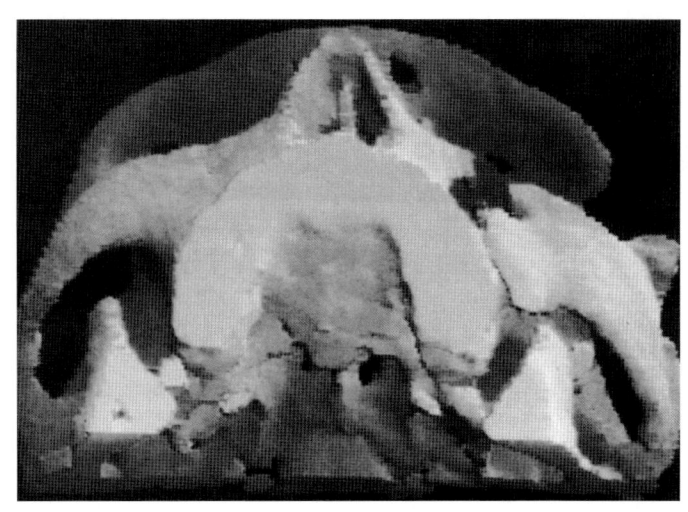

Fig. 4.**211** Tripod fracture. **a** and **b** Three-dimensional CT images showing a left tripod fracture. Note separation of left frontozygomatic suture, inferior orbital RIM fracture, and depression as well as rotation of left zygoma.

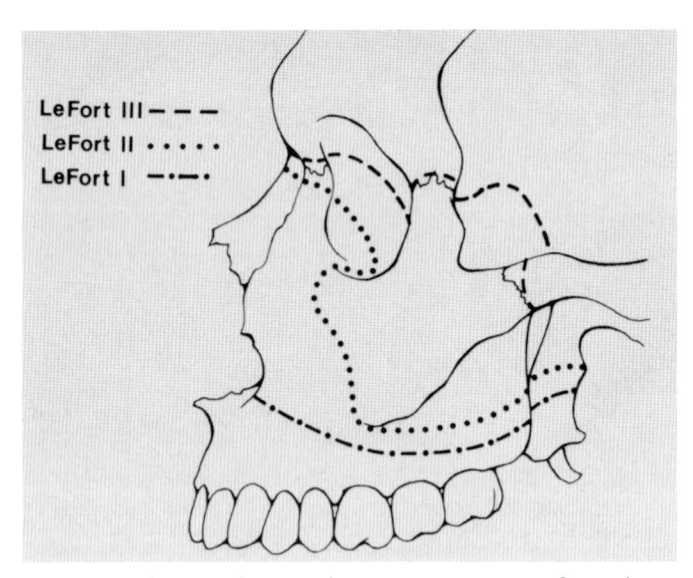

Fig. 4.**212** Schematic drawing of Le Fort type injuries. After Holt GR. Maxillofacial trauma. In: Cummings, et al, eds. Otolaryngology – Head and Neck Surgery. St. Louis: Mosby, 1986.

of the superior alveolar ridge, resulting in a "floating palate." Occasionally, a midpalatal split complicates this type of injury (Fig. 4.**213**). The Le Fort II fracture is also called a pyramidal fracture (Fig. 4.**214**) and occurs vertically through the maxilla and across the upper nasal ethmoid bone complex and back to the pterygoid plates. The zygoma is left intact with a "floating maxilla." The most severe of this group is the Le Fort III, a complete craniofacial separation (Fig. 4.**215**). The fracture line passes through the frontozygomatic sutures bilaterally, across the nose, and down to the pterygoid plates, resulting in a "floating face."[2]

Complications of Craniofacial Trauma and CSF Leak

The cribriform plate, ethmoidal arteries, optic nerve, and internal maxillary artery are all at risk of serious injury in craniofacial trauma.[1] Fractures through the orbital apex close to the optic nerve may result in blindness due to injury of the optic nerve. Trauma involving the ostium of a sinus may cause obstruction and the subsequent development of a mucocele. A fracture through the inner table of the skull may also be associated with tear of the dura and a CSF leak. Thus, an air–fluid level within the

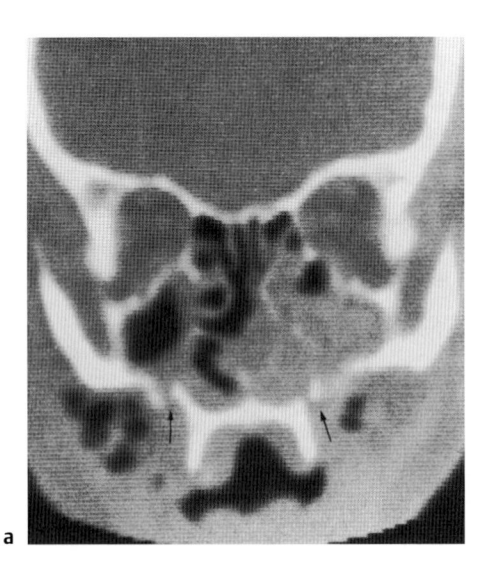

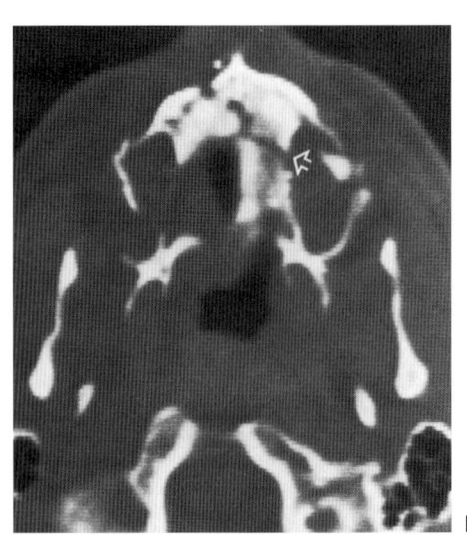

Fig. 4.**213** Le Fort I type injury. **a** Coronal and **b** axial CT images. A "floating palate" is a result of fracture just above the superior alveolar ridge (arrow). An associated fracture may extend through the palate (open arrow) as shown in **b**. From Reference 2a.

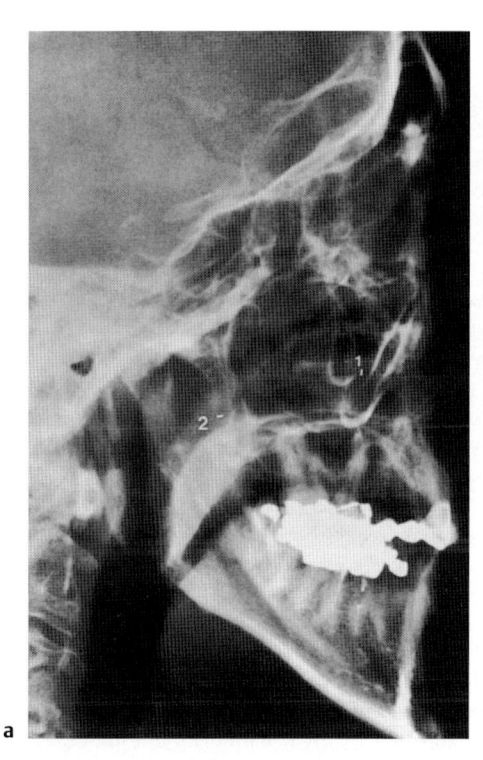

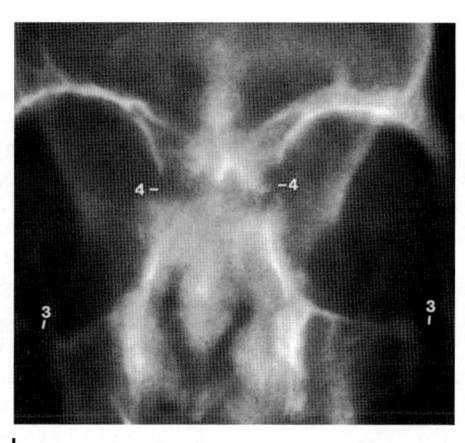

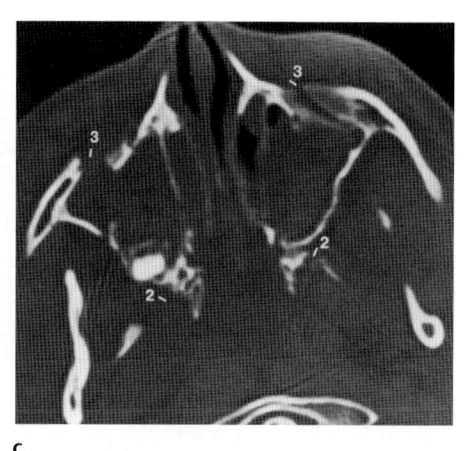

Fig. 4.**214** LeFort II type fracture. **a** Lateral projection, **b** AP tomogram, and **c** axial CT scan. Fracture through the midfacial area resulting in a "floating maxilla" can be seen through the zygoma (1) and pterygoid region (2) in **a**, through the junction of the maxilla with the zygoma (3) in **b** and **c**, and across the nasal ethmoid complex (4) in **b**. Fractures through the maxilla/zygoma area (3) and pterygoid plates (2) can be seen in **c**. From Reference 2a.

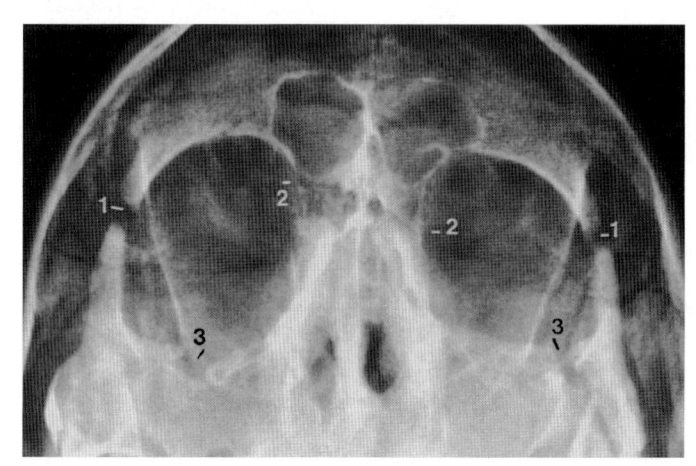

Fig. 4.**215** Le Fort III type fracture, a complete cranofacial separation, Waters projection. Fracture lines through the frontozygomatic area (1) and across the nasion (2) extend back to include the pterygoid plates (not shown here), resulting in complete separation of the facial bones from the skull. Also note the midface fracture of Le Fort II type injury (3). From Reference 2a.

sinus might be due to blood or CSF.[1] A tear in the dura may be associated with pneumocephalus caused by fracture involving the mastoid air cells, paranasal sinuses, nasal roof, or roof of the nasopharynx. It is important to establish the presence of a CSF leak because of the potential danger of meningitis. For CSF leak, CT cisternography using intrathecal injection of an appropriate iodinated contrast material is the study of choice (Fig. 4.**216**). Subcutaneous emphysema in the orbit or in the soft-tissue structures overlying the facial area is frequently seen on CT and again is indicative of a fracture of the adjacent paranasal sinus (Fig. 4.**208**). It should be noted that CSF rhinorrhea may also be a manifestation of fracture of the temporal bone with an intact tympanic membrane, caused by CSF entering the nasopharynx via the eustachian tube. Therefore, in a patient with CSF rhinorrhea, following intrathecal injection of iodinated contrast material, thin-section (3 mm) coronal CT scans should be obtained of the anterior, middle, and posterior cranial fossae while the patient is in the prone position.[1]

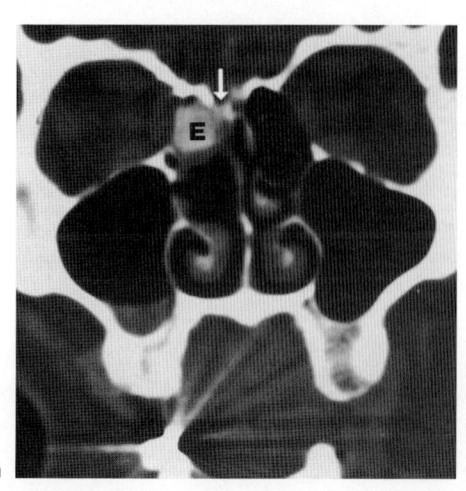

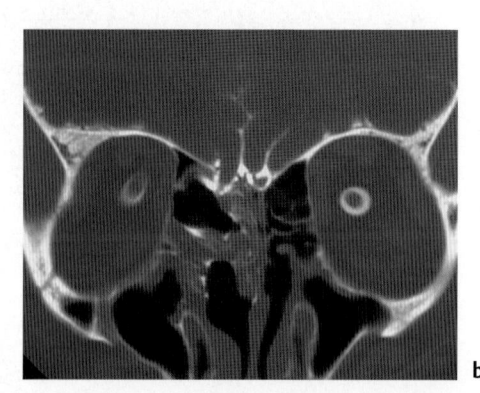

Fig. 4.**216** **a** CSF rhinorrhea. CT cisternogram shows the site of leak (arrow). Note the collection of contrast material in the ethmoid sinus (E). **b** CT cisternogram shows post-right anterior ethmoidectomy changes. Note deformity of the cribriform plate on the right side and the presence of contrast in the right ethmoid and nasal cavity.

Postoperative Changes and Complications of Sinus Surgery

There are several options for surgical treatment of sinonasal inflammatory and neoplastic disorders.[2] Sinus irrigation is contraindicated in acute sinusitis since the meatus is usually obliterated, and the penetration of the lateral nasal wall, canine fossa, or other sinuses (sinusotomy) may initiate spread of the disease.[2] If after 7–10 days' antibiotic treatment for acute sinusitis, the patient continues to have severe symptoms, a drainage procedure is usually done.[2] For maxillary sinusitis, if irrigation fails, an anterior ethmoidectomy and middle meatal antrostomy or an inferior meatal antrostomy may be performed.[2] A common procedure in the past to cure a chronic purulent maxillary sinusitis was an inferior meatal antrostomy, a so-called nasoantral window procedure (Fig. 4.**217**). This was done and still is done in an office set-up by puncturing the nasoantral wall and fracturing part of the inferior concha with a sharp curved hemostat. The opening is then enlarged in all directions with biting forceps. If there is disease within the sinus that appears irreversible, then a Caldwell–Luc operation may be performed. The Caldwell–Luc operation is a radical antrostomy and an external approach to the maxillary sinus. This was done and still is done, but less frequently, for irreversible sinus diseases such as polypoid tissue, cystic disease of the antrum, osteonecrosis, maxillary neoplasms, presence of an oroantral fistula, and complicated fractures of the maxilla.[2] The Caldwell–Luc operation requires a horizontal incision in the gingivobuccal sulcus above the dentition line (canine and second molar). The periosteum is elevated and the inferior orbital nerve is identified and protected; then the anterior wall of the sinus is fenestrated and the cutting is enlarged. Cysts and benign tumor can be removed, avoiding injury to the mucosa. During the procedure, the nasoantral wall in the inferior meatus is broken to create a nasoantral window procedure for drainage. Removal of the entire mucosal lining is rarely necessary; however, if this is done, one can see on postoperative CT scans a contracted maxillary antrum, along with calcification, periosteal thickening, or even ossification within the sinus (Fig. 4.**218**).

Today, the most common surgical approach to inflammatory diseases of sinonasal cavities is via endoscopic procedures.[3] In recent years, otolaryngologists have become interested in the ostiomeatal complex, where the frontal, ethmoidal (anterior), and maxillary sinuses drain. Abnormalities in this area, usually well seen on coronal CT scans, could explain why the patient has sinusitis (Fig. 4.**219**). Surgical treatment would then be aimed at the causative problem rather than at the resultant sinusitis. The surgical changes may be limited just to the ostiomeatal unit and few anterior ethmoid cells or may involve anterior and posterior ethmoidectomy, sphenoidotomy, and sphenoidectomy. At times, postoperative changes may be limited to uncinectomy, maxillary ostioplasty (middle meatal antrostomy),[3] frontal recess surgery, middle turbinectomy, septoplasty (Fig. 4.**220**), and "mini Caldwell Luc" procedure. Functional endoscopic endonasal sinus surgery (FESS) is a delicate operation, and surgical injury to the neighboring structures does occur (Fig. 4.**221**). Important complications include CSF leak (Fig. 4.**216b**); pneumocephalus (Fig. 4.**222**); injury to the brain parenchymal and cerebral arteries; orbital complications such as subperiosteal hematoma; injury to the extraocular muscles, particularly the medial rectus muscle (Fig. 4.**221a**); retrobulbar hematoma; blindness; and injury to the nasolacrimal duct and sac.[4–6] Any surgery on the lateral nasal wall such as endoscopic sinus surgery and rhinoplasty carries a potential risk for the lacrimal duct and sac drainage. The lacrimal drainage system is one of the structures most vulnerable to surgical trauma in the course of FESS.[6]

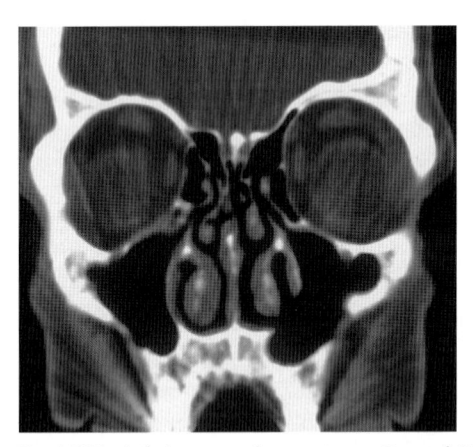

Fig. 4.**217** Inferior meatal antrostomy. Coronal CT scan shows a surgical defect along the inferior aspect of the medial wall of the left maxillary sinus due to an inferior meatal antrostomy procedure.

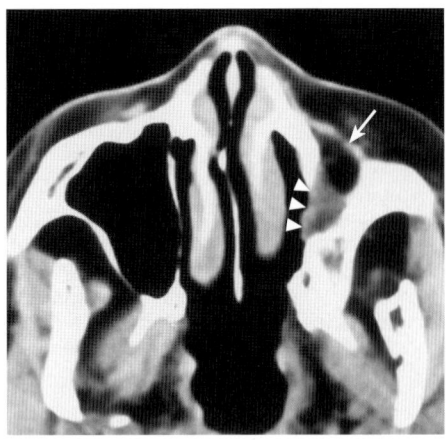

Fig. 4.**218** Caldwell–Luc procedure. Following the procedure, the CT scan shows an anterior surgical defect (arrow) and nasoantral window (arrowheads) of the left maxillary sinus. Note a contracted left maxillary antrum as well as increased reactive sclerosis of the lateral wall of the left maxillary sinus subsequent to surgical procedure.

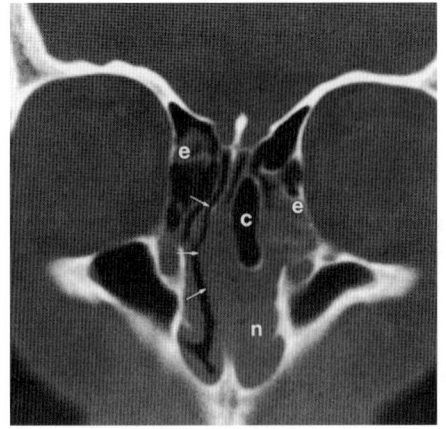

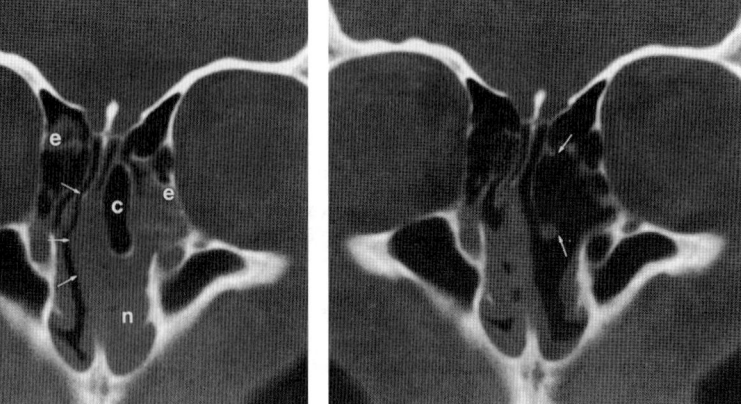

Fig. 4.**219** Chronic sinusitis and postoperative endoscopic sinus surgery.
a Coronal CT scan shows soft-tissue density in the nasal cavity (n), compatible with an inflammatory polyp. Note the anterior ethmoid disease (e), concha bullosa (c), septal deviation (arrows), and marked infundibular disease on the left side.
b The infundibular disease on the left side has been removed. The concha bullosa (arrows) has been opened, and the uncinate process on the left side has been removed.

Sinonasal Pathology   471

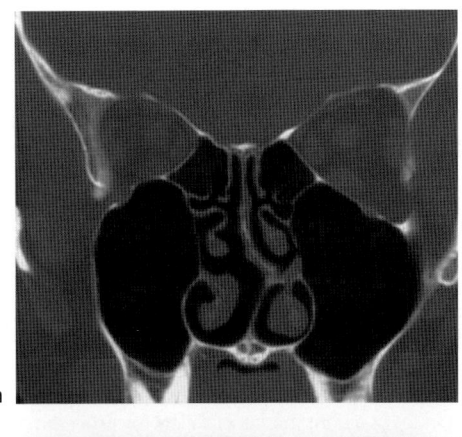

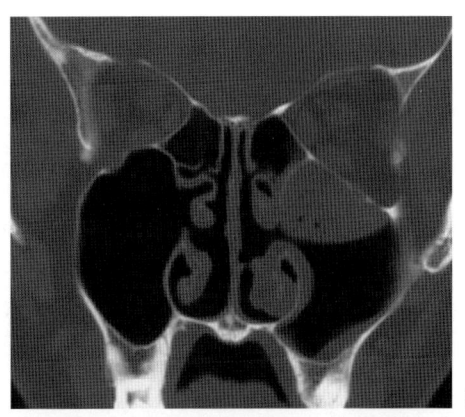

Fig. 4.**220** Status following septoplasty and middle meatal antrostomy. **a** Coronal CT scan shows deviation of the nasal septum to the left. **b** Coronal CT scan shows correction of the nasal septum deviation. **c** Coronal CT scan before surgery shows normal uncinate processes and aerated ethmoid and maxillary sinuses. Note medial position of the left middle turbinate. **d** Coronal CT scan following surgery shows bilateral uncinectomy and middle meatal antrostomy. Note lateralization of the left middle turbinate. Adhesion of the left middle turbinate to the stump of the uncinate process cannot be excluded.

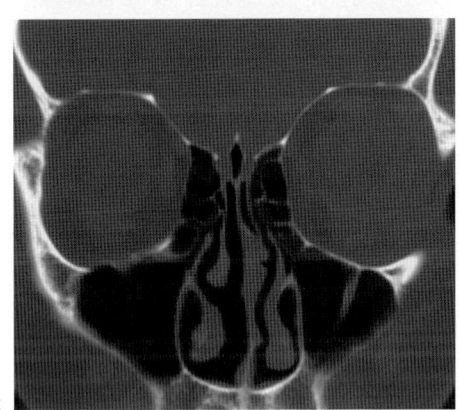

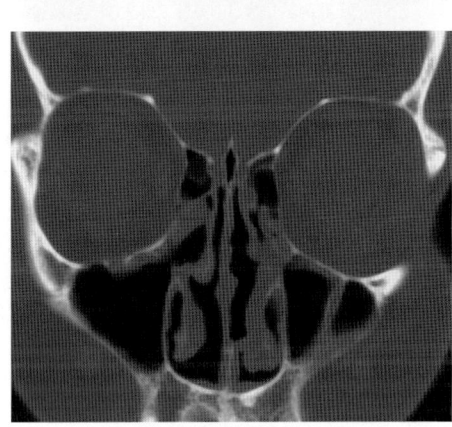

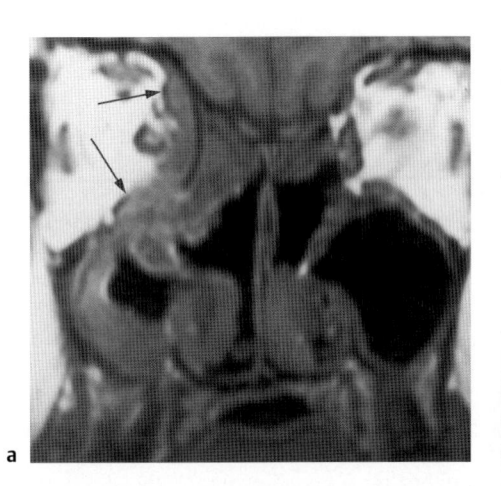

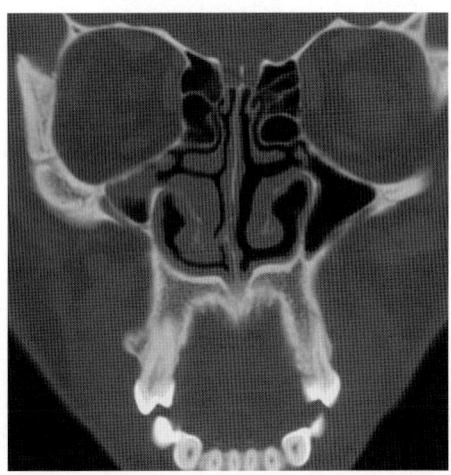

Fig. 4.**221** Complication of endoscopic endonasal surgery. **a** Coronal T1W MR scan shows postoperative changes of bilateral anterior ethmoidectomy. Note subperiosteal hematoma along the medial wall of the right orbit (arrows). **b** Coronal CT scan in another patient shows hypoplastic maxillary sinuses. Note lateral displacement of the right uncinate process. Either hypoplastic maxillary sinus or lateral attachment of the uncinate process increases the chance of intraorbital complication during uncinectomy.

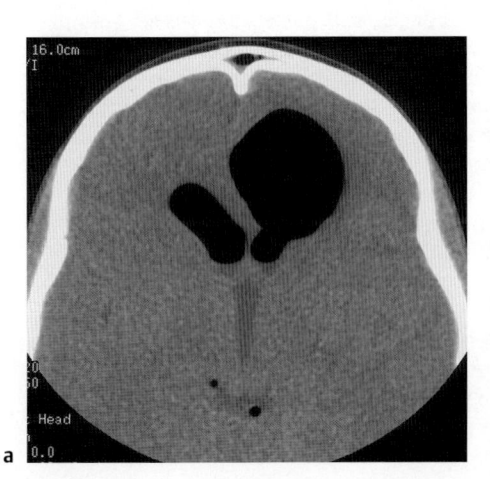

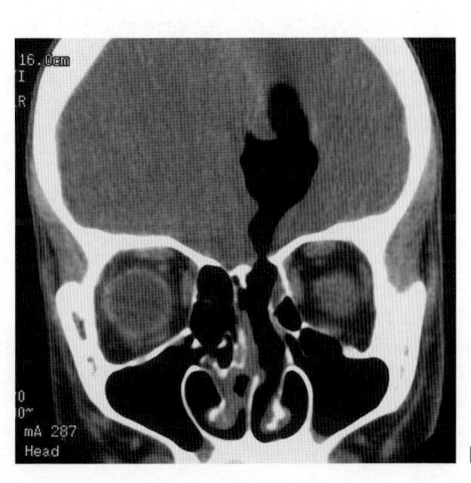

Fig. 4.**222** Pneumocephalus. **a** Axial and **b** coronal CT scans showing frontal pneumocephalus, a complication of endoscopic sinus surgery. Note the postsurgical appearance of left ethmoidectomy.

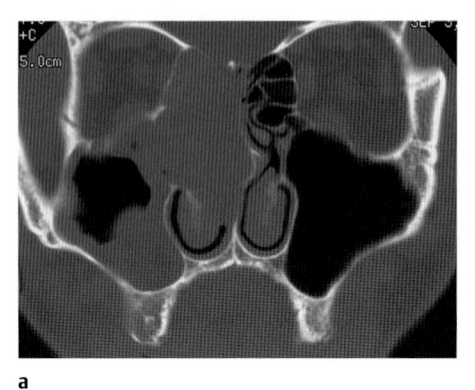

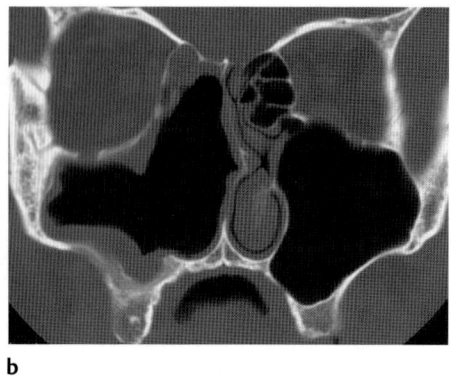

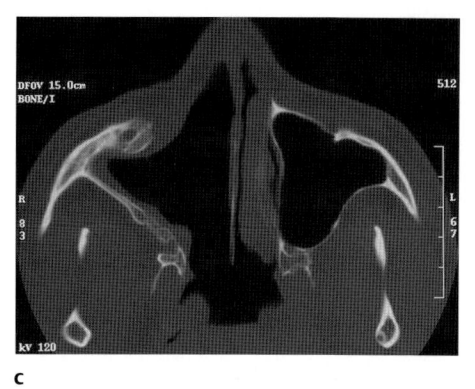

Fig. 4.**223** Status following medial maxillectomy and ethmoidectomy. **a** Coronal CT scan shows a right nasal–ethmoid papillary squamous cell carcinoma. **b** Coronal CT scan shows right ethmoidectomy and medial maxillectomy. **c** Axial CT scan shows changes of a right medial maxilletomy procedure. Note reactive/scar tissue in the surgical bed.

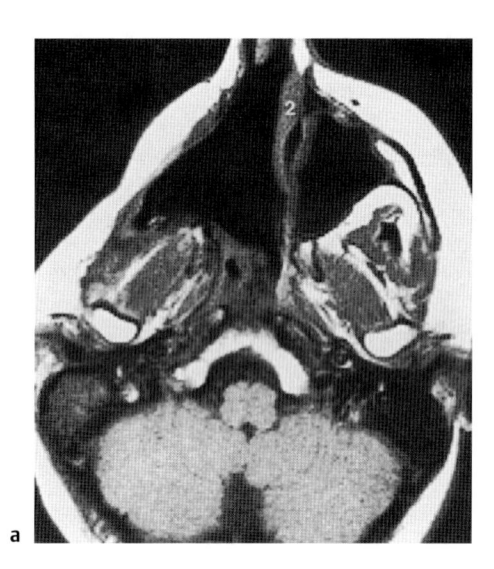

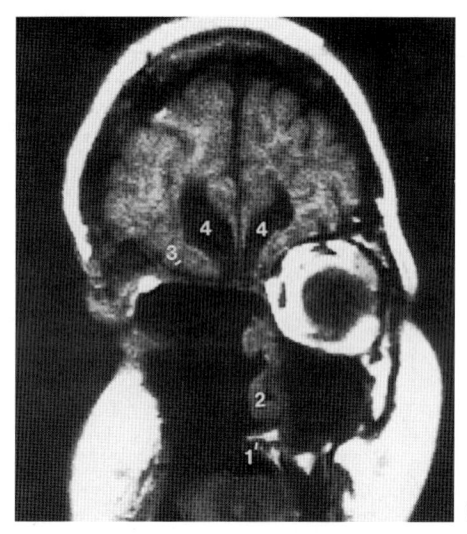

Fig. 4.**224** Total maxillectomy. Status following maxillectomy and resection of the orbit. MRI in the axial (**a**) and coronal (**b**) projections. Absence of the right zygoma, maxilla, nasal cavity, ethmoids, and right side of the hard palate, and absence of the orbit are all indicative of the radical surgery for this patient with osteogenic sarcoma of the maxillary sinus. The remaining left palate (1), the left turbinates (2), and the roof of the right orbit (3) are identifiable landmarks. Postoperative atrophy of the frontal lobe (4) occurred owing to retraction of the brain as part of the combined procedure for evaluating the roof of the ethmoid air cells and cribriform plate. From B.L. Carter, MD, 1988 Thieme.

The Maxillary Sinuses

Radiological changes of the paranasal sinuses are present following most surgical procedures in the area. For instance, a lavage of the maxillary sinus is commonly followed by the presence of an air–fluid level for several days following the procedure. If irrigation and antibiotics fail to clear an infection of the maxillary sinus, a nasal antrostomy or Caldwell–Luc procedure is performed, assuming that a dental consultation has excluded the presence of underlying apical dental disease (Figs. 4.**217**, 4.**218**). A nasal antrostomy (inferior meatal antrostomy) is the creation of an opening under the inferior turbinate to provide better drainage of the maxillary sinus to the nasal cavity (Fig. 4.**217**). If this fails, a Caldwell–Luc procedure is done in order to remove the diseased mucosa (Fig. 4.**218**). Postoperatively, the sinus may have some degree of fibrosis simulating mucosal disease. Rarely, the operated maxillary sinus appears contracted and one can see calcification, marked periosteal thickening, or even ossification within the sinus following the surgery (Fig. 4.**218**). Incomplete removal of the mucosa may result in the development of a secondary mucocele.

There are several surgical options for the treatment of the tumors of the maxillary antrum and nasal cavities. Inferior medial maxillectomy (IMM) is designed for resection of the medial wall of the antrum and the inferior turbinate. This procedure is most often used for the management of an inverted papilloma. It is done through a lateral rhinotomy incision, or through a sublabial approach. The IMM allows adequate exposure for limited tumors while preserving functional tissue and providing a very acceptable cosmetic result.[7] Medial maxillectomy is a procedure used for larger benign or intermediate tumors involving the entire lateral nasal wall but without extension to the orbit, anterior cranial fossa, lateral maxilla, or alveolus.[7] The block removed contains the lateral nasal wall, including all turbinate tissue, and the contents of the ethmoid and maxillary sinuses (Fig. 4.**223**). This is done through an extended lateral rhinotomy incision. Removal of all turbinates results in an abnormal nasal cavity, requiring chronic management of crusting.

Radical maxillectomy or total maxillectomy is the standard operation for advanced carcinoma of the maxilla. This includes removal of the maxilla along with the nasal bone, the ethmoid sinus, and, in some instances, the pterygoid plates.[7] This procedure may or may not be done with orbital exenteration (Fig. 4.**224**). Radical maxillectomy is done for the treatment of malignant tumors confined to the maxilla and those with extension to the facial soft tissue, palate, or anterior orbit but without invasion of the ethmoidal roof, posterior orbit, or pterygoid region.[7] When these areas are involved, one must decide whether to undertake craniofacial resection or use a regimen that relies on chemotherapy and radiation therapy.

The Ethmoid Sinus

Ethmoidectomy is performed for recurrent nasal obstructive polyposis, for chronic ethmoiditis, and for tumors of the ethmoid sinuses. The walls of the ethmoid air cells are removed, leaving the cribriform plate and roof of the ethmoid air cells intact. A portion of the lamina papyracea is occasionally removed with

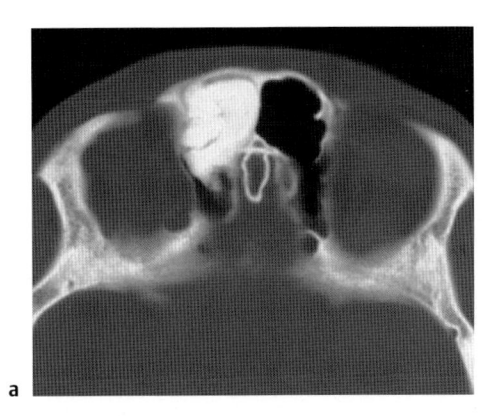

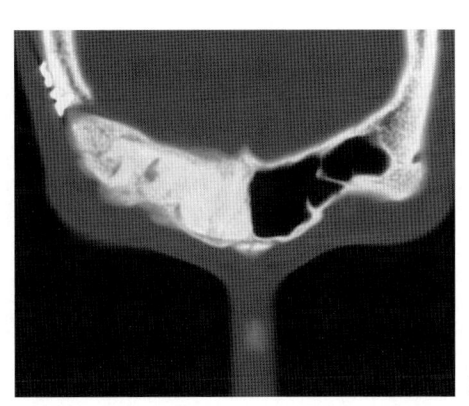

Fig. 4.**225** Frontal sinus obliteration. **a** Axial and **b** coronal CT scans showing complete obliteration of the right frontal sinus with hydroxyapatite.

the ethmoidectomy. There are three basic approaches to the ethmoid sinuses: intranasal, transantral, and external approaches. The intranasal approach may be done using various aids: an endoscope, a microscope, or a head light. The ethmoid sinus can be approached via the maxillary sinus, as can sphenoid sinuses (extended Caldwell–Luc operation) (Fig. 4.**223**). The ethmoid sinus can also be approached externally. An incision is made approximately midway between the medial canthus and the nasal dorsum down to the periosteum. The periosteum is then elevated off the nasal bone and the lamina papyracea and the ethmoid sinus is entered directly just behind the posterior lacrimal crest. The advantage of this external approach is its excellent visualization of the field. Its disadvantage is the removal of the lamina papyracea.[7]

The Frontal Sinuses

A simple drainage procedure through a trephine made in the superior medial margin of the orbit, used for drainage of the frontal sinus, has very little radiographic abnormality (see Fig. 4.**69 c**). In the case of chronic frontal sinusitis, there are two basic approaches: (1) mucosa-preserving techniques and (2) mucosa-eliminating techniques. Mucosa-preserving techniques may be performed either intranasally or externally. The intranasal approach is typically done with endoscopes and involves anterior ethmoidectomy followed by careful exenteration of the frontal recess air cells to expose the nasofrontal duct and frontal sinus ostium. Generally in this setting the frontal sinus ostium is of adequate size and nothing further needs to be done.[7] This approach may also be used for medially located frontal mucoceles. There are two types of external mucosa-preserving techniques. Both involve an approach beginning with external ethmoidectomy. This is followed either by removing a large part of the medial floor of the frontal sinus, the so-called Lynch procedure, or by enlarging the nasofrontal duct and attempting to reconstruct it with a mucosal flap, the so-called Boyden procedure.[7] A polyethylene tube (stent) is often used to hold the drainage pathway between the frontal sinus and the middle meatus. One of the disadvantages of these approaches is the fact that the soft tissues of the orbital wall tend to collapse medially in the postoperative period, obstructing the nasofrontal duct once the stent is removed.[7]

The mucosa-eliminating procedures are of three basic types. The first is the osteoplastic flap coupled with obliteration of the frontal sinus. This involves creating an anterior bone flap. Frontal sinus obliteration began in the early 1900s and although excellent results have been achieved with autogenous fat, muscle, and bone, the search for the ideal material for frontal sinus obliteration continues. The osteoplastic flap procedure has become the operation of choice since it obliterates the sinus cavity with very minimal cosmetic deformity. The osteoplastic flap is patterned from a template of the frontal sinus traced from a Caldwell projection. The anterior sinus wall margin is traced out with a saw, and the anterior wall is bent downward to expose the entire sinus cavity. The mucosa of the entire sinus is then removed first. Following this, the nasofrontal ducts are plugged and then covered with fascia and the frontal sinuses are obliterated with fat, usually from either the abdomen or the thigh. The anterior bony flap is then repositioned into its original place (Fig. 4.**225**). Another approach is the frontal sinus anterior ablation, the so-called Reidel procedure. This is rarely done today, but may be indicated for severe frontal sinusitis with osteomyelitis of the anterior table. In this technique, the anterior table is removed, then the mucosa is removed, including the mucosa of the frontonasal ducts, and the forehead skin is allowed to collapse back against the posterior table. Following six to twelve months, the anterior table may be reconstructed.[7] A third approach is the so-called cranialization procedure. This is performed in conjunction with a neurosurgical team. The procedure is done when there is infection involving the posterior table of the frontal sinus or when a severe fracture causes communication of the posterior table with the cranial space. In this case, the posterior table is removed, the mucosa is removed, the frontonasal ducts are plugged, and the brain is allowed to prolapse forward against the posterior part of the anterior table of the frontal sinus.

Techniques for frontal sinus obliteration have undergone significant evolution. Reidel, Killian, and Kichnt accomplished frontal sinus obliteration by performing variations of removal of the anterior frontal sinus wall and collapsing the overlying skin into the defect with a high rate of disease recurrence as well as significant cosmetic deformity.[8] Goodale and Montgomery[9] popularized frontal sinus obliteration with autologous fat using an anterior wall osteoplastic flap. Although frontal sinus obliteration by autologous fat continues to be the most commonly used method, a variety of other autograft materials such as autologous cancellous bone or lyophilized cartilage have been used successfully. Fat, bone, and muscle autologous grafts may have donor site morbidity and, in addition, because they are avascular grafts, they increase the risk of local infection.[7,8,9] Some authors prefer the use of pericranial flap as an effective alternative to other methods of frontal sinus obliteration.[8] The pericranial flap consists of the periosteum of the skull with its overlying loose connective tissue and the subgaleal fascia. The pericranial flap avoids donor site morbidity associated with free fat or cancellous bone grafts.[8]

Hydroxyapatite cement has recently become more popular for sinus obliteration.[10,11,12] Hydroxyapatite cement on CT scans appears as a hyperdense area, similar to the density of the cortical bone (Fig. 4.**225**). Hydroxyapatite offers the advantages of no donor site morbidity and the potential for complete osseointegration.[12]

The Sphenoid Sinus

The sphenoid sinus is generally approached through an external ethmoidectomy or through the nasal passage or the ethmoid labyrinth, or via transseptal route, opening the anterior wall of the sphenoid sinus. If transnasal and transseptal routes are not feasible, an external ethmoidectomy will allow direct access to the sphenoid. Postoperative changes are often evident in the sphenoid sinus following transphenoidal hypophysectomy. In this operation the sphenoid sinus is often packed with fat or muscle tissues. On MRI there will be evidence for fat and old blood and blood by-products.

■ References

1. Alvi A, Doherty T, Lewen G. Facial fractures and concomitant injuries in trauma patients. Laryngoscope 2003; 113: 102–106.
2. Weymuller EA, Rice DH. Surgical management of infectious and inflammatory disease: Paranasal sinuses. In: Cummings CW, Fredrickson JM, Harker LE, Krause CJ, Schuller DE, eds. Otolaryngology Head and Neck Surgery. 2nd ed. Vol. I. St. Louis: Mosby-Year Book; 1993; 955–964.
2a. Carter BL. Paranasal sinuses, nasal cavity, pterygoid fossa, nasopharynx, and infratemporal fossa. In: Valvassori GE, Buckingham RA, Carter BL, Hanafee WN, Mafee MF, eds. Head and Neck Imaging. Stuttgart: Georg Thieme Verlag; 1988: 173–250.
3. Kennedy DW, Zinreich SJ, Sharalan H, Kuhn F, et al. Endoscopic middle meatal antrostomy: theory, technique and patency. Laryngoscope 1987; 97(8 Pt 3 Suppl. 43): 1–9.
4. Silva AB, Stankiewiez JA. Perioperative and postoperative management of orbital complications in functional endoscopic sinus surgery. Oper Tech Otolaryngol Head Neck Surg 1995; 6: 231–236.
5. Unlü HH, Caylan R, Kuttu N, et al. Active transport dacryocystography in evaluating lacrimal drainage system after rhinoplasty. Am J Rhinol 1996; 10: 87–91.
6. Halis U, Goktan C, Aslan A, Tarhan S. Injury to the lacrimal apparatus after endoscopic sinus surgery: surgical implications from active transport dacryocystography. Otolaryngol Head Neck Surg 2001; 124: 308–312.
7. Weymuller EA. Paranasal sinuses neoplasms. In: Cummings CW, Fredrickson JM, Harker LA, Krause CJ, Schuller DE, eds. Otolaryngology Head and Neck Surgery. Vol. I. St. Louis: Mosby-Year Book; 1993; 941–953.
8. Parhiscar A, Har-El G. Frontal sinus obliteration with the pericranial flap. Otolaryngol Head Neck Surg 2001; 24: 304–307.
9. Goodale RL, Montgomery WW. Anterior osteoplastic frontal sinus obliterations: five years experience. Ann Otol 1961; 70: 860–863.
10. Ducic Y, Stone TL. Frontal sinus obliteration using a laterally based pedicled pericranial flap. Laryngoscope 1999; 109: 541–545.
11. Lykins CL, Friedman CD, Constantino PD, et al. Hydroxyapatite cement in craniofacial skeletal reconstruction and its effects. Arch Otolaryngol Head Neck Surg 1998; 124: 153–159.
12. Petruzzelli GJ, Stankiewicz JA. Frontal sinus obliteration with hydroxyapatite cement. Laryngoscope 2002; 112: 32–26.

Section IV Masticatory System

Chapter 5 Temporomandibular Joint

Embryology 477

Anatomy 477

Diagnostic Imaging Techniques 481

Normal Imaging Anatomy of TMJ 482

Anatomical Variations and Developmental Anomaly 484

Inflammation 486

Internal Derangements 487

Osteochondritis Dissecans 493

Arthritic Conditions 493

Chapter 6 Mandible and Maxilla

Embryology 508

Anatomy 509

Dental Anatomy 510

Imaging Techniques 511

Pathology 513

5 Temporomandibular Joint

Mahmood F. Mafee

Embryology

The temporomandibular joint (TMJ) is composed of the mandibular condyle, the glenoid fossa, and the articular eminence with the interposed disk. The glenoid fossa and articular eminence are part of the squamous portion of the temporal bone. The squamous part (squama) of the temporal bone is ossified in membranous condensed mesenchyme from a single center that appears in the region of the roots of its zygomatic process about the seventh or eighth week of intrauterine life.[1] The branchial apparatus plays an important role in the formation of the mandible, the ear, the face, and neck. The cartilage skeleton of the first pair of branchial arches, the Meckel's cartilage, which can be identified around 41 days of gestation, extends from the developing otic capsule into the first visceral (branchial) or mandibular arch, meeting its fellow at its ventral end (Fig. 5.1).[1] The dorsal end of the Meckel's cartilage becomes separated, forms the rudiments of the malleus and the incus and later on becomes ossified to form the malleus head and neck and incus body and its short process.[1] The ventral part of this cartilage is enveloped by the developing mesenchymatous mandible. The mandible eventually is formed by secondary intramembranous ossification. The intermediate part of the Meckel's cartilage disappears, but its sheath persists as the anterior ligament of the malleus and sphenomandibular ligament.[1] The mesodermal element of the mandibular arch forms the masticatory muscles (lateral and medial pterygoid muscles, masseter and temporalis muscles), tensor tympani, tensor veli palatini, mylohyoid, and anterior belly of digastric; all are supplied by the mandibular nerve, the nerve of the first arch.[1] Ossification of the mandible appears near the mental foramen about the sixth week of fetal life. A cone-shaped mass of cartilage, the condylar cartilage, appears from the head of the mandible. This contributes to the growth in height of the ramus. The articular disk embryologically originates from the same mesenchymatous component of the first branchial arch, which will also give rise to the formation of the lateral pterygoid muscle.

Anatomy

The temporomandibular joint is a diarthrodial synovial joint capable of both translation and rotation.[1–3] It is condylar in type and involves the articular eminence and the anterior portion of the mandibular fossa (glenoid fossa) of the temporal bone above and the mandibular condyle below (Fig. 5.2). The articular tubercle represents the bony protuberance on the lateral portion of the anterior eminence (Fig. 5.2). It is typically more prominent than the eminence proper.[2] The articular surfaces are covered with fibrocartilage in which collagen fibers predominate and cartilage cells are few.[1] An articular disk, composed of fibrous tissue, divides the joint into upper and lower parts (Fig. 5.3).[1–3] Cartilage is rarely a component of the disk. Chondrocytes are usually seen in pathological conditions, in which case the cartilage is metaplastic.[2] The anterior surface of the tympanic bone of the temporal bone is referred to as the *tympanic plate* (Figs. 5.2a, b). In this text, we refer to the tympanic ring as the semicircular portion of the tympanic bone that forms most of the external auditory canal. Otologists refer to the medial end of the tympanic bone as the *tympanic ring* (sulcus), where the tympanic membrane is located. The squamous portion of the temporal bone directly anterior to the tympanic plate forms the superior aspect of the TMJ. The glenoid fossa is a concave structure, and the articular eminence is a convex structure (Figs. 5.2a, b, 5.3). The glenoid fossa can also be described as being bounded by the anterior and posterior roots of the zygomatic process of the temporal bone. It is concave in both anteroposterior and mediolateral directions. The glenoid fossa blends anteriorly with the eminence (Figs. 5.2, 5.3), but it is often described anatomically as being separate.[1]

The mandibular condyle is the inferior portion of the joint. The lateral pole of the condyle is prominent and, in many cases, extends beyond the glenoid fossa. Thus, posteriorly, the condyle is often supported by cartilage and bone of the external auditory canal. Anterior and inferior to the articulating surface of the condyle is a triangular depression, the condylar fovea. This depression serves as the region of insertion for the lateral pterygoid muscle tendon. The condyle, glenoid fossa, and eminence are lined with fibrous connective tissue.[1–3] Beneath this layer of fibrous connective tissue lies hyaline cartilage.[3] Fibrocartilage has a dense layer of fibrous connective tissue on its articulating surface. The fibrocartilage surfaces are partially lined by synovium.[2] Microscopically, several tissue layers may be identified lining the condyle and temporal bone. Moving from within the joint cavity toward the bone, these layers are (1) dense fibrous connective tissue; (2) undifferentiated fibroblast (proliferative layer); (3) intermediate layer (fibroblast–chondroblast); (4) cartilage; (5) compact bone; and (6) spongy bone. Between the condyle and glenoid fossa and the eminence is the articular disk or

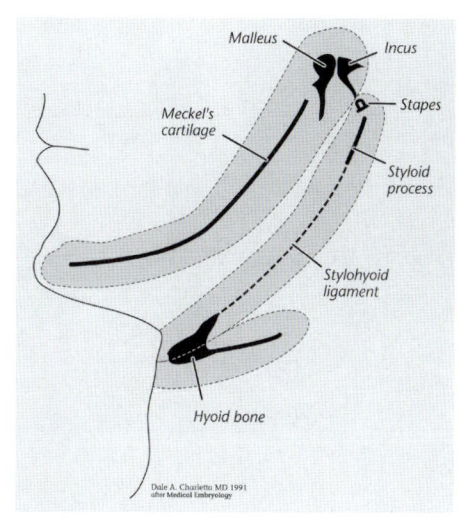

Fig. 5.1 Diagrammatic sagittal section through the regions of the face and neck, demonstrating the mandibular Meckel's cartilage and the hyoid bone.

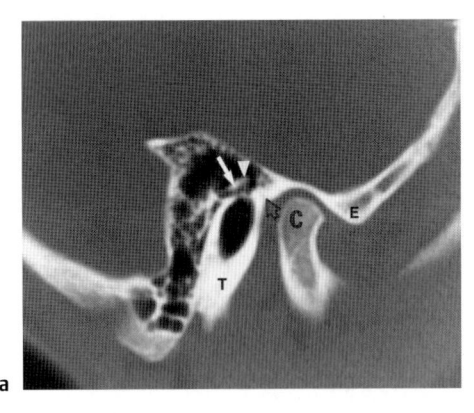

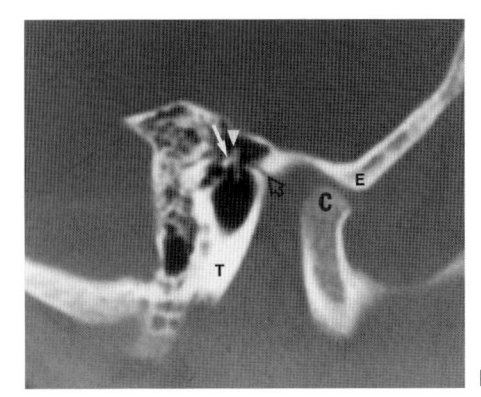

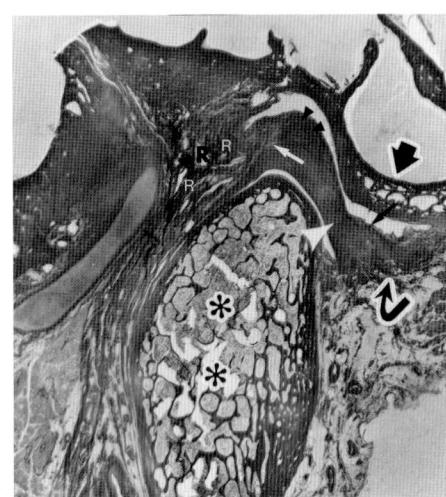

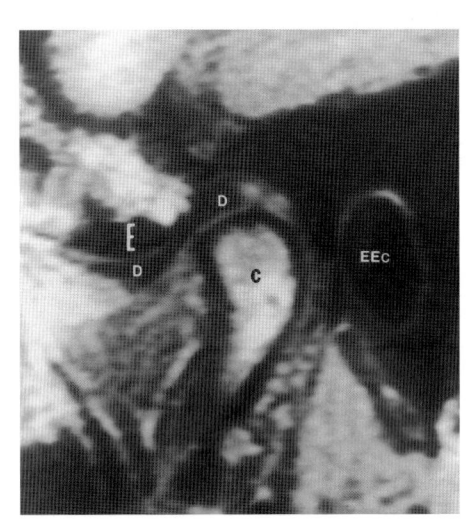

Fig. 5.2 Normal TMJ anatomy. **a, b** Sagittal CT scans show a central section of the TMJ, in the closed-mouth (**a**) and open-mouth (**b**) positions. The relationship between the normal condyle (C), glenoid fossa, and anterior articular eminence (E) is clearly seen. Note the tympanic bone (T), incus (long arrow), malleus (arrowhead), and squamotympanic fissure (open arrow). Figs **a** and **b** reproduced from Reference 4 with permission.

c Sagittal microscopic section of the right TMJ, demonstrating the posterior band (black arrowheads), intermediate zone (arrowhead), anterior band (small black arrow), anterior eminence (large black arrow), and condyle (stars). Note the anterior attachment (curved arrow), which blends with the anterior joint capsule and is composed of a looser fibrous connective tissue than the anterior band (small black arrow). The posterior attachment (white solid arrow) blends with the posterior band (black arrowheads). The disk can clearly be demarcated from the retrodiskal tissue (R). Fig. **c** courtesy of Leslie Heffez, DMD, University of Illinois at Chicago.

d Sagittal T1W MR scan demonstrating the condyle (C), disk (D), articular eminence (E), and external ear canal (EEC).

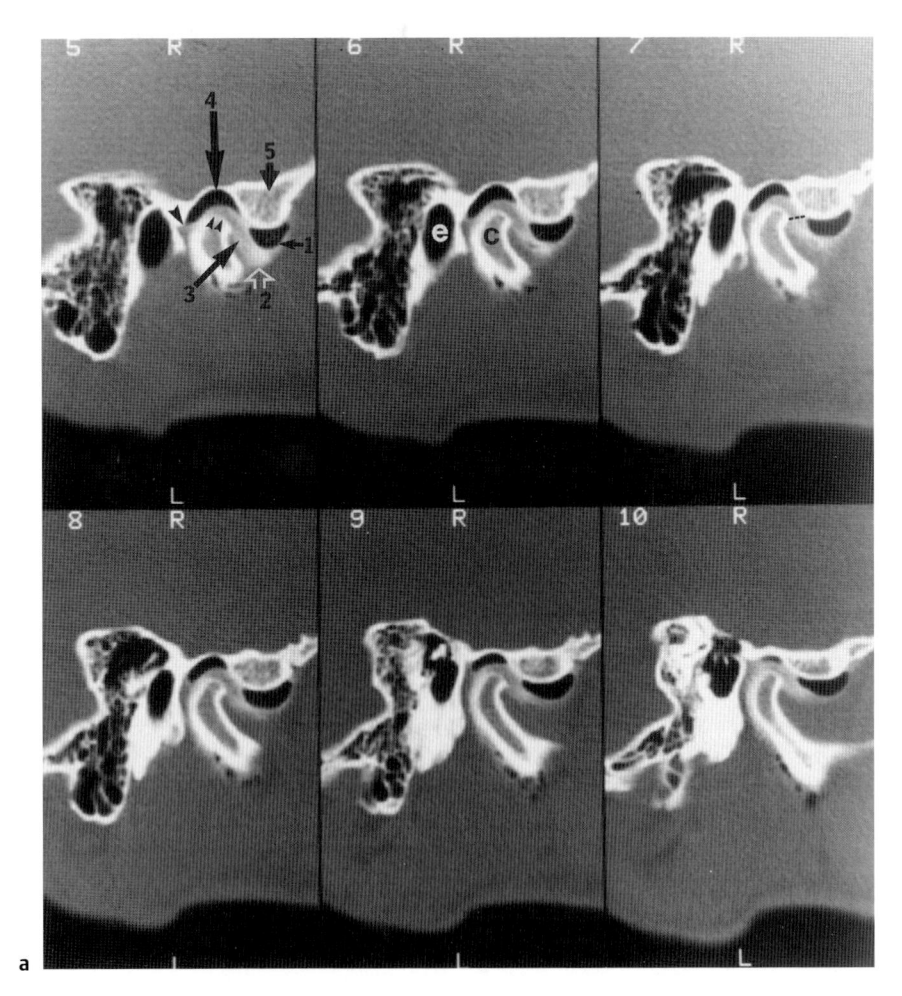

Fig. 5.3 Normal TMJ anatomy. **a** Consecutive series of double-contrast (air and iodinated contrast agent) direct sagittal images (extending medially from the section labeled 5 to that labeled 10) of a normal side TMJ, in the closed-mouth position. The images demonstrate the external auditory canal (e), retrodiskal (bilaminar) zone (single arrowhead), mandibular condyle (C), air in the anterior and posterior recesses (arrows 1 and 4) of the superior joint space, the articular eminence (arrow 5), and iodinated contrast material in the anterior recess of the inferior joint space (arrow 2). Note the anterior band (arrow 3) and posterior band (double arrowheads) of the meniscus, outlined by air and iodinated contrast in the superior and inferior joint spaces, respectively. The posterior band of the meniscus (disk) is at the top of the condyle. The intermediate zone of the disk is located between the anterior and posterior bands. A disk is said to be in the normal position when the posterior band is at the anterior portion of the superior surface of the condyle, the so-called 11- to 12-o'clock or 12- to 1-o'clock position of the condyle, depending, upon the orientation of the condyle. Alternatively, a line can be drawn from a point at the junction between the anterior and superior surfaces of the condyle to a point along the most inferior margin of the posterior slope of the articular eminence (dashed line in image 7). A disk is considered normal when this line passes through the intermediate zone of the meniscus.

Fig. 5.3 b and c ▷

meniscus (Figs. 5.**2c**, **d**, 5.**3a**), composed of fibrous connective tissue, attaching anteriorly and posteriorly in a vascular plexus.[3]

The joint cavity is supported circumferentially by a capsule. The capsule is inserted in the perimeter of the glenoid fossa (Fig. 5.**3**), inferiorly on the mandibular condyle as well as to the medial and lateral margins of the disk.[1–3] The joint cavity is completely separated by the disk into two noncommunicating compartments or spaces termed *superior* (temporodisk) and *inferior* (condylodisk) joint spaces (Fig. 5.**3**). The joint capsule has two components: an outer fibrous capsule, the stratum fibrosum, and an inner synovial layer, the stratum synovium. The articular disk, which embryologically originates from the lateral pterygoid muscle mesenchyme, has a few connections to this muscle anteromedially. These fibers, however, are not significant and do not pull the disk anteriorly.[2,4] The anterior and posterior extents of the joint spaces are termed *recesses*: (1) the anterior recess of the inferior joint space; (2) the anterior recess of the superior joint space; (3) the posterior recess of the inferior joint space; and (4) the posterior recess of the superior joint space (Fig. 5.**3**).[2–4] The synovium typically lines the posterior and anterior recesses and is located only on the very peripheral extent of the disk.[2] The synovial fluid consists of hyaluronic acid–protein complex with very few glycosaminoglycans (GAGs). Lever and Ford[5] described synovial fluid as a blood plasma dialysate.

The ligaments of the joints are essentially condensations of the fibrous connective tissue lining of the capsule.[2] The ligaments provide stability, especially in the lateral direction. The lateral temporomandibular ligament, also known as the *lateral ligament*, or temporomandibular ligament, is the principal ligament of the TMJ. The medial capsule ligament is absent in the anterior one-half to two-thirds of the joint. The medial capsule is not as strong as the lateral ligament and is oriented obliquely in an anteroposterior to posteroinferior direction.[2] The sphenomandibular and stylomandibular ligaments serve only as accessory ligaments in protecting the joint in wide excursions. The sphenomandibular ligament originates from the angular spine of the sphenoid bone and inserts on the lingula of the mandibular ramus. The stylomandibular ligament originates from the tip of the styloid process and inserts at the angle and posterior border of the mandible.

The articular disk or meniscus, composed of fibrous connective tissue, attaches anteriorly and posteriorly in a vascular plexus (Fig. 5.**3**).[2] These attachments are termed the anterior attachment and retrodiskal tissue.[2–4] Anteriorly, the disk is attached to the capsule via the anterior attachment (Fig. 5.**4**); anteromedially, the tendon of the superior head of the lateral pterygoid muscle inserts into the disk, while the inferior head of the lateral pterygoid muscle inserts into the mandibular condyle.[3] The retrodiskal tissue attaches to the posterior aspect of the disk and completes the separation of the joint cavity into two separate synovial compartments, known as superior and inferior joint spaces (Fig. 5.**5**).[3] The retrodiskal tissue is composed of fibrovascular connective tissue that appears to condense anteriorly into the disk proper. There is a general progression of vascular to less vascular to fibrous connective tissue posteroanteriorly, so that there is no clear delineation between retrodiskal tissue and the disk.[2,3] Many authors describe a posterior attachment, which refers to that portion of the retrodiskal tissue that inserts directly on the disk.[2,3] Within the retrodiskal tissue (bilaminar zone) are a dense band of fibrous connective tissue forming its most inferior portion (inferior lamina) and looser elastic tissue in the superior region (superior lamina). This arrangement is believed to facilitate the movement of the disk with the condyle and, perhaps, aid in recoil of the disk on closing to maintain a normal condyle–disk relationship. The bilaminar zone has a highly vascular component containing the branches of the

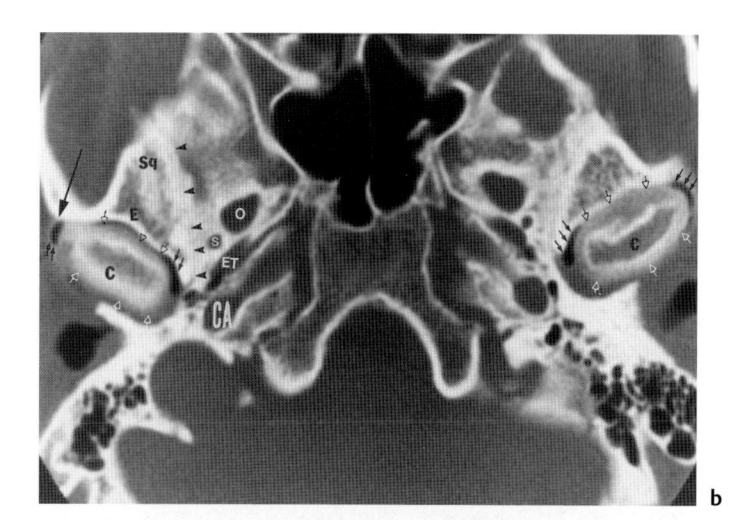

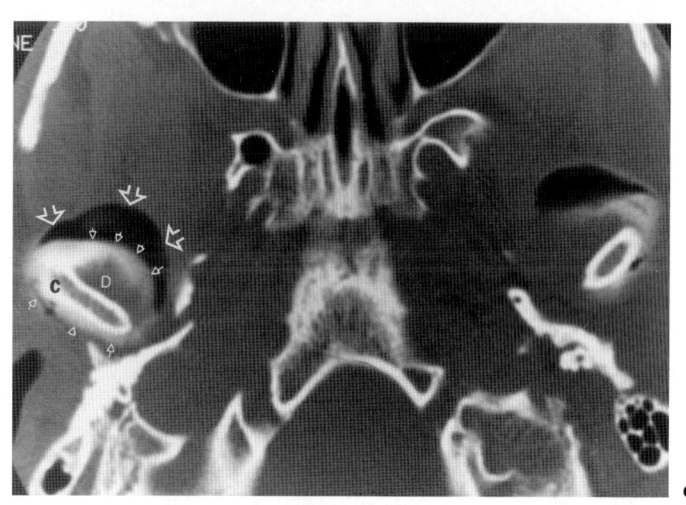

Fig. 5.**3** Normal TMJ anatomy.
b Axial section, taken at the top of the condyle, same patient as in **a**, in the closed-mouth position, demonstrating the condyle (C) and partially volumed disk, iodinated contrast material in the anterior and posterior joint spaces (white and black hollow arrows), and air in the anterior joint space (solid black short arrows). Note the articular eminence (E), articular tubercle (long arrow) and the remainder of the squamous temporal bone (Sq). The articular tubercle represents the bony protuberance on the lateral portion of the articular eminence. It is typically more prominent than the eminence proper. Oral and maxillofacial surgeons perform arthroscopy of the articular eminence and tubercle in the treatment of chronic, persistent condylar dislocation. Arrowheads = sphenosquamous suture; CA = canal for internal carotid artery; ET = eustachian tube; O = foramen ovale; S = foramen spinosum.
c Axial section, taken inferior to **b**, demonstrating condyle (C), disk (D), and air (large hollow arrows) and iodinated contrast (small arrows) within the joint spaces.
Fig. **a** reproduced from Reference 4 with permission.

auriculotemporal, masseteric, and posterior deep temporal nerves.[3] The normal disk is described as having a posterior band, intermediate zone (thin zone), and anterior band. The posterior band is more significant in size than the anterior band in the central aspect of the joint (Figs. 5.**6**, 5.**7**).

The joint spaces (compartments) only rarely communicate with each other naturally, except when a perforation of the disk occurs.[2] Typically, the perforation occurs in the remodeled retrodiskal tissue when the disk is displaced. In the normal joint, the superior joint space can accommodate a mean volume of 1.2 ml, and the inferior joint space 0.9 ml. This information, however, was derived from cadaveric studies. In clinical practice, the

480 5 Temporomandibular Joint

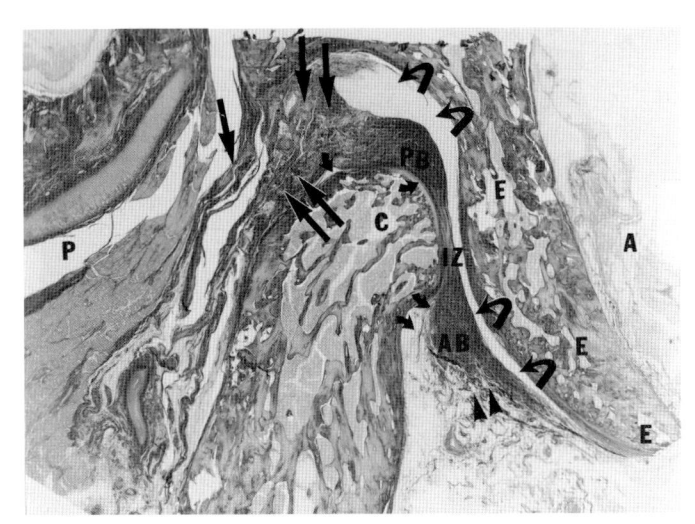

Fig. 5.**4** Normal TMJ anatomy. Sagittal microscopic section through the TMJ. The fibrous disk separates the joint into two separate compartments, the superior (long curved arrows) and inferior (short curved arrows) joint spaces. The surfaces of the glenoid fossa, articular eminence (E), and condyle (C) are lined with fibrous connective tissue; beneath lies hyaline cartilage. A vascular plexus is found posterior (straight arrows) and anterior (arrowheads) to the disk. The anterior vascular plexus is called the anterior attachment (arrowheads). The portion of retrodiskal tissue that inserts into the posterior edge of the disk is called the posterior attachment. Note the posterior band (PB), intermediate zone (IZ), and anterior band (AB) of the disk. A = anterior; P = posterior. Figure courtesy of Leslie Heffez, DMD, University of Illinois, Chicago. Reproduced from Reference 4 with permission.

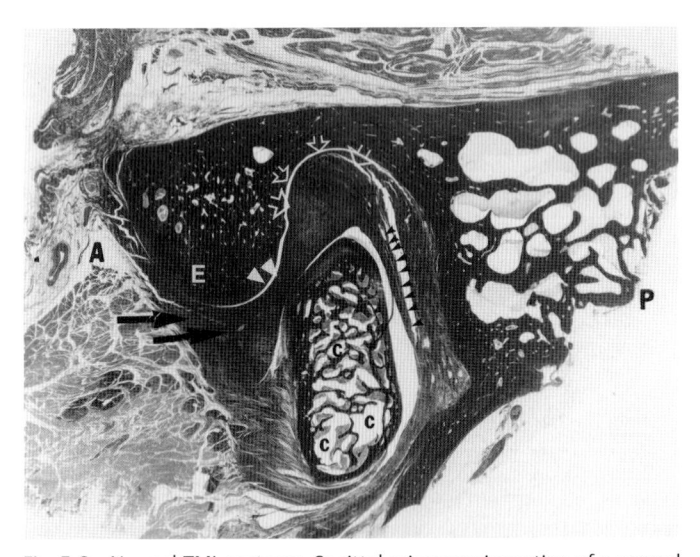

Fig. 5.**6** Normal TMJ anatomy. Sagittal microscopic section of a normal TMJ, demonstrating the posterior band (open arrows), intermediate zone (white arrowheads), anterior band (black arrows), retrodiskal tissue (black arrowheads), condyle (C), and articular eminence (E). A = anterior; P = posterior. Figure courtesy of Leslie Heffez, DMD, University of Illinois, Chicago). Reproduced from Reference 4 with permission.

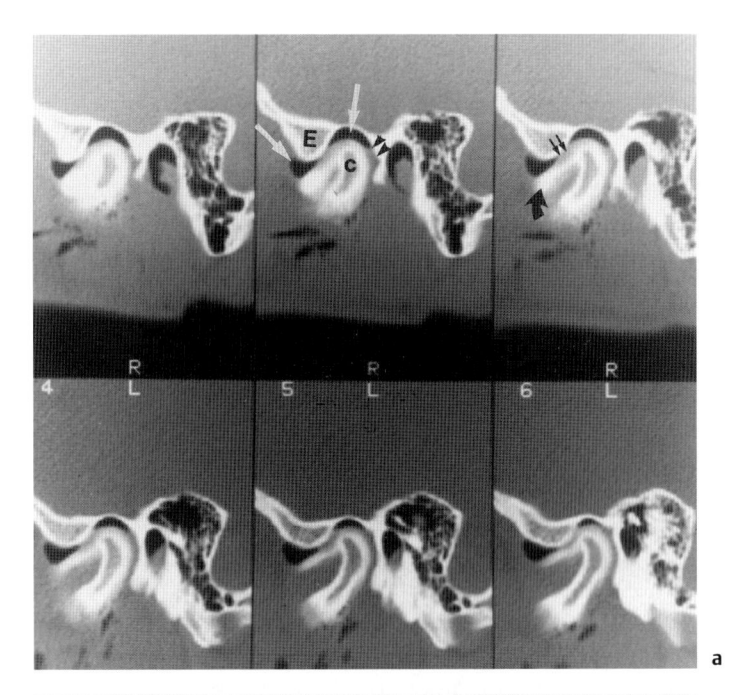

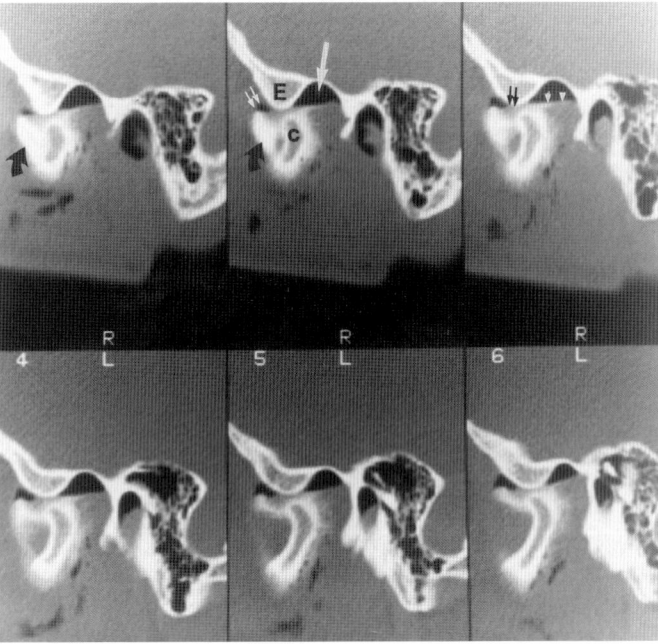

Fig. 5.**5** Normal TMJ anatomy. **a** Series of sagittal double-contrast CT images (extending from lateral to medial) of a normal right TMJ in the closed-mouth position, demonstrating the normal condyle (C), disk (black arrows), and articular eminence (E). Note the air (white arrows) in the superior joint space, iodinated contrast material (curved arrow) in the inferior joint space and retrodiskal (bilaminar) zone (double arrowheads). **b** Series of sagittal double-contrast CT images (extending from lateral to medial) of a right TMJ in the open-mouth position. The relationship between the normal condyle (C), disk (straight black arrows), and articular eminence (E) is seen. There is stretching of the retrodiskal tissue (arrowheads). There is air (white arrows) in the superior and iodinated contrast material (curved arrows) in the inferior joint spaces. Note the altered shape of the disk from the closed-mouth (**a**) to the open-mouth (**b**) position. Reproduced from Reference 4 with permission.

volumes of the joint spaces are much smaller when arthrography is performed: 0.4–0.5 ml and 0.2–0.3 ml for superior and inferior joint spaces, respectively.[2–4]

The retrodiskal tissue contains multiple endothelium-lined spaces (sinuses), which remain collapsed in the closed mouth position. When the condyle translates, the retrodiskal tissue (Fig. 5.**5a**) is expanded because of traction by the condyle on the inferior aspect of the retrodiskal tissue. This causes blood to flow within the retrodiskal tissue.[4]

The relationship of the disk to the condyle and eminence is the basis for describing disk displacement. In the normal joint the disk is located with its posterior band superior to the condyle and, on opening, the condyle rotates under the disk at the same time that the disk–condyle complex translates anteriorly and inferiorly under the articular eminence (Figs. 5.**5**, 5.**6**, 5.**7**).[2,6]

The mandibular condyle does not merely rotate in the glenoid fossa; it moves forward into and under the articular eminence of the temporal bone, taking the articular disk with it.[2,3] Closed-mouth articulation occurs between the condyle and both the posterior articular eminence and glenoid fossa (Figs. 5.**3a**, 5.**5a**). Open-mouth articulation occurs along the inferior and posterior aspect of the articular eminence (Fig. 5.**5b**).[3] The normal relationship of the disk and condyle is nearly the same at rest and during opening.[3] The retrodiskal fibroelastic and areolar tissues expand and contract in the opening and resting positions.[3] On opening, there will be some change in the shape of the disk as compared with that at rest (Fig. 5.**5**).[3] On mandibular opening, the retrodiskal vascular zone engorges with blood, partially filling the space vacated by the mandibular condyle.[3]

In the normal relationship, the intermediate (central) zone or thin zone of the disk lies between the anterior prominence of the condyle and the articular eminence, along the posterior slope of the articular eminence (Figs. 5.**6**, 5.**7**). The anterior band is located under the articular eminence and the posterior band is located at the 12-o'clock or 11-o'clock position in relation to the condylar head (Fig. 5.**7**). This definition is rather subjective and therefore does not allow for complete discrimination between a normal disk and a slightly subluxed disk. In equivocal cases, one should rely on the position of the meniscus on both the closed-mouth and open-mouth views.[2,3] This allows better evaluation of the position of the meniscus. The distribution of GAGs is primarily in the inferior aspect of the posterior band and posterior aspect of the intermediate zone. The GAGs help to resist the compressive forces by absorption and retention of water by osmosis. The GAGs determine water distribution and, thus, influence the MR characteristics of the disk. The displaced disk is often noted to be folded onto itself. In addition, the disk appears to be partly resorbed and partly condensed into the anterior capsule. As the disk is displaced, the retrodiskal tissue becomes prolonged.

Diagnostic Imaging Techniques

Progress in the management of diseases of the TMJ has been tied closely to better etiological understanding of the various conditions affecting this region as well as to improved diagnostic methods.[6,7] Several imaging techniques exist for evaluating the TMJ. Plain film and panoramic imaging can be used for initial screening for osseous abnormalities and to rule out gross pathology such as fractures and advanced degenerative joint disease.[2,6,7] Panoramic, lateral oblique, and transcranial radiographs are typically obtained. Plain radiographs can serve as a basis for obtaining more sophisticated imaging. Complex motion tomography was used extensively in the past for detection of osseous abnormality but has been replaced by computed tomography (CT).[6] CT is the study of choice for the evaluation of the osseous anatomy and lesions of the TMJ (Figs. 5.**2a, b**). Arthrography was the prime diagnostic modality for disk displacement before MRI was developed. The technique of TMJ arthrography was pioneered by Norgaard in 1944,[8] and has since been modified by several investigators.[3] Arthrography is currently used much less frequently.[2,6]

Computed tomography (CT) scanning remains the gold standard for cross-sectional anatomy of the hard tissue of the TMJ. CT can also provide useful information about the soft-tissue structures related to the TMJ. Arthrography and magnetic resonance imaging (MRI) provide optimal information about the disk and its relationships. The technique of CT air–positive contrast (double contrast) arthrography was described for the first time in 1988.[3,9,10] This technique permits reliable examination of the disk and its relationship to the condyle, the glenoid fossa, and/or the eminence (Figs. 5.**3**, 5.**5**).[3,9] This requires injection of 0.4–0.8 ml of air/contrast (60% meglumine diatrizoate) under fluoroscopic guidance in the superior and inferior joint spaces. After injection of air/contrast, the patient is transferred to the CT suite and direct sagittal sections (1.5–3 mm) are taken in both open-mouth and closed-mouth positions.[3,9,10] Conventional arthrography and CT-contrast arthrography have for the most part been replaced by MRI.

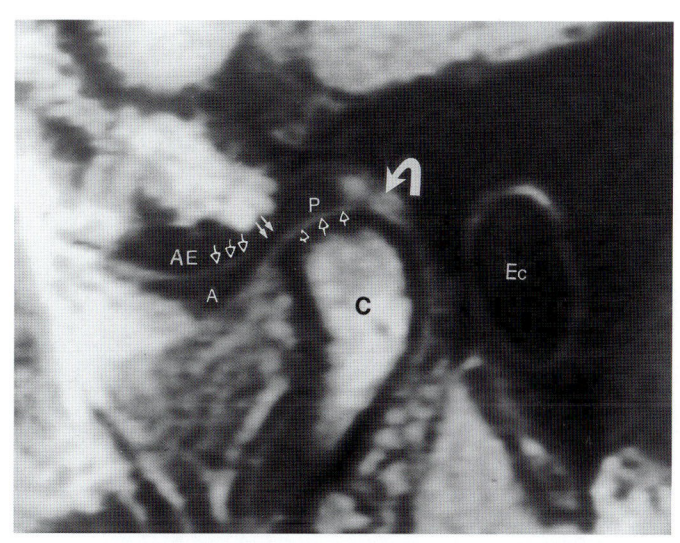

Fig. 5.**7** Normal TMJ anatomy. T1W central sagittal section of the TMJ in the closed-mouth position. Note the relationship between the normal condyle (C), articular eminence (AE), and the external auditory canal (Ec). Note the disk anatomy represented by a low signal intensity: posterior band (P), intermediate zone (straight solid double arrows), and anterior band (A). The intermediate zone is positioned between the posterior slope of the eminence and the anterior surface of the condyle. The retrodiskal tissue is represented by a heterogeneous intermediate signal intensity (curved arrow). The compact bony covering of the condyle is smooth. The mandibular condyle, glenoid fossa, and eminence are lined by fibrocartilage. The fibrocartilage surfaces are partially lined by synovium. This fibrocartilage/synovium covering is seen as an intermediate signal intensity (triple hollow arrows) on MRI. Compare the anatomy demonstrated here with that of sagittal microscopic section in Fig. 5.**6**. Reproduced from Reference 4 with permission.

Nuclear Medicine (Scintigraphy)

Nuclear medicine has been shown to be sensitive in the detection of some TMJ abnormalities, such as osteomyelitis, fibro-osseous lesions, and metastases, but this modality is nonspecific. Nuclear medicine is used occasionally in patients with growth abnormalities such as condylar hyperplasia.[6,7]

CT Technique

The CT scan of the TMJ for routine as well as arthrographic purposes should include the use of 1.5–3 mm collimation with 0.25 mm pixels and extended gray scales to 4000 for appropriate evaluation of the bony structures of the TMJ. This includes 10–16 sections in closed-mouth position, followed by selected sections with open-mouth position, with the use of a bite block. It is preferable to obtain direct sagittal/parasagittal sections if a specially constructed sagittal head holder is available.[3,9,10] Otherwise, reformatted sagittal images should be obtained. Direct coronal sections are needed as well.

In our institution, direct sagittal CT scan images were obtained using a head holder that was developed at this institution.[3,9,10] Since the introduction of spiral/helical and multidetector CT scanners, we no longer use our head holder to obtain direct sagittal/parasagittal images of the TMJ. Instead, we obtain direct axial or coronal sections. The reformatted sagittal images using the data from axial sections are of high quality and appropriate for diagnostic interpretation. The technical procedure for CT of the TMJ in our institution is as follows:

1. Obtain 1.5–3 mm axial sections with zero skip with the jaw closed with 120 kV, 170 mA, with prospective targeting for soft-tissue detail and retrospective targeting for bone detail.
2. Repeat step (1) with the jaw opened.
3. Obtain 3 mm direct coronal sections with zero skip with the jaw closed with 120 kV, 170 mA, and with prospective targeting for soft-tissue detail and retrospective targeting for bone detail.
4. Obtain reformatted sagittal/or parasagittal (oblique sagittal) images using the data from axial CT scans. At times, reformatted oblique coronal (parallel to the horizontal long axis of the mandibular condyle) images may be obtained for determining osseous abnormalities that are sometimes better seen on the oblique coronal rather than the true coronal plane.

MRI Technique

MRI provides better information on meniscal anatomy and its pathological alterations than does CT. Straight or oblique sagittal MR sections perpendicular to the long axis of the condyles satisfactorily depict the normal disk and its dislocated position (Fig. 5.**7**). For optimal quality, the images should be oriented perpendicular (sagittal) and parallel (coronal) to the horizontal long axis of the mandibular condyle rather than in the true sagittal and coronal planes.[6] Lateral or medial displacement of the disk is better assessed on coronal MR images.[2,4,6] All MR scans presented in this chapter were performed with a 1.5 T superconducting MR imager, using the body coil as the transmitter and a 7.6 cm diameter circular surface coil (or bilateral phased-array multicoils) as the receiver. An axial localizer MR image is used to determine the orientation of oblique sagittal and coronal images. Most images were obtained with a 256×256 matrix, four excitations, section thickness of 3 mm, and a field of view of 12 or 16 cm, with the jaw at rest (Table 5.**1**). A spin-echo multislice technique with a TR of 600–1000 ms and a TE of 20–30 ms was used to obtain T1-weighted images. For an open-mouth position, a 256×192 or 256×128 matrix was used, with the other factors the same as for the closed-mouth position. A disposable mouth prop was used to obtain open-mouth MR images.[4] T2-weighted images with a TR of 2000–2500 ms and a TE of 70–80 ms are obtained to evaluate fluid within the joint and/or inflammatory changes of the TMJ (see Fig. 5.**22**). Some authors believe fast spin-echo (FSE) T2-weighted MR images provide better signal-to-noise ratios than standard T2-weighted MR images.[6] In general, for MR imaging of the TMJ, it is important to keep the slice thickness around 3 mm or less.[6] A low-flip-angle, fast-scanning technique, such as gradient-echo or gradient-recalled acquisition in the steady state (GRASS), can be used to evaluate joint effusion as well as increased vascularity of the retrodiskal tissues and other parts of the TMJ. Although dynamic MR imaging with GRASS or similar sequences has been applied to the TMJ, these sequences have not proved to be valuable for routine use.[6] The use of intravenous gadolinium-based MR contrast has very little role in the imaging of the TMJ for internal derangement. Gadolinium-enhanced MR study has proved to be very effective for the evaluation of the proliferating synovium of rheumatoid arthritis of the TMJ (see Fig. 5.**32**), degenerative and infectious arthritis, and in patients with synovial chondromatosis and tumors affecting the TMJ.[2-4,6]

Table 5.1 Scanning parameters for MR imaging of the TMJ

Axial localizer	
TR/TE	400 ms/16 ms
NEX	0.5
FOV	18 cm
Thickness	3 mm
Matrix	256 × 128
Sagittal, closed mouth	
TR/TE	600–1000 ms/20–30 ms
NEX	2–4
FOV	12–16 cm
Thickness	3 mm
Interslice gap	0.3–2 mm
Matrix	256 × 192 or 256 × 256
Sagittal, open mouth	
TR/TE	600–1000 ms/20–30 ms
NEX	2–4
FOV	12–16 cm
Thickness	3 mm
Interslice gap	0.3–2 mm
Matrix	256 × 128 or 156 × 192
Coronal, closed and sagittal, open	
TR/TE	2000–2500 ms/70–80 ms
NEX	2
FOV	16 cm
Thickness	3 mm
Interslice gap	0–0.3 mm
Matrix	256 × 192

FOV, field of view; NEX, number of excitations; TE, echo time; TR, repetition time.

Normal Imaging Anatomy of TMJ

CT is an excellent means of evaluating the normal anatomy of TMJ. The normal CT imaging anatomy of the TMJ is demonstrated in Figure 5.**2a**, **b**. The relationship of the disk–condyle–eminence can be evaluated on CT double-contrast arthrography (pneumoarthrography) (Figs. 5.**3a**, 5.**5**).[3,9,10] MRI is the gold standard for the evaluation of disk and other soft-tissue structures of the TMJ (Figs. 5.**2d**, 5.**7**). Magnetic resonance imaging of the normal joint will demonstrate a low signal intensity structure (disk) conforming between the condyle and glenoid fossa (Fig. 5.**7**). The disk is often described as bow-tie-shaped. The anatomical portions of the disk, namely, posterior band, intermediate zone, and anterior band, are usually well defined (Figs. 5.**2d**, 5.**7**), but these structures are not clearly demarcated, apart from by their morphology. The bow-tie shape is not regularly seen, because of partial volume averaging, oblique sectioning, section thickness, and disk morphology and size. In a number of individuals, anatomical variations can make difficult the diagnosis of a normal disk. A combination of closed-mouth and open-mouth positions, however, always helps the imager to differentiate normal from abnormal disk position.

In the open-mouth position, the posterior band of the disk appears to protrude from the stretched retrodiskal tissue (Fig. 5.**5b**). In the closed-mouth position, the retrodiskal tissue is a thin structure portraying homogeneous intermediate signal intensity (Fig. 5.**7**). In some cases, the tissue cannot be clearly identified because it is juxtaposed to the fibrocartilage–synovium–cortical bone complex of the glenoid fossa and condyle. In the open-mouth position, the retrodiskal tissue expands under the concavity of the glenoid fossa and may demonstrate a heterogeneous signal intensity. The heterogeneity occurs because of the flow of blood into this region during opening. The retrodiskal tissue is always closely apposed to the condyle and glenoid fossa. The fibrocartilage (intermediate signal intensity) lining the glenoid fossa/eminence as well as the condyle separates the low signal intensity of the cortex of the temporal bone and condyle from the disk (Fig. 5.**7**). The fibrocartilage lining the condyle is not always apparent. Identification of the precise limits of the TMJ capsule can be difficult.

Anatomical Variations and Developmental Anomaly

Anatomical variations include the flaring or angulation of the mandibular condyle, pneumatization of the glenoid fossa and eminence, and developmental defects of the tympanic plate.[2] Pneumatization of the mastoid bone can be so extensive as to involve the glenoid fossa and eminence (Fig. 5.**8**). This finding is significant when an arthroplasty is contemplated. Pneumatized bone provides a poor anchor for screw fixation.

Developmental defects in the tympanic plate may be seen on standard tomographic and CT images. In the absence of or lack of history of neoplasm, infection, or trauma, the defects should be ascribed to the failure of the foramen of Huschke to close during growth and development. Rarely, the defect is sufficiently large to result in a deformation of the anterior wall of the external auditory meatus (Fig. 5.**9**). The tympanic part of temporal bone is ossified in collagenous fibrous tissue from a center that appears at about the third month of fetal life.[1] At birth it is represented by an incomplete ring, the tympanic ring. After birth the tympanic ring extends laterally and backward to form a more cylindrical structure, the tympanic part of the temporal bone. For a time during its development, there exists in the floor of the external meatus an opening called the foramen of Huschke.[1] With the downward and forward growth of the mastoid process, the foramen of Huschke changes its location from inferior to anterior. Typically, the foramen is closed by the fifth year of life. As the retrodiskal tissue originates from the anterior wall of the tympanic plate, a defect in the plate results in the retrodiskal tissue originating directly from the subcutaneous tissue/skin lining the meatus.[11] Patients with large defects may complain of auricular sensitivity with temperature changes. Such defects could theoretically facilitate the traumatic entry of an arthroscopic trocar into the external auditory canal. When an arthrotomy is planned with placement of an alloplast, there is always the risk of its posterior displacement and the creation of an external auditory canal fistula.[11]

■ Condylar Agenesis (Otomandibular Dysostosis, Mandibulofacial Dysostosis, Hemifacial Microsomia)

Developmental abnormalities affecting the TMJ often result in skeletal facial anomalies including facial asymmetry (Figs. 5.**10**–5.**13**). Condylar agenesis can result in severe facial deformity. In unilateral cases, lack of growth on the affected side combined with continued growth on the contralateral side produces flatness of the face on the normal side and deviation of the chin to the abnormal side.[7] In the rarely occurring bilateral cases there is no facial asymmetry, but the chin is markedly retruded.[7] Depending on the extent of involvement, there may be associated abnormalities of the external ear and middle ear. In patients with hemifacial microsomia and mandibulofacial dysostosis (Treacher-Collins syndrome), mandibular anomalies are almost always associated with anomalies of the external and middle ears.[12–14] Anomalies of inner ear, however, are far less common.[12,14] The facial nerve, as well as the parotid gland and masseter and medial and lateral pterygoid muscles, also may be partially absent (Fig. 5.**10**).[7] At times there will be moderate to marked atrophy of the masticator muscle with no significant mandibular hypoplasia (Fig. 5.**14**).

In the case of hemifacial microsomia or Goldenhar syndrome, the deformity is focused in the otomandibular region and

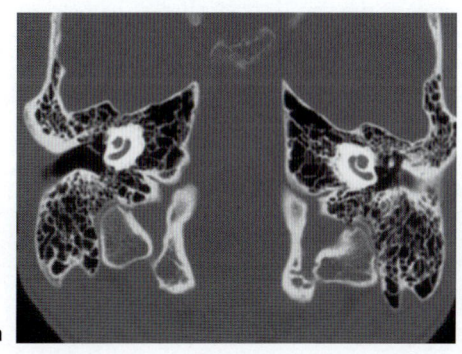

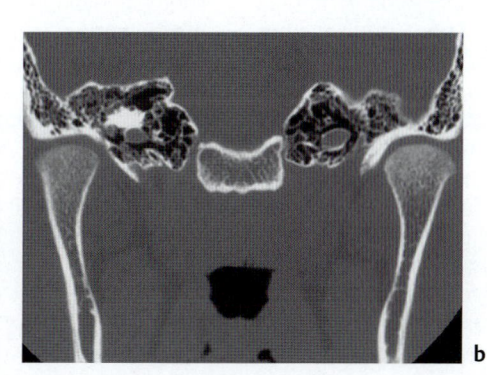

Fig. 5.**8** Pneumatization of glenoid fossa and articular eminence. **a** Axial and **b** coronal CT scans showing extensive pneumatization of temporal bones including the glenoid fossa and anterior articular eminences.

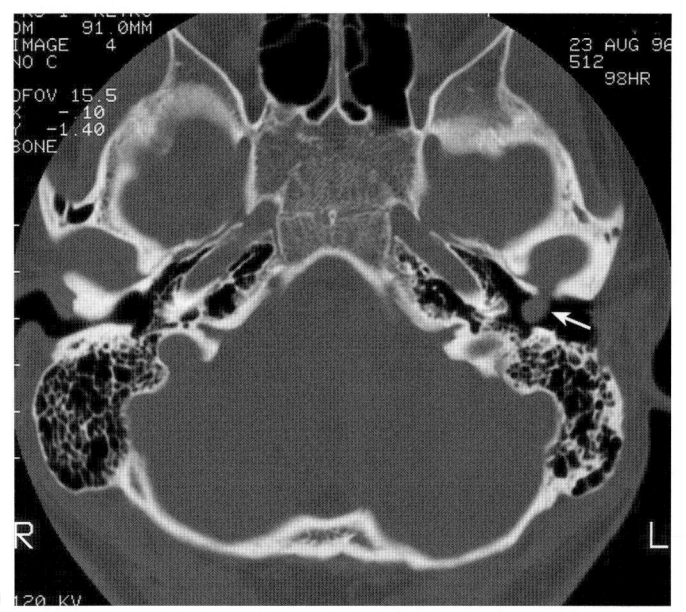

Fig. 5.9 TMJ herniation into external canal. **a** Axial CT scan shows a bony defect at the anterior wall of the left external auditory canal, due to failure of the foramen of Huschke to close during growth and development. Note herniation of the joint capsule into the external auditory canal (arrow) and exostosis of the right external auditory canal. **b** Coronal CT scans show herniation of joint capsule into the external auditory canal (arrow).

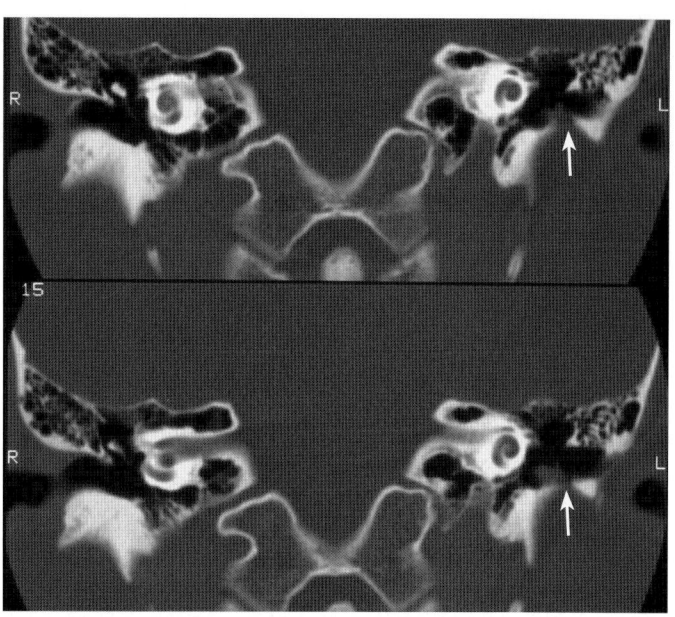

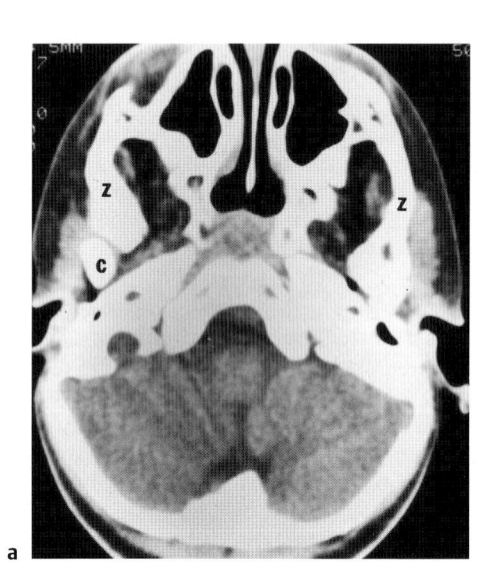

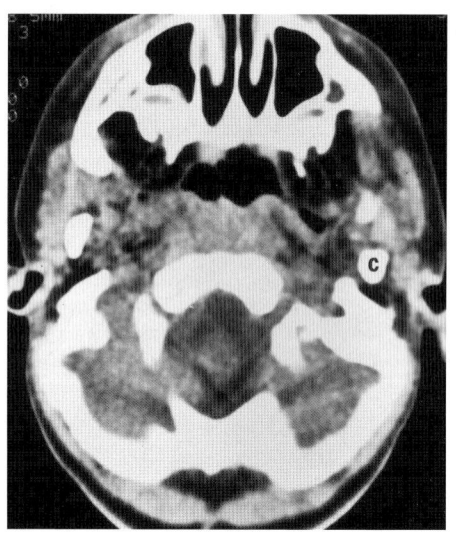

Fig. 5.10 Pierre Robin syndrome. **a, b** Axial CT scans showing hypoplastic condyles (C). Note deformity of zygomatic arches (Z) and poor development of masticator muscles.

from there radiates circumferentially to involve the middle and lower two-thirds of the facial skeleton and overlying soft tissues (Fig. 5.11). Typically, the mandible anterior to the antegonial notch is normal. The severity of the mandibular hypoplasia may be classified as grade I, when the TMJ and ramus are normal but reduced in structure; as grade II, when the TMJ and ramus are morphologically abnormal but remain functional; or as grade III, when both TMJ and ramus are absent. Other features that have been described include hypoplasia of the glenoid fossa, zygoma, maxilla, masticatory and tongue muscles, and parotid gland; reduced orotragal distance; macrostomia–enlarged philtrum; bifid uvula; cleft lip and palate; and dental malformations

Condylar agenesis or hypoplasia results in mandibular deficiency (retrognathia). Excessive condylar growth results in mandibular excess (prognathism). In many cases, the maxilla also demonstrates an abnormal growth pattern. Surgical treatment often includes the realignment of both jaws using complex osteotomies. Orthodontic treatment is integral to this treatment. The differential diagnosis of facial asymmetry includes unilateral condylar hypoplasia, unilateral condylar hyperplasia, unilateral macrognathia, neoplasm (primary or metastatic, benign or malignant), or unilateral condylar hypertrophy. Condylar hypoplasia may occur as a feature of several syndromes including hemifacial microsomia (first and second branchial arch syndrome) (Figs. 5.11, 5.12). These syndromes manifest with laterognathia to the affected side. In these patients, the condyle, the glenoid fossa, the coronoid process, portions of the ramus, and even parts of the mandibular body may be absent.[7, 12, 14]

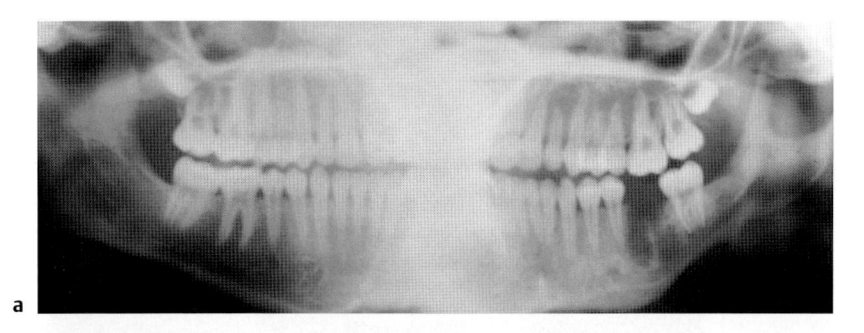

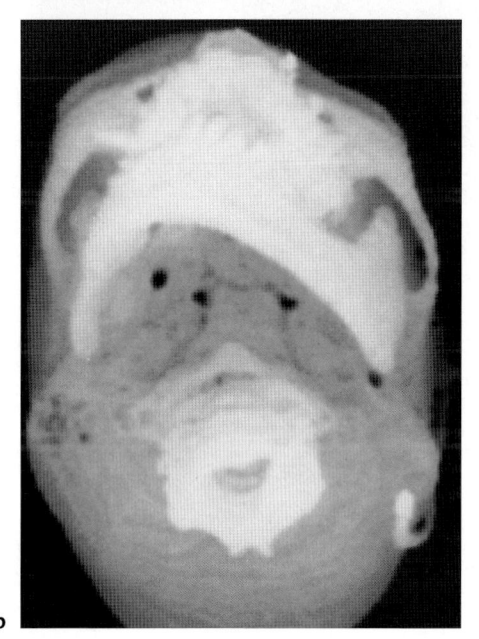

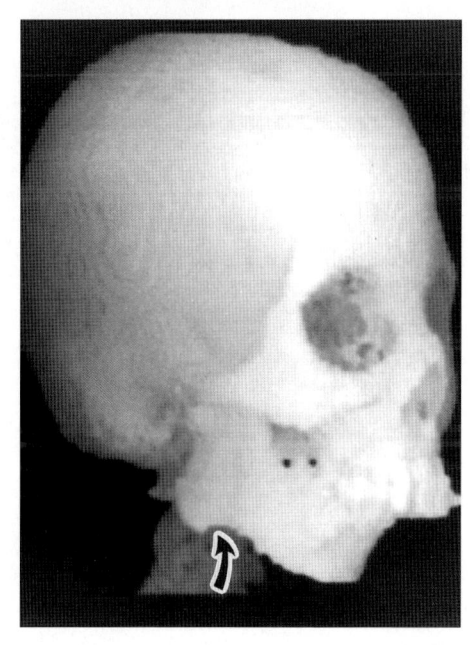

Fig. 5.11 Hemifacial microsomia. **a** Panorex view of the mandible reveals marked hypoplastic left mandible. **b, c** 3D views of another patient with hemifacial microsomia, showing hypoplastic right mandible including right condyle. Note antegonial notching (arrow) and malocclusion.

■ Condylar Hypoplasia

Condylar hypoplasia can be congenital (Figs. 5.**10**–5.**13**). However, it is more often the result of postnatal causes. The most common etiologies include trauma, infection, and radiation (Fig. 5.**15**).[7] The condition is usually unilateral, but it can occur bilaterally. Radiographically there is a small condyle, a shallow sigmoid notch, and often a shorter ramus and mandibular body, and the presence of increased antegonial notching on the affected side (Fig. 5.**11**). On the unaffected side, the mandibular body may be long and flat, with chin deviated to the affected side.[7] Patients with bilateral condylar hypoplasia demonstrate condylar morphological changes on both sides. In addition they have a short mandible and retruded chin.[7]

■ Condylar Hyperplasia

Bilateral overgrowth of the mandible, including the mandibuar condyle, has been reported in certain hereditary syndromes such as Klinefelter syndrome and angiokeratoma corporis diffusum syndrome as well as in patients with acromegaly and gigantism[7]. However, the most common form of overdevelopment of the condyle is associated with idiopathic unilateral condylar hyperplasia.[15] This condition is characterized by a slowly progressive enlargement of one side of the mandible, starting at the time when growth should normally stop.[7] Radiographically, the con-

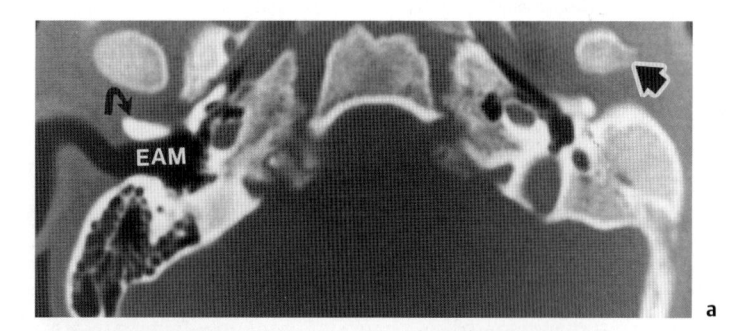

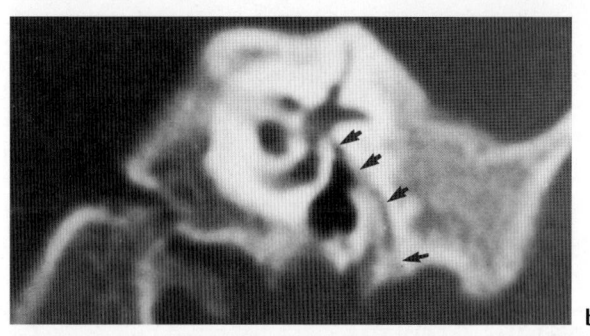

Fig. 5.**12** Hemifacial microsomia. **a** Axial CT scan shows hypoplastic left condyle (straight arrow) and absent left external auditory meatus. Note normal right tympanic bone (curved arrow) and normal right external auditory meatus (EAM). **b** Coronal CT scan shows lack of pneumatization of mastoid. Note anterior location of facial nerve canal (arrows).

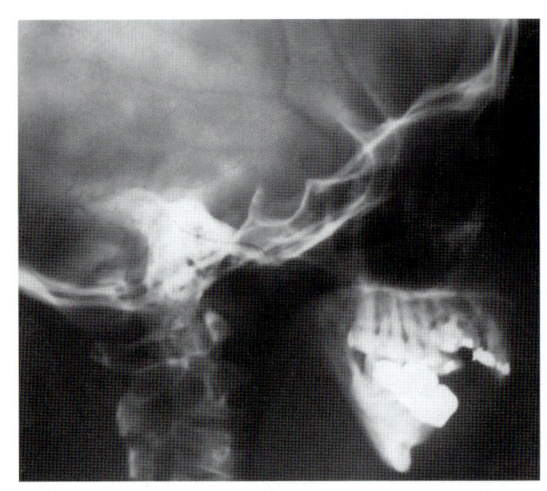

Fig. 5.**13** Mandibulofacial dysostosis. Lateral view of the head shows hypoplastic mandible with absent condyles.

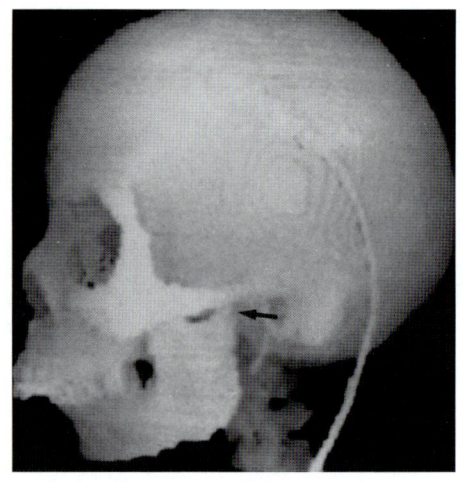

Fig. 5.**15** TMJ ankylosis and condylar hypoplasia. TMJ ankylosis following neonatal meningitis and presumed TMJ infection. Three-dimensional CT image shows deformity of the left condyle (arrow) and absence of the normal condyle–fossa relationship as a result of ankylosis. The patient has a ventriculoperitoneal shunt. Reproduced from Reference 4 with permission.

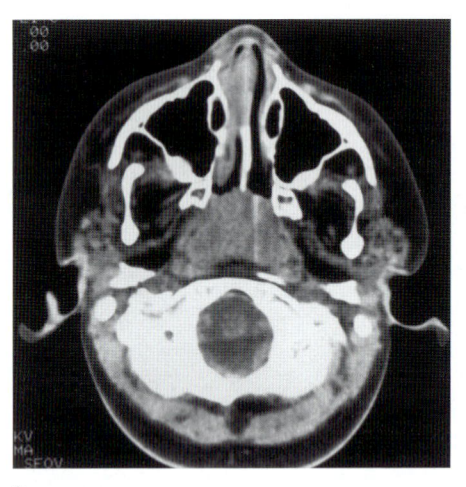

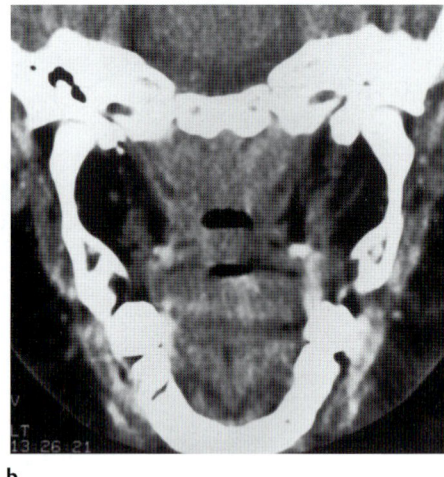

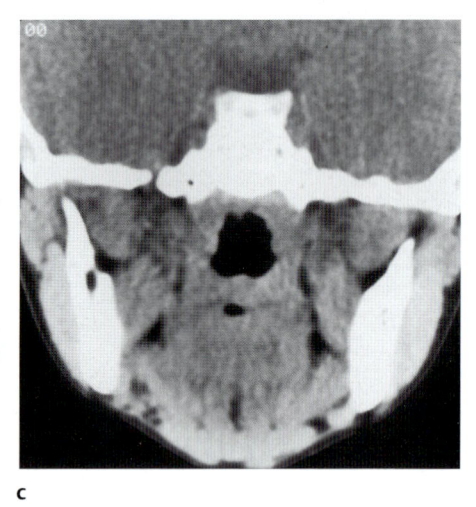

Fig. 5.**14** Idiopathic atrophy of masticatory muscles. **a** Axial and **b** coronal CT scans in a 5-year-old child showing marked atrophy of the masticatory muscles. Note deformity of the mandibular rami and condyles. **c** Normal coronal CT scan (same age as patient) for comparison.

dyle may appear asymmetrically enlarged. There will also be elongation of the ipsilateral mandibular neck and ramus and chin deviation to the unaffected side.

Condylar hyperplasia refers to overgrowth of the condyle. Unilateral macrognathia is a rare syndrome in which the entire ipsilateral mandible, including the teeth, is enlarged. Treatment of condylar hyperplasia is dependent on whether condylar growth is still occurring. In this regard, technetium bone scanning is useful to confirm active growth in the case of condylar hyperplasia.[7]

Inflammation

■ Infectious Arthritis

The TMJ may be involved as part of a systemic infection such as staphylococcal or streptococcal septicemia, gonorrhea, tuberculosis, syphilis, actinomycosis, or one of the mycoses.[16–19] A more common cause is direct extension from an adjacent infection, e.g., of parotid, otic, or dental origin.[7, 16] Infection may also arise consequent to penetrating injury of the TMJ and a complication of arthroscopy or other surgical procedures of TMJ (e.g., infection of a prostatic TMJ). The onset of infectious arthritis is usually accompanied by chills, fever, and sweating.[7, 16] This is followed by redness, swelling, and tenderness in the region of the joint, leading to accumulation of pus and inflammatory exudate within the joint capsule (Fig. 5.**16**) and to limitation of motion.[7, 16] Later, depending on the severity of the infection, various degrees of destruction, ranging from partial to complete damage of the articular disk to osteomyelitis of the condyle and glenoid fossa, may develop.[16] In the late stages of infection, fibrosis and dystrophic calcifications occur, leading to fibrous or bony ankylosis.[16] In children, the disease may affect the growth potential of the condyle, which in turn may lead to facial deformity and malocclusion. The rapid development of TMJ ankylosis requires that the treatment begin as soon as the first signs of acute infectious arthritis appear.[16–18] The findings on conventional radiographs in the early stage (days 7–10) of infectious arthritis are ordinarily insignificant owing to a lack of osseous involve-

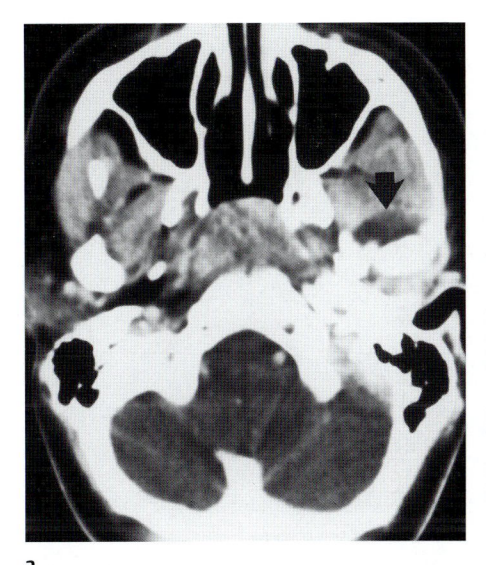

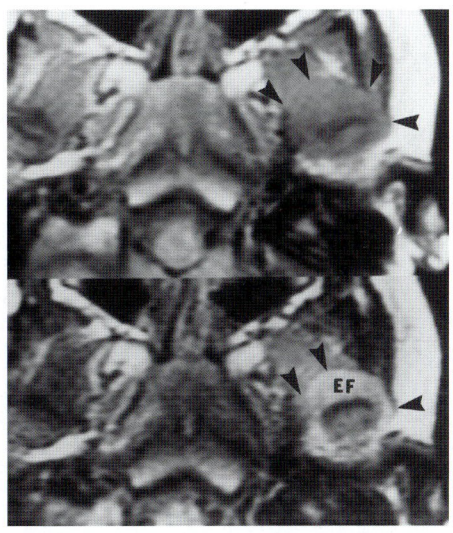

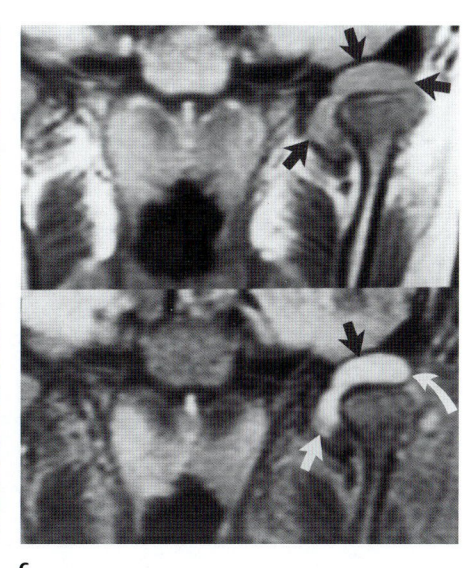

Fig. 5.16 Acute septic arthritis of the left TMJ. **a** Enhanced axial CT scan shows fluid collection (pus) in the left TMJ (arrow). **b** Proton-density (top) and T2W (bottom) axial MR scans, same patient as in **a**, demonstrating expansion of the joint capsule (arrowheads) due to presence of joint effusion (EF). **c** Proton-density (top) and T2W (bottom) coronal MR scans, same patient as in **a**, demonstrating expansion of the superior and medial portion of the left TMJ (arrows) due to fluid collection (pus and inflammatory exudate). Reproduced from Reference 4 with permission.

ment.[7,16] However, the intra-articular collection of pus or inflammatory exudate can be easily seen by CT and, especially, MRI (Fig. 5.16). In the later stage, when bone rarefaction and erosion occur, CT may be superior to MRI in delineating changes within the hard tissues of the joint.[10] Depending on the severity of the infection, varying degrees of destruction may be seen, ranging from damage to the articular surface to osteomyelitis of the condyle.[10] In the late stages, fibrous or bony ankylosis may develop. In children, infectious arthritis can affect the growth potential of the condyle and result in facial asymmetry.[7]

Necrotizing External Otitis

Necrotizing external otitis is a condition predominantly of elderly, poorly controlled diabetic patients and is usually caused by *Pseudomonas aeruginosa*.[16] The infection may spread rapidly along several routes: directly via bony erosion into the adjacent mastoid air cells and middle ear; anteriorly into the TMJ, parotid gland, and masticatory space; and frequently into the soft tissues of the parapharyngeal space and infratemporal fossa.[16] In this condition, involvement of TMJ and adjacent soft-tissue structures is best evaluated by MRI. On the other hand, bone erosions due to osteomyelitis of the external ear canal, TMJ, and base of the skull are best evaluated by CT scan.[16] For more details see Chapter 1.

Internal Derangements

Although diverse pathological conditions can affect the TMJ, the most common is the internal derangement, which represents an abnormal internal structural and functional change of the disk, as well as an abnormal relationship of the disk to the condyle, glenoid fossa, and articular eminence when the teeth are in the closed-mouth position.[3,4,6,9,16,17,20-24] This includes disk dislocation, disk perforation, and disk fragmentation.[2,3] The disk is usually displaced anteriorly (Fig. 5.17), and it may be associated with perforation of the posterior disk attachment.[3,4] TMJ dysfunction due to internal derangement is reportedly a fairly common abnormality. The clinical symptoms and signs consist of headache, periarticular pain, joint clicking, limitation of jaw movement, and tightness of facial musculature.[2,3,4,6] Patients are most frequently female and in their teens to mid-thirties.[6] The etiology of internal derangement of TMJ is unknown, but apparently involves a spectrum of traumatic conditions, including microtrauma (intubation, prolonged dental procedures, bruxism, masticatory muscle spasm, and malocclusion) and micro/macrotrauma (fracture, dislocation, and hemarthrosis), as well as degenerative and inflammatory joint diseases (e.g., osteoarthritis, rheumatoid arthritis, and psoriatic arthritis).[2,6] The pathophysiology of internal derangement of TMJ is believed to be related to loss of the ability of the posterior meniscal attachment to counteract the pulling forces of the lateral pterygoid muscle.[2,3,4] When this occurs, the meniscus remains anterior to the condyle during closure and the condyle impinges directly upon the posterior neurofibrovascular zone (Fig. 5.17). McCarty and Farrar[24] reported that more than 70% of patients with TMJ problems have some form of meniscal displacement. Internal derangement of the TMJ is usually divided into subluxation and dislocation.[2,4] The ability of the condyle to negotiate around the displaced disk is termed "reduction." Anterior meniscal displacement with reduction on opening (referred to by some authors as subluxation) (Fig. 5.18) is often accompanied by audible clicking noises. This is because a reducing disk displacement is characterized by a reciprocal clicking as the condyle jumps around the displaced disk upon opening and then slips off the posterior edge of the disk upon closing.[4] Anterior meniscal displacement without reduction on jaw opening (referred to by some authors as dislocation) implies that the condyle is unable to negotiate past the displaced disk (Figs. 5.19–5.25). This represents a more severe stage of internal derangement of the TMJ and is often accompanied by chronic pain and limitation of opening (closed lock). In internal derangements, the disk often becomes displaced forward and usually medially. The posterior attachment undergoes a remodeling process. In some cases, a distinct posterior band, intermediate zone, and anterior band are no longer discernible (Fig. 5.23). When the disk is anteriorly displaced its functional position in the joint changes so that loading is on the

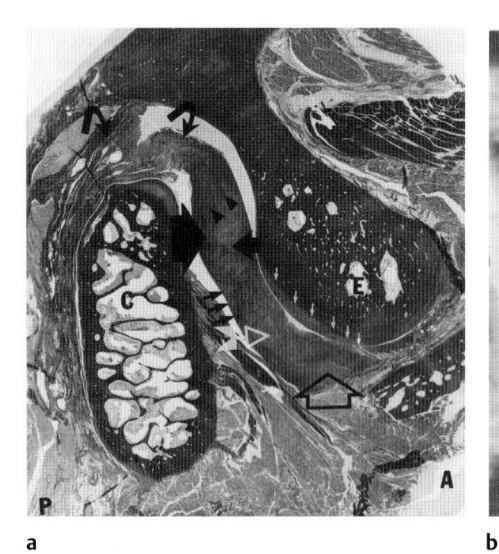

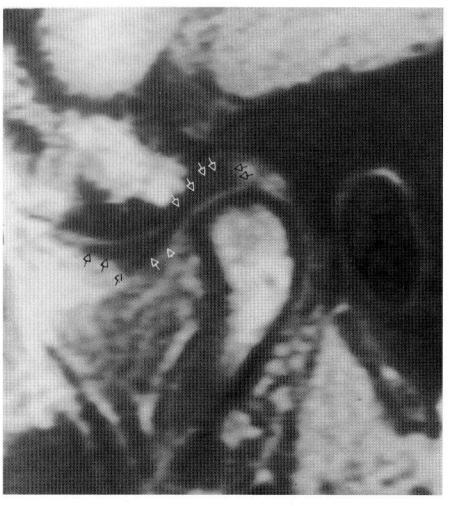

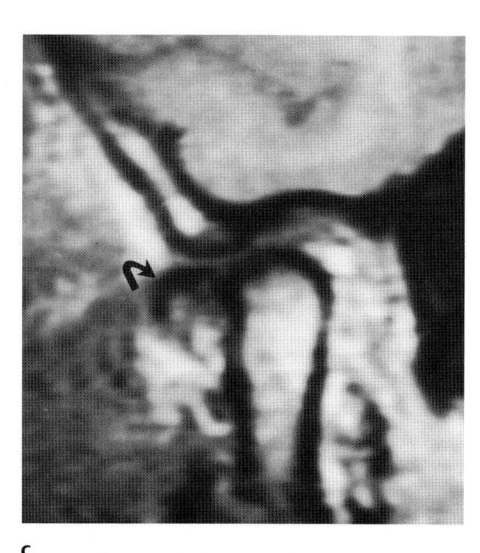

Fig. 5.**17** Internal derangement. **a** Sagittal microscopic section of a TMJ with internal derangement. In internal derangements the disk becomes displaced forward and usually medially. The posterior band (large black arrows) of the disk undergoes deformation. In some cases the posterior band, intermediate zone, and anterior band are no longer distinct. The anatomy of the disk illustrated here is still preserved, and the posterior band (large black arrows), intermediate zone (small black arrows), and anterior band (open black arrow and open white arrow) are all present. As the disk is progressively displaced forward, the retrodiskal tissue (curved arrows) is stretched forward over the condyle surface. This tissue then undergoes progressive remodeling. With advanced remodeling, this tissue can resemble the disk because it is devoid of vascularity. The approximate delineation between the deformed posterior band and remodeled retrodiskal tissue is indicated (black arrowheads). There is thickening of the fibrous connective tissue lining the eminence (series of small white arrows). A = anterior; C = condyle; E = eminence; P = posterior. Figure courtesy of Leslie Heffez, DMD, University of Illinois, Chicago. **b** Sagittal T1W MR scan in the closed-mouth position, with a normal disk, is shown. Note typical bow-tie appearance of normal disk (arrows). **c** Internal derangement and nonreduced disk dislocation. Sagittal T1W MR scan, obtained with the mouth open, shows a deformed, anteriorly displaced disk (arrow). Reproduced from Reference 4 with permission.

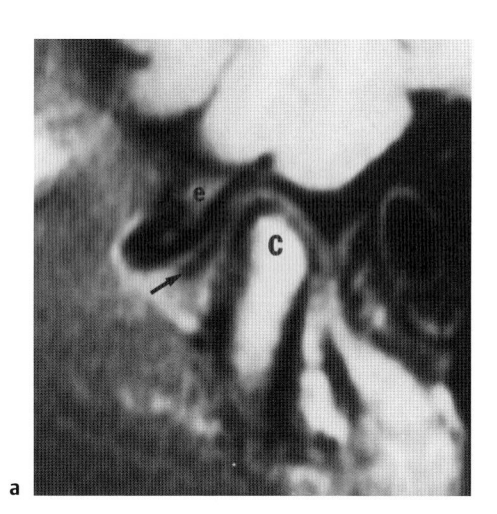

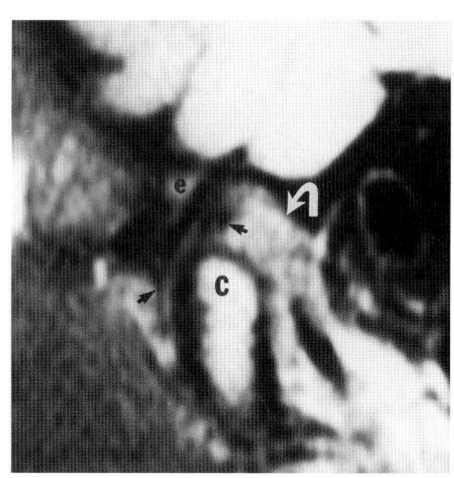

Fig. 5.**18** Anterior disk displacement with reduction. **a** Central-section, sagittal T1W MR image of the TMJ in the closed-mouth position is shown. There is slight anterior displacement with reduction (see **b**). The disk is straight (arrow) with no clear delineation of the posterior band, intermediate zone, and anterior band. The retrodiskal tissue (intermediate signal intensity) lies above the condyle (C). The cortical bone of the condyle (C), glenoid fossa, and eminence (e) is smooth. **b** Open-mouth position. With slight translation and rotation of the condyle (C), the disk, although deformed, appears to be positioned normally (black arrows). The disk shape in the open- and closed-mouth positions may be a factor in apparent deformation. Note the intermediate signal intensity of the retrodiskal tissue (curved arrow) enveloping the posterior band. e = eminence. Reproduced from Reference 4 with permission.

retrodiskal tissue rather than the disk itself.[6] Morphologically, this results in thickening of the posterior band and diminishing of the anterior two-thirds of the disk (Figs. 5.**22**, 5.**23**). The retrodiskal (bilaminar zone) tissue becomes more fibrotic and may appear as a "pseudodisk" (Figs. 5.**22**, 5.**23**). Other sequelae of disk displacement include perforation and degenerative joint disease. Perforations usually occur in the retrodiskal tissue, or at its junction with the disk, rather than in the disk itself.[6] In a normal state, there is no communication between the upper and lower joint spaces. During arthrography, leakage of contrast material from the lower joint space to the upper joint is an indication for perforation.[6] Perforation cannot be determined by MRI or routine CT study of the TMJ.

On MR imaging, the position of the disk is qualitatively described as slight displacement when the posterior band contacts the anterior-superior aspect of the condyle, moderate displacement when the posterior band is located between the condyle and apex of the eminence, and severe displacement when the posterior band is located to the apex of the eminence (Figs. 5.**23**–5.**25**). Regardless of the imaging modality used, all planes of section should be carefully evaluated to rule out localized alterations in disk shape or rotational disk displacement.[2-6]

Gradient echo images and T2-weighted images may be used to supplement the standard T1-weighted imaging to identify areas of interstitial fluid within the deformed disk and intracapsular fluid within the joint space (Figs. 5.**21**, 5.**22**). The

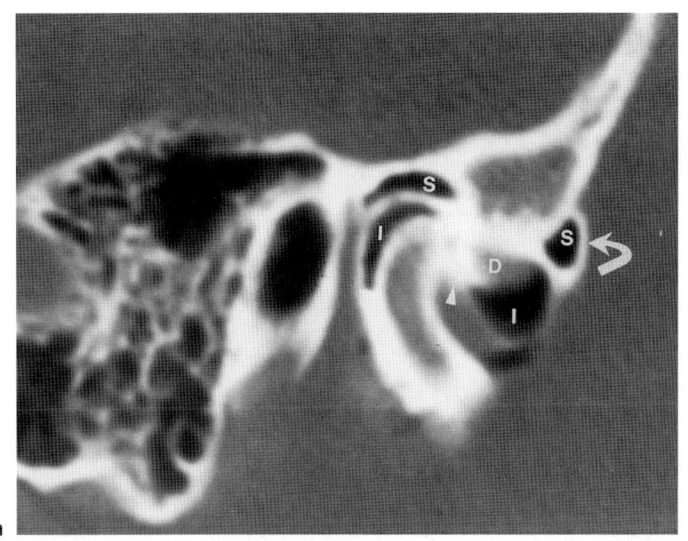

Fig. 5.19 Anterior dislocation of the left TMJ disk. **a** Double-contrast CT arthrogram of the left TMJ, obtained with the mouth closed, shows anteriorly displaced disk (D). Air is seen in the superior (S) and inferior (I) joint spaces. Note the presence of iodinated contrast (arrowhead) in the inferior joint space and along the anterior joint capsule (curved arrow). **b** Sagittal T1W MR scan, of the left TMJ, same patient as in **a**, obtained with the mouth closed, shows anterior displacement of the disk (arrows). c = condyle; E = eminence. Reproduced from Reference 4 with permission.

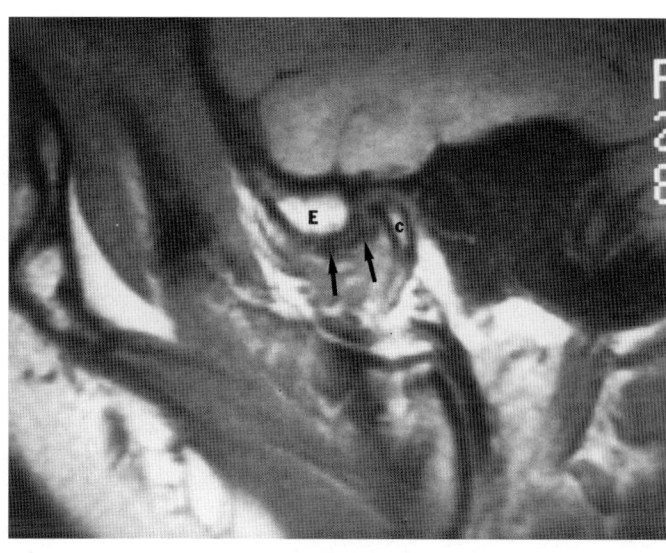

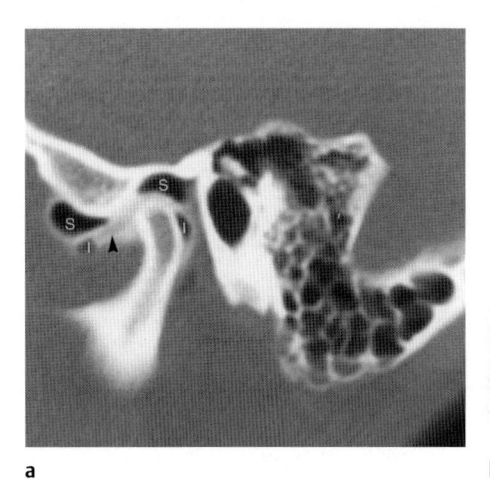

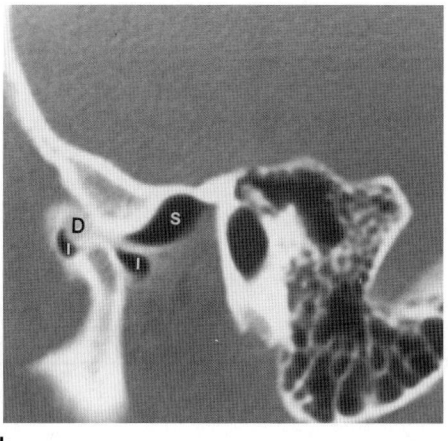

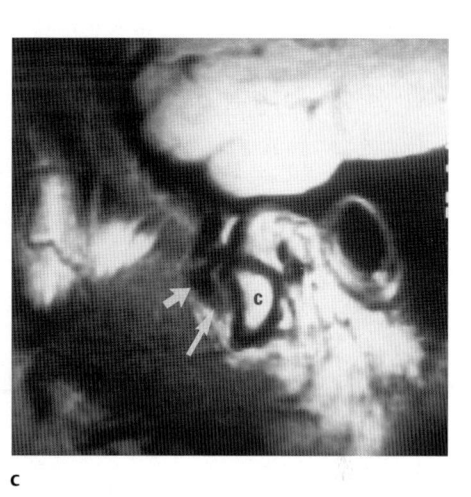

Fig. 5.20 Anterior dislocation of the right TMJ disk without reduction. **a** Double-contrast CT arthrogram of the right TMJ, obtained with the mouth closed, shows anteriorly dislocated disk (arrowhead). Air is present in the superior (S) and inferior (I) joint spaces. Iodinated contrast (arrowhead) outlines the displaced disk. **b** Double-contrast CT arthrogram of the right TMJ, obtained with the mouth open, shows anteriorly displaced disk (D). Air is present in the superior (S) and inferior (I) joint spaces. **c** Sagittal proton-weighted MR scan, same patient as in **a** and **b**, obtained with the mouth open, shows a deformed, anteriorly displaced disk (arrows). C = condyle. Reproduced from Reference 4 with permission.

gradient echo and T2-weighted imaging complements the T1-weighted images and can help in delimiting the precise limits of the capsule. Regardless of disk displacement, the retrodiskal tissue maintains its ability to expand. Its degree of expansion largely depends on the distance the condyle translates. The degree of condylar translation depends on several factors including the presence of interstitial or intracapsular fluid accumulation, muscle inflammation, and intracapsular adhesions. The disk shape alone is rarely a physical limitation to translation.[2]

Some clinicians and investigators have used the term *avascular necrosis* to describe MR findings of condylar remodeling. Avascular necrosis is clearly defined and identified in the condyle of the femoral head, where its occurrence is principally idiopathic. Currently, the pathogenesis is believed to involve the decrease of blood supply to the condyle of the femoral head, subsequent inflammation, and necrosis of the marrow. With the destruction of the marrow, the cortical bone becomes unsupported and collapses centrally within the femoral condyle. As healing occurs, the femoral condyle undergoes significant remodeling and becomes deformed and sclerotic. The blood supply to the femoral head is anatomically isolated from the blood supply of the metaphysis. Hence, the femoral condyle is susceptible to changes in blood flow. In contrast, the blood supply to the mandibular condyle is derived from the lateral pterygoid muscle as well as from the mandibular ramus marrow cavity; the mandibular condyle therefore appears to be more protected from this process.[2] The etiology of aseptic necrosis of the TMJ, is different from the same condition in the femoral head because no clear association with common etiological factors such as steroid use or sickle cell disease has been established for TMJ bone marrow alterations.[2,6] The clinical significance of bone marrow signal alterations in the mandibular condyle is unknown and the need for treatment has not been established.[6]

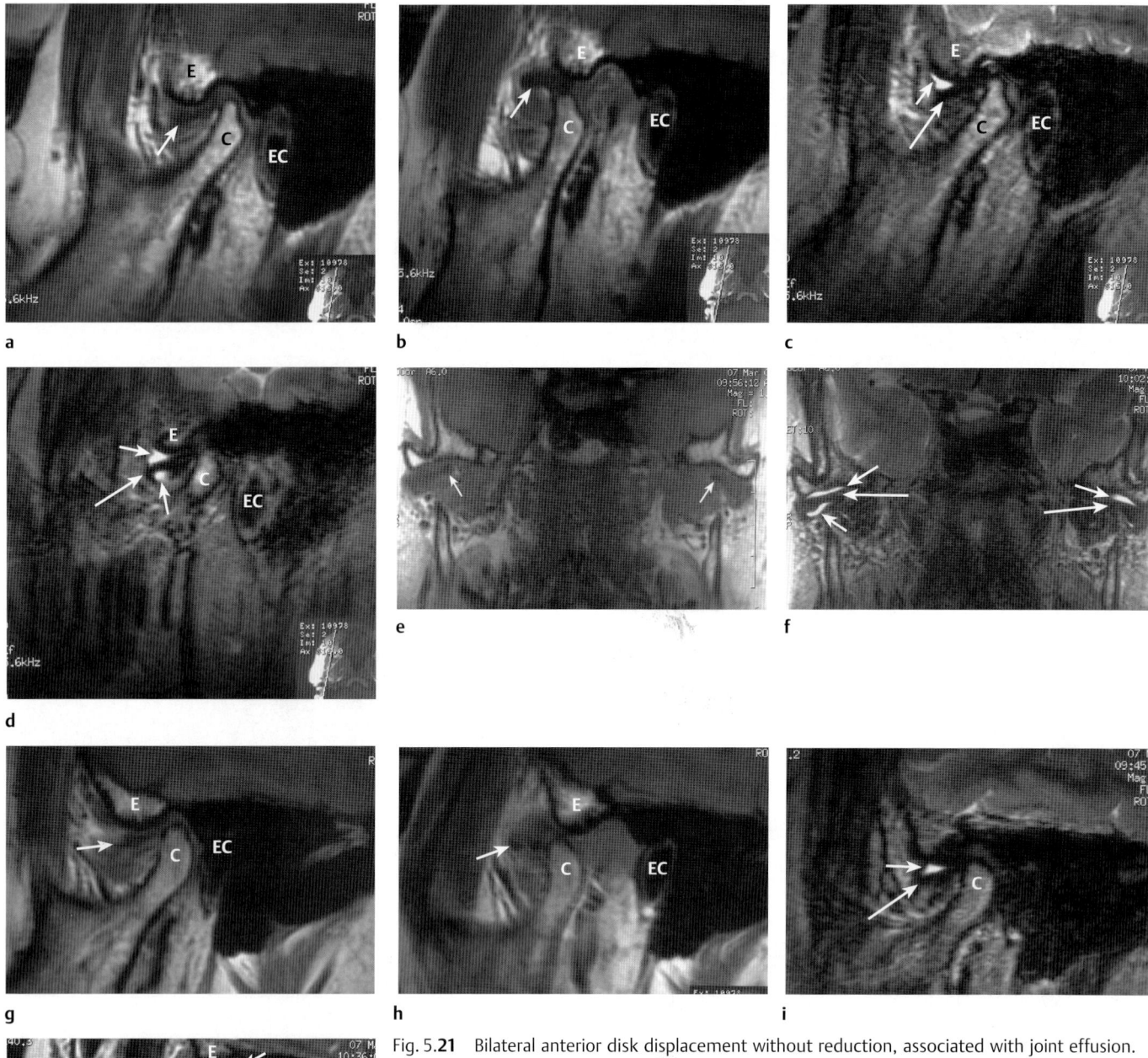

Fig. 5.21 Bilateral anterior disk displacement without reduction, associated with joint effusion. **a** Sagittal T1W MR scan of the right TMJ, obtained with mouth closed, demonstrates anterior displacement of the disk (arrow). C = condyle, E = eminence, EC = external ear canal. **b** Sagittal T1W MR scan of the right TMJ, obtained with mouth open, demonstrates nonreduced disk (arrow). **c** Sagittal T2W MR scan of the right TMJ, obtained with mouth closed. Note displaced disk (long arrow) and fluid in the anterior superior joint space (short arrow). **d** Sagittal T2W MR scan of the right TMJ, obtained with mouth closed. Note displaced disk (long arrow) and fluid in the anterosuperior and anteroinferior joint spaces (short arrows). **e** Coronal T1W MR scan, obtained with mouth closed. Note anterolateral displacement of the disks (arrows). **f** Coronal T2W MR scan, obtained with mouth open. Note the displaced disks (long arrows) and fluid in the joints (short arrows). **g** Sagittal T1W MR scan of the left TMJ, obtained with mouth closed, demonstrates anteriorly displaced disk (arrow). **h** Sagittal T1W MR scan of the left TMJ, obtained with mouth open, demonstrates nonreduced disk (arrow). **i** Sagittal T2W MR scan of the left TMJ, obtained with mouth closed. Note anterior disk displacement (long arrow) and effusion in the superior anterior joint space (short arrow). **j** Sagittal T2W MR scan of the left TMJ, obtained with mouth open. Note nonreduced disk (long arrow) and shifting fluid from anterior joint space to posterior joint space (short arrows). C = condyle, E = eminence EC = external ear canal.

Internal Derangements 491

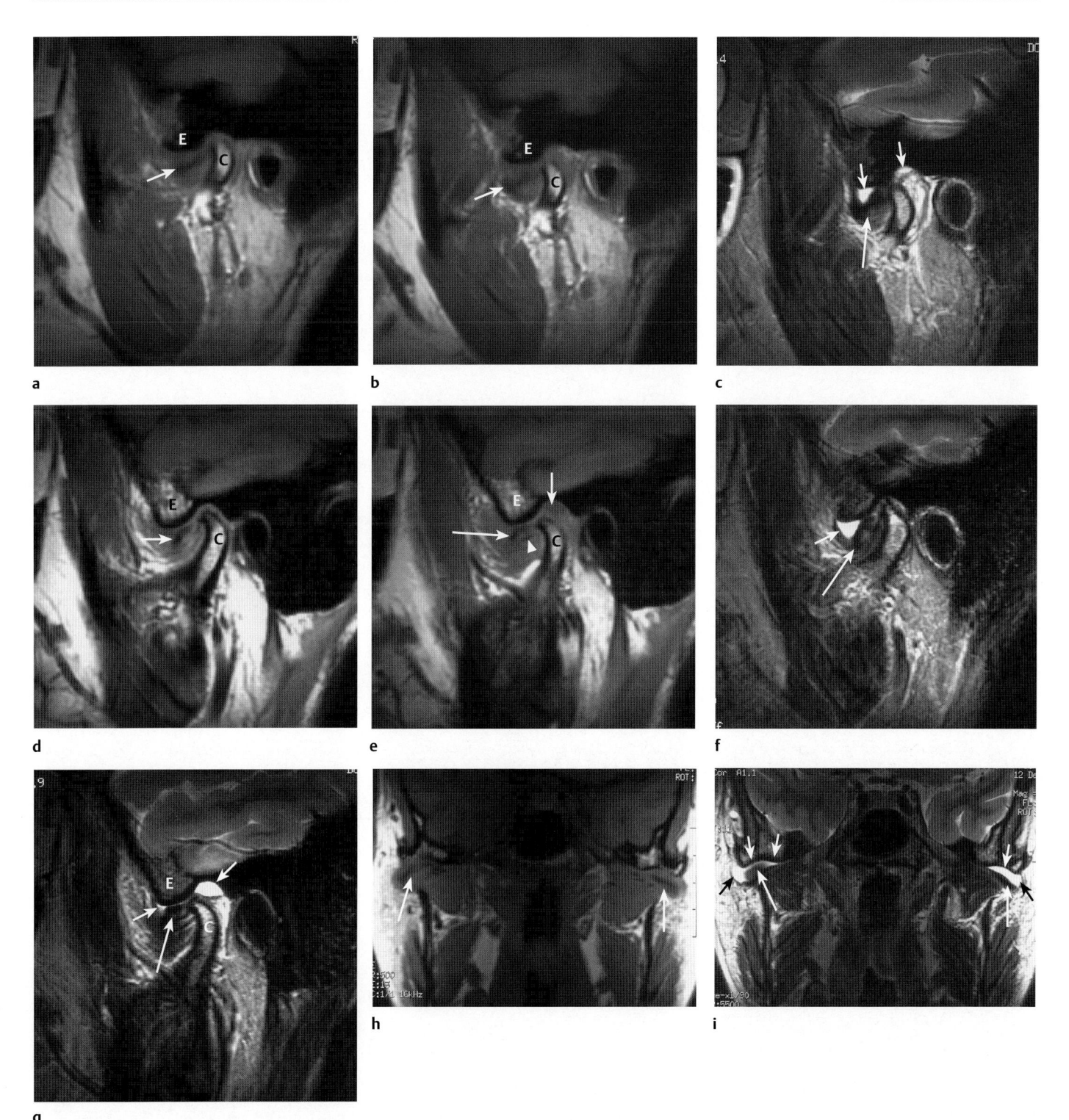

Fig. 5.22 Bilateral disk displacement and joint effusion. **a, b** Sagittal T1W MR scans of the left TMJ, obtained with mouth closed (**a**) and open (**b**) demonstrate anterior disk displacement without reduction (arrows). E = articular eminence, C = condyle. **c** Sagittal T2W MR scan of the left TMJ, with mouth open. Note anteriorly displaced disk (long arrow) and joint effusion (small arrows) in the superior joint space. **d** Sagittal T1W MR scan of the right TMJ, obtained with mouth closed, demonstrates anteriorly displaced disk (arrow). **e** Sagittal T1W MR scan of the right TMJ, obtained with mouth open, demonstrates dislocated disk (long arrow), tendon of the lateral pterygoid muscle (arrowhead), and fluid in the joint (short arrow). The effusion is better seen on T2W MR scans (**f, g**). **f** Sagittal T2W MR scan of the right TMJ, obtained with mouth closed, demonstrates displaced disk (long arrow) and joint effusion (short arrow). **g** Sagittal T2W MR scan of the right TMJ, obtained with mouth open, demonstrates displaced disk (long arrow) and joint effusion (short arrows). **h** Coronal T1W MR scan, obtained with mouth closed, demonstrates bilateral anterolateral disk displacement (arrows). **i** Coronal T2W MR scan shows bilateral displaced disks (long arrows) and joint effusions (short arrows). C = condyle, E = articular eminence.

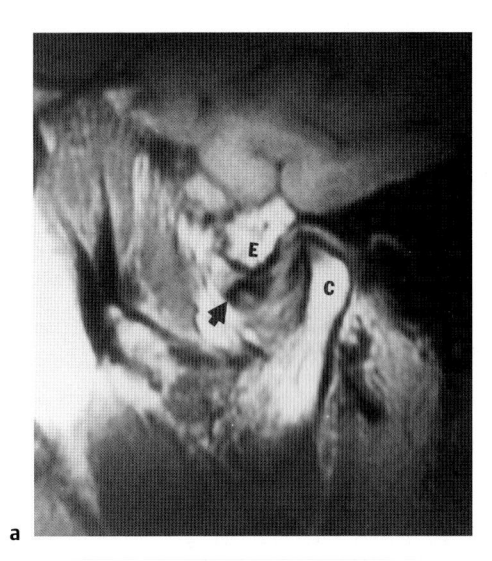

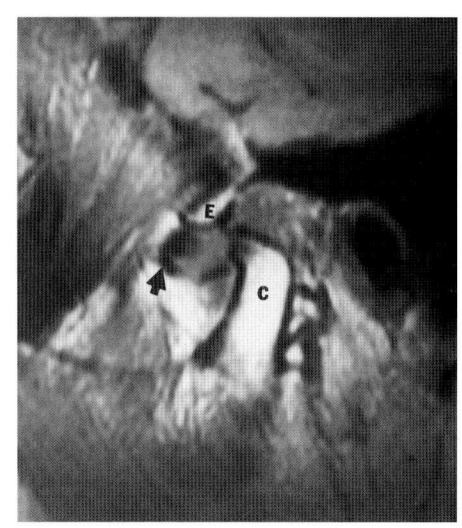

Fig. 5.23 Severe anterior disk displacement without reduction. **a**, **b** Central sagittal T1W MR scans of the TMJ in the closed-mouth (**a**) and open-mouth (**b**) positions; a deformed buckled disk (arrow) that is displaced anteriorly is shown. C = condyle, E = articular eminence. Reproduced from Reference 4 with permission.

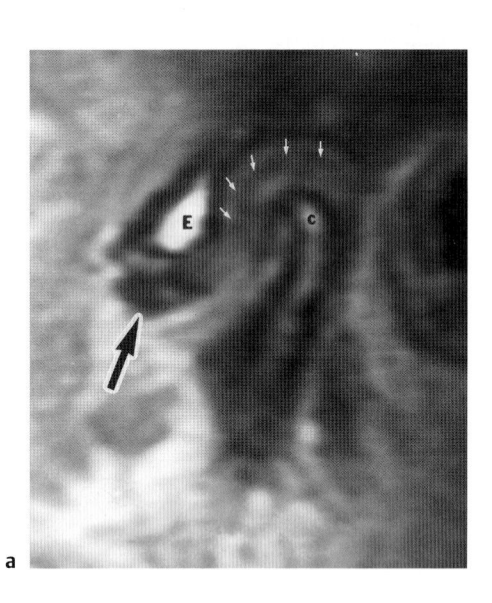

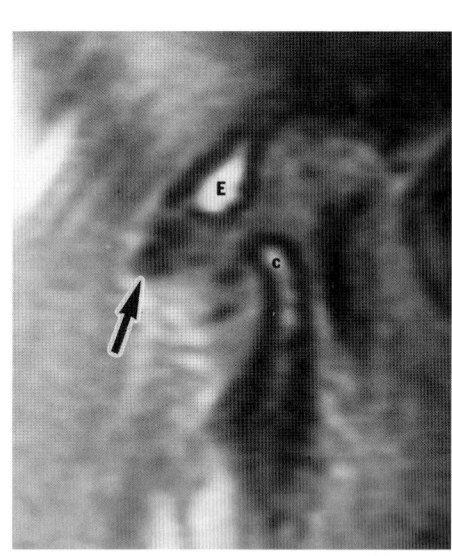

Fig. 5.24 Nonreducing severe disk dislocation with remodeled retrodiskal tissue. Sagittal T1W MR scans of the right TMJ in the closed-mouth (**a**) and open-mouth (**b**) positions, demonstrating a dislocated dumbbell-shaped disk (large arrow), located under the apex of the articular eminence (E). The condyle (C) is relatively thin. The retrodiskal tissue appears considerably thickened under the glenoid fossa. The low signal intensity image indicated by small arrows in Fig. 5.24a, is the remodeled retrodiskal tissue. The intermediate signal intensities superior and inferior to the remodeled retrodiskal tissue represent hypertrophic, reactive fibrosynovial tissue.

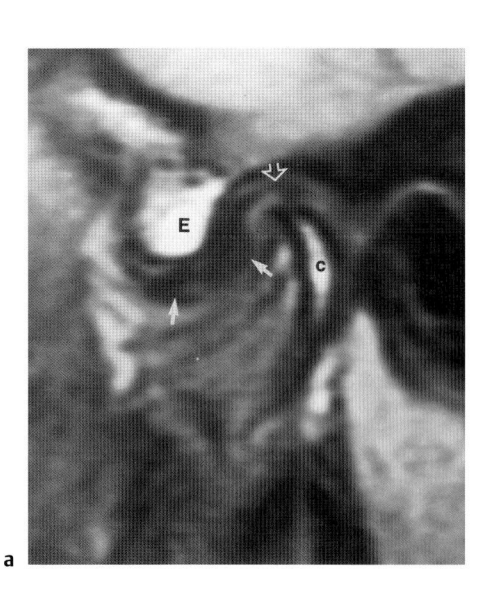

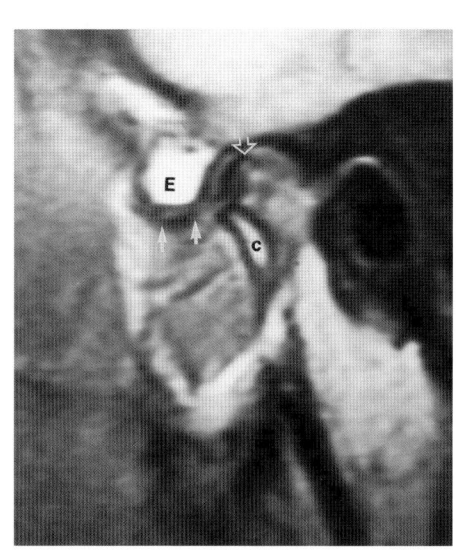

Fig. 5.25 Anterior disk displacement with remodeling of retrodiskal tissue. Central-section sagittal T1W MR scans of the TMJ in the closed-mouth (**a**) and open-mouth (**b**) positions, with a buckled, anteriorly displaced meniscus (solid arrows). The low-intensity signal at the top of the condyle (open arrow) is due to remodeled and fibrotic retrodiskal tissue. c = condyle; E = articular eminence. Reproduced from Reference 4 with permission.

Osteochondritis Dissecans

Osteochondritis dissecans implies a loose body in the joint with a corresponding defect in the condyle or temporal joint component.[6] This condition is rare and may occasionally be seen in the TMJ.[25]

Arthritic Conditions

The TMJ may be afflicted by the same arthritic processes that afflict other joints. Of these, degenerative arthritis and rheumatoid arthritis are most frequently encountered, but cases of posttraumatic arthritis, psoriatic arthritis, and metabolic arthritis (gout and pseudogout) also have been described.[7] The medical management of the arthritic conditions in many cases supersedes surgical management.[2,7]

■ Degenerative Arthritis (Osteoarthritis, Osteoarthrosis)

The diagnosis of osteoarthrosis is based primarily on the clinical and radiographic examinations. Laboratory findings are of little benefit in providing a ruling in this condition. Osteoarthrosis is the most common form of arthritis. Terms used for this condition include *degenerative joint disease* and *osteoarthritis*. It is generally felt that this condition is not inflammatory and that any inflammatory changes are secondarily superimposed as a result of microtrauma or macrotrauma.[2] Osteoarthrosis may be primary or secondary in origin. Primary degenerative osteoarthrosis is caused by the normal joint wear and tear associated with aging and usually begins in the fifth decade.[2,7] The onset is generally insidious, and symptoms are relatively mild.[7] There may be slight cracking or crepitation in the joint, but this usually is not associated with significant pain. Although the arthritic changes occur bilaterally, sometimes only one joint is involved.[7] Secondary osteoarthritis of the TMJ is often seen in 20- to 40-year-old patients and is frequently caused by acute trauma.[2,7] Osteoarthrosis predominantly affects the adult population, peaking in the fourth and fifth decades. Females are affected six times more frequently than males.[2] The disease may afflict younger populations when there are internal derangements and excessive parafunctional habits. In persons younger than 45 years, osteoarthrosis is more commonly noted in the male population. After 45, this predilection reverses.[2] Typically, osteoarthrosis affects other joints such as the hips, feet, knees, and hands. According to Blackwood[26] and Macalister,[27] osteoarthrosis of the TMJ is very common. Their random cadaveric studies confirmed an incidence of 40–69 %. In subsequent studies, however, this incidence was not repeated. Incidence data depend largely on the criteria used for identification of this disease entity. Although the disease process may often be bilateral, patients' complaints are often limited to one side.[2]

Repetitive loading of articulations may result in osteoarthrosis. The parafunctional habits of bruxism and clenching may simulate this excessive loading. The presence of an internal derangement leads to alteration of the forces applied across the condyle and glenoid fossa/eminence. These changes in forces often lead to remodeling of the bony surfaces. The pathogenesis of osteoarthrosis involves the weakening of the functional surface of the articulating elements. The proteoglycan molecules within the cartilage undergo destruction.[2] These molecules are responsible for retention of water and, therefore, indirectly confer the lubricative and protective properties to the cartilage.[2] The effect of the proteoglycan destruction results in a greater absorption of interstitial fluid, resulting in a decreased capacity to resist stress. The remodeling process that ensues results in the radiographic appearance of bone condylar and eminence flattening.[2] One hallmark of the remodeling process is the development of subarticular cysts known as Eli's cysts.[2] The proliferation of bone at the margin of bone resorption may result in osteophytes (Figs. 5.**26**–5.**29**). Rarely, the osteophytes will fracture, creating "joint mice" (Fig. 5.**28**). These are loose bodies within the synovium-lined cavity of the joint. The debris within the joint cavity may lead to secondary inflammation.

Osteoarthrosis tends to pass through several acute and chronic stages in its development.[2] Initially, the disease may demonstrate a slow onset and many patients never complain significantly enough to seek medical advice. Many clinicians have noted asymptomatic advanced condylar and eminence remodeling on routine screening radiographs.[2] During the acute phase, the patient typically demonstrates severe tenderness to palpation over the preauricular region. The masticatory muscles may also demonstrate some spasm or tenderness, secondary to parafunctional habit. The process of osteoarthrosis tends to become quiescent with age as bony remodeling becomes more significant.[2] Unlike in rheumatoid arthritis, morning stiffness is not a common feature of this disease process, and no laboratory findings are specifically indicative of the disease process.

The earliest radiographic feature of degenerative arthritis of the TMJ, whether primary or secondary, is subchondral sclerosis of the condyle.[28] If the condition progresses, flattening of the condyle, osteophytes (marginal lipping), increased sclerotic changes, narrowing of the joint space, and flattening of the eminence may be noted (Figs. 5.**26**–5.**28**).[7] Often, there are concurrent internal derangements. Intra-/extra-articular calcifications (joint mice) as well as disk calcification may be present (Fig. 5.**29**). The undermining of articular surface by the remodeling process may result in subcortical bone cysts, seen as radiolucent areas (Eli's cysts) (Fig. 5.**27**). Although the changes in the

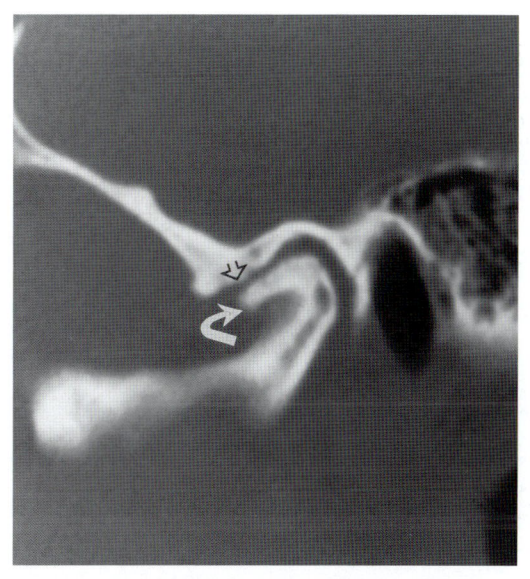

Fig. 5.**26** Degenerative arthritis of the TMJ. Direct sagittal CT scan shows flattening of the mandibular condyle, anterior lipping (curved arrow), and deformity, as well as flattening of the articular eminence (open arrow). Reproduced from Reference 4 with permission.

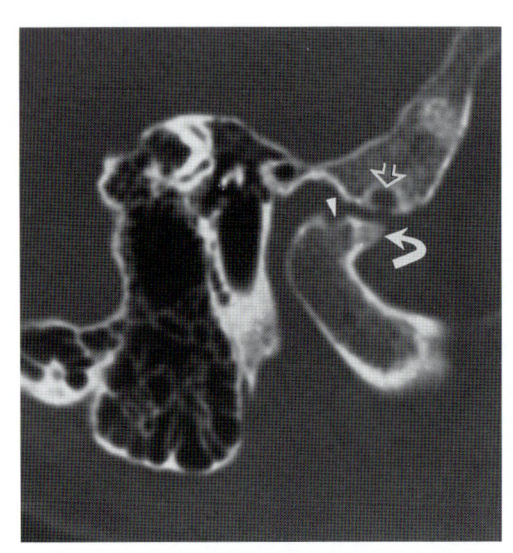

Fig. 5.**27** Degenerative arthritis of the TMJ. Direct sagittal CT scan shows subcortical erosion of the condyle (arrowhead), marginal osteophyte (curved arrow), and subcortical cyst formation (open arrow) involving the articular eminence. Reproduced from Reference 4 with permission.

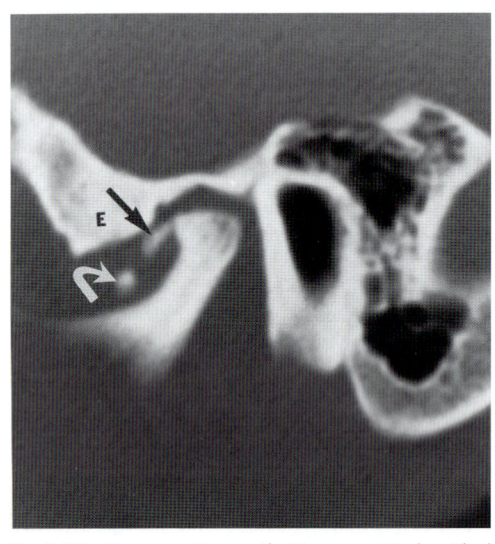

Fig. 5.**28** Degenerative arthritis associated with loose body. Direct sagittal CT scan shows flattening of the mandibular condyle and glenoid fossa, anterior marginal osteophyte (black arrow), and an intra-articular calcification (loose body) (white arrow). Note increased sclerosis of the anterior articular eminence (E). Reproduced from Reference 4 with permission.

glenoid fossa generally are not as severe as those in the condyle, cortical erosion can sometimes be present. Narrowing of the joint space usually indicates degenerative changes in the articular disk.[7] In the early stages of the disease, radiographic changes are not present, and it is believed that technetium bone scanning is a more sensitive imaging technique. Treatment of osteoarthrosis is aimed at obtaining symptomatic relief until the process essentially "burns out." The patient must be educated as to the nature of the disease process. Treatment includes medical therapy, physical therapy, appliance therapy, and, rarely, surgery.[2,6,27] Surgery may involve diskoplasty, diskectomy, and/or arthroplasty.[2] Gap arthroplasty is performed when ankylosis is present (Figs. 5.**30**, 5.**31**).

▪ Traumatic Arthritis

Traumatic arthritis represents the immediate intra-articular response to injury of the TMJ. The resultant inflammation and occasional hemarthrosis result in pain, joint tenderness, loss of tooth contact on the affected side, and limitation of jaw movement.[2] At this stage, CT is the modality of choice to evaluate the TMJ, since there may be an intracapsular fracture present.[2,4] A hemarthrosis of the TMJ is seen on CT as an increased size of the joint space.[4] The density of the blood may not be higher than the density of the periarticular soft tissues or the density of adjacent muscles.[4] MRI is more specific in detecting hemarthrosis (acute or chronic). If an internal derangement is present, MR imaging will show the anterior position of the intra-articular disk.[7] In patients who have severe TMJ trauma, evidence of degenerative arthritis may eventually be present.

▪ Rheumatoid Arthritis

Rheumatoid arthritis (RA) is a chronic systemic disease of unknown etiology, manifested primarily by inflammatory arthritis of the peripheral joints. The serum and joint fluid of the majority of patients with RA contain antibodies specific for immunoglobulin G (IgG; rheumatoid factor).[2] Rheumatoid arthritis may affect the TMJ. When it does, it typically involves other small joints of the body. The disease is usually bilateral, symmetric, and polyarticular. Rarely does the disease remain monoarticular.

According to Tabeling and Dolwick,[29] approximately 50% of patients with rheumatoid arthritis present with complaints of TMJ dysfunction, which range from mild joint stiffness to ankylosis of the joint. In the child, significant effects on skeletal facial growth patterns may result.[2] The clinical course of rheumatoid arthritis is variable and may range from a pauciarticular form to a relentless progressive polyarthritic disease. The most destructive arthritic form of the disease tends to occur in patients with high titers of rheumatoid factors. Articular involvement is typically manifested with the onset of pain, morning stiffness, limitation of joint motion, and signs of inflammation. Pain is typically exacerbated with joint motion. The stiffness secondary to rheumatoid arthritis is believed to occur secondarily to synovial membrane congestion, thickening of the joint capsule, and joint effusions. Although, initially, the limitation of motion is secondary to inflammatory changes, later fibrosis, muscle contracture, and bony or fibrous ankylosis are responsible for the restrictions in joint motion.

Steinbrocker et al.[30] classified the progression of arthritis by four stages: stage I (early), stage II (moderate), stage III (severe), and stage IV (terminal). Radiographically, stage I disease demonstrates osteoporosis. Stage II rheumatoid arthritis demonstrates soft-tissue changes such as nodules and tenosynovitis without joint deformity. Osteoporosis is present with or without slight subcondylar bone destruction. Stage III results in destruction of the cartilage and bone with joint deformity and without fibrous or bony ankylosis. Stage IV demonstrates fibrous or bony ankylosis. Condylar destruction, narrowing of the joint space, anterior positioning of the condylar head, flattening of the articular eminence, erosion of the roof of the glenoid fossa, and osteophytic formation may be noted. The mandibular rami shorten in length, and the patient may demonstrate posterior malocclusion secondary to loss of vertical dimension.[2]

The main objectives of treatment are relief of pain, preservation of joint and muscle function, and preservation of facial form.[31-33] Ankylosis of the TMJ is typically treated with a gap arthroplasty to create a pseudoarthrosis.

Juvenile rheumatoid arthritis is a chronic synovial inflammatory disease that is relatively common in children;[2] an eponym for this disease is Still disease. When juvenile rheumatoid arthritis affects the TMJ, one is principally concerned by its effect on growth. Severe micrognathia with retrogenia may develop.

Juvenile rheumatoid arthritis apparently has three subtypes: systemic onset disease (20%), polyarticular (40%), and pauciarticular (40%). There is some controversy as to the preferred mode of classification.[2] In the systemic subtype, the sex ratio is approximately equal. Rheumatoid factor and anti-nuclear antibodies are negative.[2] Children present with high fevers, rash, generalized lymphadenopathy, hepatosplenomegaly, leukocytosis, and anemia.[2] The systemic manifestations occur for several months and recur in approximately 50% of patients. Chronic polyarthritis develops in patients several months following the systemic manifestations. When the TMJ is affected, it may present as a unilateral or bilateral disease. Early intervention with joint transplantation or reconstruction is required in many patients.[2] The bone grafting is typically performed in association with a gap arthroplasty to release ankylosis.

Radiographic Findings

Because rheumatoid arthritis begins as a chronic inflammatory disease of the synovial tissues, there initially may not be any osseous changes seen radiographically.[32] As the condition progresses, however, about 50–80% of patients show bilateral evidence of demineralization, condylar flattening, and erosion.[33] The erosion occurs most frequently on the anterosuperior aspect of the condyle. Later, the cortical outlines of the condyle and glenoid fossa become increasingly irregular (Fig. 5.**32**). As the destruction progresses, the loss in vertical dimension can lead to an anterior open bite.[7] Gadolinium-enhanced MR study is very effective in demonstrating the proliferating synovium of rheumatoid arthritis of the TMJ (Fig. 5.**32c**).

■ Metabolic Arthritis

Metabolic arthritis, which can accompany gout (uric acid arthritis) or pseudogout (calcium pyrophosphate dihydrate arthropathy, chondrocalcinosis), is rare in the TMJ.[7] It occurs most frequently in men over 40 years of age. The attacks are usually sudden, and the joint becomes painful, swollen, red, and tender. Recovery may occur in a few days, and remission can last for months to years.[2,7] Calcified areas in the disk (Fig. 5.**29**), destruction of the hard tissues of the joint, exostoses, and spurring have been reported.[7] The TMJ may be affected by other arthritic conditions such as systemic lupus, Reiter syndrome, and Lyme disease. The radiographic findings may be similar in all these conditions. They include osteoporosis, erosive changes of the condyle and eminence, calcifications of the articular disk, subchondral cysts, sclerosis of the articular surfaces, narrowing of the joint space, and ankylosis.[7] These disease entities have no specific radiographic findings.

■ Rheumatoid Variants (Ankylosing Spondylitis, Psoriatic Arthritis)

Ankylosing spondylitis is a condition that typically results in spinal fusion. Males are considered to have a more symptomatic and severe presentation. Several arthritic conditions have been lumped together in a category called *seronegative spondylarthropathies*. Ankylosing spondylitis serves as the prototype of this category.[2] Other arthritic conditions included in the spondylarthropathies include psoriatic arthropathy, Reiter syndrome, reactive arthropathies, and juvenile chronic polyarthropathy.[2] Synonyms for ankylosing spondylitis include Marie–Strümpell disease and rheumatoid spondylitis.[2] Ankylosing spondylitis, however, does not demonstrate rheumatoid factor in the serum and clinically rheumatoid nodules are absent. The hallmark of this disease process is sacroiliitis. The articular symptoms result from inflammation of the synovial tissues and insertions of ligaments and tendons followed by ossification that leads to fusion of adjacent vertebrae and fixation of the back in extreme flexion, resulting in limitation of chest movement and respiratory impairment.[2,7] TMJ involvement usually occurs several years after the onset of the disease in about one-third of all patients.[34] The TMJ has been reported to be involved in as many as 50% of cases. Similar to the presentation of sacroiliitis, TMJ involvement manifests with pain, morning stiffness that improves with exercise, and ankylosis. The radiographic findings generally are similar to those seen in rheumatoid arthritis (adult), with evidence of erosive changes in the condyle and glenoid fossa.[7] When the joint is severely affected, subchondral sclerosis and narrowing of the joint space with ankylosis and florid osteophytic response may be noted.

Psoriatic Arthritis of the TMJ

Psoriatic arthritis is seen in a small percentage of patients, more often female than male, with long-standing cutaneous psoriasis. The metatarsophalangeal and interphalangeal joints of the fingers and toes are the most frequently affected. Some temporal relationship has been recognized between nail and joint involvement. When the TMJ is involved, presentation is typically unilateral.[7] Ankylosis may develop. Initially, there may be a widening of the interarticular spaces and subchondral cyst formation as a result of cartilage destruction. Later, bony ankylosis may occur.[2] The radiographic findings are generally similar to rheumatoid arthritis.[7]

Ankylosis/Hypomobility Conditions

Conditions resulting in hypomobility of the temporomandibular articulation include ankylosis (fibrous or bony) (Figs. 5.**29**, 5.**30**); postoperative scarring within the masticatory muscles following jaw reconstruction surgery; unilateral or bilateral coronoid hypertrophy; impingement of the coronoid process by a medially displaced fractured zygoma; fractured condyle; masticatory muscle spasm; acute closed lock; internal derangements; fascial space infection; and suppurative arthritis. Other arthritis-related conditions include neoplasms of the condyle or adjacent tissues; and myositis ossificans (see Fig. 5.**34c**).[2]

TMJ ankylosis is a sign of a disease rather than a specific disease entity, as it can have a number of different causes.[7] It may be partial or complete, fibrous or bony, unilateral or bilateral, and intra-articular (true) or extra-articular (false).[7] Chronic limitation of movement due to involvement of muscles of mastication or adjacent parts of the mandible is referred to as false ankylosis. Ankylosis rarely results in total inability to open the mouth. Even with complete bony ankylosis there usually is enough flexibility of the bone to permit limited opening.[7] The final distinction between fibrous and bony ankylosis therefore depends on the radiographic findings.

The treatment of TMJ ankylosis is surgical. True TMJ ankylosis is an intra-articular process characterized by fibrous or bony ankylosis between the mandibular condyle and the base of the skull (Fig. 5.**30**). Causative factors traditionally identified are

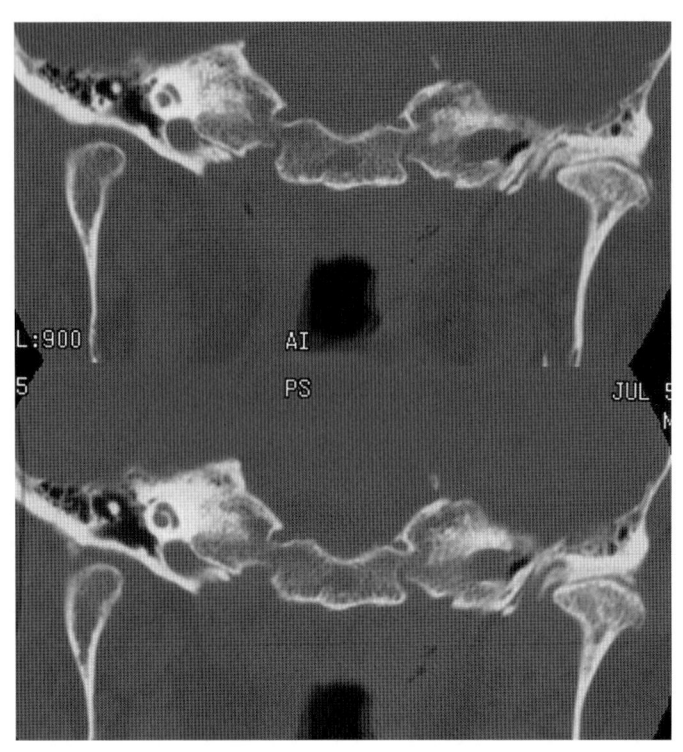

Fig. 5.**29** Degenerative arthritis associated with calcification of the TMJ disk. Coronal CT scans show degenerative changes of the left TMJ. Note marked calcification of the left disk.

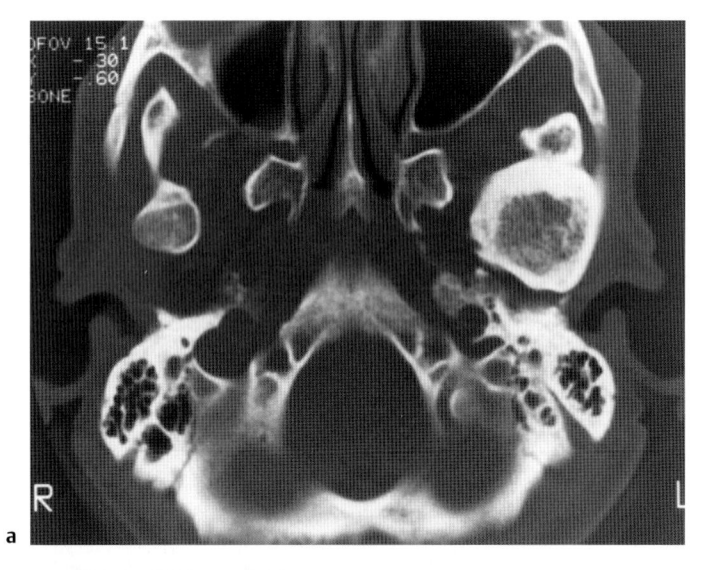

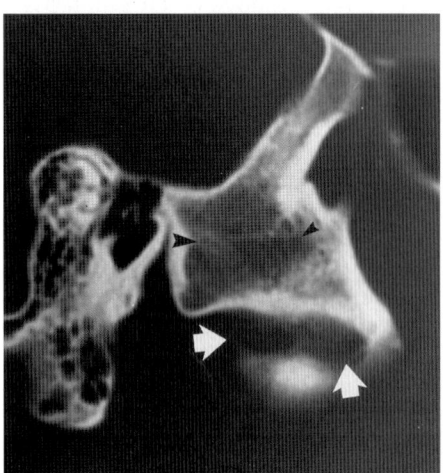

trauma, inflammation, and infection; congenital; and unknown. Accurate determination of the cause of the ankylosis is difficult because a 10-year delay usually elapses between the onset of the condition and the time the patient seeks corrective therapy.[2] This time lapse adversely affects the patient's ability to accurately recall factors involved in the initiation of the process. Trauma has been implicated as the causative factor in 26–75% of cases of ankylosis.[2] Any trauma that initiates intra-articular bleeding of the TMJ may be followed by fibrosis and eventually bony ankylosis of the joint. Bony ankylosis is more likely to occur when the disk and its attachments are disrupted. Trauma directed at the symphysis is most common.

Approximately half of rheumatoid arthritic patients experience some limitation in opening their jaws. Patients with stage IV rheumatoid arthritis will often present with bilateral ankylosis. According to Davidson et al.[35] in Marie–Strümpell disease or ankylosis spondylitis, the TMJ was involved in 11.5% of 100 patients studied.

Otitis externa, otitis media, mastoiditis, and *osteomyelitis* of the temporal bone particularly in diabetic patients with necrotizing external otitis can directly extend into the TMJ and, if not treated on time and appropriately, may result in ankylosis. Anachoresis (the preferential collection or deposits of particles at a certain site, as of bacteria or of metals that have localized out of the bloodstream in areas of inflammation; also called the *anachoretic effect*) of bacteria to an arthritic joint following scarlet fever, typhoid fever, gonorrhea, and tuberculosis has on occasion been reported, resulting in the long-term in TMJ ankylosis.[2] Congenital or infantile ankylosis has been reported. Trauma or infection in the neonatal period may be involved in these cases (Fig. 5.**15**). Patients may develop ankylosis if they do not regain normal range of motion following arthrotomy. A significant number of cases of TMJ ankylosis have an unknown cause.[2]

Ankylosis most often occurs unilaterally. Patients experience varying degrees of limitation in the mobility of the jaws. In unilateral ankylosis, deviation in opening to the affected side usually occurs. Despite even a bilateral bony ankylosis, patients may exhibit a mouth opening secondary to pull of the suprahyoid musculature and the inherent elasticity of the mandible.[2] When the ankylosis occurs in the growing child, a facial deformity occurs as a result of micrognathia of the mandible. Antegonial notching and reduced vertical ramus growth develop. Bilateral ankylosis may result in an open-bite deformity, compensatory maxillary hyperplasia, micrognathia with microgenia, and a "bird face" appearance.[2] Other common dental findings include neglected caries and/or open bite.[2]

Radiographic Findings

Ankylosis caused by fibrous union of the condyle and glenoid fossa cannot be detected radiographically, although there may be some changes in the soft tissue such as calcification, increased contrast enhancement, narrowing of joint space, changes in bone morphology, and limitation of motion during open mouth position that could make one suspect this possibility. With bony

◁ Fig. 5.**30** TMJ bony ankylosis. **a** Axial and **b** sagittal CT scans of a 34-year-old woman. Ankylosis developed following a traumatic incident at the age of 2 years. Note marked deformity of the left condyle and bilateral deformed mandibular rami. Note the surgical procedure of creation of a gap in the ramus (white arrows). The gap is incomplete anteriorly. For gap arthroplasty to be successful, it must be carried out through the ramus and be approximately 5–10 mm in width in its entirety. Note the site of fusions of deformed condyle to the hypertrophic deformed glenoid fossa (black arrowheads).

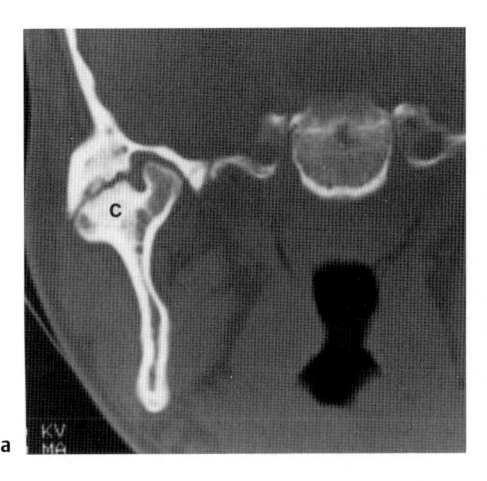

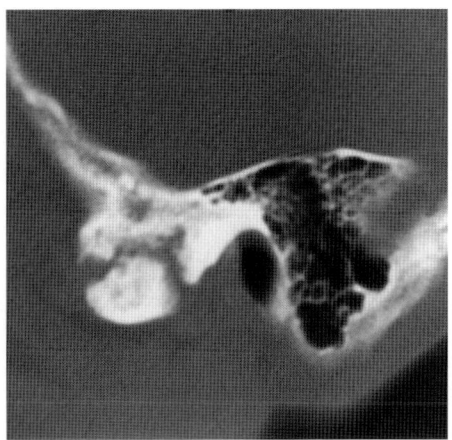

Fig. 5.**31** TMJ ankylosis. **a** Coronal and **b** sagittal CT scans showing marked deformity of right mandibular condyle (C), marked deformity of right glenoid fossa and intra-articular calcification compatible with bony ankylosis.

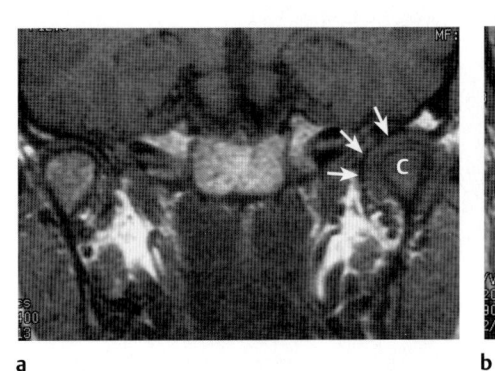

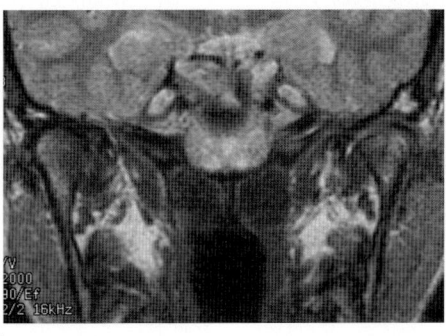

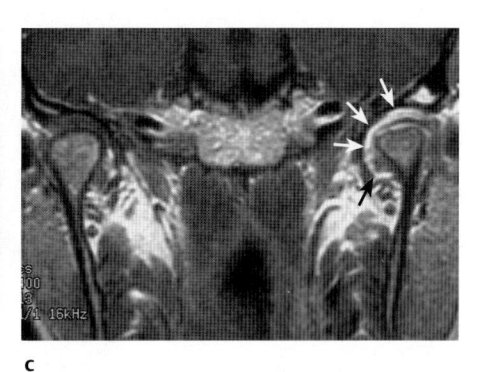

Fig. 5.**32** Rheumatoid arthritis. **a** Coronal T1W MR scan shows increased soft-tissue thickening of the left TMJ (arrows). Note hypointensity of the left mandibular condyle marrow space (C). **b** Coronal T2W MR scan shows hyperintensity of the left TMJ, related to synovial hypertrophy and inflammatory edema. **c** Coronal enhanced T1W MR scan shows increased enhancement of the left TMJ due to synovial hypertrophy and panus formation (arrows).

ankylosis, the joint space is partially or completely obliterated by calcification (Figs. 5.**30**, 5.**31**). In some cases there may be a large, bony mass with marked sclerosis of the condyle and glenoid fossa (Fig. 5.**30**).

CT images obtained in sagittal, coronal, and axial views are imperative to determine the precise extent of the ankylosis (Figs. 5.**30**, 5.**31**). From CT images one can, however, often determine reliably the precise nature of the ankylosis, fibrous or bony. The radiolucent region between the ankylosed segments may represent osteoid or immature bone. CT images are important in the evaluation of the mediolateral extent of the ankylosis and in determining the appropriate site for the arthroplasty. Three-dimensional CT offers additional advantages in obtaining a proper perspective.

The purpose of surgery is to create a gap or pseudoarthrosis at or near the site of ankylosis (Fig. 5.**30**). Immediate or secondary growth-center transplantation is necessary in the growing child. In the adult, the gap may be filled with an autograft or alloplast to maintain the gap so as to prevent re-ankylosis.[2, 36]

■ Synovial Chondromatosis

Synovial chondromatosis is a rare, benign joint disorder characterized by metaplasia of the synovium with the formation of numerous foci of cellular hyaline cartilage.[4, 37] These foci may detach from the synovium and become loose bodies within the joint space, and they may also calcify. The disease is usually monoarticular, is of unknown origin, and occurs most often in larger joints such as the knee, shoulder, and hip.[4, 37] Synovial chondromatosis of TMJ was first described by Axhausen in 1933, and it has been reported to occur in individuals ranging from age 18 to 75 years, with a mean age of 46 years.[4, 37] There is a predilection for women. It is a benign disease, although chondrosarcoma has been reported to develop in association with synovial chondromatosis. Such cases probably represent a primary tumor. None of these cases involved the TMJ. The clinical findings of synovial chondromatosis of TMJ include pain, restriction of mandibular movement, and, often, preauricular swelling.[4, 37] Radiographic findings of synovial chondromatosis of the TMJ include widening of the joint space, the presence of calcified loose bodies, and erosive and sclerotic changes in the condyle and glenoid fossa (Fig. 5.**33**). These findings are not specific for synovial chondromatosis; all or some of them may be seen in patients with degenerative arthritis (Fig. 5.**28**). Radiopaque loose bodies in the TMJ are not pathognomonic for synovial chondromatosis and can be found in patients with other disorders, such as degenerative arthritis (Fig. 5.**28**), osteochondritis dissecans,[6] condylar fracture, myositis ossificans (Fig. 5.**34c**), granulomatous (tuberculous) arthritis, rheumatoid arthritis, and neuropathic arthropathy.[4] CT has been helpful in the diagnosis of synovial chondromatosis, because it identifies intra-articular as well as extra-articular calcifications that are not seen on conventional radiography (Figs. 5.**33**, 5.**34**). Erosion and sclerosis of the condyle and glenoid fossa can best be evaluated by CT scans (Fig. 5.**33a**). Expansion of the joint capsule and the presence of fluid

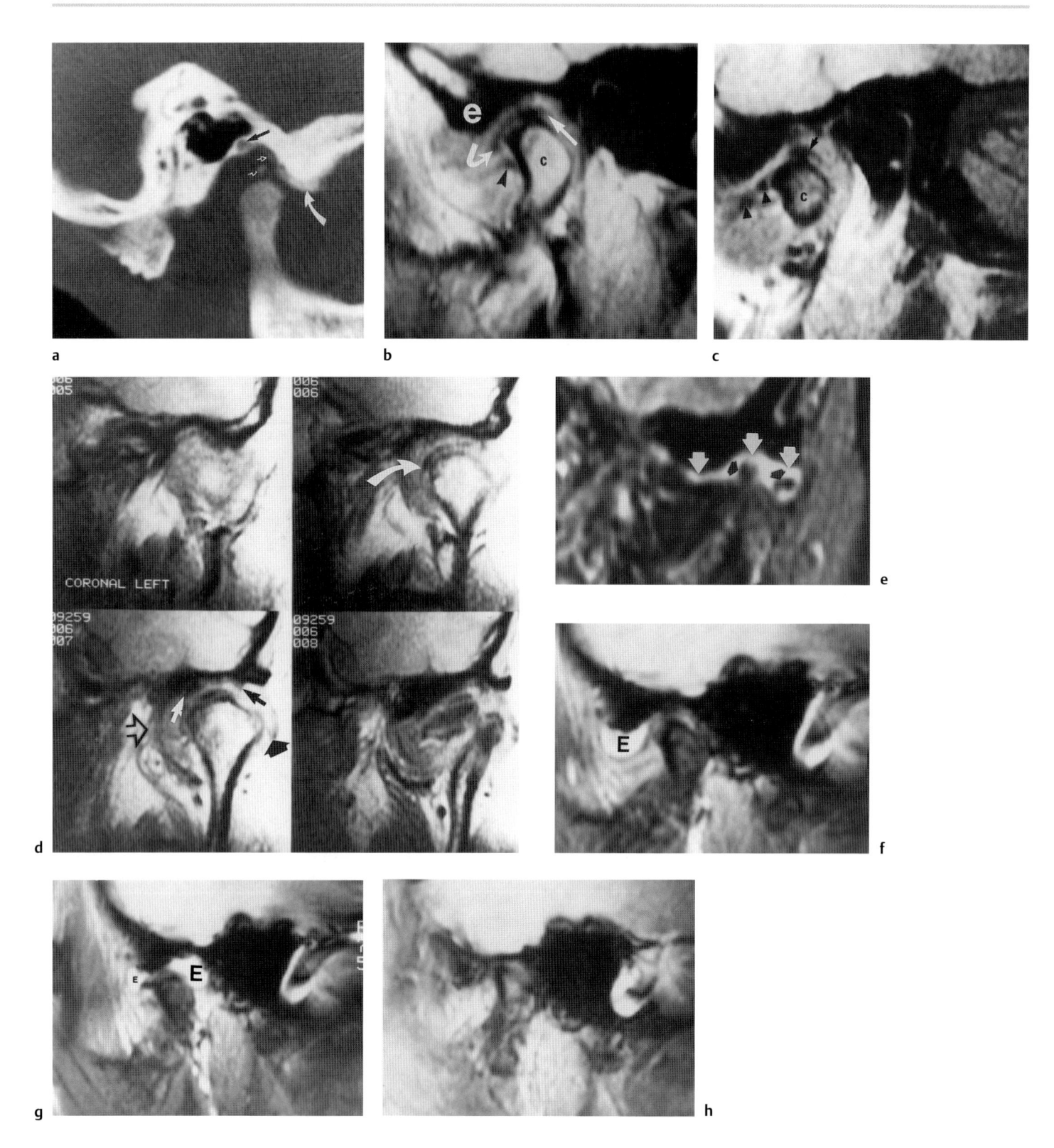

Fig. 5.**33** Synovial chondromatosis. **a** Direct sagittal CT scan of the left TMJ, obtained with the mouth closed, shows widening of the joint, apparently by a soft-tissue or joint effusion. Note irregular outline of the mandibular condyle and glenoid fossa, irregular calcifications along the inferior margin of the articular eminence (curved arrow), calcifications within the joint space (small white arrows), and focal erosion of the glenoid fossa (black arrow). **b** Sagittal T1W MR scan of the left TMJ, obtained with the mouth closed, shows moderate widening of the joint space. The disk (arrows) is irregular, but its position is normal. Note an intra-articular hypointense area (arrowhead) within the anterior joint space, related to a calcification (loose body). **c** Sagittal T1W MR scan of the left TMJ, same patient as in Fig. 5.**33a,b**, obtained with mouth open. Note the disk (arrow), and hypointense loose bodies (arrowheads). C = condyle. **d** This series of coronal T1W MR scans of the left TMJ, obtained with the mouth closed, shows marked expansion of the joint capsule (open arrow and wide black arrow) and a few areas of hypointensity in the superior joint space (small arrows), related to loose bodies. The disk is seen as a hypointense curvilinear band (curved arrow in the top right panel). **e** This coronal T2W MR scan of the left TMJ, obtained with the mouth closed, shows hyperintense fluid within the joint space (white arrows) and hypointense loose bodies (black arrows). Note the expansion of the joint capsule as a result of joint effusion. **f** Gradient-echo (GRASS) sagittal MR scan of the left TMJ, obtained with the mouth closed, shows hyperintense effusion (exudate) (E) in the anterior joint spaces. **g** Gradient-echo (GRASS) sagittal MR scan of the left TMJ, obtained with the mouth open, shows hyperintense effusion (E) in the anterior and posterior joint spaces. **h** Gradient-echo sagittal MR scan of the right TMJ shows a normal right TMJ with no evidence of significant effusion in the joint.

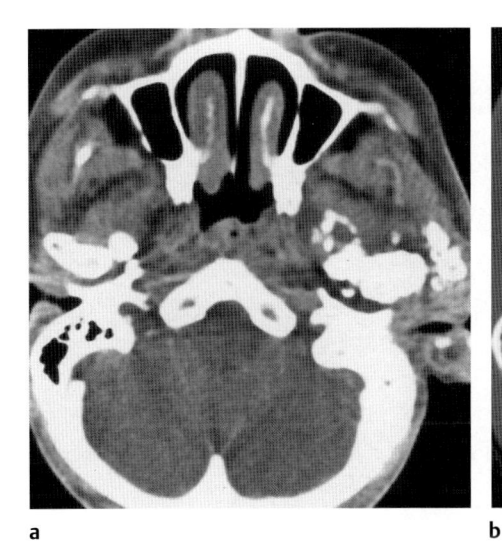

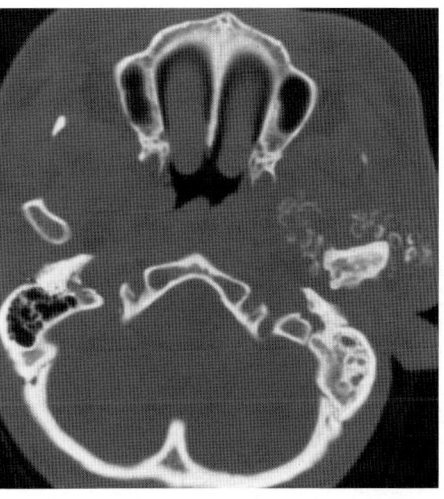

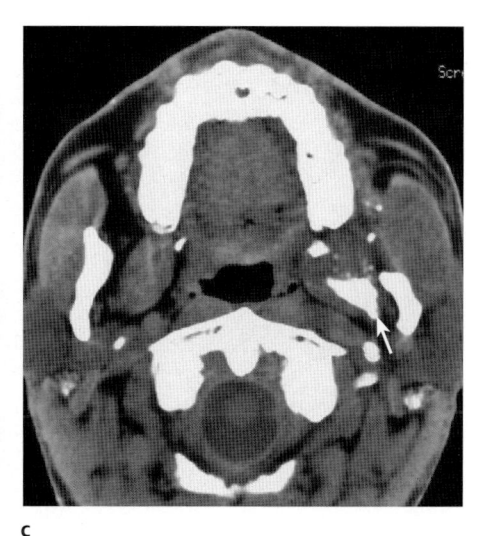

Fig. 5.**34a, b** Synovial chondromatosis. **a** Axial CT scan shows the presence of synovial/cartilage calcified loose bodies, medial, lateral, and anterior to the condyle. The condyle is irregular and sclerotic. **b** Axial CT (bone window); the irregular calcified loose bodies are more precisely delineated. **c** Myositis ossificans. Axial CT scan in another patient shows posttraumatic myositis ossificans of the left medial pterygoid muscle (arrow). Note posttraumatic deformity of the left mandibular ramus.

within the joint cavity are common findings in patients with synovial chondromatosis, and these findings can best be delineated by MRI (Fig. 5.33).

Calcified synovial bodies are best seen on CT scans. Fluid accumulation is best seen on magnetic resonance gradient echo and T2-weighted MR images (Figs. 5.33e–g). Significant joint capsular expansion can occur, corresponding to clinically observed facial swelling. The expansion is due to fluid accumulation and thickening of the capsular tissues. The expansion of the capsule can be so significant that the infratemporal fossa and middle cranial fossa are encroached on. Most cases of synovial chondromatosis have been treated with arthrotomy, disectomy, and synovectomy. It is unclear whether arthroscopy can effectively eradicate this condition.

■ Neoplasms

The TMJ is rarely affected by tumors, either benign or malignant. The actual incidence of benign and malignant tumors affecting the TMJ is difficult to determine because of the paucity of cases reported in the literature. Chondroma, osteochondroma, and osteoma are the most common benign tumors of the TMJ; however, osteoid osteoma,[38] myxoma, fibromyxoma (Fig. 5.**35a**), chondromyxoid fibroma, chondroblastoma, osteoblastoma (Figs. 5.**35b–d**), giant-cell tumor (osteoclastoma) (Figs. 5.**36**–5.**38**), central reparative giant-cell granuloma, schwannoma (see Fig. 9.**105**), Langerhans cell histiocytosis (Fig. 5.**39**), synovial hemangioma, and metastasis have also been reported.[2,7] Fibrosarcoma, chondrosarcoma (Figs. 5.**40**, 5.**41**), and synovial sarcoma are the most common malignancies that involve the TMJ;[2,7] however, malignancies of the parotid gland or adjacent structures, such as the external ear canal, may spread into the TMJ.

Malignant tumors include chondrosarcoma, synovial cell sarcoma, osteosarcoma, rhabdomyosarcoma, malignant schwannoma, lymphoma including multiple myeloma, and metastasis. The synovial cell sarcoma typically occurs remote from a synovial joint. Head and neck cases have occurred within the soft tissues of the cheek more frequently than within the TMJ proper. Multiple myeloma may present as a lytic region in the condyle or simply as an osteoporotic pattern. This latter pattern, if isolated, can be misdiagnosed for a normal condylar fovea. Metastases to the TMJ are rare. They typically affect the condyle. Most metastatic neoplasms are carcinomas, specifically, adenocarcinoma. Metastatic lesions from prostate, breast, lung, colon, and thyroid cancers have been reported.

Radiographic Findings

Benign lesions such as osteoma, osteoblastoma, and osteochondroma produce enlargement of the condyle. Osteoma affecting the condyle has been reported. This entity is difficult to differentiate from enostosis, exostosis, osteochondroma, or osteoblastoma. Lind and Hillerstrom[38] reported an osteoid osteoma in the mandibular condyle. Osteochondroma tends to demonstrate growth in a superoinferior direction. Osteoblastoma tends to demonstrate growth in a lateromedial direction. Other benign entities include chondroblastoma, chondromyxoid fibroma, benign giant-cell tumor, and central reparative giant-cell granuloma. More recently, the giant-cell lesion has been reported in association with the Proplast Teflon implants. These lesions are truly foreign body reactions to microparticulate matter.[2]

Giant-cell tumors destroy bones of the glenoid fossa and adjacent condyle (Figs. 5.**36**–5.**38**). Osteoma, osteoblastoma, and osteochondroma appear hypointense on T2-weighted MR images (Fig. 5.**35c**). The nonmineralized portion of these tumors, similar to other benign fibro-osseous lesions, such as fibrous dysplasia and ossifying fibroma, show moderate to marked contrast enhancement on enhanced T1-weighted MR images (Fig. 5.**35d**). Giant-cell tumors have heterogeneous signal characteristics, particularly on T2-weighted MR images, with areas of hypointensity and hyperintensity due to hemorrhage. The solid components of giant-cell tumors show moderate to marked contrast enhancement on enhanced T1-weighted MR images. Chondroblastoma of the TMJ, similarly to other chondroblastomas, may show significant contrast enhancement on enhanced T1-weighted MR images (Fig. 5.**42**). Malignant tumors of the TMJ usually destroy the bone and produce defects with irregular margins.

Pigmented Villonodular Synovitis

Pigmented villonodular synovitis (PVNS) is a term given to a group of benign, locally invasive lesions of the synovium of joints, bursae, and tendon sheaths.[39,40] Involvement of the TMJ is

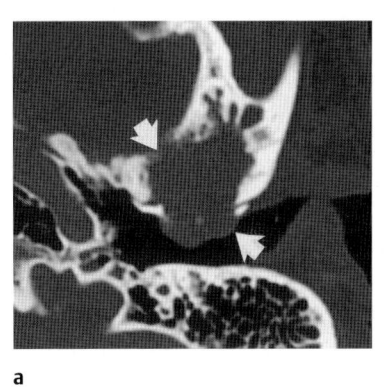

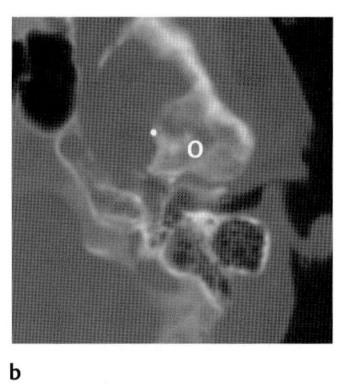

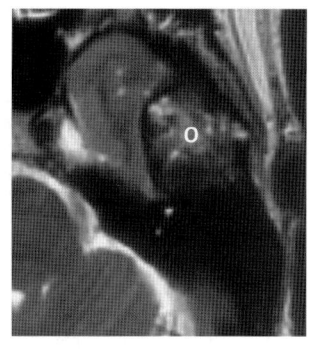

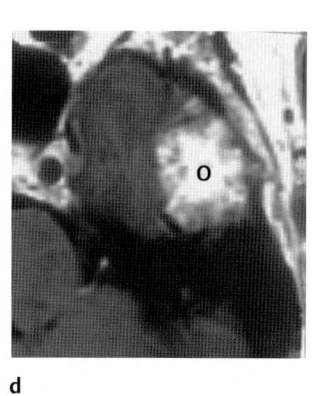

Fig. 5.35 Fibromyxoma. **a** Axial CT scan shows an expansile destructive mass (arrows), involving the left TMJ, extending into the external auditory canal. Case courtesy of Dr. G. Lee, Kansas City, MO, USA.
b–d Osteoblastoma of the temporal bone involving left TMJ. **b** Axial unenhanced CT scan shows an expansile mass involving the squamous portion of the left temporal bone (O). Note moderate mineralization within the tumor. **c, d** Axial T2W (**c**) and enhanced T1W (**d**) MR scans. The mass is heterogeneous in T2W and shows marked enhancement on enhanced T1W.

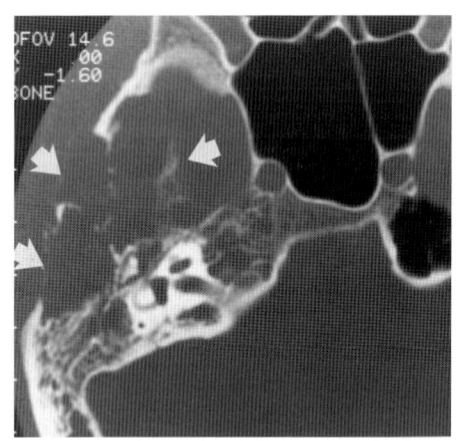

Fig. 5.36 Giant-cell tumor (osteoclastoma). Axial CT scan shows destructive lesion (arrows) involving the squamous portion of the right temporal bone, where it contributes to the TMJ region.

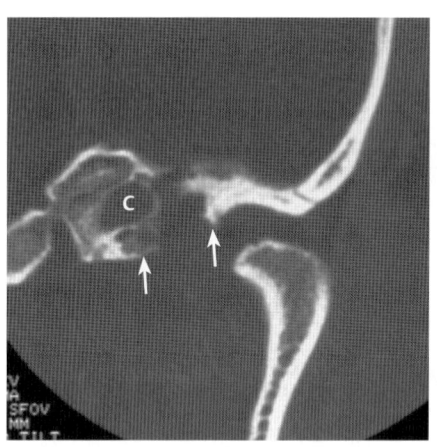

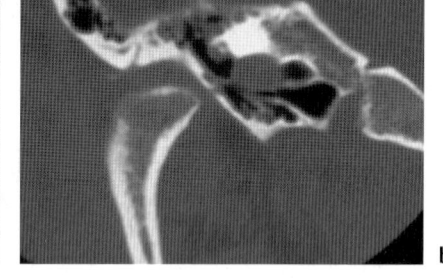

Fig. 5.37 Giant-cell tumor (osteoclastoma). **a** Coronal CT scan shows a lytic lesion (arrows), involving the undersurface of the left petrous temporal bone, adjacent to the TMJ region. C = carotid canal. **b** Coronal CT scan of the normal right side for comparison.

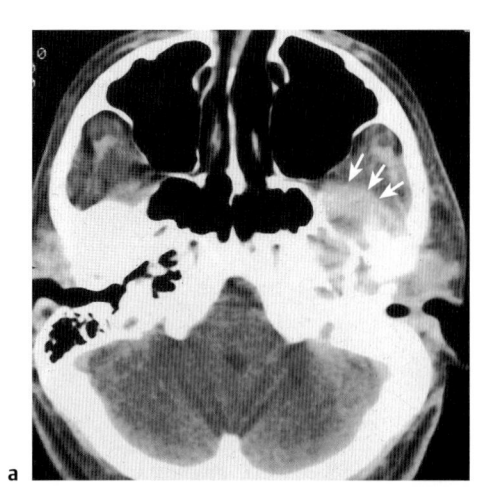

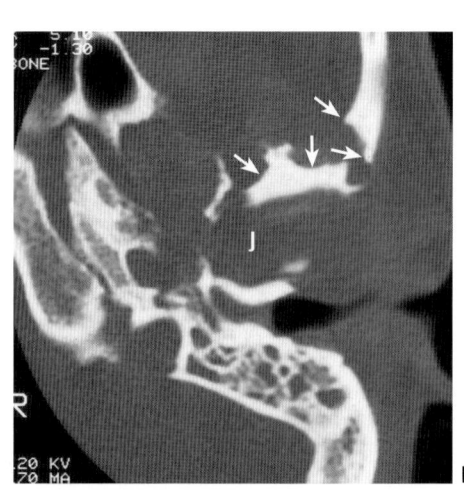

Fig. 5.38 Giant-cell tumor (osteoclastoma). **a** Enhanced axial CT scan shows an enhancing mass (arrows) involving the left skull base, adjacent to the left TMJ region. **b** Axial CT scan shows bone destruction in the region of left TMJ (arrows), along with increased soft tissue within the joint (J).

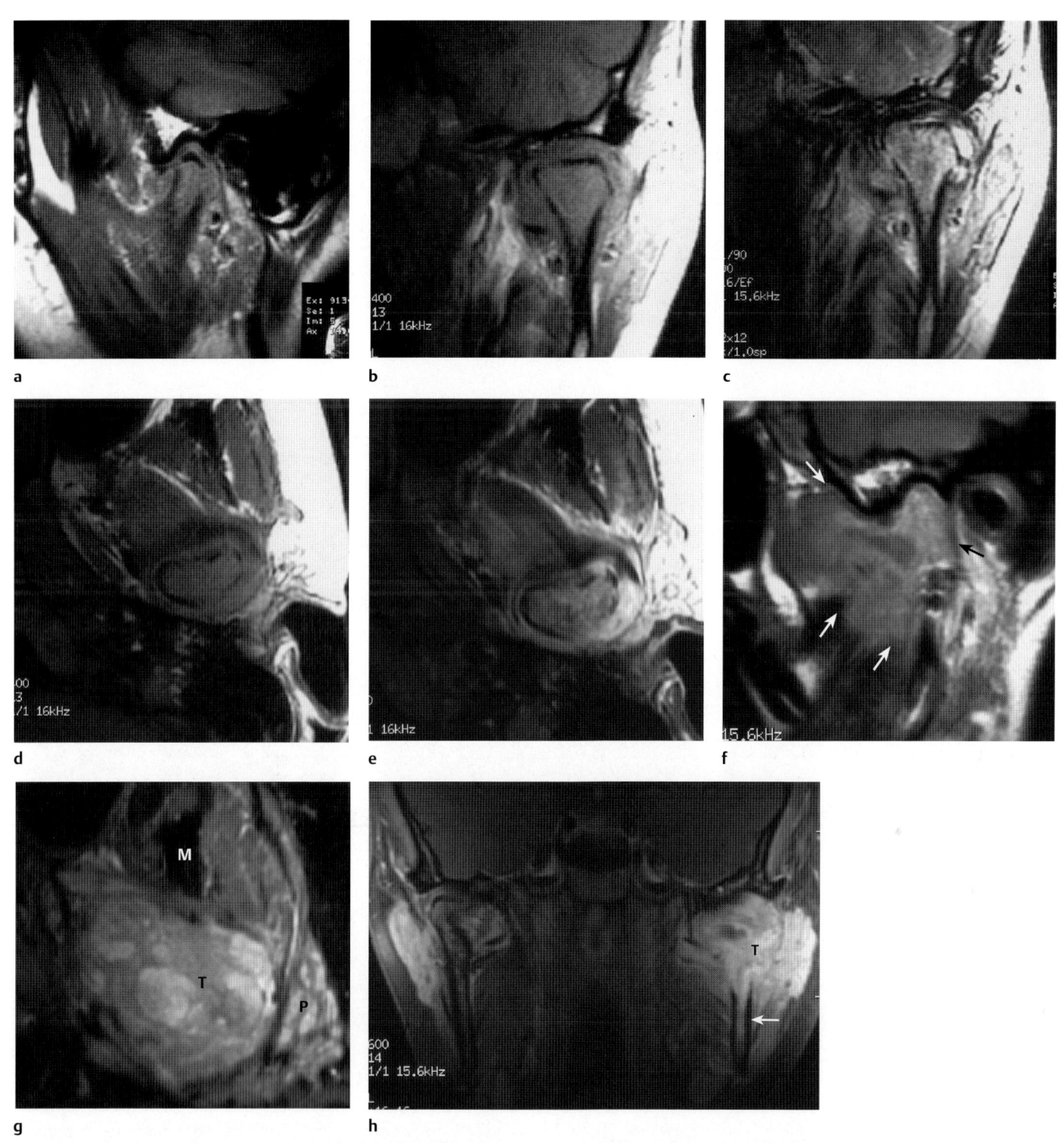

Fig. 5.**39** Langerhans cell histiocytosis. **a** Sagittal T1W MR scan shows slight expansion of the joint space, replacement of the condylar marrow by hypointense process, and normal articular disk, with distinct posterior band, intermediate zone and anterior band. **b, c** Coronal T1W (**b**) and T2W (**c**) MR scans show slight expansion of the joint capsule. Note joint effusion in the lateral aspect of the TMJ, and moderate hyperintensity of the condylar marrow, seen in **c**. **d** Axial T1W MR scan shows expansion of the left TMJ capsule and bone marrow change of the condyle. **e** Axial enhanced T1W MR scan shows marked contrast enhancement of the left TMJ and condylar marrow. **f** Sagittal T1W MR scan, obtained a month later, shows marked destruction of the left condyle along with increased soft-tissue infiltration of the joint (arrows). **g** Axial T2W MR scan shows marked hyperintense soft-tissue tumor (T) in the left TMJ region and adjacent pterygoid muscle. M = mandible, P = parotid gland. **h** Coronal fat suppression T1W scan shows marked contrast enhancement of the tumor (T) involving the TMJ and upper mandibular ramus (arrow).

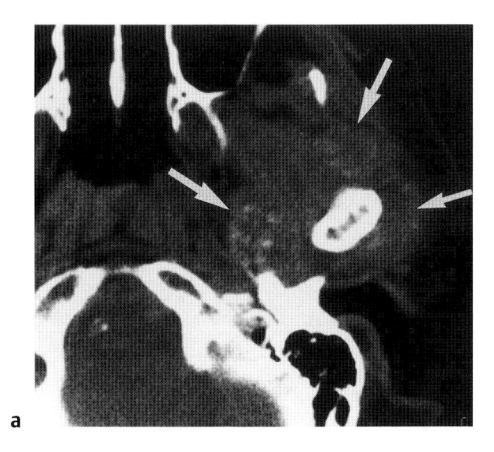

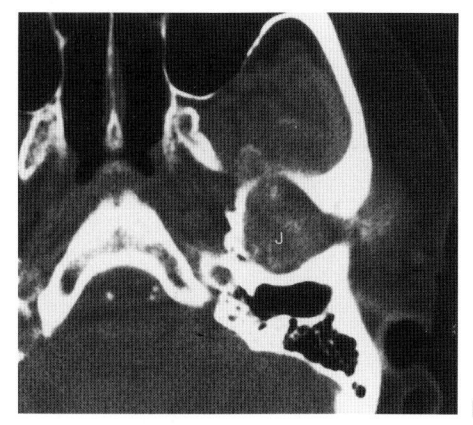

Fig. 5.40 Chondrosarcoma. **a** Axial CT scan shows a soft-tissue mass (arrows) involving the left TMJ. Note speckled calcifications characteristic of chondrogenic tumor. **b** Axial CT scan shows extension of tumor into the left TMJ (J).

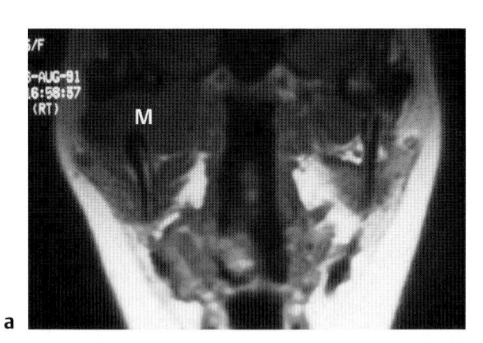

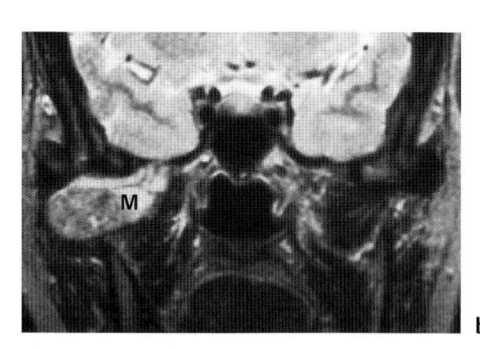

Fig. 5.41 Chondrosarcoma of the right TMJ. **a** Coronal T1W and **b** T2W MR scans showing a mass (M) involving the right TMJ. The lesion is hypointense in T1W and hyperintense in T2W MR images.

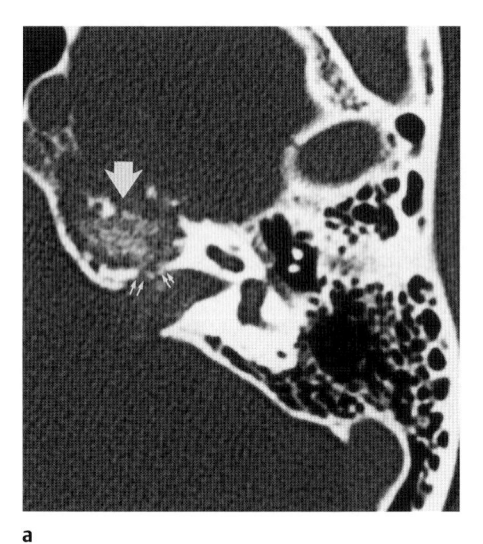

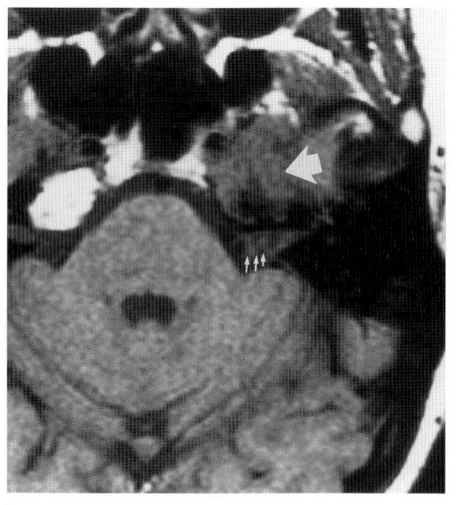

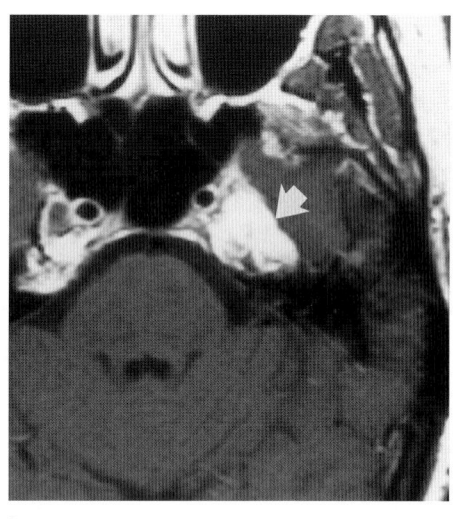

Fig. 5.42 Chondroblastoma of left temporal bone. **a** Axial CT scan shows a destructive mass involving the left petrous apex (wide arrow) and with extension into the left IAC (small arrows). Note intralesion foci of mineralization. **b** Axial T1W MR scan shows a hypointense mass (wide arrow) replacing the normal hyperintense marrow signal of the left petrous apex. Note abnormal soft tissue in the left IAC (small arrows). **c** Enhanced T1W MR scan, taken few millimeters inferior to **b**, showing marked enhancement of tumor (arrow) involving the left petrous apex. Case courtesy of Dr. G. Lee, Kansas City, MO, USA.

rare.[39] The etiology of PVNS remains unclear.[40] Microscopically, PVNS demonstrates a nonspecific inflammatory process along with proliferation of the synovial lining cells. There are many hemosiderin granules, multiple giant cells, and abundant lipid pigment, which gives a yellow coloration to the rusty brown of hemosiderin.[40] On imaging, PVNS shows its nature as a mass with a tendency toward bone erosion on both sides of the TMJ. There may be moderate expansion of the joint capsule. Hemorrhage is often present in various stages and can best be demonstrated by MR imaging. These lesions are highly vascular and therefore demonstrate increased vascularity on angiograms as well as increased contrast enhancement on enhanced CT and MR images.[39,40]

The differential diagnoses of PVNS of the TMJ on the basis of CT and MR scans include synovial chondromatosis, giant-cell granuloma, Langerhans cell histiocytosis, giant-cell tumor, chondromyxoid tumor, and chondroblastoma.

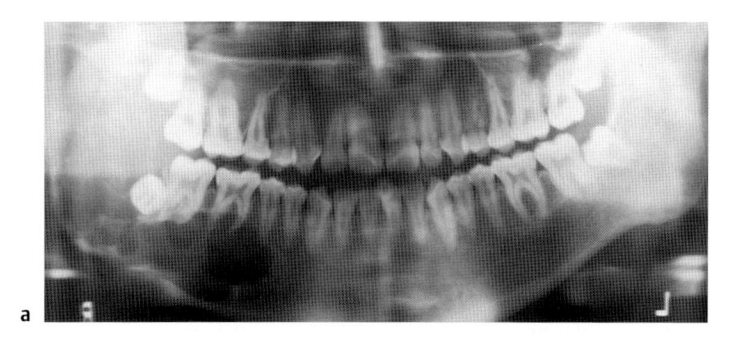

Fig. 5.43 Extension of an odontogenic keratocyst into the right condyle. **a** Panorex view of the mandible shows a large keratogenic cyst involving the entire right ramus with extension into the condyle. **b** Coronal CT scan shows a large hypodense cystic lesion involving the right ramus including the condyle.

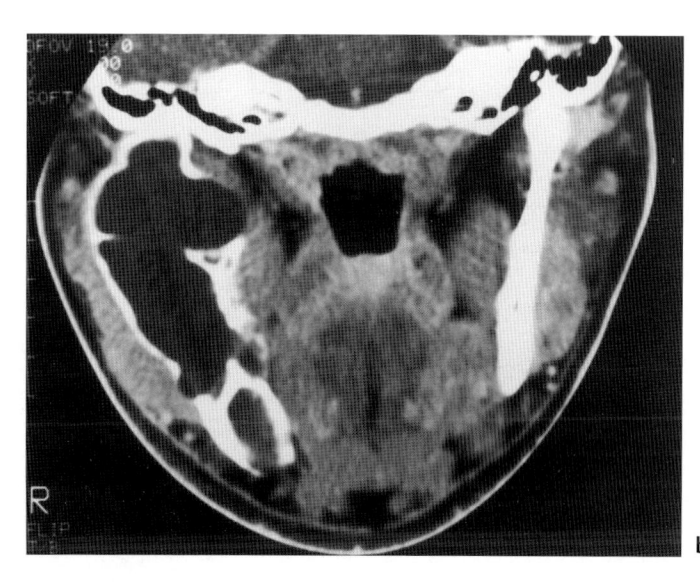

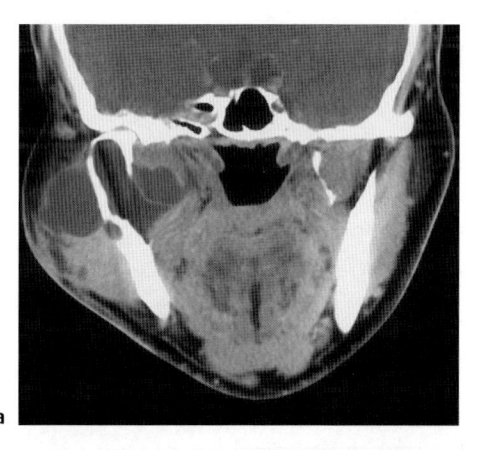

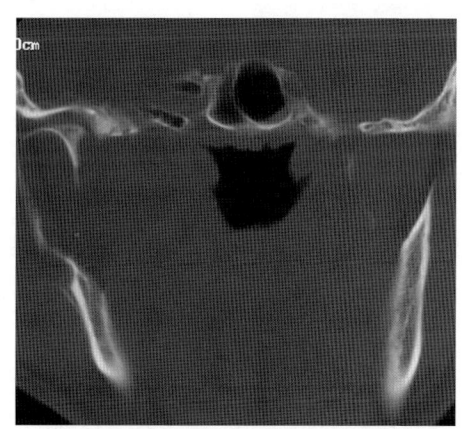

Fig. 5.44 Extension of an odontogenic keratocyst into the right condyle and masticator space. **a** Coronal (soft-tissue window) and **b** (bone window) MR scans, showing an odontogenic cyst with extension into the right condyle and masticatory space.

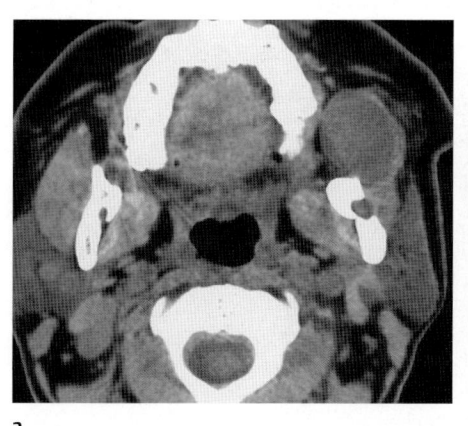

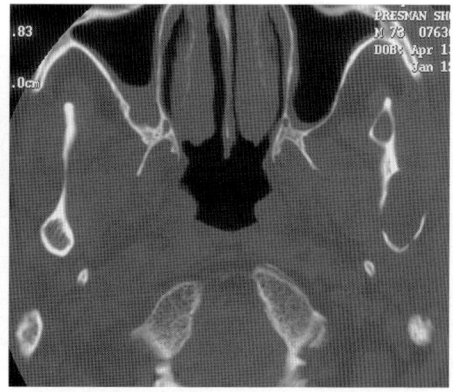

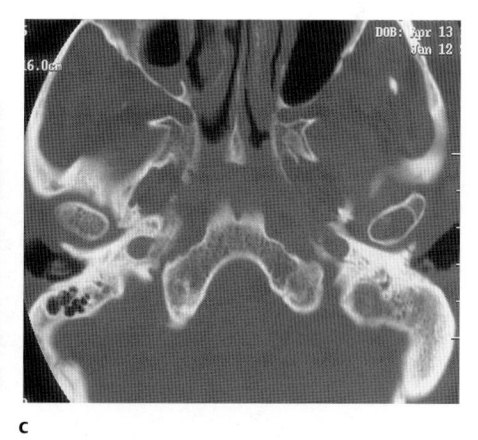

Fig. 5.45 Ameloblastoma involving the left TMJ and buccal space. **a** CT scan shows a large left buccal mass. Note deformity of the left ramus with small lytic lesion. Note marked deformity of the left masseter muscle. **b** CT scan in another patient shows expansion of the left ramus with lytic lesions involving the left ramus compatible with ameloblastoma. **c** Axial CT scan, same patient as in Fig. 5.45b, shows extension of ameloblastoma into the left condyle. Note that the normal spongy appearance of the condyle has been replaced by a uniform low-density image.

■ Miscellaneous

In this section, imaging of several conditions that can mimic the signs and symptoms of TMJ dysfunction are illustrated. Cysts and tumors of the mandible may extend superiorly to involve the condyle and glenoid fossa (Figs. 5.**43**–**45**). The differential diagnoses for TMJ dysfunction should include those pathological conditions in the head and neck that can cause pain referred to the joint and masticatory muscles. Disorders such as Eagle syndrome, atypical neuralgia, trigeminal neuralgia, carotodynia, and acute and chronic sinusitis should be ruled out. Otitis media and external auditory meatus pathology should be considered as well

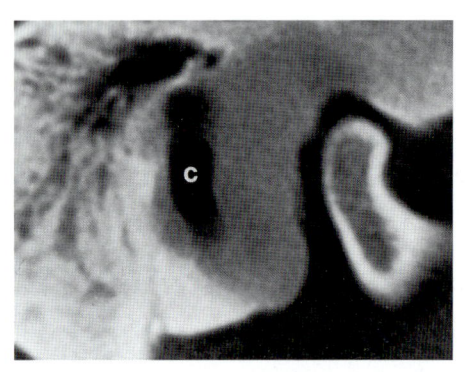

Fig. 5.46 Fibrous dysplasia involving the TMJ. Sagittal CT scan shows fibrous dysplasia involving the glenoid fossa and external ear canal. Note constriction of the ear canal (C).

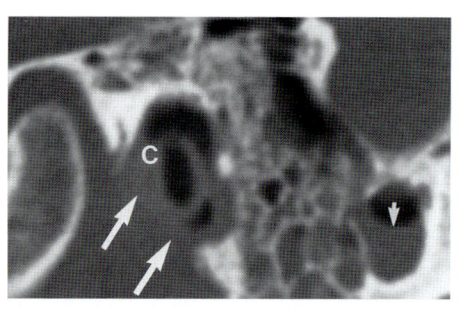

Fig. 5.47 Extension of cholesteatoma of the external canal into the TMJ. Sagittal CT scan shows an external canal cholesteatoma (C). Note erosion of the anterior wall of the external canal (large arrows) and fluid in the mastoid air cell (small arrow).

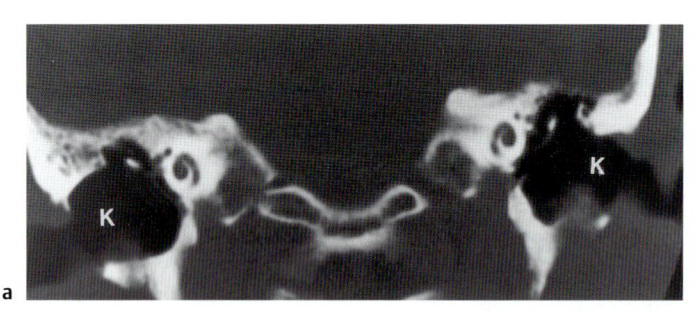

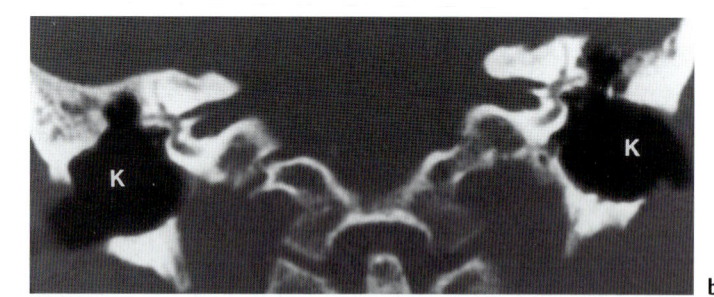

Fig. 5.48 Bilateral keratosis obliterans. Coronal CT scans (**a**, **b**) showing marked expansion of both external auditory canals due to keratosis (K). The keratomatous debris has been exteriorized. Keratosis obliterans and canal cholesteatoma have similar CT appearance to that seen in Fig. 5.**47**.

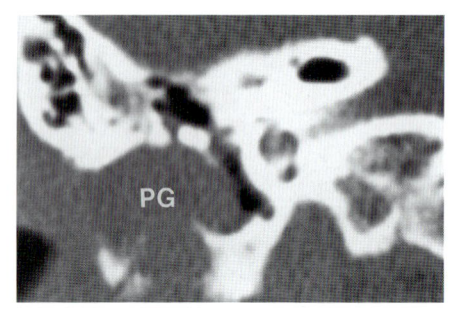

Fig. 5.49 Extension of pyogenic granuloma of external canal into the TMJ. Coronal CT scan shows a large mass in the external canal compatible with a pyogenic granuloma (PG). Note erosion of the floor of the external canal and extension into the TMJ.

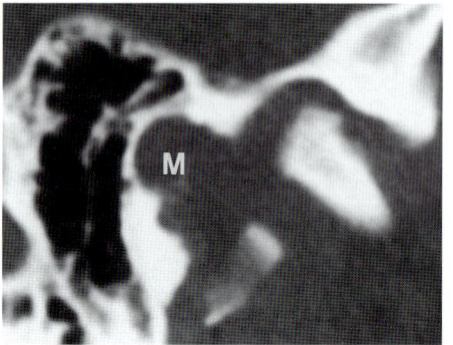

Fig. 5.50 Extension of carcinoma of the external auditory canal into the TMJ. **a** Sagittal CT scan shows a soft-tissue mass (M) within the external canal. Note erosion of the anterior wall of the external canal. **b** Sagittal T1W MR scan shows a large mass within the external ear (arrows). Note extension into the TMJ (arrowhead).

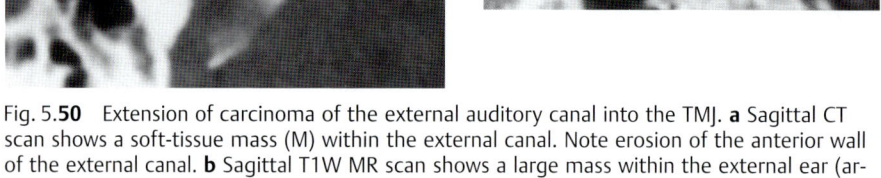

(Figs. 5.**46–50**). Malignancies of the skull base and neighboring tissues may secondarily affect the TMJ or cause referred symptoms.

■ Fractures

Fractures of the condyloid process are commonly referred to as condylar fractures. Only those fractures that involve the intracapsular portion of the condyloid process, however, are true condylar fractures (Fig. 5.**51**).[7] Most fractures occur across the neck of the condyle and are more correctly termed subcondylar fractures. Condyloid fractures may be unilateral or bilateral; the former are more common. Unilateral fractures often are associated with a fracture of the mandible in the region of the contralateral mental foramen. Blood in the external auditory canal is an indication of an associated fracture of the tympanic bone or the skull base.[7] Condylar fractures account for 25–35% of all reported facial fractures. These fractures may result in ankylosis, disturbances in masticatory function, and internal derangements, and may interfere with mandibular growth, resulting in facial asymmetry.

Most condylar fractures are displaced anteromedially (Fig. 5.**51**), which is due to the pull of the lateral pterygoid muscles. In

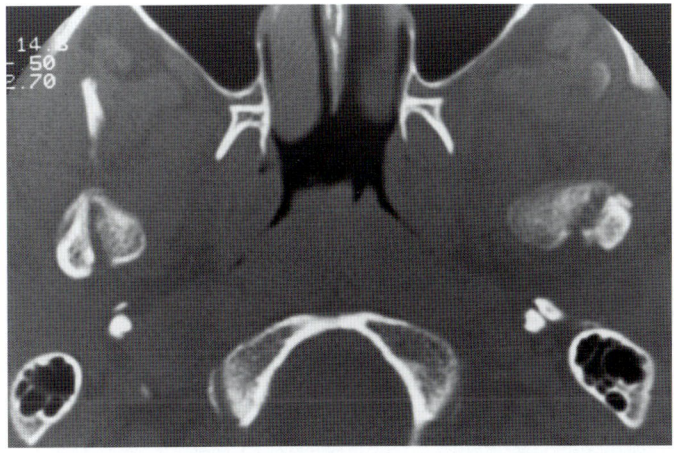

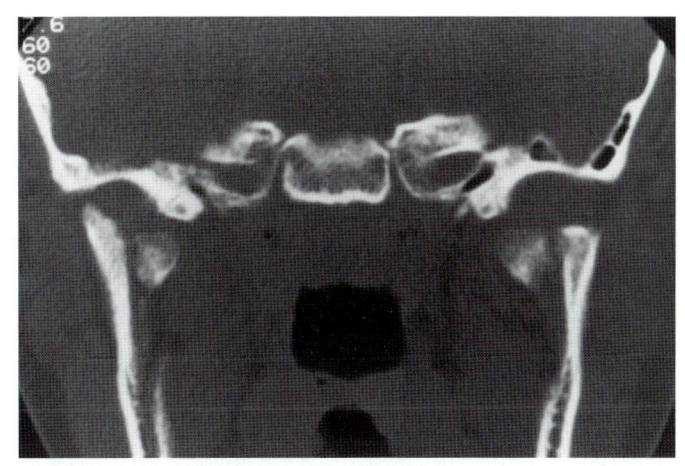

Fig. 5.51 Bilateral condylar fractures. **a** Axial and **b** coronal CT scans showing bilateral intracapsular condylar fractures.

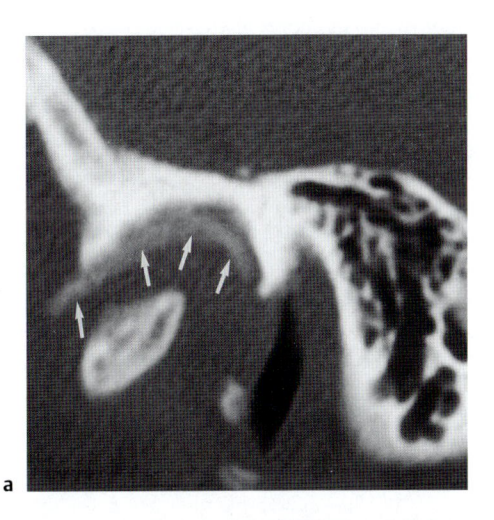

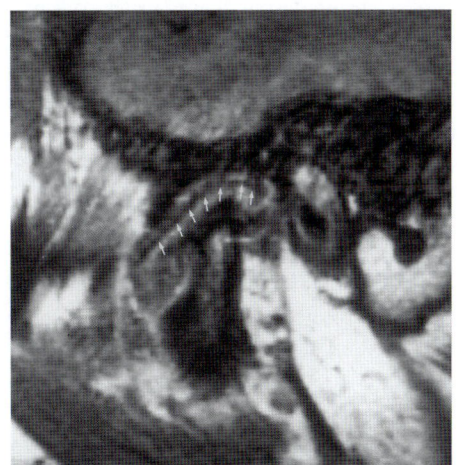

Fig. 5.52 Postoperative change of TMJ. **a** Sagittal CT scan shows a Proplast Teflon implant. The implant (arrows) is positioned within the enlarged glenoid fossa. There is close approximation of the implant to the glenoid fossa. Note reactive periosteal bone formation at the anterior aspect of the glenoid fossa. The anterior aspect of the implant is not supported by bone. **b** Sagittal T1W MR scan; the implant (arrows) appears hypointense and follows the contour of the glenoid fossa.

some instances, the condyle is displaced laterally with the destruction of the lateral capsule and ligaments. The degree of condylar damage relates to the force of impact, the direction of the blow, the presence of natural or artificial teeth to cushion the blow, and whether or not the mouth is open during the injury. Rarely, the condyle may be superiorly dislocated within the external auditory canal and even into the middle cranial fossa.[2] On imaging, fractures may also be described as occurring within the capsule (intracapsular) or at the condylar neck, inferior to the joint capsule attachment (Fig. 5.51). The terms *displacement* and *dislocation* have also been used to qualitatively describe the fracture. *Displacement* connotes an increase in the joint space; *dislocation* connotes actual dislodgment of the fragment from the glenoid fossa.[2]

Radiographic Findings

Because of the close approximation of other bony structures to the TMJ, fractures high on the mandibular neck and intracapsular fractures may be difficult to identify from plain films, and CT scan may be needed (Fig. 5.51).[7] Whenever a condylar fracture is discovered, the radiographs should be evaluated carefully to rule out accompanying fractures of the mandibular body, which occasionally may be occult.[7] Edema of the bone marrow, soft-tissue damage and intracapsular hemorrhage can best be evaluated by MRI.

■ Postoperative Conditions

The interpretation of images of the postoperative joint may be difficult. The intra-articular fibrosis that ensues can render delineation of the disk or differentiation of disk anatomy nearly impossible. After diskectomy, the intermediate-to-low signal intensity of the intra-articular scar that replaces the disk cannot be distinguished definitively from retrodiskal tissue. When metallic alloplasts are used to reconstruct the articulation, only polytomography and routine radiographs are of value in the postoperative evaluation. The artifacts observed with CT and MR imaging render most images uninterpretable.

CT is the ideal method for evaluating the position of the Proplast Teflon and silastic interarticular implants (Figs. 5.52, 5.53). The CT findings associated with long-term use of Proplast Teflon implants may vary from one case to the other. CT scans may demonstrate significant deformity of the condyle, glenoid fossa, and eminence, with superior and anterior migration of implants. Bone remodeling or destruction can be accurately evaluated on CT. MR imaging is of value in the presence of particulation or fragmentation of the implant and when inflammatory or granulomatous changes are suspected. An expanded fibrotic capsule usually develops around the implants.[6] This fibrotic change and granulation tissue around the implant can be observed on MR imaging. At times the interposed silastic implant (silastic cap prosthesis) may become displaced and become incorporated with surrounding

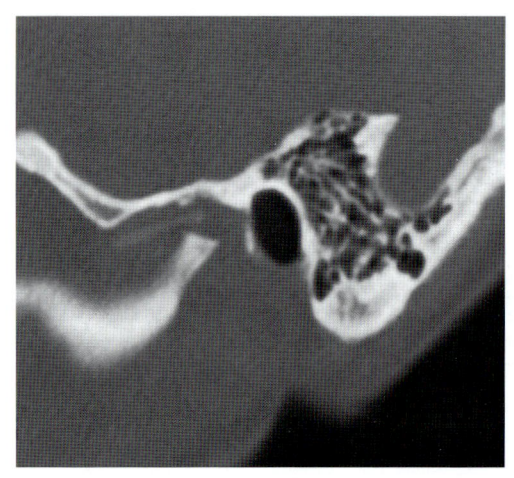

Fig. 5.**53** Postoperative changes of condylectomy and diskectomy with Proplast Teflon implant replacement. Direct sagittal CT scan shows partial condylectomy and an implant, which is positioned within an enlarged glenoid fossa.

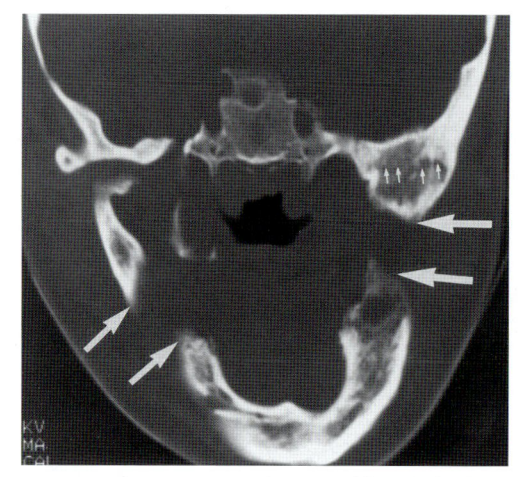

Fig. 5.**54** Postoperative changes of bilateral gap arthroplasty. Coronal CT scan shows bilateral gap arthroplasty (large arrows). The selection of gap location is usually based on surgical access and location of the inferior alveolar canal. Note the site of fusion of bony ankylosis (small arrows). For gap arthroplasty to be successful it must be carried out through the entire ramus and be approximately 5–10 mm in width in its entirety.

tissue. With time, the implant frequently fragments and the condition of the implant can be evaluated on both MR images and CT. However, CT is more precise for evaluation of the integrity of the implant. Alloplastic TMJ implants are not currently used because of the poor long-term prognosis.[6] Total joint replacements were previously used in the TMJ. The metallic condyle prostheses used to be fixed with screws to the ramus of the mandible. The Proplast Teflon glenoid fossa implants were used along with the condyle prostheses.

Gap arthroplasty is a surgical procedure used for the treatment of ankylosis of the TMJ. For the gap to be successful it must be carried out through the ramus and be approximately 5–10 mm in width in its entirety (Fig. 5.**54**). The materials placed within the gap may become displaced with time and the bone reformed at the surgical site.

References

1. Warwick R, Williams PL, eds. Gray's Anatomy, 35th British edition. Philadelphia: W.B. Saunders; 1973.
2. Heffez LB, Mafee MF, Rosenberg H, eds. Imaging Atlas of the Temporomandibular Joint. Philadelphia; Williams and Wilkins; 1995.
3. Mafee MF, Heffez L, Campos M, et al. Temporomandibular joint: role of direct sagittal CT air-contrast arthrogram and MRI. Otolaryngol Clin North Am 1988; 21: 575–588.
4. Mafee MF. Case 7: Temporomandibular joint anatomy. In: Som PM, Curtin HD, Dillon WP, Hasso AN, Mafee MF, eds. Head and Neck Disorders (Fourth Series) Test and Syllabus. Reston, VA: American College of Radiology; 1992: 144–162.
5. Lever JD, Ford HER. Histological, histochemical and electron microscopic observation on the synovial membrane. Anat Rec 1958; 123: 528.
6. Westesson P-L. Temporomandibular joint and dental imaging. Neuroimaging Clin North Am 1996; 6: 333–355.
7. Laskin DM. Diagnosis of pathology of the temporomandibular joint. Clinical and imaging perspectives. Radiol Clin North Am 1993, 31: 135–147.
8. Norgaard F. Arthrography of temporomandibular joint. Acta Radiol 1944; 174: 663–637.
9. Heffez LB, Mafee MF, Langer B. Double-contrast arthrography of the temporomandibular joint: role of direct sagittal CT imaging. Oral Surg Oral Med Oral Pathol 1988; 65: 511–514.
10. Mafee MF, Kumar A, Tahmoressi CN, et al. Direct sagittal CT in the evaluation of temporal bone disease. AJR 1988; 150: 1403–1410.
11. Heffez LB, Anderson D, Mafee MF. Developmental defects of the tympani plate. Case reports and review of the literature. J Oral Maxillofac Surg 1989; 47: 1336.
12. Mafee MF, Valvassori GE. Radiology of the craniofacial anomalies. Otolaryngol Clin North Am 1981; 14: 939–988.
13. Herring SW, Rowlatt UF, Pruzansky S. Anatomical abnormalities in mandibulofacial dysostosis. Am J Med Genet 1979; 3: 225–259.
14. Mafee MF, Schild JA, Kumar A, et al. Radiological features of the ear-related developmental anomalies in patients with mandibulofacial dysostosis. Int J Pediatr Otolaryngol 1983; 7: 229–238.
15. Obwegeser HL, Makek MS. Hemimandibular hyperplasia – hemimandibular elongation. J Maxillofac Surg. 1986, 14: 183.
16. Mafee MF. Case 15: TMJ synovial chondromatosis. In: Som P, Curtin HD, Dillon WP, Hasso AN, Mafee MF, eds. Head and Neck Disorders (Fourth Series) Test and Syllabus. Reston VA: American College of Radiology; 1992: 343–362.
17. Bounds GA, Hopkins R, Sugar A. Septic arthritis of temporomandibular joint – a problematic diagnosis. Br J Oral Maxillofac Surg 1987; 25: 61–67.
18. Wurman LH, Flannery JV, Sack JF. Osteomyelitis of the mandibular condyle secondary to dental extractions. Otolaryngol Head Neck Surg 1979; 87: 190–198.
19. Schellhas KP, Wilkes CH. Temporomandibular joint inflammation: comparison of MR fast scanning with T1 and T2-weighted imaging techniques. AJR 1987; 153: 93.
20. Heffez LB, Jordan S. A classification of temporomandibular joint disk morphology. Oral Surg 1989; 67: 11.
21. Westesson PL, Rohlin M: Internal derangement related to osteoarthrosis in temporomandibular joint autopsy specimens. Oral Surg 1984; 17: 17.
22. Katzberg RW, Bessette RW, Tallents RH, et al. Normal and abnormal temporomandibular joint: MR imaging with surface coil. Radiology 1986; 158: 183–189.
23. Rao VM, Farole A, Karasick D. Temporomandibular joint dysfunction: correlation of MR imaging, arthrography, and arthroscopy. Radiology 1990; 174: 663–667.
24. McCarthy WL, Farrar WB. Surgery for internal derangements of temporomandibular joint. J Prosthet Dent 1979; 42: 191–196.
25. Schellhas KP, et al. MR of osteochondritis dissecans and avascular necrosis of the mandibular condyle. AJR 1989; 152: 551–563.
26. Blackwood H. Arthritis of the mandibular joint. Br Dent J 1963; 115: 317.
27. Macalister A. A microscopic study of the human temporomandibular joint. NZ Dent J 1954; 50: 161.
28. Bean LR, Omnel KA, Öberg T. Comparison between radiological observations and macroscopic tissue changes in the temporomandibular joint. Dentomaxillofac Radiol 1977; 6: 90.
29. Tabeling HG, Dolwick MR. Rheumatoid arthritis: diagnosis and treatment. Fla Dent J 1985, 56: 1.

30 Steinbrocker O, Trager CH, Batterman RC. Therapeutic criteria in rheumatoid arthritis. JAMA 1949; 140: 659.
31 Katzborg RW. Temporomandibular joint imaging. Radiology 1989; 170: 297–307.
32 Syrjäneen SM. The temporomandibular joint in rheumatoid arthritis. Acta Radiol 1985; 26: 235.
33 Ogus H. Rheumatoid arthritis of the temporomandibular joint. Br J Oral Surg 1975; 12: 275.
34 Resnick D. Temporomandibular joint involvement in ankylosing spondylitis. Radiology 1974; 112: 587.
35 Davidson C, Wojtulewsky JA, Bacon PA, Winstock D. Temporomandibular joint disease in ankylosis spondylitis. Ann Rheum Dis 1975; 34: 87.
36 Schwartz L, et al. Facial pain and mandibular dysfunction. Philadelphia: WB Saunders; 1968.
37 Herzog S, Mafee MF. Synovial chondromatosis of the TMJ: MR and CT findings. AJNR 1990; 11: 742–745.
38 Lind P, Hillerstrom K. Osteoid osteoma in the mandibular condyle. Acta Otolaryngol 1963; 57: 467–470.
39 Youssef RE, Roszkowski MJ, Richter KJ. Pigmented villonodular synovitis of the temporomandibular joint. J Oral Maxillofac Surg 1996; 54: 224–227.
40 Klenoff JR, Lowlicht RA, Lesnik T, et al. Mandibular and temporomandibular joint arthropathy in the differential diagnosis of the parotid mass. Laryngoscope 2001; 111: 2162–2165.

6 Mandible and Maxilla

Alfred L. Weber
Mahmood F. Mafee

Embryology

At about the fourth week of gestation, the stomodeum, or the primitive mouth, is bounded cranially by the projection of the forebrain and caudally by the cardiac prominence. The mandibular region and the whole of the neck, which will subsequently intervene between the mouth and developing thorax, are as yet absent, but will be formed by the appearance of six paired branchial or pharyngeal arches, which develop on the lateral aspects of the head in the vicinity of the hindbrain.[1] At this stage of embryonic development (end of the fourth week), five swellings (prominences) can be identified surrounding the stomodeum. These elevations or prominences include a single frontonasal prominence, and two paired mandibular and maxillary prominences. The mandibular and maxillary prominences (processes) lie on each side of the stomodeum, inferior and superior to the stomodeum, respectively (see also Chapter 10). The frontonasal prominence gives rise to the formation of the median facial structures (see also Chapter 4). The mandibular and maxillary prominences originate from the first branchial arch and give rise to the formation of the mandible and lateral two-thirds of the upper jaw, the upper teeth (except the incisors), and the palatal shelves. The intermaxillary segment of the upper lip and the premaxillary portion of the upper jaw containing the four incisors are formed by the developing nasal placodes from the frontonasal prominence (see also Chapter 10). The first pair of branchial arches are usually referred to as the mandibular arches and the second pair of arches as hyoid arches.[1] The mandibular division of the trigeminal nerve innervates the musculature of the mandibular arch; the facial nerve supplies the hyoid arch. The cartilaginous skeleton of the first arch (Meckel's cartilage) extends from the developing otic capsule into the mandibular arch, meeting its fellow at its ventral end (Fig. 6.1). The Meckel's cartilage can be identified at six weeks of gestation. The dorsal end of the Meckel's cartilage becomes separated and is often held to form the rudiments of the malleus and incus (Fig. 6.1).[1] The ventral portion of the Meckel's cartilage gradually disappears, and the mandible is formed around it by secondary intramembranous ossification (mesenchymatous mandible). The intermediate part of the Meckel's cartilage disappears, but its perichondrial sheath persists as the anterior malleolar and sphenomandibular ligaments. The muscle mass of the mandibular arch forms the tensor tympani, the tensor veli palatini, the masticatory muscles, myelohyoid, and anterior belly of digastric; all being supplied by the mandibular nerve.[1]

The human mandibular arch (first arch) grows ventromedially in the floor of the pharynx to meet its fellow in the midline. While the mandibular process is invading the floor of the mouth and pharynx, the mesenchyme between the central aspect of the forebrain and the mouth proliferates and bulges to form the frontonasal elevation or process. During the fifth week a thickened plaque of ectoderm develops, dividing this frontonasal elevation into medial and lateral elevations or folds. These thickenings are the olfactory or nasal placodes. Extensions of mesenchyme from the medial processes into the roof of the stomodeum proliferate to form the premaxillary process. While these changes are progressing, an elevation swells ventrally from the dorsal region of the mandibular arches (first branchial or pharyngeal arch). This is the maxillary process. The maxillary process grows in a ventral direction and fuses with the nasal fold. The opposed margins of the lateral nasal and maxillary elevations growing together thus establish continuity between the side of the future nose and the cheek.[1]

■ Dental Development

At about the 8–9 mm stage of embryonic development the primitive oral epithelium begins to bulge into the underlying mesenchyme in the region that will later be occupied by the teeth. This horseshoe-shaped thickening in each jaw is called the dental lamina. The tooth buds, which later develop into the teeth, arise from this dental lamina as well as the surrounding cells.[1] At about the 20 mm embryonic stage, ectodermal outgrowths of the dental lamina can be identified as discrete elevations. An ectodermal outgrowth together with the adjacent ectomesenchyme is known as a tooth bud.[1] At this stage the ectodermal part of tooth bud is called the enamel organ, the ectomesenchymal part is called the dental papilla.[1] The growing enamel organ compresses the surrounding adjacent cells so that they assume a concentric arrangement. These cells comprise the tooth follicle. The depression in the alveolar bone of the jaw containing the tooth germ and follicle is called a tooth crypt.[1] As the jaws grow in length, the dental lamina penetrates the jaw mesenchyme and forms the buds for the permanent molars and the deciduous teeth.

■ Development of Enamel

Prior to differentiating into ameloblasts, the cells of the internal enamel epithelium of the enamel organ begin to lengthen and in

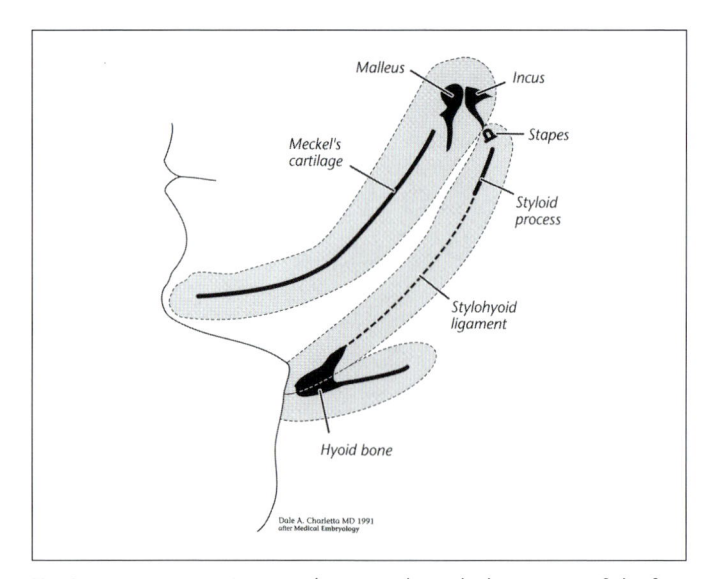

Fig. 6.1 Diagrammatic sagittal section through the regions of the face and neck, demonstrating the mandibular Meckel's cartilage and the hyoid Reichert's cartilage.

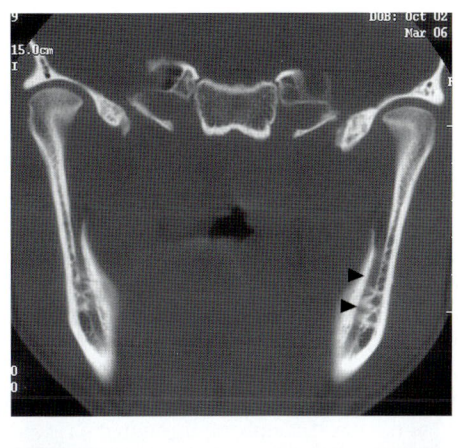

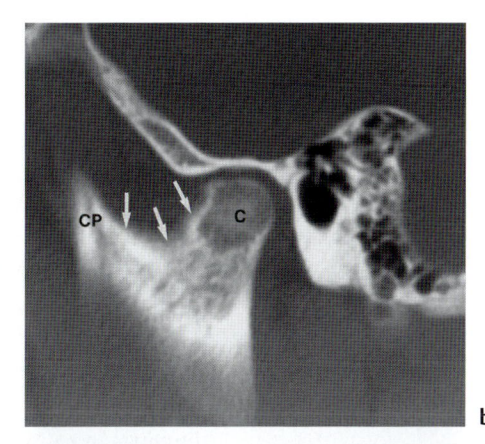

Fig. 6.2 Normal mandible. **a** Coronal and **b** sagittal CT scans demonstrating condyle (C), coronoid process (CP), sigmoid notch (arrows), and mandibular canals (arrowheads). **c, d** Reformatted 3D lateral (**c**) and basal (**d**) views of the skull, showing normal 3D anatomy of an edentulous mandible.

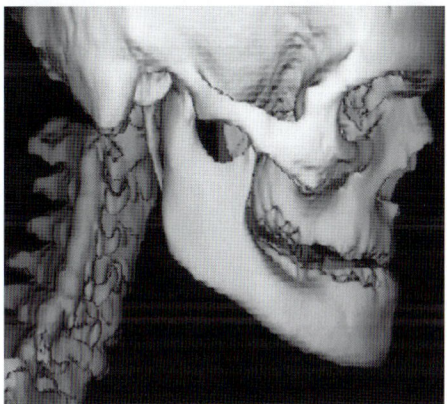

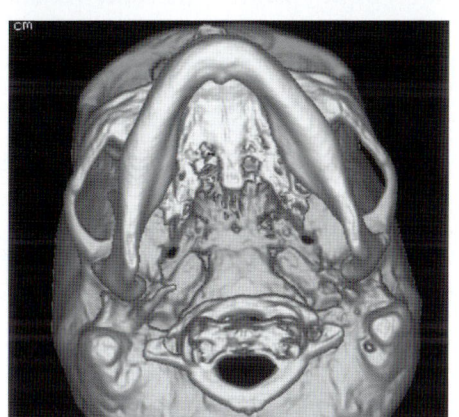

the meantime induce the differentiation of odontoblasts from cells of the dental papilla.[1] As soon as dentine has been formed and mineralized, the ameloblasts secret the enamel.

■ Ossification

The mandible is ossified in dense fibromembraneous tissue (intramembranous bone formation) that lies lateral to the inferior alveolar nerve and the lower part of the ventral portion of the Meckel's cartilage. Each half is ossified from one center, which appears near the mental foramen about the sixth week of fetal life.[1] At birth the mandible is in two separate halves, united in the median plane by fibrous tissue. The union is termed the symphysis menti.

Anatomy

■ The Mandible

The mandible, which is the largest and strongest bone of the face, has a curved horizontal body and two broad ascending rami (Fig. 6.2). The lower border of the body is termed the base of the mandible. The upper border of the body is the alveolar part (alveolus), which houses 16 sockets for the roots of the teeth. The inner aspect is divided into two areas by a shallow oblique ridge, termed the mylohyoid line.[1] Below the mylohyoid line there is a depression, called the submandibular fossa, for the submandibular gland. In front, above the mylohyoid line, is a depression, referred to as the sublingual fossa, for the sublingual gland. The mental foramen, from which emerges the mental nerve and vessels, opens on the outer surface of the body of the mandible, below the second premolar tooth. The ramus of the mandible is quadrilateral and has two surfaces, four borders, and two prominent processes. The mandibular foramen is located above the center of the medial surface of the ascending ramus of the mandible (Fig. 6.2). This opening (foramen) leads into the mandibular canal, which curves downward and forward into the body to open at the mental foramen (Fig. 6.2). In front and on the medial side, the mandibular foramen is obscured by a thin triangular process termed the lingula (Fig. 6.2).[1] The upper border of the ramus is thin and is formed by a curvilinear notch, called sigmoid notch or the mandibular incisure. The sigmoid notch is continued in front by a projection, termed the coronoid process, and behind by the condylar process. The coronoid process provides insertion for most of the fibers of the temporalis muscle. The condylar process is expanded above to form the articular part of the mandible (Fig. 6.2). It is covered with fibrocartilage and articulates with the mandibular fossa of the squamous portion of the temporal bone. The constricted portion below the head is termed the neck of the condylar process. The mandibular canal contains the inferior alveolar nerve and vessels, from which branches enter the roots of the teeth.[1]

■ The Maxillae

The maxillae are the largest bones of the face, after the mandible, and by their union form the whole of the upper jaw.[1] Each maxilla consists of a body and four processes: zygomatic, frontal, alveolar, and palatine. The body of the maxilla is roughly pyramidal. It has four surfaces—anterior, posterior or infratemporal, superior or orbital, and medial or nasal—which

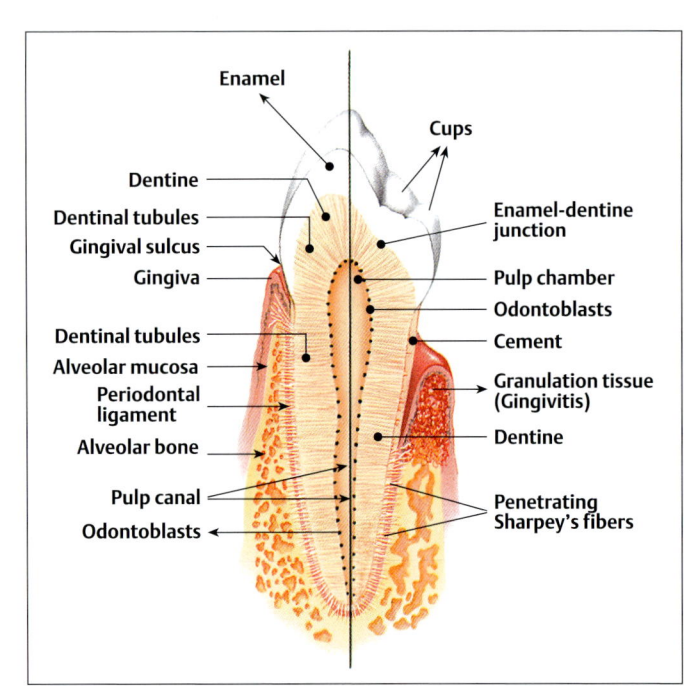

Fig. 6.3 Diagram of a longitudinal section of a tooth in situ. A buccolingual longitudinal section of a mandibular molar tooth, showing the various structures of the tooth. Note that the enamel tapers to a knife-edge at the cervical margin. The odontoblasts, represented as black dots, are arranged as cells lining the pulpal surface of the dentine. Periodontal ligament holds the tooth in its socket. The root of the tooth is covered by cement, a bonelike tissue. The Sharpey's fibers are extensions of collagen fibers that cross the periodontal ligament and insert into the alveolar bone. Courtesy of M.F. Mafee, MD.

enclose a large air-filled cavity, the maxillary sinus (antrum). The anterior surface above the incisor teeth has a slight depression, the incisive fossa. Lateral to the incisive fossa there is a larger and deeper depression, named the canine fossa. Above the canine fossa is the infra-orbital foramen, which represents the anterior end of the infra-orbital canal and transmits the infra-orbital nerve and vessels. Medially the anterior surface merges into a deeply concave border, the nasal notch, which ends below in a pointed process that, with the corresponding process of the opposite maxilla, forms the anterior nasal spine.[1] The infratemporal surface is convex anteriorly and is the anterior wall of the infratemporal fossa. It is separated from the anterior wall by the zygomatic process. It contains near its center the aperatures of two or three small alveolar canals, which transmit the posterior superior alveolar vessels and nerves.[1] At the lower and posterior part of this surface there is a round eminence, the maxillary tuberosity, the medial aspect of which articulates with the pyramidal process of the palatine bone. The orbital surface of the maxilla constitutes the greater part of the floor of the orbit. The nasal surface displays posterosuperiorly a large, irregular opening, the maxillary hiatus, which leads into the maxillary sinus. The maxillary sinus is a large pyramidal cavity in the body of the maxilla. Its walls correspond to the orbital, anterior, infratemporal, and alveolar aspects of the body of the bone. The floor is formed by the alveolar process of the maxilla, and its lowest part is usually about 1.25 cm below the level of the floor of the nasal cavity. In some cases, the floor is perforated by the roots of the molar teeth.

The zygomatic process of the maxilla articulates with the zygomatic (malar) bone. The frontal process projects upward and backward between the nasal and lacrimal bones. The medial surface of it is part of the lateral wall of the nasal cavity. The upper end of the frontal process articulates with the nasal part of the frontal bone. The maxillary alveolar process is thick and arched, being broader behind than in front, and is excavated to form sockets for the reception of the roots of the teeth.[1] The cavity for the canine tooth is the deepest; those for the molars are the widest. The palatine process of the maxilla, which is thick and strong, is horizontal and projects medially from the lowest part of the nasal surface of the bone. It forms a considerable part of the floor of the nasal cavity and the roof of the mouth. The palatine process of the maxilla joins its fellow of the opposite bone and forms the anterior three-fourths of the bony palate. The horizontal plate of the palatine bone forms, with the corresponding surface of the opposite bone, the posterior quarter of the bony palate. Immediately behind the incisor teeth, the orifices of two lateral canals are visible. These are named the incisor canals; each leads upward into the corrresponding half of the nasal cavity and through it pass the terminal branch of the greater palatine artery and the nasopalatine nerve.[1]

Dental Anatomy

■ The Teeth

An extracted tooth consists of two parts: (1) the crown, which is covered by highly mineralized enamel, a very hard translucent tissue, and (2) the root, which is invested by a thin layer of cement, a yellowish bone-like tissue (Fig. 6.3). The neck or cervical margin is located between the crown and the root. A longitudinal section of a tooth is shown in Fig. 6.3. As seen, the bulk of a tooth is composed of dentine (ivory). The enamel covering of a tooth is about 1.5 mm thick, while the cement covering is much thinner (Fig. 6.3).[1] The pulp cavity (chamber) is located in the central canal of the dentine (Fig. 6.3). At the root of a tooth, the pulp cavity becomes narrow to form the pulp canal, opening at the tip of the root into an apical foramen. The dental pulp consists of specialized connective tissue resembling primitive mesenchyme. The cemental covering of the root is separated from the socket of the alveolar bone by soft tissue, called the periodontal ligament (membrane) (Fig. 6.3). The periodontal ligament is about 0.2 mm wide. The ligament provides tough suspension for each individual tooth.[1] At the cervical margin of a tooth, the periodontal ligament is covered by the gingiva or gum (Fig. 6.3).[1]

Dental anatomists use special terms to describe the surfaces of teeth. The tooth surface adjacent to the lips or cheeks is referred to as the labial or buccal surface. The surface adjacent to the tongue is referred to as the lingual or palatal surface. Each jaw quadrant contains a central and a lateral incisor. Distal to each lateral incisor is a canine tooth, which has the longest root in the jaws. Distal to each canine are two premolars, each having a buccal and a palatal or lingual cusp. The second premolar may be congenitally absent in about 2% of individuals.[1] Distal to each second premolar are three molars; each has a four or five cusps. The incisors, canines, and premolars of the permanent dentition will replace the two deciduous incisors, a deciduous canine, and two deciduous premolars, respectively, in each jaw quadrant. The deciduous molars resemble the permanent molars.

■ Dental Blood and Lymphatic Vessels

The inferior alveolar artery (IAA) is a branch of the maxillary artery. After entering the mandibular foramen, the IAA passes anteriorly in the mandibular alveolar canal and supplies the lower teeth and body of the mandible. Veins from the mandibular alveolar bone and teeth collect either into large veins in the interdental septa or into networks of veins that pass into several inferior alveolar veins. Some of these veins join the facial vein, others pass posteriorly to join the pterygoid plexus of veins.[1] The upper jaw is supplied by the anterior and posterior superior alveolar arteries. The latter branches from the maxillary artery, which is a branch of the infraorbital artery. The periodontal ligaments are supplied by the dental branches of the alveolar arteries. The veins accompanying the superior dental arteries drain either anteriorly to join the facial vein or posteriorly to join the pterygoid venous plexus.[1]

■ Dental Lymphatics

There is little precise knowledge of the lymphatic drainage of the jaws and teeth. Because dental abscesses and osteomyelitis of the Jaws in humans lead to submandibular and upper deep cervical lymphadenopaty, this must be considered the common path for lymphatic drainage of both upper and lower teeth.

■ Dental Innervation

The upper teeth are supplied by the anterior and posterior superior alveolar nerves. These nerves arise from the maxillary nerve. The teeth are supplied by a plexus that extends from the posterior to the anterior wall of the maxillary antrum.[1] The lower jaw and alveolar bone are largely supplied by branches of the inferior alveolar (dental) nerve together with branches of the buccal nerve to the buccal gingiva of the molar and premolar teeth, and branches of the lingual nerve to the lingual gingiva of all the lower teeth.[1] The inferior alveolar nerve arises from the maxillary nerve. The buccal and lingual nerves are the sensory branches of the mandibular nerve.

■ Dental Histology

The bulk of a tooth (Fig. 6.**3**) consists of dentine, which is a hard, elastic, yellowish-white, avascular mineralized tissue; 70% of the dentine is mineralized (largely by crystalline hydroxyapatite, but some in the form of amorphous calcium phosphates). The remaining 30% is mainly water and collagen.[1] The characteristic microscopic feature of dentine is that of evenly spaced dentinal tubes (Fig. 6.**3**), about 1–2 μm in diameter; dentinal tubes extend out from the pulpal of the dentine, including to the enamel–dentine (amelodentinal) junction (Fig. 6.**3**). Each dentinal tubule contains the membrane-covered cytoplasmic process of a cell body (an odontoblast), located in the peripheral portion of the pulpal chamber.[1] The odontoblasts, the dentine forming cells, line the pulpal surface of the dentine (Fig. 6.**3**). Predentine, a layer of nonmineralized dentine, separates the odontoblasts from the mineralized part of the dentine[1]. Pulp calcifications (stones) are of unknown etiology may rarely be seen with increased age.

■ The Dental Pulp

The dental pulp is situated within the central part of the dentine. The dental surface of the pulp is covered by the odontoblasts. The central part contains the vascular pulp, sensory nerve fibres, and connective tissue (Fig. 6.**3**)[1]. The vascular pulp is a rich network of capillaries, supplied by small arteries which enter the pulp canal from the periodontal ligament via the apical foramen. The pulp is continuous with the periodontal ligament and tissue spaces of the alveolar bone via the apical foramen of the tooth (Fig. 6.**3**).

■ The Enamel, Cement, and Periodontal Ligament

The enamel, which covers the entire crown, is extremely hard. It is composed of closely packed rods or prisms. Prisms are about 3–6 μm wide and are packed with hydroxyapatite crystallites. Ameloblasts are epithelial cells responsible for enamel formation. The cement is an amorphous bonelike tissue covering the two-thirds of the roots of the teeth (Fig. 6.**3**) and is about 40% mineral by weight. The cement contains the cementocytes and is perforated by Sharpey's fibers, the extensions of collagen fibers that cross the periodontal ligament to be inserted into the alveolar bone (Fig. 6.**3**). Throughout life, new layers of cement are deposited to compensate for tooth movements. The cement is a densely calcified organic substance similar to the matrix of bone, and is generally acellular. The acellular and cellular forms of cement differ only in the absence or presence of cementocytes; either form may exist over any part of the root.[1] The periodontal ligament (Fig. 6.**3**) is about 0.2 mm wide. It is a dense fibrous tissue which forms a thin fibrous attachment between the tooth root and the alveolar bone. Its main functions are to suspend the tooth in its socket and to provide sensory information by means of pressure receptors. The main components of the ligament are the collagenous principal fibers, of which there are several named groups.[1]. The collagen fibres are referred to as Sharpey's fibres (Fig. 6.**3**).

■ The Gingivae (Gums)

The tissue surrounding the necks of the teeth is the "free" gingiva or gum (Fig. 6.**3**). The attached gingiva is the tissue providing protective covering for the alveolar bone. In a healthy mouth the gingiva can be distinguished from the rest of the oral mucosa because it is pale pink and stippled, whereas the adjacent alveolar mucosa is red, shiny, and smooth. The gingival and palatal epithelia are keratinized (or parakeratinized); the alveolar epithelium is not keratinized.[1] The inflamed mucosa becomes very red and, in long-standing gingivitis there will be associated bone resorption of the alveolar process (Fig. 6.**3**).

Imaging Techniques

Cystic lesions and benign and malignant tumors of the mandible and maxilla represent a large group of diverse lesions that are easily demonstrated with various radiological modalities,[2–9] such as intraoral dental films, conventional views of the mandible (posteroanterior, lateral, and oblique views and panoramic radiographs), CT, and MRI.[2–9] Cysts and benign tumors are easily recognized on conventional films and, in some cysts, a radiological diagnosis can be established. Large cysts and aggressive benign and malignant lesions, however, should be further assessed with CT and MRI. Intraoral dental films are used for detailed analysis of the relationship of some lesions to a tooth. Radiographic examination of the mandible can be performed on a head unit or on a horizontal x-ray table. Intensifying screens are used to obtain detail of the anatomical structures. The film cassette is placed on the tabletop or in a head holder of the head unit. The standard

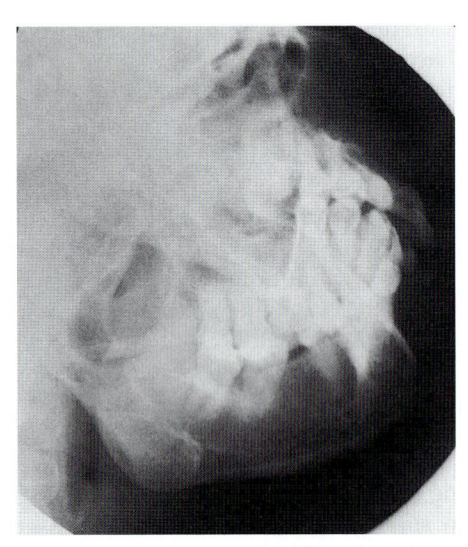

Fig. 6.4 Normal, conventional film of mandible. A lateral oblique view of the mandible demonstrates a normal body, angle, and ascending ramus of the mandible with the mandibular condyle and coronoid process.

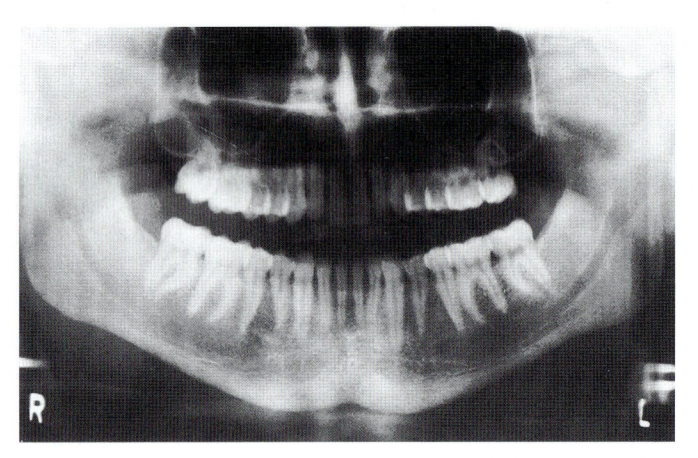

Fig. 6.5 Normal mandible and maxilla. Panorex view of the mandible and maxilla reveals normal texture and density of the mandible with normal bilateral mandibular canals, condyles, and coronoid processes, and normal alignment and position of the teeth.

routine views in the radiological evaluation of the mandible consist of (1) posteroanterior (PA) view, (2) lateral view, and (3) left and right oblique views. These radiographic techniques can be supplemented, when indicated, by views of the temporomandibular joints or occlusal radiographs.

1. **PA view**. This projection provides a good view of the ascending ramus, the angle of the mandible, and the body of the mandible seen from the front. Because of the superimposition of the cervical spine, the symphysis of the mandible is poorly delineated. This can be partially circumvented by turning the head slightly to the left or right side, depending on the area of interest. This view is obtained by having the patient place his or her forehead and nose on the cassette. The sagittal plane of the head is perpendicular to the plane of the cassette; the central ray is perpendicular to the cassette.
2. **Lateral oblique view** (Fig. 6.4). This view is the most common and useful of the conventional projections. It is obtained by placing a 5 × 7-inch film cassette at the side of the lower jaw. The x-ray tube is angled 30° cranially with the central beam at the angle of the mandible. This view depicts the body, including alveolar part, retromolar trigone, angle, ascending ramus, sigmoid notch, mandibular condyle, and coronoid process of the mandible.
3. **Lateral view**. This view provides limited information because both halves of the mandible are superimposed. The film cassette is placed on the side of the face, including the jaw. The x-ray tube points toward the face from a straight lateral position. The central beam is focused on the angle of the mandible.
4. **Panoramic radiograph** (Fig. 6.5). The panoramic x-ray machine makes a curved plane tomogram of the upper and lower jaw, including teeth. The image is obtained by a synchronous and reciprocal movement of the x-ray tube and the film cassette around the lower region of the patient's head. This single radiograph provides a survey of the entire mandible, including condyles and coronoid processes, and the maxilla, including the lower part of the nasal cavities and maxillary antra. The apices of the teeth, are well depicted, with the exception of the anterior teeth, for which the cervical spine usually interferes.

■ Intraoral Radiography

Intraoral dental radiography is performed with small dental film packets containing nonscreen high-speed x-ray film and a sheet of lead foil to reduce x-ray backscatter. The dental x-ray machine consists of a small, lightweight, freely movable tube head with a tube current of 10–15 mA and a range of 60–100 kVp. There are three basic intraoral projections: periapical, bitewing, and occlusal. For a radiologist, the periapical and intraoral views are important in the evaluation of the anatomy of the tooth apices and adjacent bone. The relationship of the tooth to pathological processes constitutes an important diagnostic parameter in many lesions. The intraoral dental view depicts the lingual and outer surface of the anterior mandible and localizes stones in the submandibular ducts. In addition, this view can be used to demonstrate the anterior hard palate.

■ Computed Tomography

CT has become an important diagnostic tool in the assessment of many mandibular and maxillary lesions, especially malignant tumors within and outside of the mandible. It is well suited for demonstrating bony abnormalities in the mandible and maxilla and for evaluating the adjacent soft-tissue structures. The examination should include: (1) bone and soft-tissue window settings; (2) 3, 4, or 5 mm axial sections parallel to the inferior bony margin of the body of the mandible from the level of the temporomandibular joint to the hyoid bone (Fig. 6.6); and (3) 3–4 mm coronal sections from the external auditory canal to the anterior margin of the symphysis of the mandible perpendicular to the orbitomeatal line (Fig. 6.7). CT (with high-resolution targeting and extended bone window setting) is especially indicated for analyzing bony abnormalities, such as expansion (especially of the lingual and outer buccal surface of the mandible), bone destruction, and extraosseous extension of benign and malignant lesions. Lesions arising in the floor of mouth and gingiva with secondary invasion of the mandible are also well seen on CT. CT improves detection of cortical thinning, pathological fracture, periosteal reaction, and degree of osseous expansion, and confirms the presence or absence of matrix mineralization in various tumors of the mandible and maxilla.[4,5,7]

■ Magnetic Resonance Imaging (MRI)

MRI has limited application for the majority of mandibular lesions. There are, however, some lesions in which MRI contributes to the diagnostic assessment, such as differentiation of solid from

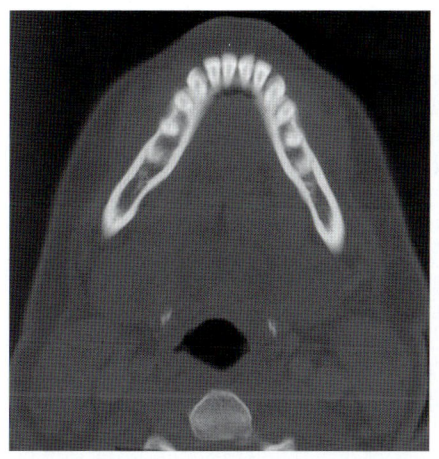

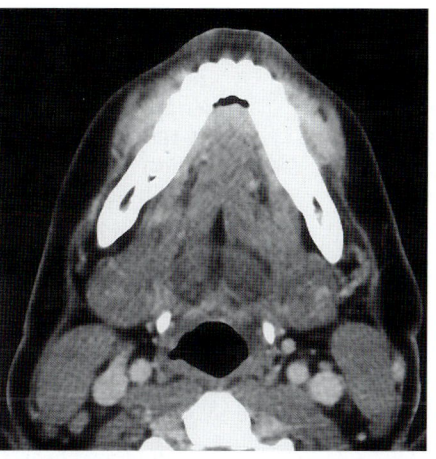

Fig. 6.6 Normal CT study of the mandible. Axial CT sections of the mandible (**a** bone window; **b** soft-tissue window setting) demonstrate a normal mandible and adjacent soft-tissue structures.

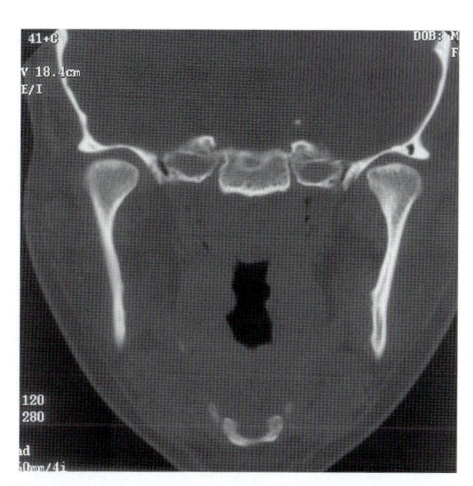

Fig. 6.7 Normal CT study of the mandible. Coronal CT projection (bone window) demonstrates normal ascending rami.

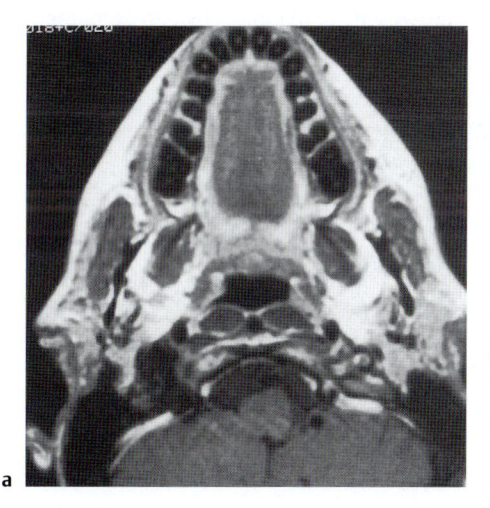

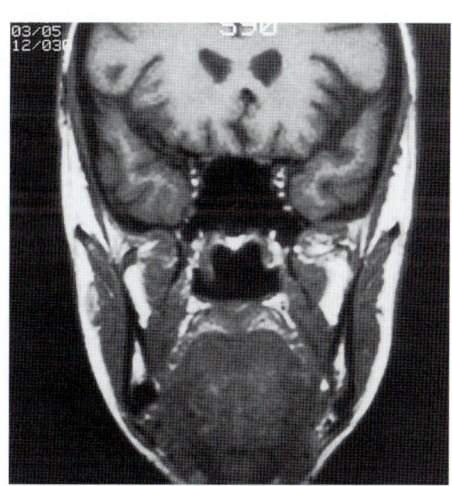

Fig. 6.8 Normal MR study of the mandible. **a** Axial T1W image reveals the normal ascending rami of the mandible and alveolar portion containing teeth of the maxilla. **b** Coronal T1W section of the mandible reveals the ascending rami. The cortex is low in signal intensity, while the marrow reveals high signal intensity. Note the masticator space adjacent to the ascending ramus of the mandible.

cystic lesions, invasion of the mandible by a malignant tumor, and bone marrow abnormalities. MRI may also provide information in the characterization of the cyst content (such as fluid, keratin, and blood). MR imaging is superior to CT in delineating soft-tissue tumor extent because of its improved contrast resolution. The examination should be performed with 3–5 mm axial and coronal projections, using T1-weighted and T2-weighted images (Fig. 6.8). Contrast material is indicated for assessing the extent of malignant lesions.

On the magnetic resonance images, a fluid-filled cyst exhibits a low, intermediate, or high signal intensity depending on the composition of the fluid. Proteinaceous fluid and subacute/chronic blood exhibit high signal intensity on T1-weighted and T2-weighted MR images. Acute hemorrhage appears very hypointense on T2-weighted MR sequences. Hemosiderin appears hypointense on T2-weighted and on gradient-echo pulse sequences. In benign as well as malignant tumors, the T1-weighted sequence most often reveals a low to an intermediate signal intensity and the T2-weighted MR images reveal high signal intensity. Tumors, unlike cystic lesions, will demonstrate enhancement on gadolinium-enhanced T1-weighted MR pulse sequences. Differentiating between cyst and tumor may be useful in younger patients with certain types of cysts, such as the hemorrhagic bone cyst, where, in some cases, surgical intervention is not indicated. Some tumors, including ameloblastoma, exhibit aggressive behavior with extraosseous extension. If the tumor is not completely removed surgically, recurrence is apt to occur in a high percentage of cases. MRI is of the utmost importance for visualizing and delineating the extraosseous extension prior to surgical extirpation. The mandible is a frequent site of erosion by carcinomas arising in the adjacent structures, such as the gingiva, floor of the mouth, and tongue. This bony erosion is characterized by loss of the signal void displayed by the cortical bone of the mandible. The medullary portion of the mandible consists of fatty marrow, which is reflected by high signal intensity on the T1-weighted MR images; therefore, obliteration of the increased signal intensity on the T1-weighted MR images often reflects tumor invasion. Tumors within the marrow, such as metastatic disease, leukemia, lymphoma, or multiple myeloma, also replace the high signal intensity on T1-weighted MR images by a low signal intensity.

Pathology

■ Congenital and Developmental Anomalies

Developmental anomalies affecting the mandible and maxilla often result in skeletal facial anomalies including facial asymmetry. Condylar agenesis or hypoplasia result in mandibular

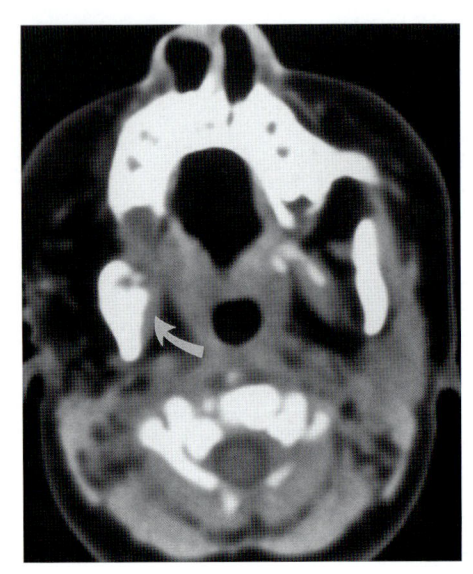

Fig. 6.9 Hemifacial microsomia. CT scan shows a hypoplastic right mandibular ramus. Note also hypoplasia of the right medial pterygoid muscle (arrow) and absence of the right parotid gland. Case courtesy of M.F. Mafee, MD.

deficiency (retrognathia). Excessive condylar growth results in prognathism. In many cases, the maxilla also demonstrates an abnormal growth pattern. Mandibular hypoplasia may occur as a feature of several syndromes including hemifacial microsomia (first and second branchial arch syndrome), Treacher–Collins syndrome (mandibulofacial dysostosis), Goldenhar syndrome, and Pierre Robin syndrome (Fig 6.9). In hemifacial microsomia, marked hypoplasia of the mandible on the affected side is seen. At times the mandibular ramus may be absent. The masticatory muscles show reduced volume ipsilateral to the side of involvement. In mandibulofacial dysostosis (MFD), moderate to marked hypoplasia of the mandibular rami and condyles is present. Pierre Robin syndrome is characterized by micrognathia, glossoptosis, and cleft palate. In Crouzon syndrome, Apart syndrome, and Saethre–Chotzen syndrome, the maxilla is hypoplastic with elongated prominent alveolar process as well as high-arched palate. In some cases, the coronoid process may be elongated, resulting in limitation of mandibular movement (Fig. 6.10).

Inflammation

A variety of inflammatory conditions can involve the mandible and maxilla. Chief among them is dental infection. Inflammatory processes can spread to the bone, causing osteomyelitis. Inflammatory changes in the mandible and maxilla have the same imaging appearance as infection in other bones. Actinomycosis and other chronic inflammatory diseases including fungal infections can involve the mandible and maxilla. Fungal infections, particularly aggressive aspergillosis and mucormycosis, are seen in immunocompromised patients. Fungal infections can invade the wall of the maxillary sinus and lead to significant bone erosion and soft-tissue involvement, followed by orbital and cranial involvement. Osteomyelitis of the mandible may present radiographically as suppurative osteomyelitis, sclerosing (chronic) osteomyelitis, or osteomyelitis with periostitis, and as osteoradionecrosis.[7] Acute suppurative osteomyelitis is sudden in onset and runs a very acute course, associated with fever and other constitutional reactions. In the first 8–10 days, plain radiographs may be negative for abnormal findings. Later, radiolucent areas will appear. Bone scintigraphy, MR and CT imaging may detect the early stage of the disease (Fig. 6.11). Sclerosing osteomyelitis of the mandible is a predominantly proliferative reaction of bone representing the reaction of bone to a low-grade infection.[7] The process may be focal or diffuse. The focal type is known as periapical osteitis, often chronic, resulting in a periapical sclerotic bone. The chronic diffuse type causes thickening of the cortical outline and sclerosis of the marrow spaces.[7] Osteomyelitis with periostitis is a variant of osteomyelitis in which a periosteal reaction predominates, leading to subperiosteal deposition of new bone.[7] This condition was erroneously described in the past as Garré osteomyelitis.[7] In osteomyelitis one should also look for formation of sequestra.

Osteoradionecrosis

Osteoradionecrosis, which occurs following high-dose irradiation of the bone, is characterized by a chronic, painful necrosis accompanied by late sequestration and permanent bone deformity (Fig. 6.12). The plain film or CT scans may show multiple radiolucent areas or a moth-eaten appearance of involved bone (Fig. 6.12).

Benign and Malignant Tumors

Despite the application of the various radiological modalities, a definitive diagnosis often cannot be made, and exploration and histological examination are mandatory. Table 6.1 provides a list of the most common cysts and benign and malignant tumors that are encountered in the mandible and maxilla. For a tentative radiological diagnosis, various parameters should be analyzed: (1) the location of the lesions within the mandible (symphysis, body, or ascending ramus) or maxilla, (2) the relationship of the cyst to the adjacent tooth structures (whether the crown of the tooth is incorporated [dentigerous cyst] or whether the apex of the tooth is part of the cyst wall [radicular, dentigerous cysts], (3) the shape of the lesions (round or oval) and the presence of interdigitation or fingerlike projections between the tooth apices (hemorrhagic bone cyst), (4) the degree of lucency manifested by the cystic cavity and the presence of calcification or bone (Pindborg tumor, cementoma, odontoma, ossifying fibroma, periapical cemental dysplasia), (5) the demarcation of the lesion (sharply delimited or less well defined), (6) sclerotic reaction or new bone formation (osteogenic sarcoma, chondrosarcoma), and (7) the presence of teeth or tooth derivatives within a lesion (odontoma). These radiological criteria should be evaluated in each case, and their analysis forms the basis for the final radiological diagnosis.

Odontogenic and Nonodontogenic Cysts of the Mandible[4, 5, 7]

Cystic lesions of the mandible and maxilla represent a diverse group of lesions that are easily visualized by radiographic means.[2, 7] Cysts are defined as epithelium-lined cavities containing fluid or semisolid material. A microscopic examination of the lining, along with the radiographic findings, is necessary for the diagnosis. Cysts present radiologically as unilocular or multilocular lucent areas of various sizes, contours, and definitions. Their relationship to a tooth provides important differential diagnostic features. They have been subdivided on the basis of development into odontogenic and nonodontogenic cysts (Table 6.1).

Odontogenic Cysts[4, 5, 7]

Odontogenic cysts arise from tooth derivatives and are differentiated according to the composition of the epithelial layer, the relationship to a tooth, and possible containment of calcifications.

Pathology 515

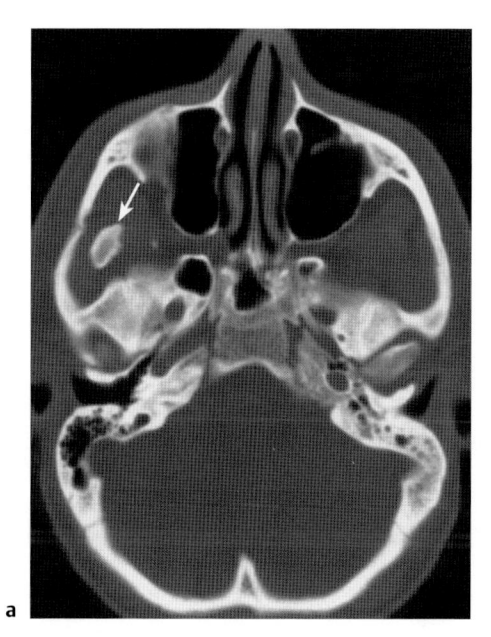

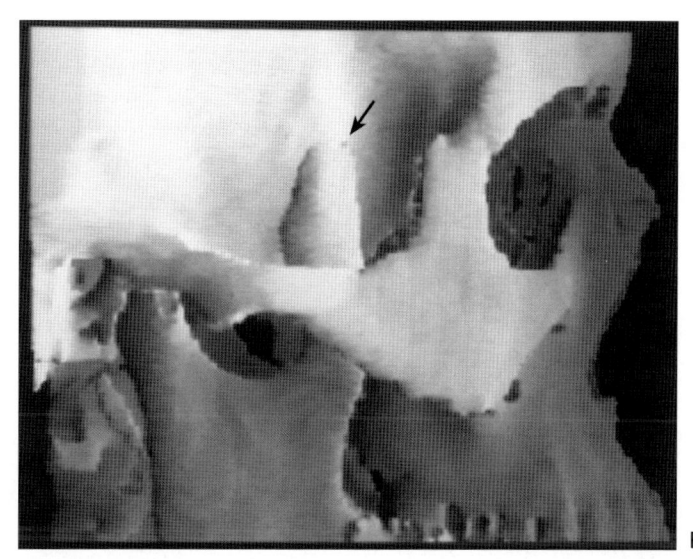

Fig. 6.**10** Elongated coronoid process. **a** Axial CT scan and **b** reformatted 3D image showing marked elongated right coronoid process (arrow).

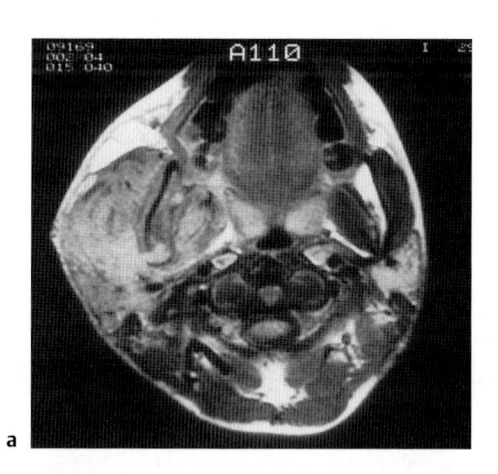

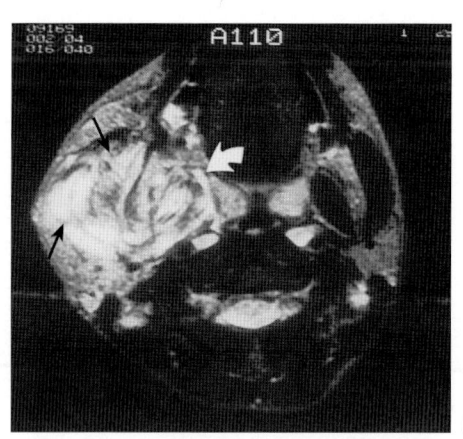

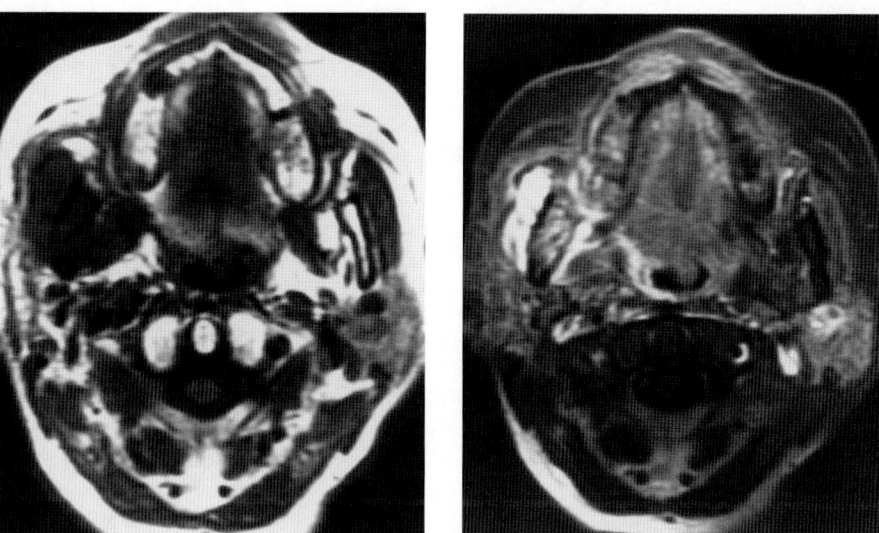

Fig. 16.**11** Osteomyelitis of the mandible associated with infection of the masticatory space.
a   Axial PW MR scan shows marked swelling of the right masseter, right medial pterygoid muscle, and involvement of the adjacent parotid space. Notice the edema of the marrow of the ipsilateral mandible, along with the periosteal reaction.
b   Axial T2W MR scan shows the extent of soft-tissue edema better than the PW MR scan; swollen masseter muscle (black arrows), swollen medial pterygoid muscle (curved arrow). Case courtesy of M.F. Mafee, MD.
c, d Osteomyelitis of the mandible. **c** Axial T1W and **d** axial enhanced fat-suppression T1W MR scans showing increased contrast enhancement, related to inflammatory changes involving the right mandibular ramus, right masseter, and right pterygoid muscles. Case courtesy of M.F. Mafee, MD.

Table 6.1 Cystic lesions and benign and malignant tumors the mandible and maxilla

I.	**Odontogenic cysts**
	Radicular cyst
	Dentigerous cyst
	Odontogenic keratocyst
	Basal cell nevus syndrome
		V	**Fibro-osseous lesions**
			Fibrous dysplasia
			   Monostotic
			   Polyostotic
			   McCune–Albright syndrome
			   Cherubism
			Ossifying fibroma
			Psammomatous ossifying fibroma (juvenile aggressive ossifying fibroma)
			Osteoblastoma
			Chondroblastoma
			Paget disease
			Osteopetrosis

II	**Nonodontogenic cysts**
	Fissural cysts
	   Nasopalatine duct cyst (incisive canal cyst)
	   Globulomaxillary cyst
	   Nasolabial cyst (nasoalveolar cyst)
	Solitary, simple, or hemorrhagic bone cyst
	Static bone cavity (Stafne cyst)		

III	**Benign odontogenic tumors**
	Epithelial odontogenic tumors
	   Ameloblastoma
	   Calcifying epithelial odontogenic tumor (Pindborg tumor)
	   Mixed tissue tumors of odontogenic origin
	   Odontoma
	      Complex composite odontoma
	      Compound composite odontoma
	      Ameloblastic odontoma
	Mesodermal odontogenic tumors
	   Odontogenic fibromyxoma
	   Cementomas
	      Periapical cemental dysplasia
	      Cementifying fibroma
	      Gigantiform cementoma
	      Benign cementoblastoma
		VI	**Vascular tumors**
			Hemangiomas
			Lymphangioma
			AVM
			Hemangiopericytoma

		VII	**Neurogenic tumors** Neurilemoma (schwannoma) Neurofibroma Malignant schwannoma and neurofibroma

		VIII	**Malignant tumors**
			Carcinoma
			   Secondary invasion by squamous cell carcinoma
			   Mucoepidermoid carcinoma (minor salivary gland)
			   Adenoid cystic carcinoma (minor salivary gland)
			   Metastases
			      Bronchogenic carcinoma
			      Breast
			      Hypernephroma
			      Prostate
			      Thyroid
			      Miscellaneous
			Sarcomas
			   Osteogenic sarcoma
			   Chondrosarcoma (maxilla, TMJ)
			   Fibrosarcoma
			   Ewing sarcoma
			   Synovial sarcoma (TMJ)
			Malignant lymphoma
			Multiple myeloma
			Burkitt lymphoma

IV	**Benign nonodontogenic tumors**
	Exostoses
	   Torus mandibularis
	   Torus palatinus
	   Multiple exostoses
	   Osteochondroma
	Osteomas
	   Single
	   Multiple (Gardner syndrome)
	Giant cell tumor
	Giant cell reparative granuloma
	Brown tumor of hyperparathyroidism
	Aneurysmal bone cyst (ABC)
	Langerhans cell histiocytosis
	   Letterer–Siwe disease
	   Hand–Schüller–Christian disease
	Eosinophilic granuloma		

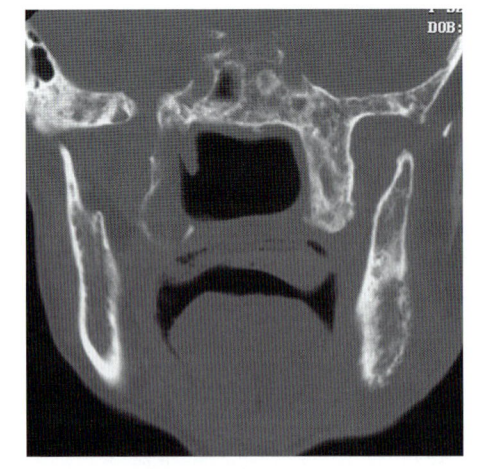

Fig. 6.12 Osteoradionecrosis. Coronal CT scan shows irregular loss of bone density of the left side of the mandible in a patient with osteoradionecrosis.

Radicular Cyst[10]

The radicular cyst is the most common cyst of the mandible and maxilla. It is a well-circumscribed radiolucency arising from the apex of a tooth. It is bounded by a thin rim of cortical bone and lined by squamous epithelium (Fig. 6.13). In larger lesions, there is expansion of the cortex. The radicular cyst causes tooth structures to be displaced, and slight root resorption may occur in the adjacent teeth. Extension into the maxillary sinus may be observed if the cyst occurs in the maxilla. Radiographically, radicular cysts cannot be differentiated from periapical granulomas, but the latter are usually less than 1.5 cm in diameter.[4,5,7]

Dentigerous (Follicular) Cyst[11]

The dentigerous cyst, after the radicular cyst, is the most common odontogenic cyst. Most are located in the mandible and are related to the crown of an unerupted tooth. Rarely, multiple dentigerous cysts may occur. They are variable in size, sharply delimited, and may expand bone if of sufficient size. They are well-defined, unilocular or rarely multilocular radiolucencies

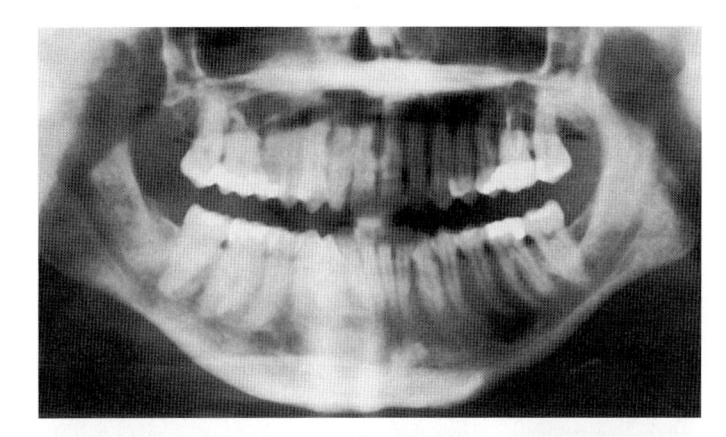

Fig. 6.**13a** Radicular cyst of the mandible. Panorex view of the mandible reveals a sharply defined cystic lesion in the body of the mandible, adjacent to the root of the left second premolar tooth.

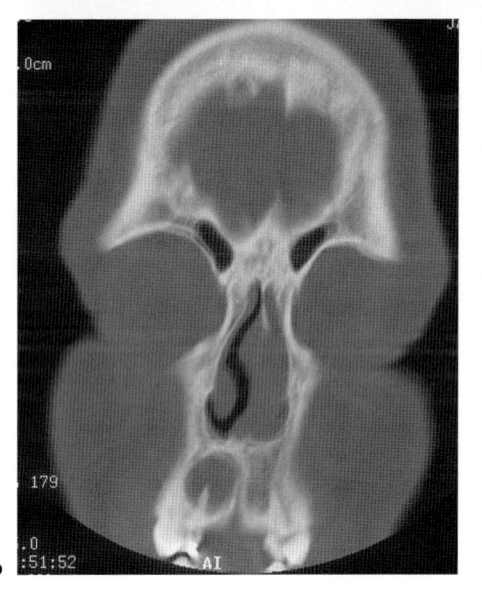

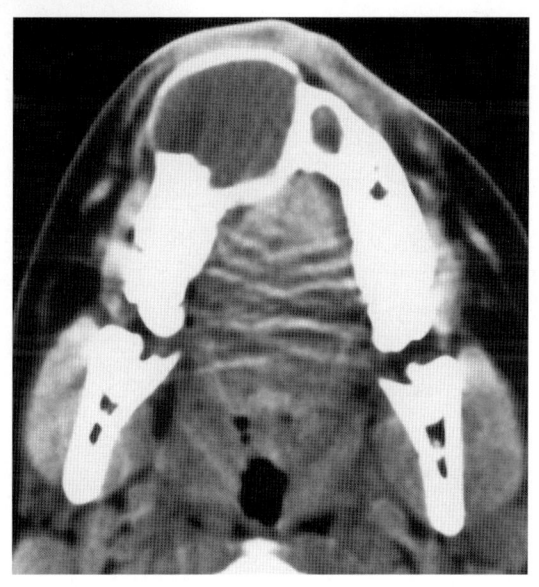

Fig. 6.**13**
b Radicular cyst. CT scan reveals a sharply defined cyst in the maxilla adjacent to the roots of the right lateral incisor and canine tooth.
c Radicular cyst of maxilla. Clinical data: 10-year-old girl with expansile right maxillary cyst, consistent with odontogenic cyst. CT scan demonstrates a large expansile cyst, involving the anterior portion of the right maxilla. Pathology report indicated squamous-lined fibrous-walled cyst with chronic inflammation, consistent with radicular cyst. Case courtesy of M.F. Mafee, MD.

that incorporate the crown of a tooth (Fig. 6.**14**). They may cause displacement of teeth, and apical resorption of adjacent tooth structures may occur. Rarely, the dentigerous cyst is the development site of ameloblastomas, mucoepidermoid tumors, and carcinomas. On MR imaging, the contents of the cyst show low signal intensity on T1-weighted and high signal intensity on T2-weighted MR images. There will be no contrast enhancement on enhanced CT and MR scans. A thin rim of enhancement may be present representing the capsule. Those lesions that involve the maxilla often extend into the maxillary antrum, displacing and remodeling the bony sinus. Unlike ameloblastoma, dentigerous cysts do not demonstrate an extracystic soft-tissue mass; not all ameloblastomas, however, demonstrate a soft-tissue component and an ameloblastoma may simulate a dentigerous cyst. On the other hand, ameloblastomas, mucoepidermoid tumors, and carcinomas may develop in a dentigerous cyst.[7]

Odontogenic Keratocyst[12–16]

The odontogenic keratocyst (OKC) arises from epithelial rests of the dental lamina and accounts for 2–11 % of all jaw cysts.[12–16] The cyst occurs in patients of all ages, with a peak incidence in the second and third decades of life.[13] This cyst has been classified as a separate type of bone cyst because of its different clinical behavior and histological composition. The odontogenic keratocyst is filled with yellow cheesy keratin and lined with multiple layers (6–8) of stratified, epithelial cells, with keratinization of the cyst lining.[6–12] The cyst may be unilocular (but often multilocular) and demonstrate an aggressive growth pattern reflected by marked thinning of bone with expansion. In cysts that have not been completely excised, recurrence has been demonstrated in 30–40 % of these lesions. The diagnosis depends on its microscopic features and is independent of its radiographic appearance (i.e., a dentigerous or radicular cyst may prove to be a keratocyst on histological examination). The keratocyst is a radiolucent lesion that is often multiloculated, has a smooth or scalloped border, and is most commonly located in the body and ramus of the mandible (Figs. 6.**15**–6.**17**). It may cause marked cortical thinning and expansion with root resorption (Fig. 6.**15**). Large keratocysts in the maxilla cause expansion of the antrum and loss of bone (Fig. 6.**14c, d**). CT shows a water-density, sharply defined cystic lesion. At times, there may be focal increased density due to dense epithelial debris (keratoma). On MR images, the cyst is low or intermediate in signal intensity on T1-weighted images, and high in signal intensity on T2-weighted images (Figs. 6.**16**, 6.**17**). Following intravenous administration of gadolinium contrast material, there will be some enhancement at the peripheral portion of the cyst (Fig. 6.**15e**). Invasion of the adjacent tissues such as masseter muscle may result in moderate to marked reactive enhancement of the involved soft tissue (Fig. 6.**16**), giving an MR appearance in favor of an ameloblastoma rather than OKC (Fig. 6.**16d**). In many instances, a keratocyst cannot be differentiated radiographically from an ameloblastoma.

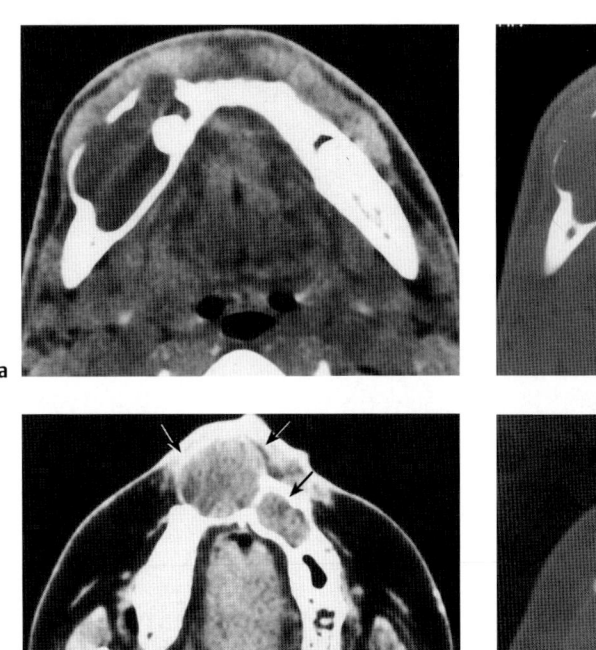

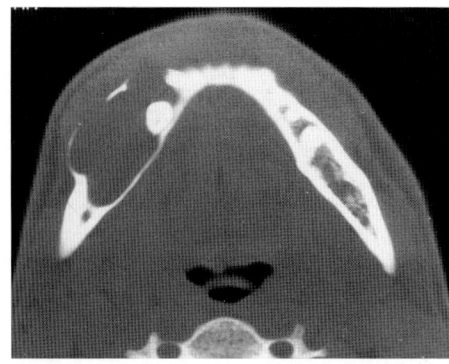

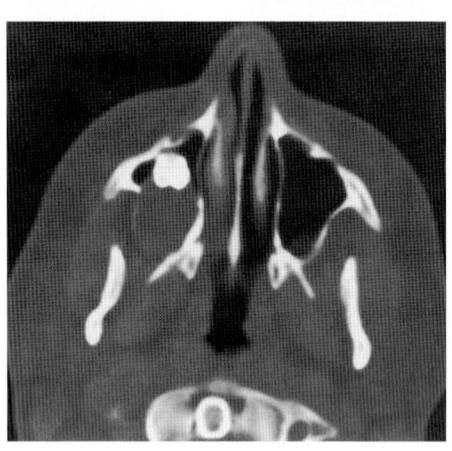

Fig. 6.**14** Dentigerous cyst. Axial (**a** soft-tissue window; **b** bone-tissue window) CT scans demonstrate an expansile cystic lesion involving the body of the right mandible. There is incorporation of the root of a tooth in the anterior portion of the cyst. Note partial erosion of the buccal cortex of the mandible. **c** Axial CT scan in another patient shows a dentigerous cyst (arrows) involving the maxilla. Cases courtesy of M.F. Mafee, MD. **d** Dentigerous cyst. Axial CT section demonstrates an expansile cystic lesion in the posterior portion of the right maxillary antrum and adjacent infratemporal fossa. There is incorporation of the root of a tooth in the anterior portion of the cyst. This cyst arose from the alveolar process of the right maxilla, which is not demonstrated.

Lesions such as OKC, dentigerous cyst, ameloblastoma, ameloblastic fibroma, adenomatoid odontogenic cyst, and traumatic cyst must all be considered when a well-circumscribed radiolucent lesion of the jaw is seen on panoramic radiographs.[14, 15] Complete excision of the cyst is the treatment of choice. The recurrence rate after incomplete surgical excision has been variously reported as between 20% and 60%.[13] Brannon's[16] well-known study of 312 OKCs demonstrated that there were no recurrences when the lesions were excised in one piece.

Basal Cell Nevus Syndrome (Gorlin or Gorlin-Goltz Syndrome)

Basal cell nevus syndrome (nevoid basal cell carcinoma syndrome) is a genetic disorder, inherited as an autosomal dominant trait with variable penetrance and expressivity.[7] Multiple keratocysts of variable size are found in basal cell nevus syndrome, along with multiple basal cell nevi that usually transform into basal cell carcinomas. In addition, there are skeletal abnormalities and ectopic excessive dural calcifications. The jaw cysts develop early in childhood; they may be either unilocular or multilocular and often prove to be keratocytes, varying in size from a few millimeters to several centimeters (Fig. 6.**18**).

Nonodontogenic Cysts[4]

Nonodontogenic cysts are developmental in origin. The fissural variety arise, as the name implies, along lines of fusion of various bones and embryonic processes. Like the odontogenic cysts, they are lined with epithelium and usually contain fluid or semisolid material. Fissural cysts are classified according to their anatomical location. Additional developmental cysts are derived from embryological rests, such as dermoid and epidermoid cysts. Cysts of other etiologies without epithelial lining include solitary bone cysts, Stafne cysts, and "aneurysmal bone cysts".

Fissural Cysts

The **nasopalatine duct cyst** ("incisive canal cyst") is located in the incisive canal near the anterior palatine papilla.[7, 17] These cysts probably arise from epithelial remnants in the incisive canal. Most of the cysts are small and are found on routine radiographic studies. The incisive canal is always located at or in close proximity to the midline. The cyst is well circumscribed and oval or round (Fig. 6.**19**). Large cysts may bulge into the nasal cavity or maxillary antra. A condensed rim of cortical bone is often seen along the periphery, and the roots of the central incisor may be divergent.

The **globulomaxillary cyst**[12] is a historical term used to describe a cyst that is located in the maxilla between the lateral incisor and the canine tooth at the site that corresponds to the incisive suture (Fig. 6.**20**). The cyst is believed to arise from epithelial rests between the medial nasal and maxillary processes during embryonic fusion.[19] It is likely that some of the lesions diagnosed as globulomaxillary cyst were in fact odontogenic cyst.[20] It usually extends toward the crest of the alveolar ridge and may produce a divergence of roots of the adjoining teeth, assuming a pear shape as it increases in size. If a globulomaxillary cyst extends over the apex of the root of one or both adjacent teeth, it is important to determine the vitality of the tooth in question to differentiate the globulomaxillary cyst from the radicular cyst.

The **nasoalveolar** (nasolabial cyst) occurs in the soft tissues of the lateral aspect of the nose and adjacent upper lip.[19, 21] These cysts are three times more common in women than in men.[19] Nasoalveolar cysts are found between the nasal ala and the maxilla and do not invade or separate bone.[19] They usually elevate the anterior nasal floor on the involved side. They may rarely be bilateral. The cyst is believed to originate from trapped epithelium in a cleft formed during the development of the

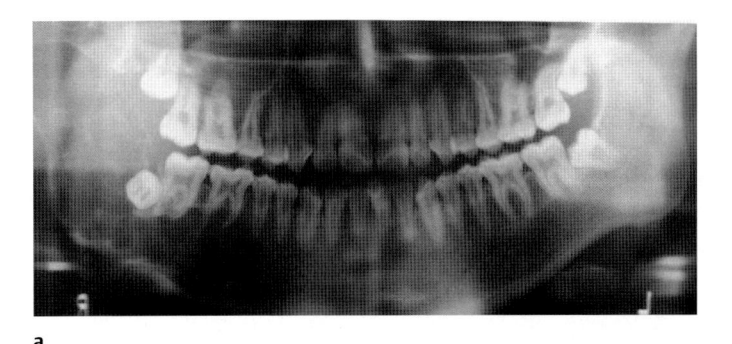

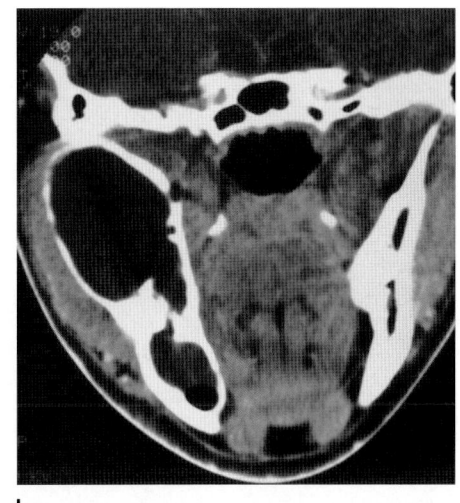

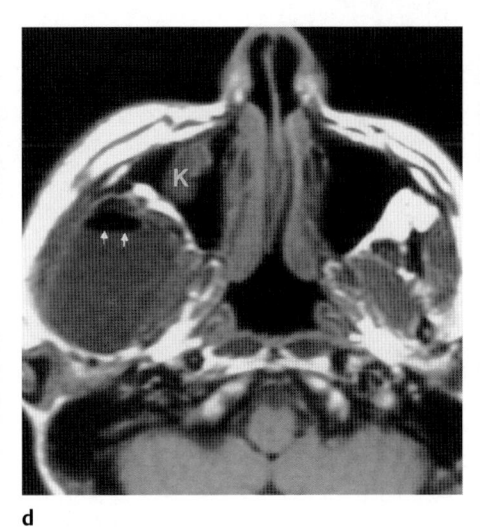

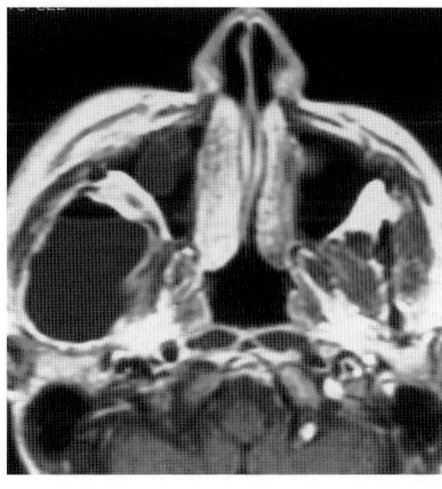

Fig. 6.15 Odontogenic keratocyst. **a** Panorex view of the mandible demonstrates a large multicompartmental cystic lesion, involving the entire ramus and part of the body of the mandible on the right side. The cysts are separated by linear septations. **b** Coronal CT scan (soft-tissue window) reveals an expansile cystic lesion in the ramus and body of the right mandible. **c** Axial CT scan (bone window), shows the expansile lesion in the right ramus, associated with some cortical scalloping (large arrows) as well as cortical thinning. Note another keratocyst (small arrows) involving the alveolar process of the right maxilla. **d** Unenhanced T1W and **e** enhanced T1W MR scans demonstrate an air–fluid level (arrows) in the mandibular cyst. Note a thin rim of contrast enhancement at the periphery of the cyst and a small maxillary keratocyst (K). Case courtesy of M.F. Mafee, MD.

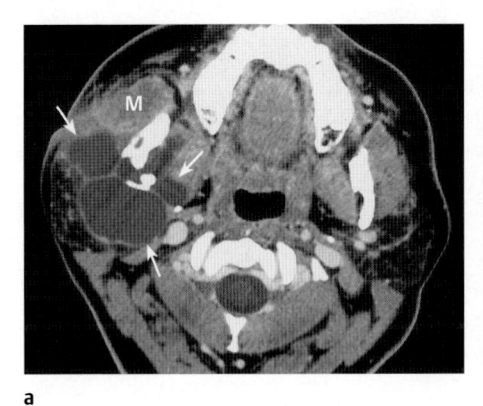

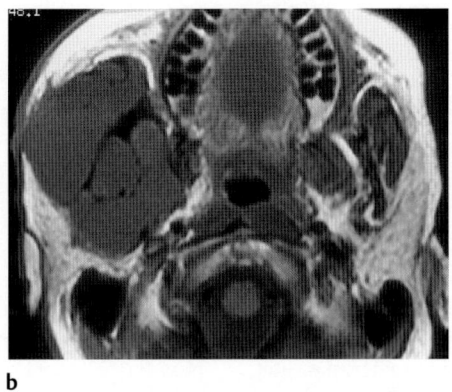

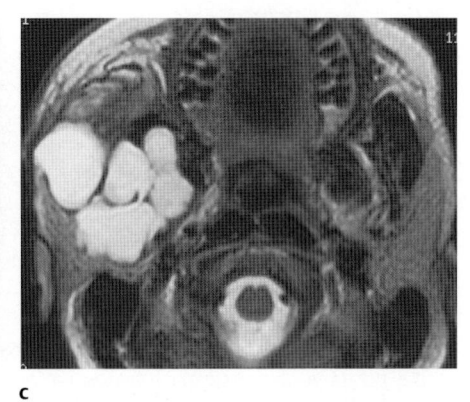

Fig. 6.16 Odontogenic keratocyst, invading the masseter muscle. **a** Enhanced axial CT scan, **b** unenhanced axial T1W, **c** axial T2W, **d** enhanced axial fat suppression T1W, and **e** enhanced coronal T1W MR scans demonstrate a large mandibular keratocyst (arrows), invading right masseter muscle (M). Note increased enhancement of the deformed right masseter muscle (M), related to inflammation. Case courtesy of M.F. Mafee, MD.

Fig. 6.**16 d, e** ▷

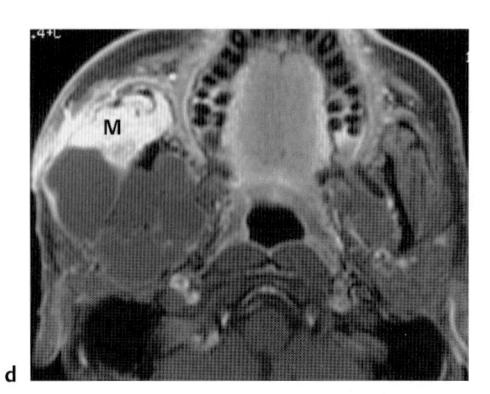

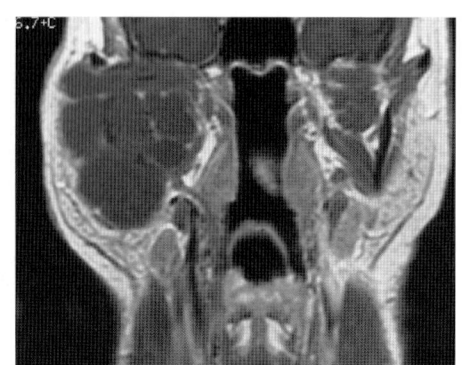

Fig. 6.**16 d, e**

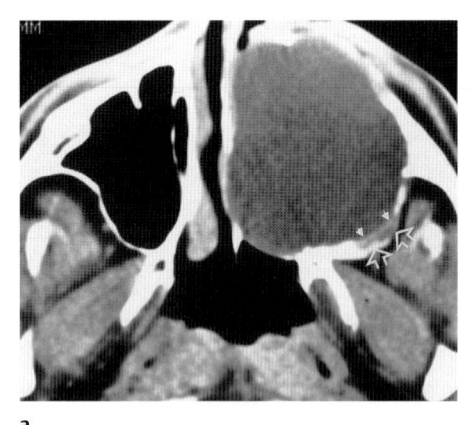

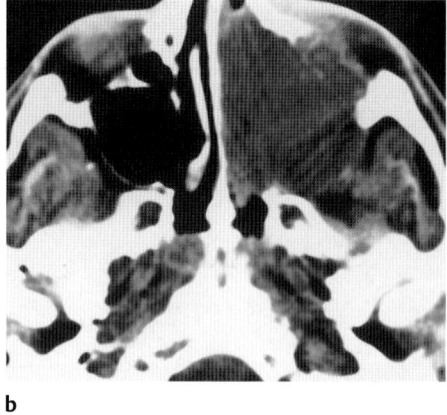

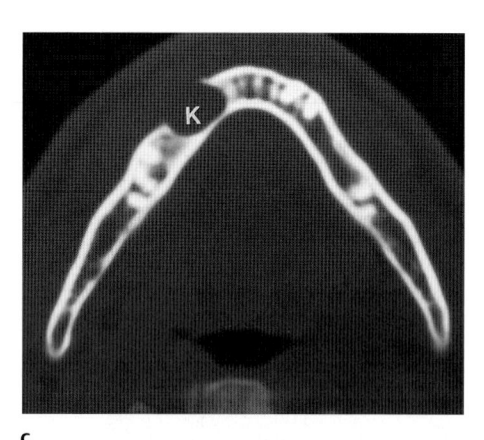

a b c

Fig. 6.**17** Multiple odontogenic keratocysts. **a** CT scan shows an expansile cystic lesion involving the left maxilla. Note remodeling of the posterior wall of the maxilla (hollow arrows) and a rim of calcification along the cyst wall (small arrows). **b** CT scan shows the cystic lesion along with erosion of the anterior and posterior wall of the left maxillary antrum. The cyst arose from the left maxillary alveolus and extended into the left maxillary antrum. **c** CT scan of the mandible shows another small keratocyst (K) involving the right mandible. Case courtesy of M.F. Mafee, MD.

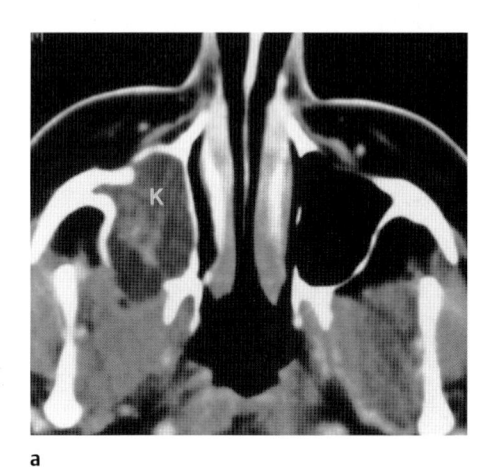

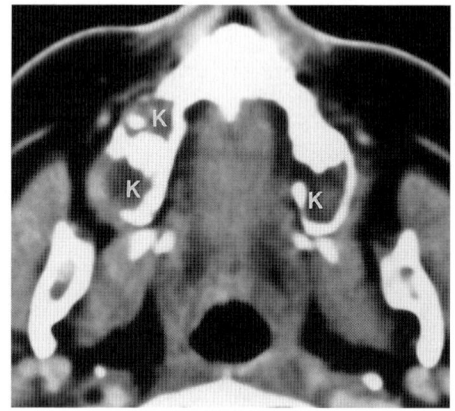

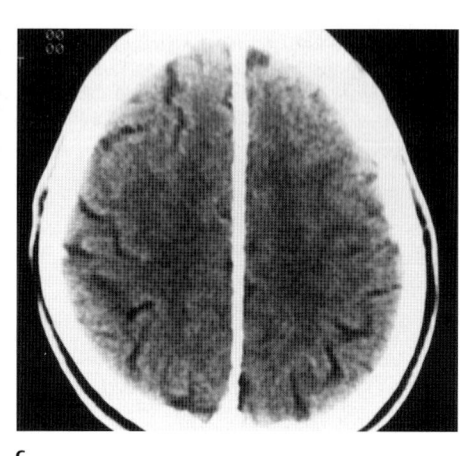

a b c

Fig. 6.**18** Basal cell nevus syndrome. **a** Enhanced axial CT scan shows an expansile mass in the right maxillary antrum, compatible with a keratocyst (K). Note increased density within the cyst, which was related to dense epithelial debris (keratoma) as well as increased enhancement. **b** Axial CT scan shows multiple keratocysts (K) involving maxillary alveolus. **c** CT scan shows marked calcification of the falx cerebri.

Fig. 6.**18 d, e** ▷

maxillary medial and lateral nasal processes.[22] Another theory is that nasoalveolar cysts arise from displaced nasolacrimal duct tissue.[19] Although these cysts are congenital, they typically present in adults.[19] These cysts are characterized by their well-defined contour and their slow expansion within the maxilla. Pressure from the cyst may cause remodeling of the adjacent maxillary bone with a hemispheric defect. On CT scan, a homogeneous, nonenhancing cystic mass is noted anterior to the piriform aperture, without erosion or separation of the underlying maxilla (Fig. 6.21).[19] If the mass has been present for a long time, there may be pressure bone atrophy and remodeling of the anterior maxilla. CT characteristics help to differentiate nasoalveolar cyst from odontogenic abscess, odontogenic cyst, globulomaxillary cyst, median palatal cyst (incisive canal cyst), fibro-osseous lesions and surgical ("postoperative") ciliated cysts (inclusion cyst) of the maxilla.[19]

Pathology 521

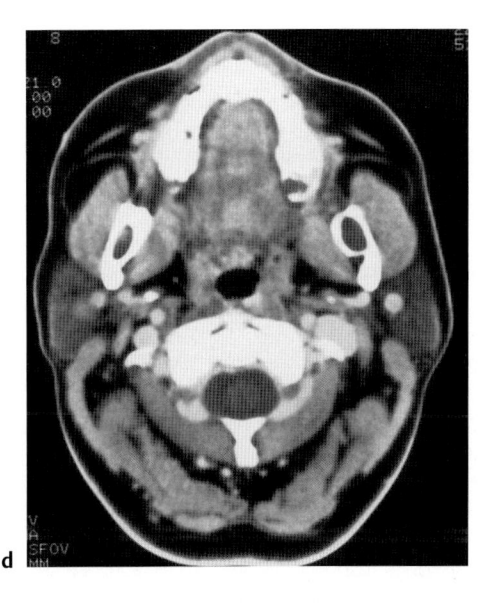

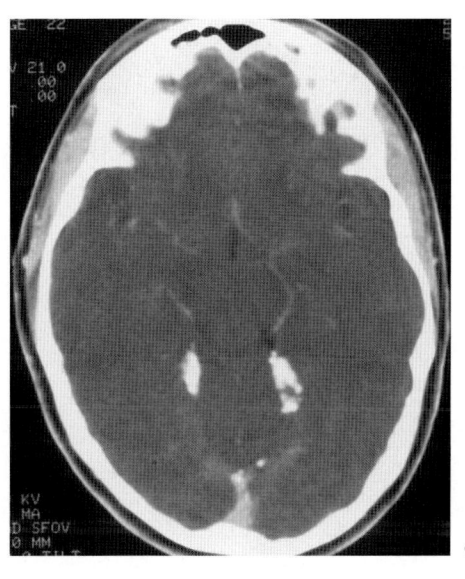

Fig. 6.**18 d** Axial CT scan shows small keratocysts involving both mandibular rami. **e** Axial CT scan shows marked calcification of the tentorium. Case courtesy of M.F. Mafee, MD.

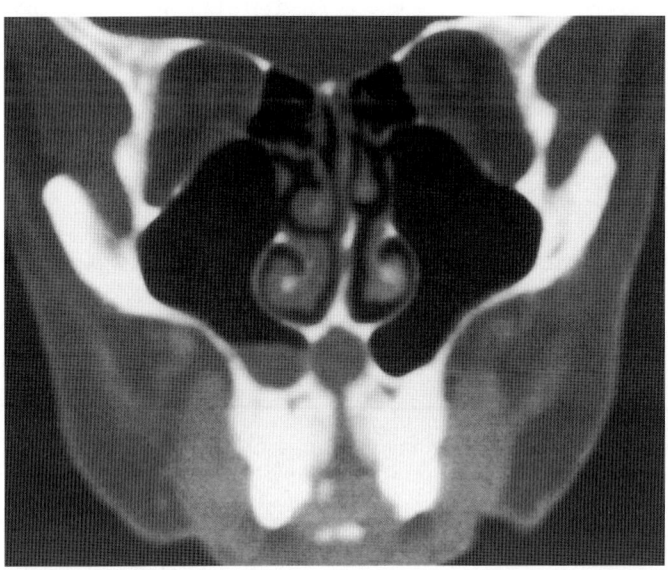

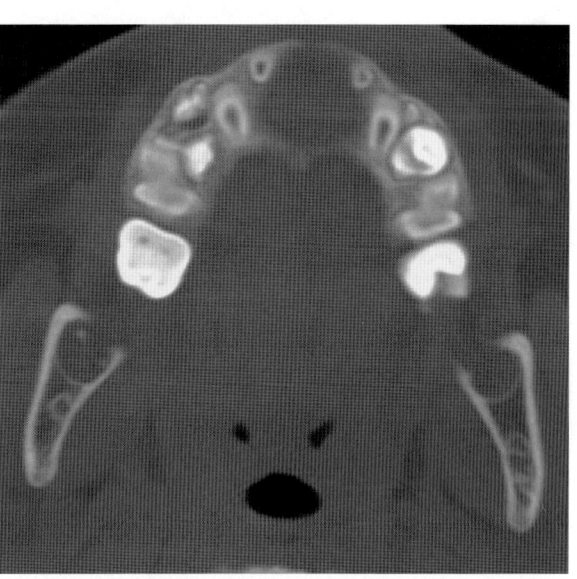

Fig. 6.**19 a** Nasopalatine cyst. Coronal CT scan shows a sharply defined, round-to-oval cystic lesion with bony expansion in the anterior incisive canal between the central incisors. **b** Axial CT scan in another patient shows a cystic lesion with bony expansion in the premaxilla compatible with an incisural cyst.

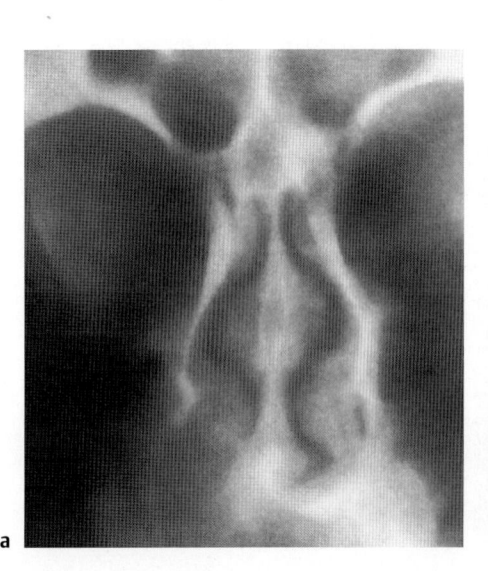

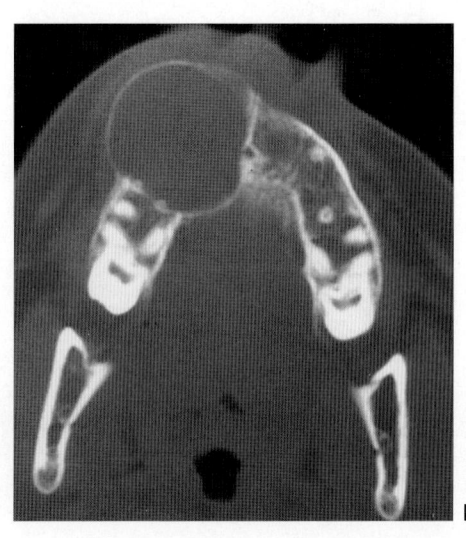

Fig. 6.**20 a** Globulomaxillary cyst. Coronal tomographic study reveals a defect in the anterior maxilla with extension into the right nasal cavity, along with a slight bulge of the lower medial wall of the right antrum laterally. **b** Axial CT scan in another patient shows a sharply defined, cystic lesion involving the right maxilla, compatible with a globulomaxillary cyst.

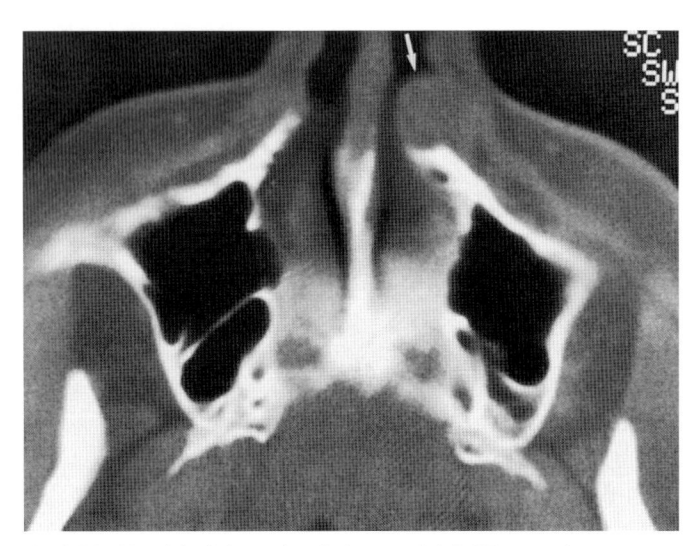

Fig. 6.21 Nasolabial (nasoalveolar) cyst. Axial CT scan shows a cyst (arrow). The cyst is displacing the nasal process of the maxilla.

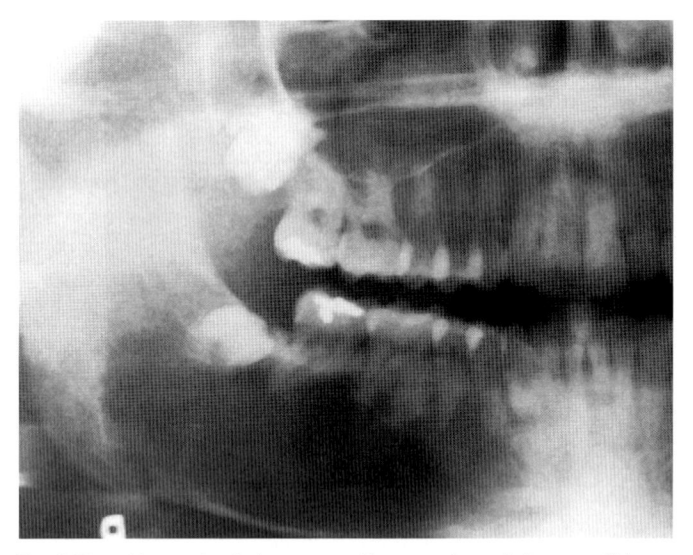

Fig. 6.22a Hemorrhagic bone cyst. Panorex view of the mandible reveals a large, oval-shaped cyst in the body, angle, and ascending ramus of the right mandible, causing slight scalloping and thinning of the inferior cortex. Note the slight encroachment with mottling on the root of the second right molar tooth.

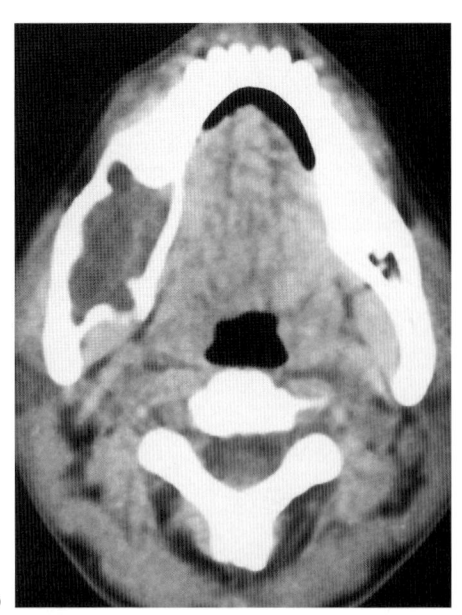

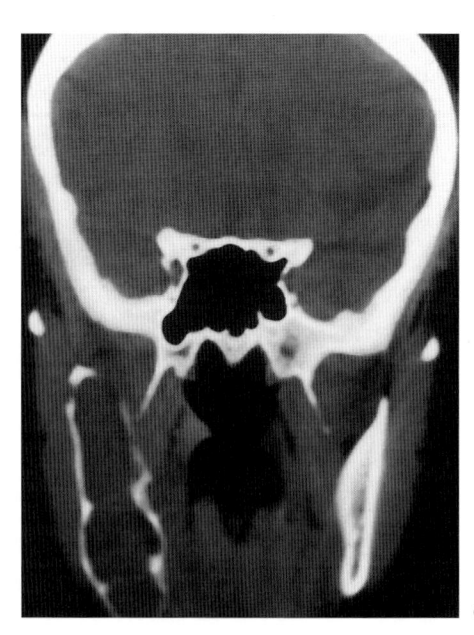

Fig. 6.22b Axial and c coronal CT scans showing a large expansile cystic lesion in the body and ramus of the right mandible, causing scalloping of the inner cortex. This was diagnosed as traumatic bone cyst. The cyst showed no epithelial lining on histological examination. Case courtesy of Berry Wenig, MD, Chicago, IL, USA.

Solitary, Simple, or Hemorrhagic Bone Cyst

The hemorrhagic bone cyst[13] is, likewise, categorized as a nonodontogenic cyst and occurs predominantly in the body of the mandible in young persons. It is usually unilocular and filled with clear or sanguinous fluid. The lining consists of loose, vascular connective tissue and no epithelial layer and may contain areas of recent or old hemorrhage. Radiographically, these cysts are slightly scalloped in shape and size and have a slightly indistinct border (Fig. 6.22). The outline of the cyst between the roots of the teeth has a scalloped appearance. Larger cysts may extend into the interdental spaces and the ramus and cause slight expansion of the mandible (Fig. 6.22b).

Static Bone Cavity (Stafne Cyst)

A Stafne cyst is a pseudocyst, seen adjacent to the medial surface of the mandible. The cortex of the mandible becomes scalloped and the bone "defect" contains fatty-areolar tissue or part of the submandibular gland tissue. Bilateral lesions have been described. The Stafne cyst[24] is usually located in the posterior mandible, often near the angle of the mandible below the mandibular canal (Fig. 6.23). It is detected incidentally on routine radiographs of the mandible and appears as an elliptic, ovoid, or round radiolucency with a well-defined border, often showing slight sclerosis of the margin.

Benign Odontogenic Tumors[25]

Odontogenic tumors result from an abnormal proliferation of the cells and tissues involved in odontogenesis. They represent a diverse group of lesions that reflect the complex development of the dental structures. The radiographic appearance varies, and many of the tumors cannot be differentiated from the cysts previously described.

Epithelial Odontogenic Tumors

Ameloblastoma

The most common benign, but aggressive, epithelial tumor is the ameloblastoma.[25,26] Ameloblastoma (synonyms: adamantinoma; adamantoblastoma) represents approximately 1% of all lesions of the jaws.[26] The tumor may occur at any age, but is most common in the third and fourth decades of life. More than 80% involve the mandible, particularly the molar–ramus area. They are often associated with unerupted third molar teeth.[26] Maxil-

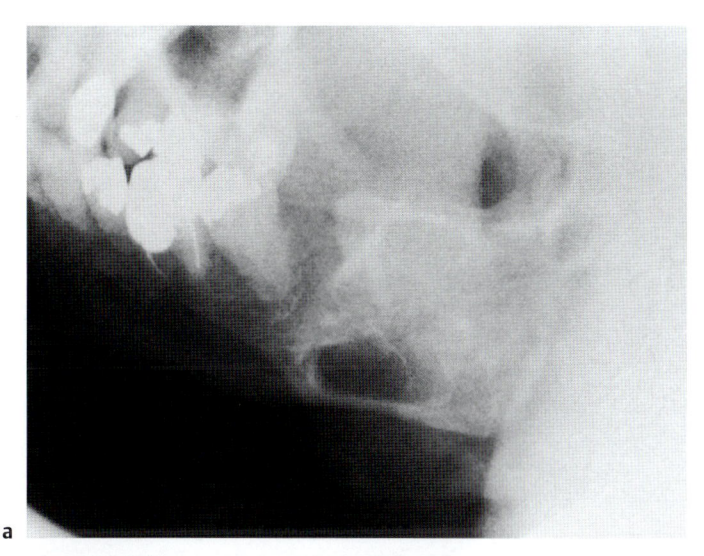

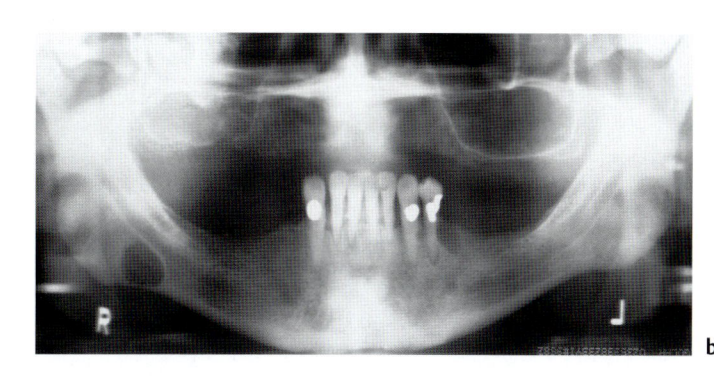

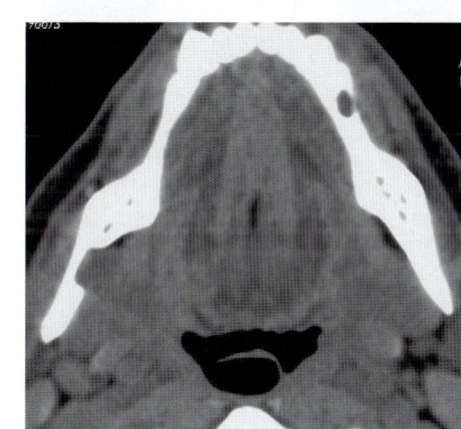

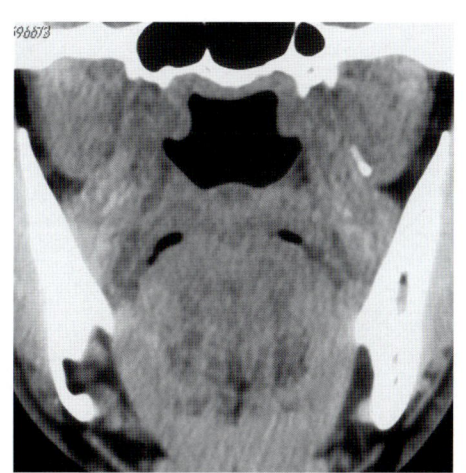

Fig. 6.23 a Stafne cyst. Oblique view of the mandible reveals a sharply defined, oval-shaped cyst in the body of the mandible inferior to the mandibular canal with a slightly sclerotic margin. b Panorex view of the mandible in another patient with presumed Stafne cyst shows a sharply defined, round cyst in the body of the right mandible inferior to the mandibular canal. c Axial and d coronal CT scans, same patient as in figure 2.23b reveal that the mandibular defect is filled with fibroneurovascular-areolar tissues, as well as part of the right submandibular gland. Case courtesy of M.F. Mafee, MD.

lary ameloblastomas primarily occur in the molar region, but the antrum and floor of the nasal cavity are often involved. The most common clinical presentation is a painless swelling of the affected area. Histologically the tumor is unencapsulated proliferating nests, islands, or sheets of odontogenic epithelium that resemble the enamel organ. Histological subtypes of ameloblastoma include follicular (solid and cystic), plexiform, acanthomatous, basal cell, and granular cell.[26] The histological subtypes of ameloblastoma have no bearing on treatment or prognosis except for the granular cell variant, which appears to be associated with an increased recurrence rate.[26] Prognosis is dependent on size, extent, and location of the tumor. Mandibular ameloblastoma tends to be confined tumors owing to the inherently thick cortical bone of the mandible. Histological malignant transformation of an ameloblastoma is referred to as ameloblastic carcinoma, which is noteworthy for predilection for the mandible and morphologically similar to squamous cell carcinoma. The tumor metastasizes to the lungs, lymph nodes, bone, and liver.[26] The differential diagnosis includes dentigerous cyst, odontogenic keratocyst, and ameloblastic fibroma. Radiographically, ameloblastomas may be unilocular or multilocular radiolucent lesions (Figs. 6.24–6.28). The unilocular variety reveals a round-to-oval configuration with distinct borders, occasional slight marginal sclerosis (Fig. 6.26), and no new periosteal bone formation. Bony expansion of various degrees, sometimes with a scalloped margin, is also observed. Loss of the lamina dura, erosion of the tooth apex, and displacement of the teeth are also encountered.[4,5,7] In the multilocular form, the lesion reveals a honeycombed or soap bubble appearance. These loculi may be oval or spherical and may vary in size. The size varies from a small cyst confined to the alveolar portion to a cyst that causes extensive expansion and destruction of the mandible or maxilla. The tumor has a tendency to penetrate the cortex of the jaw bone with subsequent formation of an extra-bony soft-tissue mass. The CT findings consist of low-attenuation cystic areas intermixed with isodense areas, reflecting the solid component of this lesion (Figs. 6.25–6.27, 6.29, 6.30). The expansile nature of an ameloblastoma is characterized by a bony shell that represents the expanded maxilla or mandible. The bony rim may be continuous or interrupted. CT is especially indicated for delineating the extraosseous component of the tumor, which is best illustrated with axial and coronal sections using bone and soft-tissue window settings (Fig. 6.25).[27] The MR appearance of ameloblastoma is similar to that of squamous cell carcinoma.[27] The lesion is low in signal intensity on T1-weighted images, and high-intensity areas are found on T2-weighted images.[27] However, ameloblastomas often show marked increase in signal intensity on T2-weighted images (Fig. 6.27). Conspicuity and edge enhancement are increased by this high signal characteristic on T2-weighted images (Figs. 6.27, 6.28).[27] On T1-weighted images, the high-intensity marrow fat is replaced by low-intensity tumor. The solid component of ameloblastoma demonstrates moderate to marked enhancement following administration of intravenous gadolinium contrast material.

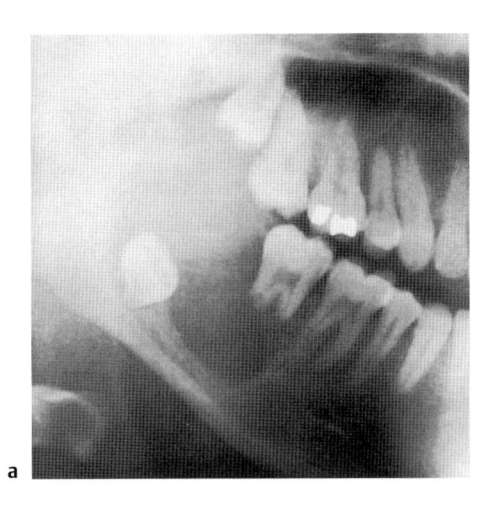

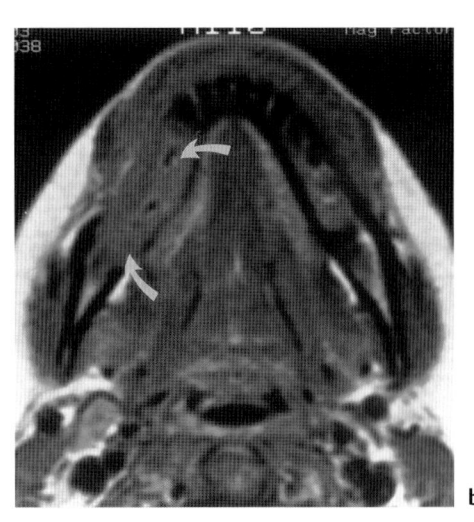

Fig. 6.**24** **a** Ameloblastoma of the right mandible. Panorex view of the mandible reveals a lucent area in the body, angle, and ascending ramus of the mandible. The lesion expands the alveolar ridge and bulges into the adjacent oral cavity. There is an impacted tooth at the posterior inferior site of the lesion and slight amputation of the posterior root of the second right molar tooth. **b** Axial CT scan in another patient showing an ameloblastoma of the left mandible (arrows). Note low signal intensity of the lesion and replacement of high-intensity fat. Case (**b**) courtesy of M.F. Mafee, MD.

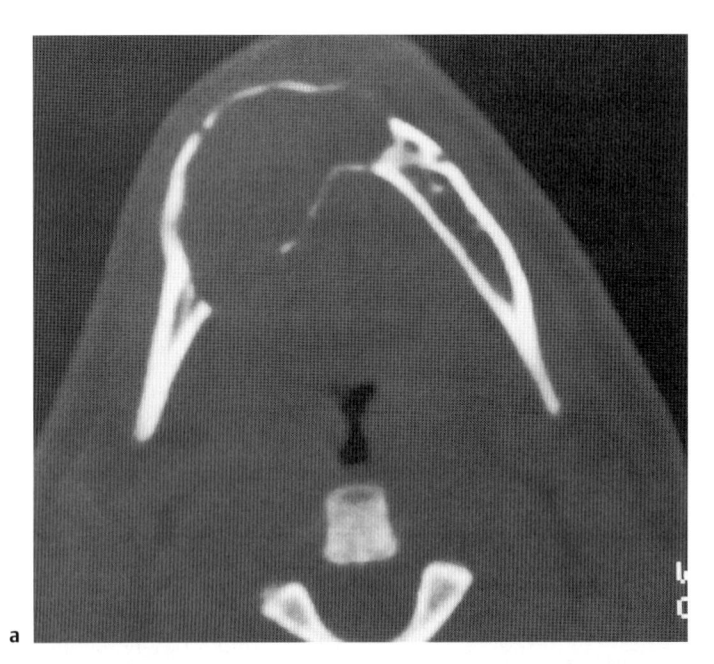

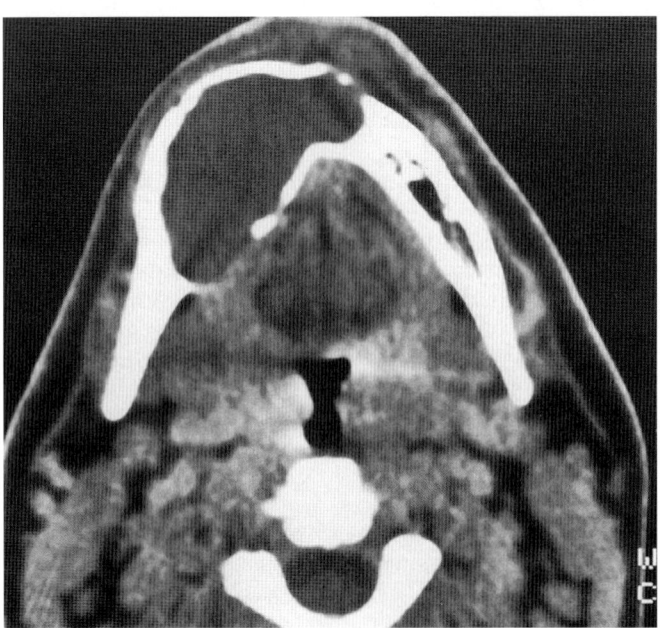

The **calcifying epithelial odontogenic tumor (Pindborg tumor)**[13, 28, 29] is a rare form of odontogenic tumor. The tumor occurs predominantly in the mandible and is most commonly encountered in the molar and premolar regions. The tumor grows slowly and extends into the extraosseous soft-tissue structures rarely. The polyhedral epithelial cells form clusters with an amyloid-like material, which may calcify. Previously, uncertainty regarding the histological characteristics of Pindborg tumor was reflected in the variety of terms for the disease, including unusual ameloblastoma, cystic odontoma, and adenoid adamantinoma.[29] Association with adenomatoid odontogenic tumor and dentigerous cyst has been reported and suggests heterogeneity in histopathogenesis.[29-31] Radiographically, they are depicted as fairly well-defined lucent areas that may be unilocular or multilocular (Fig. 6.**31**). There are often small, radiopaque, calcified foci located within the lytic lesion and found in the amyloid-like material. There is often an impacted tooth associated with the lesion. The CT appearance of Pindborg tumor includes a heterogeneous mass within the mandible and less commonly adjacent to maxillary alveolus. The lesion may contain a central tooth with surrounding amorphous calcification and moderate to marked soft-tissue elements in its peripheral portion.[29] MRI shows a heterogeneous mass that appears hypointense on T1-weighted and hyperintense on T2-weighted MR images.[29] Calcifications appear as intralesional areas of low signal on T1- and T2-weighted images. The soft-tissue component demonstrates moderate to marked enhancement following intravenous administration of gadolinium contrast material.[29]

Calcifying Odontogenic Cyst (Odontogenic Ghost Cell Tumor)

Calcifying odontogenic cyst is a rare odontogenic lesion having features of both a cyst and a solid neoplasm.[7] In the most recent WHO classification, the term odontogenic ghost cell tumor is used.[7] The ghost cell tumor designation results from characteris-

◁ Fig. 6.**25** Ameloblastoma. **a** Axial CT section (bone window) reveals an expansile lesion in the body of the right mandible with cortical thinning and possibly some loss of bone. **b** Axial CT section (soft-tissue window) again shows the expansile lesion in the right mandible. The content of the lesion exhibits a slightly low attenuation value when compared with the adjacent muscle.

Fig. 6.**25 c–g** ▷

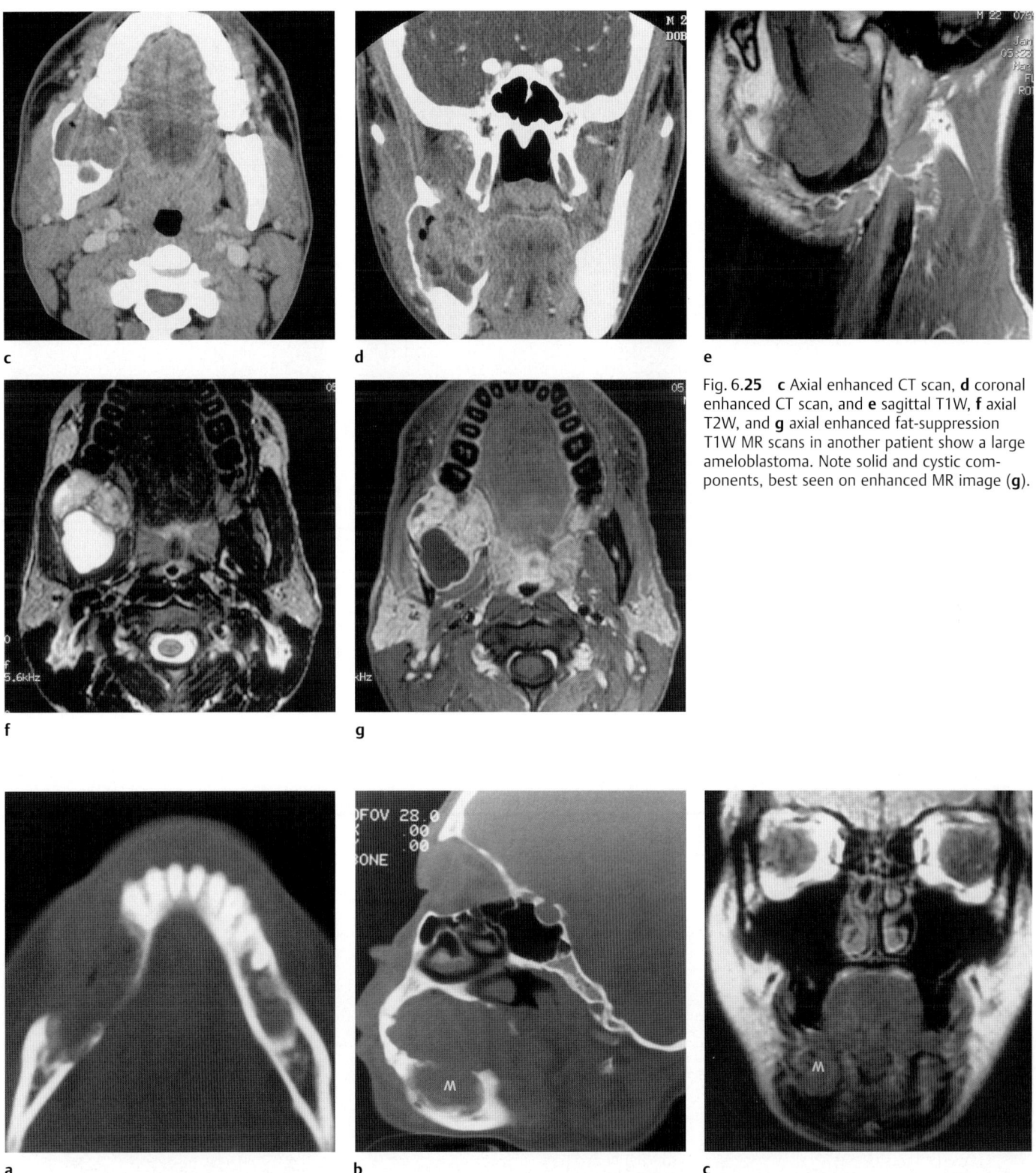

Fig. 6.25 **c** Axial enhanced CT scan, **d** coronal enhanced CT scan, and **e** sagittal T1W, **f** axial T2W, and **g** axial enhanced fat-suppression T1W MR scans in another patient show a large ameloblastoma. Note solid and cystic components, best seen on enhanced MR image (**g**).

Fig. 6.**26 a–c** Ameloblastoma of the right mandible. **a** Axial and **b** sagittal CT scans and **c** T1W MR scan show a right mandibular mass (M), compatible with ameloblastoma.

Fig. 6.**26 d–g** ▷

tic cells found in the wall of the cyst, having eosinophilic cytoplasm and no nuclei.[7] These cells can calcify. The lesion can be found in both mandible and maxilla. The cyst may be present as a unilocular or multilocular radiolucency, containing scattered irregular calcifications of various sizes. The radiographic appearance may be similar to adenomatoid odontogenic tumor, Pindborg tumor, and ameloblastic fibro-odontoma.[7]

Clear Cell Odontogenic Carcinoma

Clear cell odontogenic carcinoma (CCOC), which has been described within the past two decades, is a rare odontogenic tumor that tends to occur in the mandible of older adults, with a predilection for women. It is potentially aggressive and capable of multiple local recurrences and locoregional and distant metastases.[32] CCOC is a low-grade malignant odontogenic carcinoma. Many CCOCs were initially diagnosed either as various

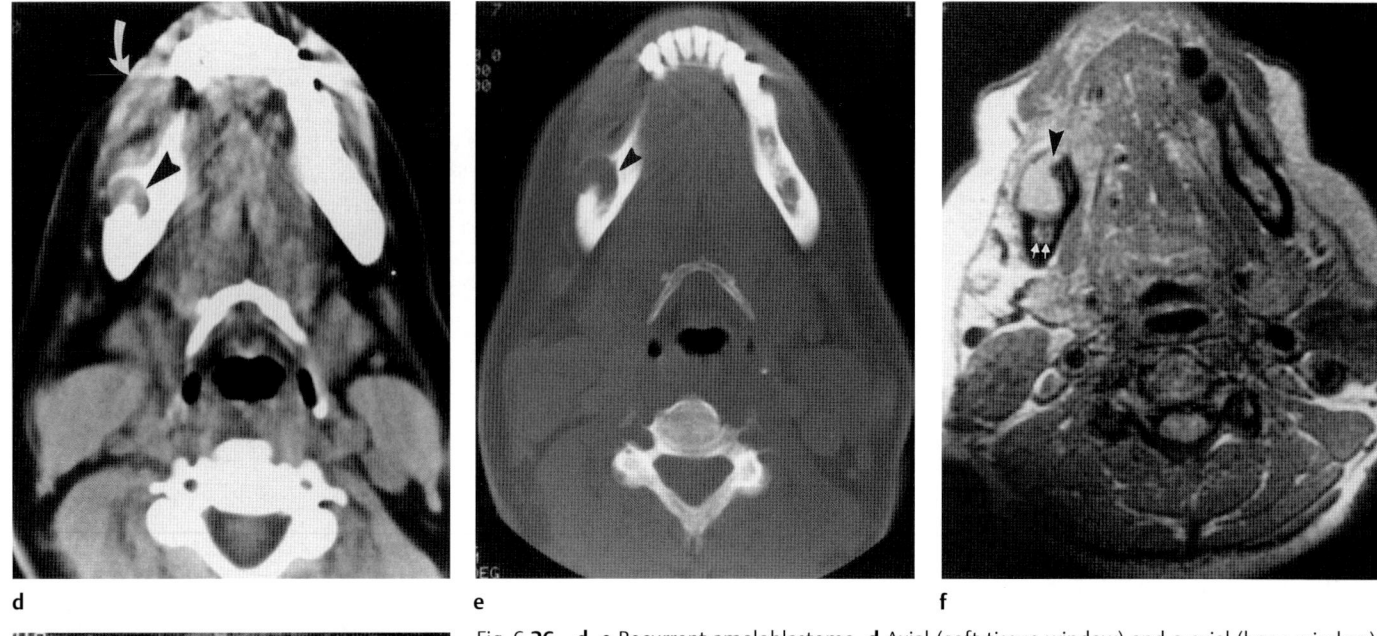

Fig. 6.**26** **d**, **e** Recurrent ameloblastoma. **d** Axial (soft-tissue window) and **e** axial (bone window) CT scans in another patient showing recurrent ameloblastoma (arrowhead). The soft-tissue density (arrow) anterior to the mandibular body proved to be fibrosis. The differentiation between tumor and fibrosis is better appreciated on MR (**f**, **g**) than CT scans. **f** Axial PW and **g** T2W MR scans, showing recurrent ameloblastoma (arrows); part of the lesion remains cystic (black arrowhead). Case courtesy of M.F. Mafee, MD.

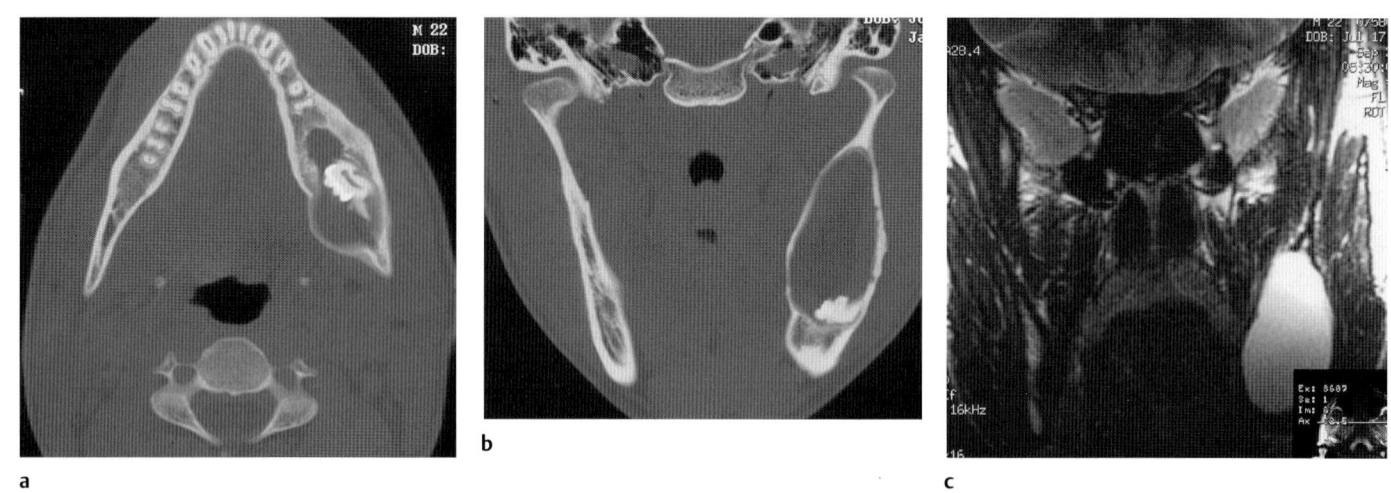

Fig. 6.**27** Ameloblastoma. **a** Axial and **b** coronal CT scans demonstrate an expansile lesion in the ramus of the left mandible. There is an impacted tooth at the inferior part of the lesion. **c** Coronal T2W MR scan; the lesion appears hyperintense and cannot be differentiated from a dentigerous cyst. Case courtesy of M.F. Mafee, MD.

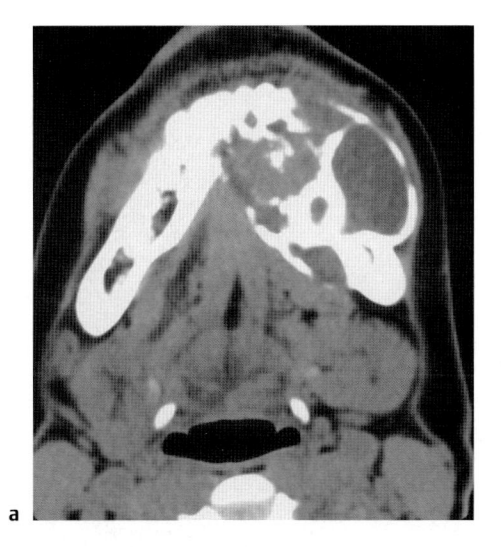

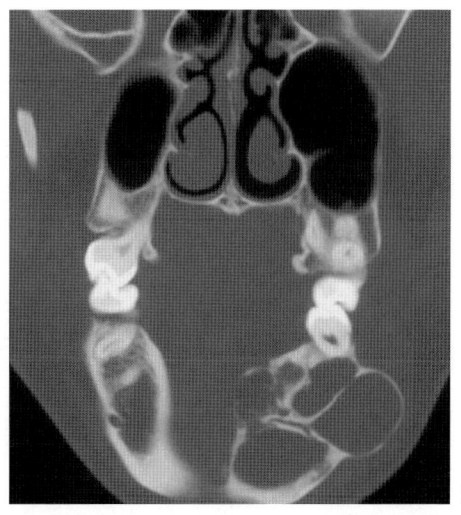

Fig. 6.28 Ameloblastoma. **a** Axial and **b** coronal CT scans demonstrate an expansile lytic lesion in the body of the left mandible. There are multiple lytic lesions, separated by thin septations. Case courtesy of M.F. Mafee, MD.

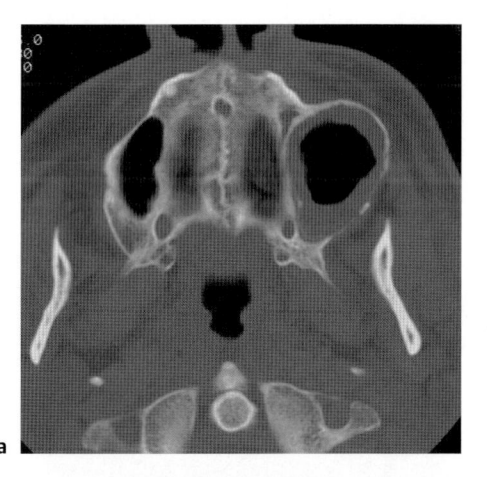

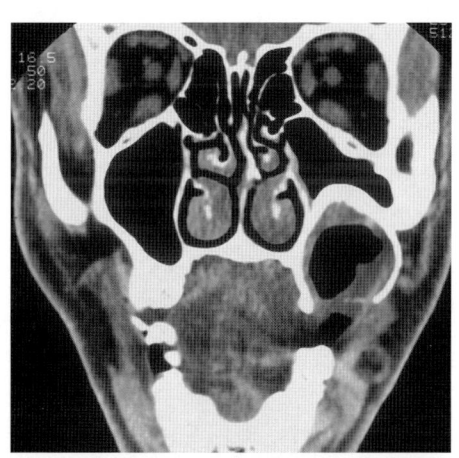

Fig. 6.29 Ameloblastoma of the maxilla. **a** Axial CT scan shows an expansile lesion involving the left maxilla. **b** Coronal CT scan shows extension of lesion into the left maxillary antrum. Note communication between the oral cavity and cystic ameloblastoma. **c, d** Coronal CT scans in another patient showing an odontogenic keratocyst of the maxilla. Note that this lesion cannot be differentiated with certainty from an ameloblastoma (**a, b**). Cases courtesy of M.F. Mafee, MD.

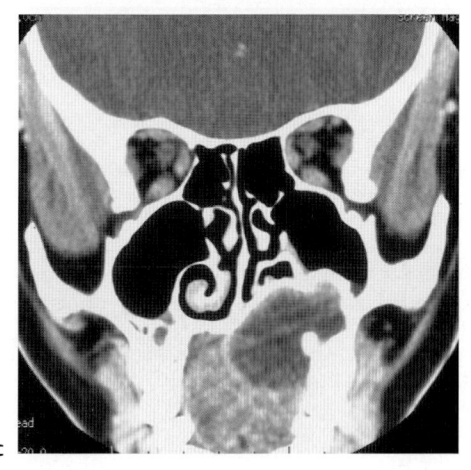

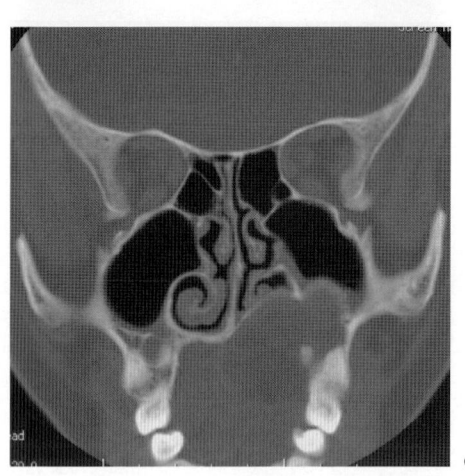

types of ameloblastoma, including atypical ameloblastoma, clear cell ameloblastoma, adenomatoid odontogenic tumor, mucoepidermoid carcinoma, or as metastatic adenocarcinoma. The term CCOC is used because of the increased understanding of the histological analysis, immunohistochemistry, electron microscopy, and low-grade malignant potential of this tumor.[32] The differential diagnosis of intraosseous clear cell tumors of the jaws includes metastatic carcinoma, particularly renal cell carcinoma, central (intraosseous) salivary gland tumor, and odontogenic tumors (which may have clear cell components, such as calcifying epithelial odontogenic tumor and ameloblastoma with clear cell change).[32] Central (primary osseous) salivary gland tumors are extremely rare. Salivary clear cell carcinoma has rarely been reported to occur in the jaw.[32] Adenoid cystic carcinoma and mucoepidermoid carcinoma (which may undergo clear cell change) are the two most common diagnoses.[32] Other salivary tumors, which can have extensive clear cell change (e.g., myoepithelioma/myoepithelial carcinoma, and oncocytoma), do

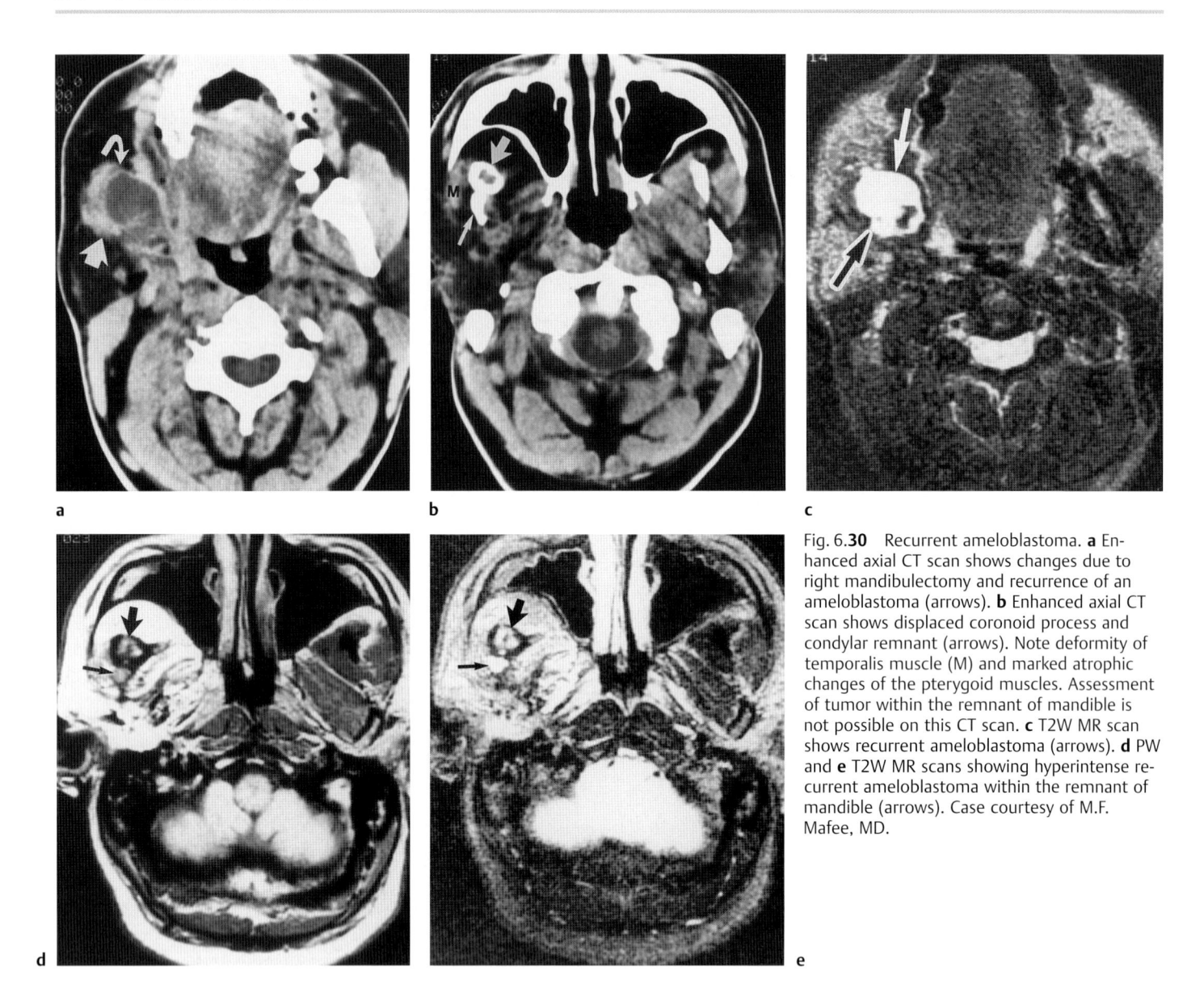

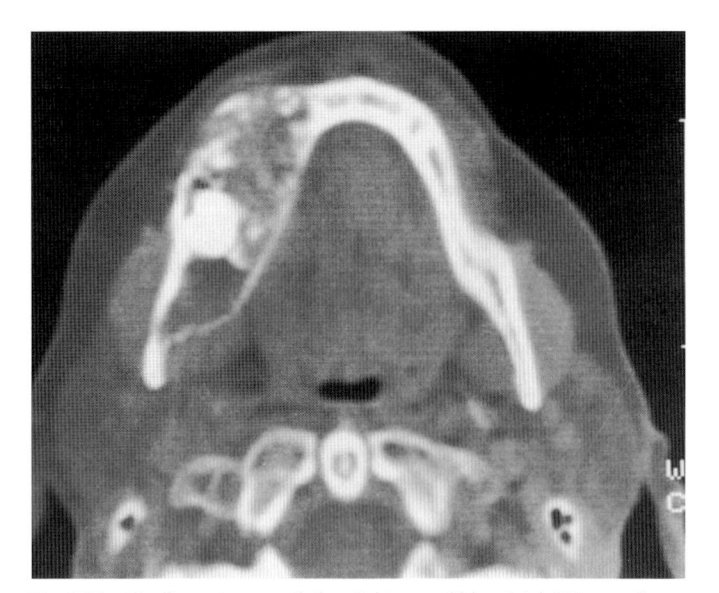

Fig. 6.**30** Recurrent ameloblastoma. **a** Enhanced axial CT scan shows changes due to right mandibulectomy and recurrence of an ameloblastoma (arrows). **b** Enhanced axial CT scan shows displaced coronoid process and condylar remnant (arrows). Note deformity of temporalis muscle (M) and marked atrophic changes of the pterygoid muscles. Assessment of tumor within the remnant of mandible is not possible on this CT scan. **c** T2W MR scan shows recurrent ameloblastoma (arrows). **d** PW and **e** T2W MR scans showing hyperintense recurrent ameloblastoma within the remnant of mandible (arrows). Case courtesy of M.F. Mafee, MD.

Fig. 6.**31** Pindborg tumor of the right mandible. Axial CT scan (bone window setting) reveals an expansile lesion in the body of the right mandible with extension toward the symphysis. There are mottled calcifications within the lesion. Note the impacted third molar tooth.

not occur as primary osseous jaw tumors. Radiographically, CCOC is seen as poorly circumscribed radiolucency in plain films, including panoramic view. On CT scans, the lesion appears as an expansile lobulated mass with moderate contrast enhancement following intravenous administration of iodinated contrast material. There may be erosion of the mandibular cortex.[32]

Mixed Epithelial Odontogenic Tumors

Odontoma

Odontoma[33] is composed of all dental tissues arranged in a disorderly pattern (i.e., enamel, dentin, cementum, and pulpal tissue). Compound odontoma (compound composite odontoma) consists of dental tissues that are similar to a normal tooth. Complex odontoma (complex composite odontoma) is composed of dental tissues, arranged in a disorderly pattern and bearing no morphological similarity to normal or rudimentary teeth.[7] Tumors that contain ameloblastic-like structures, in addition to these components, are referred to as **ameloblastic fibro-odontomas**.[7] The lesion, which is frequently asymptomatic, is often associated with unerupted teeth. Most of these lesions are small, measuring only a few millimeters, but they may reach a considerable size. Radiographically, odontomas present as well-demarcated masses with amorphous areas of calcification (**com-**

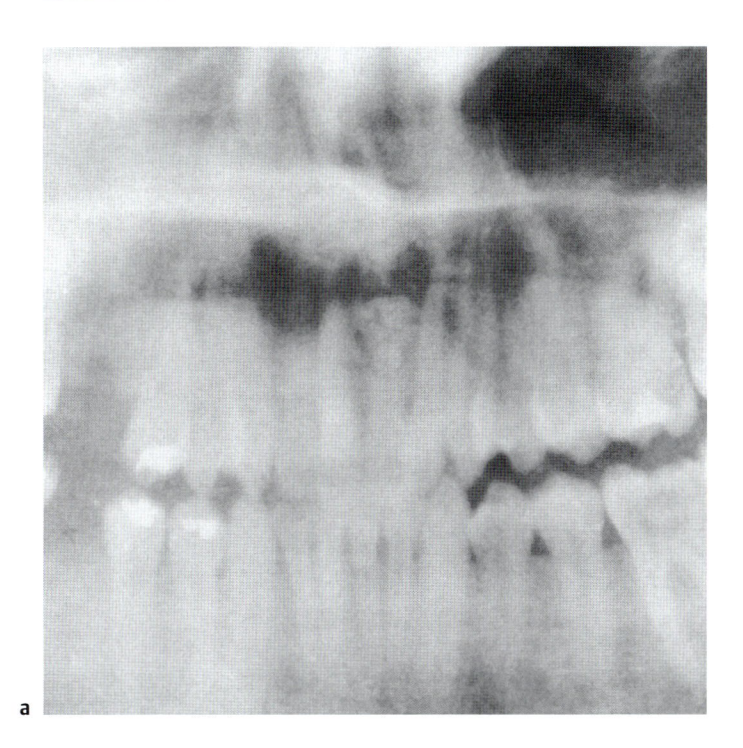

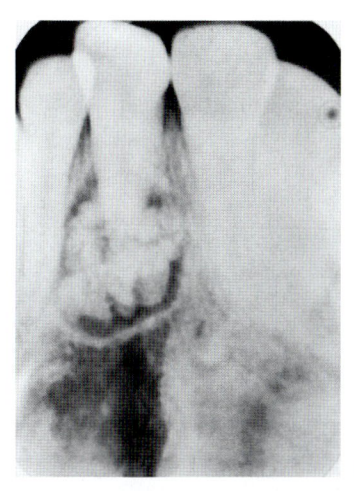

Fig. 6.32 Complex odontoma. **a** Panorex view of the maxilla reveals a poorly defined defect in the upper maxilla with multiple calcific densities. There is amputation of the root of the adjacent central incisor. **b** Dental view of the same area reveals the calcific densities in greater detail, along with a sharply defined bony rim representing the wall of the odontoma.

plex odontoma) (Figs. 6.32–6.35) and/or malformed teeth (**compound odontoma**) arranged in a disorderly pattern (Fig. 6.35). The tumor is frequently surrounded by a narrow radiolucent zone. The developing odontoma without calcification or with few calcifications may be difficult to diagnosis radiologically as it cannot be differentiated from other lesions with similar appearances. The ameloblastic fibro-odontoma is demonstrated radiologically as a well-defined osteolytic area with scattered radiopaque densities in the lumen.

Adenomatoid Odontogenic Tumor

Adenomatoid odontogenic tumor (adenoameloblastoma) is a rare tumor of odontogenic epithelium of the teeth, especially in the canine.[7] The imaging appearance of this lesion may be similar to those of calcifying odontogenic cyst, ameloblastic fibro-odontoma, and Pindborg tumor.[7]

Mesodermal Odontogenic Tumors

The **odontogenic fibromyxoma**[9] originates from the mesodermal portion of the odontogenic apparatus.[5,7] This tumor is not found in bones outside of the jaw and accounts for about 3–6% of odontogenic tumors.[5,7,34] Localization to the jaw bones has led to the belief that these tumors take origin from the primordial odontogenic mesenchyme or from an osteogenic embryonic connective tissue.[26] There are, however, rare cases of fibromyxoma arising in the temporal bone.[35,36] The odontogenic fibromyxoma involves the mandible and maxilla with about equal frequency. In the mandible, the body and ramus are most often affected. Radiographically, multiple radiolucent areas that vary in size are demonstrated, septated by straight or curved bony trabeculae forming triangular (Fig. 6.36), quadrangular, or square compartments. Unilocular lesions have also been described. The radiographic margins of the tumor may be well or poorly defined (Fig. 6.37). This tumor may simulate an ameloblastoma, central giant-cell granuloma, or cyst (Fig. 6.37). When the tumor is aggressive and grows rapidly, little encapsulation is demonstrated, and the lesion often extends through the bone into the soft tissues without any well-defined margin.

Cementomas[20] are categorized into periapical cemental dysplasia, cementifying fibroma, gigantiform cementoma, and benign cementoblastoma. **Periapical cemental dysplasia** is a rare lesion that occurs most often in the mandibular region; it always occurs at the roots of the teeth. The initial lesion is the result of connective-tissue proliferation from the periodontal membrane. It presents as a well-defined radiolucency, but it may subsequently be transformed into a radiopaque calcified mass (Fig. 6.38a). It can be divided radiographically into three stages. (1) a rather well-defined radiolucency at the apex of a tooth (osteolytic or early stage); (2) a lesion that is partly radiopaque and partly radiolucent (cementoblastic or mixed stage) with the hard-tissue formation usually initiated centrally in the lesion; and (3) a lesion that is transformed into a mineralized radiopaque mass surrounded by a narrow radiolucent zone (mature inactive stage).[4,5,7] The involved tooth is normal. Periapical cemental dysplasia does not require treatment unless it becomes infected. Florid cemental dysplasia (florid cemento-osseous dysplasia) is a diffuse form of periapical cemental dysplasia (Fig. 6.38b, c).

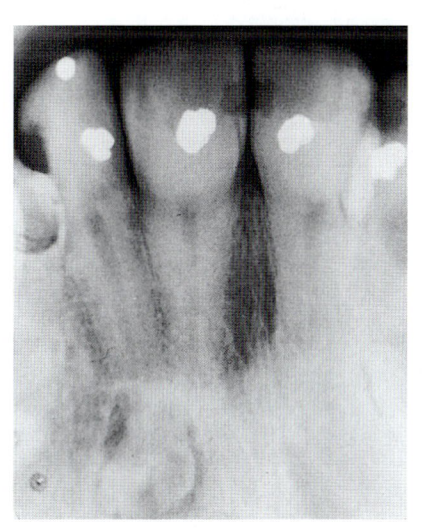

Fig. 6.33 Complex odontoma. Dental view of anterior teeth reveals a lucent area containing a malformed tooth adjacent to the root of the lateral incisor.

530 6 Mandible and Maxilla

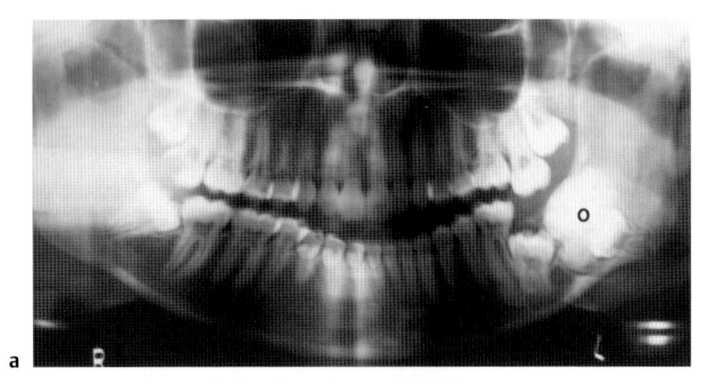

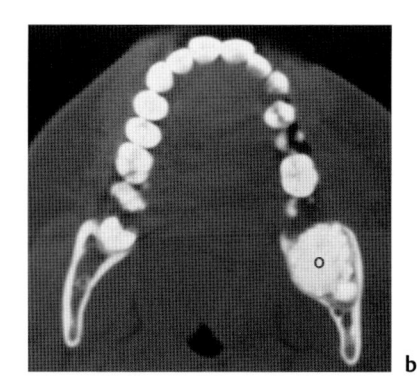

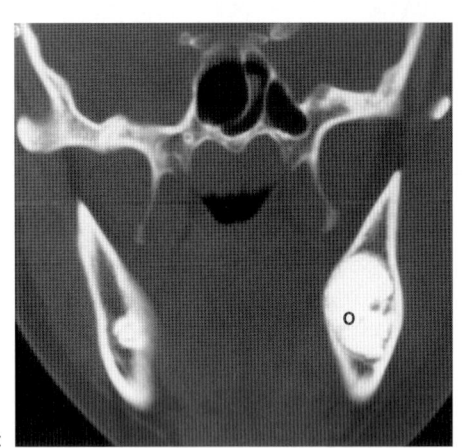

Fig. 6.**34** Complex odontoma. **a** Panorex view, **b** axial CT scan, and **c** coronal CT scan, showing an odontoma (O). Case courtesy of M.F. Mafee, MD.

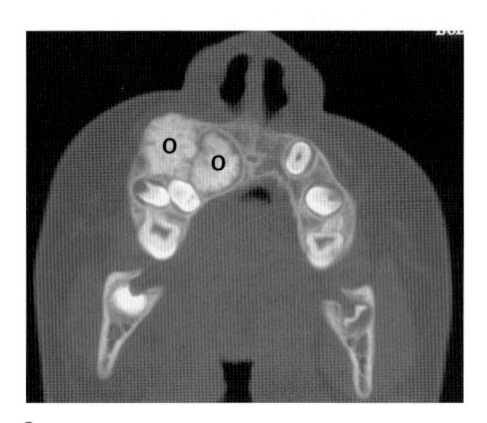

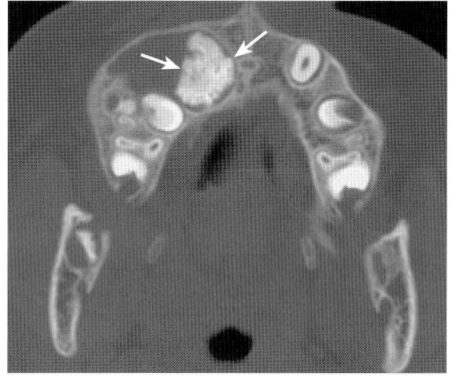

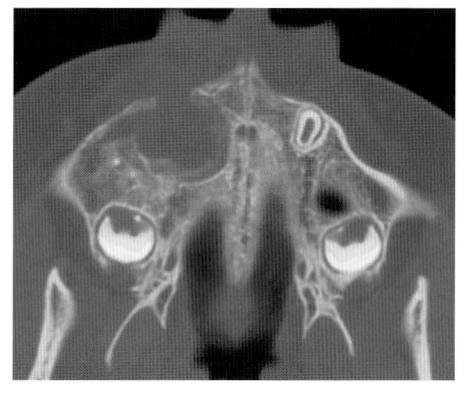

Fig. 6.**35** Complex odontoma. **a** CT scan shows a large odontoma (O) in this 4-year-old-child. **b** CT scan shows residual tumor (arrows) following surgery. **c** CT scan following second operation shows complete resection of odontoma. Case courtesy of M.F. Mafee, MD.

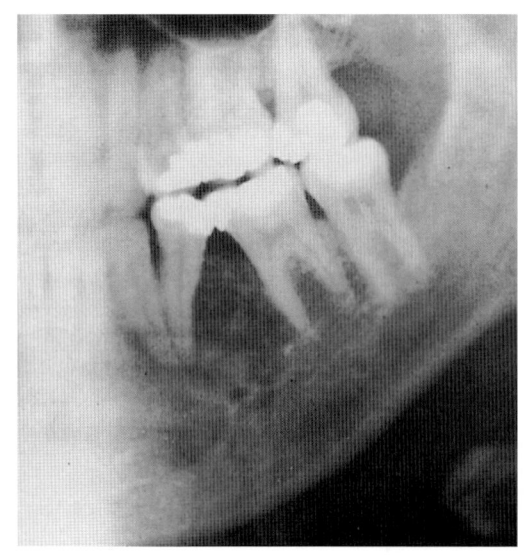

◁ Fig. 6.**36** Fibromyxoma of the left mandible. Panorex view of the mandible reveals a loculated, lucent area with multiple angulated septations in the alveolar portion and adjacent body of the left mandible between the premolar and molar teeth.

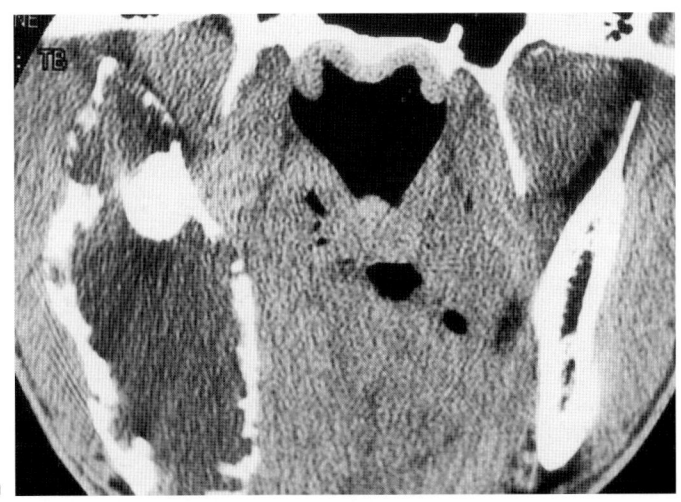

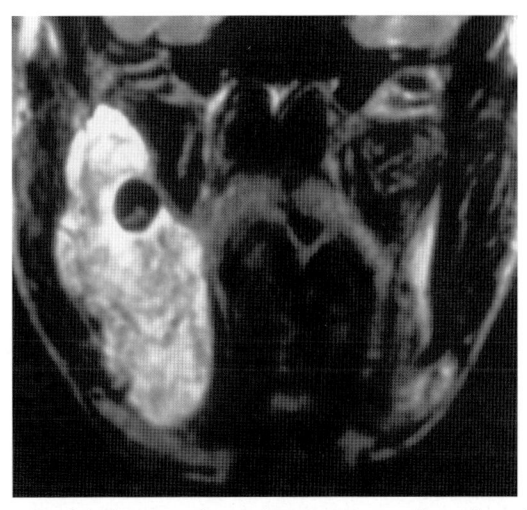

Fig. 6.**37** Fibromyxoma. **a** Coronal CT scan and **b** coronal T2W MR scan, showing a large, expansile mass involving the right mandible, compatible with a fibromyxoma. Note a displaced root of a tooth in the superior portion of the lesion. Enhanced T1W MR scans showed moderate to marked contrast enhancement (not shown here). Case courtesy of M.F. Mafee, MD.

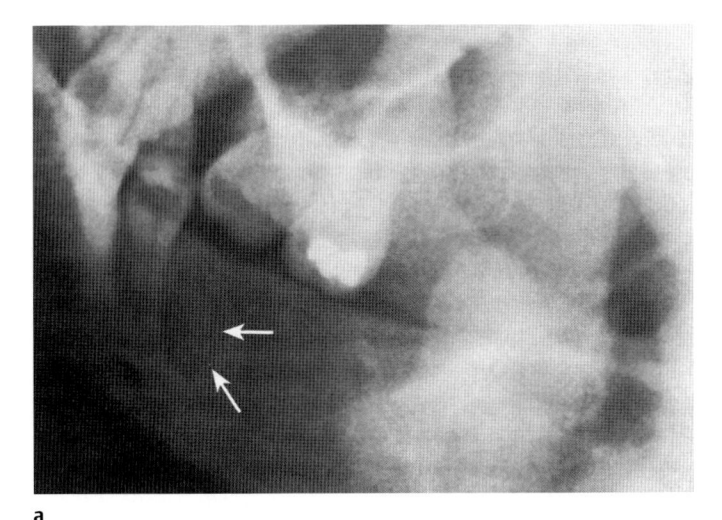

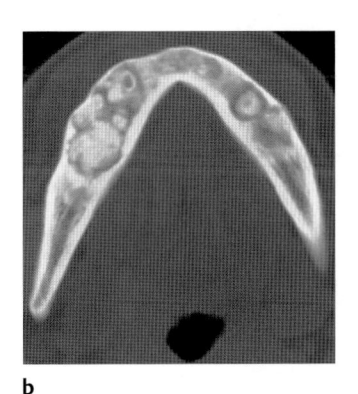

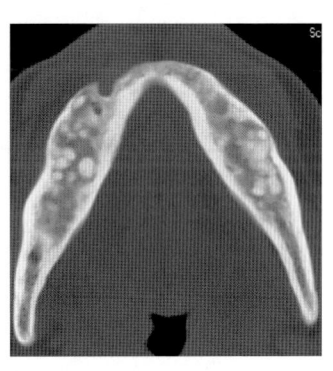

Fig. 6.**38** **a** Periapical cemental dysplasia. Oblique view of the mandible demonstrates a poorly defined, lucent area with central calcification adjacent to the root of the premolar tooth (arrows). **b, c** Presumed florid cemento-osseous dysplasia. **b** Axial CT scan shows a slightly expansile lesion of the right mandible. There are areas of mineralization of varied sizes within the lesion. The mandibular cortex is intact. There are similar changes seen on the opposite side. **c** Axial CT scan, taken 6 mm cephalad to **b** shows that the left mandible is similarly involved with several foci of mineralization within the lesion. Case courtesy of M.F. Mafee, MD.

Cementifying Fibroma

Cementifying fibroma is a slow-growing lesion of mesenchymal origin that is composed of cellular fibroblastic tissue containing basophilic masses of cementum-like tissues. The tumor involves the mandible and is usually 1–2 cm in diameter (larger lesions are rarely observed).[38] The radiographic features depend on the stage of development. In the early stage, a cementifying fibroma presents as a well-circumscribed, well-demarcated radiolucent lesion with no internal radiopacities simulating cysts. Subsequently, speckled calcifications are deposited within the lesion, forming a dense radiopaque mass surrounded by a radiolucent zone.[38]

Gigantiform Cementoma

Gigantiform cementomas, composed of largely acellular cementum, present as unilateral or bilateral symmetric masses of varied radiopacities interspersed with radiolucent zones. They are located adjacent to the roots of the teeth and occur most often in the mandible.[38]

Benign cementoblastoma is a rare lesion composed of functional cementoblasts, characterized by the formation of a cementum-like mass enveloping the apex of a tooth root (Fig. 6.**39**). (It most often involves a permanent tooth, but may be seen in a primary tooth.) The lesion is solitary, is usually located in the molar or premolar region, and it frequently involves the mandibular first molar.[38] Radiographically, the lesion is well defined, and the dense radiopaque central part is attached to the tooth root and most often surrounded by a radiolucent zone of uniform width, which represents the peripheral unmineralized tissues of the formative cellular layers. The lesion may expand the cortical bones of the jaws.[38]

Benign Nonodontogenic Tumors[39]

These tumors are not only found in the jaw bone but are also seen in other areas of the skeleton. Radiographically, the appearance of those found in the jaw does not differ significantly from those in other bones, taking into account abnormalities they impart on adjacent tooth structures.[38]

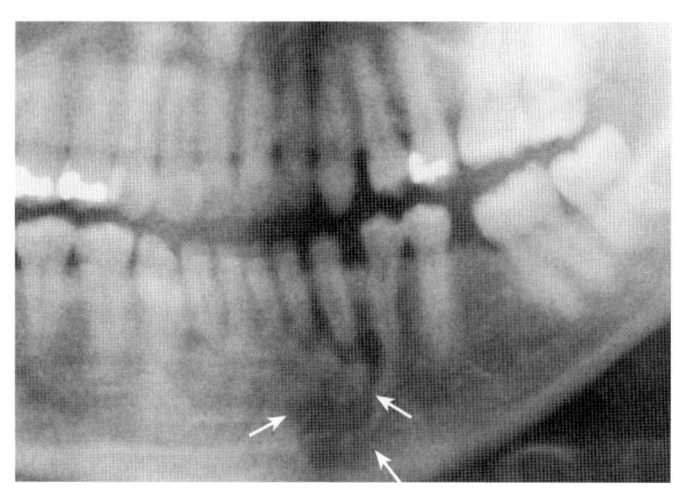

Fig. 6.39 Cementoblastoma. Panorex view of the mandible demonstrates a calcified mass in the body and symphysis of the mandible, adjacent to the roots of the incisors and canine teeth (arrows).

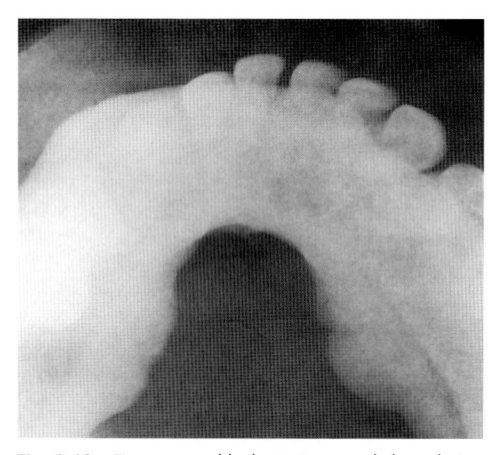

Fig. 6.40 Torus mandibularis. Intraoral dental view demonstrates bony exostoses along the anterior mandibular margin on the left and right.

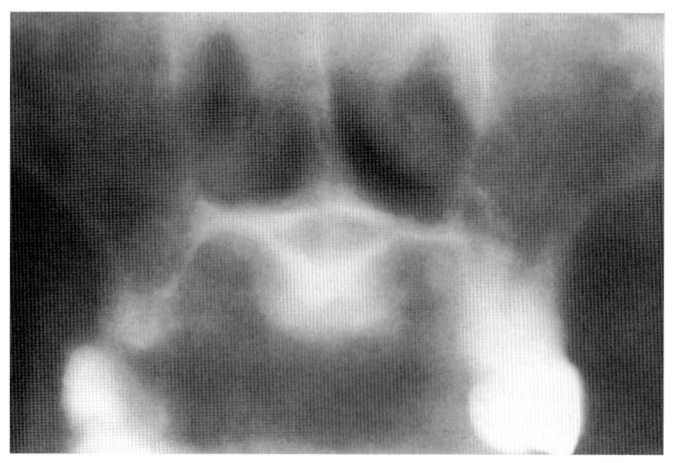

Fig. 6.41 Torus palatinus. Coronal tomographic section reveals a bony exostosis arising from the mid-portion of the hard palate.

Exostoses[40, 41]

Exostoses are localized outgrowths of bone that are variable in size and appear as flat, nodular, or pedunculated protuberances on the surface of the mandible or maxilla. There are three types of exostoses, (1) torus mandibularis, (2) torus palatinus, and (3) multiple exostoses, which must be differentiated according to their location. **Torus mandibularis** is an outgrowth of bone on the lingual surface of the mandible (Fig. 6.**40**). The size, shape, and number of the protuberances may vary. They are usually bilateral and situated above the mylohyoid line, opposite the bicuspid teeth. **Torus palatinus** is a flat, spindle-shaped, nodular, or lobular exostosis that arises in the middle of the hard palate (Fig. 6.**41**). **Multiple exostoses** arise from the buccal surface of the maxilla in the molar region and appear as small, nodular, bony masses.[38]

Radiographically, they are seen as areas of increased bony density. Exostoses that are composed of compact bone are of uniform radiopacity, whereas those that contain a marrow space have trabeculations. Exostoses are often difficult to demonstrate on plane radiographs, especially those of small size and those that are superimposed on the teeth. These can be readily visualized using high-resolution extended bone-scale CT scan.[38]

Osteochondroma

Osteochondroma is a benign lesion that is believed to arise from overgrowth of cartilage at a growth site. Within the mandible, osteochondromas have been reported most frequently in the coronoid process and the condyle. Osteochondromas are very slow-growing lesions. Radiographically, they appear as radiodense extraosseous projections. On imaging they may simulate exostosis, and at times parosteal osteogenic sarcoma. Although rare, osteochondroma may have malignant potential. Complete surgical removal is the treatment of choice.

Osteomas[38, 42]

Osteomas are benign lesions composed of compact or cancellous bone, usually in an endosteal or periosteal location (Fig. 6.**42**). They vary greatly in size from small tumors to large tumors that cause disfiguration. Radiographically, they have a characteristic appearance of well-circumscribed, sclerotic, bony masses attached with a broad base or pedicle to the surface of the mandible (Fig. 6.**43**). Root resorption may occur when the tumor is located near a tooth.

Gardner syndrome[43] consists of multiple osteomas associated with multiple polyposis of the colon, epidermoid and sebaceous cysts, desmoid tumors of the skin, and impacted supernumerary and permanent teeth. The multiple osteomas most often precede colonic polyps (which eventually become malignant in most patients older than 30 years).[38] Osteomas are most often found in the frontal bone, ethmoid bone, maxilla, and mandible, although they have been seen in any of the bones of the cranium or facial skeleton (Fig. 6.**44**).

Giant-Cell Tumor and Giant-Cell Reparative Granuloma[5, 7, 38, 44-46]

Giant-cell tumor encompasses a variety of conditions. Three distinct entities are found in the head and neck area, namely, giant-cell tumor, giant-cell reparative granuloma, and brown tumor of hyperparathyroidism.[44] Histological differentiation of the giant-cell tumor (GCT) of bone is always difficult and at times impossible. These tumors all contain two major cell types, the giant cells and the stromal cells. Interspersed among these is a varying amount of matrix.[44] The stroma of GCT is vascular and contains numerous thin-walled capillaries, often with foci of hemorrhage.[46] These lesions may be associated with secondary, aneurysmal bone cyst (ABC) formation. ABC is a radiographic description and not a pathological entity. It is a secondary process, associated with an underlying primary disease. ABC contains only hemorrhagic cystic regions. In 1953 Jaffe[45] coined the term "giant-cell reparative granuloma" (GCRG) to represent that variety of giant-cell tumor found exclusively in the jaws, where areas of osteoid deposition are seen alongside areas of destruction, giving the appearance of attempted repair.[44, 45] Jaffe believed these le-

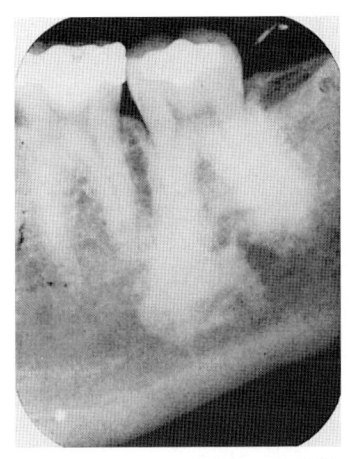

Fig. 6.**42** Osteoma of the mandible. Panorex view of the mandible demonstrates a sharply defined, bony lesion in the medullary portion of the mandible, abutting the adjacent root of the molar tooth.

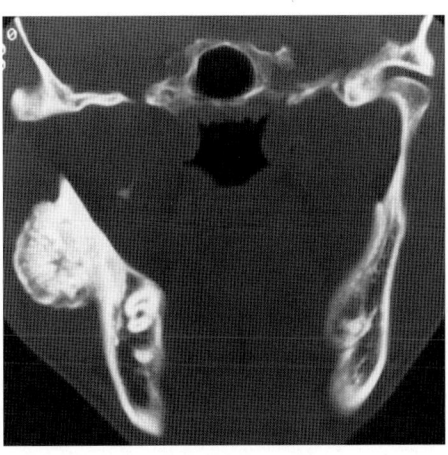

Fig. 6.**43** Osteoma of the mandible. Coronal CT scan shows an osteoma of the right mandible. Case courtesy of M.F. Mafee, MD.

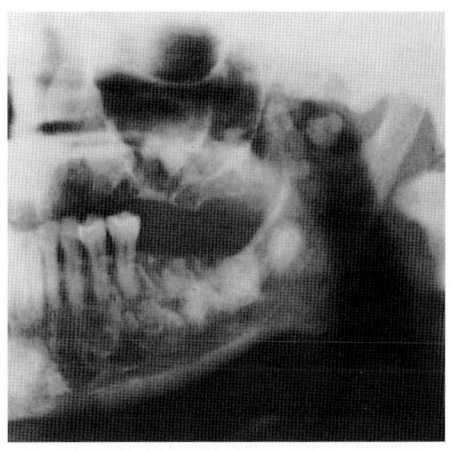

Fig. 6.**44** Gardner syndrome. Panorex view of the mandible demonstrates multiple osteomas in the mandible and maxilla.

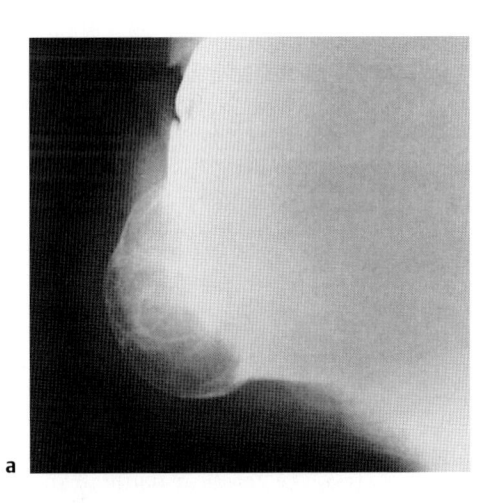

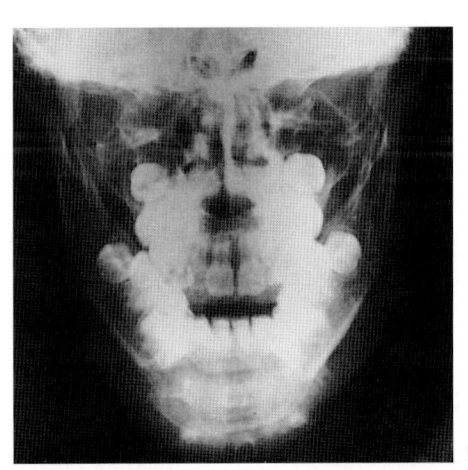

Fig. 6.**45** Giant-cell granuloma of the mandible. **a** Oblique view of the mandible demonstrates an expansile, septated lesion with a soap-bubble appearance in the symphysis of the mandible. **b** PA view of the mandible shows the expansile lesion in the symphysis of the mandible, causing slight encroachment and displacement of the adjacent anterior teeth.

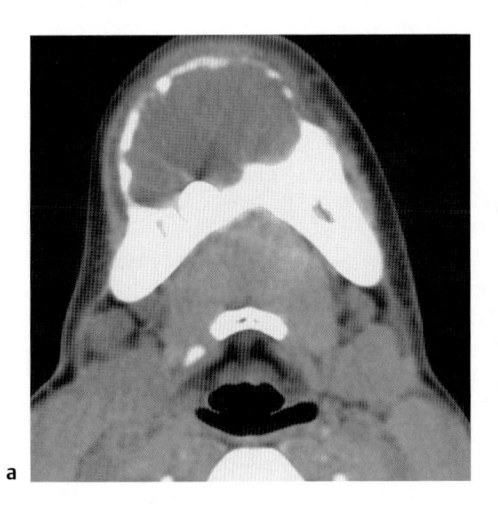

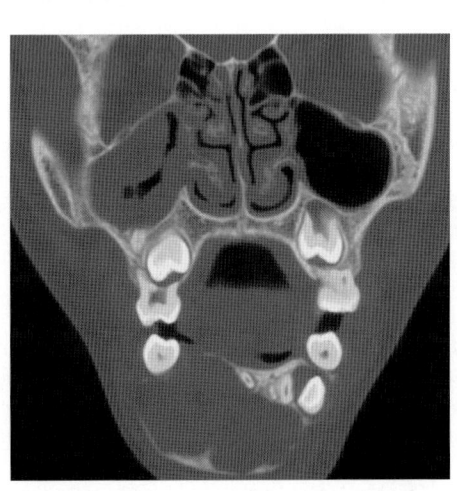

Fig. 6.**46** Giant-cell reparative granuloma. A 12-year-old boy with mandibular mass. **a** Axial and **b** coronal CT scans demonstrate a large expansile mass compatible with histologically proven giant-cell reparative granuloma. Case courtesy of M.F. Mafee, MD.

sions represented a response to intraosseous hemorrhage from jaw trauma.[45] Other researchers prefer the term giant-cell granuloma to describe this lesion, noting the inconsistent history of trauma and lack of significant elements of reparative tissue.[46] GCRG is usually readily distinguished on histological analysis from GCT. Its granulomatous appearance is produced by plump, bland fibroblasts and multinucleated giant cells surrounding foci of hemorrhage.[46] Osteoid production along hemorrhagic foci, an unusual feature in GCT, is commonly seen in these lesions.[46] Cystic degeneration and ABC components are uncommon. Gnathic cases of GCRG have been further subdivided into central (i.e., occurring in bone) (Figs. 6.**45**, 6.**46**) and peripheral (i.e., occurring in gingival soft tissues).[44,46] The peripheral soft-tissue type of GCRC is more common than the central type and involves the gingiva and alve-

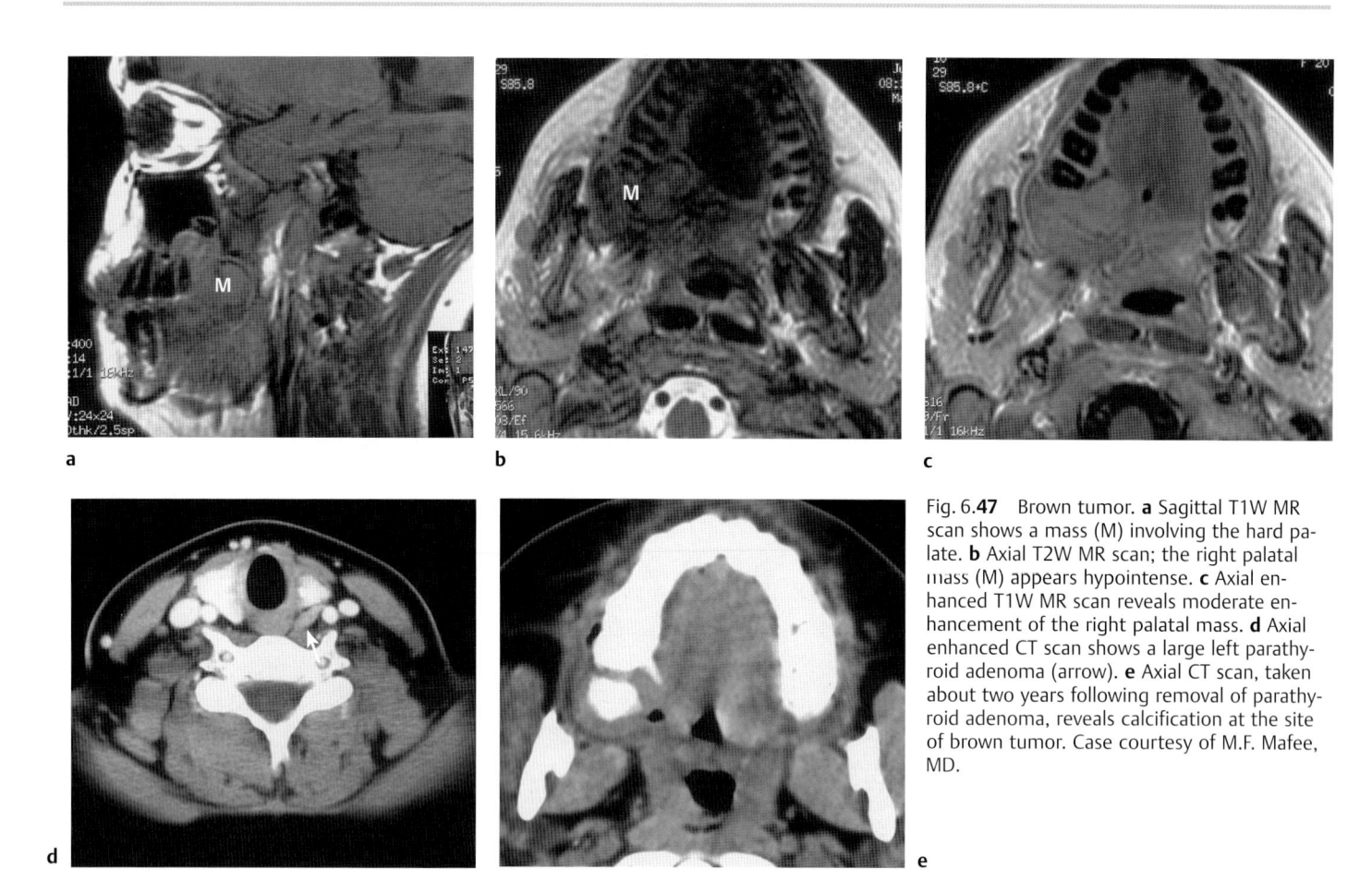

Fig. 6.47 Brown tumor. **a** Sagittal T1W MR scan shows a mass (M) involving the hard palate. **b** Axial T2W MR scan; the right palatal mass (M) appears hypointense. **c** Axial enhanced T1W MR scan reveals moderate enhancement of the right palatal mass. **d** Axial enhanced CT scan shows a large left parathyroid adenoma (arrow). **e** Axial CT scan, taken about two years following removal of parathyroid adenoma, reveals calcification at the site of brown tumor. Case courtesy of M.F. Mafee, MD.

olar mucosa. The tumor usually develops in females over 20 years of age and may be related to a prior tooth extraction. Central GCRG often seen in patients 10–20 years of age and may or may not be related to trauma. True giant-cell tumor (GCT) is a relatively common skeletal tumor. The vast majority of GCTs affect skeletally mature patients. GCTs arise on the metaphyseal side of the skeletal bone, with the most common specific locations being about the knee. GCTs occurring in the maxillofacial skeleton are rare.[26] A giant-cell lesion of the mandible and maxilla is more likely to be a GCRG or brown tumor rather than a true GCT (osteoclastoma). Whether the "true" giant-cell tumor of long bones exists in the maxillofacial skeleton continues to be a controversy.[46] Giant-cell granulomas have a predilection for the mandible and maxilla (Figs. 6.43, 6.47). They are most often located in the anterior part of the mandible (Figs. 6.45, 6.46) with extension from the premolar and molar regions, often with extension across the midline. The lesion usually has a radiolucent, multilocular, honeycombed appearance, with tiny bony septa traversing the involved area (Fig. 6.47). The loculi are irregular in shape and vary in size; however, unilocular tumors without trabeculation have been seen. There is often a rather marked expansion with thinning of the cortical plates (Fig. 6.47). When these lesions are adjacent to the teeth, displacement and root resorption occur. Giant-cell granulomas that are located in the maxilla (especially in the antral region) produce "ground glass" radiopacities.[38] As in GCT, these lesions have low to intermediate signal intensity on both T1-weighted and T2-weighted MR images. Cystic areas (ABC components) demonstrate low or high signal intensity on T1-weighted and low or high signal intensity on T2-weighted MR images, depending on the age of associated hemorrhage. The solid component of tumor demonstrates moderate to marked gadolinium contrast enhancement.

Brown Tumor[47]

Osteitis fibrosa cystica, bone cyst, brown tumor, and other giant-cell lesions are rare clinical entities that may be associated with hyperparathyroidism.[47] Brown tumors are generally part of the generalized process, including reduced bone density and generalized osteoporosis, subperiosteal bone resorption of phalangeal tufts and the clavicle, absence of lamina dura around the teeth, and demineralization of the calvarial bones. Brown tumor represents a reparative cellular process, consisting of clusters of hemosiderin-laden macrophages, giant cells, and proliferating fibroblasts.[47] Vascularity, hemorrhage, and deposits of hemosiderin impart the characteristic brown hue to the lesion, hence the name "brown tumor." Brown tumors are histologically indistinguishable from the other giant-cell-containing lesions, such as true giant-cell tumor, "aneurysmal bone cyst," and giant-cell reparative granuloma.[47] Brown tumors as part of hyperparathyroidism are commonly multiple, occurring in the ribs, clavicle, skull, and pelvic girdle. Brown tumors of both mandible and maxilla have been reported. Radiographically, brown tumor of mandible and maxilla may be seen as expansile multilocular lesions, simulating metastatic process and other fibro-osseous lesion (Figs. 6.47, 6.48).

Langerhans Cell Histiocytosis[48]

Langerhans cell histiocytosis (LH) is a spectrum of disease that has as its primary pathology a proliferation of lipid-laden Langerhans histiocytes, associated with an inflammatory response.[48] The process may be systemic, multifocal, or focal; acute or chronic; benign or malignant. Based on clinical course, three variants have been described: Letterer–Siwe disease, Hand–Schüller–Christian disease, and eosinophilic granuloma.

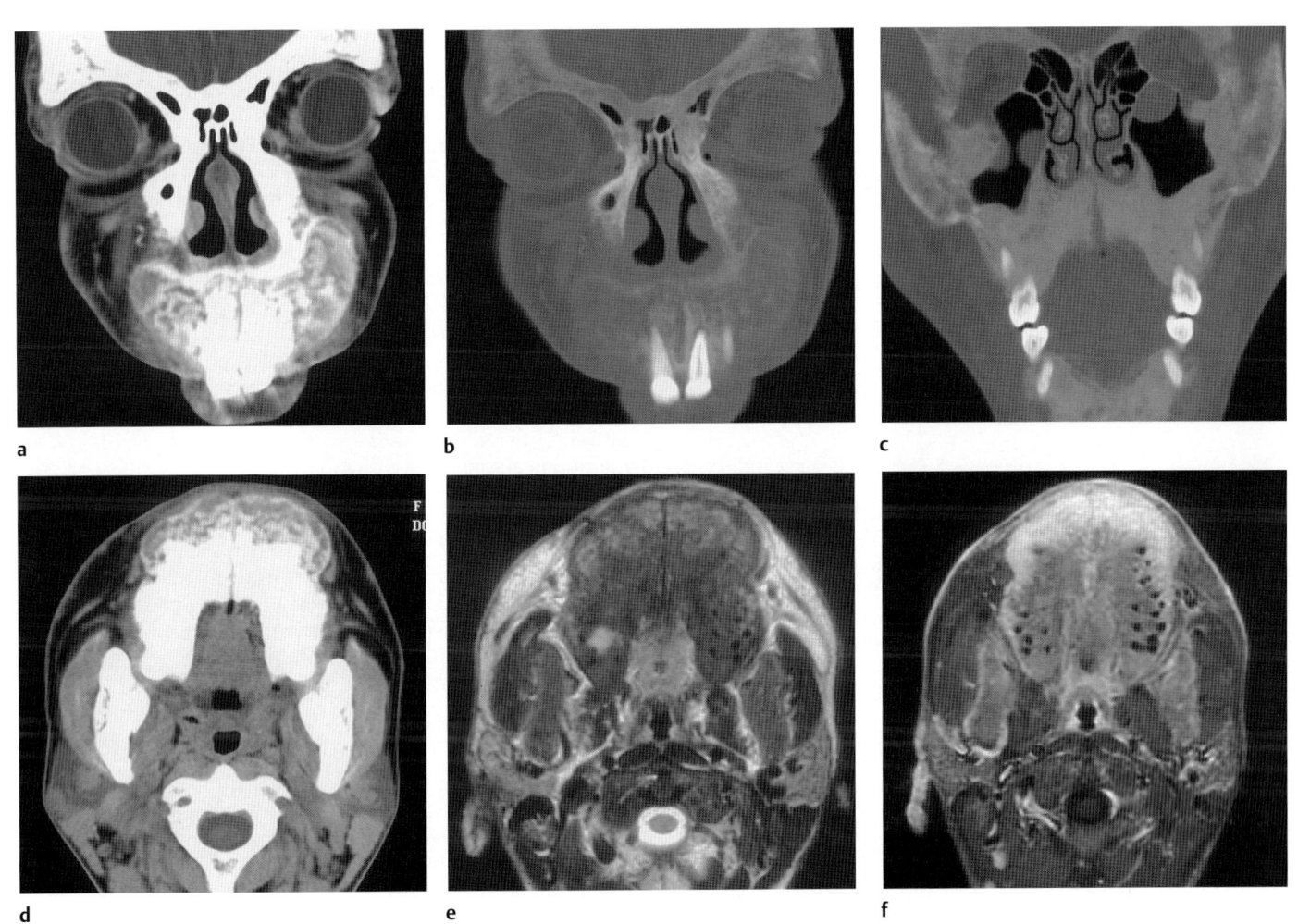

Fig. 6.**48** Brown tumor in a patient with renal osteodystrophy. **a** Coronal CT scan shows marked soft-tissue thickening of the upper gum, associated with irregular areas of mineralization. **b**, **c** Coronal CT scans show bony changes of renal osteodystrophy. **d** Axial CT scan shows marked soft-tissue thickening of the upper gum, associated with areas of mineralization. **e** Axial T2W MR scan; the gingival lesion appears heterogeneous in signal characteristics. **f** Axial enhanced T1W MR scan reveals moderate to marked enhancement of the upper gingival lesion. Biopsy of the upper gum was compatible with brown tumor. Case courtesy of M.F. Mafee, MD.

Letterer–Siwe disease is the acute, widely disseminated form of LH occurring in infants under the age of 2 years. The clinical manifestations include cutaneous lesions, hepatosplenomegaly, lymphadenopathy, and pulmonary lesions. In addition lesions are most often present in several bones and may appear as multiple, small, round radiolucencies with well-defined borders. If teeth are involved, they are frequently mobile, and there is associated gingival bleeding.[7,38]

Hand–Schüller–Christian disease [38,48] is a disseminated chronic skeletal and extraskeletal form of LH, which represents the intermediate stage between eosinophilic granuloma and Letterer–Siwe disease. It has three classic findings: (1) single or multiple, sharply defined calvarial defects; (2) unilateral or bilateral exophthalmos; and (3) diabetes insipidus noted in about 10% of patients related to involvement of the infundibulo-hypothalamic axis. Other organs (i.e., lymph nodes, liver, spleen, lungs, and skin) may be involved.[38,48] The disease may first be noted in the oral structures, either in the form of red spongy gingiva or through premature loss of teeth. Lesions present radiographically as irregular, lucent defects in the mandible and maxilla. Marked alveolar bone destruction gives the teeth the appearance of "floating in space." [38]

Eosinophilic granuloma[38,48] is the mildest form of LH and may be unifocal or multifocal. It occurs virtually in any bone in the skeleton. It is most often seen in the skull, ribs, femur, and tooth-bearing areas of the jaw, predominantly in the mandible. It may be detected incidentally on a radiographic study. The area of bone involvement, usually in the medullary cavities, is characterized as an irregular, lucent area with no reactive sclerosis (Figs. 6.**49**, 6.**50**). The tumorlike lesions are often single, but multiple areas of rarefaction simulating periapical granulomas and periodontal disease may be seen.[38] An early radiographic finding may be destruction of the crest of the alveolar bone and interdental septum, along with loss of the cortical outline of the tooth follicle or lamina dura. The teeth in the involved regions become loose, float in space, and exfoliate. CT and MRI are helpful in evaluating various forms of LH, particularly in delineating soft-tissue extension (Fig. 6.**50**). LH demonstrates low signal intensity on T1-weighted and intermediate signal intensity on T2-weighted MR images. There will be moderate to marked enhancement on post-gadolinium T1-weighted MR images (Fig. 6.**50 c**).[48]

Fibro-Osseous Lesions[47,49]

Fibrous Dysplasia

Fibrous dysplasia is an idiopathic nonheritable (except cherubism) benign bone disease in which normal bone is replaced by structurally weak fibrous and osseous tissue.[47,48] It occurs more often in the maxilla than the mandible, and usually arises in the posterior regions. It occurs in three forms: (1) monostotic, (2) polyostotic (multiple bony lesions, often bilateral), and (3)

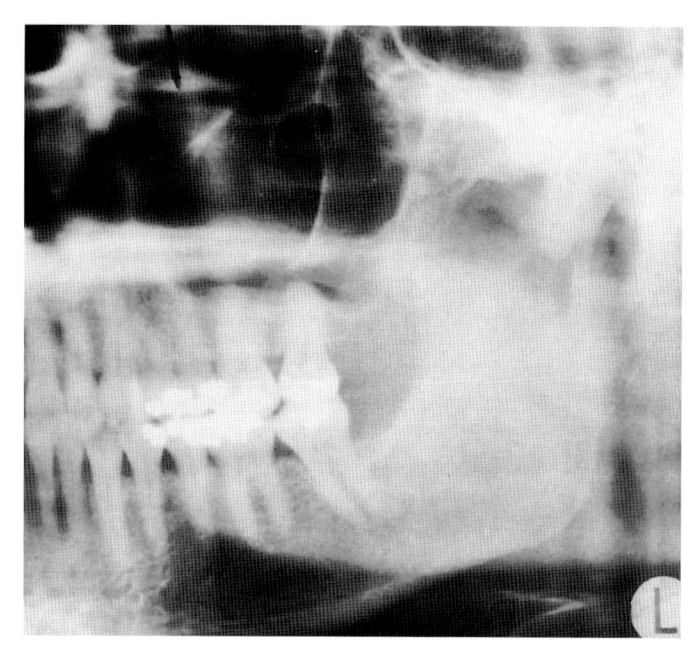

Fig. 6.49 Eosinophilic granuloma. Panorex view of the mandible. There is a slightly irregular, sharply defined, lytic lesion in the ascending ramus of the left mandible adjacent to the condylar neck.

McCune–Albright syndrome, which is a rare disease, consisting of polyostotic fibrous dysplasia associated with endocrine disorders and cutaneous hyperpigmentation.[47,48]

Monostotic fibrous dysplasia accounts for 70% of cases and is manifested by painless swelling or bulging of the jaw (usually the labial or buccal plate), along with malalignment and displacement of the teeth, protuberance of the maxilla, and involvement of the maxillary sinus, zygomatic process, and floor of the orbit; it sometimes extends to the skull base. Monostotic fibrous dysplasia occurs equally in males and females, usually in early adolescents. It stops growing at the time of growth plate closure. The monostotic form of the disease does not evolve into the polyostotic form. **Polyostotic fibrous dysplasia** occcurs in 27% of cases and is characterized by deformities of long bones, such as bowing and cortical thickening. The skull and face, including the mandible and maxilla, are frequently involved, often with obvious asymmetry secondary to bony expansion. **McCune–Albright syndrome** accounts for 3% of cases and is characterized by cutaneous pigmentation, endocrine abnormalities, precocious puberty, and multiple skeletal lesions and is most often seen in young girls.[47,48]

Histologically, fibrous dysplasia is composed of variable proportions of fibrous tissue and woven (immature) bone. Radiologically, it appears as a unilocular or multilocular, ill-defined, radiolucent lesion when fibrous tissue is predominant; however, when bony matrix predominates (Figs. 6.**51**–6.**57**), the degree of opacity depends on the amount of woven bone laid down within the lesion. Another appearance is that of a marked, homogeneous increase in bone density associated with bony expansion. Large lesions cause thinning and expansion of the cortex (Fig. 6.**51**). **Cherubism**[49] is inherited as an autosomal dominant trait and occurs between the ages of 2 and 20 years. Its name is derived from the cherubic appearance. There is post-pubertal involution of the process with jaw remodeling in adulthood. The disease is characterized by bilateral swelling of gnathic bones, usually the mandible.[49] The mandible and maxilla are involved by multiple, often bilateral fibro-osseous lesions, especially in the rami of the mandible (Figs. 6.**52**, 6.**53**). Imaging typically shows expansile lesions with cortical thinning and multilocular lucencies, with a coarse trabecular pattern (Fig. 6.**51**). Histologically the lesion is composed of fibrous tissue with numerous multinucleated giant cells.

Ossifying Fibroma[47,49]

Ossifying fibroma is a well-demarcated, benign lesion consisting of fibrous tissue that contains various amounts of irregular bony trabeculae, which is occasionally intermixed with cementum. It occurs most often in the mandible.[7,38] Radiographically, it reveals a distinct boundary (Fig. 6.**58**) as opposed to fibrous dysplasia. In its early stages, it presents as a lucent area and, as the tumor matures, bony densities are deposited, transforming the lesion into a radiopaque mass (Fig. 6.**59**).

Psammomatoid Active Ossifying Fibroma (Juvenile Aggressive Ossifying Fibroma)[47,49]

The psammomatoid active ossifying fibroma, also called the juvenile aggressive psammomatoid ossifying fibroma, is a variant of ossifying fibroma that typically occurs in the maxilla and sinonasal tract.[47,49] These lesions occur in younger age groups. The lesion has an aggressive appearance with marked expansion of the involved bone (Fig. 6.**60**). This entity has been described in more detail in Chapter 4 on Nasal Cavity and Paranasal Sinuses.

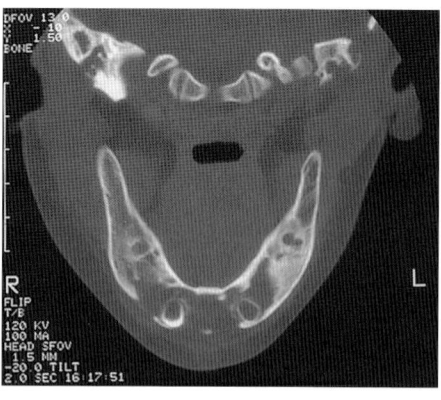

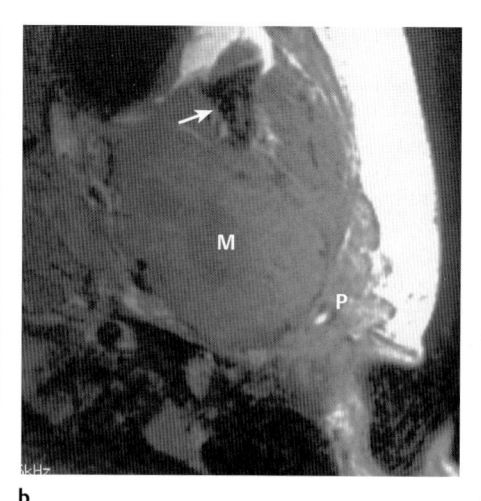

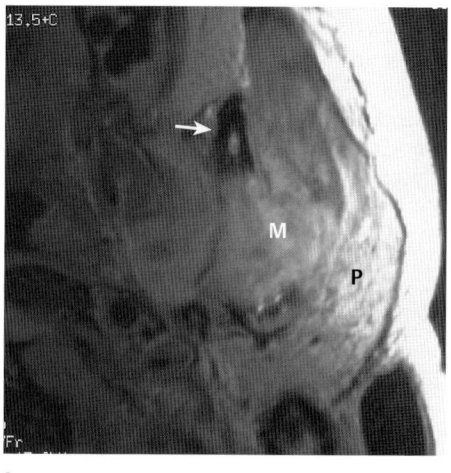

Fig. 6.50 **a** Langerhans cell histiocytosis. CT scan shows multiple lytic lesion involving the mandible; both mastoids were involved as seen. **b** Axial T1W and **c** enhanced axial T1W MR scans in another patient with Langerhans cell histiocytosis demonstrate a large mass (M) involving the mandible. Note uninvolved portion of the mandible (arrow). P = parotid gland. Case courtesy of M.F. Mafee, MD.

Pathology 537

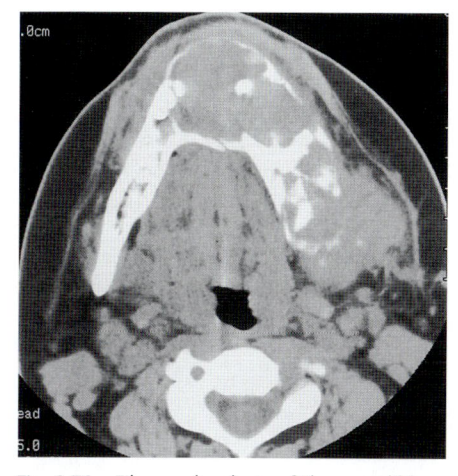

Fig. 6.**51** Fibrous dysplasia of the mandible. Axial CT section (soft-tissue window) demonstrates an expansile lesion in the left mandible including symphysis. There are multiple bony densities within the expanded mandible. The expanded contour of the bone is slightly irregular and deficient.

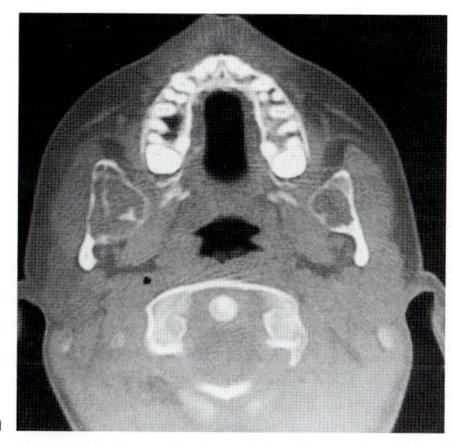

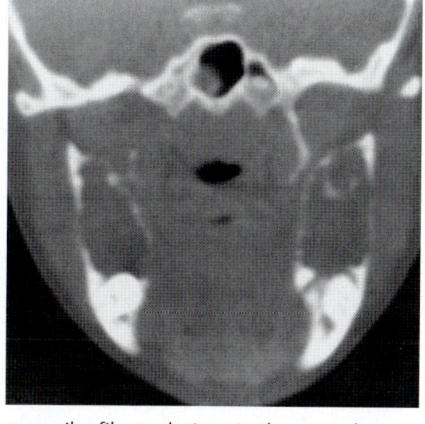

Fig. 6.**52** Cherubism. **a** Axial CT section reveals expansile, fibrous lesions in the ascending rami of the mandible. **b** Coronal CT section again demonstrates the slightly septated, expansile, cystic lesions in the left and right mandible.

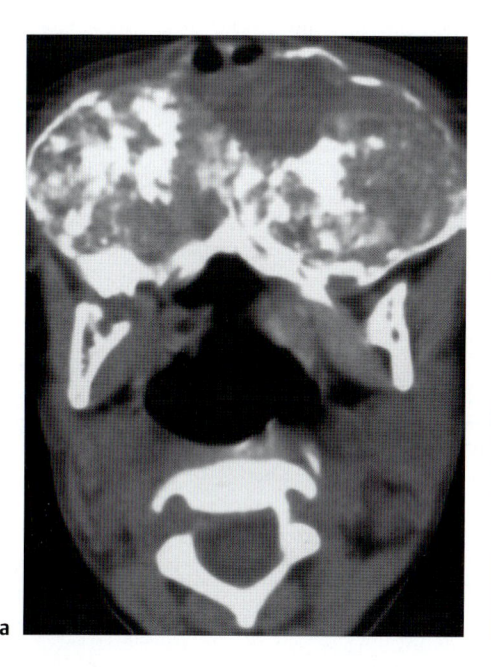

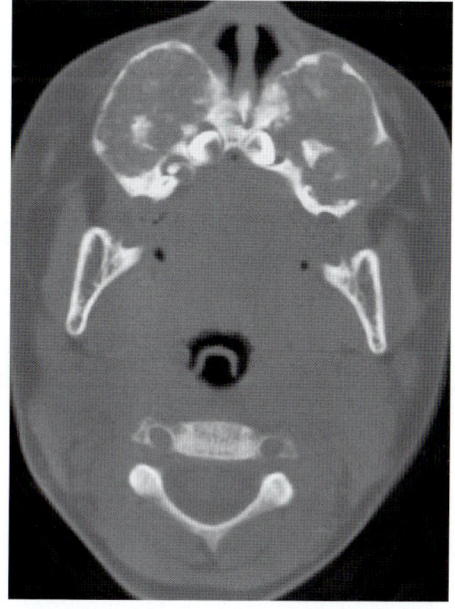

Fig. 6.**53** Cherubism. **a, b** Axial CT scans reveal marked expansion of the maxilla by a fibrous-osseous process, compatible with fibrous dysplasia. Case courtesy of M.F. Mafee, MD.

Osteoblastoma[47, 49]

Osteoblastoma is a benign osteoblastic neoplasm that occurs in the 2nd and 3rd decades of life, with males outnumbering females by 2:1. The lesion shares a histological appearance with osteoid osteoma but is of larger size (usually larger than 2 cm). Osteoblastomas are round to oval in shape, well-circumscribed and are composed of interconnecting trabeculae of woven bone rimmed prominently by osteoblasts. The stroma surrounding the tumor bone is loose connective tissue containing many capillaries. Head and neck sites of osteoblastoma include the mandible, maxilla, orbit, and temporal bone. Radiographically, osteoblastomas appear as a well-defined round expansile lesion with prominent calcified rim.[47, 49] The central portion of osteoblastoma reveals moderate to marked enhancement on T1-weighted MR images, obtained following intravenous administration of gadolinium-based contrast material (see Chapters 4 and TMJ).

Chondroma

Chondromas are slow-growing lesions that are believed to arise from cartilaginous remnants in the bone;[7] they are seen as lytic lesions in the body of the mandible and occasionally in the condyle.[7] Histologically, they are neoplasms of hyaline cartilage and therefore these lesions have high signal intensities on T2-weighted MR images.[7] They appear hypointense on T1-weighted MR scans and show contrast enhancement on T1-weighted MR images following intravenous administration of gadolinum-based contrast material.[7]

Chondroblastoma[47, 49]

Chondroblastoma is a benign cartilaginous neoplasm composed of chondroblasts that form a primitive hyaline matrix surrounding the cells. Chondroblastomas are uncommon and less than 2% of them occur in the head and neck region.[49] The most common site of involvement is the temporal bone (see Chapter 3). Chondroblastoma produce a well-defined geographic lucency that commonly has spotty calcifications.

538   6   Mandible and Maxilla

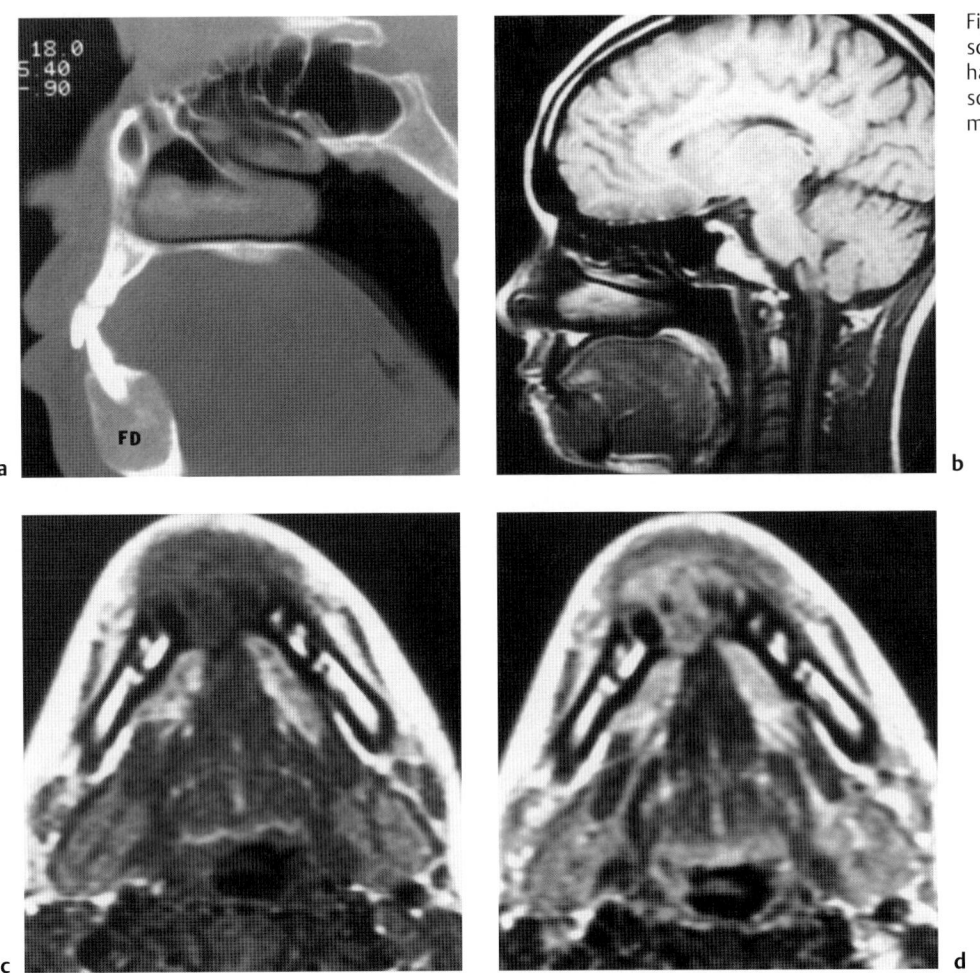

Fig. 6.54 Fibrous dysplasia. **a** Sagittal CT scan, **b** sagittal T1W MR scan, **c** axial unenhanced T1W and **d** axial enhanced T1W MR scans showing fibrous dysplasia (FD) of the mandible. Case courtesy of M.F. Mafee, MD.

Fig. 6.55 Fibrous dysplasia. Axial CT scan shows an expansile lesion of the body of the right mandible compatible with fibrous dysplasia. The lesion shows few areas of mineralization.

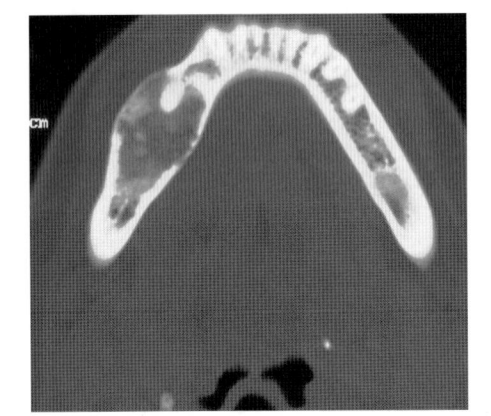

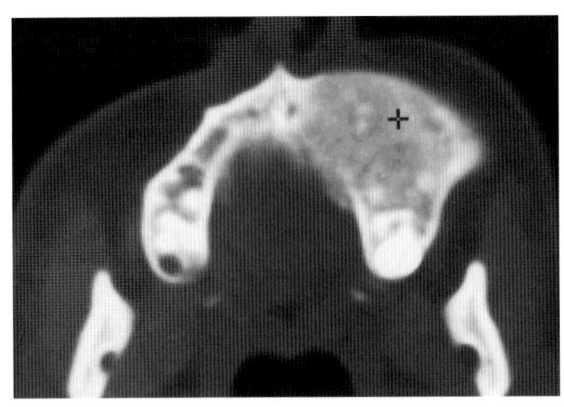

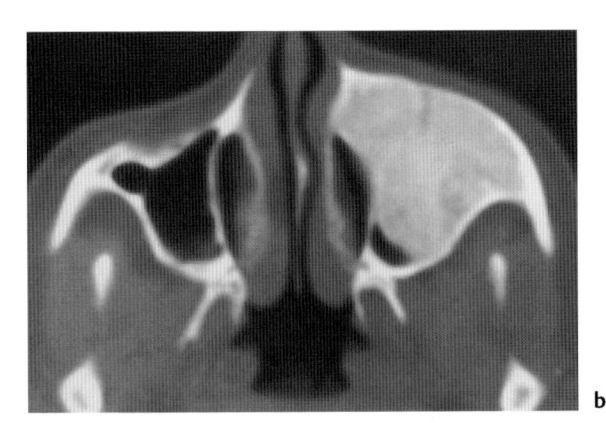

Fig. 6.56 Fibrous dysplasia. Axial CT scans (**a** and **b**) show fibrous dysplasia involving the maxilla and left maxillary antrum. Note that, unlike the lesion in Fig 6.55, there is diffuse mineralization of this fibrous dysplasia lesion, giving characteristic ground-glass appearance to the CT scans. Case courtesy of M.F. Mafee, MD.

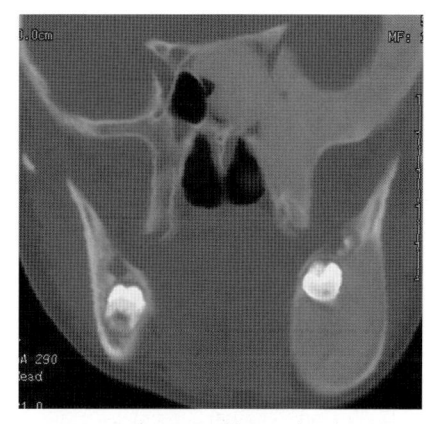

Fig. 6.57 Polyostotic fibrous dysplasia. Coronal CT scan shows fibrous dysplasia involving the left mandible, left sphenoid, and left temporal bone.

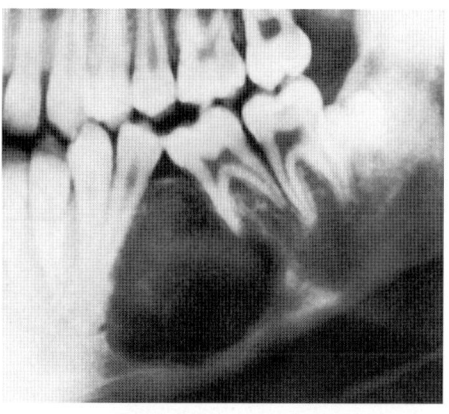

Fig. 6.58 Ossifying fibroma of the left mandible. Panorex view of the mandible demonstrates a sharply defined, lytic, slightly expansile lesion in the body of the mandible, causing encroachment with slight displacement of the molar and premolar teeth.

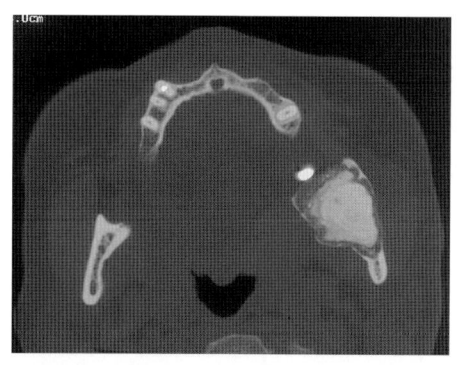

Fig. 6.59 Axial CT scan shows a presumed ossifying fibroma involving the left mandible. Case courtesy of M.F. Mafee, MD.

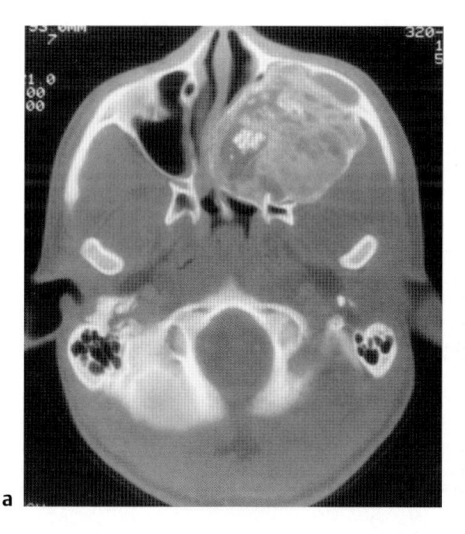

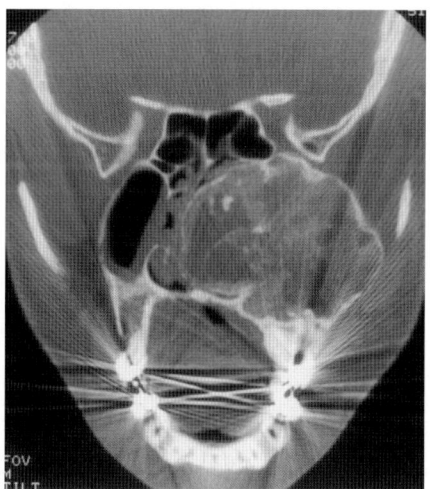

Fig. 6.60 Juvenile aggressive ossifying fibroma. Axial CT (**a**) and coronal (**b**) scans show expansile mass with foci of mineralization (psammoma bodies), involving the left maxilla, compatible with a psammomatous ossifying fibroma. Case courtesy of M.F. Mafee, MD.

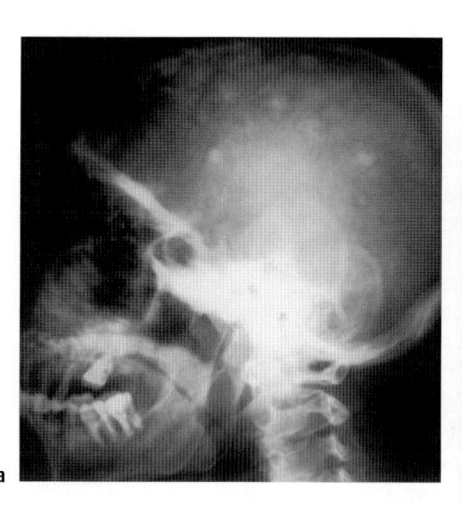

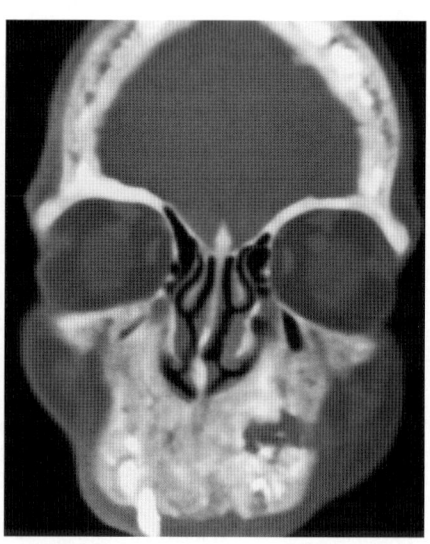

Fig. 6.61 Paget disease. **a** Lateral view of the skull shows pagetoid changes of the maxilla and skull. **b** CT scan shows marked involvement of the frontal bone, maxilla, and mandible by Paget disease. Case courtesy of Calvin Flowers, MD, Chicago, IL, USA.

Paget Disease of Bone[50]

Paget disease of bone is a common disorder affecting approximately 3–4% of the population over 40 years of age.[50] It is characterized by excessive and abnormal remodeling of bone, with both active and quiescent phases.[50] Three pathologic phases have been described; the lytic phase in which osteoclasts predominate; the mixed phase in which osteoblasts cause repair superimposed on the resorption; and the blastic phase in which osteoblasts predominate.[50] The radiographic appearance of Paget disease reflects these pathological changes. Initially, there is osteolysis with subsequent development of trabecular and cortical thickening and enlargement of bone and expansion of bone marrow (Fig. 6.61). Bone marrow changes are seen and during the active phase there is moderate to marked enhancement of bone

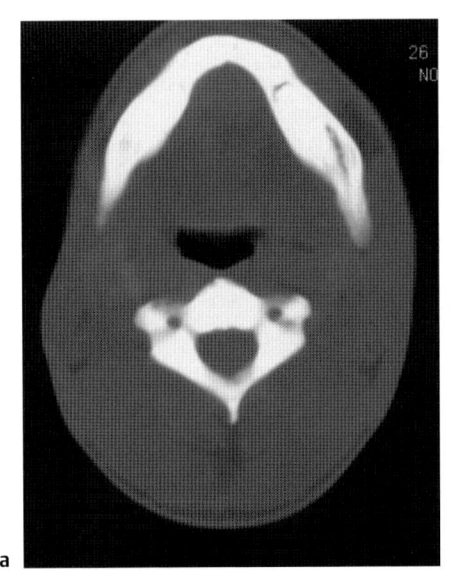

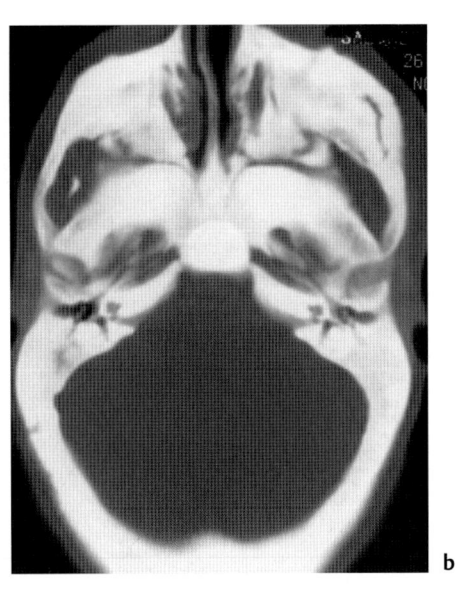

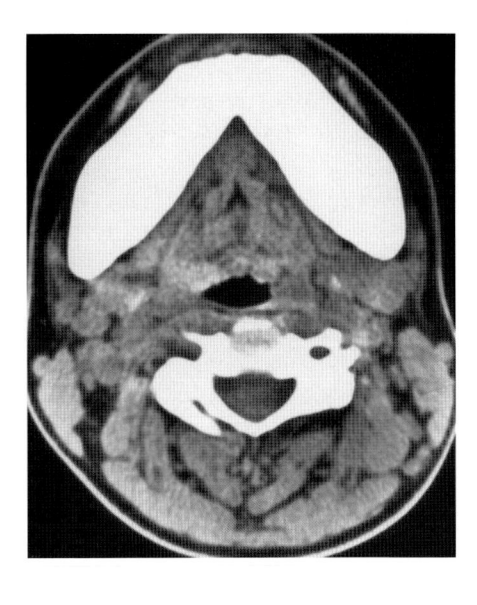

Fig. 6.**62** Osteopetrosis. CT scans (**a** and **b**) showing marked sclerosis of the mandible, maxilla and other craniofacial bones with obliteration of the marrow due to osteopetrosis. Case courtesy of M.F. Mafee, MD.

Fig. 6.**63** Presumed Engelmann disease. CT scan shows marked sclerosis and thickening of the mandible. Case courtesy of M.F. Mafee, MD.

marrow on T1-weighted MR images, obtained following intravenous administration of a gadolinium-based contrast material. Bone destruction and associated soft tissue mass should herald sarcomatous transformation.[50]

Osteopetrosis

Osteopetrosis is a heterogeneous group of conditions sharing an underlying impaired bone resorption by osteoclasts.[51, 52] Five types of disease have been described. The two most commonly seen forms are autosomal recessive (malignant) osteopetrosis and autosomal dominant (benign) osteopetrosis.[51] The different forms can easily be differentiated by mode of inheritance, clinical and imaging findings, and prognosis.[52] The autosomal recessive type presents at birth or in early life and causes death in early childhood. The benign autosomal dominant type of osteopetrosis is known as adult type and is sometimes incidentally detected on radiological examination.[52] Depending on the distribution of sclerosis, two basic phenotypes are distinguished within this group: autosomal dominant osteopetrosis type I (ADO-I) and type II (ADO-II). ADO-I is characterized by a generalized, uniform osteopetrosis mainly in the skull, the spine, and the long bones.[52] Type II is characterized by a different distribution of the sclerosis. Instead of a more uniform sclerosis, a more focal hyperostosis pattern is seen, resulting in endobones ("bones-within-bones"), and the predominant sclerosis of the skull base.[52] Plain radiographs and CT show uniform sclerosis of the craniofacial structures including the marrow space (Fig. 6.**62**). The involved bones appear hypointense in all MR pulse sequences.[51] The CT appearance of Engelmann disease may be similar to osteopetrosis (Fig. 6.**63**).

Vascular Tumors

Hemangiomas[38]

Hemangiomas are vascular tumors that rarely are located in the jaw and most often occur in the skull and vertebrae. They are benign tumors composed of newly formed blood vessels (capillary, cavernous, or mixed type) that may be found incidentally on a radiographic study. Radiographically, the lesion presents as a radiolucent area, often traversed by delicate bony trabeculae, with formation of different-sized small cavities (Fig. 6.**64**). In large hemangiomas, the cortex is thinned, expanded, and may be disrupted. A sunburst appearance results if the trabeculae are arranged in a radiating pattern. In some cases, a single radiolucent lesion with a sclerotic or ill-defined border (simulating a cyst) is encountered.[38]

Vascular Malformation

Vascular malformations are usually present at birth. Vascular malformations can be composed solely of capillary, venous, arterial, or lymphatic tissues, or can be a combination of these tissues. They are subdivided into high-flow and low-flow lesions on the basis of their clinical and angiographic patterns.[7] In the maxillo-mandibulo-facial region they frequently involve bone (Fig. 6.**65**).

Hemangiopericytoma[26]

Hemangiopericytoma is a vascular neoplasm of varying biological behavior arising from pericytic cells that function as baroreceptors and are identified within the outer portion of the capillary wall.[26] In the head and neck, hemangiopericytomas can be identified in virtually any site, but the most common site of occurrence is the nasal cavity, orbit and paranasal sinuses. Hemangiopericytomas are richly vascular and may cause bone erosion. An intraosseous hemangiopericytoma may simulate an intraosseous hemangioma (Fig. 6.**66**).

Neurogenic Tumors

Benign neurogenic tumors (neurilemoma or neurofibroma)[38] are occasionally found in the jaw, the majority occurring in the mandible. The **neurilemoma** (**schwannoma**) is usually encapsulated and contains two histological components (Antoni type A and Antoni type B tissue).

The **neurofibroma** arises from the connective tissue sheath of the nerve fibers and reveals neurites (axons) that traverse the unencapsulated tumor. These tumors may occur as a single lesion or as a part of neurofibromatosis. Radiographically, they appear as a solitary radiolucency associated with enlargement of the mandibular canal (Fig. 6.**67**), or as a unilocular or multilocular radiolucency with cortical expansion and even perforation.

Sometimes, the intraosseous tumor may perforate the cortex of the jaw bone and extend into the overlying soft tissues. A neurofibroma adjacent to the bone may produce a saucer-shaped, erosive defect on the bone surface.[38]

Malignant Tumors

Malignant tumors can be classified into (1) lesions invading the mandible and maxilla secondarily from adjacent soft-tissue structures, (2) tumors arising primarily within the mandible and maxilla, and (3) metastatic tumors from distant sites. They represent a diverse group of lesions, which predominantly consist of carcinomas and sarcomas.[38] The radiographic appearance of malignant lesions often makes it possible to differentiate them from benign tumors and cysts, although in many instances a biopsy is indicated for the final diagnosis. It is important, however, to radiologically assess the extent of the malignant tumor prior to surgery or radiation therapy. CT and MRI are the modalities of choice in the assessment of malignant tumors of the mandible and maxilla. They are complementary in that CT is better suited for bone analysis, demonstration of calcification, and assessing the tumor extent outside the mandible and maxilla, and MRI is more specific for tissue characterization, optimally defining the

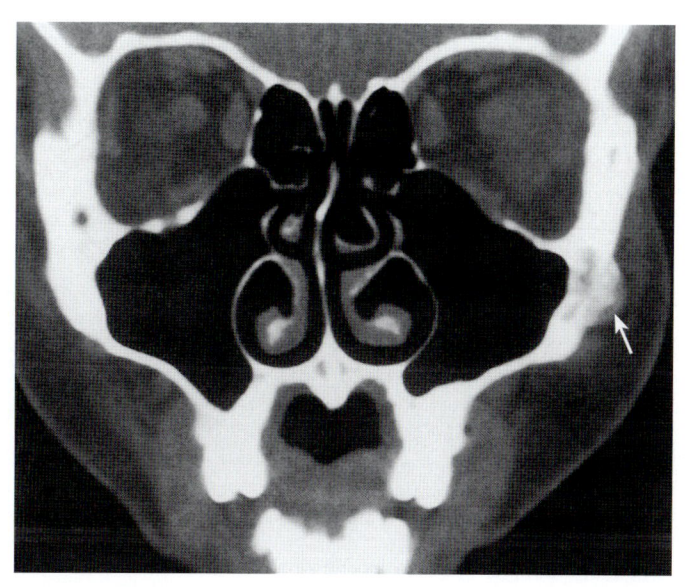

Fig. 6.**64** Hemangioma of the left maxillary bone. Coronal CT section (bone window) demonstrates an expansile lesion in the left maxillary bone (arrow). The lesion is sharply defined and has radiating bony spicules within the center.

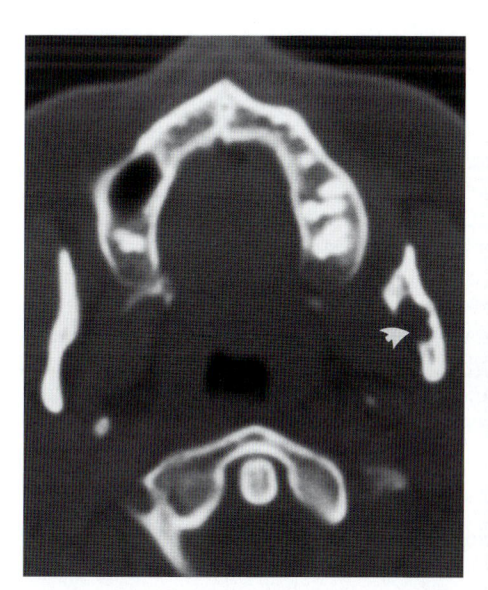

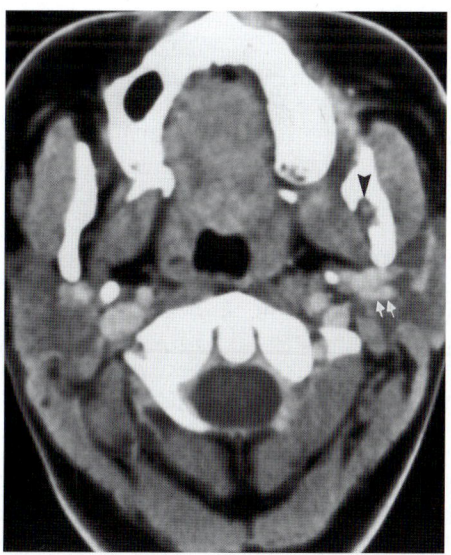

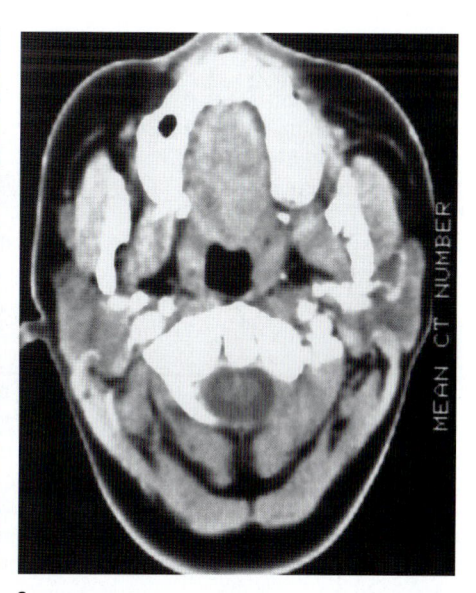

Fig. 6.**65** Facial arteriovenous malformation (AVM) with involvement of the mandible. **a** Axial CT scan shows a hypodense area (arrow) involving the left mandibular ramus. **b** Axial enhanced CT scan shows increased retromandibular vascularity (white arrows). Note a bone defect in the left mandibular ramus with a focal increased enhancement (black arrowhead). **c** Dynamic CT scan shows marked rapid enhancement of mandibular AVM. Case courtesy of M.F. Mafee, MD.

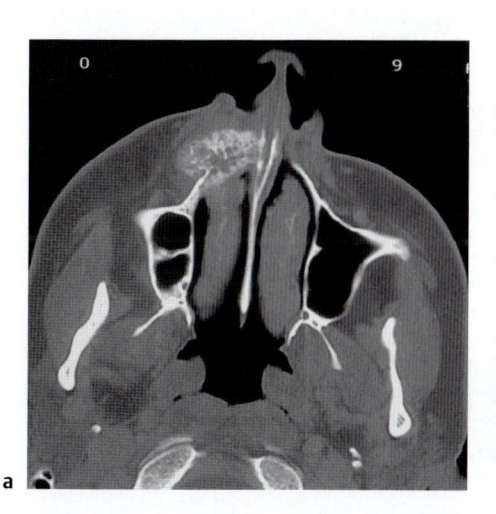

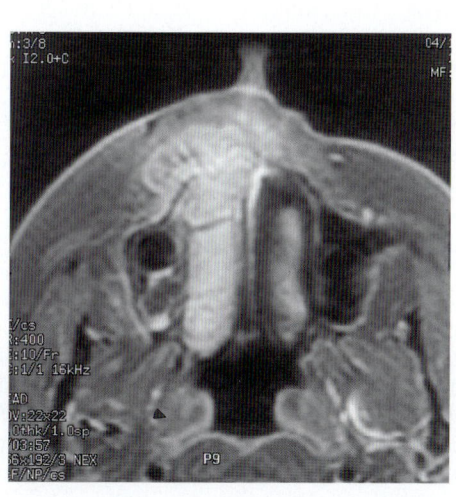

Fig. 6.**66** Hemangiopericytoma. **a** CT scan and **b** enhanced T1W MR scan showing an intraosseous hemangiopericytoma involving the maxilla.

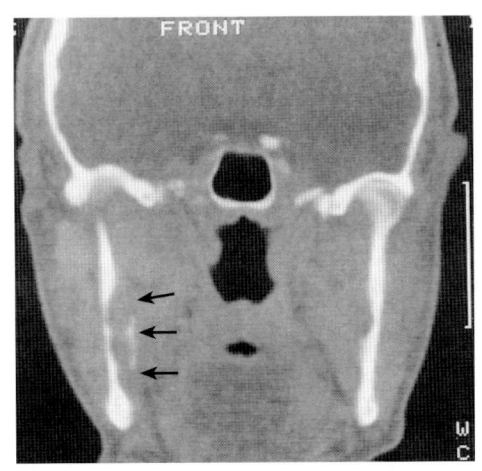

Fig. 6.**67** Neurofibroma of the right mandibular canal in a patient with neurofibromatosis. Coronal CT section reveals diffuse dilatation of the right mandibular canal (arrow). The inner margin of the canal appears scalloped.

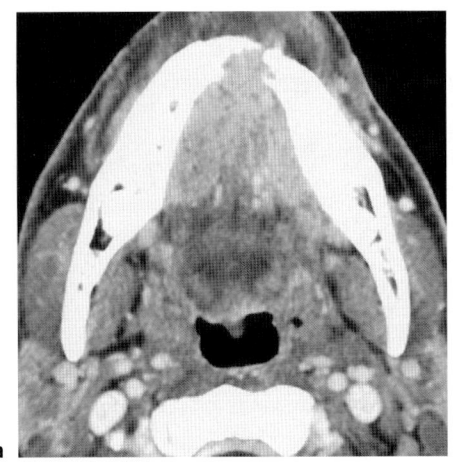

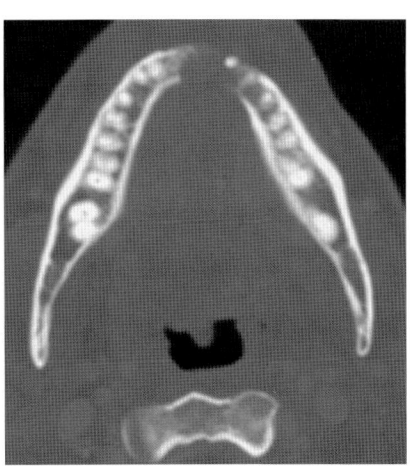

Fig. 6.**68** Carcinoma invading the mandible. CT scans (**a** soft-tissue window; **b** bone window) show invasion of the mandible by squamous cell carcinoma of the floor of mouth, seen on Fig. 6.**68a**. Case courtesy of M.F. Mafee, MD.

boundaries of extraosseous soft-tissue involvement and demonstrating marrow invasion.[5, 38]

Carcinomas[38, 53]

The majority of carcinomas occurring in the jaw originate in the oral cavity and maxillary sinuses. They invade the mandible and maxilla secondarily, and bone involvement occurs by extension through nutrient channels or direct erosion of the advancing tumor.[53] The basis for the "jaw–neck" or "commando" procedures was the long-held belief that oral cavity lymphatics passed through the mandible en route to the cervical lymphatics.[53] Thus, removal of the mandible was considered oncologically necessary. In 1964, Marchetta et al.[54] disproved this notion. Through careful anatomical and histological analyses of segmental mandibulectomy specimens, they demonstrated that oral cavity tumors invade the mandible by direct extension, not through lymphatic channels.[54] Therefore, segmental resection of bone is not always necessary in patients with oral cavity cancer, even in tumors seemingly close to the mandible on physical examination.[53] Marginal mandibulectomy, in preserving mandibular continuity, is associated with less functional and cosmetic morbidity, and can provide satisfactory oncological margins if tumor has not invaded through the entire cortical bone.[53] Preoperative knowledge of bone invasion is, therefore, critical in planning the appropriate procedure.[53] The modalities that have been used to date for studying mandibular invasion by cancer include clinical examination, panorex radiographs, CT, radionuclide scanning, DentaScan and MRI.[38, 53, 55] Mukherji et al.[55] in a series of 49 patients, calculated the diagnostic accuracy of CT as follows: sensitivity 96%; specificity 87%; positive predictive value 89%; and negative predictive value 95%. They attribute their excellent results to superior imaging technique, using 3 mm thick sections and reconstructing with both bone and soft-tissue algorithms.[55] Radiographically, the osseous involvement manifests at the alveolar ridge, causing a saucer-shaped erosive defect (Figs. 6.**68**, 6.**69**). Initially, this may be shallow and well defined (Fig. 6.**68**), but over time an irregular cavity is formed (Fig. 6.**69**). Extrinsic, cortical erosion, especially of the lingual surface of the mandible is best visualized with axial CT sections (Fig. 6.**68**). A pathological fracture is a common finding in advanced cases. Usually, there is no evidence of bony sclerosis (unless there is associated chronic osteitis) or periosteal reaction in carcinomatous involvement of the jaw.

A subgroup of carcinomas is referred to as **central epidermoid carcinoma of the jaw**.[38] This rare tumor may develop from epithelial components (which were part of the development of the teeth) or from epithelial cells (which have become enclosed within the deeper structures of the jaw during the embryonic process). The majority of these lesions are located in the mandible. The radiographic appearance is that of a radiolucent lesion with an irregular outline. Multiple small areas of bone destruction may create a moth-eaten appearance. The radiographic findings are nonspecific, and differentiation from other malignant lesions is not possible. Carcinomatous transformation of the epithelium in an odontogenic cyst is rare, but has been reported in dentigerous, radicular, and residual cysts and keratocysts.[38] Radiologically, the lesion has a cystlike appearance with a circumscribed margin. In the area of malignant degeneration, the cyst margin becomes ill-defined and irregular or moth-eaten.

Mucoepidermoid Carcinoma[7, 38]

Mucoepidermoid carcinoma is another type of carcinoma that may occur in the jaw. It is derived from aberrant salivary gland tissue within the mandible or maxilla, usually in the premolar or molar region. The radiographic findings consist of ill-defined, cystic, or multilocular cystic areas. Mucoepidermoid carcinoma and adenoid cystic carcinoma of the major and minor salivary glands may involve the mandible and maxilla (Fig. 6.**71**). Perineural extension of adenoid cystic tumor may result in enlargement of the mandibular alveolar canal, incisor foramina, and greater and lesser palatine foramina. Likewise, perineural extension of squamous cell carcinoma and lymphoma of the head and neck may result in enlargement of the mandibular canal, incisor foramina, palatine foramina, infraorbital canal, and other skull base foramina.[38]

Sarcomas

Sarcomas are rare in the mandible and maxilla and often occur in younger people. One of the most frequent sarcomas is the **osteogenic sarcoma**.[38] Radiographically, this lesion causes lytic bone destruction with indefinite margins (osteolytic type), sclerosis with increased radiopacity (osteoblastic type), or a mixed pattern (Figs. 6.**72**, 6.**73**). Some osteosarcomas present a sunray effect caused by radiating mineralized tumor spicules (Fig. 6.**72**). In advanced cases, cortical breakthrough with tumor outside the

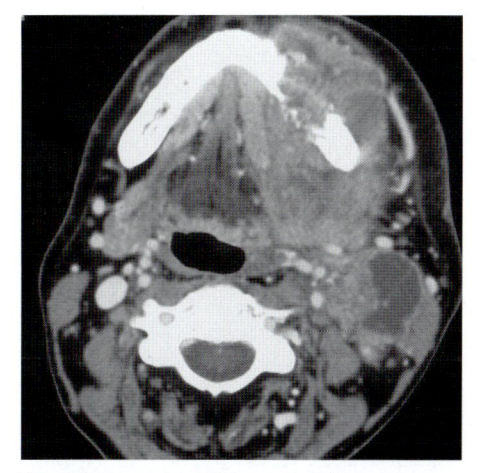

Fig. 6.69 Invasion of the mandible by squamous cell carcinoma of the alveolar ridge. Enhanced CT scan shows a large tumor involving the left mandibular alveolar ridge. Note invasion of the left mandible as well as tumor along the left floor of mouth. Note large necrotic level 2 nodes on the left side.

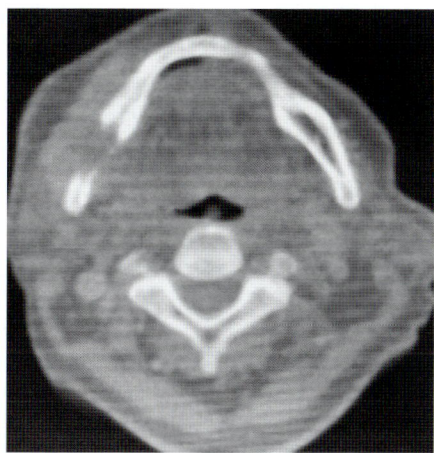

Fig. 6.70 Invasion of the mandible by carcinoma of the alveolar ridge. a Axial CT section (bone window) reveals lytic destruction of the horizontal ramus of the right mandible. b Axial CT section (soft-tissue window): again, note the destruction of the bony compartment of the right mandible with an associated soft-tissue mass.

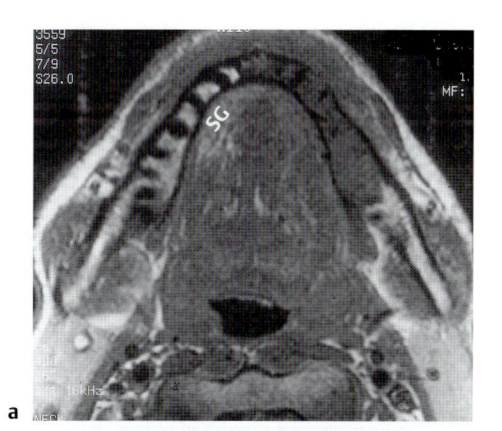

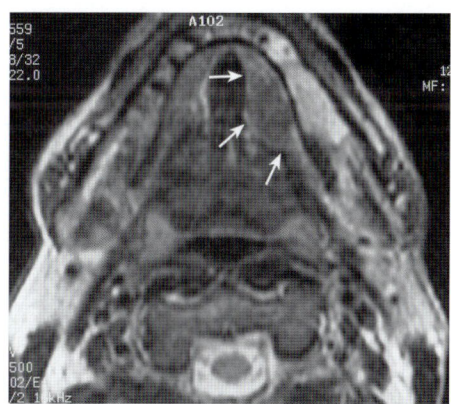

Fig. 6.71 Adenoid cystic carcinoma with perineural mandibular involvement. a T1W and b T2W MR scans, showing normal right sublingual gland (SG) and diffuse enlargement of the left sublingual gland (arrows) compatible with an adenoid cystic carcinoma. Note abnormal signal of the left ramus due to perineural extension of tumor. Case courtesy of M.F. Mafee, MD.

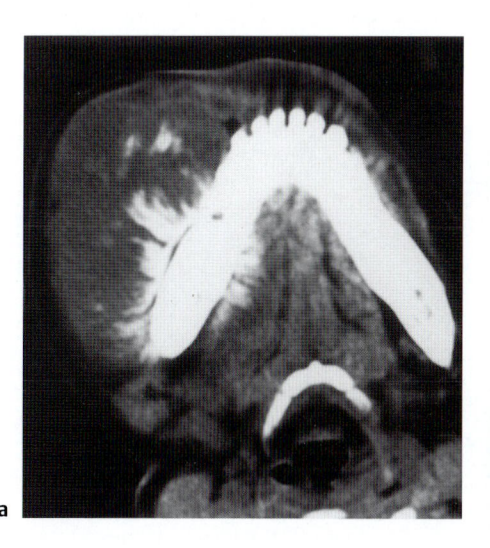

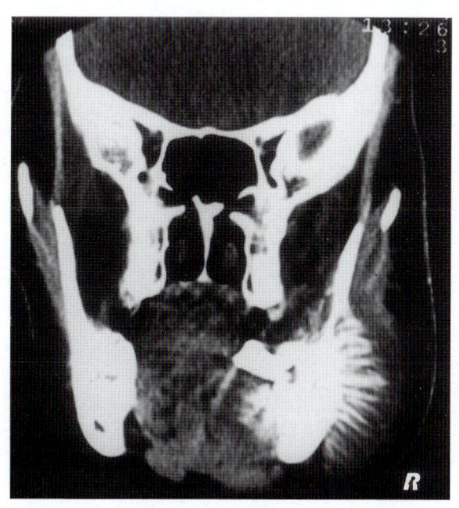

Fig. 6.72 Osteogenic sarcoma of the mandible. a Axial and b coronal CT scans showing an osteogenic sarcoma with a sunray pattern caused by radiating mineralized tumor spicules. R = right. Case courtesy of M.F. Mafee, MD.

jaw is a common finding. Lesions that contain calcium or osteoid or both are easily identified on CT (Figs. 6.74 a, b).

Chondrosarcomas

Cartilaginous neoplasms (chondroma and chondrosarcoma) of the head and neck are uncommon.[26, 47, 49] The most common sites of chondroma of the head and neck include the paranasal sinuses, nasal cavity, nasal septum, maxilla and mandible, larynx, palate, pharynx, and ear. The most common site of chondrosarcoma in the head and neck is the larynx; other sites of involvement include the mandible, maxilla, and paranasal sinuses.[26] Chondroma and chondrosarcoma are rare lesions of the jaw and at times may be seen adjacent to the TMJ (see Chapters 3, 5).

Fibrosarcoma[42] is a rare lesion of the jaw that occurs predominantly in the mandible and has been differentiated into central and peripheral fibrosarcomas. The rare, central, form

544 6 Mandible and Maxilla

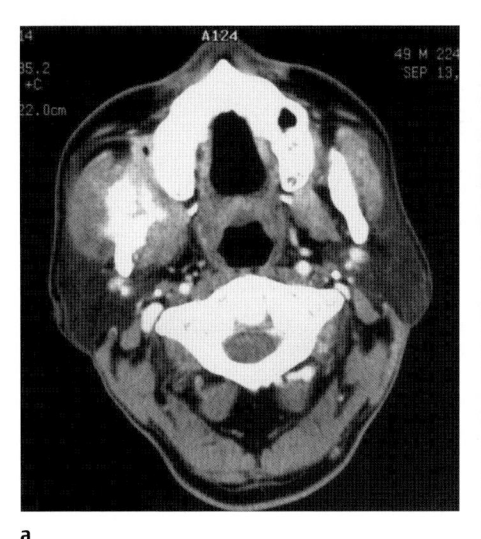

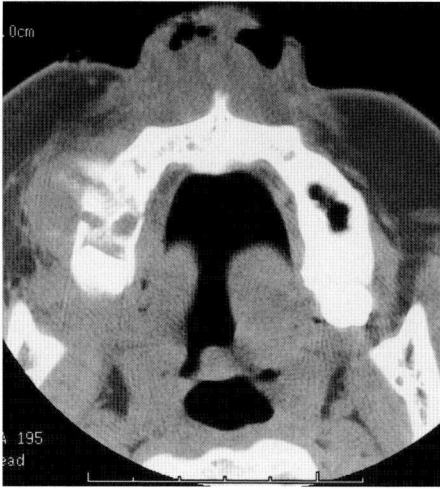

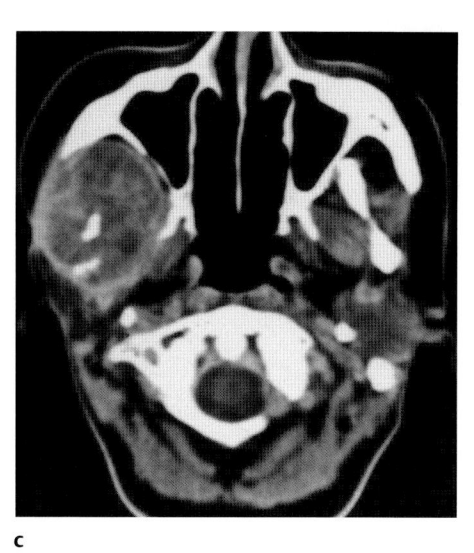

Fig. 6.**73** Osteogenic sarcoma. **a** CT scan shows an osteogenic sarcoma involving the right mandibular ramus. **b** CT scan in another patient shows chondrogenic osteosarcoma involving the right maxilla. In both cases there is marked tumor invasion of surrounding soft tissue. **c** CT scan of another patient shows recurrence of an osteogenic sarcoma of the right mandible. Cases courtesy of M.F. Mafee, MD.

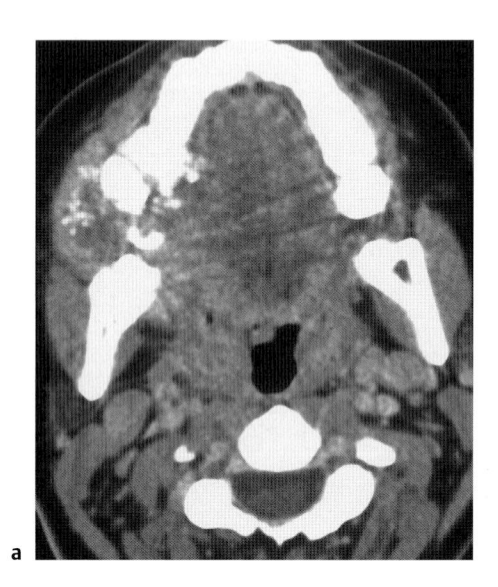

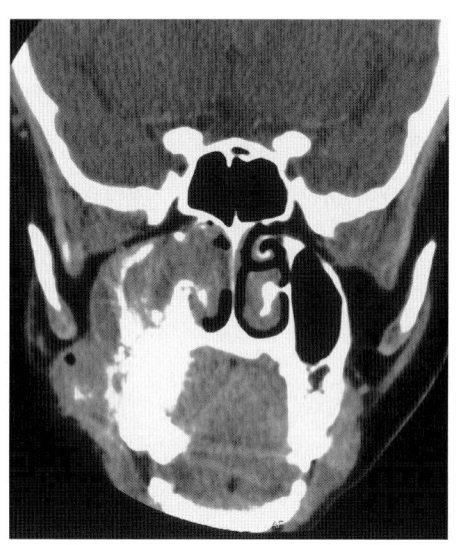

Fig. 6.**74** Osteogenic sarcoma of the maxilla. **a** Axial and **b** coronal CT scans show a soft-tissue mass involving the right maxilla. Note mineralized tumor spheres and spicules characteristic of osteogenic sarcoma. Case courtesy of M.F. Mafee, MD.

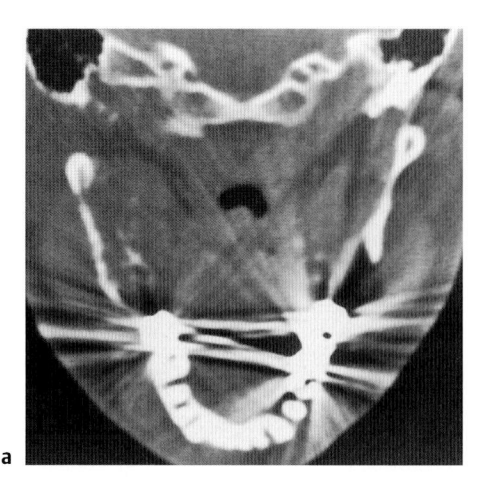

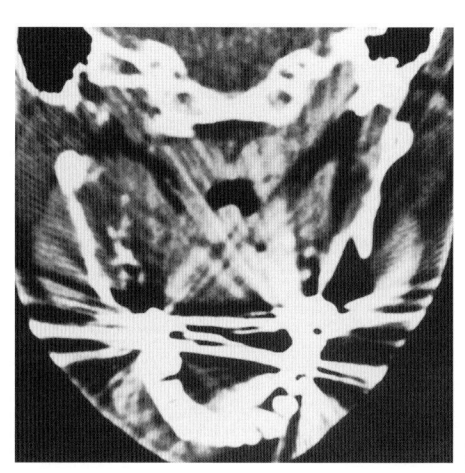

Fig. 6.**75** Ewing sarcoma of right mandible. **a** Coronal CT section of the mandible (bone window) reveals a lytic destructive lesion in the ascending ramus of the mandible. **b** Coronal CT section (soft-tissue window) demonstrates the lytic destruction with extraosseous mass component laterally and medially.

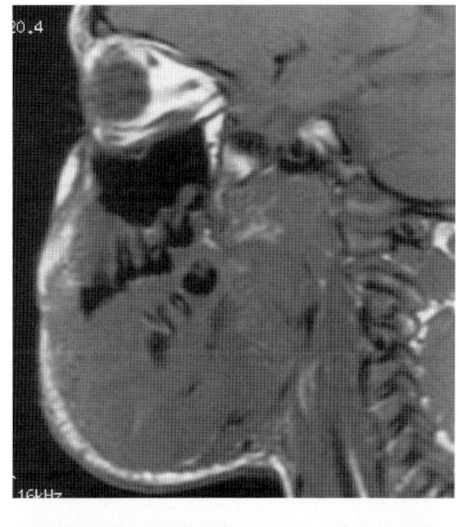

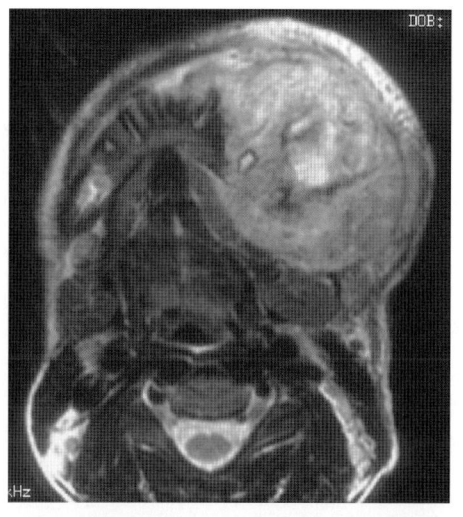

Fig. 6.**76** Ewing sarcoma. **a** Sagittal T1W, **b** axial T2W, and **c** axial enhanced T1W MR scans in a 12-year-old boy show a destructive lesion involving the left mandible. **d** CT scan shows large lytic lesion with areas of sclerosis. This cannot be differentiated from an osteogenic sarcoma or Burkitt lymphoma. Case courtesy of M.F. Mafee, MD.

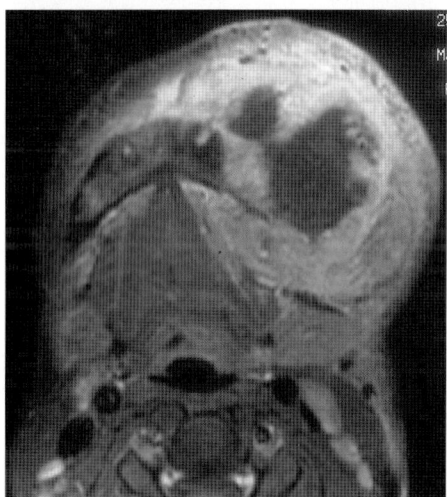

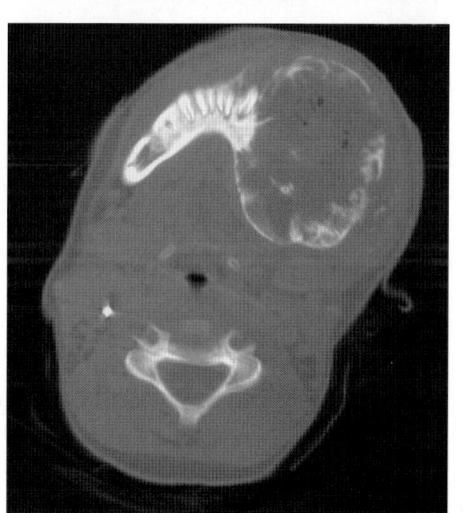

most frequently develops in the mandibular canal and causes bone destruction, which is located centrally, with gradual expansion leading to cortical erosion in larger lesions. The more prevalent, peripheral type originates from the periosteum of the mandible or the periodontal membrane, frequently in the body of the mandible. Erosive changes are seen radiographically at the alveolar ridge or at the inferior border of the mandible. The depth of the erosive defect varies depending on the state of tumor development.[7, 38]

Ewing sarcoma[38] has been found 10 times more frequently in the mandible than in the maxilla. Radiographically, the lesion has a mottled, irregular, lucent appearance with sclerosis interspersed in a small percentage of cases (Figs. 6.**75**, 6.**76**). Perpendicular bony spicules and extensive bone destruction may be found at the cortex (Fig. 6.**76**). The characteristic onion-peel layering of new subperiosteal bone is often absent in lesions affecting the mandible and maxilla.[38]

Malignant Lymphoma[7, 38]

Primary lymphoma of bone may occur in the mandible and maxilla. Radiographically, there are no pathognomonic findings (Fig. 6.**77**). Most often there are ill-defined lytic destructive areas of variable size within the mandible (see also Chapter 4).

Multiple Myeloma[7, 38]

Multiple myeloma is characterized by multiple or diffuse bone involvement, although single lesions are occasionally seen. Among multiple myelomas of the jaw, mandibular lesions are the most common (especially in the region of the angle, ramus, and molar teeth). The typical radiographic appearance is punched-out, regular, circular, or ovoid radiolucencies with no circumferential bone reaction (especially when the skull is involved) (Fig. 6.**78**). The cortex of the mandible may be perforated, but bone expansion is not demonstrated. If the lesion is extensive, the entire bone may be destroyed.

Burkitt Lymphoma[26]

Burkitt lymphoma is a high-grade non-Hodgkin malignant lymphoma with distinct clinical, pathological, and epidemiological features. Two forms are recognized: endemic or African type, and non-endemic or American type. The African type affects males more than females, most commonly in the first decade of life. The disease presents most frequently with extranodal tumor in the jaw (Fig. 6.**79**), kidneys, ovaries, retroperitoneum, orbit, and meninges. Approximately 90% of cases have elevated Epstein–Barr virus (EBV) titers and EBV DNA genome. The American type affects males more than females, most commonly in the second decade of life. The disease presents with intra-abdominal tumors in the GI tract-associated lymphoid tissue; other sites of involve-

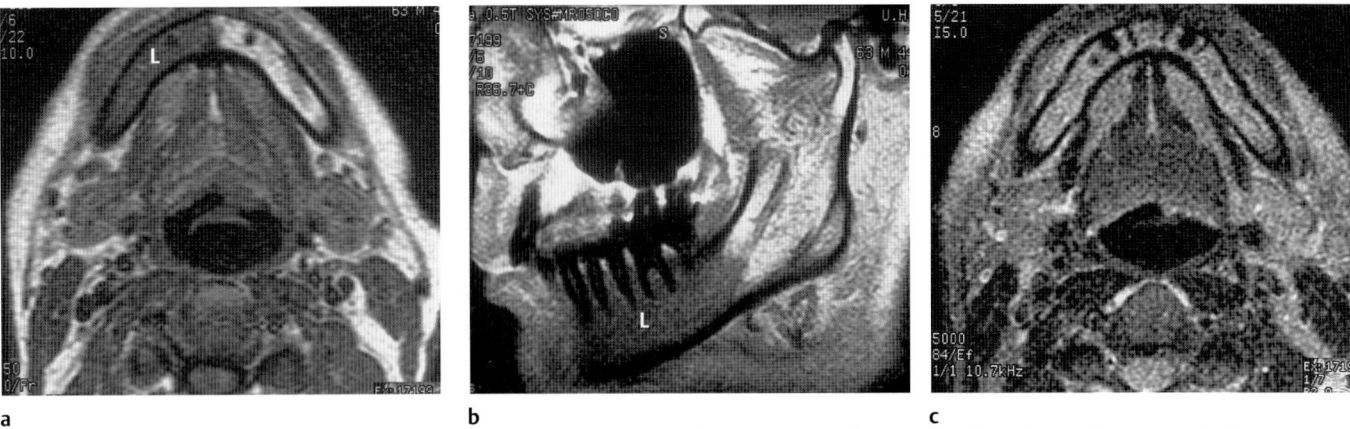

Fig. 6.77 Lymphoma of the mandible. **a** Axial T1W, **b** sagittal T1W, and **c** axial T2W MR scans show primary lymphoma (L) involving the bone marrow of the right mandible. Case courtesy of M.F. Mafee, M.D.

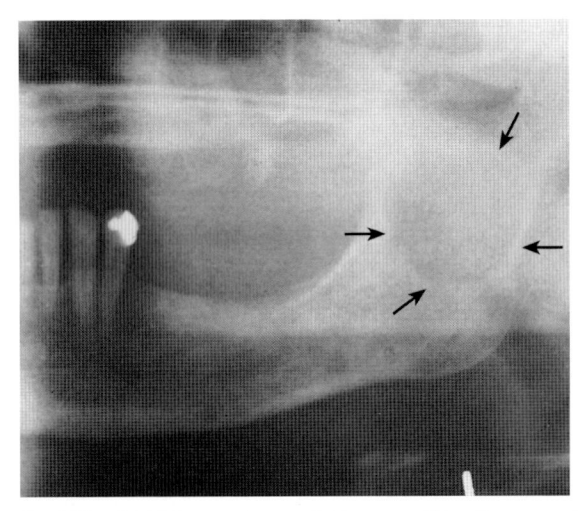

Fig. 6.78 Multiple myeloma of the mandible. Panorex view of the mandible reveals a fairly well-defined, lytic lesion in the ascending ramus of the mandible (arrows). Note the smaller, punched-out, lytic lesions in the body of the mandible.

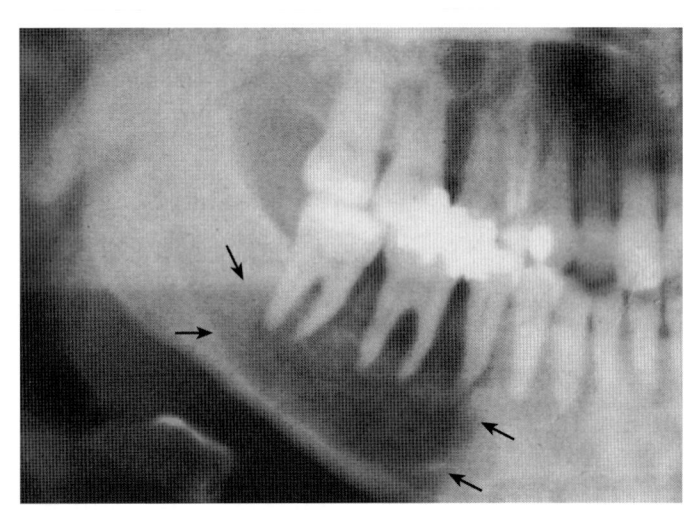

Fig. 6.79 Burkitt lymphoma of mandible. Panorex view of the right mandible reveals an ill-defined, mottled, destructive area in the body of the right mandible adjacent to the roots of the adjacent molar teeth (arrows).

ment include the ovary, nasopharynx, orbit, meninges, retroperitoneum, kidney, peripheral lymph nodes, and bone marrow. Evidence of EBV infection is seen in less than 30% of cases.[26,38]

Leukemia

Leukemia may involve the jaw bones. The initial radiographic finding is loss of the lamina dura with loosening of the teeth, which is often followed by a variable degree of lytic bone destruction.[38] MRI is very sensitive for showing bone marrow changes due to leukemic infiltration. The involved bone marrow appears moderately to markedly hypointense on T1-weighted and T2-weighted MR images.[7]

Metastases[38]

A metastatic tumor of the mandible or maxilla may be the first indication of a malignancy from an undiscovered site, or the first evidence of dissemination of a known primary tumor. Metastases to the mandible occur four times more often than to the maxilla. The most common primary tumors are from the breast, lung (bronchogenic carcinoma), kidney (hypernephroma), thyroid, prostate, and stomach. Most often the bone destruction is demonstrated radiographically as an irregular lucency with indistinct margins (Figs. 6.**80**–6.**82**). Occasionally, a mixed type of lesion (containing lytic and sclerotic areas) may be encountered, such as in carcinoma of the breast. Rarely, metastasis from carcinoma of the prostate causes diffuse osteoblastic changes (Fig. 6.**80**). The areas of destruction within the mandible may be localized, unilateral, bilateral, or diffuse through a large portion of the bone.[7,38]

DentaScan

Progressive periodontal disease will subsequently result in loss of teeth. Permanent replacement of natural teeth has been attempted unsuccessfully for many years with complications of loosening, infection, and loss of bone surrounding the implants.[56,57] In 1969, Branemark et al.[58] showed that titanium implants could be safely placed in the jaw with a low failure rate if a strict two-step operative procedure was performed. The titanium implants are placed in the bone and buried under the oral mucosa for 3–6 months before they are attached to artificial teeth during the second surgical procedure.[57] Successful endosseous implantation requires knowledge of the precise location of the mandibular canal, maxillary alveolus, and maxillary sinuses. Injury to the neurovascular bundle, within the mandibular canal, results in paresthesia of the face, whereas perforation of the maxillary sinuses increases the likelihood of implant failure and the potential for sinus infection.[56,57] The surgeon needs to

Pathology 547

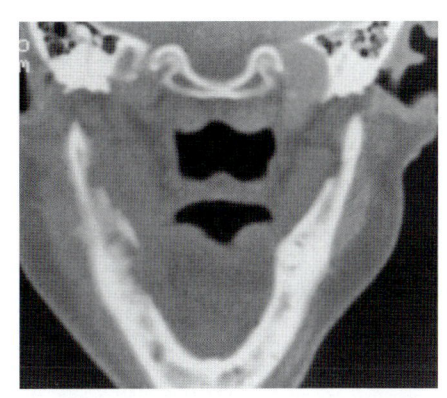

Fig. 6.80 Metastasis to the left mandible from carcinoma of the prostate. Coronal CT section (bone window) demonstrates a sclerotic metastasis in the body and ascending ramus of the left mandible.

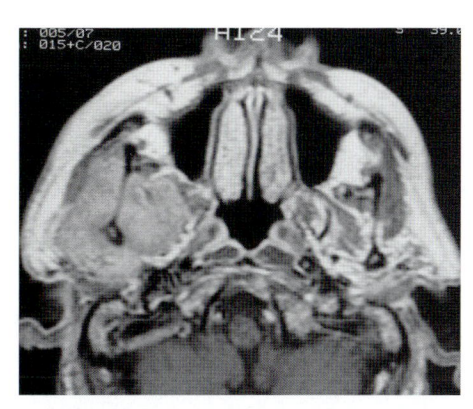

Fig. 6.81 Metastasis. Axial enhanced T1W MR scan shows metastasis to the right mandible from carcinoma of the prostate. Case courtesy of M.F. Mafee, MD.

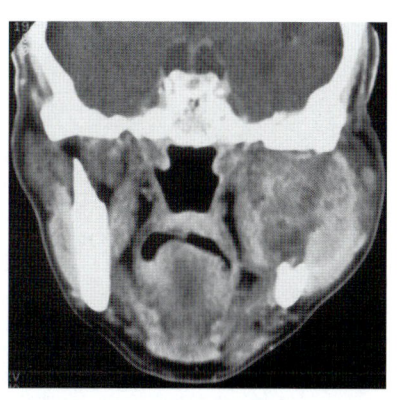

Fig. 6.82 Metastasis. Coronal enhanced CT scan shows metastasis to the left mandible from hypernephroma. Case courtesy of M.F. Mafee, MD.

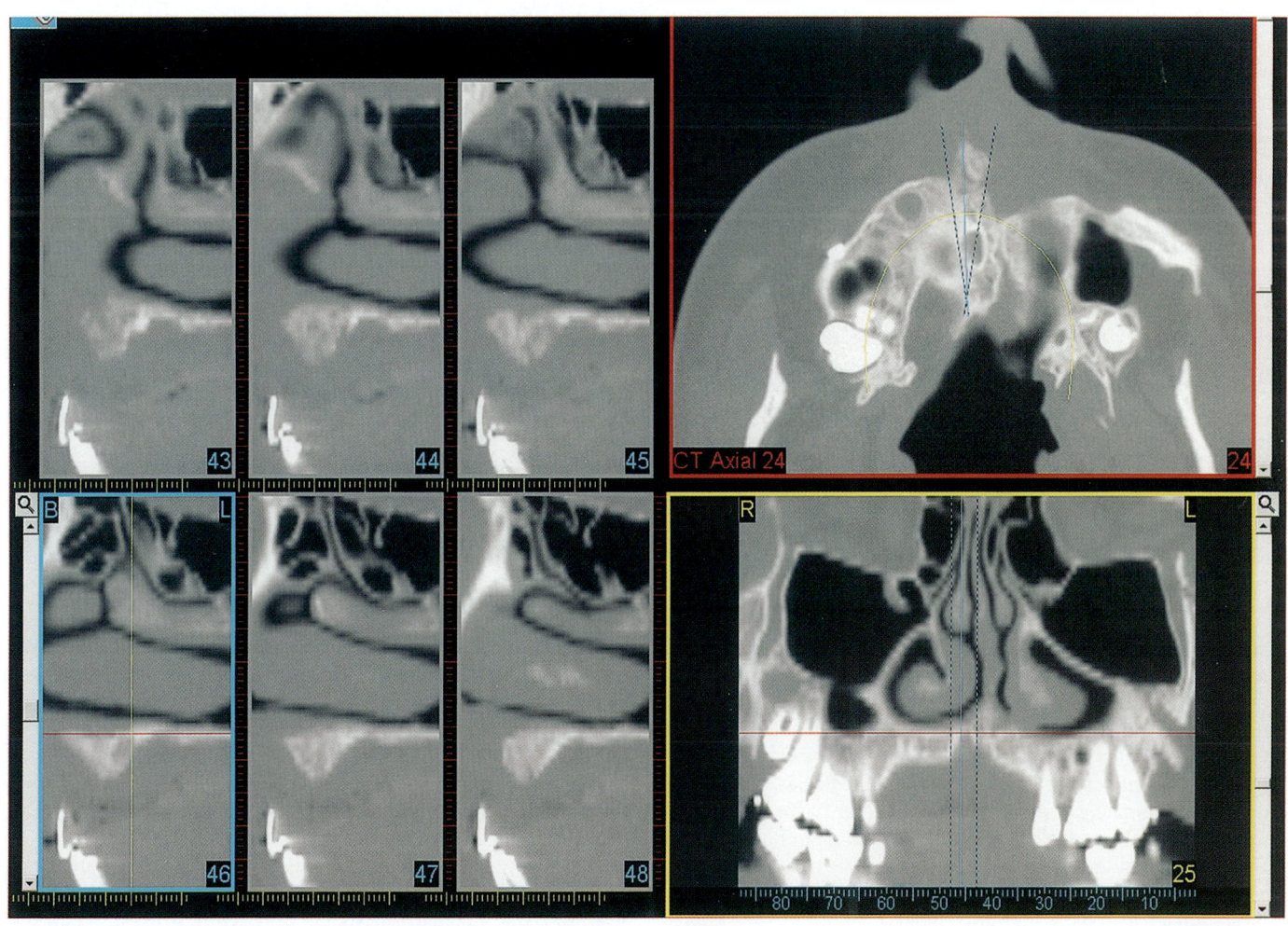

Fig. 6.83 DentaScan of the maxilla in a patient with cleft palate. One of the axial source images, numbered in the lower right corner (24), is displayed at the upper right corner. The curved yellow line that follows the curvature of the alveolar process of the maxilla references the exact location of the panoramic image displayed in the lower right corner. The blue lines perpendicular to the curved yellow line reference the exact location of the sectional reformatted images (43–48). The red horizontal line across the panoramic image references the exact location of the axial image (CT axial 24). The set of red tick marks located immediately to the left of the yellow border of the panoramic image references the position of each axial image in the CT study. The blue vertical lines in the panoramic image reference the exact position of the sectional reformatted images (43–48). The B and L markers seen in reformatted image 46 show the patient's buccal (B) and lingual (L) sites. The red horizontal line across this image references the exact position of the axial CT image. The red sets of tick marks to the right of the sectional reformatted images (43–48) reference the position of each axial source image in the CT study. The yellow vertical line seen in reformatted image 46 references the exact location of the panoramic image. The sets of yellow tick marks below the cross-sectional reformatted images (43–48) reference the position of each panoramic image in the 3D reconstruction study.

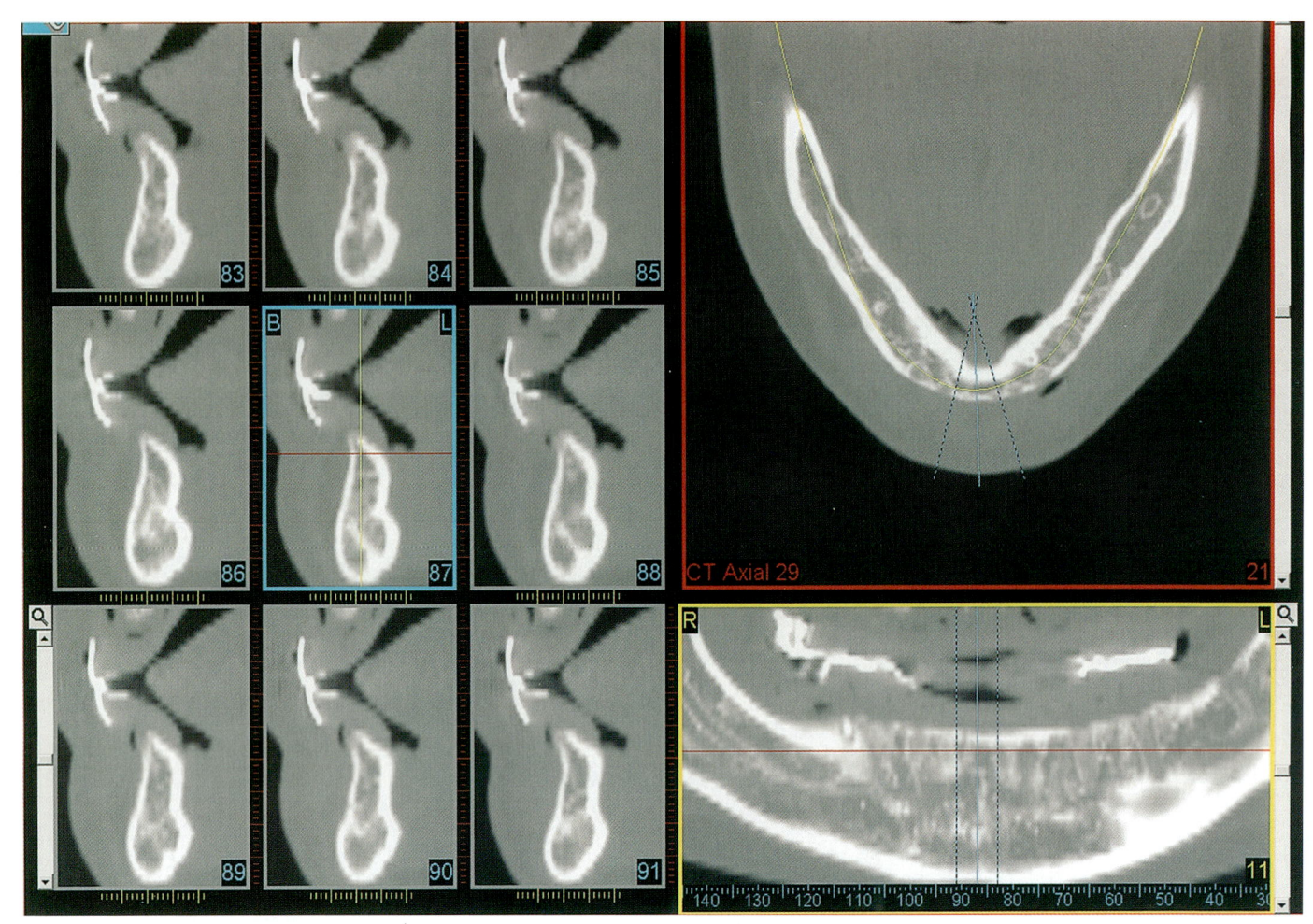

Fig. 6.84 DentaScan of the mandible. An axial image (upper right corner), a panoramic image (lower right corner), and nine reformatted images (83–91) of the mandible are displayed. One of the axial source images is surrounded by a red border and numbered in the lower right corner (21), with the numbers increasing from inferior to superior on scrolling. The axial number assigned by the CT scanner is displayed in the lower left corner (29). The numbers may not coincide for the following reason: Sometimes, as in this patient, one may not need all the images for doing 3D reconstruction as the lowermost images may not contain any bone and they are therefore discarded. The 3D reconstruction may actually start from the ninth axial image, in which case the first axial image displayed will show CT Axial 9 on the lower left hand corner and 1 in the lower right corner. Therefore, the ninth CT axial image is the first axial image used for 3D reconstruction. The DentaScan was obtained using the software package CT/MASTER (Maryland, USA).

measure the height and width of the alveolar process in order to select the proper implant and ensure adequacy of bone. A cross section of the mandible perpendicular to the mandibular canal is desirable for providing the required preoperative information. The dental implants are intraosseous and, therefore, need a certain bone volume for burial inside the bone.[57] In the lower jaw, implants can be safely placed in front of the mental foramina. For implants to be placed lateral to mental foramina, the precise location of the mandibular canal (inferior alveolar nerve) needs to be known to prevent injury to the inferior alveolar nerve. The oromaxillofacial surgeon, therefore, needs to evaluate the superoinferior dimension of the alveolar process above the mandibular canal. If this dimension is not sufficient for the length of the implant, permanent nerve damage can occur.[57] In the maxilla, extension of pneumatization into the alveolar process of the maxilla may result in too little bone for placement of intraosseous maxillary implants.[57] The implants are about 4 mm in diameter and range in length from 7 mm to 15 mm.[57]

DentaScan, a dental computed tomography software program, is a technique developed to assist oromaxillofacial surgeons in planning for endosseous implantation.[56,57] DentaScan reformats standard axial CT scans into two unique views: panelliptical (panoramic) and parasagittal (Figs. 6.83, 6.84). Reformatting images allows for close inspection of buccal and lingual cortices, and in theory should improve specificity and sensitivity of direct axial and coronal sections for the evaluation of mandibular and maxillary anatomy and pathology.[53,56,57] The DentaScan program uses data from thin-slice axial CT. The unenhanced axial images are acquired parallel to the alveolar ridge (mandibular occlusal plane), using a bone algorithm, and 1 mm slice thickness and table increment. Images obtained on the multislice scanner were obtained with a slice thickness and table increment of 1.25 mm. The CT images (source images) are postprocessed using the DentaScan program. A curve is designed from an axial image at the roots of the teeth, irrespective of the lesion location (Fig. 6.83). This axial CT scan with curved line (Fig. 6.83) defines the plane and location of the reformatted panoramic view (Fig. 6.84). Next, sectional locations are numbered in this reference axial CT scan with curved line, and then the sectional images at 2–3 mm are reformatted along multiple numbered lines that the program automatically draws perpendicular to this curve (Fig. 6.84). Panellipse images also can be obtained at 2 mm increments.[53,56] Once the axial, panelliptical, and sectional images are displayed, each can be related to the others by a series of tick marks that appear on the images. This permits precise correlation between one anatomical plane and the next.[56,57] The digital information obtained can be forwarded to the dental service for use in surgical planning.

References

1. Warwick R, Williams PL, eds. Gray's Anatomy, 35th British edition. Philadelphia: W.B. Saunders; 1973.
2. Stafne EC, Gibilisco JA. Oral Roentgen Diagnosis, 4th ed. Philadelphia: W.B. Saunders; 1975.
3. Seldin EB. Radiology of the mandible. In: Taveras JA, Ferrucci JT, eds. Radiology: Diagnosis, Imaging, Intervention, Vol. 3. Philadelphia: J.B. Lippincott; 1987.
4. Weber AL. Radiological evaluation. In: Thaller SR, Montgomery WW, eds. Guide to Dental Problems for Physicians and Surgeons. Baltimore: Williams and Wilkins; 1988.
5. Weber AL, Easter K. Cysts and odontogenic tumors of the mandible and maxilla. Part I. Contemp Diagn Radiol 1982; 5(25): 1–5.
6. Weber AL, Easter K. Cysts and odontogenic tumors of the mandible and maxilla. Part II. Contemp Diagn Radiol 1982; 5(26): 1–5.
7. Weber AL, Kaneda T, Scrivani SJ, Aziz S. Jaw: cysts, tumors, and non-tumorous lesions. In: Som PM, Curtin HD (eds). Head and Neck Imaging, 4th ed. St. Louis, MO: Mosby; 2003: 930–994.
8. Osborn AG, Hanafee WN, Mancuso AA. Normal and pathological CT anatomy of the mandible. AJR 1982; 139(3): 555–559.
9. Christianson R, Lufkin RB, Abeymayor E et al. MRI of the mandible. Surg Radiol Anat 1989; 11(2): 163–169.
10. Stafne EC, Milhorn JA. Periodontal cysts. J Oral Surg 1945; 3: 102–111.
11. Mourshed F. A roentgenographic study of dentigerous cysts. Oral Surg Oral Med Oral Pathol 1964; 18: 47–51, 54–61.
12. Donoff RB, Guralnick WC, Clayman L. Keratocysts of the jaw. J Oral Surg 1972; 30: 800–804.
13. Weber AL. Imaging of cysts and odontogenic tumors of the jaw: Definition and classification. Radiol Clin North Am 1993; 31: 101–120.
14. Meara JG, Shah S, Likk RL, Cunningham MJ. The odontogenic keratocyst: a 20-year clinicopathological review. Laryngoscope 1998; 108: 280–283.
15. Grafenberg MR, Kim S, Sorensen D. Pathology Quiz Case 2. Odontogenic keratocyst (OKC). Arch Otolaryngol Head Neck Surg 2002; 128: 1100–1102.
16. Brannon RB. The odontogenic keratocyst: a clinicopathological study of 312 cases, part II: histological features. Oral Surg Oral Med Oral Pathol 1977; 43: 233–255.
17. Abrams A, Howell FV, Bullock WK. Nasopalatine cysts. Oral Surg Oral Med Oral Pathol 1963; 16: 306–32.
18. Little JW, Jakobsen J. Origin of the globulomaxillary cyst. J Oral Surg 1973; 31: 188–195.
19. Hillman T, Galloway EB, Johnson LP. Pathology Quiz Case I. Nasoalveolar cyst. Arch Otolaryngol Head Neck Surg 2002; 128: 452–455.
20. Wysocki GP, Goldblatt LI. The so-called "globulomaxillary cyst" is extinct. Oral Surg Oral Med Oral Pathol 1993; 76: 185–186.
21. Kuriloff DB. The nasolabial cyst-nasal hamartoma. Otolaryngol Head Neck Surg 1987; 96: 268–272.
22. Klestadt WD. Nasal cysts and the facial cleft cyst theory. Ann Otol Rhinol Laryngol 1953; 62: 84–92.
23. Huebner GR, Turlington EG. So-called traumatic (hemorrhagic) bone cysts of the jaw. Oral Surg 1971; 31: 254–265.
24. Stafne EC. Bone cavities situated near the angle of the jaw. J Am Dent Assoc 1942; 29: 1969.
25. Regezi JA, Kerr DA, Courtney RM. Odontogenic tumors: analysis of 706 cases. J Oral Surg 1978; 36: 771–778.
26. Wenig BM. Atlas of Head and Neck Pathology. Philadelphia: W.B. Saunders, 1993; 175–178.
27. Heffez L, Mafee MF, Vaiana J. The role of magnetic resonance imaging in the diagnosis and management of ameloblastoma. Oral Surg Oral Med Oral Pathol 1988; 65: 2–12.
28. Franklin CD, Pindborg JJ. The calcifying epithelial odontogenic tumor. Oral Surg Oral Med Oral Pathol 1976; 42: 753–765.
29. Sik-Chung Ching A, Wai Pak U, Kew J, Metreweli C. CT and MR imaging appearances of an extraosseous calcifying epithelial odontogenic tumor (Pindborg tumor). AJNR 2000; 21: 343–345.
30. Wood NK, Goaz PW, eds. Differential diagnosis of oral and maxillofacial lesions. St. Louis, MO: Mosby; 1997: 428–431.
31. Ismail IM, Al-Talabani NG. Calcifying epithelial odontogenic tumor associated with dentigerous cyst. Int J Oral Maxillofac Surg 1986; 15: 108–111.
32. Brandwein M, Said-Al-Naief N, Gordon R, Urken M. Clear cell odontogenic carcinoma. Report of a case and analysis of the literature. Arch Otolaryngol Head Neck Surg 2002; 1281: 1089–1095.
33. Tratman EK. Classification of odontomas. Br Dent J 1951; 91: 167–173.
34. Davis RB, Baker RD, Alling CC. Odontogenic myxoma. Clinical pathological conference: Case 24: I and II. Oral Surg Oral Med Oral Pathol 1978; 36: 534–538, 610–615.
35. Pitkaranta A, Carpen O, Ramsay H. Fibromyxoma of temporal bone. Otolaryngol Head Neck Surg., 1997; 117:201–203.
36. Shaw EA, Antonelli PJ. Radiology case 1. Fibromyxoid tumor of the petrous apex. Arch Otolaryngol Head Neck Surg., 2003; 129: 129–132.
37. Zegarelli EV, Kutscher AH, Napoli N, Furono F, Hoffman P. The cementoma. A study of 230 patients with 435 cementomas. Oral Surg Oral Med Oral Pathol 1964; 17: 219–224.
38. Weber AL. Radiographic evaluation of the mandible and maxilla (cysts, benign and malignant tumors). In: Valvassori GE, Mafee MF, Carter BL (eds). Imaging of the Head and Neck. Stuttgart: Thieme; 1995. pp.; 510–526
39. Wood NK, Goaz PW. Differential Diagnosis of Oral Lesions. St. Louis, MO: C.V. Mosby; 1980: 392–393.
40. Sazuki M, Sakai T. A familial study of torus palatinus and torus mandibularis. Am J Phys Anthropol 1986; 18: 263–272.
41. Bhaskar SN, Cutright DE. Multiple exostoses; report of cases. J Oral Surg 1968; 26: 321–326.
42. Noren GD, Roche WC. Huge osteoma of the mandible: report of a case. J Oral Surg 1978; 36: 375–379.
43. Halse A, Roed-Petersen B, Lund K. Gardner's Syndrome. J Oral Surg 1975; 33: 673–676.
44. Quick CA, Anderson R, Stool S. Giant cell tumors of the maxilla in children. Laryngoscope 1980; 90: 784–791.
45. Jaffe HL. Giant cell reparative granuloma, traumatic bone cyst, and fibrous (fibro-osseous) dysplasia of the jawbones. Oral Surg 1953; 6: 159–175.
46. Murphey MD, Nomikos GC, Flemming DF, et al. From the Archives of the AFIP. Imaging of giant cell tumor and giant cell reparative granuloma of bone: radiological-pathological correlation. Radiographics 2001; 21: 1283–1309.
47. Mafee MF, Yang G, Tseng A, et al. Fibro-osseous and giant cell lesions including brown tumor of the mandible, maxilla and other craniofacial bones. Radiol Clin North Am 2003; 13: 525–540.
48. Hidayat AA, Mafee MF, Laver NV, Noujaims S. Langerhans cell histiocytosis and juvenile xanthogranuloma of the orbit. Clinicopathological, CT, and MR imaging features. Radiol Clin North Am 1998; 36: 1229–1240.
49. Wenig BM, Mafee MF, Gosh L. Fibro-osseous, osseous, and cartilaginous lesions of the orbit and paraorbital region. Correlative clinicopathological and radiographic features, including the diagnostic role of CT and MR imaging. Radiol Clin North Am 1998; 36: 1241–1259.
50. Smith SE, Murphey MD, Notamedi R, et al. From the Archives of the AFIP Radiological Spectrum of Paget disease of bone and its complications with pathological correlation. Radiographics 2002; 22: 1191–1216.
51. Curé JK, Key LL, Goltra DD, VanTussel P. Cranial MR imaging of osteopetrosis. AJNR 2000; 21: 1110–1115.
52. Van Hul W, Vanhoenacker F, Balemans W, et al. Molecular and radiological diagnosis of sclerosing bone dysplasias. Eur J Radiol 2001; 40: 198–207.
53. Brockenbrough JM, Petruzzelli GJ, Lamasney L. DentaScan as an accurate method of predicting mandibular invasion in patients with squamous cell carcinoma of the oral cavity. Arch Otolaryngol Head Neck Surg 2003; 129: 113–117.
54. Marchetta FC, Sako K, Badillo J. Periosteal lymphatics of the mandible and intraoral carcinoma. Am J Surg 1964; 108: 505–507.
55. Mukherji SK, Isaac DL, Creager A, et al. CT detection of mandibular invasion by squamous cell carcinoma of the oral cavity. AJR 2001; 177: 237–243.
56. Abrahams JJ. The role of diagnostic imaging in dental implantology. Radiol Clin North Am 1993; 31: 163–180.
57. Westesson PL. Temporomandibular joint and dental imaging. Neuroimaging Clin North Am 1996, 36: 1229–1240.
58. Branemark PI, Breine U, Adell R, et al. Intraosseous anchorage of dental prosthesis. I. Experimental studies. Scand J Plast Reconst Surg 1969; 3: 81–100.

Acknowledgement

We thank Nikhil Balakrishnan M.D. for his technical assistance with DentaScan.

Section V   Suprahyoid Neck

Chapter 7 Nasopharynx

Embryology 553

Anatomy 553

Histology 559

Imaging Techniques 559

Pathology of the Nasopharynx 560

Chapter 8 Parapharyngeal and Masticator Spaces

Anatomy 580

Normal Imaging Anatomy 589

Imaging Rationale and Techniques 592

Pathology 593

Chapter 9 Salivary Glands

Embryology 625

Anatomy 625

Histology 630

Imaging 631

Clinical Applications: Pathological Conditions 638

Chapter 10 Oral Cavity and Oropharynx

Developmental Aspects 682

Normal Anatomy 683

Imaging Techniques 687

Tumors of the Oral Cavity and Oropharynx 688

Inflammatory Lesions of the Oral Cavity and Oropharynx 711

Congenital Lesions 719

Miscellaneous Pathology 723

Chapter 7 Nasopharynx

Mahmood F. Mafee

Embryology

The pharynx is the cranial end of the foregut (the future site of the pharynx), and the branchial apparatus (branchial arches, pharyngeal pouches, branchial clefts or grooves, and branchial membranes) plays an important role in its development. The endodermal aspect of the first or mandibular pair of branchial arches in its dorsal part contributes to the formation of the lateral wall of the nasopharynx.[1] As the head of the embryo enlarges, the dorsal end of the first pharyngeal pouch deepens, and while it remains close to the ectoderm of the dorsal end of the first branchial cleft, the first and second endodermally lined pharyngeal pouches merge and together with the adjoining lateral part of the pharynx constitute the tubotympanic recess, which forms the tympanic cavity and the eustachian tube.

The endoderm of the ventral aspect of the second pharyngeal pouch does not contribute to the formation of the tubotympanic recess, but eventually contributes to the formation of the palatine tonsillar fossa and part of the palatine tonsil.

The lymphatic tissue of the palatine tonsil is derived from the mesenchyme of the second branchial arch. The epithelium and submucosal glands of the pharynx are of endodermal derivation, and the pharyngeal constrictor muscles are derived from the mesenchyme of the fourth and fifth to sixth brachial arches.[2] The mesenchyme of the first branchial arch gives rise to the muscles of mastication (lateral and medial pterygoid muscles, temporalis and masseter muscles), as well as to the tensor veli palatini, tensor tympani, anterior belly of digastric and mylohyoid muscles. All of them are innervated by the mandibular division of the trigeminal nerve (first branchial arch nerve). Those muscles arising from the mesoderm of the second branchial arch (posterior belly of the digastric muscle, stylohyoid muscle, stapedius, platysma, and muscles of facial expression) are innervated by the facial nerve (second branchial arch nerve).

The pharyngeal constrictor muscles are innervated by the pharyngeal nervous plexus (IX, X, and with branches from XI cranial nerves as well as with branches from sympathetic plexus). The levator veli palatini muscle is also a pharyngeal muscle. It is innervated by the pharyngeal nervous plexus as well.

Anatomy

The pharynx is a mucosa-lined musculomembranous tube, from 12 to 14 cm long, and continuous inferiorly with the esophagus, into which the nasal (nasopharynx), oral (oropharynx), and laryngeal (laryngopharynx or hypopharynx) cavities open (Fig. 7.1). The nasopharynx is a cuboidal structure whose anterior limits are the choanae, through which it is continuous with the nasal cavities (Fig. 7.1). Its roof is attached to the base of the skull at the prevertebral muscles and clivus and slopes downward to become the posterior pharyngeal wall, which overlies the atlas and its related ligaments and muscles (Figs. 7.1, 7.2).[1-4] The roof and the posterior wall are the vault of the nasopharynx.[4] The

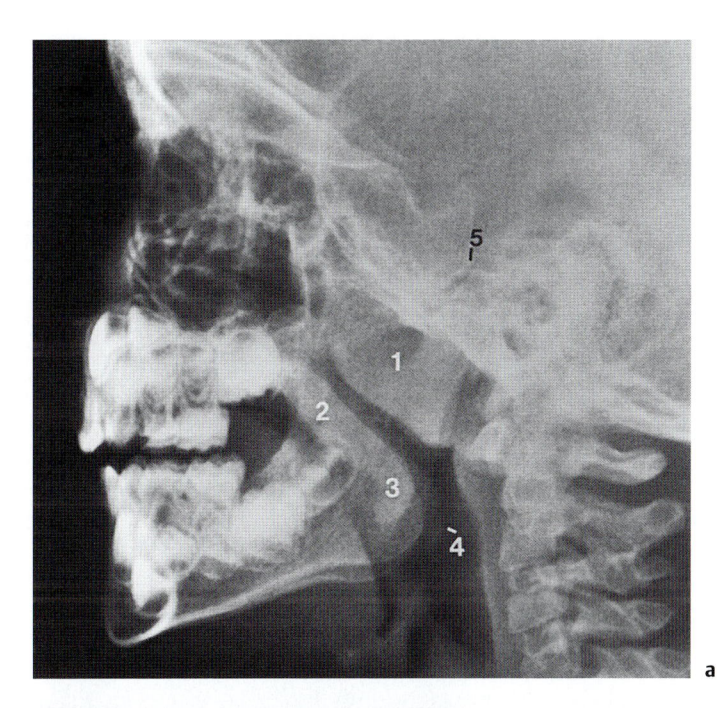

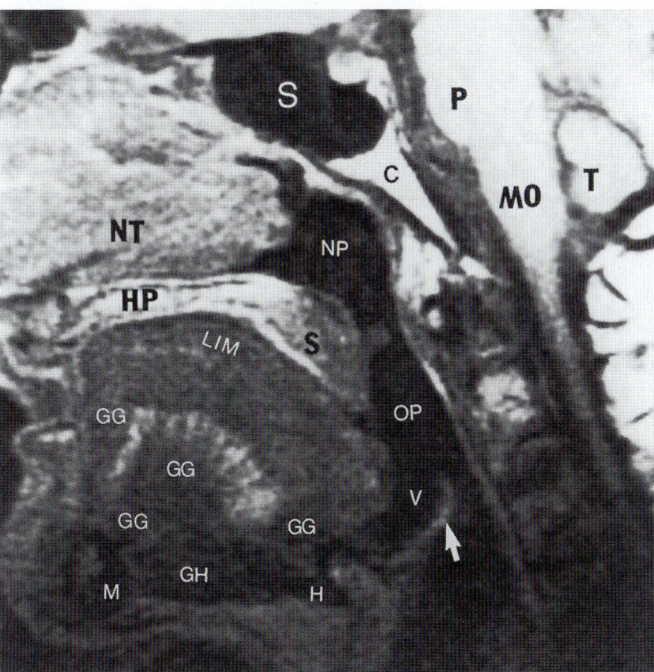

Fig. 7.1 a Normal nasopharynx; lateral film in a child. Prominent adenoid tissue (1) is evident. Also note the soft palate (2), uvula (3), palatine tonsils (4), and spheno-occipital synchondrosis (5). b Normal oral cavity and oropharynx, sagittal paramedian T1W MR section. C = clivus; GG = genioglossus muscle; GH = geniohyoid muscle; H = hyoid bone; HP = hard palate; LIM = lingual intrinsic muscle; M = mandible; MO = medulla oblongata; NP = nasopharynx; NT = nasal turbinate; OP = oropharynx; P = pons; black S = soft palate; white S = sphenoid sinus; T = cerebellar tonsil; V = vallecula; white arrow = epiglottis.

7 Nasopharynx

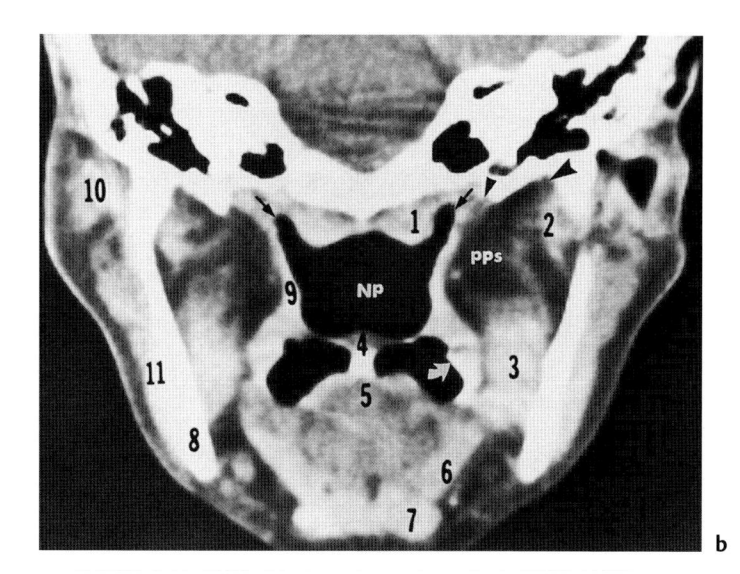

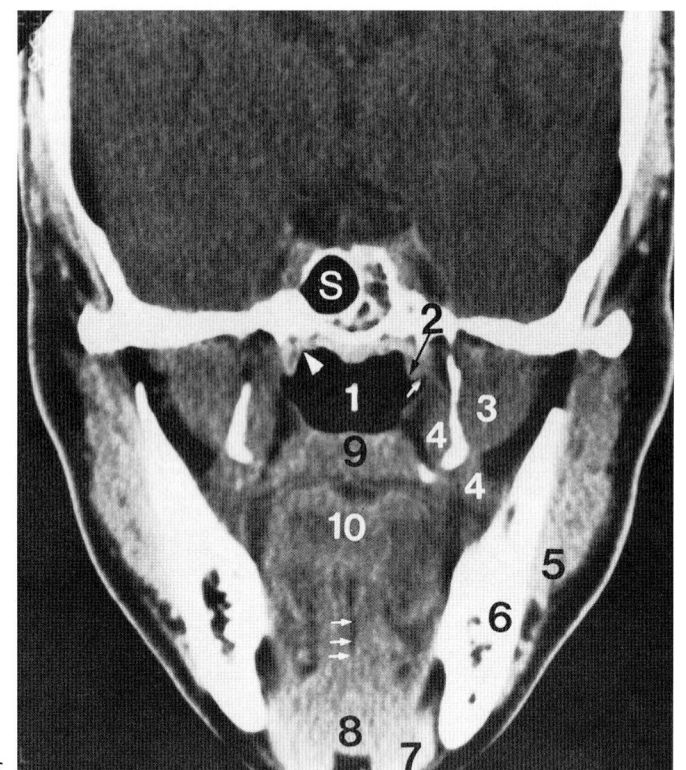

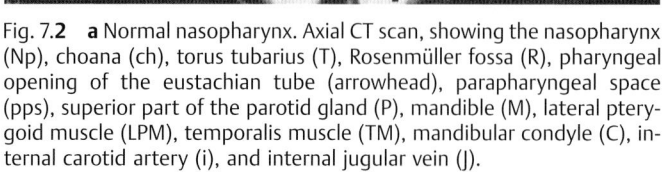

Fig. 7.2 **a** Normal nasopharynx. Axial CT scan, showing the nasopharynx (Np), choana (ch), torus tubarius (T), Rosenmüller fossa (R), pharyngeal opening of the eustachian tube (arrowhead), parapharyngeal space (pps), superior part of the parotid gland (P), mandible (M), lateral pterygoid muscle (LPM), temporalis muscle (TM), mandibular condyle (C), internal carotid artery (i), and internal jugular vein (J).
b Normal nasopharynx and parapharyngeal space. Coronal CT scan showing the nasopharynx (Np), Rosenmüller fossae (arrows), parapharyngeal space (pps), roof of the nasopharynx (longus capitis) (1), lateral pterygoid muscle (2), medial pterygoid muscle (3), soft palate (4), base of tongue (5), mylohyoid muscle (6), anterior belly of digastric (7), mandible (8), constrictor pharyngeal muscle (9), parotid gland (10), masseter muscle (11), palatoglossal arch (curved arrow) and extension of parapharyngeal fatty reticulum to the undersurface of the temporal bone (arrowheads).

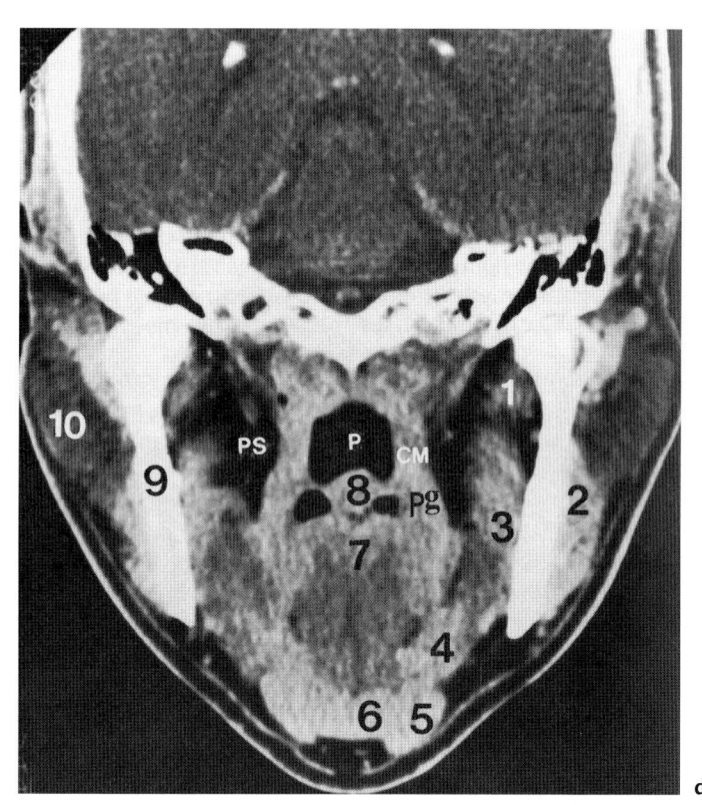

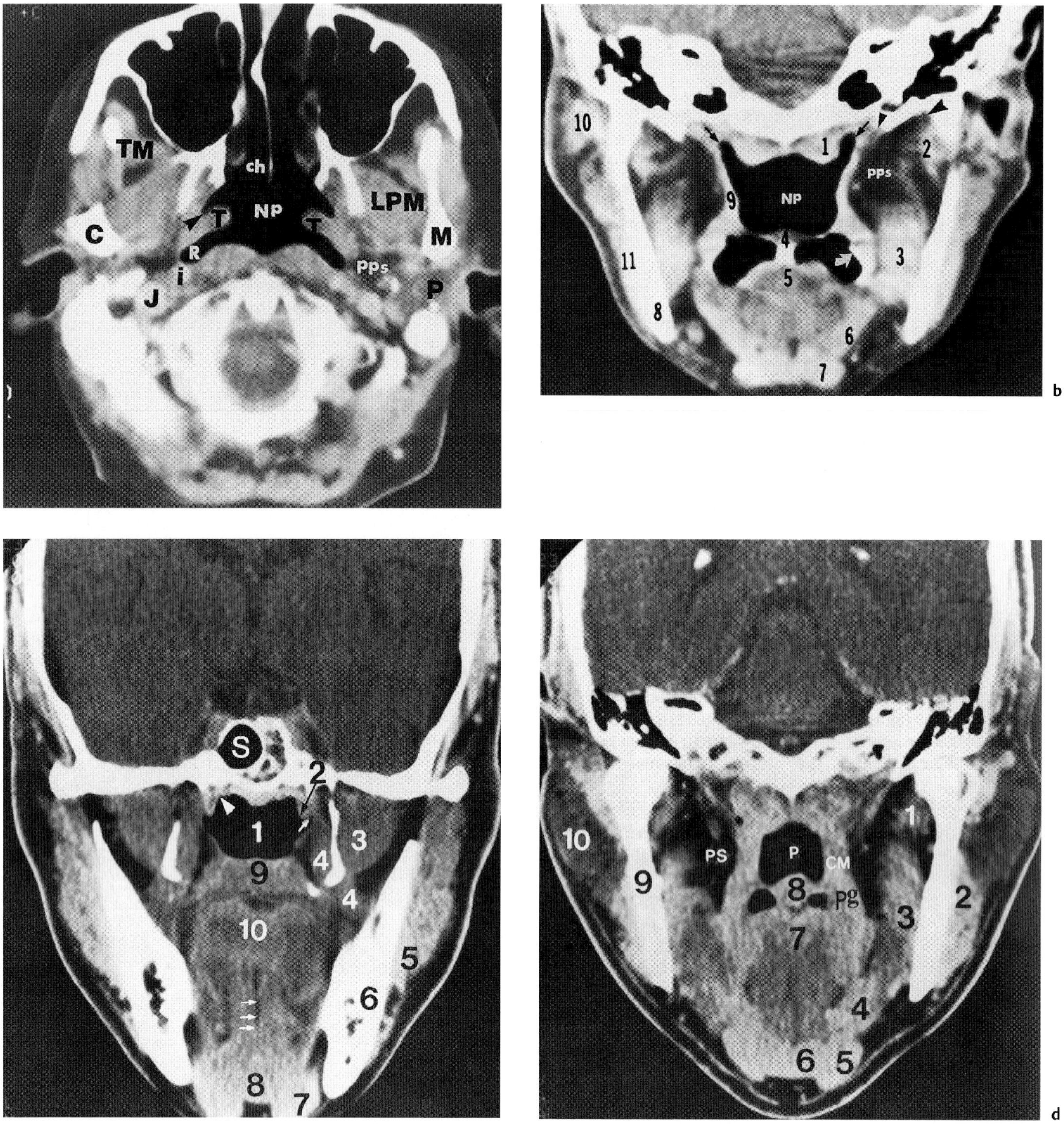

c Normal nasopharynx and parapharyngeal space. This section crosses the sphenoid sinus (S) and soft palate (9). S = sphenoid sinus; single white arrow = eustachian tube orifice; white arrows = lingual septum; white arrowhead = Rosenmüller fossa; 1 = nasopharynx; 2, with black arrow = torus tubarius; 3 = lateral pterygoid muscle; 4 = medial pterygoid muscle; 5 = masseter muscle; 6 = mandible; 7 = anterior belly of digastric muscle; 8 = genioglossus muscle; 9 = soft palate; 10 = lingual intrinsic muscles.
d This section is 6 mm posterior to **c**. CM = pharyngeal constrictor muscle; P = nasopharynx; pg = palatoglossal muscle; PS = parapharyngeal space; 1 = lateral pterygoid muscle; 2 = masseter muscle; 3 = medial pterygoid muscle; 4 = mylohyoid muscle; 5 = anterior belly of digastric muscle; 6 = genioglossus muscle; 7 = lingual intrinsic muscles; 8 = soft palate; 9 = mandible; 10 = parotid gland.

Fig. 7.2 e–i ▷

Anatomy 555

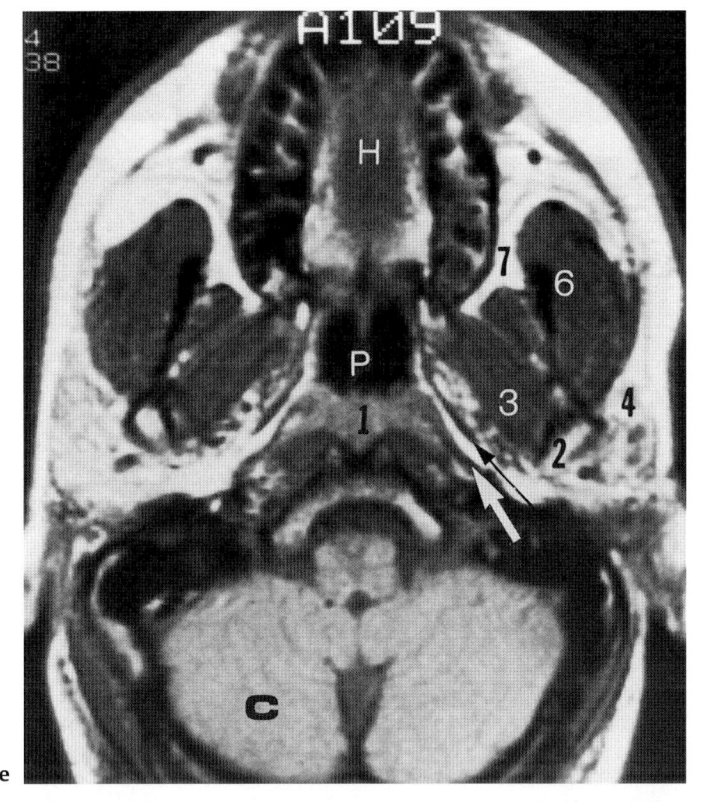

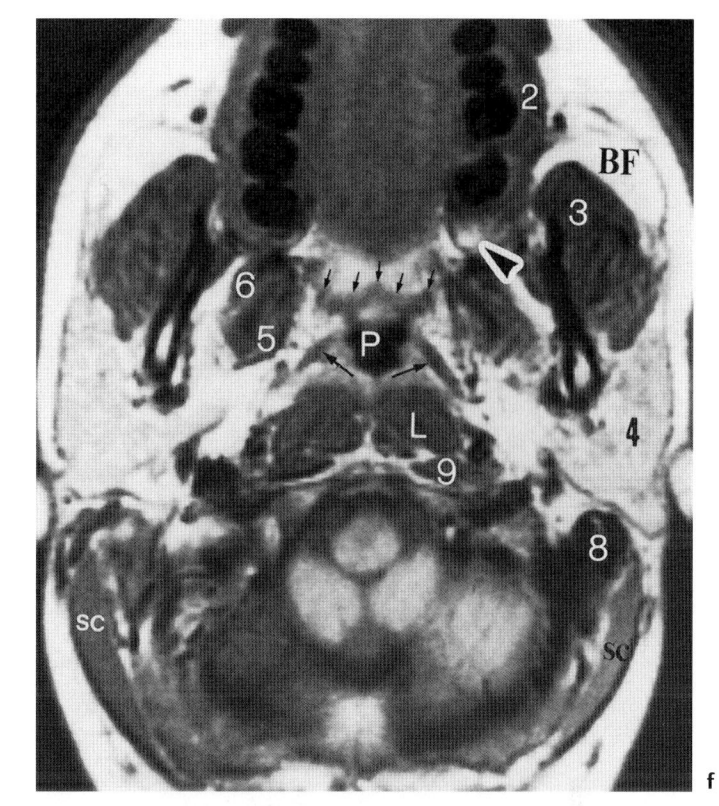

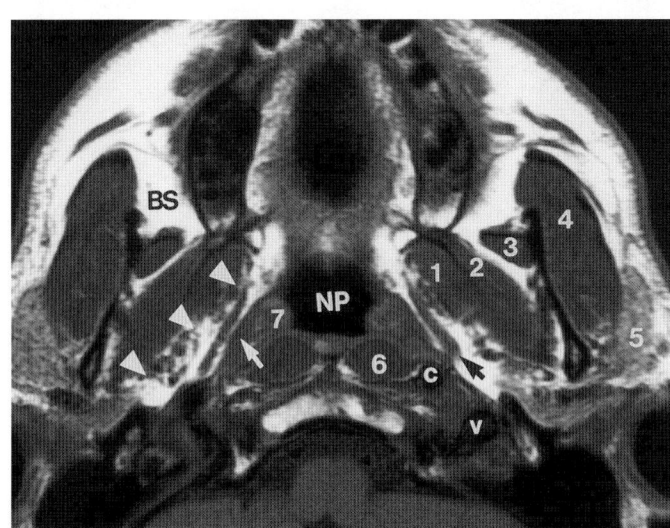

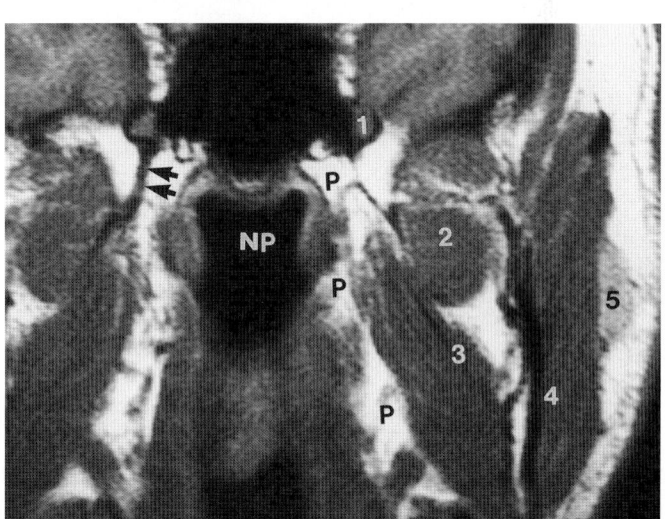

Fig. 7.2 e Normal nasopharynx and upper neck. Axial spin-density-weighted MR section. This section passes through the alveolar process of the maxilla, the nasopharynx, and the cerebellum. C = cerebellum; H = hard palate; P = nasophraynx; white arrow = levator veli palatini muscle; black arrow = tensor veli palatini muscle; 1 = adenoidal pad; 2 = mandible; 3 = lateral pterygoid muscle; 4 = parotid gland; 6 = masseter muscle; 7 = buccal fat. f This section is 6 mm inferior to e and crosses through the upper teeth, coronoid process and mastoid process. BF = buccal fat; L = longus capitis muscle; P = nasopharynx; SC = splenius capitis muscle; short black arrows = pharyngopalatine muscle; long black arrows = levator palatini muscle; black and white arrowhead = buccopharyngeal space; 2 = buccinator muscle; 3 = masseter muscle; 4 = parotid gland; 5 = medial pterygoid muscle; 6 = lateral pterygoid muscle; 8 = mastoid process; 9 = anterior rectus capitis.

g, h, i Normal nasopharynx.
g High-resolution axial T1W MR image at the lower portion of the nasopharynx (NP). 1 = Medial pterygoid muscle; 2 = lateral pterygoid muscle; 3 = temporalis muscle; 4 = masseter muscle; 5 = parotid gland; 6 = longus colli muscle; 7 = eustachian tube (torus tubarius); c = internal carotid artery; v= internal jugular vein; white arrow = levator veli palatini muscle; black arrow = tensor veli palatini muscle; BS = buccal space; arrowheads = neurovascular structures in the parapharyngeal space.
h High-resolution coronal T1W MR image showing maxillary division of trigeminal nerve (1), lateral pterygoid muscle (2), medial pterygoid muscle (3), masseter muscle (4), parotid gland (5), parapharyngeal space (P), nasopharynx (NP), and interpterygoid fascia (arrows).

Fig. 7.2i ▷

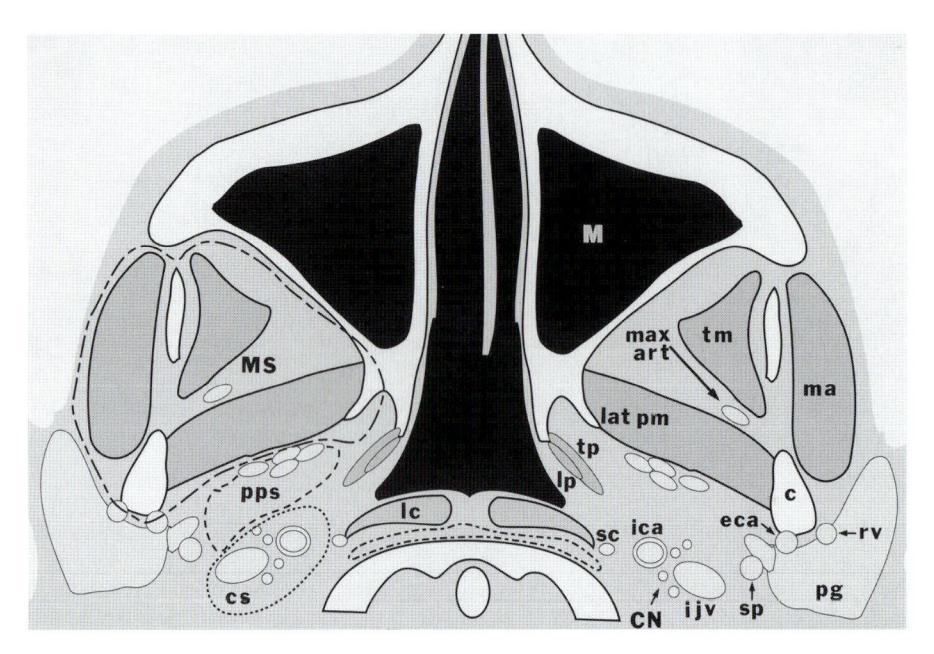

Fig. 7.2 i Schematic diagram of the nasopharynx and related spaces. M = maxillary sinus; tm = temporalis muscle; max art = internal maxillary artery; ma = masseter muscle; lat pm = lateral pterygoid muscle; tp = tensor veli palatini muscle; lp = levator veli palatini muscle; c = mandibular condyle; rv = retromandibular vein; eca = external carotid artery; pg = parotid gland; sp = styloid process; ijv = internal jugular vein; CN = cranial nerves (IX–XII); ica = internal carotid artery; SC = sympathetic chain; Lc = longus colli; cs = carotid space; pps = parapharyngeal space; MS = masticator space. Thin dotted line represents prevertebral space. Diagram by Dale Charletta, MD.

posterior wall is separated from the prevertebral muscles and clivus by the pharyngobasilar fascia, and by loose areolar tissue from the cervical portion of the vertebral column and prevertebral fascia covering the longus colli and longus capitis (Fig. 7.2 f).[1,5] The lateral wall, on each side, presents the pharyngeal opening of the eustachian tube. This opening is bounded above and behind by the tubal elevation (torus tubarius), a firm prominence that is provided by the underlying pharyngeal end of the cartilage of the eustachian tube.[1] The levator veli palatini muscle (Fig. 7.2 e), as it enters the soft palate, produces an elevation of the mucous membrane immediately below the pharyngeal opening of the eustachian tube.[1] Behind the tubal elevation, the mucous membrane lines a recess of variable depth, termed the pharyngeal recess (Rosenmüller fossa) (Fig. 7.2 a, b). The lateral wall of the nasopharynx consists of the torus tubarius, the cartilaginous medial end of the eustachian tube, surrounded by the superior pharyngeal constrictor muscle (Fig. 7.2), and is pierced by the sinus of Morgagni (weak point and the site of tumor spread), through which pass the eustachian tube (torus tubarius) and levator veli palatini muscle (Fig. 7.2).[5] The nasopharynx lies above the soft palate (Figs. 7.1, 7.2 b). During swallowing, the soft palate and uvula provide a functional floor for the nasopharynx. Inferiorly, the nasopharynx is continuous with the oropharynx (Fig. 7.3) at the level of the soft palate.

■ Pharyngobasilar Fascia

The pharynx is usually described as being composed of three tissue laminae from within, outward. These include mucous, fibrous, and muscular layers. The primary pharyngeal musculatures include three overlapping pharyngeal constrictor muscles. All of these muscles insert posteriorly on the median raphe, a thick fibrous layer that is attached to the skull base at the pharyngeal tubercle. External to the muscular layer is the thin buccopharyngeal fascia (external layer of the epimysium), which covers the external surface of the pharyngeal constrictor muscles and extends forward over the pterygomandibular raphe onto the buccinator. The fibrous intermediate layer (internal layer of the epimysium) lies between the mucous and muscular layers.[1] It is thick above (pharyngobasilar fascia) where the muscular fibers are absent. The inner surface of the pharyngeal musculature (pharyngeal constrictor muscles) is lined by the pharyngobasilar fascia (internal layer of the epimysium) (Fig. 7.3). The pharyngobasilar fascia, or pharyngeal aponeurosis (aponeurosis of superior pharyngeal constrictor muscle), superiorly, encircles the space between the upper border of the superior pharyngeal constrictor muscle and the skull base. The longus capitis and rectus capitis muscles lie between the superior pharyngeal constrictor muscle and the skull base and upper cervical vertebra (Figs. 7.2, 7.3). The pharyngobasilar fascia is firmly connected to the clivus and to the petrous part of the temporal bone medial to the carotid canal, bridging under the eustachian tube and extending forward to be attached to the posterior border of the medial pterygoid plate and to the pterygomandibular raphe.[1] As it descends, it diminishes in thickness. It is thickened posteriorly in the midline (pharyngeal raphe), which gives attachment to the constrictors. The pharyngeal muscles are described as lying external to the fibrous layer. However, the latter is in reality the thickened, deep internal epimysial layer, covering the muscles (pharyngobasilar fascia), while the thinner external layer of the epimysium constitutes the buccopharyngeal fascia.[1] On CT and MRI scans, superiorly these two fasciae are seen close together in normal subjects. The pharyngobasilar fascia demonstrates more contrast enhancement than the normal mucosa on both enhanced CT and MRI scans (Fig. 7.4). (See also Chapter 8).

The eustachian tube opens into the nasopharynx by piercing the pharyngobasilar fascia (sinus of Morgagni). Muscles affecting eustachian (pharyngotympanic) tube function are the tensor and levator veli palatini and the stylopharyngeus (Fig. 7.2 e,f). The tensor and levator palatini muscles (Fig. 7.2 e–g) originate from the inferolateral and inferomedial wall of the cartilaginous portion of the eustachian tube, respectively, and from the scaphoid fossa of the pterygoid plates. They descend vertically, medial to the pterygoid muscle, to insert on the palatine aponeurosis and palatine velum (Fig. 7.2 e, f). Elevation of the soft palate and contraction of the fibers of the superior pharyngeal constrictor muscle, the palatopharyngeal sphincter (Passavant's sphincter), close off the nasopharynx during deglutition.[1] The Passavant's muscle fibers arise from the palatopharyngeus muscle and posterolateral margin of the hard palate. The muscle fibers encircle the pharynx inside the superior pharyngeal constrictor muscle. The most prominent anatomical landmark on the lateral wall of the nasopharynx on each side is the cartilaginous medial end of

Anatomy 557

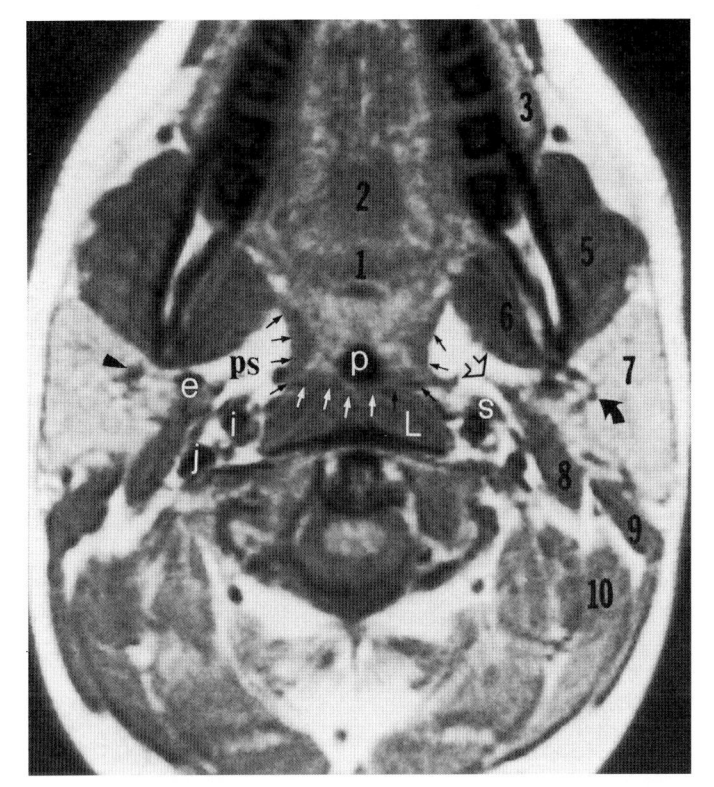

Fig. 7.3 Normal orophraynx and palatine tonsils. **a** This section is 9 mm inferior to Fig. 7.2f and crosses the lower alveolar ridge. e = external carotid artery; i = internal carotid artery; j = internal jugular vein; L = longus capitis muscle; p = oropharynx; ps = parapharyngeal space; s = stylopharyngeus muscle; small white and black arrows = superior pharyngeal constrictor muscle; hollow arrow = stylohyoid muscle; black curved arrow = facial nerve; black arrowhead = retromandibular vein; 1 = longitudinal intrinsic tongue muscles; 2 = transverse intrinsic tongue muscles; 3 = buccinator muscle; 5 = masseter muscle; 6 = internal (medial) pterygoid muscle; 7 = parotid gland; 8 = posterior belly of digastric muscle; 9 = sternocleidomastoid muscle; 10 = splenius capitis muscle.

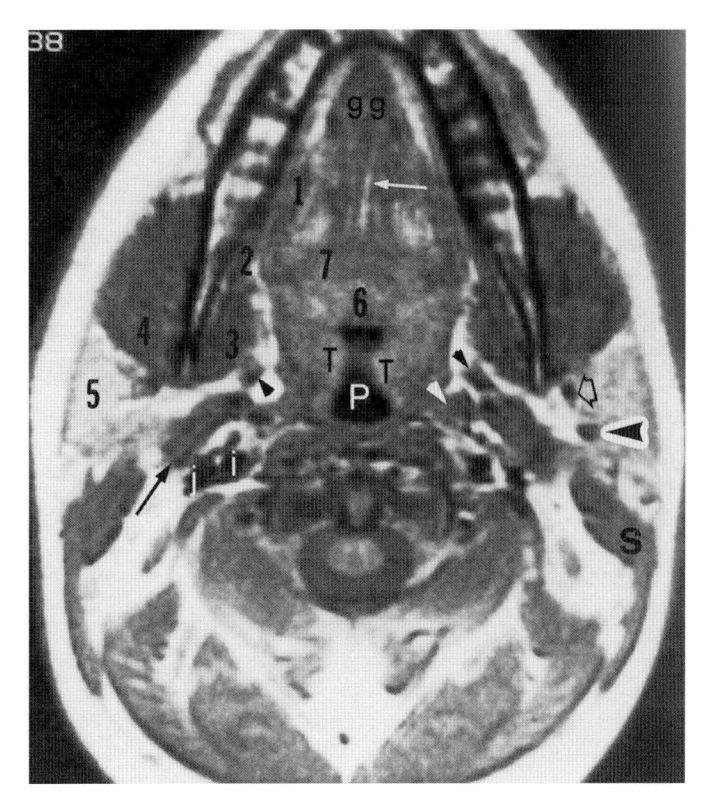

b This section is 6 mm inferior to **a**. gg = genioglossus muscle; i = internal carotid artery; j = internal jugular vein; P = oropharynx; S = sternocleidomastoic muscle; T = palatine tonsils; white arrow = lingual septum; white arrowhead = stylopharyngeus muscle; black and white arrowhead = external jugular vein; hollow arrow = retromandibular vein; black arrow = posterior belly of digastric muscle; black arrowhead = stylohyoid muscle; 1 = hyoglossus muscle; 2 = mylohyoid muscle; 3 = internal (medial) pterygoid muscle; 4 = masseter muscle; 5 = parotid gland; 6 = longitudinal intrinsic tongue muscles; 7 = transverse intrinsic tongue muscles.

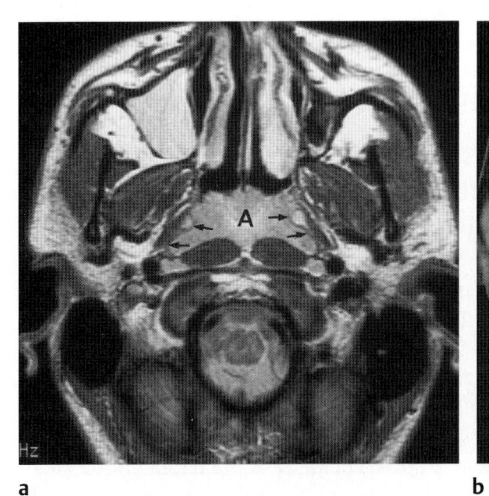

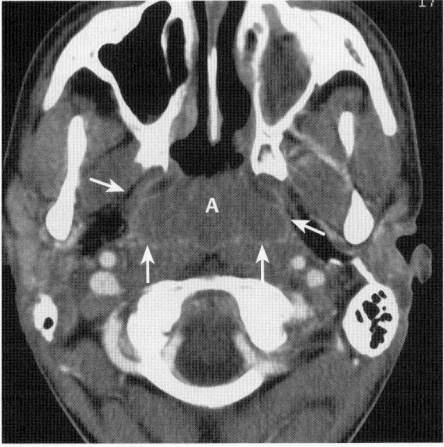

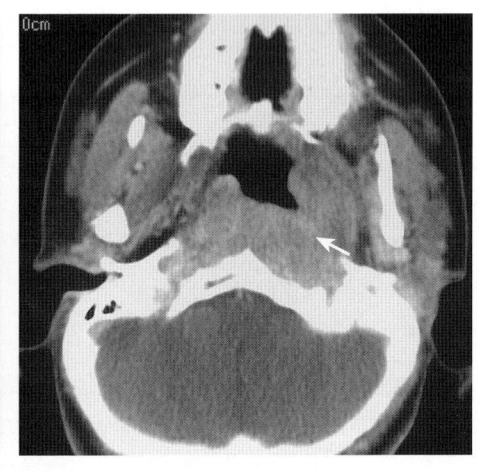

a b c

Fig. 7.4 **a** Pharyngeal tonsil (adenoid). PW axial MR scan in a 23-year-old male showing the enlarged adenoid (A). Note that the adenoidal tissue does not extend beyond the pharyngobasilar fascia (arrows). **b** Enhanced CT in a 17-year-old male patient showing hypertrophy of the adenoid (A). Note enhancement of the pharyngobasilar fascia (arrows). **c** CT scan in a 13-year-old boy showing asymmetry of the nasopharyngeal tissue due to lymphoepithelial carcinoma (arrow). Note poor delineation of the pharyngobasilar fascia on the left side.

the eustachian tube (torus tubarius) (Fig. 7.2). The pharyngeal orifice of the eustachian tube is seen just anterior to its submucosal cartilaginous elevation, the torus (Fig. 7.2a). Between the torus and the posterior wall is the fossa of Rosenmüller, a cleft-like space (Figs. 7.2a, b) whose apex reaches the anterior margin of the carotid canal (Fig. 7.2b). Nasopharyngeal carcinoma is notorious for submucosal extension. It commonly resides in the Rosenmüller fossa and may extend laterally through the sinus of Morgagni to invade the parapharyngeal space.[5] The anatomical landmarks of the nasopharynx are usually depicted better on MR images; however, at times these landmarks (torus tubarius and the Rosenmüller fossa) may not be conspicuous on CT or MR scans owing to anatomical variation (Fig. 7.2c). It is therefore important to look for the symmetry of the superficial and deep nasopharyngeal, as well as parapharyngeal, structures.

The Rosenmüller fossa remains virtually obscure to clinical examination. Its proximity to the skull base allows cancer in this region to spread into the adjacent skull base. An incomplete ring of lymphoid tissue lies in the wall of the pharynx between the mucosa and the muscles. The adenoid, or nasopharyngeal tonsil, is situated near the roof of the nasopharynx, close to the eustachian tube (Figs. 7.1, 7.4). The nasopharynx epithelium varies from stratified squamous to ciliated pseudostratified (respiratory) to transitional.[2]

The Pharyngeal Tonsil and Pharyngeal Bursa

The pharyngeal tonsil (adenoid) is small at birth and usually increases in size up to the age of 6 or 7 years, after which it, not infrequently, begins to atrophy.[1] The adenoidal tissue may remain enlarged (hypertrophic) (Fig. 7.4a) and at times be associated with serous otitis media. The adenoidal tissue appears hyperintense to muscle on proton-weighted (PW) and T2-weighted (T2W) MR scans and demonstrates moderate enhancement on enhanced CT and MRI scans (Fig. 7.4b). The hypertrophic adenoidal tissue should appear symmetric. Asymmetric appearance of nasopharyngeal adenoidal/soft tissue should be carefully investigated for more serious pathology such as cancer (Fig. 7.4c). Adenoidal tissue may be prominent in patients with AIDS. The pharyngeal tonsil/adenoidal tissue consists of a number of folds. The folds consist mainly of diffuse lymphoid tissue, but there may be some deeply placed mucous glands present. The pharyngeal bursa is an inconstant blind sac located above the nasopharyngeal tonsil in the midline of the posterior wall of the nasopharynx and cannot be delineated on CT and MRI scans. At times a small central calcification may be present at the base of the adenoid, representing the attachment of the notochord to the site of pharyngeal bursa. In the embryo, the notochord lies inferior to the base of the skull, in the region of the developing basiocciput; here it is attached to the endoderm forming the roof of the primitive pharynx, and with subsequent growth of this region the notochordal attachment draws out an angled recess of the endoderm (the pouch of Luschka), which forms the pharyngeal bursa.[1] The lateral prolongation of the nasopharyngeal tonsil behind the pharyngeal opening of the eustachian tube is known as the tubal tonsil.

Pharyngeal Isthmus, Oropharyngeal Isthmus, and Waldeyer's Ring

Between the free edge of the soft palate and the posterior wall of the pharynx, the nasal and oral parts of the pharynx communicate through an opening termed the pharyngeal isthmus. The aperture by which the mouth communicates with the pharynx is called the oropharyngeal isthmus. The palatine tonsils are two masses of lymphoid tissue situated in the lateral walls of the oropharynx. The tonsils form part of a circular band of lymphoid tissue surrounding the opening into the digestive and respiratory tubes, the so-called Waldeyer's ring. The superior part of the ring is formed by nasopharyngeal (adenoid) tonsil; the lateral portions consist of the palatine or oropharyngeal tonsils and lymphoid collections in the vicinity of eustachian tubes, and the anterior and lower part of the ring is formed by the lingual tonsil.[1] Smaller collections of lymphoid tissue are found in the intervals between these main masses (Figs. 7.1, 7.2e). The palatine tonsil (Fig. 7.3) consists of lymphoid tissue arranged in nodules or follicles. Multiplication of the lymphocytes takes place in the center (germinal layer) of the follicles.

Innervation

Motor supply and most of the sensory supply to the pharynx is via the pharyngeal plexus formed by the the pharyngeal branches of cranial nerves IX (glossopharyngeal) and X (vagus),[2,3] with branches from XI (spinal accessory) cranial nerve as well as branches from the sympathetic plexus.

Vascular Supply

Aterial supply of the pharynx is provided from various branches of the external carotid artery, including the ascending pharyngeal, facial, lingual, maxillary, and superior thyroid arteries. The pharyngeal veins form a plexus that drains into the internal jugular and facial veins directly or via a communication with the pterygoid venous plexus.[2]

Lymphatics

A rich capillary lymphatic plexus drains the nasopharynx into ipsilateral and contralateral upper deep cervical lymph nodes.[1,2,4] The lateral retropharyngeal nodes are the first echelon involved in nasopharyngeal cancer. These are deep in the neck and cannot usually be palpated.[4] Jugulodigastric (level II) and upper as well as lower accessory chain nodes (level V) are often involved by tumor spread through efferent lymphatic channels from retropharyngeal nodes or directly from the nasopharynx.[4] The lymphatics of the oropharynx, including the tonsil and base of the tongue, are drained to the upper deep cervical nodes, particularly to the jugulodigastric (level II) and jugulo-omohyoid (level III) group of lymph nodes.[2]

Regional Anatomy (Parapharyngeal Space)

The regional anatomical relationship of the nasopharynx is important for understanding of the pattern of local spread of nasopharyngeal cancer. The parapharyngeal space, masticatory space, infratemporal space, nasal cavity, orbit, as well as sphenoid sinus and the base of the skull are in close relationship with the nasopharynx. Nasopharyngeal cancer may extend to involve these structures. The parapharyngeal space (PPS) is an irregular, predominantly fat-filled space within the suprahyoid neck. Various synonyms for the PPS have been used, including lateral parapharyngeal space, pharyngomasticatory space, pterygopharyngeal space, and pharyngomaxillary space. The PPS roughly resembles an inverted pyramid, extending from the base of the skull to the level of the greater cornu of the hyoid bone (Figs. 7.2, 7.3).[6–7] The inferior boundary of the PPS ends at the junction of the posterior belly of the digastric muscle and the greater cornu of the hyoid bone.[6] The firm fascial attachments in this area limit PPS extension inferior to the hyoid bone. This fascia, however, can be weak and may be an ineffective barrier against the spread of infections.[6] Superiorly, the PPS attaches to the base of the skull at the sphenoid bone, medial to the foramen ovale, and around the foramen lacerum, as well as to the undersurface of the petrous bone in the vicinity of the carotid canal and jugular fossa (Figs. 7.2, 7.3). The PPS is further compartmentalized by thick fascial layers that direct tumor growth and the spread of inflammation. Descriptions of these fascial layers vary in anatomical, clinical, and radiological literature. The medial wall of the PPS is formed superiorly by the tensor veli palatini muscle and its fascia, the pharyngobasilar fascia, the levator veli palatini muscle, the superior pharyngeal constrictor muscle, and farther down by the tonsillar fossa (Figs. 7.2, 7.3). Its lateral wall is formed anteriorly by the medial wall of the masticator space (Fig. 7.3). The medial pterygoid muscle, along with a fascial layer extending from this muscle called the interpterygoid fascia or aponeurosis (also called the combined fascia or medial pterygoid fascia), forms the medial boundary of the masticator space and separates the masticator space from the PPS (Fig. 7.2h).[7] The PPS has been further subdivided into a prestyloid and a retrostyloid compartment. A fascia that extends from the styloid process to the tensor veli palatini muscle crosses posteriorly in the PPS fat and separates the PPS into these two areas.[6] The carotid sheath is considered anatomically to be the posterior compartment of the retrostyloid PPS (Figs. 7.2a, 7.3a). See Chapter 8 for detailed anatomy of PPS.

■ The Masticator Space

The masticator space is a separate fascial compartment, bounded by the superficial layer of deep cervical fascia, containing the pterygoid muscles, masseter muscle, inferior temporalis muscle, and posterior body and ramus of the mandible (Figs. 7.2, 7.3). The TMJ is in the upper masticator space. See Chapter 8 for further details.

■ Infratemporal Fossa

The infratemporal fossa is an irregular space behind the maxilla and lateral to the nasopharynx and pterygopalatine fossa (Fig. 7.2a). The superior extent of this fossa is the zygomatic arch. It extends inferiorly to the alveolar border of the maxilla. Its medial extent is the infratemporal surface of the greater wing of the sphenoid and lateral pterygoid plate. Medially, the fossa communicates with the pterygomaxillary fissure and pterygopalatine (sphenopalatine) fossa. The infratemporal fossa contains the masticatory muscles, the internal maxillary vessels, and the mandibular and auriculotemporal nerves. The foramen ovale (V3) and foramen spinosum (middle meningeal artery) open to its roof. See Chapter 8 for further details.

■ Applied Anatomy

Although most of the fascial layers cannot be seen as discrete layers on CT and MRI scans, the usually symmetric fat- and muscle-filled spaces define the boundaries of the PPS (Figs. 7.2, 7.3). The masticator space is readily identified by muscle-filled spaces. Nasopharyngeal carcinoma commonly extends laterally through the sinus of Morgagni to invade the PPS. Likewise, nasopharyngeal tumor can extend into the infratemporal fossa, pterygomaxillary fissure, and pterygopalatine fossa, and therefore through the inferior orbital fissure into the orbital apex. Involvement of retrostyloid PPS by carcinoma of the nasopharynx results in extension of tumor into the carotid space. Submucosal extension of tumor into the base of skull in the region of the foramen lacerum results in tumor extension into the cavernous sinus.

Histology

The superior portion of the nasopharynx is concerned with respiration and is lined by pseudostratified ciliated columnar epithelium (respiratory). Inferiorly, the pharynx is more involved with eating and the epithelium changes to a stratified squamous type. The submucosa contains mucous and minor salivary glands, as well as a prominent lymphoid component; the basement membrane of the epithelium is inconspicuous, and the lymphoid component may normally be present in the epithelium (lymphoepithelium). Adenoids are lymphoid tissue that contain germinal centers but do not have a capsule or sinusoids; nor are there epithelial crypts.[2,3]

Imaging Techniques

Superficial lesions of the nasopharynx and other parts of the aerodigestive tracts are most accurately detected by endoscopy. Deep extension of tumors or inflammatory conditions may be missed or difficult to recognize by physical examination and endoscopy. Imaging is needed to better delineate these lesions and for accurate clinical staging of cancers. CT and MRI of the nasopharynx and regional anatomy (parapharyngeal space and infratemporal fossa) provide images with significant information and exquisite anatomical detail. Axial and direct coronal plane CT scans (4–5 mm thick) are used to evaluate the nasopharynx and regional anatomy. Thinner sections (2.5–3 mm) should be obtained for smaller lesions, and for the evaluation of subtle bone invasion by nasopharyngeal carcinoma. Examination should be done with and without iodinated contrast material. Contrast is important for the evaluation of metastatic nodal disease, the base of the skull, as well as intracranial involvement. The postcontrast study should include the entire neck, the base of the skull, and part of the intracranial structures, including the cavernous sinuses and petrous apices. CT is preferred to MRI for the detection of bone invasion. MRI is the preferred modality for mapping of nasopharyngeal tumors. On CT, nasopharyngeal carcinomas often are isodense to muscle, while superior soft-tissue contrast discrimination allowed by MRI better delineates tumor boundaries and the true extent of tumor. Most magnetic resonance images in this chapter were obtained with a General Electric Horizon Echospeed 1.5 T Superconductive System Scanner (General Electric, Milwaukee, WI, USA). We use a head coil for the evaluation of the nasopharynx and infratemporal fossa, and a neck coil to evaluate the rest of the neck. The entire neck should be examined to evaluate for nodal diseases. Technical factors are as follows: sagittal, axial, and coronal planes; 4–5 mm section thickness, 256×128 or 256×192, or 256×256 matrix; a short TR of 400–800 ms, TE of 25 ms; a long TR of 2000–2500 ms, TE of 20, 25, 80, 100 ms; two excitations; 16–24 cm field of view; and a multisection acquisition technique. The standard spin-echo (SE) with long TR and short TE (TR/TE = 2000/25 ms) and long TE (TE = 80/60 ms) may be replaced by fast SE T2-weighted single echo (TE = 80 ms) pulse sequence. MRI evaluation of nasopharyngeal masses should include a combination of pre and post (Gd-DTPA) T1-weighted MR sequences. Postgadolinium axial and coronal T1-weighted images are performed with and without fat suppression. Fat-suppression pulse sequences are more prone to artifacts at air–bone interfaces (magnetic susceptibility artifact) or related to dental fillings and braces. It is our policy to obtain axial sections with and without fat suppression and coronal sections with or without fat suppression.

Pathology of the Nasopharynx

■ Congenital Anomalies

Congenital anomalies are infrequent and are associated with defects in the development of the skull base. Failure of fusion of neural elements and of bone may result in the development of an encephalocele or meningocele through the sphenoid bone into the nasopharynx or the nasal cavity. Notochord remnants, ending just caudad to the dorsal attachment of the buccopharyngeal membrane, may remain as a solid mass or as a cyst, known as Tornwaldt's (Thornwaldt's) cyst or pharyngeal bursa cyst (Fig. 7.5).[8–10] The Tornwaldt's cyst is derived from a persisting remnant of the cranial end of the embryonic notochord (pharyngeal bursa), and is present in the second or third decade of life as persistent postnasal discharge of mucous or purulent material.[10] Tornwaldt's cysts are seen as a midline nasopharyngeal cystic mass, about 1–1.5 cm in size, and usually hyperintense on both T1- and T2-weighted MR images (Fig. 7.5). On CT scans, the cyst, unless it is infected, does not show contrast enhancement. It is unusual to see a Tornwaldt's cyst larger than 2 cm in diameter. Tornwaldt's cyst is dorsal and caudad to a Rathke's pouch, which is the primordium of the anterior pituitary and lies anterior to the buccopharyngeal membrane.[3] Although usually obliterated, remnants of Rathke's pouch may persist as small epithelial cysts in the body of the sphenoid bone or in the nasopharynx. Rathke's pouch cyst is formed from residual epithelial elements of the pouch, which is an evagination of the stomodeal roof that contributes to the formation of the anterior lobe of the pituitary gland during embryogenesis. Epithelial rests from the epithelium of Rathke's pouch can be entrapped within the sphenoid bone. This occurs because the course of Rathke's pouch is through the mesenchymal anlage of the sphenoid bone before it is ossified. The epithelial rests may give rise to intrasphenoid or nasopharyngeal "extracranial craniopharyngioma" (Fig. 7.6). Epidermoid, dermoid, choristoma, teratoma, hamartoma (respiratory epithelial adenomatoid hamartoma), and neurenteric cysts are infrequently seen in the nasopharynx (Fig. 7.7a).[11, 12] Neurenteric cysts usually present in the second or third decade of life. They may be behind or within the clivus, growing out into the nasopharynx and sphenoid bone. Similarly to other neurenteric cysts in other locations (craniopharyngioma, Rathke's cyst, colloid cyst, cervical and dorsal spine neurenteric cysts), they are frequently hyperintense on T1-weighted and T2-weighted MR images (see Chapter 3). Mucous retention cysts (Fig. 7.7b) are occasionally found in the nasopharynx. A branchial cleft cyst derived from the second branchial arch,[9] thymic cyst, as well as plunging ranula (acquired cyst) may extend deep to the lateral pharyngeal wall as high as C1 (Fig. 7.8). Tornwaldt's cyst and neurenteric cyst should be differentiated from pseudocysts. Nasopharyngeal pseudocysts have been postulated to be the result of longus capitis perimyositis. Any of these cysts may become secondarily infected. Calcification is occasionally seen anterior to C1, secondary to peritendinitis of the longus colli tendon.[13] Table 7.1 outlines congenital and acquired nasopharyngeal cystic lesions.

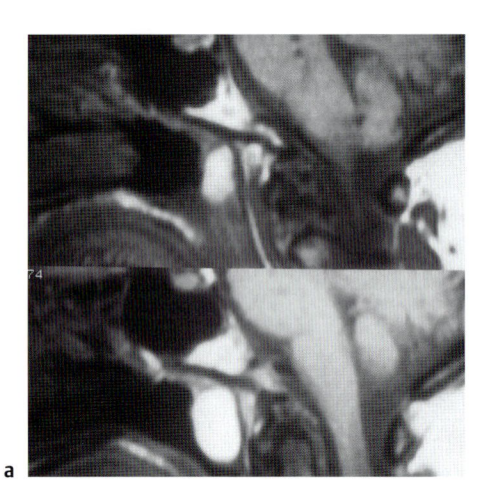

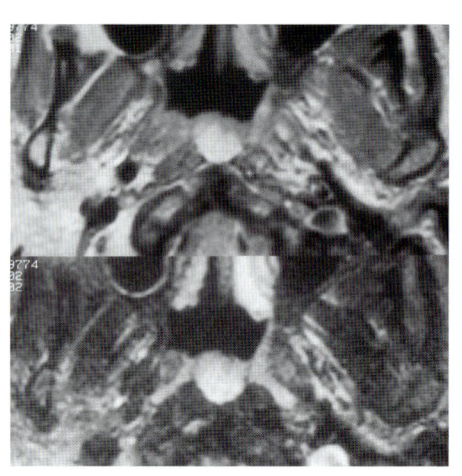

Fig. 7.5 Tornwaldt's cyst. **a** Sagittal T1W and **b** axial PW (top) and T2W (bottom) MR images showing a Tornwaldt's cyst. The lesion appears hyperintense in all pulse sequences.

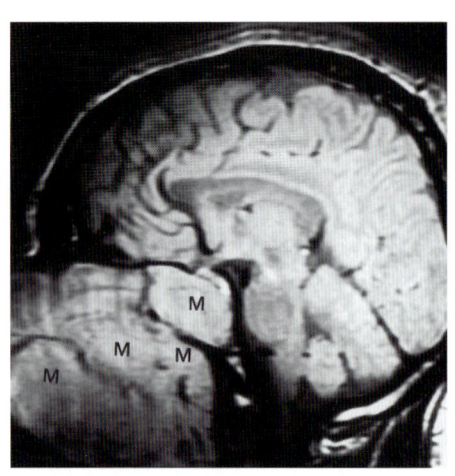

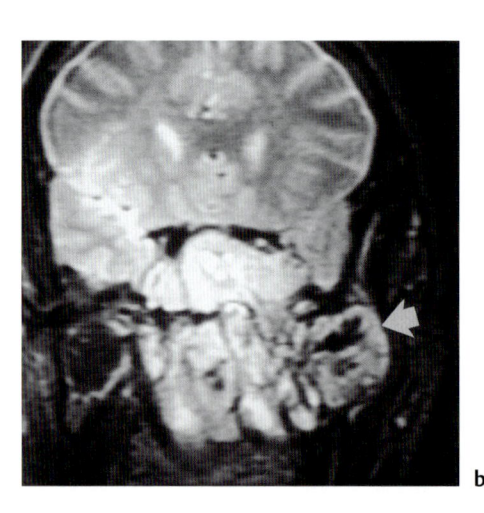

Fig. 7.6 Extracranial craniopharyngioma. **a** Sagittal T1W MR scan, showing a large mass (M), involving sphenoid sinus, nasopharynx, and palato-oral cavity. **b** T2W MR scan. The mass (M) appears hyperintense. Note extension into the infratemporal fossa (arrow). The pituitary gland and suprasellar region were normal in all MR pulse sequences.

Pathology of the Nasopharynx   561

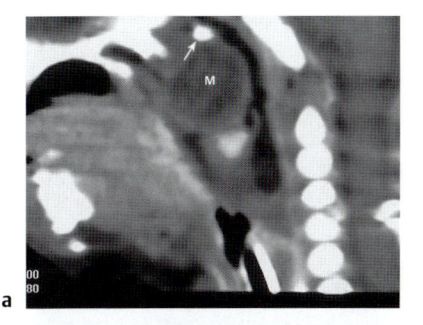

Fig. 7.7 a Nasopharyngeal teratoma. Sagittal reformatted CT image shows a large mass (M) in the nasopharynx with small calcification (arrow) compatible with teratoma. Case courtesy of Mujtaba Khan, M.D., Armed Forces Hospital Riyadh, Saudi Arabia.
b Mucous retention cyst.
1 Enhanced CT scan shows a presumed retention cyst in the central portion of the nasopharynx (arrow).
2 Axial T2W MR scan in another patient shows a hyperintense mass (arrow) in the nasopharynx.
3 Enhanced T1W MR scan shows no enhancement of this retention cyst. Enhancement of normal mucosa is present.

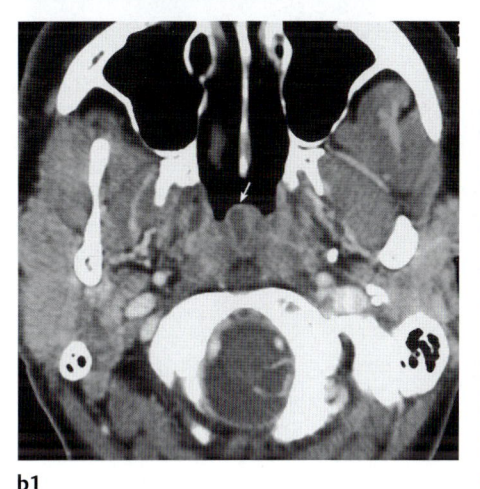

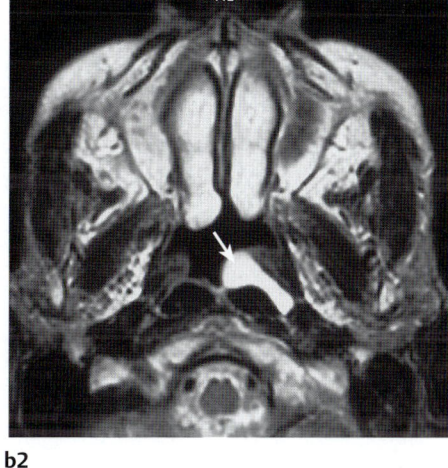

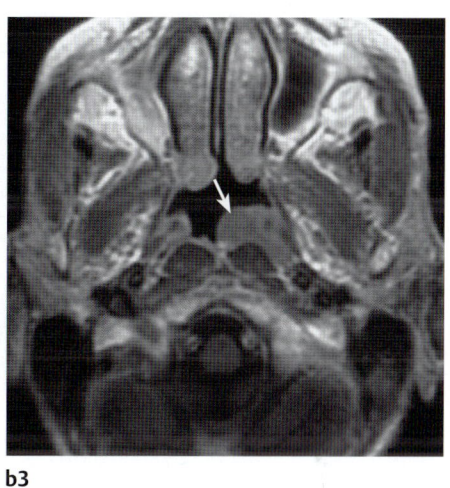

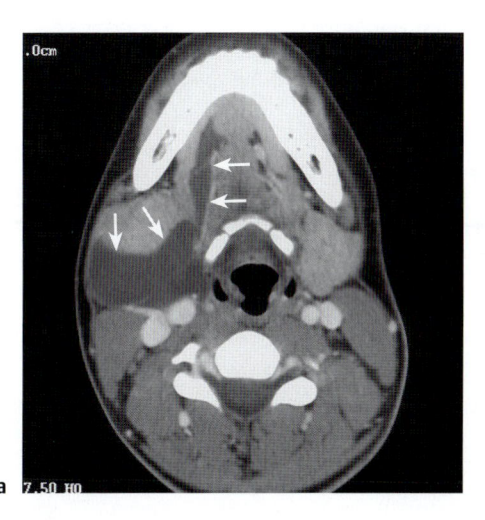

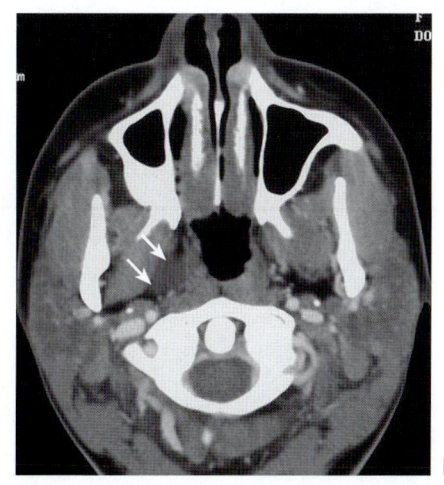

Fig. 7.8 Plunging ranula. a CT scan shows a large cystic mass (arrows) compatible with a plunging ranula. b CT scan, taken at the level of nasopharynx, showing extension of ranula to the high parapharyngeal level (arrows).

■ Inflammations

Diffuse inflammatory changes of the nasopharynx or inflammatory masses may occur with infections of the adenoid tissue and the pharyngeal and parapharyngeal spaces (Figs. 7.9–7.11), with osteomyelitis of the clivus or sphenoid bone, or with infection of the petrous apex of the temporal bone (Figs. 7.9, 7.10). The last may be secondary to chronic infection of the ear, malignant external otitis secondary to a *Pseudomonas* infection occurring in patients with poorly controlled diabetes mellitus,[14] or granulomatous disease affecting the temporal bone, such as tuberculosis. Aggressive fungal infections (mucormycosis or aspergillosis) of sinonasal cavities may rapidly spread to involve the base of the skull, nasopharynx, and adjacent structures. These changes may be identified with contrast-enhanced CT scan or with MRI. The latter has the advantage of revealing marrow changes earlier than the later bone destruction seen with CT. A case of na-

Table 7.1 Congenital and acquired cysts of the nasopharynx

A. Congenital
- Basal meningocele/meningoencephalocele
- Tornwaldt's cysts (notochord remnant)
- Neurenteric cysts (Rathke's cyst, extracranial craniopharyngioma)
- Dermoid cyst
- Epidermoid cyst
- Cystic hamartoma (choristoma)
- Cystic teratoma
- Extension of second branchial cleft cyst to the lateral pharyngeal wall
- Extension of thymic cyst to the lateral pharyngeal wall

B. Acquired
- Mucous retention cyst
- Extension of plunging ranula to the lateral pharyngeal wall
- Pseudocyst (longus capitis perimyositis), postinflammatory cyst
- Extension of C1–C2 synovial cyst (rheumatoid arthritis)
- Metastatic cystic squamous cell carcinoma of the Waldeyer's pharyngeal tissue

562   7 Nasopharynx

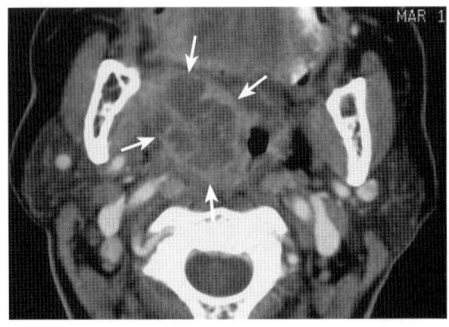

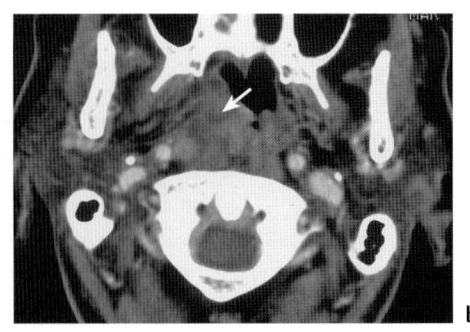

Fig. 7.9   Nasopharyngeal and oropharyngeal infection. **a** CT scan shows a paratonsillar abscess (arrows). **b** CT scan shows extension of paratonsillar infection into the nasopharynx (arrow).

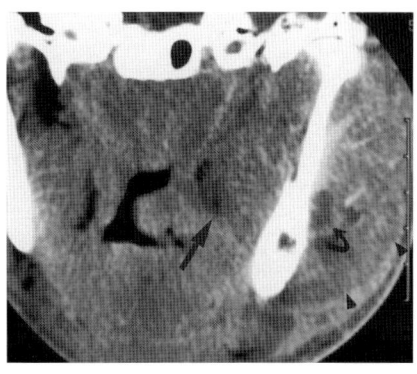

Fig. 7.10   Naso-oropharyngeal and masticator space infection. Enhanced coronal CT scan showing enlarged left palatine tonsil, paratonsillar abscess (straight arrow), parapharyngeal and nasopharyngeal inflammatory changes, and masticator space inflammatory changes (arrowheads). Note fluid collection (curved arrow) due to an abscess formation.

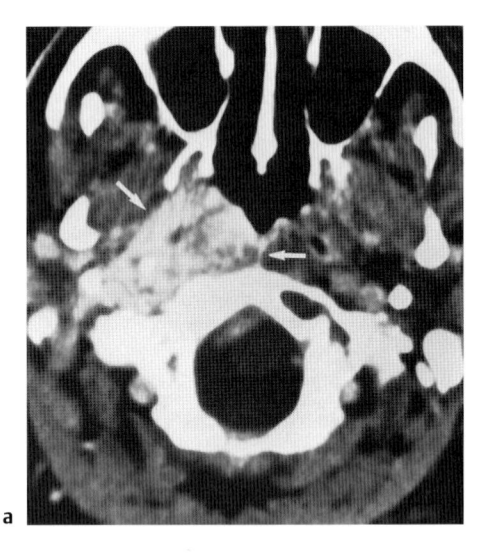

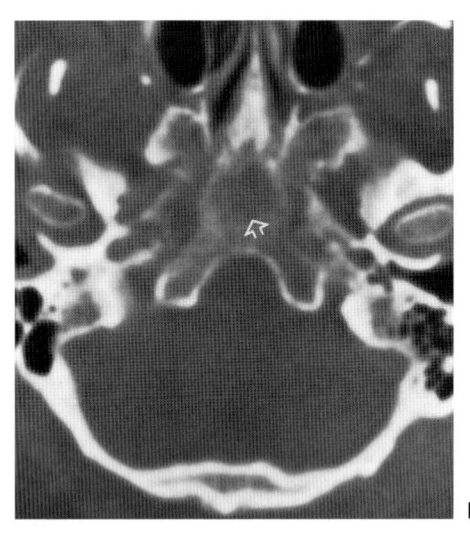

Fig. 7.11   Inflammatory mass of nasopharynx secondary to malignant external otitis (*Pseudomonas*). **a**, **b** Axial CT scan with contrast enhancament (**a** soft-tissue window; **b** bone window), and **c**, **d** MR images in axial planes. Note a mass on the right side of the nasopharynx (arrows). Bone involvement is difficult to appreciate on the CT scan **b**, but is evident (open arrow) on the MR images **c** and **d**. The osteomyelitis also resulted in increased uptake on the bone scan.

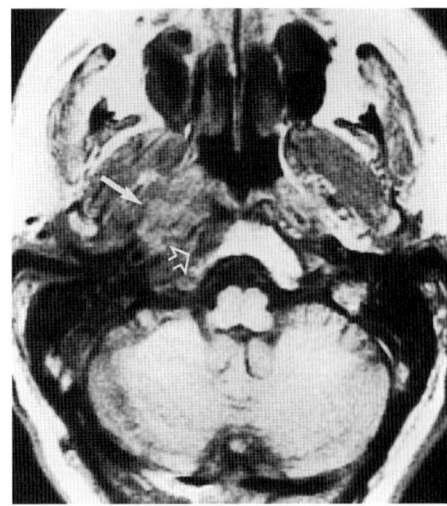

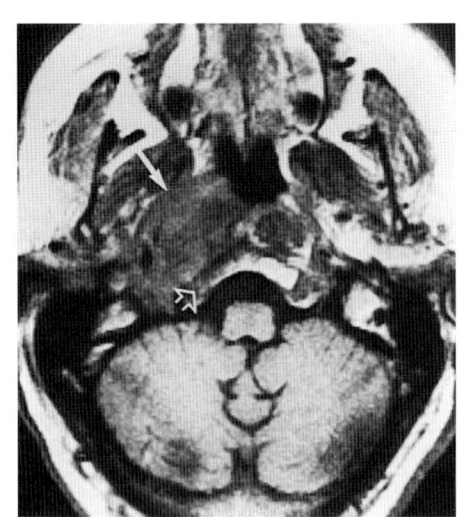

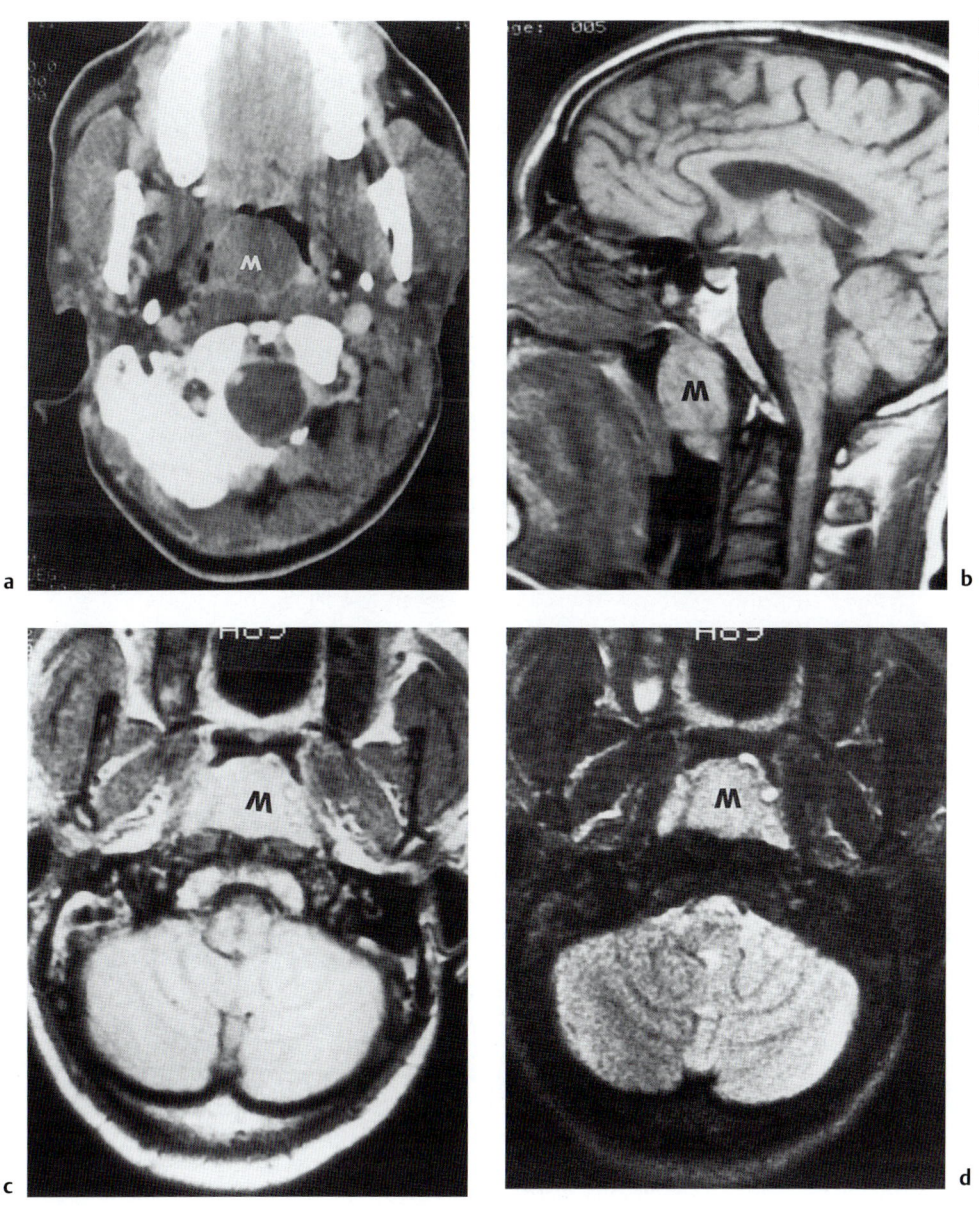

Fig. 7.**12** Rhinoscleroma of the nasopharynx. **a** Axial CT scan, and **b** sagittal T1W, **c** axial PW, and **d** axial T2W MR scans showing a mass (M) in the nasopharynx, compatible with rhinoscleroma.

sopharyngeal rhinoscleroma is shown to demonstrate the mass effect that may be seen with a chronic infection (Fig. 7.**12**). Rhinoscleroma is a chronic granulomatous disease of the respiratory tract. The organism responsible for the disease is *Klebsiella rhinoscleromatis*. The disease was initially described as a lesion involving the nose, but it is now known to involve the pharynx, trachea, and bronchi as well.

■ Infectious Mononucleosis

This is a systemic, benign, self-limiting infectious lymphoproliferative disease, caused by the Epstein–Barr virus. Clinical presentation includes acute pharyngotonsillitis, fever, malaise, lymphadenopathy, and hepatosplenomegaly. Pharyngotonsillitis is often severe and lymphadenopathy may be massive. Lymphadenopathy commonly affects the posterior cervical lymph nodes, but both anterior and posterior nodes may be involved (Fig. 7.**13**).[2]

■ Tangier Disease

Tangier disease is an autosomal disorder of lipoprotein metabolism, resulting in deposition of xanthomatous cells in the nasopharynx, tonsils, palate, liver, spleen, lymph nodes, peripheral nerves, and cornea.[2] The disease was initially observed on Tangier Island in the Chesapeake Bay of the United States. Tonsillar involvement results in symptoms of pharyngotonsillitis. Characteristically, tonsils are enlarged and yellow. Differential diagnosis includes nonspecific pharyngotonsillitis and lipid storage disease.[2]

■ Benign Tumors

Juvenile Nasopharyngeal Angiofibroma

Benign tumors of the nasopharynx are rare (Table 7.**2**), the most common being juvenile nasopharyngeal angiofibroma (JNA).[15, 16] JNA occurs in teenage boys with average age at onset of symptoms being 15 years[17] (Figs. 7.**14**–7.**18**). JNA usually originates at the superior, posterolateral wall of the nasal cavity or from the nasopharynx. Angiofibroma is a histologically benign yet locally

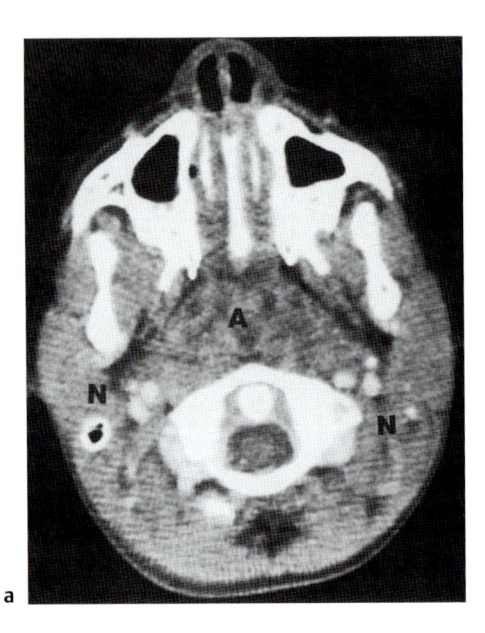

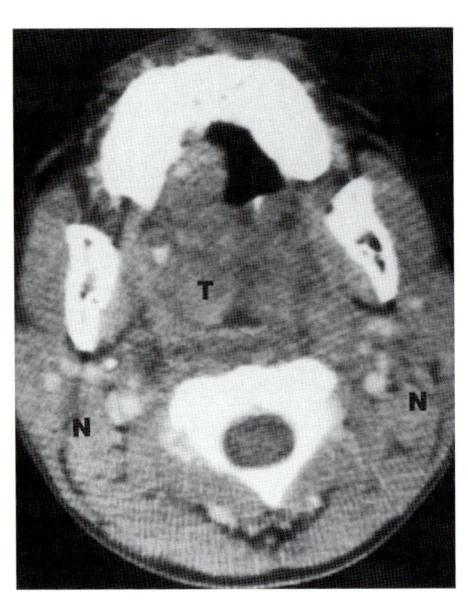

Fig. 7.13 Infectious mononucleosis. Axial CT scans of nasopharynx (**a**) and oropharynx (**b**) showing marked enlargement of the adenoids (A), palatine tonsils (T), as well as posterior triangle and jugular chain adenopathies (N).

Table 7.2 Benign tumors of the nasopharynx

- Juvenile angiofibroma
- Mucous retention cyst
- Tornwaldt's cyst (pharyngeal bursa cyst)
- Neurenteric cyst
- Meningoencephalocele
- Dermoid–epidermoid cyst
- Teratoma
- Choristoma
- Hamartoma (epithelial adenomatoid hamartoma)
- Squamous papilloma (rare)
- Nasopharyngeal polyp
- Polyp (angiomatous polyp)
- Antrochoanal polyp, extending into the nasopharynx
- Pseudotumor (inflammation)
- Granulomas (sarcoidosis)
- Benign lymphoid hyperplasia
- Pleomorphic adenoma
- Ectopic pituitary adenoma
- Hemangioma
- Lymphangioma
- Schwannoma
- Granular cell tumor
- Lipoma
- Fibroma
- Extension of jugulotympanic paraganglioma into nasopharynx
- Extension of pituitary adenoma into nasopharynx
- Extracranial craniopharyngioma (neurenteric cyst)
- Extension of craniopharyngioma into nasopharynx

aggressive vascular head and neck neoplasm.[17] The incidence of JNA is reported to occur between 1 in 6000 and 1 in 60 000 otolaryngology patients and accounts for 0.5% of all head and neck neoplasms.[17] JNA grows into the nasopharynx and often laterally out into the pterygopalatine fossa. Local extension also occurs from there to the infratemporal fossa, superiorly to the orbit via the inferior orbital fissure, and superiorly to the sphenoid sinus. It may also extend out beyond these areas to the middle cranial fossa, cavernous sinus, and sella turcica. Evidence of intracranial spread occurs in 10–20% of cases. As the tumor grows, it may be accompanied by extensive local destruction of bone. Patients typically present with nose bleeds or nasal obstruction. Although considered to be a tumor of teenage boys, these tumors have been reported in older patients.[18] A few have been reported in female patients, but the diagnosis in these instances has been questioned by some authors. The pathogenesis of JNA is unclear; suggested theories include androgens acting on embryonal cartilage, a hamartomatous nidus of inferior turbinate (Fig. 7.**17**), or normal nasopharyngeal fibrovascular stroma located in the nasopharynx.[15–17] Transforming growth factor β1 (TGF-β1) is a polypeptide that is secreted in an inactive form, cleaved to produce an active form, and then deactivated in the tissues. It activates fibroblast proliferation and is known to induce angiogenesis. TGF-β1 may play a significant role in the pathogenesis of JNA.[17] JNA, although an uncommon tumor of the head and neck, results in significant morbidity and mortality.[15–17]

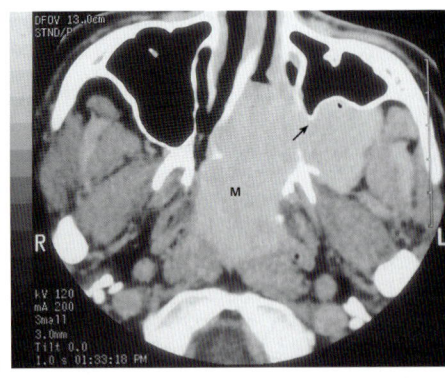

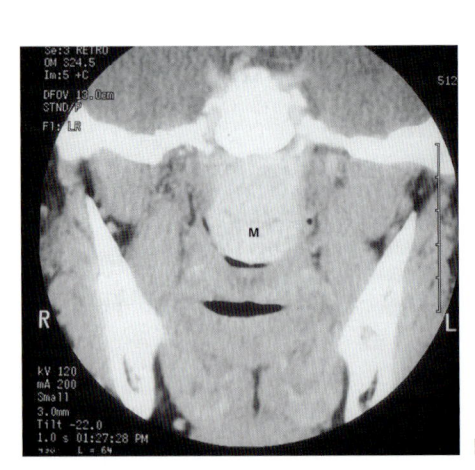

Fig. 7.14 Angiofibroma. **a** Enhanced axial CT scan, and **b** enhanced coronal CT scan, showing a nasopharyngeal mass (M) with intense enhancement. Note extension into the pterygopalatine fossa (arrow).

Fig. 7.**14 c** and **d** ▷

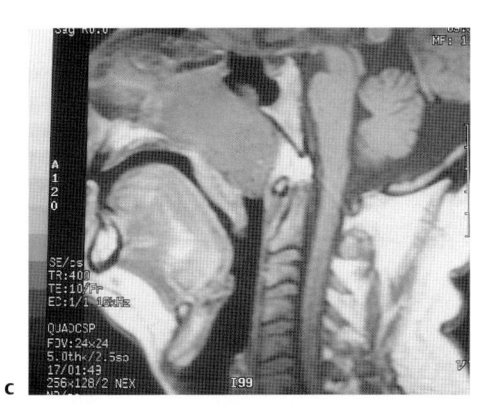

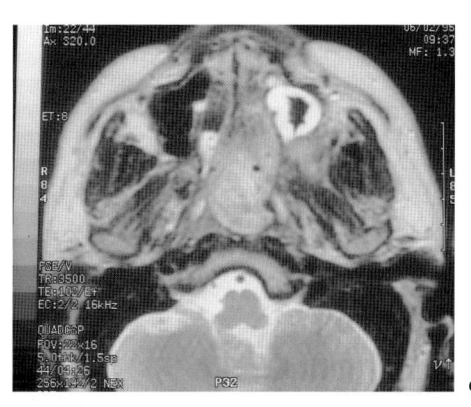

Fig. 7.14 c Sagittal T1W and d axial T2W MR scans, showing the nasopharyngeal angiofibroma.

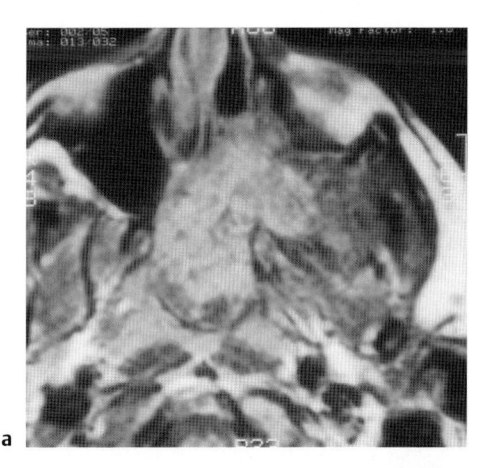

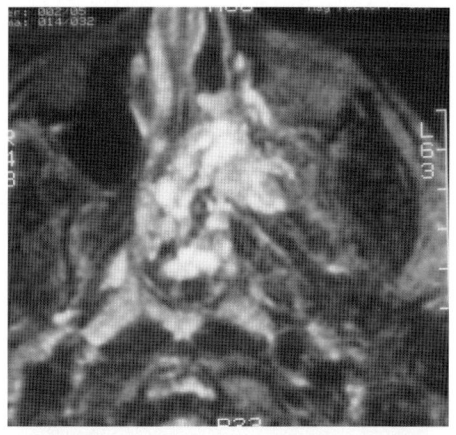

Fig. 7.15 Angiofibroma. a Axial PW, b axial T2W, c coronal T2W, and d coronal gradient-echo MR scans, showing a large nasopharyngeal angiofibroma. Note signal voids on T2W MR and increased signal on gradient-echo (d), representing hypervascular nature of this tumor.

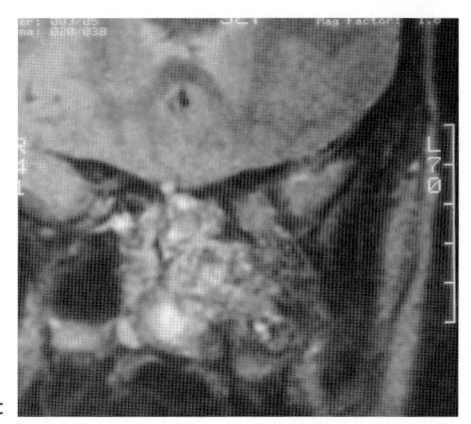

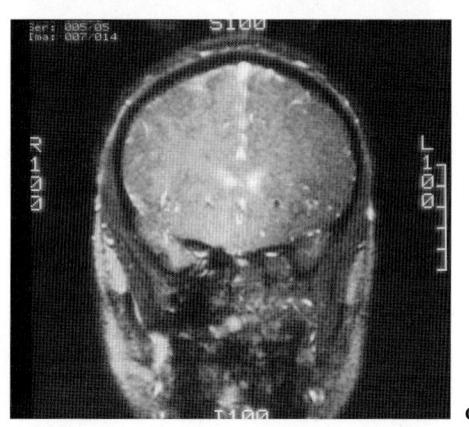

Early diagnosis of an angiofibroma is now possible with CT scan using intravenous contrast enhancement, including CT dynamic study[18] or MRI. A precise determination of the tumor extent is necessary for planning the surgical approach. JNA demonstrates intense enhancement on contrast-enhanced CT scans (Fig. 7.14 a,b). There will be an early intense enhancement on dynamic CT scans.[18] JNA appears hypointense on T1-weighted and moderately hyperintense on T2-weighted MR images (Figs. 7.14 c, d, 7.15). The lesion is hypervascular and signal voids are often seen within these lesions (Fig. 7.15). JNA, on flow sensitive pulse sequences such as gradient-echo, demonstrates flow related enhancement reflecting its hypervascularity (Fig. 7.15 d). On contrast-enhanced T1-weighted MR images, JNA demonstrates intense enhancement (Figs. 7.16, 7.17). CT and MRI play an important role for the detection of recurrent angiofibroma (Fig. 7.18). Angiomatous polyp of the nasopharynx and nasal cavity may not be differentiated from JNA by CT and MRI (Fig. 7.19).[19]

Polyp and Other Benign Tumors

Other benign growths reported in the nasopharynx include squamous papilloma, polyps including antrochoanal polyps (Figs. 7.20–7.23), hemangioma (Fig. 7.24 a), lymphangioma (Fig. 7.24 b), cystic hygromas (Fig. 7.25), lipoma, schwannoma, neurofibroma, ectopic pituitary adenoma, extension of pituitary adenoma (Fig. 7.26), hamartoma, teratomas, epidermoids, and dermoids (Table 7.2).[20,21] The term hamartoma (from the Greek word *hamartia*, meaning "defect") is used to designate nonneoplastic tumorlike proliferation or overgrowth of tissue, resulting from the development of congenital defects and characterized by

566 7 Nasopharynx

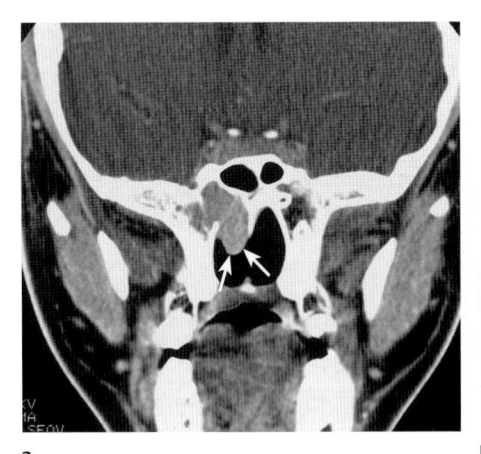

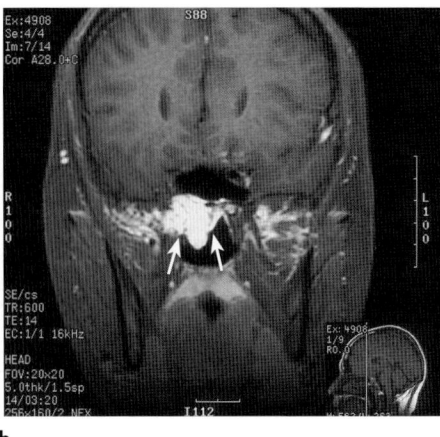

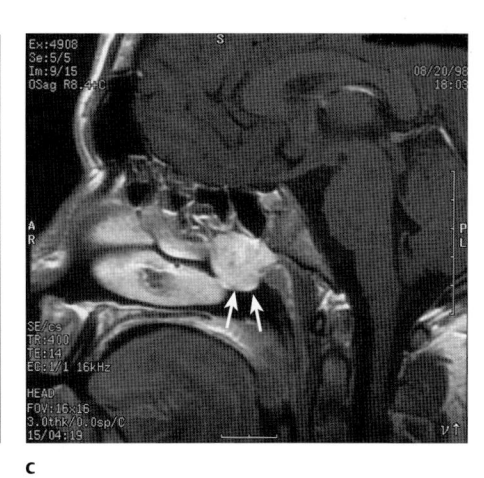

Fig. 7.16 Angiofibroma. **a** Enhanced coronal CT scan and **b**, **c** enhanced coronal and sagittal T1W MR scans showing a nasopharyngeal mass with intense contrast enhancement (arrows). Note extension of tumor into the pterygopalatine fossa.

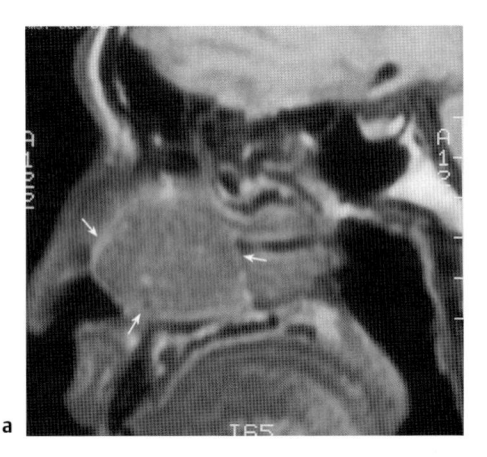

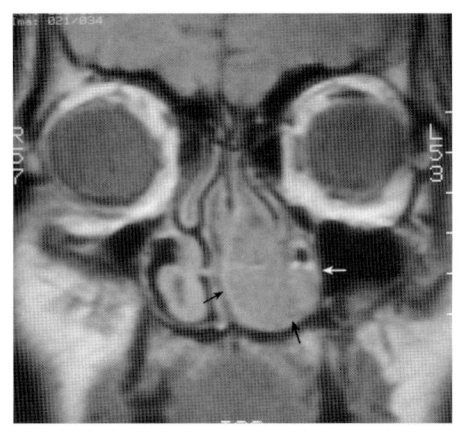

Fig. 7.17 Angiofibroma arising in the vicinity of the inferior turbinate. **a** Sagittal T1W and **b** axial PW MR scans showing an angiofibroma (arrows), arising in the vicinity of the inferior turbinate.

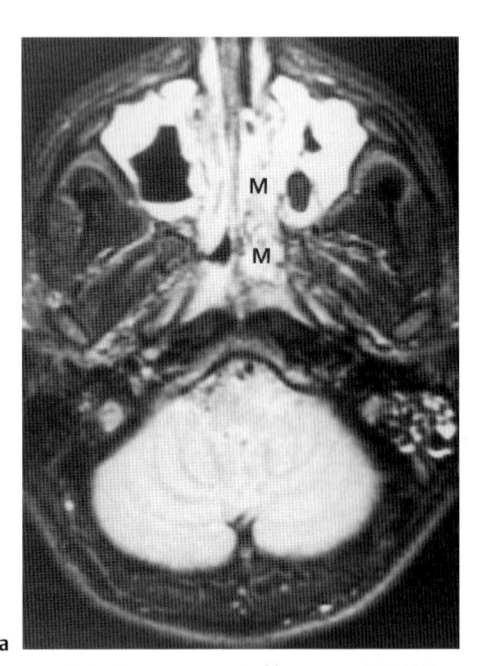

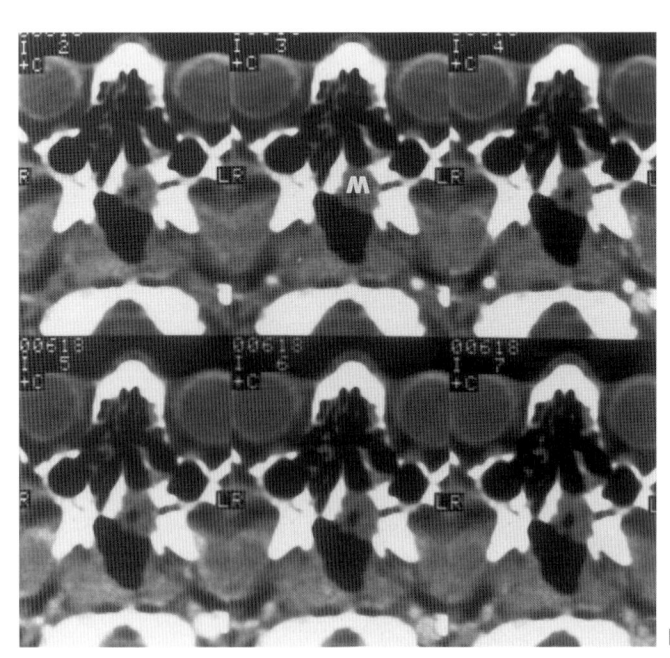

Fig. 7.18 Recurrent angiofibroma. **a** T2W MR scan showing a mass in the nasopharynx (M) and nasal cavity compatible with recurrent angiofibroma. Note inflammatory mucosal thickening of the maxillary sinuses. **b** Dynamic CT scans in another patient with history of angiofibroma, showing a nonenhancing mass (M), compatible with scar tissue.

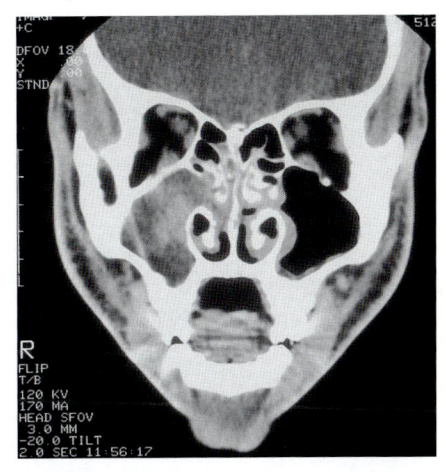

Fig. 7.19 Angiomatous polyp. Coronal enhanced CT scan shows an enhancing mass in the right maxillary antrum, extending into the nasal cavity, compatible with a vascular antronasal polyp.

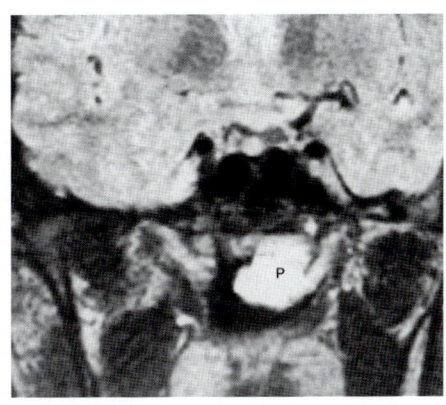

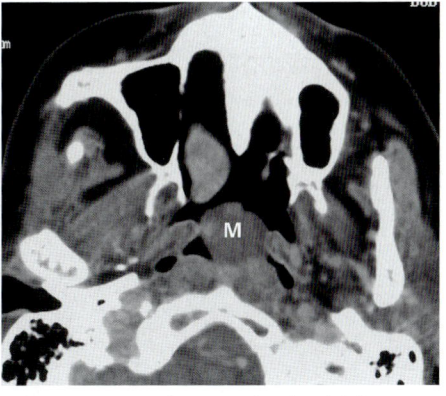

Fig. 7.20 Nasopharyngeal polyp. **a** T2W MR scan showing a nasopharyngeal polyp (P). **b** CT scan in another patient shows a mass (M) in the nasopharynx, presumed to be a polyp.

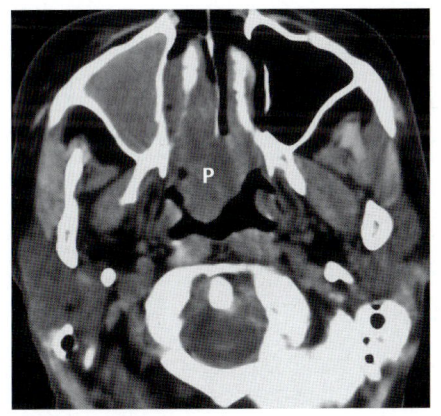

Fig. 7.21 Nasopharyngeal polyp. CT scan shows a nasal polyp, extending into the nasopharynx (P).

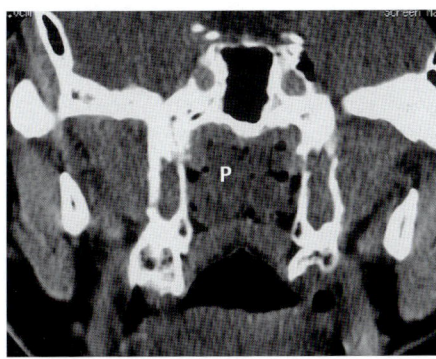

Fig. 7.22 Antrochoanal polyp with extension into the nasopharynx. **a** Coronal CT scan shows a nasopharyngeal polyp (P). **b** Coronal CT scan shows an antral polyp (AP) extending into the nasal cavity.

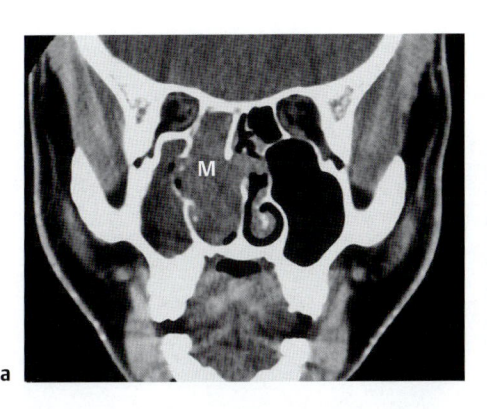

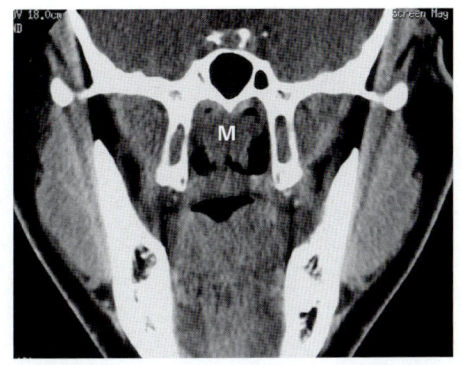

Fig. 7.23 Inverted papilloma of the nasal cavity with extension into the nasopharynx. **a** Coronal CT scan shows a mass (M) in the right nasal cavity. **b** Coronal CT scan showing extension of papilloma (M) into the nasopharynx.

the existence of cells and mature tissues common to the place of origin.[2,12] Choristomas are basically hamartomatous lesions uncommon to the place of origin. An example of choristoma is Fordyce's granules (Fordyce disease or condition), which is described as heterotopic collections of sebaceous glands at various sites in the oral cavity.[2] The term heterotopia is used to designate the presence of otherwise normal-appearing tissue in an abnormal location. Synonyms for heterotopia include choristoma, ectopia, and aberrant rests.[2] Hamartomas can be composed of multiple tissues derived from the three germ layers, but there is usually a predominance of only one of the three.[12] Teratomas, which range from benign to malignant, are autonomous, spontaneous, true neoplasms that derive from pluripotential tissues in which elements of one or more of the three germ cell layers are found.[2,12] They often include tissue that does not belong to the organ in which it is found.[12] Dermoid cysts, which are histologically similar to teratomas (well-differentiated teratoma), originate from ectoderm and mesoderm. Epidermoids originate only from ectoderm, and those that contain skin appendages such as sebaceous glands and hair follicles are considered dermoid cysts.

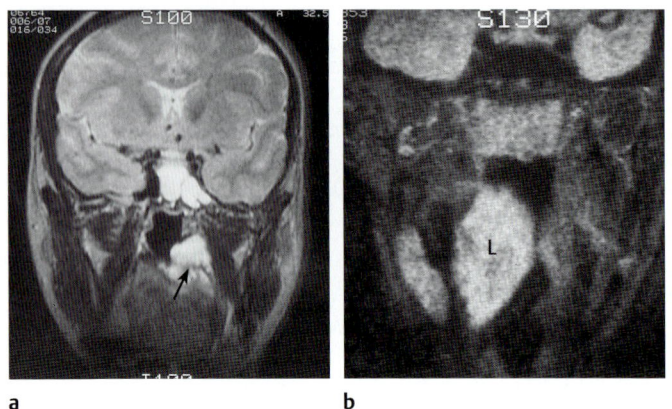

Fig. 7.24 Hemangioma of nasopharynx. **a** Coronal PW MR scan shows a nasopharyngeal hemangioma (arrow). **b** T2W MR scan in another patient with lymphangioma (L) of the tonsil. This lesion was hypointense on T1W MR scan and, unlike hemangioma, showed no contrast enhancement.

A pedunculated dermoid cyst that is covered with hair is called a hairy polyp. In 1995, Wenig and Heffner[12] reviewed the records of the Armed Forces Institute of Pathology and found 31 cases of hamartomas involving the nasopharynx, nose, sinus, and face. These authors[12] realized that inflammatory changes (polypoid growth, edema of the stroma, proliferation of seromucosal glands, vascular and fibroblastic proliferation, and mixed infiltration of inflammatory cells) were present. They therefore considered the inflammation as a component in the origin or exacerbation of such lesions, and suggested the term respiratory epithelial adenomatoid hamartoma.[12] Hamartoma, dermoid cyst, and teratoma of the nasopharynx may at times be difficult to differentiate from each other on CT and MRI scans. Hamartoma and teratoma are often heterogeneous in appearance (Fig. 7.7a). These lesions are restricted to the mucosa and may range from 1 cm to several centimeters in size. Papillomas are rare in the nasopharynx. Papillomas, especially the fungiform type, which represent 50% of the Schneiderian papillomas, usually occur in men aged 20–50 years, and the majority (95%) originate in the nasal septum.[12] Teratomas and dermoids are seen as polypoid masses, largely fatty and cystic.[8,9] Teratomas are always present at birth; they are therefore seen most often soon after birth as a cause of nasal obstruction (Fig. 7.7a). CT or MR is indicated for establishing the diagnosis and differentiating the mass from an encephalocele or identifying any intracranial tumor extension.[20] Other benign tumors to be considered in this area are pedunculated fibromas and vascular polyps.[19,21] The latter are rare, but can simulate an angiofibroma,[19] although they tend to be softer in consistency and more granular in appearance.

■ Malignant Tumors

Malignant neoplasms of the nasopharynx include nasopharyngeal carcinoma, low-grade papillary adenocarcinoma, non-Hodgkin malignant lymphoma, Burkitt lymphoma, chloroma, extramedullary plasmacytoma, rhabdomyosarcoma, malignant schwannoma, liposarcoma, Kaposi sarcoma, primary malignant mucosal melanoma, chordoma, chondrosarcoma, metastasis, etc. (see Table 7.**3**) Squamous cell carcinoma and lymphoma account for approximately 90% of nasopharyngeal malignancies.[2,4,12] The overwhelming majority of malignancies of the nasopharynx are squamous cell carcinomas with varying degrees of cellular differentiation. The histological variants include keratinizing, nonkeratinizing, and undifferentiated carcinoma.[2,4,22,23,24] The terms "lymphoepithelioma," "transitional cell carcinoma," or "Schmincke tumor" refer to undifferentiated nonkeratinizing tumors that have numerous lymphocytes. Squamous carcinomas account for 80% of nasopharyngeal cancers. The remaining malignant nasopharyngeal tumors will prove to be lymphomas including extramedullary solitary myeloma or a variety of rare conditions, including low grade papillary adenocarcinoma, other adenocarcinomas, adenocystic (adenoid cystic) carcinoma, primary mucosal melanoma, rhabdomyosarcomas, and metastasis (Table 7.**3**). The nasopharyngeal adenocarcinomas may originate from the submucosal sero-mucinous glands or from minor salivary glands scattered in the upper respiratory tract including nasopharynx.[2,4,12]

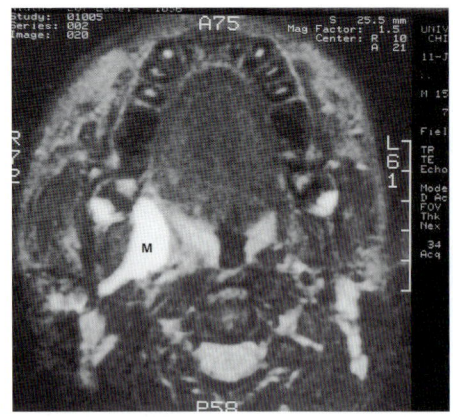

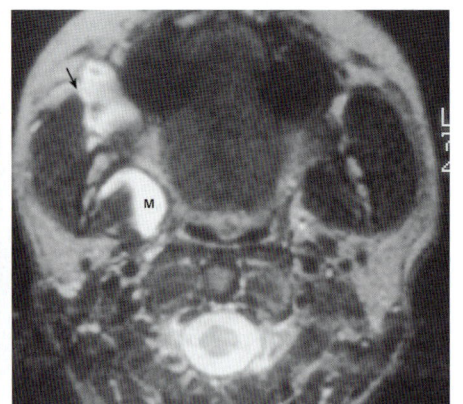

Fig. 7.25 Cystic hygroma. **a** T2W MR scan shows a hyperintense mass (M) in the right parapharyngeal space compatible with extension of a cystic hygroma of the neck. **b** T2W MR scan in another patient shows a hyperintense mass (M) in the right parapharyngeal space as well as in the right buccal space (arrow), compatible with hemangioma.

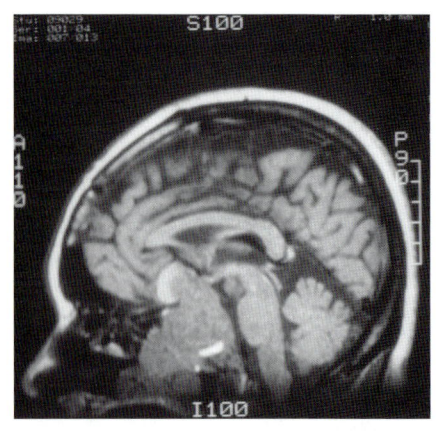

Fig. 7.26 Extension of pituitary adenoma into the nasopharynx. Sagittal T1W MR scan showing extension of a pituitary adenoma into the nasopharynx and nasal cavity.

Nasopharyngeal Carcinoma

The incidence of nasopharyngeal carcinoma (NPC) is highest among residents of the Kwangtung Province in South China.[4] In the United States, the incidence is significantly higher in patients of Southeast Asian ancestry. In China, it accounts for 15–18% of all cancers.[2,4] In the United States, it accounts for approximately 0.25% of all cancers.[2] Figures from the United States suggest an incidence of nasopharyngeal carcinoma of 0.6/100 000, with males predominating 3 : 1.[4] The peak incidence is in the 40- to 44-year-old age group in men and in the 60- to 64-year-old age group in women.[4,24] Nasopharyngeal carcinoma, in particular lymphoepithelioma can be seen in very young adults as well as in children. The youngest we have seen was in a 5-year-old girl. There appears to be a firmly established relationship between nasopharyngeal carcinoma and the Epstein–Barr virus (EBV).[2,4,24] EBV capsid antigen titers are higher in nasopharyngeal cancer patients than in normal control patients or patients with other head and neck cancers.[2,4] Elevated titers of anti-EBV antibodies are associated with nasopharyngeal carcinoma (undifferentiated and nonkeratinizing types).[2]

The World Health Organization has classified the squamous cell carcinoma of the nasopharynx into three histological variants: keratinizing, nonkeratinizing, and undifferentiated carcinoma.[2,22,25] The undifferentiated carcinoma has been described previously as a lymphoepithelioma.[23] Based on the distribution of lymphocytes among the tumor cells in undifferentiated carcinoma, two patterns have been recognized: the Regaud pattern, where the lymphocytes are present around the periphery of tumor cell aggregates; and the Schmincke pattern, where the lymphocytes are associated intimately with the tumor cells.[2] The lymphocytic infiltrate is thought to represent a local immune reaction against NPC and is beneficial in undifferentiated NPC; its presence may deter regional metastasis of cancer cells to the cervical nodes.[22] The undifferentiated type accounts for more than 60% of NPC cases.[2] The specific features of this type of NPC include absence of keratinization, prominent nonneoplastic lymphoid component, leading to the misnomer lymphoepithelioma. Other features include absent desmoplastic response to invasion, cytokeratin-positivity and leukocyte common antigen (LCA)-negativity.[2] The keratinizing subtype of NPC accounts for 25% of all NPC cases. The specific features of this subtype include conventional squamous carcinoma with keratinization and intercellular bridges, graded as well-, moderately-, or poorly differentiated.[2] Invasion typically results in a desmoplastic response. Immunohistochemically, it is cytokeratin-positive and LCA-negative.[2] The nonkeratinizing subtype of NPC is the least common, representing 1% of cases.[2] The specific features of this subtype include little to absent keratinization and growth pattern similar to transitional carcinoma of the bladder. The tumor is cytokeratin-positive and LCA-negative.[2]

Clinical Presentation

Irrespective of the histological type, the clinical presentation is similar and includes neck mass (adenopathy), hearing loss, nasal obstruction, nasal discharge, epistaxis, pain, otalgia, headache, and cranial nerve palsy (Figs. 7.**27**–7.**33**).[2,24] Occlusion of the eustachian tube may result in a middle ear effusion and hearing loss (Fig. 7.**28**). Nasopharyngeal carcinomas are the most common tumors that invade the skull base (Figs. 7.**30**, 7.**33**). The tumor often extends to involve the infratemporal fossa and sphenoid sinus (Fig. 7.**30**), and may extend into the cavernous sinus by way of the foramen lacerum. Invasion of the clivus and intracranial involvement make this cancer particularly devastating. The initial presentation of NPC may be symptoms related to 6th cranial

Table 7.**3** Malignant tumors of the nasopharynx

- Squamous cell carcinoma (most common; 80%)
- Non-Hodgkin malignant lymphomas (second most common; 10%)
- Extramedullary plasmacytoma
- Burkitt lymphoma
- Chloroma
- Low-grade nasopharyngeal papillary adenocarcinoma
- Other adenocarcinoma
- Adenoid cystic carcinoma
- Mucosal melanoma
- Malignant schwannoma
- Chordoma
- Granular cell tumor
- Rhabdomyosarcoma (children)
- Neuroblastoma (children)
- Fibrosarcoma
- Liposarcoma
- Other sarcoma
- Malignant fibrous histiocytoma
- Kaposi sarcoma
- Metastasis (kidney, lung, and breast)

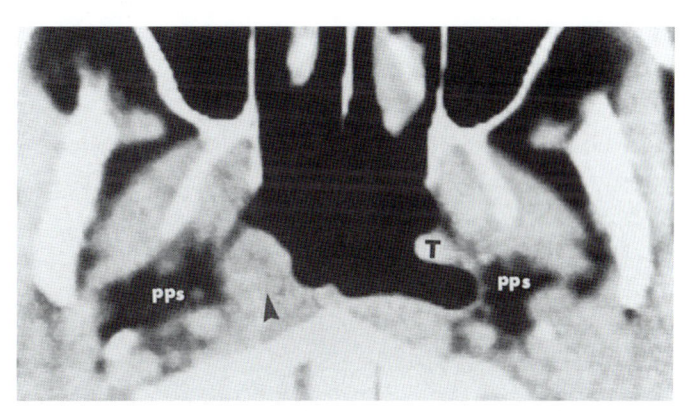

Fig. 7.**27** Carcinoma of the nasopharynx. Axial CT scan shows a mass arising from the Rosenmüller fossa (arrowhead); pps = parapharyngeal space; T = torus tubarius. Nasopharyngeal tumors extend first into the pps and then involve the base of the skull. This was an incidental finding on CT scan of head.

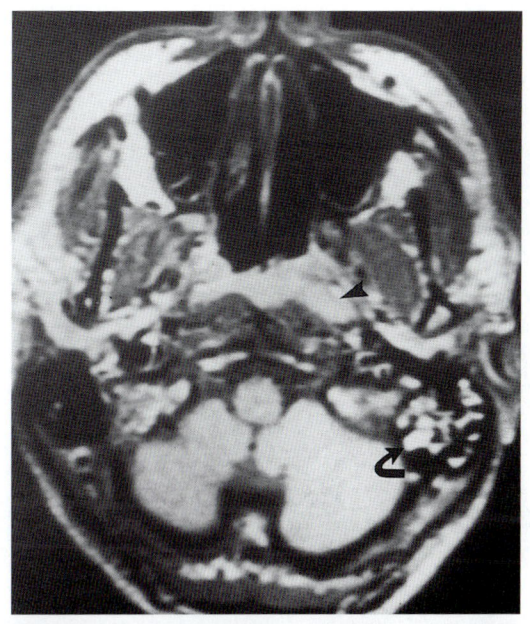

Fig. 7.**28** Carcinoma of the nasopharynx. Axial PW MR scan shows asymmetry of the Rosenmüller fossae, with increased soft tissue (arrowhead) on the left side due to cancer. Note fluid in the left mastoid air cells (curved arrow). This patient presented with unexplained left middle ear effusion.

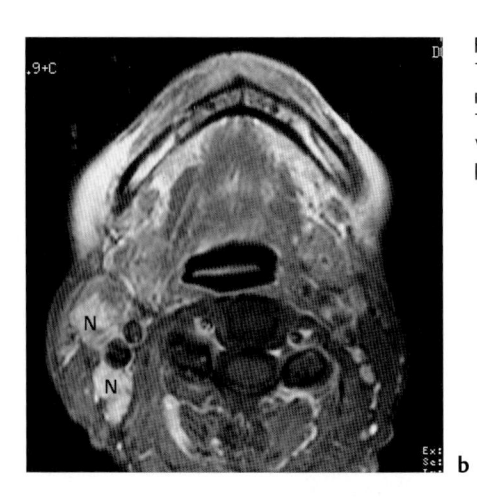

Fig. 7.29 a, b Carcinoma of nasopharynx. **a** Axial T2W MR scan shows a biopsy-proven small carcinoma (arrow). **b** Axial enhanced fat-suppression T1W MR scan shows large metastatic level II and V nodes (N) on the right side. Note hyperplastic level V nodes on the left side.

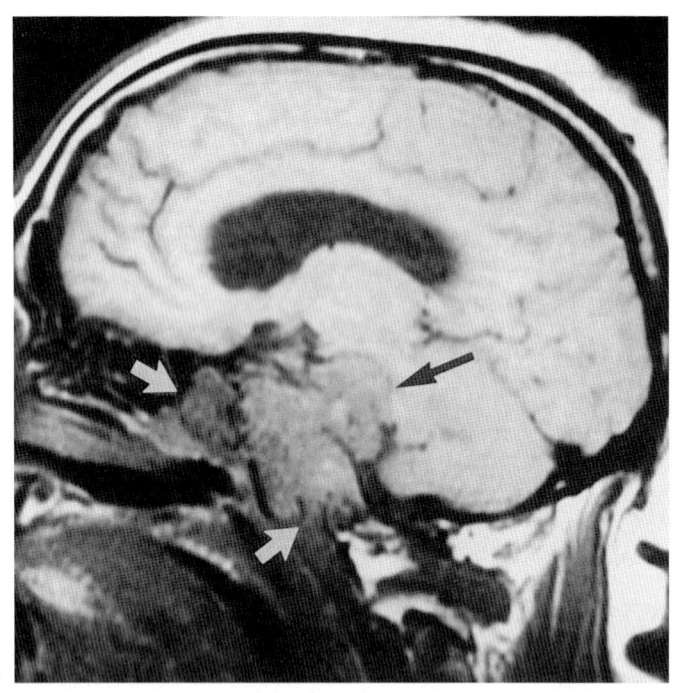

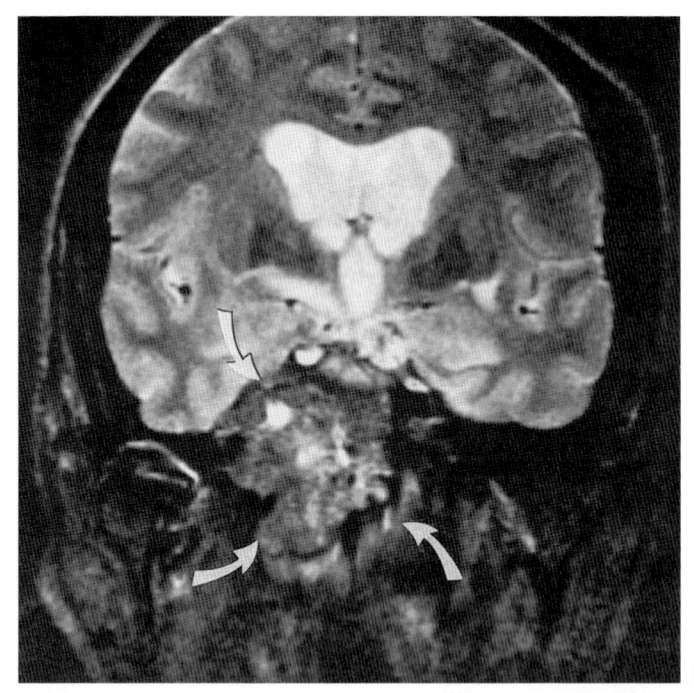

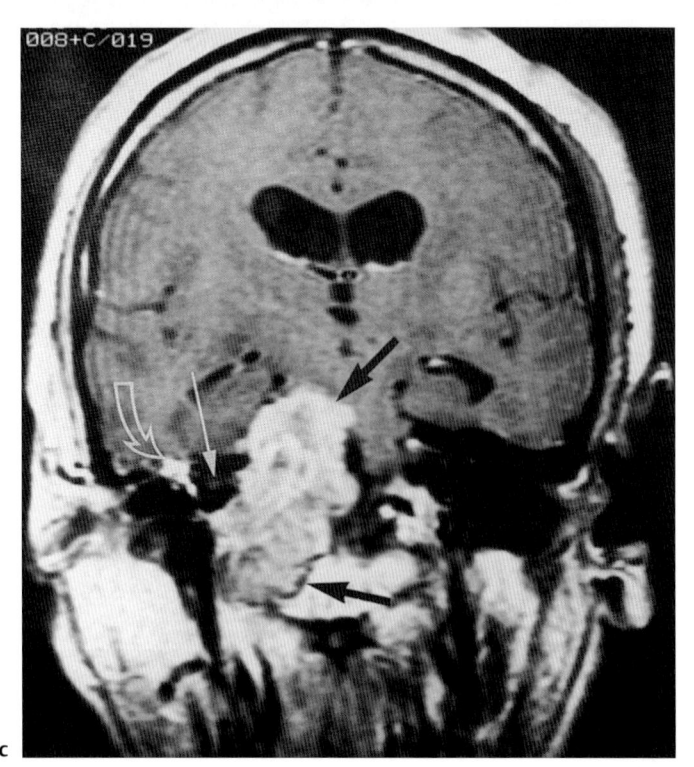

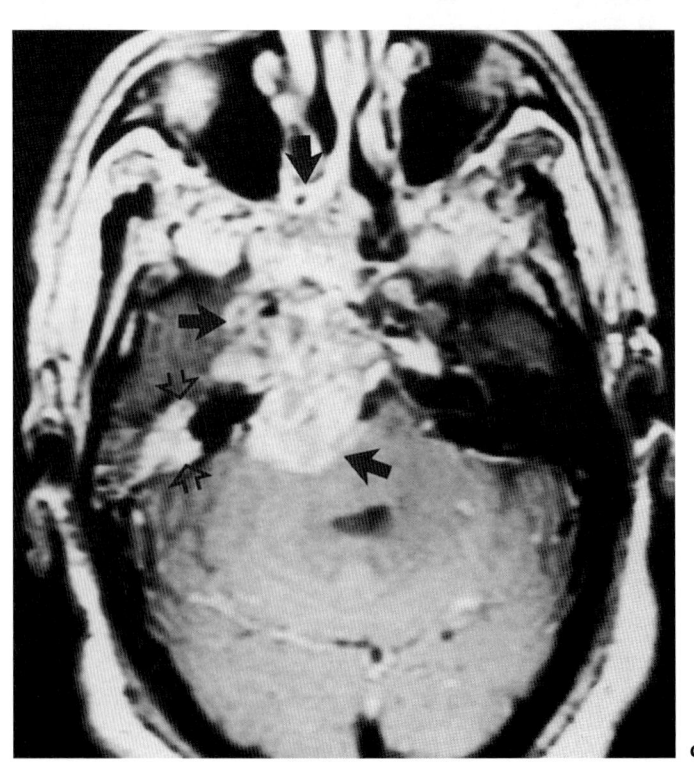

Pathology of the Nasopharynx 571

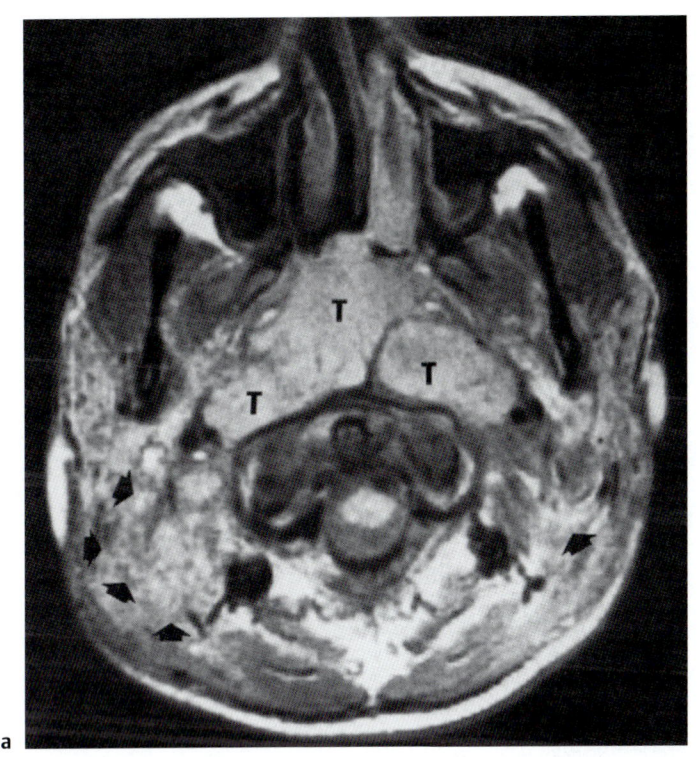

Fig. 7.31 Lymphoepithelioma of the nasopharynx with extension into the oropharynx. a, b Axial PW MR scans. This extensive tumor (T) involves the entire nasopharynx and bilateral retropharyngeal nodes, and extends inferiorly to involve the oropharynx. There are extensive nodal metastases in the posterior triangle of the neck (black arrows, N). The MR features of this tumor are similar to a non-Hodgkin lymphoma.

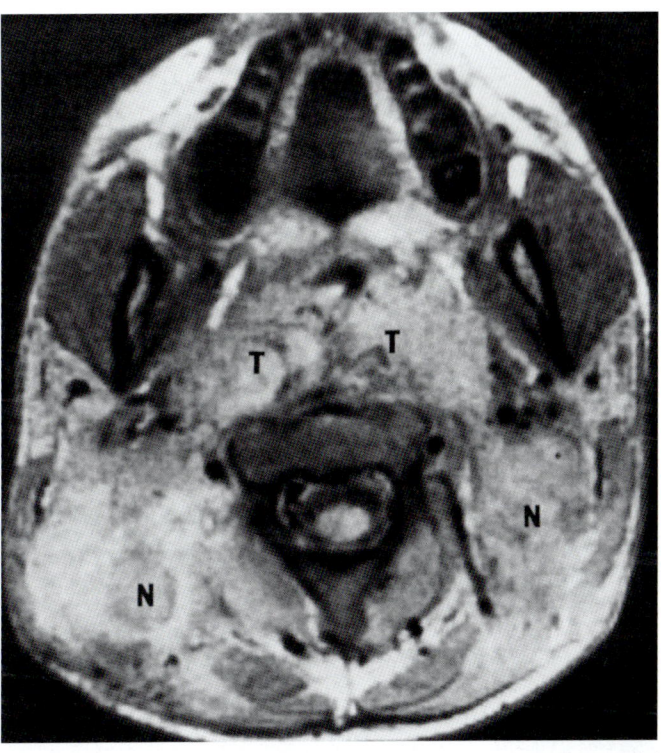

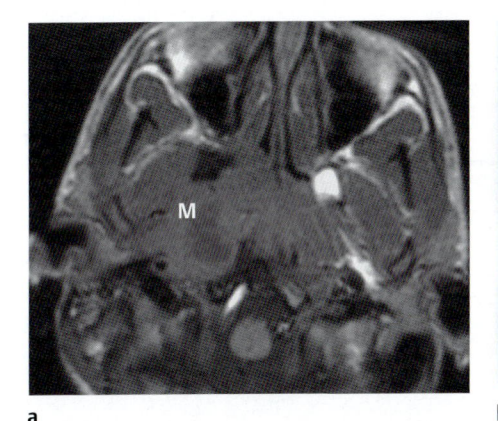

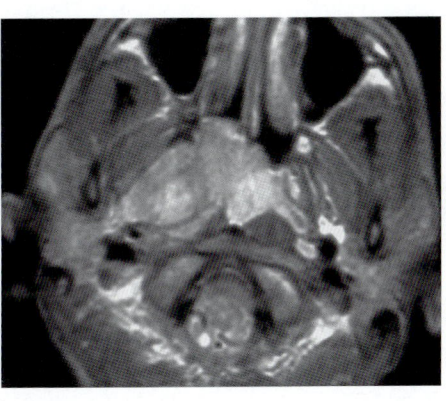

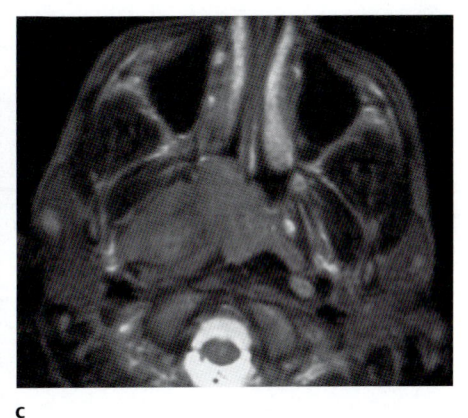

Fig. 7.32 Carcinoma (lymphoepithelioma) of the nasopharynx in a 13-year-old boy. a Axial T1W MR scan shows a large mass (M) involving the nasopharynx. b Axial PW and c axial T2W MR scans showing moderate increased signal intensity of the mass, similar to normal adenoidal tissue on the opposite side.

Fig. 7.32 d–h ▷

◁ Fig. 7.30 Carcinoma of the nasopharynx with extensive intracranial involvement.
a Sagittal T1W MR scan shows a large mass (arrows), involving the nasopharynx, sphenoid sinus, and retroclival space.
b Coronal T2W MR scan shows the mass (arrows) involving the nasopharynx and base of the skull.
c Coronal post-gadolinium contrast T1W MR scan shows marked intracranial and extracranial tumor involvement (black arrows). Note extension of tumor into the porus of the internal auditory canal (white arrow). Note extension of tumor into the middle ear (curved arrow) through the eustachian tube.
d Axial post-gadolinium contrast T1W MR scan shows extension of tumor into the prepontine region and nasal cavity (black solid arrows) and into the middle ear (hollow arrows).

nerve palsy (Fig. 7.33), and involvement of the jugular fossa (9th–11th cranial nerves), hypoglossal canal or cavernous sinuses.

The surface epithelium of the nasopharynx is richly endowed with lymphatics that freely cross the midline, so bilateral metastasis to the cervical lymph nodes is a common presentation (Figs. 7.29, 7.31).[26] The neck is thus always included in the primary radiation field. The lateral retropharyngeal nodes are the first echelon involved in nasopharyngeal cancer. These lie deep in the neck and cannot usually be palpated (Fig. 7.34). Lymph nodes are involved in about 60–80% of nasopharyngeal cancers and may be bilateral in half (Fig. 7.31). The most frequent locations of the metastatic cervical lymph nodes are level II, followed by level V, level III, then the other levels. Nodal involvement may be extensive and bilateral (Fig. 7.31). Distant (liver, bone, brain) metastasis is infrequent in nasopharyngeal cancer. We have seen liver metastases in two cases.

Fig. 7.**32 d** Enhanced coronal and **e** enhanced sagittal T1W MR scans, showing moderate enhancement of tumor. Note that tumor enhancement is more than that in normal adenoidal tissue on the opposite side. Note also that tumor has invaded the pharyngobasilar fascia (**d**) and has infiltrated the skull base. **f** Enhanced CT, taken 2½ weeks later shows mild to moderate enhancement of the tumor. **g** Enhanced CT scan shows low-density area within the tumor that was due to hemorrhage. **h** CT scan shows erosion of the clivus (arrows).

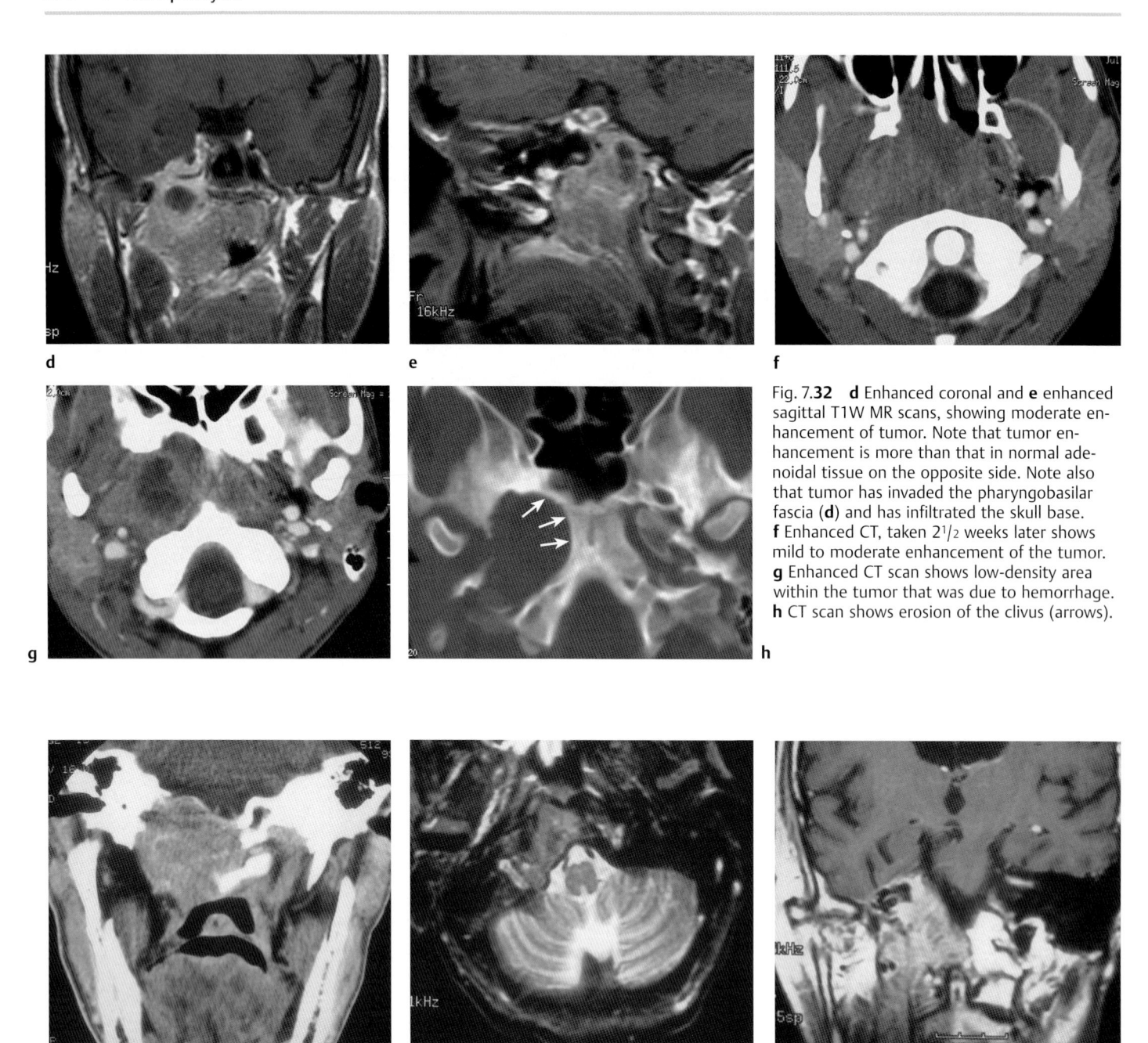

Fig. 7.**33** Submucosal nasopharyngeal carcinoma, simulating a metastatic process to the clivus. This patient presented with right sixth cranial nerve palsy. **a** CT scan shows slight asymmetry of nasopharyngeal soft tissue, but marked submucosal tumor with erosion of the clivus. **b** Axial T2W MR scan shows that the mass is isointense to brain. **c** Enhanced coronal T1W MR scan shows moderate enhancement of tumor.

Patterns of Extension of Nasopharyngeal Carcinoma

The pharyngobasilar fascia is a tough fascia and can be a strong barrier against nasopharyngeal cancer. The tumor, however, may invade the fascia to involve the clivus. Skull base extension by destruction of the pterygoid base is common, and the tumor may extend superiorly to involve the cavernous sinus and go laterally to involve the foramen ovale and foramen lacerum. Tumor may invade the dura and be present in the prepontine region. Patients may have sixth nerve palsy (Fig. 7.**33**), Horner syndrome, cavernous sinus syndrome, or jugular fossa syndrome. Regional nodal metastasis may be the first presenting symptoms and signs. Local spread of tumor to the parapharyngeal space is common. This includes the prestyloid compartment and the infratemporal fossa, which contains the auriculotemporal nerve and the inferior alveolar and lingual nerves. From here the tumor may extend to the tonsillar bed. Superior extension from this area would include the sphenoid bone, foramen lacerum, foramen ovale, and petroclival fissure. The tumor may also extend posteriorly to the posterior compartment of the parapharyngeal space and thus involve cranial nerves IX–XII, the cervical sympathetic chain, and lymph nodes in the area.[25,27] Direct posterior extension to the retropharyngeal space also occurs, including the node of Rouvière and other nodes in the area (Fig. 7.**34**). Superior extension may involve the sphenoid bone, clivus, petrous apex (including the petrous portion of the carotid artery), and intracranial cavity. CT and MRI play an important role in the diagnosis, management (staging), and postirradiation and postsurgery evaluation of patients with NPC (Fig. 7.**35**), including CT-guided biopsy, which can be performed for suspected tumor recurrence.[1,2,28,29] The nasopharyngeal soft-tissue mass as well as

Pathology of the Nasopharynx

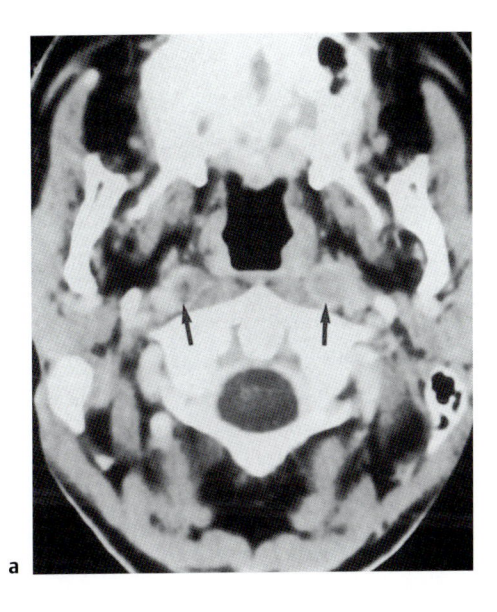

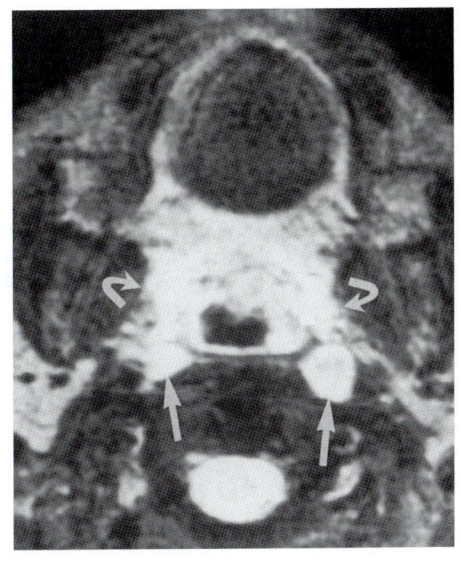

Fig. 7.34 Retropharyngeal adenopathy.
a CT scan shows retropharyngeal adenopathy (arrows) in this patient with oropharyngeal carcinoma (not shown here), which had also involved the lower part of the nasopharynx.
b Axial T2W MR scan shows the oropharyngeal carcinoma involving the palatine tonsils and soft palate (curved arrows). Note the retropharyngeal enlarged lynph nodes (straight arrows).

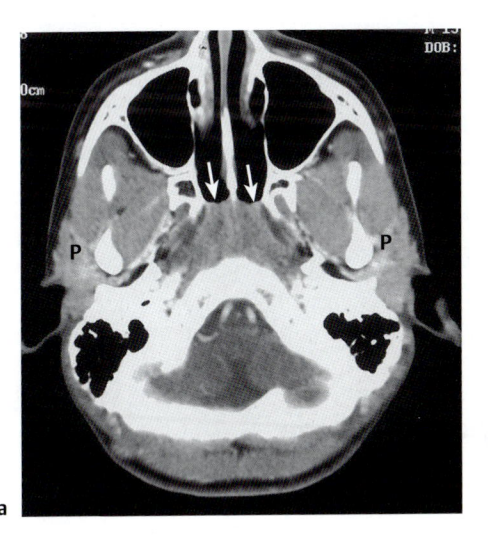

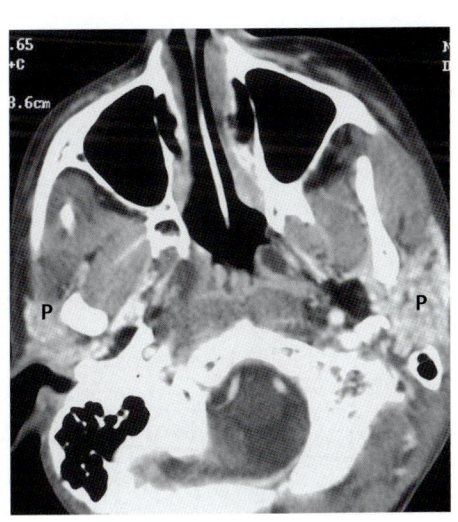

Fig. 7.35 Nasopharyngeal carcinoma. Postradiation CT scan in a 13-year-old child with lymphoepithelioma. a Following completion of radiation therapy. b Follow-up CT scan four months later. Note prominent nasopharyngeal soft tissue in a (arrows) and its reduction in b. Note increased enhancement of the mucosa of the nasopharynx as well as increased enhancement of parotid glands (P), related to radiation therapy.

the metastatic nodal disease may remain prominent for weeks following completion of radiation and chemotherapy (Fig. 7.35).

Table 7.4 shows the TNM classification of nasopharyngeal carcinoma.

Imaging Diagnosis

NPC on CT scans appears as an infiltrative mass with moderate contrast enhancement (Figs. 7.21, 7.32d, 7.33a). Early lesions are seen as increased soft-tissue thickening of the nasopharynx, particularly in the region of the Rosenmüller fossa (Fig. 7.27). The lesion may be completely submucosal with no significant deformity of the superficial landmarks of the nasopharynx, simulating a metastatic process to the clivus (Fig. 7.33). Invasion or focal increased sclerosis of the clivus and pterygoid base may be present. In our experience, the focal sclerosis is often related to a reactive process rather than tumor invasion. On MRI, NPC appears as a hypointense mass on T1-weighted and moderately hyperintense on T2-weighted MR images (Figs. 7.29, 7.30, 7.32). The more aggressive tumors, including undifferentiated types, may appear rather hypointense on T2-weighted MR images (Fig. 7.30b). NPC demonstrates moderate to marked enhancement on postcontrast T1-weighted MR images (Figs. 7.30, 7.32). The benign lesions such as nasopharyngeal polyp, benign pleomorphic adenoma, and low-grade adenocarcinoma of the nasopharynx ap-

Table 7.4 TNM classification of nasopharyngeal carcinoma

T staging	
T1	Tumor confined to nasopharynx
T2	Tumor extends to soft tissue of oropharynx and/or nasal fossa: 　T2a: Without parapharyngeal extension* 　T2b With parapharyngeal extension*
T3	Tumor invades bony structures and/or paranasal sinuses
T4	Tumor with intracranial extension and/or involvement of cranial nerves, infratemporal fossa, hypopharynx, or orbit
N staging	
N0	No regional lymph node metastasis
N1	Unilateral node(s): 6 cm or less in greatest dimension above supraclavicular fossa
N2	Bilateral node(s): 6 cm or less in greatest dimension, above supraclavicular fossa
N3	Metastasis in lymph node(s): 　N3a Greater than 6 cm in dimension 　N3b In the supraclavicular fossa
M staging	
M0	No distant metastases
M1	Distant metastases are present

* Parapharyngeal extension denotes posterolateral infiltration of tumor beyond the pharyngobasilar fascia.

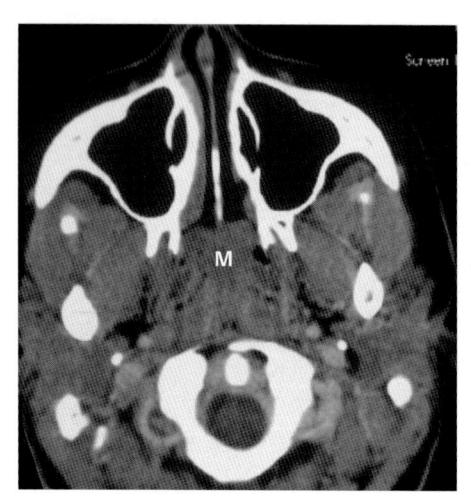

Fig. 7.36 Low-grade papillary adenocarcinoma. CT scan shows a well-defined mass (M) in the nasopharynx. This cannot be differentiated from a polyp on the basis of imaging.

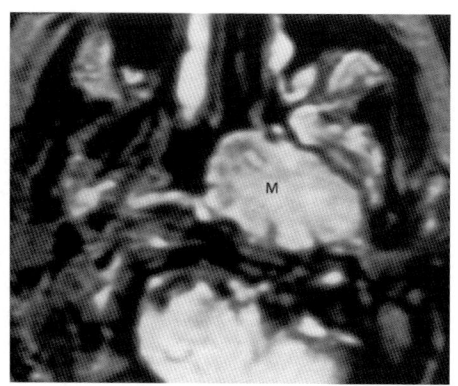

Fig. 7.37 Adenocarcinoma of the nasopharynx. T2W MR scan shows a well-defined mass (M) involving the nasopharynx.

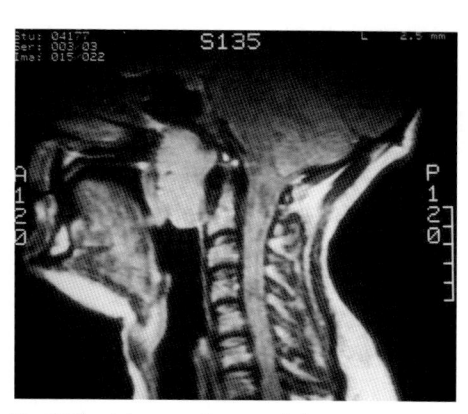

Fig. 7.38 Adenocarcinoma of the nasopharynx. PW MR scan shows a hyperintense mass involving the nasopharynx, compatible with a low-grade adenocarcinoma.

pear more hyperintense than NPC on T2-weighted and PW MR images (Figs. 7.**36**–7.**38**). The soft-tissue extent of tumor is most readily identified by MR; the degree of bone destruction is best evaluated by CT scan. The primary tumor may be so small as to be difficult to identify, yet it can cause local spread or have extensive nodal metastases (Figs. 7.**21**, 7.**29**).[28–30] In a few patients, the primary may be so small as to not be identified by either CT or MR. Such cases may require blind biopsy of the nasopharynx. CT-guided biopsies are indicated for deep-seated lesions, which are not evident by direct visualization or palpation, but which can be identified by CT.[27–29] Distant metastases are said to occur in at least 20% of patients with carcinoma of the nasopharynx. The mainstay of NPC treatment is radiotherapy.[24,26,31–35] This is because most NPCs are undifferentiated or nonkeratinizing carcinomas, which are sensitive to radiotherapy, and also because of the complexity of nasopharynx anatomy, which makes radical surgery difficult.[5] However, in recent years, advances in skull base surgery make possible the effective control of primary recurrence of NPC.[5,31,33] Currently, the contraindications for salvage surgery for recurrent NPC are (1) extensive indurated invasion, (2) cavernous sinus involvement, and (3) pharyngobasilar fascia invasion.[5] Involvement of the clivus obviously denotes tumor extension beyond the pharyngobasilar fascia. MRI remains the study of choice for preoperative evaluation to define the local extension of the primary recurrence.[5] When the primary site is controlled, neck dissection is considered an excellent choice for treating regional recurrence after radiotherapy.[34] Despite good response to radiotherapy, the incidence of isolated recurrence or persistent disease in the neck ranges from 6% to 16%.[26] Treatment outcome is often related to tumor volume.[35,36] It is generally agreed that cervical lymph node metastasis increases the risk of local–regional recurrence, as well as distant metastatic spread, and correlates with a 50% decrease in survival in head and neck cancers.[37]

Low-grade Nasopharyngeal Papillary Adenocarcinoma

Low-grade nasopharyngeal papillary adenocarcinoma is a rare malignant tumor of the nasopharynx with an indolent biological behavior (Fig. 7.**36**).[2] The tumor is composed of papillary and glandular growth pattern. Psammoma bodies and necrosis may be present.[2,37] These histological features are similar to papillary adenocarcinoma of the thyroid gland. Because of the histological similarities, thyroglobulin immunohistochemistry must be performed in order to differentiate the nasopharyngeal papillary adenocarcinoma from metastatic papillary carcinoma of the thyroid gland. Other tumors of the nasopharynx that should be differentiated from this tumor include those arising from minor salivary glands scattered within the nasopharynx, such as pleomorphic adenoma, papilloma (surface epithelial or minor salivary gland origin), mucoepidermoid carcinoma, other adenocarcinomas and metastatic papillary adenocarcinoma of the kidney (Figs. 7.**37**, 7.**38**).

Lymphoma of the Nasopharynx

Malignant lymphomas are generally divided into two major categories: non-Hodgkin and Hodgkin lymphomas. Extranodal primary Hodgkin disease occurring in the head and neck is exceedingly rare.[2] AIDS patients may develop malignant lymphomas involving the nasopharynx or originating in other parts of the head and neck. The mucosa-associated lymphoid tissue (MALT) has been implicated as giving rise to a variety of extranodal malignant lymphomas; included in this category are head and neck sites (Waldeyer's tonsillar ring, salivary glands, paranasal sinus, and others).[2,24,25,38] Lymphoma of Waldeyer's tonsillar ring (nasopharynx, tonsils, and base of tongue) accounts for approximately 50% of all extranodal lymphomas in the head and neck.[2,38] The most common sites of occurrence, in order of frequency, are tonsils, nasopharynx (Fig. 7.**39**), and base of tongue, respectively. Malignant lymphomas are classified as low-grade, intermediate-grade, and high-grade (Table 7.**5**). Although any pattern and cell type can be seen, the most common histological pattern is diffuse with large-cell or immunoblastic cytological features.[2] The large-cell and immunoblastic lymphomas can be mistaken for undifferentiated nasopharyngeal carcinoma. Lymphomas are LCA-positive and cytokeratin-negative; however, undifferentiated carcinoma is LCA-negative and cytokeratin-positive.[2] Waldeyer's ring lymphomas are predominantly B-cell in origin, demonstrating positive reactivity with B-cell markers (L-26) and negative reactivity with T-cell markers (UCHL).[2]

Lymphoma often appears bulky and less infiltrative than NPC (Fig. 7.**39**). Nasopharyngeal carcinoma and other tumors of the nasopharynx may appear bulky as well (Fig. 7.**40**). A na-

Pathology of the Nasopharynx

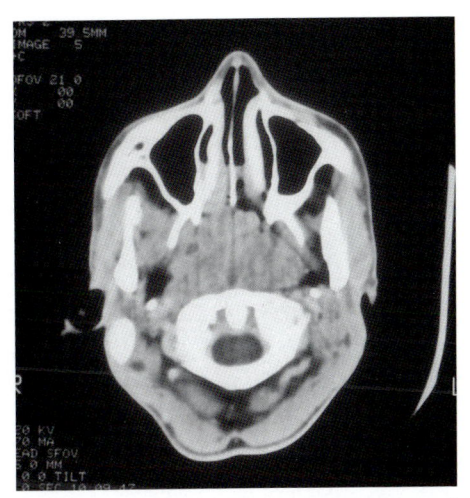

Fig. 7.39 Lymphoma. Enhanced axial CT scan shows a bulky mass in the nasopharynx, compatible with lymphoma.

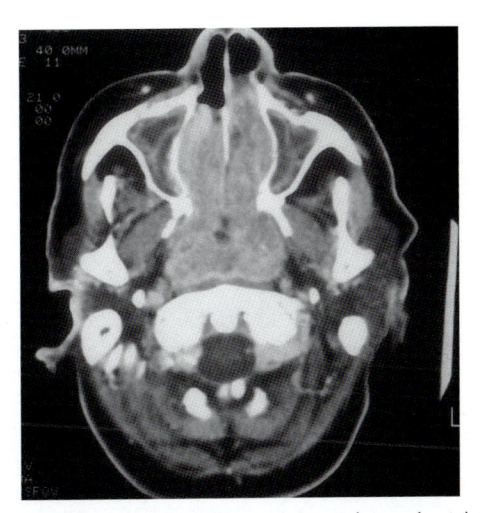

Fig. 7.40 Spindle cell carcinoma. Enhanced axial CT scan shows a bulky mass in the nasopharynx and nasal cavity, compatible with a spindle cell carcinoma.

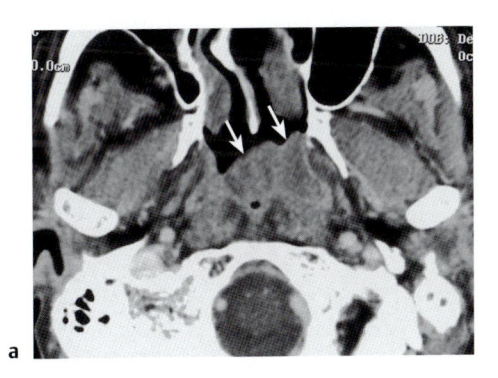

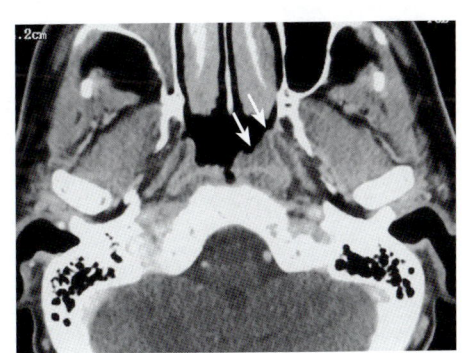

Fig. 7.41 Low-grade lymphoma. **a** Enhanced axial CT scan shows a well-defined mass (arrows) compatible with nasopharyngeal low-grade lymphoma. Note enhanced intact pharyngobasilar fascia. **b** Enhanced axial CT scan, obtained five months following treatment, showing significant decrease in the size of the tumor (arrows).

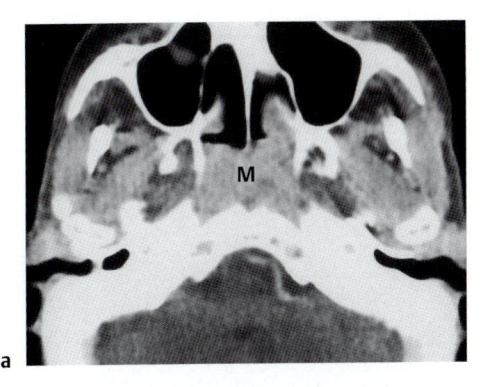

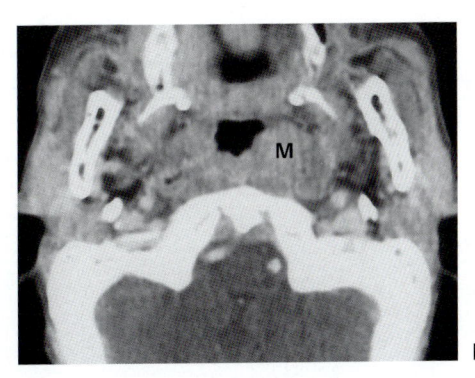

Fig. 7.42 Lymphoma. **a**, **b** Enhanced axial CT scans showing a nasopharyngeal mass (M) compatible with lymphoma. This CT appearance cannot be differentiated from a nasopharyngeal carcinoma. Lack of metastatic (necrotic) adenopathy should be used as a finding in favor of lymphoma.

sopharyngeal mass associated with intraparotid mass (node/s) should strongly raise the possibility of a systemic lymphoma. At times the CT and MRI appearance of nasopharyngeal lymphoma may simulate a benign process such as hypertrophy of adenoidal tissue (Fig. 7.41). In general the CT and MRI features of lymphoma and carcinoma of the nasopharynx are similar and cannot be differentiated from each other in most cases (Fig. 7.42). Lymphomas may not show significant contrast enhancement (Fig. 7.42). In general, a well-defined mass in the expected location of the Waldeyer's ring with clinical appearance of intact mucosa should raise the question of lymphoma (Fig. 7.43). On the other hand, an infiltrative and less-defined mass in these locations should raise the question of carcinoma (Fig. 7.44). An aggressive or less aggressive nasopharyngeal tumor in children and young adults should raise the possibility of non-Hodgkin lymphoma (Fig. 7.45), including Burkitt lymphoma, rhabdomyosarcoma (Figs. 7.46, 7.47, 7.48 a) and NPC (Fig. 7.48 b).

Table 7.5 Classification of non-Hodgkin malignant lymphomas

I		**Low-grade**
	a	Small lymphocytic
	b	Follicular, predominantly small cleaved cell
	c	Follicular, mixed small cleaved and large cell
II		**Intermediate-grade**
	d	Follicular, predominantly large cell
	e	Diffuse, small cleaved cell
	f	Diffuse, mixed small cleaved and large cell
	g	Diffuse, large cell
III		**High-grade**
	h	Large cell, immunoblastic
	i	Lymphoblastic
	j	Small noncleaved cell (Burkitt and non-Burkitt)
IV		**Others, including extramedullary plasmacytoma**

Modified from reference 2.

576   7 Nasopharynx

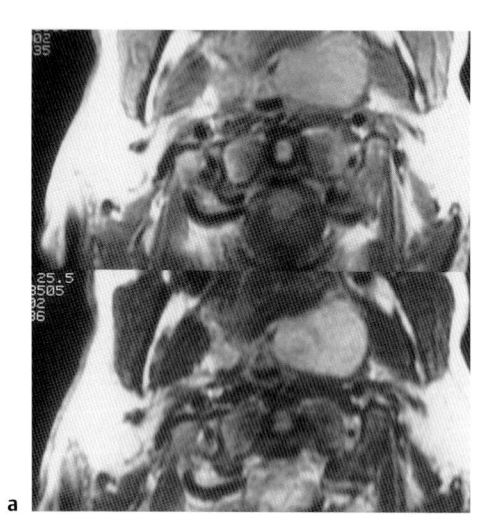

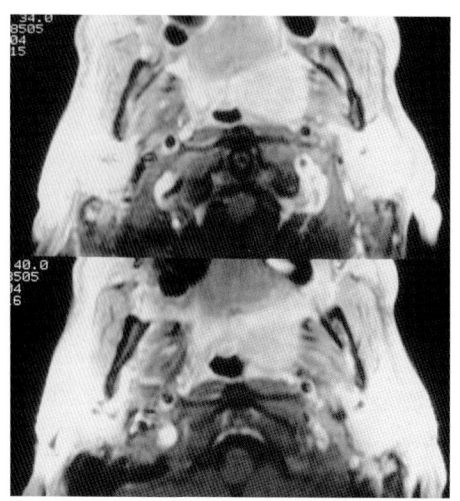

Fig. 7.43 Lymphoma. **a** PW (top) and T2W (bottom) MR scans showing a large left tonsillar mass. **b** Enhanced T1W MR scans showing moderate enhancement of tumor compatible with non-Hodgkin lymphoma.

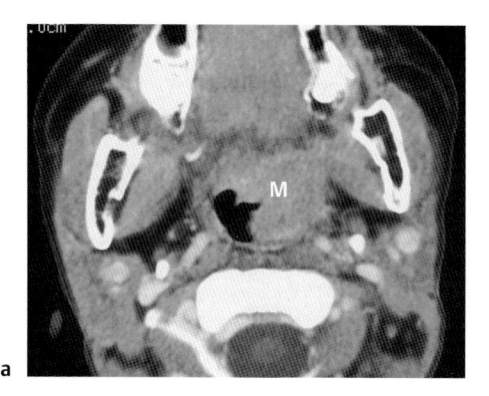

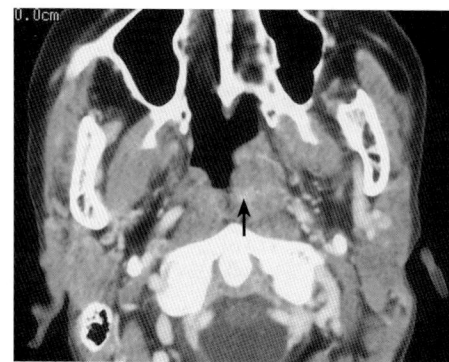

Fig. 7.44 Squamous cell carcinoma of the tonsil, extending into nasopharynx. **a** Enhanced axial CT scan showing a mass (M) involving the left palatine tonsil. **b** Enhanced axial CT scan showing extension of tonsillar carcinoma into the nasopharynx (arrow).

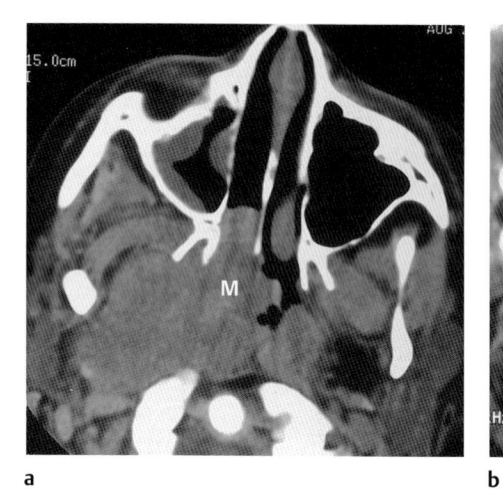

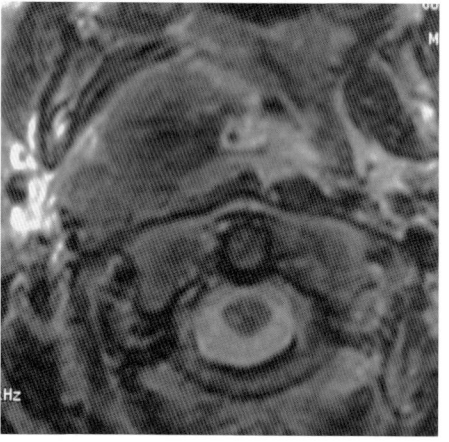

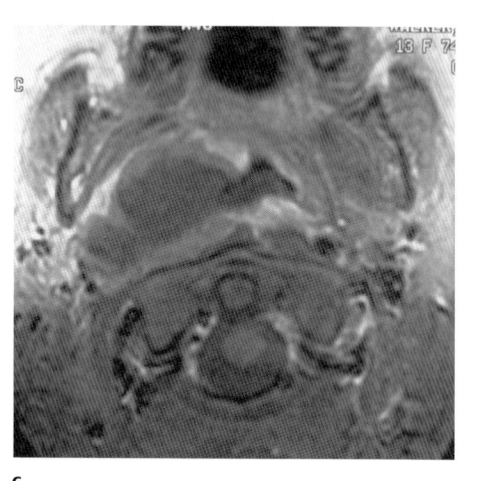

Fig. 7.45 Lymphoma in a 13-year-old girl. **a** Unenhanced axial CT scan shows a nasopharyngeal mass (M). Note marked extension into the parapharyngeal space. **b** Axial T2W MR scan. The mass is almost isointense to muscles. This is not an unusual feature of lymphomas. This is likely to be due to compact tumor cells and increased cellularity. **c** Axial fat-suppression T1W MR scan. There is only moderate peripheral enhancement present. The lack of significant enhancement in the central portion of the tumor does not necessarily indicate necrosis. This is another feature of lymphomas. Some lymphomas may show uniform contrast enhancement, as seen in Fig. 7.43.

Fig. 7.45 d, e ▷

Burkitt Lymphoma

Burkitt lymphoma is a high-grade non-Hodgkin malignant lymphoma with distinct clinical, pathological, and epidemiological features. It is discussed in Chapter 6.

Rhabdomyosarcoma of the Nasopharynx

Rhabdomyosarcoma is a malignant tumor of skeletal muscle cells (rhabdomyoblasts) in varying stages of differentiation. Rhabdomyosarcomas are the most common soft-tissue sarcoma in the

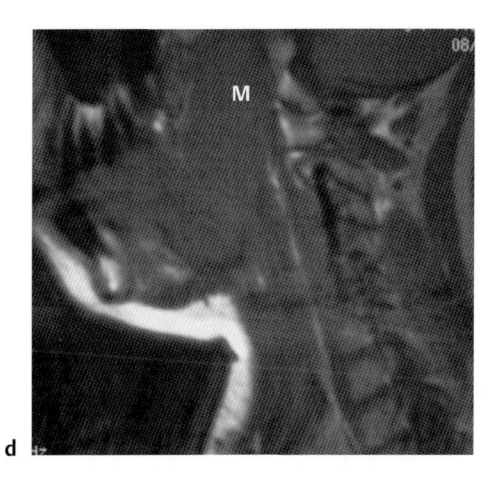

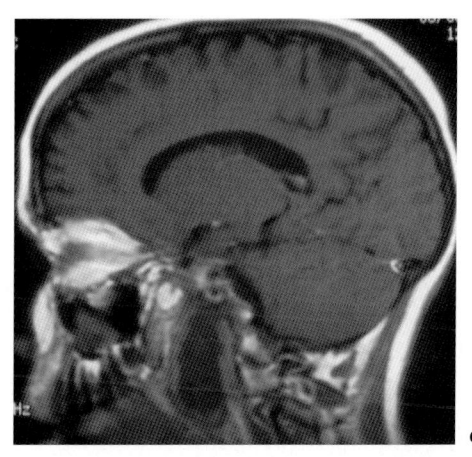

Fig. 7.45 **d** Sagittal unenhanced T1W MR scan shows the nasopharyngeal mass (M). **e** Sagittal enhanced T1W MR scan, showing peripheral enhancement of this lymphoma.

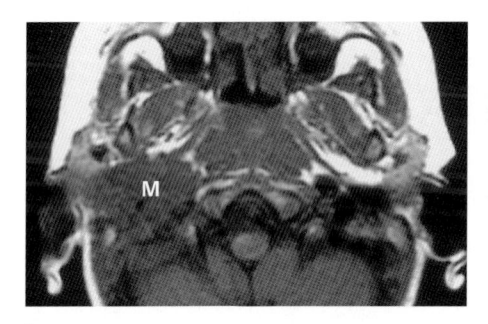

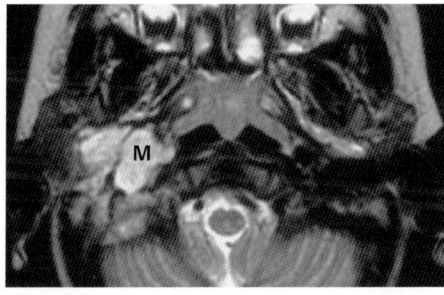

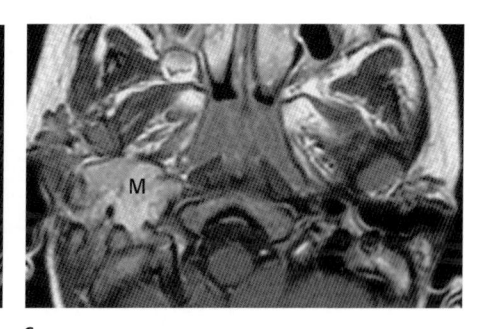

Fig. 7.46 Rhabdomyosarcoma in a 3-year-old boy. **a** Axial T1W, **b** axial T2W, and **c** axial enhanced T1W MR scans, showing a mass (M) in the base of skull, extending toward the nasopharynx.

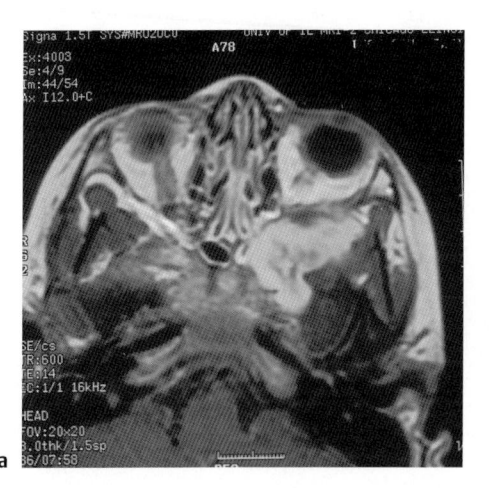

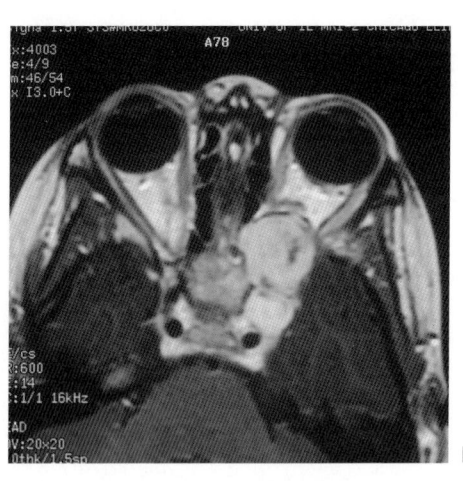

Fig. 7.47 Rhabdomyosarcoma. **a, b** Enhanced axial T1W MR scans, showing a left infratemporal mass extending into the left orbital apex.

pediatric and young adult population.[2,25] Excluding the orbit, the most common sites in the head and neck are the nasopharynx, followed by the temporal bone (ear and mastoid), sinonasal cavity, eustachian tube, and PPS.[2] Nasopharyngeal rhabdomyosarcomas may be fairly, well circumscribed, polypoid, or multinodular, and capable of attaining large size. The tumor may originate adjacent to the eustachian tube or in the parapharyngeal/pterygopalatine fossa, with extension into the nasopharynx (Figs. 7.46, 7.47, 7.48 a).

Chordoma of the Nasopharynx

Chordomas are malignant neoplasms arising from the embryonic remnants of the notochord. The notochord functions as a primitive axial skeleton in humans. Craniocervical chordomas are identified most frequently in the dorsum sella, clivus, and nasopharynx (Fig. 7.49). Nasopharyngeal chordomas often appear as a bulky soft-tissue mass, commonly associated with calcifications and destruction of the sphenoid bone (Fig. 7.49). Chordomas of the skull base are described in Chapter 3.

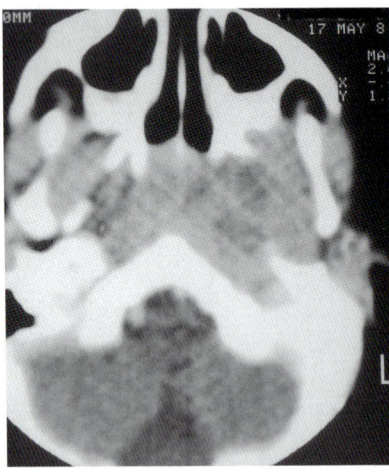

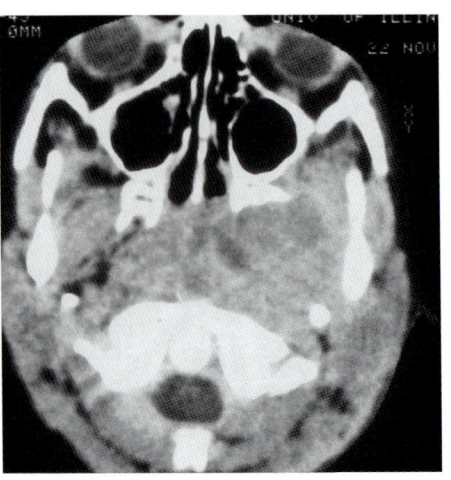

Fig. 7.48 Rhabdomyosarcoma. **a** CT scan in a 4-year-old boy, showing a nasopharyngeal rhabdomyosarcoma with extension into the base of the skull and parapharyngeal space on the left side. **b** CT scan in a 12-year-old boy, showing a nasopharyngeal carcinoma (lymphoepithelioma) with extension in the base of the skull and parapharyngeal space on the left side. Once they are diffuse and extensive, the CT and MRI features of these lesions may not be differentiated from each other in most cases.

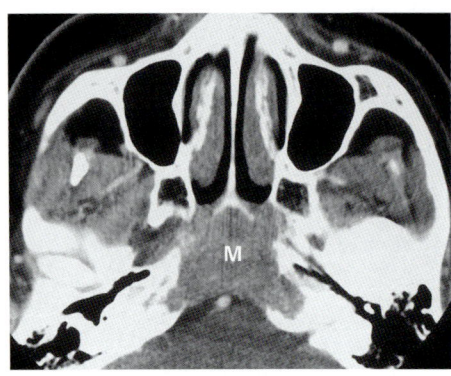

Fig. 7.49 Chordoma. Enhanced CT scan shows a destructive mass (M) in the region of the clivus, with extension into the nasopharynx.

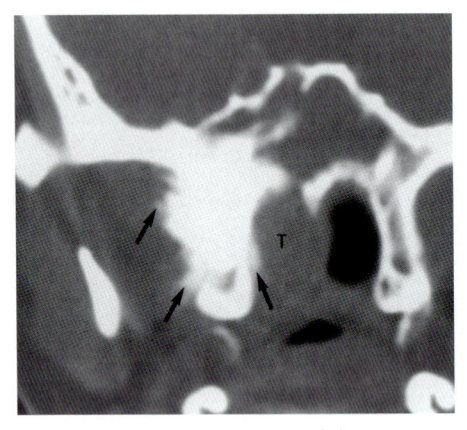

Fig. 7.50 Osteogenic sarcoma of the pterygoid plate, with extension into the nasopharynx. CT scan shows increased sclerosis of the pterygoid plate with "sunburst" tumor bone formation (arrows). Note tumor extension into the nasopharynx (T).

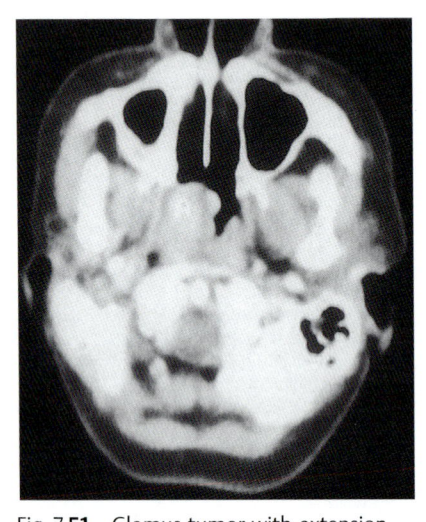

Fig. 7.51 Glomus tumor with extension into the nasopharynx. Enhanced CT scan, taken during dynamic CT scanning, shows a markedly enhanced mass in the nasopharynx. The density–time curve showed a high peak compatible with a hypervascular lesion. This jugulotympanic glomus extended via the eustachian tube into the nasopharynx.

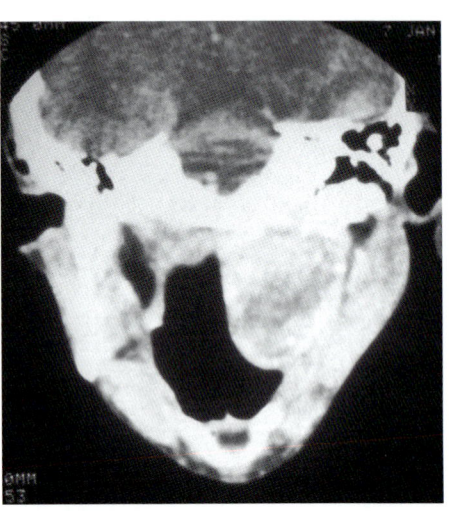

Fig. 7.52 Metastasis. Enhanced coronal CT scan shows a large enhancing mass in the right parapharyngeal and nasopharyngeal regions, compatible with a metastatic deposit from a thyroid carcinoma.

Miscellaneous Pathology

Inflammatory and neoplastic lesions of the sphenoid sinus, temporal bone, base of the skull, and parapharyngeal space may extend to involve the nasopharynx (Figs. 7.50, 7.51). Although relatively uncommon, metastasis may be seen in this region (Fig. 7.52).

Acknowledgement. We thank very much MS Jacqueline D. Jamieson for her secretarial assistance, and Hemant Shah, M.D. for his professional assistance.

References

1. Warwick R, Williams PL, eds. Gray's Anatomy, 35th British edition. Philadelphia: W.B. Saunders; 1973
2. Wenig B, ed. Atlas of Head and Neck Pathology. Philadelphia: W.B. Saunders; 1993.
3. Davies J. Embryology and anatomy of the head, neck, face, palate, nose, and paranasal sinuses. In: Paparella MM, Shumrick DA, eds. Otolaryngology. Philadelphia: W.B. Saunders; 1980; 63–123.
4. Rice DH, Spiro RH. Current Concepts in Head and Neck Cancer. The AmericanCancer Society; 1989.
5. Hao SP, Tsang NM, Chang CN. Salvage surgery for recurrent nasopharyngeal carcinoma. Arch Otolaryngol Head Neck Surg 2002; 128: 63–67.

6 Olsen KD. Tumors and surgery of the parapharyngeal space. Laryngoscope 1994; 104 (Supp.): 1–28.
7 Curtin HD. Separation of the masticator space from the parapharyngeal space. Radiology 1987; 163: 195–204.
8 Bonneville JF, Beloir A, Mawazini H, et al. Calcified remnants of the notochord in the roof of the nasopharynx. Radiology 1980; 137: 373–377.
9 Toomey JM. Cysts and tumors of the pharynx. In: Paparella MM, Shumrick DA, eds. Otolaryngology. Philadelphia: W.B. Saunders; 1980; 2323–2342.
10 James AE Jr., Macmillan AS Sr., Macmillan AS Jr., Momose JH. Tornwaldt's cyst. Br J Radiol 1968; 41: 902–904.
11 Arrat JL, Franche G, Barra MB, et al. Imaging Quiz Case 3. Hamartoma of the nasopharynx. Arch Otolaryngol Head Neck Surg 2000; 126: 1032–1036.
12 Wenig BM, Heffner DR. Respiratory epithelial adenomatoid hamartomas of the sinonasal tract and nasopharynx: a clinicopathological study of 31 cases. Ann Otol Rhinol Laryngol 1995; 104: 639–645.
13 Warrington G, Palmer MK. Retropharyngeal tendinitis. Br J Radiol 1983; 56: 52–54.
14 Curtin HD, Wolfe P, May M. Malignant external otitis: CT evaluation. Radiology 1982; 145: 383–388.
15 Chui MC, Briant TDR, Rotenberg D, Gonsalves CC. Computed tomography and angiofibroma of the nasopharynx. J Otolaryngol 1982; 11(5): 327–330.
16 Witt TR, Shah JP, Sternberg SS. Juvenile nasopharyngeal angiofibroma. Am J Surg 1983; 146: 521–525.
17 Dillard DG, Cohen C, Muller S, et al. Immunolocalization of activated transforming growth factor β1 in juvenile nasopharyngeal angiofibroma. Arch Otolaryngol Head Neck Surg 2000; 126: 723–725.
18 Michael AS, Mafee MF, Valvassori GE, et al. Dynamic computed tomography of the head and neck: Differential diagnostic value. Radiology 1985; 154: 413–419.
19 Som PM, Cohen BA, Sacker M, Choi I, Bryan NR. The angiomatous polyp and the angiofibroma: two different lesions. Radiology 1982; 144: 329–334.
20 Howell CG, Tassel PV, Gammal TE. High resolution computed tomography in neonatal nasopharyngeal teratoma. J Comput Assist Tomogr 1984; 8(6): 1179–1181.
21 Lingeman RE, Shellhamer RH. Benign neoplasms of the nasopharynx. In: Cummings CW, et al., eds. Otolaryngology Head and Neck Surgery. St. Louis, MO: Mosby; 1986; 1269–1280.
22 Jayasurya A, Bay BH, Yap WM, Tan NG. Lymphocytic infiltration in undifferentiated nasopharyngeal cancer. Arch Otolaryngol Head Neck Surg 2000; 126: 1329–1332.
23 Shanmugaratnam R, Chan SH, de-The G, et al. Histopathology of nasopharyngeal carcinoma. Cancer 1979; 44: 1029–1044.
24 Mafee MF. Nasopharynx, parapharyngeal space, and base of skull. In: Valvassori GE, Mafee MF, Carter BL, eds. Imaging of the Head and Neck. Stuttgart: Georg Thieme Verlag; 1995: 332–363.
25 Batsakis JG. Tumors of the Head and Neck. Clinical and Pathological Considerations, 2 nd ed. Baltimore: Williams and Wilkins; 1979.
26 Wei WI, Ho WK, Cheng CK. Management of extensive cervical nodal metastasis in nasopharyngeal carcinoma after radiotherapy: a clinicopathological study. Arch Otolaryngol Head Neck Surg., 2001; 127: 1457–1462.
27 Kalovidouris A, Mancuso AA, Dillon W. A CT-clinical approach to patients with symptoms related to the V, VII, IX–XII cranial nerves and cervical sympathetics. Radiology 1984; 151: 671–676.
28 Gatenby RA, Mulhern CB Jr., Richter MP, Moldofsky PJ. CT-guided biopsy for the detection and staging of tumors of the head. and neck. AJNR 1984; 5: 287–289.
29 Gatenby RA, Mu1 hern CB Jr., Strawitz J. CT-guided percutaneous biopsies of head and neck masses. Radiology 1983; 146: 717–719.
30 Curtin HD. Nasopharynx, infratemporal fossa and skull base. In: Carter BL, ed. Computed Tomography of the Head and Neck. New York: Churchill Livingstone; 1985; 59–83.
31 Fisch U. The infratemporal fossa approach for nasopharyngeal tumors. Laryngoscope 1983; 93: 36–44.
32 Janecka IP, Sen CN, Sekhar LN, Arriaga M. Facial translocation: New approach to cranial base. Otolaryngol Head Neck Surg 1990; 103: 413–419.
33 Fee WE, Moir MS, Choi EC, Goffinet D. Nasopharyngectomy for recurrent nasopharyngeal cancer: A 2-to-17-year follow-up. Arch Otolaryngol Head Neck Surg 2002; 128: 280–284.
34 Ng SH, Chang JT, Ko SF, et al. MRI in recurrent nasopharyngeal carcinoma. Neuroradiology, 1999; 41: 855–862.
35 Willner J, Baier K, Preunder L, et al. Tumor volume and local control in primary radiotherapy of nasopharyngeal carcinoma. Acta Oncol 1999; 38: 1025–1030.
36 Chong VFH, Zhou JY, Khoo JB, et al. Nasopharyngeal carcinoma tumor volume measurement. Radiology 2004; 231: 914–921.
37 Mafee MF. Discussion. Criteria for diagnosing lymph node metastasis from squamous cell carcinoma of the oral cavity: A study of the relationship between computed tomographic and histologic findings and outcome. J Oral Maxillofac Surg 1998; 56: 593–595.
37 Wenig BM, Hyams VJ, Heffner DH. Nasopharyngeal papillary adenocarcinoma: a clinicopathological study of a low-grade carcinoma. Am J Surg Pathol 1988; 12: 946–953.
38 Saul SH, Kapadia SB. Primary lymphoma of Waldeyer's ring: clinicopathological study of 68 cases. Cancer; 1985 56: 157–166.

8 Parapharyngeal and Masticator Spaces

Sherif Gamal Nour and Jonathan S. Lewin

Introduction

The pharynx is a fibromuscular tube that forms the upper part of the aerodigestive tract. It extends from the skull base down to the C6 vertebral level, serving as a conduit that conveys both air and food to the respiratory and alimentary tracts, respectively. The nasopharynx, oropharynx, and hypopharynx are the three classic pharyngeal subdivisions, which lie directly on the spine behind the nose, oral cavity, and larynx, respectively. The nasopharynx and oropharynx constitute the suprahyoid portion of the pharynx. Formed of a thin muscle layer, the pharyngeal wall is lined by mucous membrane and covered by loose fascia that permits pharyngeal movement during deglutition.[1,2]

A diverse range of pathological conditions may involve the nasopharynx and oropharynx. These may occur primarily within the layers of the pharyngeal wall, in the deep suprahyoid neck spaces adjacent to the pharynx, or they may protrude from the nose or skull base to hang into the airway as pharyngeal masses. In addition, pharyngeal disease may be a consequence of functional rather than anatomical derangement.

Prior to the modern imaging era, few tools were available to investigate pharyngeal disease. Having no more than a lateral plain radiograph, a conventional tomogram, or a contrast laryngopharyngogram, the radiologist had to depend on such signs as soft-tissue fullness, intraluminal filling defects, and abnormalities in the pharyngeal margins imaged in profile;[3] all of these signs constituted indirect evidence of pathology, yet there were no means to visualize the actual disease process.

Although amenable to clinical inspection, pharyngeal mucosal lesions may be difficult to evaluate owing to anatomical variations and patient compliance.[3] A mucosal lesion as detected by endoscopy may represent no more than the "tip of an iceberg," with the exact deep extent always remaining uncertain to the endoscopist. Moreover, associated cervical lymph nodes, unless of palpable size, may be overlooked in the clinical setting.

The advent of sectional imaging exemplified by CT, and more recently MRI, revolutionized the diagnosis of pharyngeal and deep neck diseases. For the first time, the radiologist was able to gain true insight into the actual pathology, to define its exact site of origin, to map out its extent, and to study its effect on vital neighboring neck structures. With this wealth of information, he or she could interact with the clinician in a more effective manner and could make invaluable contributions to treatment decision-making.

The improved understanding of the complex suprahyoid neck anatomy offered by these modern imaging modalities has led to the development of a new approach to the diagnosis of pathological conditions involving this region, which utilizes the concept of fascially-defined spaces rather than the classic pharyngeal subdivisions. As CT and MRI have become the basic tools for evaluating nasopharyngeal and oropharyngeal pathology, the current classifications of nasopharyngeal and oropharyngeal carcinomas adopted by the International Union Against Cancer (UICC) and the American Joint Committee on Cancer (AJCC), are now based on sectional imaging findings.

The continuing evolution of MRI has gone beyond the mere imaging of anatomical changes, and is currently approaching near-real-time recording of the functional status of the pharynx; the time nears when the radiological focus of interest broadens to include disorders of pharyngeal function, such as obstructive sleep apnea.

Finally, interventional MRI is a rapidly growing component of current radiological practice and has been successfully applied to the pharynx and adjoining deep neck spaces to guide biopsies and minimally invasive therapeutic procedures.

Anatomy

Classically, the suprahyoid head and neck is divided into the nasopharynx, oropharynx, and oral cavity (Fig. 8.**1**), with the exact contents of each compartment dependent on how much of the adjoining deep tissues are included.[4–7]

The nasopharynx is the uppermost part of the aerodigestive tract. It measures approximately 2×4 cm in anteroposterior and craniocaudal diameters, respectively. It is bounded posterosuperiorly by the basisphenoid, basiocciput, and upper two cervical vertebrae, as well as by the prevertebral muscles.[1,4–6,8] Anteriorly, it communicates with the nasal cavity through the choana, while inferiorly it is in direct continuity with the oropharynx, with the plane of division being a horizontal line drawn along the hard and soft palates and passing posteriorly to the *Passavant's ridge* (a ridge of pharyngeal musculature that opposes the elevated soft palate).[1,4–6,8,9] The features of the lateral and posterior nasopharyngeal walls are described in Chapter 7.

The oropharynx is the part of the aerodigestive tract that lies behind the oral cavity (and can be seen through the open mouth). It is separated from the oral cavity by the circumvallate papillae of the tongue, the anterior tonsillar pillars, and the soft palate. The posterior third of the tongue and lingual tonsil are therefore considered to be within the oropharynx and not part of the oral cavity.[5] Posteriorly, the superior and middle constrictor muscles separate the oropharynx from the prevertebral muscles overlying the second and third cervical vertebrae. Superiorly, the oropharynx communicates with the nasopharynx, while inferiorly it is separated from the hypopharynx by the pharyngo-epiglottic folds and from the larynx by the epiglottis and the lateral and medial glossoepiglottic folds.[5,6,10] The features of the lateral oropharyngeal walls include two faucial arches (pilars): the anterior (palatoglossus muscle) and the posterior (palatopharyngeus muscle) arch. Between them lies the tonsillar fossa that contains the "faucial" or "palatine" tonsil on each side.[10] Further discussion of the oropharynx is included in Chapter 10.

The classic compartments as described above do not take into account the fascial planes of the head and neck. Although the classic denomination of nasopharynx, oropharynx, and hypopharynx is quite effective when dealing with superficial mucosal lesions, such as squamous cell carcinoma, this "non-fascially-based" classification is much less helpful to the radiologist attempting to accurately localize deeply-seated head and neck lesions as evaluated on sectional imaging.[5,7]

The traditional classification of the suprahyoid head and neck into the nasopharynx, oropharynx, and oral cavity has thus been largely replaced by a somewhat complicated but more useful scheme dividing this region into multiple spaces defined by the layers of cervical fascia. Such a "spatial approach" has provided a satisfactory means for localizing the space of origin of a suprahyoid lesion, and consequently helped to limit the differential diagnosis to a unique set of pathological processes specific to each anatomical space.[4,5–7,11–13] Moreover, it utilizes surgically and pathologically defined terminology, thereby creating a "common language" for the radiologist and the referring surgeon.[5]

Fascial Layers of the Neck

Critical to an appreciation of suprahyoid neck spaces is a proper understanding of the fascial framework of the head and neck (Figs. 8.2–8.6).

Basically, there are two major components of the neck fasciae: the superficial and deep cervical layers:

- The **superficial cervical fascia** is a loose fibroareolar layer with the platysma muscle embedded in its deep portion.[14]
- The **deep cervical fascia** is a complex that consists of multiple fascial sheets that are generally subdivided into three layers:

Superficial Layer of the Deep Cervical Fascia (Investing Fascia)

This layer forms a complete collar around the neck, and is attached *superiorly* to the lower border of the mandibular body back to its angle and more posteriorly to the mastoid processes, the superior nuchal line, and the external occipital protuberance.

Inferiorly, this layer attaches to the acromion and spine of the scapula, to the clavicle, and to the manubrium sterni. The two halves of the investing fascia attach *posteriorly* to the ligamentum nuchae and cervical spinal processes, while anteriorly they are continuous and are attached to the hyoid bone where they converge with the middle (visceral) layer of the deep cervical fascia, dividing the neck into suprahyoid and infrahyoid portions.[1,14]

The investing fascia splits to enclose number of structures within the neck, thereby forming the following fascial spaces:

Masticator space: Above the attachment to the lower border of the mandible, a part of the investing fascia continues upward to enclose the muscles of mastication and the mandible (ramus and posterior body) by splitting into a superficial portion that covers the masseter muscle and then attaches to the zygomatic arch (this is continuous with the fascia covering the parotid gland forming the parotid-masseteric fascia) and a deep portion running deep to both pterygoid muscles to attach to the skull base, separating the masticator from the prestyloid compartment of the parapharyngeal space (Fig. 8.3).[12,14–16]

Parotid space is formed as the investing fascia splits between the mastoid process and the angle of the mandible to enclose the gland and to form its capsule.[14,16] The medial aspect of the parotid space, which contains the deep lobe of the parotid gland, extends through the stylomandibular tunnel (the gap between the styloid process and the posterior margin of the mandible) for a variable distance before it meets the prestyloid compartment of the parapharyngeal space (Fig. 8.3a).[4]

Submandibular and sublingual spaces: A layer of the investing fascia splits to line the undersurface of the submandibular gland before reattaching to the mandible at the mylohyoid line, thereby forming the capsule of the gland. In the radiological literature, the term "submandibular space" is given to the entire area superficial to the mylohyoid muscle down to the superficial layer of investing fascia as it extends from the hyoid bone to the mandible (Fig. 8.3a). The sublingual space is the area deep to the mylohyoid muscle up to the mucosa of the mouth floor (Fig. 8.3a). The relevance of these spaces to this chapter is their free communication with the prestyloid compartment of the parapharyngeal space (Fig. 8.3a).[4,16]

Muscular spaces are formed as the fascia splits to enclose the trapezius, sternocleidomastoid, digastric, and inferior belly of the omohyoid muscles.[14,16]

Suprasternal space (of Burns) is a shallow space formed just above the manubrium sterni as the investing fascia splits to attach to the anterior and posterior borders of the jugular notch.[14,16]

Deep Layer of Deep Cervical Fascia (Prevertebral Fascia)

This layer encircles the vertebral column as well as the paraspinal and prevertebral muscles, with a firm insertion on the spinous and transverse processes of the vertebral column (Figs. 8.1, 8.3a). The prevertebral fascia extends from the skull base down to the third thoracic vertebra, where it fuses with the anterior longitudinal ligament in the posterior mediastinum.[1,14] A slip of the deep layer of the deep cervical fascia, the alar fascia, lies immediately anterior to the prevertebral fascia (Figs. 8.1, 8.3a) with a similar coronal plane of orientation, and has been described by some authors.[4,14]

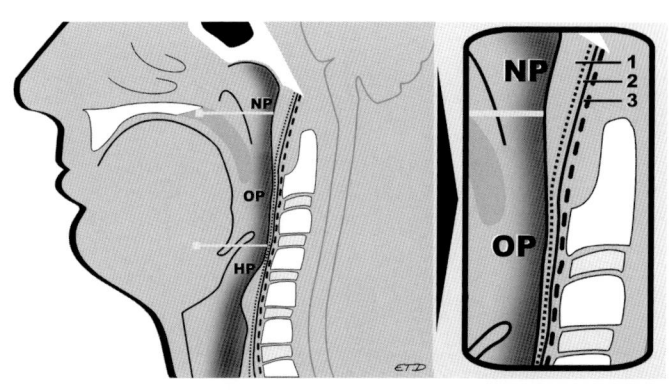

Fig. 8.1 Sagittal diagram showing pharyngeal divisions and fascial lines. NP = nasopharynx; OP = oropharynx; HP = hypopharynx; ••••• = buccopharyngeal fascia; —— = alar fascia; ---- = prevertebral fascia; 1 = pharyngeal mucosal space (PMS); 2 = retropharyngeal space (RPS); 3 = danger space (DS). Note that the soft palate belongs to the oropharynx. Reproduced and modified from Reference 4 with permission.

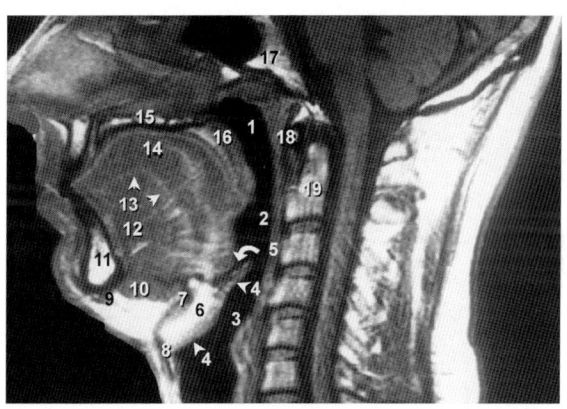

Fig. 8.2 Normal imaging anatomy of the pharynx and oral cavity on mid-sagittal nonenhanced T1W MRI. 1 = Nasopharyngeal airway; 2 = oropharyngeal airway; 3 = hypopharyngeal airway; 4 = epiglottis; 5 = vallecula; 6 = preepiglottic fat; 7 = hyoid bone; 8 = thyroid cartilage; 9 = mylohyoid muscle; 10 = geniohyoid muscle; 11 = symphysis menti; 12 = genioglossus muscle; 13 = lingual septum; 14 = body of tongue; 15 = hard palate; 16 = soft palate/uvula; 17 = clivus; 18 = anterior arch of atlas (first cervical vertebra); 19 = odontoid process (dens). Reproduced from Reference 4 with permission.

8 Parapharyngeal and Masticator Spaces

1	BFF
2	alar fascia
3	prevertebral fascia
4	fascia of the tensor veli palatini
CAR	internal carotid artery
CS	cloison sagittale
DS	danger space
JUG	internal jugular vein
LP	lateral pterygoid muscle
LVP	levator veli palatini
M	masseter muscle
Mand	mandibular condyle
MH	mylohyoid muscle
MP	medial pterygoid muscle
MS	masticator space
PBF	pharyngobasilar fascia
PPS	prestyloid compartment of parapharyngeal space
PS	parotid space
PCS	posterior cervical space
RPPS	retrostyloid compartment of the parapharyngeal space
RPS	retropharyngeal space
SLS	sublingual space
SMS	submandibular space
TVP	tensor veli palatini
V3	mandibular division of the trigeminal nerve in the masticator space
black arrow	in **b** retromandibular vein
short arrow	in **c** torus tubarius
long arrow	in **c** fossa of Rosenmüller

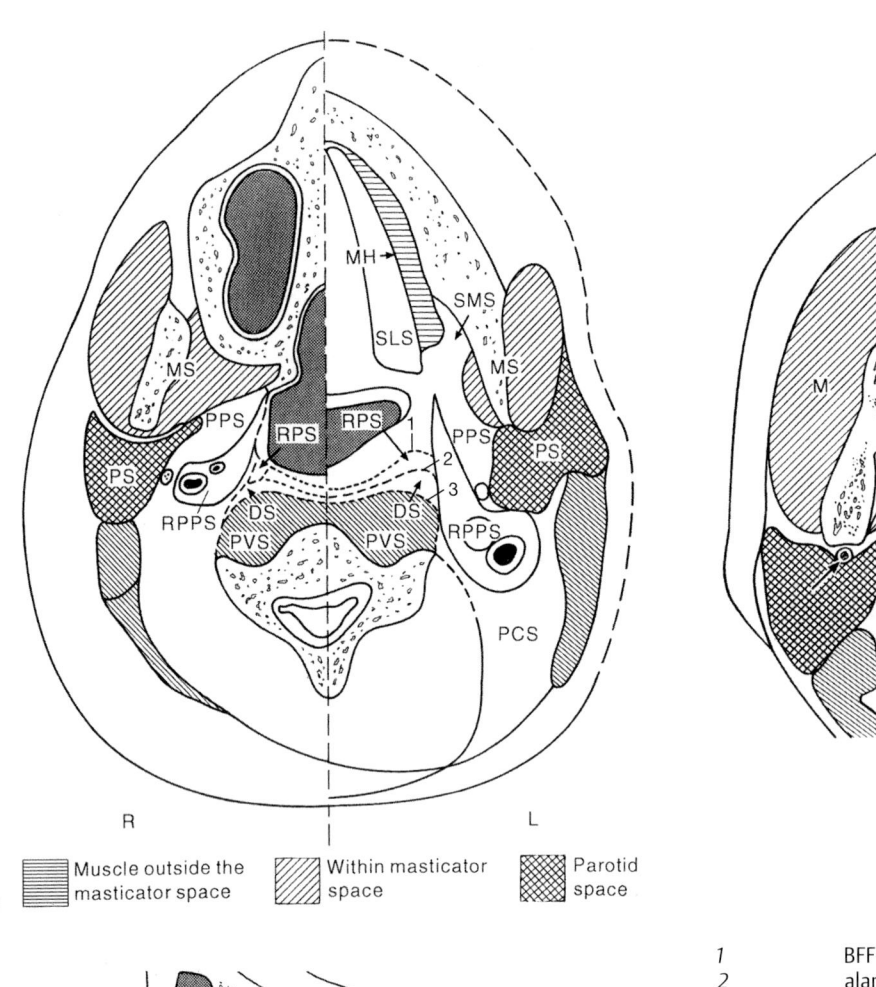

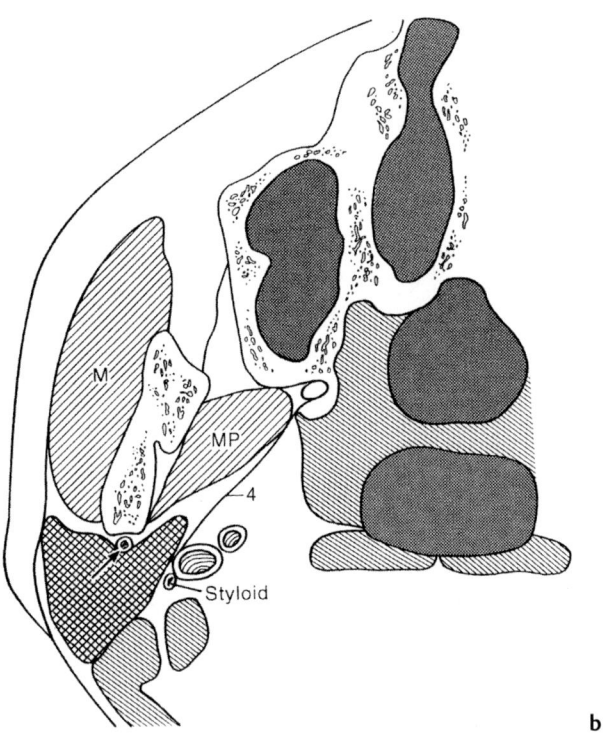

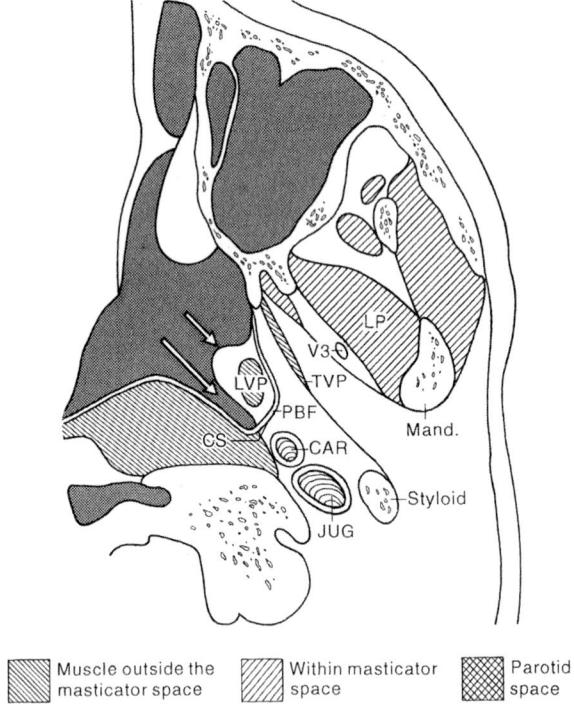

Fig. 8.3 **a** Diagram of the suprahyoid spaces at the level of the nasopharynx *(right)* and oropharynx *(left)*.

b, c Diagram of the fascial layers separating the prestyloid and retrostyloid compartments of the parapharyngeal space and the masticator space.

Fig. 8.3 d–f ▷

Anatomy 583

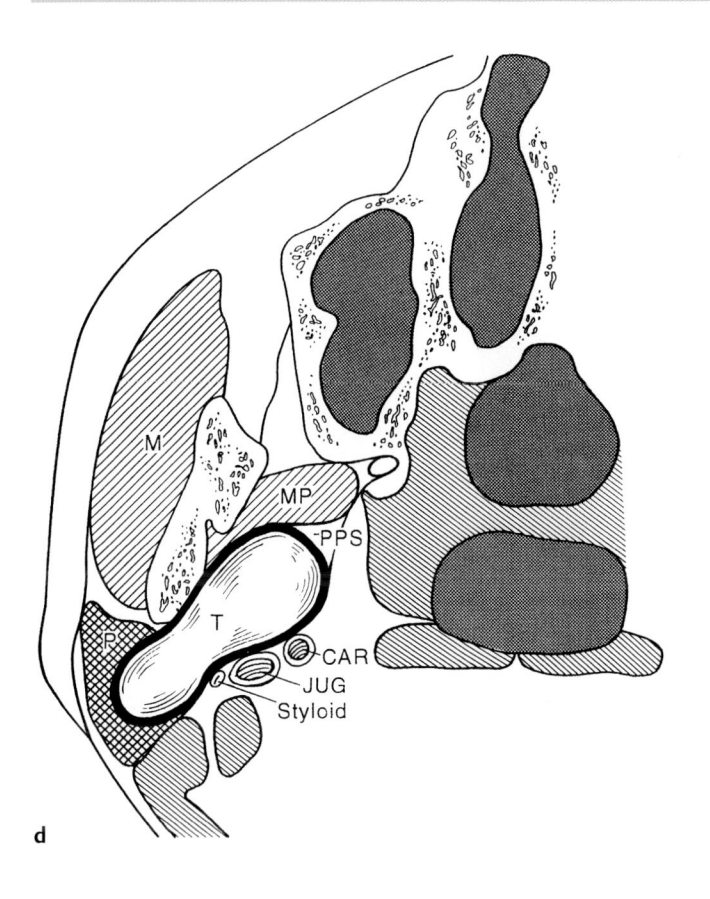

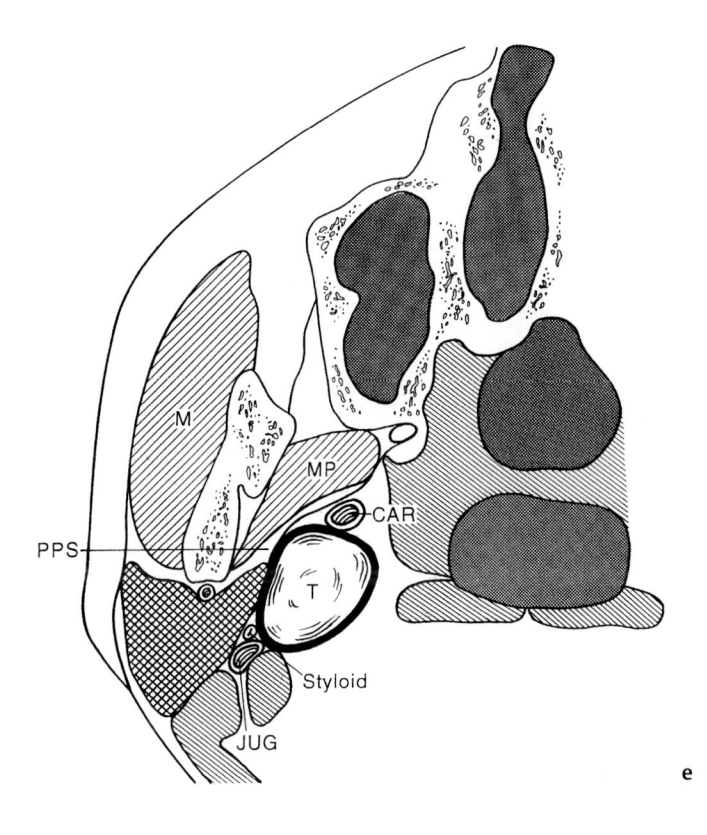

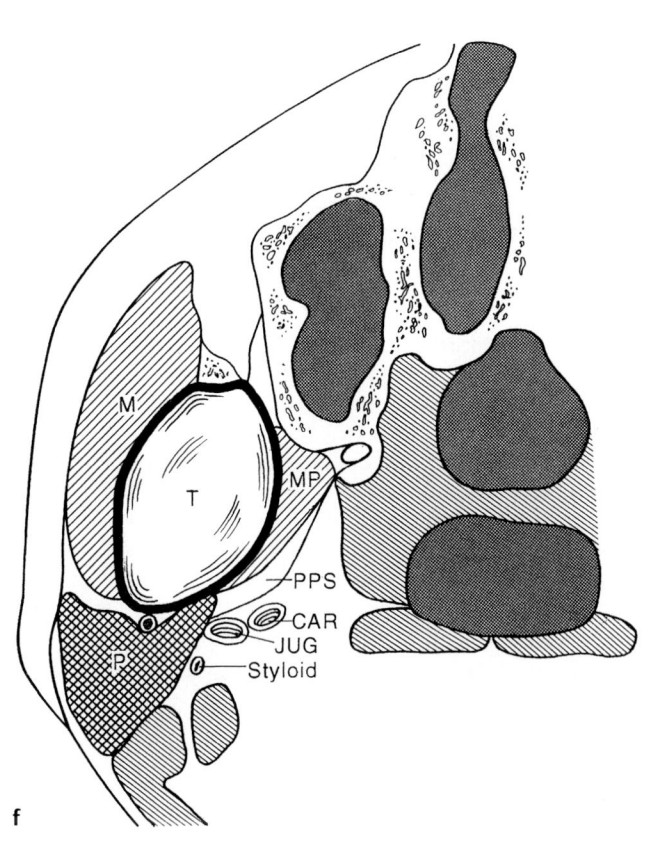

Fig. 8.**3**

- **d** Schematic diagram showing a deep lobe parotid mass. Extension of the mass through a widened stylomandibular tunnel is noted and is common with deep lobe parotid tumors. When extension through the stylomandibular tunnel is not present, careful search for an intervening fat plane between the mass and the parotid gland at every level is necessary before a mass can be considered prestyloid parapharyngeal in origin (see Fig. 8.**17 a–f**).
- **e** Schematic diagram showing a retrostyloid compartment parapharyngeal mass. Characteristic anterolateral displacement of the prestyloid parapharyngeal fat, anterior displacement of the internal carotid artery, lateral displacement of the posterior belly of digastric muscle (not shown in this diagram), and extension posterior to the styloid process are typical findings of a retrostyloid parapharyngeal mass (see Figs. 8.**21**, 8.**22**). Courtesy of Dr. H. Curtin.
- **f** Schematic diagram showing a masticator space mass. Posteromedial displacement of the prestyloid parapharyngeal fat and obliteration of the normal fat planes within the masticator space are characteristic for a masticator space mass.

CAR	internal carotid artery
JUG	internal jugular vein
M	masseter muscle
MP	medial pterygoid muscle
P	parotid gland
PPS	prestyloid compartment of parapharyngeal space
T	tumor

The perivertebral space is enclosed by the circumferential prevertebral fascia and is divided by the fascial attachment to the cervical transverse processes into the anterior prevertebral and posterior paraspinal compartments (Fig. 8.**3a**).[5,6,13] The prevertebral space extends from the skull base to the coccyx and is tight enough to resist the superoinferior spread of infection or neoplasms, because, as mentioned earlier, the prevertebral fascia fuses with the anterior longitudinal ligament at the third thoracic (T3) vertebra level.[17]

The danger space is a thin potential space lying between the prevertebral fascia posteriorly and the alar fascia anteriorly (Fig. 8.**3a**). It is so named because the space, which extends from the skull base to the level of the diaphragm, is filled with loose areolar tissue that provides a ready conduit for the spread of infection.[17]

Middle Layer of Deep Cervical Fascia (Visceral Fascia)

There has been considerable confusion in the literature concerning the layers composing this fascia, with most of the anatomical references focusing mainly on the pretracheal fascia when discussing the fascial layers between the investing and prevertebral fasciae.[1,14] However, it would be more appropriate in this context to stress the layers relevant to the suprahyoid neck in order to give the reader a full understanding of the spatial anatomy of this region. The basic fascial planes comprising the visceral fascia above the hyoid bone include the following.

Buccopharyngeal fascia: This is a thin layer of loose connective tissue, which covers the outer surface of the pharyngeal constrictor muscles (external layer of the epimesium) and permits pharyngeal movement (Figs. 8.**3a**, **c**). It attaches superiorly to the skull base, having the same attachment as the pharyngobasilar fascia (see below), and is continuous anteriorly over the buccinator muscle.[1,5,6,10,16] The buccopharyngeal fascia may not be clearly visible on CT or MR images (see also Chapter 7).[18]

Cloison sagittale: These are bilateral, small, sagittally oriented fascial slips extending from the buccopharyngeal fascia anteriorly to the prevertebral fascia posteriorly, near its attachment to the transverse processes of the cervical vertebrae (Fig. 8.**3c**). The importance of these tiny fascial slips is that they separate the medially positioned retropharyngeal space from the laterally positioned retrostyloid compartment of the parapharyngeal space.[4] These fascial slips are sometimes also termed the alar fascia, but this term is better avoided to prevent confusion with the prevertebral alar fascia described above.[4]

Fascia of tensor veli palatini: This is a relatively thick fascial sheet that envelops the styloid process and its musculature and extends anteromedially to merge with the fascia associated with the tensor veli palatini muscle (Fig. 8.**3b**). It then continues further anteriorly to fuse with the pterygomandibular raphe and buccopharyngeal fascia.[12,20] This fascial layer divides the parapharyngeal space into anterolateral (prestyloid) and posteromedial (retrostyloid) compartments (Fig. 8.**3a**).[12,20]

Pharyngobasilar fascia (pharyngeal aponeurosis): This is an important fourth fascial sheet lying between the superficial and deep layers of deep cervical fascia, but is usually described distinctly from the middle layer. It is a tough membrane that forms an almost closed, very resistant chamber, which determines the configuration of the nasopharynx.[9,18] The pharyngobasilar fascia attaches superiorly to the skull base, extending from the medial pterygoid plates, passing posteriorly to the petrous bones just anterior to the carotid foramina, and reflecting medially on either side to be continuous over the longus capitis and rectus capitis muscles (Fig. 8.**3c**). The fascia descends from the skull base, forming an elongated ring that closes the gaps above the superior constrictor muscle of the pharynx bilaterally. The anatomy references describe the fascia as then continuing lining the inner surface of the pharyngeal musculature (internal layer of the epimesium), thereby supporting the mucous membrane of most of the nasal portion of the pharynx, becoming much thinner inferiorly at about the level of the soft palate.[1,6,10,16,18,19] From the functional and imaging perspectives, the most relevant portion of the pharyngobasilar fascia is that above the superior constrictor muscle; hence the name "pharyngeal aponeurosis" (Fig. 8.**5**) (see also Chapter 7).

Formed of dense fibrous tissue, the pharyngobasilar fascia shows up on MRI images as a low-intensity line extending from the medial pterygoid plate to the carotid foramen medial to the tensor palatini (Fig. 8.**5**).[18]

Thus, the constrictor muscles of the pharynx are "sandwiched" between the pharyngobasilar fascia (inside) and the buccopharyngeal fascia (outside) (Fig. 8.**3**). Above the upper edge of the superior constrictor muscle (between it and the skull base), the two fascial layers blend to form, along with the lining mucosa, the thin wall of the lateral pharyngeal recesses (fossae of Rosenmüller).[1,18,19] Anterior to these recesses, a natural defect in the pharyngobasilar fascia (sinus of Morgagni) exists on each side, transmitting the eustachian tubes and levator veli palatini muscles from the skull base to the pharyngeal mucosal space.[6,10,18,19] The torus tubarius, the most prominent anatomical landmark on the lateral nasopharyngeal wall, is a ridge lying between the orifice of the eustachian tube anteroinferiorly and the fossa of Rosenmüller posterosuperiorly on each side. It is formed by the levator veli palatini muscle together with the cartilaginous eustachian tube and the overlying mucosa..[10,18,19]

■ Face and Neck Spaces

The deep face and neck spaces defined by the above-described layers of visceral fascia include the following.

Pharyngeal Mucosal Space (PMS)

The PMS is the area of the nasopharynx and oropharynx on the inner (airway) side of the buccopharyngeal fascia. The latter separates the PMS from the parapharyngeal space laterally and the retropharyngeal space posteriorly. The PMS is thus composed of the five layers forming the pharyngeal wall. From internal to external, they are:[1]

1 Mucous membrane: The upper part of the nasopharynx is lined by respiratory epithelium (pseudostratified ciliated columnar), while inferiorly, where food contact is more of an issue, the epithelium changes to a stratified squamous type.[19]
2 Submucosa, containing modified minor salivary glands and prominent lymphoid tissue of Waldeyer's ring (adenoids, faucial tonsils, lingual tonsils, and submucosal lymphatics). Lymphoid tissue may also normally be present in the epithelium (lymphoepithelium).[5,6,19]
3 Dense pharyngobasilar fascia.
4 Superior constrictor muscle of the pharynx, above which layers 3 and 5 are adherent and pierced by the eustachian tube (cartilaginous end) and the levator palatini muscle, which are considered within the PMS.
5 Thin buccopharyngeal fascia, forming the outer confinement of the PMS.

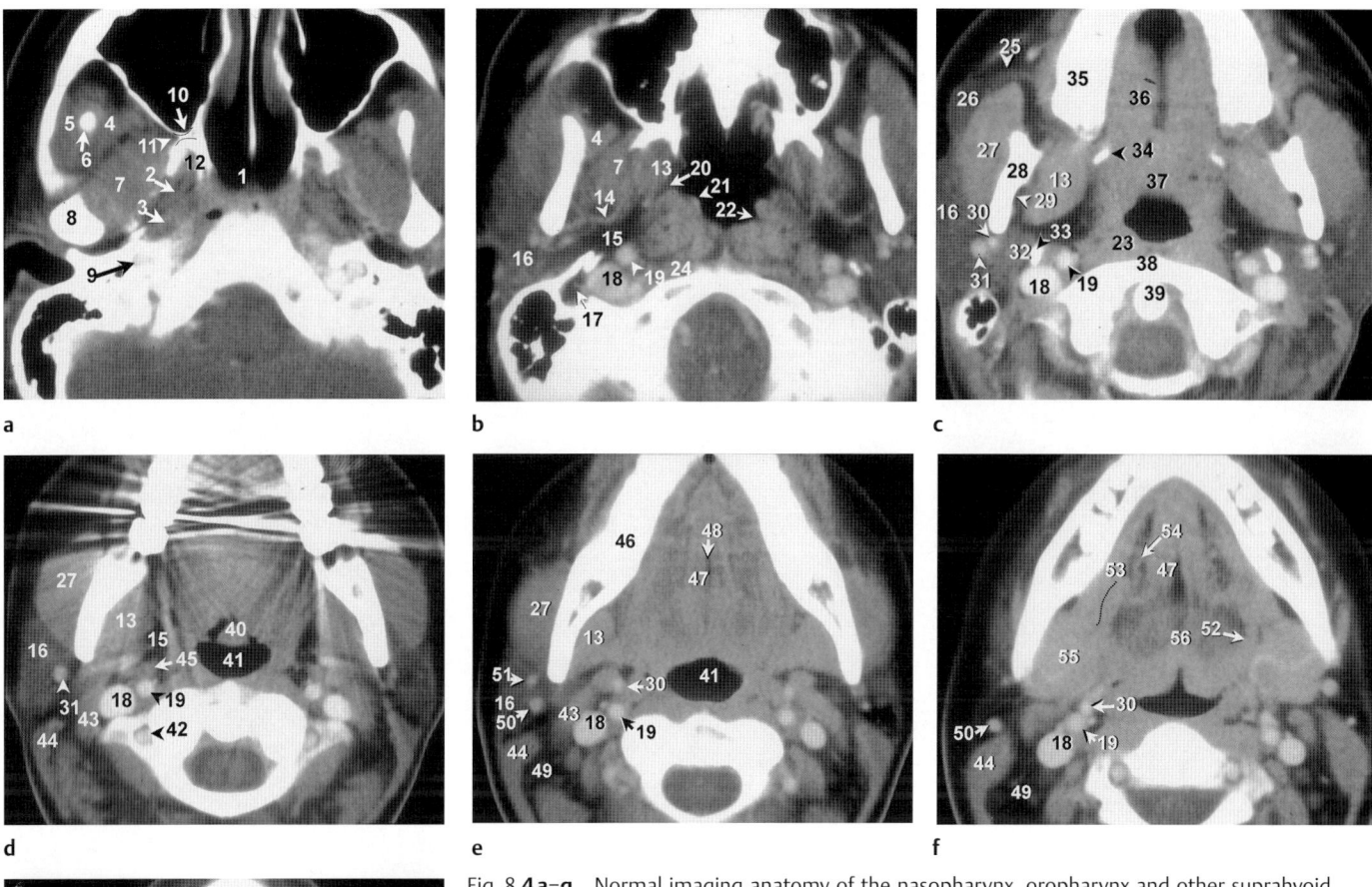

Anatomy 585

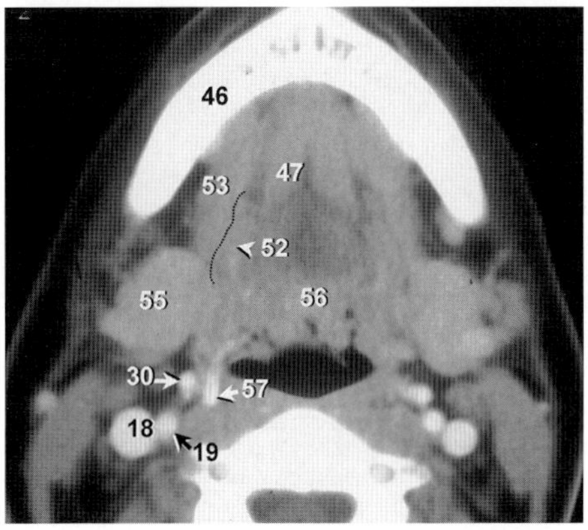

Fig. 8.**4a–g** Normal imaging anatomy of the nasopharynx, oropharynx and other suprahyoid neck structures on contrast-enhanced axial CT scan (5 mm slice thickness). 1 = Nasopharyngeal airway; 2 = tensor veli palatini muscle; 3 = levator veli palatini muscle; 4 = temporalis muscle (deep = medial head); 5 = temporalis muscle (superficial = lateral head); 6 = coronoid process of the mandible; 7 = lateral pterygoid muscle; 8 = condylar process of the mandible; 9 = internal carotid artery in the vertical segment of petrous canal; 10 = pterygopalatine fossa (basal part); 11 = pterygomaxillary fissure; 12 = pterygoid fossa between the medial and lateral pterygoid plates; 13 = medial pterygoid muscle; 14 = internal maxillary vessels; 15 = fat in prestyloid compartment of parapharyngeal space; 16 = parotid gland (superficial lobe); 17 = facial nerve surrounded by fat in stylomastoid foramen; 18 = internal jugular vein; 19 = internal carotid artery; 20 = eustachian tube orifice; 21 = torus tubarius overlying levator veli palatini muscle; 22 = lateral pharyngeal recess (fossa of Rosenmüller); 23 = longus capitis muscle; 24 = rectus capitis anterior muscle; 25 = parotid (Stensen's) duct; 26 = accessory parotid tissue; 27 = masseter muscle; 28 = ramus of the mandible; 29 = mandibular foramen; 30 = external carotid artery; 31 = retromandibular vein (lying superficial to external carotid artery); 32 = deep lobe of the parotid gland extending through the stylomandibular tunnel; 33 = styloid process; 34 = pterygoid hamulus (projecting inferiorly from the medial pterygoid plate); 35 = alveolar process of the maxilla; 36 = hard palate; 37 = soft palate; 38 = anterior arch of atlas (C1 vertebra); 39 = odontoid process (dens); 40 = uvula; 41 = oropharyngeal airway; 42 = vertebral artery in foramen transversarium; 43 = posterior belly of digastric muscle; 44 = sternocleidomastoid muscle; 45 = styloid musculature; 46 = body of the mandible; 47 = genioglossus/geniohyoid muscles; 48 = lingual septum; 49 = fat in posterior cervical space; 50 = external jugular vein; 51 = posterior facial vein (communicating the retromandibular vein with the facial vein); 52 = hyoglossus muscle; 53 = mylohyoid muscle; 54 = lingual artery within fat in sublingual space; 55 = submandibular gland; 56 = tongue base; 57 = superior cornu of hyoid bone. Reproduced from Reference 4 with permission.

Retropharyngeal Space (RPS)

The RPS is a small potential space that is bounded:[4,6]
- *Anteriorly* by the buccopharyngeal fascia, separating it from the pharyngeal mucosal space (Figs. 8.**3a, c**).
- *Posteriorly* by the prevertebral fascia, separating it from the prevertebral space.
- *Laterally* by the cloison sagittale, separating it from the retrostyloid compartment of the parapharyngeal space on each side (Fig. 8.**3c**).[4]
- *Superiorly* by the skull base.
- *Inferiorly* by the fusion of the buccopharyngeal and prevertebral fasciae between the T2 and T6 spinal levels.[21]

The RPS normally contains a small amount of fat and, in the suprahyoid region, the lateral (nodes of Rouvière) and medial retropharyngeal lymph nodes.[5,21]

The medial retropharyngeal lymph nodes are located near the midline, and are seldom seen in adults unless pathologically enlarged.[21,22] The lateral retropharyngeal (LRP) lymph nodes are found immediately medial to the internal carotid artery, adjacent

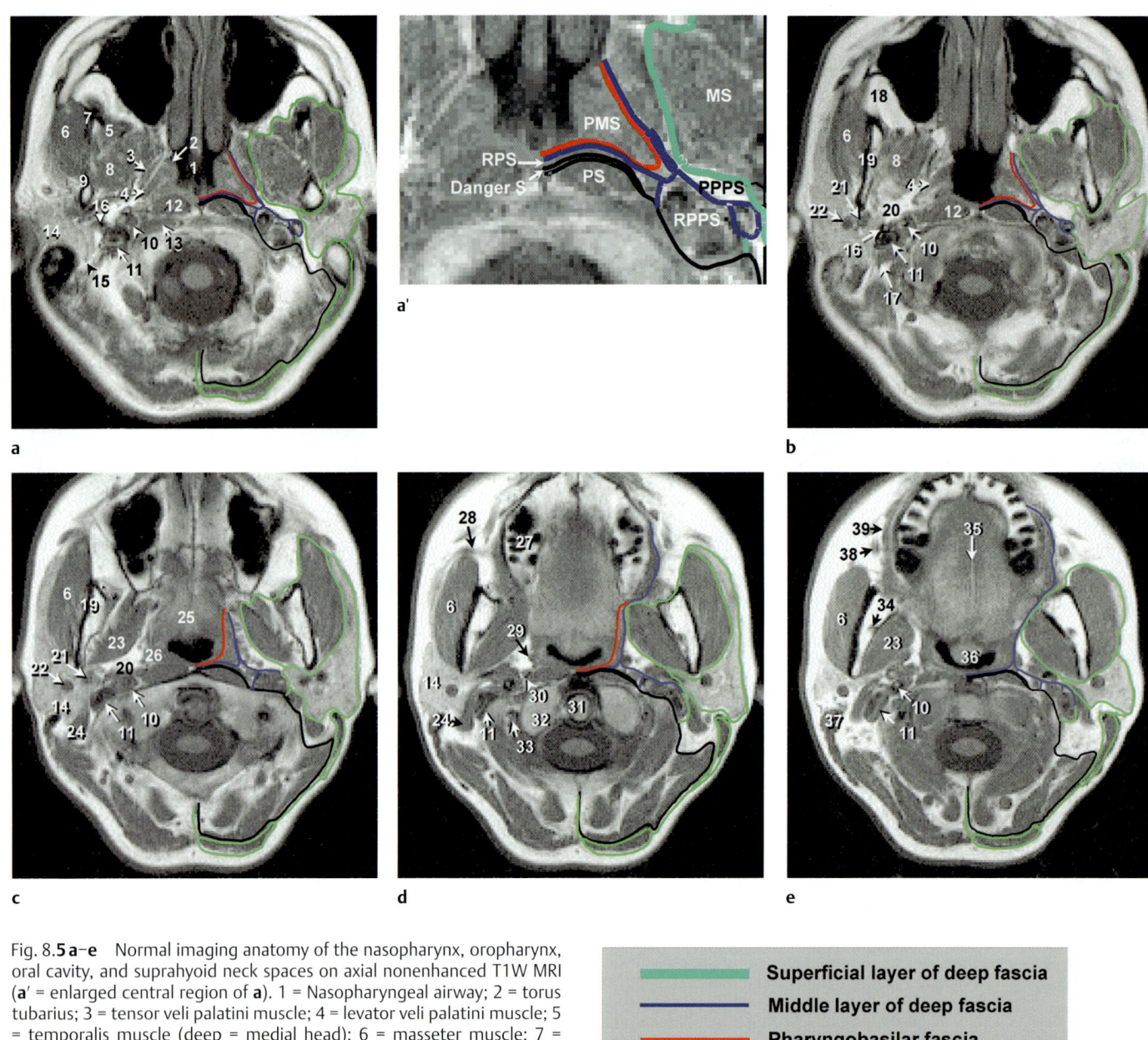

586   8 Parapharyngeal and Masticator Spaces

Fig. 8.5 a–e Normal imaging anatomy of the nasopharynx, oropharynx, oral cavity, and suprahyoid neck spaces on axial nonenhanced T1W MRI (a' = enlarged central region of a). 1 = Nasopharyngeal airway; 2 = torus tubarius; 3 = tensor veli palatini muscle; 4 = levator veli palatini muscle; 5 = temporalis muscle (deep = medial head); 6 = masseter muscle; 7 = coronoid process of the mandible; 8 = lateral pterygoid muscle; 9 = neck of the mandible; 10 = internal carotid artery; 11 = internal jugular vein; 12 = longus capitis muscle; 13 = rectus capitis anterior muscle; 14 = parotid gland (superficial lobe); 15 = facial nerve emerging from the stylomastoid foramen and entering the parotid gland; 16 = styloid process; 17 = rectus capitis lateralis muscle; 18 = fat in infratemporal fossa; 19 = ramus of the mandible; 20 = fat in prestyloid compartment of parapharyngeal space; 21 = external carotid artery; 22 = retromandibular vein; 23 = medial pterygoid muscle; 24 = posterior belly of digastric muscle; 25 = soft palate; 26 = superior constrictor muscle of the pharynx; 27 = alveolar process of the maxilla; 28 = parotid (Stensen's) duct; 29 = ascending pharyngeal artery overlying the superior constrictor muscle of the pharynx; 30 = lateral retropharyngeal lymph node (of Rouvière); 31 = odontoid process (dens); 32 = lateral mass of atlas (C1 vertebra); 33 = vertebral artery in foramen transversarium; 34 = mandibular foramen transmitting inferior alveolar nerve and vessels; 35 = lingual septum; 36 = uvula; 37 = sternocleidomastoid muscle; 38 = anterior facial vein; 39 = buccinator muscle; 40 = genioglossus/geniohyoid muscles; 41 = external jugular vein; 42 = fat in posterior cervical space; 43 = hyoglossus muscle; 44 = mylohyoid muscle; 45 = fat in sublingual space; 46 = submandibular gland; 47 = oropharyngeal airway; 48 = tongue base; 49 = body of the mandible. PMS = pharyngeal mucosal space; RPS = retropharyngeal space; PS = perivertebral space; MS = masticator space; PPPS = prestyloid parapharyngeal space; RPPS = retrostyloid parapharyngeal space (carotid space). Reproduced from Reference 4 with permission.

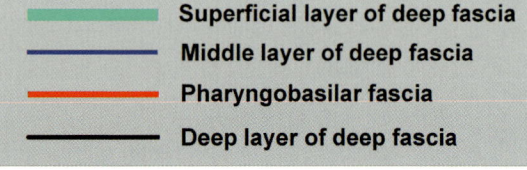

- ▬▬▬ Superficial layer of deep fascia
- ▬▬▬ Middle layer of deep fascia
- ▬▬▬ Pharyngobasilar fascia
- ▬▬▬ Deep layer of deep fascia

Fig. 8.5 f–i ▷

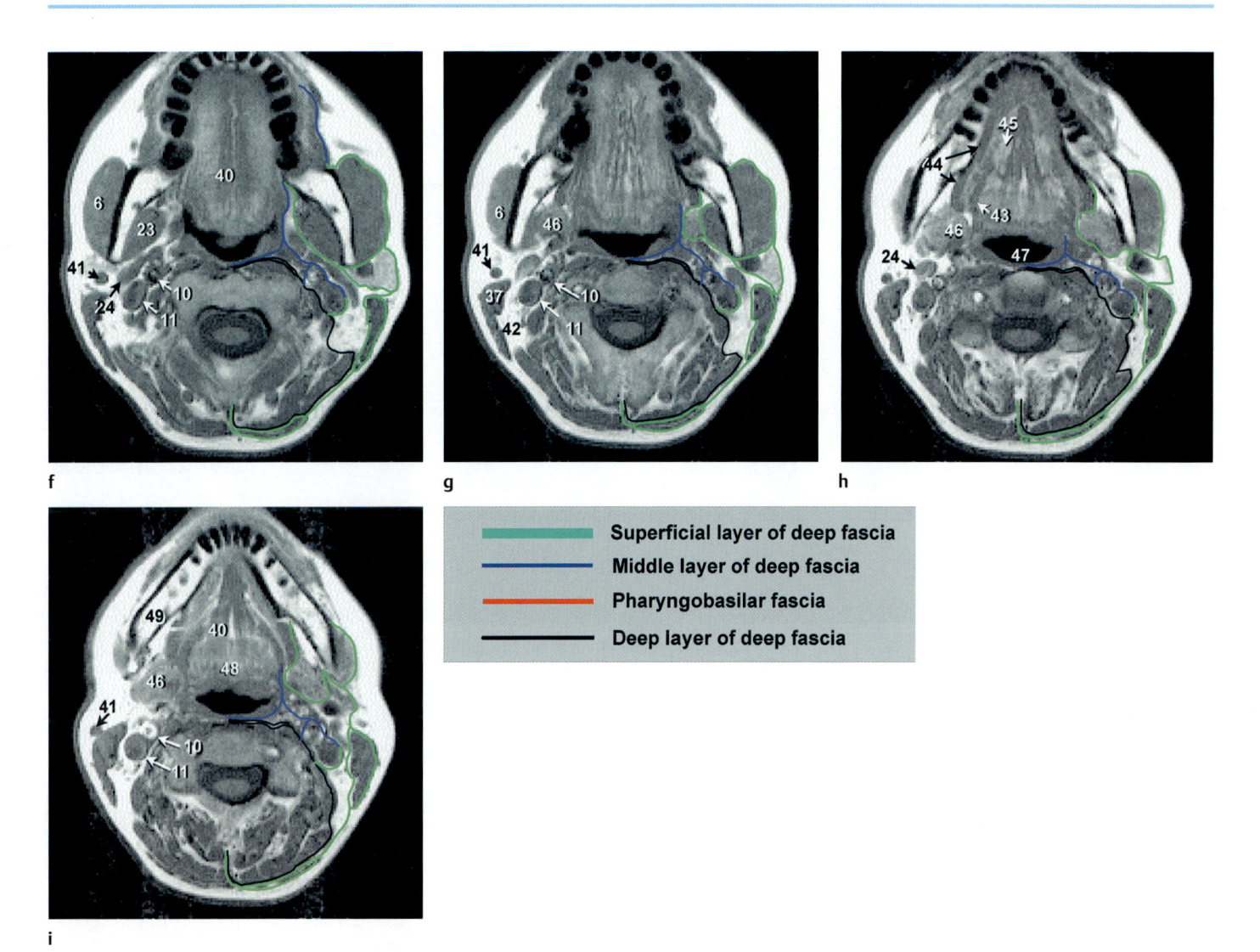

Fig. 8.5 f–i Normal imaging anatomy of the nasopharynx, oropharynx, oral cavity, and suprahyoid neck spaces on axial nonenhanced T1W MRI. 1 = Nasopharyngeal airway; 2 = torus tubarius; 3 = tensor veli palatini muscle; 4 = levator veli palatini muscle; 5 = temporalis muscle (deep = medial head); 6 = masseter muscle; 7 = coronoid process of the mandible; 8 = lateral pterygoid muscle; 9 = neck of the mandible; 10 = internal carotid artery; 11 = internal jugular vein; 12 = longus capitis muscle; 13 = rectus capitis anterior muscle; 14 = parotid gland (superficial lobe); 15 = facial nerve emerging from the stylomastoid foramen and entering the parotid gland; 16 = styloid process; 17 = rectus capitis lateralis muscle; 18 = fat in infratemporal fossa; 19 = ramus of the mandible; 20 = fat in prestyloid compartment of parapharyngeal space; 21 = external carotid artery; 22 = retromandibular vein; 23 = medial pterygoid muscle; 24 = posterior belly of digastric muscle; 25 = soft palate; 26 = superior constrictor muscle of the pharynx; 27 = alveolar process of the maxilla; 28 = parotid (Stensen's) duct; 29 = ascending pharyngeal artery overlying the superior constrictor muscle of the pharynx; 30 = lateral retropharyngeal lymph node (of Rouvière); 31 = odontoid process (dens); 32 = lateral mass of atlas (C1 vertebra); 33 = vertebral artery in foramen transversarium; 34 = mandibular foramen transmitting inferior alveolar nerve and vessels; 35 = lingual septum; 36 = uvula; 37 = sternocleidomastoid muscle; 38 = anterior facial vein; 39 = buccinator muscle; 40 = genioglossus/geniohyoid muscles; 41 = external jugular vein; 42 = fat in posterior cervical space; 43 = hyoglossus muscle; 44 = mylohyoid muscle; 45 = fat in sublingual space; 46 = submandibular gland; 47 = oropharyngeal airway; 48 = tongue base; 49 = body of the mandible. PMS = pharyngeal mucosal space; RPS = retropharyngeal space; PS = perivertebral space; MS = masticator space; PPPS = prestyloid parapharyngeal space; RPPS = retrostyloid parapharyngeal space (carotid space). Reproduced from Reference 4 with permission.

to the longus capitis muscle, and are usually most prominent at the C1–C2 level but can occasionally be visualized down to the level of the palate.[21–23] The LRP nodes are usually identified on MRI and to a lesser extent on CT. In adults, they are usually smaller than 3–5 mm, but nodes of up to 1 cm can be considered normal provided they are homogeneous.[21,23] In children, the LRP nodes may be up to 2 cm in size, particularly in those with prominent adenoids.[22] This lymph node chain provides drainage for the nasopharynx, oropharynx, middle ear, nasal cavities, and paranasal sinuses.[17,22]

588   8 Parapharyngeal and Masticator Spaces

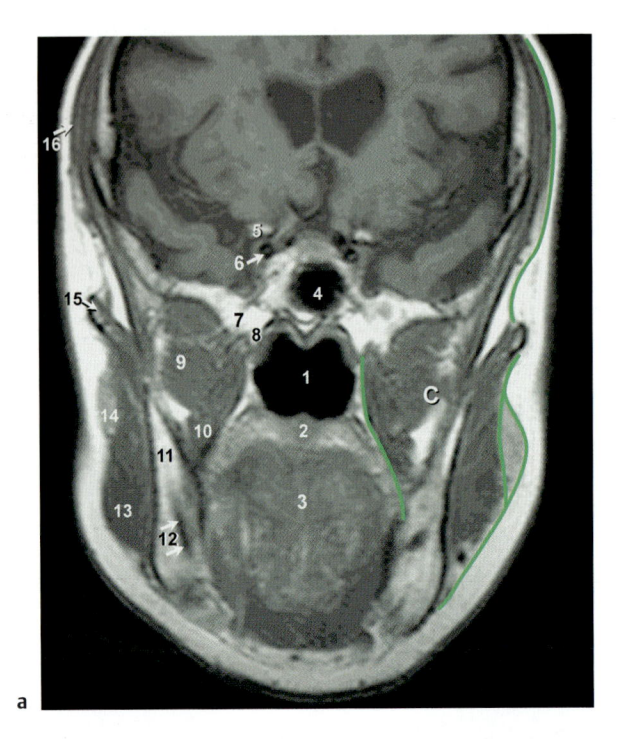

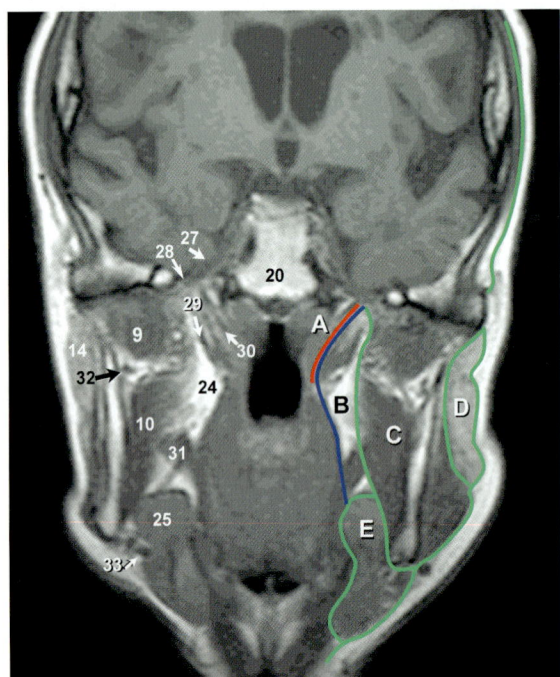

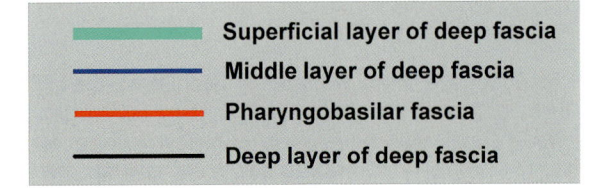

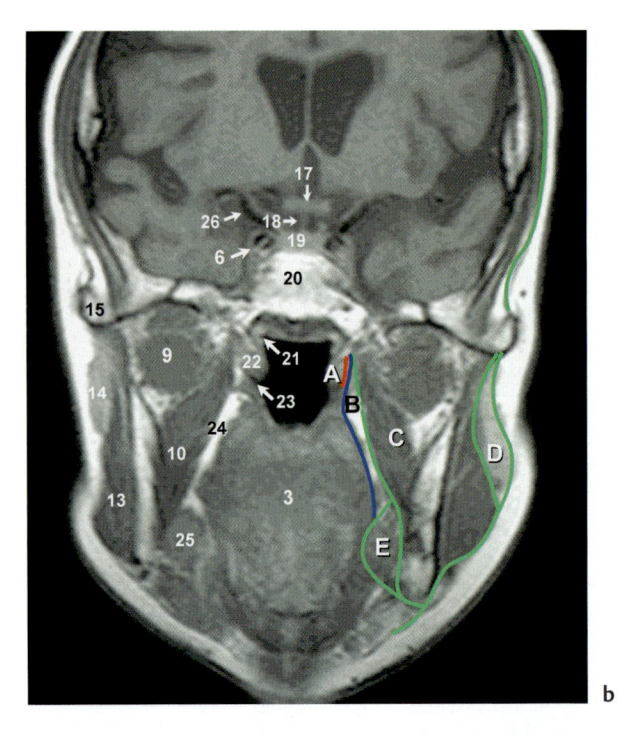

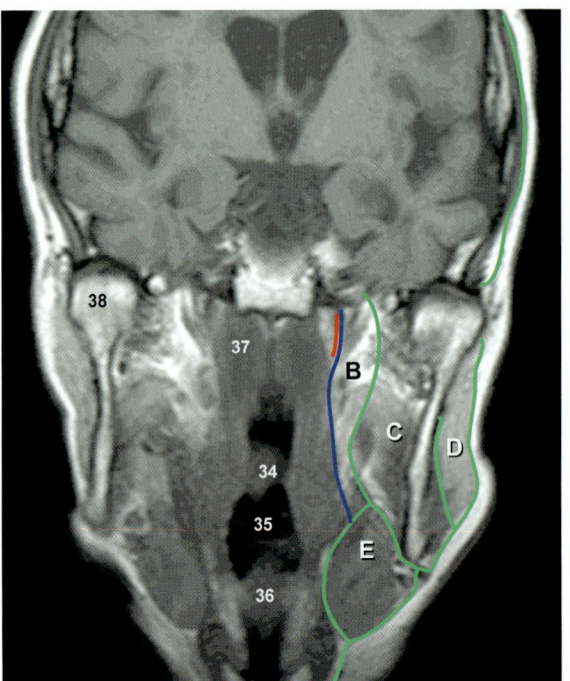

	Superficial layer of deep fascia
	Middle layer of deep fascia
	Pharyngobasilar fascia
	Deep layer of deep fascia

Fig. 8.6 a–d Normal imaging anatomy of the nasopharynx, oropharynx, oral cavity, and suprahyoid neck spaces on coronal nonenhanced T1W MRI. 1 = Nasopharyngeal airway; 2 = soft palate; 3 = tongue; 4 = sphenoid sinus; 5 = anterior clinoid process; 6 = internal carotid artery; 7 = greater wing of sphenoid bone; 8 = root of medial pterygoid plate of sphenoid bone; 9 = lateral pterygoid muscle; 10 = medial pterygoid muscle; 11 = ramus of the mandible; 12 = mandibular canal; 13 = masseter muscle; 14 = parotid gland; 15 = zygomatic arch; 16 = temporalis muscle; 17 = optic chiasm; 18 = pituitary stalk; 19 = pituitary gland; 20 = clivus; 21 = fossa of Rosenmüller (lateral pharyngeal recess); 22 = torus tubarius overlying levator veli palatini muscle; 23 = eustachian tube opening; 24 = fat in prestyloid parapharyngeal space; 25 = submandibular salivary gland; 26 = middle cerebral artery; 27 = mandibular division of trigeminal nerve; 28 = foramen ovale; 29 = tensor veli palatini muscle; 30 = levator veli palatini muscle; 31 = styloglossus muscle; 32 = internal maxillary artery; 33 = facial vein; 34 = uvula; 35 = oropharyngeal airway; 36 = epiglottis; 37 = longus capitis muscle; 38 = head of mandible. A = Pharyngeal mucosal space (PMS); B = prestyloid parapharyngeal space (PPPS); C = masticator space (MS); D = parotid space (PS); E = submandibular space. Reproduced from Reference 4 with permission.

Parapharyngeal Space (PPS)

The parapharyngeal space is an anatomical recess shaped like an inverted pyramid with its base at the base of the skull and its apex at the greater cornu of the hyoid bone. It occupies the space between the muscles of mastication and the deglutitional muscles.[12, 13, 20, 24, 25] It has the following boundaries and relations:

- **Laterally**: *Anterolaterally*: separated from the masticator space by the layer of investing fascia covering the medial aspect of the medial pterygoid muscle (Fig. 8.3).[6, 10, 19, 20]
  Posterolaterally: separated from the parotid space by the layer of investing fascia covering the deep lobe of the parotid gland (Figs. 8.3a, 8.5).[10, 20] However, this is a sparse fascial layer that does not present a barrier to the spread of disease.[4]
- **Medially**: Separated from the PMS by the buccopharyngeal fascia, while its extreme posterior part is separated from the RPS by the cloison sagittale (Fig. 8.3).[6, 20, 26]
- **Posteriorly**: Separated from the prevertebral space by the prevertebral fascia.[10, 20, 26]
- **Anteriorly**: *Anterosuperiorly* (at the level of the pterygomandibular raphe): closed by the convergence of the buccopharyngeal fascia with the fascia covering the medial aspect of the medial pterygoid muscle (Fig. 8.5).[10, 4]
  Anteroinferiorly (at the level of the mylohyoid muscle): the PPS is often continuous with the sublingual and submandibular spaces, thereby allowing lesions to pass from one space to another without crossing a fascial boundary.[5, 16, 27]
- **Inferiorly**: The PPS is generally described as extending down to the hyoid bone. However, the fusion of multiple fascial layers and muscle sheaths near the angle of the mandible limits the caudal extent of the space,[4] and the styloglossus muscle can be considered the functional inferior boundary of the PPS.[4]

The PPS as defined above is a larger area of the deep face than the fatty triangles seen on either side of the pharynx. This definition, which is supported by most authors, implies the division of the PPS by the fascia of tensor veli palatini (see above) into:[4, 25]

- **Prestyloid PPS**: anterolateral to the fascia.
- **Retrostyloid PPS**: posteromedial to the fascia. This is the suprahyoid extension of the **carotid space** (carotid sheath and its contents) (Figs. 8.3, 8.5).

The contents of the suprahyoid neck spaces along with the common disease processes involving each space are listed in Table 8.1.

Normal Imaging Anatomy

The anatomy of the normal suprahyoid neck as seen on CT and MRI is demonstrated in Figs. 8.3–8.6.

Table 8.1 Anatomical spaces of the suprahyoid neck: their contents and common disease processes.[4, 5–7, 12, 13, 24] Bold type indicates the most common lesions

Space	Contents	Differential diagnosis of lesions

1. Pharyngeal mucosal space (PMS)	1. Mucosa
	2. Submucosa containing:
	  – minor salivary glands
	  – lymphoid tissue (adenoids, faucial, and lingual tonsils)
	3. Pharyngobasilar fascia
	4. Superior and middle constrictor pharyngeal muscles
	5. Buccopharyngeal fascia (enclosing layer)
	plus originating outside PMS:
	  Cartilaginous eustachian tube
	  Levator palatini muscle
		Pseudomass
		• Asymmetric fossae of Rosenmüller
		• Pharyngitis:
		  – infectious
		  – postirradiation
		Congenital
		• Tornwaldt's cyst
		Inflammatory
		• **Adenoidal/tonsillar: hypertrophy/inflammation/abscess**
		• Postinflammatory:
		  – dystrophic calcification
		  – retention cyst
		Benign tumor
		• **Juvenile angiofibroma**
		• Hemangioma
		• Pleomorphic adenoma (benign mixed tumor) of minor salivary glands
		• Rhabdomyoma
		Malignant tumor
		• **Squamous cell carcinoma**
		• **Non-Hodgkin lymphoma**
		• Minor salivary gland malignancy
		• Rhabdomyosarcoma (pediatric)

CS, carotid space
MS, masticator space
PMS, pharyngeal mucosal space
PPPS, prestyloid parapharyngeal space
PS, parotid space
PVS, perivertebral space
RPPS, retrostyloid prapharangeal space
RPS, retropharyngeal space
ICA, internal carotid artery
IJV, internal jugular vein
AVM, arteriovenous malformation
ECA, external carotid artery

Table 8.1 Anatomical spaces of the suprahyoid neck: their contents and common disease processes.[4, 5–7, 12, 13, 24] Bold type indicates the most common lesions (continued)

Space	Contents	Differential diagnosis of lesions

2. Prestyloid parapharyngeal space (PPPS)	1. Fat
	2. Pterygoid venous plexus
	3. Internal maxillary artery
	4. Ascending pharyngeal artery
	5. Branches of the mandibular division (V3) of trigeminal nerve
		Pseudomass
		• **Asymmetric pterygoid venous plexus**
		
		Congenital
		• 2nd branchial cleft cyst
		
		Inflammatory
		• Spread of infection from adjacent spaces:
		  — PMS: pharyngitis, adenoiditis, tonsillitis, peritonsillar abscess, retromandibular vein thrombosis
		  — PS: parotid calculus disease, deep lobe parotid abscess
		  — MS: dental infection, 3rd upper molar extraction with violation of pterygomandibular raphae
		• Infection secondary to penetrating trauma to the lateral pharyngeal wall
		
		Benign tumor
		• Pleomorphic adenoma (benign mixed tumor):
		  — extending from deep lobe of parotid
		  — arising from salivary gland rests in PPS
		• Lipoma
		• Schwannoma
		
		Malignant tumor
		• Mucoepidermoid carcinoma, adenoid cystic carcinoma, malignant mixed tumor of salivary gland rest in PPS
		• Hemangiopericytoma
		• **Spread of malignancy from adjacent spaces:**
		  — PMS: sqamous cell carcinoma, non-Hodgkin lymphoma, minor salivary gland malignancy
		  — PS: mucoepidermoid carcinoma, adenoid cystic carcinoma
		  — MS : sarcoma
		• Metastases (kidney, prostate)
		  — Skull base tumor

3. Retrostyloid parapharyngeal space (RPPS) = carotid space (CS)	1. Internal carotid artery (ICA)
	2. Internal jugular vein (IJV)
	3. Lower 4 cranial nerves (IX–XII)
	4. Sympathetic chain
	5. Lymph nodes (deep cervical chain)
		Pseudomass
		• **Ectatic ICA.**
		• **Asymmetric IJVs**
		
		Inflammatory
		• Carotid space cellulitis or abscess:
		  — spread from adjacent spaces
		  — breakdown of infected internal jugular lymph nodes
		
		Vascular
		• **IJV thrombosis or thrombophlebitis**
		• **ICA thrombosis, mural thrombus, aneurysm, pseudoaneurysm, or dissection**
		
		Benign tumor
		• **Paraganglioma:**
		  — Glomus jugulare
		  — Glomus vagale.
		  — Carotid body tumor
		• Nerve sheath tumor:
		  — **Schwannoma**
		  — Neurofibroma
		• Meningioma (of jugular foramen)
		
		Malignant tumor
		• **Lymph node metastasis from squamous cell carcinoma**
		• Direct invasion by primary squamous cell carcinoma
		• Non-Hodgkin lymphoma
		• Hemangiopericytoma
		• Aggressive fibromatosis
		• Metastatic deposit (lung, breast, kidney, prostate, and thyroid) to undersurface of temporal bone

CS, carotid space
MS, masticator space
PMS, pharyngeal mucosal space
PPPS, prestyloid parapharyngeal space
PS, parotid space
PVS, perivertebral space
RPPS, retrostyloid prapharangeal space
RPS, retropharyngeal space
ICA, internal carotid artery
IJV, internal jugular vein
AVM, arteriovenous malformation
ECA, external carotid artery

Table 8.1 Anatomical spaces of the suprahyoid neck: their contents and common disease processes.[4, 5-7, 12, 13, 24] Bold type indicates the most common lesions (continued)

Space	Contents	Differential diagnosis of lesions

4. Retropharyngeal space (RPS)	1. Fat
	2. Lymph nodes:
	  – lateral retropharyngeal (of Rouvière)
	  – medial retropharyngeal
		Pseudomass
		• Tortuous ICA
		• Edema fluid or lymph spilling into the RPS secondary to venous or lymphatic obstruction
		
		Congenital
		• Hemangioma
		• Lymphangioma
		
		Inflammatory
		• **Reactive adenopathy**
		• **Suppurative adenopathy (intranodal abscess)**
		• **Cellulitis/abscess**
		
		Benign tumor
		• Lipoma
		
		Malignant tumor
		• **Nodal metastases:**
		  – **Squamous cell carcinoma of head and neck (most common: nasopharynx)**
		  – Melanoma
		  – Thyroid carcinoma
		• **Nodal non-Hodgkin lymphoma**
		• **Direct invasion from primary squamous cell carcinoma (especially posterior wall primary lesions)**
		• Direct invasion of extra-axial cranial tumors such as meningioma and chordoma

5. Masticator space (MS)	1. Mandible (ramus + posterior body)
	2. Muscles of mastication:
	  – lateral pterygoid
	  – medial pterygoid
	  – masseter
	  – temporalis
	3. Inferior alveolar and lingual nerves (branches of the mandibular division V3 of trigeminal nerve)
		Pseudomass
		• Accessory parotid gland
		• Benign masseteric hypertrophy (unilateral/bilateral)
		• Mandibular nerve (cranial nerve V3) denervation atrophy
		
		Congenital
		• Hemangioma and AVM
		• Lymphangioma/cystic hygroma
		• Developmental cysts of mandible
		
		Inflammatory
		• **Odontogenic abscess (especially lower 2nd/3rd molar)**
		• Mandibular osteomyelitis
		• Extension of necrotizing external otitis into MS
		
		Benign tumor
		• Nerve sheath tumor (schwannoma–neurofibroma)
		• Osteoblastoma.
		• Giant-cell tumor of mandible
		• Leiomyoma
		• Fibromyxoma of mandible
		
		Malignant tumor
		• **Sarcoma: chondrosarcoma/osteosarcoma/soft-tissue sarcoma**
		• Malignant schwannoma
		• **Non-Hodgkin lymphoma**
		• **Infiltrating squamous cell carcinoma from the oropharynx (retromolar trigone)**
		• **Rhabdomyosarcoma (pediatrics)**
		• Mandibular metastases (from carcinoma of lung/breast/kidney)

CS, carotid space
MS, masticator space
PMS, pharyngeal mucosal space
PPPS, prestyloid parapharyngeal space
PS, parotid space
PVS, perivertebral space
RPPS, retrostyloid prapharangeal space
RPS, retropharyngeal space
ICA, internal carotid artery
IJV, internal jugular vein
AVM, arteriovenous malformation
ECA, external carotid artery

Table 8.1 Anatomical spaces of the suprahyoid neck: their contents and common disease processes.[4, 5–7, 12, 13, 24] Bold type indicates the most common lesions (continued)

Space	Contents	Differential diagnosis of lesions

6. Parotid space (PS)	1. Parotid gland
	2. Facial nerve VII
	3. External carotid artery (ECA) (terminating in the parotid gland into internal maxillary and superficial temporal arteries)
	4. Retromandibular vein
	5. Intraparotid and periparotid lymph nodes
		Congenital
		• First branchial cleft cyst
		• Hemangioma (pediatric)
		• Lymphangioma (pediatric)
		
		Inflammatory
		• Cellulitis/abscess
		• Benign lymphoepithelial lesions (AIDS)
		• Reactive adenopathy
		• Granuloma (sarcoidosis), Kimura disease
		
		Benign tumor
		• **Pleomorphic adenoma (benign mixed tumor)**
		• **Warthin tumor (papillary cystadenoma lymphomatosum)**
		• Oncocytoma
		• Lipoma
		• Facial nerve schwannoma or neurofibroma
		
		Malignant tumor
		• *Primary*
		  — **Carcinoma:**
		    mucoepidermoid
		    adenoid cystic
		    acinous cell
		    squamous cell
		  — Non-Hodgkin lymphoma
		  — Malignant mixed tumor
		• ***Metastatic (within parotid nodes)***
		  — **Squamous cell carcinoma of scalp**
		  — **Melanoma of scalp**
		  — Non-Hodgkin lymphoma

7. Perivertebral space (PVS)	1. Prevertebral muscles
	2. Scalene muscles
	3. Vertebral arteries and veins
	4. Brachial plexus
	5. Phrenic nerve
		Pseudomass
		• **Vertebral body osteophyte**
		• Anterior disk herniation
		
		Inflammatory
		• **Vertebral body osteomyelitis (pyogenic/TB)**
		• Cellulitis/abscess
		
		Vascular
		• Vertebral artery dissection, aneurysm, or pseudoaneurysm
		
		Benign tumor
		• Schwannoma/neurofibroma (cervical nerve roots/brachial plexus)
		• Vertebral body benign bony tumors
		
		Malignant tumor
		• *Primary*
		  — **Chordoma**
		  — Non-Hodgkin lymphoma
		  — Vertebral body primary malignant tumor
		• ***Metastatic***
		  — **Vertebral body or epidural metastases**
		  — Direct invasion of squamous cell carcinoma

CS, carotid space
MS, masticator space
PMS, pharyngeal mucosal space
PPPS, prestyloid parapharyngeal space
PS, parotid space
PVS, perivertebral space
RPPS, retrostyloid prapharangeal space
RPS, retropharyngeal space
ICA, internal carotid artery
IJV, internal jugular vein
AVM, arteriovenous malformation
ECA, external carotid artery

Imaging Rationale and Techniques

CT and MRI are currently the primary modalities for investigating the suprahyoid neck. This region, which extends from the skull base to the hyoid bone, is surrounded for the most part by bones that limit external clinical examination. In addition, while the superficial extent of mucosal lesions can be readily identified by the examining physician, their deep extent and lesions confined to the deep spaces are almost totally inaccessible for clinical or endoscopic evaluation.

In many cases of suprahyoid neck masses, MRI demonstrates advantages over CT[5] because of its higher soft-tissue contrast resolution, multiplanar capability, and superiority for detecting perineural and perivascular tumor spread and intracranial invasion.

Computed Tomography

Patient Positioning

Patients are examined in the supine position for axial scans and in the prone position for direct coronal scans. The latter should be performed whenever a nasopharyngeal or palatal mass is suspected as well as when skull base erosion is in question.[10] Scanning is done during suspended respiration and attention must always be paid to proper head position.[10]

Intravenous Contrast

A confident assessment of the possible cervical lymphadenopathy associated with nasopharyngeal/oropharyngeal pathology requires optimal vascular opacification with an iodinated contrast medium. This is achieved by delivering a loading bolus (50 ml, 2 ml/s) via a power injector, followed by continuous contrast infusion (1 ml/s).[10]

Acquisition Parameters

A preliminary lateral scout is obtained. Axial scans are planned parallel to the infraorbital–meatal line and should cover the whole region from the external auditory canal to the upper border of the manubrium sterni. Such extended coverage ensures proper evaluation of the pharynx, the skull base, and all the node-bearing areas. Examination is best performed with 3–5 mm thick contiguous slices and a small field of view (FOV). An additional high-resolution bone reconstruction algorithm should be used to evaluate any pathological bone involvement.[10, 4]

Magnetic Resonance Imaging

Patient Positioning

Axial, sagittal, and coronal scans are all obtainable without the need to reposition the supine patient. A head coil is convenient for scanning the nasopharynx and oropharynx. In patients with malignancies, as the entire neck has to be evaluated for nodal disease, a dedicated neck coil must be used in addition to cover the area from the mouth floor to the supraclavicular region.[10, 18, 19] Besides head motion, pharyngeal motion, e.g., swallowing and snoring, must also be prevented in order to ensure optimal image quality.[10]

Intravenous Contrast

Post-intravenous gadolinium-DTPA T1-weighted studies are helpful for the detection of pathological lesions. Such images improve the visualization of small lesions; they provide excellent evaluation of lesion extension, subtle infiltration, and perineural spread, and they aid in the assessment of tumor recurrence following radiotherapy or surgery.[6, 8, 28, 29]

Pulse Sequences and Acquisition Parameters

In general, T1-weighted images provide the best fat/muscle and fat/tumor contrast, while T2-weighted images provide the best muscle/lymphoid tissue contrast.[10, 30, 31]

The axial plane is often most useful, and both axial T1- and T2-weighted images, encompassing at least the region from the palate to the hyoid bone, should be performed in all cases. It is recommended to acquire T2-weighted images using fast spin-echo with fat-suppression technique as this has been proven to yield very high lesion conspicuity.[6, 32]

Coronal T1-weighted images improve the evaluation of lesions adjacent to the skull base and within the submandibular or sublingual spaces; sagittal T1-weighted images are very helpful when midline lesions are evaluated.

Contrast-enhanced T1-weighted images are also best performed using fat-suppression techniques in order to obtain better definition of the enhanced areas, particularly for blocking the marrow signal when skull base or other bone involvement is being evaluated. However, it is important to realize that suboptimal fat-suppression techniques may create artifactual bright signals that mimic pathological processes, particularly in the high nasopharynx and low orbit.[6, 33]

As stated above, additional neck scanning for nodal metastases using a neck coil is required for patients with malignancies.

Slice thickness should be no more than 3–4 mm for T1-weighted images and 5 mm for T2-weighted images, with an interslice gap of 1 mm or less. For T1-weighted images, the echo time should be kept as short as possible in order to reduce the magnetic susceptibility artifact. Motion compensation gradients and spatial presaturation pulses may also be helpful to reduce flow and other motion artifacts. Phase encoding should be swept in an anteroposterior direction so that the vascular "ghost artifacts" are thrown anteroposteriorly and not across the pharyngeal tissues.[5] The optimal field of view, matrix size, and number of signal averages will depend upon the particular imaging system and field strength, but they should reflect a compromise between adequate signal-to-noise ratio, spatial resolution, and total examination length.

Several newer MRI techniques have been applied to naso/oropharyngeal imaging. These include MR angiography for evaluation of vascular occlusion or displacement by a mass;[6, 34] functional upper airway imaging to study the soft-palate function in patients with sleep apnea and cleft palate;[6, 35] perfusion imaging to assess tumor vascularity and response to treatment; and spectroscopy to determine the primary presentation of malignancy and possible tumor recurrence.[6]

Pathology

When a lesion of the suprahyoid neck is encountered, several steps are essential for its characterization and classification, based on a working understanding of the complex anatomy of this area. First, the center or presumed site of origin of the lesion must be determined. Localization of the lesion into one or more of the deep spaces of the suprahyoid neck as defined by fascial anatomy strongly guides the differential diagnosis. Second, imaging characteristics such as the presence or absence of necrosis, cystic components, calcifications, and an estimate of vascularity also enable further narrowing of the differential diagnosis. Lesion size and multiplicity, the involvement of adjacent bone, cartilage, or neurovascular structures, and the presence of perineural spread must also be carefully evaluated to allow for optimal surgical or radiation therapy planning, and to permit an accurate prognosis. Finally, both an estimate of vascularity and assessment for involvement of the internal carotid and vertebral arteries help to determine whether preoperative angiography, embolization, or balloon test arterial occlusion might be necessary.

Lesions Arising within the Pharyngeal Wall and Adjoining Deep Neck Spaces

Pharyngeal Mucosal Space (PMS) Lesions

Pseudomass

Asymmetric Fossae of Rosenmüller

Asymmetry of the lateral pharyngeal recesses may result from inflammatory debris or asymmetry in the amount of lymphoid tissue, thereby giving the impression of a mass in the PMS.[5, 6, 36] A true tumor is ruled out when:[5, 36]
1. The adjoining soft-tissue planes in the parapharyngeal and retropharyngeal spaces are maintained.
2. The nasopharyngeal mucosa is clinically intact.
3. The collapsed recess opens when rescanned using CT during the Valsalva maneuver or modified Valsalva maneuver (blowing cheeks against closed mouth).

Congenital Lesions

Tornwaldt's (Thornwaldt's) Cyst

Pathology: This is a congenital midline posterior PMS cyst lined by pharyngeal mucosa. It results from focal *adhesion* of pharyngeal mucosa to the notochord, which is then carried up as the notochord ascends to the developing skull base. A resultant nasopharyngeal diverticulum is created (pharyngeal bursa),[37] the orifice of which becomes obliterated following an attack of pharyngitis, thereby forming the cyst. Tornwaldt's cysts are present in 4% of all autopsy specimens (and head MRI).[5, 10, 36, 37–40]

Clinical presentation and imaging features: Further discussion and imaging features of this entity are included in Chapter 7.

Inflammatory Conditions

Adenoidal and Tonsillar Hypertrophy

Pathology: Hypertrophy of these lymphoid tissues represents immunological activity and not a disease process per se. It is most commonly seen in the adenoids[5] where it begins to be prominent by the age of 2–3 years and begins to regress from adolescence onward. Failure to visualize adenoidal tissue in a young child should raise the possibility of an immune deficiency state.[10] In adults, smoking not uncommonly induces nasopharyngeal lymphoid hyperplasia.[41]

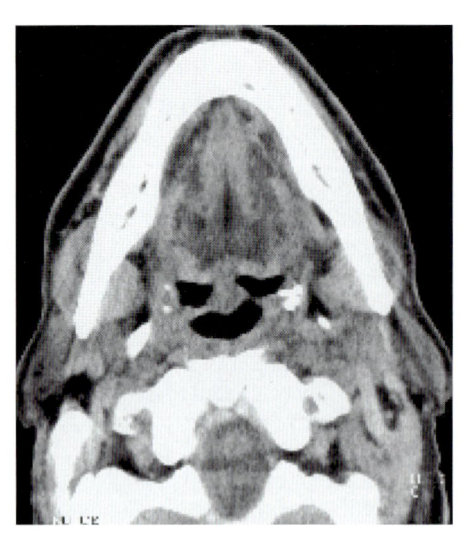

Fig. 8.7 Dystrophic calcification of the faucial tonsils. CT scan at the level of the oropharynx showing bilateral clusters of tonsillar calcification (tonsilloliths), more evident on the left side. Reproduced from Reference 4 with permission.

Clinical presentation: Infants present with difficult feeding, while older children present with other symptoms of nasal obstruction such as mouth breathing and snoring. Otitis media may result from encroachment upon the orifice of the eustachian tube.[5] Dysphagia may be caused by faucial tonsillar hypertrophy.[42, 43] Adenoidectomy or tonsillectomy is indicated when hypertrophy results in nasopharyngeal airway obstruction, chronic otitis media or serous middle ear effusion.[42, 44, 45]

Imaging features: The imaging features of hypertrophic adenoid tissue are described in Chapter 7.

Nevertheless, it is important to realize that it may be impossible to differentiate between hypertrophic adenoids and nasopharyngeal lymphoma on the basis of CT or MRI,[46] and a definitive diagnosis can only be made by biopsy.

Hypertrophic faucial tonsils are less common than adenoidal hypertrophy and present as bilateral smooth, oval, or rounded soft-tissue masses encroaching upon either side of the oropharyngeal air column. Hypertrophic lingual tonsils are the least common. They occur at the tongue base and encroach posteriorly upon the valleculae. CT and MRI appearances of both are similar to those of adenoidal hypertrophy.[47]

Tonsillitis and Peritonsillar Abscess

Pathology: Acute tonsillitis or adenotonsillitis may be caused by viral or bacterial infection. The disease is usually self-limited but, when it is severe, infection may suppurate, resulting in a peritonsillar abscess (quinsy) or rarely in a tonsillar abscess. Peritonsillar abscess constitutes 49% of head and neck space infections in children.[48] When secondary to infectious mononucleosis, acute pharyngotonsillitis is associated with cervical lymphadenopathy and hepatosplenomegaly.[19]

Clinical presentation and imaging features: Further discussion as well as the imaging features of tonsillitis and peritonsillar abscess are included in Chapter 10.

Postinflammatory Dystrophic Calcification

Clumps of tonsillar calcification (tonsilloliths) may be incidentally detected on CT (Fig. 8.7) and indicate previous healed granuloma or chronic tonsillitis. Less commonly, they are seen in the adenoids or lingual tonsil.[5, 6, 49]

Postinflammatory Retention Cyst

Pathology: Postpharyngitis sequelae also include the formation of mucous retention cysts in the inflamed obstructed mucous glands. These cysts are quite similar to those that develop within the paranasal sinuses.[7, 49]

Clinical presentation and imaging features: Cysts are usually asymptomatic but may be large enough to present by a superficial pharyngeal mass or otitis media secondary to compromise of the eustachian tube orifice.[5] Further discussion as well as imaging features of this entity are included in Chapters 7 and 10.

Benign Tumors

Juvenile Nasopharyngeal Angiofibroma

Pathology: This is a highly vascular, benign yet locally invasive, noncapsulated mesenchymal tumor[8, 50, 51–54] believed to arise near the sphenopalatine foramen[37, 49] at the junction between the nose and the nasopharynx at the root of the medial pterygoid plate. It represents 0.5% of all head and neck neoplasms,[36] with the incidence being higher in the Far East than in the United States.[9]

Clinical presentation and imaging features: Juvenile angiofibroma occurs almost exclusively in adolescent boys[37, 49], with the mean age at presentation being 15 years.[36] The most common presenting symptom is nasal speech due to nasal obstruction

(91%); the next is severe recurrent epistaxis (59%); and the least common is facial deformity.[36] On examination, a dark red, often ulcerating, mass is seen in the nasal fossa and postnasal space.[51] Further discussion as well as imaging features of this entity are included in Chapters 3 and 7.

An imaging-based grading system of juvenile angiofibromas has been proposed that would predict the prognosis and recurrence rate and would indicate the optimal surgical approach:[37,49,54,55]

Grade 1: Tumor confined to the nasopharynx.
Grade 2: Tumor extends into the pterygopalatine fossa or masticator space.
Grade 3: Tumor extends into the orbit or intracranially.

The high tumor vascularity contraindicates biopsy and requires preoperative embolization. The primary supply is through the maxillary artery. Minor contributors include the ascending pharyngeal and ascending palatine branches of the ECA, and sometimes the tumor may have a supply from the internal carotid artery.[36,49,50]

Benign Mixed Tumor of Minor Salivary Glands

Pathology: Benign mixed tumor (pleomorphic adenoma) may arise in the minor salivary glands located in the submucosal layer of the PMS, palates (most common minor salivary gland site), or tongue base. Extrapharyngeal sites include the mouth, nose, paranasal sinuses, larynx, and trachea.[10]

Clinical presentation: The presentation varies from a small submucosal nodule to a large pedunculated mass compromising the pharyngeal airway.[5]

Imaging features: When small, the tumor is best detected by MRI as a sharply demarcated, rounded, homogeneous PMS mass of low to intermediate T1-weighted and very high T2-weighted signal intensities.[49,56] A larger tumor presents on CT and MRI as a pedunculated mass encroaching upon the nasopharyngeal, oropharyngeal or oropalatal airway. The appearance is rather nonspecific, and a biopsy will usually make the diagnosis.[5,10] The imaging features of these tumors are described in Chapters 4, 7, and 10.

Malignant Tumors

Squamous Cell Carcinomas: Nasopharyngeal Carcinoma

Pathology: Squamous cell carcinoma (SCC) constitutes 70% of adult nasopharyngeal malignancies.[8,10,57] These are further subdivided into:[58]

Type 1: Keratinized squamous cell carcinoma (25%).
Type 2: Nonkeratinized carcinoma (12%) (sometimes referred to as transitional cell carcinoma).
Type 3: Undifferentiated carcinomas (63%).

Several etiological factors interact to predispose to the development of nasopharyngeal squamous cell carcinoma. These include genetic susceptibility, environmental factors (including chemical carcinogens), and exposure to Epstein–Barr virus,[59] which is very strongly associated with types 2 and 3 of nasopharyngeal SCC.[49,60,61,62-74]

Imaging features: There is a general agreement that MRI is the modality of choice for diagnosing primary as well as recurrent nasopharyngeal carcinoma.[59,60,73,75,76,79,80,81] The imaging appearance is usually nonspecific for a particular type of malignancy, and CT and MRI images of squamous cell carcinoma may be identical to those of nasopharyngeal lymphoma or minor salivary gland malignancies.[5,10] The imaging plays an important role in evaluating the extent of the nasopharyngeal carcinoma, local and intracranial tumor spread (Fig. 8.**8**), and metastatic lymph nodes (Figs. 8.**8**, 8.**10**), and therefore in establishing appropriate TNM classification.[82-106]

Evaluation of follow-up scans after radiotherapy is one of the most challenging parts of the radiological work-up of nasopharyngeal carcinoma. The clinician expects the radiologist to differentiate residual/recurrent tumor from postirradiation granulation tissue, as endoscopy that is already hampered by radiation-induced mucositis cannot detect deep recurrence. Furthermore, biopsy needs to be guided to suspect areas and is rather limited by the poor capacity of tissues to recover.[96]

Such evaluation is primarily the function of MRI, as the CT attenuations of tumor and fibrous tissue are similar.[96] On MRI, mature scar tissue (formed from dehydrated hypocellular collagen) does not enhance with contrast and exhibits dark signal on T2-weighted images, an appearance that is readily distinguishable from tumor tissue.[59,91,96] On the other hand, immature scar tissue (formed from well-hydrated hypercellular granulation tissue) cannot be differentiated from recurrent tumor on the basis of MR signal characteristics as both show contrast enhancement and intermediate to high T2-weighted signal.[59,96,100] In the latter case, the following measures may help in making the diagnosis:

- Ideally, a postradiotherapy baseline MRI is performed for comparison with future studies. This should be delayed for 3–4 months after completion of radiotherapy to allow for total resolution of slowly regressing tumors and acute postirradiation reactive changes (including thickening of the posterior pharyngeal wall and retropharyngeal edema). Progressively growing masses or tissue thickening should be deemed recurrent tumor. Unchanging lesions do not exclude the possibility of tumor recurrence, while a regressive change points to a resolving postirradiation reaction or a contracting scar.[10,96,101]
- When previous scans are unavailable, detection of an obviously positive lymph node is a reliable sign of recurrence.[10] Otherwise, study of the lesion morphology may be helpful. It has been proposed that a recurrent tumor usually presents as a lobulated lump with mass effect, while postirradiation changes are usually a more diffuse process giving rise to nasopharyngeal asymmetry with straight margins.[102] These should, however, be used as suggestive criteria and not as the sole determinant of tumor recurrence.
- When feasible, some techniques can measure the metabolic activity of the mass in question, thus distinguishing a recurrent tumor by its high metabolic rate from postirradiation scar tissue. These techniques include positron emission tomography (PET) with (^{18}F)fluorodeoxyglucose (FDG), thalium-201 scanning, and MR spectroscopy.[10,103-106]

This entity, its clinical presentation, and imaging features are described in greater detail in Chapter 7.

Squamous Cell Carcinomas: Oropharyngeal Carcinoma

Pathology: As in the nasopharynx, squamous cell carcinomas constitute the vast majority (90%) of all malignant neoplasms involving the oropharynx.[8,107-110] Spread pattern and lymphatic drainage vary according to the site of origin,[10] yet the overall incidence of cervical metastatic lymphadenopathy is 50–70%, which renders the prognosis unfavorable in most cases.[108-112]

Clinical presentation and imaging features: Further discussion of clinical and imaging features of oropharyngeal carcinomas is included in Chapter 10. Some features of their perineural spread as well as spread along fascial planes of the neck are reviewed here.

Spread of carcinoma of the palatine tonsils and faucial arches may occur laterally to invade the superior constrictor muscle into the parapharyngeal and then the masticator space, with the potential risk of extension to the skull base, as described formerly in nasopharyngeal carcinoma. Posterolateral extension

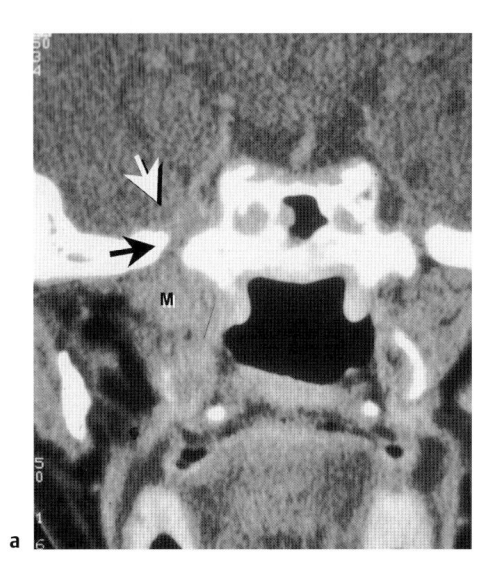

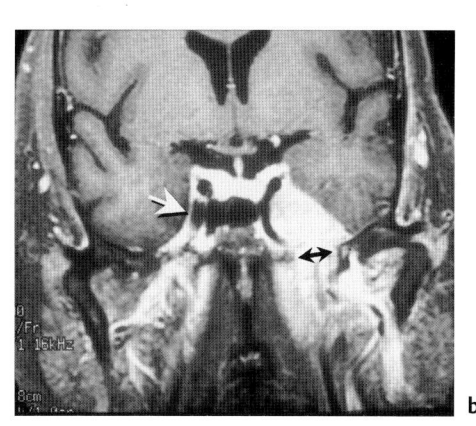

Fig. 8.8 Intracranial extension of nasopharyngeal carcinoma through foramen ovale. **a** Postcontrast coronal CT scan showing mildly enhancing right-sided soft-tissue mass lesion (M) responsible for the asymmetry of the nasopharyngeal airway and extending intracranially as evidenced by (**1**) the presence of a small enhancing soft-tissue mass (white arrow) obliterating the normal CSF density of Meckel's cave, (**2**) the widening of the right-sided foramen ovale (black arrow). **b** Post-gadolinium coronal fat-suppressed T1W MRI of another case showing an intensely enhancing left-sided parapharyngeal and masticator space mass lesion that extends intracranially through the widened ipsilateral foramen ovale (double arrow) to attain an extra-axial location within the middle cranial fossa, involving the cavernous sinus and elevating the left temporal lobe of the brain (white arrow = normal cavernous sinus).

These two cases demonstrate a common route of intracranial extension of nasopharyngeal carcinoma through the foramina ovale while the skull base is intact. Such tumor extension occurs along the mandibular division of the trigeminal nerve and is evidence that the tumor has already violated the masticator space. Reproduced from Reference 4 with permission.

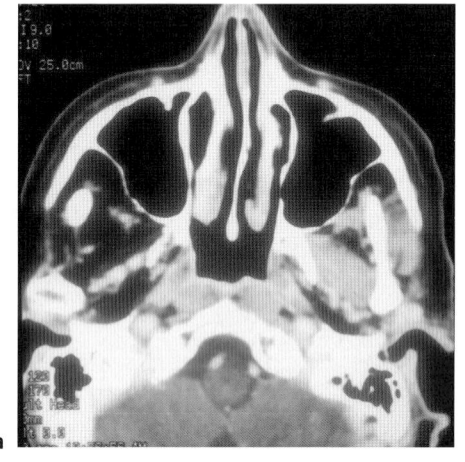

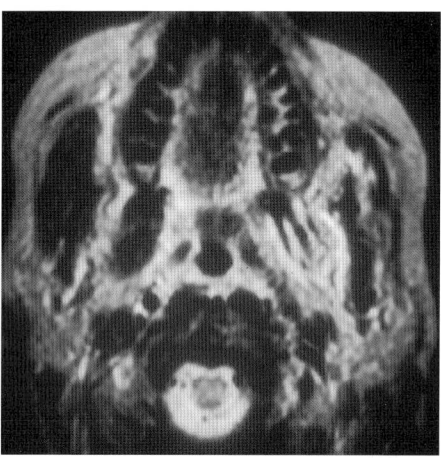

Fig. 8.9 Atrophy of muscles of mastication. **a** Enhanced axial CT scan at the level of the nasopharynx, and **b** axial T2W MR image in another patient at the level of the oropharynx showing atrophy of the right and left masticator spaces, respectively, with consequent abundance of intermuscular fat planes. Reproduced from Reference 4 with permission.

into the retrostyloid parapharyngeal space may lead to encasement of the internal carotid artery.[113]

Although the tonsillar regions may normally appear asymmetric, they should be regarded with suspicion whenever associated with obliteration of the peritonsillar tissue and parapharyngeal space or cervical lymphadenopathy.[111, 114, 115]

Carcinoma of the soft palate usually spreads first to the tonsillar pillars and hard palate. Other potential pathways include lateral infiltration along the tensor and levator palatini muscles into the parapharyngeal space and up the skull base. Superior spread occurs to the nasopharynx and/or through the greater and lesser palatine foramina into the pterygopalatine fossa then into the cavernous sinus.[10]

A problem-oriented radiological assessment of oropharyngeal carcinoma should include specific comments on issues having direct impact on the type and extent of subsequent surgery.[116–125] These can be detailed as follows:

- *Invasion of Deep Fascial Spaces, Perineural Infiltration, and Skull Base/Intracranial Extension*

As described above, oropharyngeal carcinomas can spread to invade the various fascial spaces about the pharynx. Perineural infiltration occurs primarily along the mandibular and maxillary divisions of the trigeminal nerve up to the skull base and intracranially.

Direct imaging signs of perineural spread include (Fig. 8.**8**):
1 Thickening and enhancement of the affected nerves (attention should be paid also to possible skip lesions)
2 Abnormal enhancement in Meckel's cave
3 Lateral bulging of the cavernous sinus dural membrane

Indirect signs include:
1 Foraminal enlargement on CT (Fig. 8.**8a**)
2 Atrophy of muscles of mastication (in mandibular nerve infiltration) (Fig. 8.**9**)

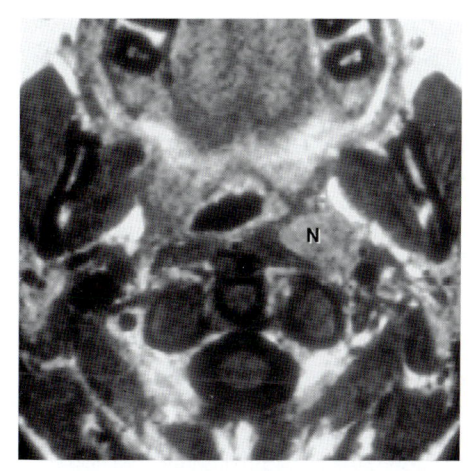

Fig. 8.10 Enlarged lateral retropharyngeal lymph node (of Rouvière). Nonenhanced axial T1W MRI at the level of the oropharynx showing the typical appearance of enlarged left-sided node of Rouvière (N) in a case of nasopharyngeal carcinoma. The enlarged node appears as a well-defined paramedian retropharyngeal nodule of intermediate T1W signal intensity. It effaces and displaces the parapharyngeal fat anterolaterally and mildly rotates the oropharyngeal airway in a counterclockwise direction. Reproduced from Reference 4 with permission.

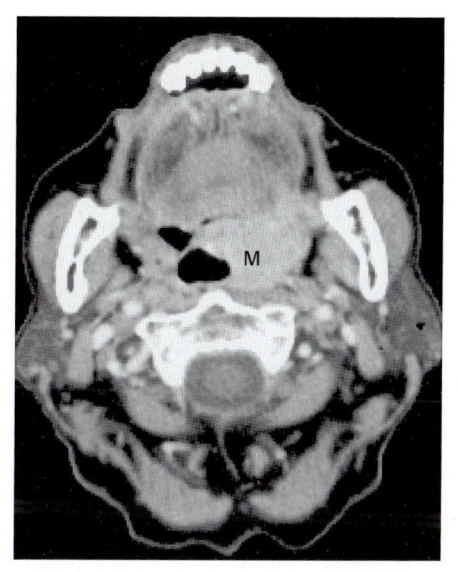

Fig. 8.11 Squamous cell carcinoma of the left palatine tonsil sparing the parapharyngeal space. Axial CT scan obtained during bolus intravenous contrast administration revealing a rather ill-defined, mildly enhancing soft-tissue mass (M) centered on the left tonsillar fossa, and extending along the anterior tonsillar pillar (palatoglossus muscle) into the soft palate and tongue base. Extension along the posterior pillar (palatopharyngeus muscle) into the posterior pharyngeal wall is also noted. The lost definition of prevertebral fat plane on the left side suggests prevertebral space invasion, but may be due to mere compression. The parapharyngeal space is intact. Reproduced from Reference 4 with permission.

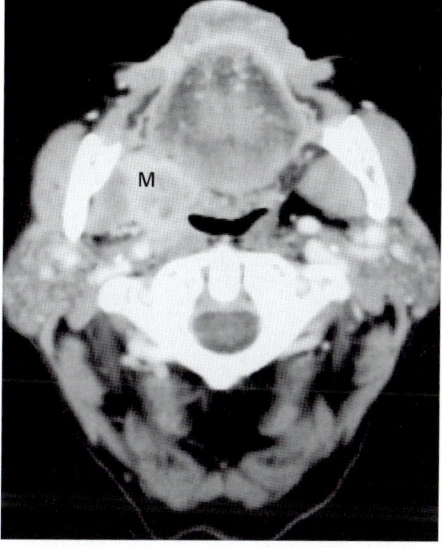

Fig. 8.12 Squamous cell carcinoma of the right palatine tonsil infiltrating the parapharyngeal space. Enhanced axial CT scan at the level of the oropharynx showing a well-defined intensely enhancing mass lesion (M) involving the right tonsillar region, with central nonenhancing areas suggestive of tumor necrosis. The tumor infiltrates the anterior tonsillar pillar into the right tongue base, the posterior tonsillar pillar into the posterior pharyngeal wall with possible involvement of the prevertebral space, the prestyloid and poststyloid parapharyngeal spaces where it abuts but does not completely encase the ICA, as well as the masticator space where the tumor is seen inseparable from the medial pterygoid muscle. Given such lateral extension, perineural spread along the mandibular nerve (V3) intracranially should be of concern. Reproduced from Reference 4 with permission.

3 Obliteration of the normal fat plane in the pterygopalatine fossa (in maxillary nerve infiltration)[49, 90, 118]

Reporting of such tumor extension changes the management of tonsillar and palatal carcinomas from wide local excision through an intraoral approach to more extensive surgery depending on the structures infiltrated. At many institutions, imaging evidence of bulky tumor abutting the skull base will preclude surgery.[119]

- *Prevertebral Muscle Invasion*
Late cases of pharyngeal carcinoma, particularly those arising in the posterior pharyngeal wall, may invade the prevertebral muscles. Findings such as obliteration of the retropharyngeal fat stripe, irregular muscle contour, bright T2-weighted muscle signal or postcontrast muscle enhancement on MRI or CT (Figs. 8.**10**–8.**12**), should prompt the radiologist to report possible prevertebral muscle invasion. The definite extent will, however, be determined by surgical evaluation as these imaging findings may also be due to peritumoral edema without actual muscle invasion. If proven to be fixed at the time of surgery, the tumor is deemed unresectable.[49, 108, 126, 127, 128]

- *Perineural Extension*
Adenoid cystic carcinoma, squamous cell carcinoma and lymphoma of the oropharynx may spread along the perineural tissue.[129, 130–132] Adenoid cystic carcinoma has the highest incidence of perineural spread among all malignant naso/oropharyngeal neoplasms.[49, 90, 118, 131, 132] Such spread is diagnosed histologically in about 50% of adenoid cystic carcinomas; when missed at initial evaluation, treatment failure may result.[10]

Retropharyngeal Space (RPS) Lesions

Pseudotumors

The clinical appearance of a retropharyngeal space mass may result from:
- A tortuous internal carotid artery that extends medially and results in a bulge in the posterior pharyngeal wall.
- Retropharyngeal hematoma, or edema due to jugular vein or lymphatic obstruction. Edema of the retropharyngeal space most commonly involves both its suprahyoid and infrahyoid portions and demonstrates on CT scans low-attenuation enlargement of the space.[21]

Congenital Lesions

Hemangioma/Lymphangioma/Vascular Malformations

These are usually infiltrative lesions that do not respect the fascial boundaries (i.e., transspacial diseases) and may extend into the retropharyngeal space as a part of multiple space involvement.

Hemangiomas and other low-flow malformations appear on CT as relatively dense lesions and typically demonstrate intense enhancement.[133] On MRI, they display intermediate signal intensity on T1-weighted and intermediate-weighted images, with heterogeneous increased signal intensity on T2-weighted im-

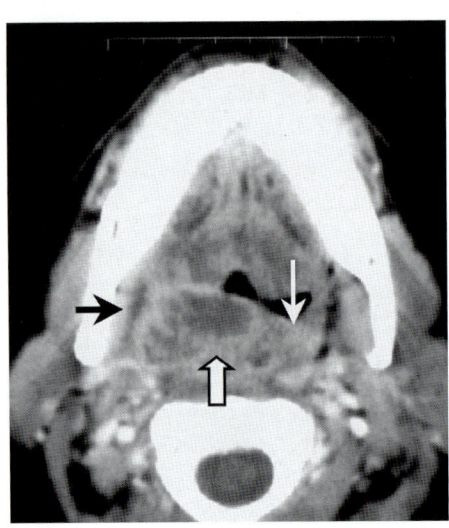

Fig. 8.13 Retropharyngeal infection. Axial contrast-enhanced CT scan through the oropharynx demonstrates enhancing thickened retropharyngeal soft-tissue consistent with cellulitis (thin white arrow) and a low attenuation collection on the right suggesting abscess formation (thick white arrow) that causes significant airway compromise. Note the abscess starting at the region of the lateral retropharyngeal lymph node (of Rouvière). Associated inflammation results in increased attenuation of the prestyloid parapharyngeal fat on the right (black arrow).

ages.[134, 135] Enhancement following gadolinium administration is usually intense.[133, 135] Areas of signal void from associated vascular structures may be identified, but are much more common with high-flow lesions.[135]

Lymphangiomas typically appear on both CT and MRI as unilocular, well-demarcated lesions when small or as multiloculated, poorly circumscribed lesions when large.[136] They exhibit fluid attenuation on CT and signal intensity on MR scans and have imperceptible, nonenhancing rims.[136] Hemorrhage may occur into a lymphangioma and manifest clinically as rapid enlargement of the lesion; this may be identified as an area of high attenuation values (acute) on CT and bright signal (chronic) on T1-weighted MRI.[129, 130] Hemorrhage-fluid levels may also be seen.[135]

Congenital vascular anomalies are currently classified as:[137, 138]

1 True capillary hemangiomas, which often involute with age. Involuting hemangiomas show focal areas of bright T1-weighted signal due to fatty replacement.[135] Hemangiomas may look identical to venous malformations unless the latter contain phleboliths.[135]
2 Vascular malformations (arterial, capillary, venous, lymphatic, and combined), which remain stable or grow slowly with the patient. These lesions typically require some form of therapy when cosmetic disfigurement, bleeding, or functional impairment occurs.[139]

From a therapeutic perspective, the most important issue is to classify these lesions into "low-flow" vascular malformations, which are often successfully treated with percutaneous sclerotherapy,[140] and "high-flow" vascular malformations, which are often treated with transarterial embolization.[139, 141] T2-weighted MRI can elegantly differentiate between these by showing the low-flow lesions to be predominantly bright and the high-flow lesions to be predominantly signal void.[139, 140, 142]

Inflammatory Conditions

Retropharyngeal Infections

Pathology: Infection of the retropharyngeal space is uncommon in adults, in whom it is most often due to direct posterior pharyngeal wall trauma as may occur during endoscopy or attempted insertion of a nasogastric tube.[143] This decreased incidence is most likely related to atrophy of the retropharyngeal lymph node chains following puberty.[17, 143] Infection is most common in patients aged 4 years or less in whom pharyngitis or infection of the adenoids or faucial tonsils, most often with streptococci or staphylococci, spreads to the retropharyngeal lymph node chains. Typically, retropharyngeal space infections progress in four successive phases, and can be stopped at any stage by appropriate treatment:

1 *Reactive lymphadenopathy:* This represents the first response of the retropharyngeal lymph nodes to spread of infection. The nodes react by hyperplasia without disruption of their internal architecture.
2 *Suppurative lymphadenitis:* The infected nodes suppurate with consequent development of an intranodal abscess.
3 *Retropharyngeal cellulitis/abscess:* Early spread of the organism outside an affected lymph node may result in cellulitis, causing the tissues to swell without focal fluid collection.[5] When the enlarged suppurated nodes eventually rupture into the retropharyngeal space, an abscess is formed that typically starts at the location of the lateral retropharyngeal lymph node chains lateral to the midline and above the level of the hyoid bone.[138] Infection then spreads to involve the entire retropharyngeal space from side to side.[21]
4 *Complicated retropharyngeal abscess:* When untreated, retropharyngeal abscess can further spread locally into adjacent neck spaces, track downward into the superior mediastinum, or penetrate the alar fascia into the danger space, where it may spread down to the level of the diaphragm.[17]

Clinical presentation: Patients present with swelling adjacent to the soft palate, which may be displaced anteriorly, along with fever, sore throat, dysphagia, mild to moderate neck stiffness, and occasionally a muffled voice. Breathing may become strained or noisy if compromise of the airway develops.[144]

Imaging features:

1 *Reactive lymphadenopathy:* At this phase, enlarged lateral retropharyngeal lymph nodes (greater than 1 cm in diameter) can be seen, keeping the configuration of normal nodes (oval or kidney-shaped), and usually presenting a homogenous texture.[5]
2 *Suppurative lymphadenitis:* Suppurated lymph nodes appear enlarged and demonstrate central low attenuation on CT or fluid signal intensity on MRI.[21, 138] However, these central changes can also be seen in early liquefying nodes without complete suppuration. Frankly suppurated nodes can be identified by their enhancing rims (Figs. 8.13, 8.14) and the associated edema of the retropharyngeal space.[5]
3 *Retropharyngeal cellulitis/abscess:* The most common finding in patients with retropharyngeal space infection is that of cellulitis localized to the retropharyngeal space at the level of the nasopharynx or oropharynx[21], and seen as diffuse thickening (more than three-quarters of the AP diameter of the vertebral body[36]) and enhancement of the retropharyngeal soft tissues (Fig. 8.13).

When an abscess forms, it appears as an area of fluid collection marginated by an enhancing rim, with possible air or air-fluid level seen within.[36] As stated above, it starts at the region of lateral retropharyngeal nodes but may spread to involve the entire retropharyngeal space (Fig. 8.14), where it may attain a characteristic "bow tie" appearance.[5] Significant mass effect is often present,[10] and the degree of pharyngeal airway compromise should always be looked for.

It is also important to distinguish a true retropharyngeal abscess, which necessitates surgical drainage, from both suppu-

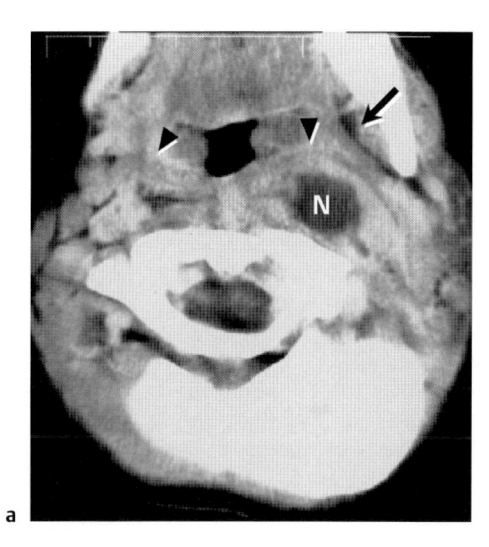

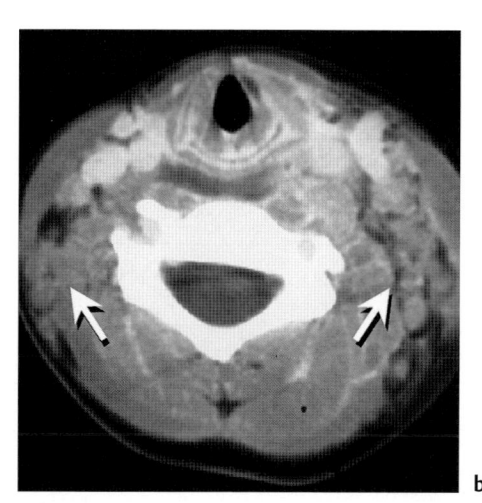

Fig. 8.**14** Retropharyngeal infection. A 5-year-old boy presenting with left upper neck swelling. **a** Postcontrast CT scan reveals enlarged left-sided lateral retropharyngeal lymph node (of Rouvière) (N), displaying central low attenuation values and thick enhancing margin; a picture consistent with suppurative lymphadenitis (intranodal abscess). The associated enlargement of faucial tonsils (arrowheads) suggests the source of infection. Note the integrity of the ipsilateral prestyloid parapharyngeal space (arrow). **b** Section at a lower level in the same patient showing fluid density filling the entire retropharyngeal space. The presence of a thin enhancing rim marginating the collection suggests a retropharyngeal abscess, rather than a mere associated edema, and may necessitate the establishment of drainage. Note the bilateral posterior cervical space lymphadenopathy (arrows). Reproduced from Reference 4 with permission.

rative adenitis (with surrounding edema) and cellulitis, as the latter two conditions may respond to conservative treatment without the need for intervention.[5, 10]

4 *Complicated retropharyngeal abscess:* The parapharyngeal fat may appear dense because of associated inflammation (Fig. 8.**13**), but when suppuration extends into this space, external drainage is indicated rather than the transoral approach used with most retropharyngeal abscesses.[143] Although axial CT usually demonstrates the full extent of retropharyngeal infection, sagittal MRI may occasionally be helpful to better define the superoinferior extent of disease and associated displacement or compression of the pharynx, larynx, trachea or esophagus.[144]

Extension of retropharyngeal space infection into the danger space cannot be differentiated from a retropharyngeal space process unless abscess or cellulitis extends below the T2 to T6 vertebral level.

Benign Tumors

Retropharyngeal Lipoma

Benign tumors of the retropharyngeal space are rare, although lipoma has been reported.[21, 145] This is readily identifiable on both CT and MRI as a retropharyngeal soft-tissue mass with characteristic low CT density (−50 to −100 HU), bright T1-weighted signal, and diminished signal on T2-weighted images.

Malignant Tumors

Malignant tumors of the retropharyngeal space are much more common and are most often secondary to:[21]
1 Direct extension of primary squamous cell carcinoma of the nasopharynx, posterior oropharyngeal wall, or hypopharynx.
2 Metastatic involvement of retropharyngeal lymph nodes:
   * Most commonly from a nasopharyngeal primary squamous cell carcinoma, but may also be seen with an oropharyngeal carcinoma.[21] Enlarged nodes may show central necrosis.
   * Metastases from other areas, such as thyroid carcinoma and malignant melanoma, can also occur.[21] Involved nodes may present bright T1-weighted signals in melanotic melanoma owing to the paramagnetic effect, and in thyroid carcinoma owing to the high protein (thyroglobulin) content[5] or hemorrhage.

In addition, the retropharyngeal lymph node chains may be involved by non-Hodgkin lymphoma, either as an initial site or as a part of a multiple chain involvement. Involved nodes initially appear unilateral and homogeneous, but later extranodal progression may cause the lymphomatous tissue to fill the entire retropharyngeal space.[5]

Prestyloid Parapharyngeal Space (PPPS) Lesions

Pseudotumor

Asymmetric Pterygoid Venous Plexuses

Occasionally, the pterygoid venous plexus (overlying the inner surface of the lateral pterygoid muscle) is larger on one side than on the other. The vascular nature of this anatomical variant can be depicted by its serpentine enhancement on postcontrast CT and contrast-enhanced fat-suppressed axial T1-weighted MRI.[5]

Congenital Lesions

Atypical (Parapharyngeal) Second Branchial Cleft Cyst

Pathology: The lower face and neck are formed from six pairs of branchial arches. Between them lie five endodermal pharyngeal pouches on the inner aspect and five ectodermal clefts on the outer aspect.[146, 147] The second pharyngeal pouch forms the tonsillar fossa and faucial tonsils, whereas the second branchial cleft (together with the third and fourth clefts) forms an ectoderm-lined tract called the cervical sinus[148], which obliterates at a later stage of development.

Failure of the cervical sinus to completely obliterate results in a second branchial cleft sinus or fistula, or, more commonly, a cyst anywhere along a line from the oropharyngeal tonsillar fossa to the supraclavicular region of the neck.[148] Although the most common location for a second branchial cleft cyst is the submandibular space,[27] they can atypically present in the parapharyngeal space arising from the parapharyngeal portion of the embryonal tract (Fig. 8.**15**).[148]

Clinical presentation: Although congenital, the cysts most commonly present in young adults and are often precipitated by respiratory tract infection or trauma.[148] Small cysts are asymptomatic. When large, a cyst in the parapharyngeal location may present with parotid gland bulge, dysphagia, or vague neck discomfort.[149] On examination, the posterolateral oropharyngeal wall appears to bulge internally.[5]

Imaging features: In its atypical (parapharyngeal) location, the cyst appears on CT and MRI as a thin, smooth-walled structure of fluid attenuation values or signal intensity extending from the

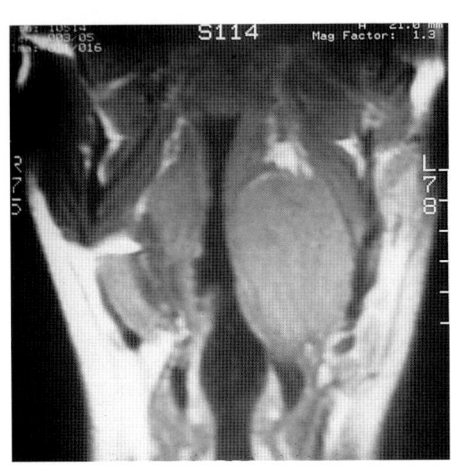

Fig. 8.**15** Atypical branchial cleft cyst. Coronal T1W MR scan shows a parapharyngeal branchial cleft cyst. Case courtesy of M.F. Mafee, M.D.

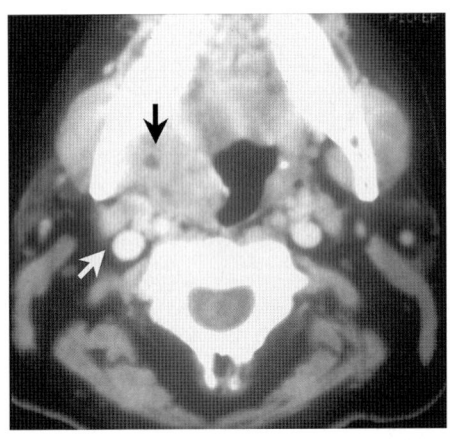

Fig. 8.**16** Prestyloid compartment parapharyngeal space infection from spread of tonsillitis. Axial contrast-enhanced CT scan at the level of the oropharynx demonstrates enlargement of the right faucial tonsil with obliteration of the prestyloid parapharyngeal fat on the right. One small area of decreased attenuation is noted within the inflammatory process, which may represent a small abscess cavity (black arrow). Fat planes surrounding the contents of the retrostyloid compartment of the parapharyngeal space remain intact (white arrow).

deep margin of the faucial tonsil into the parapharyngeal fat toward the skull base (Fig. 8.**15**).[5] Occasionally, T1 hyperintensity may result from high protein content or intracystic hemorrhage.[149] When infected, the cyst wall may become thickened and irregular and the surrounding fat planes may become obscured.[148]

Imaging features of typical second branchial cleft cysts are discussed below under "Submandibular and Sublingual Space Lesions."

Inflammatory Conditions

Parapharyngeal Space Infection

Pathology: Infection of the prestyloid compartment of the parapharyngeal space most commonly arises from spread of peritonsillar abscesses, retrotonsillar vein thrombophlebitis, third molar extractions with violation of the pterygomandibular raphe, penetrating injury to the lateral pharyngeal wall, or extension of deep lobe parotid abscesses, or as a complication of local anesthesia for tonsillectomy or dental surgery.[143, 144] Inflammation may also spread from the submandibular glands, branchial cleft or thyroglossal duct cysts, or temporal bone infections through petrous apex air cells.[143]

Patterns of spread of inflammatory changes within the parapharyngeal and adjacent spaces depend upon individual differences in fascial anatomy that may arise from normal variation, previous trauma, surgery, infection, or radiation therapy.[17] The virulence and antibiotic sensitivity of the invading organism as well as the general health and immunological status of the host may also affect the spread of infection.[17] Once inside the prestyloid parapharyngeal space, infection can readily extend into the parotid, masticator, submandibular, or retrostyloid compartment of the parapharyngeal space.[143]

Clinical presentation: Clinical presentation of infection of the parapharyngeal and adjacent spaces includes the sudden onset of fever and chills. Dysfunction of cranial nerves IX through XII or the sympathetic plexus may also occur with extension into the retrostyloid compartment, and trismus may occur with masticator space involvement. Painful swelling of the gingival tissues of the maxilla and of the cheek on the involved side may also be noted.[144] On clinical examination, a medial bulge of the lateral pharyngeal wall is commonly seen.[143, 144]

Complications of parapharyngeal space infection include erosion of the adjacent carotid artery with fatal hemorrhage or pseudoaneurysm formation, as well as extension to the retropharyngeal space with possible asphyxia or dysphagia from the resulting mass effect and inflammation.[144] Paranasal sinus and orbital involvement, intracranial extension, and osteomyelitis may also result.[134]

Imaging features: Imaging of the parapharyngeal and adjacent spaces may be of great assistance in detecting complications of deep neck infections and determining the optimal timing and approach for surgical drainage.[143] Imaging is most useful when infection is complex, widespread, or difficult to assess clinically.[134] On CT, cellulitis may present as a soft-tissue mass with obliteration of adjacent fat planes. It is often ill-defined, enhancing, and extending along fascial planes (Fig. 8.**16**) and into subcutaneous tissues.[134, 144] Involved muscles may enhance and appear enlarged, and overlying subcutaneous tissues often demonstrate linear or mottled increased attenuation beneath thickened skin.[144]

Abscesses of the deep neck spaces, reported to represent up to 9% of masses within the parapharyngeal space, often appear as uniloculated or multiloculated cystic lesions with air or fluid attenuation centers. They may have somewhat irregular enhancing walls or surrounding tissue edema and may conform to the surrounding fascial boundaries.[26, 143, 144] Occasionally, pus formation is incomplete or may be delayed by antibiotic therapy, and an area of low attenuation on CT, suggesting an abscess cavity, may not yield pus on aspiration or exploration.[144]

While axial and coronal CT may determine the extent of disease and presence of complications, MRI often provides better localization with its multiplanar capabilities and better soft-tissue contrast resolution. Inflammatory exudate is of low to intermediate signal intensity on T1-weighted images and is often isointense with adjacent muscle.[144] Both cellulitis and abscess cavities exhibit increased signal intensity on T2-weighted images. Gadolinium contrast agents may be helpful to differentiate abscess from cellulitis by demonstration of an enhancing abscess wall. Neither MR nor CT findings are typically able to differentiate a bacterial versus a granulomatous origin of inflammation.[144]

Benign Tumors

The majority of prestyloid parapharyngeal space tumors are benign and, of these, most are of salivary gland origin with pleomorphic adenoma representing the most common histology.[150]

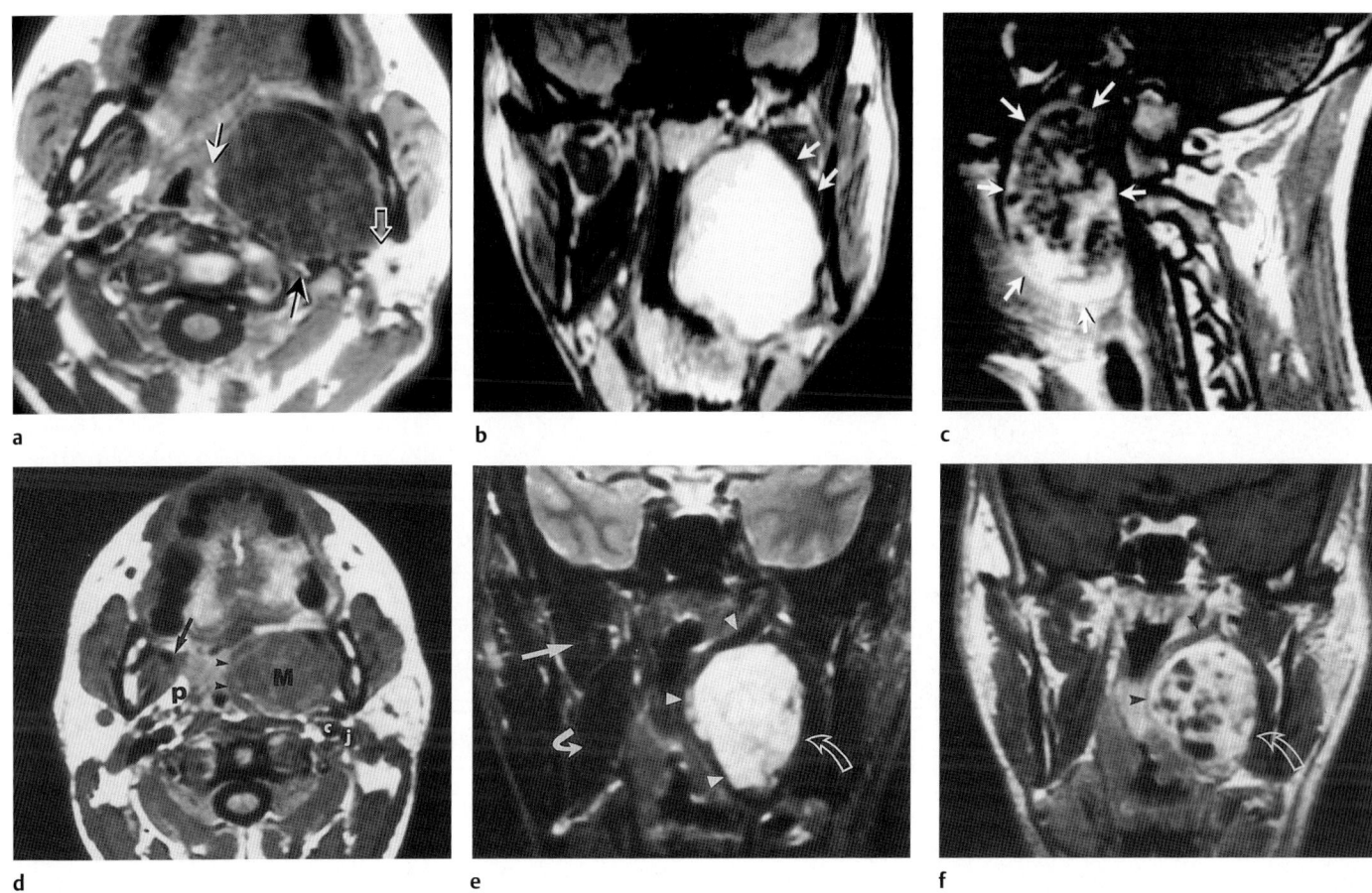

Fig. 8.17 Pleomorphic adenoma. **a** Nonenhanced T1W axial image (500/12) demonstrates a well-defined mass of lower signal intensity than adjacent muscle, replacing the prestyloid parapharyngeal fat with minimal residual fat displaced medially (straight white arrow) and the internal carotid artery displaced posteriorly (straight black arrow). No intact fat plane can be demonstrated between the lesion and the deep lobe of the parotid gland (open arrow). **b** Intermediate-weighted (2500/30) coronal image demonstrates the mass as relatively homogeneous, of increased signal intensity relative to adjacent muscles and lymphoid tissue, and well-defined, with displacement of the oropharyngeal mucosa medially. The left medial pterygoid muscle is compressed and displaced superolaterally (arrows). **c** Contrast-enhanced T1W (500/15) sagittal image demonstrates marked heterogeneity of the mass, with multiple low signal intensity regions that may represent areas of calcification or fibrosis. Both sagittal and coronal images are useful to demonstrate the craniocaudal extent of the lesion, which fills the majority of the prestyloid parapharyngeal space (arrows). The mass is inseparable from the deep lobe of the parotid gland, and must be considered as arising from the deep lobe for surgical planning. However, the deep lobe of the parotid gland was compressed and displaced laterally with no visible connection to the mass at surgery. **d** Axial T1W MR scan shows a mass (M) involving the PPS. Note the medial displacement of the superior pharyngeal constrictor muscle (arrowheads) and lateral displacement of the left medial pterygoid muscle. Note the normal right pterygoid muscle (arrow) and normal right PPS (p); internal carotid artery (c), internal jugular vein (j). **e** Coronal T2W MR scan shows the pleomorphic adenoma, located between medially displaced pharyngeal constrictor muscles (arrowheads) and left medial pterygoid muscle (curved hollow arrow). Note the normal right lateral (straight arrow) and medial (curved solid arrow) pterygoid muscles. **f** Coronal post-gadolinium-contrast T1W MR scan shows heterogeneous enhancement characteristic of pleomorphic adenomas. Note displaced pharyngeal constrictor (arrowheads) and medial pterygoid muscles (arrow). The heterogeneous enhancement is often seen in pleomorphic adenoma. At times, neurogenic tumors may show similar contrast enhancement. Figs. 8.17 **d–f** courtesy of M.F. Mafee, M.D.

Benign Mixed Salivary Gland Tumor (Pleomorphic Adenoma)

Pathology: Salivary gland tumors in this space commonly arise from the deep lobe of the parotid gland and extend into the parapharyngeal space through the stylomandibular tunnel (see Chapter 9).[150] However, salivary gland tumors can also arise primarily within the prestyloid compartment from congenital rests of salivary gland tissue.[11, 150]

Clinical presentation: The patient typically presents with a painless mass, as benign salivary gland tumors seldom result in other symptoms.[151]

Imaging features: The CT appearance of benign salivary gland tumors is usually that of an ovoid soft-tissue mass. They are typically homogeneous when small, but when larger may show variable areas of low attenuation values representing sites of cystic degeneration or seromucinous collections. Focal areas of high attenuation values representing calcification, although uncommon, may also be present (see Chapter 9).[11]

The MR appearance of a benign salivary gland tumor is that of a well-defined mass with low to intermediate signal intensity on T1-weighted and proton-weighted (long TR, short TE) MR images, and increased signal on T2-weighted MR images (Fig. 8.17). Smaller lesions are typically homogeneous in appearance, whereas lesions greater than 2.5 cm in diameter are often heterogeneous on all pulse sequences and may have internal foci of low signal or signal void, corresponding to areas of calcification or fibrosis (Fig. 8.17).[11] Areas of high signal intensity on T1-weighted and proton-weighted images may also occur in larger tumors and correspond to areas of local hemorrhage.[11] With the prevalence of such findings, mass heterogeneity is not a useful predictor of benign versus malignant neoplasm.[11] The best predictors of a benign pleomorphic adenoma are the presence of dystrophic calcifications, best detected with CT, or a well-defined, smoothly lobulated tumor contour, best seen on MRI.[11] However, it is important to realize that calcification can be seen

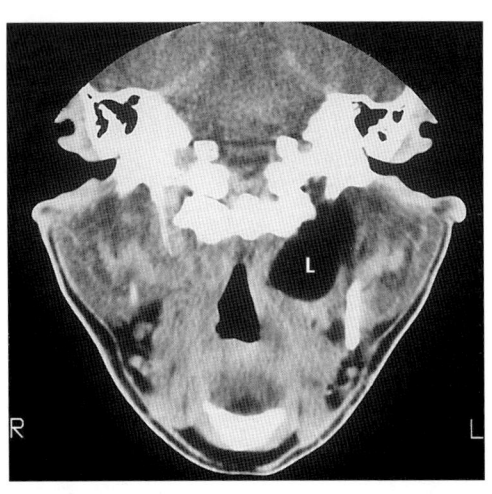

Fig. 8.18 Parapharyngeal lipoma. Coronal CT scan shows a left parapharyngeal lipoma (L), displaying characteristic fat attenuation. Case courtesy of M.F. Mafee, M.D.

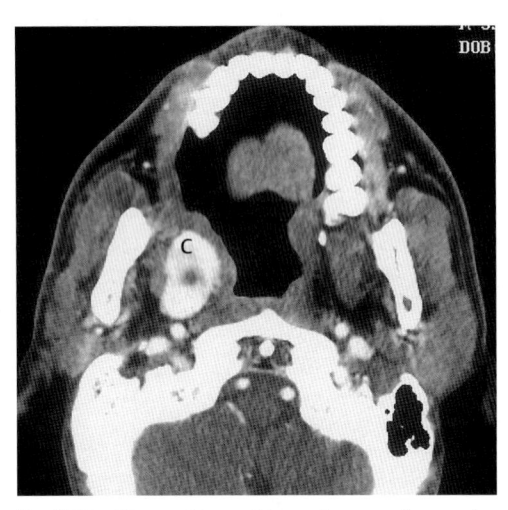

Fig. 8.19 Mucoepidermoid carcinoma of parapharyngeal space. Enhanced CT scan shows a recurrent right parapharyngeal mucoepidermoid carcinoma (c). Note unusual vivid contrast enhancement. Case courtesy of M.F. Mafee, M.D.

in Warthin tumor, acinic cell carcinoma, adenoid cystic carcinoma, and malignant degeneration of benign mixed tumor (see Chapter 9).

The site of origin of prestyloid compartment salivary neoplasms is of importance in the surgical management of these patients, as a lesion arising within the deep lobe of the parotid gland is usually treated with operative control of the facial nerve in order to prevent nerve damage, while a lesion totally confined to the prestyloid parapharyngeal space without connection to the parotid gland may be treated with little concern for facial nerve injury (Fig. 8.17 d–f).[152] At some institutions, a submandibular approach without control of the facial nerve is also used for deep lobe parotid masses when the tumor does not approach the stylomandibular tunnel.

To diagnose an extraparotid origin of a prestyloid parapharyngeal tumor, an intact fat plane between the posterolateral margin of the tumor and the deep portion of the parotid gland must be clearly demonstrated (Fig. 8.17 d). Careful attention is necessary, as this connection may be a very thin isthmus of tissue that is best detected on high-resolution, thin-section axial T1-weighted MR images (Fig. 8.17 d). When lesions are greater than 4 cm in diameter, the intervening fat plane may be obliterated by mass effect alone, and distinction between intraparotid and extraparotid origin may be impossible (Fig. 8.17 a).[11] In such cases,

the surgical approach for a tumor of parotid origin is often used in order to minimize the risk of facial nerve damage.[11,152]

Parapharyngeal Lipomas

These are uncommon lesions that are readily identified by their characteristic low attenuation on CT and characteristic signal intensity paralleling that of fat on all MR pulse sequences (Fig. 8.18).

Malignant Tumors

Malignant tumors of the prestyloid compartment of the parapharyngeal space are much less common than benign lesions, and include malignancies of salivary gland origin, such as mucoepidermoid (Fig. 8.19), adenoid cystic, and acinic cell carcinomas, along with direct invasion of malignancies of the adjacent spaces (see Chapter 9).[11,24] Differentiation from benign tumors may be difficult as approximately two-thirds of salivary gland malignancies have smooth, well-defined margins.[11] However, an irregular, ill-defined margin or infiltration of surrounding tissues may be present, suggesting a more aggressive lesion. Unfortunately, an inflammatory reaction surrounding a benign tumor may occasionally result in a similar appearance.[153]

Retrostyloid Parapharyngeal Space (RPPS) Lesions

Pseudotumors and Vascular Abnormalities

Several nonsurgical vascular pseudotumors may occur, including a redundant, ectatic, or tortuous internal carotid artery, which may present clinically as a pulsatile parapharyngeal space mass.[152] On CT, thrombosis of the internal carotid artery or internal jugular vein may mimic a necrotic mass in this region.[5] This potential pitfall may be avoided by noting the tubular configuration of the abnormality, MR signal intensity characteristics suggesting thrombus, or the absence of a normal internal carotid artery or internal jugular vein. Aneurysm or pseudoaneurysm formation of the internal carotid artery within the space is of particular importance, as palpation of a pulsatile mass may clinically mimic a paraganglioma. Preoperative diagnosis of this abnormality is essential for surgical planning to prevent potentially catastrophic hemorrhagic complications. This abnormality should be suggested when a markedly enhancing mass on CT is inseparable from the internal carotid artery in this region, or when flow void or signal intensity suggesting thrombus is noted on MR.[5] If the diagnosis is in question, MR angiography, CT angiography, or radiographic angiography can be performed for confirmation.

Inflammatory Conditions

Carotid Space Cellulitis or Abscess

Pathology: Infection of the retrostyloid compartment of the parapharyngeal space often results from extension of cellulitis or abscess from adjacent spaces; it may also result from suppuration and breakdown of internal jugular chain lymph nodes draining areas of submandibular, tonsillar, or pharyngeal infection.[144,154] Infection of this space may result in a septic thrombophlebitis of the internal jugular vein, which was relatively common in the preantibiotic era, or it may result in internal carotid artery erosion, thrombosis, or pseudoaneurysm formation.[154]

Clinical presentation: Findings of cellulitis and abscess are discussed above in the section on the prestyloid compartment of the parapharyngeal space.

Imaging features: MR is very useful in the assessment of retrostyloid compartment inflammation, as loss of the normal flow void within the internal carotid artery and internal jugular vein assists in the diagnosis of vascular thrombosis.[144] As with the prestyloid compartment, extension to the adjacent deep spaces is common. Extension into the infrahyoid carotid space is relatively uncommon, as there is little room for distension of the fascial space surrounding the vessels. However, inferior extension may occur in the presence of septic thrombosis.

Benign Tumors

Benign tumors represent the most common cause of masses within the retrostyloid compartment of the parapharyngeal space. The most common benign tumors are paragangliomas and schwannomas.

Paragangliomas

Pathology: Paragangliomas of the head and neck, also known as chemodectomas (nonchromaffin paraganglioma), or glomus tumors, are slow-growing hypervascular tumors composed of nests of cells with characteristic cellular Zellballen pattern, separated by numerous vascular channels within a fibrous matrix.[155, 156] They most commonly arise at the carotid artery bifurcation (carotid body tumor), followed by lesions within the jugular foramen (glomus jugulare) or middle ear (glomus tympanicum), and from the ganglion nodosum of the vagus nerve (glomus vagale).[156] However, paragangliomas may also arise anywhere along the cervical course of the vagus nerve and its branches to the larynx and trachea, as well as within the mediastinum at the level of the aortic arch and pulmonary artery bifurcation.[156, 157] Rarely, they arise along the facial nerve (glomus faciale) or within the orbit or nasal cavity.[156] The cell of origin acts as a homeostatic chemoreceptor, with tissue hyperplasia at the level of the carotid body and ganglion nodosum of the vagus nerve under hypoxic conditions. This hyperplasia is associated with a markedly increased incidence of paragangliomas in high-altitude regions such as Peru, Colorado, and Mexico City.[151, 156] Paragangliomas of the retrostyloid compartment of the parapharyngeal space arise most commonly at or just below the ganglion nodosum of the vagus nerve and are termed "glomus vagale" tumors; they may also be secondary to inferior extension of a paraganglioma arising within the jugular foramen (glomus jugulare), or to superior extension of a carotid body tumor.[150, 152, 156–158] Occasionally, paragangliomas also arise from other chemoreceptor tissue located within the parapharyngeal space.[151]

Clinical presentation: Glomus vagale tumors may present as an asymptomatic mass, but more commonly present with symptoms of vagus nerve dysfunction, such as vocal cord paralysis, or with symptoms from involvement of the hypoglossal or glossopharyngeal nerves.[151, 156] This presentation is in contrast to carotid body paragangliomas, which seldom result in symptoms.[151] The age of patients presenting with paragangliomas varies widely, with the majority being less than 40 years old.[158] These lesions are multicentric in approximately 3% of all patients and approximately one-quarter of patients with a family history of paragangliomas.[155] While malignant features with local nodal or distant metastasis are seen in approximately 6% of carotid body tumors, the incidence of malignancy may rise to as high as 16% for glomus vagale tumors.[156] However, in the author's experience, malignant paragangliomas are very rare.

Imaging features: On CT examination, a glomus vagale tumor presents as a well-marginated mass within the retrostyloid compartment of the parapharyngeal space, almost always displacing the internal carotid artery anteriorly. Enhancement is intense following contrast administration and is homogeneous in the majority of cases.[11, 152] Occasionally, focal nonenhancing areas are noted internally that are thought to represent areas of hemorrhage or necrosis.[11, 152] With dynamic CT scanning during bolus administration of contrast, rapid initial accumulation of contrast material consistent with a hypervascular mass is strongly suggestive of paragangliomas (Figs. 8.**20a**, **b**).[11, 152, 155] Without this dynamic information, a paraganglioma cannot be reliably differentiated with CT from other tumors that may enhance intensely, including approximately one-third of schwannomas.[11, 152, 159] When paragangliomas arise within the jugular foramen and extend inferiorly into the parapharyngeal space, a CT scan with high-resolution bone algorithm reconstruction best demonstrates the subtle or gross osseous changes and relationship of the tumor to the middle ear, and typically reveals a permeative pattern of bone involvement (see Chapter 1).[11] In addition, the remainder of the neck must be carefully evaluated to exclude multicentric involvement whenever a paraganglioma is suspected (Fig. 8.**20b**).

On MR evaluation, paragangliomas are clearly outlined and distinguished from adjacent soft tissues, and are typically ovoid in shape with slight lobulation of the largest lesions (Figs. 8.**20d–f**, 8.**21**, 8.**22**).[11] Again, the internal carotid artery is usually anteriorly or medially displaced. The tumors are of approximately equal or slightly higher signal intensity compared with adjacent muscle on T1-weighted and proton-weighted MR images (Figs. 8.**20d**, **f**, 8.**21a**, 8.**22a**).[153, 155] On T2-weighted MR images the lesions are of moderately high signal intensity, greater than that of adjacent muscle (Figs. 8.**21c**, 8.**22b**).[153, 155] The most characteristic finding of paraganglioma on MR is the presence of serpentine or punctate very low-signal intensity regions, or "signal voids," which are thought to be secondary to high-velocity flow and resultant signal loss (Fig. 8.**22b**).[153, 155, 160, 161] These vary in number and distribution within the tumor and may not be present on every slice.[153] However, some areas of signal void should be seen in any lesion greater than 1.5–2.0 cm in maximal diameter.[153, 155] Tumor vascularity is best demonstrated on flow-sensitive pulse sequences, such as gradient echo sequence (Figs. 8.**20e**, 8.**21e**, 8.**22c**). Areas of high signal thought to be secondary to slow flow may also be seen interspersed with the areas of signal void.[153, 155] The adjacent high- and low-intensity regions have been termed by several authors as having a "salt-and-pepper" appearance.[153, 155] This appearance is highly suggestive of a hypervascular tumor, with the glomus vagale and carotid body tumors by far the most common lesion giving rise to this appearance in this location.[153] This characteristic pattern of signal intensity, excellent tissue contrast and anatomical detail, and good delineation of adjacent vascular structures makes MR the imaging modality of choice in evaluation of suspected paragangliomas of the suprahyoid neck (Figs. 8.**20**–8.**22**).[155, 162]

Prior to dynamic contrast-enhanced CT scanning (Fig. 8.**20b**) and MR imaging, the diagnosis of paraganglioma was established by its characteristic angiographic appearance (Fig. 8.**20c**).[156] The angiographic diagnosis of a glomus tumor was suggested by its profuse vascularity, with tortuous, well-defined nutrient vessels of relatively uniform caliber in the arterial phase (Fig. 8.**20c**) and a dense tumor blush in the capillary phase.[156, 163] Characteristically, glomus vagale tumors demonstrate anterior and medial displacement of the internal carotid artery without involvement of the bifurcation, and without direct involvement of the adjacent vessels (Fig. 8.**21e**). The external carotid artery may be displaced laterally or medially.[156, 163] The tumor blush may be less homogeneous than that typical for a carotid body tumor or jugulotympanic paraganglioma; this may be due to the greater degree of sclerosis noted histologically in some glomus vagale tumors.[156] While no longer necessary for diagnosis, angiography continues to have a role in the treatment of paragangliomas, permitting palliative or preoperative embolization and outlining the vascular supply prior to surgical resection.[155, 156] The preferred treatment of a glomus vagale tumor is complete surgical resection; adjunctive radiation therapy may also be useful if complete resection is impossible due to involvement of critical neurovascular structures at the skull base.[156]

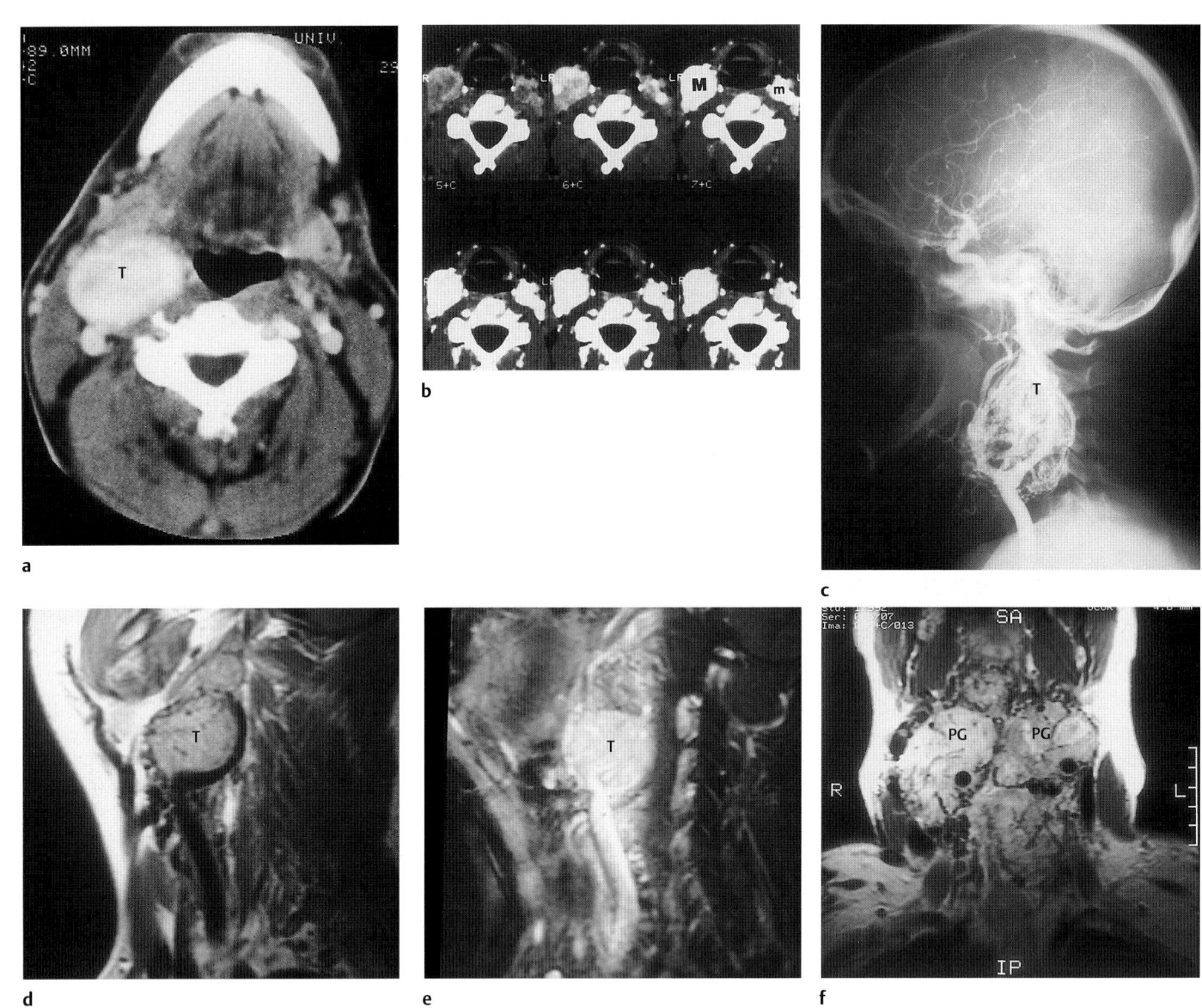

Fig. 8.20 Carotid body tumor. **a** Axial enhanced CT scan shows a right carotid body tumor (T). **b** Bilateral carotid body paragangliomas. Dynamic CT scans in another patient show right (M) and left (m) carotid body tumors. **c** Lateral angiogram in another patient shows a large carotid body tumor (T). **d** Sagittal T1W MR scan in another patient showing a large carotid body tumor (T). **e** Sagittal gradient echo MR scan showing hypervascular mass compatible with carotid body tumor. **f** Coronal T1W MR scan, same patient as **d**, **e**, showing bilateral paragangliomas (PG). Cases courtesy of M.F. Mafee, M.D.

Nerve Sheath Tumors

Pathology: The second major category of benign retrostyloid parapharyngeal space tumors consists of tumors of nerve sheath origin. Of these, the schwannoma is the most common tumor, followed by the neurofibroma.[150] Schwannomas arise from the Schwann cells of the nerve sheath and typically have both a solid fibrous component (Antoni type A) and a gelatinous component (Antoni type B), with both patterns typically present in the same tumor.[151] The schwannomas of this space most commonly arise from the vagus nerve but may arise from the sympathetic trunk or, less commonly, from other adjacent nerves (see Chapter 3).[150,151]

Clinical presentation: While these tumors may present as asymptomatic masses, the nerves of origin are commonly paralyzed, with ipsilateral vocal cord paralysis representing the most common symptom of a vagus nerve schwannoma.[151] Pain and rapid growth are unusual in a schwannoma and suggest malignant change and a poor prognosis.[151] When below the angle of the mandible, these tumors are usually mobile from side-to-side but not in the superior–inferior direction on clinical examination.[192] As with paraganglioma, there is a wide age range at the time of detection, with the majority of patients in their fourth or fifth decade of life.[187]

Imaging features: Schwannomas are usually ovoid or fusiform masses within the retrostyloid parapharyngeal space, and typically displace the internal carotid artery anteriorly when arising from the vagus nerve (Fig. 8.23).[191] This tumor typically has well-delineated margins. It is most commonly higher in attenuation than adjacent muscle on contrast-enhanced CT scan, but may be isodense or, less commonly, of lower attenuation than adjacent muscle (Fig. 8.24a).[191] Approximately one-third of schwannomas enhance significantly on CT (Fig. 8.23).[164] However, neurogenic lesions typically demonstrate a hypovascular enhancement time course on dynamic bolus-enhanced CT, differentiating them from hypervascular paragangliomas.[191] When the tumor extends to the level of the jugular foramen, CT typically demonstrates smooth scalloping of the bony margins, as opposed to the permeative changes noted with paraganglioma (see Chapter 3).[5]

MR evaluation typically demonstrates a mass of intermediate signal intensity on T1-weighted and intermediate-

Pathology 605

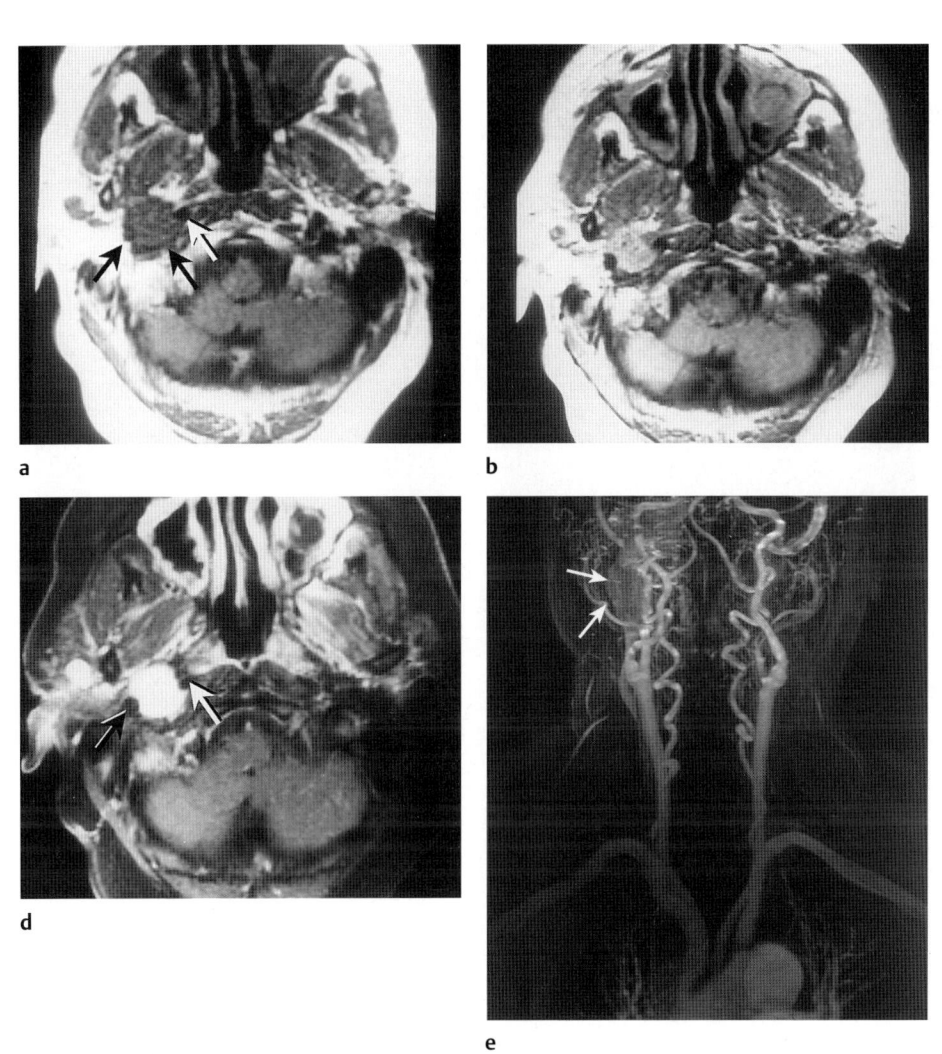

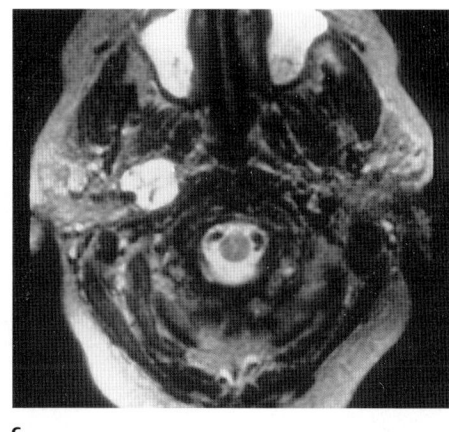

Fig. 8.21 Glomus vagale tumor. **a** T1W (570/15) axial MR image demonstrates lesion (black arrows), approximately equal to adjacent muscle in signal intensity, which is displacing the prestyloid parapharyngeal fat and internal carotid artery (white arrow) anteromedially. **b** Proton-weighted (2500/15) image demonstrates signal intensity higher than that of adjacent muscle, with few punctuate areas of decreased signal intensity consistent with flow voids. **c** T2W (2500/90) MR image better demonstrates multiple curvilinear signal voids that likely represent flow within vessels. The lesion has well-defined margins and is much higher in signal intensity than the surrounding tissues. **d** Contrast-enhanced T1W (600/15) MR image with fat suppression demonstrates marked enhancement of the lesion. Flow void within the anteromedially displaced internal carotid artery is again noted (white arrow) and the styloid process is visualized (black arrow). **e** 2D time-of-flight MR angiogram, different patient. Note the increased vascularity of the paraganglioma (arrows).

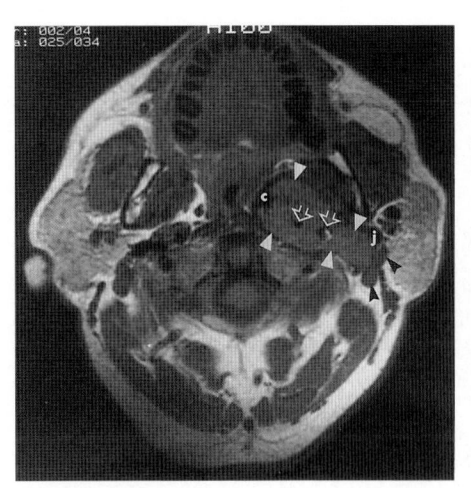

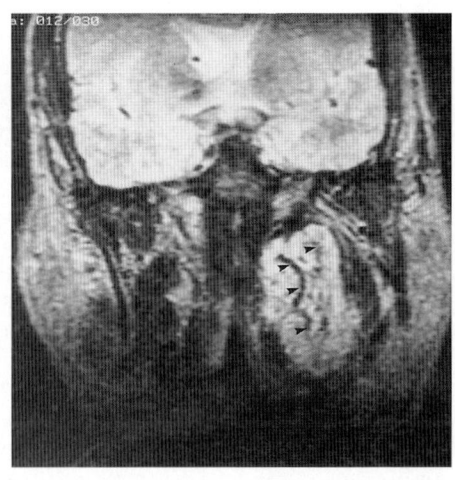

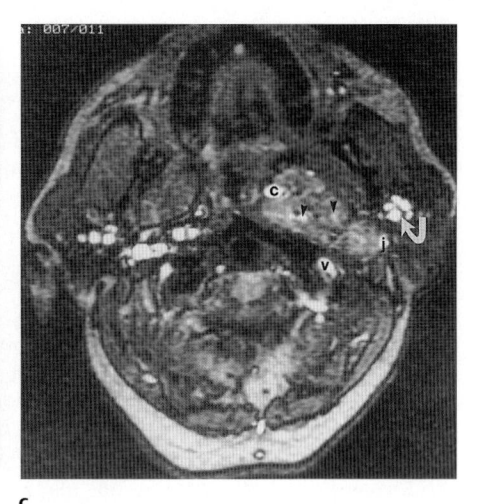

Fig. 8.22 Vagal paraganglioma. **a** Axial PW MR scan shows a large parapharyngeal mass (white arrowheads) compatible with a vagal paraganglioma. Notice anterior displacement of the internal carotid (c) and lateral displacement of the jugular vein (j) and the posterior belly of the digastric muscle (black arrowheads). Note the increased vascularity of the tumor (hollow arrows). **b** Coronal T2W MR scan. The mass is predominantly hyperintense and shows marked curvilinear images (arrowheads) representing increased vascularity characteristics of paragangliomas. **c** Axial gradient-echo MR scan. Note increased vascularity within the tumor (arrowheads); internal carotid (c) vertebral artery (v), internal jugular vein (j), retromandibular vessels (external carotid and external jugular vein branches) (curved arrow). Case courtesy of M.F. Mafee, M.D.

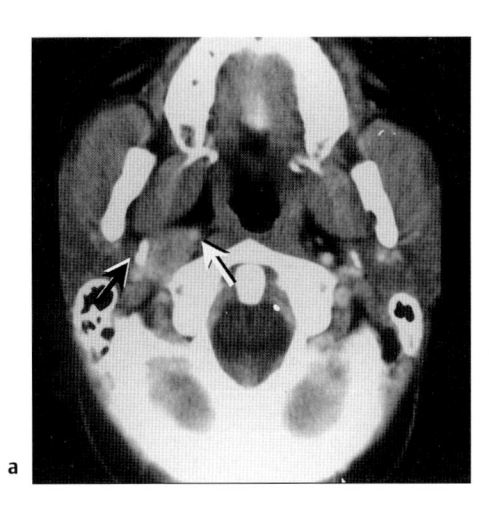

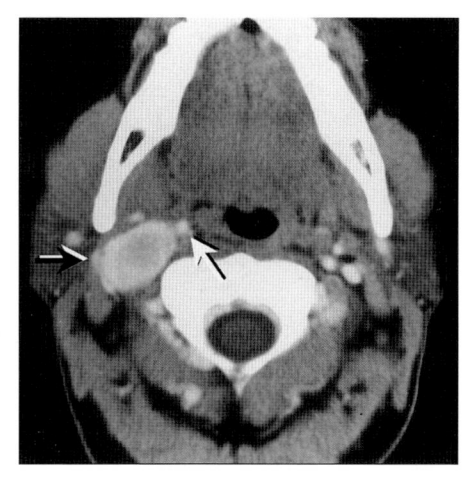

Fig. 8.23 Vagus schwannoma. a Axial CT scan at the onset of bolus contrast administration demonstrates an ovoid mass displacing the prestyloid parapharyngeal fat and internal carotid artery (white arrow) anteromedially and the styloid process (black arrow) slightly anterolaterally. The mass has relatively well-delineated margins and is slightly higher in attenuation values than adjacent muscle on this early contrast-enhanced scan. b A slightly lower image again demonstrates displacement of the internal carotid artery medially (white arrow) and internal jugular vein laterally (black arrow). The mass enhances densely on this image acquired later in the course of bolus contrast enhancement.

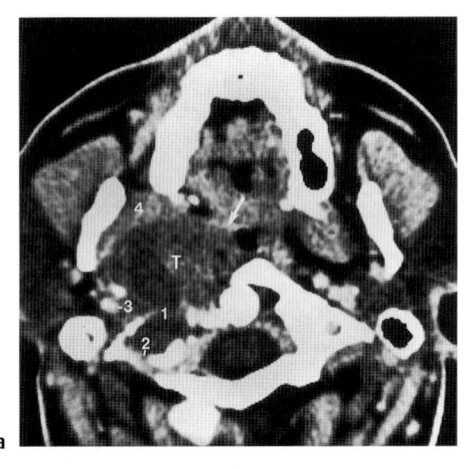

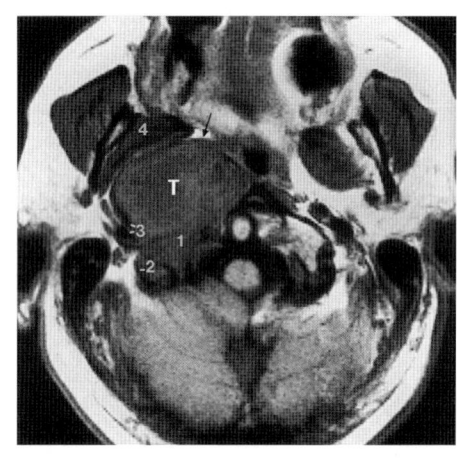

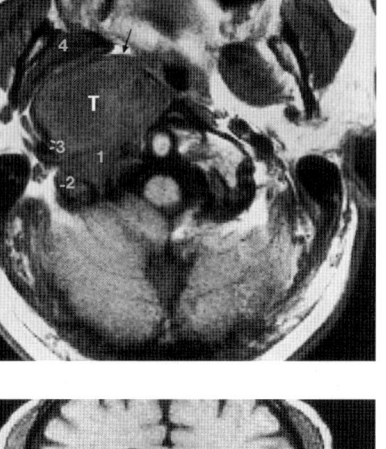

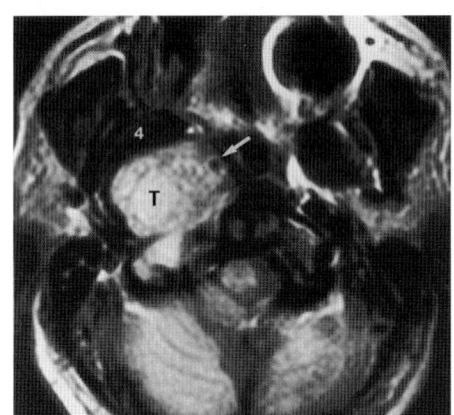

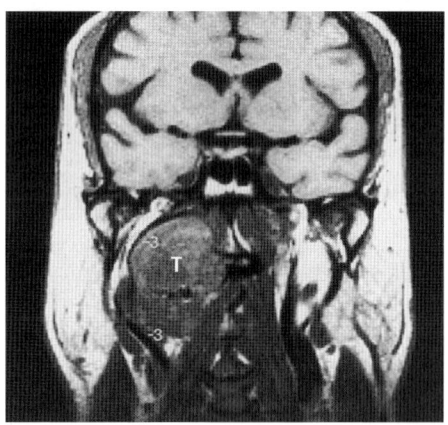

Fig. 8.24 Benign schwannoma encroaching on the right parapharyngeal space. a Enhanced CT scan and b axial TW1, c axial TW2, and d coronal T1W MR images. Recurrent right otitis media due to obstruction of the eustachian tube by a tumor mass (arrow) was noted clinically and on CT scan of temporal bone. The Tumor (T) was noted to be causing destruction of the lateral mass of C1 (1) displacing the vertebral artery posteriorly (2), carotid artery, and jugular vein posterolaterally (3). This extended forward to encroach on the lateral pterygoid muscle (4). MRI scans show similar findings. The coronal image d also showed posterolateral displacement of the vessels by this large tumor, proven to be a schwannoma apparently arising from C1. Case courtesy of Barabara L. Carter, M.D.

weighted images (Figs. 8.24b, 8.26a) and increased signal intensity on T2-weighted images, again with smooth well-delineated contours and often a homogeneous overall appearance (Figs. 8.24c, 8.25, 8.26b).[153] Although areas of signal void may occasionally be detected, these lesions do not have the salt-and-pepper appearance noted with paragangliomas (Figs. 8.20d, 8.22a).[153] Occasionally, schwannomas may appear cystic on CT and MR; histologically, these lesions may demonstrate a coalescence of interstitial fluid forming cystic spaces with prominent Antoni B tissue, or an abundance of lipid-rich Schwann cells.[165]

Neurofibromas also occur within the retrostyloid compartment of the parapharyngeal space and, while often multiple in patients with neurofibromatosis, may present as a solitary lesion without a history of von Recklinghausen disease.[150] Medium to large neurofibromas can have significant fatty infiltration and necrosis, and can appear on CT as a single mass or as multiple low-attenuation masses that may have either no apparent rim or a very thin rim of enhancement.[152] Histologically, the low attenuation appears to be due to the presence of adipocytes (transformed fibroblasts), entrapment of perineural adipose tissue by plexiform neurofibromas, or cystic degeneration secondary to infarction or necrosis.[165]

On MR, neurofibromas typically have an intermediate signal intensity on T1-weighted and proton-weighted images, similar to that of adjacent muscle, and may be somewhat heterogeneous on T2-weighted images.[153] Scattered focal areas of low signal intensity may be seen in larger lesions and may be due to dystrophic calcification, fibrosis, or flow.[153] A salt-and-pepper appearance

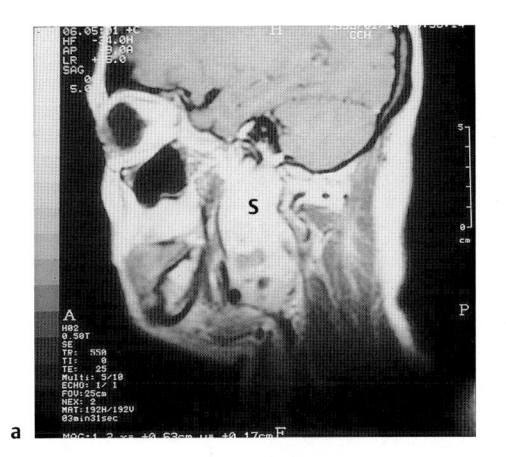

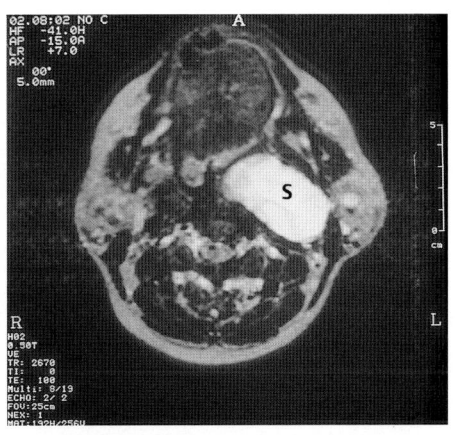

Fig. 8.**25** **a** Sagittal postcontrast T1W and **b** axial T2W MR scans showing a parapharyngeal vagal schwannoma (S). Case courtesy of M.F. Mafee, M.D.

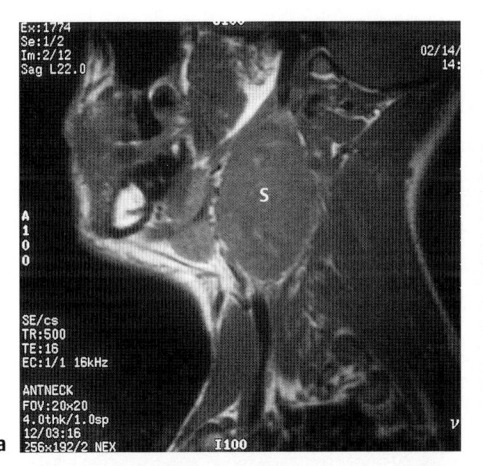

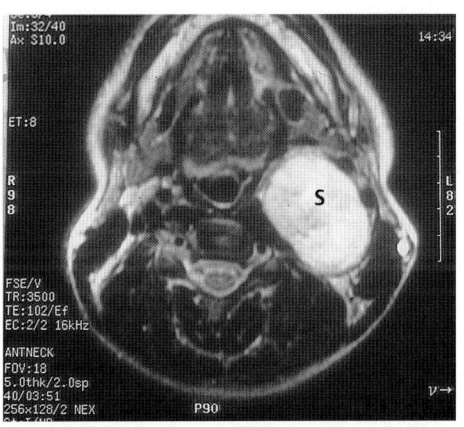

Fig. 8.**26** **a** Sagittal T1W, **b** axial T2W, **c** coronal enhanced T1W, and **d** MR angiogram, showing a parapharyngeal sympathetic schwannoma (S). Compare with Fig. 8.**21 e**; here there is lateral displacement of the ICA but no significant increased vascularity is present. Note anterolateral displacement of internal carotid artery (ICA) on MR images. Case courtesy of M.F. Mafee, M.D.

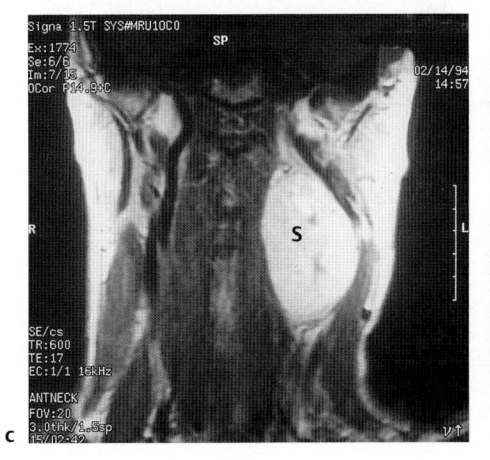

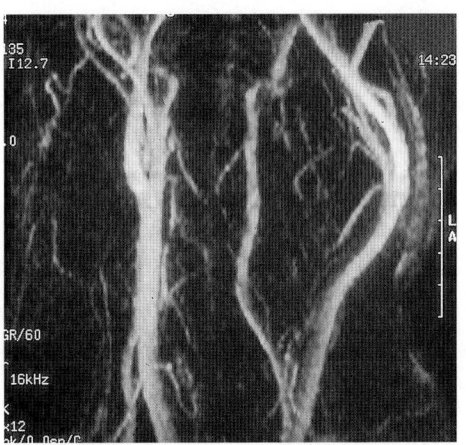

has been reported in one lesion, but this is atypical for a neurofibroma.[153] On CT, the presence of multiple low-attenuation, well-defined masses is highly suggestive of this abnormality.

On angiography, neurogenic tumors may present either as avascular or as hypervascular lesions.[192] Typically, the vascular stain of a neurogenic tumor is less dense than that of a paraganglioma and is generally more patchy, with interspersed hypovascular and hypervascular areas.[192] In addition, the vascular stain of a neurogenic tumor is generally noted later in the angiographic run than is the early arterial stain of a paraganglioma.[192] As with paragangliomas, the preferred method of treatment is total surgical resection.[166]

Other Benign Tumors

Other benign tumors of the retrostyloid compartment of the parapharyngeal space are uncommon. Of note, extracranial extension of meningiomas, while rare, may extend into this space, and typically demonstrate a dumbbell configuration with a small intracranial and larger extracranial component.[152] On CT scan, the presence of scattered flecks or larger dense areas of calcification is typical, as is significant enhancement following contrast administration.[152] Smooth, scalloped enlargement of the jugular foramen or hyperostosis of the adjacent bone may also occasionally be identified.

608   8 Parapharyngeal and Masticator Spaces

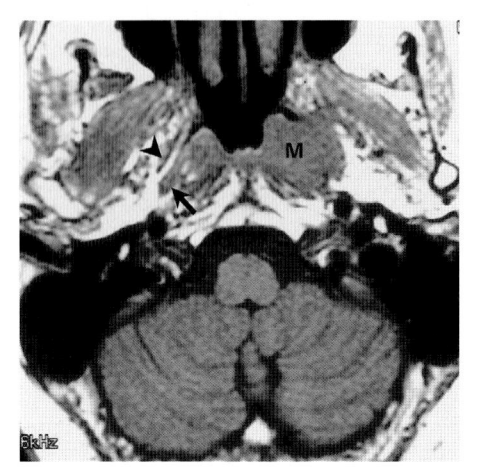

Fig. 8.**27** Nasopharyngeal carcinoma. Axial nonenhanced T1W MR image of the nasopharynx demonstrating a small left-sided isointense nasopharyngeal pharyngeal mucosal space mass lesion (M) that infiltrates the ipsilateral prestyloid parapharyngeal fat and barely touches the adjacent lateral pterygoid muscle, raising the possibility of masticator space invasion as well. Note the preserved fat stripe between the levator (arrow) and tensor (arrowhead) veli palatini muscles on the normal right side. Reproduced from Reference 4 with permission.

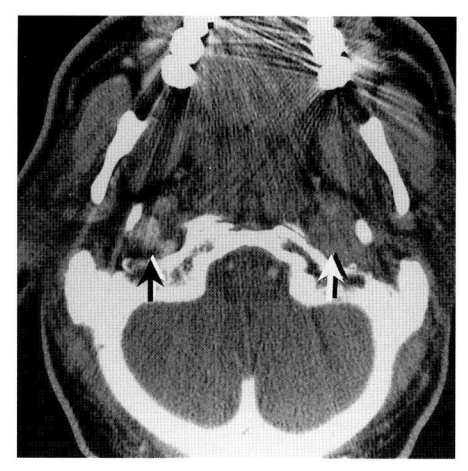

Fig. 8.**29** Carcinoma metastasis to the retrostyloid compartment of the parapharyngeal space. This patient presented with glossopharyngeal neuralgia and syncope several years following treatment for a squamous cell carcinoma of the hypopharynx. Axial contrast-enhanced CT demonstrates a soft-tissue mass within the retrostyloid compartment of the parapharyngeal space on the left (white arrow), obliterating the normal fat planes and enhancing vessels. The normal neurovascular structures and surrounding fat planes can be seen on the right (black arrow).

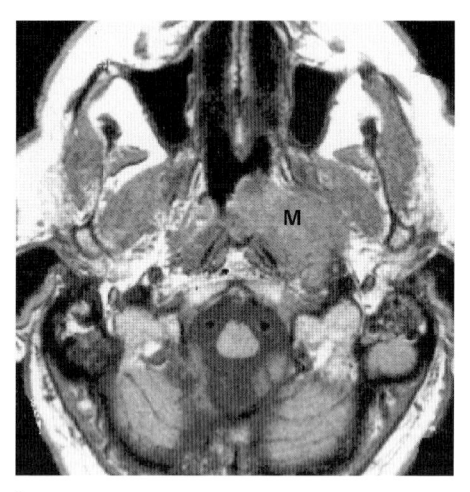

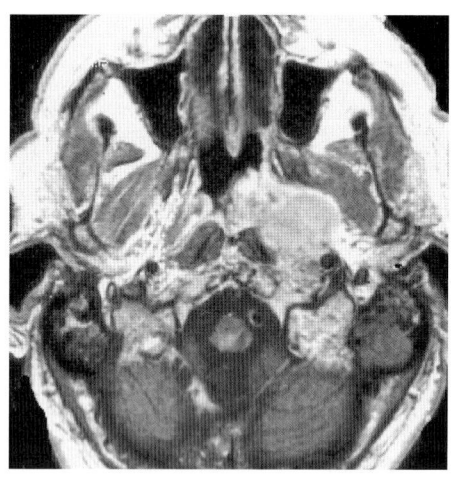

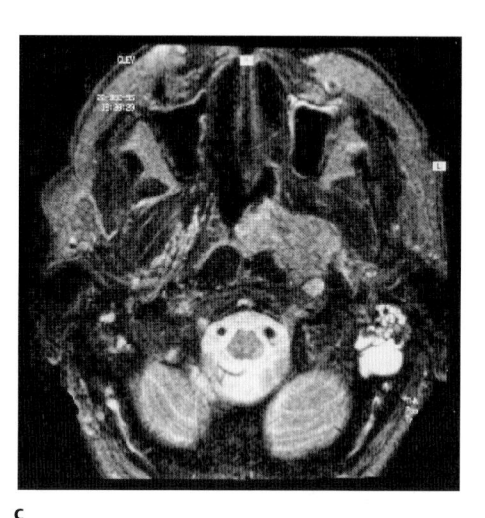

Fig. 8.**28** Nasopharyngeal carcinoma infiltrating the left parapharyngeal space. **a** Axial nonenhanced T1W MR image demonstrating an approximately 4×2.5 cm soft-tissue mass (M) involving the left aspect of the pharyngeal mucosal space, bulging into the nasopharyngeal airway, and extending deeply into the ipsilateral prestyloid parapharyngeal space (compare the size and shape of parapharyngeal fat on both sides). The imperceptible fat planes between the tumor and the lateral pterygoid muscle anteriorly and prevertebral muscles posteriorly raise the possibility of masticator and prevertebral space involvement. **b** Axial post–gadolinium T1W MR image shows considerable tumor enhancement and delineates the exact tumor boundaries except in relation to parapharyngeal fat; an issue that is already observed on the nonenhanced scan. **c** Axial T2W MR image of the same case shows intermediate signal of the tumor. Note the associated fluid signal within the left mastoid air cells secondary to eustachian tube obstruction. Reproduced from Reference 4 with permission.

Malignant Tumors

The most common malignant processes involving the parapharyngeal space are metastatic disease and direct extension from nasopharyngeal or tonsillar carcinoma.[150,195] In particular, nasopharyngeal carcinoma typically extends superiorly through the sinus of Morgagni, the only lateral opening within the tough pharyngobasilar fascia, and along the course of the eustachian tube into the parapharyngeal space (Figs. 8.**11**, 8.**12**, 8.**27**–8.**29**).[167]

Metastasis to the internal jugular lymph node chain is also common, with demonstration of pathologically enlarged lymph nodes anterolateral to the internal carotid artery and internal jugular vein at or below the level of the posterior belly of the digastric muscle. Although these are generally considered to be below the retropharyngeal compartment of the parapharyngeal space, extranodal spread of malignancy from the uppermost lymph nodes may extend superiorly and present as a mass in this region. Lymph nodes in the upper internal jugular chain are considered abnormal when greater than 1.5 cm in diameter or when there is evidence of central hypodensity suggesting necrosis, frequently encountered with metastatic squamous cell carcinoma.[152] Other primary carcinomas may metastasize to this region as well. In particular, hypervascular metastases from primary lesions of the thyroid gland or kidney may have similar signal intensity characteristics as paragangliomas, with intermediate signal intensity on T1-weighted and proton-weighted images and relatively high signal intensity on T2-weighted images.[153] Multiple areas of flow void with a salt-and-pepper appearance may also be noted on T2-weighted images.[153] However, the poorly defined, infiltrative mar-

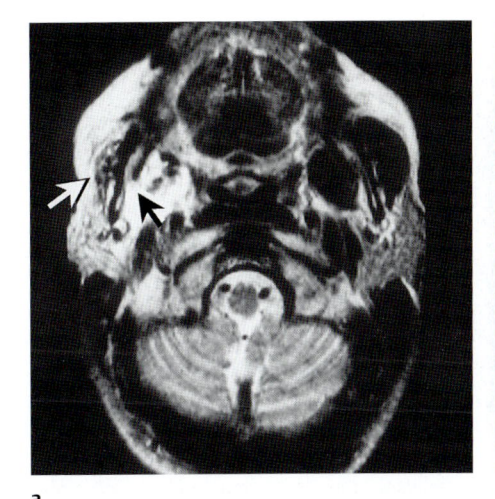

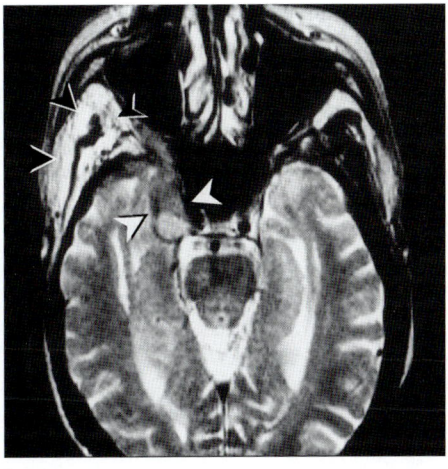

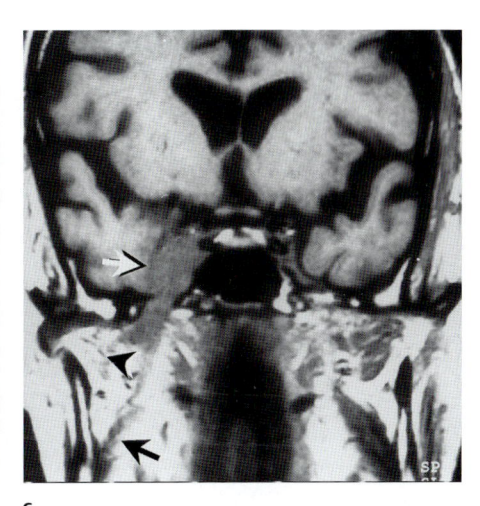

Fig. 8.**30** Denervation atrophy associated with a malignant schwannoma of the trigeminal nerve. **a, b** Axial T2W (3230/90) FSE MR images demonstrate intermediate signal and volume loss of the right masseter (white arrow), medial pterygoid (black arrow), and temporalis muscles. The temporalis tendon and residual muscle tissue are seen outlined by increased signal intensity (black arrowheads). The intermediate signal intensity malignant schwannoma is noted enlarging the right cavernous sinus and extending through the foramen rotundum and into the inferior orbital fissure (white arrowheads). **c** T1W (600/15) coronal MR image demonstrates the mass within the cavernous sinus extending inferiorly through a widened foramen ovale (white arrow) along the mandibular division of the trigeminal nerve. Fatty replacement of the lateral pterygoid (black arrowhead) and medial pterygoid (black arrow) muscles is also noted.

gins and loss of definition of adjacent fat and muscle planes helps to distinguish hypervascular metastasis from paraganglioma.[153] Angiographic findings may also suggest a hypervascular mass with these metastases; an irregular arterial caliber suggestive of tumor encasement may be observed and can help to differentiate between vascular metastasis and paraganglioma.[192] Occasionally, a malignant paraganglioma or malignant schwannoma may be encountered as well.

This upper internal jugular lymph node chain may also be involved by lymphoma, which typically demonstrates abnormal lymph nodes anterolateral to the vessels within the high internal jugular lymph node chain. The lymph nodes are typically homogeneous on CT scan and may enhance.[152] On MR, lymphoma has an intermediate signal intensity on T1-weighted and proton-weighted images that is similar to muscle, and is moderately higher in signal intensity than muscle on T2-weighted images.[153] The lymph nodes are typically smooth and have homogeneous internal signal intensity.[153] The signal intensity of lymphomatous nodes is usually identical to that of normal lymphoid tissue within the adenoids and faucial tonsils.[153] Most commonly, the diagnosis is suggested by the presence of other involved lymph node chains.

Masticator Space (MS) Lesions

Pseudotumors

Accessory Parotid Gland

Asymmetric accessory parotid tissue may mimic a mass on clinical examination. Accessory parotid tissue is present along the course of Stenson's duct in approximately 21% of the general population.[5] On palpation, this may suggest a mass within the masseter muscle; however, imaging studies will clearly define tissue overlying the masseter outside of the masticator space that is identical to the parotid gland on CT and MR examination (Fig. 8.**4c**).[5]

Benign Masseteric Hypertrophy

Benign masseteric hypertrophy is an unusual entity causing a diffuse, homogeneous enlargement of the masseter that is unilateral in half of patients and bilateral in the rest.[168, 169] This may be familial or acquired through habitual grinding of the teeth during sleep; malocclusion may also contribute.[169] In addition to hypertrophy of the masseter, a rough bony projection of cortical bone may be observed along the anterior surface of the mandible at the site of the masseter insertion.[169] Smooth margins, attenuation and signal intensity identical to normal muscle, and lack of abnormal enhancement differentiate this entity from a soft-tissue tumor of the masseter.[169]

Denervation Atrophy

Denervation atrophy of the muscles of mastication may result from lesions affecting the brainstem nuclei, trigeminal nerve or ganglion, or peripheral divisions and branches of the trigeminal nerve; it may also occur in association with underlying systemic diseases, such as myasthenia gravis, polymyositis, progressive systemic sclerosis, or rheumatoid arthritis.[170] While long-standing denervation results in loss of muscle volume and fatty replacement (Fig. 8.**9**), acute denervation can result in muscle edema during the active phase of muscle resorption that can be observed on CT or MR images (Fig. 8.**30**).[170] Care must be taken to avoid confusion of this entity with tumor arising within the masticatory muscles. In addition, reflex sympathetic dystrophy can be seen involving the muscles of mastication following skull fracture or craniotomy.[170] Localized edema and inflammation can also be seen associated with contusion, laceration, or temporomandibular joint inflammation.[170]

Congenital Lesions

Hemangioma

Pathology: Hemangiomas of the face and neck may be of the capillary or cavernous forms, commonly involve the masseter muscle, and may be associated with bony deformity of the adjacent mandible.[133, 135, 168, 171]

Clinical presentation: Capillary hemangiomas typically present in early infancy with rapid growth and undergo fatty replacement and involution by adolescence, while cavernous angiomas and other congenital vascular malformations grow at a similar rate as the patient, do not involute or regress, and may not present until late infancy or childhood.[135]

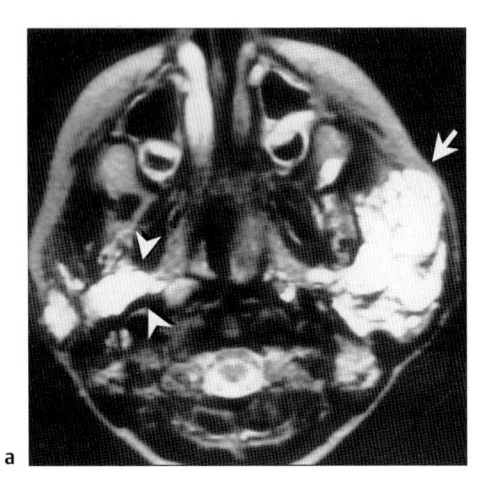

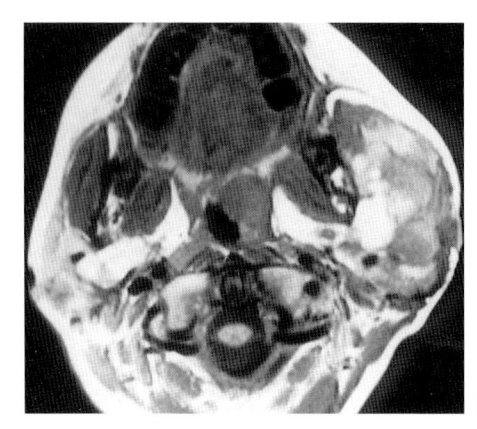

Fig. 8.31 Lymphangiomas of bilateral parotid spaces and left masticator space. **a** T2W (5400/90) FSE axial MR image demonstrates a multiloculated mass involving the superficial and deep portions of the left parotid space, extending anteriorly to replace the bulk of the left masseter muscle (arrow). A similar multiloculated mass is noted within the right parotid space, extending through the stylomandibular tunnel into the prestyloid parapharyngeal space (arrowheads). Both lesions are similar to cerebrospinal fluid in signal intensity and extend through adjacent fascial spaces with an infiltrative appearance. **b** T1W (750/15) axial MR image at the same level demonstrates varying signal intensity within the loculations of the masses, with many demonstrating increased signal intensity suggesting methemoglobin or highly proteinaceous fluid from prior hemorrhage. The combination of multiloculated fluid-filled masses with areas of internal hemorrhage is highly characteristic for lymphangioma.

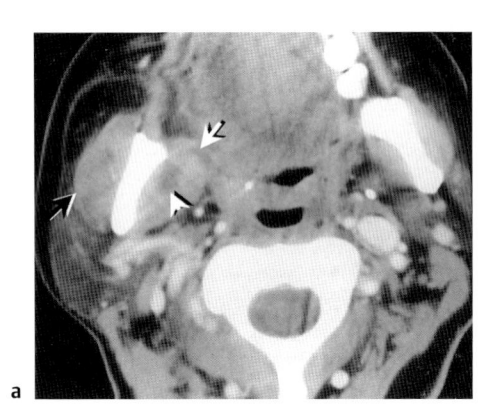

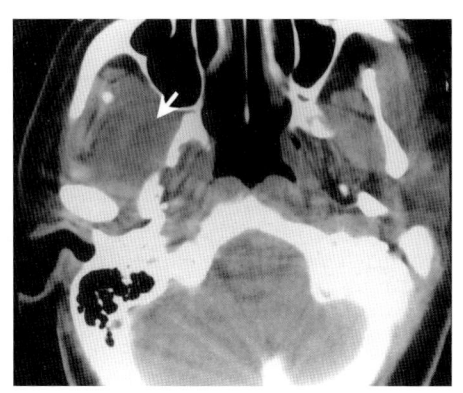

Fig. 8.32 Masticator space infection following wisdom tooth extraction. **a** Axial contrast-enhanced CT image at the level of the mandibular ramus demonstrates marked enlargement of the right medial pterygoid muscle (white arrow) with a central region of decreased attenuation suspicious for abscess formation (arrowhead). The posterior aspect of the masseter is also decreased in attenuation and swollen (black arrow). **b** Axial contrast-enhanced CT image through the level of the mandibular condyle demonstrates involvement of the right lateral pterygoid muscle, which is markedly enlarged and decreased in attenuation (white arrow).

Imaging features: Hemangiomas may be well-defined on imaging studies or may infiltrate along fascial planes; satellite lesions may also be noted.[135] While the CT appearance may be characteristic for a cavernous or venous lesion when phleboliths are identified within a neck mass, MR is usually better than CT in defining vascular malformations because of superior contrast between the lesion and normal surrounding tissues.[135, 168, 171] CT and MR imaging features of hemangiomas and other vascular malformations are described above under Congenital Lesions in the section "Retropharyngeal Space (RPS) Lesions."

Lymphangioma

Lymphangiomas are composed of anomalous lymphatic channels and cysts that often extend along the fascial planes of the head and neck, and typically infiltrate around rather than compress adjacent structures.[135, 136] MR imaging features of lymphangioma are illustrated above (Fig. 8.**31**). As mentioned above, lymphangiomas, like hemangiomas and other vascular malformations, frequently do not respect fascial boundaries and commonly involve more than one deep fascial space.

Inflammatory Conditions

Infection of the masticator space typically follows dental extraction of a lower second or third molar tooth or curettage of a dental socket or infected root.[144] Osteomyelitis of the mandible or the zygomatic or temporal bones following trauma can also secondarily involve the masticator space.[168]

Pathology: Typically, odontogenic infection results in a subperiosteal abscess, cellulitis, or localized osteomyelitis of the mandible. The infection may then extend to involve the masseter, temporalis, and pterygoid muscles, as well as the fat within the masticator space.[144] While infection may be confined initially, it tends to spread along fascial and muscle planes, vessels, nerves, salivary gland ducts, and fat pads, and can rapidly involve multiple contiguous spaces, following the path of least resistance.[168] Infection typically spreads most easily toward the skull base and suprazygomatic portion of the masticator space.[183] Infection may spread downward as well, into the floor of the mouth and adjacent spaces.[171]

Clinical presentation: Pain, fever, marked trismus, and induration over the angle and ramus of the mandible are often present.[144] When an abscess is confined to the masticator space, intraoral drainage may provide adequate treatment.[143] However, when infection has spread to contiguous areas, such as the floor of mouth, parotid, or parapharyngeal spaces, external drainage may be necessary.[168]

Imaging features: Radiological examination begins with a panorex view to search for periapical abscesses or granulomas, and to evaluate evidence of osteomyelitis.[144] CT examination may demonstrate a loss of fat planes with cellulitis or fluid collections suggesting drainable abscesses (Fig. 8.**32**).[171] In addition to demonstrating involvement of spaces other than those clinically suspected, coronal and axial CT scans with bone algorithm reconstruction are helpful to detect osteomyelitis of the mandible or skull base.[144, 171] Osteomyelitis is characterized by a loss of

a **b** **c**

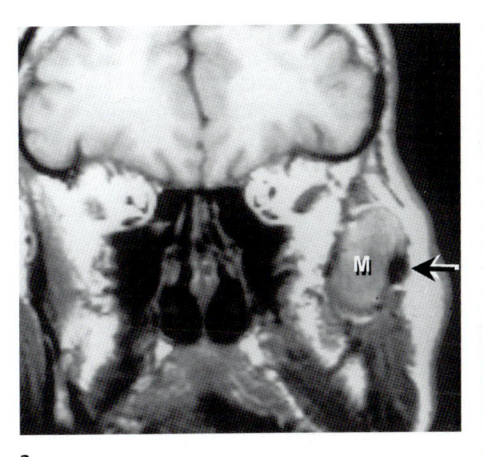

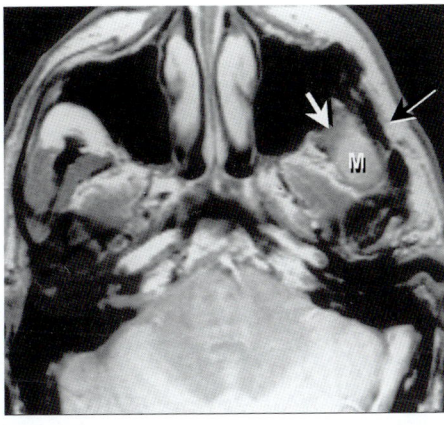

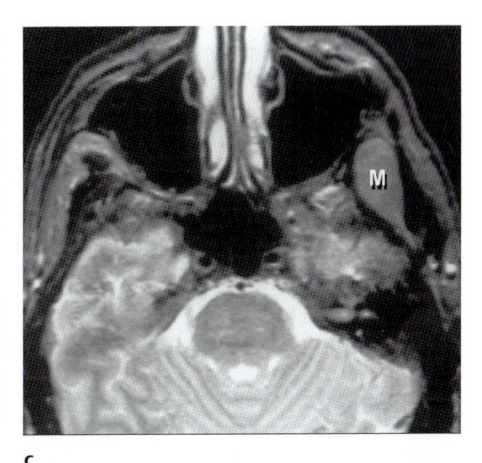

Fig. 8.**33** Schwannoma of the masticator space. **a** T1W (600/15) coronal MR and **b** intermediate-weighted (2500/22) axial MR images demonstrate a lesion of intermediate signal intensity slightly higher than that of adjacent muscle that is well-defined and involves the junction of the suprazygomatic and infrazygomatic compartments of the left masticator space, medial to the zygomatic arch (black arrows). The mass (M) is well-delineated and displaces the adjacent temporalis muscle (white arrow). **c** T2W (2500/90) axial MR image reveals the lesion (M) to be of intermediate signal, approximately equal in intensity to white matter.

definition of the bone cortex associated with increased attenuation within the medullary cavity and poorly defined lucencies within the bone.[144] Bony sequestra and sclerosis may be seen if the infection is long-standing.[144] On MR, disruption of fat planes, multispace involvement, and fluid collections suggesting abscess may be identified. In addition, osteomyelitis may be detected as loss of the normal signal-void of cortical bone with obliteration of the normal signal from medullary fat on T1-weighted images.[144] T2-weighted images may demonstrate subperiosteal abscess or increased signal intensity within the medullary cavity of the mandible.[144]

Benign Tumors

Nerve Sheath Tumors

Benign tumors within the masticator space are most commonly of nerve sheath origin, as the mandibular division of the trigeminal nerve and its major branches pass through the masticator space (Fig. 8.**33**). The mandibular division of the trigeminal nerve enters through the foramen ovale immediately lateral to the fascial layer separating the prestyloid compartment of the parapharyngeal space from the masticator space.[12] Imaging characteristics of nerve sheath tumors within the masticator space are identical to those arising within the retrostyloid compartment of the parapharyngeal space, as discussed above.

Other Benign Tumors

Other benign tumors such as osteoblastoma (see Chapter 3), rhabdomyoma (Fig. 8.**34**), and meningioma may occasionally be encountered (Fig. 8.**35**).

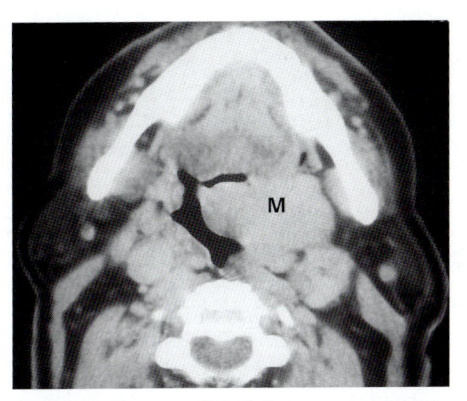

Fig. 8.**34** Pharyngeal rhabdomyoma. Axial CT scan shows a large mass (M), compatible with leiomyoma of the oropharynx, extending into the left parapharyngeal space. Case courtesy of M.F. Mafee, M.D.

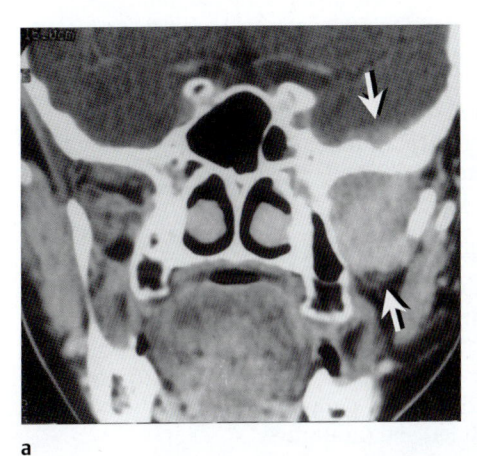

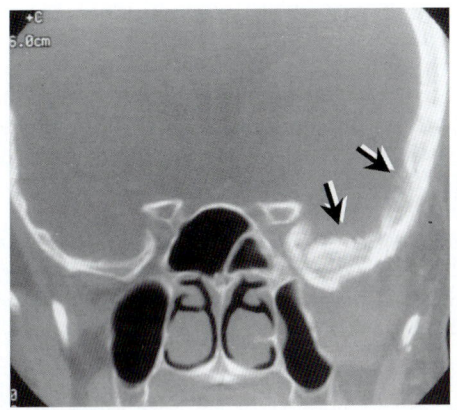

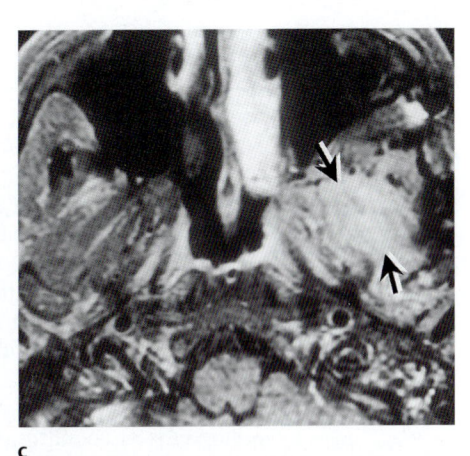

a **b** **c**

Fig. 8.**35** Meningioma of the masticator space. **a** Coronal CT scan demonstrates enhancing mass of the left masticator space that obliterates the upper and lower heads of the lateral pterygoid muscle and their surrounding fat planes. Thickening of the greater wing of the sphenoid is noted, with abnormal enhancing soft tissue extending slightly above the sphenoid bone into the middle cranial fossa (arrows). **b** Coronal CT scan with bone reconstruction demonstrates thickening of the greater wing of the sphenoid bone, consistent with meningioma (arrows). **c** Gadolinium-enhanced T1W (450/20) axial MR image with fat suppression demonstrates enhancing mass replacing the lateral pterygoid muscle (arrows).

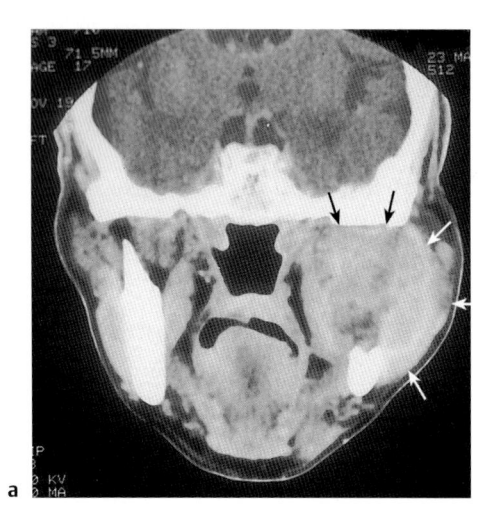

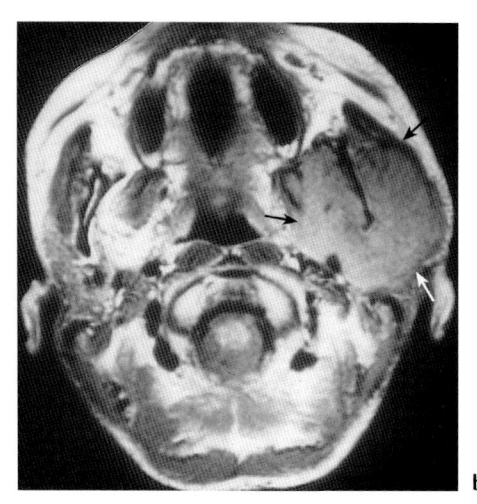

Fig. 8.36 a Coronal CT scan shows metastatic hypernephroma to the left mandible and masticator space (arrows). b Axial pw MR scan shows metastatic squamous cell carcinoma to the left masticator space (arrows). Case courtesy of M.F. Mafee, M.D.

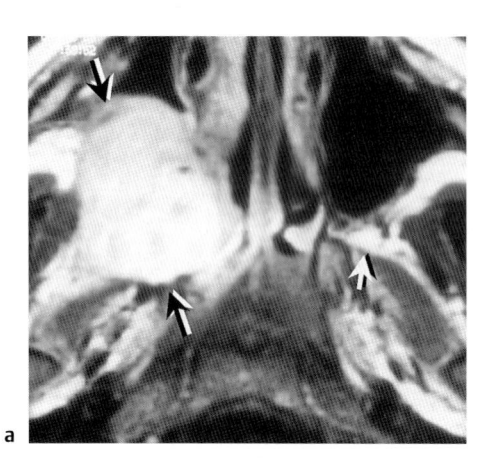

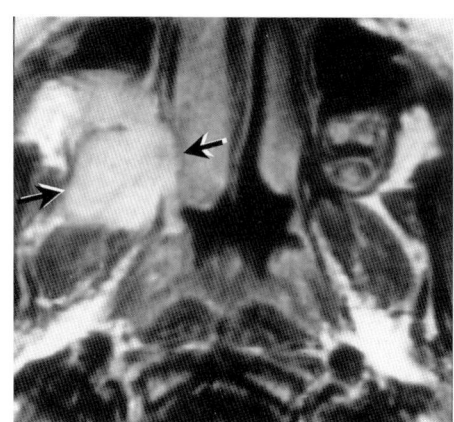

Fig. 8.37 Ten-year-old patient with rhabdomyosarcoma of the pterygopalatine fossa and inferior orbital fissure with masticator space extension. a, b T1W (540/15) contrast-enhanced axial MR images at the level of the nasopharynx demonstrate an enhancing, slightly heterogeneous mass invading the anterior aspect of the lateral pterygoid muscle (black arrows) and extending anteriorly into the maxillary sinus. The mass obliterates the right pterygopalatine fossa, which is normally seen as a fat-filled cleft at this level, as noted on the left (white arrow). Extension into the orbital apex through the inferior orbital fissure was noted on higher images.

Malignant Tumors

Malignant tumors of the masticator space may arise directly from the contents of the space, extend from adjacent spaces, or represent metastatic carcinoma (Fig. 8.36a, b). The most common primary malignancies of the masticator space are sarcomas (see Chapter 5).[171]

Sarcomas

Sarcomas within the masticator space include chondrosarcomas, which arise from the mandible near the temporomandibular joint; osteosarcomas, which may originate anywhere along the mandible; malignant schwannomas, which develop in the mandibular division of the trigeminal nerve and its branches; or less commonly, soft-tissue sarcomas.[171,172] Rhabdomyosarcoma may also involve the masticator space and is more commonly seen in younger patients (Fig. 8.37) (see Chapters 2 and 3).[153]

Sarcomas of the masticator space present as lesions with intermediate-attenuation values on CT scans, often demonstrating destruction of the adjacent mandible. The different cell types are generally indistinguishable on imaging studies, although the presence of nonossified osteoid with high attenuation values or tumor bone formation within osteosarcoma can aid in the diagnosis of this lesion.[136] Identification of chondroid calcification on CT may suggest the diagnosis of chondrosarcoma (see Chapter 5).[5] Bone fragments within tumors may be seen within any sarcoma in the presence of significant mandibular invasion. The MR appearances of the different sarcomas are also often indistinguishable, with intermediate signal intensity on T1-weighted and proton-weighted images and moderately increased signal intensity relative to muscle on T2-weighted images.[153]

Other primary or secondary lesions of the mandible, such as ameloblastoma or fibrosarcoma, are occasionally seen and may extend into the masticator space. The mandibular origin of these lesions is usually evident (see Chapter 6).

Malignant Schwannoma

Malignant schwannoma of the masticator space appears similar to that in the retrostyloid compartment of the parapharyngeal space, often presenting as a tubular mass following the mandibular division of the trigeminal nerve and its primary branches. Extension through the foramen ovale to involve the gasserian ganglion is not uncommon with this lesion, and evaluation of the entire trigeminal nerve to the level of the root entry zone of the pons should be performed to avoid inadequate surgical resection or radiation therapy.[172]

Non-Hodgkin Lymphoma

Non-Hodgkin lymphoma may also occur in this site and may present with better-defined, smooth margins as compared to the other malignancies of this space.[153] However, preoperative diagnosis is difficult unless other sites of extranodal or nodal involvement are present to suggest lymphoma.[172] Lymphomas may sometimes be ill-defined and infiltrative.

Carcinomas

Carcinoma involving the masticator space may be metastatic from a distant primary, such as the lung, breast, prostate, or kidney, or may represent spread by squamous cell carcinoma of the oral cavity, or salivary gland carcinoma, or external auditory canal carcinoma.[171] Hypervascular metastases, such as renal cell and thyroid carcinoma, are usually indistinguishable from other malignancies of this region, but may demonstrate a "salt-and-pepper" appearance on MR, similar to that noted with paragangliomas.[153] The presence of malignant features such as infiltration of adjacent fat planes and muscles and bone destruction differentiates the hypervascular metastasis from a paraganglioma.

When the masticator space is involved by malignant tumor, particularly with adenoid cystic carcinoma or recurrent squamous cell carcinoma of the oral cavity or oropharynx, perineural spread of tumor is relatively common and the course of the mandibular division of the trigeminal nerve and its branches should be carefully examined as detailed above under "Squamous Cell Carcinomas: Oropharyngeal Carcinoma" (see Chapter 6).[13,90,171,173] Perineural spread may also occur into the masticator space and through the foramen ovale from parotid malignancies along the auriculotemporal branch of the trigeminal nerve and result in similar imaging findings (see Chapter 3). In addition to detecting perineural spread, imaging allows preoperative evaluation of tumor extent, thereby providing better presurgical prediction of resectability and assisting in surgical and radiation therapy planning.[171]

Parotid Space (PS) Lesions

The vast majority of pathological processes originating within the parotid space arise from the parotid gland itself, which is covered elsewhere in the text. However, there are several entities found within the parotid space that may not arise from the gland. These include congenital lesions, infection, and tumor arising within the periparotid and intraparotid lymph nodes.

Congenital Lesions

First Branchial Cleft Cyst

Pathology: While anomalies of the first branchial cleft are unusual, representing only 8% of all branchial cleft abnormalities, this diagnosis should be considered whenever a cystic lesion is detected within or adjacent to the parotid gland.[148] First branchial cleft cysts arise from failure to completely obliterate the first branchial cleft during the eighth to ninth weeks of fetal development.[174] Normally, the external auditory canal is derived from the first branchial cleft. The tympanic cavity, mastoid air cells, and eustachian tube form from the first branchial pouch.[148] A cyst of the first branchial cleft can form anywhere along the course of the potential first branchial cleft fistula. This begins as a cutaneous opening superolateral to the hyoid bone within the submandibular space, ascends through the parotid gland (see Chapter 9) with variable interaction with the gland and facial nerve, and terminates at the cartilaginous–bony junction of the external auditory canal.[148,174]

Clinical presentation: Clinically, these cysts are most common in middle-aged women and typically present as enlarging masses within the lower pole of the parotid gland or within the external auditory canal.[148,174]

Imaging features: The CT appearance of first branchial cleft cysts is that of an oval to round cystic mass either within or adjacent to the parotid gland[148] (see Chapter 9). Cyst wall thickness and enhancement are variable and increase with recurrent infections. The differential diagnosis for a cyst in this region also includes the more common parotid gland entities such as retention cyst, sialocele, necrotic lymphadenopathy, lymphangioma, Warthin tumor, ganglion cyst of the temporomandibular joint, lymphoepithelial parotid cyst associated with the human immunodeficiency virus, and sebaceous cyst.[174] The possibility of a first branchial cleft cyst should be communicated preoperatively, as diagnosis may be difficult for the pathologist owing to its relative rarity and the fact that associated inflammatory changes may obscure the epithelial lining.[148]

Hemangiomas and Lymphangiomas

Low-flow vascular malformations, including hemangiomas and lymphangiomas, occur in the parotid space, often presenting in the young infant (Fig. 8.**38**). Imaging characteristics are similar to those in the retropharyngeal and masticator spaces, as discussed above. Further discussion of both entities as well as their imaging features is included in Chapter 9.

Inflammatory Conditions

Infection of the parotid space typically arises within a dehydrated gland from coagulase-positive staphylococci ascending from the oral cavity through Stenson's duct.[154] Suppuration of infected intraparotid or periparotid lymph nodes may also lead to infection of the parotid space, as can severe external otitis extending through the fissures of Santorini of the external auditory canal.[154] When infection arises within the gland itself, multiple glandular septae often result in an abscess with a multiloculated appearance.[154] As noted above, the boundary between the parotid space and prestyloid compartment of the parapharyngeal space provides little barrier to the spread of infection into the deep neck; parotid infection can also originate from, or lead to, infection of the adjacent masticator space (Fig. 8.**39**).

Malignant Tumors

Lymph nodes within and adjacent to the parotid gland may harbor malignancy of the parotid space other than that of parotid gland origin. The intraparotid and periparotid lymph nodes drain the external auditory canal and scalp, and both squamous cell carcinoma and malignant melanoma arising within the skin around the parotid external auditory canal and in the scalp may metastasize to these nodes and present as a parotid space mass.[5] In addition, non-Hodgkin lymphoma can arise either within these nodal groups (Fig. 8.**40**) or, less commonly, within the parotid gland itself.[175]

Submandibular and Sublingual Space Lesions

The submandibular and sublingual spaces are divided by the mylohyoid muscle, but are continuous posteriorly around its posterior margin. Much of the pathology encountered in the sublingual space is related to direct extension of oropharyngeal carcinoma, which is discussed in detail earlier in this chapter. In addition, many abnormalities involving the submandibular or sublingual space are related to salivary gland pathology, which is also covered elsewhere in this text. A variety of congenital, inflammatory, and neoplastic processes unrelated to the salivary glands may also present within these spaces, and are discussed in Chapters 9 and 12.

Congenital Lesions

The majority of these lesions present within the first two years of life, but may manifest at any age.[176]

Typical Second Branchial Cleft Cyst

Pathology: Second branchial cleft abnormalities comprise 95% of all branchial cleft anomalies and may be found, as mentioned earlier, in the prestyloid parapharyngeal space, anywhere along a potential tract from the oropharyngeal tonsillar fossa to the supraclavicular fossa, with cysts more common than either fistulae or sinuses.[148,174]

Clinical presentation: Although they arise from a congenital abnormality, typical second branchial cleft cysts most commonly

614   8 Parapharyngeal and Masticator Spaces

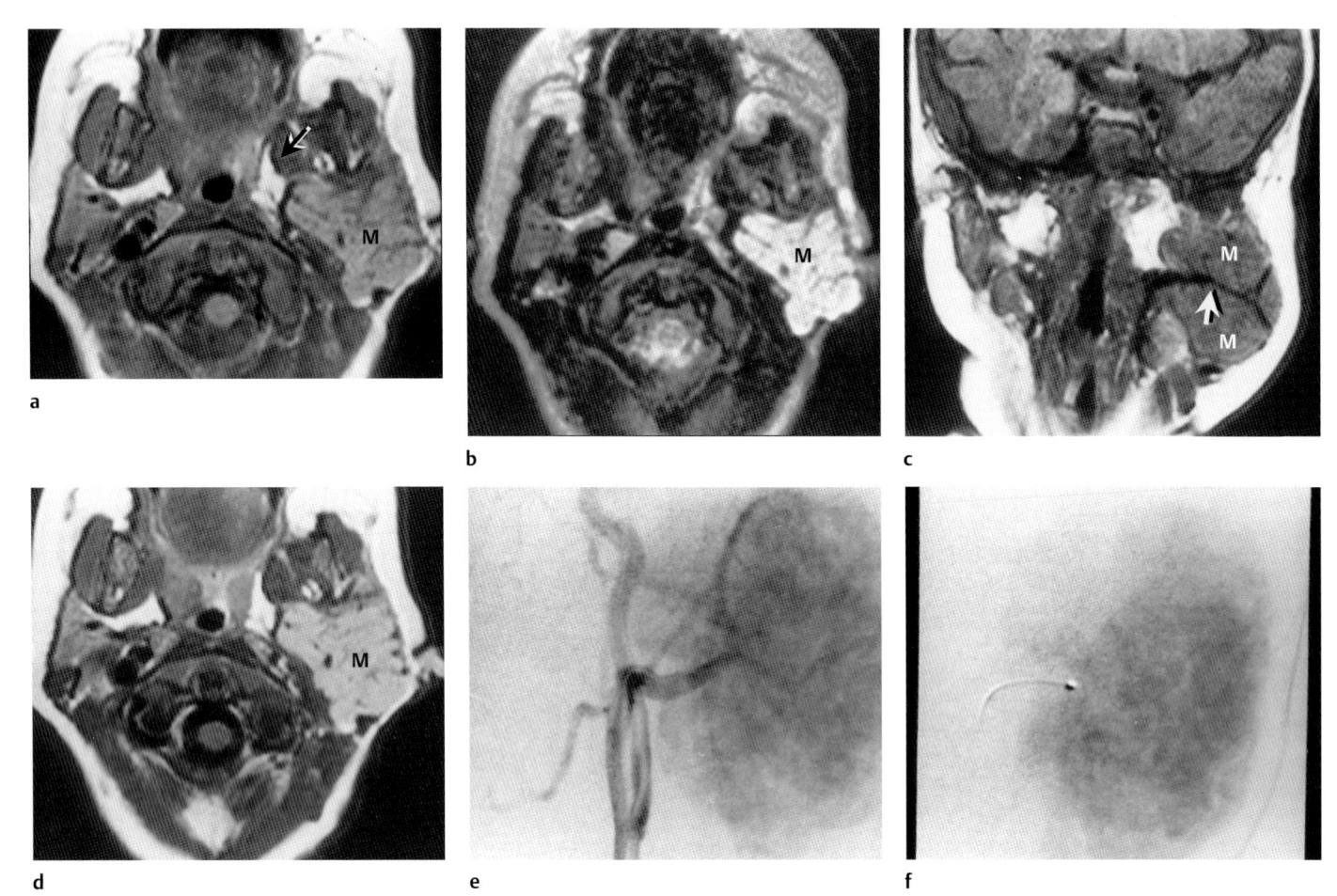

Fig. 8.38 Hemangioma of the parotid space in a 7-month-old infant. **a** Proton-weighted (2200/20) and **b** T2W (2200/100) axial MR images demonstrate a slightly lobulated mass (M) of increased signal intensity relative to muscle on the proton-weighted image and of signal intensity similar to cerebrospinal fluid on the T2W image, which fills the parotid space and extends through a widened stylomandibular tunnel to displace the prestyloid parapharyngeal fat (arrow) anteromedially. **c** T1W (800/20) coronal MR image demonstrates the mass (M) to be of similar signal intensity to adjacent muscle, with a markedly enlarged central feeding vessel (arrow). **d** T1W (800/20) contrast-enhanced MR image demonstrates marked diffuse enhancement, with the mass much higher in signal intensity than adjacent muscle following contrast administration. **e** Late arterial phase of a conventional contrast angiogram also shows the large feeding vessel along with tumor blush. **f** Late capillary phase demonstrates persistent tumor stain, characteristic of hemangioma.

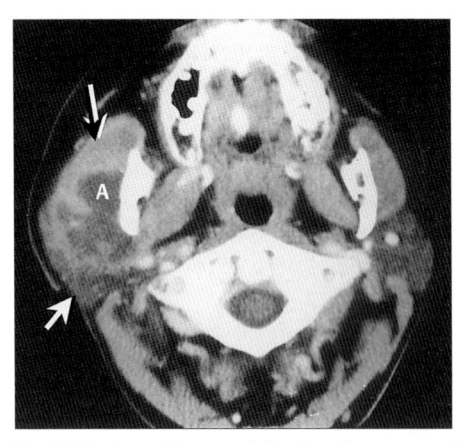

Fig. 8.39 Parotid space infection from extension of an odontogenic masseter muscle abscess. Axial contrast-enhanced CT scan at the level of the oropharynx demonstrates enlargement of the right masseter (black arrow) with a large, low-attenuation collection consistent with abscess formation (A). The abscess appears to bulge posteriorly into the parotid space, with increased attenuation of the adjacent parotid gland parenchyma consistent with inflammation (white arrow).

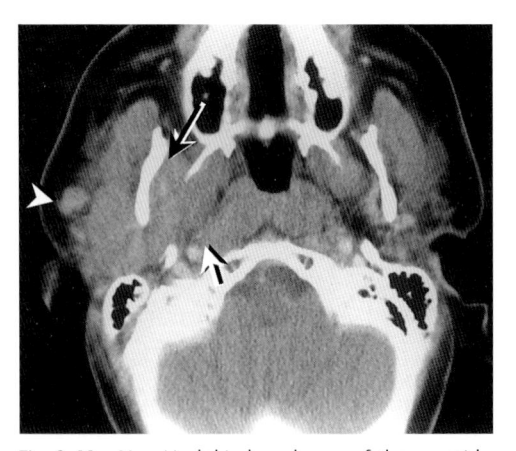

Fig. 8.40 Non-Hodgkin lymphoma of the parotid space. Axial contrast-enhanced CT scan demonstrates an intermediate-attenuation mass infiltrating through the right parotid gland with extension into the masticator space and obliteration of the normal fat plane between the lateral pterygoid muscle and mandibular ramus (black arrow). Ill-defined increased attenuation is noted, obscuring the fat planes medial to the right internal carotid artery within the retrostyloid compartment of the parapharyngeal space (white arrow). A prominent periparotid lymph node is also noted (arrowhead).

present as a mass at the mandibular angle in the young adult, which is often precipitated by a respiratory tract infection or trauma.[148]

Imaging features: As discussed above, the most common location for a second branchial cleft cyst is within the submandibular space, characteristically displacing the submandibular gland anteriorly, the sternocleidomastoid muscle posterolaterally, and the carotid and jugular vessels posteromedially (Fig. 8.41).[176] Occasionally, the cyst may extend between the internal and external carotid arteries.

On imaging studies, this lesion typically appears as an oval mass with low attenuation values on CT and fluid signal intensity on MR scans, with wall thickness and surrounding soft-tissue edema dependent upon the presence and severity of associated infection.[148] When a thin-walled cyst is seen in a young adult with this characteristic pattern of displacement of adjacent structures, the diagnosis can be suggested with confidence (Fig. 8.41).[148]

At this location, it is important to consider cystic metastasis of papillary thyroid carcinoma in the differential diagnosis. An enhancing soft-tissue nodule in the latter may provide a clue to the diagnosis (Fig. 8.42). Other cystic lesions of the submandibular space (but rarely giving the characteristic pattern of displacement of adjacent structures) include submandibular gland cysts, lymphangiomas, necrotic or cystic nerve sheath tumors, epidermoid or dermoid cysts, and metastatic cystic node of primary squamous cell carcinoma[31] (see Chapters 10 and 12).

Lymphangioma

As discussed above, lymphangiomas present as thin-walled unilocular or multilocular masses of fluid attenuation values or fluid signal intensity.[176] The submandibular space is a common site for lymphangiomas, which often extend into adjacent fascial spaces. At times, lymphangiomas appear hyperintense on T1-weighted and T2-weighted MR images owing to proteinaceous fluid or old hemorrhage.

Thyroglossal Duct Cyst

Thyroglossal duct cysts, representing approximately 70% of congenital neck abnormalities, are the most common nonodontogenic neck cysts.[177, 178] During embryogenesis, the thyroglossal duct passes from the foramen cecum in the midline through the tongue musculature and mylohyoid muscle in the floor of the mouth, and then continues deep to the platysma muscle and anterior to the hyoid bone. The duct loops around the inferior border of the hyoid bone and passes slightly upward into the concavity of the posterior surface of the hyoid bone before resuming its inferior course anterior to the thyrohyoid membrane and strap muscles.[178] Ultimately, the duct terminates at the level of the thyroid gland isthmus. The thyroglossal duct is lined with secretory epithelium, and cysts can form anywhere along its course if involution is incomplete.[178] Remnants of thyroid tissue may occasionally be found within these cysts, and migration of the thyroid gland itself can be arrested anywhere along the course of the thyroglossal duct.[178] Only 20% of thyroglossal duct cysts are within the suprahyoid neck, with 15% at the level of the hyoid bone and 65% below.[174, 178] When suprahyoid and within the submandibular space, thyroglossal duct cysts typically separate the anterior bellies of the two digastric muscles and are in the midline (Fig. 8.43).[176] However, up to 25% of suprahyoid thyroglossal duct cysts may be paramedian.[174] Further discussion of thyroglossal duct cysts is included in Chapter 12.

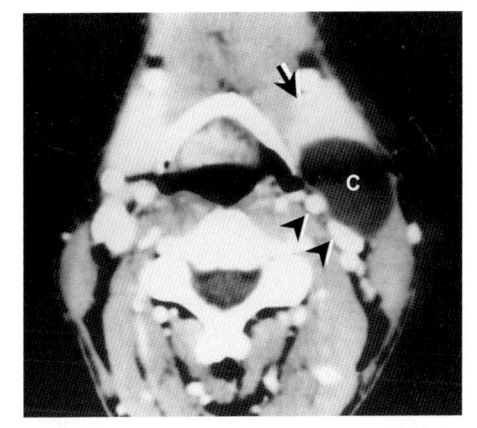

Fig. 8.41 Second branchial cleft cyst. Axial contrast-enhanced CT scan demonstrates a low-attenuation thin-walled well-defined cyst (C) that displaces the submandibular gland anteriorly (arrow), the sternocleidomastoid muscle posterolaterally, and the carotid artery and internal jugular vein posteromedially (arrowheads). This is the characteristic appearance for a second branchial cleft cyst in its most common location.

Ranulas

Although ranulas arise from the salivary glands (sublingual, submandibular) and are discussed in the appropriate chapter (Chapter 9), their place in the differential diagnosis of cystic lesions of the sublingual and submandibular spaces merits additional brief description. The simple ranula represents a mucous retention cyst of the sublingual gland and appears as a sharply marginated lesion of low attenuation values or fluid signal intensity conforming to the fascial boundaries of the sublingual space (Fig. 8.44).[176] If the ranula ruptures through its capsule, it may extend from the sublingual space into the submandibular space and is then termed a "diving" or "plunging" ranula. At this stage, the cystic lesion typi-

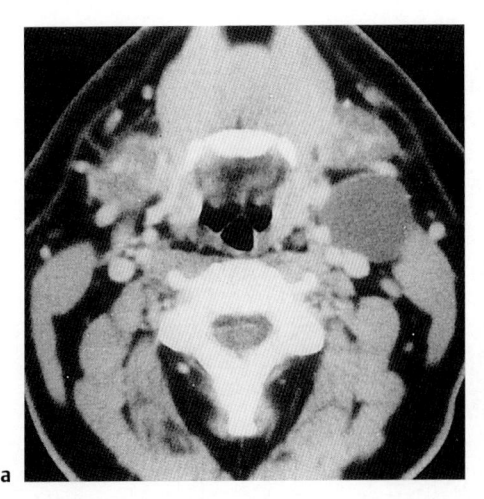

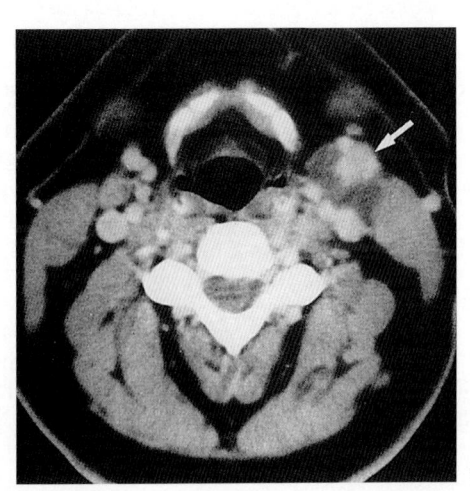

Fig. 8.42 Cystic thyroid carcinoma metastasis mimicking a second branchial cleft cyst. **a** Axial contrast-enhanced CT scan demonstrates a thinned walled, well-defined mass of fluid-attenuation in a characteristic location for a second branchial cleft cyst. **b** Axial contrast-enhanced CT scan at a lower level demonstrates an enhancing soft-tissue nodule (arrow) within the cystic lesion, which excludes an uncomplicated branchial cleft cyst from the differential diagnosis. Excisional biopsy demonstrated papillary thyroid carcinoma.

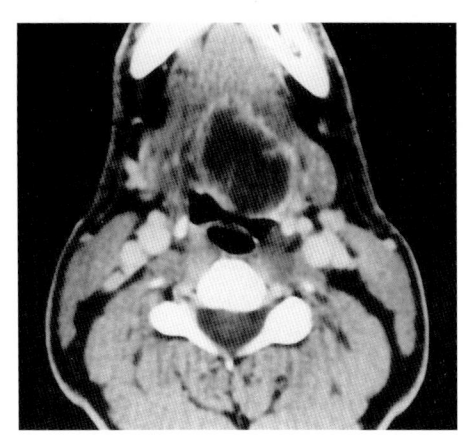

Fig. 8.43 Infected thyroglossal duct cyst. Axial contrast-enhanced CT scan at the level of the tongue base in a patient with fever and dysphagia demonstrates a fluid attenuation mass near the midline immediately above the hyoid bone. The irregular, slightly thickened rim is consistent with associated infection.

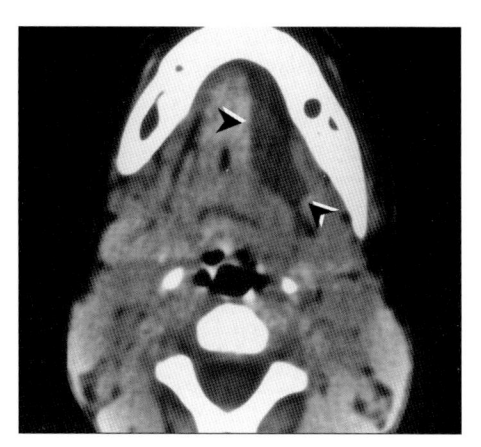

Fig. 8.44 Ranula. Axial CT scan demonstrates a fluid-attenuation mass filling and expanding the left sublingual space, without a visible wall (arrowheads).

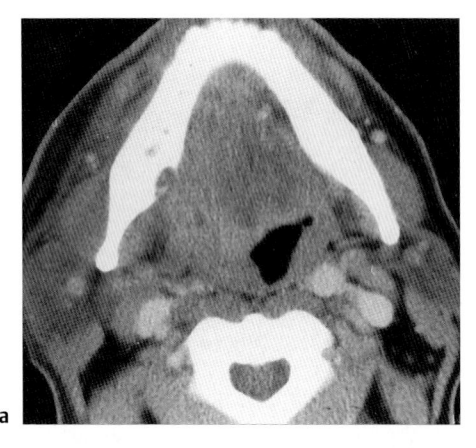

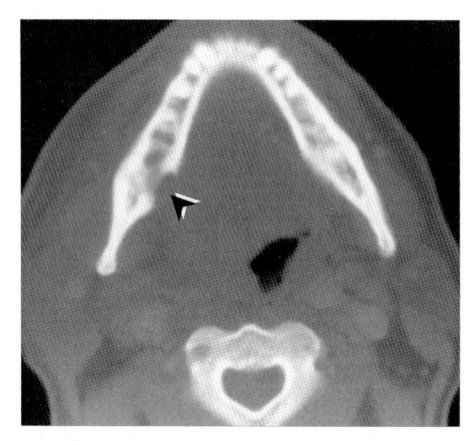

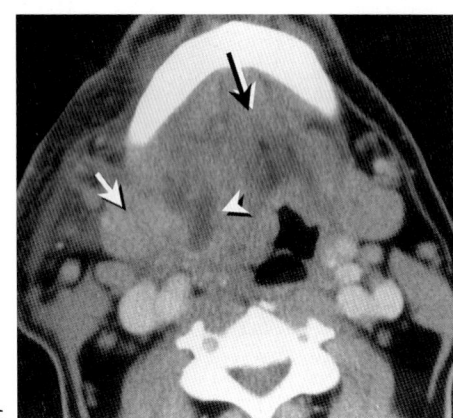

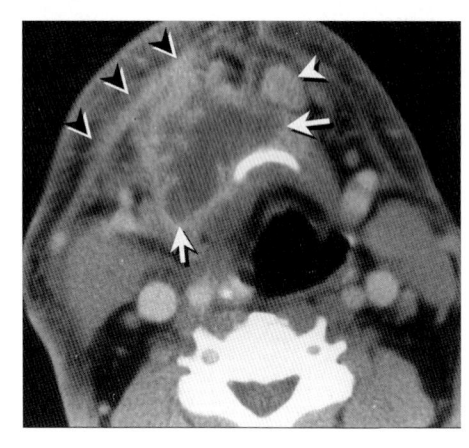

Fig. 8.45 Submandibular and sublingual space infection and mandibular osteomyelitis following wisdom tooth extraction. **a** Axial contrast-enhanced CT scan demonstrates an erosion within the inner margin of the posterior mandible, with abnormal increased attenuation obscuring the fat planes of the sublingual space on the right and resulting in displacement of the oropharynx. **b** Bone window at the same level better demonstrates abnormal lucency within the mandibular cortex extending to the level of the third molar root socket (arrowhead). **c** Axial contrast-enhanced CT scan at a lower level demonstrates displacement of the geniohyoid muscles toward the left (black arrow) and extension of the inflammatory process posteriorly into the submandibular space adjacent to the submandibular gland (white arrow). An area of decreased attenuation is noted, suggesting abscess formation (arrowhead). **d** Axial contrast-enhanced CT scan at a lower level demonstrates extension into the submandibular space inferiorly to the level of the hyoid bone, with a large low-attenuation collection with slightly enhancing rim consistent with abscess formation (white arrows). Marked edema is noted within the overlying subcutaneous tissues, along with thickening of the skin and thickening of the overlying platysma muscle (black arrowheads). A prominent submental lymph node is present, displaced toward the left (white arrowhead).

cally conforms to the boundaries of the submandibular space, but may also extend into the prestyloid compartment of the parapharyngeal space.[176] Typically, diving ranulas demonstrate a "tail" of low attenuation values on CT or fluid signal intensity on MR extending around the posterior margin of the mylohyoid muscle into the sublingual space.[5] Occasionally, the communication may be through the mid-anterior aspect of the mylohyoid muscle.[176] The presence of this tail differentiates the ranula from an epidermoid cyst or lymphangioma.[176] Simple ranulas may infrequently become large and extend over the posterior margin of the mylohyoid muscle without rupturing, appearing similar to a diving ranula. When a history of previous infection or surgery is present, the typical imperceptibly thin wall may thicken.[176] Further discussion of ranulas is included in Chapters 9 and 10.

Inflammatory Conditions

Infection of the submandibular and sublingual spaces is common and can easily pass from one space to the other around the posterior margin of the mylohyoid muscle. If the process is not controlled, the infection may spread into the masticatory and parapharyngeal spaces. Infections of the submandibular space most commonly occur from dental, floor of mouth, or buccal infections draining to the submandibular lymph nodes; extension of infections of the submandibular glands, often resulting from ductal obstruction by stones, may also lead to submandibular space inflammation.[144] Cellulitis and abscess of the submandibular space readily extends posteriorly into the prestyloid parapharyngeal space. Submandibular space infection may also result directly from odontogenic infection (Fig. 8.**45**). Typically, the roots of the second and third molars extend beneath the mylohyoid attachment, and infection can directly involve the submandibular space. Infection of roots anterior to the second molar extends above the mylohyoid muscle and leads to sublingual space involvement.[154] The responsible organisms are usually streptococci or staphylococci, although mixed infections including anaerobic bacteria are common and tend to spread to multiple adjacent spaces.[176, 179]

One potentially lethal form of acute infection of the sublingual space, termed Ludwig angina, deserves special attention.[179] Ludwig angina is defined as a cellulitis of the floor of the mouth that usually results from dental infection, trauma, or tooth extraction.[154] Ninety percent of reported cases are related to infection of the mandibular molars.[179] By definition, the cellulitis always involves both sublingual glands and spreads rapidly throughout the suprahyoid soft tissues of the neck, resulting in edema with posterior and superior displacement of the tongue.[154, 179] If it is untreated, extension may occur to involve the prestyloid and retrostyloid compartments of the parapharyngeal space, retropharyngeal space, and, infrequently, the mediastinum and subphrenic areas.[179] Ludwig angina represents a clinical emergency since, if it is not recognized and treated promptly, suffocation may result from compromise of the airway.[179] Further discussion of Ludwig angina and its imaging features is included in Chapter 10.

Benign Tumors

Benign tumors of the submandibular and sublingual spaces include dermoid and epidermoid tumors, lipomas, and benign tumors of salivary gland origin. The salivary glands are covered elsewhere (Chapter 9). Lipomas are uncommon and are diagnosed by their characteristic appearance identical to that of subcutaneous fat on CT and MR (Fig. 8.**46**).

Both dermoid and epidermoid cysts are included in the differential diagnosis of midline or near-midline cystic masses of the sublingual and submandibular spaces, along with suprahyoid thryoglossal duct cysts and necrotic lymph nodes. Dermoid cysts are rare in the neck, but may account for up to 22% of midline or near-midline neck lesions.[134] They may occur in either the submandibular or the sublingual space and have an epithelial lining composed of both ectodermal and mesodermal components.[134, 176] CT and MR typically demonstrate a thin-walled cystic lesion. The presence of internal fat can help differentiate dermoid tumors from other cysts of this region.[134, 176] Further discussion of dermoid and epidermoid cysts is included in Chapter 10.

Malignant Tumors

Malignant tumor outside of the salivary glands most commonly arises from the submandibular and submental lymph node chains, which represent the primary drainage for neoplasms occurring in the lower lip, anterior buccal mucosa, alveolar ridge, oral tongue, and sublingual space.[176] Sublingual and submandibular space involvement can also result from direct extension of oral cavity or tongue carcinoma (Fig. 8.**47**). As with malignant lymphadenopathy elsewhere in the neck, malignant lymph nodes are typically thick-walled and irregular and demonstrate moderate contrast enhancement following intravenous administration of contrast media. Metastatic nodes may be cystic (Fig. 8.**42**) or extend into adjacent tissues (extranodal extension).

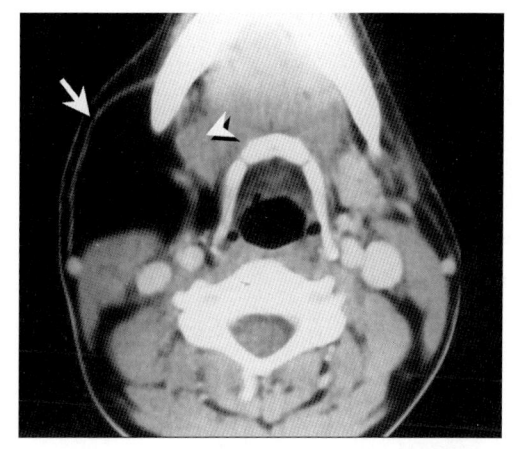

Fig. 8.**46** Lipoma of the submandibular space. Axial contrast-enhanced CT scan at the level of the hyoid bone demonstrates a mass displacing the right submandibular gland anteromedially (arrowhead) and the platysma muscle laterally (arrow). The mass is identical in attenuation to subcutaneous fat and is well-defined and homogeneous.

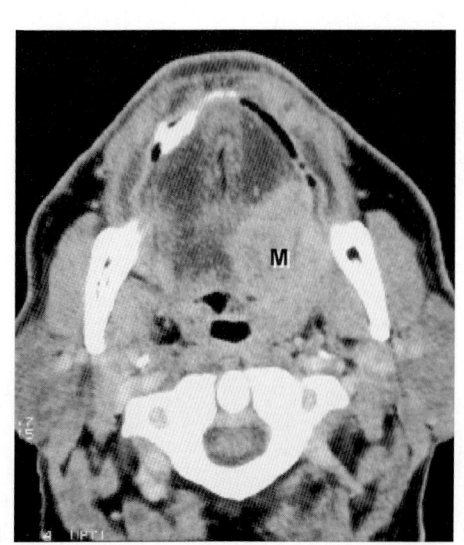

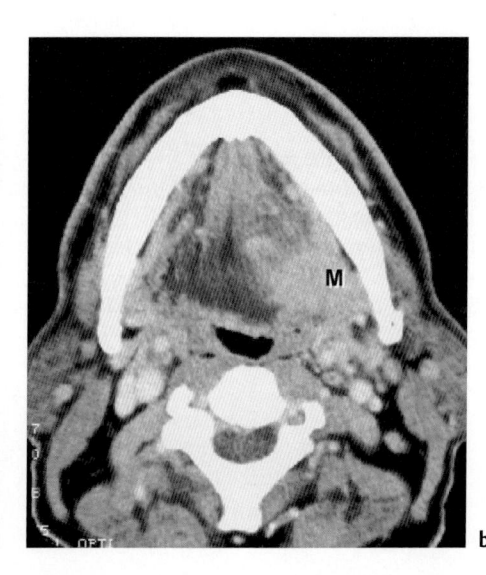

Fig. 8.**47** Squamous cell carcinoma of the tongue base. **a** Enhanced axial CT scan demonstrates a large, fairly enhancing mass lesion (M) involving the left root of the tongue, obliterating the normal fat plane between the pharynx and the medial pterygoid muscle, and extending posteriorly to infiltrate the anterior tonsillar pillar (palatoglossus muscle). **b** Section at the level of the floor of the mouth in the same case, showing the tongue base mass to be violating the left sublingual space (harboring the left neurovascular bundle of the tongue) and infiltrating the ipsilateral genioglossus/geniohyoid muscles, but stopping short of the midline. Reproduced from Reference 4 with permission.

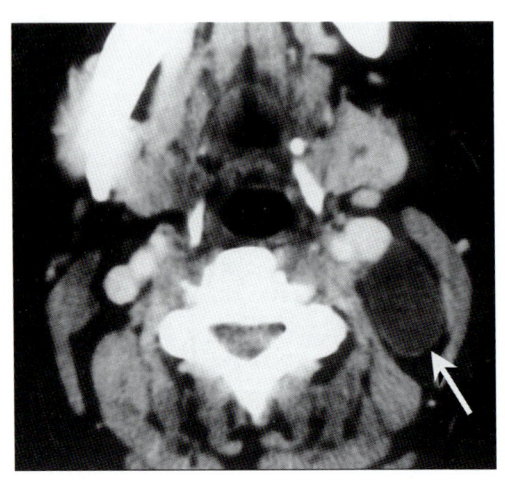

Fig. 8.**48** Lymphangioma (cystic hygroma) of the posterior cervical space. Axial contrast-enhanced CT scan at the level of the hyoid bone demonstrates a well-defined unilocular fluid-attenuation mass with a thin, uniform wall, which expands the posterior cervical space (arrows). A metastatic cystic nodal disease from papillary thyroid carcinoma and squamous cell carcinoma may simulate this lymphangioma.

Posterior Cervical Space

The posterior cervical space, between the paraspinal muscles and sternocleidomastoid muscle, is relatively small in the suprahyoid neck but becomes much larger below the hyoid bone. This space can be involved by a number of processes, including congenital lesions such as lymphangioma cystic hygroma (Fig. 8.**48**), hemangiomas, and branchial cleft cysts, or tumors such as lipomas, neurofibromas, schwannomas, lymphoma, aggressive fibromatosis and other rare sarcomas.[180] However, most disease of the posterior cervical space relates to the spinal accessory chain of lymph nodes, including inflammatory adenopathy, metastatic carcinoma, and lymphoma.[21,180,181] The majority of these processes are more common below the level of the hyoid bone.

The posterior cervical space is the most common location for lipomas of the head and neck, which comprise 13% of all lipomas.[134] They are rare in the first two decades of life and are usually detected during the fifth and sixth decades.[134] Lipomas are usually readily diagnosed on CT or MR as masses of attenuation values or signal intensity identical to those of subcutaneous fat that displace and compress contiguous structures but rarely infiltrate.[134]

■ Suprahyoid Neck Trauma

The suprahyoid portions of the pharynx, i.e., the nasopharynx and oropharynx, are less vulnerable to trauma than the infrahyoid pharynx (hypopharynx) or the larynx,[10] with the vast majority of radiologically documented nasopharyngeal or oropharyngeal injuries being described in the literature as case reports.[187-199]

The clinicopathological outcome and the imaging findings expected after trauma to this part of the pharynx are to a large extent dictated by the mechanisms of trauma. By convention, these are classified into blunt (closed) and penetrating (open) types.

Blunt Trauma

Blunt head and neck trauma, such as that caused by motor vehicle accidents, may result in the formation of retropharyngeal hematoma, a condition that may progress rapidly into a life-threatening airway obstruction.[21,200]

Once posttraumatic prevertebral soft-tissue fullness is seen on the emergency radiographs, the primary concern should be directed toward securing and maintaining the patient's airway.[187] A CT scan should then be performed to evaluate for potential cervical spine fractures. Sections should start as high as the skull base in order to detect possible occipital condyle fractures[191] and should cover as low as the inferior extent of the hematoma, which may reach down to the mediastinum.

Retropharyngeal hematomas have also been reported following minor blunt trauma,[187] minor hyperextension injuries,[190] and airbag deployment in a minor motor vehicle accident.[188]

Nontraumatic causes of retropharyngeal hematoma include anticoagulant therapy and complications of aneurysms, tumors, and infections.[190]

Penetrating Trauma

Trauma leading to pharyngeal perforation may be accidental or iatrogenic. Accidental perforations usually involve the oropharynx and may be caused by foreign bodies,[21] fish bones,[197] gunshots,[198] and direct injuries by intraoral sharp objects. The latter is particularly common in children falling with objects, e.g., tooth brushes, in their mouths.[199] Iatrogenic perforations more commonly involve the nasopharynx and may complicate upper GI endoscopy,[194] assisted ventilation,[21] neonatal pharyngeal suction catheters, and nasogastric or tracheal intubation during resuscitation of newborns.[193]

The results of pharyngeal perforation may include any or a combination of the following:

- Surgical emphysema, caused by air dissecting its way through the torn pharyngeal wall. Retropharyngeal free air is the most common sequel of perforation and is readily identified on CT. Occasionally, quite large amounts of interstitial air may cause multiple deep fascial spaces and may extend downward, giving rise to pneumomediastinum.[21,192,194,201]
- Retropharyngeal abscess occurs less often and is due to the spread of organisms from the oral bacterial flora. Uncontrolled infection may spread into the deep fascial planes, resulting in fasciitis or parapharyngeal abscess,[10] may extend downward along the retropharyngeal space to cause mediastinitis, and may even enter the danger space to reach down to the diaphragm.[192] The imaging features of retropharyngeal abscess have been described earlier in this chapter.
- Vascular injury. Internal carotid artery (ICA) thrombosis and cerebral ischemia may complicate posterolateral oropharyngeal injury, particularly in children falling with sharp objects in their mouths. The ICA is typically injured 1–3 cm above the common carotid bifurcation, where it is separated from the oropharyngeal airway only by the tonsil and superior constrictor pharyngeal muscle. The patient classically presents, after a lucid interval of occasionally more than 24 hours, with disturbed consciousness, hemiplegia, and possibly expressive aphasia if ischemia involves the dominant cerebral hemisphere.[199]

Carotid artery thrombosis has also been reported following blunt intraoral[195] and minor pharyngeal injuries.[196]

Obstructive Sleep Apnea Syndrome (OSA)

Pathophysiology: OSA is episodic upper airway obstruction during sleep, most commonly occurring at the pharyngeal level.[202] The condition may be considered, in part, a neuromuscular disorder. Normally, the neural output to the pharyngeal muscles decreases with the onset of sleep, thus reducing their tone. With inspiration, the negative pressure created in the upper airway has the potential to collapse the hypotonic pharyngeal wall if the pharyngeal airway is originally smaller or more compliant than normal.[203]

Clinical presentation: The condition is more common among obese males. The incidence of OSA also increases with age, snoring, tobacco and alcohol use, and use of sedatives, as well as with genetic and familial risks.[202]

The repetitive episodes of apnea during sleep, lasting from 10 to more than 60 seconds[202], result in arterial oxygen desaturation and recurrent awakening, leading to the syndrome characterized by daytime somnolence, morning headache, and poor concentration.[203, 204] Other associated conditions that have been linked to OSA include gastroesophageal reflux, impotence, cardiac arrhythmias, hypertension, and increased risk of stroke and myocardial infarction.[166, 168]

Role of imaging: Currently, the diagnosis of OSA is a clinical one supported by overnight polysomnography (continuous recording of relevant physiological changes during sleep) to determine the physiological severity, and transnasal fiberoptic endoscopy to estimate the actual grade of airway narrowing.[202]

With the emergence of new imaging technology, dynamic imaging of the pharynx in near real time has become a reality, permitting the noninvasive assessment of functional pharyngeal abnormalities. Many reports have described the use of ultrafast CT (electron beam computed tomography)[203, 205–208] and MR fluoroscopy[204, 209–213] for the dynamic evaluation of upper airways in OSA patients.

Ultrafast CT scanning utilizes an electron gun to produce a fast-moving electron beam that hits multiple detector rings in the gantry, permitting the simultaneous acquisition of multiple image sections. This results in a superior temporal resolution with images obtained in as little as 50–100 ms.[214] Other than the utilization of ionizing radiation, the disadvantage of using ultrafast CT in evaluating patients with OSA is the inability to obtain primary images in the midsagittal plane.[204]

The term "MR fluoroscopy" has been introduced with the development of numerous rapid gradient-echo sequences capable of acquiring MR images at rates as high as 0.3–7 seconds per frame.[215, 216] Fluoroscopic MR imaging has been used for functional imaging of the upper airways utilizing GRASS (gradient-recalled acquisition in the steady state)[204, 209, 210] and FLASH (fast low-angle shot)[204, 211, 213] sequences. Images are obtained in the sagittal and axial planes during quiet nasal respiration, simulation of snoring, and performance of the Müller maneuver (inspiratory effort with the mouth and nose closed).[204] Axial scans are obtained at the levels of the oropharynx and velopharynx (lowest part of nasopharynx opposite the soft palate, which is one of the narrowest sites in OSA patients[218]).

Two fundamental imaging abnormalities are sought when evaluating patients with OSA:[203, 204]
1. Narrowing of the luminal cross-sectional area of the pharynx, as seen on axial images. The length of narrowing is determined on the sagittal images.
2. Increased compliance of the pharyngeal walls. The mobility of the uvula, tongue base, and posterior pharyngeal wall is assessed on sagittal images, whereas the mobility of the lateral pharyngeal walls is assessed on axial images.

Suprahyoid Neck Biopsy and Interventional MRI

Interventional MRI is the use of MR techniques to guide radiological interventions, including both diagnostic and minimally invasive therapeutic procedures.

In areas of complex anatomy, the tissue contrast, spatial resolution, and multiplanar capabilities peculiar to MRI provide the obvious advantages for its use to guide interventional procedures. This is particularly true for sampling suprahyoid neck lesions,[216, 219, 220] where CT guidance is limited by several factors, including the inability to maintain a confident localization of the vascular anatomy throughout the procedure, the inability to go beyond a single imaging plane (usually axial), the frequent improper definition of pharyngeal submucosal lesions on CT, and the beam hardening artifacts inherent in CT at the skull base.

The major benefits of using MRI for procedure guidance in this region are[216, 219, 220] (Fig. 8.**49**):

- The ability to continuously visualize the internal carotid, vertebral, and major branches of the external carotid arteries during the entire needle insertion (Fig. 8.**49**). The high vascular conspicuity is due to flow-related enhancement effects inherent in the gradient-echo sequences used for procedure guidance.
- The multiplanar imaging capabilities that ensure precise needle centralization along the axial as well as the craniocaudal dimensions of the lesion. In addition, imaging in any arbitrary plane allows the needle trajectory to be tailored according to the individual case.
- The ability to guide needle insertion with continuous, near-real-time imaging so that the needle can be redirected in order to avoid critical structures in a time-efficient manner.
- The ability to shift between T1-weighted and T2-weighted contrast during the procedure to maximize the lesion conspicuity. T2-weighted techniques also allow sampling of the nonnecrotic regions of complex masses, thus increasing the diagnostic tissue yield.

An additional use of the interventional MR imaging techniques that form the basis for biopsy guidance is application of these methods for the guidance and monitoring of direct intralesional drug injection, including injection for sclerotherapy of vascular malformations. The same rapid image updates used for interactive needle placement can be used to monitor the injection of sclerosing agents for the treatment of low-flow vascular malformations.[139] The multiplanar images obtained with MR allow the injection of alcohol or other sclerosing agents to be monitored during administration, to ensure filling of the entire targeted portion of the malformation and to exclude extravasation or dissipation of the agent through venous egress.[139]

The use of radiofrequency thermal energy to induce tongue base scarring and subsequent shrinkage has been reported for the treatment of selected patients with OSA syndrome.[221] Recently, a new technique of percutaneous MR-guided radiofrequency ablation of the tongue base has been described.[222]

The accuracy and safety of MR-guided procedures depend on proper needle visualization. Achieving this requires a sound understanding of a number of user-defined imaging parameters as well as needle trajectory decisions, which are beyond the scope of this chapter.[215, 216, 219, 223]

Three basic components combine to form the foundation of the modern interventional MR suite:
1. The availability of an "open" magnet imaging system to facilitate the patient access necessary for performing the procedures (Fig. 8.**50**).

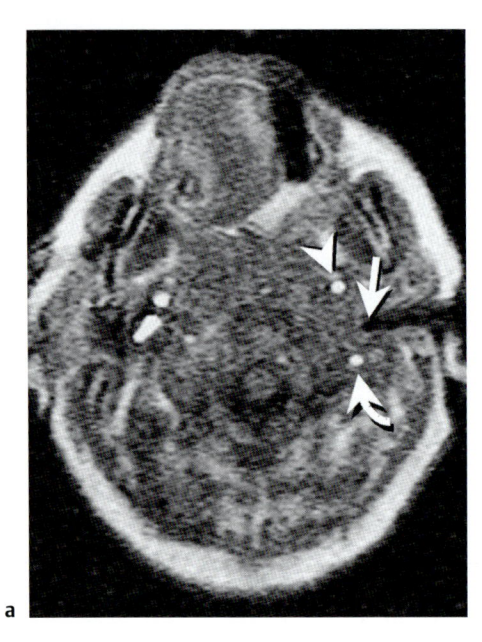

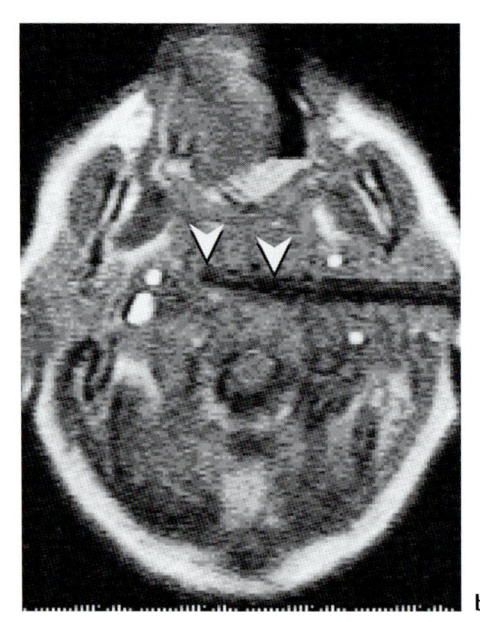

Fig. 8.**49** Interventional near-real-time MR-guided suprahyoid neck biopsy. Images from continuous series obtained at 7 seconds/image with fast imaging with steady-state precession (FISP) sequence (18/7/4/90°, TR/TE/number of signal averages/flip angle) obtained during guidance of needle insertion in a 68-year-old man with C1–2 vertebral and prevertebral mass. A previous attempt at surgical transoral biopsy had been unsuccessful. **a** Image early during insertion demonstrates needle tip passing through the left parotid space. An ill-defined mass can be seen in the prevertebral space. High vascular conspicuity resulting from 2D Fourier transform technique allows ready visualization of flow-related enhancement within the internal carotid (arrowhead) and vertebral (curved arrow) arteries. The needle tip (straight arrow) can be interactively directed to avoid these major vascular structures. **b** The needle is redirected more anteriorly once safely beyond the internal carotid artery (ICA). The location of the needle's side notch is shown as an area of thinning of the distal needle tip (between arrowheads). Histology demonstrated chronic osteomyelitis and cellulitis and the offending organism was successfully isolated. Reproduced from Reference 4 with permission.

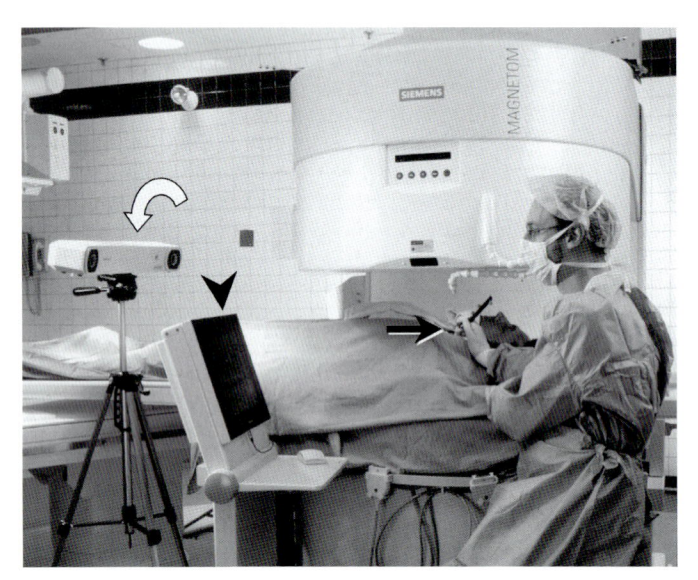

Fig. 8.**50** Interventional MRI suite. MR suite set up for radiological intervention has an open magnet design to provide easy access for the patient, and a video camera sensor array (curved arrow) that detects the location and orientation of a hand-held probe (black arrow). The system automatically acquires continuous MR images based on the probe position, and automatically updates the display of four images on a shielded LCD monitor adjacent to the scanner (arrowhead). A computer mouse on the LCD console and foot pedals (not shown) allow the scanner to be operated by the radiologist throughout the procedure. Reproduced from Reference 4 with permission.

2 The application of new fast gradient-echo pulse sequences that allow a wide range of tissue contrast in a time frame sufficient for device tracking (between 0.3 and 7 seconds per image) even at the low field strengths of open magnets and with the suboptimal coil position sometimes necessary for accessing the puncture site.[215,217,219,224,225]

3 The ability to view images in near real time at the scanner side through an in-room high-resolution radiofrequency-shielded monitor (Fig. 8.**50**).[36,215,216]

With these three components, the entire procedure can be performed with the operator sitting next to the patient and without the need to remove the operator's hand from the interventional device at any time. This manner of intervention, analogous to an angiographic or sonographically-guided procedure, is well-suited to the skill set developed by radiologists during more conventional types of image-guided intervention.

References

1. Moore KL. The neck. In: Clinically Oriented Anatomy 3d ed. Baltimore: Williams and Wilkins; 1992: 783–852.
2. Mukherji SK, Castillo M. Normal cross-sectional anatomy of the nasopharynx, oropharynx, and oral cavity. Neuroimaging Clin North Am. 1998; 8: 211–8.
3. Seaman WB. Pharynx. radiology. In: Margulis AR, Burhenne HJ, eds. Alimentary Tract Radiology, 3d ed. St Louis, MO: Mosby; 1983: 491–518.
4. Nour SG, Lewin JS. Nasoparynx/oropharynx. In: Haaga JR, Lanzieri CF, eds. CT and MR Imaging of the Whole Body, 4th ed. St. Louis, MO: Mosby; 2002: 619–662.
5. Harnsberger HR. Head and neck imaging. In: Osborne AG, Bragg DC, eds. Handbooks in Radiology, 2d ed. St Louis: Mosby-Year Book; 1995
6. Norbash AM. Nasopharynx and deep facial spaces. In: Eldman RR, Hesselink JR, Zlatkin MB, eds. Clinical Magnetic Resonance Imaging, 2d ed. Philadelphia: W.B. Saunders; 1996: 1079–1109.
7. Barakos JA. Head and neck imaging. In: Brant WE, Helms CA, eds. Fundamentals of Diagnostic Radiology, 2d ed. Philadelphia: Lippincott Williams and Wilkins; 1999: 211–232.
8. Mendenhall WM, Million RR, Mancuso AA, et al. Nasopharynx. In: Million RR, Cassisi NJ, eds. Management of Head and Neck Cancer: A Multidisciplinary Approach. Philadelphia: Lippincott; 1994: 599–626.
9. Ryan SP, McNicholas MMJ. Head and neck. In: Anatomy for Diagnostic Imaging. London: W.B. Saunders; 1994: 1–44.
10. Mukherji SK, Holliday RA. Pharynx. In: Som PM, Curtin HD, eds. Head and Neck Imaging, 3d ed. St Louis, MO: Mosby; 1996: 437–487.
11. Som PM, Sacher M, Stollman AL, Biller HF, Lawson W. Common tumors of the parapharyngeal space: refined imaging diagnosis. Radiology 1988; 169: 81–85.
12. Curtin HD. Separation of the masticator space from the parapharyngeal space. Radiology 1987; 16: 195–204.

13 Harnsberger HR, Osborn AG. Differential diagnosis of head and neck lesions based on their space of origin. 1. The suprahyoid part of the neck. AJR 1991; 157: 147–154.
14 Clemente CD, ed. Muscles and fasciae. In: Gray's Anatomy, 30th American edition. Philadelphia: Lea and Febiger; 1985: 429–605.
15 Hardin CW, Harnsberger HR, Osborn AG, Doxey GP, Davis RK, Nyberg DA. Infection and tumor of the masticator space: CT evaluation. Radiology 1985;157: 413–417.
16 Hollinshead WH, Rosse Cornelius. Pharynx and larynx. In: Textbook of Anatomy, 4th ed. Philadelphia: Harper and Row; 1985; 987–1006.
17 Paonessa DF, Goldstein JC. Anatomy and physiology of head and neck infections (with emphasis on the fascia of the face and neck). Otolaryngol Clin North Am 1976; 9: 561–580.
18 Lanzieri CF, Lewin JS. Oropharynx and Nasopharynx. In: Stark DD, Bradley WG, eds. Magnetic Resonance Imaging, 3d ed. St. Louis, MO: Mosby; 1999.
19 Mafee MF. Nasopharynx, parapharyngeal space, and skull base. In: Valvassori GE, Mafee MF, Carter BL, eds. Imaging of the Head and Neck. Stuttgart: Georg Thieme Verlag; 1995: 332–363.
20 Som PM, Biller HF, Lawson W. Tumors of the parapharyngeal space: preoperative evaluation, diagnosis and surgical approaches. Ann Otol Rhinol Laryngol Suppl 1981; 90: 3–15.
21 Davis WL, Harnsberger HR, Smoker WR, Watanabe AS. Retropharyngeal space: evaluation of normal anatomy and diseases with CT and MR imaging. Radiolog. 1990; 174: 59–64.
22 Cross RR, Shapiro MD, Som PM. MRI of the parapharyngeal space. Radiol Clin North Am 1989; 27: 353–378.
23 Mancuso AA, Harnsberger HR, Muraki AS, Stevens MH. Computed tomography of cervical and retropharyngeal lymph nodes: normal anatomy, variants of normal, and applications in staging head and neck cancer. Part I: normal anatomy. Radiology 1983; 148: 709–714.
24 Silver AJ, Mawad ME, Hilal SK, Sane P, Ganti SR. Computed tomography of the carotid space and related cervical spaces. Part I: Anatomy. Radiology 1984; 150: 723–728.
25 Olsen KD. Tumors and surgery of the parapharyngeal space. Laryngoscope 1994; 104: 1–28.
26 Maran AG, Mackenzie IJ, Murray JA. The parapharyngeal space. J Laryngol Otol 1984; 98: 371–380.
27 Coit WE, Harnsberger HR, Osborn AG, Smoker WRK, Stevens MH, Lufkin RB. Ranulas and their mimics: CT evaluation. Radiology 1987; 163: 211–216.
28 Vogl T, Dresel S, Bilaniuk LT, Grevers G, Kang K, Lissner J. Tumors of the nasopharynx and adjacent areas: MR imaging with Gd-DTPA. AJR 1990; 154: 585–592.
29 Robinson JD, Crawford SC, Teresi LM, Schiller VL, Lufkin RB, Harnsberger HR, Dietrich RB, Crim JR, Duckwiler GR, Spickler EM, et al. Extracranial lesions of the head and neck: preliminary experience with Gd-DTPA-enhanced MR imaging. Radiology 1989; 172: 165–170.
30 Unger JM. The oral cavity and tongue: magnetic resonance imaging. Radiology 1985; 155: 151–153.
31 Lufkin RB, Wortham DG, Dietrich RB, Hoover LA, Larsson SG, Kangarloo H, Hanafee WN. Tongue and oropharynx: findings on MR imaging. Radiology 1986; 161: 69–75.
32 Lewin JS, Curtin HD, Ross JS, Weissman JL, Obuchowski NA, Tkach JA. Fast spin-echo imaging of the neck: comparison with conventional spin-echo, utility of fat suppression, and evaluation of tissue contrast characteristics. AJNR 1994; 15: 1351–1357.
33 Anzai Y, Lufkin RB, Jabour BA, Hanafee WN. Fat-suppression failure artifacts simulating pathology on frequency-selective fat-suppression MR images of the head and neck. AJNR 1992; 13: 879–884.
34 Vogl TJ, Dresel SH. New developments in magnetic resonance imaging of the nasopharynx and face. Curr Opin Radiol 1991; 3: 61–66.
35 McGowan JC 3d, Hatabu H, Yousem DM, Randall P, Kressel HY. Evaluation of soft palate function with MRI: application to the cleft palate patient. J Comput Assist Tomogr 1992; 16: 877–882.
36 Dähnert W. Ear, nose, and throat disorders. In: Radiology Review Manual, 4th ed. Baltimore: Williams and Wilkins; 1999: 314–335.
37 Chong VF, Fan YF. Radiology of the nasopharynx: pictorial essay. Australas Radiol 2000; 44: 5–13.
38 Ikushima I, Korogi Y, Makita O, Komohara Y, Kawano H, Yamura M, Arikawa K, Takahashi M. MR imaging of Tornwaldt's cysts. AJR 1999; 172: 1663–1665.
39 Battino RA, Khangure MS. Is that another Thornwaldt's cyst on M.R.I.? Australas Radiol 1990; 34: 19–23.
40 Boucher RM, Hendrix RA, Guttenplan MD. The diagnosis of Thornwaldt's cyst. Trans Pa Acad Ophthalmol Otolaryngol 1990; 42: 1026–1030.

41 Finkelstein Y, Malik Z, Kopolovic J, Bernheim J, Djaldetti M, Ophir D. Characterization of smoking-induced nasopharyngeal lymphoid hyperplasia. Laryngoscope 1997; 107: 1635–1642.
42 Brodsky L, Koch RJ. Anatomic correlates of normal and diseased adenoids in children. Laryngoscope 1992; 102: 1268–1274.
43 Potsic WP. Assessment and treatment of adenotonsillar hypertrophy in children. Am J Otolaryngol 1992; 13: 259–264.
44 Gates GA, Avery CA, Prihoda TJ, Cooper JC Jr. Effectiveness of adenoidectomy and tympanostomy tubes in the treatment of chronic otitis media with effusion. N Engl J Med. 1987; 317: 1444–1451.
45 Gates GA, Avery CA, Prihoda TJ. Effect of adenoidectomy upon children with chronic otitis media with effusion. Laryngoscope 1988; 98: 58–63.
46 Dillon WP, Mills CM, Kjos B, DeGroot J, Brant-Zawadzki M. Magnetic resonance imaging of the nasopharynx. Radiology 1984; 152: 731–738.
47 Hudgins PA, Jacobs IN, Castillo M. Pediatric airway disease. In: Som PM, Curtin HD, eds. Head and Neck Imaging, 3d ed. St Louis, MO: Mosby, 1996; 545–611.
48 Ungkanont K, Yellon RF, Weissman JL, Casselbrant ML, Gonzalez-Valdepena H, Bluestone CD. Head and neck space infections in infants and children. Otolaryngol Head Neck Surg 1995; 112: 375–382.
49 Yousem DM, Chalian AA. Oral cavity and pharynx. Radiol Clin North Am 1998; 36: 967–981.
50 Weissleder R, Rieumont MJ, Wittenberg J. Head and neck imaging. In: Primer of Diagnostic Imaging, 2d ed. St. Louis, MO: Mosby, 1997; 547–594.
51 Phelps PD. The pharynx and larynx: the neck. In Sutton D, ed. Textbook of Radiology and Imaging, 6th ed. New York: Churchill Livingstone; 1998: 1273–1295.
52 Gullane PJ, Davidson J, O'Dwyer T, Forte V. Juvenile angiofibroma: a review of the literature and a case series report. Laryngoscope 1992; 102: 928–933.
53 Reddy M, Anton JV, Schoggl A, Reddy B, Matula C. Recurrent angiofibroma invading the skull base—case report. Neurol Med Chir (Tokyo) 2002; 42(10): 439–442.
54 Ungkanont K, Byers RM, Weber RS, Callender DL, Wolf PF, Goepfert H. Juvenile nasopharyngeal angiofibroma: an update of therapeutic management. Head Neck 1996; 18: 60–66.
55 Radkowski D, McGill T, Healy GB, Ohlms L, Jones DT. Angiofibroma. Changes in staging and treatment. Arch Otolaryngol Head Neck Surg 1996; 122: 122–129.
56 Maroldi R, Battaglia G, Farina D, Maculotti P, Chiesa A. Tumours of the oropharynx and oral cavity: perineural spread and bone invasion. JBR-BTR. 1999; 82: 294–300.
57 Neel HB, Slavitt DH. Nasopharyngeal cancer. In: Baily BJ, ed. Head and neck surgery—otolaryngology. Philadelphia: J.B. Lippincott; 1993: 1257–1260.
58 Shanmugaratnam K, Sobin LH. Histological typing of upper respiratory tract tumors. In: International Histological Classification of Tumors, No. 19. Geneva, Switzerland: World Health Organization; 1978.
59 Chong VF, Fan YF, Mukherji SK. Carcinoma of the nasopharynx. Semin Ultrasound CT MR 1998; 19: 449–462.
60 Chong VF, Fan YF, Khoo JB. Nasopharyngeal carcinoma with intracranial spread: CT and MR characteristics. J Comput Assist Tomogr 1996; 20: 563–569.
61 Chong VF, Fan YF, Toh KH, Khoo JB, Lim TA. Magnetic resonance imaging and computed tomography features of nasopharyngeal carcinoma with maxillary sinus involvement. Australas Radiol 1995; 39: 2–9.
62 Yu MC, Yuan JM. Epidemiology of nasopharyngeal carcinoma. Semin Cancer Biol 2002; 12(6): 421–429
63 Dickson RI. Nasopharyngeal carcinoma: an evaluation of 209 patients. Laryngoscope 1981; 91: 333–354.
64 Easton JM, Levine PH, Hyams VJ. Nasopharyngeal carcinoma in the United States. A pathological study of 177 US and 30 foreign cases. Arch Otolaryngol 1980; 106: 88–91.
65 Chia KS, Lee HP, Seow A, et al. Trends in Cancer Incidence in Singapore 1968–1992. Singapore: Singapore Cancer Registry; 1996.
66 King AD, Kew J, Tong M, Leung SF, Lam WW, Metreweli C, van Hasselt CA. Magnetic resonance imaging of the eustachian tube in nasopharyngeal carcinoma: correlation of patterns of spread with middle ear effusion. Am J Otol 1999; 20: 69–73.
67 Chong VF, Fan YF. Jugular foramen involvement in nasopharyngeal carcinoma. J Laryngol Otol. 1996; 110: 987–90.
68 Su CY, Lui CC. Perineural invasion of the trigeminal nerve in patients with nasopharyngeal carcinoma. Imaging and clinical correlations. Cancer 1996; 78: 2063–2069.

69 Wakisaka M, Mori H, Fuwa N, Matsumoto A. MR analysis of nasopharyngeal carcinoma: correlation of the pattern of tumor extent at the primary site with the distribution of metastasized cervical lymph nodes. Preliminary results. Eur Radiol 2000; 10: 970–977.
70 Mesic JB, Fletcher GH, Goepfert H. Megavoltage irradiation of epithelial tumors of the nasopharynx. Int J Radiat Oncol Biol Phys 1981; 7: 447–453.
71 Chong VF, Fan YF, Khoo JB. Retropharyngeal lymphadenopathy in nasopharyngeal carcinoma. Eur J Radiol 1995; 21: 100–105.
72 Mancuso AA, Hanafee WN. Nasopharynx and parapharyngeal space. In: Computed Tomography and Magnetic Resonance Imaging of the Head and Neck, 2d ed. Baltimore, MD: Williams and Wilkins, 1985; 428–498.
73 Sievers KW, Greess H, Baum U, Dobritz M, Lenz M. Paranasal sinuses and nasopharynx CT and MRI. Eur J Radiol 2000; 33: 185–202.
74 King AD, Lam WW, Leung SF, Chan YL, Teo P, Metreweli C. MRI of local disease in nasopharyngeal carcinoma: tumour extent vs tumour stage. Br J Radiol 1999; 72: 734–741.
75 Ng SH, Chang TC, Ko SF, Yen PS, Wan YL, Tang LM, Tsai MH. Nasopharyngeal carcinoma: MRI and CT assessment. Neuroradiology 1997; 39: 741–746.
76 Barakos JA, Dillon WP, Chew WM. Orbit, skull base, and pharynx: contrast-enhanced fat suppression MR imaging. Radiology 1991; 179: 191–198.
77 Crawford SC, Harnsberger HR, Lufkin RB. The role of gadolinium-DTPA in the evaluation of extracranial head and neck lesions. Radiol Clin North Am 1989; 27: 219–242.
78 Hillsamer PJ, Schuller DE, McGhee RB Jr, Chakeres D, Young DC. Improving diagnostic accuracy of cervical metastases with computed tomography and magnetic resonance imaging. Arch Otolaryngol Head Neck Surg 1990; 116: 1297–1301.
79 Hunink MG, de Slegte RG, Gerritsen GJ, Speelman H. CT and MR assessment of tumors of the nose and paranasal sinuses, the nasopharynx and the parapharyngeal space using ROC methodology. Neuroradiology 1990; 32: 220–225.
80 Ng SH, Chong VF, Ko SF, Mukherji SK. Magnetic resonance imaging of nasopharyngeal carcinoma. Topics Magn Reson Imaging 1999; 10: 290–303.
81 Xie C, Liang B, Lin H, Wu P. Influence of MRI on the T, N staging system of nasopharyngeal carcinoma. Zhonghua Zhong Liu Za Zhi 2002; 24(2): 181–184.
82 Union Internationale Contre le Cancer; Sobin L, Wittekind C, eds. TNM Classification of Malignant Tumors, 5th ed. New York: Wiley-Liss; 1997.
83 American Joint Committee on Cancer. Fleming I, Cooper J, Henson D, et al., eds. Manual for Staging of Cancer, 5th ed. Philadelphia: Lippincott-Raven; 1997.
84 Sham JS, Cheung YK, Choy D, Chan FL, Leong L. Nasopharyngeal carcinoma: CT evaluation of patterns of tumor spread. AJNR 1991; 12: 265–270.
85 Sham JS, Choy D. Prognostic value of paranasopharyngeal extension of nasopharyngeal carcinoma on local control and short-term survival. Head Neck 1991; 13: 298–310.
86 Yu ZH, Xu GZ, Huang YR, Hu YH, Su XG, Gu XZ. Value of computed tomography in staging the primary lesion (T-staging) of nasopharyngeal carcinoma (NPC): an analysis of 54 patients with special reference to the parapharyngeal space. Int J Radiat Oncol Biol Phys 1985; 11: 2143–2147.
87 Su CY, Hsu SP, Chee CY. Electromyographic study of tensor and levator veli palatini muscles in patients with nasopharyngeal carcinoma. Implications for eustachian tube dysfunction. Cancer 1993; 71: 1193–1200.
88 Chong VF, Fan YF. Radiology of the masticator space. Clin Radiol 1996; 51: 457–465.
89 Chong VF. Masticator space in nasopharyngeal carcinoma. Ann Otol Rhinol Laryngol 1997; 106: 979–
90 Laine FJ, Braun IF, Jensen ME, Nadel L, Som PM. Perineural tumor extension through the foramen ovale: evaluation with MR imaging. Radiology 1990; 174: 65–71.
91 Olmi P, Fallai C, Colagrande S, Giannardi G. Staging and follow-up of nasopharyngeal carcinoma: magnetic resonance imaging versus computerized tomography. Int J Radiat Oncol Biol Phys 1995; 32: 795–800.
92 Chong VF, Fan YF. Skull base erosion in nasopharyngeal carcinoma: detection by CT and MRI. Clin Radiol 1996; 51: 625–631.
93 Chong VF, Fan YF. Meningeal infiltration in recurrent nasopharyngeal carcinoma. Australas Radiol 2000; 44: 23–27.
94 Mineura K, Kowada M, Tomura N. Perineural extension of nasopharyngeal carcinoma into the posterior cranial fossa detected by magnetic resonance imaging. Clin Imaging 1991; 15: 172–175.
95 Chong VF, Fan YF. Maxillary nerve involvement in nasopharyngeal carcinoma. AJR 1996; 167: 1309–1312.
96 Ng SH, Chang JT, Ko SF, Wan YL, Tang LM, Chen WC. MRI in recurrent nasopharyngeal carcinoma. Neuroradiology 1999; 41: 855–862.
97 Chong VF, Fan YF. Pterygopalatine fossa and maxillary nerve infiltration in nasopharyngeal carcinoma. Head Neck 1997; 19: 121–125.
98 Chong VF, Fan YF, Khoo JB, Lim TA. Comparing computed tomographic and magnetic resonance imaging visualisation of the pterygopalatine fossa in nasopharyngeal carcinoma. Ann Acad Med Singapore 1995; 24: 436–441.
99 Daniels DL, Rauschning W, Lovas J, Williams AL, Haughton VM. Pterygopalatine fossa: computed tomographic studies. Radiology 1983; 149: 511–516.
100 Mancuso AA. Imaging in patients with head and neck cancer. In: Million RR, Cassisi NJ, eds. Management of Head and Neck Cancer: A Multidisciplinary Approach. Philadelphia: Lippincott; 1994: 43–59.
101 Sham JS, Wei WI, Kwan WH, Chan CW, Kwong WK, Choy D. Nasopharyngeal carcinoma. Pattern of tumor regression after radiotherapy. Cancer 1990; 65: 216–220.
102 Chong VF, Fan YF. Detection of recurrent nasopharyngeal carcinoma: MR imaging versus CT. Radiology 1997; 202: 463–470.
103 Mukherji SK, Drane WE, Tart RP, Landau S, Mancuso AA. Comparison of thallium-201 and F-18 FDG SPECT uptake in squamous cell carcinoma of the head and neck. AJNR 1994; 15: 1837–1842.
104 Mukherji SK, Gapany M, Phillips D, Neelon B, O'Brien S, McCartney W, Buejenovich S, Parekh JS, Noordzij JP, Castillo M. Thallium-201 single-photon emission CT versus CT for the detection of recurrent squamous cell carcinoma of the head and neck. AJNR 1999; 20: 1215–1220.
105 Fischbein NJ, AAssar OS, Caputo GR, Kaplan MJ, Singer MI, Price DC, Dillon WP, Hawkins RA. Clinical utility of positron emission tomography with 18F-fluorodeoxyglucose in detecting residual/recurrent squamous cell carcinoma of the head and neck. AJNR 1998; 19: 1189–1196.
106 Kao CH, ChangLai SP, Chieng PU, Yen RF, Yen TC. Detection of recurrent or persistent nasopharyngeal carcinomas after radiotherapy with 18-fluoro-2-deoxyglucose positron emission tomography and comparison with computed tomography. J Clin Oncol 1998; 16: 3550–3555.
107 Lenz M, Greess H, Baum U, Dobritz M, Kersting-Sommerhoff B. Oropharynx, oral cavity, floor of the mouth: CT and MRI. Eur J Radiol 2000; 33: 203–215.
108 Becker M. Oral cavity, oropharynx, and hypopharynx. Semin Roentgenol 2000; 35: 21–30.
109 Franco RA, Har-El G. Cancer of the head and neck. In: Lucente FE, Har-EL G, eds. Essentials of Otolaryngology, 4th ed. Philadelphia: Lippincott Williams and Wilkins; 1999: 326–335.
110 Sheman LJ. Diseases of the oropharynx. In: Lee KJ, ed. Textbook of Otolaryngology and Head and Neck Surgery. New York: Elsevier; 1989; 407–414.
111 Gale DR. CT and MRI of the oral cavity and oropharynx. In: Valvassori GE, Mafee MF, Carter BL, eds. Imaging of the Head and Neck. Stuttgart: Georg Thieme Verlag; 1995: 445–474.
112 Gromet M, Homer MJ, Carter BL. Lymphoid hyperplasia at the base of the tongue. Spectrum of a benign entity. Radiology 1982; 144: 825–828.
113 Yousem DM, Hatabu H, Hurst RW, Seigerman HM, Montone KT, Weinstein GS, Hayden RE, Goldberg AN, Bigelow DC, Kotapka MJ. Carotid artery invasion by head and neck masses: prediction with MR imaging. Radiology 1995; 195: 715–720.
114 Muraki AS, Mancuso AA, Harnsberger HR, Johnson LP, Meads GB. CT of the oropharynx, tongue base, and floor of the mouth: normal anatomy and range of variations, and applications in staging carcinoma. Radiology 1983; 148: 725–731.
115 Nigauri T, Kamata SE, Kawabata K, Hoki K, Mitani H, Yoshimoto S, Yonekawa H, Miura K, Beppu T, Fukusima H. Squamous carcinoma of the posterior oropharyngeal wall. Nippon Jibiinkoka Gakkai Kaiho 2002; 105(8): 882–886.
116 Leslie A, Fyfe E, Guest P, Goddard P, Kabala JE. Staging of squamous cell carcinoma of the oral cavity and oropharynx: a comparison of MRI and CT in T- and N-staging. J Comput Assist Tomogr 1999; 23: 43–49.
117 Beahrs OH, Henson DE, Hutter RVP, Kennedy BJ, eds. Manual for Staging of Cancer: American Joint Committee on Cancer, 5th ed. Philadelphia: J.B. Lippincott; 1997.

118 Curtin HD, Williams R, Johnson J. CT of perineural tumor extension: pterygopalatine fossa. AJR 1985; 144: 163–169.
119 Mukherji SK, Castelijns J, Castillo M. Squamous cell carcinoma of the oropharynx and oral cavity: how imaging makes a difference. Semin Ultrasound CT MR 1998; 19: 463–475.
120 Becker M, Hasso AN. Imaging of malignant neoplasms of the pharynx and larynx. In: Taveras JM, Ferrucci JT, eds. Radiology: Diagnosis–Imaging–Intervention. Philadelphia: J. B. Lippincott; 1996: 1–16.
121 Mukherji SK, Mancuso AA, Mendenhall W, Kotzur IM, Kubilis P. Can pretreatment CT predict local control of T2 glottic carcinomas treated with radiation therapy alone? AJNR 1995; 16: 655–662.
122 Mukherji SK, Weeks SM, Castillo M, Yankaskas BC, Krishnan LA, Schiro S. Squamous cell carcinomas that arise in the oral cavity and tongue base: can CT help predict perineural or vascular invasion? Radiology 1996; 198: 157–162.
123 Keberle M, Hoppe F, Dotzel S, Hahn D. Prognostic value of pretreatment CT regarding local control in oropharyngeal cancer after primary surgical resection. RoFo. Fortschritte auf dem Gebiete derRontgenstrahlen und der neuen bildgebenden Verfahren 2003; 175(1): 61–66.
124 Chung TS, Yousem DM, Seigerman HM, Schlakman BN, Weinstein GS, Hayden RE. MR of mandibular invasion in patients with oral and oropharyngeal malignant neoplasms. AJNR 1994; 15: 1949–1955.
125 Sigal R, Zagdanski AM, Schwaab G, Bosq J, Auperin A, Laplanche A, Francke JP, Eschwege F, Luboinski B, Vanel D. CT and MR imaging of squamous cell carcinoma of the tongue and floor of the mouth. Radiographics 1996; 16: 787–810.
126 Loevner LA, Ott IL, Yousem DM, Montone KT, Thaler ER, Chalian AA, Weinstein GS, Weber RS. Neoplastic fixation to the prevertebral compartment by squamous cell carcinoma of the head and neck. AJR 1998; 170: 1389–1394.
127 Hudgins PA, Burson JG, Gussack GS, Grist WJ. CT and MR appearance of recurrent malignant head and neck neoplasms after resection and flap reconstruction. AJNR 1994; 15: 1689–1694.
128 Sugimura K, Kuroda S, Furukawa T, Matsuda S, Yoshimura Y, Ishida T. Tongue cancer treated with irradiation: assessment with MR imaging. Clin Radiol 1992; 46: 243–247.
129 Wong DS, Fuller LM, Butler JJ, Shullenberger CC. Extranodal non-Hodgkin's lymphomas of the head and neck. Am J Roentgenol Radium Ther Nucl Med 1975; 123: 471–481.
130 Chong VF, Fan YF. The retropharyngeal space: route of tumour spread. Clin Radiol 1998; 53: 64–67.
131 Conley J, Dingman DL. Adenoid cystic carcinoma in the head and neck (cylindroma). Arch Otolaryngol 1974; 100: 81–90.
132 Kim KH, Sung NW, Chung PS, et al. Adenoid cystic carcinoma of the head and neck. Arch Otolaryngal Head and Neck Surg 1994; 120: 721–726.
133 Rossiter JL, Hendrix RA, Tom LW, Potsic WP. Intramuscular hemangioma of the head and neck. Otolaryngol Head Neck Surg 1993; 108: 18–26.
134 Faerber EN, Swartz JD. Imaging of neck masses in infants and children. Crit Rev Diagn Imaging 1991; 31: 283–314.
135 Baker LL, Dillon WP, Hieshima GB, Dowd CF, Frieden IJ. Hemangiomas and vascular malformations of the head and neck: MR characterization. AJNR 1993; 14: 307–314.
136 Reede DL, Holliday RA, Som PM, Bergeron RT. Nonnodal pathological conditions of the neck. In: Som PM, Bergeron RT, ed. Head and Neck Imaging. St. Louis, MO: Mosby-Year Book; 1991.
137 Mulliken JB, Glowacki J. Hemangiomas and vascular malformations in infants and children: a classification based on endothelial characteristics. Plast Reconstr Surg 1982; 69: 412–422.
138 Robertson RL, Robson CD, Barnes PD, Burrows PE. Head and neck vascular anomalies of childhood. Neuroimaging Clin North Am 1999; 9: 115–132.
139 Lewin JS, Merkle EM, Duerk JL, Tarr RW. Low-flow vascular malformations in the head and neck: safety and feasibility of MR imaging-guided percutaneous sclerotherapy—preliminary experience with 14 procedures in three patients. Radiology 1999; 211: 566–570.
140 Govrin-Yehudain J, Moscona AR, Calderon N, Hirshowitz B. Treatment of hemangiomas by sclerosing agents: an experimental and clinical study. Ann Plast Surg 1987; 18: 465–469.
141 Yakes WF, Haas DK, Parker SH, Gibson MD, Hopper KD, Mulligan JS, Pevsner PH, Johns JC Jr, Carter TE. Symptomatic vascular malformations: ethanol embolotherapy. Radiology 1989; 170: 1059–1066.
142 Meyer JS, Hoffer FA, Barnes PD, Mulliken JB. Biological classification of soft-tissue vascular anomalies: MR correlation. AJR 1991; 157: 559–564.
143 Stiernberg CM. Deep-neck space infections. Diagnosis and management. Arch Otolaryngol Head Neck Surg 1986; 112: 1274–1279.
144 Weber AL, Baker AS, Montgomery WW. Inflammatory lesions of the neck, including fascial spaces—evaluation by computed tomography and magnetic resonance imaging. Isr J Med Sci 1992; 28: 241–249.
145 Hockstein NG, Anderson TA, Moonis G, Gustafson KS, Mirza N. Retropharyngeal lipoma causing obstructive sleep apnea: case report including five-year follow-up. Laryngoscope 2002; 112(9): 1603–1605.
146 Benson MT, Dalen K, Mancuso AA, Kerr HH, Cacciarelli AA, Mafee MF. Congenital anomalies of the branchial apparatus: embryology and pathological anatomy. Radiographics 1992; 12: 943–960.
147 Chandler JR, Mitchell B. Branchial cleft cysts, sinuses, and fistulas. Otolaryngol Clin North Am 1981; 14: 175–186.
148 Harnsberger HR, Mancuso AA, Muraki AS, Byrd SE, Dillon WP, Johnson LP, Hanafee WN. Branchial cleft anomalies and their mimics: computed tomographic evaluation. Radiology 1984; 152: 739–748.
149 Cerezal L, Morales C, Abascal F, Usamentiaga E, Canga A, Olcinas O, Bustamante M. Pharyngeal branchial cyst: magnetic resonance findings. Eur J Radiol 1998; 29: 1–3.
150 Lawson VG, LeLiever WC, Makerewich LA, Rabuzzi DD, Bell RD. Unusual parapharyngeal lesions. J Otolaryngol 1979; 8: 241–249.
151 Heeneman H, Maran AG. Parapharyngeal space tumours. Clin Otolaryngol 1979; 4: 57–66.
152 Som PM, Biller HF, Lawson W, Sacher M, Lanzieri CF. Parapharyngeal space masses: an updated protocol based upon 104 cases. Radiology 1984; 153: 149–156.
153 Som PM, Braun IF, Shapiro MD, Reede DL, Curtin HD, Zimmerman RA. Tumors of the parapharyngeal space and upper neck: MR imaging characteristics. Radiology 1987; 164: 823–829.
154 Paonessa DF, Goldstein JC. Anatomy and physiology of head and neck infections (with emphasis on the fascia of the face and neck). Otolaryngol Clin North Am 1976; 9(3): 561–880.
155 Olsen WL, Dillon WP, Kelly WM, Norman D, Brant-Zawadzki M, Newton TH. MR Imaging of pragangliomas. AJNR 1986; 7: 1039–1042.
156 Duncan AW, Lack EE, Deck MF. Radiological evaluation of paragangliomas of the head and neck. Radiology 1979; 132: 99–105.
157 Cook PL. Clinical records bilateral chemodectoma in the neck. J Laryngol 1977; 91: 611–618.
158 McIlrath DC, ReMine WH, Devine KD, Dockerty MB. Tumors of the parapharyngeal region. Surg Gynecol Obstet 1963(Jan.): 88–94.
159 Shugar MA, Mafee MF. Diagnosis of carotid body tumors by dynamic computerized tomography. Head Neck Surg 1982(Jul./Aug.): 518–521.
160 Axel L. Blood flow effects in magnetic resonance imaging. AJR 1984; 143: 1157–1166.
161 Bradley WG, Waluch V. Blood flow magnetic resonance imaging. Radiology 1985; 154: 443–450.
162 Som PM, Sacher M, Stollman AR, Biller HF, Lawson W. Common tumors of the parapharyngeal space: Refined imaging diagnosis. Radiology 1988; 169(1): 81–85.
163 Tsai FY, Goldstein JC, Parhad IM. Angiographic features of lateral cervical masses. Trans Am Acad Ophthalmol Otol 1977; 84: 840–850.
164 Som PM. Parapharyngeal Space. In Som PM, Bergeron RT, eds. Head and Neck Imaging. St. Louis, MO: Mosby-Year Book; 1991.
165 Kumar AJ, Kuhajda FP, Martinez CR, Fishman EK, Jezic DV, Siegelman SS. Computed tomography of extracranial nerve sheath tumors with pathological correlation. J Comput Assist Tomogr 1983; 7(5): 857–865.
166 Shoss SM, Donovan DT, Alford BR. Tumors of the Parapharyngeal Space. Arch Otolaryngol 1985; 111: 753–757.
167 Teresi LM, Lufkin RB, Vinuela F, Dietrich RB, Wilson GH, Bentson JR, Hanafee WN. MR imaging of the nasopharynx and floor of the middle cranial fossa. Part II. Malignant tumors. Radiology 1987; 164: 817–821.
168 Braun IF, Hoffman JC, JR. Reede D, Grist W. Computed tomography of the buccomasseteric region: 2. Pathology. AJNR 1984; 5: 611–616.
169 Braun IF, Torres WE, Landman JA, Davis PC, Hoffman JC Jr. Computed tomography of benign masseteric hypertrophy. J Comput Assist Tomogr 1985; 9(1): 167–170.
170 Schellhas KP. MR imaging of muscles of mastication. AJNR 1989; 10: 829–837.
171 Hardin CW, Harnsberger HR, Osborn AG, Doxey GP, Davis K, Nyberg DA. Infection and tumor of the masticator space: CT 3 valuation. Radiology 1985; 157: 413–417.
172 Som PM, Biller HF. The combined CT-sialogram. Radiology 1980(May); 135: 387–390.
173 Curtin HC, Williams R, Johnson J. CT of perineural tumor extension: pterygopalatine fossa. AJNR 1984; 5: 731–737.

174 Miller MB, Rao VM, Tom BM. Cystic masses of the head and neck: pitfalls in CT and MR interpretation. AJR 1992; 159: 601–607.

175 Harnsberger HR, Bragg DG, Osborn AG, Smoker WRK, Dillon WP, Davis RK, Stevens MH, Hill DP. Non-Hodgkin's lymphoma of the head and neck: CT evaluation of nodal and extranodal sites. AJR 1987; 149: 785–791.

176 Coit WE, Harnsberger HR, Osborn AG, Smoker WRK, Stevens MH, Lufkin RB. Ranulas and their mimics: CT evaluation. Radiology 1987; 163: 211–216.

177 Ayala C, Healy GB, Robson CD, Vargas SO. Psammomatous calcification in association with a benign thyroglossal duct cyst. Arch Otolaryngol Head Neck Surg 2003; 129(2): 241–243.

178 Reede DL, Bergeron RT, Som PM. CT of thyroglossal duct cysts. Radiology 1985; 157: 121–125.

179 Nguyen VD, Potter JL, Hersh-Schick MR. Ludwig angina: an uncommon and potentially lethal neck infection. AJNR 1992; 13: 215–219.

180 Parker GD, Harnsberger HR. Radiological evaluation of the normal and diseased posterior cervical space. AJR 1991; 157: 160–165.

181 Parker GD, Harnsberger HR, Smoker RK. The anterior and posterior cervical spaces. Semin Ultrasound CT MR 1991; 12(3): 257–273.

182 Chung SK, Chang BC, Dhong HJ. Surgical, radiological, and histological findings of the antrochoanal polyp. Am J Rhinol 2002; 16(2): 71–76.

183 Som PM, Brandwein M. Sinonasal cavities: inflammatory diseases, tumors, fractures, and postoperative findings. In: Som PM, Curtin HD, eds. Head and Neck Imaging, 3 d ed. St Louis, MO: Mosby; 1996: 126–315.

184 Mafee MF, Carter BL. Nasal cavity and paranasal sinuses. In: Valvassori GE, Mafee MF, Carter BL, eds. Imaging of the Head and Neck. Stuttgart: Georg Thieme Verlag; 1995: 248–331.

185 Weissman JL, Tabor EK, Curtin HD. Sphenochoanal polyps: evaluation with CT and MR imaging. Radiology 1991; 178: 145–148.

186 Hughes ML, Carty AT, White FE. Persistent hypophyseal (craniopharyngeal) canal. Br J Radiol 1999; 72: 204–206.

187 Daniello NJ, Goldstein SI. Retropharyngeal hematoma secondary to minor blunt head and neck trauma. Ear Nose Throat J 1994; 73: 41–43.

188 Tenofsky PL, Porter SW, Shaw JW. Fatal airway compromise due to retropharyngeal hematoma after airbag deployment. Am Surg 2000; 66: 692–694.

189 Mazzon D, Zanatta P, Curtolo S, Bernardi V, Bosco E. Upper airway obstruction by retropharyngeal hematoma after cervical spine trauma: report of a case treated with percutaneous dilational tracheostomy. J Neurosurg Anesthesiol 1998; 10: 237–240.

190 O'Donnell JJ, Birkinshaw R, Harte B. Mechanical airway obstruction secondary to retropharyngeal haematoma. Eur J Emerg Med 1997; 4: 166–168.

191 Mariani PJ. Occipital condyle fracture presenting as retropharyngeal hematoma. Ann Emerg Med. 1990; 19: 1447–1449.

192 Siou G, Yates P. Retropharyngeal abscess as a complication of oropharyngeal trauma in an 18-month-old child. J Laryngol Otol 2000; 114: 227–228.

193 Pumberger W, Bader T, Golej J, Pokieser P, Semsroth M. Traumatic pharyngo-oesophageal perforation in the newborn: a condition mimicking oesophageal atresia. Paediatr Anaesth 2000; 10: 201–205.

194 Verron P, Grandpierre G, Vergeau B, Cornudet B, Salf E, Cudennec YF. Nasopharyngeal perforation: an exceptional accident during digestive endoscopy. Ann Otolaryngol Chir Cervicofac 1998; 115: 27–28.

195 Moriarty KP, Harris BH, Benitez-Marchand K. Carotid artery thrombosis and stroke after blunt pharyngeal injury. J Trauma 1997; 42: 541–543.

196 Sidhu MK, Shaw DW, Roberts TS. Carotid artery injury and delayed cerebral infarction after minor pharyngeal trauma. AJR 1996; 167: 1056.

197 Tsai YS, Lui CC. Retropharyngeal and epidural abscess from a swallowed fish bone. Am J Emerg Med 1997; 15: 381–382.

198 Hung T, Huchzermeyer P, Hinton AE. Air rifle injury to the oropharynx. The essential role of computed tomography in deciding on surgical exploration. J Accid Emerg Med 2000; 17: 147–148.

199 Rayatt SS, Magennis P, Hamlyn PJ. Carotoid artery thrombosis following a penetrating oro-pharyngeal injury of unusual aetiology. Injury 1998; 29: 320–322.

200 Chin KW, Sercarz JA, Wang MB, Andrews R. Spontaneous cervical hemorrhage with near-complete airway obstruction. Head Neck 1998; 20: 350–353.

201 Schoem SR, Choi SS, Zalzal GH, Grundfast KM. Management of oropharyngeal trauma in children. Arch Otolaryngol Head Neck Surg 1997; 123: 1267–1270.

202 Maniglia AJ, Davis JA, Maniglia JV. Obstructive sleep apnea syndrome. In: Lee KJ, ed. Essential Otolaryngology. Head and Neck Surgery, 7 th ed. Stamford: Appleton and Lange; 1999: 859–874.

203 Galvin JR, Rooholamini SA, Stanford W. Obstructive sleep apnea: diagnosis with ultrafast CT. Radiology 1989; 171: 775–778.

204 Jager L, Gunther E, Gauger J, Reiser M. Fluoroscopic MR of the pharynx in patients with obstructive sleep apnea. AJNR 1998; 19: 1205–1214.

205 Stein MG, Gamsu G, de Geer G, Golden JA, Crumley RL, Webb WR. Cine CT in obstructive sleep apnea. AJR 1987; 148: 1069–1074.

206 Ell SR, Jolles H, Galvin JR. Cine CT demonstration of nonfixed upper airway obstruction. AJR 1986; 146: 669–677.

207 Brasch RC, Gould RG, Gooding CA, Ringertz HG, Lipton MJ. Upper airway obstruction in infants and children: evaluation with ultrafast CT. Radiology 1987; 165: 459–466.

208 Ergun GA, Kahrilas PJ, Lin S, Logemann JA, Harig JM. Shape, volume, and content of the deglutitive pharyngeal chamber imaged by ultrafast computerized tomography. Gastroenterology 1993; 105: 1396–1403.

209 Shellock FG, Schatz CJ, Julien PM, Silverman JM, Steinberg F, Foo TK, Hopp ML, Westbrook PR. Dynamic study of the upper airway with ultrafast spoiled GRASS MR imaging. J Magn Reson Imaging 1992; 2: 103–107.

210 Shellock FG, Schatz CJ, Julien P, Steinberg F, Foo TK, Hopp ML, Westbrook PR. Occlusion and narrowing of the pharyngeal airway in obstructive sleep apnea: evaluation by ultrafast spoiled GRASS MR imaging. AJR 1992; 158: 1019–1024.

211 Suto Y, Matsuo T, Kato T, Hori I, Inoue Y, Ogawa S, Suzuki T, Yamada M, Ohta Y. Evaluation of the pharyngeal airway in patients with sleep apnea: value of ultrafast MR imaging. AJR 1993; 160: 311–314.

212 Schoenberg SO, Floemer F, Kroeger H, Hoffmann A, Bock M, Knopp MV. Combined assessment of obstructive sleep apnea syndrome with dynamic MRI and parallel EEG registration: initial results. Invest Radiol 2000; 35: 267–276.

213 Jager L, Gunther E, Gauger J, Reiser M. Fluoroscopic MR of the pharynx in patients with obstructive sleep apnea. AJNR 1998; 19: 1205–1214.

214 Huda W, Slone RM. Computers and computed tomography. In: Review of Radiological Physics. Philadelphia: Lippincott Williams and Wilkins; 1995: 93–109.

215 Lewin JS, Petersilge CA, Hatem SF, Duerk JL, Lenz G, Clampitt ME, Williams ML, Kaczynski KR, Lanzieri CF, Wise AL, Haaga JR. Interactive MR imaging-guided biopsy and aspiration with a modified clinical C-arm system. AJR 1998; 170: 1593–1601.

216 Lewin JS. Interventional MR imaging: concepts, systems, and applications in neuroradiology. AJNR 1999; 20: 735–748.

217 Mahfouz AE, Rahmouni A, Zylbersztejn C, Mathieu D. MR-guided biopsy using ultrafast T1- and T2-weighted reordered turbo fast low-angle shot sequences: feasibility and preliminary clinical applications. AJR 1996; 167: 167–169.

218 Caballero P, Alvarez-Sala R, Garcia-Rio F, Prados C, Hernan MA, Villamor J, Alvarez-Sala JL. CT in the evaluation of the upper airway in healthy subjects and in patients with obstructive sleep apnea syndrome. Chest 1998; 113: 111–116.

219 Merkle EM, Lewin JS, Aschoff AJ, Stepnick DW, Duerk JL, Lanzieri CF, Strauss M. Percutaneous magnetic resonance image-guided biopsy and aspiration in the head and neck. Laryngoscope 2000; 110: 382–385.

220 Lewin JS, Nour SG, Duerk JL. Magnetic resonance image-guided biopsy and aspiration. Topics Magn Reson Imaging 2000; 11: 173–183.

221 Powell NB, Riley RW, Guilleminault C. Radiofrequency tongue base reduction in sleep-disordered breathing: A pilot study. Otolaryngol Head Neck Surg 1999; 120(5): 656–664.

222 Nour SG, Lewin JS, Gutman M, Hillenbrand C, Wacker FK, Wong JW, Mitchell IC, Armstrong CB, Hashim MM, Duerk JL, Strauss M. Percutaneous MR imaging-guided radiofrequency interstitial thermal ablation of tongue base in porcine models: implications for obstructive sleep apnea syndrome. Radiology 2004; 230: 359–368.

223 Lewin JS, Duerk JL, Jain VR, Petersilge CA, Chao CP, Haaga JR. Needle localization in MR-guided biopsy and aspiration: effects of field strength, sequence design, and magnetic field orientation. AJR 1996; 166: 1337–1345.

224 Duerk JL, Lewin JS, Wendt M, Petersilge C. Remember true FISP? A high SNR, near 1-second imaging method for T2-like contrast in interventional MRI at .2 T. J Magn Reson Imaging 1998; 8: 203–208.

225 Chung YC, Merkle EM, Lewin JS, Shonk JR, Duerk JL. Fast T(2)-weighted imaging by PSIF at 0.2 T for interventional MRI. Magn Reson Med 1999; 42: 335–344.

9 Salivary Glands

Mahmood F. Mafee

Embryology

The salivary glands arise from solid local proliferations or buds from the epithelial lining of the primitive mouth (stomatodeum). The parotid glands are first to appear as an ectodermal ingrowth of local surface ectoderm of the mouth, extending into the adjacent mesenchyme. The submandibular and sublingual glands are believed to develop probably from the endodermal germ layer.[1] The parotid gland is recognizable in human embryos 8 mm long (fourth to sixth weeks of gestation). The anlagen of submandibular gland can be recognized in human embryos 13 mm long as an epithelial outgrowth from the floor of the linguogingival groove. The sublingual glands are the last to develop and are identifiable in human embryos 20 mm long as a small epithelial thickening in the linguogingival groove (paralingual sulcus). Branching epithelial cords from the enlarging buds become excretory ducts; the distal ends (saccules) differentiate into the acini.[1] The adjacent surrounding mesenchyme forms the capsule and septae between lobes and lobules. The minor salivary glands are developed later and cannot be recognized until late in the twelfth week (62 mm long) of embryonic life.[2] The secretary cells of the salivary glands do not produce secretion during embryonic development. The encapsulation of parotid glands takes place after submandibular and sublingual glands become encapsulated. It is important to realize that the development of the lymphatic system of the neck occurs after encapsulation of the submandibular and sublingual and before the encapsulation of the parotid glands. This explains why the parotid glands have a lymphatic system, while the other major salivary glands do not. During the encapsulation process of the parotid glands, "ectopic" salivary gland tissue may be included within the intraparotid as well as periparotid lymph nodes. This rare embryonic development explains the unusual situation of salivary gland tumor arising within cervical lymph nodes while major salivary glands appear normal.

Anatomy

The salivary glands consist of two groups: the three paired major glands (parotid, submandibular, and sublingual) and various minor salivary glands scattered throughout the oral cavity and pharynx.[1-4] The major glands are tubuloacinar in type.[5] The minor salivary glands consist of approximately 600–1000 small, independent aggregations of glandular tissue, situated beneath the oral mucosa and scattered throughout the mouth and to a lesser extent in the pharynx, parapharyngeal space, nasal cavity, paranasal sinuses, larynx, and trachea.[1-6]

■ Parotid Gland

The parotid gland, the largest of the salivary glands, is located predominantly in the subcutaneous tissues superficial to the masseter muscle and mandibular ramus. Its inferior portion, the "tail," is separated from the submandibular gland by the stylomandibular ligament. The gland is invested with a well-defined fibrous connective-tissue capsule, derived from the superficial layer of the deep cervical fascia. The parotid gland (Fig. 9.1)

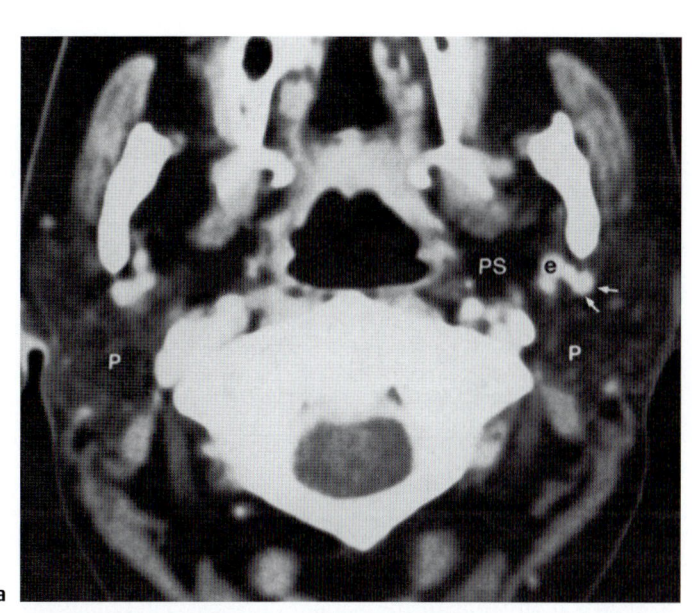

Fig. 9.1 Normal CT anatomy of the parotid gland.
a CT image. Axial contrast-enhanced CT scan shows normal parotid glands (P), external carotid artery (e), retromandibular veins (arrows), and parapharyngeal space (PS).
b Normal submandibular and parotid glands. Coronal contrast enhanced CT scan at the level of styloid processes.

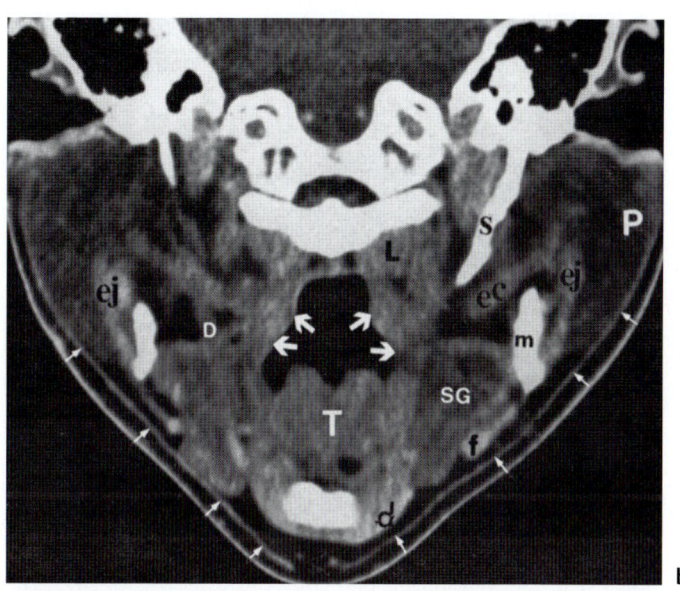

d = anterior belly of the digastric muscle; D = partially volumed posterior belly of digastric muscle; ec = external carotid artery; ej = external jugular vein; f = facial vein; L = longus colli muscle; m = mandible; P = parotid gland; S = styloid process; SG = submandibular gland; T = tongue; small white arrows = platysma muscle; large white arrows = pharynx. Enhanced carotid sheaths are seen medial to the styloid processes (S).

9 Salivary Glands

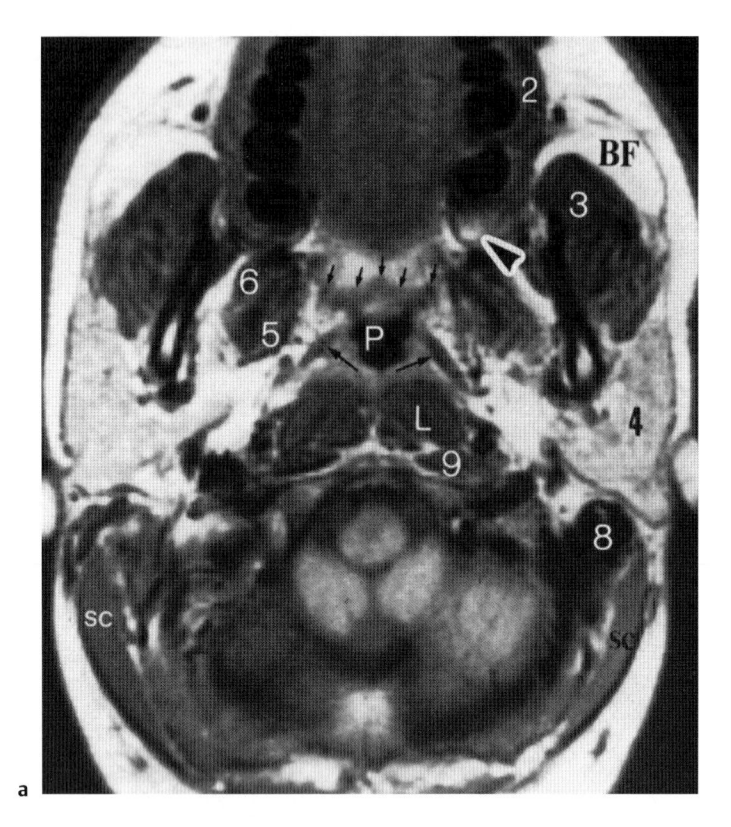

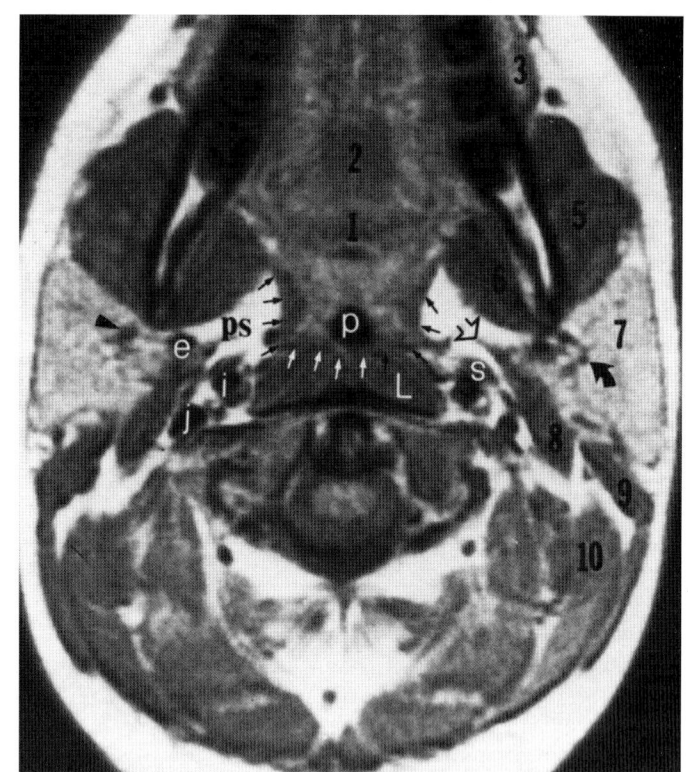

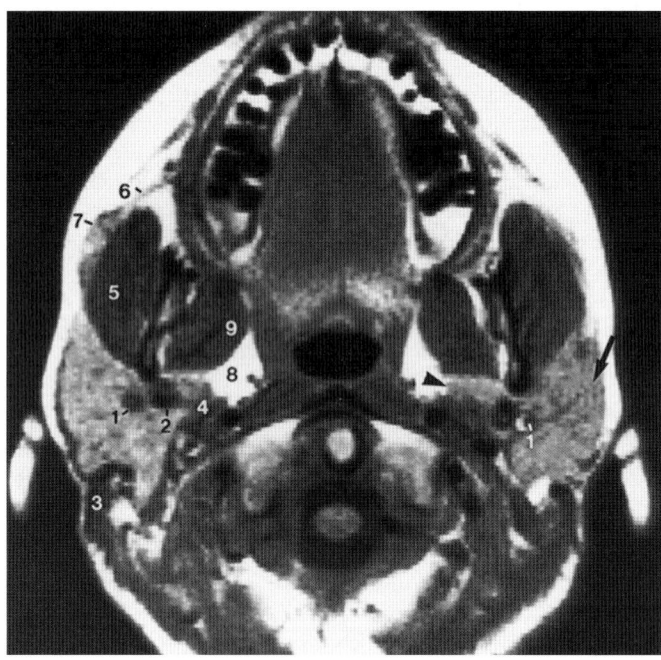

Fig. 9.2 Normal MR anatomy of the parotid gland.
a Axial MR sections, spin density weighted. This section crosses through the upper teeth, coronoid and mastoid processes.
BF = buccal fat; L = longus capitis muscle; P = nasopharynx; SC = splenius capitis muscle; short black arrows = pharyngopalatine muscle; long black arrows = levator palatini muscles; black and white arrowhead = buccopharyngeal space; 2 = buccinator muscle; 3 = masseter muscle; 4 = parotid gland; 5 = medial pterygoid muscle; 6 = lateral pterygoid muscle; 8 = mastoid process; 9 = anterior rectus capitis.
b This section is 9 mm inferior to a and crosses the lower alveolar ridge.
e = external carotid artery; i = internal carotid artery; j = internal jugular vein; L = longus capitis muscle; p = oropharynx; ps = parapharyngeal space; s = stylopharyngeus muscle; small white and black arrows = superior pharyngeal constrictor muscle; hollow arrow = stylohyoid muscle; black curved arrow = facial nerve; black arrowhead = retromandibular vein; 1 = longitudinal intrinsic tongue muscles; 2 = transverse intrinsic tongue muscles; 3 = buccinator muscle; 5 = masseter muscle; 6 = internal pterygoid muscle; 7 = parotid gland; 8 = posterior belly of digastric muscle; 9 = sternocleidomastoid muscle; 10 = splenius capitis muscle.
c Axial MR image showing parotid gland with normal retromandibular vein (1); external carotid artery (2); sternocleidomastoid muscle (3); posterior belly of digastric muscle (4); masseter muscle (5); Stensen's (parotid) duct (6); and overlying masseter muscle. Facial nerve position (arrow) is lateral to retromandibular vein. Its main trunk separates the superficial portion from the deep portion of the parotid gland. Note the accessory lobe (7) of the parotid, the parapharyngeal space (8), extension of parotid gland (arrowhead) into parapharyngeal space. 9 = Medial pterygoid muscle.

is bounded superiorly by the zygomatic arch; posteriorly by the mastoid process, the styloid process, and the bony and cartilaginous portions of the external auditory canal; inferiorly and posteriorly by the sternocleidomastoid muscle and the posterior belly of the digastric muscle; and medially by the styloid group of muscles, internal jugular vein, internal carotid artery, and cranial nerves IX, X, XI, and XII (Fig. 9.2). The parotid (Stensen's) duct is approximately 5 cm long and passes forward from the gland in the surrounding adipose tissue, superficial to the masseter muscle, in a course inferior and parallel to the zygomatic arch (Fig. 9.2c). The parotid duct then turns medially, penetrating the buccinator muscle to open on a papilla in the oral cavity opposite the second maxillary molar tooth[6] (Fig. 9.2c). In approximately 20% of the population, an accessory parotid gland can be found immediately adjacent to the parotid duct and anterior to the parotid gland (Fig. 9.2c).[3,5]

Additional normal structures that pass through the substance of the parotid gland are (1) branches of the external carotid artery, including the posterior auricular, maxillary, and superficial temporal arteries; (2) the posterior facial vein (retromandibular vein) (Figs. 9.1, 9.2);[1,7] (3) the auriculotemporal branch of the fifth cranial nerve; and (4) the extracranial facial nerve. The retromandibular vein formed in the upper part of the gland by the union of the maxillary and superficial temporal veins is superficial to the intraglandular part of the external carotid artery (Fig. 9.3). The parotid gland is the only salivary gland that contains several small lymph nodes.[8]

Although there is no anatomical division of the parotid gland, a plane created by the trunk of the intraparotid facial nerve is used to arbitrarily divide the parotid into deep and superficial lobes (Fig. 9.2c). This artificial division has practical significance: a neoplasm located superficial to the main trunk facial nerve is treated by a superficial parotidectomy; a neoplasm located deep to the nerve requires a total parotidectomy.[7] The facial nerve exits the skull base through the stylomastoid foramen posterior to the styloid process (Fig. 9.4). It passes through the deep and posterior aspects of the parotid gland prior to dividing into its branches to the face. The proximal portion of the extracranial facial nerve may be enveloped by a small amount of fatty tissue before entering the parotid gland.[9] Effacement of this fat pad can sometimes be used as a sign of perineural extension of tumor.[9,10] The facial nerve then courses anterolateral to the posterior belly of the digastric muscle and posterolateral to the styloid process (Fig. 9.4). The facial nerve then enters the upper part of the parotid gland from the posterior medial aspect of the parotid gland (Figs. 9.2c, 9.4) and divides within the substance of the gland into two major branches, the temporofacial (superior portion) and cervicofacial (inferior portion). These main branches anastomose, forming a plexus that gives rise to the major branches responsible for motor innervation to facial expression.[8,9]

The smaller deep lobe of the parotid gland extends through a gap between the styloid process and the mandibular ramus (stylomandibular tunnel) to lie within the prestyloid parapharyngeal space (PPS) (Figs. 9.1, 9.2). The parapharyngeal space (PPS) is the area containing fat and areolar tissue lateral to the naso-oropharynx and pharyngobasilar fascia (Figs. 9.1, 9.2). The prestyloid PPS is limited anterolaterally by the medial pterygoid fascia and posteromedially by the tensor veli palatini fascia (Fig. 9.2). Neoplasms arising from the prestyloid PPS are predominantly of salivary gland origin. The PPS is further divided into the poststyloid PPS, located posteromedial to the tensor veli palatini fascia (Fig. 9.2a). The poststyloid PPS contains the carotid artery, jugular vein, lymph nodes, and cranial nerves IX to XII (Fig. 9.2b, c). Neoplasms arising from the poststyloid PPS are predominantly nerve sheath tumors, paragangliomas, or metastatic lymph nodes.

Vascular Supply and Lymphatic Drainage

Arterial supply of the parotid gland is via branches of the external carotid artery and includes the posterior auricular, internal maxillary, superficial temporal, and transverse facial arteries. Venous structures empty into the external jugular vein.

Lymphatic drainage is to the superficial and deep cervical lymph nodes via the intraparotid and periparotid lymph nodes.[8]

Parotid Space

The parotid space is formed as the superficial layer of the deep cervical fascia splits anterior to the sternocleidomastoid muscle into the medial and lateral leaves, which enclose the parotid gland, intraparotid and periparotid lymph nodes, and the facial nerve, retromandibular vein, distal external carotid artery, and origin of several of its branches. The anterior aspect of the parotid space is contiguous with the masticator space; its superior aspect

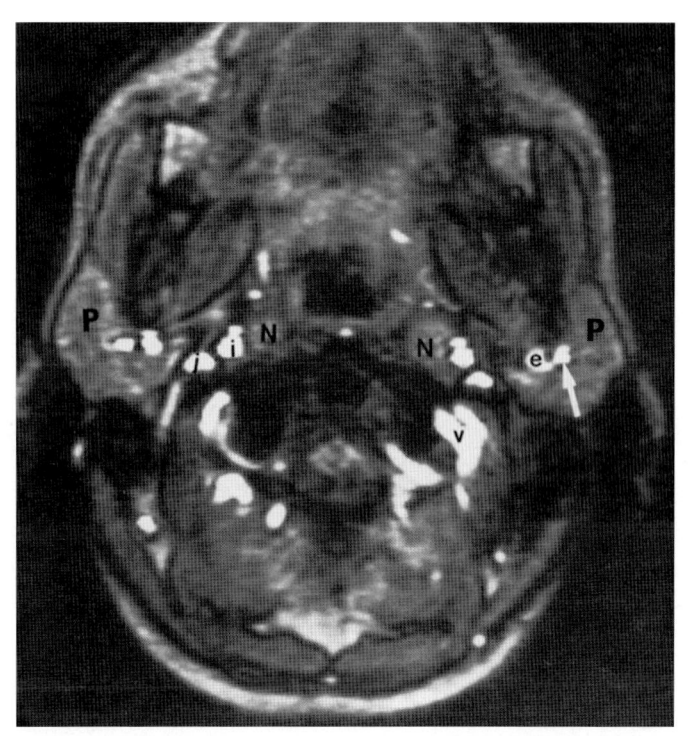

Fig. 9.3 Normal MR vascular anatomy of the parotid gland. Normal parotid gland in a patient with carcinoma of the nasopharynx; axial MR scan. Scan obtained with a narrow flip angle (GRASS, TR-30, TE-12 ms, Θ = 30°) shows parotid glands (P), with medium signal intensity similar to muscle. The normal vascular structures are hyperintense. e = external carotid artery branch; i = internal carotid artery; j = internal jugular vein; v = vertebral artery; arrow = retromandibular vein; N = enlarged retropharyngeal nodes, metastatic from the nasopharyngeal carcinoma.

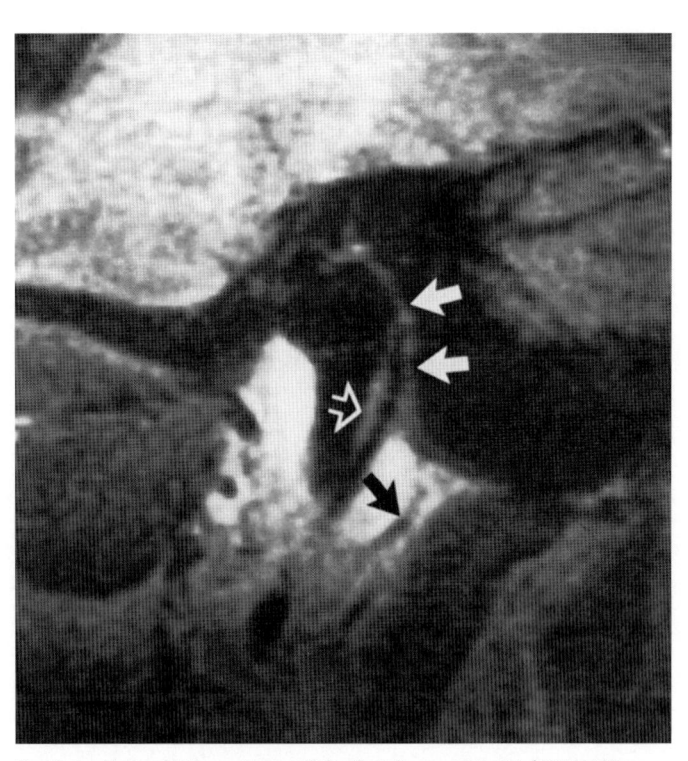

Fig. 9.4 Normal MR anatomy of the facial nerve. Sagittal T1W MR scan. This scan shows the tympanic, mastoid and parotid segments of the facial nerve (arrows), and the stapedius muscle (hollow arrow).

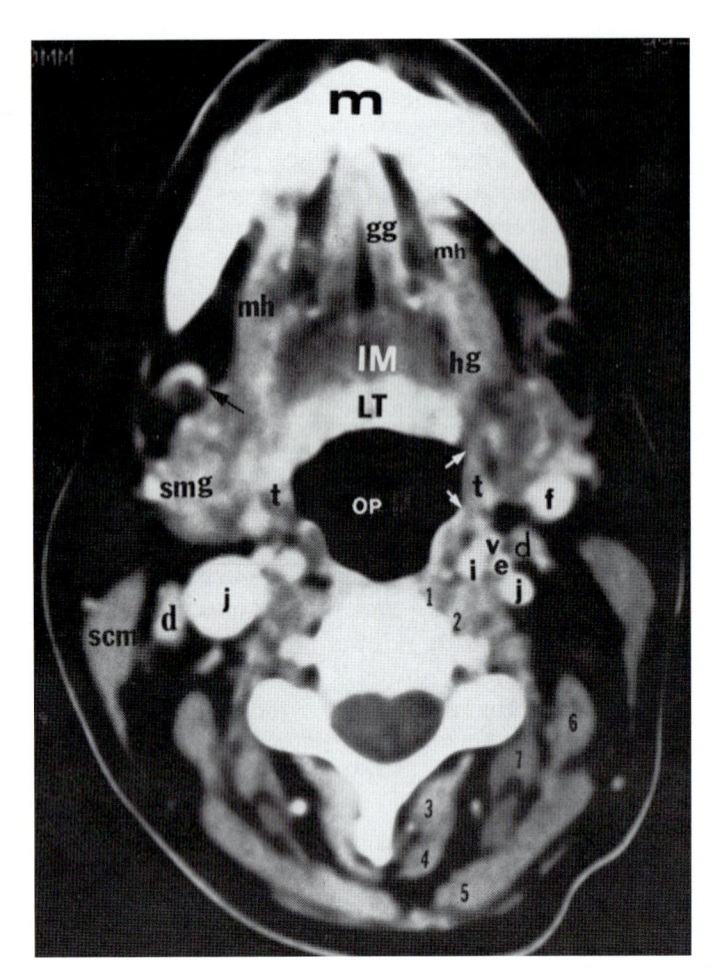

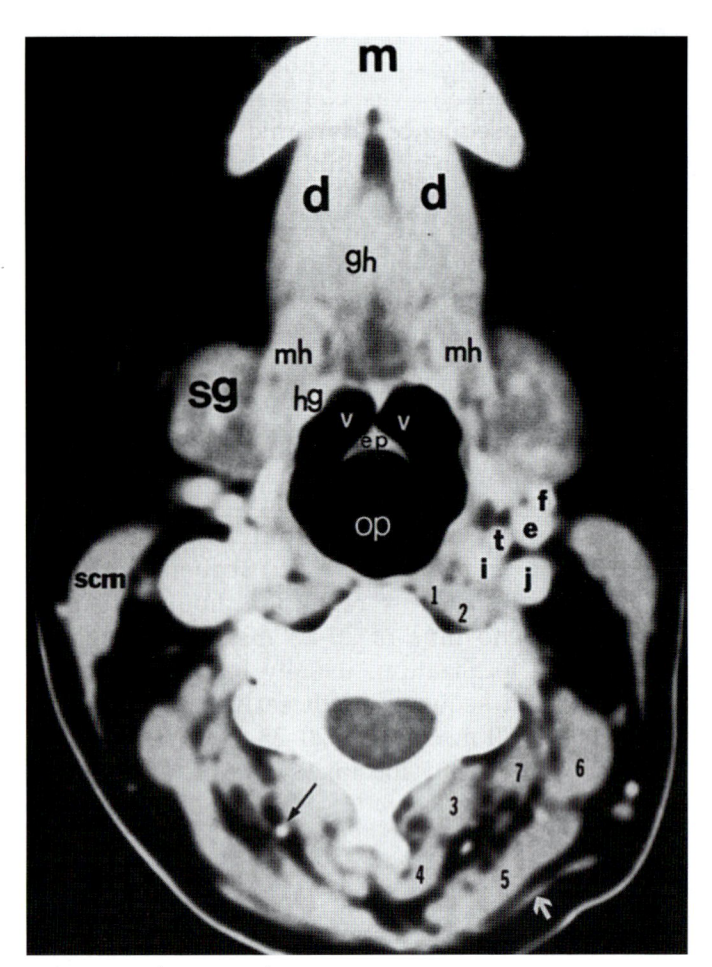

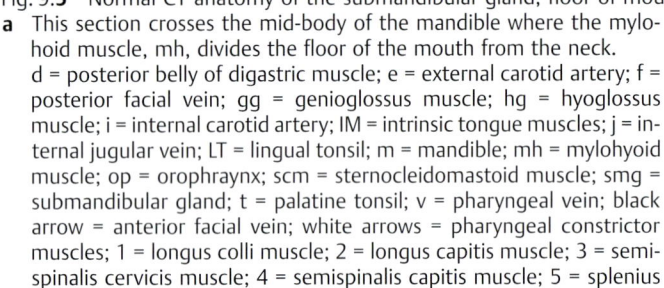

Fig. 9.5 Normal CT anatomy of the submandibular gland, floor of mouth, oropharynx, and upper neck.

a This section crosses the mid-body of the mandible where the mylohoid muscle, mh, divides the floor of the mouth from the neck.
d = posterior belly of digastric muscle; e = external carotid artery; f = posterior facial vein; gg = genioglossus muscle; hg = hyoglossus muscle; i = internal carotid artery; IM = intrinsic tongue muscles; j = internal jugular vein; LT = lingual tonsil; m = mandible; mh = mylohyoid muscle; op = orophraynx; scm = sternocleidomastoid muscle; smg = submandibular gland; t = palatine tonsil; v = pharyngeal vein; black arrow = anterior facial vein; white arrows = pharyngeal constrictor muscles; 1 = longus colli muscle; 2 = longus capitis muscle; 3 = semispinalis cervicis muscle; 4 = semispinalis capitis muscle; 5 = splenius capitis muscle; 6 = levator scapulae muscle; 7 = longissimus capitis muscle.

b This section crosses the lower mandible, m, and the inferior body of the third cervical vertebra.
d = anterior belly of digastric muscle; e = external carotid artery; ep = epiglottis; f = posterior facial vein; gh = geniohyoid muscle; hg = hyoglossus muscle; i = internal carotid artery; j = internal jugular vein; m = mandible; mh = mylohyoid muscle; op = oropharynx; scm = sternocleidomastoid muscle; sg = submandibular gland; t = superior thyroid artery; v = valleculae; black arrow = deep cervical vein; white arrow = trapezius muscle; 1 = longus colli muscle; 2 = longus capitis muscle; 3 = semispinalis cervicis muscle; 4 = semispinalis capitis muscle; 5 = splenius capitis muscle; 6 = levator scapulae muscle; 7 = longissimus capitis muscle.
(The submandibular gland is visualized in coronal section in Fig. 9.**1b**.)

is contiguous with the external auditory canal, whereas its inferior margin reaches to the angle of the mandible. The medial aspect of the parotid space, the so-called parapharyngeal aspect of the parotid space, contains the deep lobe of the parotid and extends toward the prestyloid PPS. The interposed fascial boundary in this region is very thin and at times deficient, resulting in the spread of neoplasm or infection from the parotid space to the PPS.

■ Submandibular and Sublingual Glands

The submandibular glands are the second largest paired salivary glands and consist of both superficial and deep lobes. The larger superficial lobe is located in the submandibular space, posterior and inferior to the mylohyoid muscle (Fig. 9.**5**). The smaller superior portion (deep lobe) extends superiorly over the posterior margin of mylohyoid muscle with a fingerlike projection (uncinate process) to enter the sublingual space (Fig. 9.**6**). The facial artery indents the lateral aspect of the submandibular gland. The submandibular (Wharton's) duct courses from the deep lobe, over the mylohyoid muscle in the sublingual space along the floor of the mouth, opening near the midline in the sublingual papilla on the ipsilateral side of the frenulum of the tongue.[1–3]

The sublingual glands, the smallest of the paired salivary glands, are located in the submucosa of the floor of the mouth, superior to the mylohyoid muscle and lateral to the geniohyoid/genioglossus muscle complex to lie within a sublingual depression on the medial margin of the mandible near the symphysis menti (Fig. 9.**6**). The sublingual glands are immediately anterior to the deep portion of the submandibular gland. Unlike the other major salivary glands, sublingual glands do not have a discrete capsule. There are approximately 8–20 individual minor ducts (of Rivinus) of the sublingual gland that open independently along the summit of the sublingual fold (sublingual papilla). Some of these minor ducts may be fused and form Bartholin's duct, which opens into the submandibular duct near its orifice.[1–3] The sublingual and hypoglossal nerves extend through the sublingual space, providing a potential pathway of perineural extension of tumor.[1, 3, 10]

Innervation of Submandibular and Sublingual Glands

The facial nerve through the chorda tympani provides the sensory and secretomotor function of the submandibular and sublingual glands. The lingual nerve, a branch of the mandibular division of the trigeminal nerve which passes through the submandibular ganglion, accompanies the chorda tympani.[8]

Vascular Supply and Lymphatic Drainage

Arterial supply to the submandibular gland is via branches of the external carotid artery including the facial and lingual arteries. The sublingual gland is supplied by the sublingual and submental arteries, branches of the lingual and facial arteries, respectively.[8]

Lymphatic drainage is to the superficial and deep cervical lymph nodes via submandibular and sublingual lymph nodes.[8]

■ Applied Anatomy

The definition and boundaries of the fascial planes are important not only because fascial planes tend to regulate the spread of tumors and infections, but also because the type of tumor arising in a specific space depends on the types of predominant tissues found in that region. The deep lobe of the parotid gland is in the prestyloid PPS (Fig. 9.2), and most lesions in this space are of salivary gland origin (Fig. 9.7). The poststyloid compartment contains lesions related to the great vessels, cranial nerves, and lymph nodes (e.g., paragangliomas, nerve sheath tumors, and lymphadenopathy) (Fig. 9.8). Although neoplasms originating from the prestyloid PPS predominately arise within the parotid gland, extraparotid primordial salivary gland rests or minor salivary gland tissue within the PPS may also give rise to salivary neoplasms within the prestyloid PPS.[11] The PPS masses may clinically simulate a parotid tumor (Fig. 9.8). The superior portion of the deep lobe of the submandibular gland is related to the anteroinferior wall of the PPS (Fig. 9.5 b). Therefore, submandibular tumors or inflammatory processes can extend into the PPS. The distinction between a parotid mass and a PPS tumor is important surgically (Figs. 9.9, 9.10), since intraparotid neoplasms are removed by transparotid approach with careful manipulation of the facial nerve, whereas extraparotid neoplasms can be approached via a transoral or transcervical operation, avoiding manipulation of the facial nerve.[11] Identification of a complete fat plane between the mass and the deep lobe of the parotid gland suggests an extraparotid lesion (Fig. 9.7 a). Deformity, as well as lateral displacement of the deep lobes of the parotid, along with normal appearance of the stylomandibular tunnel should support an extraparotid PPS mass (Fig. 9.7). MRI may be superior to CT in making this distinction;[11] however, this distinction may not be possible in large masses. As seen in Figures 9.1 a and 9.2 b, a tumor of the deep lobe of the parotid gland can be inferred by observing extension through the stylomandibular tunnel and/or medial displacement of the posterior belly of digastric muscle, and medial displacement of parapharyngeal fat. Prestyloid PPS masses can be inferred by observing location anterior to the sty-

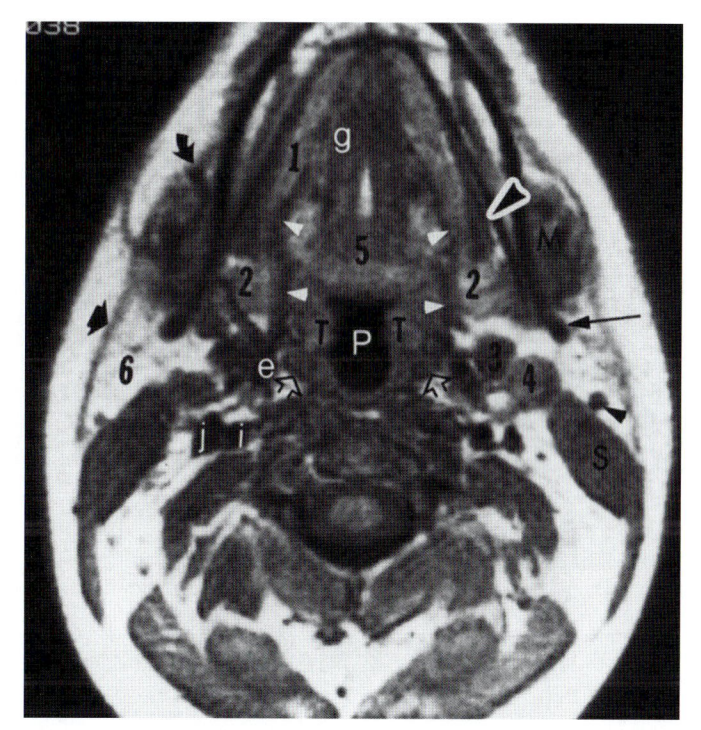

Fig. 9.6 Normal MR anatomy of sublingual gland. Axial MR section, spin density weighted. This section through the oropharynx and upper neck crosses the body of the mandible just above the mental foramina.
e = external carotid artery; g = genioglossus muscle; i = internal carotid artery; j = internal jugular vein; M = masseter muscle; P = pharynx; S = sternocleidomastoid muscle; T = palatine tonsils; white arrowheads = styloglossus muscle posterior to hyoglossus muscle; black and white arrowhead = mylohyoid muscle; black arrow = retromandibular vein; short black curved arrow = anterior facial vein; hollow arrows = pharyngeal constrictor muscles; black arrowhead = external jugular vein; 1 = sublingual gland; 2 = submandibular gland; 3 = stylohyoid muscle; 4 = posterior belly of digastric and partially volumed lymph node; 5 = intrinsic tongue muscles; 6 = parotid gland.

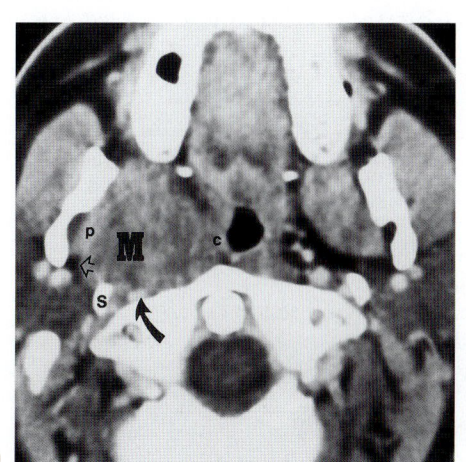

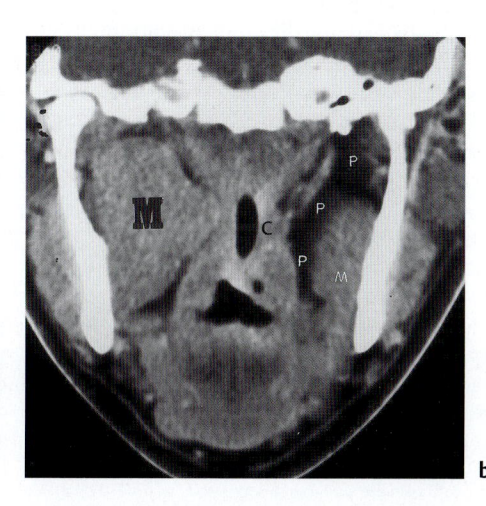

Fig. 9.7 Benign mixed tumor of the parapharyngeal space. a Enhanced axial CT scan shows a round mass (M) in the right parapharyngeal space. Note that the internal carotid artery (curved arrow) is posterior to the mass. The mass has displaced the medial pterygoid muscle (p) laterally and the constrictor pharyngeal muscle (c) medially. There is a clear fatty-areolar tissue (hollow arrow) between the mass and laterally displaced deep lobe of the parotid. S = styloid process. b Coronal CT scan shows the right parapharyngeal mass (M) between the constrictor pharyngeal and medial pterygoid muscles. Note normal left parapharyngeal space (P), constrictor (c), and medial pterygoid muscles (m).

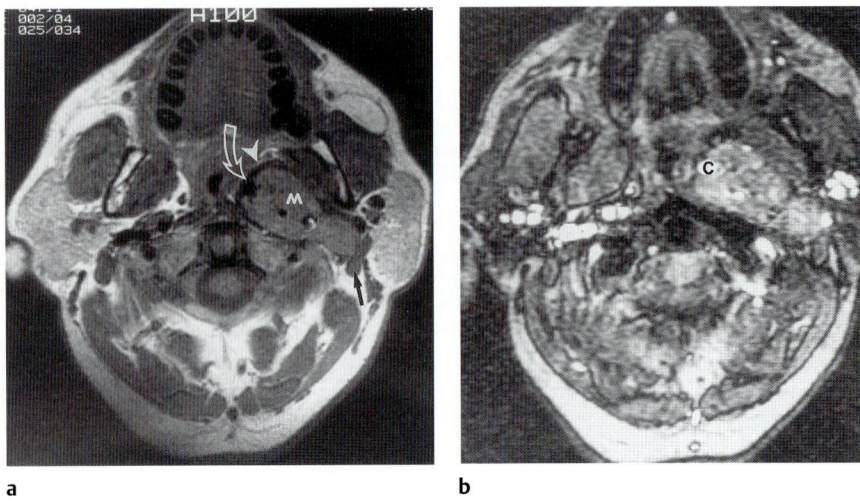

Fig. 9.8 Chemodectoma. **a** Enhanced axial MR scan shows a parapharyngeal mass (M) compatible with a vagal chemodectoma. Note anteriorly displaced internal carotid artery (curved arrow), laterally displaced posterior belly of digastric muscle (black arrow), and medially displaced parapharyngeal fat (arrowhead). Note prominent arteries (signal void) within the mass characteristic of chemodectoma. **b** Gradient echo scan confirms the hypervascularity of the tumor. C = internal carotid artery. Clinical diagnosis in this patient was a left parotid gland tumor.

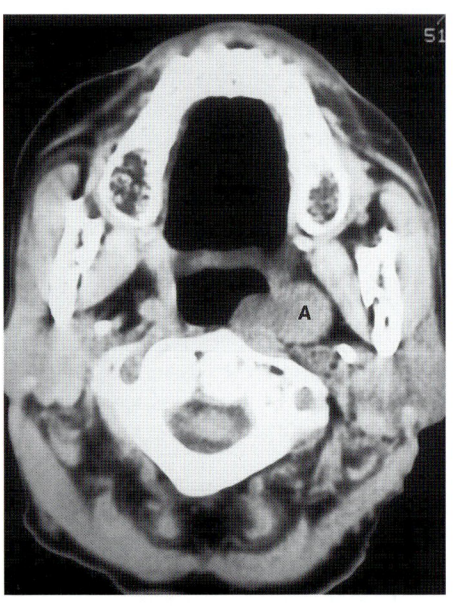

Fig. 9.9 Parapharyngeal lymphadenopathy. Axial CT scan shows a prestyloid parapharyngeal mass compatible with an adenopathy (A).

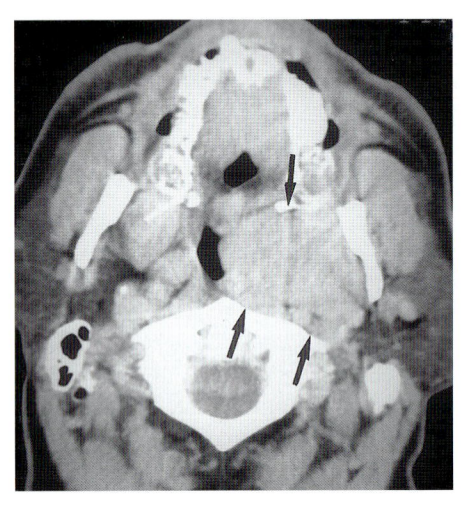

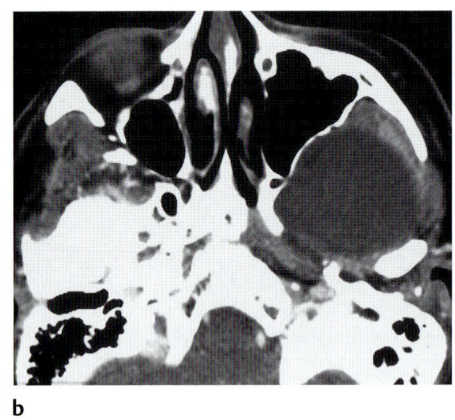

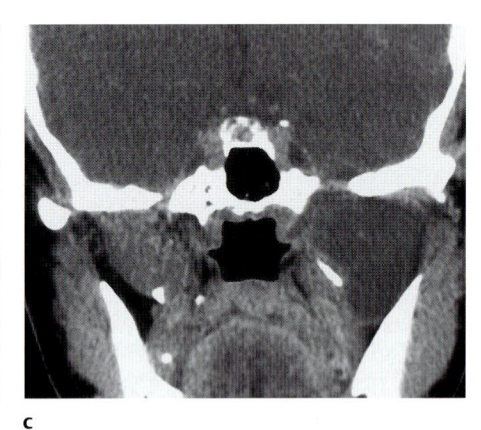

Fig. 9.10 a Rhabdomyoma. CT scan shows a large parapharyngeal mass (arrows) compatible with a rhabdomyoma. The mass is separated from the parotid gland by a thin layer of fatty-areolar tissue. **b, c** Schwannoma. **b** Enhanced axial and **c** coronal CT scans in another patient show a large mass in the left infratemporal space, associated with enlargement of the left foramen ovale, presumed to be a schwannoma. Some schwannomas may not demonstrate significant contrast enhancement.

loid process (Fig. 9.1 a), displacement of the internal carotid artery posteriorly (Figs. 9.1 a, 9.2 b), displacement of the posterior belly of the digastric muscle laterally (Fig. 9.2 c), and/or displacement of PPS fat posteromedially (Figs. 9.7, 9.9, 9.10). Poststyloid PPS masses can be inferred by observing anterior displacement (anterolateral or anteromedial) of the internal carotid artery (Figs. 9.2 b, 9.8), anterolateral displacement of the posterior belly of the digastric muscle (Figs. 9.2 b, 9.8), location posterior to the styloid process (Fig. 9.1 a), and extension posteromedial to the posterior belly of the digastric muscle (Figs. 9.2 b, 9.8). Failure to appreciate the regional anatomical relationships can result in the selection of an incorrect surgical approach, resulting in difficult removal of the tumor, damage to vital structures, or tumor spillage.[11] Anterolateral to the prestyloid PPS is the masticator space, which contains the medial and lateral pterygoid, masseter, and temporalis muscles (Fig. 9.2); the mandibular ramus; and V3. V3 exits the foramen ovale lateral to the medial pterygoid fascia and extends inferiorly within the masticator space. As a result, pathological processes arising within the masticator space have a high incidence of perineural extension through the foramen ovale. Lesions that can be localized to the masticator space are not likely to be of salivary gland origin (Fig. 9.10 b, c).[11]

Histology

Histologically, the salivary glands consist of multiple acini and ducts divided by connective-tissue septa. Variable numbers of adipocytes are noted in all salivary glands,[6,7] and accumulations of fat cells in connective-tissue septa are characteristic of the parotid gland.[5] The amount of fat within the connective tissue is related to body habitus of the individual and increases with age.

The acini consist of a combination of mucous and serous secreting cells that comprise approximately 85–90% of the cell volume of the major salivary glands.[3,6] The parotid gland consists almost exclusively of serous secreting cells. The submandibular and sublingual glands have mixed secretory units, with serous secreting cells predominating in the submandibular gland and mucous secreting cells predominating in the sublingual glands.[3,5] The acini drain into intercalated ducts, which drain into striated ducts, which ultimately drain into the excretory duct. Myoepithelial cells which are of epithelial origin and contain intracellular contractile elements (myofilaments) surround the acini and intercalated ducts and promote active secretion by contraction. Oncocytes, which have no known function, are found throughout the salivary glands and tend to increase in numbers as an individual ages. Oncocytes may be present in many organs (thyroid gland, liver, kidney, nasal cavity, trachea, etc.) and represent a form of cellular regression/degeneration with loss of specific cellular function.[3,5] The parotid glands are the only salivary glands that contain lymphatic tissue. This is due to the relatively late embryological encapsulation of the parotid gland, resulting in incorporation of adjacent lymphatic tissue. Conversely, salivary gland tissue may be incorporated into intraparotid and periparotid lymph nodes.[7]

Imaging

Imaging studies of the salivary glands provide useful information that enables the physician to establish a diagnosis and select appropriate therapy.[1-5] In the history and examination, it is important to establish whether the symptoms are acute or chronic, whether the disease is uniglandular or multiglandular, and whether there is swelling, involvement of the overlying skin, facial nerve paralysis, and pain. It is important to rule out the presence of systemic disease, such as sarcoidosis, lymphoreticular proliferative diseases, immunodeficiency, and metabolic and endocrine disorders.

Conventional radiography, plain film sialography, radionuclide scan, CT, CT sialography, MRI, MR sialography, ultrasonography, and at times angiography are used:
- To determine the accurate location and map extension of the salivary gland lesions and to differentiate them from parapharyngeal masses.
- To identify neoplastic from inflammatory and other pathologic processes.
- To differentiate, if possible, benign from malignant neoplasms.[1-5, 11-21]

■ Conventional Radiography

Calculi in the submandibular and parotid glands may be demonstrated by standard views such as oblique lateral films of the mandibular region or intraoral occlusal views or by panoramic radiography (Fig. 9.11).[1-5, 12] Occlusal films are very useful for calculi within the anterior two-thirds of the submandibular ducts (Fig. 9.11 c). Parotid stones are best demonstrated by an anteroposterior or axial tangential view (Fig. 9.11 d, e). Most (80%) salivary calculi are radiopaque.[1] Preexisting calcifications, which may be present in lymph nodes, tonsils, tumors, and phleboliths, must be differentiated from salivary calculi. CT is more reliable than conventional radiography in the detection and delineation of calculi and a variety of calcifications (Fig. 9.11 f). With 1–2.5 mm helical or axial CT scanning, even 1–2 mm calculi maybe observed within the salivary ductal system (Fig. 9.11 g).[1]

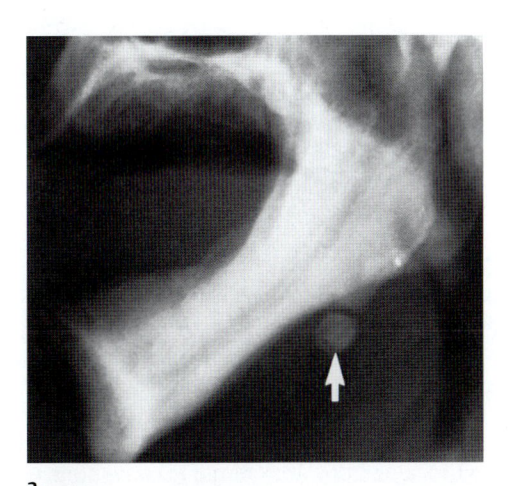

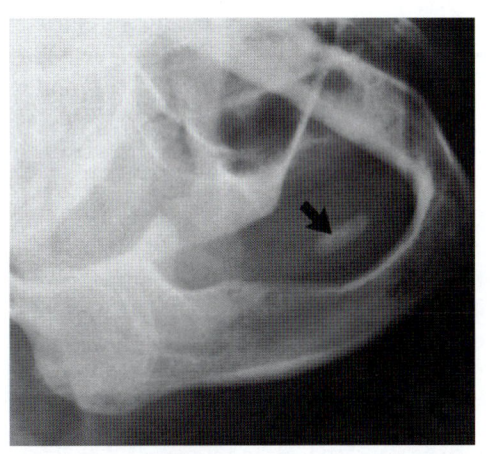

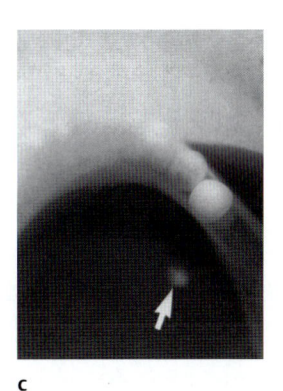

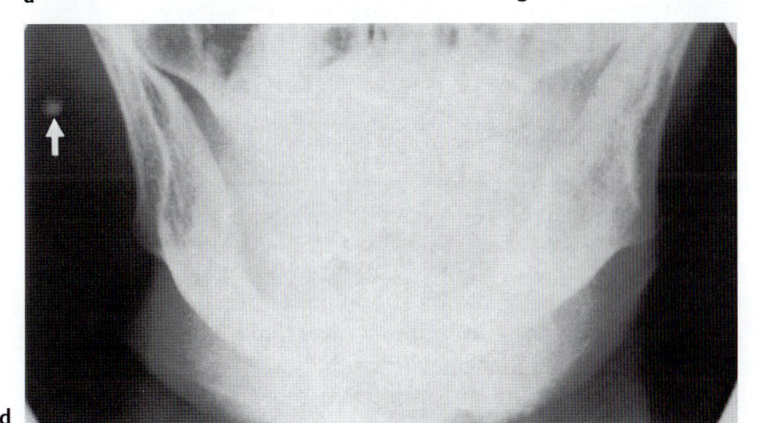

Fig. 9.11 Sialolithiasis.
a Lateral conventional view of the mandibular region shows an opaque stone in the right submandibular gland (arrow).
b Lateral oblique of the mandibular region shows a stone in the Wharton's duct (arrow).
c Occlusal view shows a Wharton's duct stone (arrow).
d AP view of the parotid and cheek region shows a calculus in the Stensen's duct (arrow).

Fig. 9.11 e–g ▷

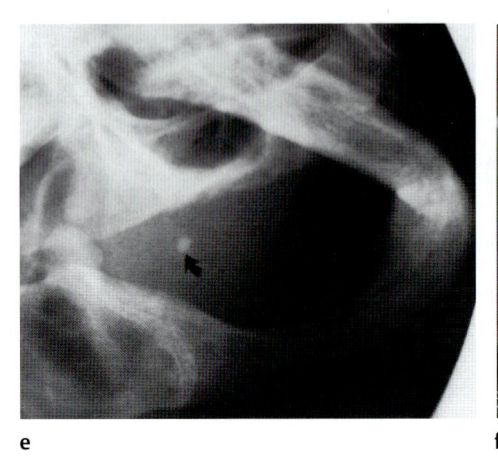

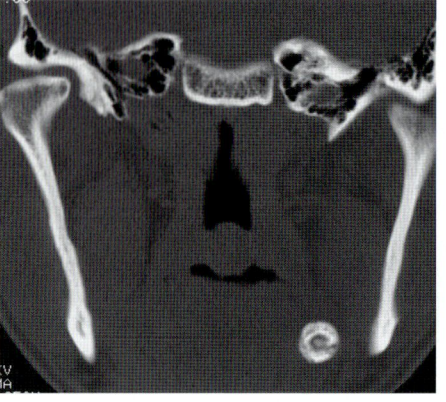

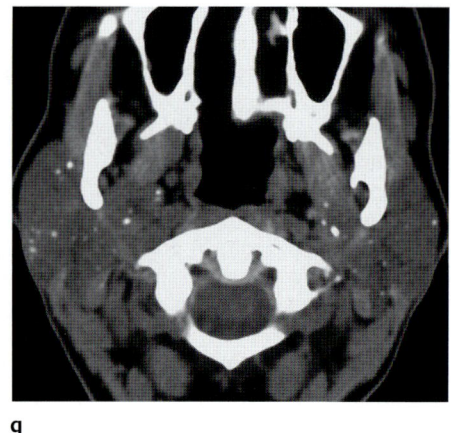

Fig. 9.**11 e–g** Sialolithiasis.
e Oblique view of the parotid and cheek area shows a calculus in the Stensen's duct (arrow).
f Coronal CT scan shows a left Wharton's duct stone.
g Axial CT scan shows multiple calcifications in the parotid glands due to chronic sialadenitis.

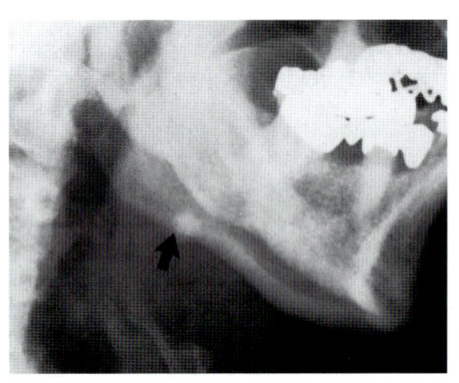

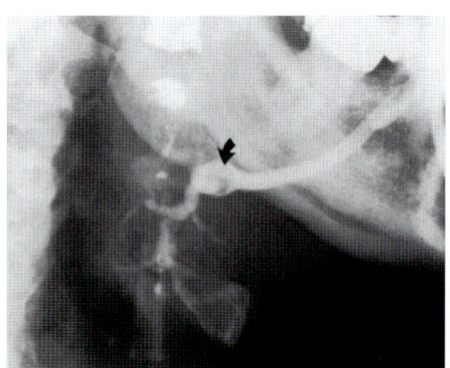

Fig. 9.**12** Submandibular duct calculus.
a Lateral view of the mandibular region shows a calculus (arrow).
b Sialogram showing the filling defect caused by the stone in the proximal portion of the Wharton's duct. There is moderate sialectasia behind the obstruction caused by the stone, and there is irregularity of the intraglandular ductal system due to inflammatory sialadenitis.

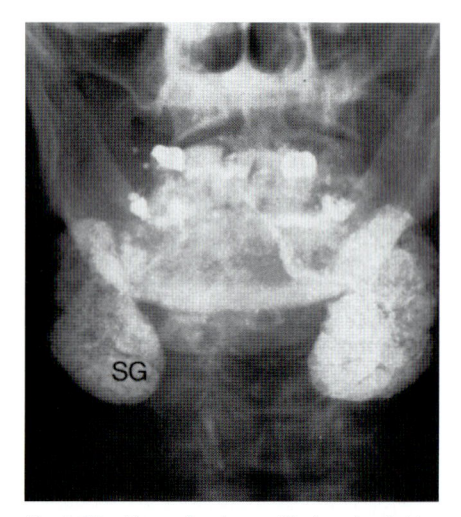

Fig. 9.**13** Normal submandibular gland, bilateral conventional sialograms. Frontal view, acinar opacification phase. The submandibular glands (SG) are opacified and Wharton's ducts are seen.

■ Conventional Sialography

Sialography, which can resolve the intraglandular ductal system, provides very useful information and leads to accurate diagnosis of intraductal pathology (Figs. 9.**12**, 9.**13**).[1–5, 12] Although both CT and MRI procedures permit remarkable accuracy, in both anatomical and pathological diagnosis, and have largely replaced plain film sialography, conventional sialography still has an important role for evaluating ductal disease,[12] sialosis, chronic inflammatory disease of the salivary glands, and noncalcified calculi, but this technique is no longer applied in the diagnosis of salivary gland masses and tumors.[12] CT and MRI with and without contrast infusion and CT sialography demonstrate anatomy and tumors of the salivary glands far more clearly and accurately than conventional sialography (Figs. 9.**14**, 9.**15**). It has recently been suggested that the diagnosis of chronic sialadenitis and Sjögren syndrome can be established with MRI and MR sialography, if typical imaging and clinical features are present, obviating the need for sialography or biopsy in selected cases (see Figs. 9.**45**, 9.**46**).[18, 20] The three main indications for sialography are:

1. Sudden acute swelling suggesting obstruction by calculus, not identified on CT scans (noncalcified calculus). Sialography in this situation unlike MR sialography may at times have a therapeutic effect of stone release.
2. Gradual progression or chronic recurrent enlargement of one or more of the salivary glands, suggesting chronic infection, ductal stenosis/strictures, or sialosis.
3. A palpable mass in the salivary glands, not identified on CT or MRI. In this setting CT sialography is preferred to conventional sialography or both can be combined.

Conventional sialography is preferred by some authors to MR and CT sialography for sialodochitis and evaluation of salivary duct after sialodochoplasty.[12] It is not indicated in acute suppurative or other acute inflammatory conditions of the salivary glands, previous reaction to contrast material with sialography, and anticipated thyroid function test.[1]

Conventional Sialography Technique

A blunt needle should be used to avoid laceration of the papillae and perforation of the duct wall. When the papilla is too small, the orifice is dilated with graduated probes. For the injection, a slightly curved blunt needle with an olive-shaped dilatation 1 cm

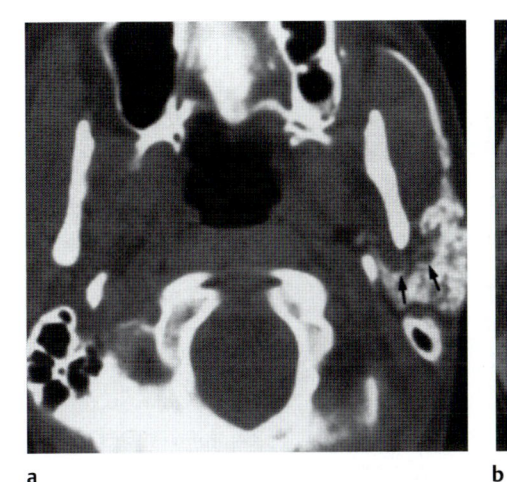

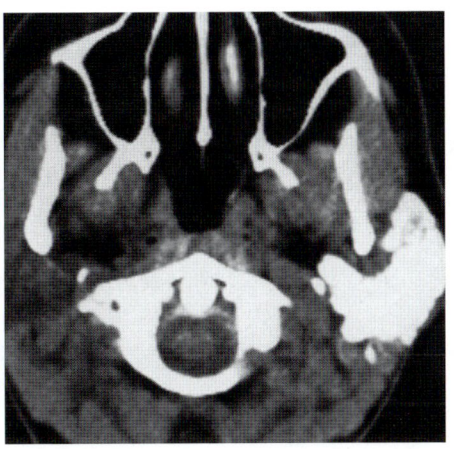

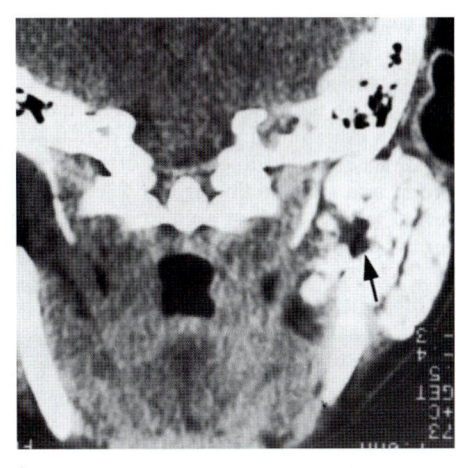

Fig. 9.**14 a-c** Normal parotid CT sialograms.
a The left parotid gland and Stensen's duct are opacified with contrast. The retromandibular vasculatures are indicated by the arrows.
b The left parotid gland is densely opacified with contrast. The deep lobe of the parotid gland extends medially behind the mandible into the pharyngeal space.
c Coronal sialogram shows good filling of the superficial and deep portions of the gland. Note the intraparotid vasculature (arrow).

from the tip is preferred.[3] The olive prevents overpenetration of the cannula and, when the olive is pressed against the orifice, backflow of the contrast media will not occur. Cannulation may be done with the patient seated or supine. The parotid duct orifice is usually easily identified in the buccal mucosa opposite the upper second molar tooth. With careful massage of the parotid gland, a droplet of saliva can be seen at the orifice of the duct. The orifice of the submandibular duct is smaller than that of the parotid, and magnifying spectacles are often needed to identify the opening. The duct opens into the sublingual caruncle on the floor of the mouth lateral to the frenulum of the tongue.[1,3] Fat-soluble contrast materials such as Pantopaque and water-soluble iodinated organic compounds have been used for conventional sialography (Figs. 9.**12**, 9.**13**). Water-soluble contrast material (0.5–1.5 ml) with high iodine content, such as Sinografin (38% bound iodine, diatrizoate meglumine, Squibb), is preferable when available.[1] Ethiodol (39% bound iodine, ethiodized poppyseed oil, Savage Laboratories) and an esterized form of poppyseed oil have been used in the past and may occasionally produce a better visualization of the ducts.[1] Water-soluble contrast materials do not produce images of the ductal system as clear as those made with the oily contrast media. This is because of the rapid diffusion and dilution by saliva and absorption of the contrast in the bloodstream. Either water-soluble or oily contrast materials are satisfactory if only the ducts are to be studied.[3]

There are three phases of sialography: duct filling, acinar filling, and postevacuation (Figs. 9.**12**, 9.**13**). Parenchymal opacification observed during sialography is due to normal filling of the acini with contrast material and is useful in outlining parenchymal masses.[1,3] Failure of the acini to opacify is abnormal but is not specific. Any process that causes marked swelling or edema of the glands or that fills the acinar lumina or causes destruction, infiltration, or replacement of the acini may prevent acinar opacification.[1,3] Postevacuation films taken one hour or longer after the injection are an important part of the sialographic examination. The postevacuation film is taken to record any extravasation of contrast material and to evaluate the pattern of emptying. Delayed evacuation of the contrast may be due to inflammation, obstruction, or processes associated with parenchymal destruction, such as autoimmune sialosis, chronic infection, the effects of radiation, or tumor infiltration.[1,3] Sialography is contraindicated in acute infections, since the injection of contrast material aggravates the acute symptoms. Sialography also should not be performed in iodine-sensitive patients. In patients who are planning to have thyroid function studies, sialography should be postponed until the thyroid work-up is completed.[1]

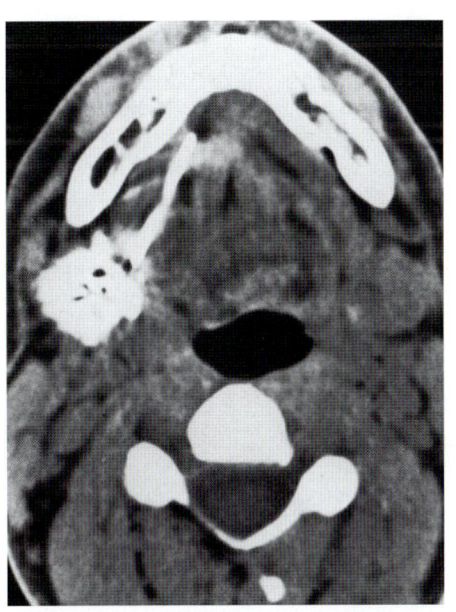

Fig. 9.**15** Normal submandibular gland CT sialogram. There is opacification of the deep lobe and Wharton's duct by contrast.

■ Computerized Tomography (CT) and Magnetic Resonance Imaging (MRI)

Tumors of all the salivary glands including the minor salivary glands can be demonstrated by CT and MRI. However, often neither CT scans nor MR images obtained with various pulse sequences permit a specific diagnosis of salivary gland lesions. Both MRI and CT can be used to determine location and extension of salivary gland masses. MRI is preferred for differentiating parapharyngeal space lesions from deep-lobe parotid lesions and is useful in determining the relationship of parotid masses to the facial nerve.[3,5,9,10,11] Conventional or MR sialography are preferred for the diagnosis of autoimmune sialopathy, sialodochitis,

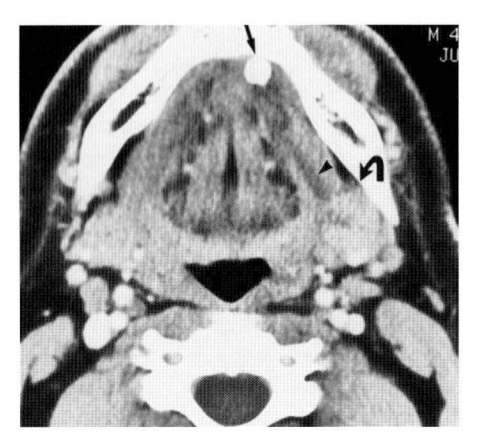

Fig. 9.**16** Submandibular calculus. Axial CT scan. The stone (arrow) is obstructing the duct (arrowhead). The superior (deep) portion of the submandibular gland (curved arrow) is also visible.

and salivary ductal strictures as well as chronic inflammatory salivary gland disease due to ductal stenosis.[12] Conventional sialography in these patients may demonstrate ductal strictures, dilatation and sacculation of the intraglandular ductal system, and delayed filling or emptying, changes that cannot be confidently diagnosed by CT scan and MRI. However, CT is the method of choice for the evaluation of acute inflammatory processes and abscesses and can easily detect radiodense stones in the ducts and within the glands (Fig. 9.16).

CT Technique and CT Appearance of the Salivary Glands

Salivary glands are well imaged in axial sections obtained with the chin slightly elevated (Fig. 9.**1 a**). Whenever dental fillings are present, which distort the images, the semiaxial projection with the head extended and the gantry tilted 15–20° should be used. The tilting angle to avoid dental fillings can be easily determined on a lateral digital scout view. CT scans are obtained using the following scanning parameters: 3 mm spiral acquisition reconstructed at contiguous 3 mm intervals; a pitch of 1; 170–280 mA; and 120 V. Axial scans are obtained from the skull base at the level of external auditory canal to the level of the mid-thyroid cartilage. The direct coronal projection is often obtained for parotid and submandibular gland lesions (Fig. 9.**1 b**). At times some parotid lesions may be better delineated in coronal images. Our routine scanning protocol consists of precontrast and postcontrast sequences. The contrast study begins with an initial intravenous bolus injection of 50 ml, followed by the injection of 100 ml of iodinated contrast material at a rate of 1.0 ml/s. Parotid CT performed too early after intravenous administration of iodinated contrast material could result in markedly decreased lesion conspicuity of pleomorphic adenoma.[22] The addition of coronal projection will solve this problem because of the time delay between administration of contrast and coronal CT acquisition. The normal parotid gland is lower in density than the adjacent masseter muscle as a result of saliva and variable amounts of fatty reticulum within the gland (Fig. 9.**1 a**). The submandibular glands are generally denser than the parotid (Fig. 9.**5**). Most intraparotid masses are visualized by plain CT scanning since they are denser than the normal glandular parenchyma. Some parotid glands are denser, which can decrease the conspicuity of soft-tissue-density lesions within the gland. Intravenous contrast enhancement results in better visualization of vascular structures and is essential for diagnosing hemangiomas and rare cases of hemangiopericytoma. Enhanced CT scans also often result in increased conspicuity of various salivary gland tumors. Pleomorphic adenomas often demonstrate delayed CT contrast enhancement.[22] This improved lesion conspicuity through delayed enhancement is an important imaging finding to improve diagnostic certainty for pleomorphic adenoma. Ring enhancement may be seen in inflammatory masses. Submandibular masses may not be recognizable in plain CT sections, since they can be isodense to the gland parenchyma. Contrast-enhanced CT scan is therefore necessary in evaluation of submandibular gland masses. At times salivary gland tumors, in particular mucoepidermoid carcinoma, adenoid cystic carcinoma, and acinic cell carcinoma may not demonstrate significant contrast enhancement on CT or on MR images (see Fig. 9.**92**). These lesions may also demonstrate no soft-tissue-density (intensity) conspicuity on unenhanced CT and MR scans. CT sialography may be required to evaluate these salivary gland masses which are not well delineated by CT and MR scans.

MRI Technique

The majority of images in this chapter were obtained with a Horizon Echospeed 1.5 T superconductive magnet scanner (GE Medical Systems, Milwaukee, WI, USA). The MR sialographic images were performed with a Picker unit (Picker International). Our protocol for imaging the salivary glands utilizes the quadrature head coil or a neurovascular head coil manufactured by MEDRAD, Inc. (Indianola, PA, USA) for GE Medical Systems. The pulse sequences and imaging options include sagittal T1-weighted images (TR = 600 or 800 ms, TE = 20 or 25 ms) followed by fast or conventional axial spin-echo (2000 ms TR and 20 ms TE = spin density or proton-weighted and 2000 ms TR, 80 ms TE = T2-weighted) sequences. In some cases, additional T1-weighted coronal images are obtained for further evaluation of the salivary gland masses. Sagittal T1-weighted images may be obtained to further evaluate the facial nerve and its relationship to the parotid masses. T1-weighted images provide the best spatial resolution and best anatomical details and T2-weighted images provide better contrast resolution. The short tau inversion recovery (STIR) pulse sequence can be used in the assessment of salivary gland pathology. At times lesions may be more conspicuous in the STIR sequences.

Currently there are no well-established indications for intravenous gadolinium (Gd) contrast administration for evaluating salivary gland masses.[23] Paradoxically, Gd enhancement may diminish contrast between the mass and the parotid gland.[23] A recent study[23] demonstrated that Warthin's tumors are characterized by the absence of Gd enhancement and thus the lack of enhancement may be used as a criterion to support the diagnosis of Warthin's tumor. There is, however, conflicting evidence that other benign and even malignant tumors may not enhance[23] and therefore the use of Gd enhancement remains controversial. We routinely use Gd-DTPA, obtaining T1-weighted MR images with and without fat-suppression for the evaluation of major and minor salivary gland masses. In our experience, Gd contrast enhancement has been useful for evaluating benign and malignant tumors of the salivary glands, as well as for the detection of intracranial extension of aggressive neoplasms and perineural spread of salivary gland tumors. We have found that the solid component of Warthin's tumor may demonstrate mild to moderate and at times marked contrast enhancement on both CT and MR scans.

Magnetic resonance (MR) imaging, having superior soft-tissue contrast resolution and multiplanar imaging capability, is considered the procedure of choice for evaluating suspected neoplasms of the salivary glands.[23–26] Since a mass of salivary gland origin will usually undergo excisional biopsy,[4,5,11] the primary

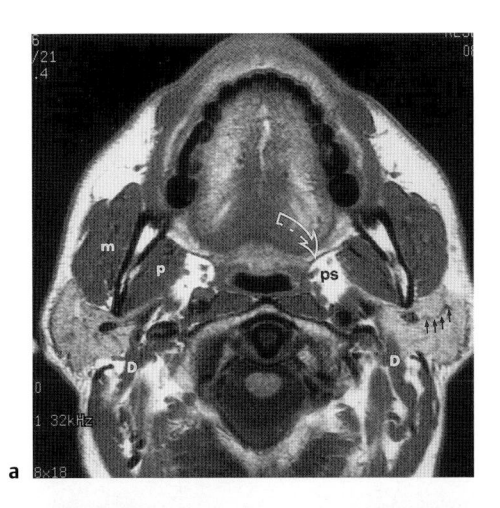

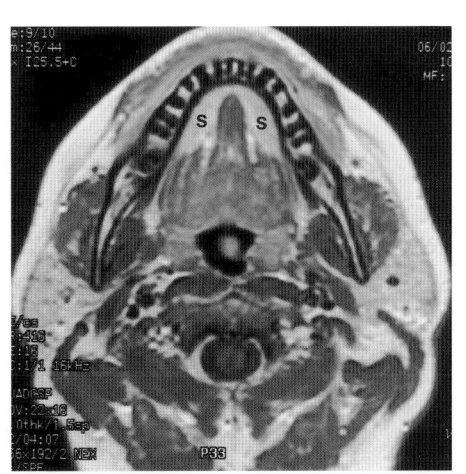

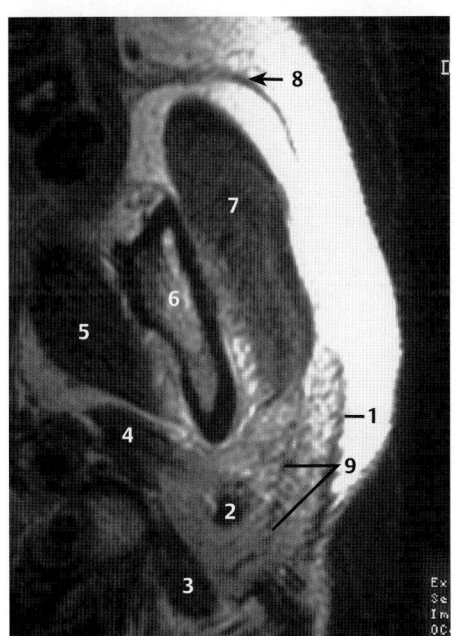

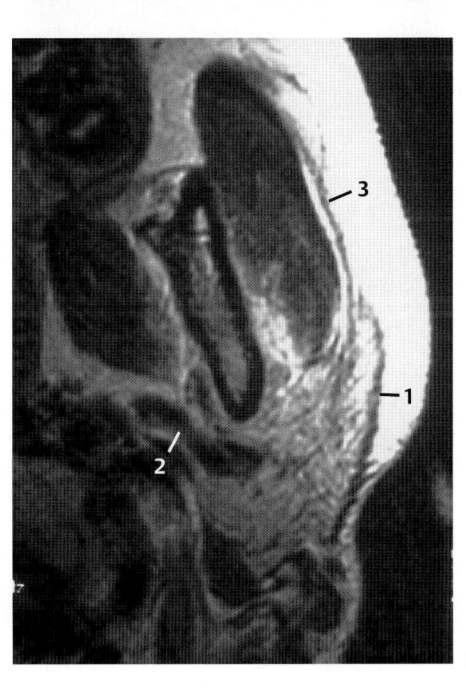

Fig. 9.**17** Normal MRI of the salivary glands.
a Axial unenhanced T1W MR scan shows normal parotid glands and a segment of facial nerve (black arrows). D = digastric muscle; m = masseter muscle; P = medial pterygoid muscle; ps = parapharyngeal space; curved arrow = presumed pterygomandibular raphe. The raphe is the junction of oral cavity and oropharynx, lying between the anterior pillar and the retromolar region.
b Axial enhanced T1W MR scan. Note moderate enhancement of parotid glands and sublingual glands (S).
c Axial T2W (3000/89, TR/TE) MR scan, taken with surface coil, shows normal parotid gland, parotid gland capsule (1), retromandibular vein (2), posterior belly of digastric muscle (3), stylomastoid group of muscles (4), medial pterygoid muscle (5), mandible (6), masseter muscle (7), parotid duct (8), and facial nerve (9). Note numerous delicate fibrous septae throughout the parotid gland.
d Axial T2W (3000/89, TR/TE) MR scan, taken with surface coil, shows normal parotid gland, parotid gland capsule (1), retromandibular vein (2), and parotid duct (3). Note numerous delicate fibrous septae throughout the parotid gland.

Fig. 9.**17** e–g ▷

role of MR imaging is therefore to confirm the location of the mass and determine its relationship to surrounding normal structures. Specifically, in the parotid gland, the goal is to determine the relationship of the mass relative to the facial nerve in an effort to preserve facial nerve function.[5,7,24,25] Direct imaging of the intraparotid facial nerve using MR has been reported in this regard.[9] However, in clinical practice, depiction of the facial nerve is not always possible and potential confusion with the parotid ductal system and branches of the facial vein can occur (Fig. 9.**17**).[3,5,9,27]

MR evaluation of suspected inflammatory or ductal disease is limited by the inability to accurately identify calcifications or to resolve the intraglandular ductal system. Detection of calcifications or radiopaque sialoliths associated with a salivary gland pathological process often supports the diagnosis of inflammatory disease. Therefore, computed tomography (CT), having the ability to discriminate subtle density differences, remains the procedure of choice for evaluating suspected acute inflammatory disease or abscesses.[22]

MR Appearance of the Normal Salivary Glands

Signal intensity of the parotid gland is slightly less than that of subcutaneous fat and hyperintense relative to muscle on T1-weighted, proton density, and T2-weighted images (Fig. 9.**17**).

There will be mild to moderate homogeneous enhancement following administration of Gd-DTPA contrast material (Fig. 9.**17b**). The submandibular gland has signal intensity hypointense relative to the parotid gland on T1-weighted, proton density, and T2-weighted images (Fig. 9.**6**). Furthermore, the submandibular gland has lower signal intensity than the sublingual gland on proton density and T2-weighted sequences (Fig. 9.**6**), making possible distinction of the deep lobe of the submandibular gland from the sublingual gland. On blood flow-sensitive pulse sequences such as gradient-echo MR images, there will be more increased intensity of the submandibular and sublingual glands compared with that of parotid gland (Fig. 9.**3**). The high signal intensity of the parotid gland on T1-weighted images is believed to result from its relatively high fat content.[25] On T1-weighted images, the facial nerve has intermediate signal intensity that contrasts with the high signal intensity of the fat-laden parotid gland (Figs. 9.**2c**, 9.**17**). Small branches of the retromandibular vein may parallel the intraparotid branches of the facial nerve (Fig. 9.**2b**). Numerous delicate fibrous septa are present throughout the parotid gland but do not approach the diameter of the major trunks of the facial nerve (Fig. 9.**17 a, c, d**).[9] The main trunk of the facial nerve is best visualized by T1-weighted sagittal images, particularly if a surface coil is used (Fig. 9.**4**). Major branches of the facial nerve are best demonstrated with high-resolution T1-weighted and T2-weighted oblique-axial sections

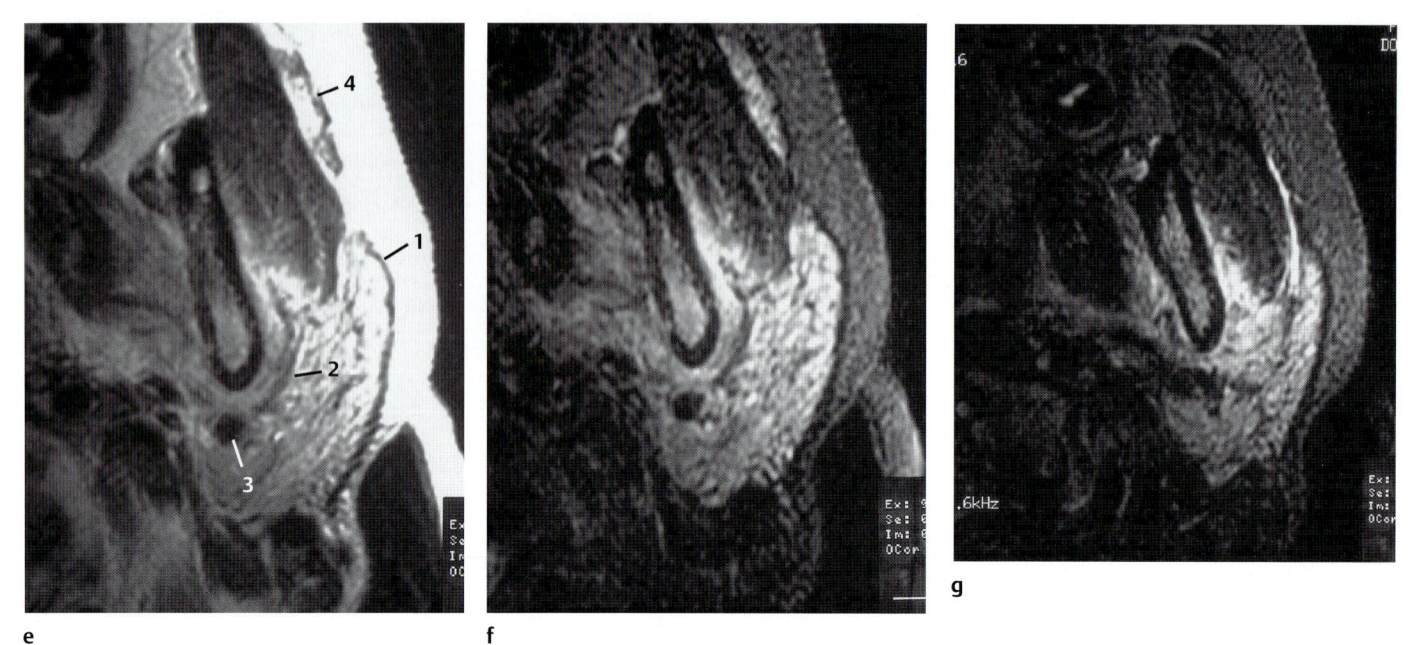

Fig. 9.**17 e–g** Normal MRI of the salivary glands.
e Axial T2W (3000/89, TR/TE) MR scan, taken with surface coil, shows normal parotid gland, parotid gland capsule (1), intraparotid facial nerve (2), retromandibular vein (3), and accessory lobe of the parotid gland (4).
f Axial FSEIR (3900/75/140, TR/TE/TI) MR scan, taken with surface coil (same level as **e**), shows normal parotid gland, parotid gland capsule, intraparotid facial nerve, retromandibular vein, and accessory lobe of the parotid gland.
g Axial FSEIR (3900/75/140, TR/TE/TI) MR scan, taken with surface coil (same level as **d**), shows normal parotid gland, parotid gland capsule, retromandibular vein, and parotid duct, which appears hyperintense.

(Fig. 9.**17 c, e, f**) (i.e., angling 35° caudal to the orbitomeatal line improves visualization of the cervicofacial division;[9,27] angling 15° cephalad to the orbitomeatal line improves visualization of the temporofacial division).[9] However, the facial nerve is not consistently identified in all cases and can be simulated by small branches of the facial vein[9] as well as the parotid ductal system as previously mentioned.[27] Typically, if a large intraparotid mass is present, visualization of the facial nerve is often difficult because of effacement of the perineural tissue and reduced contrast between the facial nerve and the tumor. More reliably, if tumor extension is medial to the retromandibular vein and mandibular ramus, then deep lobe involvement is indirectly suggested.[11]

■ MR Sialography Technique

M. Becker

Similarly to MR cholangiopancreatography, MR sialography is based on the principle that stationary fluids are hyperintense on heavily T2-weighted images. Following a preliminary report by Lomas et al. in 1996,[15] subsequent investigators have evaluated different sequences in the attempt to improve conspicuity of the ducts[16,17] and have reported MR sialography findings of ductal displacement by mass lesions,[17] intraglandular collections of saliva in the context of Sjögren syndrome,[18,19] and intraductal calculi and stenoses.[20,21] MR sialography uses an exceptionally long TE and long echo train length to obtain heavily T2-weighted images within a reasonable acquisition period. Because of the T2 decay during data acquisition, tissues with a short T2 produce practically no signal in the echoes at the end of the pulse train. Different types of sequences have been used for MR sialography, such as a standard rapid acquisition with relaxation enhancement (RARE) sequence, a single-shot turbo spin-echo (HASTE) technique, a T2-weighted gradient and spin-echo (GRASE) sequence, a 2D fast spin-echo sequence (2D FSE), a 3D fast spin-echo sequence (3D FSE), a 3D extended phase symmetry rapid spin-echo sequence (3D EXPRESS), and a constructive interference in steady state (CISS) sequence.[15] 3D techniques have the advantage of allowing acquisition of very thin slices (0.6 mm) for the detection of small stones, and maximum intensity projection (MIP) images for visualization of the overall ductal anatomy. Most of the signal related to vascular motion, as well as most of the adjacent tissue signal, is removed. Additional spectral fat suppression to improve background suppression may be used, but some authors have found that discrete background visualization of anatomical structures on MIP reconstructions may be helpful as it facilitates orientation with respect to surrounding structures. Using 3D FSE, CISS, and 3D EXPRESS sequences, images of diagnostic quality may be obtained in all cases; the only failures are due to claustrophobia on the part of the patient.

From the results of recent series, several advantages of MR sialography become evident. As we are dealing with a relatively young population with benign salivary gland diseases, the lack of ionizing radiation appears as an important advantage. In addition, MR sialography can be performed in the acute stage and may also be performed in patients with known reaction to iodinated contrast material. Even in experienced hands, conventional sialography is technically not feasible in 4% of cases because of failure to cannulate the ductal orifice.[20,21] In addition, in as many as 16% of all patients MR sialography may reveal additional information by allowing better visualization of the upstream portion of the salivary ducts and by enabling the definitive diagnosis in those cases where conventional sialography shows only displacement of normal ducts (such as in salivary gland tumors, cysts, and ranulas). Therefore, in almost 20% of cases, MR sialography appears to be clearly superior to conventional sialography.[20,21]

Disadvantages of MR sialography include general MR contraindications, and distortion artifacts by dental amalgam may impair visualization of calculi or stenoses located near the main ductal orifice. Despite inferior resolution of MR sialography compared to conventional sialography, especially for the assessment of secondary and tertiary ducts, diagnosis often is not affected.[21]

Imaging 637

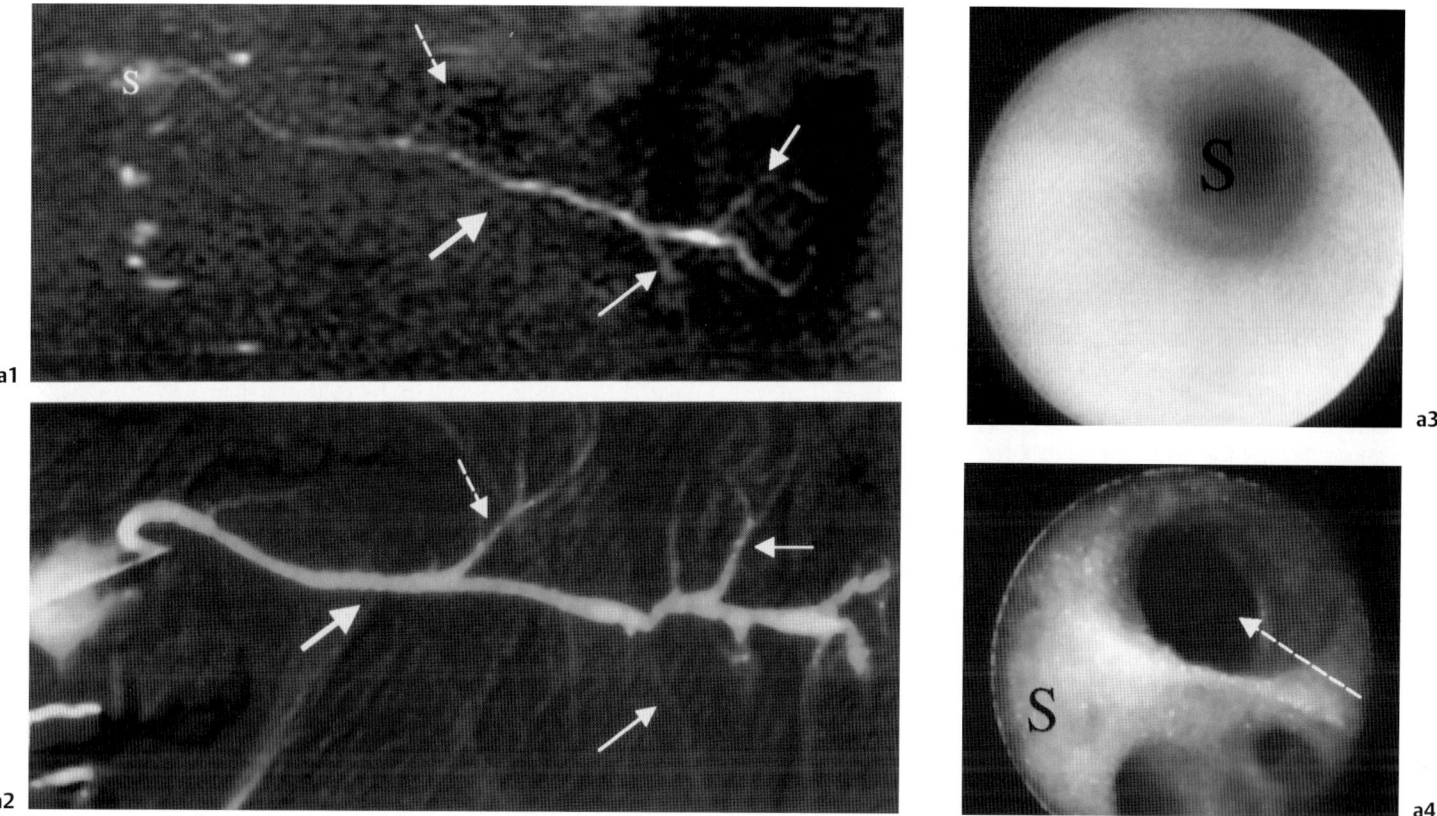

Fig. 9.18 a Normal conventional sialography, MR sialography, and normal sialendoscopy of the parotid gland. 1, MIP reconstruction of a sagittal oblique 3D-EXPRESS sequence shows a normal main parotid duct with a diameter of 1–2 mm (thick arrow), normal primary branches (thin arrows), and a normal accessory duct (dashed arrow), which has a diameter of less than 1 mm. Hyperintense saliva (s) within the oral cavity. 2, Conventional sialography performed after MR sialography confirms the diagnosis of normal ducts. The main parotid duct (thick arrow), the accessory duct (dashed arrow), and the primary and secondary branches (thin arrows) appear slightly larger than on MR sialography images because of active filling with contrast material. 3, 4, Diagnostic sialendoscopy was performed to rule out a small mucous plug. Sialendoscopy confirmed a normal appearance of Stensen's duct (S), primary branches (dashed arrow), and secondary branches (not shown). Case provided by M. Becker, MD.

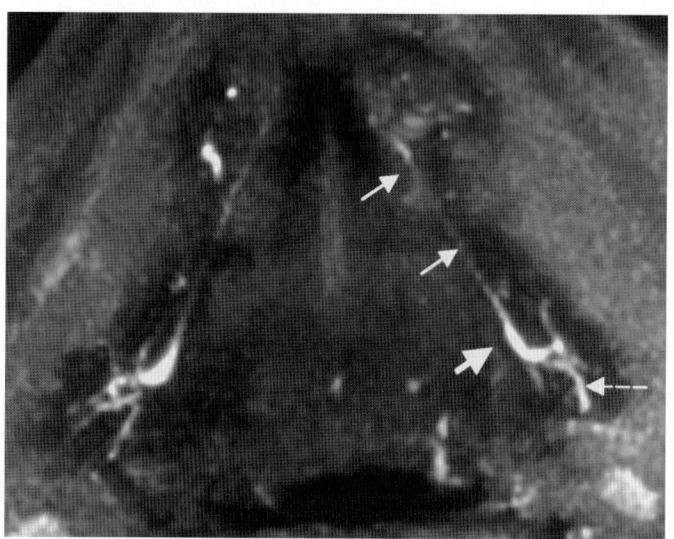

Fig. 9.18 b Normal appearance of the submandibular ductal system as seen on axial MR sialography (MIP reconstruction) and on sialendoscopy. 1, On MR sialography Wharton's duct appears to be thinner in its anterior portion at the level of the floor of the mouth, as it is physiologically collapsed (thin arrows). The most posterior portion widens progressively (thick arrow) and the primary intraglandular branches (dashed arrow) are even larger than the most anterior portion of Wharton's duct. 2, Sialendoscopic view of Wharton's duct at the level of the floor of the mouth shows its flattened appearance. Arrow points to the emergence of an accessory duct. 3, Sialendoscopy of intraglandular ducts shows their rounded shape and wider size (dashed arrow). Case provided by M. Becker, MD.

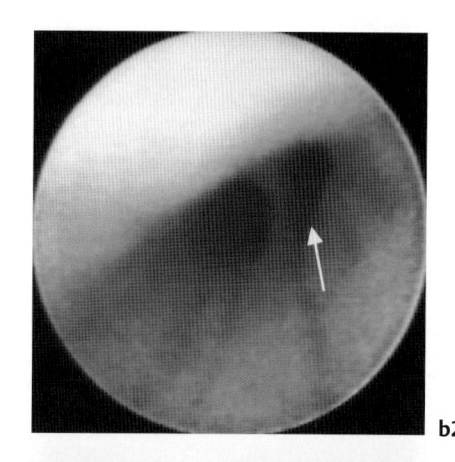

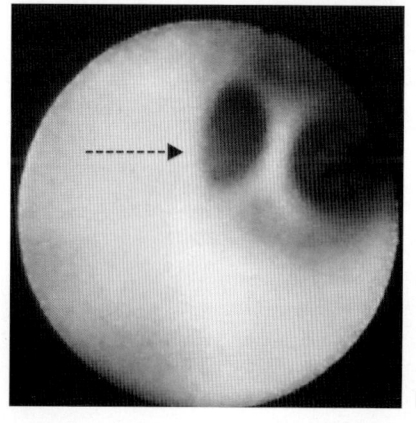

Protocol for a 3D EXPRESS Sequence

The patients do not undergo any specific preparation and they are asked to breathe quietly and refrain from coughing or vigorous swallowing during image acquisition. Rapid sagittal, coronal, and axial localizers are obtained to facilitate slice positioning. MR sialography images are obtained in an axial plane parallel to the hard palate and in a sagittal oblique plane parallel to either Wharton's or Stensen's duct. MR sialography is performed with a three-dimensional extended-phase conjugate-symmetry rapid spin-echo (3D EXPRESS) sequence, a heavily T2-weighted single-shot fast spin-echo sequence with half-Fourier analysis. The imaging parameters are: repetition time (TR) 6000–10 000 ms; echo time (TE) 190 ms; echo-train length (ETL) 136; interecho spacing 8.5 ms; 2×RAM (reduced-acquisition matrix); field of view (FOV) 16×16 cm; matrix size 256×256 pixels; slice thickness 0.6–1.5 mm; imaging time 5–6 minutes, 30 seconds per sequence. In all patients, postprocessing of the MR sialographic images was performed on a separate workstation (Picker International). Maximum intensity projection (MIP) reconstructions are obtained in all cases.

■ Ultrasound Technique

Ultrasonography (US) of the salivary glands can be used for evaluation of calculi, inflammatory diseases, and congenital lesions; in combination with fine-needle aspiration cytology, it is a powerful tool for characterizing salivary gland tumors. However, US is operator-dependent and does not enable complete, sectional imaging of the parotid and submandibular glands. Visualization of the deepest portion of the submandibular gland may be difficult and assessment of the deep lobe of the parotid gland may be impossible because of the adjacent mandible. US of the salivary gland is best performed using linear-array broadband transducers with a frequency of about 7–12 MHz. As in other parts of the body, the selection of the transducer's frequency depends on the depth of the lesion to be examined and on the attenuation of the interposed tissues. To examine very superficial lesions, a standoff pad made of silicone elastomer may be used. Although Doppler and power Doppler imaging are often useful in the examination of the salivary glands, most diagnoses are made with the standard gray-scale technique.

■ Nuclear Medicine

Radioisotope scanning with ^{99}Tc-pertechnetate is not as accurate as contrast sialography, CT, or MR in demonstrating lesions of the salivary glands. This technique is of value, however, in establishing the diagnosis of Warthin's tumors and oncocytomas, since these are the only tumors that regularly show an increased uptake of the isotope. It may also help in identifying subclinical involvement of the salivary gland with such systemic diseases as sarcoidosis and collagen disorders.

Clinical Applications: Pathological Conditions

■ Congenital Lesions

Congenital lesions of the salivary glands are uncommon. In the first and second branchial arch syndrome, the parotid gland is sometimes absent (Fig. 9.**19a, b**). These cases are to be differentiated from those with atrophy and/or fatty replacement of the glands. Branchial cleft anomalies as well as cystic hygroma may involve the parotid gland. Cystic hygroma may involve all major salivary glands. Rarely ectopic thymic tissue may be present adjacent to the major salivary glands (Fig. 9.**19c, d**).

Branchial Apparatus Anomalies

Developmental alterations of the branchial apparatus result in cysts, sinuses, or fistulae. A branchial pouch sinus has an internal opening; a branchial cleft sinus has an external opening. A branchial fistula has both internal and external openings, representing persistence of the pouch and cleft, with obliteration of the epithelial plate in between.[28] A branchial cleft cyst is related to residual trapped pouch or cleft.[28] Sinuses and fistulae are associated with discharge of mucoid or purulent secretions from the tract opening. Up to 10% of cases may be bilateral.[8]

Branchial cleft anomalies are congenital lesions caused by incomplete regression of the cervical sinus of His during the sixth and seventh weeks of embryogenesis (see Chapters 10 and 11).[16,28,29] First branchial anomalies often appear as cysts (68%), sinuses (16%), and fistulae (16%).[8,29] The parotid gland, pinna, and facial nerve are variably influenced by a first branchial cleft cyst. The first branchial groove is an anlage to the external auditory canal (EAC). Arrested development or cell remnants in the area may result in cysts within or adjacent to the parotid gland, or in fistulae associated with the EAC, posterior auricle, lobule, or angle of the mandible.[1,8,16,29] On examination, the cyst is a smooth, round, nontender, fluctuant mass in the periauricular/parotid region. There may be an external opening present along the floor of the external auditory canal.[1] If infected, the patient may represent with swelling of the parotid gland, otitis externa, and neck abscess.[29] First branchial cleft cysts occur in or adjacent to the salivary glands and commonly in the parotid gland (Fig. 9.**20**). Other development cysts such as dermoid (Fig. 9.**21a, b**) and epidermoid (Fig. 9.**21c, d**) cysts may simulate parotid gland, submandibular gland, or branchial cleft cysts.[29] Congenital cystic dilatation of the major ductal system with formation of the multilocular cystic areas (polycystic or dysgenetic cysts) are even more rare, may be unilateral or bilateral, and may manifest in infancy or appear later.[17] If the ducts into the cyst are patent, sialography may outline the cystic spaces.

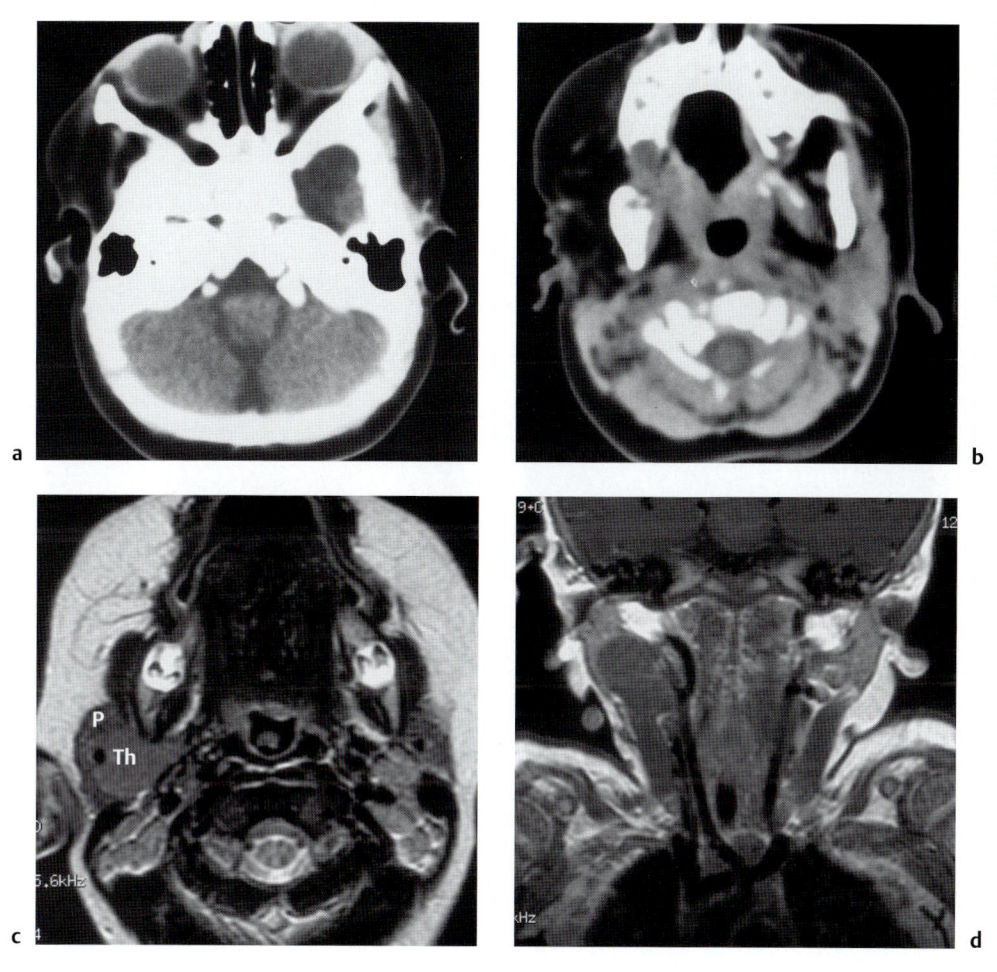

Fig. 9.**19** Right hemifacial microsomia and absent right parotid gland. **a, b** Axial CT scans show deformed right external ear and hypoplastic right temporalis muscle, foreshortening of right lateral orbital wall, hypoplastic right pterygoid muscles, and absent right parotid gland. **c** Axial T2W and **d** coronal T1W MR scans in another patient, an 8-month-old girl, showing an ectopic thymic tissue (Th) replacing part of the right parotid gland (P).

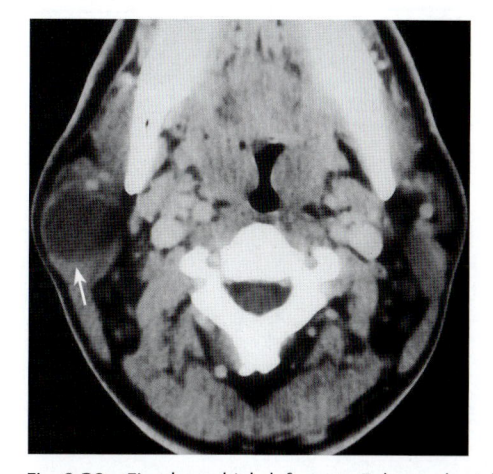

Fig. 9.**20** First branchial cleft cysts. Enhanced axial CT scan shows a cyst (arrow) compatible with first branchial cleft cyst.

Other Cystic Lesions of Salivary Gland Regions

Other cystic lesions of the salivary glands and salivary gland regions include dermoid (Fig. 9.**21 a, b**), epidermoid (Fig. 9.**21 c, d**), ranula, and cystic hygroma. Ranulas are mucous retention cysts, acquired secondarily to obstructed sublingual or minor salivary glands, and arise within the sublingual space.[1] Extravasation of fluid from an obstructed sublingual duct into the floor of the mouth results in formation of a ranula. A ranula is not lined by epithelium and thus is just a pseudocyst. Ranulas can herniate through or around the mylohyoid muscle to lie within the low parapharyngeal space or submandibular space, and these are referred to as plunging ranulas (Fig. 9.**22 a, b**).[1] Ranulas are thin-walled, unilocular, and homogeneous cystic lesions arising from the sublingual space. They have uniform low to intermediate signal intensity on T1-weighted MR images and high signal intensity on T2-weighted MR images (Fig. 9.**23**). Epidermoid and dermoid cysts are often in the floor of the mouth or submandibular space and can present as a mass near the submandibular or sublingual glands (Fig. 9.**21**). Dermoid and epidermoid cysts may be located within the parotid (Fig. 9.**21 a, b**) and submandibular (Fig. 9.**21 c, d**) glands. Cystic hygromas are cystic lymphangiomas presumed to develop from congenital obstruction of lymphatic drainage. The majority of cystic hygromas occur within the posterior triangle of the neck and may involve the salivary glands directly or by extension.[1, 29] Cystic hygroma of the parotid gland is an uncommon congenital lesion that presents as an asymptomatic, soft, fluctuant mass. Cervical ultrasonography, CT, and MRI are used to assess the size and extent of the lesion and to assist in planning the surgical approach. Cystic hygromas appear hypodense on CT scans (Fig. 9.**24**) and demonstrate low or intermediate signal intensity on T1-weighted and high signal intensity on T2-weighted MR images (Fig. 9.**25**). Cysts sometimes contain a high protein-to-fluid ratio or hemorrhage, resulting in T1-weighted hyperintensity. In contrast to branchial cleft cysts and ranulas, most cystic hygromas contain visible low-intensity

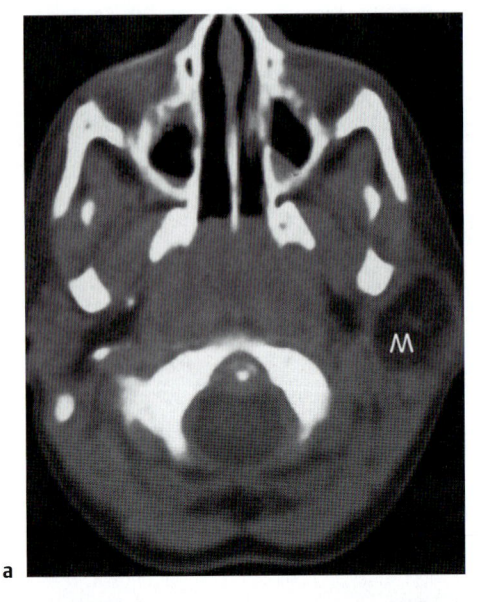

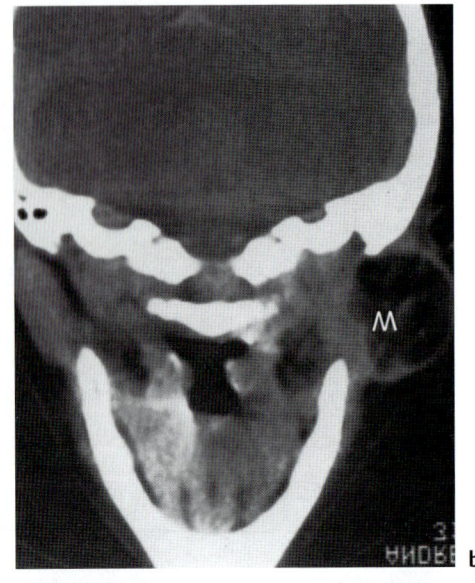

Fig. 9.21 a, b Dermoid cyst of the parotid gland. **a** Axial, **b** coronal contrast-enhanced CT scans. The left parotid gland is enlarged by an inhomogeneous low density mass (M). **c, d** Epidermoid cyst of the floor of the mouth. Axial enhanced CT scans, at levels 1 cm apart. There is a large-low density lesion compatible with an epidermoid cyst (EC) in the right side of the neck surrounded by a thin capsule. ad = anterior belly of the digastric muscle; gg = genioglossus muscle; mh = mylohyoid muscle; S = sternocleidomastoid muscle; sg = submaxillary (submandibular) gland; sl = sublingual gland.

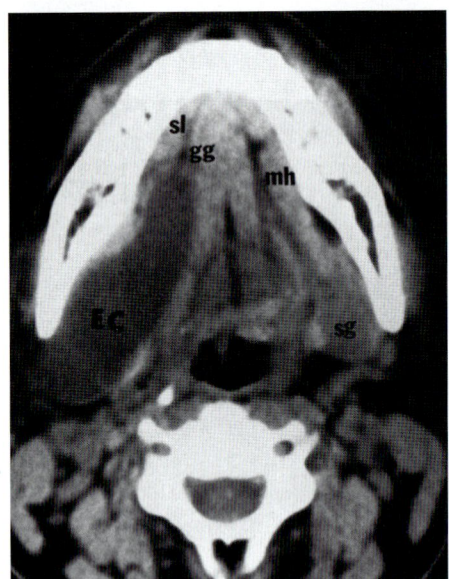

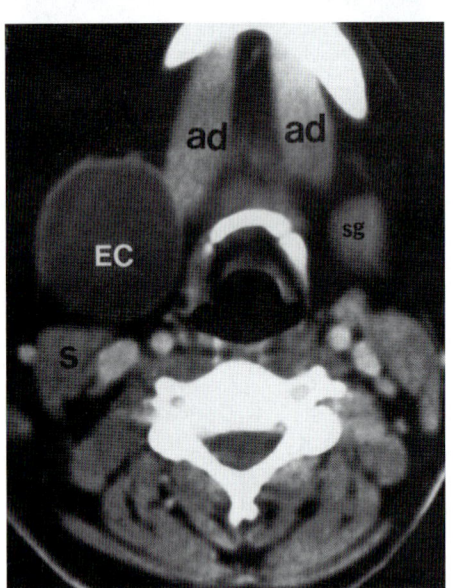

Fig. 9.22 Ranula, plunging type.
a Axial CT scan shows a large ranula (R) in the floor of the mouth and neck displacing the right submandibular gland (sg) laterally. There is marked deformity of the mylohyoid muscle on the involved side as compared to normal left side (Mh).
b The coronal CT scan at the level of the rami of the mandible shows the plunging ranula (R), which has displaced the tongue to the left and mylohyoid muscle (MH) inferiorly. ad = anterior belly of the digastric muscle.

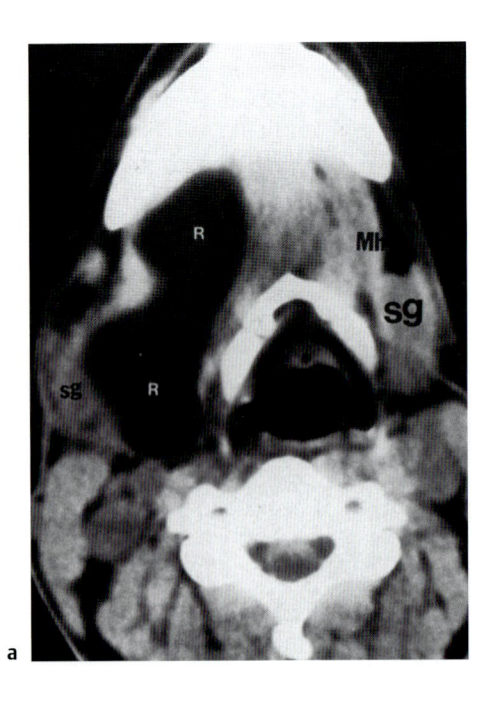

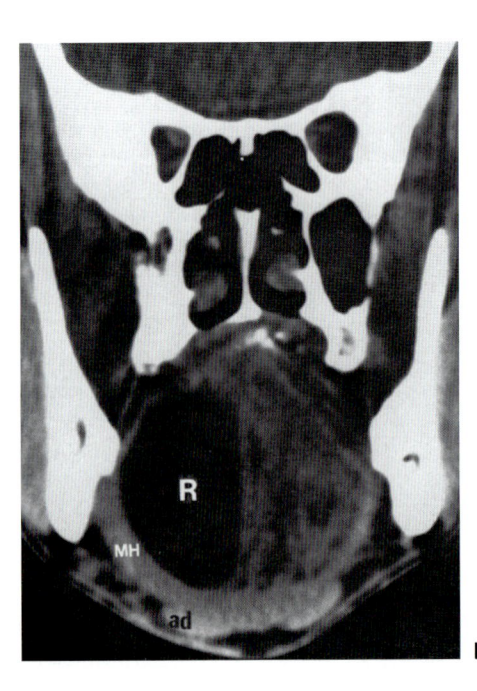

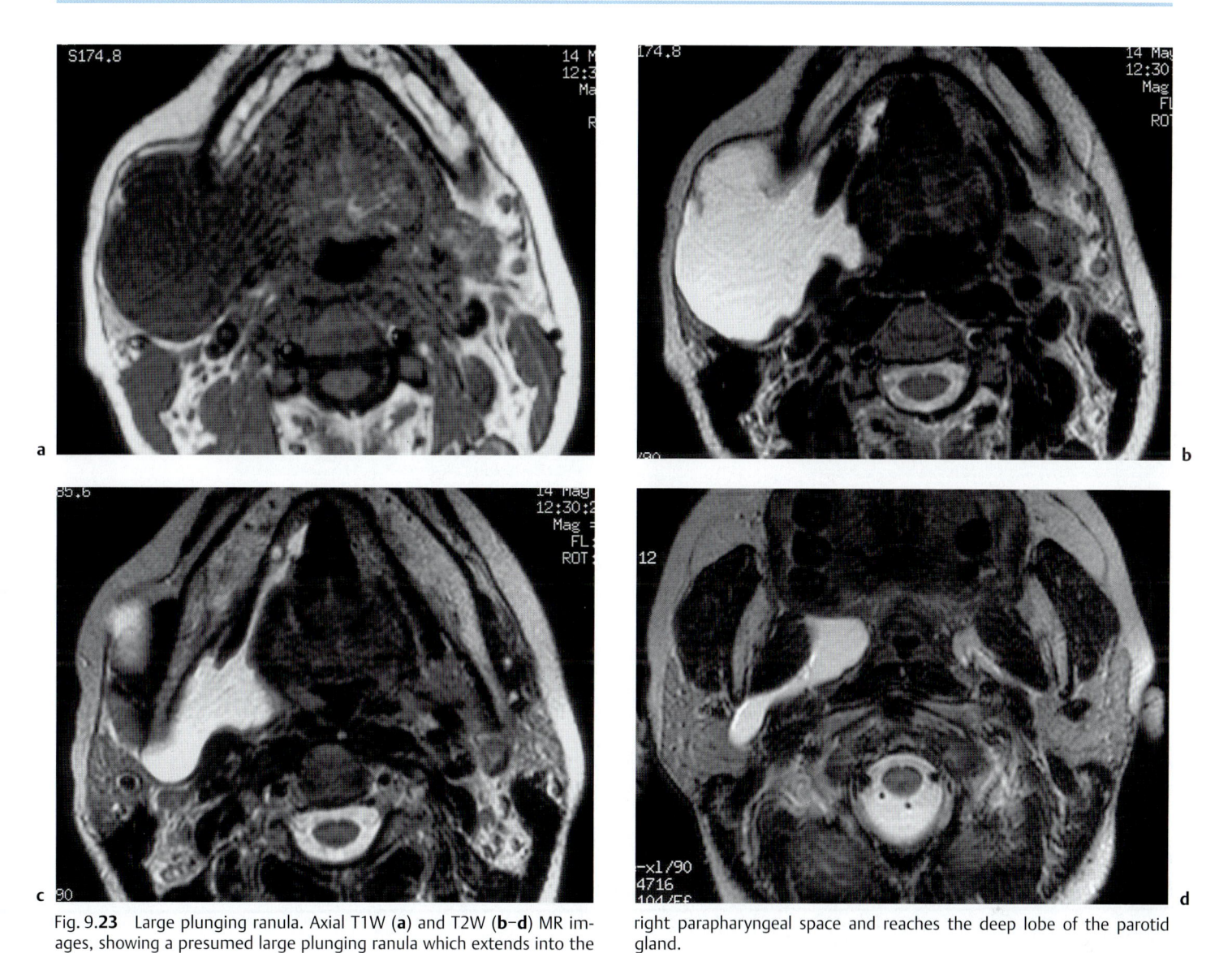

Fig. 9.23 Large plunging ranula. Axial T1W (a) and T2W (b–d) MR images, showing a presumed large plunging ranula which extends into the right parapharyngeal space and reaches the deep lobe of the parotid gland.

septations corresponding to fibrous septa. Fluid levels within cystic spaces may sometimes be observed.[30] Multiple sebaceous cysts adjacent to the parotid gland can simulate a parotid gland cysts or tumors.

Inflammatory Diseases of the Major Salivary Glands

Inflammatory diseases of salivary glands may be classified as acute or chronic. Acute inflammatory disease includes viral infections such as epidemic parotitis or mumps, and bacterial infections such as acute suppurative sialoadenitis. Imaging studies are not indicated in mumps unless sialoadenitis appears to be persistent (Fig. 9.26). Diffuse enlargement of one or both parotid and/or submandibular glands due to mumps is to be differentiated from other viral etiologies such as Coxsackie virus A and B, ECHO (echovirus, Rhinovirus type 1), Epstein–Barr, herpes, influenza type A, cytomegalovirus, and choriomeningitis virus.[1] Sialography is contraindicated in the presence of an acute infection because of the danger of spreading the infection. CT or MRI with contrast enhancement should be performed if clinically indicated. Diffuse enhancement of a swollen gland is characteristic of inflammation (Fig. 9.26). Chronic inflammatory diseases include chronic recurrent sialoadenitis, chronic sialectasis, chronic granulomatous disease (i.e., sarcoidosis, tuberculosis, syphilis, actinomycosis), lymphoepithelial sialadenopathy, Kimura disease, and sialolithiasis.

Acute Suppurative Sialadenitis with Abscess Formation

Acute suppurative sialadenitis is a bacterial infection, and the parotid gland is more frequently involved in abscess formation than the submandibular gland. The most common bacterial organisms are *Staphylococcus aureus* and *Streptococcus viridans*.[1] CT and MR are both useful in showing the inflammation or abscess (Figs. 9.27, 9.28). There is diffuse swelling of the gland, and the abscesses are seen as unilocular or multilocular collections of fluid. Abscesses of the submandibular gland are usually secondary to obstruction from a stone or stricture of the duct. Parotid abscesses may be complicated by inflammation of the mastica-

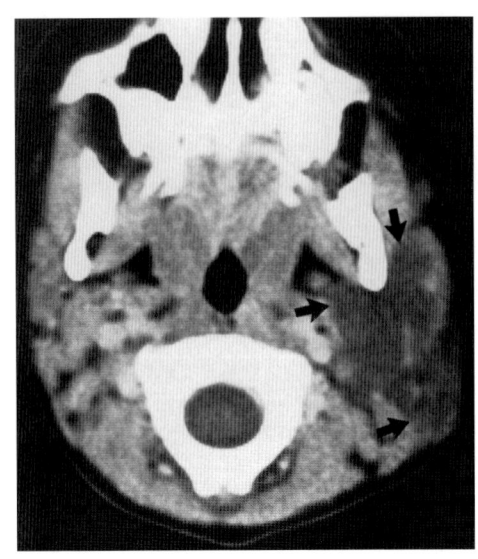

Fig. 9.24 Cystic hygroma involving the parotid gland. Contrast-enhanced axial CT scan. A large low-density mass involves the left parotid gland and posterior triangle of the neck (arrows).

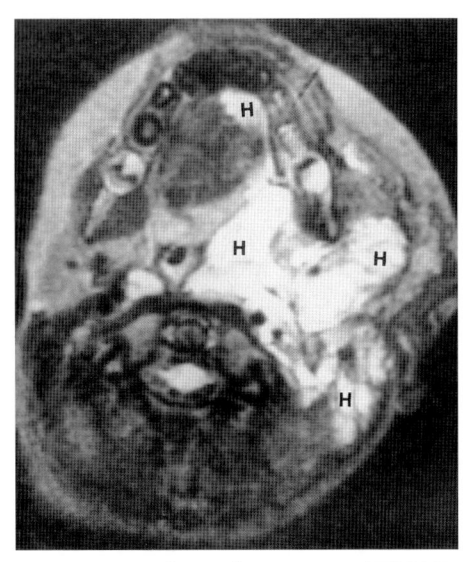

Fig. 9.25 MRI of cystic hygroma. Axial T2W MR scan shows a large cystic hygroma (H), involving the left parotid gland, parapharyngeal space, oral cavity, and posterior neck.

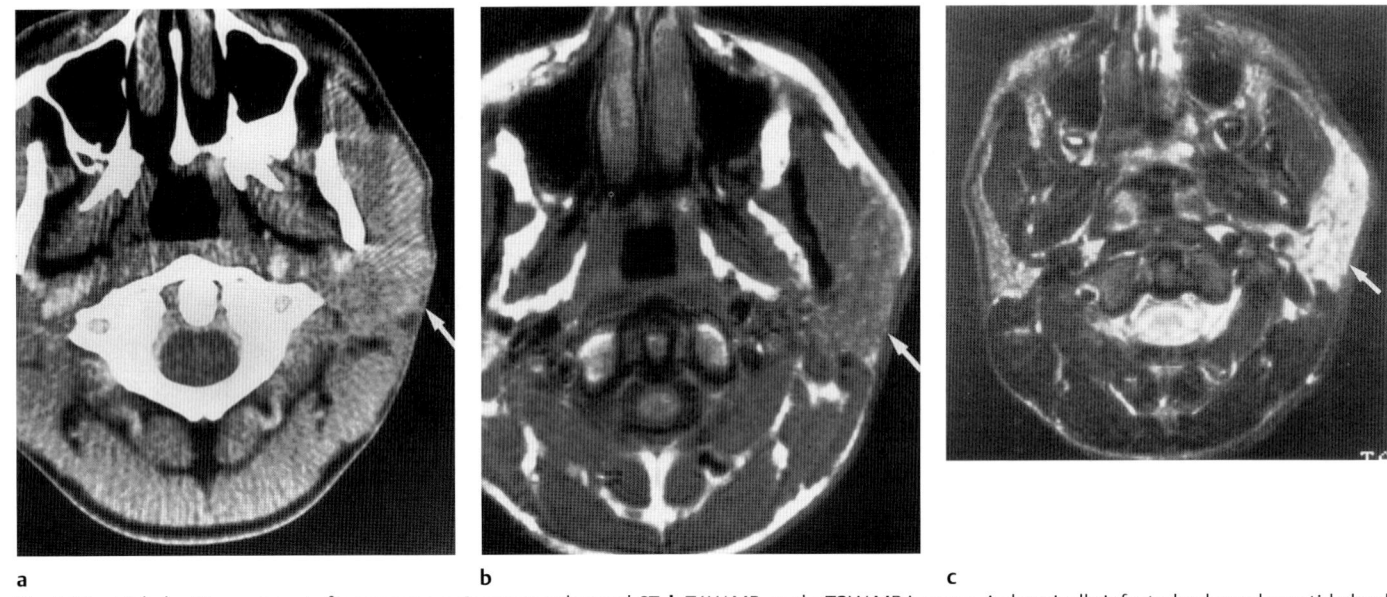

a b c

Fig. 9.26 Sialadenitis persistent after mumps. **a** Contrast-enhanced CT, **b** T1W MR, and **c** T2W MR images. A chronically infected enlarged parotid gland (arrow) developed in this patient as a persistent swelling following mumps. Note hyperintense enlarged left parotid gland (arrow) on T2W MR inmage (**c**). From Reference 1.

tory space (Fig. 9.28). Unfortunately, inflammatory processes, particularly chronic sialadenitis, may at times mimic neoplastic processes on CT and MR (Fig. 9.29). In contrast to malignancies, acute inflammatory masses tend to be associated with thickening of the superficial cervical fascia as well as the superficial layer of the deep cervical fascia and infiltration of the subcutaneous fat. Diffuse increased signal intensity on T2-weighted MR images and contrast enhancement may be observed in acute infections of salivary glands. Identification of associated calcifications/sialoliths is additional supportive evidence for infection, since calcifications are rare in parotid neoplasms.[3] Calcification, however, can be present in pleomorphic adenoma, Warthin's tumor, acinic cell carcinoma, and adenoid cystic carcinoma (Table 9.1). The end result of chronic obstruction of a salivary gland will be atrophy and fatty replacement of the gland (see Fig. 9.43c).

Chronic Recurrent Sialadenitis

Strictures, calculi, or both within the main salivary gland duct may result in chronic infection of the duct (sialodochitis) and the gland (sialadenitis). Pools of purulent material accumulating within the intraglandular ducts and associated with chronic infection of the gland itself result in persistent swelling of the gland. Chronic recurrent sialadenitis is characterized by a recurrent salivary gland enlargement (Figs. 9.30, 9.31) associated with pain, tenderness, and often frank pus that can be expressed from

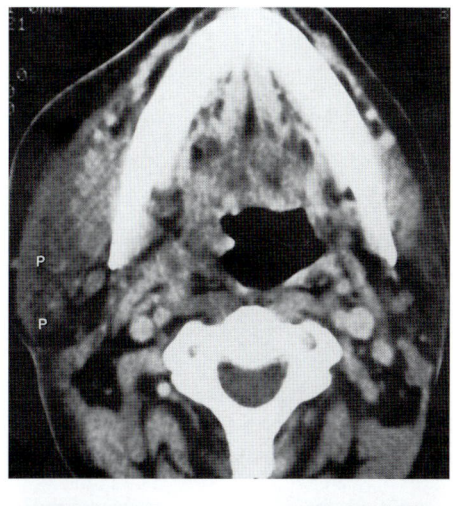

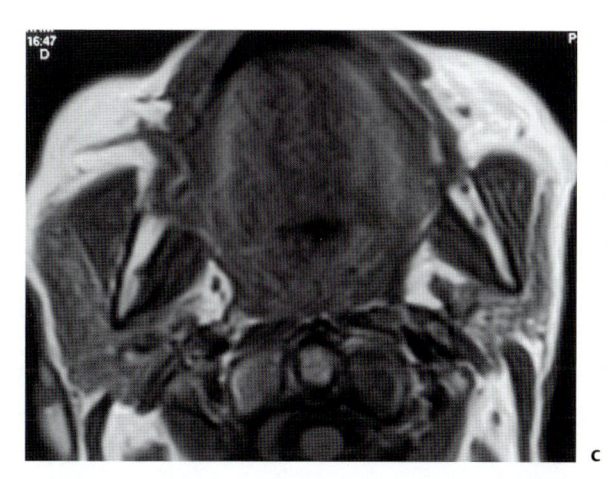

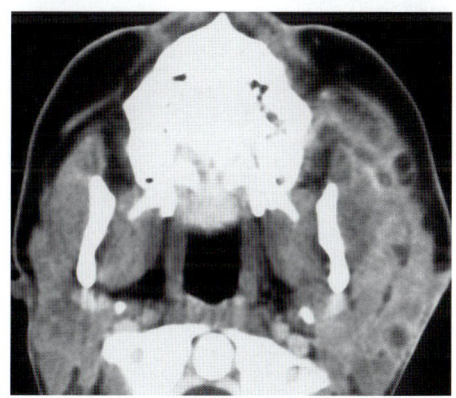

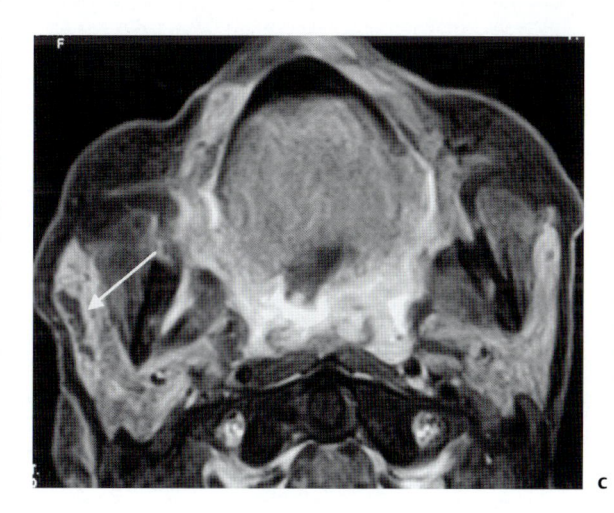

Fig. 9.**27 a** Acute parotitis. Contrast-enhanced axial CT scan shows diffuse swelling of the right parotid gland (P). There is associated subcutaneous edema.
b Acute parotitis. Enhanced axial CT scan in another patient shows diffuse enlargement of the left parotid gland. Note small abscesses within the paroid gland and along the course of the dilated Stensen's duct. There is also swelling of the left masseter muscle.
c Marantic (wasting) parotitis with abscess formation. MRI findings. This 70-year-old diabetic patient presented with acute right parotid swelling, renal failure, and laboratory findings consistent with bacterial infection. *Top:* Unenhanced T1W MR image shows low signal intensity of the superficial lobe of the right parotid gland and rather atrophic left parotid gland. *Bottom:* On the fat-suppressed T1W MR image, after IV injection of contrast material, an abscess within the superficial lobe of the parotid gland is seen (arrow). The abscess was drained surgically and the patient recovered uneventfully. Case provided by M. Becker, MD.

the duct. CT is preferable to MRI for evaluation of patients with inflammatory diseases of the salivary glands. Diffuse enlargement of a swollen gland, with or without dystrophic calcifications (Fig. 9.**30**), associated with low-density areas representing pus or dilated intraglandular ducts are characteristic of chronic sialadenitis. Chronic sialectasis is usually the end stage of chronic recurrent sialadenitis (Fig. 9.**30**). Sialography in early stages may reveal a near-normal ductal system with normal emptying time. In more advanced cases, sialography shows dilatation and sacculation of the intraglandular ductal system (Fig. 9.**30c**) with marked delay in emptying time (see Fig. 9.**45b**). Congenital sialectasis is found in young children. Chronic inflammatory disease of the salivary glands can result in loss of parenchymal as well as fatty matrix and subsequent shrinkage of the gland. Hypointensity (relative) on T1-weighted and T2-weighted images related to chronic inflammatory changes has been observed (Fig. 9.**29c**).[1,3]

Chronic Progressive Disorders of the Salivary Glands (Granulomatous Lesions)

Granulomatous lesions of the salivary glands usually present as chronic progressive, localized or diffuse painless enlargement of the gland. Granulomas that affect the salivary glands include sarcoidosis, tuberculosis, atypical mycobacterial infections, cat scratch disease, lymphogranuloma venereum, leprosy, tularemia, brucellosis, fungal infection, actinomycosis, syphilis,[31–33] and toxoplasmosis. Associated cervical lymphadenopathy is a common finding.[1] Tuberculosis might be secondary to primary infection of the palatine tonsil or a break in the buccal mucosa. This may represent a cystic or solid mass in the salivary gland. There may be multiple masses in the parotid gland (enlarged nodes). Three-quarters of tuberculous infections of the salivary glands affect the parotid gland.[1] Cat scratch disease is due to pleomorphic Gram-negative non-acid-fast bacilli *(Bartonella henselae)*, which are transmitted from healthy cats or kittens.[1] Symptoms include enlarged and often tender lymph nodes with potential involvement of the submental, submandibular, cervical, occipital, and supraclavicular lymph nodes.[8] It resolves spontaneously in 2–3 months. Salivary glands are involved in about

Table 9.**1** Differential diagnosis of salivary gland calcification

- Sialolithiasis
- Chronic sialadenitis (dystropic calcification)
- Chronic granulomatous sialadenitis (sarcoidosis, tuberculosis)
- Chronic stage of autoimmune sialosis (punctate calcifications)
- Postradiation chronic sialadenitis
- Pleomorphic adenoma
- Warthin tumor
- Acinic cell carcinoma
- Adenoid cystic carcinoma
- Malignant degeneration (osteochondrosarcoma) in an ex-pleomorphic adenoma
- Extension of synovial chondromatosis of TMJ into parotid space
- Extension of chondrosarcoma of TMJ into the parotid space

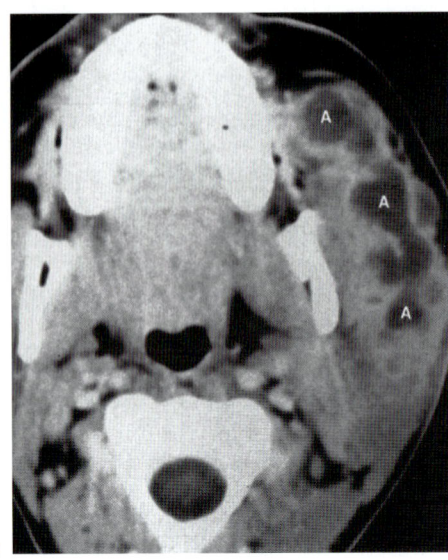

Fig. 9.28 a Parotid and masseter abscesses. Contrast enhanced axial CT scan reveals a large inflammatory mass occupying the left side of the face. The infected masseter muscle merges with the adjacent parotid gland. Multiple low-density areas with ring enhancement are produced by loculated abcesses (A).

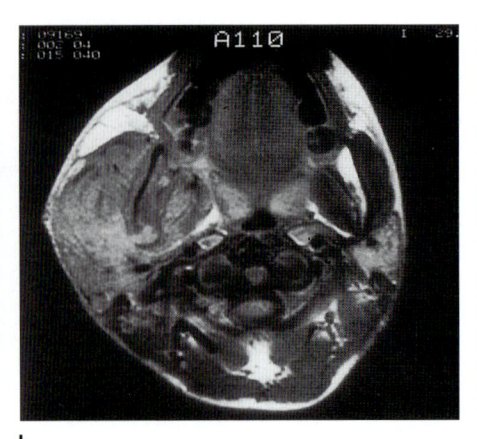

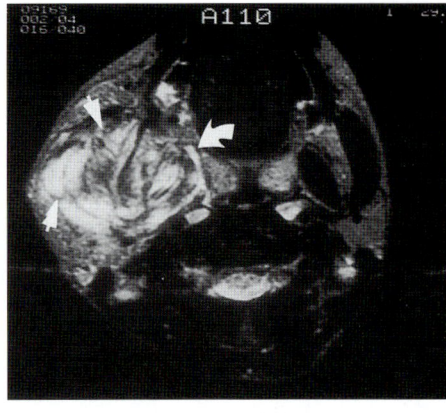

b, c Osteomyelitis of the mandible associated with infection of the masticator and parotid spaces.
b Axial PW MR scan shows marked swelling of the right masseter and right medial pterygoid muscles, and involvement of the adjacent parotid space. Note the edema of the marrow of the ipsilateral mandible, along with the periosteal reaction.
c Axial T2W MR scan shows the extent of soft-tissue edema including parotid gland better than the PW MR scan (**b**); swollen masseter muscle (arrows), swollen medial pterygoid muscle (curved arrow). Note marked edema of the marrow of the right mandible and subperiosteal fluid collection over the outer cortex of the right mandible.

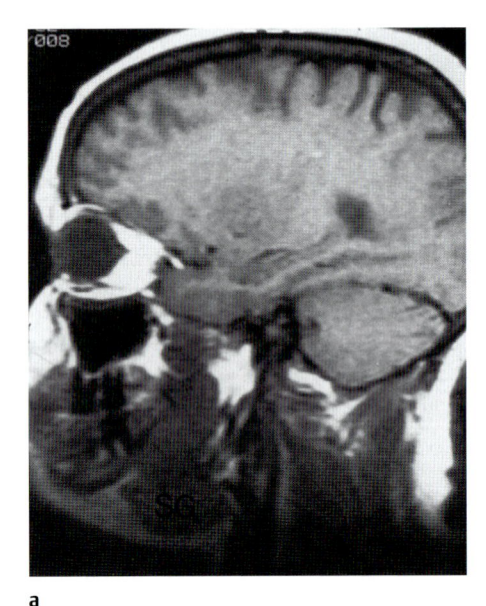

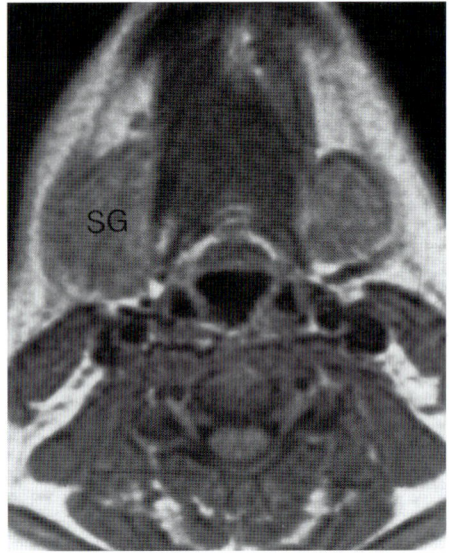

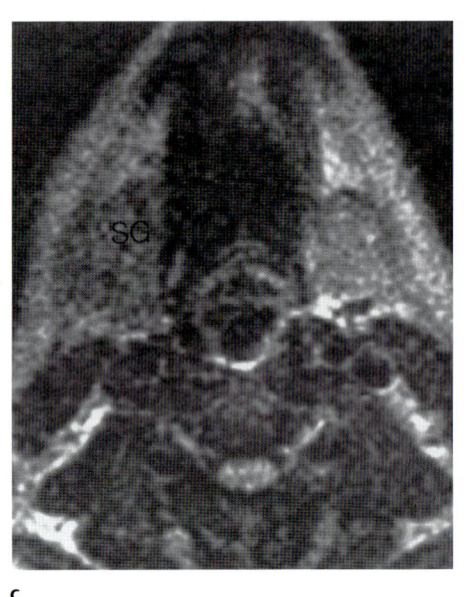

Fig. 9.29 Chronic sialadenitis of the right submandibular gland and associated carcinoma. **a** Sagittal T1W, **b** axial spin-density-weighted, and **c** axial T2W MR scans. There is enlargement of the right submaxillary (submandibular) gland. The lesion is hypointense in T1W (**a**) and isointense in spin density (**b**) images. In T2W image (**c**), the lesion is hypointense to normal gland, indicating a chronic inflammation. At surgery, chronic inflammation was confirmed. In addition a mass was found in the superior portion of the gland. The mass was isointense to the remainder of the gland in all pulse sequences and therefore could not be differentiated from the inflamed portion of the gland.

Table 9.2 Differential diagnosis of parotid gland enlargement

- Infectious diseases (mumps, cat-scratch disease, suppurative parotitis, actinomycosis)
- Granulomas (sarcoidosis, tuberculosis, etc.)
- Kimura disease
- Immunological diseases
- Collagen vascular autoimmune diseases (e.g., Sjögren syndrome)
- Metabolic and endocrine-related sialopathy
- Vasculogenic (hemangioma, vascular malformation)
- Lymphangioma (cystic hygroma)
- Lymphoepithelial disorder (AIDS sialopathy)
- Lymphoma
- Parotid neoplasms (epithelial, mesenchymal)
- Metastasis (kidney, lung, breast, thyroid, malignant melanoma)

4–6% of patients with sarcoidosis[31] (Fig. 9.32). Sarcoidosis is a systemic granulomatous disease of unknown etiology.[31–33] It is confined to the parotid glands in approximately 6% of patients; however, 10–30% of patients with systemic disease have parotid involvement.[31] Unilateral parotid gland involvement may also occur. Concomitant parotid gland, lacrimal gland, eye (chorioretinitis), and cranial nerve (facial) involvement may occur, known as uveoparotid fever or Heerfordt syndrome.[31] Patients with disease limited to the parotid glands usually present with bilateral, nontender, diffusely enlarged parotid glands and/or dryness of the mouth.[3,31–33] Table 9.2 outlines the differential diagnosis of parotid gland enlargement. Serum angiotensin con-

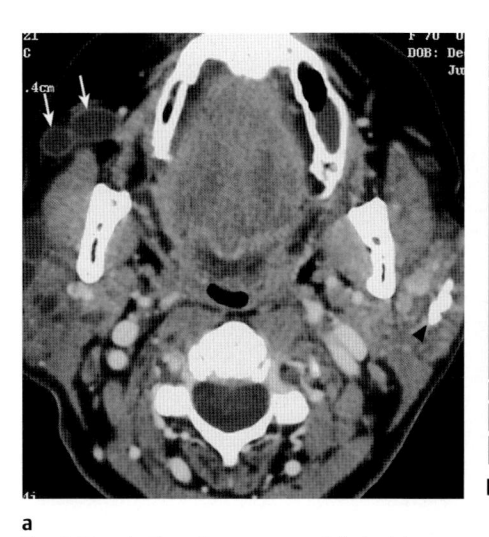

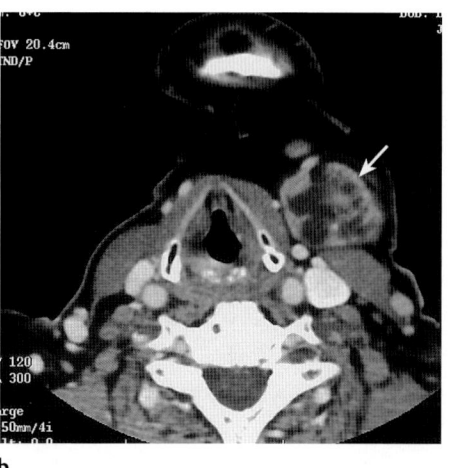

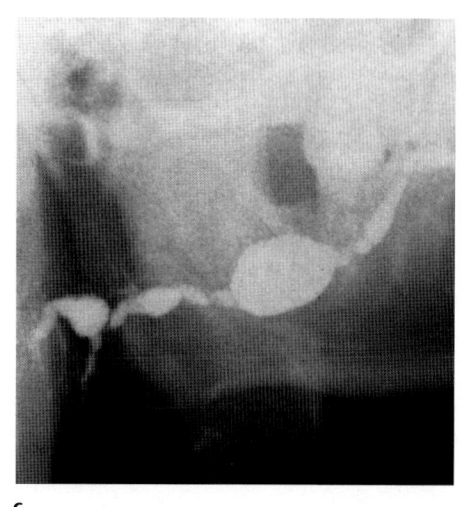

Fig. 9.**30a, b** Chronic recurrent sialadenitis.
a Enhanced CT scan shows cystic changes in the right parotid, sialectasis of the right Stensen's duct (arrows) and dystrophic calcification (arrowhead) in the left parotid gland.
b Enhanced CT scan, same patient as in **a**, shows enlarged left submandibular gland (arrow) with multiple cysts. The right submandibular gland is missing. This 70-year-old woman had a long-standing history of sialadenitis with a history of removed calculi.
c Chronic sialadenitis with sialectasis. A lateral sialogram of the left parotid gland in another patient shows dilatation of the main duct and some of the branches. There are segments of narrowing between the dilated segments.

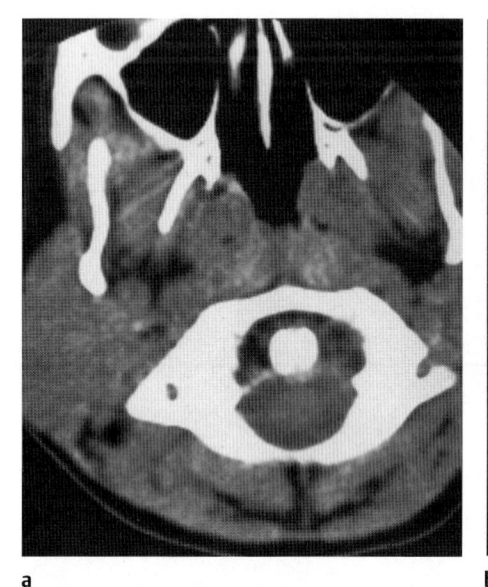

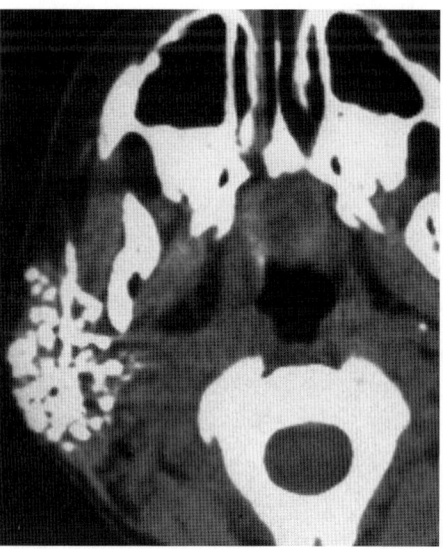

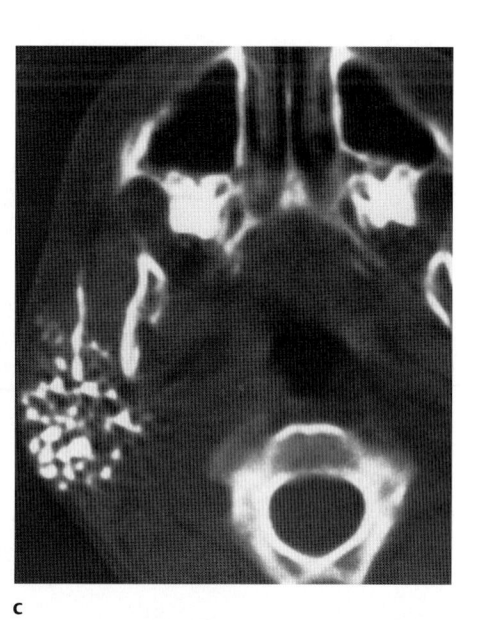

Fig. 9.**31** Recurrent sialadenitis in a 7-year-old boy with intermittent swelling of the right parotid gland.
a Plain axial CT scan shows marked enlargement of the right parotid gland.
b, c CT sialograms show saccular dilatation of the acini and ducts. There are several filling defects, which are better appreciated in the wide window setting of **c**. These are produced by inflammatory changes and probably fibrosis in the stroma.

verting enzyme (ACE) levels are elevated in 50–80% of patients with sarcoidosis.[31] The ACE levels may be increased in other disorders, including diabetes, cirrhosis, silicosis, and hypersensitivity pneumonitis.[31] Sialography, CT, and MRI are diagnostic adjuncts that can be very helpful in patients who may have sarcoidosis of the parotid glands (Figs. 9.**32–35**).[33] Sialographic and CT findings include diffuse enlargement of the salivary gland, multiple small nodular densities distributed throughout the gland, or a solitary mass. In patients with parotid gland sarcoidosis, the intraparotid segment of the facial nerve may be thickened and irregular. This can be best demonstrated on MR images of the gland (Fig. 9.**35**).

Kimura Disease

Kimura disease is an idiopathic inflammatory disease, affecting the parotid and submandibular glands, with regional lymphadenopathy. The disease is more common in orientals and is to be differentiated from tumor and inflammatory conditions of the salivary glands. The pathological characteristics include abnormal proliferation of lymphoid follicles as well as vascular endothelium. There will be scattered infiltrates of eosinophils and histiocytoid cells. The patient may have peripheral eosinophilia.[1,34] The CT and MRI findings are nonspecific (Fig. 9.**36**). Angiolymphoid hyperplasia with eosinophilia (histocytoid hemangioma) may be as-

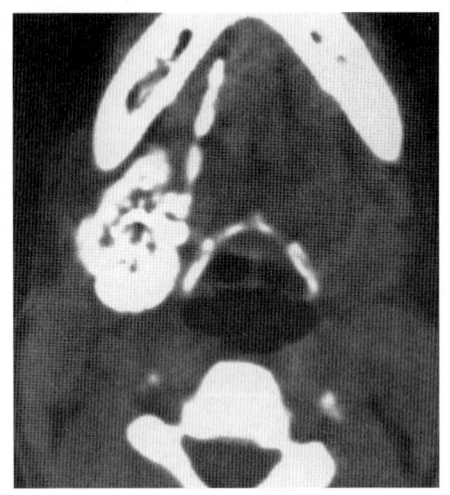

Fig. 9.**32** Sarcoidosis of the right submandibular gland. Axial CT sialogram shows enlargement of the right submandibular gland. Several filling defects are seen due to sarcoid granulomas.

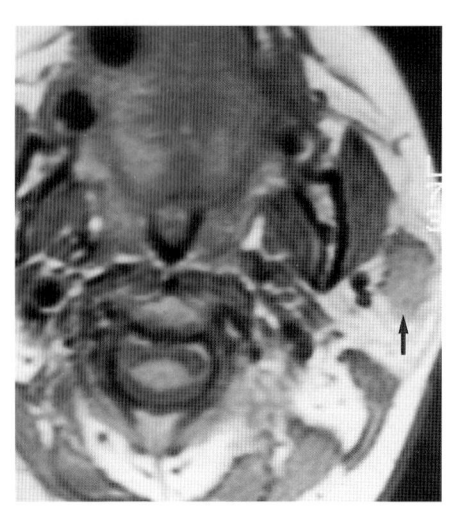

Fig. 9.**33** Sarcoidosis. Axial PW MR scan shows an intraparotid mass (arrow), compatible with sarcoid granuloma.

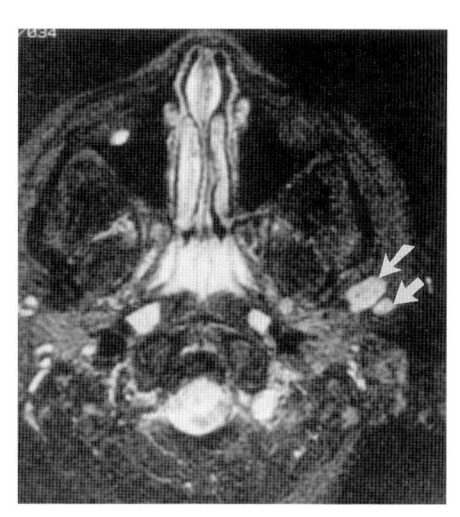

Fig. 9.**34** Axial T2W MR scan shows presumed parotid sarcoid granulomas (arrows).

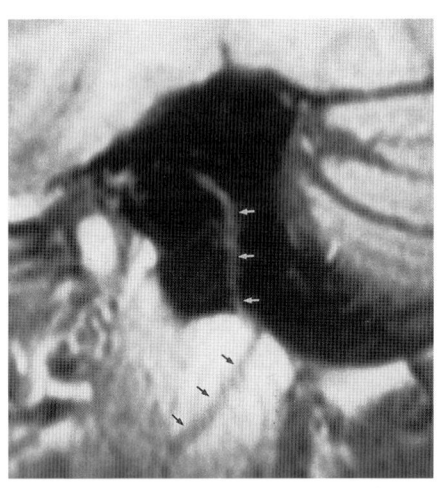

Fig. 9.**35** Sarcoidosis with facial paralysis. Sagittal T1W MR scan shows enlarged parotid gland as well as irregular thickening of the parotid segment of the facial nerve (arrows) in a patient with presumed sarcoidosis.

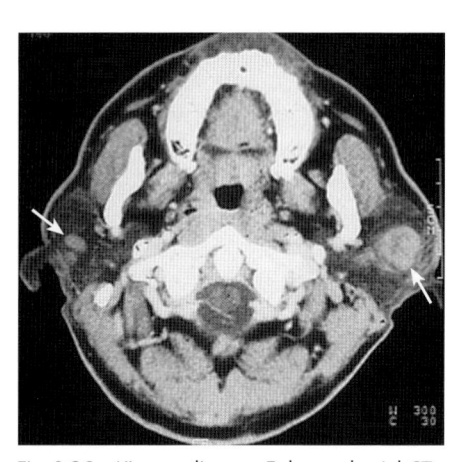

Fig. 9.**36** Kimura disease. Enhanced axial CT scan shows bilateral parotid masses (arrows). There is slight thickening of the capsule of the left parotid gland and overlying skin.

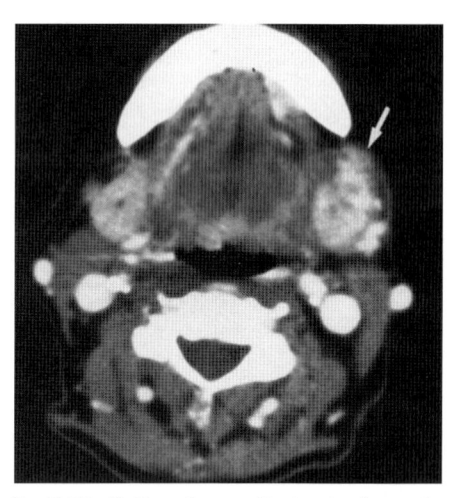

Fig. 9.**37** Kuttner tumor. Contrast-enhanced CT scan. A slightly enlarged left submandibular gland (arrow) related to chronic inflammation simulates a tumor. From Reference 1.

sociated with regional lymphadenopathy and peripheral eosinophilia. The etiology of the disease is unknown. Many authors believe that Kimura disease and angiolymphoid hyperplasia with eosinophilia represent two different disease processes.[8]

Kuttner Tumor

The name Kuttner tumor has been used to refer to a chronic sclerosing sialadenitis with fibrous encasement of the gland and ductal system.[1] The gland appears clinically firm and somewhat enlarged (Fig. 9.**37**).[1]

Recurrent Sialadenitis of Childhood

The exact etiology of recurrent sialadenitis of childhood is not well understood. In this condition, intermittent swelling of the parotid glands may be unilateral or bilateral, and each episode lasts several days to several weeks.[1] Sialography shows punctate or globular collections of contrast material throughout the swollen gland (Figs. 9.**31**, 9.**38**). Some of the cases resolve spontaneously, whereas some may require antibiotics.[1] Most cases subside at puberty,[1] but a few patients develop secondary infections progressing throughout adulthood.

Postirradiation Sialadenitis

This condition is characterized by acute swelling, tenderness, and pain, which subside within a few days. The irradiated gland usually remains more dense on plain CT and will show increased enhancement following contrast infusion (Fig. 9.**39**). The increased enhancement will remain for a long period following irradiation and may be related to radiation-induced vasculitis and mucositis.

Iodide Mumps

Intravenous contrast material (iodinated) has rarely been reported to cause salivary gland enlargement, called iodide mumps, which is an inflammatory reaction due to the high concentration of iodide in the saliva.[15]

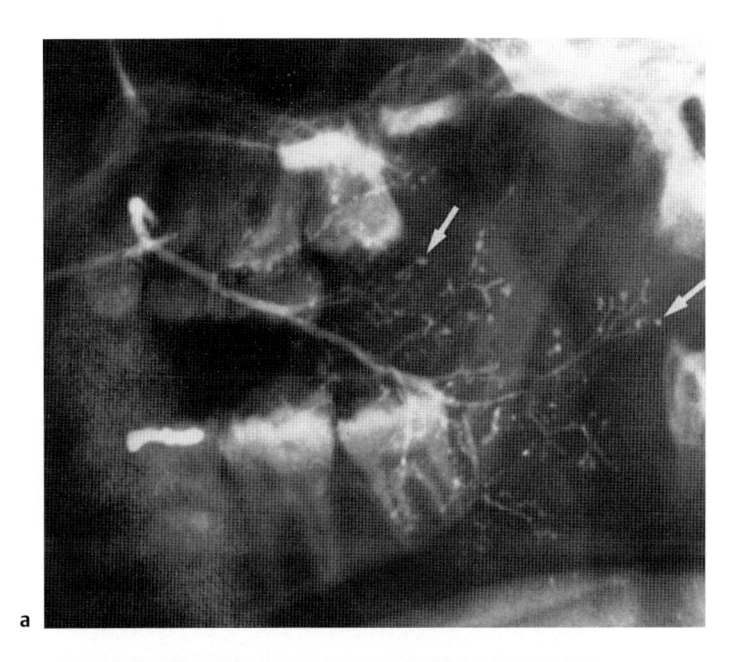

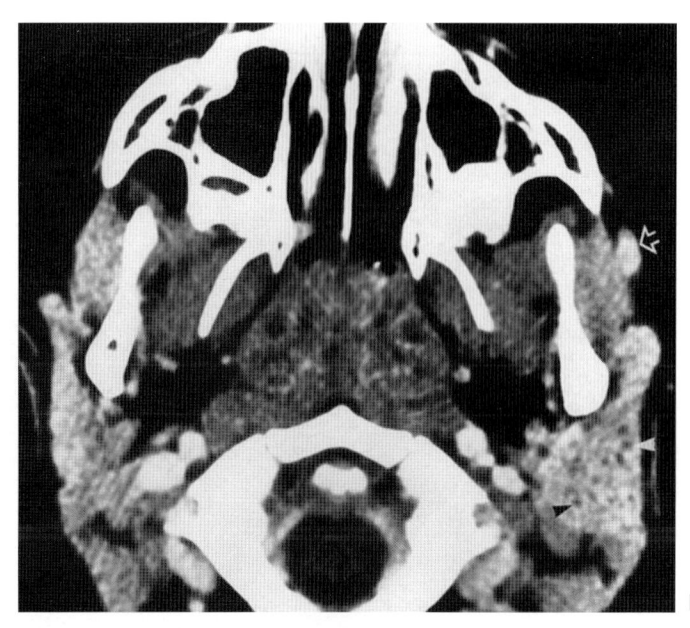

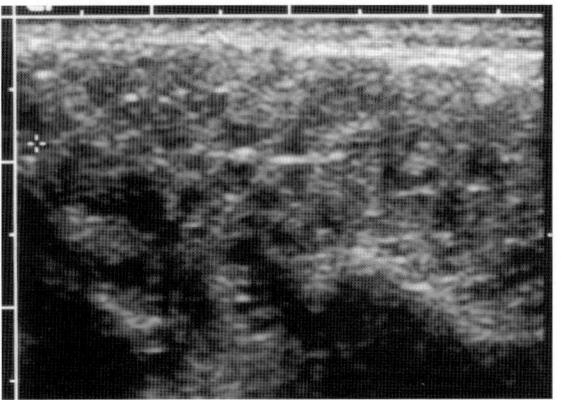

Fig. 9.**38 a**, **b** Recurrent sialadenitis of childhood.
a Sialogram. Punctate collections of contrast material (arrows) are typical for this manifestation of sialadenitis by sialography.
b Contrast enhanced CT scan. Note multiple pockets of low attenuation (arrowheads) representing small collections of fluid in the left enlarged parotid gland, which is enhanced. Also note the enhancement of the accessory lobe of the parotid (open arrow). From Reference 1.

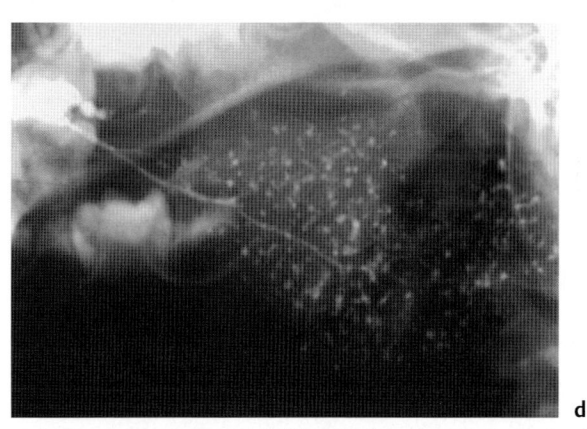

c, d Recurrent parotitis in childhood. Characteristic US and sialographic appearances. **c** US of the parotid gland shows characteristic hypoechoic small lesions measuring a few millimeters in size and scattered homogeneously throughout the gland. The finding was bilateral.
d Conventional sialography (lateral view) shows the same imaging findings as in Sjögren syndrome seen in adults. The central ductal system is normal and multiple punctate collections of contrast material are evenly distributed throughout the gland. Case (**c** and **d**) provided by M. Becker, MD.

Necrotizing Sialometaplasia

This is a rare benign, self-healing (reactive) inflammatory process of salivary gland tissue that clinically and histologically mimics a malignant neoplasm.[8] The disease most commonly involves the minor salivary glands of the palate. It presents as ulceration of the palate, attributed to ischemic necrosis of the minor salivary glands of the palate.[1]

Sialolithiasis and Chronic Sialadenitis

Sialolithiasis is a relatively frequent occurrence, affecting up to 1% of salivary glands according to autopsy studies.[35] It leads to recurrent painful swelling of the involved gland. Swelling and pain usually occur during meals, when salivary secretion is stimulated.[18, 35] Sialolithiasis is sometimes associated with frank infectious sialadenitis.[35] The thicker and more alkaline nature of the submandibular secretions predisposes to precipitation of salts.[3] Mucous plugs and debris in the lumen of the duct due to exfoliated ductal epithelium are associated with dehydration and may serve as a nidus for the calculus.[1] About 85–90% of salivary gland calculi occur in the submandibular gland, while 10% occur in the parotid. Sublingual and minor salivary glands are rarely affected.[8] Sialoliths are composed of organic and inorganic substances, in varying ratios.[35] The organic substances are glycoproteins, mucopolysaccharides, and cellular debris.[36] The inorganic substances are mainly calcium carbonates and calcium phosphates.[35] Calcium, magnesium, and phosphate ions each make up between 20% and 25% of the mass, with other minerals (manganese, iron, and copper) comprising the rest.[35] The chemical composition consists mainly of microcrystalline apatite ($Ca_5[PO_4]_3OH$) or whitlockite, tribasic calcium phosphate ($Ca_3[PO_4]_2$).[35, 36]

The exact pathogenesis of sialolithiasis is unknown, and various hypotheses have been proposed.[36] One theory is based on the existence of intracellular microcalculi that, when excreted in the canal, become a nidus for stone formation. A second theory is based on formation of a "mucous plug" in the ductal system, which becomes a nidus. Another hypothesis is that substances or bacteria within the oral cavity might migrate in the salivary ducts

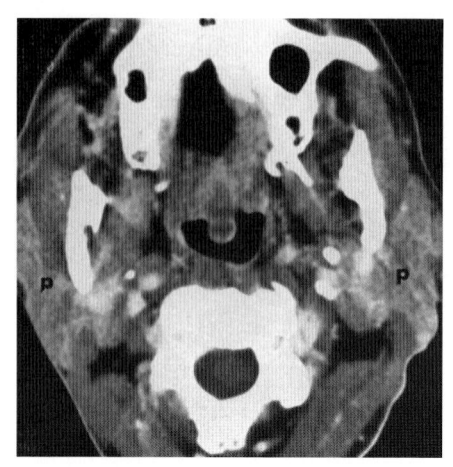

Fig. 9.39 Postradiation sialadenitis. Contrast-enhanced axial CT scan shows diffuse increased enhancement of the parotid glands (p) enhanced owing to mucositis and vasculitis.

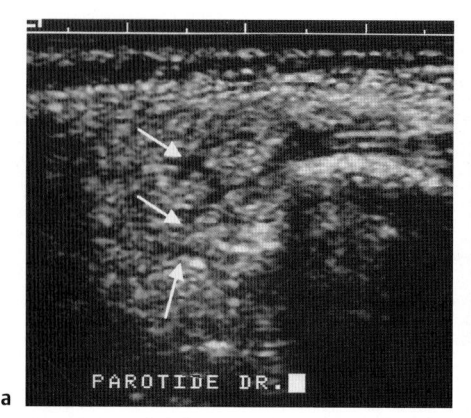

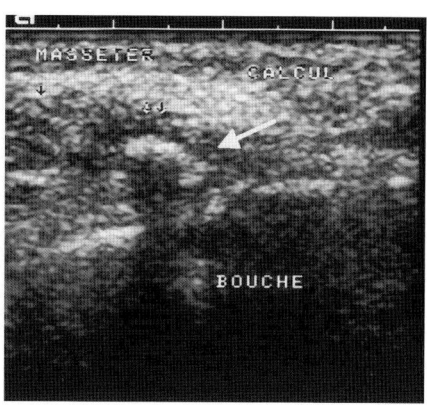

Fig. 9.40 Sialolithiasis and acute sialadenitis as seen on US. **a** Transverse US scan through the parotid gland shows swelling of the gland and dilatation of the intraglandular ductal system (arrows). **b** A 4 mm calculus with an acoustic shadow is seen in Stensen's duct (arrow). Case provided by M. Becker, MD.

and become the nidus for stone formation.[35] Stones in the sublingual glands are rare. In the submandibular gland, the calculi usually form at the hilum of the gland or are found in the ductal system.

The traditional treatment for salivary stones has been surgical intraoral extraction, usually associated with meatotomy, whereas recurrent postobstructive sialadenitis was usually treated with sialadenectomy. Several new minimally invasive, organ-preserving techniques have recently been developed to treat sialolithiasis, such as extracorporeal sialolithotripsy and percutaneous and endoscopic stone removal.[12] Current treatment strategies stress the need to diagnose salivary gland calculi in early stages of the disease process, when they have not caused significant parenchymal damage and fibrosis, and when endoscopic or percutaneous retrieval is easier.[21]

Imaging techniques for the detection of salivary gland calculi include plain films, US, CT, conventional sialography, digital sialography, and, more recently, MR sialography.[1, 2, 12, 15–21] Digital sialography is currently considered the modality of choice for assessing the presence or absence of ductal abnormalities, including calculi, although its role is increasingly being challenged by MR sialography.[20, 21] Advantages of digital sialography include assessment of ductal function as a response to sialogogue and occasional therapeutic success of stone release after a retrograde injection of contrast material. Disadvantages include irradiation, dependence on the operator's technical skills for successful cannulation, and the need for retrograde injection of contrast material. Injection of contrast material may also result in displacement of an anterior ductal stone into a posterior position where it can no longer be reached by an intraoral surgical approach or where endoscopic removal is more difficult (Fig. 9.**41 b**).[20, 21]

High-resolution US is widely used as a first-line examination to assess the presence or absence of salivary gland calculi, because it is noninvasive, easily available, and of lower cost. The diagnosis of calculi by US is made in the presence of hyperechoic oval or round images casting an acoustic shadow below them (Fig. 9.**40 a**, **b**). The sensitivity of US for the detection of sialolithiasis depends mainly on the size of the calculi. While all calculi larger than 3 mm may be diagnosed by US, half of the calculi less than 3 mm may be missed by US.[20, 21] Calcified nodes, vascular calcifications, and stenoses may mimic salivary gland calculi on US. Another problem with US is the difficulty of correctly assessing the total number of calculi. A precise pretherapeutic assessment of the number and location of calculi is, however, very important when planning endoscopic procedures (duration of the procedure; local versus general anesthesia).

On MR sialography, calculi are diagnosed when round, ovoid, or irregularly shaped signal void images are identified within or immediately next to a dilated or nondilated salivary duct (Fig. 9.**41**). The sensitivity of MR sialography for the detection of calculi is excellent, provided that a 3D acquisition technique with very thin slices (0.6 mm) is used. Although most small calculi may be reliably diagnosed using MR sialography, false-negative readings may occur in patients with 2–3 mm stones causing no ductal dilatation[20, 21] (Fig. 9.**41 c**, **d**). MR sialography does not enable one to distinguish solid calculi from inspissated mucus and/or debris, since the latter may also cause signal void intraductal images. From a practical point of view, however, this distinction has probably no significant impact on the clinical management, since in a symptomatic patient endoscopic removal would usually be indicated in both situations. Small calculi are best displayed on axial MR source images (Fig. 9.**43 g**). On MIP reconstructed images, small calculi may be obscured because of volume averaging with surrounding hyperintense saliva.[21] It is important to realize that normal MR sialography and US examination do not exclude 2–3 mm calculi causing no ductal dilatation. Therefore, in such patients with persistent symptoms, conventional sialography should be performed.[21]

Symptoms of a salivary gland stone may include intermittent swelling and colicky pain on eating. The symptoms of sialolithiasis and salivary stricture are similar. Infection and sialadenitis are common complications. The diagnosis is made by manual palpation, probing of the duct, and imaging studies. Most (80–90%) submandibular gland duct calculi are radiopaque owing to the higher calcium salt content and are visible on plain films and CT scans. CT is more sensitive than plain film and permits identification of tiny calculi: 25% of patients may have multiple calculi. If no calculus is demonstrated on plain film or CT, conventional sialography will reveal radiolucent stones. There is dilatation of the duct proximal to the obstruction and delayed emptying of contrast material. If there is complete obstruction, the ductal system beyond the calculus will of course not fill. In patients with history of chronic and recurrent sialadenitis, standard sialography or MR sialography is imperative, especially to diagnose the presence of several calculi or to detect one or several strictures (Figs. 9.**42**, 9.**43**).[18]

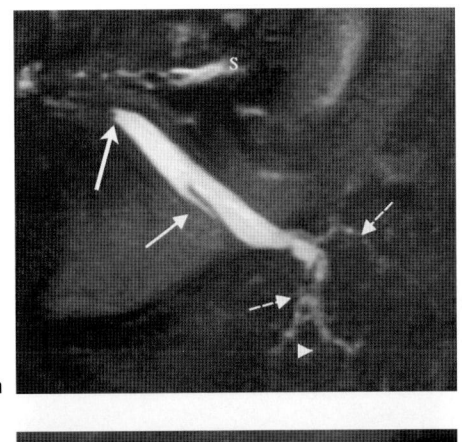

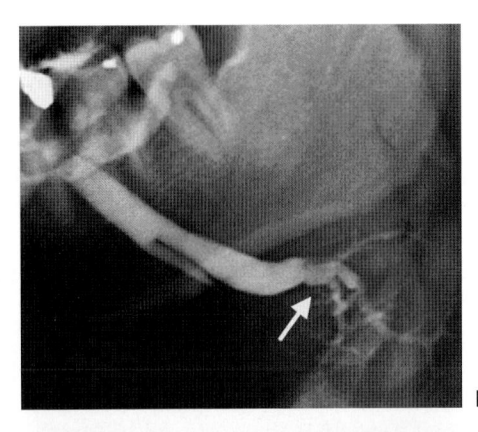

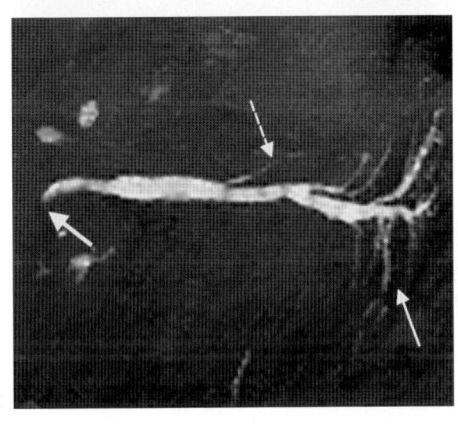

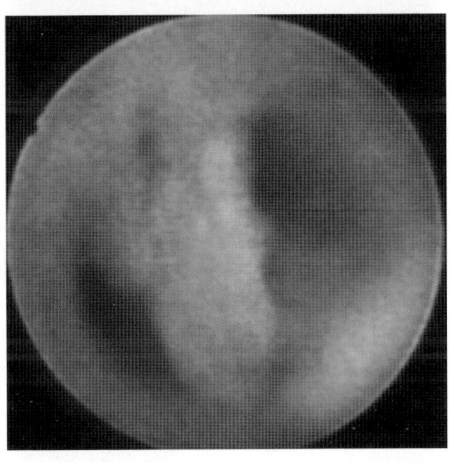

Fig. 9.**41a, b** True-positive MR sialography for lithiasis. **a** MIP reconstruction of a sagittal oblique MR sialography sequence shows a suspected 4 mm stone situated near the orifice of Wharton's duct (thick arrow). Note slight dilatation of Bartholin's duct (thin arrow), primary branches (dashed arrows), and secondary intraglandular branches (small arrowhead) Hyperintense saliva within the oral cavity (s). **b** Conventional sialography performed after MR sialography confirms the diagnosis of sialolithiasis. Note, however, distal displacement of the calculus (arrow) caused by active filling of the ductal system. The calculus was removed endoscopically. From Reference 21.

c, d False-negative MR sialography for lithiasis. **c** MIP reconstruction of a sagittal oblique MR sialography sequence shows dilatation of Stensen's duct in its entire course from the orifice (thick arrow) to its intraglandular branches (thin arrow). A short stenosis at the orifice was suspected. Dashed arrow points to an accessory duct. **d** Sialendoscopy performed after MR sialography shows a 3×1 mm calculus located near the orifice of Stensen's duct and causing ductal dilatation. No stenosis was seen. The calculus was removed endoscopically. From Reference 21.

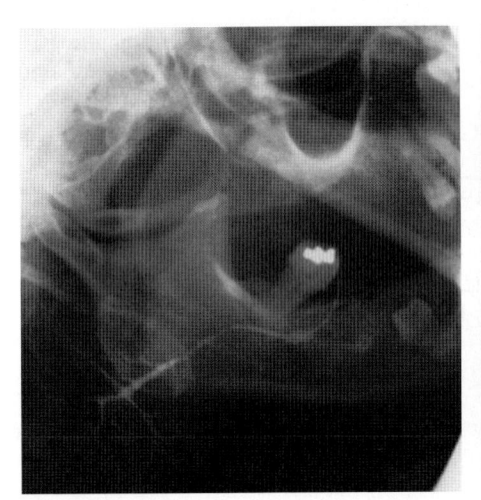

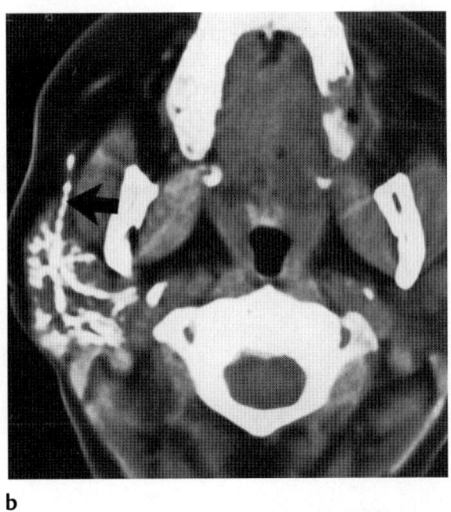

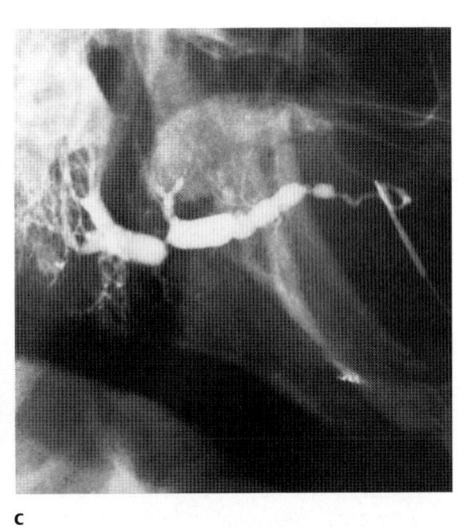

Fig. 9.**42a, b** Chronic sialadenitis.
a Sialogram shows irregularity of the Stensen's duct and intraglandular ductal system. The intraparenchymal ducts appear narrowed and stretched.
b CT sialogram shows irregularity and beading of the Stensen's duct (arrow) and intraglandular ductal system. The filling defects are due to obstruction of some of the intraglandular ducts and parenchymal inflammatory reaction.
c Sialodochitis with multiple strictures of the parotid duct as shown by sialography. Fig. 9.**42c** from Reference 1.

Stones of the parotid duct are much less common. Calcifications may be seen within the duct or the parotid gland itself secondary to chronic disease (autoimmune disease, Sjögren syndrome, chronic granuloma) or to tumor. Sialodochitis, a chronically infected, dilated duct, may be associated with multiple strictures (Fig. 9.**30c**). Dilated ducts may be visible on MR or CT scans (Fig. 9.**43**). The surgical approach to intraglandular parotid calculi would involve parotidectomy.[18] For submandibular calculi, the surgical approach is influenced by the location of the stone. Palpable stones anterior to the posterior border of the mylohyoid muscle are usually extracted using a transoral incision. When the stone is posterior to the mylohyoid muscle, removal of the entire gland is recommended.[18] Extracorporeal sialolithotripsy, endoscopic stone removal, and mechanical removal of calculi and sialodochoplasty by balloon catheter are alternatives to surgery for the treatment of patients with sialoliths as well as salivary duct strictures.[18, 21]

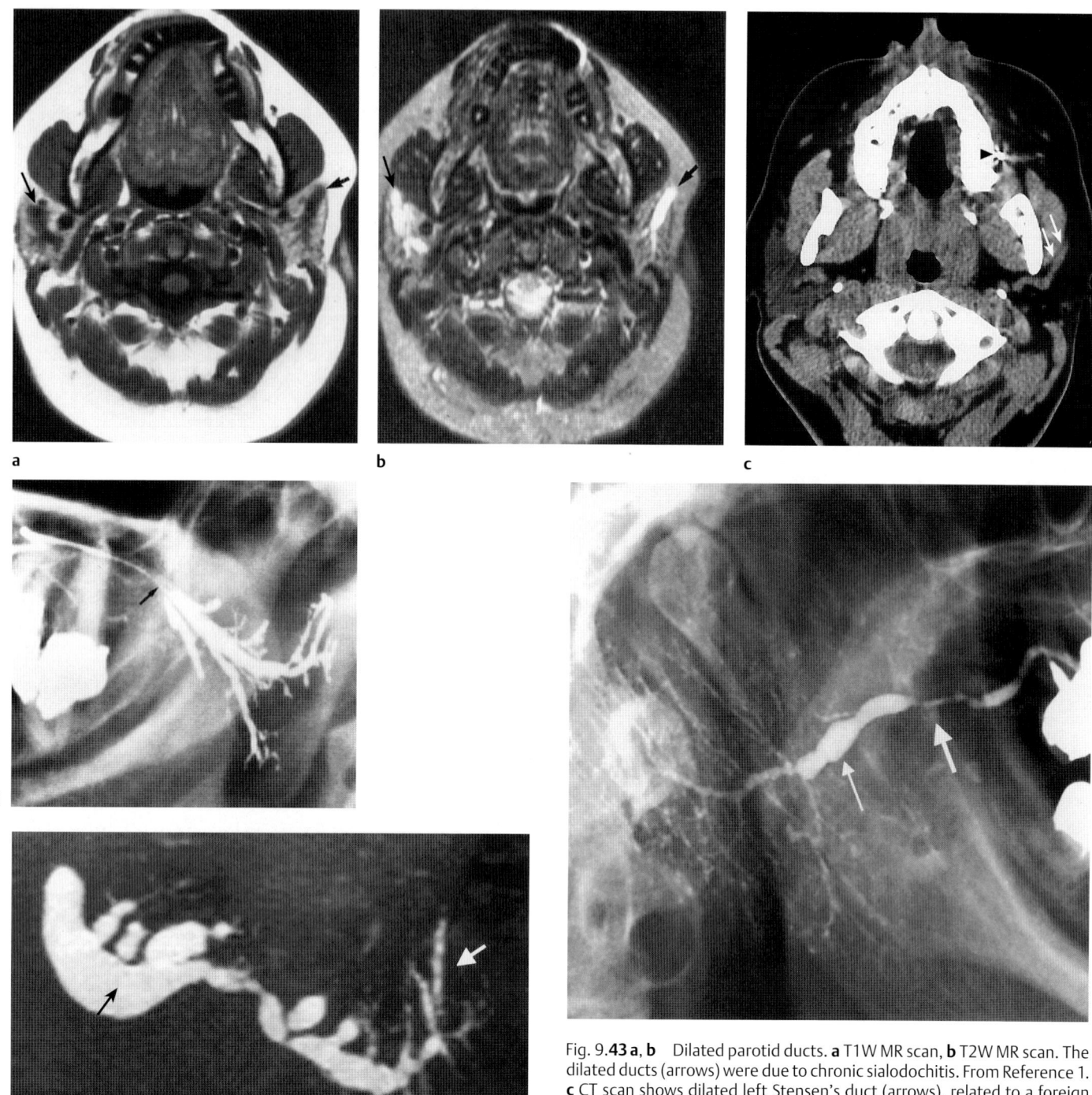

Fig. 9.**43 a, b** Dilated parotid ducts. **a** T1W MR scan, **b** T2W MR scan. The dilated ducts (arrows) were due to chronic sialodochitis. From Reference 1.
c CT scan shows dilated left Stensen's duct (arrows), related to a foreign body (arrowhead) at its orifice. Note fatty replacement of the left parotid gland.
d Sialodochitis with elongated stricture (arrow) of the parotid duct. From Reference 1.
e Chronic sialodochitis and sialadenitis as seen on MR sialography and conventional x-ray sialography. **1** MIP reconstruction of a sagittal oblique 3D-EXPRESS sequence shows a dilated and lobulated main duct with stenotic areas and diverticular outpouchings. Note variation in caliber of primary and secondary intraglandular branches corresponding to dilated areas (black arrow) and stenotic areas (white arrows), respectively. **2** Conventional sialography of the left parotid gland confirms MR sialography findings: marked dilatation of the main duct with stenotic areas and diverticular outpouchings. Variation in caliber of primary and secondary intraglandular branches corresponding to dilated (thick arrow) and stenotic areas (thin arrow), respectively. Note better visualization of secondary and tertiary branches due to active filling with contrast material. From Reference 21.
f Chronic sialadenitis of the parotid gland as seen on conventional sialography. Sialodochitis involving Stensen's duct, which shows areas of stenoses (thick arrow) and dilatation (thin arrow). Note irregular caliber of the intraglandular branches and scattered collections of contrast material, which represent small abscesses and dilated ductal branches.

Fig. 9.**43 g** ▷

Fig. 9.**43 g** Recurrent sialadenitis of the parotid gland caused by multiple calculi. Complementary role of source and MIP images. **1** Axial source image from a 3D-EXPRESS sequence shows multiple hypointense calculi within Stensen's duct (arrows). **2** Sagittal oblique MIP reconstruction better shows stenotic areas of an accessory duct (arrow) as well as strictures of primary and secondary branches (dashed arrows). Note that the calculi are less well visualized on the MIP image as compared to the axial source image.
Cases 43**e–g** provided by M. Becker, MD.

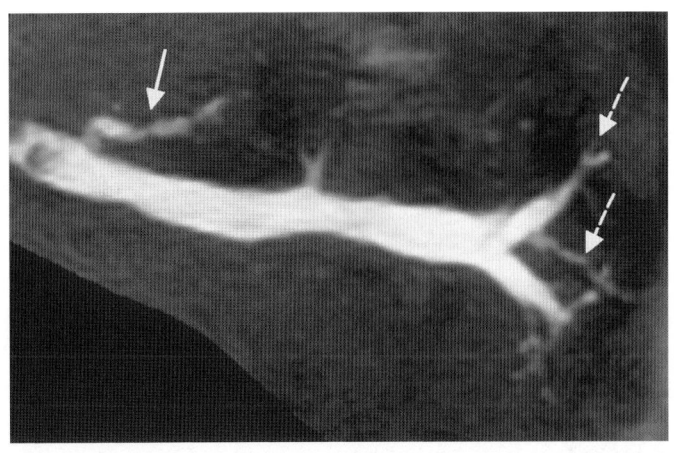

Stricture of the Salivary Gland Ducts

Stricture of the parotid or submandibular gland duct can be congenital or caused by calculus, trauma, infection, or neoplasm (see Fig. 9.**42**). The symptoms are similar to those of salivary gland calculi, with intermittent swelling, pain with eating, and superimposed infection secondary to stasis. Diagnosis is made by conventional or CT/MR sialography. Complete obstruction of the duct by stone, stricture, ligation, or trauma leads to atrophy of the gland. Current trends in the treatment of strictures and stenoses consist of either endoscopic or percutaneous dilation. On MR sialography, stenoses are diagnosed when an abrupt transition from ductal dilatation or a tapered appearance of salivary duct is seen. It is important to realize that nonvisualization of Wharton's duct in its anterior third at the level of the floor of the mouth and of Stenson's duct in its position overlying the masseter muscle on MIP reconstruction MR images is a physiological finding and should not be considered as indicative of stenosis in the absence of ductal dilatation. Although sialolithiasis may be detected by US or CT, 30% of salivary glands with lithiasis have associated single or multiple stenoses. In these cases, the diagnosis of stenoses can be made only with either MR sialography or conventional sialography.[21] Although conventional sialography allows better visualization of peripheral ducts as compared with MR sialography, the sensitivity of MR sialography for detecting stenoses is excellent.[21]

■ Acquired Immunodeficiency Syndrome and Parotid Lymphoepithelial Lesions/ Cysts

Cysts of the salivary glands are of two general types: congenital and acquired. Congenital cysts include those of branchial cleft origin (Fig. 9.**20**), epidermoid, dermoid (Fig. 9.**21 a–d**), and rare dysgenetic polycystic type.[1, 16, 17, 29] The acquired cysts include those of lymphoepithelial origin and those secondary to obstruction (sialocele), to infection, and to tumors. The term "lymphoepithelial" lesion was first introduced by Bernier in 1958,[37] who identified this as a distinct entity separate from the branchial cleft cyst. Benign lymphoepithelial lesion (BLL) encompasses a group of diseases with diverse clinical presentation but overlapping histological features. These clinical and histological features may be found independently of or in association with these diseases. The diseases associated with the term BLL include Sjögren syndrome and Sicca complex, Mikulicz disease/syndrome, and chronic punctate parotitis.[8]

Some of the manifestations of acquired immunodeficiency syndrome (AIDS) include cervical lymphadenopathy, periparotid and intraparotid lymphadenopathy, and parotid enlargement. Bilateral multicentric parotid cysts have been associated with patients infected with the human immunodeficiency virus (HIV) (Fig. 9.**44**).[32, 38–41] There is a high correlation between HIV seropositivity and the presence of multicentric parotid benign lymphoepithelial cysts associated with cervical lymphadenopathy.[11, 38–41] MRI and CT are both sensitive in detecting these changes (Fig. 9.**44**), and the radiologist should alert the referring physician to the possibility of asymptomatic HIV infection when such changes are recognized.[38] Parotid gland enlargement in these patients is predominantly related to intraparotid lymphadenopathy. Histologically, follicular hyperplasia or benign lymphoepithelial infiltrates with cystic areas of degeneration are demonstrated within intraparotid lymph nodes.

Diffuse lymphoid infiltration of the salivary gland with cystic dilatation of the salivary ducts may also be present. Parotid enlargement may also be due to viral or bacterial parotitis or neoplasia.[39] Although comparatively rare, parotid neoplasms have been reported in AIDS patients and include adenoid cystic carcinoma in a patient with HIV-induced persistent generalized lymphadenopathy, Kaposi sarcoma within an intraparotid lymph node, and large cell lymphoma in the submandibular gland.[40] Parotid gland lymphoepithelial cysts are not unique to HIV infection. These cysts may be associated with chronic infection, such as sarcoidosis, or be related to an autoimmune disease such as Sjögren syndrome (Figs. 9.**45–9.47**), or be unrelated to an immune deficiency syndrome, or they may be idiopathic.[41] The primary distinction between AIDS-related lymphoepithelial parotid cysts and other benign lymphoepithelial lesions of the parotid gland is that in the former the cyst(s) occurs within a lymph node, whereas in the latter the cyst(s) occurs within the parotid parenchyma.

Benign lymphoepithelial lesions (BLL) may be unilateral or bilateral. These cysts have smooth walls[1] and may vary in size from a few millimeters to few centimeters (Figs. 9.**44, 9.45**). Cystic Warthin's tumors, unlike BLL, have focal wall nodularity.[41] At times focal wall nodularity may be seen in BLL (Fig. 9.**44b**). The distinguishing feature between AIDS-related lymphoepithelial

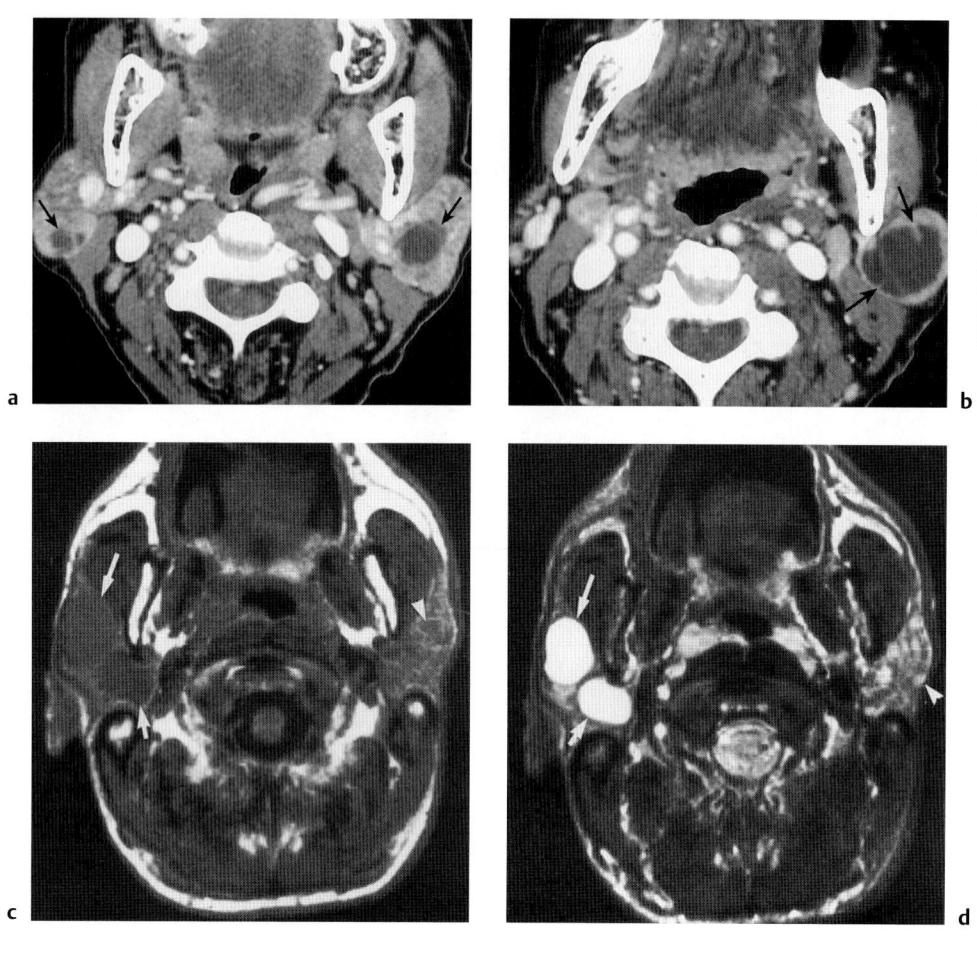

Fig. 9.**44 a–d** AIDS-related lymphoepithelial cysts and lesions. **a** Enhanced CT scan shows bilateral parotid cysts (arrows). **b** Enhanced CT scan shows a large cystic mass (arrows) involving the left parotid gland. Note peripheral nodularity with moderate enhancement. This lesion cannot be differentiated on CT scan from a Warthin's tumor. **c** T1W MR and **d** T2W MR scans, a different patient from the one in **a** and **b**. Multiple cysts (arrows) and lymphoepithelial lesions (arrowheads) are present throughout the parotid glands. Figs. 9.**44 c, d** from Reference 1.

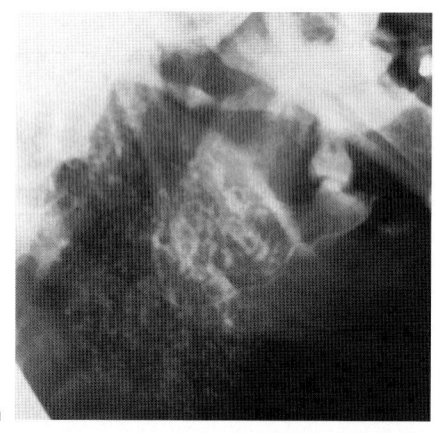

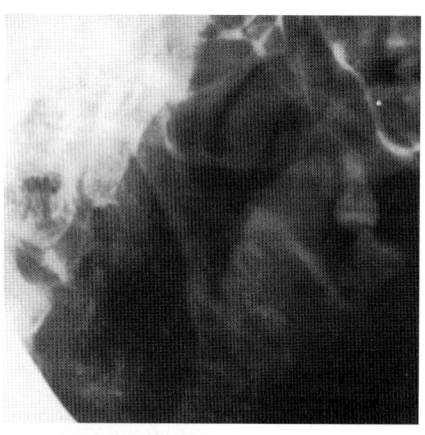

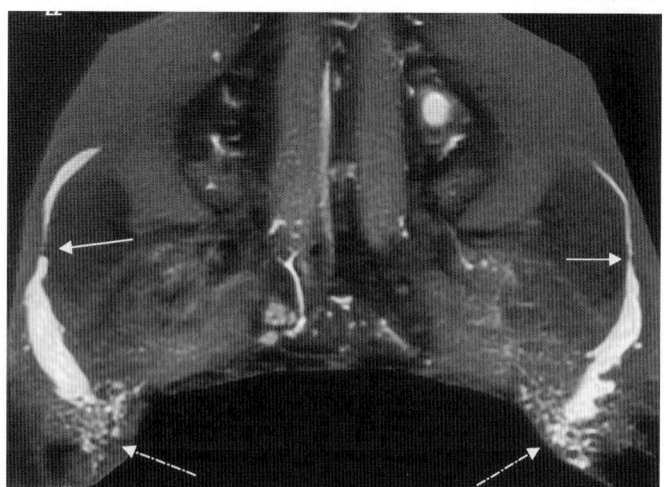

Fig. 9.**45 a, b** Sjögren syndrome. Conventional sialogram.
a Lateral sialogram immediately after injection.
b Delayed sialogram, lateral view. There are multiple, small globular collections of contrast material within the parotid gland in **a**, and delayed emptying of the acini in **b**.
c Sjögren syndrome with superimposed bilateral sialodochitis. Axial MIP reconstruction MR sialogram shows bilateral marked stenoses of Stensen's ducts (arrows), marked dilatation of the ductal system, and punctate collections of saliva scattered homogenously throughout both glands (dashed arrows). Case provided by M. Becker, MD.

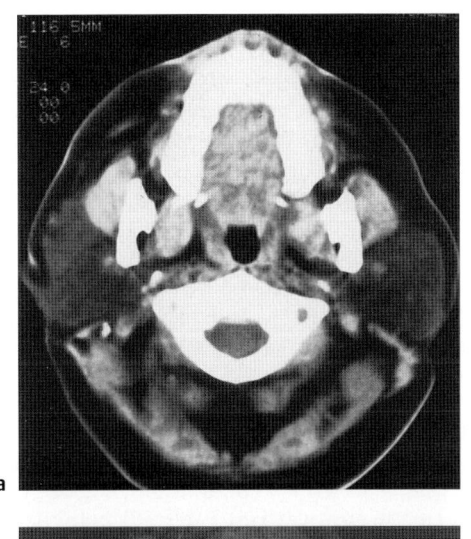

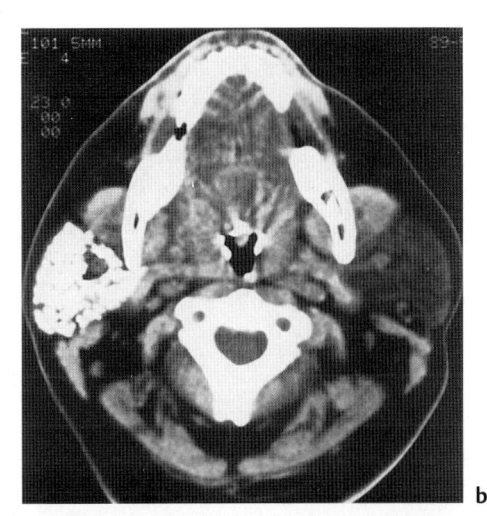

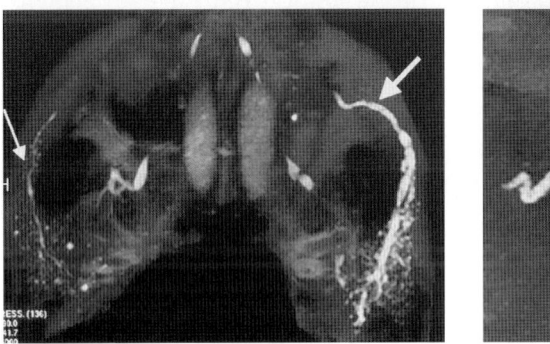

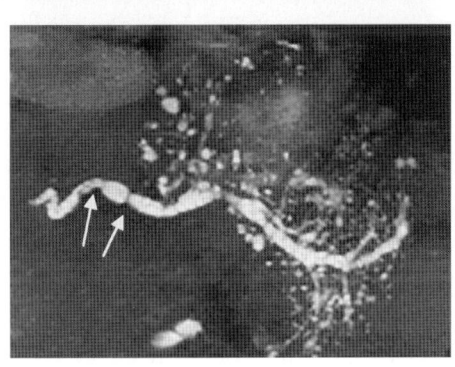

Clinical Applications: Pathological Conditions 653

Fig. 46 **a** Sjögren syndrome. Axial unenhanced CT scan shows enlargement of parotid glands. **b** CT sialogram shows globular filling of the parotid gland on the right side.
c, **d** Sjögren syndrome and superimposed sialodochitis of the left parotid gland. **c** MIP reconstruction MR sialogram of an axial 3D-EXPRESS sequence shows bilateral disease with 1–2 mm intraglandular collections of saliva in the left parotid gland and multiple intraglandular collections of saliva that are 1 mm or smaller in the right parotid gland. Note normal right Stensen's duct (thin arrow). Marked dilatation and multiple stenoses of the left main parotid duct (thick arrow) are seen, suggesting sialodochitis.
d Sagittal oblique MIP reconstruction MR sialogram of the left parotid gland shows multiple 1–2 mm-high signal intensity areas within gland parenchyma, as well as a dilated and lobulated main duct with stenotic areas (arrows). (From Reference 21.)

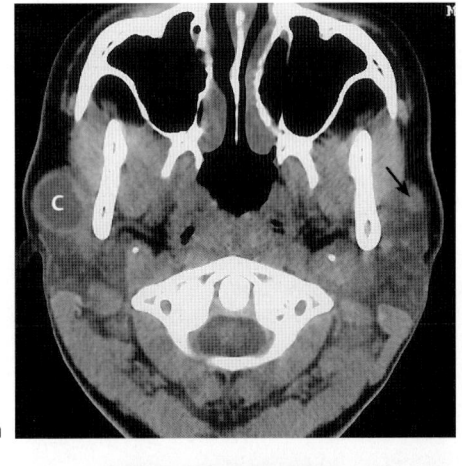

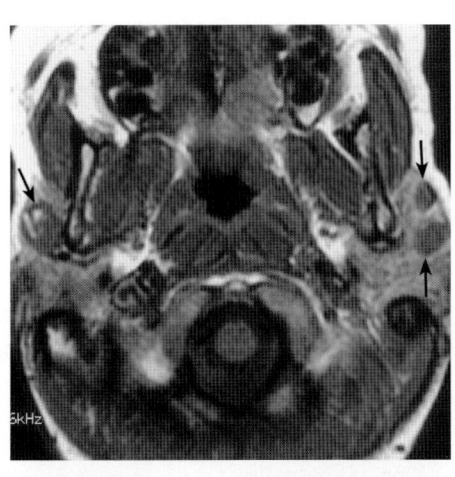

Fig. 9.47 A 22-year-old woman with Sjögren syndrome. **a** Unenhanced CT scan shows a large cystic mass (c) in the right parotid gland and a small nodule (arrow) in the left parotid gland. Note increased density of the glands with fine nodular pattern. **b** Unenhanced T1W MR scan shows bilateral parotid masses (arrows). **c** Enhanced T1W and **d** enhanced fat-suppression T1W MR scans, showing slight enhancement of parotid masses.

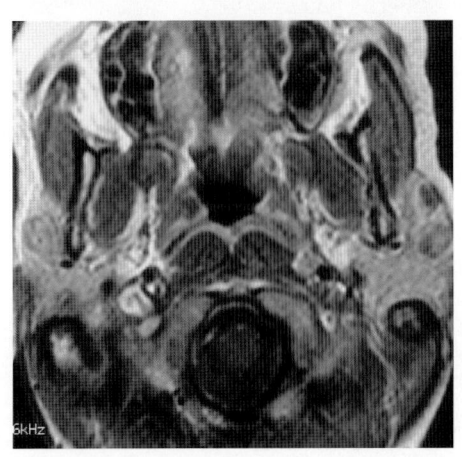

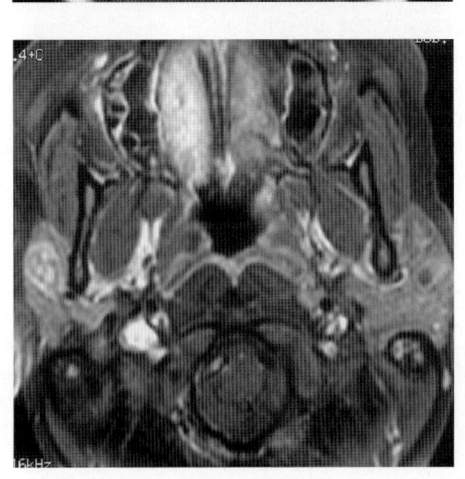

cysts and other causes is the presence of diffuse cervical adenopathy in patients with AIDS. In BLL related to sarcoidosis, associated cervical adenopathy may be present. In Sjögren syndrome, the presence of cervical lymphadenopathy should raise the possibility of associated lymphoma.

Microscopic examination of benign BLL demonstrates diffuse collection of small lymphocytes centered around the intralobular ducts and their basement membranes.[7, 8, 41] As the lymphoid infiltration increases, acinar atrophy occurs and eventually will be replaced by collection of lymphocytes. As the process goes on, there will be associated proliferation of ductal epithelium, and ultimately ductal narrowing, dilatation, and cyst formation. Some authors[41] suggest that AIDS-related lymphoepithelial cyst is most likely the result of cystic dilation of intranodal (parotid lymph node) ductal epithelial inclusions, analogous to the development of Warthin's tumors, albeit lacking papillary hyperplasia seen in Warthin's tumor.[41]

■ Benign Lymphoepithelial Sialadenopathy (Autoimmune Sialosis)

Nonneoplastic unilateral or bilateral enlargement of the major or minor salivary or lacrimal glands associated with or occurring independently of an autoimmune disease may present as a clinical entity. This specific lesion affecting the salivary glands can be distinguished by clinical, radiological, and pathological criteria. The disease is usually seen in women beginning at the age of 40–50 years. Clinically there is recurrent diffuse swelling of the salivary glands, associated with mild pain and tenderness. The disease is usually multiglandular, although often only the parotid gland is affected. Typically, there are no systemic signs, but there may be superimposed acute bacterial infections secondary to stasis of secretion. The disease process is also known as autoimmune sialosis, benign lymphosialadenopathy, chronic lymphoepithelial sialadenopathy, nonobstructive sialectasis, and punctate parotitis. The etiology of this disease is most likely an autoimmune process. The specific entity in this group is Sjögren syndrome, although chronic sarcoidosis may have similar manifestation in the parotid glands.

Sjögren Syndrome

Sjögren syndrome is an autoimmune disease (autoimmune sialosis).[20, 43] Current evidence indicates that Sjögren syndrome is the result of a lymphocyte-mediated destruction of exocrine glands, which in turn leads to diminished or absent glandular secretion and mucosal dryness.[7] The term Mikulicz disease has been used clinically for instances in which parotid and lacrimal gland enlargement, keratoconjunctivitis sicca, and xerostomia are present without systemic symptoms.[1] Mikulicz disease has been used synonymously with benign lymphoepithelial cyst and represents asymptomatic enlargement of the major salivary glands or the lacrimal glands. The terminology is appropriate for use clinically, but is not appropriate as a morphological term.[8]

Sjögren syndrome is characterized by lymphocyte-mediated destruction of the exocrine glands resulting in keratoconjunctivitis sicca and xerostomia. There may also be associated systemic autoimmune disease such as rheumatoid arthritis or less commonly systemic lupus erythematosus.[20, 43] Sjögren syndrome predominantly affects women with an average age of onset around 50 years. One-third of patients have unilateral or bilateral salivary gland swelling, with the parotid gland usually involved. The specific autoimmune antibodies (SS-A and SS-B) may be elevated only during active disease or not elevated at all.[41] A biopsy of the minor salivary glands is required for a definitive diagnosis. In the parotid gland, periductal mononuclear and dense lymphocytic cell infiltration is present.[41, 43] Epimyoepithelial islands surrounded by lymphocytic infiltration are also noted, which obstruct intercalated ducts, resulting in dilatation of the intraglandular ductal system. There have been rare reports of benign lymphoepithelial cyst in Sjögren syndrome.[41] These cysts, unlike AIDS-related lymphoepithelial cysts, are located in the parotid parenchymal tissue and not within the parotid nodes.[19, 41] Other collagen disorders may also be associated with benign lymphoepithelial sialadenopathy, including systemic lupus erythematosus, scleroderma, polyarteritis nodosa, and polymyositis. There is a high incidence of non-Hodgkin lymphomas in patients with Sjögren syndrome.[7]

Imaging studies that have been used for the diagnosis of Sjögren syndrome include plain-film sialography, radionuclide scintigraphy, sonography, CT, MRI (Figs. 9.**45**–9.**48**), and MR sialography. Plain-film sialography is more sensitive than CT and MRI for the detection of Sjögren syndrome.[1] Sialography demonstrates punctate to globular contrast collections (Fig. 9.**45**). The disadvantage of plain-film sialography is that it may exacerbate the inflammatory process, resulting in increased pain and discomfort.[19] Ultrasound has also proved to be very valuable for the diagnosis of this syndrome. In the early stage of the disease, CT demonstrates nonspecific enlargement of the parotid glands (Fig. 9.**46**). In later stages of the disease, CT may demonstrate increased density of the gland with the nodularity (Fig. 9.**47a**) or fat-replaced parotid glands with multiple nodular densities and punctate calcifications. MR imaging of Sjögren syndrome demonstrates an enlarged parotid gland with an inhomogeneous speckled or nodular pattern (salt-and-pepper appearance) of increased and decreased T2-weighted signal intensity. There is an overall decrease in T2-weighted signal intensity of the parotid gland compared to normal controls. (Figs. 9.**47**, 9.**48**).[19, 42] This pattern is considered suggestive of Sjögren syndrome and when identified in a patient with the clinical suggestion of Sjögren syndrome may obviate further evaluation.[19] These areas of hypointensity are believe to represent focal accumulation of lymphocytes accompanied by increased collagenous fibrous tissue. Hyperintense areas of T2-weighted images probably represent dilated intraglandular ducts.[19] Salivary gland involvement in Sjögren syndrome can be confirmed by plain-film sialography or by MR sialography (Fig. 9.**45**). This new technique[44] is capable of demonstrating characteristic changes that include diffuse areas of punctate high signal intensity, representing a dilated intraglandular ductal system. In later stages of the disease, MR sialography, similarly to conventional sialography, may demonstrate marked dilatation and irregular branching of the intraglandular ductal system (Figs. 9.**42c**, 9.**45b**, 9.**46c**).[20, 43] Complications include acute sialadenitis, chronic sialadenitis, cysts, calculi, glandular atrophy, and punctate calcifications throughout the parotid gland.[1]

■ Neoplasms of Salivary Glands

General Considerations

Salivary gland neoplasms are rare and represent 0.3% of all malignant neoplasias and less than 3% of all head and neck neoplasms.[5, 46, 47] Most tumors of the salivary glands are asymptomatic masses. The salivary glands demonstrate a greater variety of neoplasms than any other organ system in the body.[5] Fortunately, most salivary gland tumors are low-grade malignancies or benign neoplasms. High-grade malignancies are uncommon. Seventy to eighty percent of all salivary gland neoplasias are at the parotid gland, with a reported malignancy varying from 17% to 34%.[5, 46, 47] Patients with acinic cell carcinoma and mucoepider-

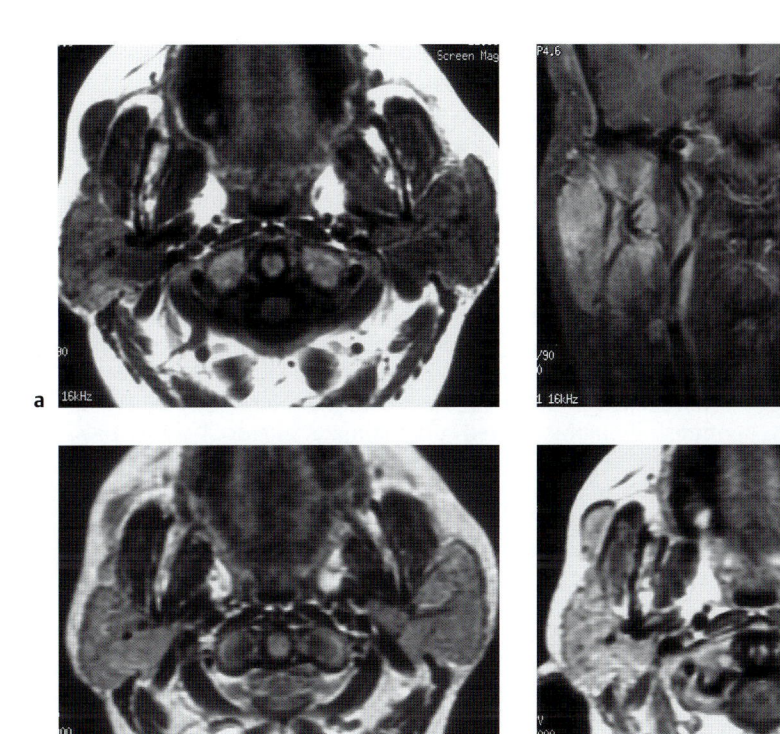

Fig. 9.**48** Sjögren syndrome. **a** Axial unenhanced T1W, **b** enhanced coronal fat-suppression T1W, **c** T2W, and **d** PW MR scans showing moderate enlargement of the parotid glands. The glands appear heterogeneous on unenhanced T1W, T2W, and PW MR scans (**a, c, d**).

moid carcinoma have a better prognosis compared with adenocarcinoma, malignant mixed tumor, adenoid cystic carcinoma, squamous cell carcinoma, and undifferentiated carcinoma.[46] The incidence of lymph node metastases in parotid carcinomas at the time of initial presentation varies from 12% to 24%.[46]

Clinically, symptoms are unreliable with regard to predicting the benign or malignant nature of a lesion. Benign lesions of low-grade malignancies may be seen initially as slow-growing, painless masses. Aggressive malignancies or inflammatory lesions may be associated with rapid growth and pain. However, facial nerve paralysis associated with a parotid mass is highly suspicious for a malignant neoplasm and dictates a poor prognosis.[47,48] We have seen a case of benign mixed tumor presented with facial paralysis. The lesion was located high up, compressing the facial nerve at its exit from stylomastoid foramen (see Fig. 9.**61 a, b**). Other authors have also reported facial paralysis with benign tumor of the parotid gland. Some authors recommend that if a mass is clearly confined to the superficial lobe of the parotid gland and a fine-needle aspiration biopsy demonstrates benign histology, then a superficial parotidectomy may be performed without imaging.[49,50] Otherwise, imaging is indicated prior to surgical extirpation. However, one has to consider the possibility of recurrence and seeding due to needle aspiration.

Preoperatively, a mass should be localized as intrinsic or extrinsic to the salivary glands (see Figs. 9.**7**–9.**10**); involvement of the deep or superficial parotid gland should be defined; if possible, its relationship with respect to the facial nerve should be carefully defined;[2,5,7,24,27,51] the possibility of high-grade malignancy should be noted.[48] The presence of a high-grade malignancy should alert the surgical team to the possibility of a more radical surgery.[48]

The primary neoplastic disorders of the salivary glands may be divided as follows: (a) neoplasms of epithelial tissue origin (Tables 9.**3**, 9.**4**); (b) neoplasms of supporting tissue origin such as hemangioma, lymphangioma, lipoma, schwannoma, fibroma, malignant lymphoma, and various sarcomas (Tables 9.**3**, 9.**4**). Rare lesions such as angiolipoma, hemangiopericytoma, lymphoepithelioma-like carcinoma, giant-cell tumor, carcinosarcoma, aggressive fibromatosis, and metastases including metastatic meningioma of the parotid gland have been reported (Tables 9.**3**, 9.**4**).

Table 9.**3** Benign tumors of the salivary glands

Epithelial
1 Pleomorphic adenoma (benign mixed tumor) (cylindroma), most common tumor
2 Monomorphic adenoma
   a Warthin tumor (papillary cystadenoma lymphomatosum, second most common
   b Oncocytoma (acidophilic cell adenoma), or oxyphilic adenoma
   c Myoepithelioma
   d Canalicular adenoma
   e Basal cell adenoma
   f Clear cell adenoma
   g Glycogen-rich adenoma
3 Ductal papillomas
   a Sialadenoma papilliferum
   b Intraductal papilloma
   c Inverted ductal papilloma

Nonepithelial
- Hemangioma, capillary type, cavernous type
- Lymphangioma
- Lymphangiohemangioma
- Schwannoma/neurofibroma
- Lipoma
- Fibroma

Modified from references 1 and 8.

CT Appearance of Salivary Gland Tumors

Most benign neoplasms or low-grade malignancies of the salivary glands are encapsulated or pseudoencapsulated and consist of a single mass with fairly well-defined margins. Malignant neoplasms are unencapsulated and have poorly defined margins.[1,3,5,63–68] Benign neoplasms can sometimes demonstrate poorly circumscribed borders, related to surrounding inflammatory reaction.[4] The capsule of benign mixed tumor may be ir-

Table 9.4 Malignant tumors of the salivary glands

Epithelial
- Mucoepidermoid carcinoma, most common (adults and children)
- Adenoid cystic carcinoma
- Adenocarcinoma (mucin-producing)
- Clear cell adenocarcinoma (nonmucinous, glycogen-containing or non-glycogen-containing)
- Adenocarcinomas, not otherwise specified
- Acinic cell carcinoma (second most common in children)
- Oncocytic carcinoma (malignant oncocytoma)
- Malignant mixed cell tumor (true malignant mixed tumor or carcinosarcoma)
- Carcinoma ex-pleomorphic adenoma (carcinoma arising in a benign mixed tumor)
- Primary squamous carcinoma (rare)
- Basal cell adenocarcinoma
- Undifferentiated carcinoma
- Epithelial-myoepithelial carcinoma (rare)
- Lymphoepithelioma-like carcinoma (carcinoma ex-lymphoepithelial lesion)
- Stensen's duct carcinoma (rare)
- Sebaceous carcinoma

Nonepithelial
- Lymphoma
- Sarcoma (liposarcoma, fibrosarcoma, angiosarcoma, etc.)
- Sarcoma in ex-pleomorphic adenoma (osteogenic–chondrogenic sarcoma)
- Fibrohistiocytoma
- Hemangiopericytoma
- Synovial sarcoma
- Giant-cell tumor
- Malignant schwannoma
- Neurofibrosarcoma

Metastatic
- Melanoma
- Squamous cell carcinoma
- Renal cell carcinoma
- Lung
- Thyroid
- Meningioma (unusual case reported).

Modified from references 1 and 8.

regular in thickness. This is because tumor cells may be on the surface or occur as excrescences outside of the capsule. Invasion of the muscles of mastication appears to be a more consistent indicator of malignancy.[67,68] Perineural extension is a characteristic feature of adenoid cystic tumor (see Figs. 9.**68**, 9.**85**–9.**90**).

In general, differentiation of benign and malignant tumors by CT or MRI is not the primary goal of CT and MRI. Rather, CT and MRI become important in defining the anatomical localization, total extent of disease, local lymphadenopathy, and distant metastasis.[5,45,51] In a series of 32 consecutive parotid tumors, preoperative CT scans resulted in the discovery of detail not revealed by clinical examination.[47] The CT appearance of cysts is similar to that of cysts in other organs of the body.[45] Generally, cysts have thin walls, are well circumscribed, and contain water-density material or proteinaceous fluid; the cyst may appear rather dense. Hemangiomas demonstrate marked contrast enhancement (Figs. 9.**49**–9.**51**) and may have a characteristic dynamic CT appearance (Fig. 9.**50b**). Lymphangiomas have a characteristic MR appearance (Figs. 9.**52a, b**). Benign mixed tumors are typically sharply circumscribed, lying in an otherwise normal gland (Figs. 9.**53**, 9.**54**).[1–5,22,45] Intraparotid facial neuroma may not be differentiated from benign mixed tumor. In the parotid, the mass is usually of higher CT density than the generally low-density parotid gland. Some parotid glands may be relatively dense and therefore the mass may be isodense with gland tissue. Identification may then require CT sialography or MRI to outline the tumor mass.

Benign parotid pleomorphic adenomas demonstrate mild to moderate enhancement following intravenous administration of contrast medium (Fig. 9.**55**). The enhancement pattern may be homogeneous or heterogeneous, related to their mixed histology (mixed tumor). Larger pleomorphic adenomas often appear as a nonhomogeneous image, characterized on CT scans by low-attenuation foci of necrosis, old hemorrhage, and cystic changes.[2,22] Other benign or malignant salivary gland lesions, however, may also have similar imaging characteristics.[4,5] Some authors[22] have demonstrated that the enhancement characteristics of pleomorphic adenomas may be a function of the time delay between administration of iodinated contrast material and CT scan acquisition. In one series, for seven of the eight pleomorphic adenomas, the degree of lesion enhancement increased with time, becoming more uniform and homogeneous.[22] For nine of the ten nonpleomorphic adenomas, no significant change was found in either the degree or pattern of contrast enhancement between the early and delayed CT scans.[22] The improved lesion conspicuity through delayed enhancement is an important imaging finding for improving diagnostic certainty for pleomorphic adenoma. At many institutions, fine-needle aspiration biopsy of potential pleomorphic adenomas is thought to be unnecessary. This increases the chance of violating the capsule and therefore of seeding. Excisional biopsy is preferred for lesions presenting as typical pleomorphic adenomas. Submandibular masses have similar CT appearances to those of the parotid (Fig. 9.**56**); however, the normally high density of the submandibular gland at times necessitates MRI. Some tumors, and especially submandibular gland masses, may hardly be recognized on CT and MRI, including in contrast-enhanced studies (see Fig. 9.**29**). These lesions may easily be confused with chronic sialadenitis. In the appropriate clinical set-up, the detection may necessitate CT or MRI sialography.

Malignant tumors may be similarly sharply circumscribed, or they may have indistinct margins. Invasive tumors are poorly marginated and extend beyond the glandular tissue into the fat and fascial planes. These tumors invade adjacent anatomical structures and may extend into the external auditory canal, middle ear, base of the skull, lateral pharyngeal space, and infratemporal fossa. Localized inflammatory lesions within the salivary glands may mimic mass lesions. Inflammatory disease usually results in a relatively diffuse, irregular, radiodense lesion in an enlarged gland.[2,4] It is not possible by CT alone to differentiate a benign lesion from malignant one whenever a well-defined tumor is present in the salivary glands. Although an infiltrating mass is most likely to be a malignant lesion, an inflammatory reaction around a benign mass can simulate a similar appearance to malignant tumor. It should also be noted that masses arising in a salivary gland may be entirely or almost entirely surrounded by salivary tissue, or they may extend outside the salivary gland and be only partly buried in the gland (see Fig. 9.**56a**).[4] In this situation, the intraglandular component abuts the salivary gland tissue directly without an intervening fat layer.[4] Calcification may be present in Warthin's tumor and acinic cell tumor. Calcification is rare in mixed tumors. Irregular calcifications in a mixed tumor, associated with pain or rapid growth, should raise the possibility of malignant degeneration (see Fig. 9.**64c**).

MR Appearance of Salivary Gland Tumors

MRI and CT are both useful in the evaluation of salivary gland masses.[2,22,45,48,64] They can help to differentiate intrinsic from extrinsic lesions, such as a cervical node and a parapharyngeal

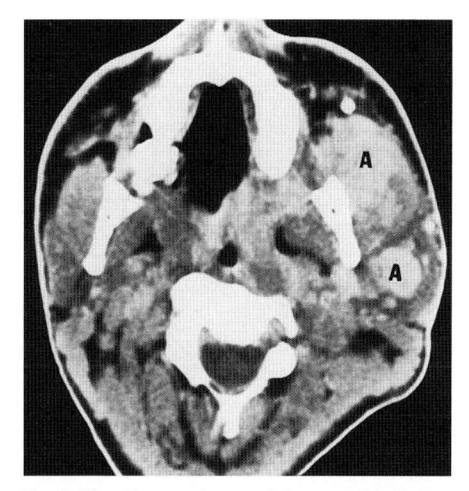

Fig. 9.**49** Hemangioma of the parotid. Contrast enhanced CT scan. There are enhancing masses involving the left masseter muscle and parotid gland, compatible with hemangioma (A). Note calcification anterior to the left masseter.

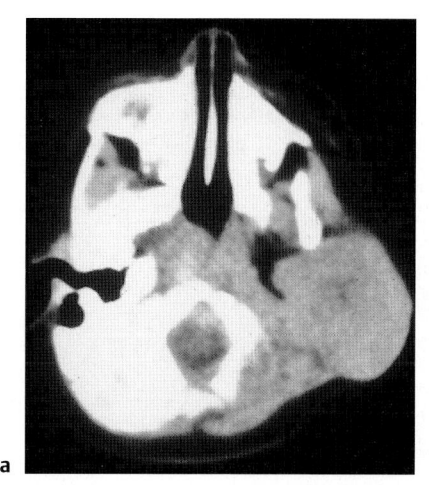

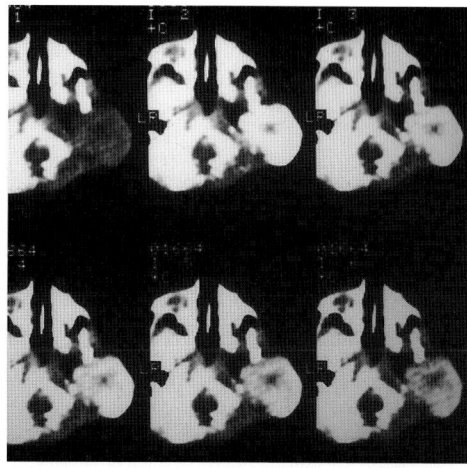

Fig. 9.**50** Capillary hemangioma of the parotid. **a** Enhanced CT and **b** dynamic CT scans showing a capillary hemangioma involving the entire left parotid gland. Note intense rapid enhancement as well as rapid washout of contrast on the dynamic CT scans.

mass from a parotid mass.[2,4] MRI may give some indication of the relationship of a parotid mass to the facial nerve. Although MRI, like CT scan, cannot give a histological diagnosis, it can give an indication of the general morphology of the tumor. Rounded, sharply marginated, well capsulated tumors tend to be benign, whereas irregular, diffuse tumors tend to be malignant. In a study using MRI, the finding of a complete capsule together with a lobulated contour had a positive predictive value of 100% for the diagnosis of pleomorphic adenoma.[45] Lipomas, lymphangiomas, and hemangiomas may be specifically differentiated from other salivary tumors.

Benign lesions and low-grade malignancies typically demonstrate low signal intensity on T1-weighted MR images and high signal intensity on T2-weighted MR images, presumably related to the presence of serous and mucoid materials with high water content.[2,64] In contrast, high-grade malignancies often demonstrate low signal intensity on T1-weighted and relatively lesser signal intensity on T2-weighted MR images, presumably related to the high ratio of tumor cellularity to free water content, the high mitotic ratio, and the presence of paramagnetic materials.[2,48] Large-cell tumors, which can be highly malignant, and necrotic tumors appear to be an exception to this rule. Large-cell tumors are composed of large cells containing varying amounts of cytoplasm, resulting in relative T2 hyperintensity. Intravenous Gd-DTPA contrast administration scanning, similar to enhanced CT scanning, may result in mild to moderate to marked contrast enhancement of various salivary gland lesions. Adenoid cystic carcinoma, acinic cell carcinoma, and Warthin's tumors may at times demonstrate no appreciable contrast enhancement compared to enhancement of normal gland (see Figs. 9.**91**, 9.**92**).

Vascular Lesions

Hemangioma

Hemangiomas, benign tumors of endothelial cell origin, may involve the salivary glands (Fig. 9.**49**). Hemangiomas are classified by the type of vascular channels formed as capillary, cavernous, or sclerosing. Congenital capillary hemangioma is the most common cause of parotid swelling in the newborn. Hemangiomas (capillary type) are the most common (90%) parotid gland neoplasm of infants,[8] occurring most commonly in females,[3,26] and are the most common cause of parotid swelling in the newborn (Fig. 9.**50**). They can occur in the submandibular gland.[1] Spontaneous involution occurs in 50% of capillary hemangiomas, particularly during the second and third years of life. An overlying cutaneous angioma may be present. Cavernous hemangiomas are seen in a slightly older age group; these may contain phleboliths and are less apt to regress.[1] Hemangiomas may be well circumscribed (Fig. 9.**50**) or infiltrative and can involve the adjacent musculature (Fig. 9.**49**). Cavernous hemangiomas may be identified in salivary glands and are noted as being seen in older children and adults, as primarily involving the parotid gland, and as being characterized by the presence of dilated, thin-walled vessels lined with flattened endothelial cells. Unlike capillary hemangioma, the cavernous hemangioma does not regress and therefore requires complete surgical excision.[8] Hemangioma and arteriovenous malformation (AVM) demonstrate intermediate signal intensity on T1-weighted MR images and high signal intensity on T2-weighted MR images (Fig. 9.**51**). Signal voids representing large vessels or calcification (phleboliths), often in a scattered pattern, are characteristic of AVM[51] and differentiate them from lymphangiomas, if present. Calcification may be seen in lymphangio-hemangiomas.

Lymphangioma

Lymphangiomas and cystic hygromas are benign congenital lesions of lymphatic vessels. The salivary glands are involved either directly or by encroachment of a hygroma in the neck (Figs. 9.**24**, 9.**25**, 9.**52**). Lymphangiomas are seen as multilocular low-density, nonenhancing images on CT and as hyperintense images on T1-weighted MRI, with high signal intensity on spin density and T2-weighted MR images. Some of the lymphangiomas may appear hypointense on T1-weighted MR images. Lymphangiomas may be extensive, involving several compartments, including the orbit; they may be bilateral. Lymphangiomas may demonstrate varying signal intensity related to hemorrhage. The combination of multiloculated fluid-filled masses with areas of internal hemorrhage is highly suggestive of lymphangioma and cystic hygroma. Lymphangiomas do not show significant contrast enhancement.

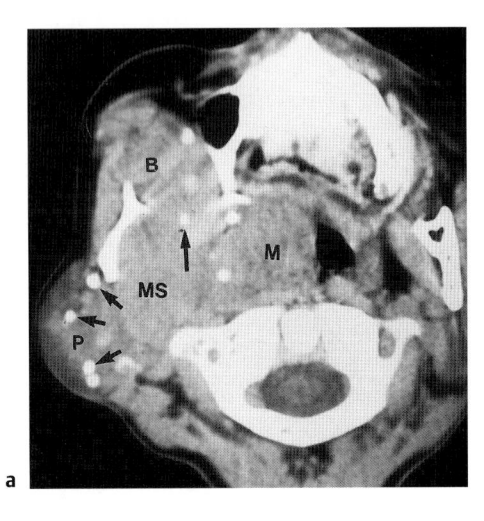

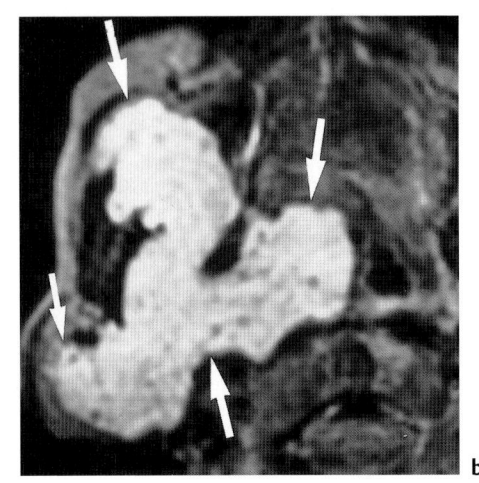

Fig. 9.51 Hemangioma. **a** CT scan shows a large mass involving the parapharyngeal space (M), masticator space (MS), buccal space (B), and parotid space (P). Note multiple vascular calcifications (arrows). **b** T2W MR scan demonstrates the various components of the hemangioma seen in **a** (arrows).

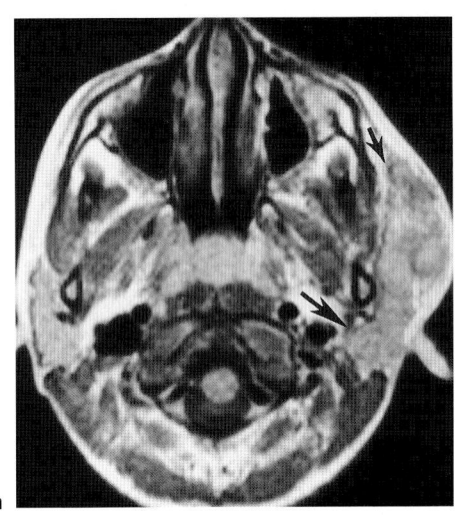

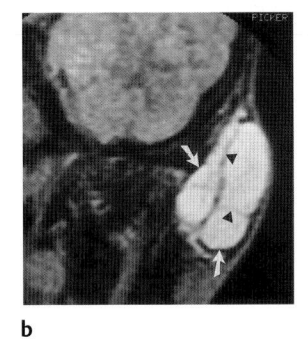

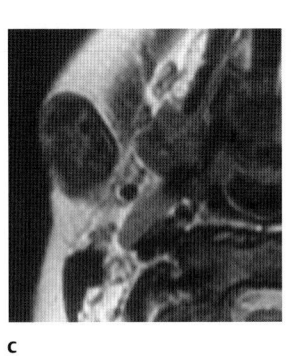

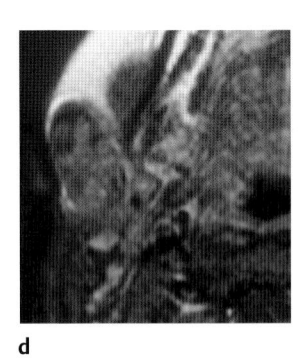

Fig. 9.52 Lymphangioma. **a** Axial proton-weighted and **b** coronal T2W MR scans, showing a multiseptated mass (arrows), involving the left parotid gland and lateral face. The septae (arrowheads), which are characteristic of lymphangiomas, are demonstrated better on the T2W MRI scan (**b**).
c, d Pilomatrixoma. **c** Axial T2W MR scan shows a hypointense mass (M) in the subcutaneous region of the right submandibular space. **d** Axial enhanced T1W MR scan shows heterogeneous enhancement of the mass.

Sebaceous Gland Cysts

Sebaceous gland cysts seen in the submandibular space or in the cheek and peri-/para-parotid regions can clinically simulate a submandibular gland or parotid cyst or tumor respectively. Sebaceous cysts and tumors appear on CT scans as isodense to muscle. These lesions appear hypointense on T1-weighted and hyperintense on T2-weighted MR images. At times hypointense areas may be present, related to dense secretions as well as calcifications.

Pilomatrixoma

Pilomatrixoma is a benign skin neoplasm of hair follicle origin, first reported by Malherbe and Chenantais in 1880 as a calcified tumor originating from the sebaceous gland.[52] The tumor was eponymously labeled "calcified epithelioma of Malherbe." Those lesions seen in the cheek and periauricular region can clinically simulate a hemangioma or superficial parotid cyst or solid mass. In 1961, Forbis and Helwig[53] introduced the term pilomatrixoma when further ultrastructural studies established the outer root sheath cell of the hair follicle as the cell of origin. Clinically these lesions present as solitary, firm, painless dermal or subcutaneous masses.[54,55] The overlying skin may have a reddish or blue hue in 24% of cases.[53] The lesions are more commonly seen in the cheek, neck, periorbital, and scalp. They have a characteristic histopathological appearance consisting of basaloid cells, ghost cells, foreign body giant cells, and intralesional calcifications. CT in pilomatrixoma will demonstrate a well-circumscribed and often calcified subcutaneous mass. The lesions appear hypointense on T1-weighted and T2-weighted MR images, related to calcification (Fig. 9.**52c**). Lesion demonstrates heterogeneous enhancement (Fig. 9.**52d**).[54]

Neoplasms of Epithelial Tissue Origin

General Considerations

1 Benign lesions of salivary glands include benign mixed tumors (pleomorphic adenoma), papillary cystadenoma lymphomatosum (Warthin's tumor), acidophilic cell adenoma (oncocytoma, oncocytosis), and the monomorphic tumors, which include basal cell adenoma, glycogen-rich adenoma, clear cell adenoma, and myoepithelioma.[3,5,51,56] Other benign tumors of the salivary gland include papillary ductal adenoma (papilloma); benign lymphoepithelial lesion; sebaceous gland adenoma, and lymphadenoma.[50,51,56]

2 Malignant lesions of salivary glands include malignant mixed tumor; malignant ex-pleomorphic adenoma (carcinoma arising in a benign mixed tumor); primary squamous cell carcinoma;

adenoid cystic adenocarcinoma; mucoepidermoid carcinoma (low-grade, high-grade); acinic cell (acinous) adenocarcinoma (low-grade, high-grade); oncocytic carcinoma (malignant oncocytoma); adenocarcinoma (mucus-producing); clear cell adenocarcinoma (nonmucinous and glycogen-containing or non-glycogen-containing) and other adenocarcinomas; and miscellaneous tumors, which include sebaceous adenocarcinoma, Stensen's duct tumors, melanoma, carcinoma ex-lymphoepithelial lesion, carcinosarcoma, undifferentiated carcinoma, unclassified lesions, and metastasis.[5,50,51,56] Epithelial-myoepithelial carcinoma (EMC) is a rare malignant salivary gland neoplasm. EMC is thought to represent about 1% of all salivary gland tumors.[57] EMC is a low-grade adenocarcinoma, but recurrences and metastases to cervical nodes, as well as distant sites, have been reported.[57] EMC is predominantly a tumor of the parotid, but a few cases have arisen in the submandibular gland and intraoral minor salivary gland.[57] The significant risk factors for neck metastasis in parotid carcinoma are histological type, T-stage (T3 and T4), and severe desmoplasia.[46] The adenocarcinoma, undifferentiated carcinoma, high-grade mucoepidermoid carcinoma, squamous cell carcinoma, and salivary duct carcinoma are considered high-risk histological types.[46] The acinic cell carcinoma, malignant mixed tumor, and myoepithelial carcinoma are considered moderate-risk histological types.[58,59] The low-risk histological types are adenoid cystic carcinoma, low-grade mucoepidermoid carcinoma, and intermediate-grade mucoepidermoid carcinoma (Table 9.**5**).[46]

The prerequisite for adequate treatment of parotid malignant tumors is an accurate histopathological diagnosis, since the biological aggressiveness and outcome of these tumors appear to correlate with the histology.[2,48] The correlation of histopathology with behavior has allowed these tumors to be divided into two or sometimes three groups: low-grade, intermediate-grade, and high-grade cancers (Table 9.**5**).[14,56] It is not unusual for a single carcinoma to have all multiple histological patterns present, making classification quite subjective.[46,56] In general the biological nature of salivary gland tumors may not be determined through the analysis of frozen sections. The use of adjuvant radiation therapy or chemotherapy may be indicated when permanent section analysis demonstrates high-grade histological patterns.[58,59] Seventy to eighty percent of parotid tumors are benign.[46,47] On the other hand, 50% of tumors of the submandibular gland and minor salivary glands are malignant.[5,59] Approximately 90% of sublingual gland tumors are malignant and account for 0.5–4.5% of all salivary gland malignancies. Half of the tumors are adenoid cystic carcinomas (see Fig. 9.**87**) and the remainder are mucoepidermoid carcinomas with a small percentage of squamous cell cancers.[5] Sixty to sixty-five percent of solitary parotid masses are benign mixed tumors. Warthin's tumor, or papillary cystadenoma lymphomatosum, the second most frequent benign tumor in the parotid gland, makes up about 8% of all parotid gland tumors.[5,14,41] Facial nerve paralysis associated with a parotid mass indicates malignancy and carries a poor prognosis.[60–62] Occasionally a benign mixed tumor may cause facial paralysis. Eneroth[60] found no cases of facial nerve paralysis in a series of 1790 benign parotid tumors, but in 378 malignant parotid tumors he found 46 cases of facial paralysis. In the latter group the mortality was 100% at 5 years. In another review, Eneroth and co-workers[60,61] studied 1029 cases of malignant parotid tumors and found an incidence of facial paralysis of 14% and a 5-year survival rate of 9% for these patients. Conley and Hamaker[62] reviewed 279 malignant parotid tumors and did not find that facial nerve paralysis was quite as hopeless a prognostic indicator: 9 of 34 patients were free of disease at 5 years, and 4 of 26 patients who were available for 10-year follow-up were free of disease at 10 years.

Table 9.**5** Histological type of salivary gland tumors and their risk for neck metastasis and prognosis

High risk	a	Undifferentiated carcinoma
	b	High-grade mucoepidermoid
	c	Adenocarcinoma
	d	Squamous cell carcinoma
	e	Salivary duct carcinoma
Intermediate risk	f	Acinic cell carcinoma
	g	Ex-pleomorphic carcinoma (malignant mixed tumor)
	h	Myoepithelial carcinoma
Low risk	i	Adenoid cystic carcinoma
	j	Low-grade mucoepidermoid carcinoma
	k	Intermediate-grade mucoepidermoid carcinoma
	l	Epithelial-myoepithelial carcinoma

Skin involvement in salivary gland tumors indicates advanced malignancy and adverse prognosis. Ninety percent of parotid tumors originate in the superficial lobe.[47] Tumors may arise in any portion of the parotid gland. If tumor originates in the superficial portion of the parotid gland, a swelling develops anterior to or above or below the tragus of the ear.[47] Tumors of the tail arise in the region of the angle of the mandible or in the upper portion of the neck. If the deep retromandibular portion of the gland is the site of origin, the tumor may pass through the stylomandibular tunnel and enter the parapharyngeal space, producing a bulge in the soft palate.[49,63] These are the so-called dumbbell tumors (see Figs. 9.**63**, 9.**70**). On the other hand, salivary gland tumor only in the parapharyngeal area, the so-called round tumor (see Fig. 9.**69**), may also present as an asymptomatic soft-palate mass. Benign mixed tumors arising in the submandibular gland are also usually asymptomatic. Any portion of the submandibular gland may be the site of origin, but the outer portion is the most frequently affected.[47]

Some authors advocate that biopsy by needle or incision is usually contraindicated in benign mixed tumors. Although most parotid tumors are benign pleomorphic adenomas, there is still a definite association with carcinoma ex-pleomorphic adenoma occurring in a preexisting benign parotid mass.[47] Implantation of tumor cells is always a danger. The capsule of benign mixed tumors varies considerably in thickness and continuity.[2] Tumor cells may be on the surface or occur as excrescences outside the capsule.[2] This multicentric growth accounts for the dictum of wide surgical excision including normal gland.[2,48] In rare instances, multiple sites of origin may occur (multicentric pleomorphic adenoma) that are widely scattered in the parotid gland.[45] As a general rule, surgical excision is the treatment of choice in all benign mixed tumors regardless of gland or site of origin. The total submandibular gland is usually excised. In the parotid gland, excision usually includes a wide margin of normal parotid tissue with preservation of the facial nerve. Mixed tumors usually recur in patients who have undergone inadequate primary surgery. It is not common for a malignancy to develop in a benign mixed tumor. If malignancy occurs, it may be adeno- or squamous or sarcomatous cell type.[5,51]

Benign Epithelial Neoplasms

The majority of salivary gland neoplasms that occur in the parotid gland arise from the superficial lobe and are benign. Less commonly, neoplasms occur within the deep lobe of the parotid or in the submandibular, sublingual, or minor salivary glands. These are more likely to be malignant (Figs. 9.**53**–9.**56**).[4,5]

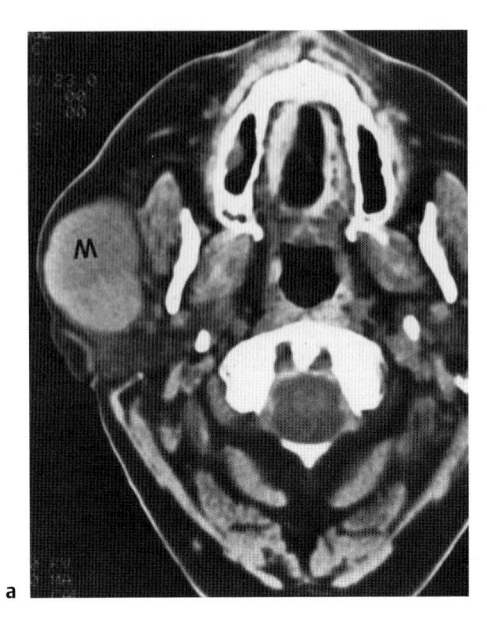

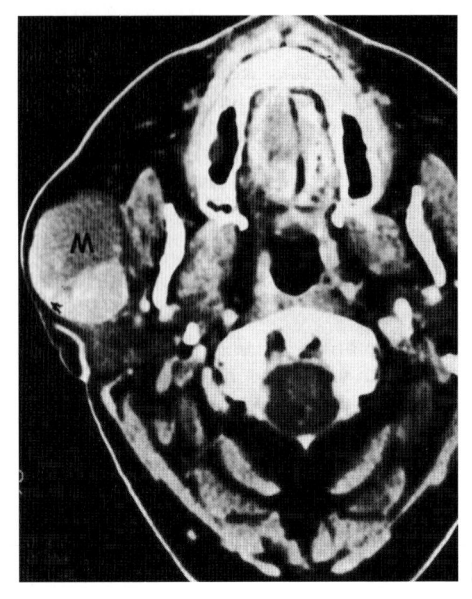

Fig. 9.**53** Benign pleomorphic adenoma of right parotid gland. **a** Plain and **b** enhanced CT scans. In **a** the right parotid gland is enlarged by a large inhomogeneous mass (M). **b** Following IV contrast infusion, the irregular enhancement of the tumor is apparent. The presumptive diagnosis in this patient was pleomorphic adenoma.

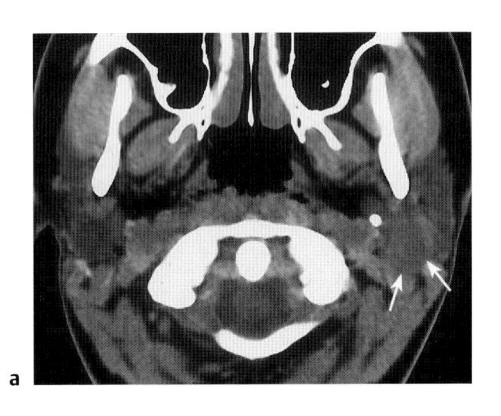

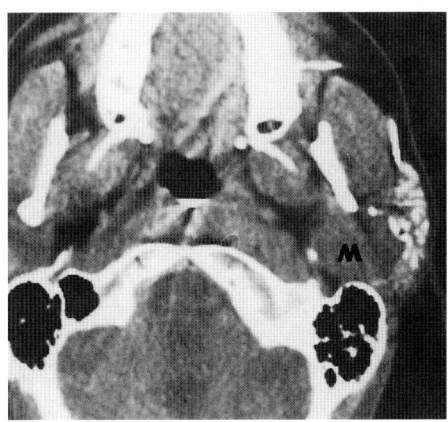

Fig. 9.**54** **a** Benign pleomorphic adenoma of the parotid gland in a 17-year-old female patient. Unenhanced CT scan, showing a nearly isodense mass (arrows), involving left parotid gland.
b Pleomorphic adenoma, parotid gland. Axial CT sialogram in another patient shows a well-circumscribed mass (M) in the deep lobe of the left parotid gland.

Pleomorphic Adenoma (Benign Mixed Tumor)

Pleomorphic adenoma, also known as benign mixed tumor, is the most common salivary gland tumor, accounting for 40–70% of all neoplasms involving the major salivary glands,[8] with the majority (85%) occurring within the parotid gland.[1-5] Pleomorphic adenomas of the sublingual glands are rare.[5] The frequency of benign mixed tumors in the submandibular gland is about 40%.[5] They are more common in the outer portion of the submandibular gland (Fig. 9.**56**). In the parotid gland they are found most often in the lateral portion, but they may occur in any portion of it (Fig. 9.**53**). Tumors of the salivary glands in children are not as common as in adults and they are mostly benign (Fig. 9.**54a**).

Pleomorphic adenomas histologically contain a mixture of ductal, myoepithelial, and mesenchymal cells arranged within a pleomorphic stroma consisting of admixtures of mucoid, myxoid, chondroid, hyaline tissues, and in rare cases, bone and fat, thus giving rise to the name "mixed tumor."[5] The benign mixed tumors appear grossly encapsulated, but microscopically visible tumor cells and small projections may be outgrowing on the outside surface. This accounts for the high incidence of recurrence if the tumor is merely shelled out.[5] Bilateral (Fig. 9.**57**) and multicentric lesions are rare.[5] Most reported cases of multiple pleomorphic adenomas result from dissemination of tumor cells at the time of surgery (see Fig. 9.**62**). Malignant degeneration can occur and is manifested by a period of rapid growth in a patient with a long-standing history of benign mixed adenoma[67] (see Fig. 9.**66**). The vast majority of these tumors are solid, but rare examples have been associated with cystic degeneration or hemorrhage.

Spontaneous and tumor-associated infarction of the parotid gland tumors has been reported.

Pleomorphic adenomas usually appear as well-circumscribed, relatively homogeneous masses, having increased density relative to normal gland on unenhanced CT scan (Fig. 9.**53**). Some of the benign pleomorphic adenomas may be isodense with parotid gland tissue (Fig. 9.**54a**). Calcification, although not common, may be seen in pleomorphic adenoma. Benign mixed tumors demonstrate mild to moderate enhancement on enhanced CT scans (Figs. 9.**53**, 9.**55**). The enhancement may be homogeneous or heterogeneous (Figs. 9.**53**, 9.**55**). In benign pleomorphic adenomas, the degree of contrast enhancement will increase with time, becoming more uniform and homogeneous.[22] In the submandibular gland, the enhancement of benign pleomorphic adenoma may be far less than that of the normal gland tissue (Fig. 9.**56**). Bilateral and multicentric pleomorphic adenomas are rare (Fig. 9.**57**). Benign pleomorphic adenomas on MRI have low signal intensity on T1-weighted images, intermediate signal on proton-weighted images and high signal intensity on T2-weighted images (Figs. 9.**58**, 9.**59**). Some tumors may be less homogeneous on various pulse sequences (Fig. 9.**60**). Benign pleomorphic adenomas not uncommonly demonstrate marked

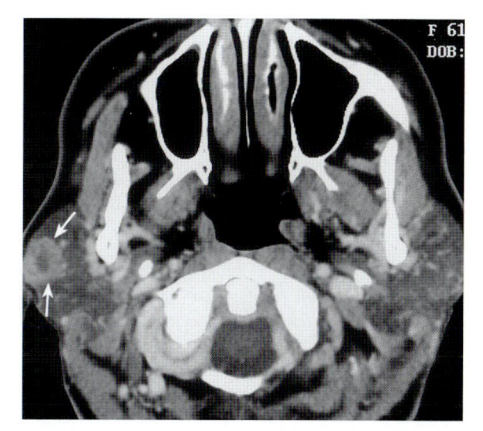

Clinical Applications: Pathological Conditions   661

Fig. 9.**55** Benign pleomorphic adenoma of the parotid gland. Enhanced CT scan, showing a heterogeneously enhanced pleomorphic adenoma (arrows).

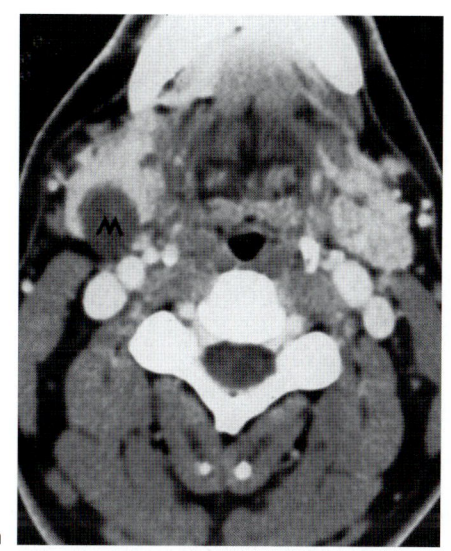

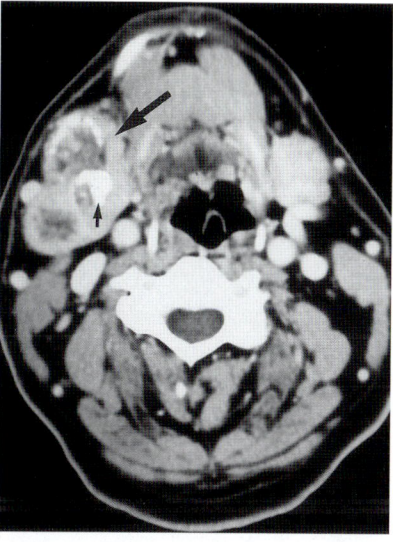

Fig. 9.**56** **a** Benign pleomorphic adenoma of the submandibular gland. Enhanced axial CT scan shows a well-defined nonenhancing mass (M) replacing the posterior portion of the right submandibular gland. Note marked enhancement of the normal submandibular glands. **b** Benign pleomorphic adenoma of the submandibular gland. Enhanced CT scan in another patient, showing a heterogeneous mass (large arrow), involving the right submandibular gland. Note prominent calcification (small arrow).

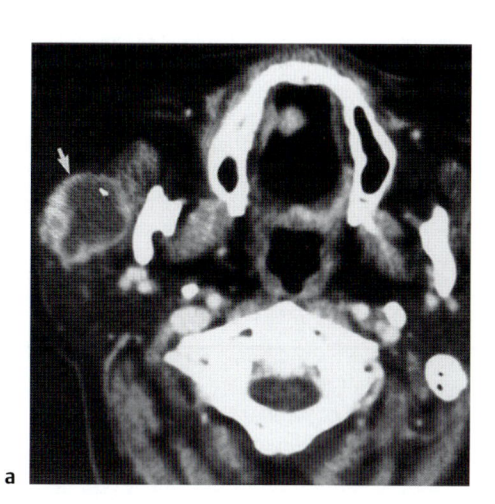

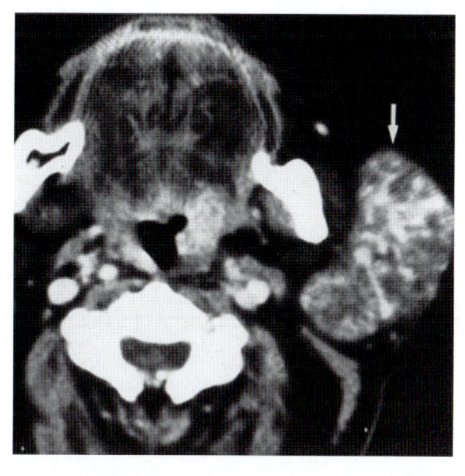

Fig. 9.**57** Bilateral parotid gland pleomorphic adenomas. Contrast-enhanced CT scans: **a** is cephalad to **b**. The pleomorphic adenomas (arrows) are sharply defined, heterogeneous, and located in the superficial lobe. The tumor on the left was excised; the tumor on the right was proven by biopsy. Bilateral pleomorphic adenomas are very unusual. From Reference 1.

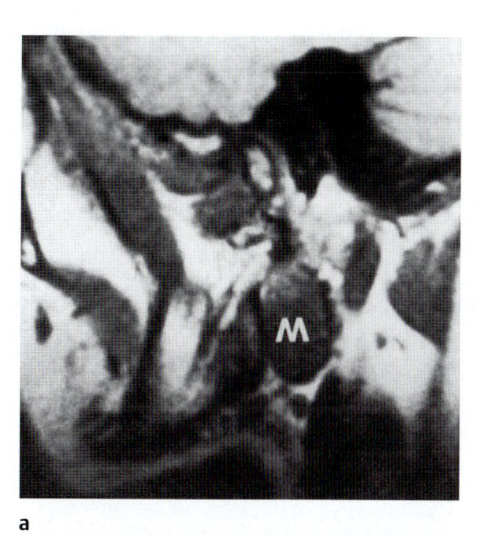

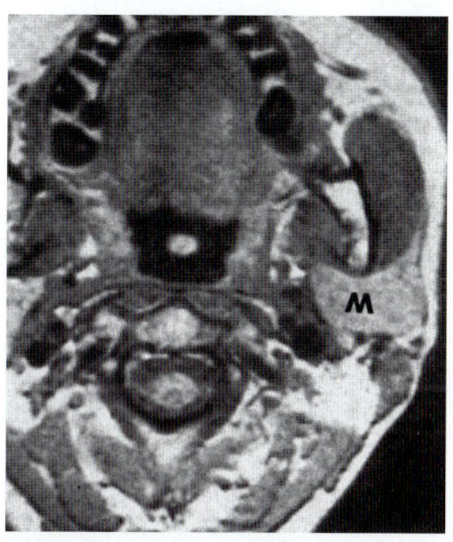

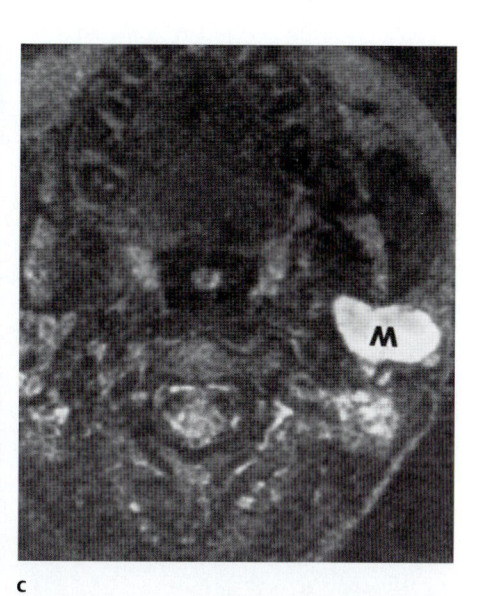

Fig. 9.**58** Benign pleomorphic adenoma. **a** Sagittal T1W, **b** axial spin-density-weighted, and **c** axial T2W MR scans. A well-defined mass (M) lies in the left parotid gland. The tumor is of low signal intensity in the T1W image (**a**), intermediate intensity in the spin density image (**b**), and high intensity in the T2W image (**c**). The retromandibular vasculatures are displaced posteriorly.

662   9 Salivary Glands

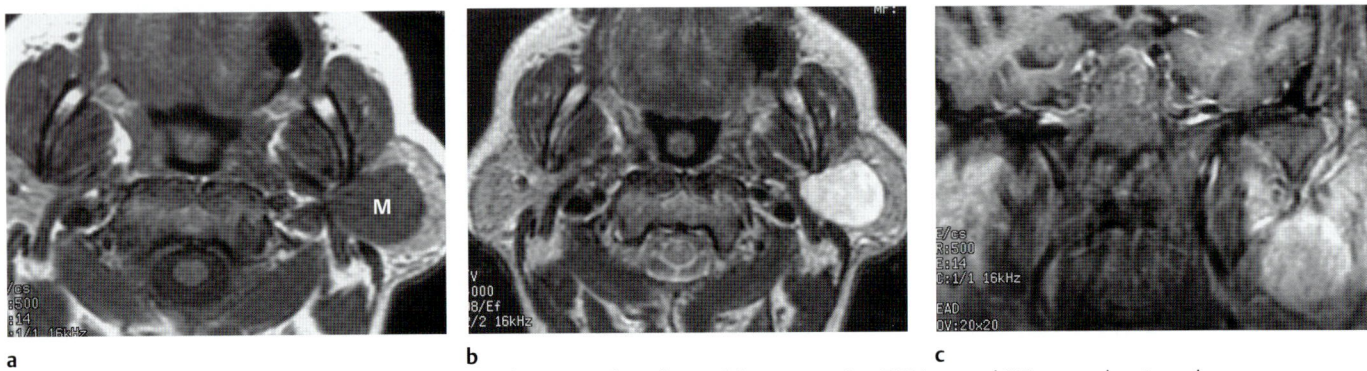

Fig. 9.59 Benign pleomorphic adenoma. **a** Axial T1W, **b** T2W, and **c** enhanced fat-suppression T1W coronal MR scans showing a homogeneous mass (M) involving the superficial lobe of left parotid gland compatible with benign pleomorphic adenoma.

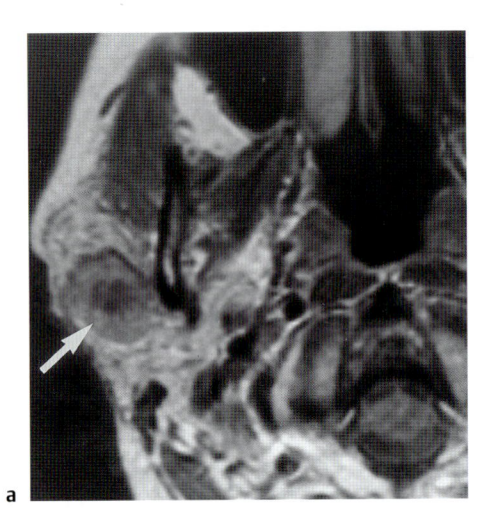

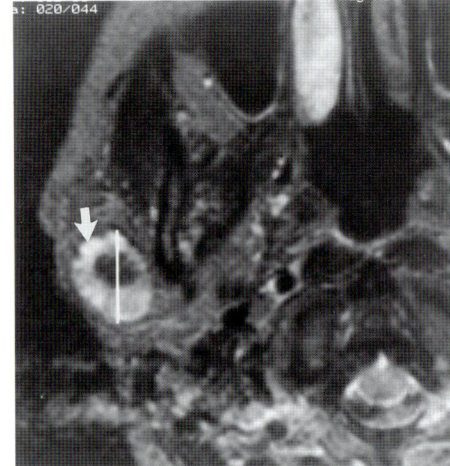

Fig. 9.**60**   Benign pleomorphic adenoma. **a** Axial PW and **b** T2W MR scans, showing a heterogeneous mass (arrow), involving the right parotid gland. The heterogeneity is a feature of pleomorphic adenoma (mixed tissues, epithelial–mesenchymal) related to epithelial and various mesenchymal tissues, cystic areas, and at times hemorrhage. Note the irregular outline of the margins of this tumor, a finding that is more in keeping with the diagnosis of a more infiltrative tumor such as mucoepidermoid or adenocarcinoma than that of a benign tumor such as this case. This is because the capsule of benign mixed tumor varies in thickness and continuity. Tumor cells may be on the surface or occur as excrescences outside the capsule.

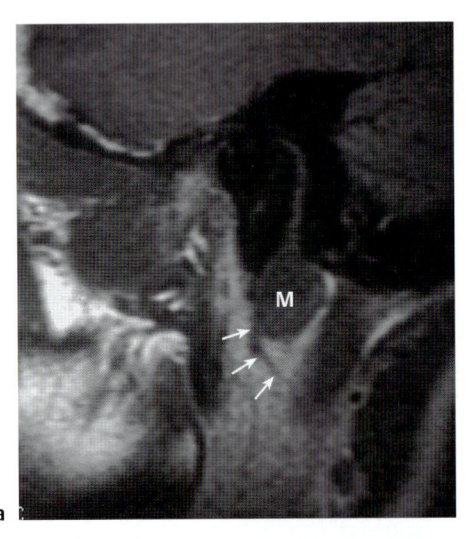

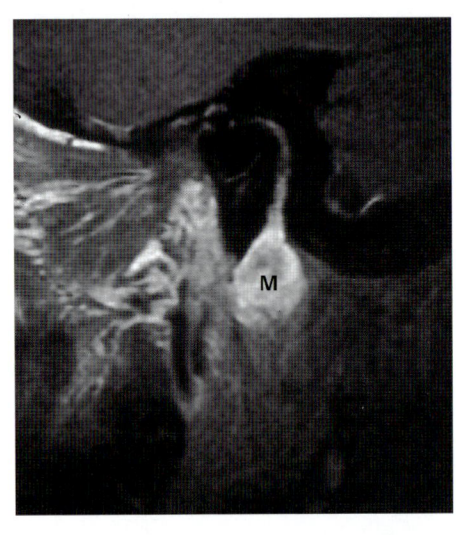

Fig. 9.**61 a, b**   Pleomorphic adenoma in a patient with facial paralysis. **a** Unenhanced and **b** enhanced sagittal T1W MR scans showing a mass (M) compatible with an adenoma, displacing facial nerve (arrows).
c–e Facial nerve neuroma. **c** Coronal T1W, **d** axial spin-density-weighted, and **e** T2W MR scans, in another patient showing a well defined mass (M) within the left parotid gland. The intensity of the mass is low in T1W (**c**), medium in spin-density-weighted (**d**), and high in T2W (**e**) images.

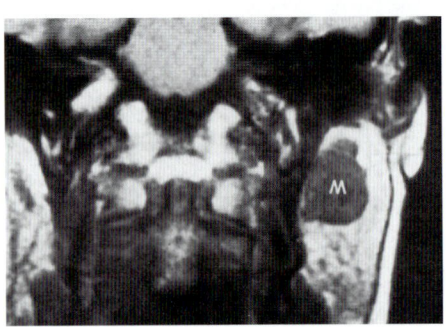

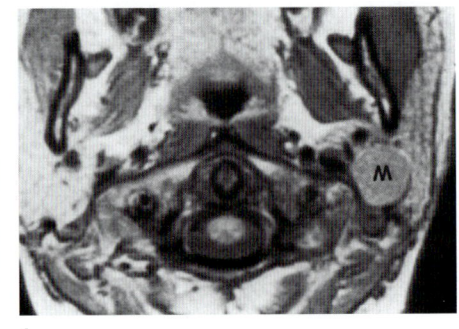

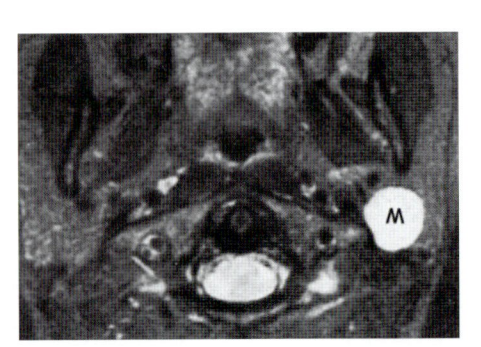

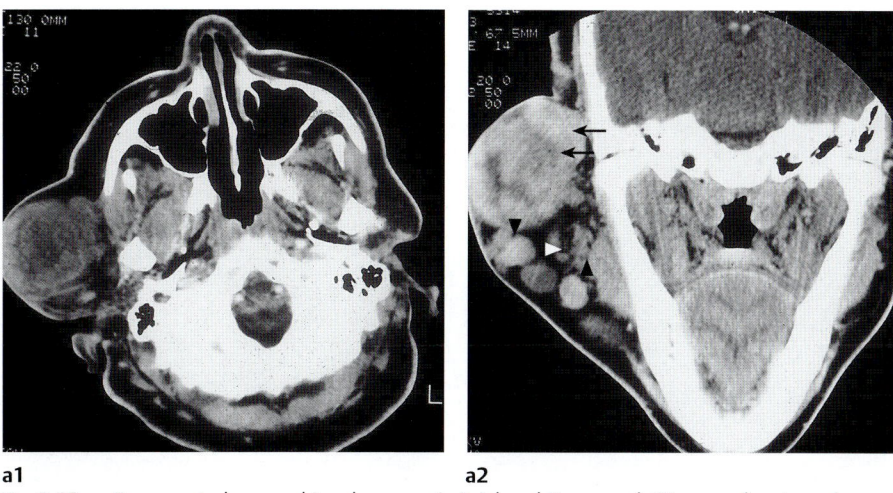

Clinical Applications: Pathological Conditions 663

Fig. 9.62a Recurrent pleomorphic adenoma. 1, Axial and 2, coronal CT scans showing a large mass (arrows) and several smaller masses (arrowheads) compatible with recurrent disease.

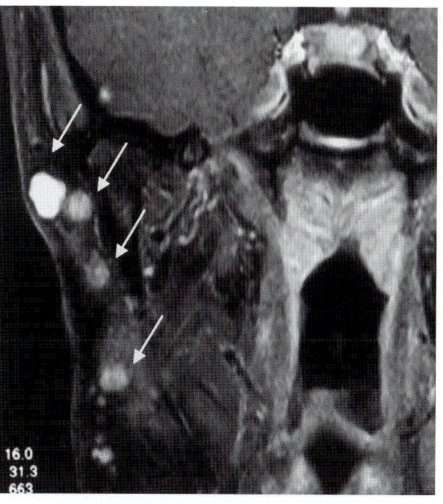

b Enhanced fat-suppression T1W coronal MR scan in another patient shows multifocal recurrent pleomorphic adenoma (arrows) after superficial parotidectomy. Fig. 9.62b provided by M. Becker, MD.

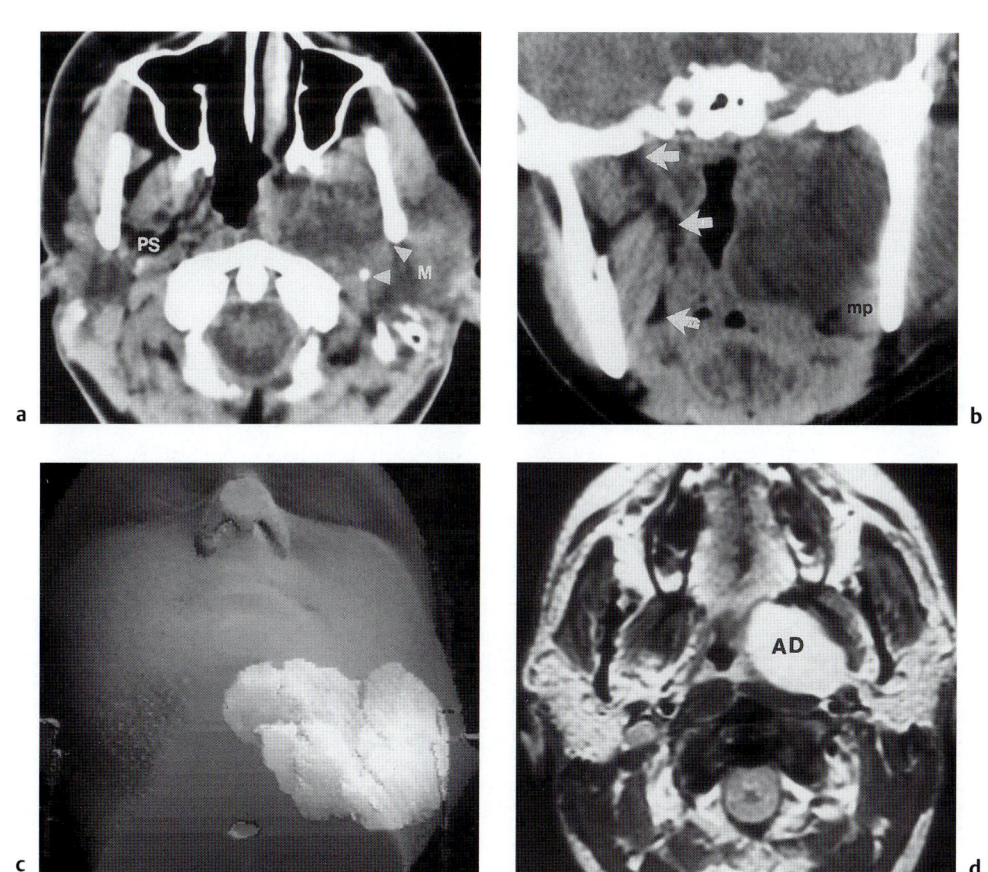

Fig. 9.63 Recurrent pleomorphic adenoma of the parotid gland. a Axial, b coronal, and c 3D CT scans, showing a large mass (M) involving the entire region of the left parotid gland ("dumbbell tumor"). Note widening of the stylomandibular tunnel (arrowheads). mp = medial pterygoid muscle. PS = parapharyngeal space. The mass has replaced the entire parapharyngeal space. Note normal parapharyngeal space in coronal section (arrows). This patient developed lung metastasis due to malignant transformation of the tumor. d T2W MR scan in another patient showing a benign pleomorphic adenoma (AD) in the parapharyngeal space. The mass is well-defined, fairly round ("round tumor"), and separated from the deep lobe of the parotid gland.

heterogeneous enhancement on enhanced MR images. Some tumors may appear homogeneous on T1-weighted and T2-weighted images but become heterogeneous on enhanced T1-weighted MR images (see Fig. 9.69). Less frequently, these lesions have lobulated, poorly circumscribed margins. Foci of low signal intensity may represent areas of calcification or fibrosis (Fig. 9.60).[4,5,51] Areas of intense signal may be present on T2-weighted MR images related to myxoid matrix. These myxoid areas can be distinguished from cystic spaces due to enhancement of myxoid areas as opposed to cyst on Gd-DTPA-enhanced T1W MR scans. In very rare cases, benign pleomorphic adenoma may cause facial paralysis (Fig. 9.61a, b). The identification of calcium in a suspected parotid neoplasm favors the diagnosis of a pleomorphic adenoma (calcification may be seen with acinic cell carcinoma as well as adenoid cystic carcinoma and Warthin's tumor), since calcifications are rare in other neoplasms.[48] Therefore, in selected cases, increased specificity for pleomorphic adenomas is possible with CT. The CT and MRI appearance of intraparotid facial neuroma may be identical to that of a benign mixed tumor (Fig. 9.61c, d, f).[3,5,51]

Some of the parotid gland facial nerve tumor may be extensive, multilobulated, and with areas of cystic formation. The

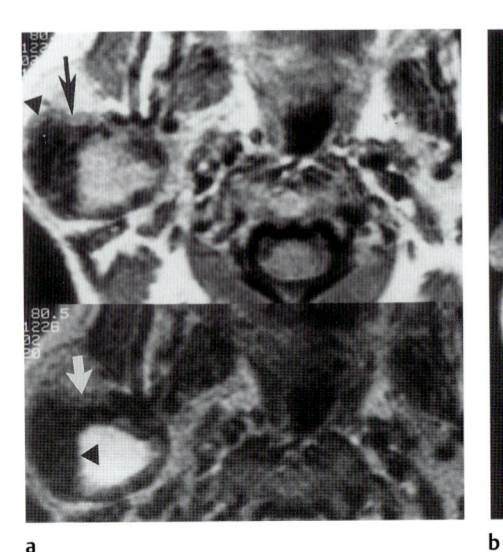

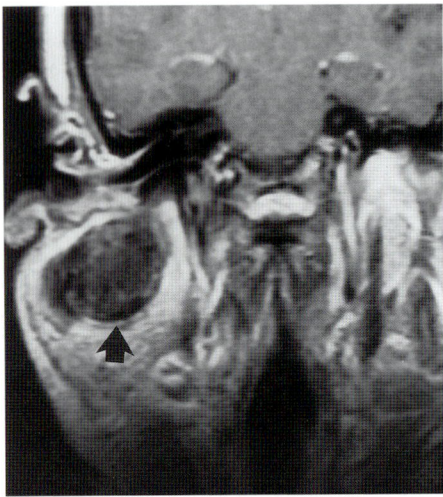

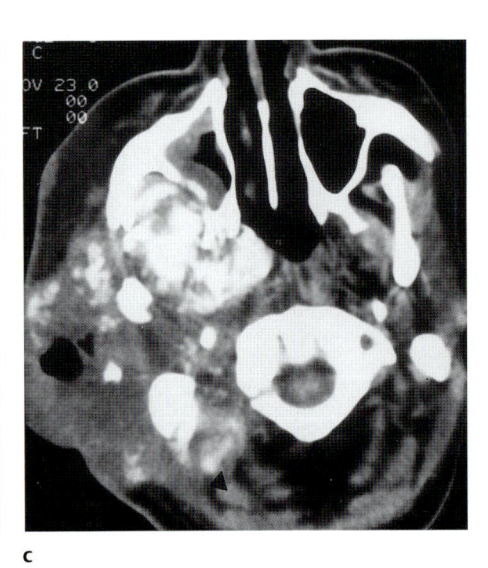

Fig. 9.64 Osteogenic sarcoma transformation in an ex-pleomorphic adenoma. **a** Axial PW (*top*) and T2W (*bottom*) and **b** enhanced coronal T1W MRI scans, showing a heterogeneous mass involving the right parotid gland (arrows). The hypointense area (arrowheads in **a**) is related to bone formation. **c** Follow-up CT scan shows massive tumor in the parotid and masticator space with foci of tumor bone formation.

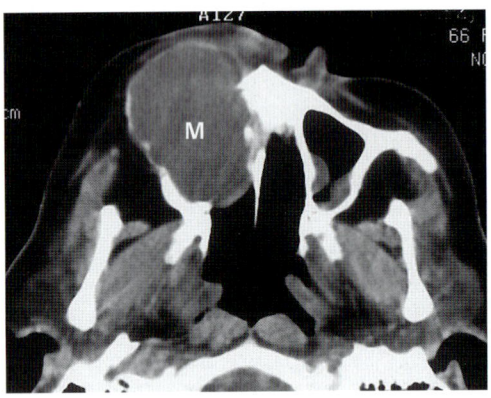

Fig. 9.65 Benign mixed tumor of minor salivary gland. CT scan shows a large, well-defined, expansile mass (M), involving the hard palate and maxilla.

standard surgical management of benign tumors of the parotid gland requires superficial, subtotal, or, rarely, total parotidectomy.[69,70] In a series of 256 consecutive patients who underwent parotid surgery, there was a 46.1% incidence of immediate facial dysfunction but no incidence of long-term paresis and only a 3.9% incidence of long-term paresis in nerve-sparing surgery.[69] Pleomorphic adenomas must be completely resected. Biopsy before resection may cause the risk of recurrence (Fig. 9.**62**).[5] Incomplete resection results in recurrence, and the recurrence may increase the risk of malignant degeneration (Fig. 9.**63**). Recurrent pleomorphic adenomas are often seen as clusters of multiple nodules in the surgical bed. Recurrent tumors are best seen on T2-weighted MR images as areas of high signal intensity. Although malignant degeneration has been reported to be as low as 2–5%, by some accounts, up to 25% of pleomorphic adenomas, left untreated, will undergo malignant transformation to carcinoma ex-pleomorphic adenoma.[1–5,14] Because of this development of carcinoma ex pleomorphic adenoma as well as sarcomatous transformation (Fig. 9.**64**), pleomorphic adenomas must be completely resected.

Benign Mixed Tumor of Minor Salivary Glands

Benign pleomorphic adenoma or benign mixed tumor may arise from minor salivary glands, situated beneath the oral mucosa and scattered throughout the mouth and upper respiratory tract. Involvement of minor salivary glands occurs most frequently on the palate, followed by the lip; the most common site of pleomorphic adenomas in the upper respiratory tract is by far the nasal cavity, followed by the nasopharynx and larynx.[8] According to Auclair,[74] "for every 100 parotid tumors there are about 40 minor gland tumors, 15 submandibular gland tumors, and less than 1 sublingual gland tumor." About 50% of minor salivary gland tumors are malignant.[1] Most malignant tumors are adenoid cystic carcinoma. The CT and MRI characteristics of minor salivary gland tumors are similar to those involving major salivary glands (Figs. 9.**65**, 9.**66**). Exophytic ameloblastoma may be mistaken on imaging for minor salivary gland tumors (Fig. 9.**67**). Adenoid cystic carcinomas are the most common malignancy to involve the minor salivary glands. These tumors have a high propensity for perineural and perivascular invasion (Fig. 9.**68**). Benign pleomorphic adenomas may arise from ectopic minor salivary glands in the parapharyngeal space (Fig. 9.**69**). These tumors should be differentiated from those arising from the deep lobe of the parotid gland (Fig. 9.**70**).

Warthin's Tumor (Papillary Cystadenoma Lymphomatosum)

Warthin's tumors (adenolymphoma or papillary cystadenoma lymphomatosum), although comprising the second most common benign neoplasm of the salivary gland, account for 5–8% of all salivary gland tumors[8] and up to 12–10% of all benign parotid neoplasms.[2,5,41,71–73] They almost exclusively involve the parotid gland, although they may arise in the adjacent lymph nodes as well.[3,4] Rare cases are reported in submandibular gland, palate, lip, tonsil, larynx, and maxillary sinus.[8] As many as 10% of cases have bilateral involvement.[41] Warthin's tumor is also the most common lesion to occur as multifocal unilateral disease. The tumor is benign; only very rarely has disputed malignant transformation been reported. Warthin's tumor presents as multiple masses within one or both parotid glands more frequently than any other salivary neoplasm. Bilateral acinic cell carcinoma, and few examples of bilateral benign mixed tumors, have been reported.[1] Warthin's tumor usually occurs in the tail of the parotid gland and is characterized by a painless, slow-growing asymptomatic mass.[5,51]

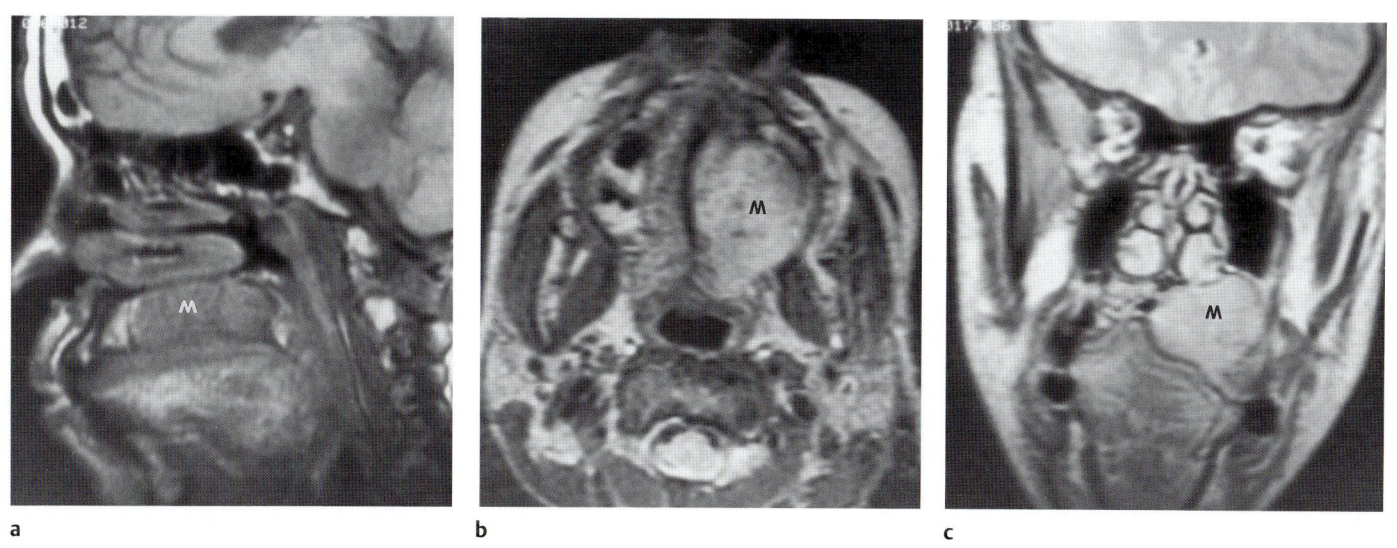

Clinical Applications: Pathological Conditions 665

Fig. 9.66 Benign mixed tumor of minor salivary gland. **a** Sagittal T1W, **b** axial T2W, and **c** coronal enhanced T1W MR scans, showing a large mass (M) involving the hard palate.

Warthin's tumor consist of a proliferation of salivary ducts within the embryologically incorporated parotid gland lymph nodes.[2,41] Histologically its characteristics include a double-layered epithelium having a tubulopapillary cystic pattern within lymphoid matrix or a lymph node.[2,5,41,51] Facial paralysis in patients with Warthin's tumor is very rare but has been reported.[71] The pathogenesis of facial nerve paralysis in benign parotid tumors has been thought to be due to sudden increase in the size of the tumor.

The CT appearance of Warthin's tumor is nonspecific, usually appearing as a well-circumscribed isodense or hyperdense mass within or on the surface of the parotid gland.[2] Although histologically these tumors often have cystic components and some mucoid fluid within, the CT characteristics are not specific because the cystic spaces are very small (Fig. 9.71). When a Warthin's tumor is cystic or partially cystic, the cyst wall may be smooth, but at times the cyst wall shows nodularity with some degree of contrast enhancement of variable thickness. Warthin's tumor may originate within the accessory lobe of the parotid gland (Fig. 9.72). Warthin's tumors may tend to have multiple lobules

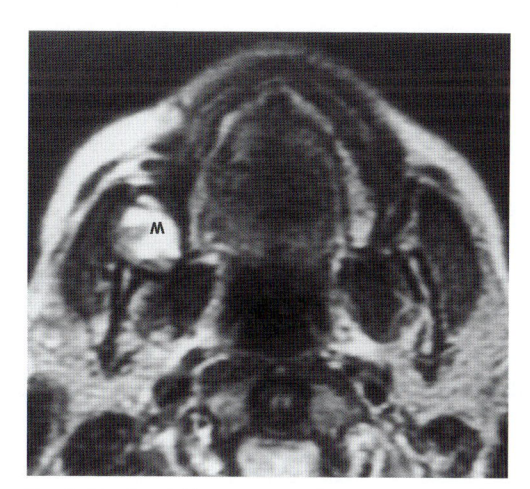

Fig. 9.67 Ameloblastoma. Axial T2W MR scan shows a right hyperintense buccal mass (M), simulating a pleomorphic adenoma of minor salivary gland.

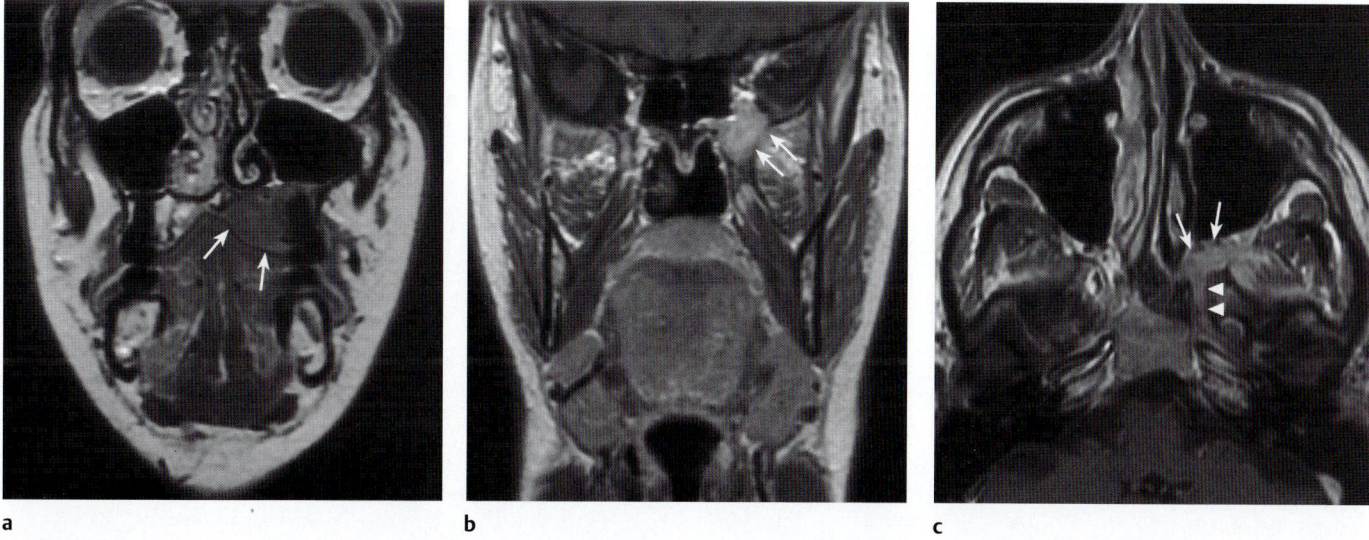

Fig. 9.68 Adenoid cystic carcinoma of the hard palate with perineural extension. **a** Coronal T1W MR scan shows a left hard-palate mass (arrows). **b** Coronal T1W enhanced MR scan shows a mass in the left pterygopalatine fossa (arrows). **c** Axial T1W fat-suppression enhanced MR scan shows a mass in the left pterygopalatine fossa (arrows), extending along the vidian canal (arrowheads).

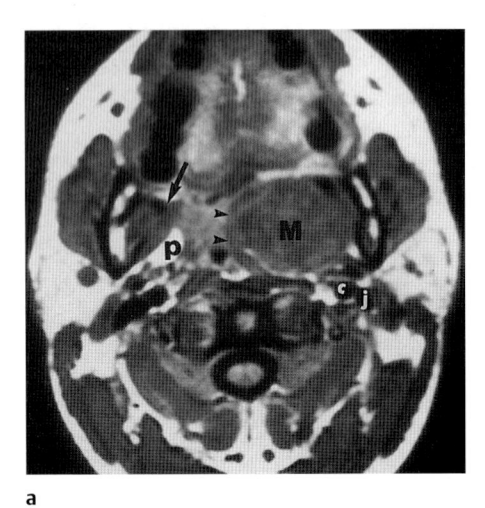

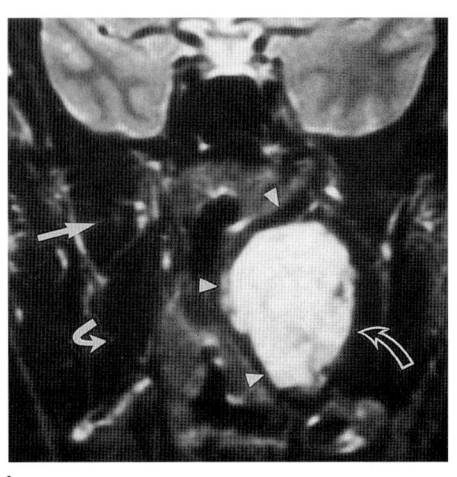

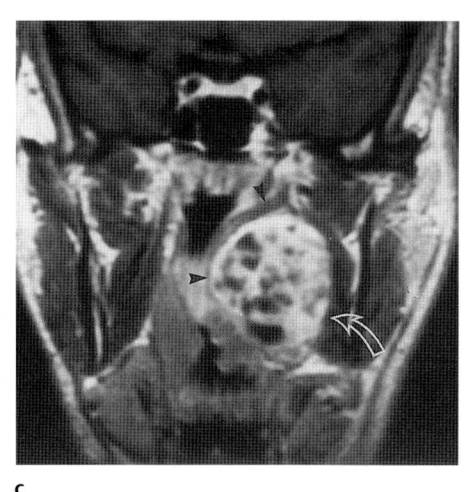

Fig. 9.69 Pleomorphic adenoma of the parapharyngeal space.
a Axial T1W MR scan shows a mass (M) involving the parapharyngeal space. Note the medial displacement of the superior pharyngeal constrictor muscle (arrowheads) and the lateral displacement of the left medial pterygoid muscle. Note the normal right pterygoid muscle (arrow) and normal right pps (p); c = internal carotid artery; j = internal jugular vein.
b Coronal T2W MR scan shows the pleomorphic adenoma, located between medially displaced pharyngeal constrictor muscles (arrowheads) and left medial pterygoid muscle (curved hollow arrow). Note the normal right lateral (straight arrow) and medial (curved solid arrow) pterygoid muscles.
c Coronal post–gadolinium contrast T1W MR scan shows heterogeneous enhancement characteristic of pleomorphic adenomas. Note displaced pharyngeal constrictor (arrowheads) and medial pterygoid (arrow) muscles. The heterogeneous enhancement is often seen in pleomorphic adenoma. At times, neurogenic tumors may show similar contrast enhancement.

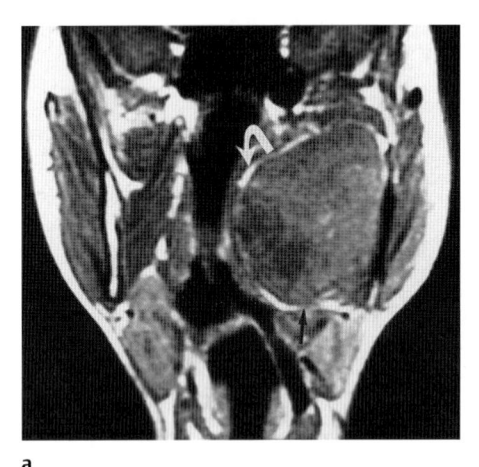

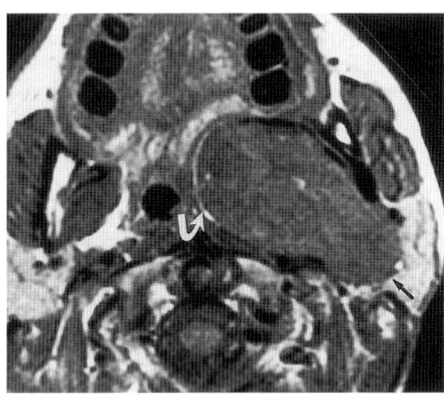

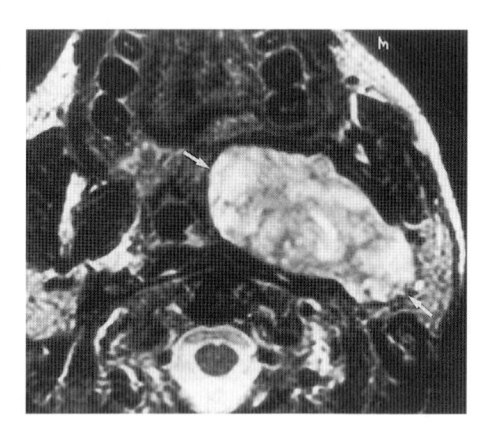

Fig. 9.70 Pleomorphic adenoma of the deep lobe of the parotid gland. **a** Coronal T1W, **b** axial T1W, **c** axial T2W MR images. This large tumor (arrows) is an exophytic lesion arising from the deep portion of the parotid. Note the medial displacement of parapharyngeal fat (curved arrows). The patient noted a slight swelling of his face but refused surgery until he started having some difficulty swallowing. From Reference 1.

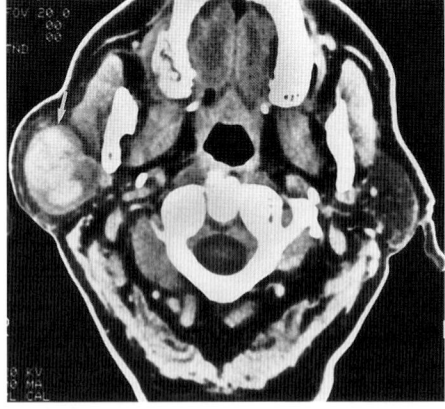

Fig. 9.71 Warthin's tumor. Enhanced CT scan. A lobulated tumor (arrow) in the superficial portion of the right parotid gland is sharply defined, and enhances with contrast. Courtesy of Merric Landy, Salem Hospital, Salem, MA, USA.

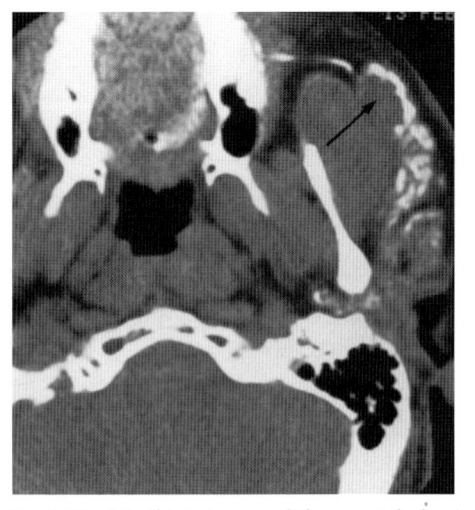

Fig. 9.72 Warthin's tumor of the parotid gland. CT sialogram shows a tumor mass (arrow) within the superficial portion of the left parotid gland, displacing Stensen's duct laterally.

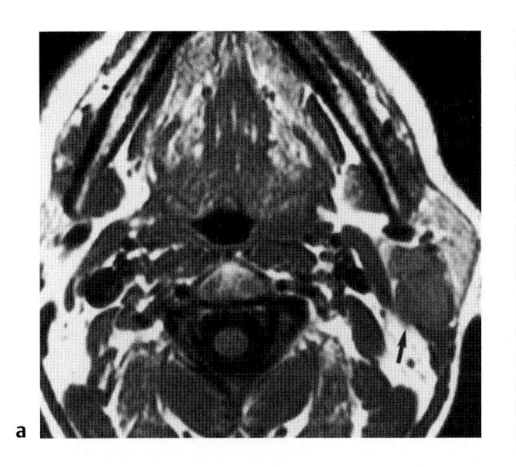

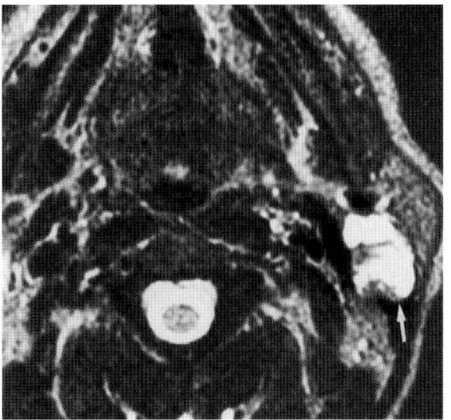

Fig. 9.**73** A lobulated lesion (arrows), showing low signal intensity on T1W and high signal intensity on T2W MR images is seen, involving the posterior portion of the left parotid gland, compatible with Warthin's tumor. From Reference 1.

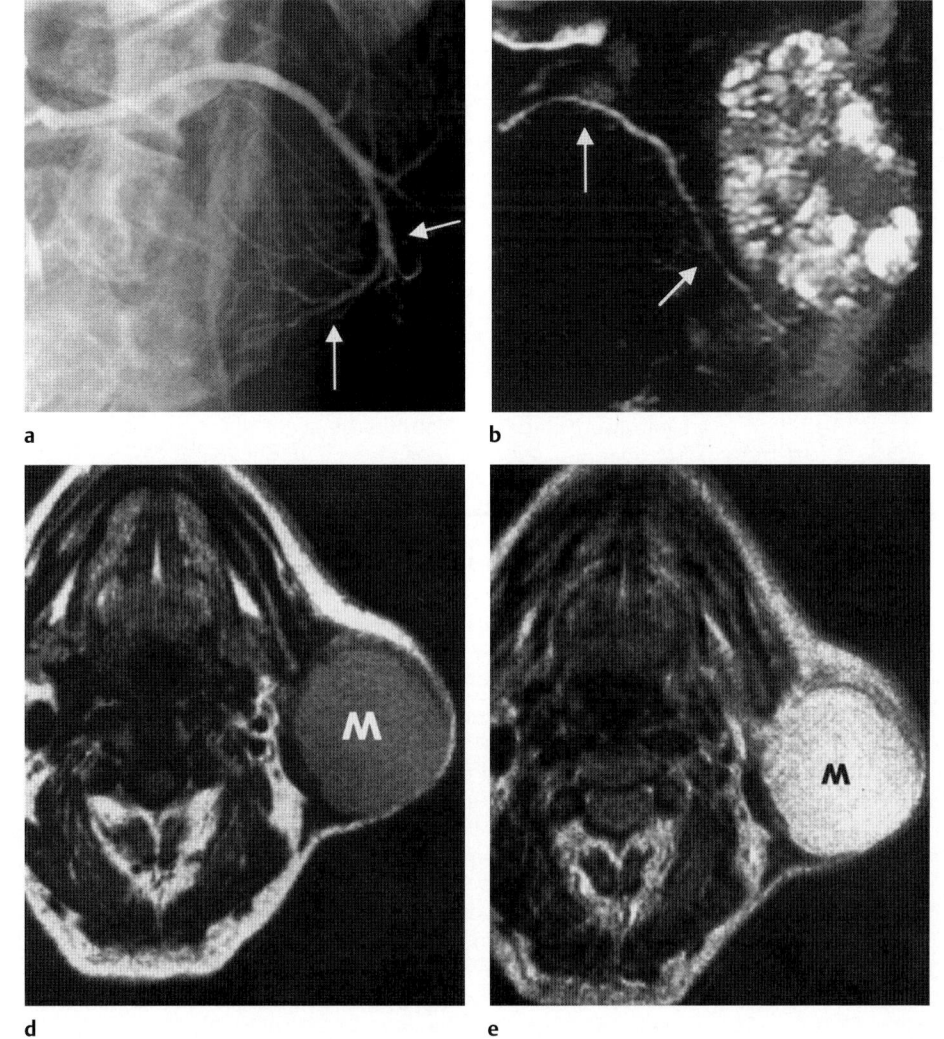

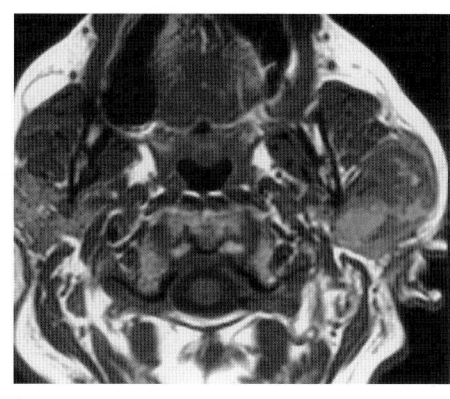

Fig. 9.**74a–c** Warthin's tumor presenting as an acute parotid gland swelling. **a** Conventional sialography of the left parotid gland shows an abnormal course of the left main parotid duct and of its intraglandular branches, which are displaced in an inferolateral direction (arrows). Intraparotid ducts have a normal caliber. The patient underwent MRI. **b** MIP reconstruction MR sialogram of a sagittal oblique 3D-EXPRESS MR sequence shows inferior displacement of a normal main parotid duct (arrows) by a large mass with hyperintense and hypointense areas. **c** T1 SE MR image depicts large hypointense (cystic) and hyperintense (hemorrhagic) areas suggesting the diagnosis of Warthin's tumor. Surgery confirmed the findings of a Warthin's tumor with acute hemorrhage. Case provided by M. Becker, M.D; Figs. **a** and **b** from Reference 21.
d, e Large parotid cyst. **d** T1W and **e** T2W axial MR scans show a large homogeneous mass (M) enlarging the left parotid gland. The mass has a low signal intensity in the T1W image, and high signal intensity in the T2W image.

and may originate from relatively small intraglandular components with larger extraglandular components, with or without foci of calcifications, and an appearance that has been compared to a bunch of grapes.[5,51] Calcifications may be diffuse and a prominent feature. The solid component of Warthin's tumor shows mild to moderate enhancement on enhanced CT scan.

Warthin's tumors are, in general, inhomogeneous,[2,22] well-circumscribed or lobulated masses having low or intermediate signal intensity on T1-weighted MR images and high signal intensity on T2-weighted MR images, similarly to a benign mixed tumor (Fig. 9.73). Some Warthin's tumors may be hypointense or low in conspicuity on T2-weighted MR images. Occasional areas of hyperintensity and hypointensity on T1-weighted images likely related to proteinaceous cysts[7] may be seen, or hemorrhage and fibrous stroma,[24,72] (Fig. 9.**74c**). Warthin's tumor may not be differentiated from other parotid cyst (Fig. 9.**74d**). War-

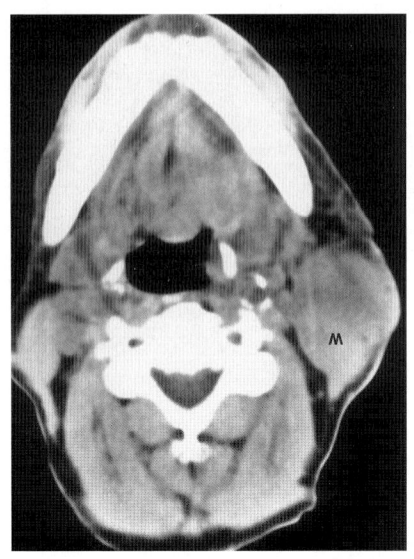

Fig. 9.75 Low-grade mucoepidermoid carcinoma. Plain CT scan shows a large mass (M), involving the tail of the left parotid gland.

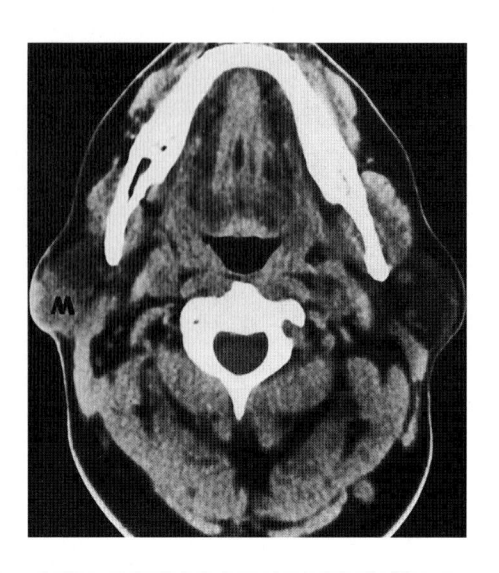

Fig. 9.76 High-grade mucoepidermoid carcinoma. Plain axial CT scan shows a high-density mass (M) involving the posterior portion of the right parotid gland. There is involvement of the subcutaneous tissue evident by comparison with the normal subcutaneous tissue on the opposite side. Except for the subcutaneous invasion, which is strongly suggestive of an aggressive lesion, the CT appearance of the lesion is identical to that of a benign parotid mass.

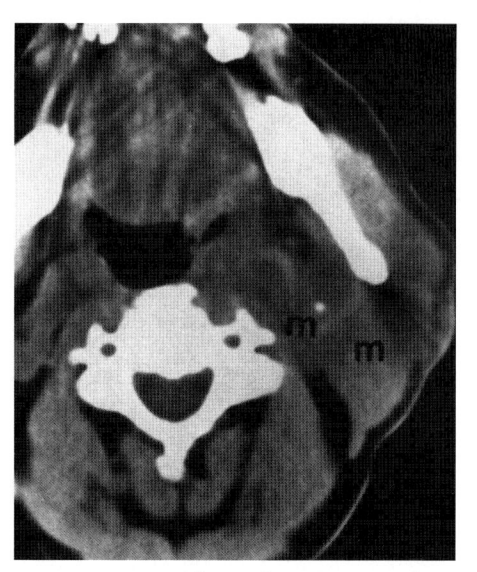

Fig. 9.77 Mucoepidermoid carcinoma. A plain axial CT scan shows a large inhomogeneous mass (m) involving the superficial and deep lobes of the parotid gland. The tumor extends into the parapharyngeal space, distorting and displacing the lateral wall of the pharynx medially.

thin's tumors demonstrate minimal or moderate contrast enhancement (Fig. 9.71).[22,72] The differential diagnosis of bilateral nonenhancing or minimally enhancing cystlike lesions includes Warthin's tumor, autoimmune sialosis, lymphoepithelial cysts and lesions associated with HIV infection, and inflammatory or idiopathic cysts.[2,53] There may be foci of fine or coarse calcification present within the parotid, particularly in Warthin's tumor, autoimmune sialosis, and inflammatory cysts.

Technetium-99m scans may aid in preoperative diagnosis because Warthin's tumors can concentrate the radionuclide, and bilateral lesions are often demonstrated. Oncocytomas may also accumulate the radionuclide; however, they are less common and are predominantly unilateral lesions. Pleomorphic adenomas, metastases, squamous cell carcinoma, and abscesses do not accumulate the radionuclide.[73]

Oncocytoma or Oxyphilic Adenoma (Oncocytosis)

Oncocytoma is a rare tumor of glandular tissue that occurs predominantly in the major salivary glands, though these tumors have been reported to occur in thyroid gland, liver, kidney, trachea, the nasal cavity, and virtually anywhere along the seromucous lining of the respiratory tract.[58] Most oncocytomas are benign. This benign lesion is believed to arise from ductal epithelium.[5,8] The characteristic cell of the oncocytoma is the oncocyte. This cell is characterized by an excessive number of mitochondria and is best determined by electron microscopy.[58] Oncocytoma, like Warthin's tumor, has the ability to concentrate ^{99m}Tc, and therefore a "hot" area on ^{99m}Tc scan will indicate the possible presence of either a Warthin's tumor or an oncocytoma. The CT and MRI appearances of oncocytoma cannot be differentiated from benign mixed tumor and solid Warthin's tumor.

Malignant Epithelial Neoplasms

Mucoepidermoid Carcinoma

Malignant epithelial neoplasms can be divided into well-differentiated (low-grade), poorly differentiated (high-grade), or intermediate-grade malignancies on the basis of histological appearance and degree of anaplasia (Table 9.5).[14] A common malignant tumor of the salivary glands is the mucoepidermoid carcinoma. Fifty-four percent of these tumors were found at the AFIP to be in the major salivary glands (primarily parotid), whereas 46% were present in the intraoral minor salivary glands.[59] The low-grade form contains more cysts, which can make up a large portion of the tumor. They may appear to be benign, but show up with metastasis years later.[1] The more malignant form of this tumor is more cellular, solid, and infiltrative. These have a high recurrence rate,[59] and may spread to regional lymph nodes or to the lungs, bones, and brain.[59] The CT and MRI appearances also vary with the grade of malignancy. The lower-grade tumors appear to exhibit benign features, are cystic, and may be hemorrhagic with well-defined margins, even though they are infiltrative microscopically.[1] They may appear very similar to the pleomorphic adenoma. Fewer cysts are seen with the intermediate-grade malignancy, and more solid tumors with the higher-grade malignancy, which may appear as low-to-intermediate signal intensities on T1-weighted and T2-weighted MR images.[1] The most common low-grade malignancies are mucoepidermoid and adenocystic carcinomas, although clinically adenocystic tumors often have poor outcome. Mucoepidermoid carcinoma (the most common salivary gland malignancy) occurs predominantly within the parotid gland[1-5,48,51] and has the highest prevalence in the fifth decade of life.[5] Although less common in children, mucoepidermoid carcinomas remain the most common malignant salivary gland

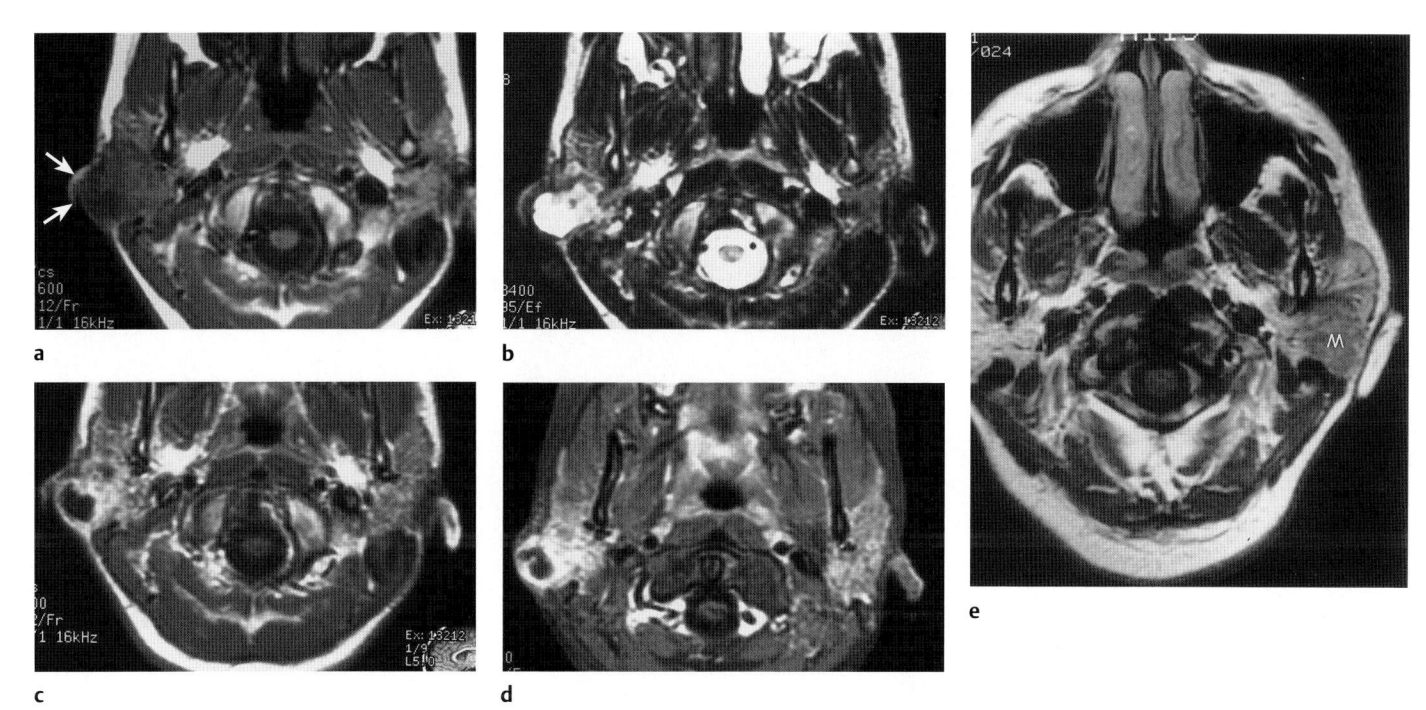

Clinical Applications: Pathological Conditions 669

Fig. 9.**78** High-grade mucoepidermoid carcinoma in a 12-year-old girl. **a** Axial T1W, **b** T2W, **c** enhanced T1W, and **d** enhanced fat-suppression T1W MR scans showing a mucoepidermoid carcinoma of the right parotid gland (arrows). **e** High-grade mucoepidermoid carcinoma. Enhanced T1W MR scan in another patient showing an ill-defined mass (M) that shows less enhancement compared to normal parotid gland tissue.

tumor in children. Mucoepidermoid carcinoma may be low-grade (Fig. 9.**75**) or high-grade (Fig. 9.**76**). Mucoepidermoid carcinoma not infrequently appears isodense or even of low density on CT scan (Fig. 9.**77**); it demonstrates mild to moderate to marked enhancement on CT and MR scans (Fig. 9.**78**). Mucoepidermoid carcinoma may be small, may be limited to the superficial lobe of the parotid, and may demonstrate CT and MRI appearances of a benign mixed tumor.[1] Recurrent mucoepidermoid carcinoma appears as infiltrative and poorly defined and with moderate to marked contrast enhancement (Fig. 9.**79**). Acinic cell carcinomas (Fig. 9.**80**) may not be differentiated from mucoepidermoid carcinoma and benign or malignant mixed tumors (Fig. 9.**81**). Undifferentiated carcinomas appear infiltrative and aggressive, with tumor spreading in various directions, often associated with facial nerve involvement (Fig. 9.**82**). Primary squamous cell carcinomas of the parotid gland are very rare and have similar CT and MRI characteristic

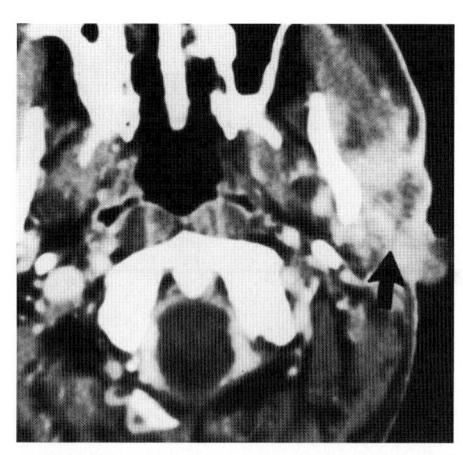

Fig. 9.**79** Recurrent mucoepidermoid carcinoma. Contrast-enhanced axial CT scan shows inhomogeneous enhancement of the enlarged left parotid gland (arrow) with infiltration of the adjacent masseter muscle.

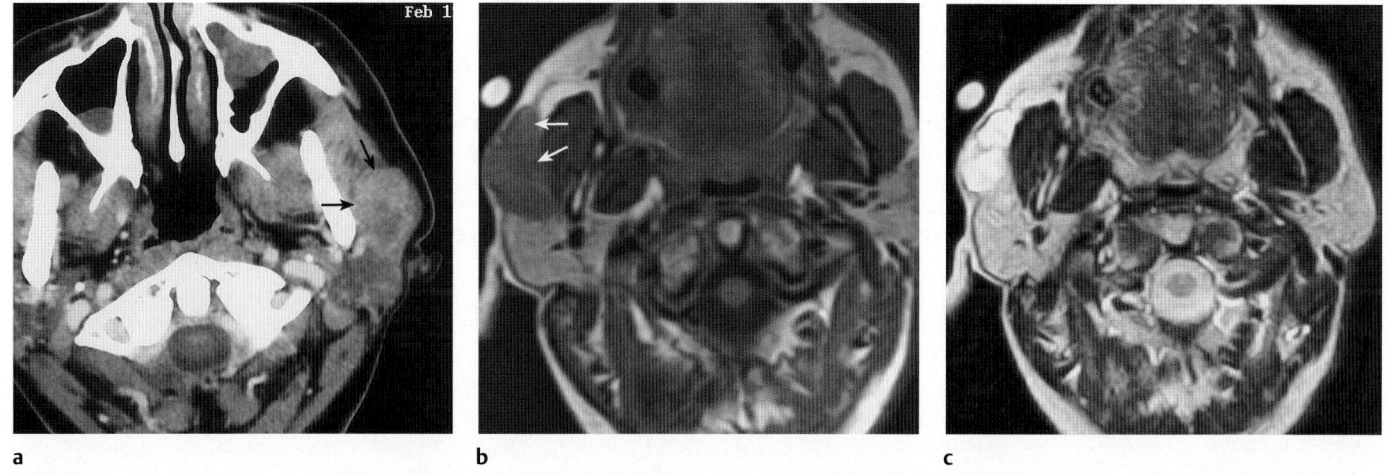

Fig. 9.**80** **a** Acinic cell carcinoma of the parotid gland. Enhanced CT scan shows a moderately enhancing mass (arrows), involving the superficial lobe of left parotid gland. **b**, **c** Myoepithelial carcinoma. **b** Axial T1W and **c** T2W MR scans in another patient, showing a mass (arrows) involving right parotid gland compatible with a myoepithelial carcinoma.

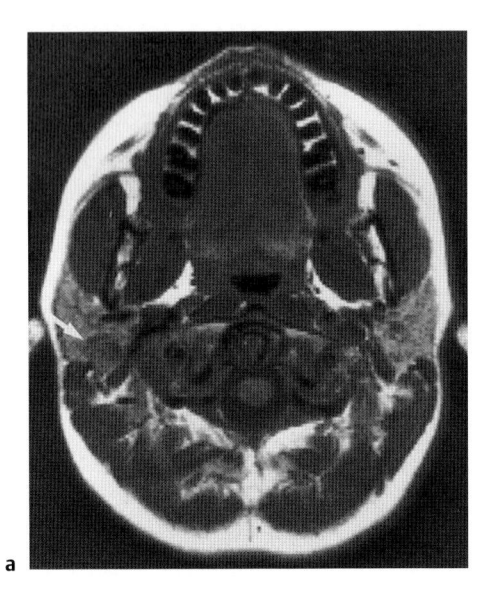

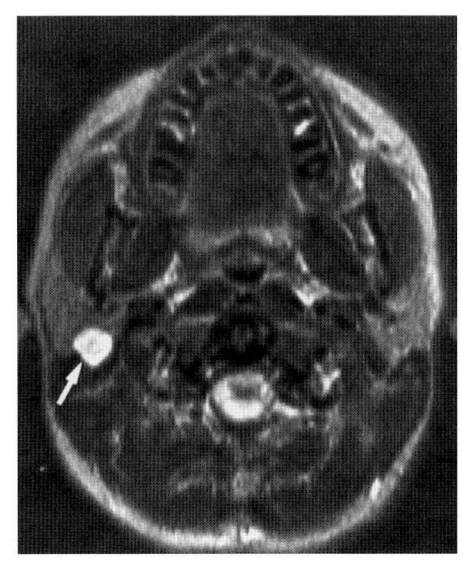

Fig. 9.81 Acinic cell carcinoma. **a** T1W and **b** T2W MR scans. A sharply defined tumor (arrow) is seen in the high posterior portion of the parotid gland with a somewhat low signal on the T1W image (**a**) and a bright signal on the T2W image (**b**). From Reference 1.

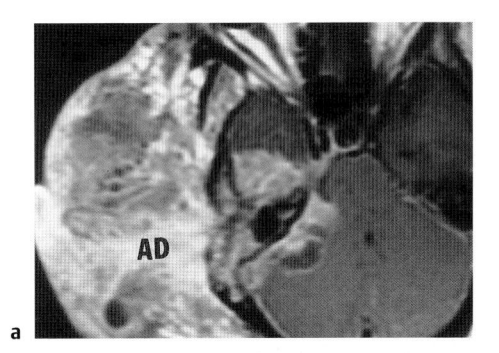

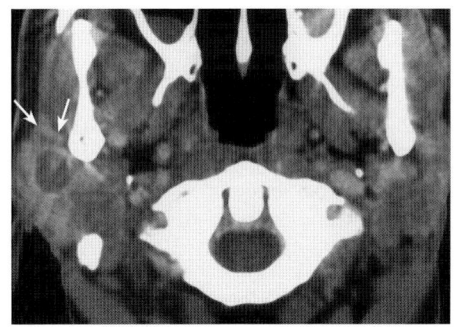

Fig. 9.82 a Undifferentiated adenocarcinoma in a 25-year-old woman. Enhanced T1W MR scan, showing an extensive right parotid mass. Note extension of this aggressive parotid adenocarcinoma (AD) into the temporal bone and cranial cavity. **b** Adenocarcinoma of the parotid gland. Axial enhanced CT scan in another patient shows a poorly defined mass (arrows) with a cystic component involving the right parotid gland, compatible with an adenocarcinoma.

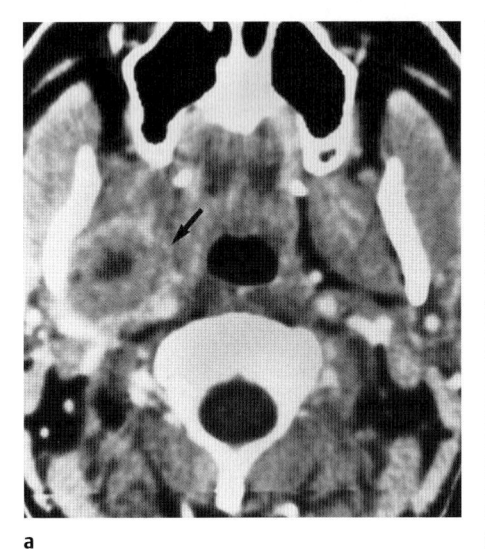

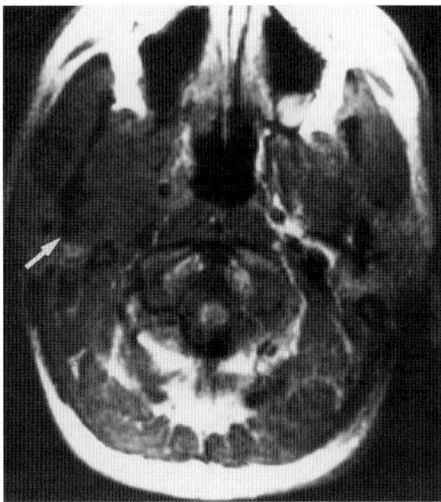

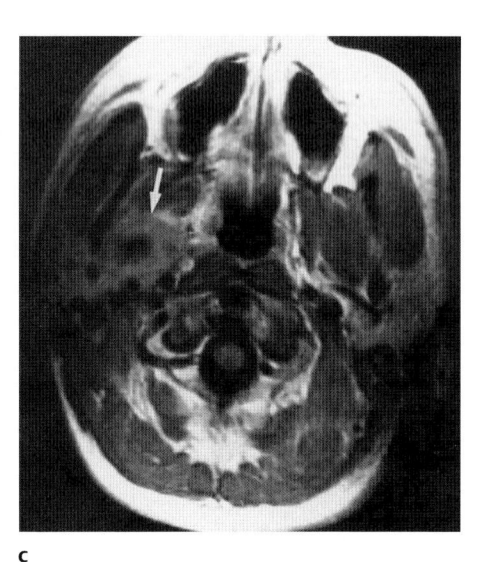

Fig. 9.83 Carcinoma ex-pleomorphic adenoma. **a** Contrast-enhanced CT scan, **b** T1W pre–gadolinium enhancement MR image, **c** T1W post–gadolinium enhancement MR image.

Fig. 9.83 d–f ▷

to high-risk adenocarcinomas. The most common high-risk salivary neoplasms include high-grade mucoepidermoid carcinomas (Fig. 9.78), undifferentiated carcinomas (Fig. 9.82), adenocarcinomas, squamous cell carcinomas, and salivary duct carcinoma (Table 9.5). In contrast to benign and low-grade malignant neoplasms, these lesions are highly cellular, form solid nests of cells, have high nuclear-to-cytoplasmic ratios, and contain minimal or no serous and mucoid material. These lesions exhibit more local invasion, lymph node metastasis, and perineural invasion.[3,4]

As previously discussed, high-grade neoplasms, in contrast to benign and low-grade malignant neoplasms, have low signal

d **e** **f**

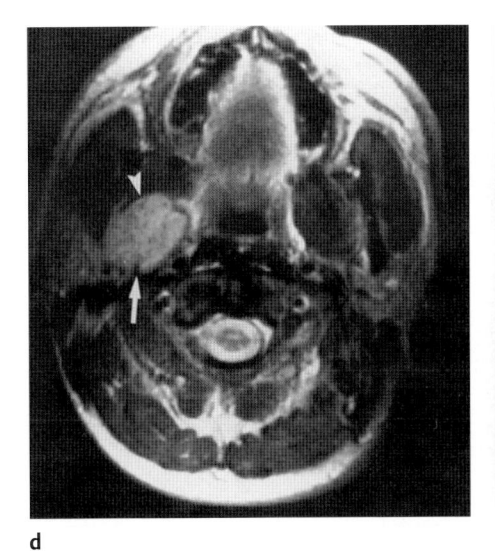

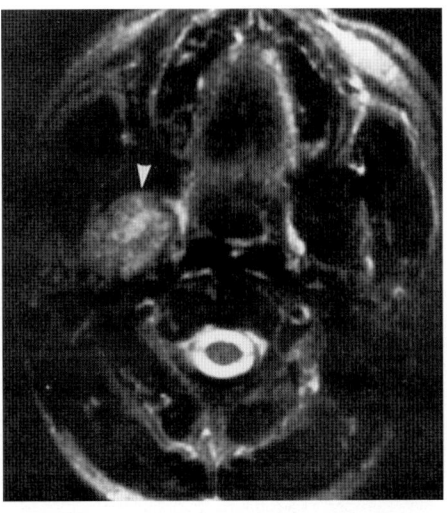

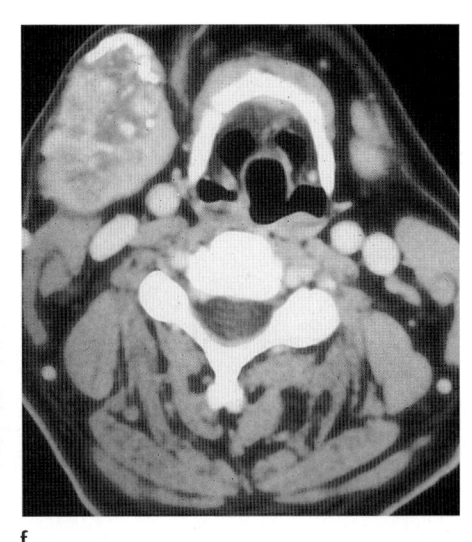

Fig. 9.83 d–f **d** Proton-weighted MR, and **e** T2W MR scans. This tumor (arrow) arising from the deep portion of the parotid enhances somewhat with gadolinium (**c**) and has fuzzy borders on CT (**a**) but sharply defined borders on MR (**c–e**). The patient presented with TMJ symptoms, had a normal TMJ MR study, and was later found to have this tumor encroaching on the parapharyngeal space and the medial pterygoid muscle (arrowhead). **f** Enhanced CT scan in another patient shows a mass involving right submandibular gland, compatible with malignant ex-pleomorphic adenoma. Figs. 9.83 a–e from Reference 1.

intensity on T1-weighted and relatively low signal intensity on T2-weighted images.[2,48] Therefore the identification of low signal intensity within a mass, regardless of clinical presentation and tumoral margins, should result in suspicion of a possible aggressive malignancy.[48] However, some aggressive tumors may be hyperintense on T2-weighted MR images (Fig. 9.**78**).

Malignant mixed salivary tumors are rare, accounting for 2–10% of all mixed salivary tumors (Fig. 9.**83**). Metastasis is usually to the lung. Bone metastases from malignant mixed tumors have been reported. Malignant parotid gland tumors are rare in the first two decades of life but may occur more often among patients who have received radiation therapy and/or chemotherapy.

Adenoid Cystic Tumors

Adenoid cystic carcinomas represent approximately 12% of all malignant salivary gland tumors. Adenoid cystic carcinomas (cylindromatous carcinoma) are uncommon in the parotid gland (Fig. 9.**84**), but are the most common malignant neoplasms that arise from the minor salivary, submandibular, and sublingual glands (Figs. 9.**85**–9.**87**). This tumor may also arise in the lacrimal gland (50% of all lacrimal gland neoplasm) as well as ceruminal

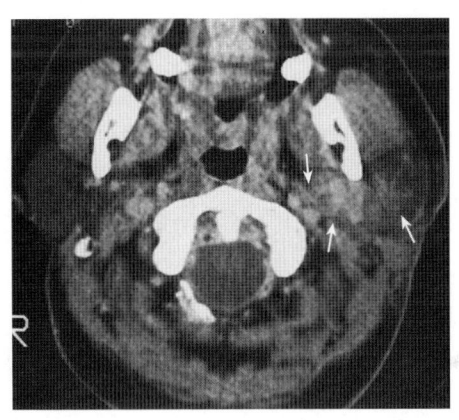

Fig. 9.**84** Adenoid cystic carcinoma of parotid gland with facial paralysis. Axial enhanced CT scan shows infiltration and enlargement of the left parotid gland, including the deep lobe, by a nonhomogeneous mass (arrows). This lesion was not palpable clinically.

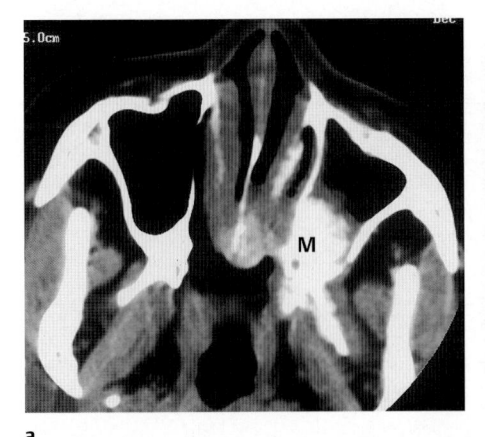

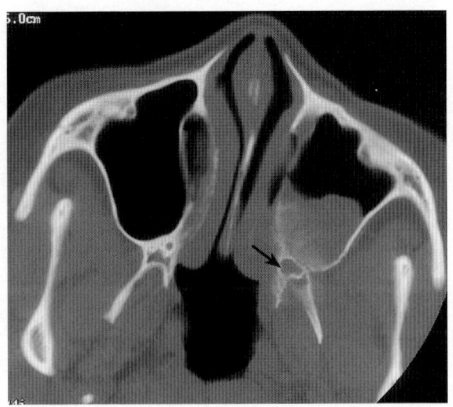

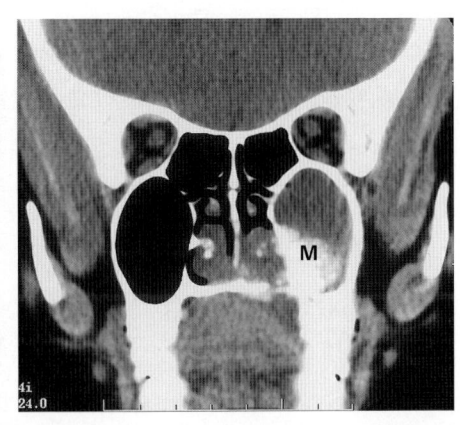

a **b** **c**

Fig. 9.**85** Adenoid cystic carcinoma of minor salivary gland with perineural extension. **a** Axial CT scan shows a partially calcified mass (M) in the posterior left maxillary sinus. **b** Axial CT scan shows enlargement of the greater palatine foramen (arrow) due to perineural extension. **c** Coronal CT scan, showing the mass (M). Note erosion of adjacent hard palate. This mass has arisen either from the minor salivary gland of the mucosa of the maxillary sinus or from the hard palate.

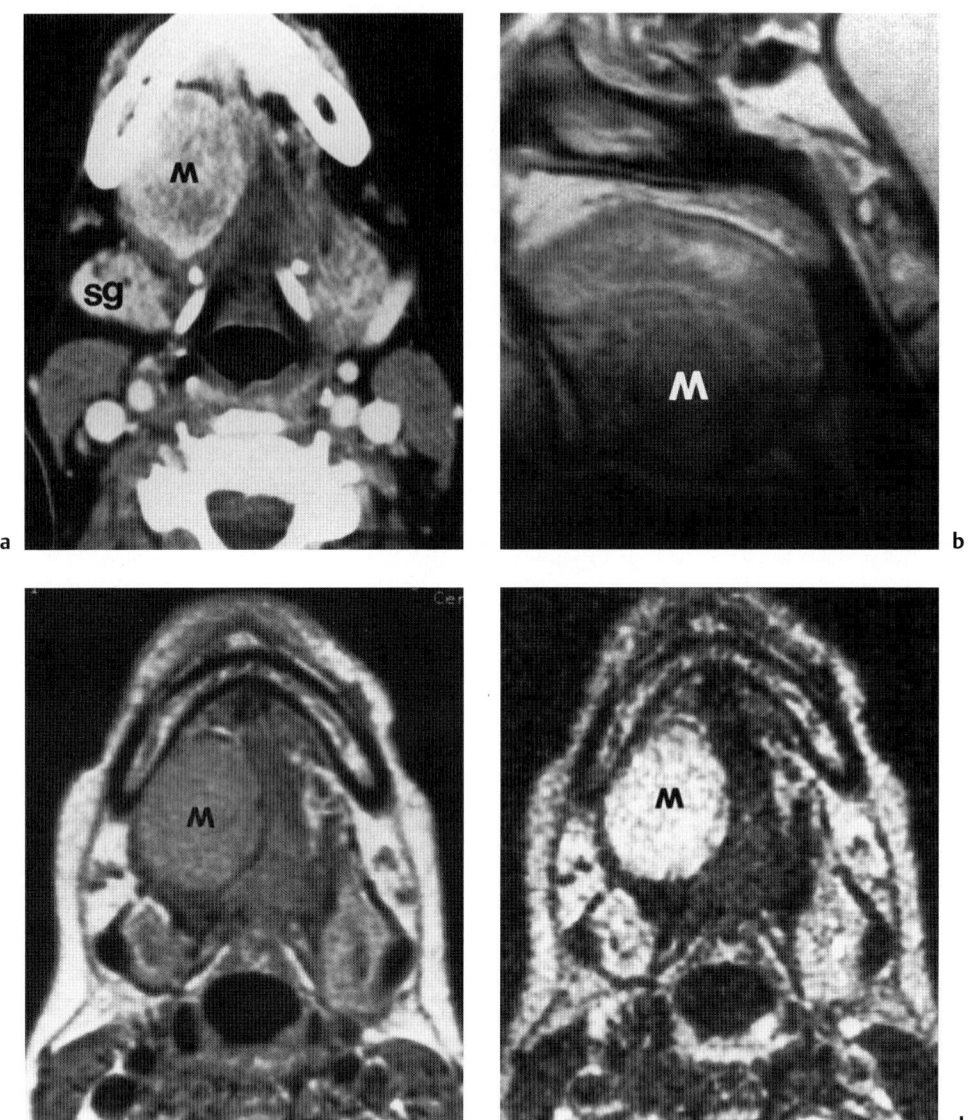

Fig. 9.**86** Adenoid cystic carcinoma of minor salivary gland of the floor of the mouth. **a** Contrast-enhanced axial CT scan shows a large enhancing mass (M) anterior to the submandibular gland (sg). **b** Sagittal T1W, **c** axial spin-density-weighted, and **d** axial T2W MR scans show a large mass (M) in the floor of the mouth. The mass is hypointense to muscle in T1W, isointense to muscle in spin-density-weighted, and hyperintense in T2W MR images.

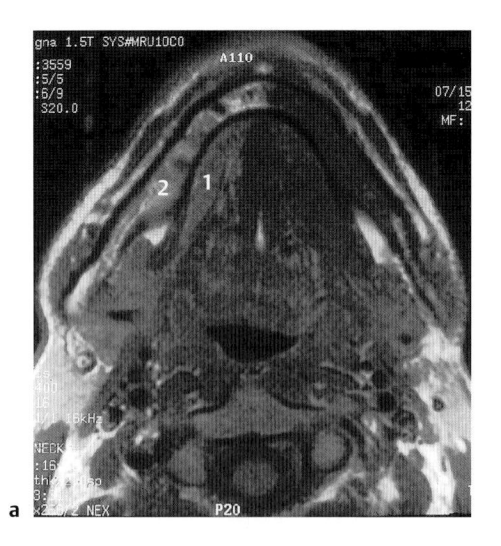

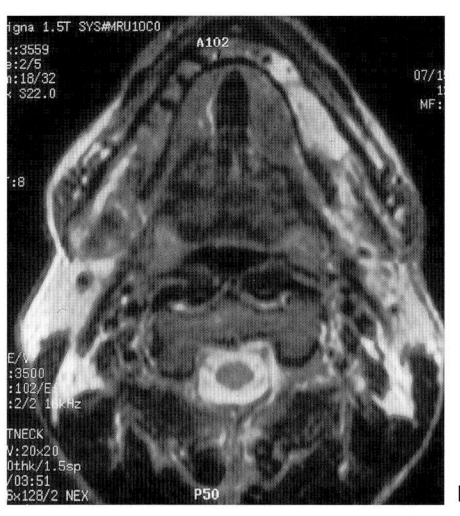

Fig. 9.**87** Adenoid cystic carcinoma of the left sublingual gland with perineural extension. **a** Axial T1W and **b** T2W MR scans, showing enlargement as well as signal alteration of the left sublingual gland. Note perineural extension along the mandibular inferior alveolar nerve as depicted by signal alteration of the left mandibular marrow.
1 = Normal right sublingual gland
2 = Normal right mandible

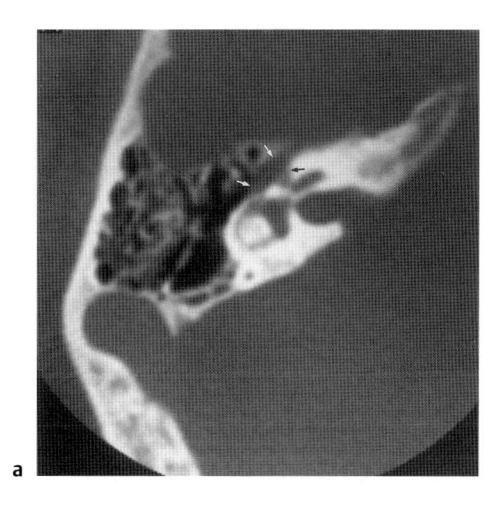

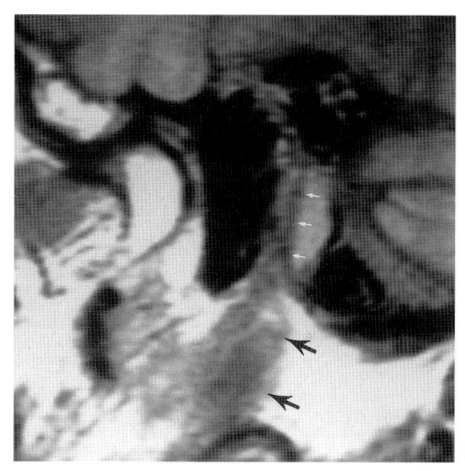

Fig. 9.88 Adenoid cystic carcinoma of the parotid in a patient with a two-year history of facial palsy related to carcinoma of the parotid tumor. **a** CT scan shows enlarged facial nerve canal (arrows). **b** Sagittal T1W MR scan shows an irregular mass in the parotid (large arrows). Note perineural extension along the facial nerve (small arrows). The parotid tumor was diagnosed on MR scan, and confirmed by surgery.

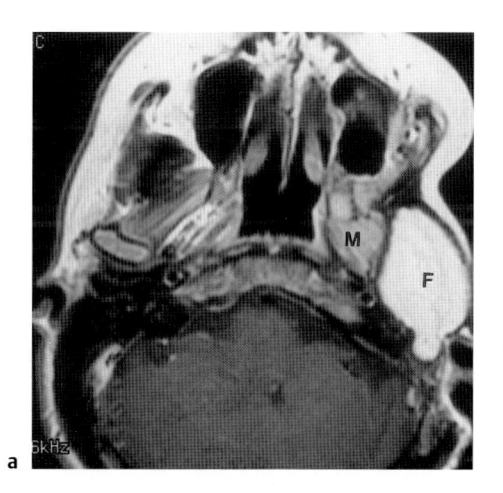

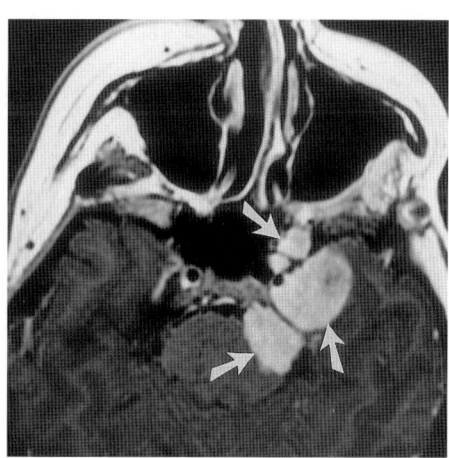

Fig. 9.89 Adenoid cystic carcinoma and perineural extension of the tumor. **a** Enhanced axial T1W MR scan shows fat (F) in the surgical bed of the parotid gland resected years age for an adenoid cystic carcinoma. Note abnormal mass with enhancement in the left parapharyngeal space (M). **b** Enhanced axial T1W MR scan shows tumor enhancement (arrows) along the fifth cranial nerve.

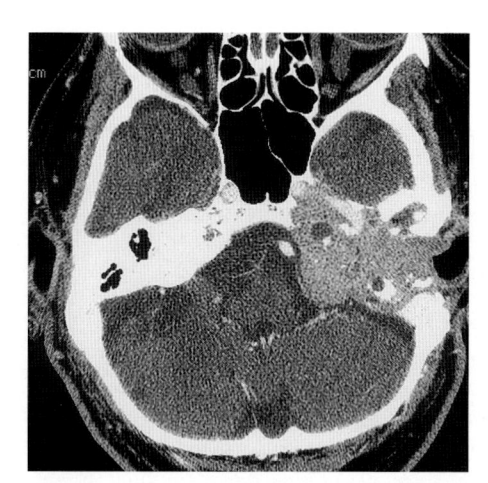

Fig. 9.90 Total replacement of petrous bone due to an adenoid cystic carcinoma of the parotid gland. CT scan shows tumor replacement of the left petromastoid bone.

glands of the external ear canal and upper airways.[8] The tumor is also variously named as adenocystic adenocarcinoma, cylindroma, pseudoadenomatous basal cell carcinoma, and adenocarcinoma.[5,51] It occurs most frequently from the minor salivary gland and commonly occurs in women of early middle age (Figs. 9.**85**–9.**87**). Adenoid cystic carcinoma may show irregular calcification and sometimes changes that may simulate osteogenic sarcoma (Fig. 9.**85**). Pain is common and may be a prominent symptom. The mass grows slowly and encapsulation of the lesion is not common. An important feature of adenoid cystic carcinomas is their strong tendency to invade the perineural lymphatics and perivascular space,[1–5,51] which can be observed at the time or long after the primary lesion is removed (Figs. 9.**68**, 9.**87**, 9.**88**, 9.**89**). Perineural and endoneural tumor spread occurs from adenoid cystic carcinoma of the major and minor salivary glands as well as squamous cancer of facial skin. Direct extension as well as perineural extension of adenoid cystic tumor of the parotid gland may result in total replacement of temporal bone (Fig. 9.**90**). Adenoid cystic carcinoma (Fig. 9.**91**) and other adenocarcinomas of salivary gland origin such as acinic cell carcinoma (Fig. 9.**92**) may originate from major or minor salivary glands or, in rare cases, from ectopic salivary gland tissue within the cervical lymph nodes. These lesions often appear infiltrative and may demonstrate minimal enhancement on enhanced CT and MRI scans (Figs. 9.**91**, 9.**92**), mimicking a cystic lesion such as plunging ranula (Fig. 9.**92**). The histological appearance of adenoid cystic carcinoma includes an eosinophilic hyaline to mucinous myxoid stroma arranged with characteristic small basaloid cells that form cylindrical or other shapes.[5,51] Lymph node spread is usually by direct extension rather than via lymphatics.[51] More common spread is by the bloodstream to liver, lungs, brain, and bone. The primary treatment of this tumor is radical removal of tumor. Adenoid cystic carcinoma may grow slowly from months to years,

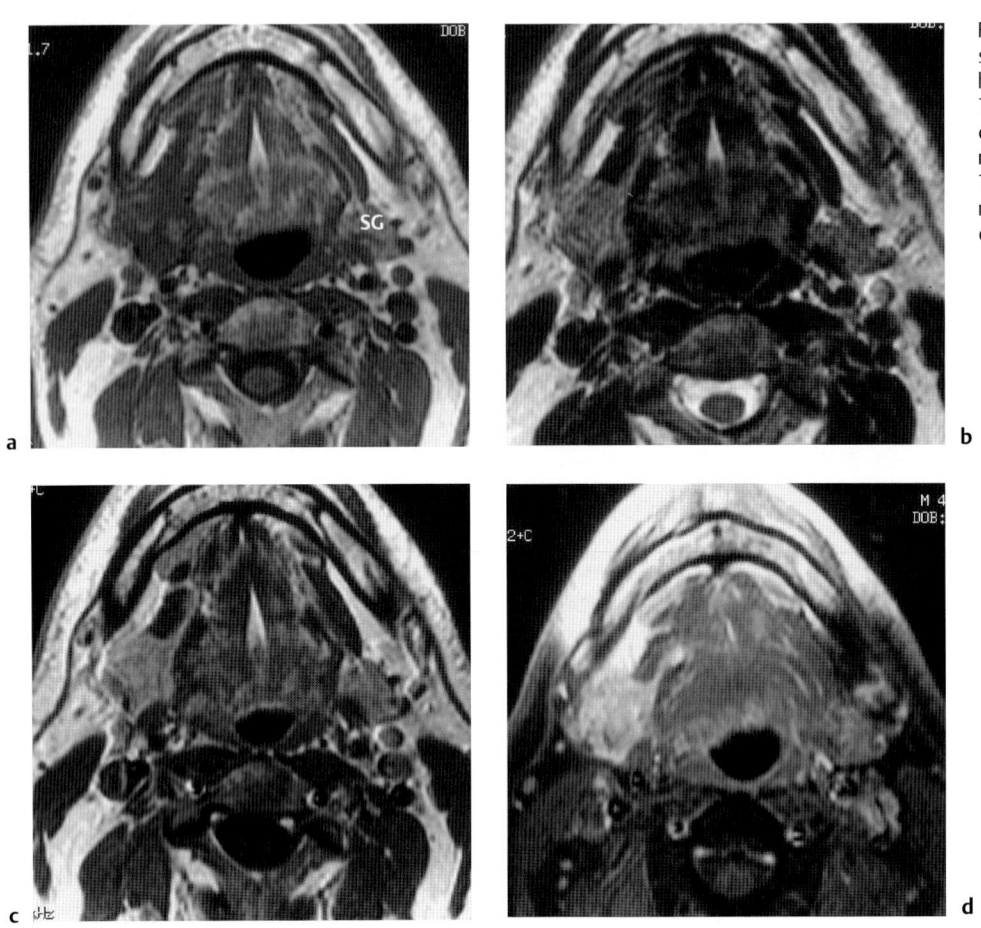

Fig. 9.**91** Adenoid cystic carcinoma of the submandibular gland. **a** T1W, **b** T2W, **c** enhanced T1W, and **d** enhanced fat-suppression T1W MR scans. Note normal left submandibular gland (SG) and enlargement of the right submandibular gland due to carcinoma. The appearance of this infiltrative tumor cannot be differentiated from a subacute or chronic inflammatory process.

eventually causing pain, tenderness, and fixation to skin and/or deeper structures including the facial nerve. The overall survival rate is reported to be 69%, and the 15-year survival rate 38%. The low signal on T2-weighted MR images correlates with the dense cellular tumors (Fig. 9.**91**) and with poor outcome. Distant metastases to lungs and bones are seen in 20–50% of cases.[1] The tumor may be sharply marginated (Fig. 9.**86**) or show poor margin along with invasion of adjacent structures (Figs. 9.**87**, 9.**91**).

Malignant Mixed Tumors

Although relatively uncommon, this group of tumors includes primary (true) malignant mixed cell tumor or carcinosarcoma and carcinoma ex-pleomorphic adenoma. Carcinoma ex-pleomorphic adenoma represents a carcinoma arising from or within a preexisting (primary or recurrent) pleomorphic adenoma.[8] Malignant mixed tumors account for approximately 7% of all malignant salivary neoplasms, 4–6% of all mixed tumors (benign and malignant combined), and 2–4% of all salivary gland neoplasms. They occur most commonly in parotid gland; they are uncommon in the minor salivary glands (Fig. 9.**83**).[1]

Acinic Cell Adenocarcinoma

Acinic cell adenocarcinoma is a low-grade malignant salivary gland neoplasm that represents approximately 18% of all malignant salivary gland neoplasms and 6.5% of all salivary gland neoplasms.[8] Tumor affects females more than males and occurs most frequently in the fourth and fifth decades of life. More than 90% arise in the parotid gland and have a 5-year survival rate of 82%, and 10-year survival rate of 68%.[1] Tumor may also be identified in the submandibular and sublingual glands (Fig. 9.**92**), as well as in minor salivary glands throughout the upper respiratory tract.[5]

In the pediatric age group, acinic cell adenocarcinoma represents the second most common malignant salivary gland neoplasm next to mucoepidermoid carcinoma (Table 9.**4**).[8] Bilateral parotid gland involvement may occur in up to 3% of cases.[5] Tumor is thought to arise from distal portions of the salivary duct system. Pathologically, tumor is well-demarcated or encapsulated, round or multilobulated. Most tumors have a homogeneous appearance, but may be cystic and hemorrhagic. On CT and MRI the tumor may be fairly well circumscribed (Figs. 9.**80a**, 9.**81**) or less defined and infiltrative (Fig. 9.**92**). The imaging characteristics of acinic cell carcinoma may not be differentiated from myoepithelial carcinoma (Fig. 9.**80b, c**) or other benign or malignant tumors (Figs. 9.**81**, 9.**82b**).

Primary Squamous Cell Carcinoma

Primary squamous cell carcinoma of the parotid gland is a rare tumor. The diagnosis is contingent on the absence of clinical or historical evidence of a squamous cell carcinoma in another head and neck site. Metastatic squamous cell carcinomas are more common than primary ones. Squamous cell carcinomas, adenocarcinomas, poorly differentiated carcinomas, and lymphoepithelial carcinomas have the imaging characteristics of high-grade malignant infiltrating tumors. Metastatic carcinoma and sarcoma must be considered in the differential diagnosis.[1,5]

Nonepithelial Neoplasms

Nonepithelial neoplasms arise from intraglandular or contiguous mesenchymal tissue elements and are less common than epithelial neoplasms.[1] Common nonepithelial neoplasms include hemangiomas (Figs. 9.**49**, 9.**50**), lipomas (Fig. 9.**93**), and

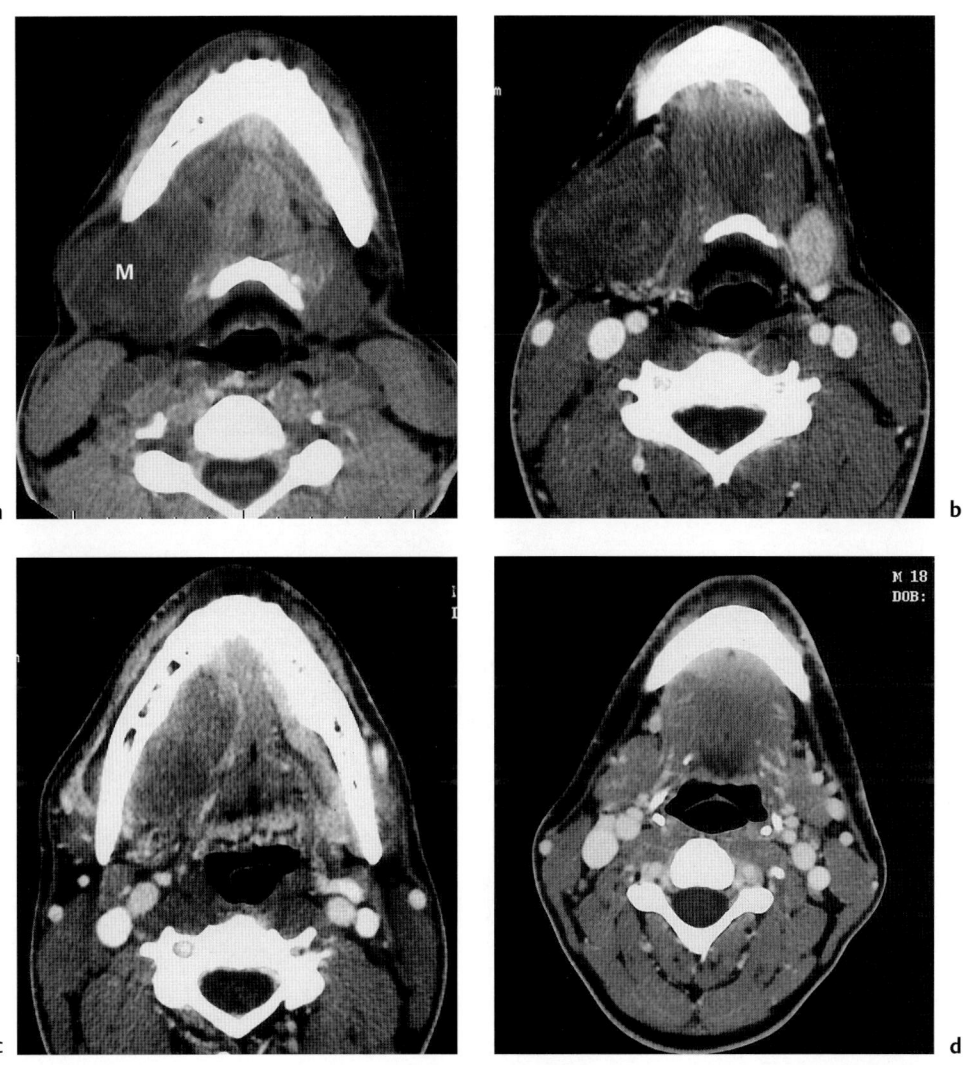

Fig. 9.**92** Acinic cell carcinoma. **a** Unenhanced CT scan, showing a submandibular space mass (M). **b** Enhanced CT scan shows mild enhancement within the mass. Note normal enhancement of the left submandibular gland. **c** Enhanced CT scan, showing extension of tumor along the floor of the mouth. The right jugulodigastric node is slightly enlarged. **d** Enhanced CT scan following surgery demonstrates normal submandibular glands. The right submandibular gland, which was compressed by tumor, could not be visualized on preoperative scans (**a**, **b**, **c**). This tumor is presumed to have arisen from ectopic salivary gland tissue, minor salivary glands, or the sublingual gland.

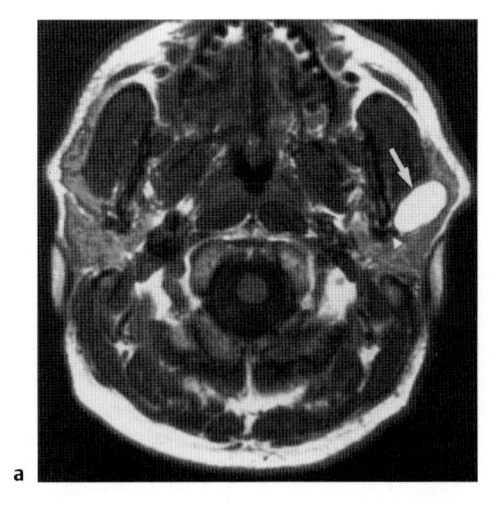

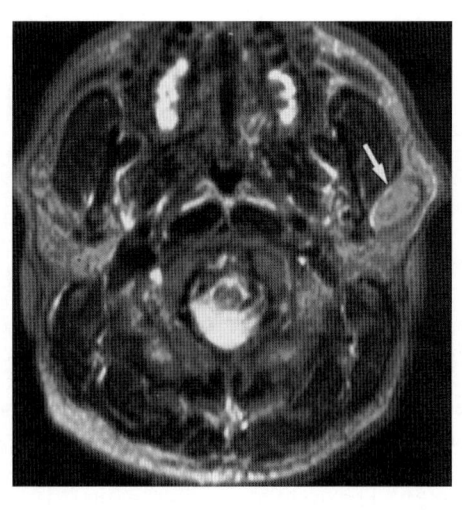

Fig. 9.**93** Lipoma of parotid gland. **a** T1W, **b** T2W MR scans. This benign, fat-containing tumor (arrows) is lateral to the retromandibular vein (arrowhead) and yet was found deep to the facial nerve. From Reference 1.

neurogenic tumors (Fig. 9.**61 c–e**).[1–5] Neurogenic tumors of the salivary glands are usually seen in middle-aged individuals; they frequently occur in the parotid gland and less often in the submandibular gland. In general, these lesions have low signal intensity on T1-weighted, intermediate signal intensity on proton density, and high signal intensity on T2-weighted MR images (Fig. 9.**61 c–e**). Scattered focal areas of low signal intensity may be related to dystrophic calcifications (rare), flow voids, or cystic changes. The presence of multicentric lesions is considered supportive evidence for neurofibromatosis.[3,5,51] Neurogenic tumors demonstrate moderate to marked contrast enhancement. It is not uncommon that part of the tumor shows less or no enhance-

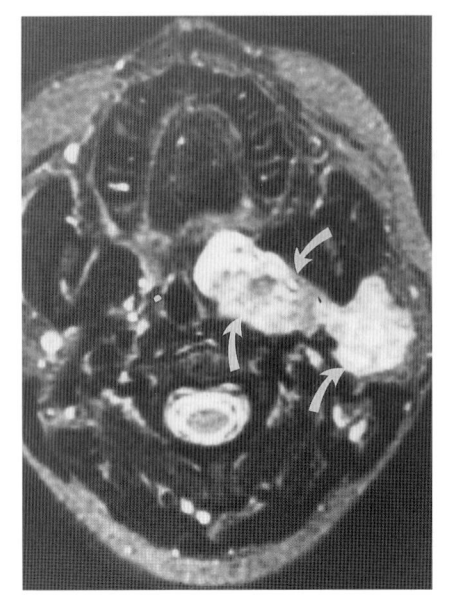

Fig. 9.**94** Liposarcoma of parotid gland. Axial T2W MR scan shows a hyperintense mass (arrows). This might not be differentiated from a malignant or large benign parotid tumor.

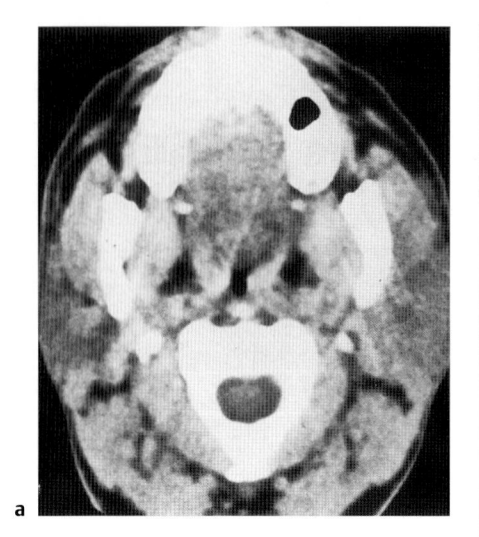

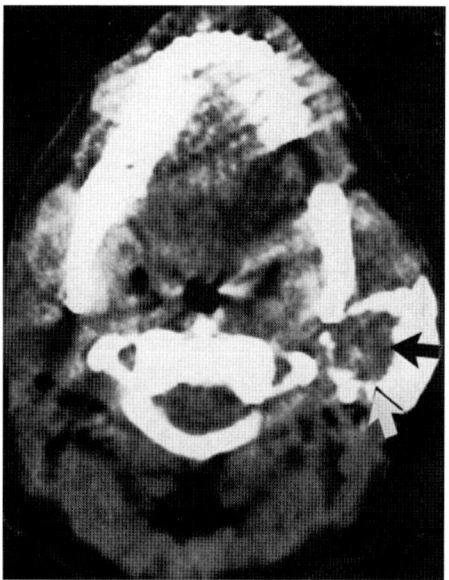

Fig. 9.**95** Sarcoma of the left parotid gland.
a Contrast-enhanced axial CT scan shows a nonspecific enlargement of the left parotid gland. The tumor is isodense with the remainder of the gland and, therefore, could easily be overlooked. There is effacement of the posterior aspect of the masseter muscle.
b CT sialogram outlines an irregular mass compatible with a sarcomatous lesion (arrows).

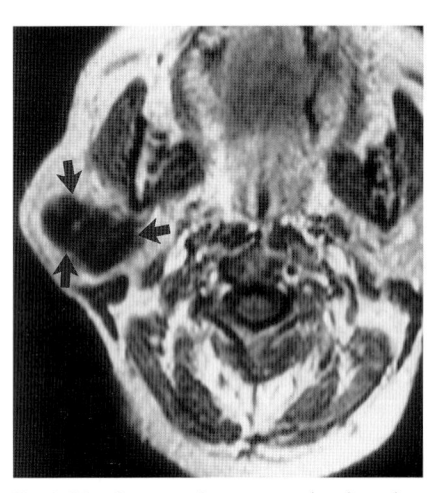

Fig. 9.**96** Osteogenic sarcoma developed in an ex-pleomorphic adenoma. Enhanced MR scan shows a hypointense mass (arrows) compatible with an osteogenic sarcoma. The hypointensity is related to tumor bone formation.

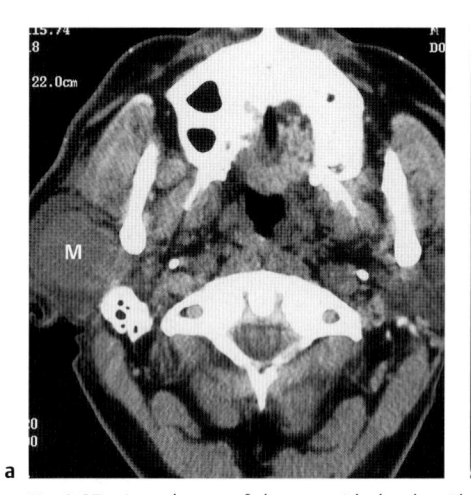

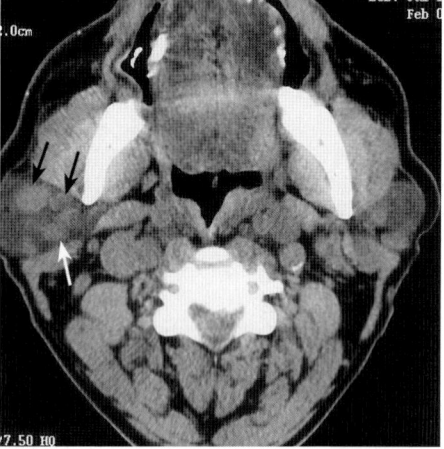

Fig. 9.**97** Lymphoma of the parotid gland. **a** Plain CT scan shows a large mass (M), involving the right parotid gland. **b** Plain CT scan shows multiple intraparotid masses (arrows), representing involved lymph nodes. There is an enlarged superficial node within the left parotid.

ment. Lipomas are less common but occur in all age groups. Lipomas, as well as neurofibromas, invade deeply into the intraglandular septa and have a tendency to recur.[4] The MR appearance is similar to fat, having high signal intensity on T1-weighted images and diminished signal intensity on T2-weighted images (Fig. 9.**93**).[7] Lipomas should not be confused with pleomorphic adenomas, which on rare occasions can contain fat.[66] Liposarcoma of the parotid gland may have similar CT and MR characteristics of malignant epithelial tumors (Fig. 9.**94**). Some of the sarcomas may be poorly delineated on plain as well as enhanced CT scans. At times, CT sialography may be performed to delineate the mass (Fig. 9.**95**). Other sarcomas (rhabdomyosarcomas, fibrohistiocytoma, fibrosarcomas, angiosarcoma, neurosarcomas, osteo/chondrosarcoma and synovial sarcomas) may arise in the major salivary glands (Fig. 9.**96**) (Table 9.**4**). Sarcomas can occur in all age groups but are more common in patients under 40 years of age. The MR signal intensities and morphological appearance of sarcomas are nonspecific, similar to those of the malignant tumors and lymphomas.[3,5,65]

Lymphoma

Primary malignant lymphomas arising from the salivary gland are rare, whereas secondary involvement is common. An increased incidence of malignant lymphomas is noted in chronic autoimmune sialadenitis, being 40 times higher in Sjögren syndrome than in the normal population.[2,5,51] Intraparotid lymph-

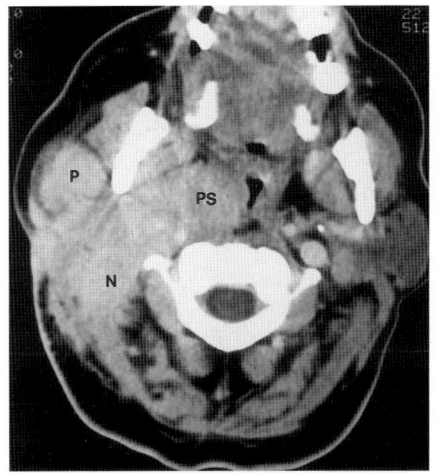

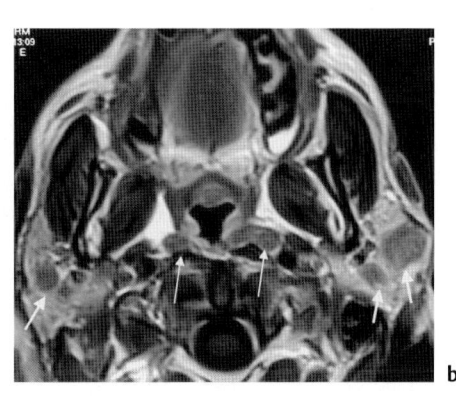

Fig. 9.98 a Lymphoma of the parotid gland. Enhanced CT scan shows an infiltrative process, involving the entire right parotid gland (P) with extension into the parapharyngeal space (PS). Note an enlarged node (N) and infiltration of extraparotid fascial planes as well as sternocleidomastoid muscle. b Non-Hodgin lymphoma with bilateral parotid gland involvement (arrows) and involvement of the retropharyngeal lymph nodes (thin arrows) in an HIV-positive patient, consistent with non-Hodgkin lymphoma. Case provided by M. Becker, MD.

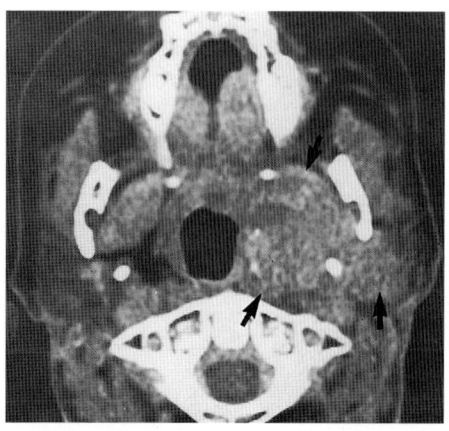

Fig. 9.99 Squamous cell carcinoma of the left tonsil. Contrast-enhanced axial CT scan shows a left tonsillar and parapharyngeal mass (arrows) infiltrating the left tonsillar and parotid gland.

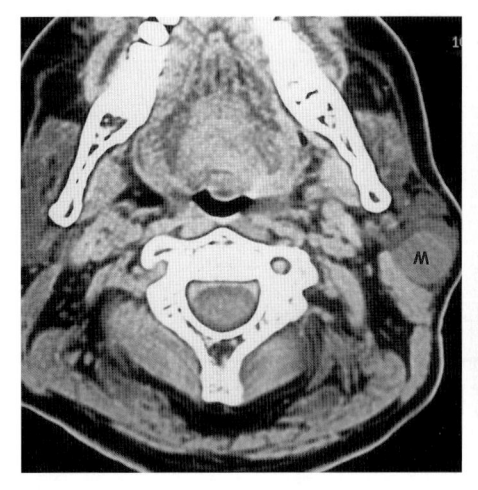

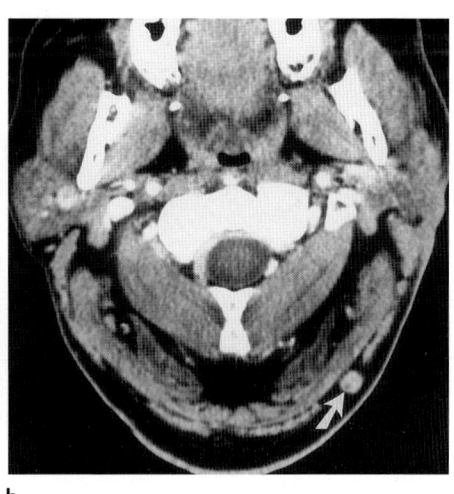

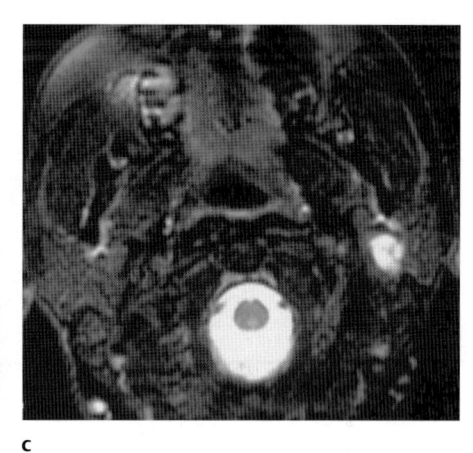

Fig. 9.100 Metastatic malignant melanoma. a CT scan shows a well-defined mass (M) involving the left parotid gland. Preoperative diagnosis was a benign mixed tumor. b CT scan at higher level shows a node (arrow) that was positive for metastasis. c Axial T2W MR scan in another patient shows a metastatic lymph node involving left parotid gland, from a primary Merkel cell tumor of the left cheek.

adenopathy may also be the result of lymphadenitis, tuberculosis, sarcoidosis, toxoplasmosis, HIV lymphadenitis, or metastatic disease.[2,4,5,51] Primary lymphoma of the parotid gland demonstrates moderate to high density on CT, and intermediate signal intensity on T1-weighted and decreased or increased signal intensity on T2-weighted MR images (Figs. 9.97, 9.98).[2] The lesion may appear well defined (Fig. 9.97) or diffuse and infiltrative (Fig. 9.98).

Metastasis

Metastatic disease or direct extension of head and neck carcinoma involving the salivary glands is not unusual (Fig. 9.99). Parotid glands removed for primary neoplasms reveal a 4% incidence of metastatic disease from a primary malignancy outside the parotid gland. The parotid gland is more susceptible to metastatic disease because of its extensive intercommunicating network of lymph nodes and vessels not found in other salivary glands. Cutaneous squamous cell carcinomas and melanomas account for the majority of lymphatic metastases to the parotid gland (Fig. 9.100). Less common hematogenous dissemination of metastatic disease from primary disease of the kidney (Fig. 9.101), prostate (Fig. 9.102), lung (Fig. 9.103), breast, and gastrointestinal tract has been reported.[4,7] Although metastatic tumors to the head and neck from the primary sites below the clavicles are uncommon, a significant number of these cases are from the urogenital tract.[74] The parotid metastasis may be the first clinical evidence of the primary tumor. The metastasis may only become apparent as a parotid mass more than 10 years after a nephrectomy.[74] Although parotid metastasis is a rare condition, one should be aware of the possibility when a clear cell neoplasm is disclosed in the parotid specimen or the patient has a history of renal cell carcinoma.[74] For solitary parotid metastasis, parotidectomy with facial nerve preservation should be considered a

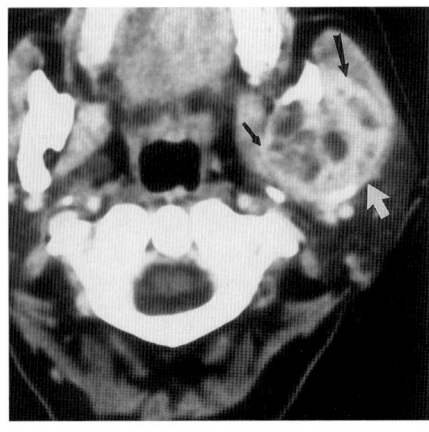

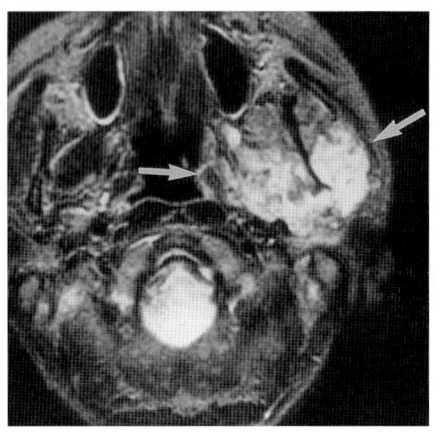

Fig. 9.**101** Metastatic hypernephroma to the mandible with involvement of the parotid space. **a** Axial enhanced CT scan shows a large partially necrotic mass (arrows) involving the mandible and adjacent masticator and parotid spaces. **b** T2W MR scan in another patient shows metastatic tumor involving parotid and masticator spaces.

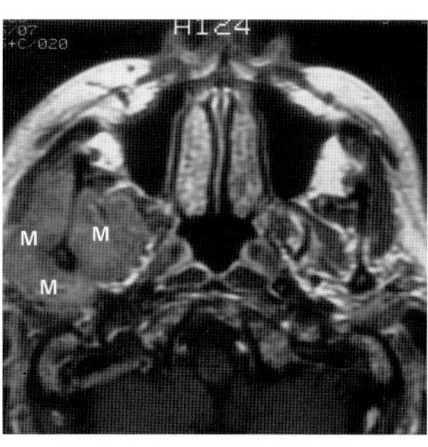

Fig. 9.**102** Metastatic prostate carcinoma to the mandible with involvement of the parotid and masticator spaces. Enhanced T1W MR scan shows a large mass (M) that involves the right parotid and masticator spaces.

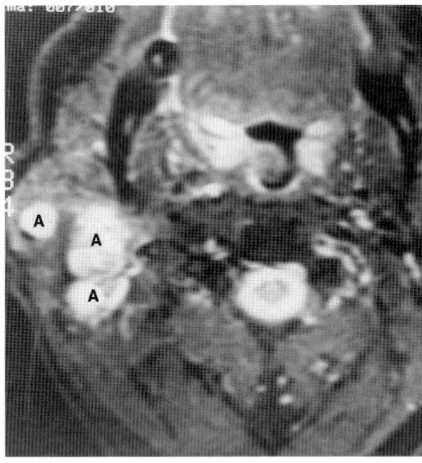

Fig. 9.**103** Parotid gland metastases from an undifferentiated adenocarcinoma of the lung. T2W MR scan shows enlargement of right parotid gland with large hyperintense metastatic adenocarcinoma (A). This might not be differentiated from a primary parotid undifferentiated carcinoma.

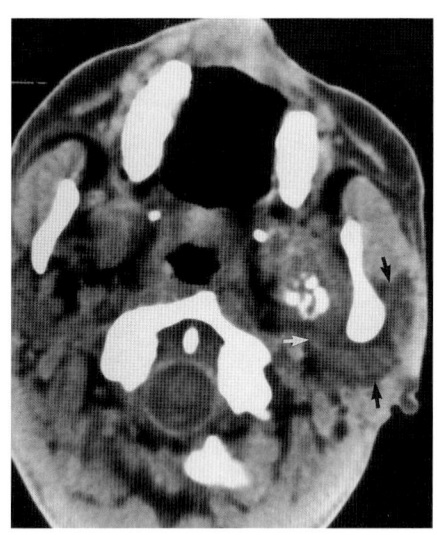

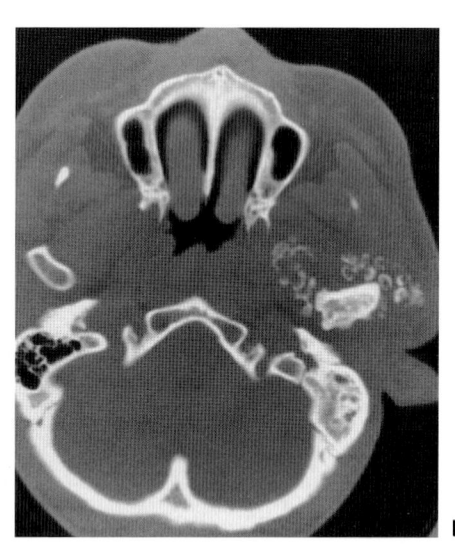

Fig. 9.**104** Synovial chondromatosis of the TMJ. **a** CT scan shows marked soft-tissue enlargement of the left TMJ and parotid region (arrows). Note calcification involving the pterygoid muscle. **b** CT scan shows multiple para-articular calcifications (loose bodies).

definitive therapeutic option.[74] Metastatic tumors to the mandible and temporomandibular disorders may clinically be mistaken for parotid masses (Figs. 9.**101**, 9.**102**, 9.**104**, 9.**105**).[77]

Miscellaneous Lesions

Synovial Chondromatosis

Lesions of the temporomandibular joint (TMJ) such as synovial chondromatosis may extend to involve the parotid space. Synovial chondromatosis is a rare, benign disorder characterized by metaplasia of the synovium with the formation of numerous foci of cellular hyaline cartilage. These foci may detach from the synovium and become loose bodies within the joint space, and also may calcify. Extra-articular extension can occur, simulating a parotid mass or a parapharyngeal mass.[75,76] CT may demonstrate multiple calcifications within the joint space as well as within the extracapsular component. MR may reveal striking expansion of the joint capsule as well as the loose bodies.[75] The presence of a large volume of fluid within the joint space can be confirmed by the T2-weighted as well as gradient-echo pulse sequences.[75] Delineation of the boundaries of the lesion is important owing to the proximity of vital structures and the possibility of extra-articular extension, of which several cases have been reported (Fig. 9.**104**).[75,76] Tumors of the TMJ and masticator space such as chondrosarcoma, chondromyxoid fibroma, synovial sarcoma, and malignant schwannoma, may extend to involve the parotid space (Fig. 9.**105**). Similarly, lesions of the external auditory canal such as necrotizing external otitis and squamous cell carcinoma of the ear can extend into the parotid space.

Metabolic and Endocrine-related Salivary Gland Disorders (Sialadenosis)

Sialadenosis, or sialosis, is a nonneoplastic, noninflammatory, parenchymatous disease of the salivary glands whose origin is based in metabolic and secretory disorders of the functional salivary parenchymas and which is clinically manifested by recurrent, painless swelling of the salivary glands, principally the

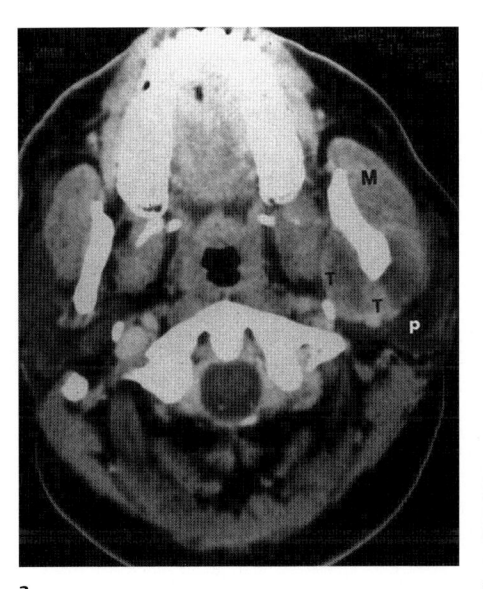

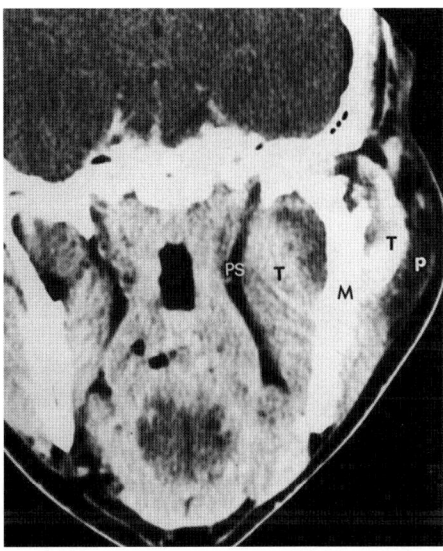

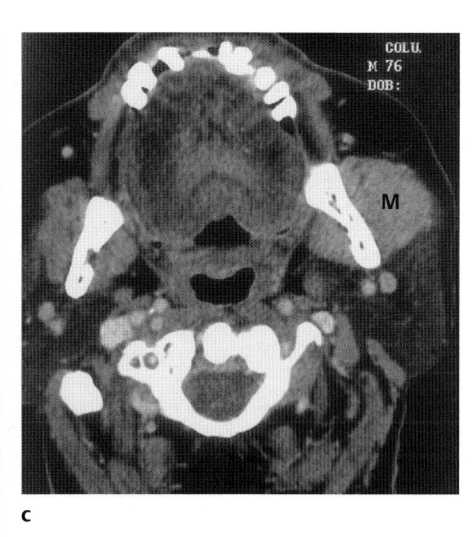

Fig. 9.**105 a, b** Malignant schwannoma of masticator space.
a Axial postcontrast CT scan shows a large retromandibular tumor (T); M = masseter muscle; p = parotid gland.
b Coronal postcontrast CT scan shows the malignant schwannoma within masticator space (T); M = mandible, p = parotid gland; PS = parapharyngeal space.

c Malignant fibrous histiocytoma of masticator space. Axial enhanced CT scan shows a moderately enhancing mass (M), involving the left masseter muscle, compatible with a malignant fibrous histiocytoma.

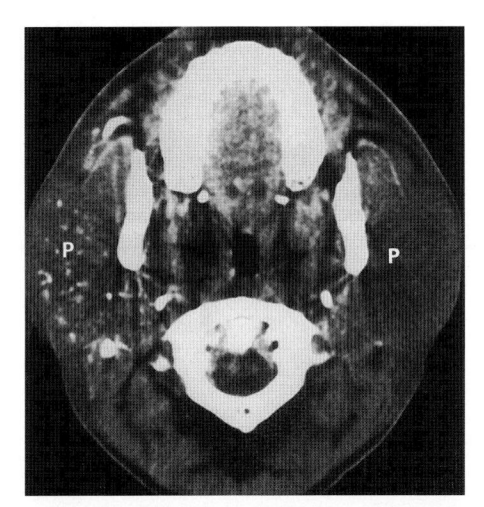

Fig. 9.**106** Metabolic sialadenitis. Axial CT scan in a diabetic patient shows enlargement of both parotid glands (P). The CT sialography on the patient's right parotid shows multiple irregular collections of contrast.

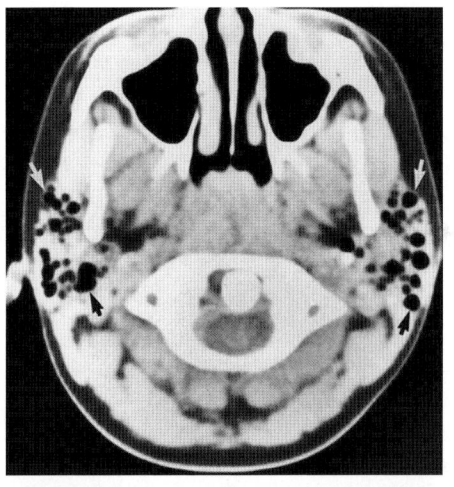

Fig. 9.**107** Pneumoparotitis. Contrast-enhanced CT scan. Multiple pockets of air (arrows) can be seen in both parotid glands in a child with recurrent swelling. The child had been shown to have recurrent sialadenitis. From Reference 1.

parotid.[7,8] Noninflammatory salivary gland enlargement has been associated with a variety of metabolic and endocrine disorders such as diabetes mellitus (Fig. 9.**106**), gout, celiac disease, vitamin deficiency, malnutrition, alcoholism, in children with cystic fibrosis, in dysfunction of the autonomic nervous system (neurogenic sialadenosis),[7] and in patients who take various medications, such as thiourea drugs, reserpine, phenylbutazone, heavy metals, etc.[1]

Kussmaul Disease

Inspissated mucus due to cystic fibrosis may result in ductal stenosis, microliths, and interstitial fibrosis, especially in the sublingual gland.[1] Kussmaul disease is an unusual cause of parotid or submandibular gland enlargement due to a mucous plug obstructing the duct seen in dehydrated or debilitated patients.[1]

Pneumoparotitis

Inflation of the parotid gland ducts by air has been reported in glass blowers, trumpet players, and malingerers.[1] Pneumoparotitis is demonstrable on plain film and on CT scans (Fig. 9.**107**).

(Special appreciation to Jacqueline Jamieson for transcription of this chapter.)

References

1. Carter BL. Salivary glands. In: Valvassori GE, Mafee MF, Carter BL, eds. Imaging of the Head and Neck. Stuttgart: Georg Thieme Verlag;1995: 475–509.
2. Som PM, Brandwein M. Salivary glands. In: Som PM, Curtin HD, eds. Head and Neck Imaging. St. Louis, MO: Mosby; 1996: 823–915.
3. Mafee MF. Oral cavity, oropharynx, upper neck and salivary glands. In: Valvassori GE, Buckingham RA, Carter BL, Hanafee WN, Mafee MF, eds. Head and Neck Imaging. Stuttgart: Georg Thieme Verlag; 1988: 253–309.
4. Mafee MF. Imaging of the oral cavity, pharynx, larynx, trachea, salivary glands, and neck. In: Ballenger JJ, Snow JB, eds. Ballanger's Otorhinolaryngology Head and Neck Surgery, Chapter 5a. Ontario, Canada: BC Decker; 2002; 1353–1391.
5. Mafee MF, Venkatesan TK, Ameli N, et al. Tumors of parotid gland and parapharyngeal space: role of CT and MRI. Oper Techn Otolaryngol Head Neck Surg 1996; 7(4): 348–357.
6. Ghaney DO, Jacobs JR, Kern R. Salivary Glands; Anatomy. In: Cummings CW, Fredrickson JM, Harker LA, Krause CJ, Schuller DE, eds. Otolaryngology Head and Neck Surgery. St. Louis, MO: Mosby-Year Book; 1993: 977–985.
7. Batsakis JG. Salivary glands; physiology. In: Cummings CW, Fredrickson JM, Harker LA, Krause CJ, Schuller DE, eds. Otolaryngology Head and Neck Surgery. St. Louis, MO: Mosby-Year Book; 1993: 986–996.
8. Wenig BM, ed. Atlas of Head and Neck Pathology. Philadelphia: W.B. Saunders; 1993.
9. Teresi LM, Kolin E, Luffkin RB, et al. MR imaging of the intraparotid facial nerve: normal anatomy and pathology. AJNR 1987; 8: 253.
10. Tabor EK and Curtin HD. MR of the salivary glands. Radiol Clin North Am 1989; 27(2): 379–392.
11. Olson KD. Tumors and surgery of the parapharyngeal space. Laryngoscope 1994; 104 (Supp.): 1–28.
12. Kim RH, Strimling AM, Grosch T, et al. Nonoperative removal of sialoliths and sialodochoplasty of salivary duct strictures. Arch Otolaryngol Head Neck Surg 1996; 122: 974–976.
13. Olsen RD, Maragos NE, Weiland LH. First branchial cleft anomalies. Laryngoscope 1980; 90: 423–436.
14. Seifert G, Thomson ST, Donath K. Bilateral dysgenetic polycystic parotid glands. Virchows Arch. Pathol Anat 1981; 390: 273–288.
15. Lomas DJ, Carroll NR, Johnson G, Antoun NM, Freer CE. MR sialography. Work in progress. Radiology 1996; 200: 129–133.
16. Murakami R, Baba Y, Nishimura R, et al. MR sialography using half-Fourier acquisition single-shot turbo spin-echo (HASTE) sequences. AJNR 1998; 19: 959–961.
17. Jungehülsing M, Fischbach R, Schröder U, et al. Imaging case study of the month: MR sialography. Ann Otol Rhinol Laryngol 1998; 107: 530–535.
18. Takashima S, Takeuchi N, Morimoto S, et al. MR imaging of Sjögren syndrome: correlation with sialography and pathology. J Comput Assist Tomogr 1991; 393–400.
19. Tonami H, Ogawa Y, Matoba MI, et al. MR sialography in patients with Sjögren's syndrome. AJNR 1998; 19: 1199–1203.
20. Jager L, Menauer F, Holzknecht N, Scholz V, Grevers G, Reiser M. Sialolithiasis: MR sialography of the submandibular duct—an alternative to conventional sialography and US? Radiology 2000; 216: 665–671.
21. Becker M; Marchal F; Becker CD, et al. Sialolithiasis and salivary ductal stenosis: diagnostic accuracy of MR sialography with a three-dimensional extended-phase conjugate-symmetry rapid spin-echo sequence. Radiology 2000; 217: 347–358.
22. Lev MH, Khanduja K, Norris P, Curtin HD. Parotid pleomorphic adenomas: delayed CT enhancement. AJNR 1998; 19: 1835–1839.
23. Sharafuddin MJA, Diemer DP, Levine RS, Thomasson JL, Williams AL. A Comparison of MR sequences for lesions of the parotid gland. AJNR 1995; 16: 1895–1902.
24. Casselman JW, Mancuso AA. Major salivary gland masses: comparison of MR imaging and CT. Radiology 1987; 165: 183.
25. Mandelblatt SM, Braun IF, and Davis PC: Parotid Masses: MR imaging. Radiology 1987; 163: 411.
26. George CD, Ng YY, Hall-Craggs MA, Jones BM. Parotid haemangioma in infants: MR imaging at 1.5 T. Pediatr Radiol 1991; 21: 483–485.
27. Thibault F, Halimi P, Bely N, et al. Internal architecture of the parotid gland at MR imaging: facial nerve or ductal system? Radiology 1993; 188: 701–704; discussion 705.
28. Cunningham MJ. The management of congenital neck masses. Am J Otolaryngol 1992; 13(2): 78–92.
29. Ho S, Lee D, Bluestone C. Imaging Quiz Case 2: First branchial cleft cyst. Arch Otolaryngol Head Neck Surg 2000; 126: 793–797.
30. Siegel MJ, Glazer HS, St Amour TE, et al. Lymphangiomas in children: MR imaging. Radiology 1989; 170: 467.
31. Baumgartner BJ, Sorensen DM, Willard CC, et al. Pathology Quiz Care. Sarcoidosis of the parotid glands. Arch Otolaryngol Head Neck Surg 2002; 128: 195–196.
32. Newman LS, Rose CS, Maier LA. Sarcoidosis. N Engl J Med 1997; 336: 1224–1234.
33. Som PM, Shugar JM, Biller HF. Parotid gland sarcoidosis and the CT sialogram. J Comput Assist Tomogr 1981; 5: 674–677.
34. Som PM, Biller HF. Kimura disease involving parotid gland and cervical nodes. CT and MR findings. J Comput Assist Tomogr 1992; 16: 320–322.
35. Marchal F, Kurt AM, Dulguerov P, Lechman W. Retrograde theory in sialolithiasis formation. Arch Otolaryngol Head Neck Surg 2001; 127: 66–68.
36. Ashby RA. The chemistry of sialoliths: stones and their homes. In: Norman JED, McGurk M, eds. Color Atlas and Text of the Salivary Glands. Diseases Disorders and Surgery. London, UK: Mosby-Wolfe 1995; 243–251.
37. Bernier JL, Bhaskar SN. Lymphoepithelial lesions of salivary glands. Cancer 1958; 11: 1156–1178.
38. Holiday RA, Cohen WA, Schinella RA, et al. Benign lymphoepithelial parotid cyst and hyperplastic cervical adenopathy in AIDS-risk patients: a new CT appearance. Radiology 1988; 168: 439.
39. Shugaar JM, Som PM, Jacobsen AL, et al. Multicentric parotid cysts and cervical adenopathy in AIDS patients: a newly recognized entity: CT and MR manifestations. Laryngoscope 1988; 98: 772.
40. Tunkel DE, Loury MC, Fox CH, et al. Bilateral parotid enlargement in HIV-seropositive patient. Laryngoscopy 1989; 99: 590.
41. Som PM, Brandwein MS, Silvers A. Nodal inclusion cysts of the parotid gland and parapharyngeal space: A discussion of lymphoepithelial, AIDS related parotid, and branchial cysts, Cystic Warthin's tumors, and cysts in Sjögren's syndrome. Laryngoscope 1995; 105: 1122–1128.
42. Elliott JN, Oertel YC. Lymphoepithelial cysts of the salivary glands. Am J Clin Pathol 1990; 93: 39–43.
43. Spath M, Kruger K, Dresel S, Grevers G, Vogl T, Schattenkirchner M. Magnetic resonance imaging of the parotid gland in patients with Sjögren's syndrome. J Rheumatol 1991; 18(9): 1372–1378.
44. Ohbayashi N, Yamada I, Yoshino N, Sasaki T. Sjögren syndrome: comparison of assessments with MR sialography and conventional sialography. Radiology 1998; 209: 683–688.
45. Ikeda K, Tasutoma K, H-Kawa S, et al. The usefulness of MR in establishing the diagnosis of parotid pleomorphic adenoma. AJNR 1996; 17: 555–559.
46. Brito Santos IR, Kowalski LP, Araujo VC, et al. Multivariate analysis of risk factors for neck metastases in surgically treated parotid carcinomas. Arch Otolaryngol Head Neck Surg 2001; 127: 56–60.
47. Urquhart A, Hutchins LG, Berg RL. Preoperative computed tomography scans for Parotid tumor evaluation. Laryngoscope 2001; 111: 1984–1988.
48. Som PM, Biller HF: High-grade malignancies of the parotid gland: identification with MR imaging, Radiology 1989; 173: 823–826.
49. Myssiorek D. Removal of the inferior half of the superficial lobe is sufficient to treat pleomorphic adenoma in the tail of the parotid gland. Arch Otolaryngol Head Neck Surg 1999; 125: 1164–1165.
50. Helmus C. Subtotal parotidectomy: A 10-year review (1985 to 1994). Laryngoscope 1997; 107: 1024–1027.
51. Kramer LA, Mafee MF. Salivary glands. In: Stark DD, Bradley WG, eds. Magnetic Resonance Imaging, 3rd ed. St. Louis: Mosby; 1999: 1771–1784.
52. Malherbe A, Chemantais J. Note Sur L'epithelioma calcific des glands sebacees. Prog Med 1880; 8: 826–828.
53. Forbis R, Helwig EB. Pilomatrixoma (calcified epithelioma). Arch Dermatol 1961; 83: 606–618.
54. Agarwal RP, Handler SD, Mathews MR, et al. Pilomatrixoma of the head and neck. Otolaryngol Head Neck Surg 2002; 125: 510–515.
55. Fink AM, Berkowitz RG. Sonography in preauricular pilomatrixoma of childhood. Ann Otol Rhinol Layngol 1997; 106: 167–169.
56. Seifert C, Sobin LH. The World Health Organization's histological classification of salivary gland tumors. Cancer 1992; 70: 379–386.
57. Amin KS, McGuff HS, Cashman SW, et al. Recurrent epithelial-myoepithelial carcinoma of the parotid with direct intracranial extension. Otolaryngol Head Neck Surg 2002; 126: 83–84.

58. Hamdan AI, Kahwagi G, Farhat F, Tawii A. Oncocytoma of the nasal septum: a rare cause of epistaxis. Otolaryngol Head Neck Surg 2002; 126: 440-441.
59. Auclair PL, Ellis GL. Mucoepidermoid carcinoma. In: Ellis GL, Auclair PL, Gnepp DR, eds. Surgical Pathology of the Salivary Glands. Philadelphia: W.B. Saunders; 1991: 269-298.
60. Eneroth CM. Facial nerve paralysis: A criterion of malignancy in parotid tumors. Arch Otolaryngol 1972; 95(4): 300-304.
61. Eneroth CM, Andreasson L, Beran M, et al. Preoperative facial paralysis in malignant parotid tumors. ORL J Otorhinolaryngol Relat Spec 1977; 39(5): 272-277.
62. Conley J, Hamaker RC. Prognosis of malignant tumors of the parotid gland with facial paralysis. Arch Otolaryngol 1975; 101: 39.
63. Rabinov K, Kell T, Gordon P. CT of the salivary glands. Radiol Clin North Am 1985; 22: 145-159.
64. Casselman JW, Mancuso AA. Major salivary gland masses: comparison of MR imaging and CT. Radiology 1987; 165: 183-189.
65. Lampe HB, Savoury L, Nicholson RL, et al. Evaluation of parotid lesions by magnetic resonance imaging, J Otolaryngol 1988; 17(4): 183.
66. Som PM, Braun IF, Shapiro MD, et al. Tumors of the parapharyngeal space and upper neck: MR imaging characteristics, Radiology 1987; 164: 823.
67. Som PM, Shugar JM, Sacher M, et al. Benign and malignant parotid pleomorphic adenomas: CT and MR studies, J Comput Assist Tomogr 1988; 12(1): 65.
68. Freling NJ, Molenaar WM, Vermey A, Mooyaart EL, Panders AK, Annyas AA, Thijn CJP. Malignant parotid tumors: clinical use of MR imaging and histologic correlation. Radiology 1992; 185: 691-696.
69. Mehle ME, Kraus DH, Wood BG, et al. Facial nerve morbidity following parotid surgery for benign disease: The Cleveland Clinic Foundation experience. Laryngoscope 1993; 103, 386-388.
70. Watanabe Y, Ishikawa M, Shojaku H, et al. Facial nerve palsy as a complication of parotid surgery and its prevention. Acta Otolaryngol (Stockh) 1993; Supp 504: 137-139.
71. Rinkel RNPM, Manni JJ, Quiz Care 2. Warthin tumor. Arch Otolaryngol Head Neck Surg 1999; 125: 1271-1273.
72. Minami M, Tanioka H, Oyama K, Ital Y, Eguchi M, Yoshikawa K, Murakami T, Sasaki. Warthin tumor of the parotid gland: MR-pathologic correlation. AJNR 1993; 14: 209-214.
73. Bocchini T, Graham A, Williams W, et al. Bilateral Warthin's tumor. Clin Nucl Med 1988; 13: 892.
74. Auclair PL, Ellis GL, Gnepp DR, Wing BM, Janney CG. Salivary gland neoplasms—general considerations. In: Ellis GL, Auclair PL, Gnepp DR, eds. Surgical Pathology of the Salivary Glands. Philadelphia: W.B. Saunders; 1991: 135-164.
75. Herzog S, Mafee MF. Synovial chondromatosis of the TMJ: MR and CT findings. AJNR 1990; 11: 742-745.
76. Klenoff JR, Lowlicht RA, Lesnik T, et al. Mandibular and temporomandibular joint arthropathy in the differential diagnosis of the parotid mass. Laryngoscope 2001; 111: 2162-2165.
77. Park YW, Hlivko TJ. Parotid gland metastasis from renal cells carcinoma. Laryngoscope 2002; 112: 453-456.

10 Oral Cavity and Oropharynx

M. Becker

Introduction

The main reasons for imaging the oral cavity and oropharynx are: (1) to evaluate and stage squamous cell carcinoma, as well as other non-squamous cell tumors; (2) to search for the site of an unknown head and neck primary in patients with metastatic nodal disease; (3) to image inflammatory and infectious diseases and their complications; and (4) to evaluate congenital/developmental lesions of this area. Diagnostic evaluation of the oral cavity and oropharynx is primarily done by clinical examination, endoscopy and clinically directed biopsy. While small oral cavity and oropharyngeal tumors are usually not imaged radiographically, sectional imaging will be performed in those cases where there is a clinical suspicion of deep invasion or metastatic disease or whenever the etiology of the lesion is not clear from the clinical presentation. In addition, because tumors in this area may spread submucosally without always disrupting the normal mucosa, sectional imaging may be extremely helpful in directing the endoscopist to the most promising site for biopsy, thus reducing the number of false-negative biopsies. In patients with suspected inflammatory or infectious diseases, imaging is mainly performed to assess potential complications, thereby assisting the otorhinolaryngologist or maxillofacial surgeon in making pertinent therapeutic decisions. Therefore, close cooperation between the otorhinolaryngologist, the maxillofacial surgeon, and the radiologist is required. Radiological diagnosis, however, requires a thorough knowledge of the relatively sophisticated anatomy of the region.

Developmental Considerations

The branchial or pharyngeal arches, which contribute to the formation of the head and neck, appear in the fourth and fifth weeks of development.[119b] They are separated from each other by branchial clefts. Simultaneously with the development of arches and clefts, the pharyngeal pouches appear along the lateral walls of the pharyngeal gut, which is the cranial portion of the primitive gut. At the end of the fourth week, the center of the face is formed by the stomodeum (depression of the surface ectoderm), which in turn is surrounded by the first pair of pharyngeal arches. At this point five mesenchymal swellings can be distinguished: two mandibular swellings (first pharyngeal arch), two maxillary swellings (dorsal portion of the first pharyngeal arch), and the frontal prominence (Fig. 10.1). Later the nasal swellings form (Fig. 10.1). Initially, the stomodeum is separated from the primitive pharynx by the oropharyngeal membrane. The membrane ruptures at 24–26 days, bringing the primitive gut into communication with the amniotic cavity.

Each branchial arch consists of mesenchyme and neural crest. This mesenchyme gives rise to muscles, cartilages, bone, and blood vessels, while the nerves grow into the arches from the brain.[119b]

The first branchial arch cartilage gives rise to the maxilla, zygomatic bone, parts of the temporal bone, and mandible. The musculature derived from the first pharyngeal arch includes the muscles of mastication, the anterior belly of the digastric muscle, the mylohyoid, the tensor tympani, and the tensor palatini muscle (see Normal Anatomy). Sometimes, the muscles of the different arches migrate into surrounding regions. Therefore, they do not always attach to the bony component of their own arch. However, the nerve supply of these muscles always comes from the arch of origin. The nerve supply to the muscles of the first arch is provided only by the mandibular branch of the trigeminal nerve which is the nerve of the first arch (see Normal Anatomy).

The second branchial arch cartilage gives rise to the stapes, the styloid process, the stylohyoid ligament, the lesser horn, and the upper part of the body of the hyoid bone. The muscles derived from the second pharyngeal arch include the stapedius, the stylohyoid, the posterior belly of the digastric muscle, and the muscles of facial expression. All these muscles are supplied by the facial nerve, which is the nerve of the second arch.

The cartilage of the third pharyngeal arch forms the lower part of the body and the greater horn of the hyoid bone. The muscles derived from the third arch include the stylopharyngeus muscle and the upper constrictor muscle. They are innervated by the glossopharyngeal nerve, which is the nerve of the third arch.

The epithelial lining of the second pharyngeal pouch forms buds, which in turn form the palatine tonsils. During the third to

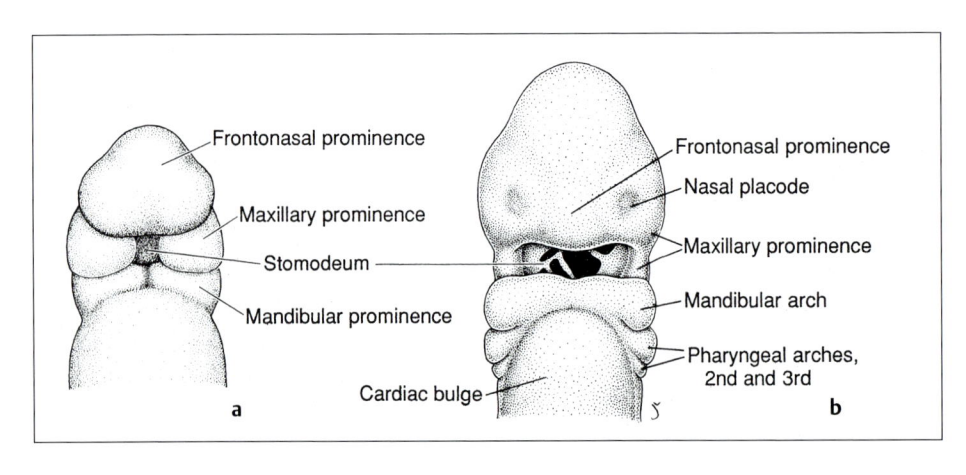

Fig. 10.1 **a** Frontal view of an embryo at about 24 days. The stomodeum, temporarily closed by the buccopharyngeal membrane, is surrounded by five mesenchymal swellings. **b** Frontal view of a slightly older embryo, showing the rupture of the buccopharyngeal membrane. Reproduced from Reference 119b with permission.

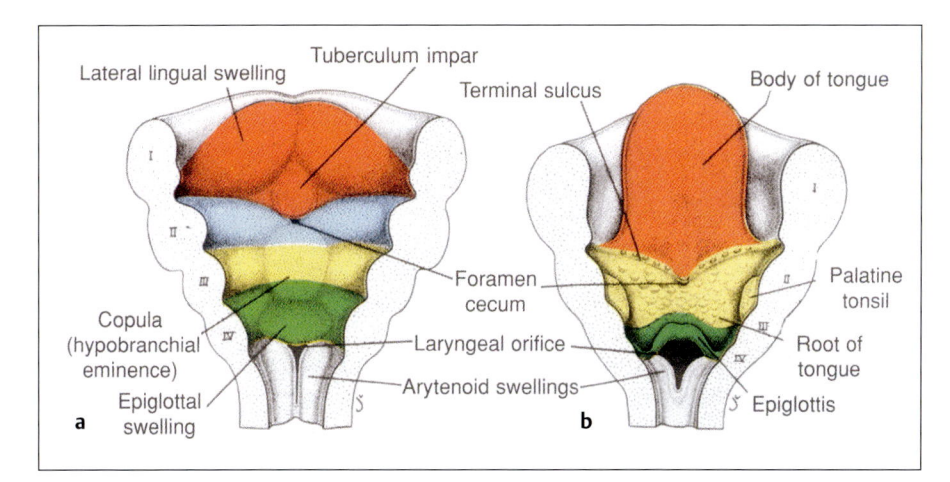

Fig. 10.2 The ventral portions of the pharyngeal arches seen from above, to show development of the tongue. The cut pharyngeal arches are indicated by numbers I to IV, respectively. **a** At 5 weeks. **b** At 5 months. Note the foramen cecum, the site of the thyroid primordium, and the terminal sulcus, which forms the dividing line between the first and second pharyngeal arches. Reproduced from Reference 119 b with permission.

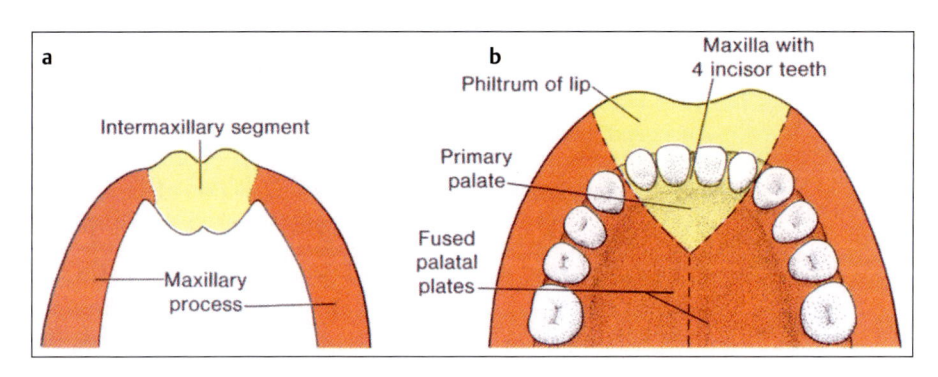

Fig. 10.3 **a** Schematic drawing of the intermaxillary segment and maxillary processes. **b** The intermaxillary segment gives rise to the philtrum of the upper lip, the median part of the maxillary bone and its four incisor teeth, and the triangular primary palate. Reproduced from Reference 119 b with permission.

fifth months, the tonsils are gradually infiltrated by lymphatic tissue.

The tongue appears in embryos at approximately 4 weeks in the form of two lateral lingual swellings and one medial swelling, the so-called tuberculum impar. These three swellings originate from the first pharyngeal arch (Fig. 10.2). A second median swelling (the copula) is formed by mesoderm of the second, third, and fourth arches. The lateral tongue swellings overgrow the tuberculum impar and merge with each other, forming the anterior two-thirds of the tongue (body of the tongue, mobile tongue, or oral tongue). Therefore, the sensory innervation of the anterior two-thirds of the tongue is by the mandibular branch of the trigeminal nerve (see Normal Anatomy). The posterior third of the tongue (fixed portion, base of the tongue, or pharyngeal tongue) originates from the second, third, and fourth pharyngeal arches. The third branchial arch overgrows tissue of the second arch. Therefore, the sensory innervation of this tongue portion is supplied by the glossopharyngeal nerve, which is the nerve of the third branchial arch. The extreme posterior part of the tongue (which is derived from the fourth branchial arch) is innervated by the superior laryngeal branch of the vagus, which is the nerve of the fourth arch. The anterior two-thirds of the tongue are separated from the posterior third by a V-shaped groove called the terminal sulcus. The foramen cecum, the remnant of the proximal end of the thyroglossal duct is located at the apex of the terminal sulcus (see also Chapter 12). Most tongue muscles develop from myoblasts originating in the occipital somites. Therefore, the tongue musculature is innervated by the hypoglossal nerve.

The upper lip is formed by fusion of the two maxillary swellings (Figs. 10.1, 10.3) and two lateral nasal swellings. The hard and soft palate are formed by fusion of the deeper portions of the two maxillary swellings and the derivatives of the so-called intermaxillary segment, which represents the two merged maxillary swellings (Fig. 10.3).

Normal Anatomy

The oral cavity and oropharynx are completely lined with squamous epithelium. The *oral cavity* includes the lips, the hard palate, the upper and lower alveolar ridges, the anterior two-thirds of the tongue, the buccal mucosa, the retromolar trigones, and the floor of the mouth. The upper alveolar ridge is referred to the mucosa covering the maxillary alveolar process. This extends from the line of the attachment of the mucosa in the upper gingivo-buccal gutter to the junction with the hard palate. The lower alveolar ridge is referred to the mucosa covering the mandibular alveolar process, which extends from the line of the attachment of the mucosa in the lower gingivo-buccal gutter to the mucosa of the floor of the mouth. The oral cavity is separated from the oropharynx by a line connecting the anterior tonsillar pillars, the circumvallate papillae, and the junction of the hard and soft palate (Fig. 10.4). From a clinical point of view this division is useful because squamous cell carcinomas in the oral cavity and oropharynx differ in their presentation, histological grade, and prognosis.[9–11, 13, 32] The hard palate separates the oral cavity from the nasal cavity (Fig. 10.4). It is bounded anteriorly and laterally by the upper alveolar ridge. In the midline, there is a raphe that terminates anteriorly at the incisor canal. Numerous minor salivary glands are located between the mucosal surface and the underlying bone.

The tongue is composed of paired intrinsic and extrinsic muscles. There are four pairs of intrinsic muscles—inferior longitudinal, superior longitudinal, vertical, and transverse fibers; and there are four pairs of extrinsic muscles—hyoglossus, styloglossus, genioglossus, and palatoglossus (Figs. 10.5–10.8). Both the intrinsic and the extrinsic tongue muscles are innervated by cranial nerve XII (hypoglossus). Superior and inferior longitudi-

10 Oral Cavity and Oropharynx

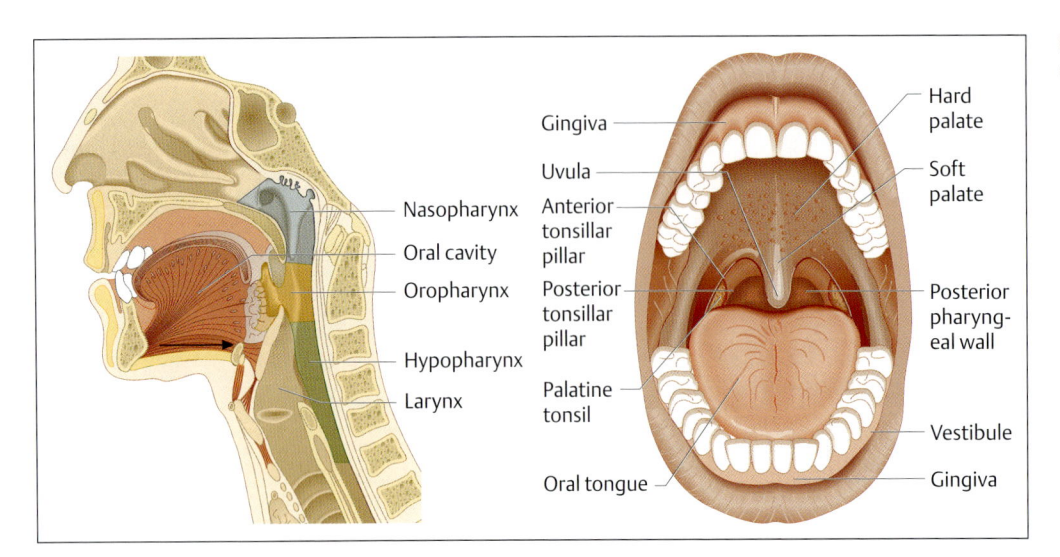

Fig. 10.4 Schematic drawing of the oral cavity and oropharynx.

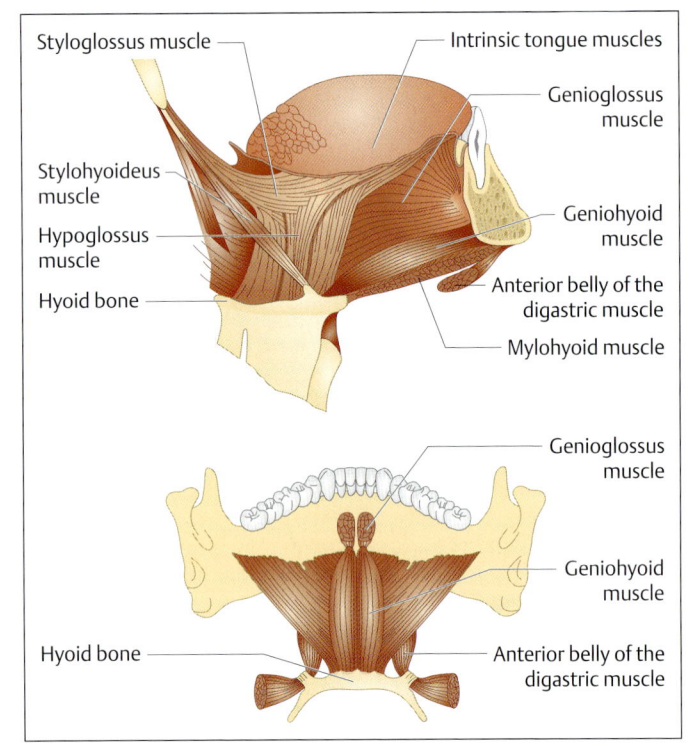

Fig. 10.5 Schematic drawing of the intrinsic and extrinsic tongue muscles.

nal groups may be separated from transverse and vertical elements by fibrous septae, the strongest of which lies in the midline and is called the septum lingue. The intrinsic muscles of the tongue are best seen on MRI with low signal intensity bundles surrounded by high signal intensity fat as well as submucosal mucous glands on T1-weighted and fast spin echo (FSE) T2-weighted sequences. On MRI, the intrinsic muscles of the tongue demonstrate greater signal intensity than the extrinsic muscles, but less than squamous cell cancers.[13, 14, 51, 77, 78] The extrinsic muscles of oral tongue may be seen on both CT and MRI and they show a low signal intensity on T1 and FSE T2-weighted MRI sequences (Fig. 10.6). The hyoglossus muscle attaches to the hyoid bone and ascends superiorly, blending with the styloglossus muscle (Figs. 10.5, 10.7). The styloglossus muscle arises from the stylohyoid ligament and styloid process and radiates anteri-

orly and inferiorly. The hyoglossus and styloglossus muscles together form the lateral border of the tongue.

The circumvallate papillae lie at the junction of the anterior two-thirds and posterior one-third of the tongue. At the apex of the chevron shape formed by the circumvallate papillae lies the foramen cecum, from which the embryological thyroid tissue begins its descent. The frenulum attaches the tongue to the floor of the mouth. Wharton's ducts open on either side of the frenulum.

The sensory innervation of the tongue is different in its anterior and posterior portions. In the anterior two-thirds of the tongue, the lingual nerve (branch of the mandibular division of the trigeminal nerve, V3) provides sensation, while the chorda tympani (which joins with the facial nerve) supplies taste. The intracranial course of the taste fibers is geniculate ganglion – intermediary nerve – nucleus solitarius of the pons. In the posterior third of the tongue, the glossopharyngeus nerve (IX) provides taste, touch, and gag.

The vascular supply of the tongue includes the lingual artery (branch of the external carotid artery) and the lingual vein, which runs along with the hypoglossal nerve and two separate lymphatic systems. The anterior tongue is drained by both a central and a marginal system. While the central system drains into ipsilateral and contralateral submandibular lymph nodes, the marginal system drains into ipsilateral submandibular nodes only. The posterior tongue lymphatic system drains into ipsilateral and contralateral deep cervical (jugulodigastric) nodes.[10, 56]

The *sublingual spaces* are situated lateral to the paired genioglossus muscle and superomedial to the mylohyoid muscle (Figs. 10.6, 10.7). The genioglossus muscle arises from the anterior mandible and fans out posteriorly into the tongue. Each sublingual space contains the anterior extension of the hyoglossus muscle, the lingual gland, the neurovascular bundles (lingual artery, vein, and nerve; and hypoglossal nerve), and the deep portion of the submandibular gland with Wharton's duct. The lingual septum, which contains fat, separates the left and right genioglossus muscles (Figs. 10.6, 10.7). Because the lingual septum is not a fascial barrier, there is free communication between the sublingual spaces.

The floor of the mouth is the semilunar region over the mylohoid and hyoglossus muscles. It extends from the undersurface of the anterior two-thirds of the tongue to the inner surface of the lower alveolar ridge. The bases of the anterior tonsillar pillars mark the posterior boundaries of the floor of the mouth. The *floor of the mouth* is composed of the extrinsic muscles of the tongue

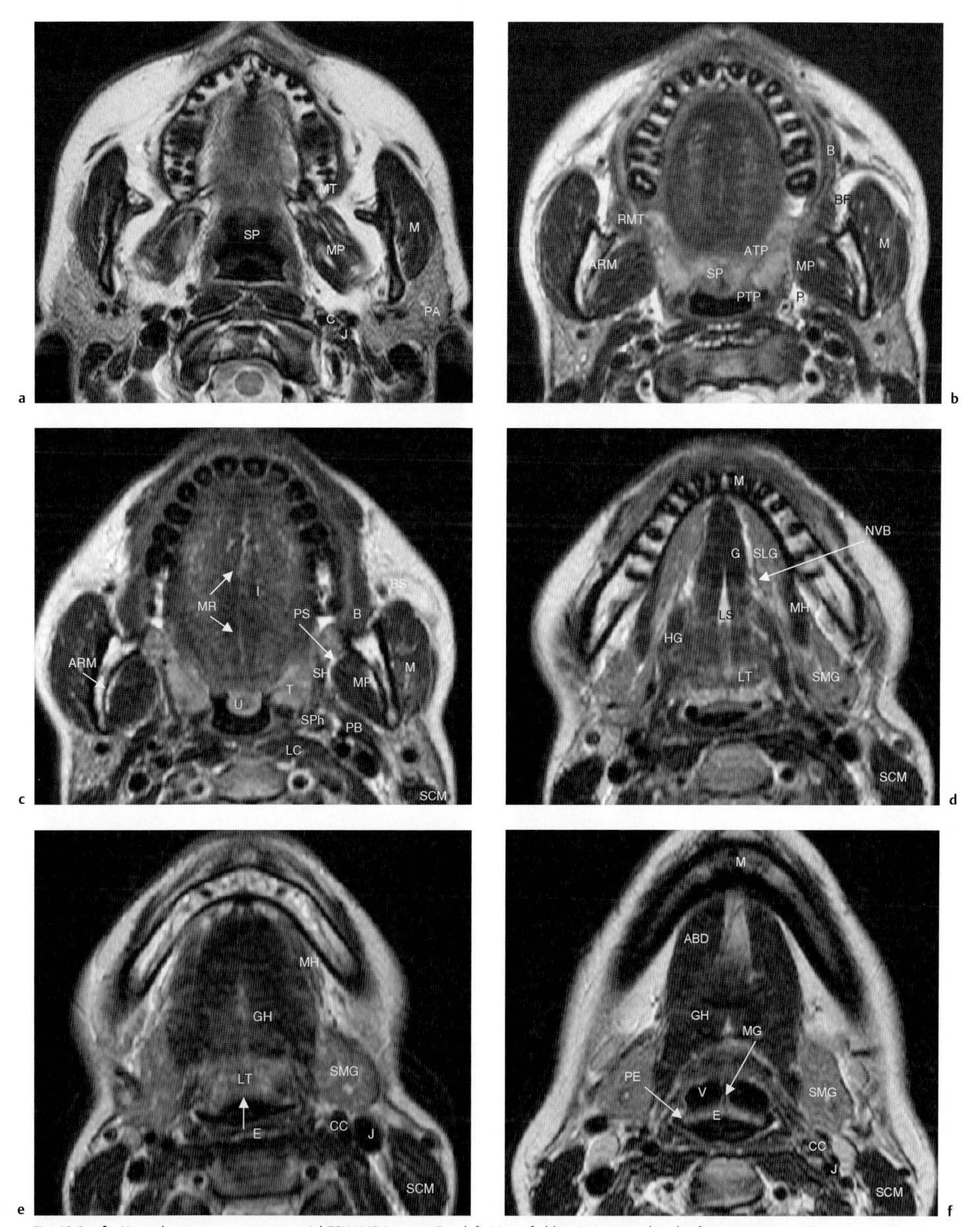

Fig. 10.**6 a–f** Normal anatomy as seen on axial T2W MR images. For definition of abbreviations used in this figure, see Fig. 10.**7**.

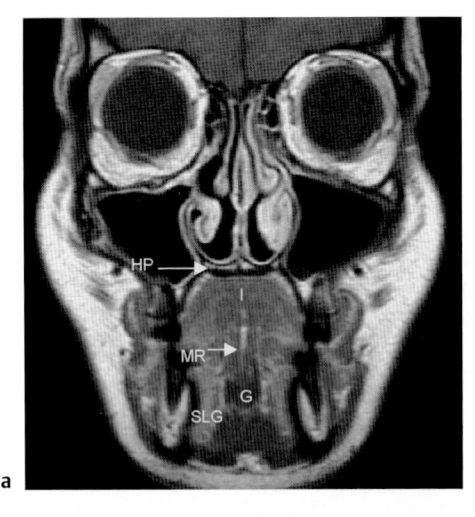

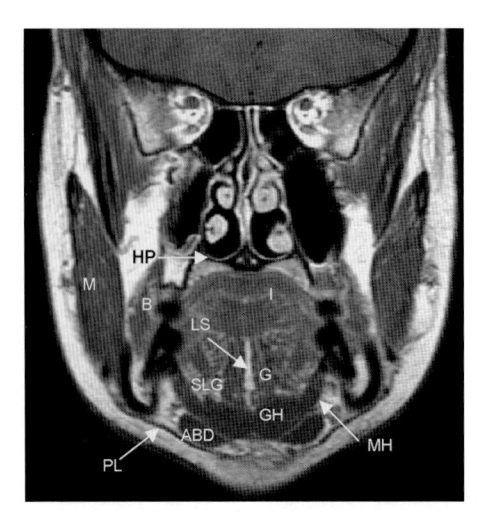

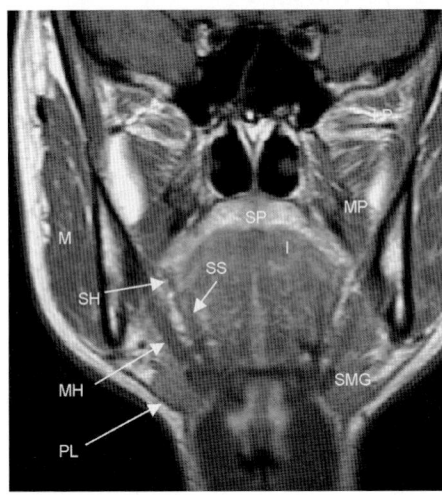

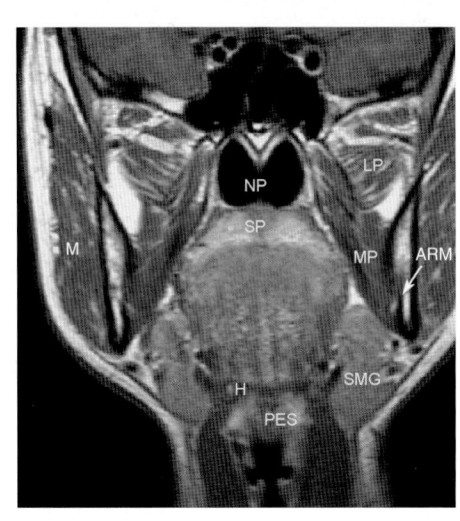

Fig. 10.7 a–d Normal anatomy as seen on coronal contrast-enhanced T1W MR images. ABD = anterior belly of the digastric muscle; ARM = ascending ramus of the mandible; ATP = anterior tonsillar pillar; B = buccinator muscle; BF = buccal fat pad; C = internal carotid artery; CC = common carotid artery; E = epiglottis; G = genioglossus muscle; GH = geniohyoideus muscle; H = hyoid bone; HG = hyoglossus muscle; HP = hard palate; I = intrinsic muscles of the tongue; J = internal jugular vein; LC = longus colli muscle; LP = lateral pterygoid muscle; LS = lingual septum; LT = lingual tonsils; M = masseter muscle; MG = median glossoepiglottic fold; MH = mylohyoid muscle; MP = medial pterygoid muscle; MR = median raphe; MT = maxillary tuberosity; NP = nasopharynx; NVB = neurovascular bundle; P = parapharyngeal space; PA = parotid gland; PB = posterior belly of the digastric muscle; PE = pharyngoepiglottic fold; PES = preepiglottic space; PL = platysma; PS = pterygomandibular space; PTP = posterior tonsillar pillar; RMT = retromolar trigone; SCM = sternocleidomastoid muscle; SLG = sublingual gland; SMG = submandibular gland; SH = stylohyoid muscle; SP = soft palate; SPh = stylopharyngeus muscle; SS = styloglossus hyoglossus muscles; T = palatine tonsil; U = uvula; V = vallecula.

along with the mylohyoid and geniohyoid muscles. It is best evaluated on coronal images. The mylohyoid muscle forms a sling that serves as the main supporting structure. The sling is formed as a result of its attachment along the inner aspect of the mandible. The posterior free edge of the mylohyoid muscle provides a pathway for both neoplastic and infectious processes to extend from the sublingual space (situated above the mylohyoid muscle) to the submandibular space (situated below the mylohyoid muscle) and vice versa (Figs. 10.**6**, 10.**7**). The geniohyoid muscle lies below the genioglossus muscle and inserts into the hyoid bone. The anterior belly of the digastric muscle lies lateral and inferior to the mylohyoid muscle. The mylohyoid muscle and the anterior belly of the digastric muscle are innervated by the mandibular nerve (V3).[56,97]

The *submandibular space* is located inferolateral to the mylohyoid muscle and superior to the hyoid bone. No fascial margin separates the posterior submandibular space and sublingual space from the inferior parapharyngeal space. The submandibular space contains the anterior belly of the digastric muscle, the superficial portion of the submandibular gland, facial artery and vein, the inferior loop of the hypoglossal nerve, some fat, and the submandibular and submental lymph nodes.[56,72]

The *oropharynx* lies posterior to the circumvallate papilla of the tongue. It comprises the posterior third (base) of the tongue, the valleculae (medial and lateral glossopharyngeal folds), the anterior and posterior tonsillar pillars (palatoglossal and palatopharyngeal arches), the soft palate, the pharyngeal constrictors from the level of the hard palate to the level of the hyoid bone (posterior and lateral walls of the oropharynx), and the palatine and lingual tonsils (Figs. 10.**6**–10.**8**).

The *soft palate*, which forms a functional floor for the nasopharynx, separates the oropharynx from the nasopharynx. Anteriorly the soft palate attaches to the posterior portion of the hard palate, and laterally it merges with the palatoglossal and palatopharyngeal arches and with the pharyngeal constrictor muscles. The soft palate is a fibromuscular shelf composed of the palatoglossus muscle, palatopharyngeus muscle, musculus uvulae, tensor veli palatini muscle, and levator veli palatini muscle. The mandibular nerve (V3) innervates the tensor veli palatini muscle. The remainder of the palatal muscles are innervated via the sphenopalatine ganglion. Vascular supply to the palate includes the maxillary artery, and its venous drainage is via the venous pterygoid plexus (which drains into the internal jugular vein). Its lymphatics drain into the upper deep cervical nodes and retropharyngeal nodes. The CT appearance of the soft palate is similar to that of muscle, and mucosal enhancement on enhanced CT scans is variable. On T1-weighted MR images, the mucosal signal is either hyperintense or isointense relative to muscle; after intravenous administration of gadolinium-based contrast material, the soft palate mucosa, as well as mucosal membranes of the oral cavity and oropharynx, demonstrate moderate to marked contrast enhancement.[13,27,31,126] On T2-weighted MR images, the mucosal membrane demonstrates high signal intensity likely related to numerous submucosal mucous glands.

The *retromolar trigone* is a triangular region bordered anteriorly by the posterior surface of the last mandibular molar tooth, posteromedially by the anterior tonsillar pillar, and laterally by the buccal mucosa. Its apex superiorly is attached to the pterygoid hamulus. The pterygomandibular raphe is a band of connective tissue situated beneath the mucosal surface of the retromolar trigone. It attaches superiorly at the medial pterygoid plate and interiorly to the posterior aspect of the mylohyoid line of the mandible. The mucosa of the retromolar trigone is separated from the adjacent ascending mandibular ramus by the buccal fat pad (Fig. 10.**6b**).

The palatine tonsils are paired structures located laterally in the oropharynx. They are situated in a fossa formed by the anterior and posterior tonsillar pillars, formed by the palatoglossus and palatopharyngeus muscles, respectively (Fig. 10.**6**). The palatoglossus muscle elevates the tongue and narrows the oropharyngeal opening, and the palatopharyngeus raises the larynx and pharynx and narrows the oropharyngeal opening. Laterally, the tonsils are bordered by the superior constrictor pharyngeal muscles. On CT scanning, the tonsils are difficult to differentiate from the anterior and posterior tonsillar pillars because of their similar attenuation coefficients. Similarly, on T1-weighted MR images, the tonsils are difficult to separate from muscle because the two are nearly isointense. On T2-weighted MR sequences, the tonsils have a higher signal intensity than muscle because the lymphoid tissue and submucosal glands within the tonsils have a longer T2 relaxation time relative to the adjacent muscles (Fig. 10.**6**). On T2-weighted MR images, lymphoid tissue throughout Waldeyer's ring (palatine, lingual, and pharyngeal tonsils) has a high signal intensity. Because the tonsils may vary in size, resulting in an asymmetric size of the tonsillar fossae, small neoplasms within the tonsillar fossa may be very difficult to detect with both CT and MRI scans unless there is evidence of deep invasion. On unenhanced T1-weighted and T2-weighted MR images, signal characteristics of normal tonsillar tissue can overlap those of neoplasms. However, on fat-suppressed gadolinium (Gd)-enhanced T1-weighted MR images, tumors can be better recognized because of their increased enhancement and improved contrast resolution of fat-suppression pulse sequences. (Fig. 10.**9**).

The lingual tonsil is of variable appearance and is located submucosally at the tongue base. The *valleculae* lie on either side of the median glossoepiglottic fold and, on each side, the valleculae are bordered by the lateral glossoepiglottic folds (Figs. 10.**6**, 10.**8**). The median glossoepiglottic fold extends from the base of the tongue to lingual surface of the epiglottis. At the base of the glossoepiglottic fold lies the hyoepiglottic ligament, which forms the superior border of the preepiglottic space (Fig. 10.**8**).

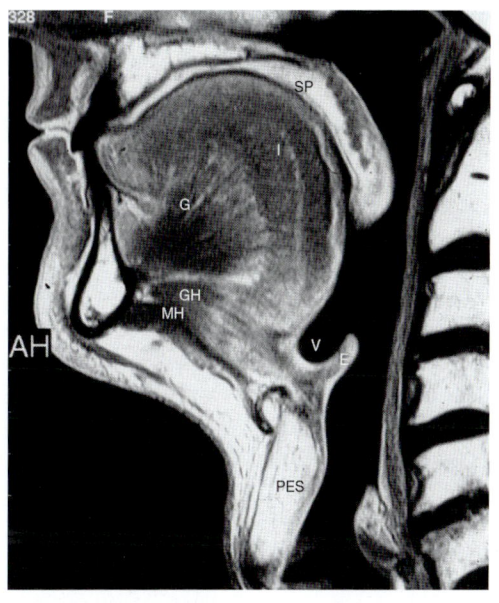

Fig. 10.**8** Midsagittal contrast-enhanced T1W MR image through the oral cavity and oropharynx. SP = soft palate; I = intrinsic muscles of the tongue; G = genioglossus muscle; GH = geniohyoid muscle; MH = mylohyoid muscle; V = vallecula; E = epiglottis; PES = preepiglottic space.

Imaging Techniques

■ CT

The main advantages of CT in comparison with MR imaging are rapid image acquisition, availability, and cost. Inherent disadvantages of CT are radiation exposure, the need for relatively high doses of iodinated contrast materials to obtain adequate soft-tissue contrast, and artifacts originating from dental implants. Scanning protocols may vary, depending on the technical capabilities of hardware and software. *Helical scanning* enables complete data sets to be obtained from axial acquisitions in less than 20 seconds and reconstruction of overlapping slices at any level. Helical acquisitions with 2–3 mm collimation and 1–1.5 pitch produce images of adequate quality to answer most clinically relevant questions. High-detail work or high-quality 2D-reconstructions in the coronal or sagittal plane may require acquisitions with 1–1.3 mm collimation and 1–1.5 pitch. Depending on

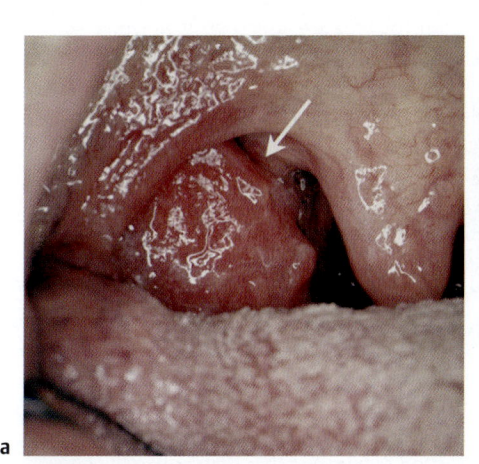

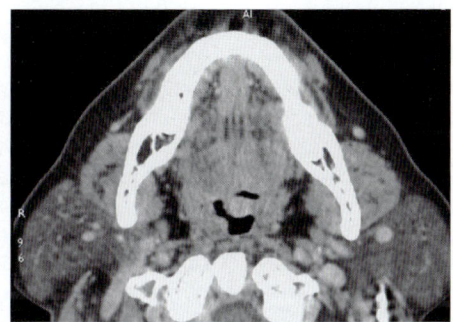

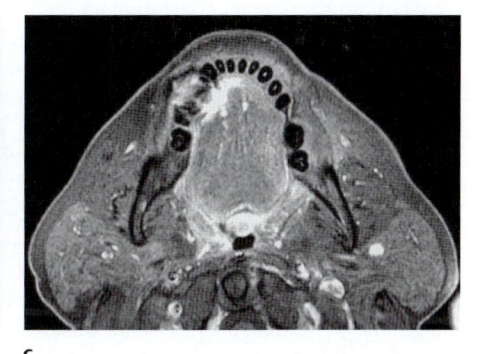

Fig. 10.**9** **a** Clinical examination of an elderly patient with oropharyngeal pain shows enlargement of the right tonsil (arrow). No obvious mucosal abnormality is seen. **b** Contrast-enhanced CT image at the level of the oropharynx shows only slight asymmetry of the tonsillar fossae, the right tonsil being slightly larger than the left. Note that there is no abnormal tonsillar enhancement on CT. **c** Contrast-enhanced, fat-suppressed T1W MR image shows abnormal enhancement of the right tonsil indicating the presence of a possible tumor. No involvement of the parapharyngeal space. Tonsillectomy proved squamous cell cancer of the right tonsil.

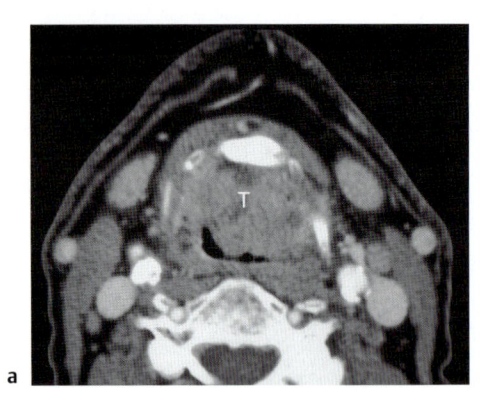

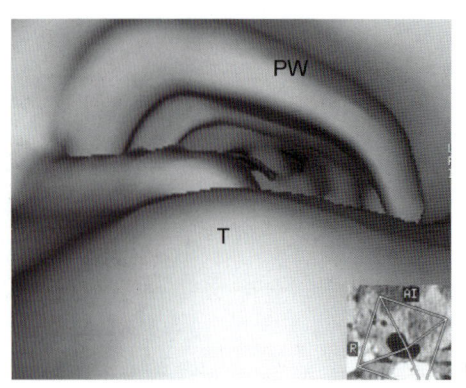

Fig. 10.**10 a** Contrast-enhanced CT image at the level of the oropharynx shows a large base of the tongue tumor (T) extending into the valleculae. **b** Virtual endoscopy image obtained from the volumetric data set shows the abnormal bulge of the posterior tongue caused by the large tumor (T). PW = posterior wall of the pharynx.

vendor-related software options, such data sets also enable 3D volume reconstructions and so-called "virtual endoscopy" images (Fig. 10.**10**). Since the advent of multidetector helical scanning, 2D coronal and sagittal reconstructions of excellent quality may be obtained routinely. Parameters used with 16-row multidetector scanners include 1.3–2 mm collimated sections overlapped in 0.6–1 mm intervals and a pitch setting of 1–1.5. Regardless of the acquisition technique, a CT examination of the oral cavity and oropharynx should always include reconstruction algorithms for both soft tissue and bone detail. The area to be examined should extend from the skull base to the thoracic inlet. Ideally, axial images at the level of the oral cavity and oropharynx should be parallel to the plane of the hard palate, and coronal images should be perpendicular to the hard palate.[87, 124] In the presence of dental amalgam, care should be taken to modify scan angles in order to avoid artefacts. Particular attention should also be paid to patient positioning, as poor positioning may result in apparent loss of normal symmetry, thus mimicking pathology. Because oral cavity cancer is associated with coexisting tumors of the pharynx, larynx, or tracheobronchial tree in one-sixth of cases, extended imaging into the thorax may be justified.[27, 52, 94, 107]

■ MR Imaging

Superior soft-tissue contrast is the most striking advantage of MR imaging in comparison with CT. Drawbacks are the relatively long examination time, limited availability, and cost. MR imaging demands more patient cooperation than CT and cannot be done in patients with claustrophobia, severe dyspnea, or odynophagia, or in the presence of electronic implants. MR imaging of the oral cavity and oropharynx is best done at high field strength and requires a head and neck volume coil, thin sections, and at least a set of T1- and T2-weighted MR images and contrast-enhanced T1-weighted MR images. Typical image parameters for a standard examination include a slice thickness of 3 or 4 mm with a 0–1 mm intersection gap, a field of view of 20 × 20 cm or less, and two averages. The acquisition matrix should be at least 256 × 256, but 512 × 256 or 512 × 512 should be used whenever possible. Fat-suppression techniques after intravenous administration of gadolinium-based contrast material are extremely useful in delineating tumor extent and short tau inversion recovery (STIR) images are particularly sensitive for marrow infiltration or detection of small lesions. As with CT, the area to be examined should extend from the skull base to the thoracic inlet, and axial images at the level of the oral cavity and oropharynx should be parallel to the plane of the hard palate, while coronal images should be perpendicular to the hard palate.[13, 14, 87, 97, 143] Although dental artifacts can occur with both CT and MR images, they are usually less disruptive on MR studies.

■ Ultrasonography

Ultrasonography (US) can be used for dedicated evaluation of certain pathological conditions of the floor of the mouth and tongue, such as salivary calculi, inflammatory and congenital lesions, and tongue motility disorders. However, US is operator-dependent and does not enable complete, sectional imaging of the anatomical structures of the region as CT or MR imaging. Ultrasonography of the oral cavity is best performed using curved-array or linear-array broadband transducers with a frequency of about 5–12 MHz. As in other parts of the body, the selection of the transducer frequency depends on the depth of the lesion to be examined and on the attenuation of the interposed tissues. For examination of very superficial lesions, a standoff pad made of silicone elastomer may be used. However, this is rarely needed with modern high-frequency transducers, which enable good visualization of the key anatomical structures of this area. Although color Doppler and power Doppler imaging are often useful in the examination of the oral cavity, most diagnoses are made with the standard gray-scale technique.

Tumors of the Oral Cavity and Oropharynx

■ Squamous Cell Carcinoma

Squamous cell carcinomas involving the oral cavity and oropharynx present major therapeutic challenges because of the poor prognosis of advanced disease, and the adverse effect of treatment on oral and pharyngeal function.[107] Squamous cell carcinomas represent a little over 90 % of all malignant neoplasms of the oral cavity and oropharynx. In the United States, this form of neoplasm accounts for 3–7 % of all malignancies, whereas in certain countries of the East and Far East these carcinomas account for almost half of all malignant neoplasms.[9, 10] Squamous cell carcinomas of the oral cavity and oropharynx affect males more than twice as often as females, occurring most commonly between the sixth and eighth decades.[11] However, a recent study has shown a tendency toward an increase of the incidence of squamous cell carcinoma in patients younger than 40 years.[86] The two most common risk factors for squamous cell cancers are smoking and alcohol abuse. Other conditions associated with an increased risk of developing squamous cell carcinoma of the oral cavity and oropharynx include use of snuff, tertiary syphilis, dystrophic epidermolysis bullosa, lichen planus, dyskeratosis congenita, oral submucous fibrosis as a result of chewing betel nut,

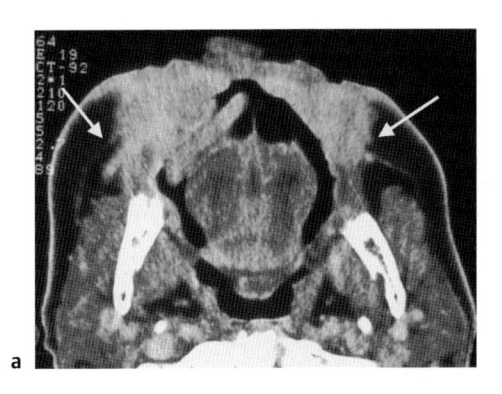

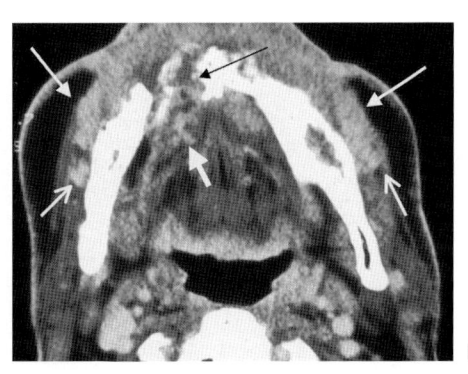

Fig. 10.**11** Two different patients with advanced squamous cell cancer of the lip as seen on contrast-enhanced CT images. **a** Infiltrative cancer of the upper lip, extending into the vestibule and invading the buccal space fat bilaterally (arrows). **b** Advanced ulcerative cancer of the lower lip invading the perioral musculature (arrows) and with massive mandibular invasion (black arrow). Note extension of the tumor into the floor of the mouth (thick arrow) and bilateral spread of tumor into the anteroinferior portion of the masseter muscle (open arrows).

and occupational exposures (leather and textile manufacturing industries). The increased risk associated with therapeutic radiation has at least a 10-year latency period.[32,52,107] It has recently been suggested that Epstein–Barr virus (EBV) and human papillomavirus (HPV) type 16 may play an important etiological role in squamous cell cancers of Waldeyer's tonsillar ring.[69,111] HPV-positive patients tend to have larger tumors at initial presentation and a higher incidence of lymph node metastases than HPV negative patients.[111]

Although squamous cell carcinomas in the oral cavity and oropharynx tend to present earlier than elsewhere owing to ease of direct inspection, the majority are, nevertheless, advanced at presentation. The mucosa of the oropharynx differs from that in the oral cavity, being derived from endoderm, and consequently squamous cell lesions in the oropharynx tend to be more undifferentiated, more aggressive, and associated with a poorer outcome than squamous cell lesions of the oral cavity.[35,107,129] Persistent ulceration in the mouth or ulceration as a result of an ill-fitting denture, bleeding within the mouth, the presence of a mass, halitosis, dysarthria, sore throat, odynophagia, dysphagia, and otalgia are characteristic symptoms of oral cavity and oropharyngeal neoplasms. Nevertheless, extensive tumors, especially when originating from the base of the tongue, may remain entirely asymptomatic despite their size and it is not uncommon for a patient to present with a large neck mass as the first sign of primary neoplasia within the oropharynx. Clinically, early superficial mucosal lesions are detected on visual inspection as either patches of leukoplakia or patches of erythroplakia. Leukoplakia is a white patch of mucosa and 10% of leukoplakic lesions develop cancers. Because an area of leukoplakia may harbor dysplasia, carcinoma in situ, or even invasive carcinoma, persistent leukoplakic lesions of unknown cause should be biopsied and evaluated histologically. Erythroplakia is a relatively rare red, velvety, plaquelike lesion most commonly found in the floor of the mouth, ventral and lateral aspects of the tongue, anterior tonsillar pillars, and soft palate.[35,107,129] Erythroplakia carries an 80% risk of developing malignancy.

Pretherapeutic staging of squamous cell carcinoma is the most common indication for sectional imaging. MRI is undoubtedly more sensitive, specific, and elegant than CT in the oral cavity and oropharynx. However, the larger numerical presence of CT scanners in most hospitals and the high speed (especially with multidetector CT scanners) and relatively lower cost determine that many patients with suspected oral cavity or oropharyngeal neoplasia will undergo initial CT scanning rather than MRI. Most oropharynx and oral cavity squamous cell cancers larger than 1.5 cm are easily identified by their bulk or distortion of fascial planes. Because the specific diagnostic issues may differ considerably from one primary tumor site to another, squamous cell cancers of the oral cavity and oropharynx need to be discussed individually.

Regions and Patterns of Tumor Spread

Carcinoma of the Lip

Carcinoma of the mucous membrane of the vermillion area of the lips is the most common malignant neoplasm of the oral cavity.[9-11] These cancers, as they present in the United States, are most common in white men aged 50–70 years. Elsewhere, particularly in Scandinavia, women manifest a significant number of carcinomas of the lip in contrast to their US counterparts. Risk factors include fair or ruddy complexion, excessive exposure to sun, tobacco use (especially pipe smoking), alcohol use, poor dental hygiene, chronic immunosuppression (e.g., renal transplantation), and syphilis. As many as 95% of all lip carcinomas originate in the lower lip at a point about halfway between the midline and commissure.[10,51,52] Despite the relatively high frequency for this anatomical region, carcinomas of the lower lip constitute only 0.6% of all cancers in man.[9,10] The upper lip is an uncommon site for carcinoma to develop, but when it is primary there, the neoplasm is near the midline and as a general rule it will grow more rapidly and will behave more aggressively than carcinoma of the lower lip. Surprisingly, in view of its exposed position, carcinoma of the lip is not often diagnosed early, many patients relating a delay of up to two years before seeking medical attention. Nearly half of the patients with carcinoma of the lip have a lesion measuring more than 1.5 cm in diameter at initial examination (Fig. 10.**11**). Three morphological types of squamous cell carcinomas are seen: exophytic, ulcerative, and verrucous. The ulcerative form tends to be more infiltrative than the exophytic variety and verrucous carcinomas are extremely rare. Many of the labial carcinomas arise in areas of clinical leukoplakia and may present as exophytic outgrowths or begin as small ulcers. Carcinomas of the lip have an indolent and often protracted clinical course. In general, metastases to lymph nodes are late and relatively infrequent (less than 10% in lower lip cancers), as compared to squamous cell cancers of other regions. However, advanced lower lip lesions may spread to the submental and submandibular lymph nodes, while upper lip lesions metastasize to the preauricular, submental, and submandibular lymph nodes.

Early lesions are difficult to differentiate from the normal orbicularis oris muscle and they will only rarely be imaged. The lesions that will usually undergo imaging are already advanced and the margin of the tumor cannot be evaluated clinically. On CT and MR images the primary tumor may appear as a mass with or without areas of ulceration (Fig. 10.**11**). Subtle bone erosion usually occurs along the buccal surface of the mandibular or maxillary alveolar ridge and is best detected with CT, which may be supplemented by using dental CT software. Large tumors may also extend directly into the mandible or involve the mental nerve without cortical bone destruction (Figs. 10.**11**, 10.**12**) Because of the presence of bone erosion these lesions are considered as T4 in the TNM classification, thereby necessitating

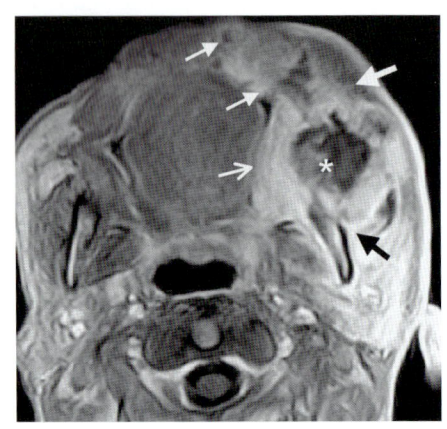

Fig. 10.12 Patient with extensive lower lip cancer presenting with trismus. T1W MR image obtained after injection of contrast material on a low-field MR unit (0.2 T) shows a tumor mass involving the left lower lip (arrows) and the left buccal mucosa (open arrow) and with extension into the masticator space and buccal space (thick arrows). Note large area of necrosis (asterisk) and invasion of the ascending ramus of the mandible.

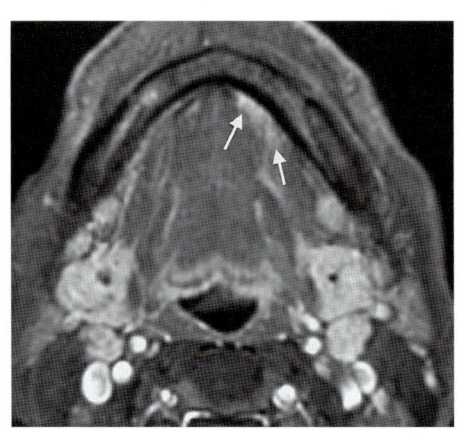

Fig. 10.13 Small histologically proven squamous cell cancer of the left floor of the mouth (T1) seen as a discrete area of increased enhancement on a fat-suppressed T1W MR image (arrows).

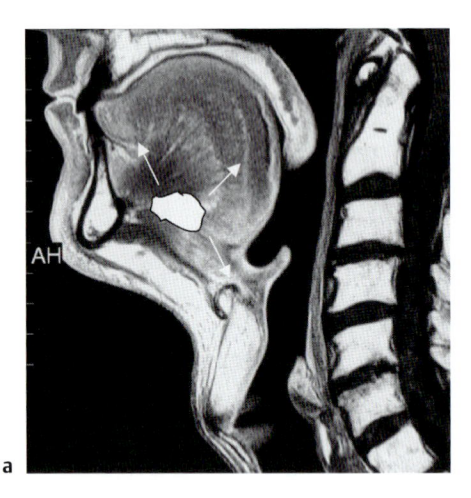

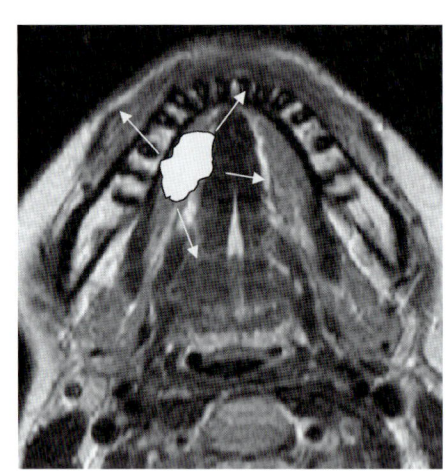

Fig. 10.14 a, b Patterns of tumor spread in floor of the mouth carcinoma (see text also).

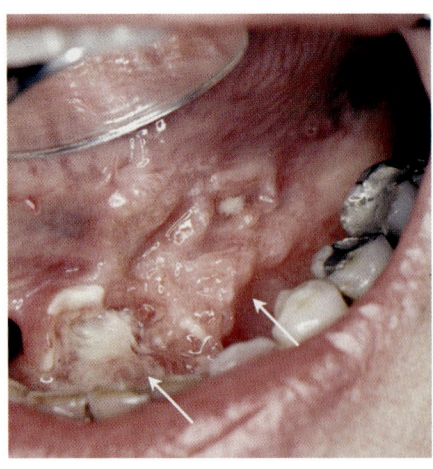

Fig. 10.15 Clinical presentation of a floor of the mouth cancer. This elderly patient presented with a painful exophytic lesion of the left floor of the mouth (arrows), which is easily seen at clinical inspection. On palpation, the entire left floor of the mouth and the anterior floor of the mouth were indurated, suggesting submucosal spread. Biopsy proved well-differentiated squamous cell carcinoma.

either a partial mandibulectomy (in lower lip tumors) or partial maxillectomy (in upper lip tumors).[98, 100]

Most carcinomas of the lip are treated by surgical excision, although small carcinomas my be treated by either surgery or radiation therapy. While small lesions are usually excised with primary closure, defects not amenable to primary closure are reconstructed with local or regional flaps.

Carcinoma of the Floor of the Mouth

Squamous cell carcinoma of the floor of the mouth arises from the mucosa covering the U-shaped area between the lower gum (inner surface of the lower alveolar ridge) and the undersurface of the anterior two-thirds of the tongue (Figs. 10.13–10.15). It accounts for approximately 10–15% of all oral carcinomas and it occurs primarily in males with an average age of 60 years. It is the third most common carcinoma of the oral cavity and it is the most common intraoral site in Africans.[10, 52] The usual association with tobacco and alcohol use has been noted. The majority of tumors originate in the anterior portion of the floor of the mouth at the midline and lateral to or involving the frenulum.[3–6] At its onset, the lesion may be very small (Fig. 10.13), but with progression of time the characteristic exophytic or papillary appearance is obtained. The lesion begins only very rarely as an ulcer. Tumors of the floor of the mouth may spread in a variety of directions

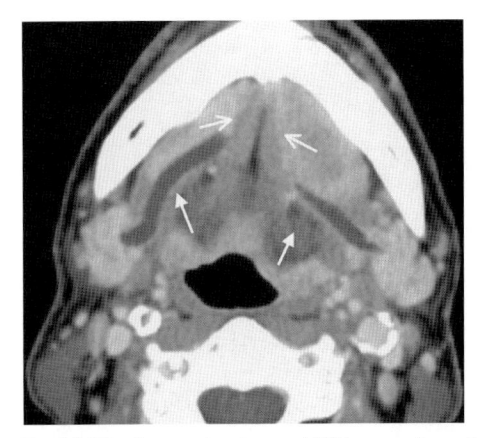

Fig. 10.16 Contrast-enhanced CT image of a patient presenting with bilateral, painful submandibular masses. Note a large bilobar anterior floor of the mouth tumor invading both sublingual spaces and neurovascular bundles and with bilateral obstruction of Wharton's duct (arrows). Invasion of the geniohyoid muscles (open arrows).

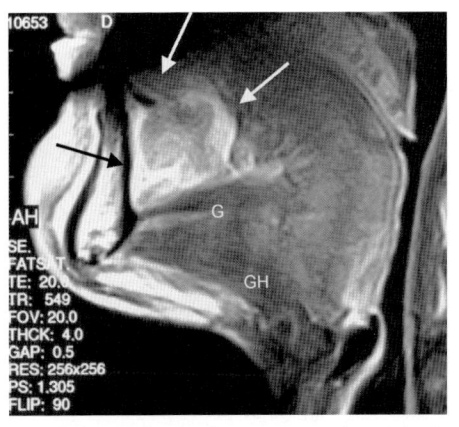

Fig. 10.17 Midsagittal, contrast-enhanced, fat-suppressed T1W MR image shows an anterior floor of the mouth tumor spreading mainly into the ventral surface of the tongue (arrows). Invasion of the genioglossus muscle (G) and sparing of the geniohyoid muscle (GH). The tumor also abuts the lingual surface of the anterior mandible (black arrow). Note that there is some inhomogeneous fat saturation in the chin area caused by dental amalgam.

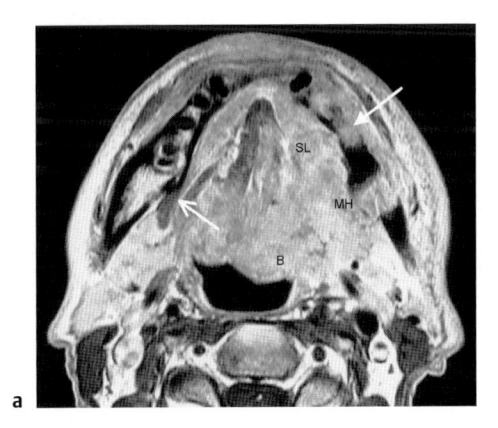

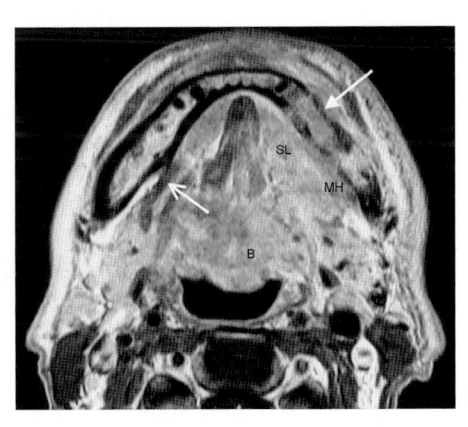

Fig. 10.18 a, b Contrast-enhanced T1W MR images of an extensive floor of the mouth squamous cell cancer. Involvement of the left sublingual (SL) space, left mylohyoid muscle (MH), left base of the tongue (B), and mandible (arrows). Note normal appearance of the contralateral mylohyoid muscle (open arrow). The left neurovascular bundle is embedded in the tumor.

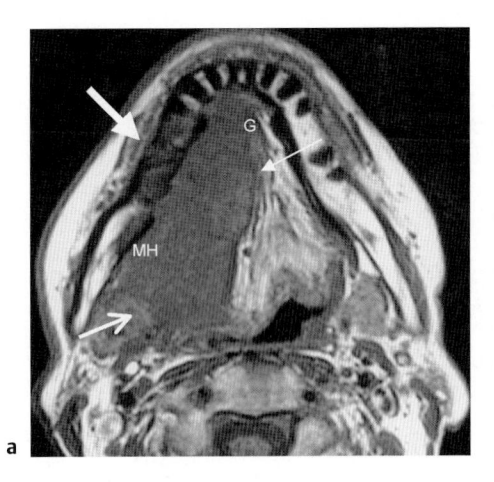

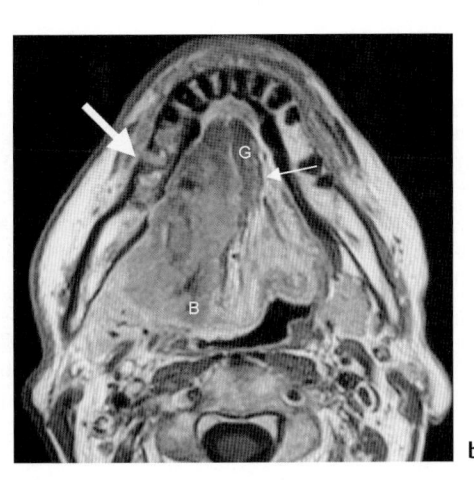

Fig. 10.19 Squamous cell carcinoma of the floor of the mouth with invasion of the base of the tongue and mandible. **a** Unenhanced and **b** contrast-enhanced T1W MR images obtained at the same level show a large tumor crossing the midline (thin arrows), with invasion of the genioglossus muscles (G), right mylohyoid muscle (MH), right submandibular space (open arrow), and base of the tongue (B), and with invasion of the mandible (thick arrows). Note the presence cortical erosions, abnormal signal intensity on the unenhanced T1W image and abnormal enhancement within the marrow space.

(Fig. 10.14). Inferior spread occurs into the sublingual spaces and may result in obstruction of the submandibular duct and chronic inflammation or infection of the submandibular gland (Fig. 10.16). Inferior spread may also occur into the genioglossus and hyoglossus muscles and eventually through the mylohyoid muscle into the anterior bellies of the digastric muscles, as well as into the submandibular spaces. Superiorly and posteriorly the tumors tend to involve the ventral surface of the tongue, the adjacent lingual neurovascular bundle, the base of the tongue, and the glossotonsillar sulcus[13, 14, 100, 124, 143] (Figs. 10.17–10.19). The relationship of a floor of the mouth cancer with the midline lingual septum and with the contralateral lingual neurovascular bundle must be determined either by CT or by MRI before surgery. Anteriorly and laterally, the neoplasm may advance into the adjacent

10 Oral Cavity and Oropharynx

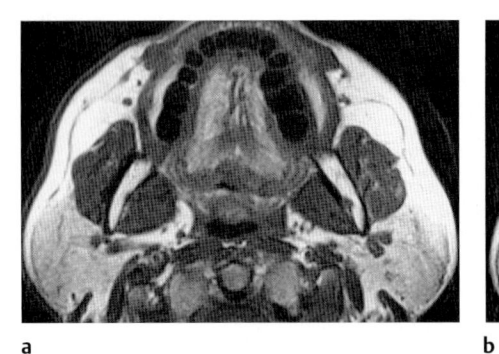

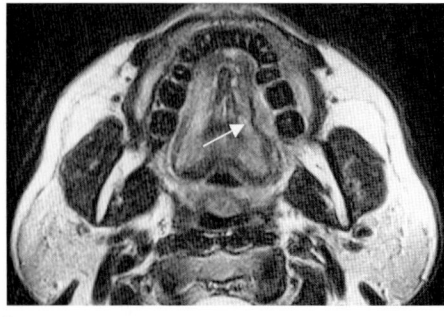

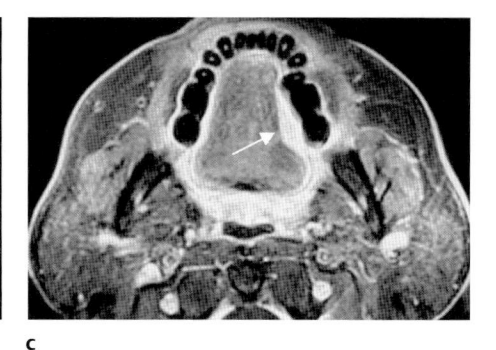

Fig. 10.20 Small squamous cell carcinoma of the tongue originating along the left lateral border. The tumor is hardly seen on the T1W MR image (**a**). It is somewhat better seen on the T2W MR image (arrow in **b**) and is most accurately identified on the contrast-enhanced, fat-suppressed T1W MR image (arrow in **c**).

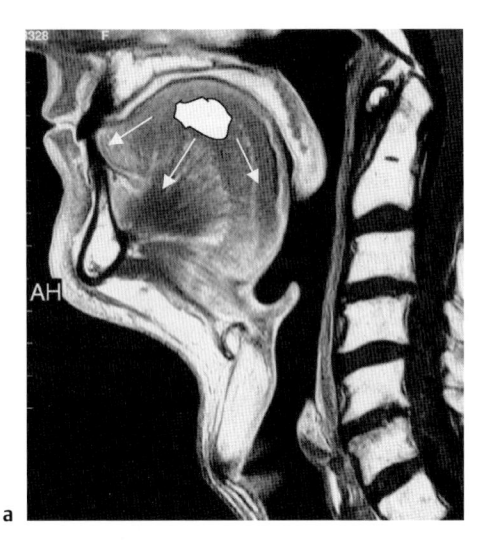

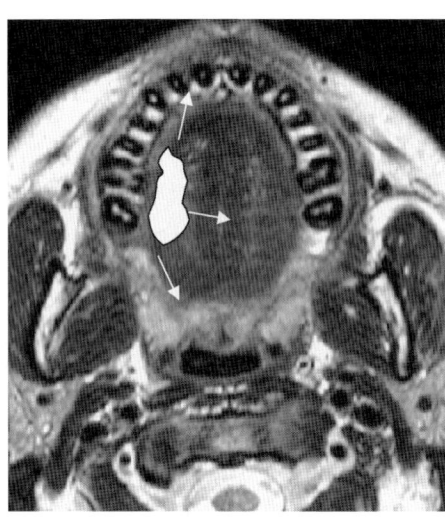

Fig. 10.21 a, b Patterns of tumor spread in carcinoma of the oral tongue (see text also).

gingival mucosa, may then spread along the periosteum and may destroy the lingual cortex of the mandible and involve the marrow space of the mandible (Figs. 10.**18**, 10.**19**). The location and amount of mandibular invasion alters the prognosis and surgical approach (see below).

The prevalence of lymph node metastases in floor of the mouth cancers is between 30% and 70%; however, metastases to cervical lymph nodes are usually a later manifestation than that observed in carcinoma of the tongue. Lymphatic drainage is either into the submandibular region or into the high jugulodigastric chain, depending upon the precise location of the primary neoplasm. Bilateral involvement is not uncommon.

Early carcinomas of the floor of the mouth can be treated by radiation therapy or surgery with equal effectiveness. A combination of surgery and radiation therapy is usually recommended for advanced cancers. While small lesions are usually excised with primary closure, defects not amenable to primary closure are reconstructed with skin grafts, regional flaps, or microvascular free flaps.

Carcinoma of the Oral Tongue

As many as 75% of squamous cell carcinomas of the tongue arise in the oral portion of the tongue (anterior two-thirds). Carcinoma of the oral tongue is the second most common site of oral cavity cancer (approximately 20% of oral carcinoma).[10,52,107] Carcinoma of the tongue is a disease of men. It is most commonly found in the sixth to eighth decades, but the disease may also be seen in the young. Because of the association with preexisting Plummer–Vinson syndrome, Scandinavian women have a higher incidence than American women. Poor oral hygiene and habits, tobacco and alcohol use, and the coincidence of syphilis are important predisposing factors. As with other forms of oral cancer, there is a wide geographical variation; for example, in India there is a disproportionately high occurrence of carcinoma of the tongue. Squamous cell carcinomas involving the *anterior two-thirds of the tongue* usually originate along the lateral border (middle third) or ventral surface of the tongue (Fig. 10.20). The tip and dorsum of the tongue are infrequent sites of origin. In general, the prognosis of carcinoma of the anterior tongue is more favorable than that of carcinoma of the tongue base, which tends to be histologically less well differentiated. The growth pattern of tongue cancers is usually infiltrative, ulcerative, and exophytic, and most lesions are more than 2 cm in diameter at the time of first clinical examination. Large tumors arising from the lateral border of the tongue tend to grow into the glossotonsillar sulcus, base of the tongue, tonsillar fossa, floor of the mouth, and subsequently the submandibular space (Figs. 10.**21**–10.**24**). The neoplasms arising from the ventral surface extend directly toward the floor of the mouth, and in many instances it is difficult to determine the exact site of origin. Large anterior tongue lesions may extend into the base of the tongue and vice versa. Neoplastic involvement of the lingual nerve is responsible for the pain in the ear on the affected side in patients with advanced carcinoma of the tongue or floor of the mouth.

On initial presentation, 40% of anterior tongue cancers present with regional adenopathy, half of these bilaterally. In addi-

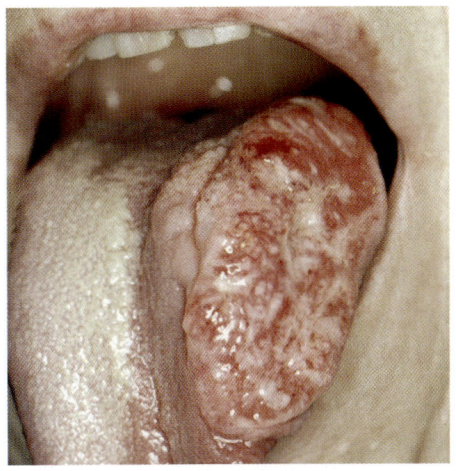

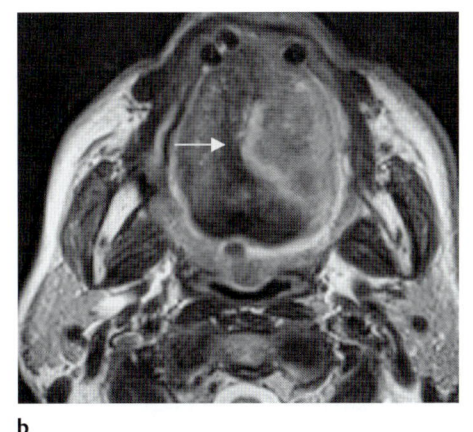

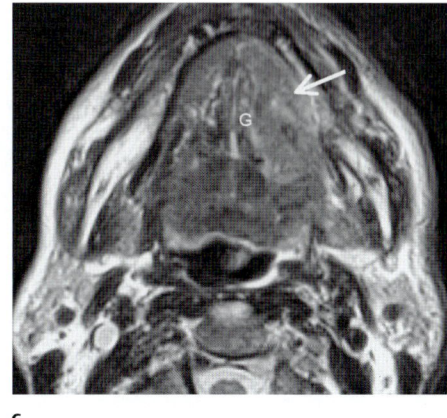

Fig. 10.22 Squamous cell carcinoma of the tongue originating along the left lateral border. **a** Clinical presentation. Note a large exophytic tumor involving almost the entire left hemitongue and with an abnormal mucosal surface with ulcerations. Clinically, the tumor did not cross the midline. **b**, **c** T2W FSE images show that the tumor crosses the midline (arrow) and that there is invasion of the left floor of the mouth (open arrow). The left neurovascular bundle is compromised, the left genioglossus muscle (G) is invaded.

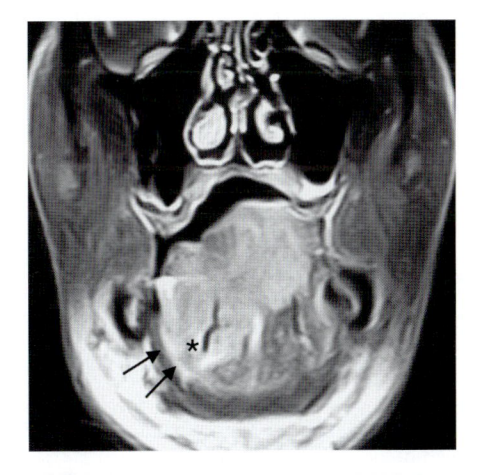

Fig. 10.23 Large tongue tumor seen on a coronal fat-suppressed T1W MR image obtained after injection of contrast material. The bilateral tumor involves nearly the entire intrinsic musculature. Both genioglossus muscles are invaded, the right sublingual space (asterisk) and the right mylohyoid muscle (arrows). Both neurovascular bundles are invaded by tumor. Note nonhomogeneous fat saturation in the chin area.

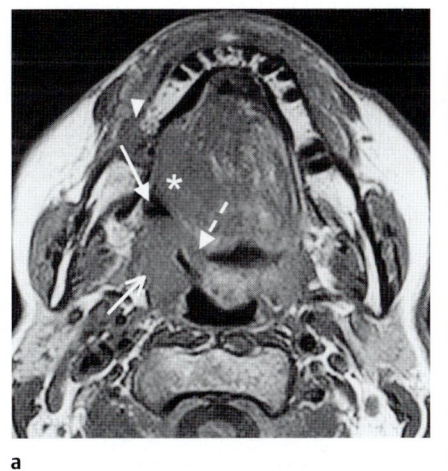

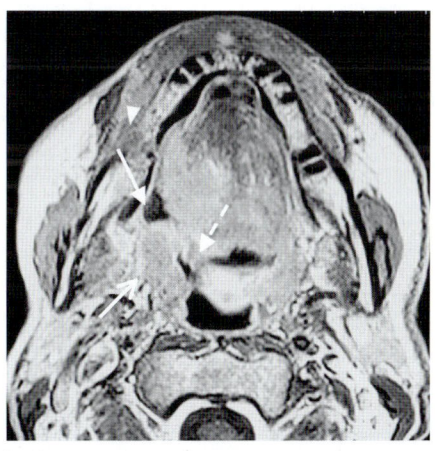

Fig. 10.24 **a** Unenhanced and **b** contrast-enhanced T1W MR images show a squamous cell cancer arising from the lateral border of the tongue (asterisk) growing into the glossotonsillar sulcus (arrows), tonsillar fossa (open arrow), and anterior tonsillar pillar (dashed arrow). Note associated mandibular invasion on the right (arrowheads).

tion to routine axial images, coronal CT or MR images may provide additional information about the exact extent of tongue neoplasms and their relationship to the neurovascular bundle. Therapeutic options (local excision, partial or total glossectomy, radiation therapy) depend upon tumor extent, bilaterality, and involvement of the ipsilateral and contralateral neurovascular bundle.

Carcinoma of the Buccal Mucosa and Gums

The cheek forms the lateral wall of the oral cavity and is made up of the buccal mucosa, buccinator muscle, external fibroadipose tissue, and skin. The mucosal surface connected with the cheek extends from the upper to the lower gingivobuccal gutters, where the mucosa reflects itself to cover the upper and lower alveolar ridges and forms the commissures of the lips and the related ramus of the mandible. Squamous cell carcinomas are typically encountered at the commissure of the mouth, along with the occlusal plane of the teeth, at the retromolar areas, or along the gums. Most **buccal carcinomas** are encountered in men in their seventh decade and tobacco or betel nut chewing, in particular, appear to play an important role in the pathogenesis of buccal carcinoma.[10,52,107] Buccal carcinomas are also divided into three subtypes: exophytic, ulcerative, and verrucous. Squamous cell carcinoma of the buccal mucosa tends to invade the masticator space, the buccinator muscle with subsequent involvement of the skin, the anterior tonsillar pillars, and the soft palate.[13,87,100] (Figs. **10.25**, **10.26**). Infiltration of the medial pterygoid muscle causes trismus and this may be the first presenting symptom.

Pathways of lymphatic spread in buccal carcinoma are variable and include the submandibular, facial, intraparotid, and preauricular nodes. Lymph node metastases are seen early and are present in approximately 50% of cases. Early buccal cancers may be difficult to visualize on sectional imaging, as they may be indistinguishable from the orbicularis oris muscle. Large tumors are easily seen on CT and MRI. Low-volume lesions may be treated by a transoral excision. However, tumors that extend to

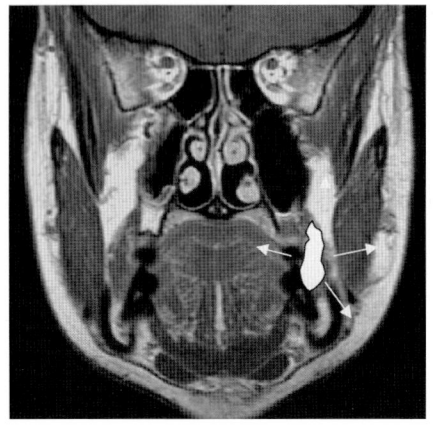

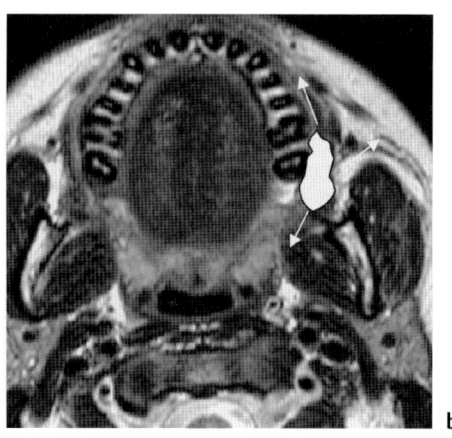

Fig. 10.25 a, b Patterns of tumor spread in carcinoma of the buccal mucosa.

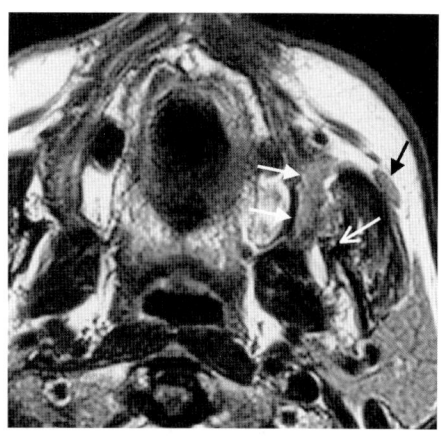

Fig. 10.26 T2W MR image shows a buccal carcinoma that extends posteriorly along the buccinator muscle (arrows). The tumor abuts the anterior portion of the ascending ramus of the mandible (open arrow). Note also the presence of an enlarged facial lymph node (black arrow).

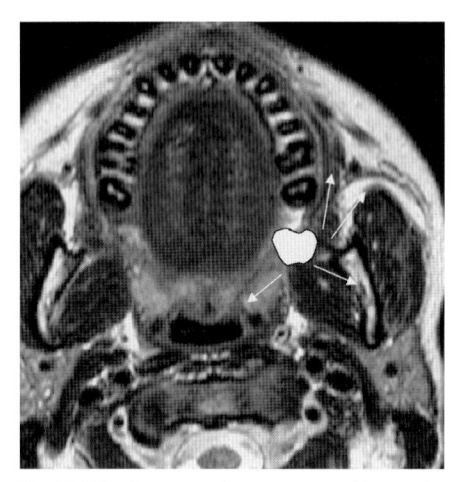

Fig. 10.27 Patterns of tumor spread in carcinoma of the retromolar trigone.

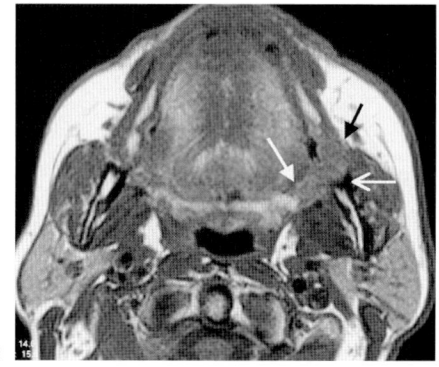

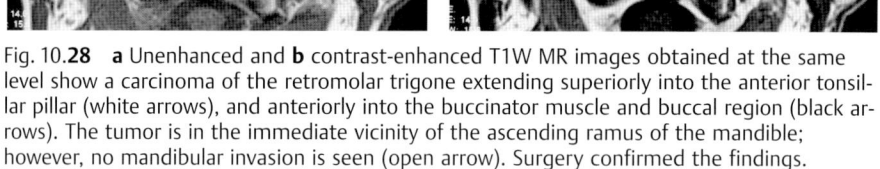

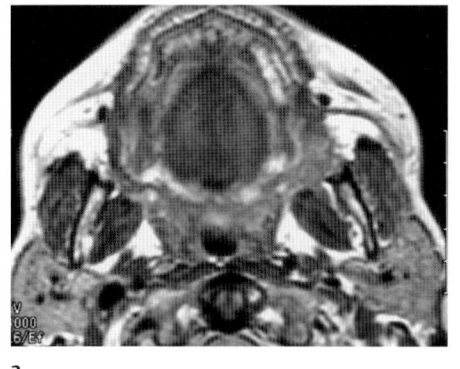

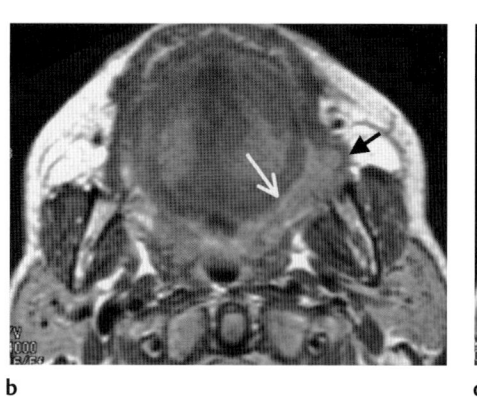

Fig. 10.28 **a** Unenhanced and **b** contrast-enhanced T1W MR images obtained at the same level show a carcinoma of the retromolar trigone extending superiorly into the anterior tonsillar pillar (white arrows), and anteriorly into the buccinator muscle and buccal region (black arrows). The tumor is in the immediate vicinity of the ascending ramus of the mandible; however, no mandibular invasion is seen (open arrow). Surgery confirmed the findings.

Fig. 10.29 T2W MR images at various levels (**a–c**) show a retromolar trigone cancer arising posterior to the maxillary tuberosity. The tumor extends anterolaterally along the buccinator muscle, invades the buccal fat (arrow), extends posteriorly into the anterior tonsillar pillar (open arrow) and inferiorly into the floor of the mouth (arrow), and invades the ascending ramus of the mandible (dashed arrow). Note for comparison the normal aspect of the right mandible with a high-signal intensity fatty marrow.

the pterygomandibular raphe require a more extensive resection and bone invasion requires additional partial mandibulectomy or maxillectomy.[100]

Cancers originating in the *retromolar trigone* may grow anteriorly into the buccal region, and thus mimic a buccal carcinoma (Figs. 10.27, 10.28). They may grow posteriorly along the superior constrictor pharyngeal muscle into the tonsil. Superior growth along the pterygomandibular raphe allows for access to the skull base and nasopharynx, whereas inferior growth results in invasion of the floor of the mouth. Owing to the close vicinity of the ascending branch of the mandible, osseous invasion is common (Fig. 10.29). Low-volume superficial lesions may be treated by a

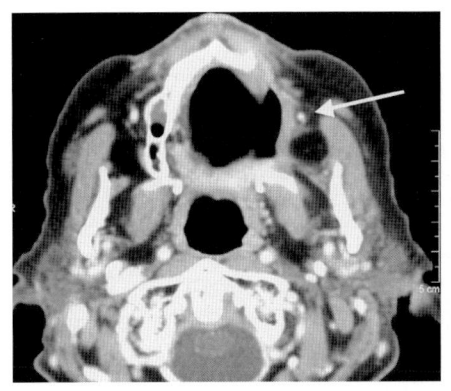

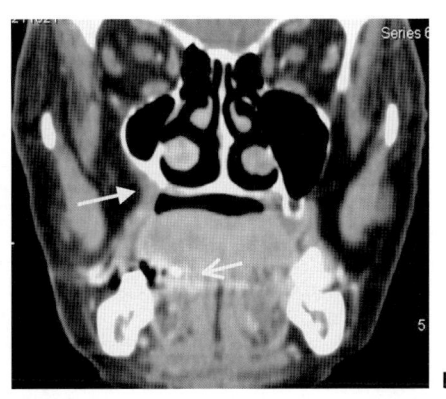

Fig. 10.**30** Squamous cell carcinoma of the hard palate. **a** Contrast-enhanced axial CT image and **b** coronal 2D reconstruction from volumetric data set show an advanced tumor of the hard palate originating from the left lateral border and with extensive invasion of the maxilla (arrows). The patient had a second primary neoplasm arising from the left lateral tongue border (open arrow).

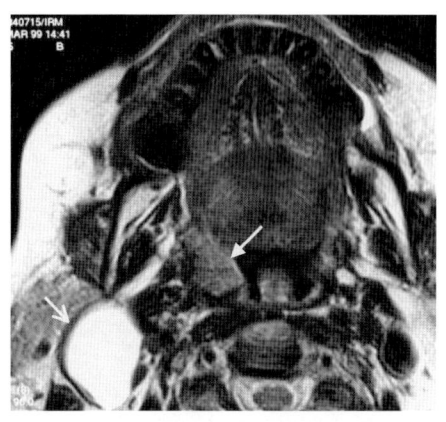

Fig. 10.**31** Squamous cell carcinoma of the right tonsil with a large "cystic" lymph node metastasis. On the T2W MR image the right tonsillar fossa is larger than the left, suggesting the presence of a tumor mass (arrow). Open arrow points to a large upper jugular lymph node metastasis that is entirely necrotic ("cystic").

transoral surgical approach. Large tumors with invasion of adjacent structures at imaging will undergo either surgery including partial mandibulectomy/maxillectomy or organ-preserving combined radiation therapy and chemotherapy.[100, 124, 143]

Squamous cell carcinoma of the gums (gingiva and alveolar mucosa) frequently occurs in the molar and premolar regions along the gingival margin of a tooth or tooth socket with the lower jaw affected more often than the upper jaw.[10, 52, 107, 124, 143] The clinical diagnosis may be difficult, since the signs and symptoms may be confused with benign inflammatory or reactive lesions so commonly seen in this location. Clinically, these tumors may present as ulcerating, plaque-like or nodular lesions. Destruction of the underlying bone is a frequent finding occuring in nearly 50% of carcinomas of the gums.[61, 139] The usual route of invasion is through the edentulous alveolar ridge. Bone destruction is in many cases clinically occult and is seen only at imaging. Radiographs, including dental views, Panarex view, CT, DentaScan or MRI augment the evaluation. Nearly 50% of patients have submandibular lymph node metastases at initial presentation and, as a general rule, metastases tend to be less differentiated than the primary tumor. Cervical metastases from the lower alveolar ridge are more common than from the upper alveolar ridge. Both sites tend to metastasize to the submandibular lymph nodes; however, upper alveolar ridge cancers may also metastasize to the upper deep cervical lymph nodes.

Carcinoma of the Hard Palate

In the western hemisphere, malignant tumors arising from the hard palate are of minor salivary gland origin in approximately 50% of cases and of squamous cell origin in the remaining 50%.[10, 52, 107] Squamous cell carcinoma of the hard palate usually occurs in elderly men and is related to smoking. A high incidence of hard palate carcinomas occurs in those countries where reverse smoking is practiced. Necrotizing sialometaplasia and follicular lymphoid hyperplasia are two benign lesions that can be confused with carcinoma of the hard palate.

Squamous cell carcinoma of the hard palate may arise in the midline or to one side or the other of the hard palate close to the upper gingiva. The neoplasm is only rarely localized and is often surrounded by areas of leukoplakia. Although the tumor is often confined to its site of origin at the time of diagnosis, advanced tumors may invade the maxilla, nasal cavity, buccal mucosa, tongue, or retromolar trigone (Fig. 10.**30**). Perineural extension via the greater and lesser palatine nerves into the pterygopalatine fossa is a common pathway not only for adenoid cystic carcinoma but also for squamous cell carcinoma. Therefore, perineural tumor spread should be sought with MRI to evaluate the pterygopalatine fossa and foramen rotundum. Small tumors may be very difficult to see on CT, as they may appear only as a slight asymmetry. However, CT is the ideal modality to evaluate subtle bone erosion. On T2-weighted MR images, tumors of the hard palate may show high signal intensity, allowing easier detection. Coronal sections (CT or MRI) are extremely useful for evaluating these tumors. Approximately 30% of patients with squamous cell carcinoma of the hard palate present with cervical lymph node metastases. Lymphatic spread occurs along the facial and retropharyngeal lymph nodes and along the upper jugular chain.

The management of squamous cell carcinoma of the hard palate is similar to that of other oral tumors. Low-volume superficial lesions without bone erosion may be excised through an intraoral approach, while extensive tumors with bone erosion may require partial maxillectomy.

Carcinoma of the Tonsils and Palatine Arches

Oropharyngeal squamous cell carcinomas are usually poorly differentiated and locally advanced at the time of clinical presentation. The overall incidence of cervical lymph node metastasis is 50–70%. Therefore, the prognosis is often unfavorable.[10, 52, 107, 129]

Carcinomas of the tonsil accounts for 1.5–3% of all cancers and are second in frequency only to carcinomas of the larynx among the malignancies of the upper aerodigestive tract. A sore throat may be the only symptom, and the first indication of a neoplasm may be a lymph node metastasis. Furthermore, occult and small carcinomas situated in the tonsillar crypts tend to produce cystic metastases in the jugulodigastric region and the primary lesion has to be looked for thoroughly (Fig. 10.**31**). Tonsillar carcinomas, in their early stages, are usually found arising near the upper pole of the tonsil. The tumor is prone to spread anteriorly and posteriorly to the tonsillar pillars, thereby acquiring the potential spread pattern associated with these sites (Fig. 10.**32**). These lesions may extend posterolaterally to the lateral pharyngeal wall, parapharyngeal space, and pterygoid muscles; inferiorly to the glossotonsillar sulcus, base of the tongue, and floor of the mouth; and superiorly to the soft palate and nasopharynx.[13, 14, 51] (Figs. 10.**33**–10.**35**). Bone erosion is an unusual finding and is present only in advanced stages. Extensive inva-

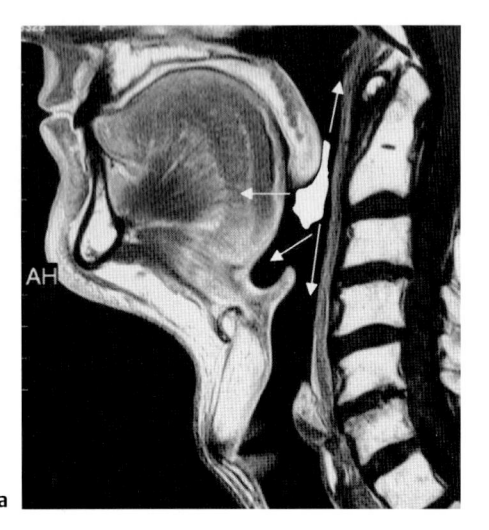

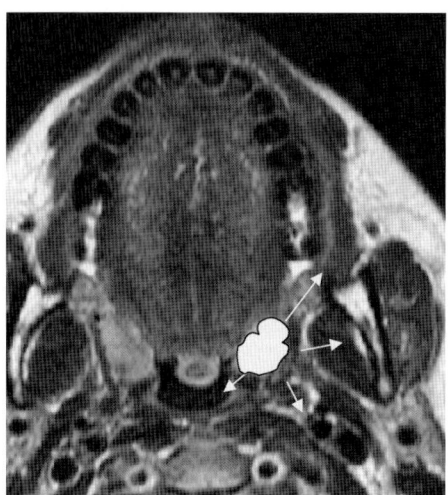

Fig. 10.**32a, b** Patterns of tumor spread in carcinoma of the tonsil.

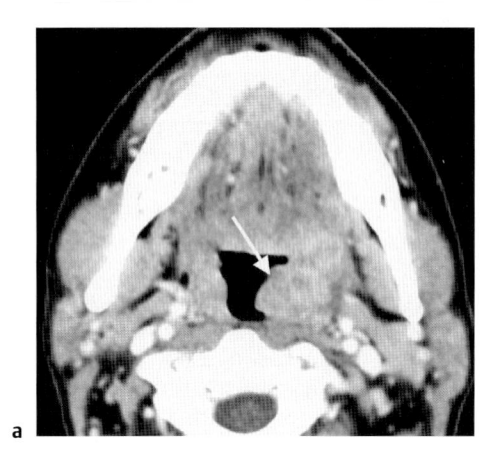

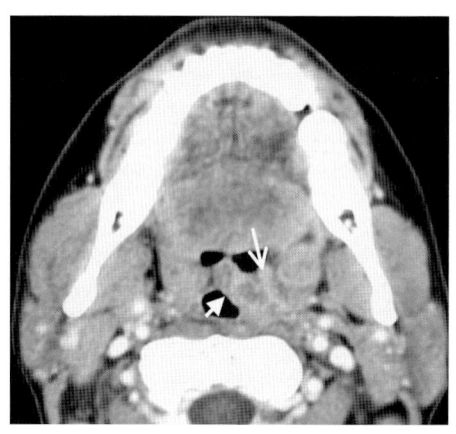

Fig. 10.**33a, b** Axial contrast-enhanced CT images. Squamous cell carcinoma of the left tonsil (arrow) with invasion of the anterior tonsillar pillar (open arrow) and soft palate (short arrow).

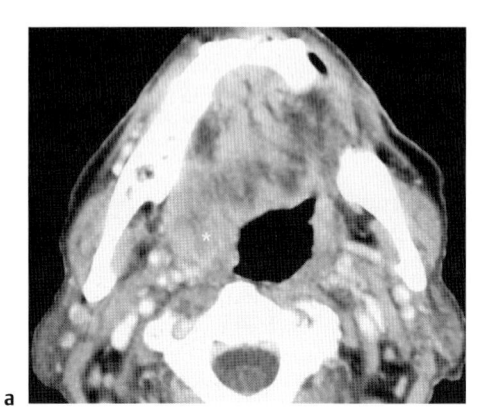

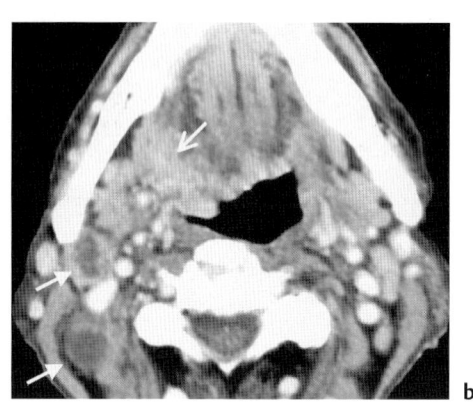

Fig. 10.**34a, b** Axial contrast-enhanced CT images show a squamous cell carcinoma of the right tonsil (asterisk) with inferior spread into the glossotonsillar sulcus and floor of the mouth (open arrow) and invasion of the parapharyngeal space. Note for comparison the normal appearance of fat within the left parapharyngeal space. Upper jugular lymph node metastases with central nodal necrosis are seen on the left (arrows).

sion of the parapharyngeal and masticator spaces may be associated with carotid artery encasement or extension superiorly along the fascial and muscle planes into the skull base. If the tumor encompasses more than 270° of the circumference of the carotid artery on axial images, it becomes unlikely that it can be removed without resecting the vessel.[144] Although the normal tonsillar fossae may be asymmetric, asymmetry of the tonsillar region should be viewed with strong suspicion when there is metastatic adenopathy in the neck from an unknown primary. Obliteration of the parapharyngeal space should be viewed with suspicion regardless of the nodal status in the neck.

Lymph node metastases occur primarily in the upper jugular or retropharyngeal nodes, but the spinal accessory and submandibular nodes are also at risk. Squamous cell cancers arising within the tonsillar fossa have an overall 70% chance of having clinically positive nodal metastases at initial presentation. Early tumors localized in the tonsillar fossa may undergo a wide local excision through an intraoral approach. Advanced lesions extending to the parapharyngeal and masticator spaces require resection of portions of the tongue base, mandible, or maxilla. In many institutions these large tumors will be treated with combined radiation therapy and chemotherapy.

Distant metastases constitute a significant problem in patients with tonsillar cancers, occurring in approximately 15–20% of all patients over the course of the disease. Distant spread occurs most commonly to the lungs in patients with advanced

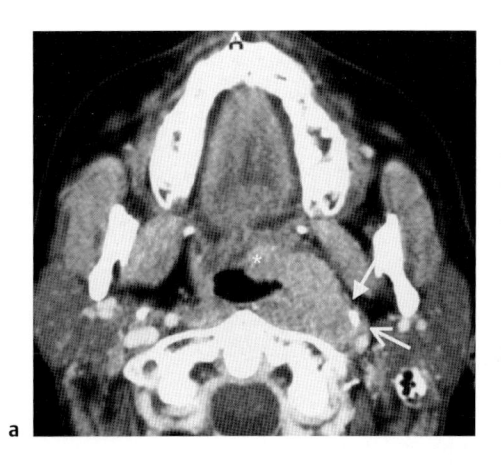

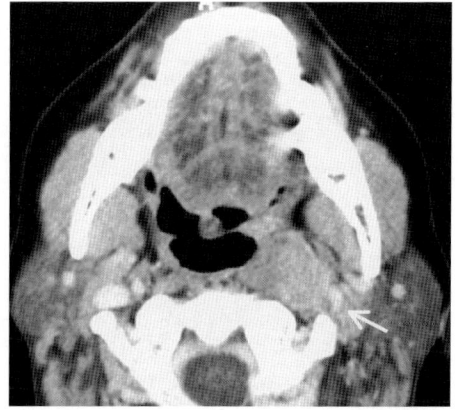

Fig. 10.**35 a**, **b** Axial contrast-enhanced CT images. Squamous cell carcinoma of the left tonsil extending into the posterior tonsillar pillar (asterisk) and parapharyngeal space (white arrow). Note displacement and encasement of the left internal carotid artery (open arrows).

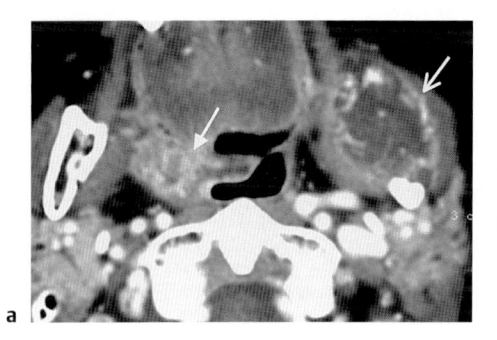

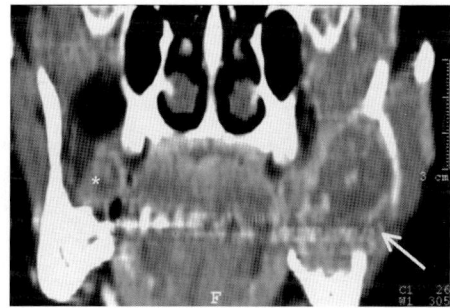

Fig. 10.**36 a** Axial contrast-enhanced CT image and **b** 2D coronal reconstruction from volumetric data set. Squamous cell carcinoma of the right tonsil (asterisk) extending into the soft palate (arrow). The patient also has a large osteolytic lesion within the ascending ramus of the left mandible (open arrows). Histology confirmed that it was a metastasis from his squamous cell cancer. Thoracic CT showed further metastases to the lungs (not shown).

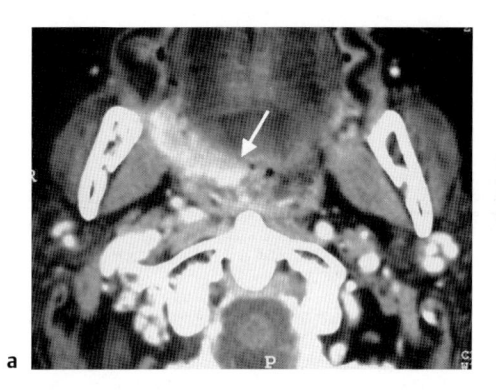

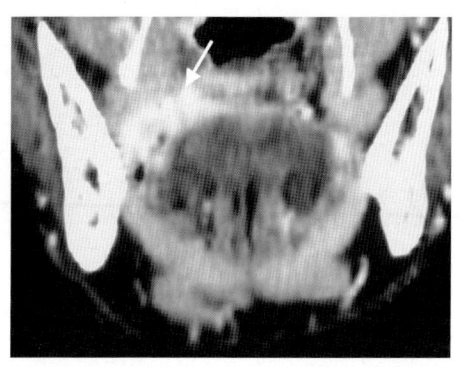

Fig. 10.**37 a** Axial contrast-enhanced CT image and **b** 2D coronal reconstruction from volumetric data set show a strong enhancing lesion arising from the right anterior tonsillar pillar and spreading superiorly into the soft palate (arrows). Histology confirmed squamous cell cancer.

disease or with pathologically proven lymph nodes at multiple levels in the neck or in the lower neck.[52,94,107] (Fig. 10.**36**).

Superficial tumors involving the palatine arches typically demonstrate multifocality, commonly known as "sick mucosa."[10,51,52,107] Tumors arising on the *anterior tonsillar pillars* are much more common than tumors arising on the posterior tonsillar pillars. **Squamous cell cancers of the anterior tonsillar pillar** tend to spread superiorly to invade the soft palate, and from there anteriorly into the hard palate or further superiorly into the nasopharynx, pterygoid muscles, and skull base[87,100] (Fig. 10.**37**). Anterior spread of anterior tonsillar pillar lesions occurs along the pterygomandibular raphe into the buccinator muscle and inferior spread occurs along the palatoglossus muscle into the base of the tongue. Lymph node metastases occur primarily in the submandibular and in the upper jugular lymph nodes. Squamous cell cancers arising within the anterior tonsillar pillar have an overall 45% chance of having clinically positive nodal metastases at initial presentation.

Squamous cell cancers of the posterior tonsillar pillar tend to spread superiorly into the soft palate, posteriorly into the posterior pharyngeal wall, or inferiorly into the pharyngoepiglottic fold. The primary lymphatic drainage is to the upper jugular nodes. However, the retropharyngeal and spinal accessory nodes are at risk in the presence of posterior pharyngeal wall involvement.

Carcinoma of the Base of the Tongue

Twenty-five percent of tongue neoplasms occur in the posterior one-third (base of the tongue), which is the oropharyngeal portion of the tongue. **Squamous cell carcinoma of the base of the tongue** is an aggressive, deeply infiltrative tumor with a 75% incidence of lymph node metastases at presentation and with nearly 30% of patients having bilateral lymph node metastases.[10,107] Base of the tongue cancers may extend laterally to involve the mandible and medial pterygoid muscles; superiorly to involve the tonsillar fossa and soft palate; anteriorly to involve the mobile tongue and floor of the mouth; and inferiorly to involve the vallecula, preepiglottic space, and epiglottis (see below) or portions of the hypopharynx.[13,98,100,126] (Figs. 10.**38**–10.**40**). Neoplasms and normal lymphoid tissue at the base of the tongue can be confused on both CT and MR imaging because of their enhancement patterns and T2 signal characteristics. Deep

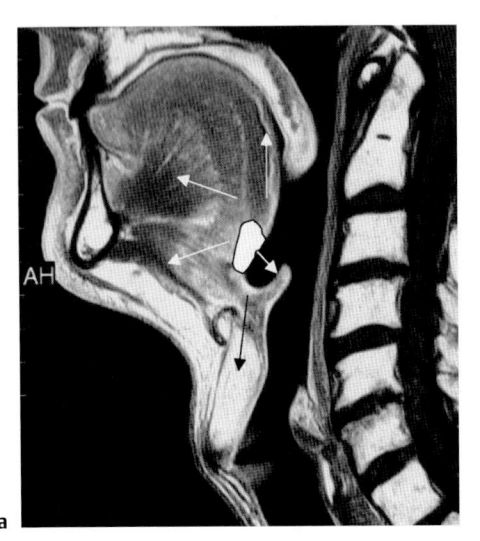

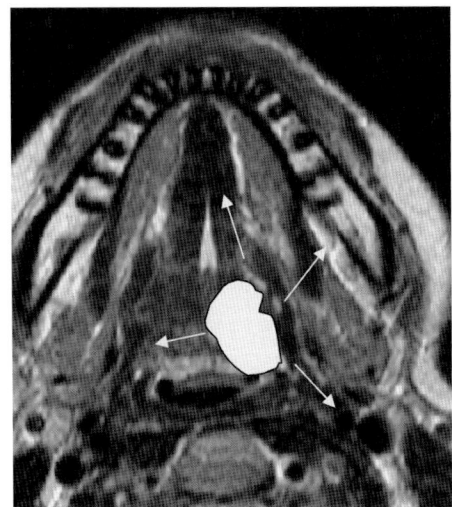

Fig. 10.**38 a**, **b** Patterns of tumor spread in carcinoma of the base of the tongue.

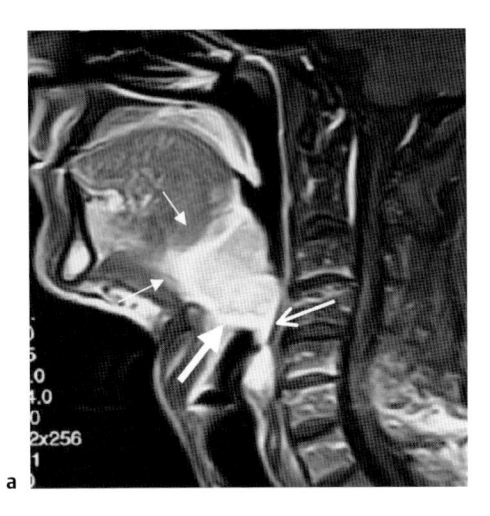

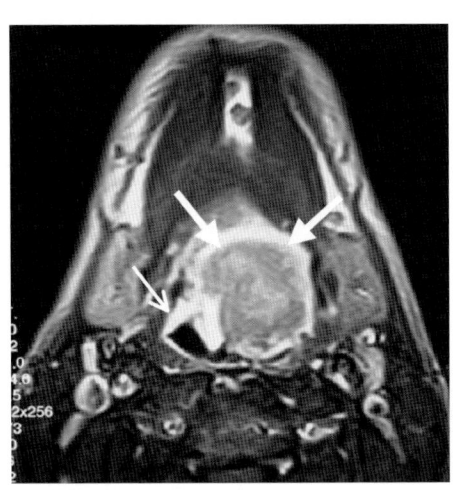

Fig. 10.**39** **a** Sagittal and **b** axial fat-saturated T1W MR images obtained after injection of contrast material show a large base of the tongue tumor spreading anteriorly into the genioglossus and geniohyoideus muscles (thin arrows) and inferiorly into the valleculae (thick arrows). The epiglottis is displaced to the right and inferiorly (open arrows). There is no invasion of the preepiglottic space. Note significant airway compromise.

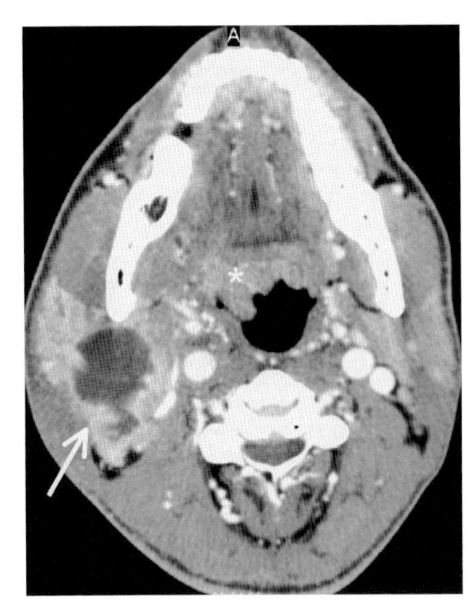

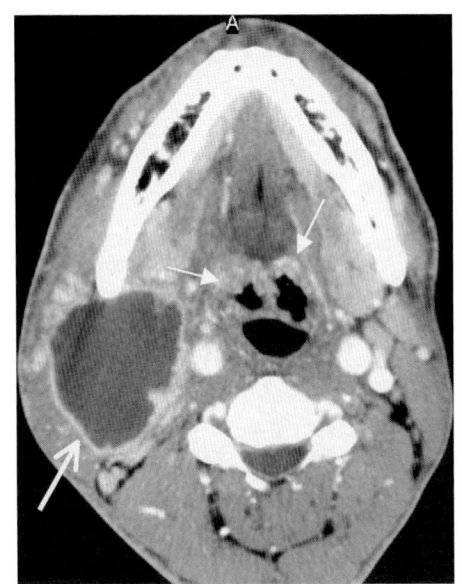

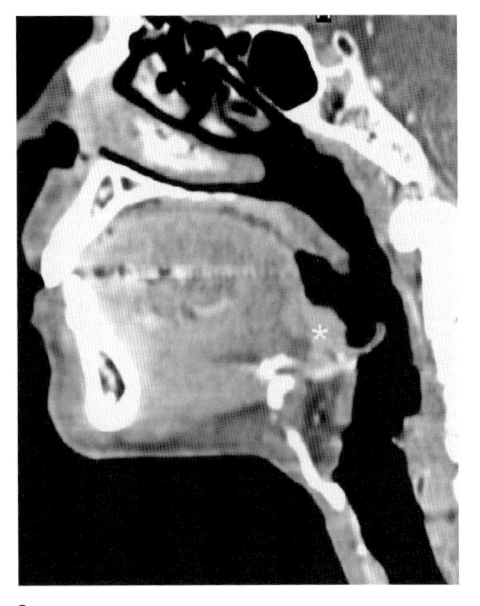

Fig. 10.**40 a**, **b** Axial contrast-enhanced CT images and **c** 2D sagittal reconstruction from volumetric data set show a base of the tongue tumor (asterisks) invading the valleculae (arrows), the median glossoepiglottic fold, and the lingual surface of the epiglottis, which appears irregular Clinically, the tumor was not visible as the mucosa appeared intact. However, deep biopsy revealed undifferentiated carcinoma of nasopharyngeal type. Note the large necrotic lymph node metastasis on the right (open arrow).

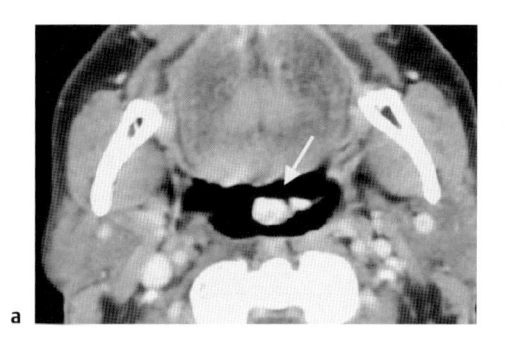

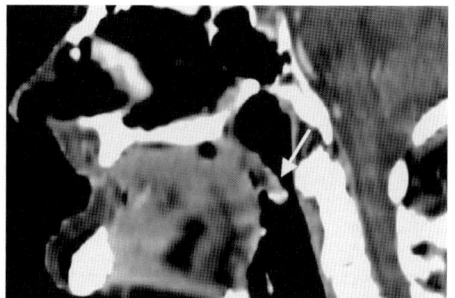

Fig. 10.**41** **a** Axial contrast-enhanced CT image and **b** 2D sagittal reconstruction from volumetric data set show a relatively small soft palate tumor extending into the uvula, which has an increased size and is irregular (arrows).

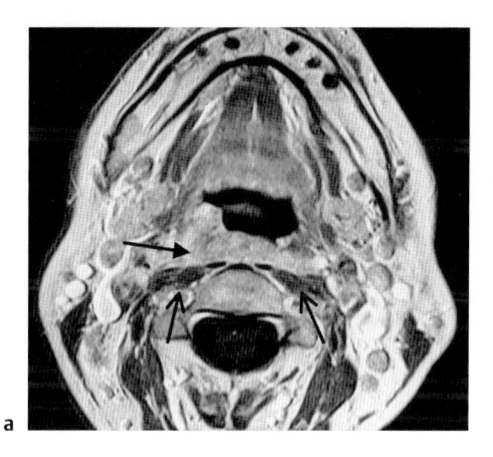

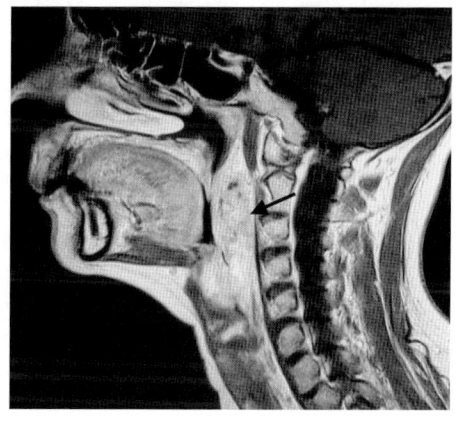

Fig. 10.**42** Squamous cell carcinoma of the posterior pharyngeal wall. **a** Axial and **b** sagittal contrast-enhanced T1W MR images show a large exophytic tumor arising from the posterior pharyngeal wall invading the pharyngeal constrictors and the retropharyngeal space (arrows), The tumor does not invade the prevertebral muscles, which show no enhancement (open arrows) Note extensive craniocaudal spread, best appreciated on the sagittal MR image (**b**).

endoscopic biopsies are the only way to differentiate between the two. In addition to routine axial images, sagittal and coronal images may provide an excellent appreciation of the volume of the tumor in the tongue base. Therapeutic options depend upon tumor volume, bilaterality, and invasion of the ipsilateral and contralateral neurovascular bundle (see below).

Carcinoma of the Soft Palate

Most soft-palate tumors are squamous cell carcinomas; however, minor salivary gland cancers may typically be seen in the posterior soft palate.[10,12,68] Squamous cell carcinomas of the soft palate have the best prognosis of all oropharyngeal carcinomas. They usually affect the oral aspect of the soft palate. Tumor extension may occur anteriorly to the hard palate, laterally to the tonsillar pillars and fossa, and from there extend further laterally into the parapharyngeal space, nasopharynx, and base of the skull. Lymph node metastases are seen in 60% of cases at initial presentation. Coronal and sagittal CT scans and MRI images are essential to evaluate soft-palate tumors, as smaller lesions may be missed on the axial plane. On CT, the attenuation values and enhancement pattern of the soft palate and tumor may be similar, and unless there is obvious fullness at imaging, the tumors may be missed (Fig. 10.**41**). Because the palate intrinsically has a high signal intensity on T1-weighted images (abundant mucous glands and fat), tumors are easily identified on T1-weighted images because of their lower signal intensity.

Carcinoma of the Posterior Oropharyngeal Wall

Carcinomas of the posterior oropharyngeal wall have the worst prognosis of all squamous cell oral cavity and oropharyngeal carcinomas. These tumors spread both in a caudal direction into the hypopharynx and in a cephalad direction into the nasopharynx[10,13,14,100,126] (Fig. 10.**42**). They commonly spread submucosally, invading the retropharyngeal fat, but owing to the presence of the prevertebral fascia, which acts as a barrier to tumor spread, invasion of the prevertebral muscles is uncommon at initial presentation. Treatment of these lesions is often by radiation therapy.

The Role of Sectional Imaging for the Pretherapeutic Workup

Some anatomical key areas and structures that are crucial for treatment planning of oral cavity and oropharyngeal carcinoma cannot be assessed reliably by means of clinical evaluation and endoscopic biopsy alone and sectional imaging therefore plays a crucial role for pretherapeutic evaluation. These key areas include bilateral or deep tongue base and neurovascular bundle; the preepiglottic space; the mandible and the maxilla; the pterygopalatine fossa and the skull base; and the prevertebral muscles.

Invasion of the Bilateral or Deep Tongue Base and Neurovascular Bundle

Low-volume superficial lesions of the anterior and posterior tongue that have no imaging findings indicative of perineural spread may be treated with wide local excision or localized radiotherapy. Advanced lesions that do not cross the midline may be adequately treated with a partial glossectomy.[100,143] From the standpoint of swallowing, as well as of speech, most individuals are able to maintain an acceptable quality of life with half of their tongue present. Tumor extension across the midline and involvement of the contralateral neurovascular bundle requires total glossectomy. Total glossectomy is a mutilating procedure that leaves the patient without any possibility of speaking intelligibly or swallowing. At many institutions, this radical form of resection is often considered an unacceptable alternative and nonsurgical organ preservation therapy consisting of combined chemotherapy and radiation therapy is performed. If a small mobile portion of the base of the tongue is preserved, functional recovery with flap reconstruction is much improved.

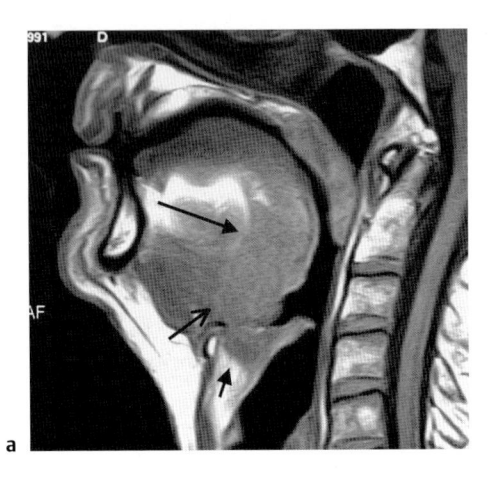

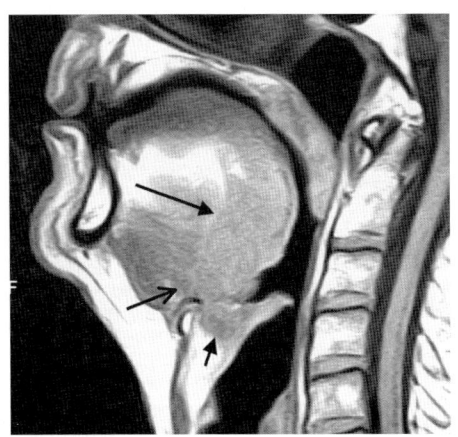

Fig. 10.**43** **a** Unenhanced and **b** contrast-enhanced sagittal T1W MR images show a large base of the tongue tumor invading the genioglossus muscle (long arrows), the geniohyoid muscle (open arrows), the valleculae, and the preepiglottic space (short arrows). Note only mild enhancement of the tumor mass.

Important surgical planning information is derived from the observation of displacement or breach of the lingual septum by tumor centered on one half of the tongue at CT or MRI. The demonstration of this feature indicates contralateral extension. Invasion of the neurovascular bundle may be well appreciated on CT by observing the margin of the tumor versus the enhancing vessels in the sublingual space.[101] T2-weighted MR images and enhanced T1-weighted MR images are also very useful in assessing the exact extent of tongue cancers and their relationship to the neurovacular bundle.

Recently it has been shown that CT may also be quite helpful in predicting whether the hypoglossal nerve (XII) will be sacrificed in floor of mouth, oral tongue, and tongue base tumor resections. Hypoglossal nerve "sacrifice" may be predicted on the basis of CT images if the fat planes surrounding the takeoff of the proximal lingual artery are obliterated by tumor. The negative predictive value of CT to assess the ability of the surgeon to spare the hypoglossal nerve is 87% with a specificity of 80%.[42]

Invasion of the Preepiglottic Space

The preepiglottic space is composed of fatty tissue and loose elastic and collagenous fibers. It is bounded anteriorly by the thyrohyoid membrane and thyroid cartilage; posteriorly by the infrahyoid epiglottis; cranially by the hyoepiglottic ligament; and caudally by the petiole of the epiglottis. The preepiglottic space is best displayed on axial and sagittal images. Owing to its high content of fatty tissue, the preepiglottic space has a low attenuation value on CT and a high signal intensity on T1-weighted and FSE T2-weighted MR images.

The preepiglottic space may be invaded by oral cavity and oropharyngeal cancer, extending into the base of the tongue and from there into the preepiglottic space. Invasion of the preepiglottic space implies supraglottic or even total laryngectomy.[52, 81, 100, 126, 143] Consequently, a base of the tongue tumor without invasion of the preepiglottic space may be resected without requiring a portion of the supraglottic larynx to be included in the resection specimen. Because combined resection of the base of the tongue and the larynx often leads to a poor quality of life with compromised swallowing and speaking, correct diagnosis is very important. Both CT and MRI are well suited to demonstrate replacement of the normal fatty tissue by tumor tissue within the preepiglottic space (Fig. 10.**43**). Although sagittal images are best suited to delineate the extent of craniocaudal tumor spread within the preepiglottic space, standard axial images are sufficient to establish the diagnosis. The reported sensitivity of CT and MRI to detect invasion of the preepiglottic space is 100%, and the corresponding specificities are 93% and 84–90%, respectively[13, 81, 146] (see also Section VI).

Invasion of the Mandible and Maxilla

Tumors tend to enter the mandible at the point of abutment, which in both the dentate and the edentulous jaw is often at the junction of the reflected and attached mucosa.[26] Invasion of the mandible is usually a late manifestation of squamous cell carcinoma of the oral cavity and oropharynx and is difficult to assess clinically. The surgical procedure will differ depending on the extent of involvement.[31, 100, 126, 143] If tumor abuts the periosteum without invading it, the periosteum is resected for margin control. Tumors with periosteum invasion or bone erosion limited to the inner or outer cortex of the mandible may be treated with a marginal mandibulectomy (cortex resection, rim mandibulectomy), thereby preserving the continuity of the mandible.[24, 25, 139] However, tumors that invade the lingual or labial cortex and extend into the marrow space necessitate treatment with segmental mandibulectomy followed by reconstruction, because primary irradiation incurs the risk of osteoradionecrosis at doses high enough to sterilize the bone disease.[24, 25] Following mandibular resection, microvascular free flaps are used to replace the bone and to achieve a satisfactory cosmetic result. Recently, it has been suggested that the degree of mandibular invasion may influence the survival rate of patients with squamous cell carcinoma of the oral cavity, but this difference is not due to local failure. While the local failure rate may be similar in both mandibulectomy groups (29% in rim mandibulectomy versus 25% in segmental mandibulectomy), vital outcome, as 5-year survival, is only 25% after rim mandibulectomy, compared to 40% after segmental mandibulectomy. The poorer prognosis in patients with segmental mandibulectomy (and more advanced mandibular infiltration) is caused by an increased incidence of metastases and second primary tumors.[130]

Subtle cortical erosion is best detected by thin-sectional CT (1 mm contiguous sections with bone algorithm), which may be supplemented by using dental CT software (Fig. 10.**44**). In general, both axial and coronal images are often required, especially in gingival tumors. The reported diagnostic accuracy of a dental computed tomographic software program, DentaScan, in assessing mandibular bone invasion in patients with squamous cell carcinoma of the oral cavity clinically fixed to the mandible is sensitivity 95%, specificity 79%, and negative predictive value 92%.[23] Recently, it has been shown that in patients with squamous cell carcinoma of the oral cavity that is clinically fixed to the mandible, 3 mm contiguous sections reconstructed with bone algorithm may yield similar results (sensitivity 96%; specificity 87%; positive predictive value 89%; negative predictive value 95%).[98] In tumors of the retromolar trigone, however, CT is a useful but potentially inaccurate predictor of bone invasion (sensitivity of only 50% with a negative predictive value of 61%).[74]

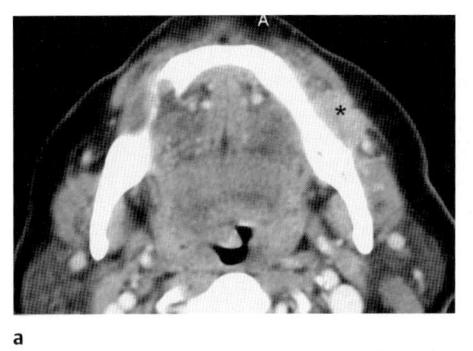

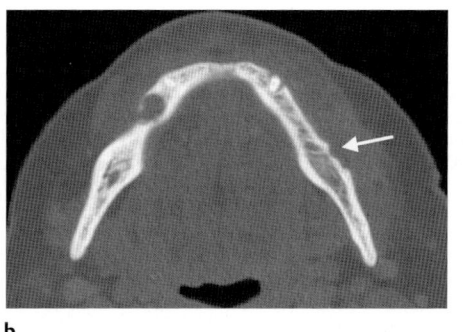

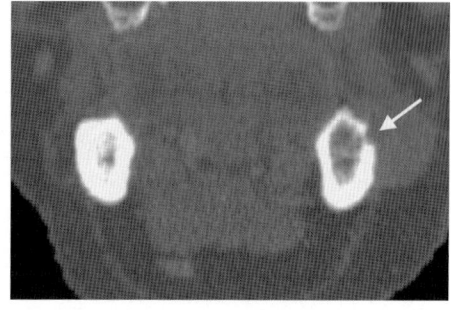

Fig. 10.**44 a, b** Axial contrast-enhanced spiral CT images acquired with 1 mm thin sections with soft-tissue (**a**) and bone algorithm (**b**). **c** Coronal 2D reconstruction image with bone algorithm from volumetric data set. A tumor of the lower right vestibular gingiva is seen (asterisk) with subtle cortical mandibular erosions (arrows).

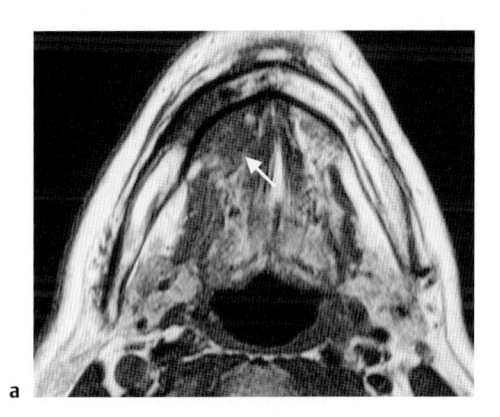

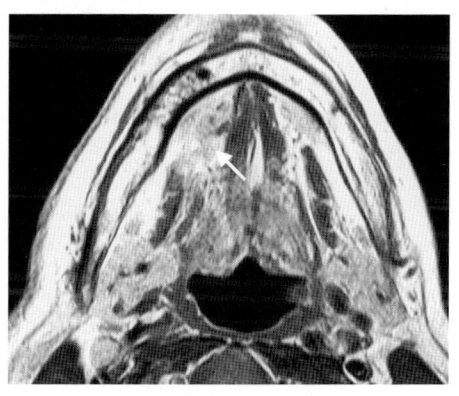

Fig. 10.**45** False-positive MRI for mandibular invasion. **a** Unenhanced and **b** contrast-enhanced axial T1W MR images show a tumor of the right floor of the mouth abutting the adjacent mandible. Clinically, the tumor was fixed to the mandible. The marrow cavity of the mandible has an abnormally low signal intensity on the T1W image and enhances after injection of contrast material. The finding were regarded as indicative of mandibular invasion, However, surgery revealed only inflammatory findings within the marrow cavity and no tumor.

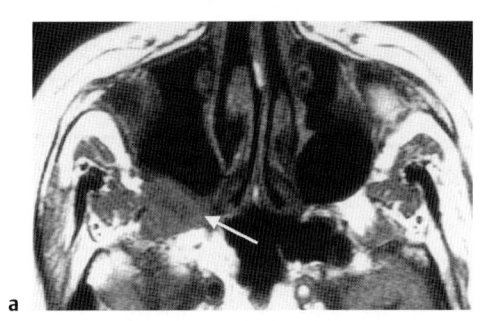

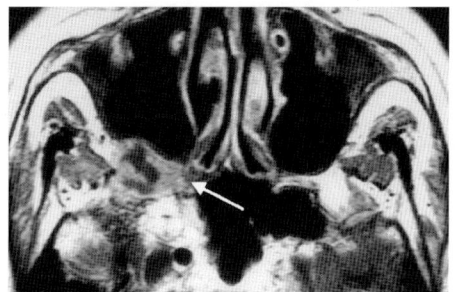

Fig. 10.**46** Perineural tumor spread along V2 to the pterygopalatine fossa in a patient with a squamous cell carcinoma of the soft palate. **a** Unenhanced and **b** contrast-enhanced axial T1W MR images show a tumor mass with central areas of necrosis within the right pteryopalatine fossa (arrows).

Invasion of the mandibular marrow is best detected with MRI. A low signal intensity on unenhanced T1-weighted MR images, high signal intensity on T2-weighted MR images or STIR images, and enhancement after administration of contrast material may be considered as indicative of mandibular invasion. However, these findings are not always specific and may also be caused by peritumoral edema and inflammation, coexisting periodontal disease, osteomyelitis, and—following radiation therapy—radiation fibrosis and osteoradionecrosis (Fig. 10.**45**). The reported sensitivity of MRI to detect invasion of the mandible is 96%, and the specificity is 84–90%.[13, 31, 143]

Invasion of the maxilla is most often seen in retromolar trigone cancers and cancers of the hard palate. Bone erosion implies resection through a partial maxillectomy rather than wide local excision. Partial maxillectomies are well tolerated by patients provided appropriately tailored obturators are constructed that separate the oral cavity from the nasal cavity and oropharynx. Otherwise, velopharyngeal insufficiency with phonation difficulties and regurgitation of food products into the nasal cavity may arise. Thin sectional (1–2 mm) coronal CT is ideal for identifying subtle erosions of the maxilla.

Pterygopalatine Fossa Invasion and Perineural Spread

Perineural tumor spread is typically seen in squamous cell carcinomas, adenoid cystic carcinomas, and lymphomas originating in the oral cavity and oropharynx (see also Chapters 3 and 4). The recognition of perineural tumor spread is critical to the complete resection of the primary tumor.

Perineural tumor spread results in increased gadolinium contrast enhancement and/or enlargement of the involved nerve on MR imaging, and enlargement of the respective neural foramen on CT scans. In a normal-sized nerve, enhancement of the nerve is suggestive of perineural tumor spread until proven otherwise.[37, 100] Because each of the major neural trunks that may serve as pathways for perineural spread are surrounded by fat as they emerge from the skull base, obliteration of this fat is suggestive of perineural tumor spread. Conversely, in the presence of normal perineural fat, perineural tumor spread can be excluded quite reliably. Perineural tumor spread may occur in both retrograde or antegrade fashion. For example, a tumor of the hard palate may spread in a retrograde fashion to the pterygopalatine fossa (Fig. 10.**46**). From the pterygopalatine fossa it may spread in an antegrade fashion to the infraorbital nerve.

Table 10.1 TNM staging of oral cavity cancer

T: Primary tumor	
TX	Primary tumor cannot be assessed
T0	No evidence of primary tumor
Tis	Carcinoma in situ
T1	Tumor diameter 2 cm or less
T2	Tumor diameter between 2 and 4 cm
T3	Tumor diameter greater than 4 cm
T4a	(lip) Tumor invades through cortical bone, inferior alveolar nerve, floor of the mouth, or skin (chin or nose)
T4a	(oral cavity) Tumor invades through cortical bone, into deep/extrinsic muscles of tongue (genioglossus, hyoglossus, palatoglossus, and styloglossus), maxillary sinus, or skin of the face
T4b	(lip and oral cavity) Tumor invades masticatoe space, pterygoid plates, or skull base, or encases internal carotid artery.
N: Regional lymph nodes	
NX	Regional lymph nodes cannot be assessed
N0	No regional lymph node metastasis
N1	Metastasis in a single ipsilateral lymph node, less than 3 cm
N2	Metastasis in a single ipsilateral lymph node between 3 and 6 cm; or in multiple ipsilateral lymph nodes, none more than 6 cm in greatest dimension; or in bilateral or contralateral lymph nodes, none more than 6 cm in greatest dimension
N2a	Metastasis in a single ipsilateral lymph node between 3 and 6 cm
N2b	Metastasis in multiple ipsilateral lymph nodes, none more than 6 cm in greatest dimension
N2c	Metastasis in bilateral or contralateral lymph nodes, none more than 6 cm in greatest dimension
N3	Metastasis in a lymph node greater then 6 cm
M: Distant metastasis	
MX	Distant metastasis cannot be assessed
M0	No distant metastasis
M1	Distant metastasis

Table 10.2 TNM staging of oropharyngeal cancer

T: Primary tumor	
TX	Primary tumor cannot be assessed
T0	No evidence of primary tumor
Tis	Carcinoma in situ
T1	Tumor diameter 2 cm or less
T2	Tumor diameter between 2 and 4 cm
T3	Tumor diameter greater than 4 cm
T4a	Tumor involves any of the following: larynx, deep/extrinsic muscles of the tongue (genioglossus, hyoglossus, palatoglossus, and styloglossus), medial pterygoid, hard palate, and mandible
T4b	Tumor involves any of the following: lateral pterygoid muscle, pterygoid plates, lateral nasopharynx, skull base, or encases the carotid artery
N: Regional lymph nodes	
NX	Regional lymph nodes cannot be assessed
N0	No regional lymph node metastasis
N1	Metastasis in a single ipsilateral lymph node, less than 3 cm
N2	Metastasis in a single ipsilateral lymph node between 3 and 6 cm; or in multiple ipsilateral lymph nodes, none more than 6 cm in greatest dimension; or in bilateral or contralateral lymph nodes, none more than 6 cm in greatest dimension
N2a	Metastasis in a single ipsilateral lymph node between 3 and 6 cm
N2b	Metastasis in multiple ipsilateral lymph nodes, none more than 6 cm in greatest dimension
N2c	Metastasis in bilateral or contralateral lymph nodes, none more than 6 cm in greatest dimension
N3	Metastasis in a lymph node greater then 6 cm Midline nodes are considered ipsilateral nodes.
M: Distant metastasis	
MX	Distant metastasis cannot be assessed
M0	No distant metastasis
M1	Distant metastasis

The trigeminal nerve is the main route for perineural spread of tumors of the oral cavity and oropharynx. The maxillary nerve is the common pathway of perineural spread from tumors of the palate and tonsillar pillars. If tumor follows the palatine nerves to the pterygopalatine fossa, the fat within the fossa is obliterated. From the pterygopalatine fossa, the tumor extends through the foramen rotundum and vidian canal to the region of the cavernous sinus and foramen lacerum, respectively. In advanced tonsillar, retromolar trigone, and buccal cancers with invasion of the pterygoid muscles, the mandibular nerve can carry tumor through the foramen ovale, reaching the cavernous sinus, gasserian ganglion, and petrous apex. Finally, the tumor can grow posteriorly from the cavernous sinus and gasserian cisterns following the preganglionic fibers of the trigeminal nerve toward the brainstem. As tumor follows the nerve, the nerve usually enlarges. Perineural spread alters the therapeutic approach considerably. Extension below the skull base may be treated surgically, but intracranial extension will be treated with radiation therapy and chemotherapy at many institutions.

Invasion of the Prevertebral Muscles

Invasion of the prevertebral muscles (longus capiti and longus colli) usually occurs with posterior spread of posterior pharyngeal wall cancers and precludes surgical resection. Because the prevertebral musculature is so close to the spinal canal and spinal cord, special attention has to be paid to radiation portals so as to avoid major radiation-induced complications, such as transverse myelitis.[11] Irregular muscle contours, a high signal intensity on T2-weighted MR images, and enhancement after administration of contrast material on T1-weighted MR or on CT images suggest the possibility of prevertebral muscle invasion. However, these findings are nonspecific and may also be caused by peritumoral edema and inflammation.[82, 143]

Imaging and Tumor Classification According to the TNM System

The guidelines of the Union Internationale Contre le Cancer (UICC) and the American Joint Committee on Cancer (AJCC)[11, 57, 127a] recommend the use of sectional imaging and several studies have shown that the use of sectional imaging greatly improves the accuracy of pretherapeutic T-classification. In spite of an improved diagnosis of T1 stages, no clear improvement in the staging of carcinoma of the oral cavity and oropharynx can be expected by spiral CT as compared to conventional dynamic incremental CT.[67] The reported overall staging accuracy of CT for oral cavity cancer is 81–85% and the staging accuracy for oropharyngeal cancer is 84–90%.[67, 77, 78] The reported overall staging accuracy of MRI is similar and varies between 81% and 90% for both regions.[77, 78, 134]. However, owing to its superior soft-tissue contrast, MRI generally offers a higher sensitivity than CT in the evaluation of small tumors of the oral cavity and oropharynx. Particularly in the oral cavity, MRI has an advantage over CT since tooth fillings or dense bone cause fewer or no artifacts.

The TNM classification of oral cavity and oropharyngeal cancer is given in Tables 10.1 and 10.2.

Atypical Forms of Squamous Cell Carcinoma

"Atypical forms of squamous cell carcinoma" are variants of squamous cell carcinoma with distinct histological and immunohistochemical characteristics. Atypical forms of squamous cell carcinoma include verrucous carcinoma, undifferentiated carcinoma of nasopharyngeal type, spindle cell carcinoma, basaloid cell carcinoma, adenoid squamous cell carcinoma and giant-cell carcinoma.[9–11, 18] According to the literature, 5–12% of all oral cavity and oropharyngeal tumors are atypical forms of squamous cell carcinoma.[4, 9–11]

Verrucous Carcinoma

Verrucous carcinoma or Ackerman tumor is typically seen in the buccal mucosa and lower gingiva of elderly men who have a history of tobacco chewing.[9, 10, 64] The prognosis of verrucous carcinoma of the oral cavity is excellent provided patients undergo surgery from the beginning. Clinically, the tumor presents as a warty, bulky outgrowth with multiple filiform projections and it may be confused with verruca vulgaris. Although verrucous carcinoma may be locally aggressive and advanced forms may invade the mandible, it almost never metastasizes to the lymph nodes. Surgery alone is considered by most authors as the treatment of choice and in most cases the lesion is amenable to local excision. Because superficial biopsies may lack the characteristic histological signs, full-thickness biopsies or, when possible, excisional biopsy are necessary to establish the diagnosis.[9, 10, 18, 64] Although verrucous carcinoma of the larynx (see Chapter 11) may display characteristic radiological features, no data on the radiological characteristics of verrucous carcinoma in the oral cavity and oropharynx have yet been published.

Undifferentiated Carcinoma of Nasopharyngeal Type

Undifferentiated carcinoma of nasopharyngeal type is an unusual variant of squamous cell carcinoma with a distinct lymphoid component.[9, 10, 18] The tumor mainly affects men between 60 and 70 years of age. Infection with the Epstein–Barr virus (EBV) appears to play an important etiological role. The tumor most commonly arises in the base of the tongue and tonsils because these regions are very rich in lymphatic tissue (Fig. 10.**40**). Patients with undifferentiated carcinoma of nasopharyngeal type present with tumors that are more aggressive than the common form of squamous cell cancer. The frequency of distant and nodal metastases in undifferentiated carcinoma of nasopharyngeal type is higher than in the common form of squamous cell cancer. Cervical lymph node metastases, metastases to the contralateral nodes and large lymph node conglomerates, may be the first presenting symptom.[9, 10, 52, 62] Similarly to what has been reported in the larynx, these tumors have the same imaging features as the common form of squamous cell carcinoma. Radiotherapy alone or in combination with chemotherapy is effective in eradicating localized disease.[75, 211, 230]

Basaloid Squamous Cell Carcinoma

Basaloid squamous cell carcinoma of the oral cavity and oropharynx is more frequent in men in their sixth and seventh decades of life and with a history of heavy smoking and alcohol abuse. Clinically, the tumor appears as an ulcerated, exophytic firm mass.[4] The main histological features include a basaloid pattern in intimate association with squamous cell carcinoma. On biopsy, basaloid squamous cell carcinoma may have some similarities with other histological types of tumors, such as adenoid cystic carcinoma, or adenosquamous carcinoma. Electron microscopy and immunohistochemical investigations are helpful in establishing the correct diagnosis. The predilection sites in the oral cavity and oropharynx are the floor of the mouth and the tonsils. The prognosis of basaloid squamous cell carcinoma is very poor and unpredictable.[4, 9, 10] The tumor has frequently been observed in advanced stages, and it shows an aggressive behavior with perineural invasion, cervical lymph node metastases, and distant spread to lungs, liver, bones, brain, and skin.[4] When compared with the common type of squamous cell carcinoma of the same region, basaloid squamous cell carcinoma demonstrates higher rates of local recurrence, of distant metastases, and of mortality and a shorter mean survival.[4]

Table 10.**3** Unusual squamous and non-squamous cell neoplasms of the oral cavity and oropharynx

Atypical forms of squamous cell carcinoma
- Verrucous carcinoma or Ackerman tumor
- Undifferentiated carcinoma of nasopharyngeal type
- Basaloid squamous cell carcinoma of the oral cavity and oropharynx

Malignant non-squamous cell neoplasms
- Minor salivary gland neoplasms
  - Mucoepidermoid carcinoma
  - Adenoid cystic carcinoma
  - Acinic carcinoma
  - Adenocarcinoma
- Primary lymphoma
  - Hodgkin
  - Non-Hodgkin
- Liposarcoma
- Rhabdomyosarcoma
- Leiomyosarcoma
- Malignant fibrous histiocytoma
- Fibrosarcoma
- Synovial sarcoma

Benign non-squamous cell neoplasms
- Pleomorphic adenoma (benign mixed tumor)
- Lipoma
- Schwannoma
- Neurofibroma
- Aggressive fibromatosis (extra-abdominal desmoid tumor)
- Rhabdomyoma
- Leiomyoma
- Hemangiopericytoma

■ Non-Squamous Cell Neoplasms

Malignant Non-Squamous Cell Neoplasms

Non-squamous cell neoplasms of the oral cavity and oropharynx are listed in Table 10.**3**.

Minor Salivary Gland Neoplasms

Minor salivary gland neoplasms represent the next most common tumors of the oral cavity and oropharynx, excluding Hodgkin and non-Hodgkin lymphoma. There are an estimated 500–1000 minor salivary glands within the oral cavity and oropharynx. The hard and soft palates are the most common locations for the salivary glands and, hence, for minor salivary gland neoplasms. Nevertheless, minor salivary gland neoplasms may arise from any other region of the oral cavity and oropharynx, such as the base of the tongue, the tonsils, and the valleculae.[12, 56, 68] The frequency of minor salivary gland neoplasms in the palate approaches that of squamous cell carcinoma in the palate. Tumors of minor salivary gland origin differ from squamous cell carcinomas in that they occur in younger patients, from the fifth to sixth decades, having an equal male to female ratio, and they grow slowly. Early minor salivary gland neoplasms are usually confined to their site of origin. Later in the course, there may be involvement of adjacent structures, such as the hard palate, maxilla, sinuses, and buccal mucosa. The most common benign tumor of minor salivary gland origin is **pleomorphic adenoma**, and the most common malignant tumor is **adenoid cystic carcinoma** (cylindroma). Together they comprise 70% of minor salivary gland neoplasms.[10, 51]

Adenoid cystic carcinoma is the most frequent malignant tumor of the minor salivary glands. The tumor can be located beneath a completely intact mucosa and clinical examination may reveal only a submucosal bulge (Figs. 10.**47**, 10.**48**). In these patients, deep submucosal biopsies are mandatory to make the

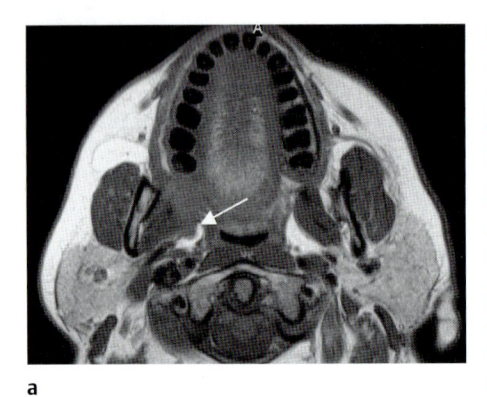

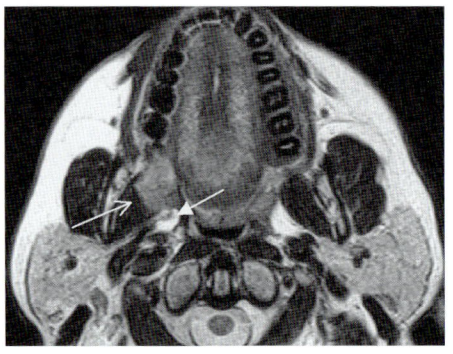

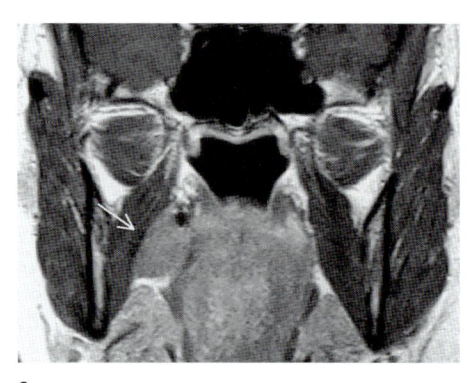

Fig. 10.47 Young female patient with trismus. At clinical examination, no mucosal lesion was seen; however, a submucosal bulge in the region of the retromolar trigone could be palpated. **a** Axial T1W MR image, **b** axial T2W MR image, and **c** coronal contrast-enhanced T1W MR image demonstrate a sharply marginated mass extending into the parapharyngeal space (arrows) and invading the internal pterygoid muscle (open arrows). Deep submucosal biopsy revealed adenoid cystic carcinoma grade 2.

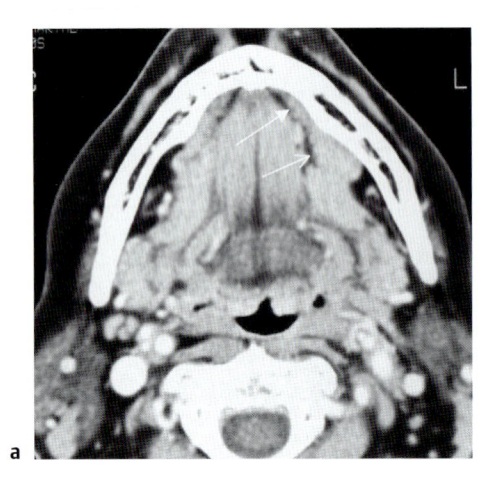

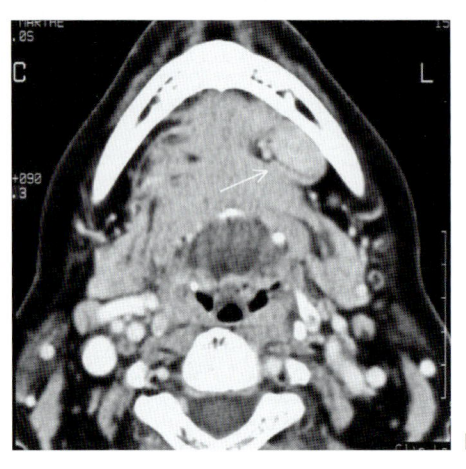

Fig. 10.48 Male patient presenting with a palpable submental mass on the left. **a, b** Contrast-enhanced CT images at the level of the floor of the mouth demonstrate a well-defined mass (open arrows) arising posterolaterally from the sublingual gland (arrow) and extending inferiorly into the submandibular space. Although the mass is homogeneous and has a sharp margin, surgery revealed an adenoid cystic carcinoma arising from an accessory salivary gland or from a minor salivary gland.

histological diagnosis. Histologically, adenoid cystic carcinoma can be subdivided into three distinct types: cribriform (grade 1), tubular (grade 2), and solid (grade 3).[63] Adenoid cystic carcinoma may display a characteristic pathway of perineural spread along the second and third divisions of the trigeminal nerve[37] (see above). Survival of patients with adenoid cystic carcinoma is longer than with squamous cell carcinoma, namely, 8 years on average, ranging up to 15–18 years.[10,125] Regional metastases to the cervical lymph nodes are rare; however, metastases to the lungs, bone, and brain almost always occur in the terminal stage. The treatment options are surgery and radiation therapy combined with chemotherapy. Both MRI and CT typically display submucosal tumor spread at the time of diagnosis (Fig. 10.**47**). Signal intensity on T1-weighted and T2-weighted sequences and patterns of contrast enhancement on MRI and CT are not specific in differentiating adenoid cystic carcinoma from other types of tumors. Nevertheless, a low signal intensity on T2-weighted MR images appears to correspond to highly cellular tumors (solid subtype, grade 3) with a poor prognosis, while a high signal intensity on T2-weighted images appears to correspond to less cellular tumors (cribriform or tubular subtype, grade 1 and 2) with a better prognosis.[125]

Mucoepidermoid and **acinic carcinoma** have varying biological behavior, whereas **adenocarcinoma** has a more lethal prognosis.[10,47] Imaging findings on CT and MRI are nonspecific and do not allow differentiation from other malignant tumors of the oral cavity and oropharynx (Figs. 10.**49**, 10.**50**). However, very coarse calcifications may be seen in adenocarcinoma (Fig. 10.**50**). Although uncommon, sublingual gland and submandibular gland tumors may spread in a cranial direction and secondarily invade the floor of the mouth, the adjacent subcutaneous fat, and sometimes the skin (Fig. 10.**51**). Clinically, these patients will present with an intact oral mucosa and a localized or diffuse swelling of the floor of the mouth (Fig. 10.**51**) Further cranial spread may occur into the parapharyngeal space and masticator space, resulting in trismus (Fig. 10.**50**).

Lymphoma

Both **Hodgkin** and **non-Hodgkin lymphoma** most commonly present in the head and neck area with lymph node enlargement. Although Hodgkin lymphoma is predominantly nodal with extranodal involvement seen only uncommonly (4%), non-Hodgkin lymphoma frequently involves extranodal sites (23%).[132] Nevertheless, **primary lymphoma** of the oral cavity and oropharynx is rare, accounting for 3.5% of all malignancies in these two regions, Lymphoma of the oral cavity and oropharynx usually involves Waldeyer's ring. The most common sites of involvement of Waldeyer's ring are the palatal tonsils followed by the lingual and pharyngeal tonsils (Figs. 10.**52**, 10.**53**). The prognosis is relatively poor with a 30% mortality rate within 3 years after diagnosis.[46] Unlike squamous cell carcinoma, lymphoma tends to lack deep invasion despite the bulky size of most lesions (Figs. 10.**52**, 10.**53**) and cervical lymphadenopathy frequently accompanies these primary lymphomas. Involved lymph nodes range in size from 1 to 10 cm.[76] Their most striking feature on CT and MRI is homogeneity and thin, peripheral rim-enhancement. Unlike squamous cell carcinoma, central nodal necrosis is very rarely seen in patients with lymph node involvement in Hodgkin and non-Hodgkin lymphoma.[15,76]

Tumors of the Oral Cavity and Oropharynx

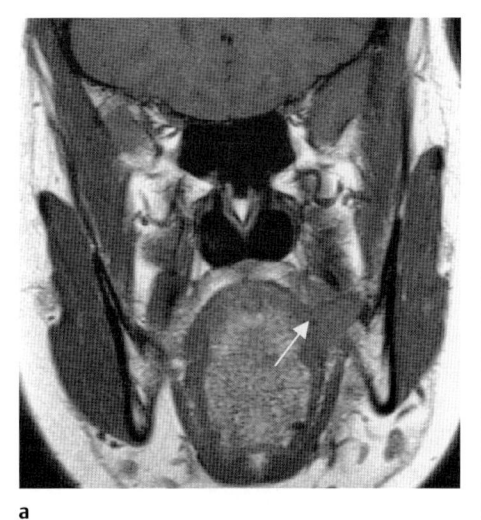

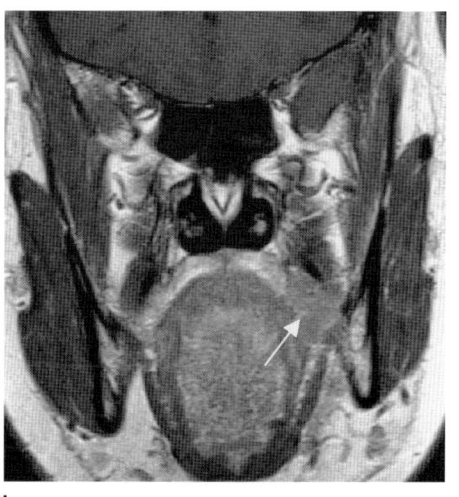

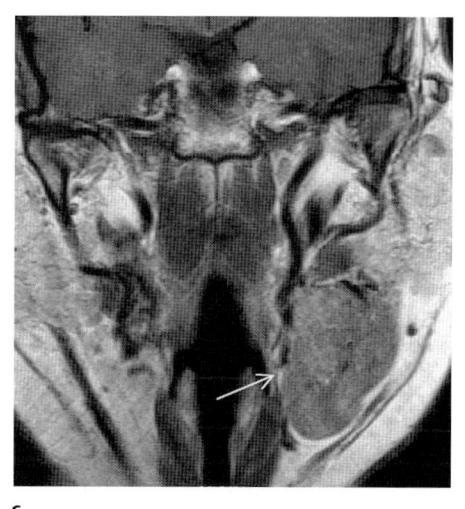

Fig. 10.**49** Young female patient presenting with a large palpable neck mass. Coronal (**a**) and contrast-enhanced T1W images (**b** and **c**) demonstrate a tumor involving the left anterior tonsillar pillar (arrow) and extending inferiorly into the glosssotonsillar sulcus. Moderate enhancement is seen. A very large homogeneously enhancing lymph node metastasis (open arrow) is equally seen on the left. Biopsy revealed mucoepidermoid carcinoma.

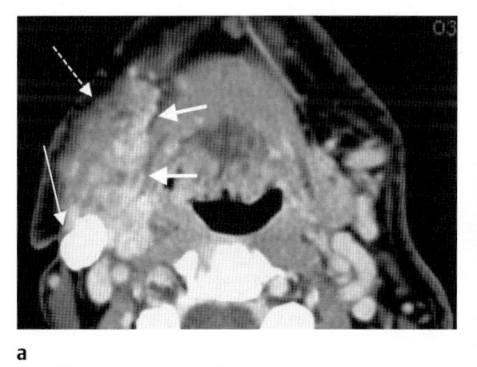

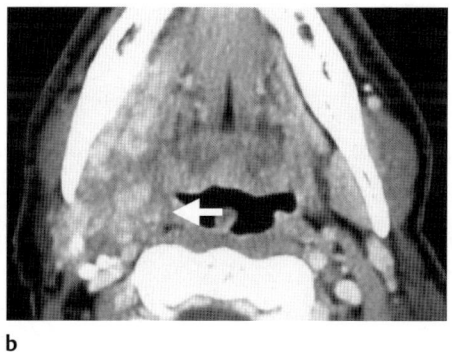

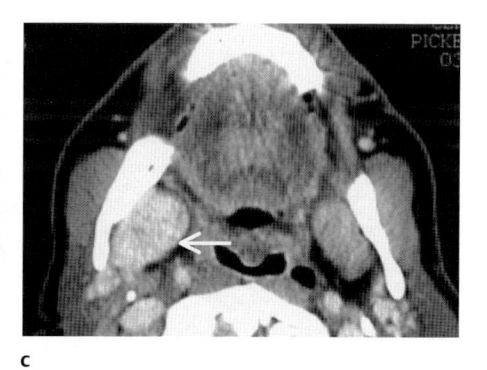

Fig. 10.**50** Young male patient with trismus presenting with a diffusely indurated submental region at clinical examination. Contrast-enhanced CT images (**a–c**) demonstrate a diffusely infiltrating mass arising from the right submandibular gland (arrows) extending superiorly into the parapharyngeal space (thick arrow) and into the internal pterygoid muscle (open arrow). Note very coarse calcifications (long thin arrow) as well as invasion of the subcutaneous fat on the right (dashed arrow). Histology revealed adenocarcinoma.

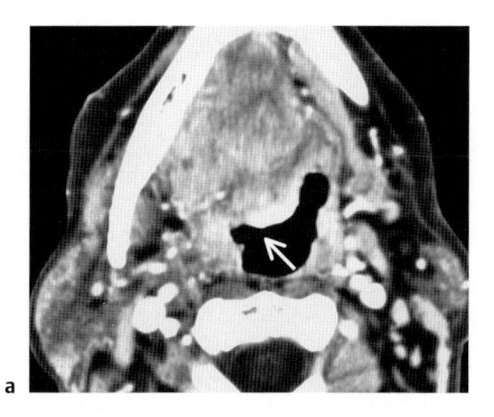

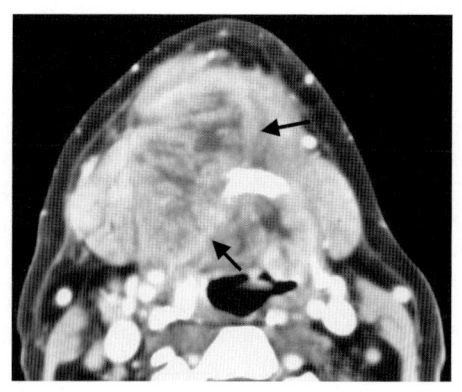

Fig. 10.**51** Elderly woman presenting with a diffusely indurated floor of the mouth and submental region at clinical examination. The mucosa was intact. Contrast-enhanced CT images (**a** and **b**) demonstrate a diffusely infiltrating mass arising from the right submandibular gland (arrows) and extending superiorly into the extrinsic tongue muscles, as well as into the base of the tongue (open arrow). Histology revealed mucoepidermoid carcinoma.

Liposarcoma

Liposarcomas are very rare in the head and neck, with fewer than 50 cases reported in the oral cavity. Within the oral cavity, liposarcomas have been reported in the cheek, palate, floor of the mouth, and submental regions.[104] Liposarcomas of this region show no gender predilection and they may occur in all age groups (median age, 50 years). They originate de novo from lipoblasts around the fascial planes and not from preexisting lipomas.[10, 104] Histologically, liposarcomas can be subdivided into four types: well-differentiated and myxoid tumors with a good prognosis and pleomorphic and round-cell lesions with a poor prognosis. Wide surgical excision is mandatory. On CT, well-differentiated liposarcomas are inhomogeneous lesions with attenuation values above those of subcutaneous fat. They typically display a mix of fat and soft-tissue elements. Very often, unsharp, infiltrating borders are seen, as well as areas of inhomogeneous contrast enhancement. On T1-

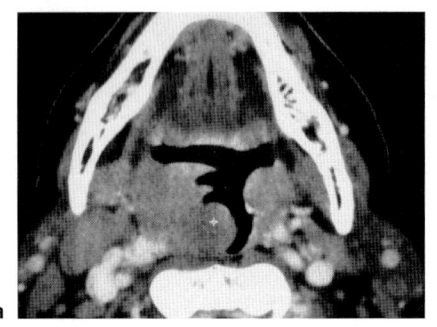

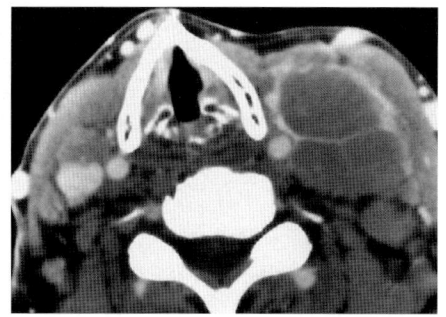

Fig. 10.**52** Contrast-enhanced CT images (**a** and **b**) in a patient with non-Hodgkin lymphoma with involvement of the Waldeyer's ring, as well as nodal involvement. Note the homogeneously enlarged tonsils, as well as the homogeneously enlarged bilateral middle jugular lymph nodes with a characteristic thin, peripheral rim enhancement.

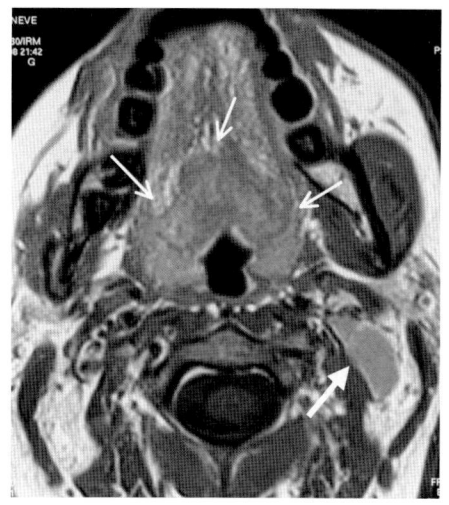

Fig. 10.**53** Contrast-enhanced T1W MR image in a patient with non-Hodgkin lymphoma. Note involvement of the lymphoid tissue in the base of the tongue (open arrows), as well as the homogeneously enlarged upper jugular lymph node with a characteristic thin, peripheral rim enhancement (arrow).

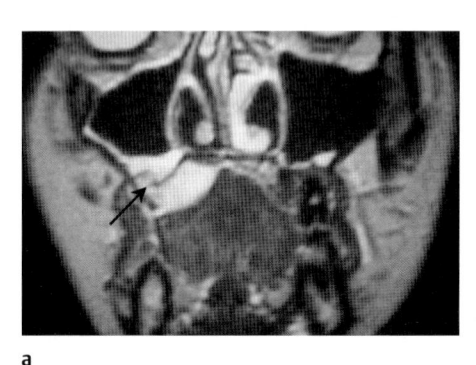

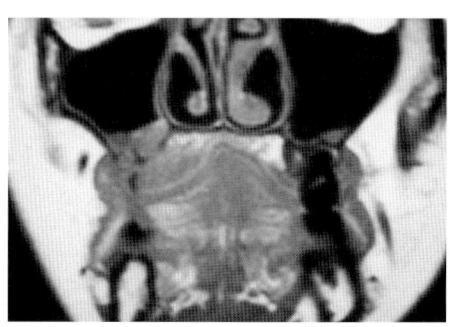

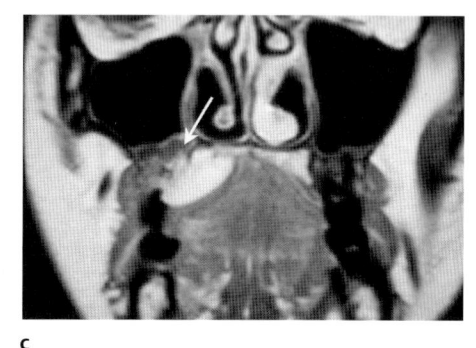

Fig. 10.**54** Myxoid liposarcoma. **a** Coronal T2W MR image obtained in a patient with submucosal swelling of the hard palate demonstrates a hyperintense lesion on the right with osseous destruction (arrow). Note thickening of the mucosa of the right maxillary sinus. **b** Coronal T1W MR image obtained at the same level shows a slightly hypointense mass on the right with osseous destruction. **c** After intravenous administration of contrast material, the tumor enhances tremendously. Note the area of bone invasion (arrow) covered by mucosal thickening of the right maxillary sinus. Based on the MRI findings, the diagnosis of a malignant tumor, possibly of salivary gland origin, was made. Surgery revealed myxoid liposarcoma. Courtesy of Dr. Jan Casselman (Sint Jan Hospital, Bruges, Belgium).

weighted MR images, well-differentiated liposarcomas appear as primarily fatty lesions but with signal intensities lower than that of the subcutaneous fat. On fat-suppressed contrast-enhanced T1-weighted MR images, liposarcomas display patchy, inhomogeneous enhancement. In the other histological forms of liposarcoma (myxoid, pleomorphic, and round cell lesions), no larger fat areas may be seen on imaging. In the absence of a fat signal (or fat attenuation value), liposarcoma cannot be differentiated from other soft-tissue tumors (Fig. 10.54).

Tumors of Muscular Tissue and Fibrous Tissue Origin

Rhabdomyosarcoma

Although **rhabdomyosarcoma** has a predilection for the head and neck region, involvement of the oral cavity and oropharynx is rare. In the oropharynx, the base of the tongue is the predilection site. The tumors, which tend to occur in children and adolescents, have attenuation values of muscle on CT and a signal intensity similar to muscle on T1-weighted MR images. On T2-weighted images, the tumors very often show an increased signal intensity (Fig. 10.55) and a variable amount of enhancement after injection of contrast material.

Malignant Fibrous Histiocytoma

Three to ten percent of all **malignant fibrous histiocytomas** (MFH) occur in the head and neck, and 10–15% of all malignant fibrous histiocytomas of the head and neck arise in the oral cavity and oropharynx.[113] MFH typically shows a 3 : 1 male predominance and the affected patients are most often older than 50 years of age. Previous radiation therapy of the oral cavity is a predisposing factor for MFH, the latency period ranging from 5 to 15 years.[21,138,141] The prognosis of radiation-induced MFH is very poor. Clinically and endoscopically, the tumor typically presents as a submucosal sessile or polypoid ill-defined, yellowish mass. As with other submucosal lesions, deep biopsies are mandatory. Since MFH is relatively resistant to radiation and chemotherapy, surgery remains the treatment of choice. Metastases to the lungs are not unusual. The histological diagnosis of MFH is based on the presence of histiocyte-like cells, fibroblasts, multinucleated giant cells, tumor giant cells, normal and/or abnormal mitoses, and collagen production. On the basis of histological criteria, MFH can be divided into several types: storiform-pleomorphic myxoid, inflammatory, giant-cell, and angiomatoid.[138,141] The storiform-pleomorphic type is the most common variant seen in the oral cavity. The differentiation from spindle cell carcinoma may be impossible without immunohistochemistry and electron microscopy. On CT scans and MRI, a large, homogeneously enhancing soft-tissue mass without evidence of necrosis or gross ulceration may be seen. While endoscopy shows an intact but yellowish mucosa, imaging typically demonstrates a solid homogeneously enhancing tumor mass, therefore suggesting an etiology other than squamous cell carcinoma.

Other, less common, malignant tumors involving the oral cavity and oropharynx include leiomyosarcoma, synovial sarcoma, and fibrosarcoma. The clinical/endoscopic and imaging findings in these tumors are noncharacteristic.

Benign Non-Squamous Cell Neoplasms

Pleomorphic Adenoma

Pleomorphic adenoma (benign mixed tumor) is the most common benign tumor of salivary gland origin seen in the oral cavity and oropharynx. Although the majority of pleomorphic adenomas are seen in the parotid gland, 8% arise within the submandibular gland, less than 1% arise within the sublingual gland, and as many as 7% occur in the minor salivary glands.[10] The CT imaging characteristics of pleomorphic adenoma include no significant enhancement and well-delineated margins (Fig. 10.**56**), although occasionally the margins may be poorly defined, suggesting a more aggressive tumor. Large tumors undergo cystic degeneration and sometimes calcifications may be seen. When the hard palate is involved, the slow tumor growth typically results in remodeling rather than bone destruction. Pleomorphic adenomas are usually isointense to muscle on T1-weighted MR images and hyperintense on T2-weighted MR images. Cystic changes, necrosis, and hemorrhage lead to varying signal intensities within these tumors on T2-weighted images. Although fine-needle aspiration cytology with or without US guidance may reveal the benign nature of the tumor, pleomorphic adenomas are—as a rule—always removed surgically because of an increased risk of undergoing malignant degeneration (see also Chapter 9).

Lipoma

Although **lipomas** are the most common tumors of mesenchymal origin, only 13% arise in the extracranial head and neck.[9,10,18]

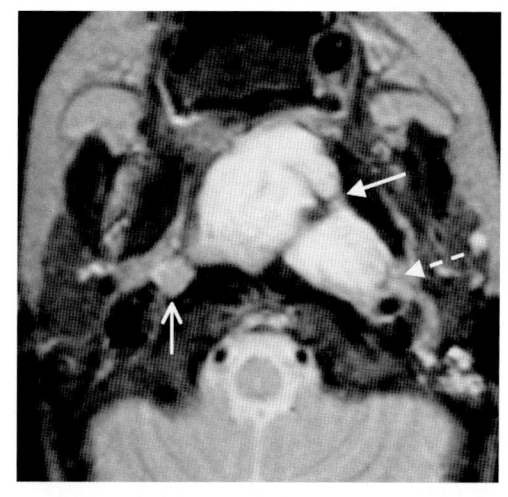

Fig. 10.**55** Rhabdomyosarcoma of the oropharynx in a young boy. T2W MR image shows a bulky mass with near total obstruction of the oropharynx. Note invasion of the internal pterygoid muscle (arrow) as well as invasion of the parapharyngeal space (dashed arrow). A retropharyngeal lymph node metastasis is seen on the right (open arrow). Courtesy of Dr. Alexandra Borges (Cancer Institute, Lisbon, Portugal).

Most head and neck lipomas are located in the posterior cervical triangle and in the retropharyngeal space (see also Chapter 12). Within the oral cavity and oropharynx, lipomas—which constitute only 1–4% of all benign tumors—are found in order of decreasing frequency in the cheek, tongue, floor of the mouth, palate, and submental region.[44,49,84,104,109] Peak age of occurrence is 40 years and above and the male-to-female ratio is 2.5 : 1. Histologically, lipoma is composed of mature adipose tissue arranged in lobules, separated by fibrous tissue septae. Most tumors are well-circumscribed and encapsulated, although infiltrating nonencapsulated lipomas have been reported especially in the tongue.[44,75,104] Surgical excision is the treatment of choice. The radiological diagnosis of lipoma is straightforward. Both CT and MRI provide a definitive diagnosis in virtually all cases. The typical CT characteristics are a homogeneous and nonenhancing lesion with attenuation values from –65 to –125 HU (Fig. 10.**57**) On MRI, lipoma has the same signal intensity as subcutaneous fat on all pulse sequences (hyperintense on T1-weighted MR images, hypointense on T2-weighted MR images and very low intensity on fat-suppressed T1-weighted MR im-

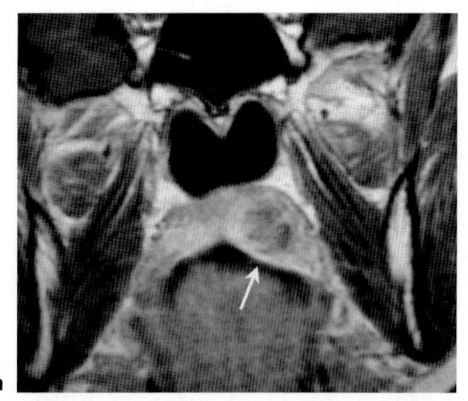

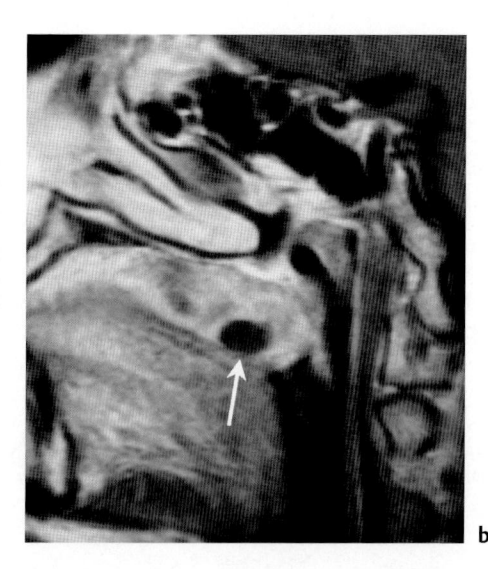

Fig. 10.**56** Pleomorphic adenoma of the soft palate. **a** Coronal and **b** sagittal contrast-enhanced T1W MR images show a well-delineated ovoid tumor mass located in the left soft palate (arrows). The central area displays cystic degeneration. Histology revealed pleomorphic adenoma. Courtesy of Dr. Jan Casselman (Sint Jan Hospital, Bruges, Belgium).

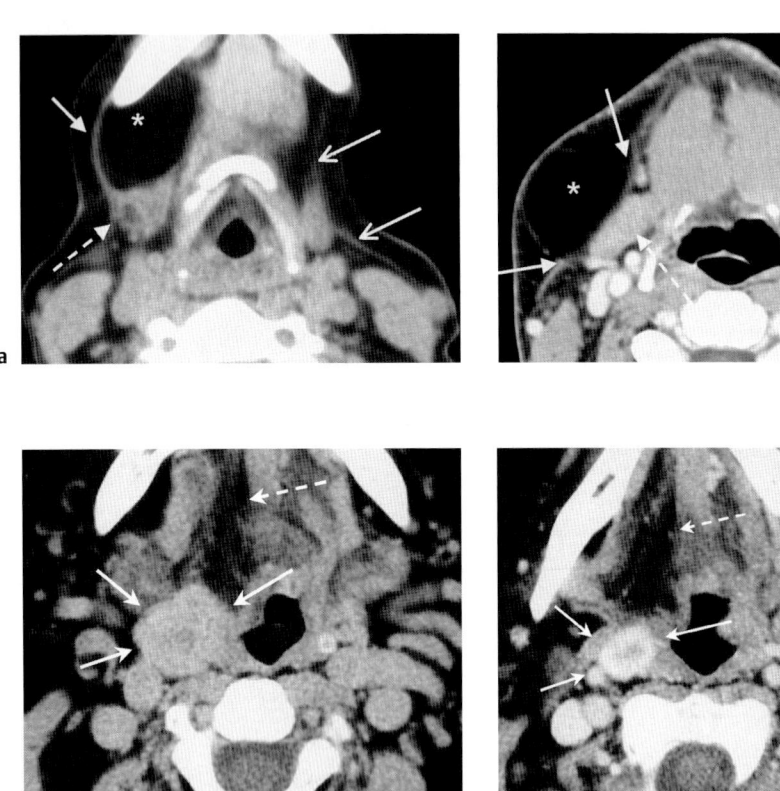

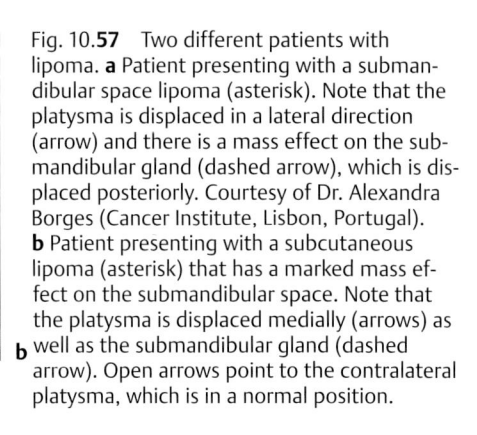

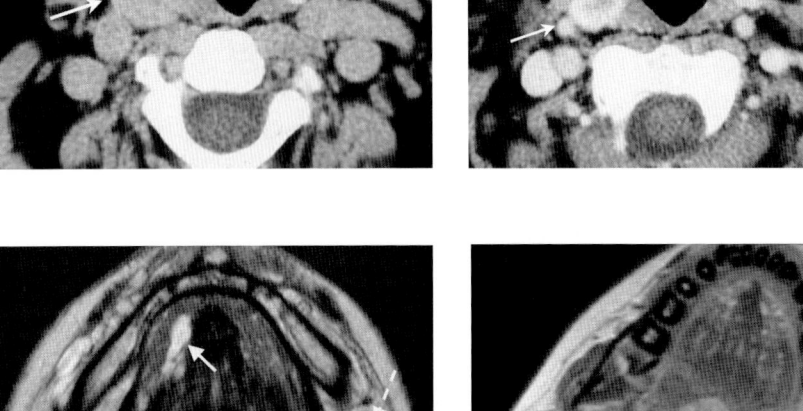

Fig. 10.57 Two different patients with lipoma. **a** Patient presenting with a submandibular space lipoma (asterisk). Note that the platysma is displaced in a lateral direction (arrow) and there is a mass effect on the submandibular gland (dashed arrow), which is displaced posteriorly. Courtesy of Dr. Alexandra Borges (Cancer Institute, Lisbon, Portugal). **b** Patient presenting with a subcutaneous lipoma (asterisk) that has a marked mass effect on the submandibular space. Note that the platysma is displaced medially (arrows) as well as the submandibular gland (dashed arrow). Open arrows point to the contralateral platysma, which is in a normal position.

Fig. 10.58 Schwannoma of the oropharynx. **a** Unenhanced and **b** contrast-enhanced axial images at the level of the floor of the mouth show a right-sided mass located within the oropharyngeal constrictors, base of the tongue, and parapharyngeal space (arrows). The mass shows a ringlike contrast enhancement. Note associated hypoglossal nerve paralysis with fatty infiltration of the right hemitongue (dashed arrow). Surgery confirmed the radiological findings and revealed a schwannoma of the hypoglossal nerve at the level of the arch of the hypoglossal nerve. Courtesy of Dr. Fernando Torrhina and Dr. David Coutinho (Imagens Medicas Integradas, Lisbon, Portugal).

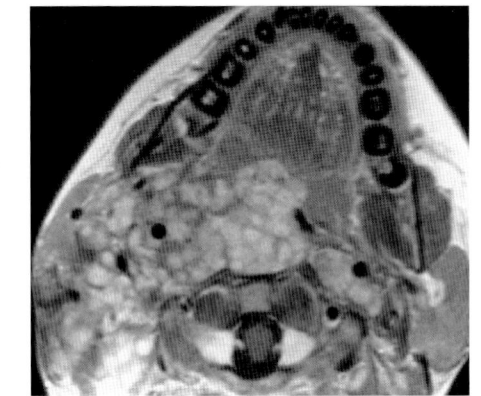

Fig. 10.59 Neurofibromas involving the oral cavity and oropharynx, as seen on MRI. **a** Axial T2W FSE image in a patient with neurofibromatosis type 1. Note multiple characteristic neurofibromas involving the sublingual space (arrow), the submandibular space (dashed arrow), the retropharyngeal space (short arrows), and the parapharyngeal space (open arrows). **b** Axial contrast-enhanced T1W MR image obtained in a different patient shows a large plexiform neurofibroma involving the subcutaneous fat, the parotid gland on the right, and the oropharynx, leading to major pharyngeal obstruction. Note encasement of the carotid arteries and internal jugular vein on the right. There is also involvement of the paravertebral muscles. Case **b** courtesy of Dr. Jan Casselman (Sint Jan Hospital, Bruges, Belgium).

ages). As in other parts of the body, if portions of the lipoma have the attenuation value or signal intensity characteristics of other soft-tissue on CT or MRI, and if contrast enhancement is observed within these strands of connective tissue, the diagnosis of a liposarcoma should be considered (see above).

Schwannomas and Neurofibromas

Nerve sheath tumors include **schwannomas** and **neurofibromas**. Only 13% of schwannomas occur in the extracranial head and neck.[10,66,85,62,123] Most schwannomas in the extracranial head and neck are seen—in order of decreasing frequency—along the sympathetic chain, brachial plexus, vagus nerve, and cervical nerve roots. Schwannomas of the oral cavity and oropharynx are rare.[60,66,89] In the oral cavity, schwannomas arise in as many as 50% of cases within the tongue.[10] Less often, schwannomas may affect the palate and floor of the mouth.[36,85,123] Schwannomas may be solitary or multiple. Females in the third and fourth decades of life are most commonly affected. On CT scans, schwannomas appear as homogeneous soft-tissue density masses with variable enhancement after intravenous administration of contrast material. Large lesions may undergo cystic degeneration and, therefore, present with central unenhancing and peripheral enhancing areas. On T2-weighted MR images schwannomas are hyperintense to muscle, and on T1-weighted images they are isointense to muscle. After intravenous administration of contrast material, homogeneous enhancement is seen in smaller lesions, whereas a "targetlike" appearance may be seen in larger lesions (hypointense center and hyperintense rim) (Fig. 10.58). This is due to central areas of cystic degeneration, which do not enhance and which are surrounded by peripheral enhancing tissue. Neurofibromas involving the oral cavity and oropharynx are almost always associated with neurofibromatosis.[10,123] Their diagnosis is straightforward in the appropriate clinical setting. On CT scans and MRI, neurofibromas may present as solitary or multiple rounded masses. Alternatively, they may appear as more infiltrative lesions, plexiform neurofibroma (Fig. 10.59).

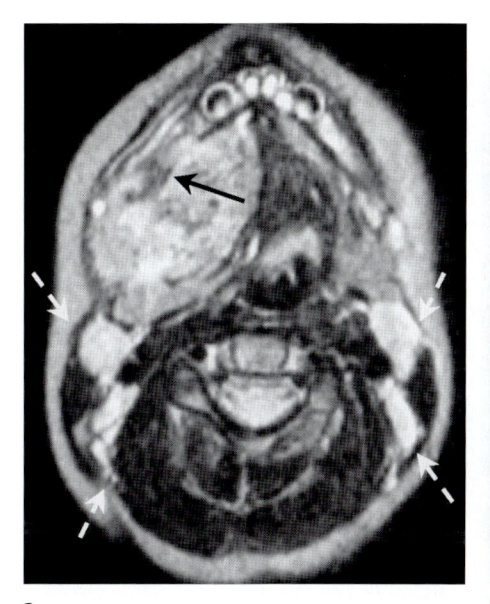

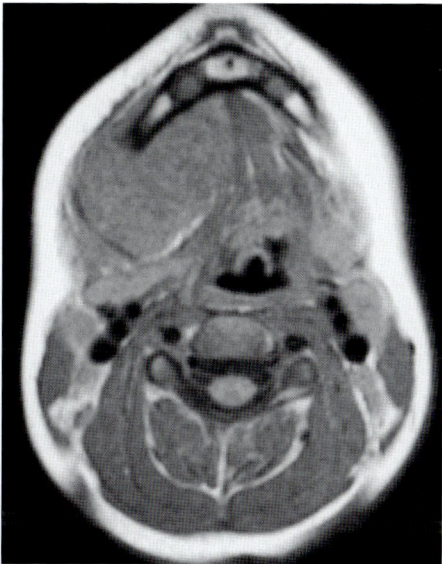

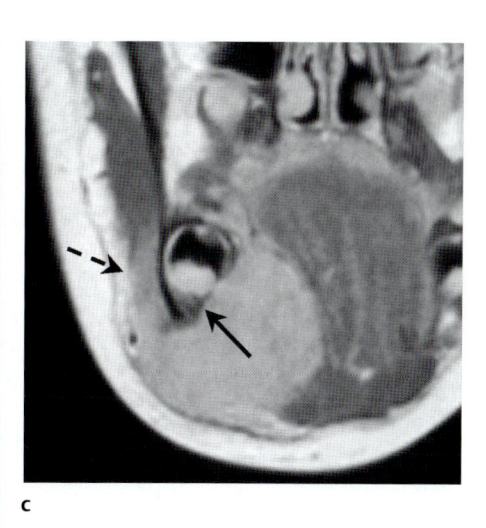

Fig. 10.60 Aggressive fibromatosis. **a** Axial T2W SE image obtained in a child shows a large hyperintense mass arising from the right floor of the mouth and invading the mandible (arrow). Note bilateral reactive lymph nodes (dashed arrows). **b** T1W image obtained at the same level shows that the mass is homogeneous and slightly hyperintense compared to muscle. **c** Coronal contrast-enhanced image clearly shows invasion of the submandibular space, mylohyoid muscle, lateral portion of the right geniohyoid muscle, and the anterior belly of the digastric muscle on the right. Note erosion of the mandible (arrow) and invasion of the inferior portion of the right masseter muscle (dashed arrow). Surgery revealed aggressive fibromatosis. Courtesy of Dr. Jan Casselman (Sint Jan Hospital, Bruges, Belgium).

Aggressive Fibromatosis

Aggressive fibromatosis, also called extra-abdominal desmoid tumor, differentiated fibrosarcoma, or fibrosarcoma-like fibromatosis, represents a group of fibrous tumors showing clinical and biological features between benign fibrous lesions and fibrosarcoma. These locally aggressive tumors are frequently seen in children and young adults.[54, 115, 117, 120] They have high recurrence rates (20–70%) but no metastasizing potential. In the head and neck area, aggressive fibromatosis typically affects the supraclavicular region and face. Involvement of the oral cavity, in particular the tongue, is very rare.[54, 115, 117] Aggressive fibromatosis lesions enhance only very slightly on CT, and are most often inseparable from adjacent muscles. Aggressive fibromatosis has variable signal intensity on T1-weighted and T2-weighted MR images and demonstrates some degree of enhancement following intravenous contrast administration (Fig. 10.**60**). Infiltration into adjacent structures is common.

Rhabdomyoma

Benign extracardiac **rhabdomyomas** are rare neoplasms of skeletal muscle origin.[1, 2, 30–39] Extracardiac rhabdomyomas have been arbitrarily subclassified into "adult" and "fetal" and can present as either solitary or multifocal lesions.[8, 10, 33, 34, 103] Fetal rhabdomyomas typically occur in children under the age of 3 years, while adult rhabdomyomas preferentially occur in the fourth to fifth decades. Adult rhabdomyomas affect men more commonly than women. The predilection sites for adult rhabdomyoma are in the tongue base, floor of the mouth, pharynx, and larynx.[19, 95] In the oral cavity and oropharynx, the tumor presents endoscopically as a submucosal, apparently well-circumscribed lesion. As with other submucosal lesions, deep biopsies are mandatory. Microscopic examination in adult rhabdomyoma reveals large, rounded or polygonal cells with deeply eosinophilic, occasionally vacuolated cytoplasm. A few of the cells show definite cross striations and some cells contain intracytoplasmic crystals (jackstraw crystals), which are thought to represent Z-band material.[9, 10] Microscopically, rhabdomyoma may be difficult to distinguish from granular cell myoblastoma without PTAH staining. The treatment of choice is surgery. Because local recurrence is common, even after a period as long as 12 years, ample excision is mandatory. CT scans show a single mass or multiple homogeneous masses with muscle density on unenhanced images and with minimal enhancement after intravenous administration of contrast material. Rhabdomyomas are isointense to muscle on T1-weighted MR images and hyperintense on T2-weighted MR images. They enhance slightly following intravenous administration of contrast material.

Tumors Originating in Adjacent Spaces

Owing to the close proximity of the oral cavity and oropharynx to the masticator space, parapharyngeal space, carotid space, and retropharyngeal space, tumors originating in these adjacent spaces may displace or secondarily involve the tonsils, the posterior pharyngeal wall, the floor of the mouth, and the cheek area. Large paragangliomas or carotid space schwannomas typically displace the tonsil and lateral oropharyngeal wall medially, causing dysphagia, dyspnea, odynophagia, and obvious asymmetry at clinical evaluation (Fig. 10.**61**). Retropharyngeal and prevertebral tumors displace the posterior pharyngeal wall anteriorly, thereby shortening the anteroposterior pharyngeal diameter. This shortened anteroposterior pharyngeal diameter may lead to snoring or sleep apnea syndrome (Fig. 10.**62**). Benign tumors of the mandible may displace the structures of the floor of the mouth, leading to slowly progressing functional impairment and facial deformity (Fig. 10.**63**), while malignant tumors may show an aggressive invasive pattern. These "perioral and perioropharyngeal" tumors are discussed in detail in other chapters in Section V and in Chapter 6.

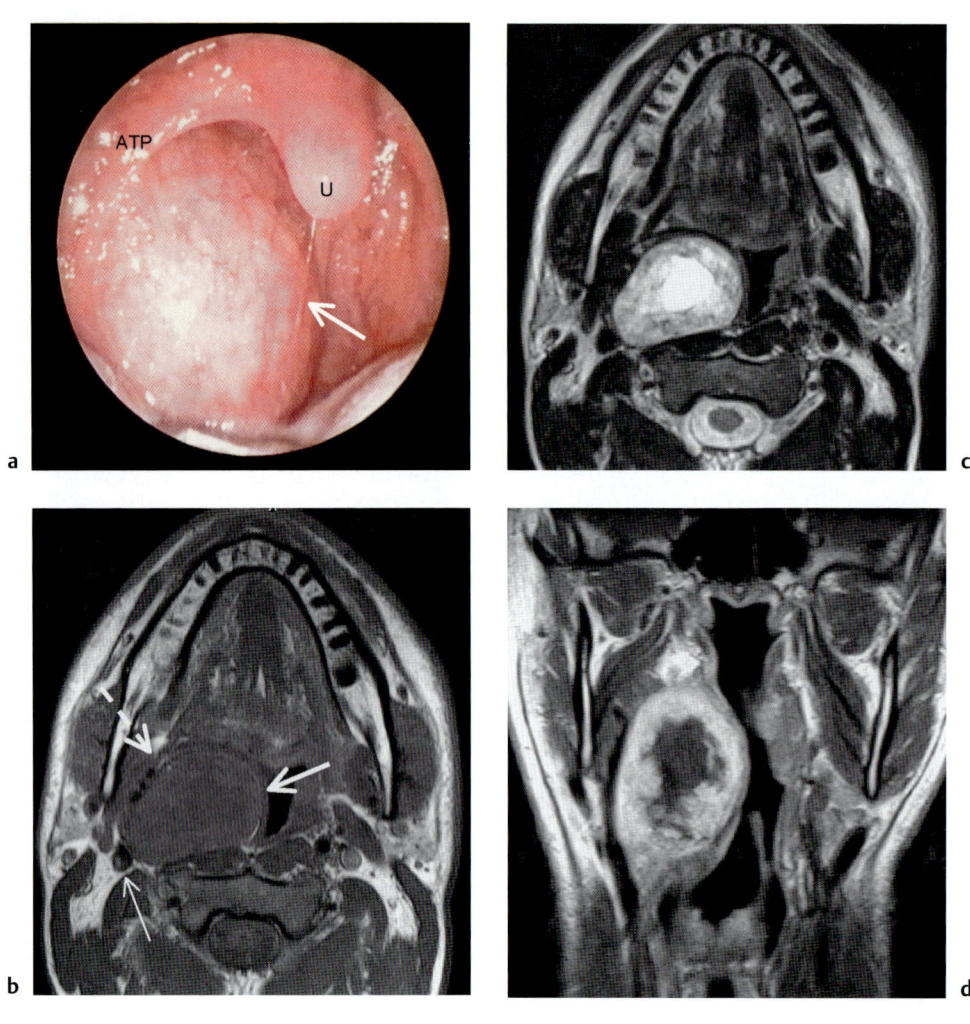

Fig. 10.**61** Schwannoma of the sympathetic chain causing major oropharyngeal displacement. **a** Young patient presenting with progressive dysphagia and with obvious asymmetry of the oropharynx at clinical evaluation. The mucosa is intact but there is major medial displacement of the lateral oropharyngeal wall (arrow). ATP = anterior tonsillar pillar, U = uvula. **b** Axial T1W MR image shows a large mass that is isointense to muscle. The mass displaces the oropharyngeal mucosa medially (arrow), the carotid arteries anteriorly (dashed arrow), and the internal jugular vein slightly laterally (thin arrow). **c** T2W MR image obtained at the same level shows that the mass has a targetlike appearance with a thick, moderately hyperintense rim and a central area with very high signal intensity. **d** Contrast-enhanced coronal T1W MR image shows massive narrowing of the oropharynx by a mass with a large necrotic center. The MR appearance of this carotid space mass suggests a neurogenic tumor. Surgery confirmed a schwannoma of the sympathetic chain.

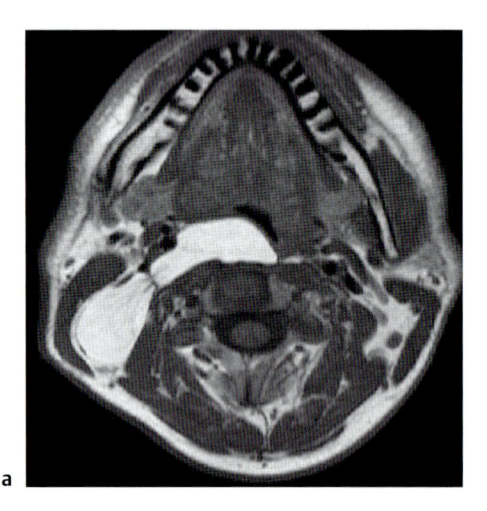

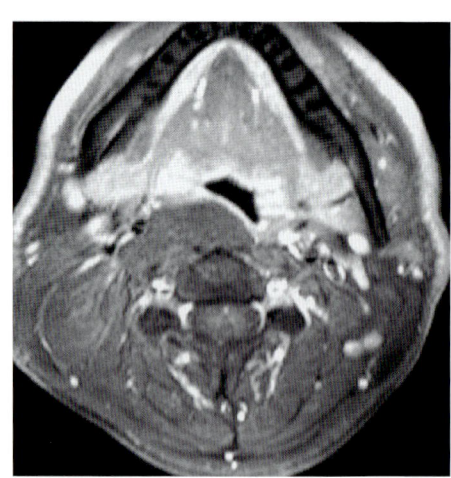

Fig. 10.**62** Young male patient presenting with snoring and with obvious asymmetry of the oropharynx at clinical evaluation. The mucosa was intact. **a** Unenhanced T1W image and **b** contrast-enhanced fat-suppressed T1W image show massive anteromedial displacement of the right tonsil by a large mass, which is hyperintense on the T1W image and hypointense on the fat-suppressed image. There is no significant enhancement present. The diagnosis is consistent with a lipoma involving the retropharyngeal space and the posterior cervical triangle. Surgery confirmed the radiological findings.

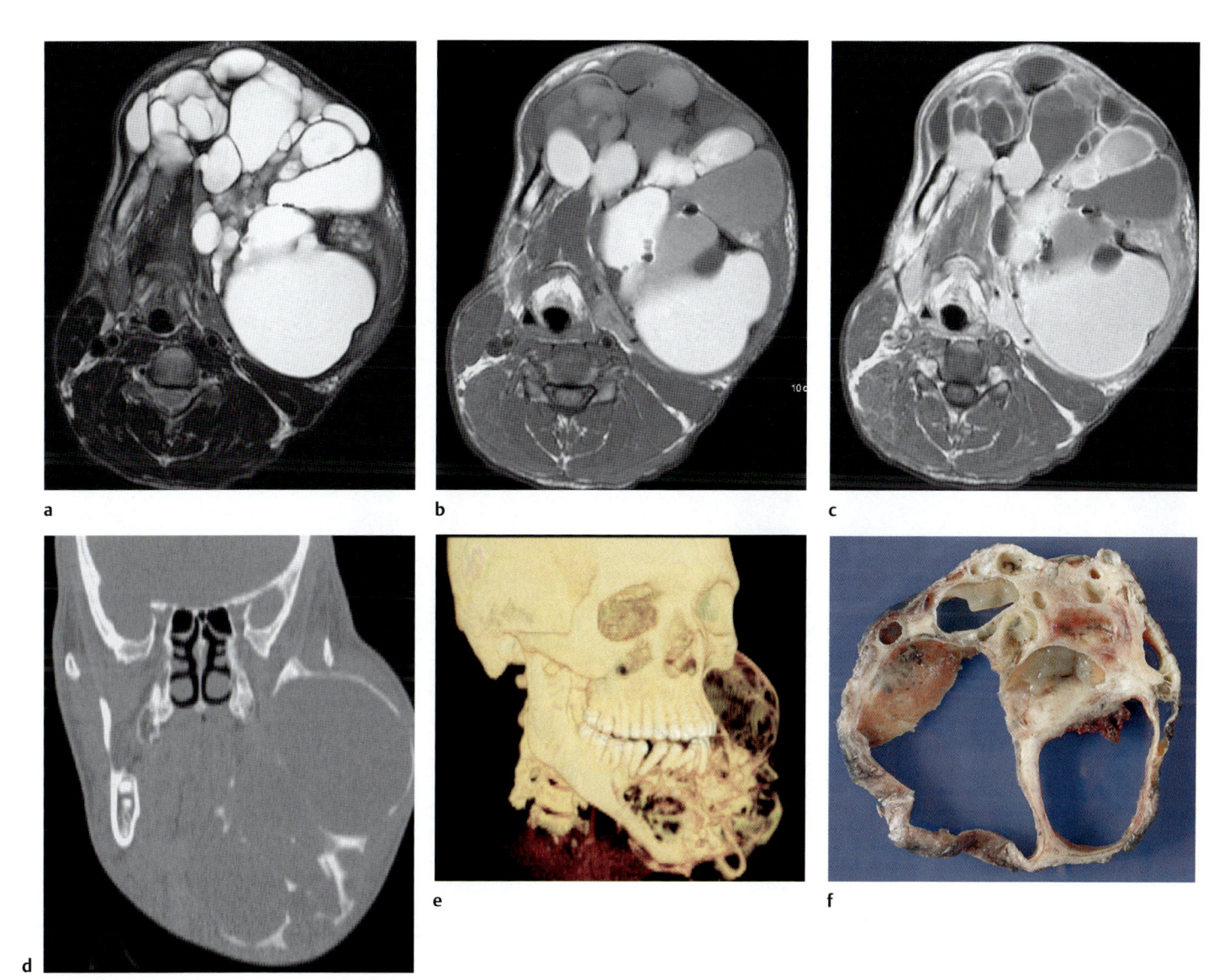

Fig. 10.**63** Giant ameloblastoma of the mandible with major facial deformity and distortion of the floor of the mouth in a young man. **a** Axial T2W image and **b** axial T1W MR image demonstrate a large multilocular lesion arising from the left mandible with major mass effect on the floor of the mouth. The cysts within the mass contain fluid with various protein contents. **c** After injection of contrast material, enhancement of the thin internal septae is seen. **d** Coronal CT image with bone window settings and **e** 3D reconstruction from volumetric data set show that the internal septae are composed of thin bony material. Note the characteristic bubblelike appearance of the mass. The patient underwent surgical resection and histology revealed follicular type ameloblastoma. **f** Macroscopic cross section through the resected specimen shows characteristic cystic formation. Mucoid material was found within the cysts.

Inflammatory Lesions of the Oral Cavity and Oropharynx

The most common inflammatory lesions to affect the oral cavity and oropharynx are of odontogenic and tonsillar origin or result from obstruction and secondary infection of the salivary ductal system.[13, 124, 126, 143] Most patients present with acute symptoms and sometimes rapid clinical deterioration. Although patients with suspected infection of the salivary ductal system will often undergo ultrasound (US) as the initial examination, CT is now considered the evaluation method of choice at most institutions. Recently it has been shown that MRI is superior to CT in the initial evaluation of acute infections of the neck with regard to lesion conspicuity, number of anatomical spaces involved, extension, and source of origin of the infectious process.[96] For practical and logistic reasons, MR imaging is currently still reserved for selected patients with inflammatory lesions in whom the use of iodinated contrast material must be limited or is contraindicated.

Odontogenic Infections

Odontogenic infection is most often caused by periapical or periodontal disease related to poor oral hygiene or by extraction of a carious tooth. Odontogenic infection may result in cellulitis, myositis, fasciitis or osteomyelitis, and abscess formation.[20, 40, 140] The first three forms of infection are difficult to diagnose with US, since displacement of structures and distortion of the anatomy are unusual. The characteristic CT features of **cellulitis** include thickening of the cutis and subcutis and increased density of fatty tissue with streaky, irregular enhancement (edematous, "dirty" fat). **Fasciitis** appears as thickening and enhancement of fasciae. **Myositis** appears as thickening and enhancement of muscles, On MRI, cellulitis, myositis, and fasciitis tend to have ill-defined margins with diffusely increased signal intensity on T2-

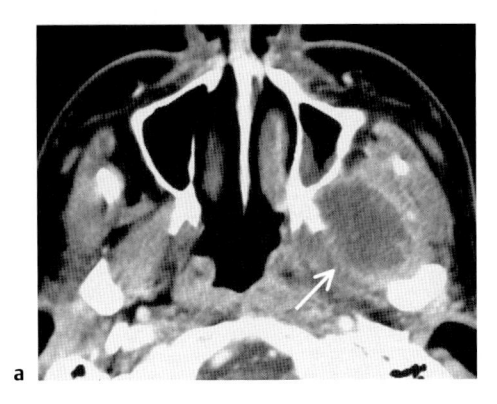

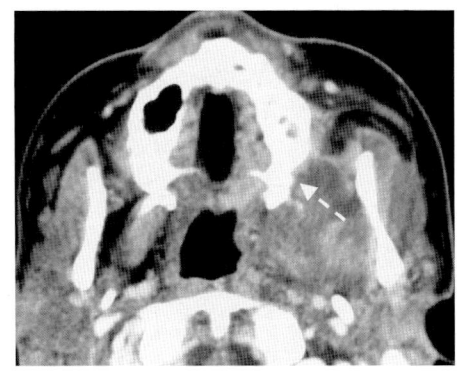

Fig. 10.**64a, b** Contrast-enhanced CT images obtained in a patient with a history of dental extraction. Odontogenic abscess within the internal pterygoid muscle (arrow) after extraction of a carious third upper molar (dashed arrow).

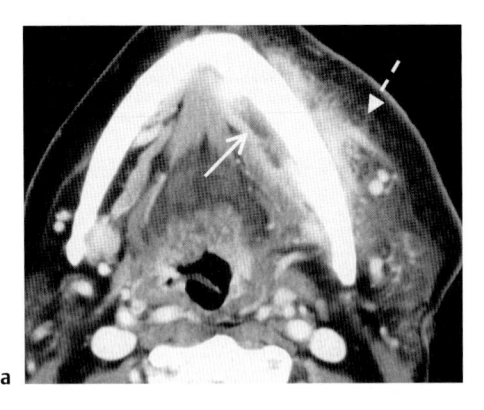

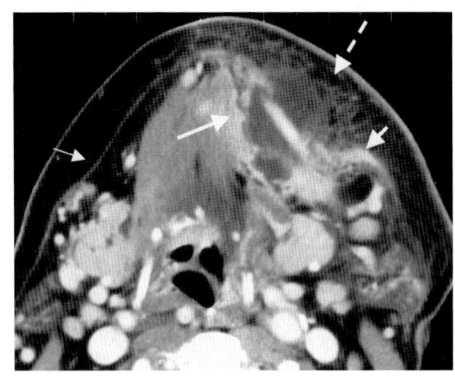

Fig. 10.**65a, b** Contrast-enhanced CT images. Odontogenic abscess after extraction of a carious premolar. Note the presence of an abscess within the sublingual space (open arrow), as well as secondary extension of the abscess along the free border of the mylohyoid muscle into the submandibular space (arrow). Associated cellulitis (dashed arrows) and myositis of the platysma (short arrow). Note for comparison the normal contralateral platysma (thin arrow).

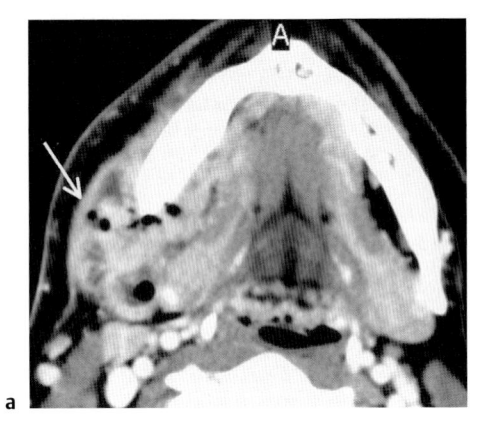

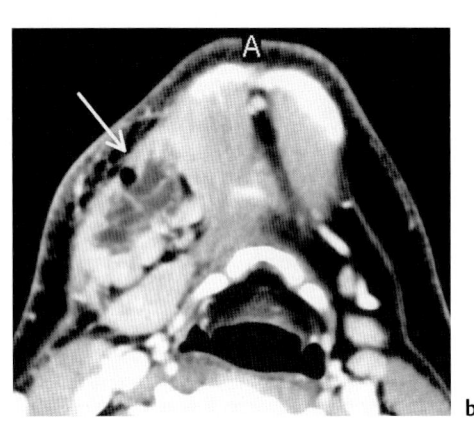

Fig. 10.**66a, b** Contrast-enhanced CT images. Odontogenic abscess caused by a third molar. Note the presence of an abscess within the submandibular space (open arrows). Air is equally present within the abscess.

weighted sequences and streaky, ill-defined enhancement on contrast-enhanced T1-weighted images. Depending on their size, **abscesses** are detectable with US, CT, or MRI. On US examination, an abscess appears as a more or less hypoechoic lesion with no perfusion in the fluid-filled center and a surrounding area of hyperperfusion on color Doppler imaging. Sometimes, hyperechoic debris may be seen within the abscess cavity. The MRI features of abscess include a high signal intensity on T2-weighted images and a low signal intensity on unenhanced T1-weighted images, with a typical rim enhancement after intravenous administration of contrast material. On CT, abscesses appear as single or multiloculated low-density areas, with or without gas collections, that usually conform to fascial spaces and demonstrate peripheral rim enhancement (see also Chapter 12).

Depending on their origin, **odontogenic abscesses** spread in a variable fashion. Odontogenic infections of the maxillary molars may produce abscesses in the buccal space and masticator space (Fig. 10.**64**). From the masticator space the abscesses may spread into the retromolar trigone, parapharyngeal space, submandibular space, and floor of the mouth. Unlike the roots of the lower second and third molars, the roots of the mandibular first molar and premolar teeth do not reach below the attachment of the mylohyoid muscle, As a result, infections arising from the lower second and third molar teeth spread into the submandibular space, while infections arising from the first molar and premolar teeth tend to involve the sublingual space[45,46] (Figs. 10.**65**, 10.**66**). Further spread from the sublingual and submandibular space occurs into the parapharyngeal space and from there to the retropharyngeal space.

The term **Ludwig angina** refers to a variety of inflammatory conditions affecting the sublingual and the submandibular spaces.[20,40,124,126,140,143] The infection most commonly affects patients between the ages of 20 and 30 years, but it has rarely been observed in children. Patients often present with facial swelling, oral pain, fever, dysphagia, and dyspnea. The source of the infection is usually odontogenic, but sublingual or subman-

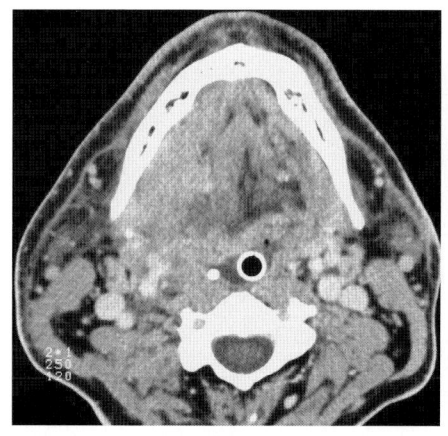

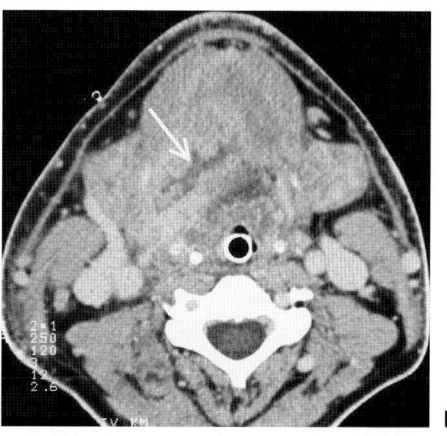

Fig. 10.**67** Ludwig angina of odontogenic origin. **a, b** Contrast-enhanced CT images obtained in an intubated patient show massive edema and cellulitis of the floor of the mouth, especially on the right. Incipient abscess formation is seen in the region of the base of the tongue (arrow).

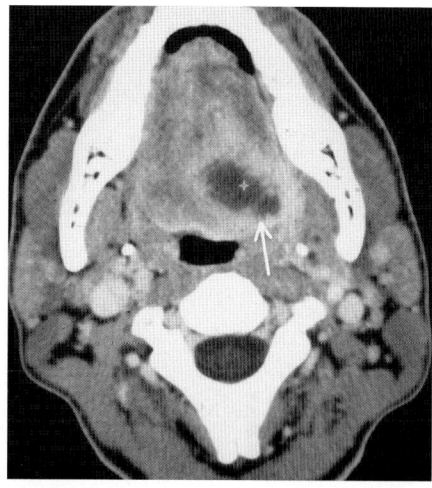

Fig. 10.**68** Contrast-enhanced CT image obtained in a patient presenting with dysphagia and dyspnea shows an abscess located in the posterior oral tongue (arrow).

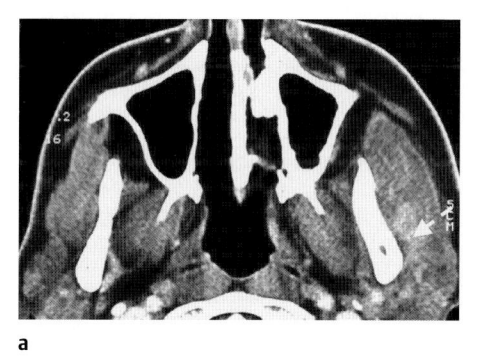

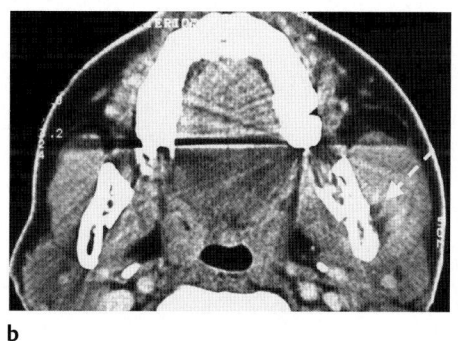

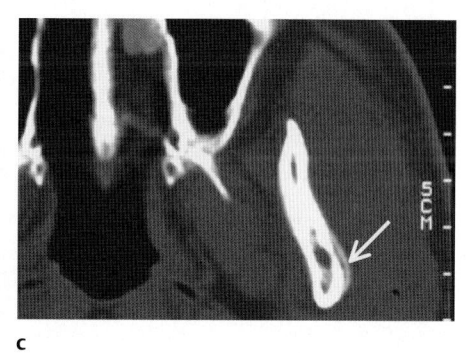

Fig. 10.**69a, b** Contrast-enhanced CT images with soft-tissue settings and **c** bone settings in a patient with a history of extraction of a carious third upper molar tooth. An abscess is seen within the masseter muscle (dashed arrows) as well as a periosteal reaction of the mandible (open arrow). The findings are consistent with osteomyelitis of the mandible. Surgery confirmed the radiological findings.

dibular sialadenitis, trauma, or surgical procedures of the floor of the mouth, e.g., resection of cancer with subsequent reconstruction by means of a skin flap, are also causes of infection. Typically, the infection originates in the form of cellulitis in the submandibular space and then propagates—via the mylohyoid cleft—to the sublingual space. The inflammation involves muscle, fascia, and connective tissue, but not the minor salivary glands. It typically spreads in a contiguous pattern via muscle and fascial planes into both submandibular spaces. On CT, cellulitis, edema, and myositis of the floor of the mouth are seen, sometimes associated with abscess formation (Fig. 10.**67**). In Ludwig angina as well as other infectious processes involving the floor of the mouth, the tongue is often elevated superiorly and displaced posteriorly, with the potential to severely compromise the airway. Although much less common than infections of the floor of the mouth, tongue infections with abscess formation (Fig. 10.**68**) may also lead to severe acute airway compromise necessitating emergency tracheotomy. Treatment of infections of the floor of the mouth and tongue infections includes antibiotics, airway management, and surgical drainage, if necessary. Because these types of infections are very dangerous, delay in correct radiological diagnosis may have serious consequences for the patient's outcome.

Infections of the *submandibular space* may spread into the parapharyngeal space, or mediastinum. Severe complications include erosion and rupture of the internal carotid artery, internal jugular vein thrombosis, necrotizing fasciitis, mediastinitis, pleural empyema, and septic shock with multiorgan failure.[20, 127] These complications are also discussed in Chapter 12.

Acute osteomyelitis of the mandible most often results from tooth infection and less often from dental manipulation, or following various surgical procedures or penetrating trauma. During the first 7–14 days of acute osteomyelitis, plain films may be normal or they may show subtle generalized osteoporosis or widening of the periodontal space around a root. Between 7 and 14 days, poor definition of trabeculae and multiple ill-defined radiolucent areas may be seen on CT scans, and bone marrow edema may be delineated on T2-weighted and STIR MR images. Because acute osteomyelitis is often accompanied by extension of infection into the adjacent spaces, a CT study is usually performed at this stage. The CT examination should always include injection of contrast material, and both soft-tissue and bone windows should be obtained. Thin slices (1–3 mm) are essential. CT findings include periosteal new bone formation, localized osseous breakdown, sequestra, sinus tracts, myositis, fasciitis, cellulitis, and abscess formation[38] (Fig. 10.**69**). On MRI, inflammatory changes involving both the marrow and soft tissues demonstrate an increased signal intensity on T2-weighted images, a decreased signal intensity on T1-weighted images and enhancement after intravenous administration of contrast material.

Chronic osteomyelitis is a persisting infection of bone, resulting from either an inadequately treated acute osteomyelitis or a long-term reaction to a subclinical infection. Chronic osteomyelitis of the jaws may be subdivided into three types: chronic

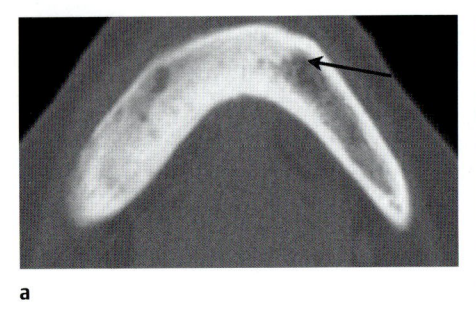

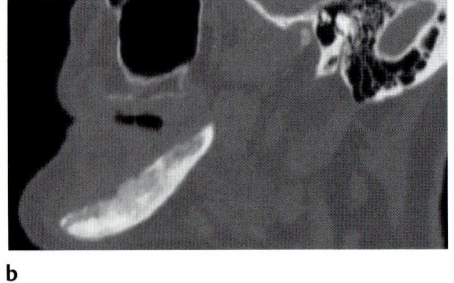

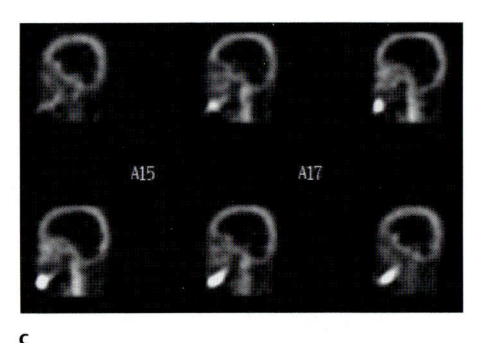

Fig. 10.70 a Axial thin-slice (1 mm) CT with bone algorithm and **b** sagittal 2D reconstruction from a volumetric data set obtained in a patient with a history of pain of several months duration show the characteristic features of chronic sclerosing osteomyelitis. Areas of sclerosis and irregular contours are seen in the right mandible. There is also obvious involvement of the contralateral side (arrow). **c** Gallium scintigraphy performed in the same patient to evaluate the activity of the inflammatory process shows major tracer uptake in the same areas as those seen on the CT examination. Surgery confirmed chronic sclerosing osteomyelitis.

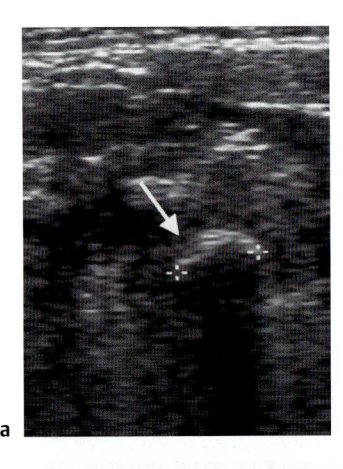

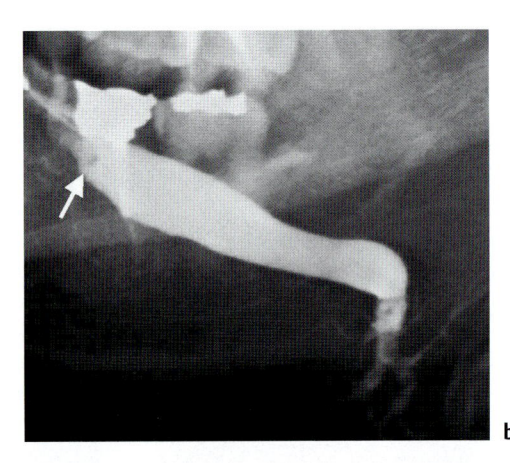

Fig. 10.71 Patient with recurrent submandibular gland swelling. True positive findings of sialolithiasis with US (**a**), conventional sialography (**b**), and MR sialography (**c**). On US a 4 mm calculus (arrow) with an acoustic shadow was detected within the floor of the mouth. On conventional sialography and MR sialography the calculus (arrows) is seen as a filling defect in the anterior portion of Wharton's duct and is causing ductal dilatation. Note the discrepancy between the size of the ductal system as seen on conventional sialography and MR sialography. This is because the ductal system is actively filled during conventional sialography, resulting in distension of the ductal system, whereas MR sialography depicts only the saliva that is present within the ducts. The calculus was retrieved endoscopically. **d** Sialendoscopy image of the 4 mm calculus (arrow) prior to retrieval.

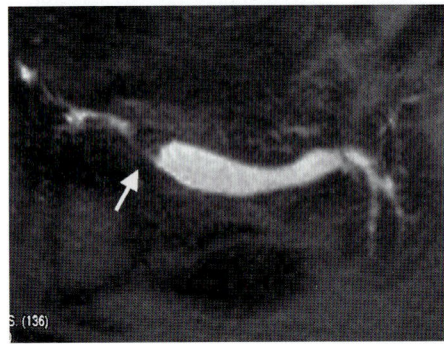

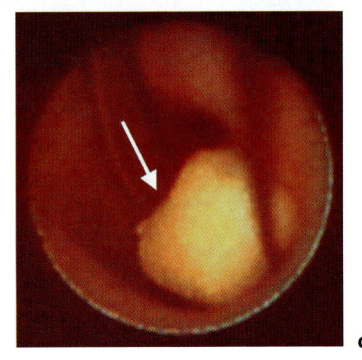

sclerosing osteomyelitis, chronic suppurative osteomyelitis, and chronic osteomyelitis with proliferative periostitis (Garré osteomyelitis). Chronic sclerosing osteomyelitis may be either focal or diffuse (Fig. 10.**70**). The focal form is characterized by a well-defined area of uniform opacity, whereas in the diffuse form extensive areas of sclerosis, poorly demarcated from noninvolved bone, are seen. Chronic suppurative osteomyelitis is characterized by multiple areas of bone destruction, abscess formation, sequestra, sclerotic changes throughout the involved bone, periosteal new bone formation including the formation of an osseous shell (involucrum), sinus tracts, cellulitis, myositis and abscess formation. Garré osteomyelitis typically occurs in the posterior mandible, resulting from a periapical abscess, a postextraction infection, or an infection associated with a partially erupted tooth. Radiologically, ill-defined marrow lesions are associated with a distinctive periosteal reaction resulting in onion-skin reduplication of the cortex.[38]

Infections of Salivary Gland Origin

Inflammatory processes involving the submandibular gland and—less often—the sublingual gland result from obstructing intraductal calculi or fibrous strictures.[17,18] Calculi and strictures may lead to dilatation of the submandibular duct, subsequent ductal infection (sialodochitis), parenchymal infection (sialadenitis), and abscess formation.

The submandibular gland duct (Wharton's duct) is seen routinely on CT and MR images. Whenever Wharton's duct is larger than 2 mm, there should be a thorough evaluation to exclude small calculi. Because only 60–80 % of salivary gland calculi are calcified, CT may miss small noncalcified sialoliths. Calculi that are larger than 3 mm are detected easily with both ultrasound and MR sialography[16,17] (Fig. 10.**71**). However, when the diameter of a calculus is smaller than or equal to 2 mm, calculi may be often missed with ultrasound (Fig. 10.**72**) and sometimes even with MR sialography. To date, however, MR sialography is the most sensitive noninvasive technique for assessing sialolithiasis provided a 3D acquisition technique is used, such as 3D FSE, EXPRESS (extended phase symmetry rapid spin echo) or CISS. The reported sensitivity of MR sialography to detect calculi is 91%, the corresponding specificity is 94–97%, the positive predictive value is 94–97%, and the negative predictive value is 91%[16] (see also Chapter 9).

The features of **acute sialodochitis** on CT and MR imaging include dilatation of the ductal system, as well as enhancement of the ductal wall (Fig. 10.**73**). In **acute submandibular sialadenitis**, the gland is enlarged because of parenchymal edema, and hyperemia. On ultrasound, the enlarged gland is "fuzzy" and inhomogeneous. Hypervascularity is typically seen on color and power Doppler images. On MRI, an increased signal intensity on T2-weighted images, a lower signal intensity on T1-weighted images, and strong enhancement after administration of contrast material are characteristic findings. Sometimes, the borders of the affected gland are unsharp and associated periglandular cellulitis or myositis may be seen (Fig. 10.**73**). Similarly to the findings on MRI, CT scan typically shows enlargement of the involved glands and marked contrast enhancement after administration of contrast material.

In **chronic recurrent sialadenitis**, MR sialography and x-ray sialography typically show ductal stenoses and sialectasia (Fig. 10.**74**). MR sialography is an excellent tool for detecting stenoses of the salivary ductal system. Its reported sensitivity is

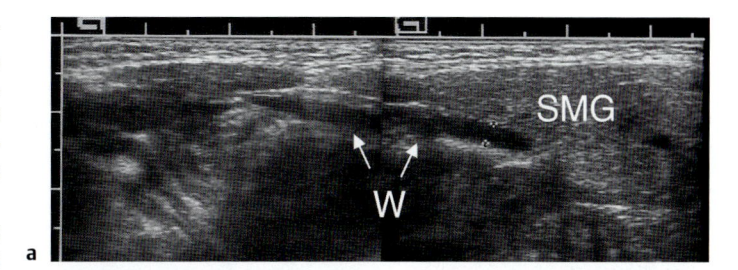

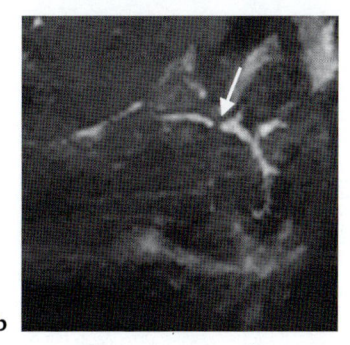

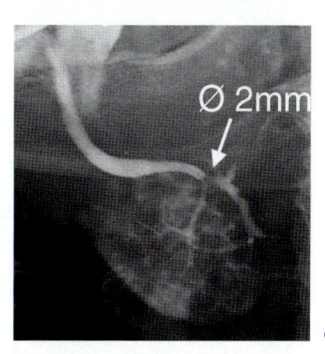

Fig. 10.**72 a** Patient with recurrent submandibular gland swelling and with a normal US examination of the submandibular gland. W = Wharton's duct; SMG = submandibular gland. **b** MR sialography and **c** conventional sialography demonstrate a 2 mm calculus (arrows), which was missed on the US examination. The calculus was afterward retrieved endoscopically. Parts **b** and **c** reproduced from Reference 16 with permission.

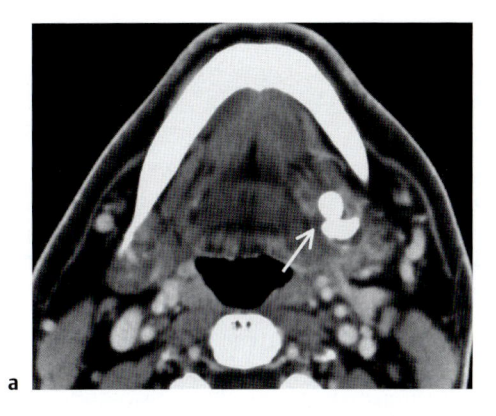

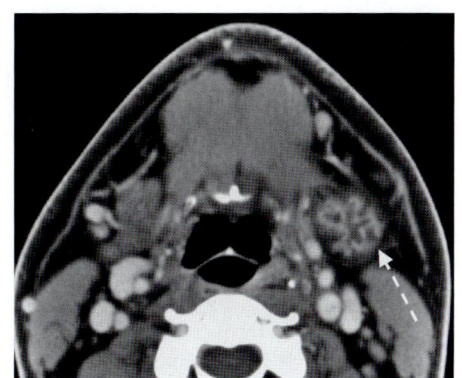

Fig. 10.**73 a, b** Contrast-enhanced CT images obtained in a patient with acute submandibular swelling show the characteristic imaging findings of sialadenitis and sialodochitis caused by obstructive calculi (arrow). Note dilated intraglandular ducts with enhancing walls (dashed arrow), as well as an edematous right submandibular gland. Discrete cellulitis around the submandibular gland is equally present on the right.

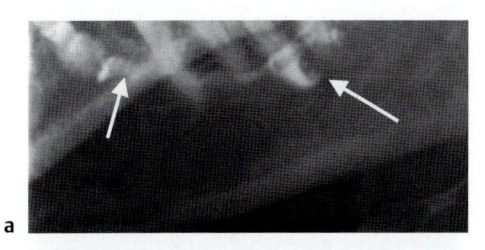

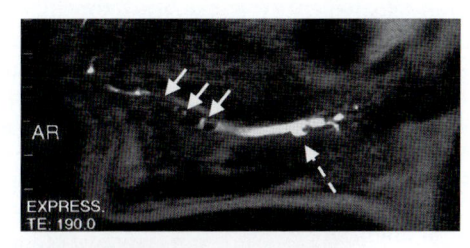

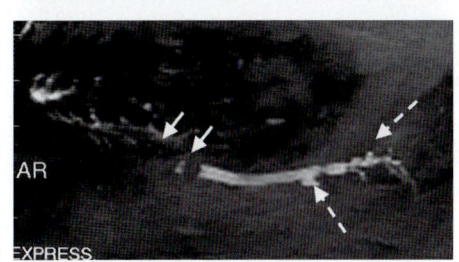

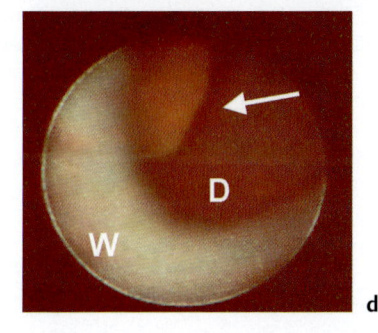

Fig. 10.**74** Female patient presenting with recurrent submandibular gland swelling during mastication. **a** Conventional sialography (lateral oblique view) shows incomplete filling of the ductal system (arrows) caused by distal displacement of calculi. The remainder of the ductal system could not be visualized despite an increased injection pressure. **b** Source image from a sagittal oblique MR sialography sequence shows multiple 2–4 mm stones (arrows) within the anterior third of Wharton's duct. Associated sialodochitis with small diverticular outpouching (dashed arrow). **c** MIP reconstruction depicts less well the calculi (arrows) situated near the orifice of Wharton's duct. However, the diverticular outpouchings (dashed arrows) and the irregular ductal caliber with areas of focal narrowing caused by sialodochitis are better depicted than on the source image. **d** Sialendoscopy confirmed the presence of calculi, stenotic areas, and diverticular outpouchings. W = Wharton's duct; D = proximal diverticulum. Arrow points to a 3 mm stone that has been displaced during conventional sialography into the proximal diverticulum. Reproduced from Reference 16 with permission.

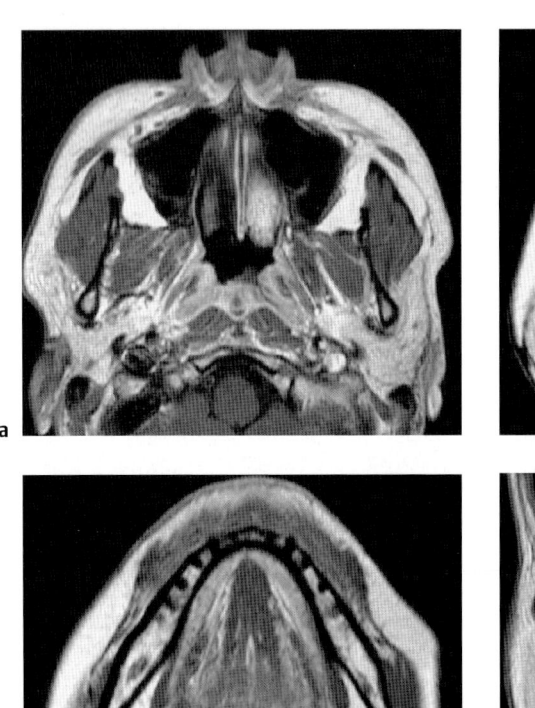

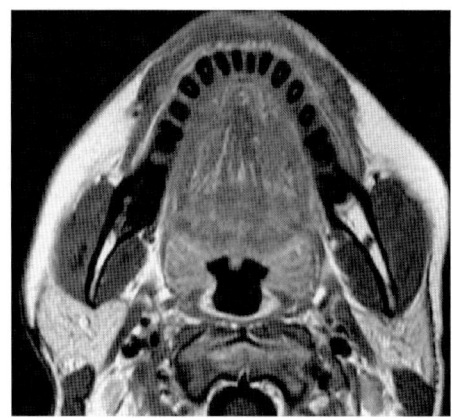

Fig. 10.**75 a–d** Contrast-enhanced T1W MR images obtained in a young patient with marked lymphoid hyperplasia. Note the characteristic appearance on MRI with symmetric involvement of the lymphatic tissue in the nasopharynx and oropharynx. Areas of enhancement are mixed with streaky areas of no enhancement.

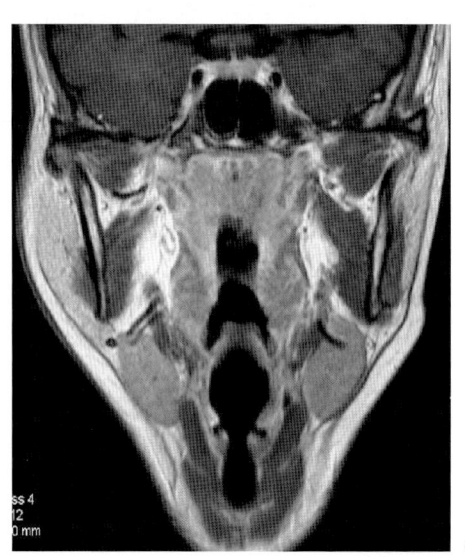

100%, the corresponding specificity is 97%, the positive predictive value is 87–95%, and the negative predictive value is 100% (see also Chapter 9).[16] In some cases of chronic recurrent submandibular sialadenitis the gland becomes indurated (Küttner tumor) and may be confused clinically with a salivary gland neoplasm. CT shows a small, homogeneously enhancing gland with sharply defined borders and on MRI a decreased signal intensity on T2-weighted images, suggesting fibrosis, may be seen. In the absence of ductal dilatation, stenoses, or calculi, differentiation from a submandibular gland neoplasm may be impossible on the basis of sectional imaging alone. Image-guided fine-needle aspiration cytology is very useful in differentiating between the two entities.[29]

Tonsillar and Peritonsillar Inflammation and Infection, and Tonsilloliths

Adenoidal and **tonsillar hyperplasia** are the morphological expressions of marked immunobiological activity rather than disease entities. This overactivity results in hypertrophy of the lymphoepithelial tissue in the pharynx, most commonly the adenoid (pharyngeal tonsil) component and less commonly the faucial (palatine) tonsils. The diagnosis is straightforward on CT or MRI. The nasopharyngeal and oropharyngeal mucosal space is full of hypertrophic adenoidal tissue with preservation of the middle layer of the deep cervical fascia. Tonsillar hyperplasia is usually symmetric (Fig. 10.**75**).

Tonsillitis presents clinically with sore throat and fever. It is caused by infection with beta-streptococci, staphylococci, *Streptococcus pneumoniae*, and *Haemophilus*. Although tonsillitis and pharyngitis are very common infections, especially in children, imaging is reserved for potential complications. Increasing difficulty in swallowing, torticollis, ear pain, trismus, and protrusion of the pharyngeal wall suggesting a submucosal mass are characteristic clinical signs of a tonsillar (peritonsillar) abscess.[88] CT scan may currently be considered to be the imaging method of choice. A **tonsillar abscess** is usually confined laterally by the superior constrictor pharyngeal muscle (Fig. 10.**76**). If the constrictor muscle is penetrated, the abscess is no longer localized to the tonsillar fossa, and the inflammation may spread to the parapharyngeal space or retropharyngeal space. The infection may also spread to the pterygoid muscles, causing trismus, and to the submandibular space. Septic thrombosis of the internal jugular vein or life-threatening septic aneurysm of the carotid artery are rare complications.[114, 131, 143] Most often, CT shows an abscess pocket that is confined by the pharyngeal constrictor muscle to the pharyngeal mucosal space. Infrequently, CT may show rupture of the abscess into the adjacent parapharyngeal space and beyond.

Tonsilloliths as sequelae of previous or chronic tonsillitis are identified as solitary or multiple calcifications within the tonsils in as much as 10% of the population (Fig. 10.**77**). Very large tonsilloliths may be mistaken clinically for tonsillar abscesses.[44]

Mucous Retention Cyst and Ranula

Mucous retention cysts due to inflamed mucus-secreting glands may occur anywhere along the oral cavity and pharynx. In the pharynx, mucous retention cysts arise from the minor salivary glands. If the mucous retention cyst is located at the level of the

Inflammatory Lesions of the Oral Cavity and Oropharynx 717

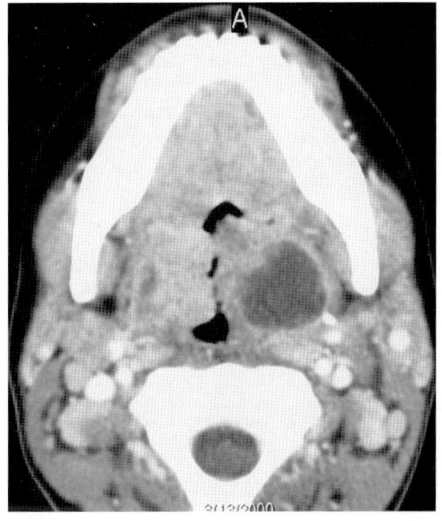

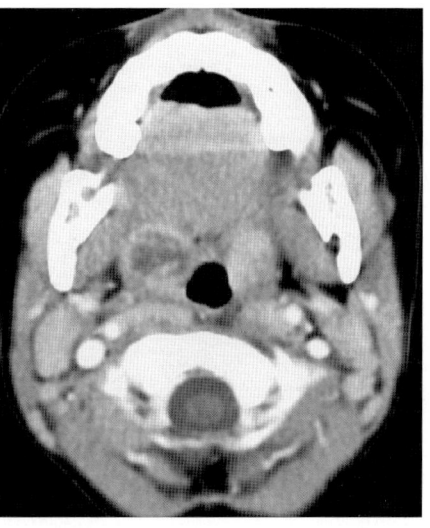

Fig. 10.**76** **a** Contrast-enhanced CT image obtained in an adult. **b** Contrast-enhanced CT image obtained in a 2-year-old boy. Both CT scans show the characteristic features of a peritonsillar abscess. Note that the abscess is limited to the tonsillar fossa without disrupting the constrictor muscles.

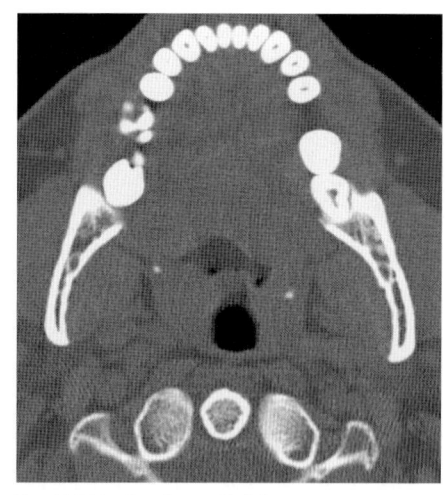

Fig. 10.**77** Small tonsilloliths seen as an incidental finding on a thin-slice CT image.

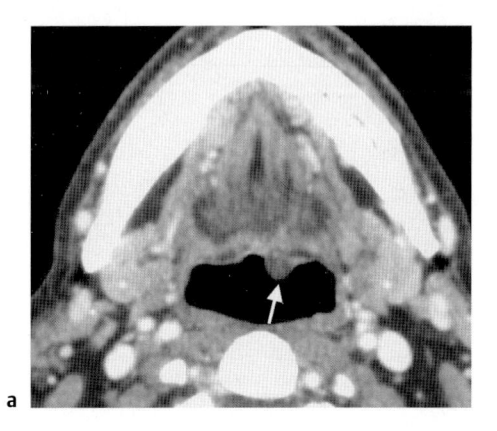

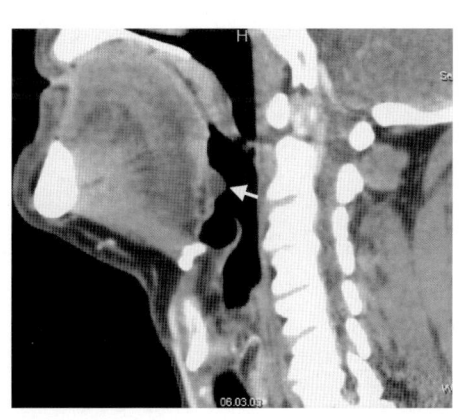

Fig. 10.**78** **a** Axial contrast-enhanced CT image and **b** sagittal 2D reconstruction from a volumetric data set show a small mucous retention cyst in the base of the tongue arrows).

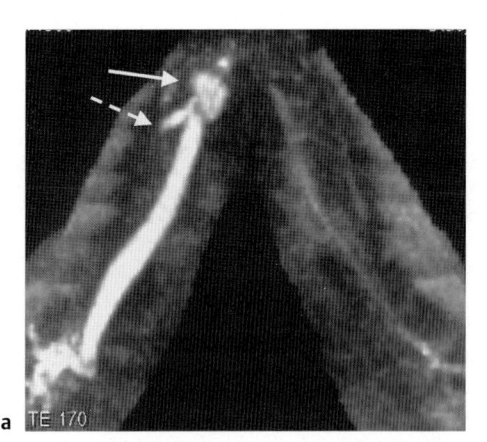

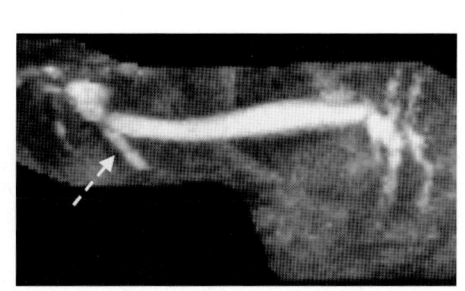

Fig. 10.**79** Posttraumatic simple ranula as seen on axial (**a**) and sagittal oblique (**b**) MIP projections of an MR sialography sequence. The ranula (arrow) is located in the sublingual space and is obstructing Wharton's duct as well as Bartholin's duct (dashed arrows).

tonsil, it is named tonsillar retention cyst. If it is located in the vallecular region, it is named vallecular retention cyst. On CT, mucous retention cysts have attenuation values between 0 and 20 HU (Fig. 10.78). On T1-weighted MR images they have a low signal intensity, whereas on T2-weighted MR images they display variable signal intensities depending on their protein content. Rim enhancement may be observed after intravenous administration of contrast material on both CT and MRI.

Mucous retention cysts of the floor of the mouth, also termed mucoceles or *ranulas*, are of two varieties. The simple ranula is caused by obstruction or trauma (including surgery) of the sublingual gland ductal system[30,55] (Fig. 10.79). It is located above the mylohyoid muscle, whereas a diving or plunging ranula results following extravasation of mucous retention along the free edge of the mylohyoid muscle into the submandibular space. Congenital atresia of the orifice of the submandibular duct

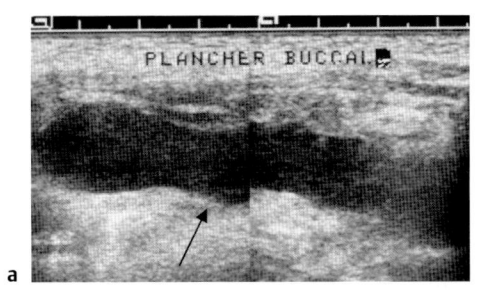

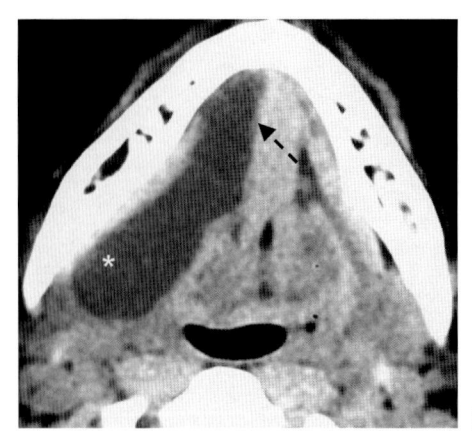

Fig. 10.80 Plunging ranula in a 3-year-old girl. Characteristic aspect on US and CT. **a** US examination of the floor of the mouth (sagittal oblique view) shows a cystic lesion located within the submandibular space (arrow), suggestive of a ranula. **b** Unenhanced CT image obtained at the level of the floor of the mouth demonstrates a plunging ranula on the right (asterisk). The bulk of the ranula is located within the deep submandibular space with a tail extending anteriorly into the sublingual space (dashed arrow). Surgery revealed a plunging ranula caused by congenital atresia of the orifice of Wharton's duct.

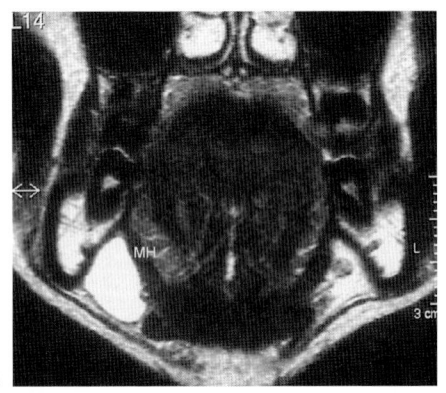

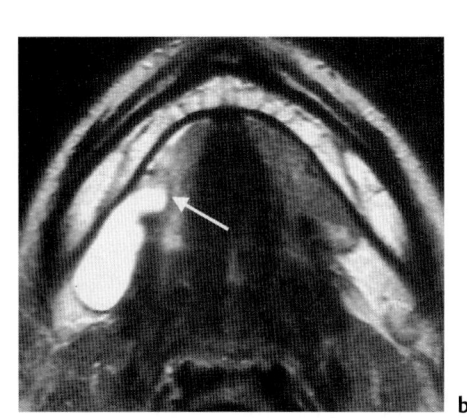

Fig. 10.81 Plunging ranula. Characteristic aspect on MRI. **a** Coronal and **b** axial T2W FSE MR images at the level of the floor of the mouth show a cystic mass located below the mylohyoid muscle (MH). The bulk of the ranula is located within the deep submandibular space with a tail extending anteriorly into the sublingual space (arrow). Courtesy of Dr. Nicole Freling (Department of Radiology, Academic Medical Center Amsterdam, The Netherlands).

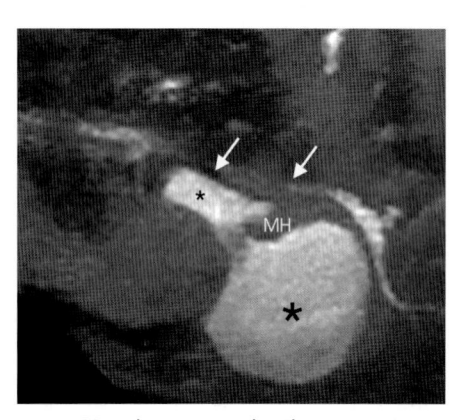

Fig. 10.82 Plunging ranula. Characteristic aspect on MR sialography. Sagittal oblique MIP projection shows a cystic mass located partly below the mylohyoid muscle (MH) and partly above the mylohyoid muscle. The bulk of the ranula is located within the submandibular space (asterisk) with a tail extending anteriorly into the sublingual space (small asterisk). Wharton's duct is displaced superiorly (arrows) by the ranula.

has been reported as a rare cause of plunging ranula.[5] On CT and MRI, ranulas are usually thin-walled, unilocular cystic-appearing lesions confined to the sublingual region (simple ranula) or to both the submandibular and sublingual regions (plunging ranula)[71] (Figs. 10.**80**–10.**82**). The importance of distinguishing between a simple ranula and a plunging ranula is that the former is treated surgically from a transoral incision, whereas the latter is treated by an incision below the mandible.[135]

Unusual Infections of the Oral Cavity and Oropharynx

Rare infections of the oral cavity and oropharynx include tuberculosis, actinomycosis, blastomycosis, cysticercosis, histoplasmosis, syphilis, and noma.[2,3]

Primary and secondary extralaryngeal head and neck **tuberculosis** is exceptional.[2,48,59] It typically has a chronic course. Rarely, the oral cavity and oropharynx, the salivary glands, the ear, the paranasal sinuses, and the orbit may be involved. Clinical manifestations in primary orofacial tuberculosis comprise oral ulcers, mandibular involvement, and salivary gland involvement.[90] Lymphadenitis may be present in 50% of the primary oral cavity and oropharyngeal cases. Patients with secondary disease may have pulmonary lesions with or without clinical and radiological signs of activity. The diagnosis is, in general, difficult owing to the common absence of lung involvement, and usually requires biopsy procedures. The outcome is usually favorable with antituberculous drugs alone.

Actinomycosis is an infectious disease caused by certain *Actinomyces* species. Actinomyces are Gram-positive organisms characterized by anaerobic rods that normally inhabit anaerobic niches of the human oral cavity. Cervicofacial, abdominal, pelvic, and thoracic infections with actinomyces are not uncommon. Although the oral mucosa is often the site of entry of actinomyces into the deeper tissues, actinomycosis in the oral mucosa is extremely rare.[3] Actinomycotic lesions are usually described as either single or multiple abscesses or indurated masses with hard fibrous walls and soft central loculations. Actinomycosis may also present primarily as a long-standing ulcer of the oral mucosa mimicking a squamous cell carcinoma.

Noma is an acute necrotizing gingivitis that spreads rapidly into adjacent soft tissue. It is most commonly seen in Third World countries, with the highest incidence in children. *Borrelia* and fusiform bacilli are always present. The CT scan features of noma are characteristic and include large soft-tissue defects due to sharply marginated ulceration, as well as "clear-cut" bony defects. The diagnosis of noma is made clinically, and CT scan with 3D reconstructions is in general used only prior to reconstructive surgery.

Congenital Lesions 719

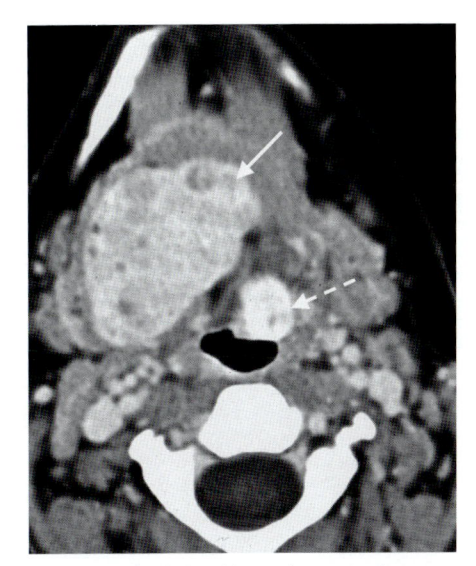

Fig. 10.83 Multifocal lingual goiter. Characteristic aspect on contrast-enhanced CT. Note strongly enhancing hypertrophic thyroid nodules at the level of the base of the tongue (dashed arrow) and at the level of the floor of the mouth (arrow).

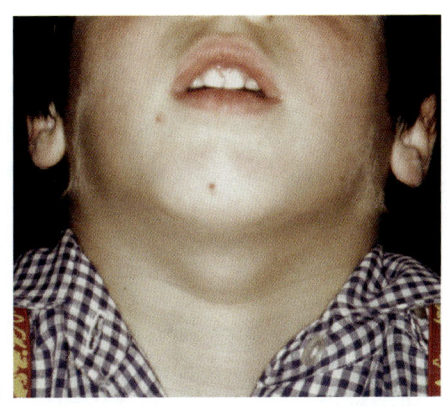

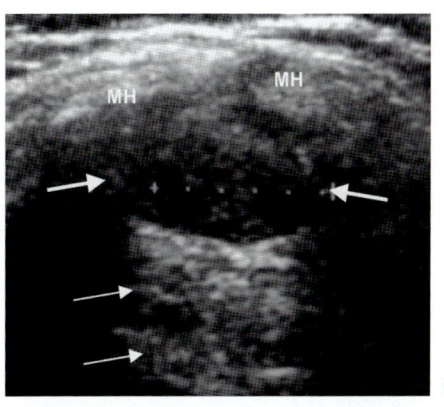

Fig. 10.84 Thyroglossal duct cyst located in the floor of the mouth. Characteristic clinical presentation, and US appearance. **a** Photograph of a young boy presenting with a submental midline swelling. The swelling was soft at palpation, strongly suggesting a thyroglossal duct cyst. **b** Coronal US view through the floor of the mouth shows an anechoic midline lesion (arrows) with a characteristic acoustic enhancement (thin arrows) suggesting a cyst. The cyst is located above the mylohyoid muscle (MH).

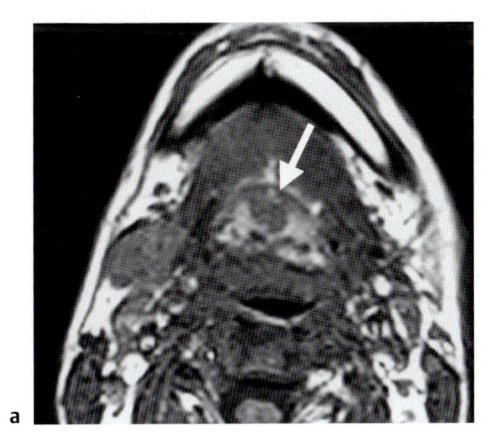

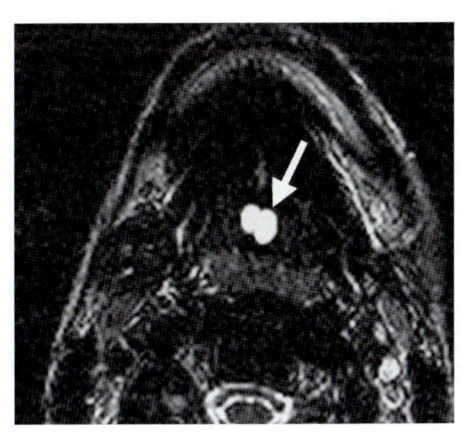

Fig. 10.85 Thyroglossal duct cyst. Characteristic aspect on MRI. **a** Axial T1W and **b** heavily T2W MR images at the level of the base of the tongue show a cystic midline lesion located at the level of the foramen cecum (arrows).

Congenital Lesions

Congenital lesions of the oral cavity and oropharynx include thyroglossal duct anomalies, dermoid cysts, epidermoid cysts, vascular malformations, and branchial cleft cysts.[65]

Thyroglossal Duct Cysts and Lingual Thyroid Tissue

During embryogenesis, the anlage of the thyroid/parathyroid glands descends from the foramen cecum at its origin from the apex of the circumvallate papillae, through the tongue base and floor of the mouth, to its final position in the lower neck.[15, 126, 143] During this caudal migration, the anlage passes just anterior to the precursor tissue of the hyoid bone, leaving behind a tract of epithelial tissue called the thyroglossal duct. The normal thyroglossal duct involutes by the eighth fetal week. **Thyroglossal duct remnants** may give rise to cysts, fistulae, or solid nodules of thyroid tissue within the base of the tongue, the floor of the mouth, or the anterior neck.

A clinically significant lingual thyroid is rare. However ectopic thyroid tissue less than 3 mm in size is found within the tongue base at autopsy in 10% of the population.[126, 143] Ectopic thyroid tissue has a high female to male preponderance, which is attributed to hormonal effects during puberty and pregnancy. Most ectopic thyroid tissue is asymptomatic and is discovered incidentally. However, dysphagia and dyspnea may occur in large ectopic thyroid masses (Fig. 10.**83**). Thyroid carcinoma has been reported to occur both in lingual thyroid and in thyroglossal duct cysts.[35] The CT and MRI characteristics of lingual thyroid tissue mimic normal thyroid tissue and intense enhancement of a lingual thyroid may be present (Fig. 10.**83**). Because this may be the only functioning thyroid tissue in the patient's body, a thyroid scintigram to search for other thyroid tissue should be performed prior to planned resection. The imaging characteristics of pathological lingual thyroid tissue are similar to those of pathology involving the thyroid gland, such as multinodular goiter, carcinoma, thyroiditis, etc.

Although most thyroglossal duct cysts (65%) occur in the infrahyoid neck, 25% are located in the tongue base or oral cavity.[3, 23] In the oral cavity, thyroglossal duct cysts are most often located in the midline. On CT or MRI, a midline or paramedian cystic mass with or without rim enhancement is typically seen. On ultrasound, a midline or paramedian cystic mass involving the floor of the mouth or the base of the tongue is easily seen, allowing the correct diagnosis (Figs. 10.**84**, 10.**85**).

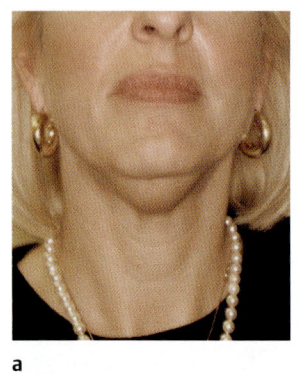

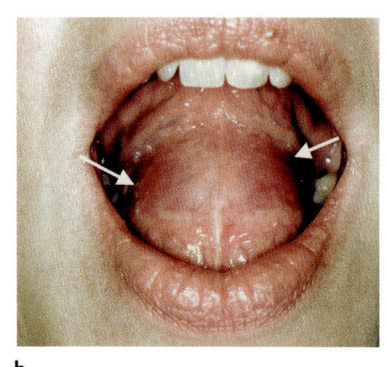

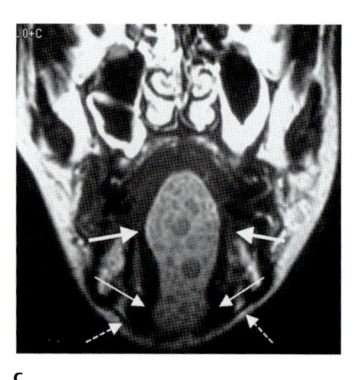

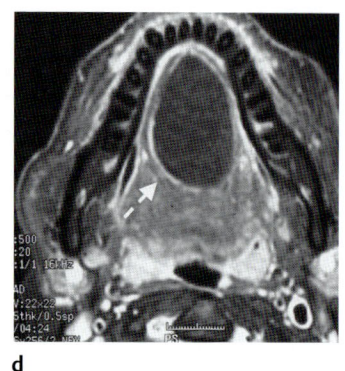

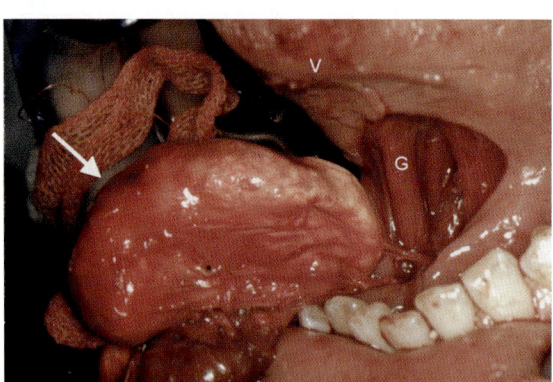

Fig. 10.86 Dermoid cyst: clinical and MRI presentation. **a** This middle-aged woman presented with a long-standing submental midline swelling. **b** On clinical inspection a well-delineated midline submucosal lesion is seen bellow the ventral tongue surface (arrow). The mucosa overlying this lesion is intact. **c** Coronal T2W and **d** axial contrast-enhanced, fat-suppressed T1W MR images show a large cystic mass located in the midline between the genioglossus muscles (arrows) and the geniohyoid muscles (thin arrows), which are displaced laterally. The mass shows inhomogeneous signal intensity on T2W imaging with multiple fat globules. Thin peripheral rim enhancement is seen on the contrast-enhanced T1W image (dashed arrow). Dashed arrows in **c** point at the mylohyoid muscle. Based on the MR imaging findings the diagnosis of a dermoid cyst was suggested. As the lesion was located above the mylohyoid muscle, an intraoral approach was chosen. **e** Intraoperative view shows a large cystic lesion with smooth walls (arrow). V = ventral tongue surface; G = genioglossus muscle. Pathology confirmed the diagnosis of a dermoid cyst.

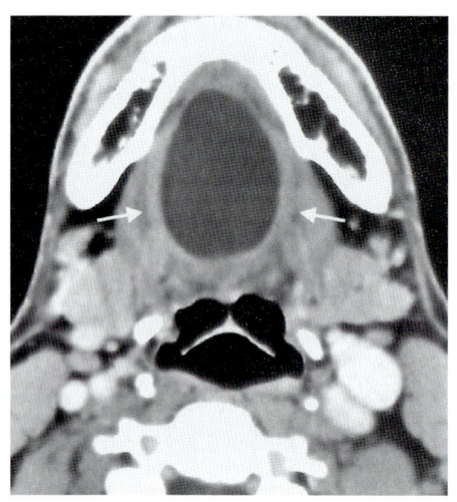

Fig. 10.87 Epidermoid cyst as seen on CT. Axial contrast-enhanced image shows a large unilocular cystic mass located in the midline between the genioglossus muscles, which are displaced laterally (arrows). The mass shows homogeneous low attenuation values. From the imaging point of view this appearance would be consistent with either a dermoid or an epidermoid cyst. Surgery confirmed the diagnosis of an epidermoid cyst.

Developmental Cysts

Developmental cysts are thought to arise from epithelial rests that become enclaved during midline closure of the first and second branchial arches. Developmental cysts may be classified into epidermoid, dermoid, and teratoid forms (see Chapter 2, Section II). Epidermoid cysts consist of simple squamous epithelium with a fibrous wall.[39,50,73] Dermoid cysts contain skin appendages, such as sebaceous glands, hair follicles, and fat tissue, and teratomas contain tissue derived from all three germ cell layers. Dermoid cysts that contain fat may be considered as well-differentiated teratomas (two germ cell layers). Dermoid cysts are very rare lesions in the oral cavity.[50] When they do occur, they are usually located in the midline or slightly off the midline within the floor of the mouth, the sublingual or submandibular space, and the tongue.[91,92,137] Carcinomatous transformation of sublingual dermoid cysts has been reported.[41] Therapy consists of surgical excision. For those lesions located above the mylohyoid muscle, an intraoral approach is preferred because it avoids a conspicuous scar and because the surgical intervention is associated with a shorter recovery time. Those lesions that lie inferior to the mylohyoid muscle are usually removed by an external approach. Therefore, the identification of the cyst location in relationship to the mylohyoid muscle on CT or MRI is extremely helpful in surgical planning.[91,135] Axial imaging and, especially, coronal imaging are essential in this regard (Fig. 10.**86**). Dermoid cysts may have the typical MRI signal intensity characteristics of these lesions elsewhere in the body. Fluid attenuation in epidermoid cysts and fat in dermoid cysts may differentiate the two (Figs. 10.**86**, 10.**87**). However, in the absence of fat, differentiation between dermoid and epidermoid cysts may be impossible at imaging. On both CT and MRI, the thin wall of the cyst usually enhances following intravenous administration of contrast material.

Vascular Malformations

According to Mulliken and Glowacki, vascular lesions of the head and neck may be divided into hemangiomas and vascular malformations.[102] **Hemangiomas** are neoplastic conditions characterized by an increased proliferation and turnover of endothelial cells, and typically display a rapid proliferation phase during the first year of life followed by an involution phase.[25–28] As opposed to hemangiomas, **vascular malformations** are not tumors but true congenital vascular anomalies with a normal proliferation rate of endothelial cells. They do not regress and may enlarge rapidly in association with trauma or endocrine changes. Vascular malformations are further subdivided into capillary, venous, arterial, and lymphatic malformations.[53] A subgroup of patients demonstrates combined vascular malformations that share either features of both high-flow and low-flow lesions or features of low-flow and lymphangiomatous lesions.

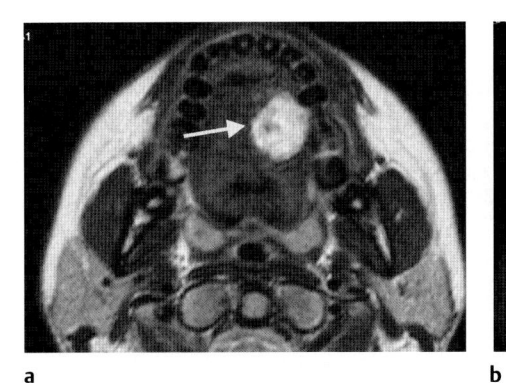

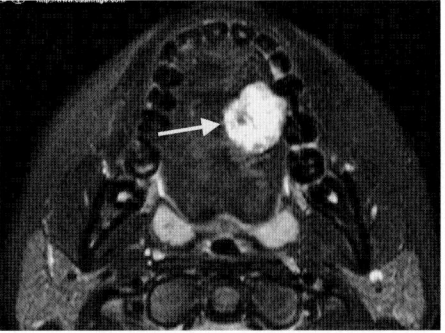

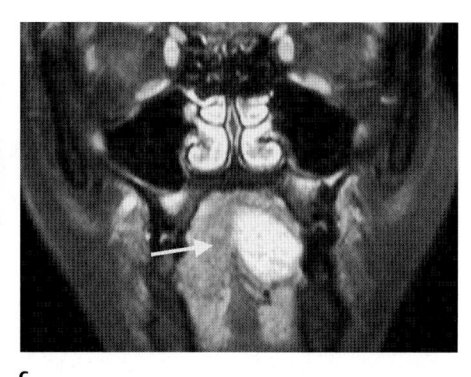

Fig. 10.**88** Venous malformation of the tongue. Characteristic MR imaging findings. **a** Axial T2W, **b** axial STIR, and **c** coronal contrast-enhanced fat-suppressed T1W MR images. The well-delineated lesion located in the left hemitongue is hyperintense on T2W and STIR MR images and shows intense enhancement after administration of contrast material. No serpiginous signal voids are seen and the small hypointense dot seen on the axial images probably corresponds to a small phlebolith or a small area of thrombosis.

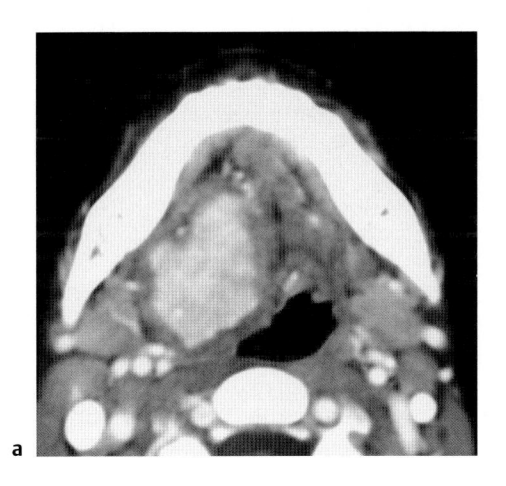

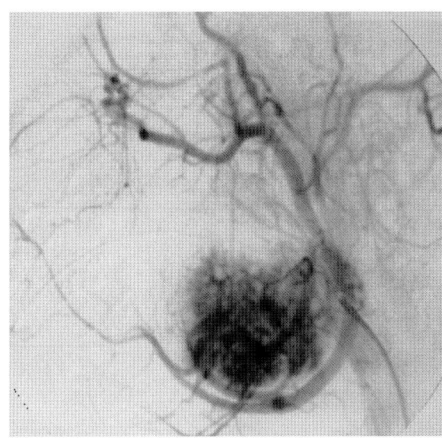

Fig. 10.**89** Venous malformation of the tongue. **a** Axial contrast-enhanced CT image shows a mass with intense enhancement located in the floor of the mouth and with extension into the base of the tongue. **b** Angiography performed in this patient prior to embolization shows an intense parenchymal stain that persisted late into the venous phase.

Arterial malformations are high-flow malformations that result from abnormal blood vessel morphogenesis.[53,102,142] Arteriovenous malformations and fistulae are included in this category. **Capillary** and **venous malformations** are low-flow lesions. In the head and neck, capillary malformations tend to involve the skin and subcutaneous tissue, while venous and arterial malformations tend to involve deeper structures. The most common locations for venous and arterial malformations include the tongue, lip, and cheek. Arterial and venous malformations are usually treated conservatively, although surgical excision and embolization are possible. On MRI, venous malformations are isointense or hyperintense to muscle on T1-weighted images, become very hyperintense on T2-weighted images, and typically enhance significantly following administration of contrast material (Fig. 10.**88**). Phleboliths may be present and are seen as round areas of signal voids on T1-weighted and T2-weighted MR images. Areas of thrombosis correspond to high signal intensity areas on T1-weighted MR images and venous lakes correspond to discrete areas of homogeneous high signal intensity on T2-weighted MR images.[142] On CT scans, venous malformations show variable degrees of enhancement (Fig. 10.**89**), and the presence of phleboliths is pathognomonic. Angiography, which may be performed prior to embolization, typically shows a deep parenchymal stain persisting late after the arterial phase (Fig. 10.**89**). Arterial malformations are composed of large tortuous arteries and draining veins, which are easily identified on angiography. These lesions typically do not show parenchymal staining on angiography. On MRI, serpiginous flow voids are seen on T1-weighted and T2-weighted MR images owing to the enlarged arterial components (Fig. 10.**90**). MRI is reported to be superior to CT in demonstrating the extent and complexity of vascular malformations.

Lymphangioma is a benign, nonencapsulated lesion that is believed to arise from sequestrations of primitive embryonic lymph sacs. On the basis of the size of the abnormal lymphatic spaces, lymphangiomas are classified into three histological types: capillary, cavernous, and cystic (cystic hygroma). Cystic hygromas contain hugely dilated cystic spaces typically occurring in the posterior cervical triangle, in the superior mediastinum, and within the oral cavity and submandibular and sublingual spaces. Involvement of the submandibular space is more common than involvement of the sublingual space. In the oral cavity, lymphangiomas can occur in the tongue, floor of the mouth, cheek, and lips[22] (Figs. 10.**91**, 10.**92**). The anterior tongue is the most common location for oral cavity lymphangiomas, commonly presenting as an enlarged tongue.[7] Cystic hygromas are difficult to remove at surgery as they often wrap around and adhere to adjacent structures, such as the neurovascular pedicle of the tongue in the case of a submandibular space lesion. Cavernous lymphangiomas contain intermediate cysts and typically occur in the tongue and salivary glands, whereas capillary lymphangiomas contain very small cysts and appear as vesicles in the skin. Cystic hygromas are the most common type of lymphangioma. Sixty-five percent of cystic hygromas are present at birth, and most cases are clinically apparent by the age of 2 years. Their CT and MR characteristics include a multiseptated cystic

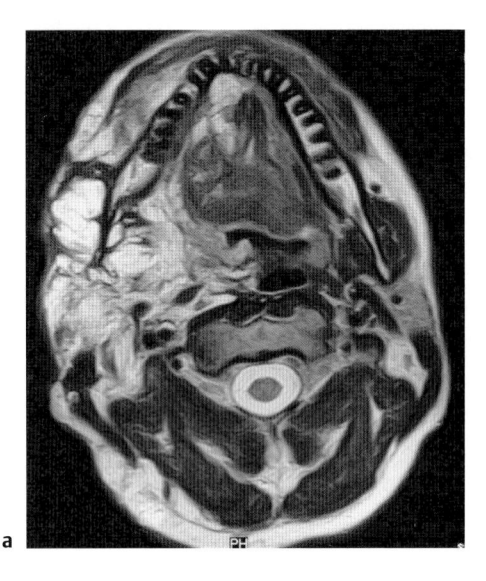

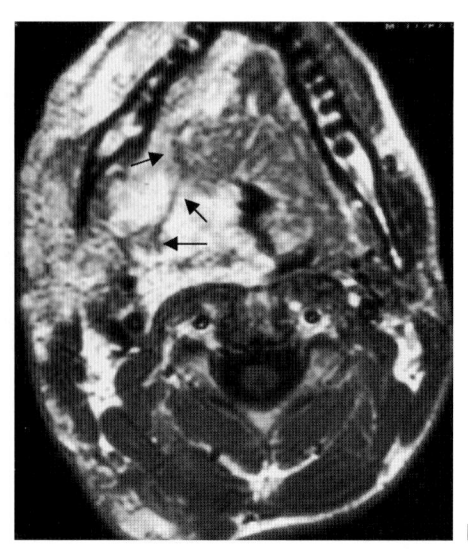

Fig. 10.**90** Extensive arteriovenous malformation. Characteristic MRI aspect. **a** T2W image. **b** Contrast-enhanced T1W MR image. A large hyperintense lesion is seen on the T2W MR image. After injection of contrast material, an intense enhancement is seen. The lesion involves the soft tissues of the face, the muscles of mastication, the parotid gland, the floor of the mouth, the oropharynx, the retropharyngeal space, and the lateral cervical region. Multiple curvilinear signal voids are seen (arrows), indicating vessels with a high flow.

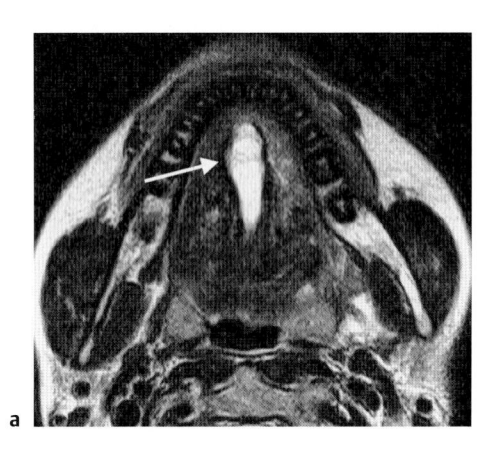

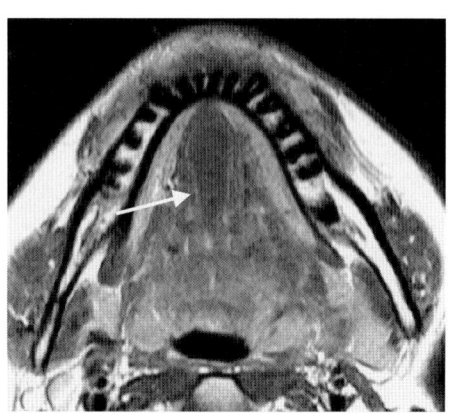

Fig. 10.**91** Lymphangioma of the floor of the mouth. **a** T2W axial MR image. **b** T1W axial MR image after injection of contrast material. A cystic lesion (arrow) is located in the midline displacing the genioglossus muscles laterally. Very thin septations are seen on the T2W image. The lesion is consistent with a lymphangioma. Surgery confirmed the diagnosis of a lymphangioma.

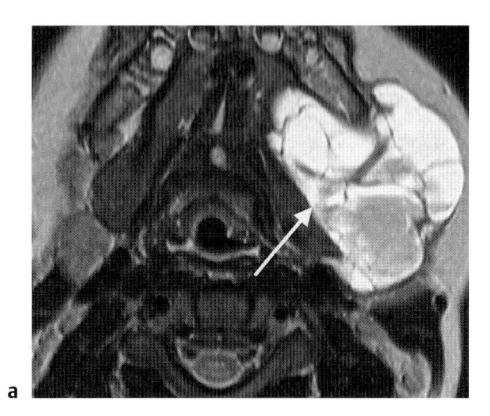

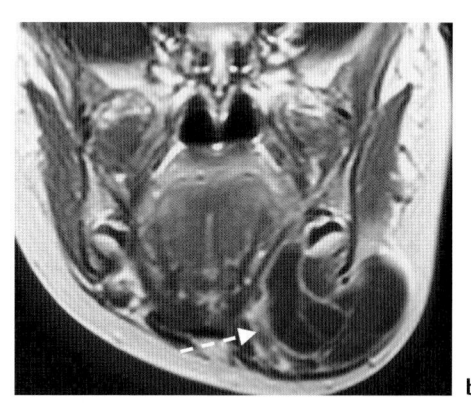

Fig. 10.**92** Lymphangioma in a 6-year-old boy presenting with rapid enlargement of a submandibular mass. **a** Axial T2W and **b** coronal T1W MR images show a multiseptated cystic mass isointense to CSF located in the submandibular space (arrow) and insinuating around the angle of the mandible. Fluid–fluid levels represent layering of blood (slightly hypointense, arrow) and lymph. Discrete enhancement of the thin septae is seen on the T1W MR image (dashed arrow).

mass that may insinuate in and around normal structures, making surgical resection very difficult. On T2-weighted MR images, cystic hygromas are typically isointense to cerebrospinal fluid, while they have a variable signal intensity on T1-weighted images owing to the variable protein content (Fig. 10.**92**). Rapid enlargement of a cervical cystic hygroma is usually due to hemorrhage into the cystic spaces of the mass. Multiple fluid–fluid levels, representing layering of blood and lymph, are characteristic. Fluid–fluid levels may be identified at CT, but the conspicuity of this finding is more apparent on MR images.

Branchial Cleft Anomalies

Of all **branchial cleft anomalies**, 95% arise from the remnant of the second branchial apparatus. Normally, the second branchial cleft apparatus involutes by the ninth fetal week.[6,99] When the involution phase is incomplete, the remnant tissue has the potential to grow into a branchial cleft anomaly. The most common form of second branchial cleft anomaly is a cystic mass without sinus or fistula. However, any permutation of cyst, sinus, or fistula may be possible. **Second branchial cleft cysts** occur either in infants or in the young adult. Typically, patients with a second branchial cleft cyst present with a painless mass in the

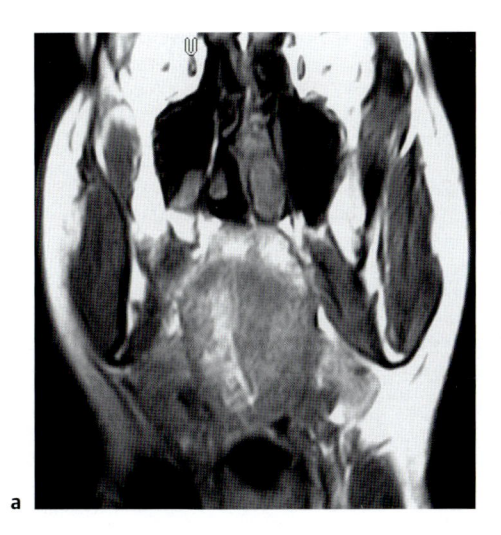

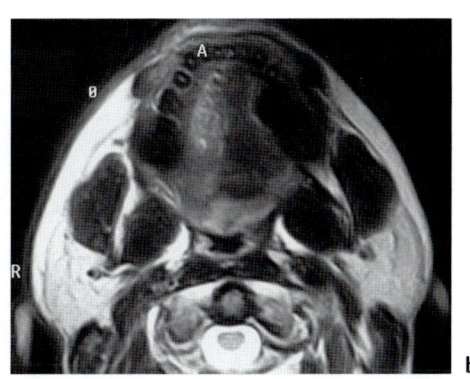

Fig. 10.**93** Hypoglossal nerve paralysis after oral intubation for abdominal surgery. Imaging was performed three weeks after onset of symptoms. MRI findings are consistent with subacute/early chronic denervation. **a** T1W coronal MR image shows an increased signal intensity of the right hemitongue due to deposition of fat. Note also slight loss of volume and displacement of the lingual septum to the right. **b** Axial T2W MR image shows an increased signal intensity in the right hemitongue consistent with edema.

submandibular space.[70] A history of a change in the size of the cyst, usually after an upper respiratory tract infection, is common. The most common location of a second branchial cleft cyst is in the posterior submandibular space. The cyst lies at the angle of the mandible posterolateral to the submandibular gland, lateral to the carotid artery, and anteromedial to the sternocleidomastoid muscle. When present on the cyst, a beak that points medially between the internal and external carotid artery is pathognomonic of a second branchial cleft cyst. CT typically reveals a unilocular cystic mass essentially isoattenuating with cerebrospinal fluid (CSF). A uniformly thin peripheral capsular enhancement is characteristic. Infection of the cyst may, however, result in thickening and irregular capsular enhancement. Depending on the relative protein concentration within the cyst, second branchial cleft cysts are typically isointense to CSF on T2-weighted MR images, while they have a variable appearance on T1-weighted MR images. The differential diagnosis includes large necrotic lymph nodes (see also Chapter 12). Rarely, second branchial cleft cysts may be seen within the oropharynx at the level of the tonsils (atypical second branchial cleft cyst). At imaging, a cystic mass is seen projecting from the deep margin of the oropharyngeal faucial tonsil up the parapharyngeal space toward the skull base (see Chapter 8).[56]

Miscellaneous Pathology

Denervation Muscle Atrophy

The hypoglossal nerve, the mylohyoid nerve (branch of the inferior alveolar nerve), and fibers from C1 supply the motor innervation of the tongue and floor of the mouth. Damage to these nerves anywhere along their course may produce denervation atrophy. Insult to the hypoglossal nerve may be seen in a variety of conditions such as brainstem and basal cistern lesions, skull base tumors, neck nodes, internal carotid artery dissection, after tonsillectomy, after submandibulectomy, as a complication of oral intubation, and after radiation therapy[1, 43, 79, 121, 122, 128, 110] (Figs. 10.**93**–10.**96**). Insult to the mandibular nerve may be seen in brainstem and basal cistern lesions, cavernous sinus/skull base lesions, mandibular space abscesses and mandibular osteomyelitis, schwannoma and neurofibroma of V3, perineural spread from squamous cell carcinoma, adenoid cystic carcinoma and lymphoma, and after retrogasserian rhizotomy and trauma.

In hypoglossal nerve injury, the intrinsic and extrinsic tongue muscles are affected.[37, 83, 118] In proximal mandibular nerve injury, the following muscles are affected: muscles of mastication (masseter, temporalis, medial and lateral pterygoid); the tensor tympani and tensor veli palati muscles (which are innervated via the masticator branch); the mylohyoid muscle and the anterior belly of the digastric muscle (which are innervated via the mylohyoid branch). In distal injury involving only the mylohyoid branch of the inferior alveolar nerve, selective atrophy of the mylohyoid muscle and anterior belly of the digastric muscle is seen. Isolated injury of the motor fibers of C1 producing selective atrophy of the geniohyoid muscle is extremely rare.

Imaging findings in hypoglossal (XII) and mandibular (V3) denervation depend on the chronicity of the process.[83, 118] Both hypoglossal and mandibular denervation can be described in terms of chronic, subacute, or acute denervation, each with a distinctive set of imaging findings. Long-standing chronic denervation is manifested by marked loss of volume of the affected musculature and extensive fatty replacement. No abnormal enhancement is seen in the affected muscles and no increased signal intensity on T2-weighted MR images. Volume loss, fatty replacement, and absence of enhancement are easily identified on both CT and MR images (Figs. 10.**95**, 10.**96**). A characteristic finding in chronic hypoglossal denervation is the prolapse of the affected hemitongue into the oropharynx on axial supine images. This finding is consistent with loss of the normal tongue muscle tone. Ipsilateral asymmetry of the torus tubarius and fluid in the mastoid due to loss of regulation of the eustachian tube related to tensor veli palatini denervation are additional findings observed in chronic V3 denervation.[118]

In early or mild chronic denervation, muscle volume is relatively preserved and fatty replacement of the denervated musculature is less extensive than in long-standing chronic denervation. Typically, there is no edemalike increased signal intensity on T2-weighted images and no abnormal muscle enhancement.[118]

Acute/subacute denervation results in edemalike signal changes and in abnormal contrast enhancement of the denervated musculature. The edemalike signal changes are seen as an increase in signal intensity on T2-weighted MR images or on STIR (short tau inversion recovery) MR images (Fig. 10.**93**, 10.**94**). Occasionally, an increased muscle volume may accompany acute denervation signal changes, suggesting that there may be a component of true edema as well. Fatty replacement may be additionally observed in acute hypoglossal denervation but it is not observed until the subacute stage in V3 denervation.[118]

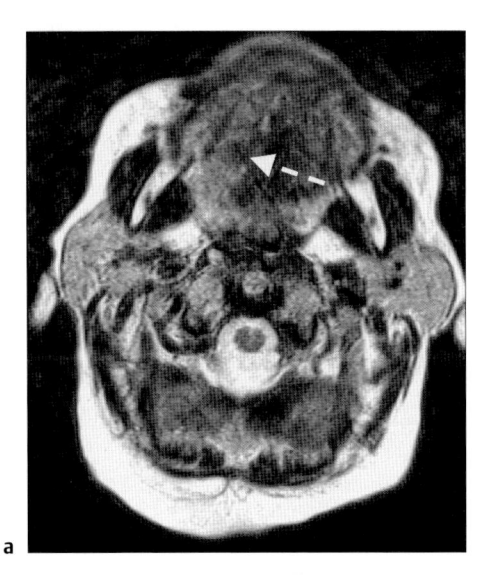

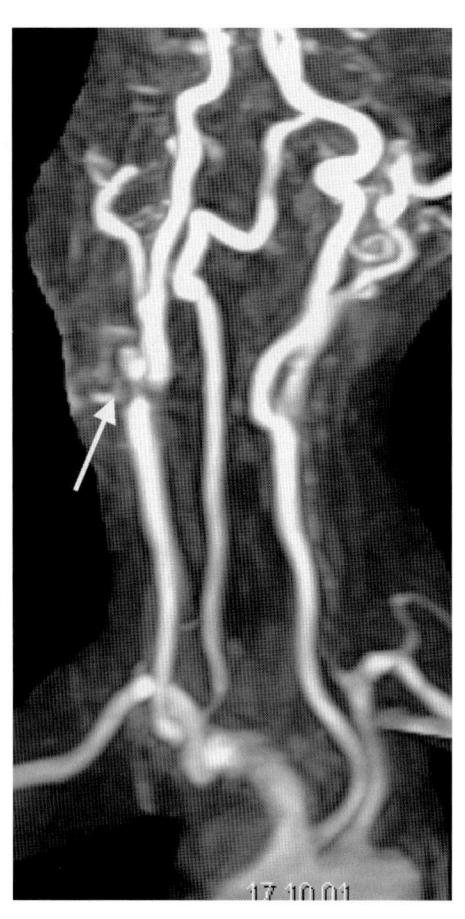

Fig. 10.**94** Hypoglossal nerve paralysis caused by an aneurysm of the internal carotid artery compressing the hypoglossal nerve. MRI findings are consistent with subacute/early chronic denervation. **a** Axial T2W image shows an increased signal intensity in the right hemitongue consistent with edema (dashed arrow), **b** Contrast-enhanced MR angiography of the carotid arteries revealed an aneurysm of the internal carotid artery on the right (arrow). Surgery confirmed compression of the hypoglossal nerve by an aneurysm of the internal carotid artery as the nerve bends anteriorly along the submandibular gland.

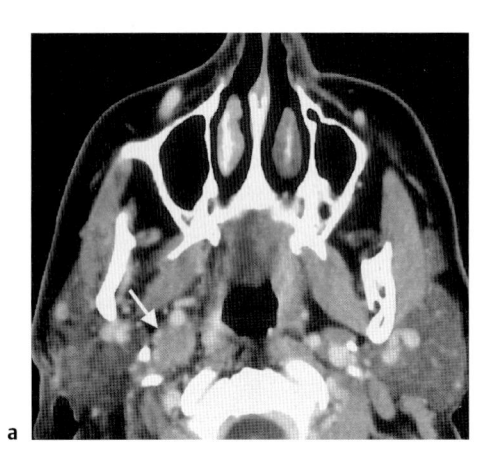

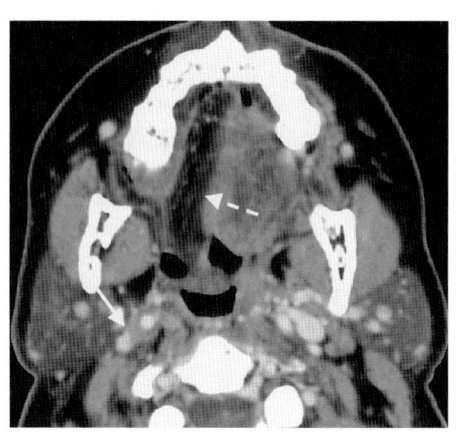

Fig. 10.**95a, b** Axial contrast-enhanced CT images of long-standing hypoglossal nerve paralysis caused by a schwannoma of the hypoglossal nerve seen at the level of the carotid space (arrows). Dashed arrow points to fatty infiltration of the right hemitongue.

Identification of hypoglossal or mandibular motor denervation should prompt an exhaustive search along the entire course of the nerve back to its origin in the brainstem, in an attempt to identify the site of pathology.

Macroglossia and Acute Tongue Swelling

Macroglossia, or tongue enlargement, may occur in a variety of congenital, endocrine, and metabolic conditions, such as Down syndrome and Pierre Robin syndrome, amyloidosis, mucopolysaccharidosis, acromegaly, cretinism, and cysts and lymphangioma of the tongue.[112] In amyloidosis of the tongue, there is symmetrical enlargement of both the extrinsic and intrinsic muscles without identification of any focal masses. The enlarged, infiltrated muscles display normal signal intensities on T1-weighted and T2-weighted MR images and no abnormal contrast enhancement.

Massive, acute **tongue swelling** causing obstruction of the airway is seen in anaphylactic reactions or as a severe complication of spinal surgery.[93, 116] Swelling results from the position of the spine during surgery (flexed thoracic–cervical position), fixation of the endotracheal tube, and compression of the base of the tongue. Swelling is the result of massive edema involving all tongue muscles. Once swelling of the tongue occurs, administration of a corticosteroid is effective in preventing airway obstruction.

Both macroglossia and acute tongue swelling are clinical diagnoses. However, imaging may be performed in exceptional situations to exclude other underlying pathologies.

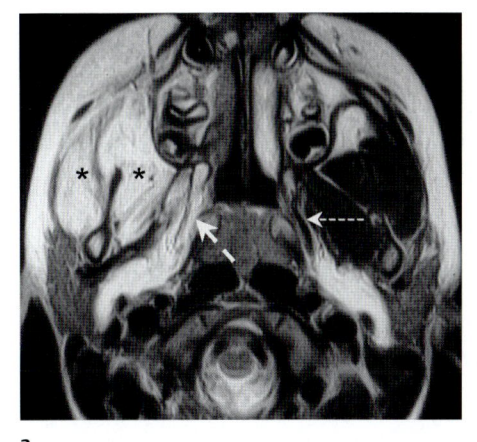

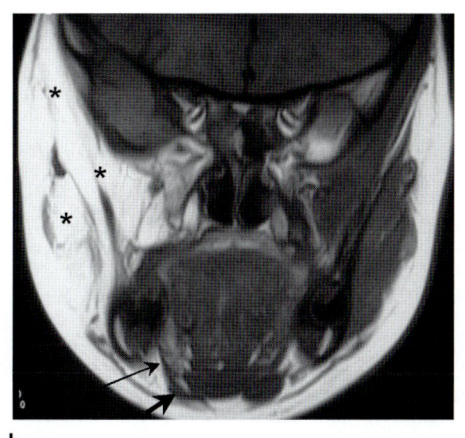

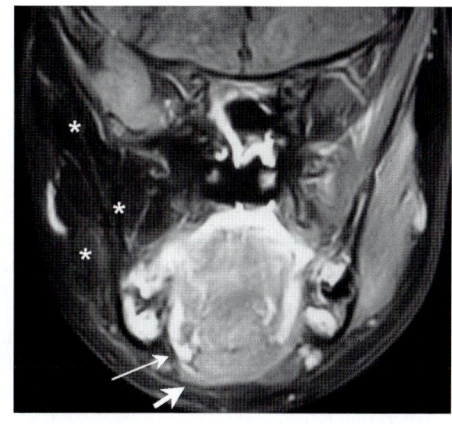

Fig. 10.**96** Long-standing paralysis of V3 in a 6-year-old girl. Characteristic MRI findings. **a** Axial T2W MR image, **b** coronal T1W MR image, and **c** coronal contrast-enhanced, fat-suppressed MR image show atrophy and fatty infiltration of the muscles of mastication on the right (asterisks), atrophy of the right mylohyoid muscle (thin arrows), right anterior belly of the digastric muscle (thick short arrows), and atrophy of the right tensor veli palatini muscle (thick dashed arrow). Thin dashed arrow points at the normal left tensor veli palatini muscle. Note normal size, as well as normal signal intensities, of the contralateral muscles of mastication, contralateral mylohyoid muscle, and anterior belly of the digastric muscle.

Acknowledgments

Many thanks to Willy Lehman M.D., Francis Marchal M.D., and Pavel Dulguerov M.D., Department of Otorhinolaryngology and Cervico-Facial Surgery, and to Paulette Mhawech M.D., Department of Clinical Pathology, Geneva University Hospital, for their valuable contributions.

References

1. Adams H, Verhoff MA, Hagemeyer TP, Muller KM. Arachnoid cyst with consecutive brainstem atrophy, hypoglossal nerve paresis and tongue atrophy. Pathologe 2001; 22(4): 266–269.
2. Aktogu S, Eris FN, Dinc ZA, Tibet G. Tuberculosis of the tongue secondary to pulmonary tuberculosis. Monaldi Arch Chest Dis 2000; 55(4): 287–288.
3. Alamillos-Granados FJ, Dean-Ferrer A, Garcia-Lopez A, Lopez-Rubio F. Actinomycotic ulcer of the oral mucosa: an unusual presentation of oral actinomycosis. Br J Oral Maxillofac Surg 2000; 38(2): 121–123.
4. Altavilla G, Mannara GM, Rinaldo A, Ferlito A. Basaloid suamous cell carcinoma of the oral cavity and oropharynx. ORL 1999; 61; 169–172.
5. Amin MA, Bailey BM. Congenital atresia of the orifice of the submandibular duct: a report of 2 cases and review.Br J Oral Maxillofac Surg 2001; 39(6): 480–482.
6. Ang AH, Pang KP, Tan LK. Complete branchial fistula. Case report and review of the literature. Ann Otol Rhinol Laryngol 2001; 110(11): 1077–9.
7. Bakaeen G, Winkler S, Bakaeen L, Rehani LA, Katsetos CD. Congenital macroglossal angiodysplasia ("lymphangioendotheliomatosis"). Arch Pathol Lab Med 2000; 124(9): 1349–1351.
8. Ballester F, Polo I, Papi M, Lafarga J, Espuch D, Niveiro M. Rhabdomyoma in the adult. Acta Otorrinolaringol Esp 2000; 51(4): 361–363.
9. Batsakis JG. Tumors of the Head and Neck. Clinical and Pathologic Considerations, 2 d ed. Baltimore: Williams and Wilkins; 1979.
10. Batsakis JG. Tumors of the Head and Neck. 2 d ed. Baltimore: Williams and Wilkins; 1979.
11. Beahrs OH, Henson DE, Hutter RVP, Kennedy BJ, eds.: Manual for Staging of Cancer: American Joint Committee on Cancer, 5 th ed. Philadelphia: J.B. Lippincott; 1997.
12. Beckhardt RN, Weber RS, Zane R, et al. Minor salivary gland tumors of the palate: Clinical and pathologic correlates of outcome. Laryngoscope 1995; 105: 1135.
13. Becker M. Oral cavity, oropharynx and hypopharynx. Semin Roentgenol 2000; 35(1): 21–30.
14. Becker M, Hasso AN. Imaging of malignant neoplasms of the pharynx and larynx. In: Taveras JM, Ferruci JT, eds. Radiology: Diagnosis-Imaging-Intervention. Philadelphia: J.B. Lippincott; 1996: 1–16.
15. Becker M, Kurt AM. Infrahyoid neck: CT and MR imaging versus histopathology. Eur Radiol 1999; 9 (Suppl. 2): 53–68.
16. Becker M, Marchal F, Becker CD, Dulguerov P, Georgakopoulos G, Lehmann W Terrier F. MR-sialography: diagnostic accuracy for assessing sialolithiasis and salivary duct stenosis using a 3D extended phase conjugate symmetry rapid spin echo (EXPRESS) sequence. Radiology 2000; 217: 347–358.
17. Becker M, Marchal F, Dulguerov P, Georgakopoulos G, Lehmann W, Terrier F. How reliable is US in the assessment of sialolithiasis? Eur Radiol 2004. [In press].
18. Becker M, Moulin G, Kurt AM et al. Atypical squamous cell carcinoma of the larynx and hypopharynx: radiologic features and pathologic correlation. Eur Radiol 1998; 8: 1541–1551.
19. Becker M, Moulin G, Kurt AM et al. Non-squamous cell neoplasms of the larynx: radiologic-pathologic correlation. Radiographics 1998; 18(5): 1189–1210.
20. Becker M, Zbären P, Hermans R, et al. Necrotizing fasciitis of the head and neck: role of CT in diagnosis and management. Radiology 1997; 202: 471–476.
21. Bonetta A, Gelli MC, Zini G, Iotti C, Barbieri V, Pedroni C, Armaroli L. Postradiation sarcoma of head and neck: report of two cases. Tumori 1996; 82(3): 270–272.
22. Brennan TD, Miller AS, Chen SY. Lymphangiomas of the oral cavity: a clinicopathologic, immunohistochemical, and electron-microscopic study. J Oral Maxillofac Surg 1997; 55(9): 932–935.
23. Brockenbrough JM, Petruzzelli GJ, Lomasney L. DentaScan as an accurate method of predicting mandibular invasion in patients with squamous cell carcinoma of the oral cavity. Arch Otolaryngol Head Neck Surg 2003; 129: 113–117.
24. Brown JS, Kalavrezos N, D'Souza J, Lowe D, Magennis P, Woolgar JA. Factors that influence the method of mandibular resection in the management of oral squamous cell carcinoma. Br J Oral Maxillofac Surg 2002; 40(4): 275–284.
25. Brown JS, Lewis-Jones H. Evidence for imaging the mandible in the management of oral squamous cell carcinoma: a review. Br J Oral Maxillofac Surg 2001; 39(6): 411–418.
26. Brown JS, Lowe D, Kalavrezos N, D'Souza J, Magennis P, Woolgar J. Patterns of invasion and routes of tumor entry into the mandible by oral squamous cell carcinoma. Head Neck 2002; 24(4): 370–383.
27. Carr RJ, Langdon JD. Multiple primaries in mouth cancer- the price of success. Br J Oral Maxillofac Surg 1989; 27: 394–399.
28. Cavicchi O, Santini D, Chiodo F. Invasive mycotic and actinomycotic oropharyngeal and craniofacial infection in two patients with AIDS. Mycoses 1994; 37(5–6): 209–215.
29. Cheuk W, Chan JK. Kuttner tumor of the submandibular gland: fine-needle aspiration cytologic findings of seven cases. Am J Clin Pathol 2002; 117(1): 103–108.

30. Cholankeril JV, Scioscia PA. Post-traumatic sialoceles and mucoceles of the salivary glands. Clin Imaging 1993; 17(1): 41–45.
31. Chung TS, Yousem DM, Seigerman HM, et al. MR of mandibular invasion in patients with oral and oropharyngeal malignant neoplasms. AJNR 1994; 15: 1949.
32. Clark JR, Vaugham CW, Fitzgerald TJ, Costello R. Cancer of the head and neck. In: Osteen RT, ed. Cancer Manual, 8th ed. Boston: American Cancer Society; 1990: 145–160.
33. Cleveland DB, Chen SY, Allen CM, Ahing SI, Svirsky JA. Adult rhabdomyoma. A light microscopic, ultrastructural, virologic, and immunologic analysis. Oral Surg Oral Med Oral Pathol 1994; 77(2): 147–153.
34. Corio RL, Lewis DM. Intraoral rhabdomyomas. Oral Surg Oral Med Oral Pathol 1979; 48(6): 525–531.
35. Datar S, Patanakar T, Armao D, Mukherji SK. Papillary carcinoma in a giant thyroglossal duct cyst. Clin Imaging 2000; 24(2): 75–77.
36. de Bree R, Westerveld GJ, Smeele LE. Submandibular approach for excision of a large schwannoma in the base of the tongue. Eur Arch Otorhinolaryngol 2000; 257(5): 283–286.
37. Delavelle J, Becker M, Megret M, Pizzolato G, Rüfenacht D A. The trigeminal nerve: diagnostic features of intracranial and extracranial pathology. Int J Neuroradiol 1998; 4(6): 445–465.
38. DelBalso AM. An approach to the diagnostic imaging of jaw lesions, dental implants, and the temporomandibular joint. Radiol Clin North Am 1998; 36: 855–890.
39. De Ponte FS, Brunelli A, Marchetti E, Bottini DJ. Sublingual epidermoid cyst. J Craniofac Surg 2002; 13(2): 308–310.
40. Deroux E. Complications of dental infections. Rev Med Brux 2001; 22(4): A289–295.
41. Devine JC, Jones DC. Carcinomatous transformation of a sublingual dermoid cyst. A case report. Int J Oral Maxillofac Surg 2000; 29(2): 126–127.
42. Dubin MG, Ebert CS, Mukherji SK, Pollock HW, Amjadi D, Shockley WW. Computed tomography's ability to predict sacrifice of hypoglossal nerve at resection. Laryngoscope 2002; 112(12): 2181–2185.
43. Dziewas R, Ludemann P. Hypoglossal nerve palsy as complication of oral intubation, bronchoscopy and use of the laryngeal mask airway. Eur Neurol 2002; 47(4): 239–243. [Review.]
44. Elidan J, Brama I, Gay I. A large tonsillolith simulating tumor of the tonsil. Ear Nose Throat J 1980; 59(7): 296–297.
45. Epivatianos A, Markopoulos AK, Papanayotou P. Benign tumors of adipose tissue of the oral cavity: a clinicopathologic study of 13 cases. J Oral Maxillofac Surg 2000; 58(10): 1113–1117.
46. Epstein JB, Epstein JD, Le ND, Gorsky M. Characteristics of oral and paraoral malignant lymphoma: a population-based review of 361 cases. Oral Surg Oral Med Oral Pathol Oral Radiol Endod 2001; 92: 519–525.
47. Evans HL. Mucoepidermoid carcinoma of salivary glands: a study of 69 cases with special attention to histologic grading. Am J Clin Pathol 1984; 81: 696–701.
48. Fortun C, Barros J Melcon C, Condes E, Cobo E, Perez-Martinez C, Ruiz-Galiana J, Martinez-Vidal A, Alvarez F. Extra-laryngeal head and neck tuberculosis. Clin Microbiol Infect 2000; 6(12): 644–648.
49. Friedman M, Chow J, Toriumi DM, Strorigl T, Grybauskas V. Benign neoplasms of the oral cavity. Clin Plast Surg 1987; 14(2): 223–231.
50. Fuchshuber S, Grevers G, Issing WJ. Dermoid cyst of the floor of the mouth—a case report. Eur Arch Otorhinolaryngol 2002; 259(2): 60–62.
51. Gluckman JL, Thompson R. Cancer of the oropharynx. In: Paparella MM, Shumrick DA, eds. Otorhinolaryngology. Philadelphia: W.B. Saunders; 1991: 2167–2187.
52. Gold L, Nazarian LN, Johar AS, Rao VM. Characterization of maxillofacial soft tissue vascular anomalies by ultrasound and color Doppler imaging: an adjuvant to computed tomography and magnetic resonance imaging. J Oral Maxillofac Surg 2003; 61(1): 19–31.
53. Graziani M, Logoluso G, Boldrini R, Fasanelli S. Aggressive fibromatosis in childhood. Radiol Med (Torino) 1995; 89(3): 364–367.
54. Harrison HD. Sublingual gland is origin of cervical extravasation mucocele. Oral Surg Oral Med Oral Pathol Oral Radiol Endod 2000; 90(4): 404–405.
55. Hattori H. Atypical lipomatous tumor of the lip with pleomorphic lipoma-like myxoid area, clinically simulating mucocele. J Oral Pathol Med 2002; 31(9): 561–564.
56. Hermanek P, Scheibe O, Spiessl B, Wagner G. TNM Classification of Malignant Tumors, 4th ed. Berlin: Springer; 1992.
57. Horn G, Werner JA, Schmidt D, Beigel A. Rhabdomyoma of the mouth floor—a case report. HNO 1992; 40(8): 322–324.
58. Iype EM, Ramdas K, Pandey M, Jayasree K, Thomas G, Sebastian P, Nair MK. Primary tuberculosis of the tongue: report of three cases. Br J Oral Maxillofac Surg 2001; 39(5): 402–403.
59. Gale DR. CT and MRI of the oral cavity and oropharynx. In: Valvassori GE, Mafee MF, Carter BL Imaging of the Head and Neck. Stuttgart: Georg Thieme Verlag; 1995: 445–4741. Smoker WRK. Oral cavity. In: Som PM, Curtin HD. Head and Neck Imaging, 3d ed. St. Louis, MO: Mosby-Year Book; 1996: 488–544.
60. Go JH. Benign peripheral nerve sheath tumor of the tongue. Yonsei Med J 2002; 43(5): 678–680.
61. Gomez D, Faucher A, Picot V, Siberchicot F, Renaud-Salis JL, Bussieres E, Pinsolle J. Outcome of squamous cell carcinoma of the gingiva: a follow-up study of 83 cases. J Craniomaxillofac Surg 2000; 28(6): 331–335.
62. Kapila K, Mathur S, Verma K. Schwannomas: a pitfall in the diagnosis of pleomorphic adenomas on fine-needle aspiration cytology. Diagn Cytopathol 2002; 27(1): 53–59.
63. Kim KH, Sung MW, Chung PS, et al. Adenoid cystic carcinoma of the head and neck. Arch Otolaryngol Head and Neck Surg 1994; 120: 721–726.
64. Koch BB, Trask DK, Hoffman HT, et al. National survey on head and neck verrucous cainoma. Patterns of presentation, care, and outcome. Cancer 2001; 92; 110–120.
65. Koeller KK, Alamo L, Adair CF, Smirniotopoulos JG. Congenital cystic masses of the neck: radiologic–pathologic correlation. Radiographics 1999; 19(1): 121–146.
66. Koizumi Y, Utsunomiya T, Yamamoto H. Cellular schwannoma in the oral mucosa. Acta Otolaryngol 2002; 122(4): 458–462.
67. Kosling S, Schmidtke M, Vothel F, Hahn S, Weidenbach H, Oeken J. The value of spiral CT in the staging of the oral cavity and of the oro- and hypopharynx. Radiologe 2000; 40: 632–639.
68. Kraitrakul S, Sirithunyaporn S, Yimtae K. Distribution of minor salivary glands in the peritonsillar space. J Med Ass Thai 2001; 84(3): 371–378.
69. Kruk-Zagajewska A, Szkaradkiewics A, Wierzbicka M, Joseph A, Wozniał A. The role of Epstein–Barr virus (EBV) infection in carcinogenesis of palatine tonsil carcinoma. Otolaryngol Pol 2001; 55: 267–272.
70. Kumara GR, Gillgrass TJ, Bridgman JB. A lymphoepithelial cyst (branchial cyst) in the floor of the mouth. NZ Dent J 1995; 91(403): 14–15.
71. Kurabayashi T, Ida M, Yasumoto M, Ohbayashi N, Yoshino N, Tetsumura A, Sasaki T. MRI of ranulas. Neuroradiology 2000; 42(12): 917–922.
72. Laine FJ, SmokerWR. Anatomy of the cranial nerves. Neuroimaging Clin North Am 1998; 8(1): 69–100. [Review.]
73. Lalwani AK, Engel TL. Teratoma of the tongue: a case report and review of the literature. Int J Pediatr Otorhinolaryngol 1992; 24(3): 261–268.
74. Lane AP, Buckmire RA, Mukherji SK, Pillsbury HC 3rd, Meredith SD. Use of computed tomography in the assessment of mandibular invasion in carcinoma of the retromolar trigone. Otolaryngol Head Neck Surg 2000; 122(5): 673–677.
75. Lawoyin JO, Akande OO, Kolude B, Agbaje JO. Lipoma of the oral cavity: clinicopathological review of seven cases from Ibadan. Niger J Med 2001; 10(4): 189–191.
76. Lee YY, Van Tassel P, Nauert C, et al. Lymphomas of the head and neck: CT findings at initial presentation AJNR 1987; 8: 665–671.
77. Lenz M. Computertomographie und Kernspintomographie bei Kopf-Hals-Tumoren. Methoden, Leitkriterien, Differentialdiagnosen und klinische Ergebnisse. Stuttgart: Georg Thieme Verlag; 1992.
78. Lenz M, Hermans R. Imaging of the oropharynx and oral cavity. Part II: Pathology. Eur Radiol 1996; 6: 536–549.
79. Lin YS, Jen YM, Lin JC. Radiation-related cranial nerve palsy in patients with nasopharyngeal carcinoma. Cancer 2002; 15(95 Pt 2): 404–409.
80. Lobitz B, Lang T. Lymphangioma of the tongue. Pediatr Emerg Care 1995; 11(3): 183–185.
81. Loevner LA, Yousem DM, Montone KT et al. Can radiologists accurately predict preepiglottic space invasion with MR? AJR 1997; 169: 1681–1688.
82. Loevner LA, Ott IL, Yousem DM, et al. Neoplastic fixation to the prevertebral compartment by squamous cell carcinoma of the head and neck. AJR 1998; 170: 1389–1394.
83. Loh C, Maya MM, Go JL. Cranial nerve XII: the hypoglossal nerve. Semin Ultrasound CT MR 2002; 23(3): 256–265.
84. Louis PJ, Hudson C, Reddi S. Lesion of floor of the mouth. J Oral Maxillofac Surg 2002; 60(7): 804–807.
85. Manfredi R, Mazzoni A, Amir R, Altman KW, Zaheer S. Neurilemmoma of the hard palate. J Oral Maxillofac Surg 2002; 60(9): 1069–1071.
86. Martin-Granizo R, Rodriguez-Campo F, Naval I, Diaz Gonzalez VJ. Squamous cell carcinoma in the oral cavity in patients younger than 40 years. Otolaryngol Head Neck Surg 1997; 117; 268–275.

87. Mancuso AA, Hanafee WN. Oral cavity and oropharynx including tongue base, floor of the mouth and mandible. In: Computed Tomography and Magnetic Resonance Imaging of the Head and Neck, 2nd ed. Baltimore: Williams and Wilkins; 1985: 358–427.
88. Mehanna HM, Al-Bahnasawi L, White A. National audit of the management of peritonsillar abscess. Postgrad Med J 2002; 78(923): 545–548.
89. Menko FH, van der Luijt RB, de Valk IA, Toorians AW, Sepers JM, van Diest PJ, Lips CJ. Atypical MEN type 2B associated with two germline RET mutations on the same allele not involving codon 918. J Clin Endocrinol Metab 2002; 87(1): 393–397.
90. Mignogna MD, Muzio LL, Favia G, Ruoppo E, Sammartino G, Zarrelli C, Bucci E. Oral tuberculosis: a clinical evaluation of 42 cases. Oral Dis 2000; 6(1): 25–30.
91. Miles LP, Naidoo LC, Reddy J. Congenital dermoid cyst of the tongue. J Laryngol Otol 1997; 111(12): 1179–1182.
92. Mitchell TE, Girling AC. Hairy polyp of the tonsil. J Laryngol Otol 1996; 110(1): 101–103.
93. Miura Y, Mimatsu K, Iwata H. Massive tongue swelling as a complication after spinal surgery. J Spinal Disord 1996; 9(4): 339–341.
94. Mohadjer C, Dietz A, Maier H, Weidauer H. Distant metastasis and incidence of second carcinomas in patients with oropharyngeal and hypopharyngeal carcinomas. HNO 1996; 44; 134–139.
95. Moriniere S, Sibel JP, Marlier F, Guerrier B. Basilingual rhabdomyoma treated by endoscopy. Ann Otolaryngol Chir Cervicofac 2001; 118(4): 245–248.
96. Munoz A, Castillo M, Melchor MA, Gutierrez R. Acute neck infections: prospective comparison between CT and MRI in 47 patients. J Comput Assist Tomogr 2001; 25(5): 733–741.
97. Muraki AS, Mancuso AA, Harnsberger HR et al. CT of the oropharynx, tongue base and floor of the mouth: normal anatomy and variations, and applications in staging carcinoma. Radiology 1983; 148: 725–731.
98. Mukherji SK, Isaacs DL, Creager A, Shockley W, Weissler M, Armao D. CT detection of mandibular invasion by squamous cell carcinoma of the oral cavity. AJR 2001; 177(1): 237–243.
99. Mukherji SK, Fatterpekar G, Castillo M, Stone JA, Chung CJ. Imaging of congenital anomalies of the branchial apparatus. Neuroimaging Clin North Am 2000; 10(1): 75–93, viii. [Review.]
100. Mukherji SK, Pillsbury HR, Castillo M. Imaging squamous cell carcinoma of the upper aerodigestive tract: what clinicians need to know. Radiology 1997; 205: 629–646.
101. Mukherji SK, Weeks S, Castillo M, Krishnan LA. Squamous cell carcinomas that arise in the oral cavity and tongue base: can CT help redict perineural or vascular invasion? Radiology 1996; 198: 157–162.
102. Mulliken JB, Glowacki J. Hemangiomas and vascular malformations in infants and children: a classification based on endothelial characteristics. Plast Reconstr Surg 1982; 69: 412–420.
103. Napier SS, Pagni CG, McGimpsey JG. Sublingual adult rhabdomyoma. Report of a case. Int J Oral Maxillofac Surg 1991; 20: 201–203.
104. Nascimento AF, McMenamin ME, Fletcher CD. Liposarcomas/atypical lipomatous tumors of the oral cavity: a clinicopathologic study of 23 cases. Ann Diagn Pathol 2002; 6(2): 83–93.
105. Nigam S, Singh T, Mishra A, Chaturvedi KU. Oral cysticercosis—report of six cases. Head Neck 2001; 23(6): 497–499.
106. Norman JE, Head K. Ranula—this term is probably one of the oldest in surgery, and its etymology is not very obvious. Br J Oral Maxillofac Surg 2002; 40(5): 455–456.
107. Norris CM Jr., Cady B. Head and neck, and thyroid cancer. In: Holleb AI, Fink DJ, Murphy GP, eds. American Cancer Society Textbook of Clinical Oncology. Atlanta, GA: American Cancer Society, 1991: 306–327.
108. Omura S, Nakajima Y, Kobayashi S, Ono S, Fujita K. Oral manifestations and differential diagnosis of isolated hypoglossal nerve palsy: report of two cases. Oral Surg Oral Med Oral Pathol Oral Radiol Endod 1997; 84(6): 635–640.
109. Parkins GE. Large sublingual lipoma. Br J Oral Maxillofac Surg 1997; 35(5): 377.
110. Pavithran K, Doval DC, Hukku S, Jena A. Isolated hypoglossal nerve palsy due to skull base metastasis from breast cancer. Australas Radiol 2001; 45(4): 534–535.
111. Paz JB, Cook N, Odom-Maryon T, Xie Y, Wilczynski SP. Human papillomavirus (HPV) in head and neck cancer. An association of HPV 16 with squamous cell carcinoma of Waldeyer's tonsillar ring. Cancer 1997; 79: 595–604.
112. Penna KJ, Verveniotis SJ. Lymphangiomatous macroglossia. Medical and surgical treatment. NY State Dent J 1995; 61(10): 30–33.
113. Poli P, Floretti G, Tessitori G. Malignant fibrous histiocytoma of the floor of the mouth: case report. J Laryngol Otol 1995; 109(7): 680–682.
114. Pulcini C, Vandenbos F, Roth S, Mondain-Miton V, Bernard E, Roger PM, De Salvador-Guillouet F, Hyvernat H, Girard-Pipau F, Mattei M, Dellamonica P. Lemierre's syndrome: a report of six cases. Rev Med Interne 2003; 24(1): 17–23.
115. Pulec JL. Aggressive fibromatosis (fibrosarcoma) of the facial nerve. Ear Nose Throat J 1993; 72(7): 460–467, 470–472.
116. Renehan A, Morton M. Acute enlargement of the tongue. Br J Oral Maxillofac Surg 1993; 31(5): 321–324.
117. Roychoudhury A, Parkash H, Kumar S, Chopra P. Infantile desmoid fibromatosis of the submandibular region. J Oral Maxillofac Surg 2002; 60(10): 1198–1202.
118. Russo CP, Smoker WR, Weissman JL. MR appearance of trigeminal and hypoglossal motor denervation. AJNR 1997; 18(7): 1375–1383.
119a. Quraishi HA, Ortiz O, Wax MK. Dermoid cyst of the floor of the mouth. Otolaryngol Head Neck Surg 1998; 118(4): 562–563.
119b. Sadler TW. Head and Neck. In: Sadler TW, ed. Langman's Medical Embryology, 5th ed. Baltimore: Williams and Wilkins; 1985: 281–310.
120. Schwartz HE, Ward PH. Aggressive fibromatosis of the tongue. Ann Otol Rhinol Laryngol 1979; 88(1 Pt 1): 12–15.
121. Shahab R, Savy LE, Croft CB, Hung T. Isolated hypoglossal nerve palsy due to internal carotid artery dissection. J Laryngol Otol 2001; 115(7): 587–589.
122. Sharp CM, Borg HK, Kishore A, MacKenzie K. Hypoglossal nerve paralysis following tonsillectomy. J Laryngol Otol 2002; 116(5): 389–391.
123. Shimoyama T, Kato T, Nasu D, Kaneko T, Horie N, Ide F. Solitary neurofibroma of the oral mucosa: a previously undescribed variant of neurofibroma. J Oral Sci 2002; 44(1): 59–63.
124. Sigal R. Oral cavity, oropharynx and salivary glands. Neuroimaging Clin North Am 1996; 6: 379.
125. Sigal R, Monnet O, de Baere T, Micheau C, Shapeero LG, Julieron M, Bosq J, Vanel D, Piekarski JD, Luboinski B, Masselot J. Adenoid cystic carcinoma of the head and neck: evaluation with MR imaging and clinical–pathologic correlation in 27 patients. Radiology 1992; 184: 95–101.
126. Sigal R, Zagdanski A-M, Schwaab G, et al. CT and MR imaging of squamous cell carcinoma of the tongue and floor of the mouth. Radiographics 1996; 16: 787–810.
127. Skitarelic N, Mladina R, Morovic M, Skitarelic N. Cervical necrotizing fasciitis: sources and outcomes. Rev Med Brux 2001; 22(4): 289–295.
127a. Sobin LH, Wittekind C, eds. TNM Classification of Malignant Tumours, 6th ed. Hoboken, NJ: Wiley; 2002:22–36.
128. Spitzer C, Mull M, Topper R. Isolated hypoglossal nerve palsy caused by carotid artery dissection the necessity of MRI for diagnosis. J Neurol 2001; 248(10): 909–910.
129. Sygula M, Skladowski K, Wydmanski J, Sasiadek W, Wygoda A. Comparison of natural history of squamous cell carcinoma and nondifferentiated carcinoma localized in the oro- and nasopharynx. Otolaryngol Pol 2000; 54 (Suppl. 31): 286–290.
130. Tankere F, Golmard JL, Barry B, Guedon C, Depondt J, Gehanno P. Prognostic value of mandibular involvement in oral cavity cancers. Rev Laryngol Otol Rhinol (Bord) 2002; 123: 7–12.
131. Thomas JA, Ware TM, Counselman FL. Internal carotid artery pseudoaneurysm masquerading as a peritonsillar abscess. J Emerg Med 2002; 22(3): 257–261.
132. Urquhart A, Berg R. Hodgkin's and non-Hodgkin's lymphoma of the head and neck. Laryngoscope 2001; 111: 1565–1569.
133. Urquhart AC, Hutchins LG, Berg RL. Distinguishing non-Hodgkin lymphoma from squamous cell carcinoma tumors of the head and neck by computed tomography parameters. Laryngoscope 2002; 112: 1079–1083.
134. Vogl TJ, Bruning R, Grevers G, Mees K, Bauer M, Lissner J. MR imaging of the oropharynx and tongue: comparison of plain and Gd-DTPA studies. J Comput Assist Tomogr 1988; 12(3): 427–433.
135. Vogl TJ, Steger W, Ihrler S, Ferrara P, Grevers G. Cystic masses of the floor of the mouth: value of MR imaging in planning surgery. AJR 1993; 161: 183–186.
136. Vuong PN, Pham-Thominet L, Neveux Y, Balaton A, Houissa-Vuong S, Fombeur JP, Soudan P. Adult type rhabdomyoma of the soft palate: pathology of 2 cases with review of the medical literature. Arch Anat Cytol Pathol 1990; 38(4): 152–158.
137. Walstad WR, Solomon JM, Schow SR, Ochs MW. Midline cystic lesion of the floor of the mouth. J Oral Maxillofac Surg 1998; 56(1): 70–74.
138. Wanebo HJ, Koness RJ, MacFarlane JK, Eilber FR, Byers RM, Elias EG, Spiro RH. Head and Neck Sarcoma: Report of the Head and Neck Sarcoma Registry. Society of Head and Neck Surgeons Committee on Research. Head Neck 1992; 14(1): 1–7.

139 Werning JW, Byers RM, Novas MA, Roberts D. Preoperative assessment for and outcomes of mandibular conservation surgery. Head Neck 2001; 23(12): 1024–1030.
140 Wiese KG, Merten HA, Wiltfang J, Luhr HG. Clinical studies on the pathophysiology of odontogenic abscesses. Mund Kiefer Gesichtschir 1999; 3(5): 242–246.
141 Wiesmiller K, Barth TF, Gronau S. Early radiation-induced malignant fibrous histiocytoma of the oral cavity. J Laryngol Otol 2003; 117(3): 224–226.
142 Yonetsu K, Nakayama E, Miwa K, Tanaka T, Araki K, Kanda S, Ohishi M, Takenoshita Y, Yoshida K, Katsuki T. Magnetic resonance imaging of oral and maxillofacial angiomas. Oral Surg Oral Med Oral Pathol 1993; 76(6): 783–789.
143 Yousem DM, Chalian AA. Oral cavity and pharynx. Radiol Clin North Am 1998; 36(5): 967–981.
144 Yousem DM, Hatabu H, Hurst MD, et al. Carotid artery invasion by head and neck masses: prediction with MR imaging. Radiology 1995; 195: 715–720.
145 Zadvinskis DP. Congenital malformations of the cervicothoracic lymphatic system: embryology and pathogenesis. RadioGraphics 1992; 12: 1175–1189.
146 Zbären P, Becker M, Laeng H. Pretherapeutic staging of laryngeal cancer: cinical findings. Computed tomography and magnetic resonance imaging versus histopathology. Cancer 1996; 77(7): 1263–1273.
147 Ziegler CM, Schwarz W, Grau A, Buggle F, Hassfeld S, Muhling J. Odontogenic focus as the etiology of cerebral ischemia. Mund Kiefer Gesichtschir 1998; 2(6): 316–319.

Section VI Infrahyoid Neck

Chapter 11 Larynx and Hypopharynx
Developmental Considerations 731

Normal Anatomy 732

Imaging Techniques 738

Squamous Cell Carcinoma 739

Non-Squamous Cell Neoplasms 755

Morphological Changes Induced by Tumor Treatment and Detection of Tumor Recurrence 761

Cystic Lesions, Pouches, Diverticula, and Webs 768

Infectious and Inflammatory Conditions 772

Congenital Lesions 774

Vocal Cord Paralysis 775

Trauma 775

Chapter 12 Other Infrahyoid Neck Lesions
Anatomy 780

Imaging Techniques 787

Neoplastic Lesions 788

Imaging of the Neck after Treatment 813

Infectious and Inflammatory Conditions 823

Miscellaneous Pathology 840

11 Larynx and Hypopharynx

M. Becker

Introduction

Although diagnostic evaluation of the larynx and hypopharynx is primarily done with endoscopy, sectional imaging plays an indispensable complementary role because it enables evaluation of the deep structures of the larynx. Both computed tomography (CT) and magnetic resonance imaging (MRI) can provide images with excellent detail of the larynx and hypopharynx. Computed tomography, the standard modality for more than two decades, has recently become further enhanced by the introduction of multidetector acquisition techniques that enable much faster image acquisition and excellent multiplanar or three-dimensional image reconstruction. Nonetheless, the role of CT is increasingly being challenged by magnetic resonance imaging. Many investigators already consider MRI as the method of choice for imaging of the larynx and hypopharynx because it provides superior resolution and superior soft-tissue contrast. However, some relative drawbacks of MRI persist, including long acquisition time, motion artifacts, claustrophobia on the part of the patient, and lack of availability. Therefore, both CT and MRI are currently used widely, with preferences being based mainly on local and individual factors.

The complementary role of endoscopy and sectional imaging demands a close, regular interdisciplinary cooperation. The radiologist who performs and interprets CT and MRI studies of the larynx and hypopharynx must be familiar not only with the normal anatomy and pathological conditions but also with the clinical relevance and therapeutic implications of the imaging findings. This appears of particular importance in the context of pretherapeutic and posttherapeutic evaluation of squamous cell carcinoma, which constitutes the most important indication for performing CT and MRI. The purpose of this chapter is to review the current role of imaging in the larynx and hypopharynx with an emphasis on neoplastic disease and other pathological conditions.

Developmental Considerations

The branchial or pharyngeal arches, consisting of bars of mesenchymal tissue, appear in the fourth and fifth weeks of development.[101b] They are separated from each other by branchial clefts. Simultaneously with the development of arches and clefts, the pharyngeal pouches appear along the lateral walls of the pharyngeal gut, which is the cranial portion of the primitive gut (see also Chapter 10). Each branchial arch contains its own cartilage/skeletal element, and its own artery, nerve, and muscle element. Because the muscles of the different arches sometimes migrate into surrounding regions, they do not always attach to the bony component of their own arch. However, the nerve supply of these muscles always comes from the arch of origin.

During the fourth week of development, a longitudinal groove, called the laryngotracheal groove, appears on the floor of the primitive pharynx, caudal to the pharyngeal pouches. Later, the laryngotracheal groove evaginates, forming a laryngotracheal diverticulum (Fig. 11.1). Then the distal end enlarges and forms a globular lung bud. The inlet of the larynx (also called the laryngeal aditus) is the opening of the laryngotracheal tube into the primitive pharynx. Initially, the laryngotracheal diverticulum widely communicates with the foregut. As the diverticulum expands in caudal direction, the esophagotracheal ridges form. They then fuse and form the esophagotracheal septum, which divides the foregut into a dorsal portion (the esophagus) and a ventral portion (the trachea and lung buds) (Fig. 11.1). The endoderm of the laryngotracheal diverticulum gives rise to the epithelium of the larynx, trachea, bronchi, bronchioles, and the pulmonary lining epithelium. The connective tissue, cartilage, and muscles of all of these structures develop from the mesenchyme surrounding the laryngotracheal diverticulum. As the embryo grows, the arytenoid swellings formed by the mesenchyme around the cranial end of the laryngotracheal tube grow rostrally toward the tongue (Fig. 11.2). The slitlike laryngeal opening is thereby converted into a T-shaped aperture, called the inlet of the larynx. The epithelium of the primitive larynx proliferates rapidly and temporarily occludes its lumen. By the tenth week, recanalization takes place and the lumen is restored. During this process, the laryngeal ventricles, the vocal folds, and

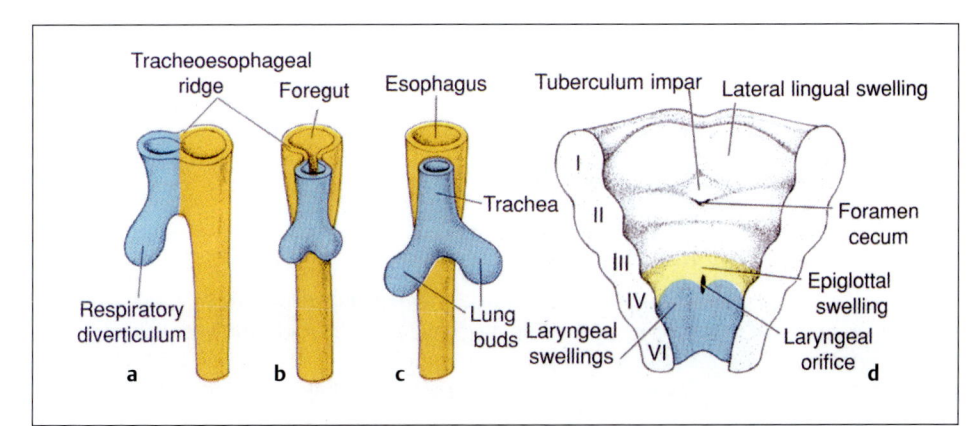

Fig. 11.1 a–c Successive stages in the development of the laryngotracheal diverticulum. Note the esophageal ridges and the formation of the septum, splitting the foregut into the esophagus and trachea with lung buds. d The ventral portion of the larynx seen from above. Note the laryngeal orifice and the surrounding swellings. Reproduced from Reference 101b with permission.

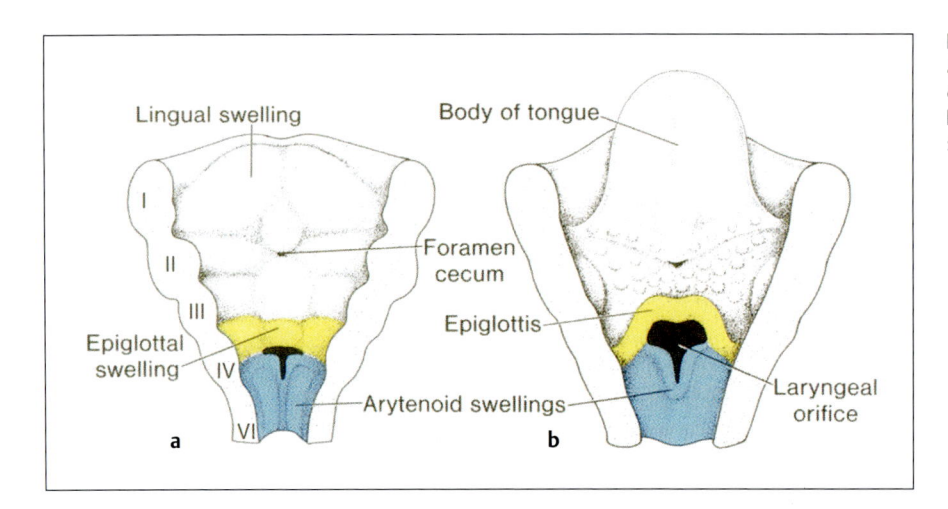

Fig. 11.2 Drawings showing the laryngeal orifice and surrounding swellings at successive stages of development. **a** At 6 weeks, **b** at 12 weeks. Reproduced from Reference 101 b with permission.

the vestibular folds form. The epiglottis develops from the most caudal portion of the copula (hypobranchial eminence; see also Chapter 10).

The cartilages of the fourth and sixth pharyngeal arches fuse and form the hyaline cartilages of the larynx (thyroid, cricoid, arytenoid) as well as the corniculate and cuneiform cartilages, which are fibroelastic cartilages. The fourth arch forms the cricothyroid, levator palati, and pharyngeal constrictor muscles. Therefore, these muscles are innervated by the superior laryngeal branch of the vagus, which is the nerve of the fourth arch. The intrinsic muscles of the larynx are derived from the sixth arch. Therefore, they are innervated by the recurrent laryngeal branch of the vagus, which is the nerve of the sixth arch.

Normal Anatomy

■ Larynx

The larynx has a framework consisting of a cartilaginous skeleton connected by muscles and ligaments. This framework supports the mucosa-covered surfaces of the larynx, which are crucial to voice generation. The most important mucosa-covered structures of the larynx are the false vocal cords, the ventricles, and the true vocal cords.

Mucosal Anatomy

The true vocal cords stretch from anterior to posterior across the airway. Anteriorly the true vocal cords converge at the anterior commissure, and posteriorly they converge at the posterior commissure. The false cords are slightly more cranial in position than the true vocal cords and they are parallel to the true vocal cords. The ventricle is a slit separating the false vocal cords from the true vocal cords. From the false cords, the laryngeal mucosa sweeps upward to the aryepiglottic folds, which separate the larynx from the hypopharynx (Fig. 11.3).

Cartilages

The thyroid cartilage is the largest of all laryngeal cartilages (Fig. 11.4). It has two large alae that meet at an angle anteriorly. Superior horns extend upward from the most posterior portion of the superior margin of each ala. Similarly, inferior horns extend downward, articulating with the cricoid cartilage. The cricoid cartilage forms a complete ring and has a shape similar to that of a signet ring (Fig. 11.4). The posterior portion of the cricoid cartilage, also called the lamina, is higher than the anterior portion. The superior border of the lamina reaches the posterior commissure and posterior true vocal cords, while the anterior portion of the cricoid cartilage lies well below the anterior commissure. The inferior margin of the cricoid cartilage is the junction between the larynx and the trachea. The pyramidal-shaped arytenoid cartilages are located on the superior margin of the cricoid lamina, contributing to the cricoarytenoid joints (Fig. 11.4). The upper portion of the arytenoid cartilages is located at the level of the false vocal cords, while each vocal ligament attaches at the vocal process of the lower arytenoids. Therefore, the lower portion of the arytenoid cartilage with the vocal process can be used as a landmark structure for determining the level of the true vocal cords at sectional imaging. The corniculate and cuneiform cartilages are located on top of the arytenoid cartilage (Fig. 11.4).

The thyroid, cricoid, and arytenoid cartilages of adults consist of three components: (1) nonossified nonmineralized hyaline cartilage; (2) cortical bone; and (3) a marrow cavity containing fatty tissue and scattered bony trabeculae. Although in young adults laryngeal cartilages are still entirely composed of hyaline cartilage, enchondral ossification normally sets in during the third decade and increases with age. The ossification process follows specific patterns in each cartilage, but the degree of ossification is quite variable.[61] The epiglottis, the vocal processes of the arytenoids, and the corniculate and cuneiform cartilages are composed of yellow fibrocartilage, which does not usually ossify.

Muscles

The muscles of the larynx are the thyroarytenoid, anterior and posterior cricoarytenoid, interarytenoid, and cricothyroid muscles. The thyroarytenoid muscle, which makes up the bulk of the true vocal cord, stretches from the thyroid cartilage anteriorly to the vocal process of the arytenoid cartilage posteriorly (Figs. 11.5–11.8). It parallels the true vocal cord–ventricle–false cord complex. The medial fibers are often referred to as the vocalis muscle.

Regions

The larynx may be subdivided into three regions: supraglottic, glottic, and subglottic (Fig. 11.5). The glottic region is the true vocal cord region. The upper border of the glottic region is the lower margin of the ventricle. The lower border of the glottic region is defined arbitrarily as a line 1 cm inferior to the ventricle.

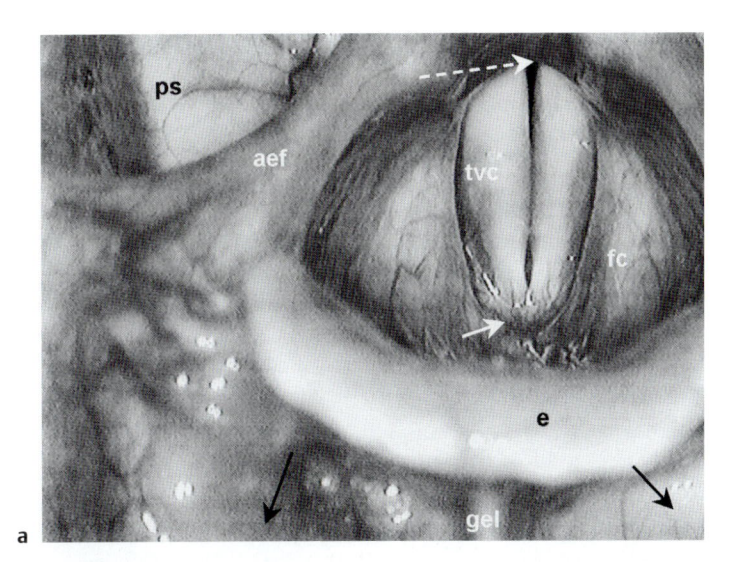

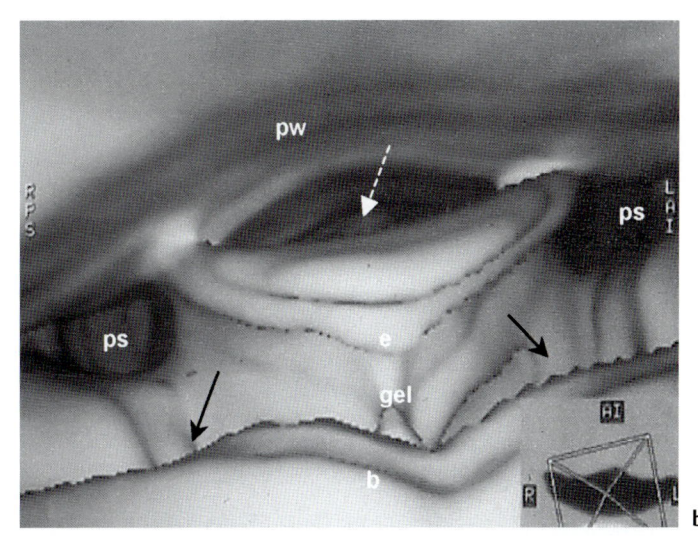

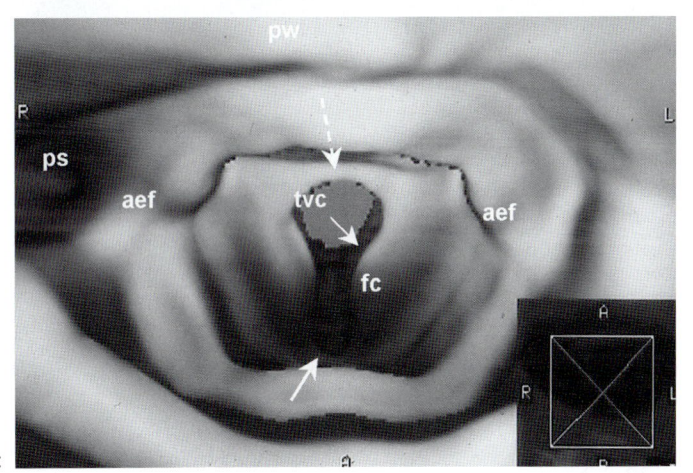

Fig. 11.3 Appearance of the larynx at endoscopy and virtual endoscopy. **a** Endoscopic image obtained during phonation. e = epiglottis; ps = piriform sinuses; gel = glossoepiglottic ligament; black arrows = vallecules; fc = false cord; tvc = true vocal cord; white arrow = anterior commissure; dashed arrow = posterior commissure; aef = aryepiglottic fold. **b**, **c** Virtual endoscopy images obtained during quiet respiration from a helical CT acquisition. **b** Image obtained at the level of the base of the tongue (b) looking from above on the epiglottis (e), piriform sinuses (ps), posterior hypopharyngeal wall (pw), glossoepiglottic ligament (gel), vallecules (arrows), and laryngeal vestibule (dashed arrow). **c** Image obtained farther caudally, after "passing" through the laryngeal vestibule. fc = false cord; tvc = true vocal cord; arrow = anterior commissure; dashed arrow = posterior commissure; aef = aryepiglottic folds; ps = piriform sinus; pw = posterior hypopharyngeal wall.

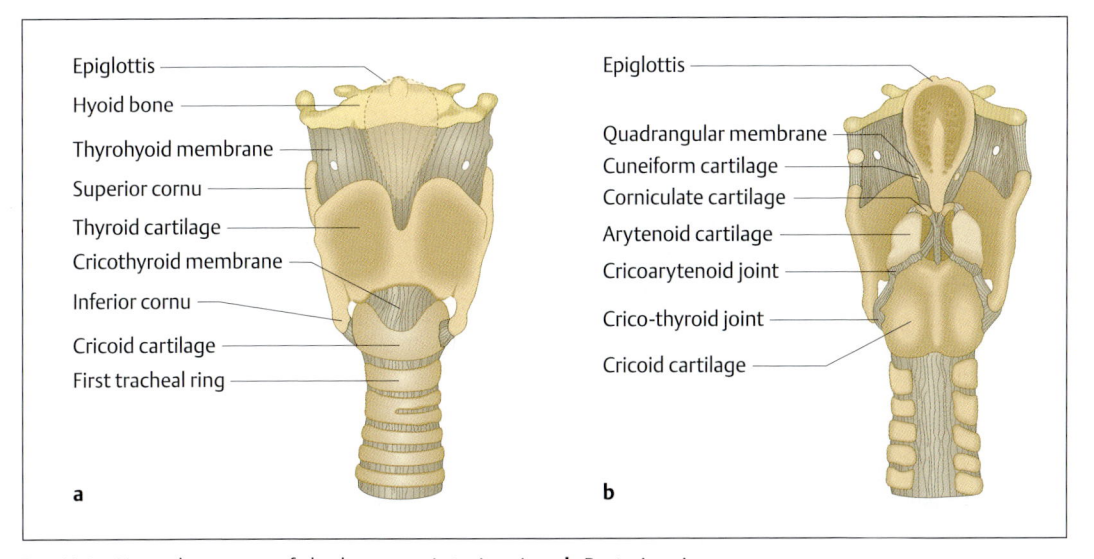

Fig. 11.4 Normal anatomy of the larynx. **a** Anterior view. **b** Posterior view.

The portion of the larynx superior to the ventricle is the supraglottic region. It extends upward to the level of the aryepiglottic folds and upper epiglottic cartilage. The false cord is in the lower part of the supraglottic region. The subglottic region extends from the inferior border of the glottic region to the inferior edge of the cricoid cartilage.

Deep Spaces

The chief laryngeal spaces are the preepiglottic space and the paraglottic space (Figs. 11.5–11.7). Both of these spaces are important pathways for spread of carcinoma within the larynx. The preepiglottic space plays an important role for the T-classification of laryngeal cancer according to the guidelines of the UICC.[55] The preepiglottic space is composed of fatty tissue and loose

11 Larynx and Hypopharynx

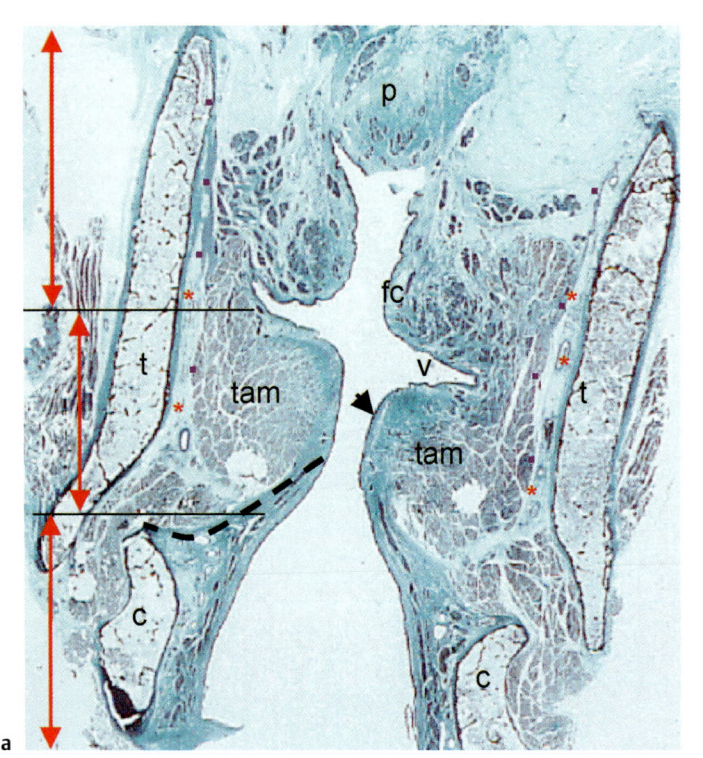

Fig. 11.5 Regional and spatial anatomy of the larynx. **a** Midcoronal whole-organ histological slice from normal autopsy specimen. Asterisks = paraglottic space containing fat; p = petiole of the epiglottis; t = thyroid cartilage; c = cricoid cartilage; tam = thyroarytenoid muscle; fc = false cord; v = laryngeal ventricle; short arrow = true vocal cord; dots = thyroglottic ligament; dashed line = conus elasticus. **b** Coronal contrast-enhanced T1W MR image obtained in a healthy volunteer shows the typical intermediate to low signal intensity of the thyroarytenoid muscle at the level of the true vocal cords (arrowhead). Thick arrow = false cord; thin arrow = laryngeal ventricle; block arrows = paraglottic space. Note that the thyroglottic ligament and the elastic cone cannot be visualized on routine MRI. c = cricoid cartilage; t = thyroid cartilage; p = petiole of the epiglottis.

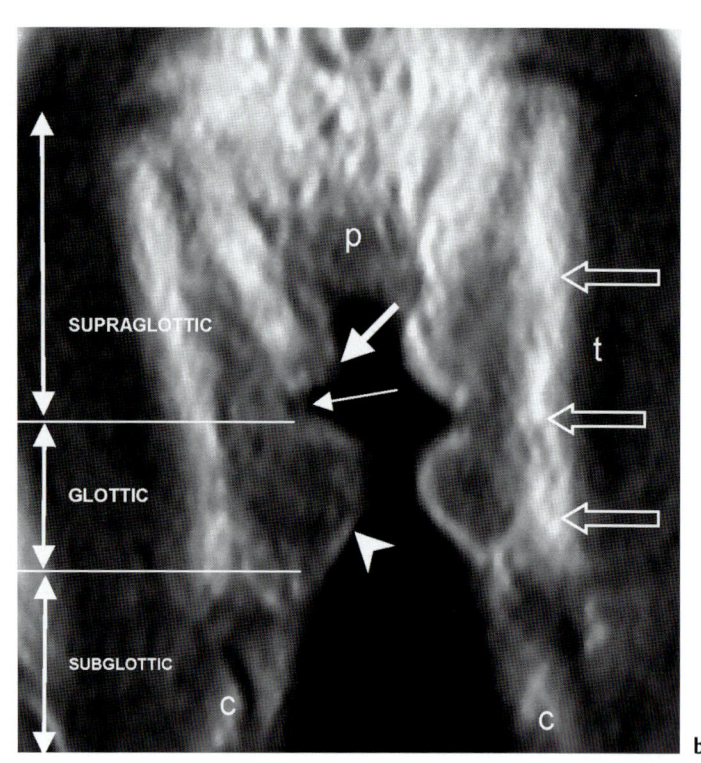

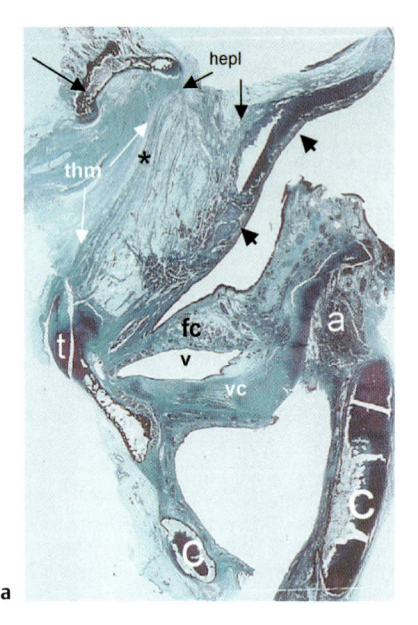

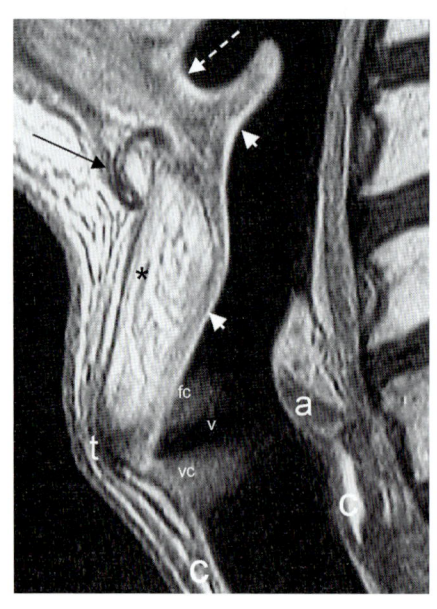

Fig. 11.6 Normal anatomy of the preepiglottic space. **a** Parasagittal whole-organ histological slice from normal autopsy specimen. **b** Parasagittal, contrast-enhanced T1W MR image obtained in a healthy volunteer. Asterisk = preepiglottic space; short arrows = epiglottis; long thin arrow = hyoid bone; t = thyroid cartilage; c = cricoid cartilage; a = arytenoid cartilage; thm = thyrohyoid membrane; hepl = hyoepiglottic ligament; v = laryngeal ventricle; fc = false cord; vc = true vocal cord; dashed arrow = vallecula.

elastic and collagenous fibers. It is bounded anteriorly by the thyrohyoid membrane and thyroid laminae, posteriorly by the infrahyoid epiglottis, cranially by the hyoepiglottic ligament, and caudally by the petiole of the epiglottis[11, 101a, 103] (Fig. 11.6). The preepiglottic space is best displayed on axial and sagittal images.

The paraglottic (paralaryngeal) space lies between the mucosa and the laryngeal framework and is paired and symmetrical. In the supraglottic region it surrounds the laryngeal ventricle and continues cephalad posterolateral to the preepiglottic space.[33, 75, 100, 101a, 103] The laryngeal ventricles and the paraglottic spaces are best displayed in the coronal plane. The preepiglottic space is adjacent posteroinferiorly to the paraglottic space and is separated from it by fibrous tissue (the so-called thyroglottic ligament), whereas the two spaces are not separated from each other posterosuperiorly.[101a, 103] The thyroglottic ligament is, however, a variable structure, being found only in some anatomical specimens.[101a] The thyroglottic ligament cannot be identified on current standard CT or MR images.

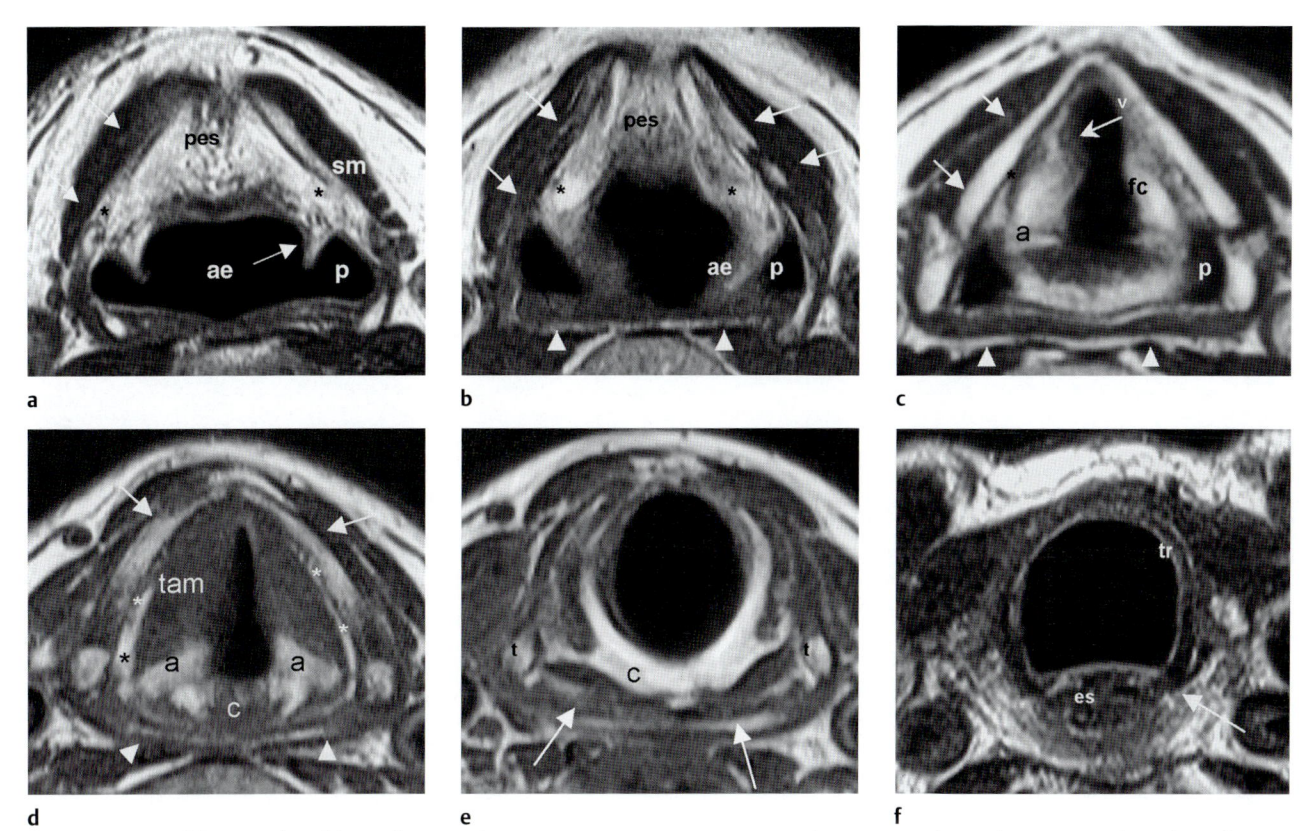

Fig. 11.7 Normal laryngeal and hypopharyngeal anatomy as seen on axial unenhanced T1W MR images. **a–c** Supraglottic level. pes = preepiglottic space; asterisks = paraglottic space; ae = aryepiglottic folds; fc = false cords; v = ventricle; p = piriform sinus; arrows = thyroid cartilage; a = arytenoid cartilage; arrowheads = pharyngeal constrictor muscles; sm = strap muscles. **d** Glottic level. Asterisks = paraglottic space; tam = thyroarytenoid muscle; arrows = thyroid cartilage; a = arytenoid cartilages; c = cricoid cartilage; arrowheads = pharyngeal constrictor muscles. **e** Subglottic level. c = cricoid cartilage; arrows = esophageal verge; t = inferior cornu of the thyroid cartilage; **f** Level of the cervical trachea (tr). es = cervical esophagus; arrow = tracheo-esophageal groove.

The paraglottic space contains adipose and loose connective tissue, as well as blood vessels with a craniocaudal orientation.[100, 101a] The absence of a horizontal anatomical subdivision at the glottic level may facilitate transglottic tumor spread. Laterally, the paraglottic space is bordered by the thyroid cartilage. Dorsally, the paraglottic space extends into the aryepiglottic folds, which separate the endolarynx anteriorly from the piriform sinuses posteriorly. Therefore, the paraglottic space is immediately adjacent to the mucosal lining of the piriform sinus. This favors tumor spread from the hypopharynx into the larynx and vice versa[64, 100] Medially, in the supraglottic region either the paraglottic space may be separated from the preepiglottic space by the thyroglottic ligament or the two spaces may communicate freely. The thyroarytenoid muscle forms the bulk and shape of the vocal cord and occupies most of the volume of the glottis (Figs. 11.5–11.8). At the glottic level, the paraglottic adipose tissue extends medially between the caudal fibers of the thyroarytenoid muscle. Inferomedially, the paraglottic space is bordered by the conus elasticus (Fig. 11.5). The conus elasticus, which extends from the vocal ligament to the upper edge of the cricoid cartilage, blends with the cricothyroid membrane anteriorly. Anteroinferior extensions of the paraglottic space extend beyond the larynx lateral to the median cricothyroid ligament through the gap between the cricoid and thyroid cartilage. At this site the cricothyroid membrane is deficient. Posteroinferiorly, the paraglottic adipose tissue is in close proximity to the adipose tissue surrounding the cricoarytenoid joint.

The subglottic region lies medial to the conus elasticus, which represents a significant boundary to tumor spread. As the mucosa is closely adjacent to the cricoid cartilage, there is normally no radiographically visible tissue layer between the cricoid cartilage and the airway and, therefore, no barrier to contralateral spread of tumor (Figs. 11.7, 11.8)[11, 75] This region is best evaluated in the axial plane.

■ Hypopharynx

Regions

The hypopharynx (laryngopharynx) is the most caudal portion of the pharynx and extends from the level of the hyoid bone and valleculae to the upper esophageal sphincter. It is formed for the most part by the inferior pharyngeal constrictor muscles. The hypopharynx has three distinct regions: the piriform sinuses, the postcricoid or retrocricoarytenoid region, and the posterior hypopharyngeal wall[11, 55, 68] (Figs. 11.3, 11.7, 11.8).

The *piriform sinus* is an anterolateral recess of the hypopharynx situated on each side of the hypopharynx between the inner surface of the thyrohyoid membrane and thyroid cartilage laterally and the aryepiglottic fold medially (Figs. 11.7, 11.8). The mucosa of the anterior portion of the piriform sinus abuts on the posterior paraglottic space. The most caudal portion of the piriform sinus (apex) lies at the level of the true vocal cords. The posterior or lateral aspect of the aryepiglottic fold forms the medial wall of the piriform sinus, while the anterior or medial aspect of the aryepiglottic fold belongs to the endolarynx. Therefore, a tumor confined to the medial aspect of the aryepiglottic fold will behave as a supraglottic tumor, while a tumor confined to the lateral aspect of the aryepiglottic fold will behave more aggressively as a hypopharyngeal tumor. The lateral wall of the piriform sinus may be subdivided into a membranous portion, which is formed by the thyrohyoid membrane, and a cartilaginous portion, which is formed by the thyroid cartilage.

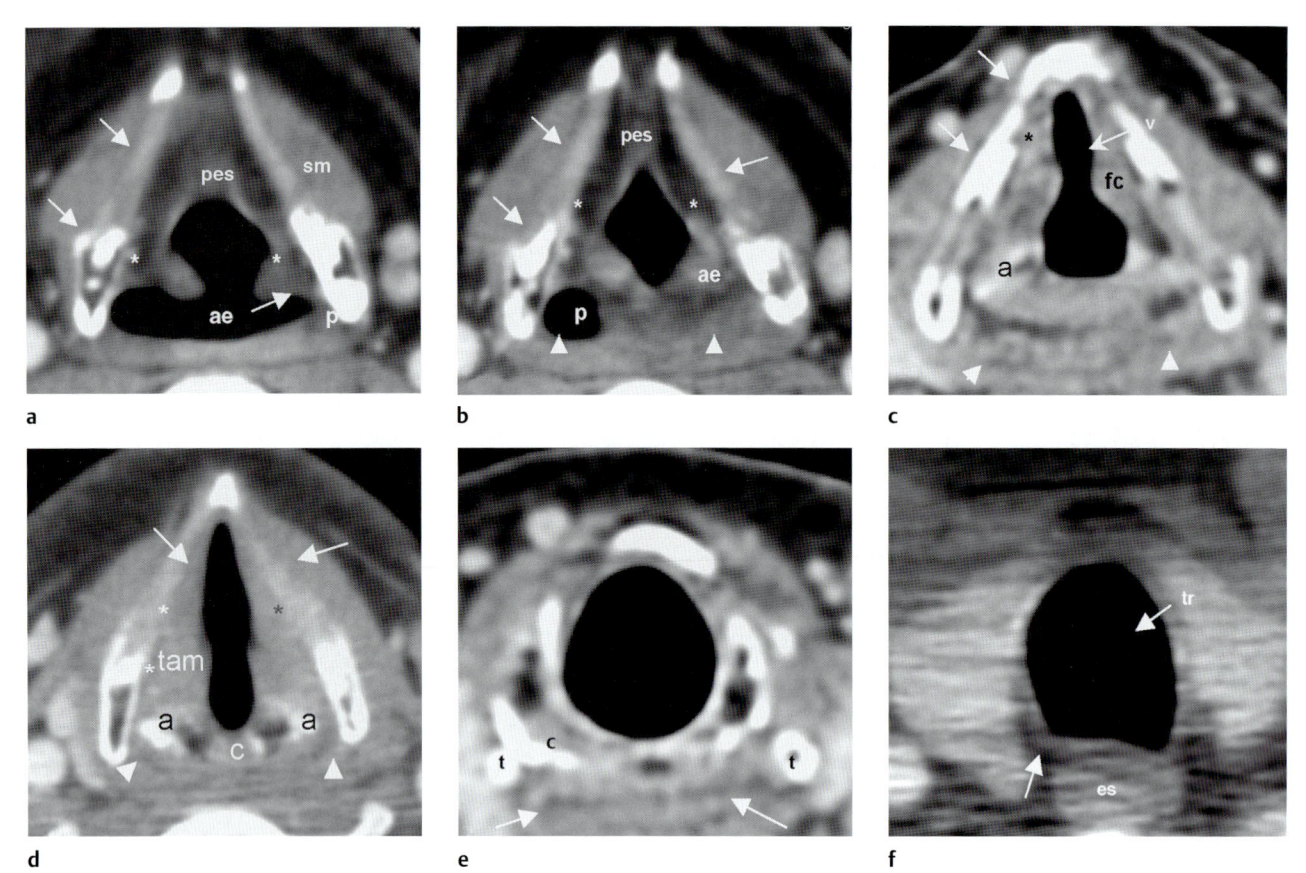

Fig. 11.8 Normal laryngeal and hypopharyngeal anatomy as seen on axial contrast-enhanced CT images. **a–c** Supraglottic level. pes = preepiglottic space; asterisks = paraglottic space; ae = aryepiglottic folds; fc = false cords; v = ventricle; p = piriform sinus; arrows = thyroid cartilage; a = arytenoid cartilage; arrowheads = pharyngeal constrictor muscles; sm = strap muscles. **d** Glottic level. Asterisks = paraglottic space; tam = thyroarytenoid muscle; arrows = thyroid cartilage; a = arytenoid cartilages; c = cricoid cartilage; arrowheads = pharyngeal constrictor muscle. **e** Subglottic level. c = cricoid cartilage; arrows = esophageal verge; t = inferior cornu of the thyroid cartilage. **f** Level of the cervical trachea (tr). es = cervical esophagus; arrow = tracheo-esophageal grove.

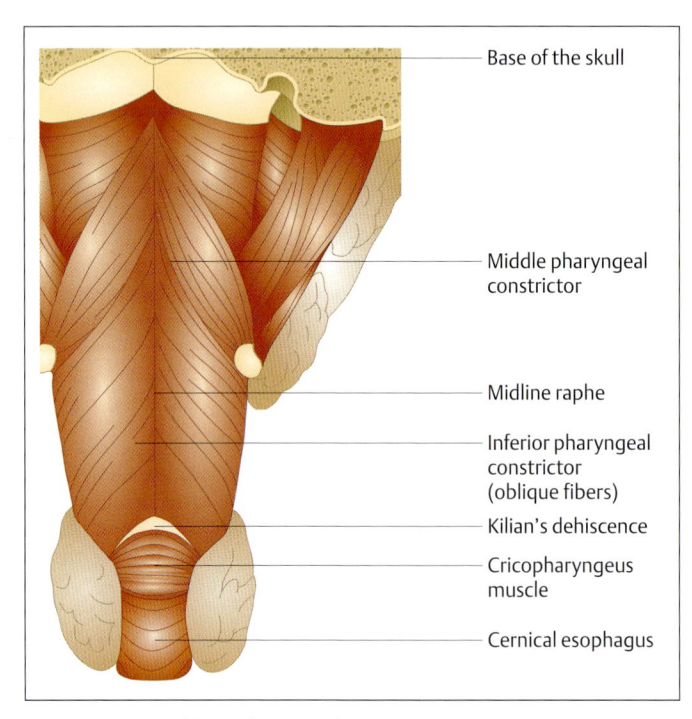

Fig. 11.9 Normal hypopharyngeal anatomy.

The *postcricoid* or *retrocricoarytenoid region* extends from the level of the arytenoid cartilages down to the lower edge of the cricoid cartilage. It forms the anterior wall of the lower hypopharynx (Figs. 11.7, 11.8).

The *posterior hypopharyngeal wall* is the continuation of the posterior wall of the oropharynx. Caudally, the posterior hypopharyngeal wall merges with the posterior wall of the cricopharyngeus muscle and then the cervical esophagus (Figs. 11.7, 11.8).

Muscles

The inferior pharyngeal constrictor muscle has a superior component and an inferior component (Fig. 11.9). The fibers of the superior component are obliquely oriented, being highest in the posterior midline. They arise from the posterior midline raphe and insert on the thyroid cartilage. The fibers of the inferior component of the inferior pharyngeal constrictor are also referred to as the "cricopharyngeus muscle." They arise from either side of the cricoid cartilage and are horizontally oriented. They blend with the circular muscles of the cervical esophagus.[59] Between the upper portion of the cricopharyngeus muscle and the lower portion of the oblique fibers of the inferior pharyngeal constrictor muscle is a small triangular space located posteriorly in the hypopharynx referred to as "Killian's dehiscence" or "Lannier's dehiscence." During swallowing, the superior, middle and inferior pharyngeal constrictors contract in a coordinated fashion. The cricopharyngeus muscle is normally closed. However, rela-

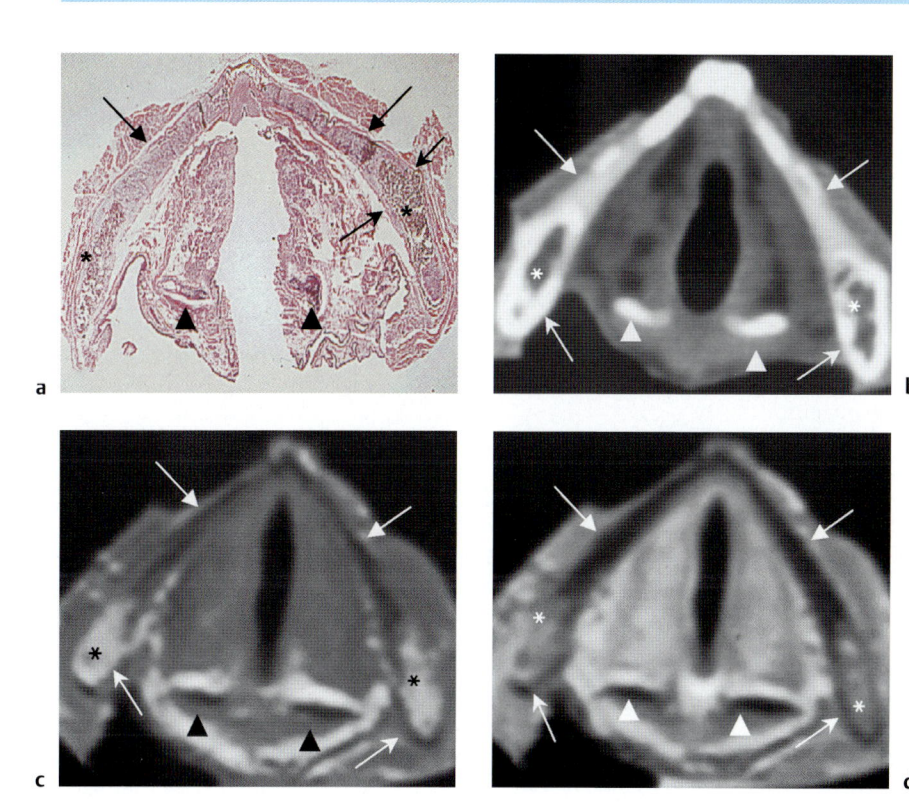

Fig. 11.10 Tissue characteristics of the laryngeal cartilages on CT and MRI. **a** Axial whole-organ histological slice from normal autopsy specimen at the level of the false cords. The thyroid cartilage is composed of nonossified hyaline cartilage (arrows) and ossified cartilage. Ossified cartilage is composed of a medullary cavity (asterisks) containing bone trabeculae and fatty tissue, and of an inner and outer cortex (stealth arrows). Arrowheads point to the arytenoid cartilages. **b** Axial CT image at the same level obtained in the same autopsy specimen. Nonossified hyaline cartilage (arrows) has attenuation values of soft tissues. The medullary cavity of ossified cartilage (asterisks) has low attenuation values and cortical bone (stealth arrows) has high attenuation values. Arrowheads point to the arytenoid cartilages. **c** Axial T1W SE image at the same level obtained in the same autopsy specimen. Nonossified hyaline cartilage (arrows) has a low signal intensity. The medullary cavity of ossified cartilage (asterisks) has a high signal intensity due to the high content of fatty tissue and cortical bone (stealth arrows) has a very low signal intensity. Arrowheads point to the arytenoid cartilages. **d** Axial T2W SE image at the same level obtained in the same autopsy specimen. Nonossified hyaline cartilage (arrows) has a low signal intensity. The medullary cavity of ossified cartilage (asterisks) has an intermediate signal intensity and cortical bone (stealth arrows) has a very low signal intensity. Arrowheads point to the arytenoid cartilages.

tively early during the pharyngeal phase of deglutition, the cricopharyngeus muscle relaxes, allowing the hypopharyngeal bolus to enter the esophagus. It then closes to prevent esophagopharyngeal reflux.[59]

Tissue Characteristics on Sectional Imaging

CT

On contrast-enhanced CT, the mucosal surface of the larynx usually shows no enhancement, whereas the hypopharyngeal mucosa is frequently seen as an enhancing, layer. The hypopharynx may be filled with air or may be collapsed, with its mucosal surfaces touching. In particular, on a CT examination a collapsed piriform sinus may mimic a tumor. A modified Valsalva maneuver may distend this region and rule out the presence of a tumor. At the level of the cricopharyngeus muscle on axial CT scans, the pharynx is oval, being wider from side to side than from front to back. Below the cricopharyngeus muscle, the cervical esophagus has a round sectional configuration and the point at which the oval shape of the pharynx changes into the round shape of the esophagus marks the transition from hypopharynx to cervical esophagus (Fig. 11.**8**). All structures that predominantly contain fat (e.g., false cords, aryepiglottic folds, preepiglottic space, and paraglottic space) are hypoattenuating on CT images (Fig. 11.**8**). Thin layers of connective tissue, e.g., the conus elasticus and the thyroglottic ligament, cannot usually be seen as a distinct structure on CT images. Similarly, the connecting membranes of the larynx (thyrohyoid membrane and thyrocricoid membrane) are not distinctly visualized on CT images. Their location can, however, be estimated by the position of the infrahyoid strap muscles.

On CT, ossified cartilage shows a high-attenuating outer and inner cortex and a central low-attenuating medullary space due to fatty tissue. Nonossified hyaline cartilage and nonossified fibroelastic cartilage have attenuation values of soft tissue[11, 16, 18, 27, 33, 73, 76] (Fig. 11.**10**). Cortical bone, fatty marrow, and nonossified hyaline cartilage show no enhancement on CT after intravenous administration of iodinated contrast material.

MR Imaging

On MRI, both the hypopharyngeal and the laryngeal mucosa display a low to intermediate signal intensity on T1-weighted images (Fig. 11.**7**), a higher signal intensity on T2-weighted images and a distinct enhancement after intravenous administration of gadolinium-based contrast material.[8, 80] Muscular tissue, e.g., the true vocal cords and the pharyngeal constrictors, displays an intermediate to low signal intensity on both T1-weighted and T2-weighted MR images and no relevant enhancement is observed after intravenous administration of gadolinium chelates. Therefore, on T2-weighted and contrast-enhanced T1-weighted MR images the mucosa can be easily differentiated from the underlying muscular tissue (Fig. 11.**5**). All structures that predominantly contain fat (e.g., false cords, preepiglottic space, and paraglottic space) display a high signal intensity on T1-weighted SE MR images and an intermediate signal intensity on T2-weighted SE MR images (Fig. 11.**7**). On T1-weighted and T2-weighted FSE MR images, fatty tissue displays a high signal intensity. Thin layers of connective tissue, e.g., the conus elasticus and the thyroglottic ligament, cannot be seen on MR images as a distinct structure even if a high-resolution matrix (512×512) and a small field of view are used. Similarly, the connecting membranes of the larynx (thyrohyoid membrane and thyrocricoid membrane) cannot currently be visualized with MR imaging as a separate structure.

On MRI, nonossified hyaline cartilage has an intermediate to low signal intensity on T1-weighted and on T2-weighted MR images. Cortical bone has a very low signal intensity on T1-weighted and T2-weighted images, whereas the medullary cavity of ossified cartilage has a high signal intensity on T1-weighted SE MR images and an intermediate signal intensity on T2-weighted SE MR images owing to the high content of fatty tissue[18, 26, 27, 39] (Fig. 11.**10**). On T1-weighted and T2-weighted FSE

MR images the medullary cavity displays a high signal intensity owing to its high content of fatty tissue. Cortical bone, fatty marrow, and nonossified hyaline cartilage show no relevant enhancement after administration of gadolinium chelates on MRI.

Imaging Techniques

■ Computed Tomography

Computed tomography (CT) was uncontested as the imaging modality of choice until the mid-1990s and has been further enhanced by the introduction of helical scanning. The technical advances of helical CT, namely, faster image acquisition and multiplanar or three-dimensional image reconstruction, have been particularly beneficial to diagnostic imaging of the larynx and hypopharynx. Rapid acquisition helps to avoid respiratory artifacts, and the new imaging algorithms have greatly improved overall image quality and spatial resolution. Multiplanar reconstruction from helical data sets may help to demonstrate tumor infiltration with regard to the complex and subtle anatomy of this region. Standard CT protocols are relatively easy to perform, which generally leads to imaging studies of reproducible, consistent quality. Access to CT imaging is easily and rapidly available. Recently introduced multidetector acquisition techniques with even faster scanning algorithms have shown that the speed and resolution of CT continue to improve considerably. Although radiation exposure is a concern with CT in general, this is only a relative disadvantage in the context of neoplastic disease, which is the main indication for imaging of the larynx and hypopharynx. The main drawbacks of CT are the relatively high doses of iodinated contrast material, with their associated potential side effects, and nephrotoxicity.

Regardless of the acquisition technique (single-slice helical scanning, multidetector technique), a standard examination is done in the supine position with the neck hyperextended, and the patient is instructed to resist swallowing or coughing. Following acquisition of a lateral scout view, axial slices are obtained from the base of the tongue to the upper trachea with a scan orientation parallel to the laryngeal ventricle or the true vocal cords. Iodinated contrast material (total dose, 35–40 g iodine) is given intravenously with an automated power injector. Most investigators prefer to obtain images during quiet breathing rather than during apnea because the abducted position of the true vocal cords facilitates evaluation of the anterior and posterior commissures.[8,9,68,75–80,96,104] In selected cases, additional scans may be obtained with phonation or modified Valsalva maneuvers, for example, to evaluate the hypopharynx and the laryngeal ventricle.

The superiority of *helical scanning* in the larynx has been shown by Suojanen et al.[111] The helical technique is routinely used in the larynx because current standard equipment enables a complete data set through the larynx to be acquired in less than 20 seconds and reconstruction of overlapping slices at any level. Acquisitions with 3 mm collimation at pitch 1 and overlapping reconstruction intervals of 2 mm are the minimum necessary to evaluate the larynx. High-detail work or high-quality 2D reconstructions in the coronal or sagittal plane may require additional acquisitions with 1 mm collimation and 1–1.5 pitch. Depending on vendor-related software options, such data sets also enable 3D volume reconstructions[84] and so-called "virtual endoscopy" images to be obtained. The latter are surface renderings that, by means of computer-generated ray casting, simulate endoscopic views of the inner surface of the larynx (Fig. 11.**3**). This image format may serve as a useful roadmap for endoscopic examination of difficult anatomical areas, e.g., the subglottis, or for evaluation of airway stenoses. Owing to its rapid image acquisition, helical scanning also greatly facilitates acquisitions during phonation or respiratory maneuvers. Regardless of the acquisition technique, standard soft-tissue algorithms for reconstructions of CT scans of the larynx are used routinely; bone algorithms may be used as an option to improve cartilage detail but rarely make a difference in accuracy of diagnosis. However, when neoplastic cartilage invasion is suspected, the images should be viewed using both soft-tissue and bone window settings.[16,79,95]

■ Magnetic Resonance Imaging

The key advantage of MRI compared with CT is its inherently superior resolution of soft-tissue contrast, which enables much better visualization of subtle tissue-specific abnormalities. In addition, contrast materials used with MR imaging have far less toxic side effects than those used with CT.

Unfortunately, MRI of the head and neck region has long been hampered by several inherent technical limitations. Long acquisition and image reconstruction times resulted in unacceptable motion and breathing artifacts. Impractical coils required the radiologist to change coils during the examination in order to obtain a complete examination, thus resulting in very long overall examination times that were intolerable for many patients with head and neck tumors. Over the past decade, these technical problems have been gradually overcome by stronger MRI gradients, faster sequences, faster reconstruction algorithms, and the new volume coils for the head and neck sequences. All these improvements have resulted in much better image quality and, although overall examination time is still longer than with helical CT, susceptibility to motion artifacts has been greatly reduced because acquisition of the individual sequences is faster. Since the mid-1990s MR imaging has therefore increasingly been able to challenge the role of CT, and many investigators consider MRI as the method of choice for imaging of most head and neck tumors, including the larynx and hypopharynx.

Today, the remaining inherent disadvantages of MRI are its inability to examine patients with certain medical implants (pacemakers, certain vascular clips and valves, neurostimulators, etc.); the narrow design of the tunnel and coils giving rise to claustrophobic reactions in a minority of patients; and, not least, the restricted access to MR imaging due to overbooking of MRI equipment.

To date, MR imaging of the larynx and hypopharynx has mainly been done at middle or high field strength (0.6–1.5 T).[18,27,33,68,118,125] Current standard equipment includes dedicated surface neck coils in phased array (multicoil) configuration. Mounted to the patient's neck in the supine position and with the neck hyperextended, these coils enable examination of the entire region from the skull base to the clavicles while offering good signal-to-noise characteristics.

The basic principle of a standard MRI examination of the head and neck region is to perform multiple MR experiments with changing parameters, in order to obtain image sequences with varying T1-weighting and T2-weighting, and other varying factors such as fat saturation and contrast enhancement, from the same region. Therefore, despite many recent technical improvements, a standard MRI examination of the larynx still takes a relatively long time (approximately 30 minutes) and requires more cooperation from the patient than does a standard helical CT examination. Dyspnea is a frequent problem in patients undergoing imaging studies of the larynx and hypopharynx and predisposes to motion artifacts. In the literature, up to 16% of MRI studies of the laryngo-hypopharyngeal region have been reported to be nondiagnostic owing to claustrophobia or motion artifacts.[18, 27, 118] Nonetheless, experience with current standard techniques at our institution indicates that good-quality MR images of the laryngo-hypopharyngeal region may now be obtained in 98% of patients provided that they are instructed carefully before and during the examination by the technical and medical staff and motivated to breathe quietly and to resist swallowing or coughing. Interaction with the patient appears particularly important for avoiding nondiagnostic images. If patients cannot avoid coughing during the acquisition, they may activate a bell, indicating that the sequence needs to be interrupted for a few seconds and continued thereafter.

The MRI protocols used for the larynx and hypopharynx are subject to the same rapid technical evolution that is currently taking place everywhere in the field of magnetic resonance imaging. Considerable differences exist among investigators that are related to vendor-related variations in hardware and software. Nonetheless, two basic pulse sequences are currently used by most investigators, namely, T1-weighted SE or T1-weighted fast spin-echo (FSE) sequences, and T2-weighted fast spin-echo (FSE) sequences. The axis of the larynx is usually identified with a rapid sagittal localizer, and axial T2-weighted FSE and T1-weighted SE or T1-weighted FSE images are obtained from the base of the tongue to the upper trachea with a scan orientation parallel to the laryngeal ventricle or the true vocal cords. Typical image parameters for a standard examination include a slice thickness of 3 or 4 mm with a 0–1 mm intersection gap, and a field of view of 20×20 cm or less. The acquisition matrix should be at least 256×256 but, whenever possible, a 256×512 or a 512×512 matrix should be used as the increased spatial resolution greatly enhances the diagnostic information. Although the use of two excitations increases imaging time, this is far outweighed by the improved image quality achieved as a result of averaging of swallowing or coughing artifacts. Respiratory compensation is an additional option to reduce motion artifacts. Additional axial T1-weighted images after intravenous administration of gadolinium chelates are obtained routinely. In order to move flow artifacts away from the larynx, especially after intravenous administration of gadolinium chelates, phase-encoding gradients are placed in the anteroposterior direction in the axial plane, and in the superoinferior direction in the coronal plane. Fat-saturated T1-weighted SE images, with or without contrast-material enhancement, and fat-saturated T2-weighted FSE images are optional.[114] Images in the coronal or sagittal plane may be obtained in order to evaluate certain anatomical spaces, e.g., the preepiglottic space in the sagittal plane, or the paraglottic space and the ventricle in the coronal plane.[8, 33, 75]

Dynamic sequential acquisition techniques may be used for differential diagnostic purposes in other areas of the head and neck (e.g., to differentiate paragangliomas from other tumors).[112] Because these sequences hold promise for the demonstration of tumor angioneogenesis and for the differentiation between tumor recurrence and scar tissue in other parts of the body, e.g., the breast, it is conceivable that they may eventually become useful to detect primary or recurrent tumors of the laryngo-hypopharyngeal region. To date, however, the superiority of these techniques over standard SE sequences or FSE sequences for clinical use in the larynx has not been shown. Subtraction techniques facilitate delineation of tumor margins and areas of mild enhancement, and they provide an increased contrast between tumor and adjacent fatty tissue. However, subtraction techniques are very susceptible to misregistration artifacts due to normal physiological respiratory motion.

Other Imaging Modalities

Ultrasonography cannot be considered as an alternative to CT or MRI for routine clinical imaging of the larynx or hypopharynx in adults, although it is a useful technique for evaluating mass lesions of this region in children.

Conventional radiographic techniques continue to play a major role, complementary to endoscopy, for the evaluation of the hypopharynx. *Barium swallow studies* are well-suited to demonstrating diverticula, webs, strictures, tumors, and postoperative and postradiation changes. Videofluorography and cineradiography are well-established and are indispensable for the functional evaluation of the hypopharynx in the context of dysphagia. Barium is routinely used, but water-soluble iodinated contrast material is preferable when a perforation or fistula is suspected. In patients with a high risk of aspiration and a suspected perforation or fistula, low-osmolarity water-soluble iodinated contrast material should be employed.

Positron emission tomography with 2-(^{18}F)fluoro-2-deoxy-D-glucose (FDG-PET) is a relatively recent technique and is based on the demonstration of increased metabolic activity of neoplastic cells as opposed to the cells within physiological tissue or cells within mature scar tissue. It may therefore help to localize small foci of tumor tissue, although the spatial resolution is relatively low. In the head and neck area, including the larynx and hypopharynx, FDG-PET is currently under investigation for the detection of recurrence of squamous cell carcinoma after radiotherapy.[53] Fusion of FDG-PET images with CT or MR images may facilitate the anatomical localization of suspected neoplastic foci.

Squamous Cell Carcinoma

Epidemiology and Rationale for Imaging

Squamous cell carcinoma of the larynx is primarily related to cigarette smoking. The predisposing role of alcohol in the etiology of laryngeal cancer is less important than it is in cancer of other locations in the head and neck region.[9, 10, 67, 125] Studies from several European countries and from the United States show that the incidence of laryngeal cancer in heavily industrialized cities is two to three times higher than in rural populations. The male-to-female ratio for laryngeal cancer is approximately 10 : 1.[67] The distribution of carcinomas within the larynx is subject to great geographic variation.

Squamous cell carcinoma of the hypopharynx is less frequent than laryngeal cancer. Predisposing factors are tobacco and alcohol use. Although the distribution of carcinomas within the hypopharynx is also subject to great geographic variation, 65–75% of hypopharyngeal carcinomas arise from the piriform sinus. Postcricoid carcinoma is very rare in most countries, although it is relatively common in England, Wales, and India, probably secondary to the Plummer–Vinson syndrome.[8, 11, 12, 67]

Only 5–10% of neoplastic lesions in the laryngohypopharyngeal region are non–squamous cell tumors, originating from a variety of tissue components and unrelated to tobacco and alcohol. Their biological behavior and prognosis are quite variable and range from entirely benign (e.g., lipoma) to very aggressive (e.g., undifferentiated sarcoma). These uncommon neoplasms must therefore be seen in a different clinical and therapeutic context than squamous cell cancers.

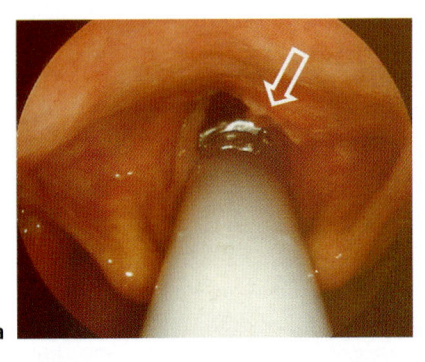

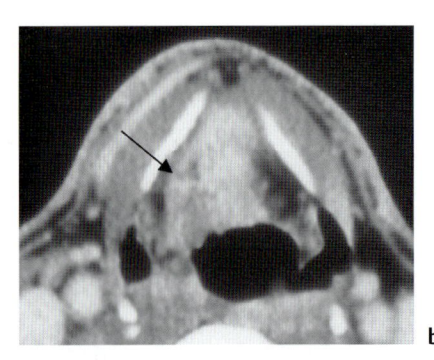

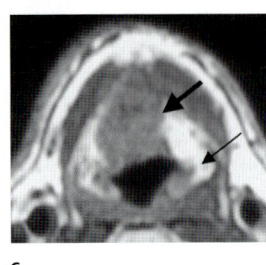

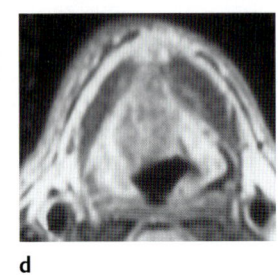

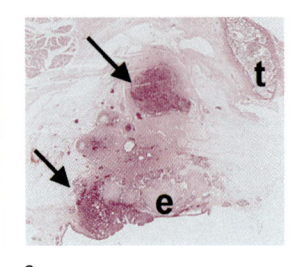

Fig. 11.**11** Invasion of the preepiglottic space due to ventral supraglottic cancer. **a** Endoscopy shows a small mucosal cancer arising from the fixed portion of the epiglottis (arrow). **b** Axial contrast-enhanced CT image in the same patient shows an enhancing tumor mass as it invades the preepiglottic space (arrow). **c** Axial unenhanced T1W SE image obtained in the same patient at the same level shows a tumor mass with an intermediate signal intensity as it extends into the preepiglottic space (thick arrow). Note the high signal intensity of the noninvaded paraglottic space due to the high content of fatty tissue (thin arrow). **d** Axial Gd-enhanced T1W SE image at the same level shows enhancement of the tumor mass invading the preepiglottic space. **e** Whole-organ axial histological slice from supraglottic horizontal laryngectomy specimen confirms tumor invasion of the preepiglottic space (arrows). e = epiglottis; t = thyroid cartilage.

The most common leading clinical symptoms are hoarseness in laryngeal squamous cell carcinoma and dysphagia, often associated with palpable cervical lymph nodes, in hypopharyngeal squamous carcinoma. Because squamous cell carcinoma almost always originates at the mucosal surface, it is usually first detected endoscopically and then confirmed with endoscopic biopsy. Neither CT nor MRI can be used to detect and delineate superficially situated squamous cell carcinoma. The attenuation values of squamous cell carcinoma on CT scans and its signal characteristics on unenhanced and contrast-enhanced MR images are very similar to those of normal mucosa. On the other hand, endoscopy cannot be used to detect tumor infiltration into the submucosal structures, whereas the different characteristics on CT and MR imaging of neoplastic tissue and the adjacent fatty, muscular, and cartilaginous tissues often allow delineation of the deep tumor infiltration in the horizontal (anterior–posterior) or longitudinal (cranial–caudal) directions. Because the prognosis and treatment of squamous cell carcinoma depends on the depth of submucosal infiltration and on the anatomical structures that are involved, sectional imaging with either CT or MR imaging may thus be considered complementary to endoscopy and plays an indispensable role in the pretherapeutic work-up of laryngeal and hypopharyngeal cancer.

Interpretation of CT and MRI studies of patients with laryngeal and hypopharyngeal cancer requires an understanding of the typical pathways of tumor spread from the different primary sites and subsites and knowledge of the criteria for neoplastic invasion of the adjacent structures, particularly the cartilaginous framework of the larynx. In addition, it is appropriate for the radiologist to be familiar with the implications of imaging findings with regard to the T-classification and options of treatment.

■ Tumor Sites and Patterns of Tumor Spread

Larynx

Supraglottic Carcinoma

According to their subsite of origin, supraglottic tumors display typical patterns of spread.[8,64,75,79] Tumors originating from the laryngeal surface of the epiglottis (ventral supraglottic carcinomas) may be subdivided into tumors arising from the suprahyoid or free margin of the epiglottis, and tumors arising from the infrahyoid or fixed portion of the epiglottis. Tumors arising from the fixed portion of the epiglottis primarily invade the preepiglottic space, either along the border of the epiglottic cartilage or through its preexisting natural perforations, or by frank cartilage destruction[31] (Fig. 11.**11**). Tumors that originate in the region of the petiole often invade the low preepiglottic space, and, via the anterior commissure, extend at first to the glottis and then the subglottis, thus becoming "transglottic" tumors (Fig. 11.**12**) (see below). These low, ventral supraglottic lesions may also spread horizontally to involve the thyroid cartilage anteriorly, and the false cords and laryngeal ventricles posteriorly. Although invasion of the preepiglottic space cannot be detected endoscopically, it plays an important role for tumor staging, treatment, and prognosis.[9,12,55,71,80] If the preepiglottic space is invaded, the tumor will be staged T3 according to the UICC and AJCC (American Joint Committee on Cancer) guidelines.[55] In the presence of extensive neoplastic infiltration of the preepiglottic space by supraglottic laryngeal carcinoma, surgical management may involve a more extensive horizontal supraglottic laryngectomy and sometimes supracricoid laryngectomy with cricohyoidopexy (see below)[71,83] Finally, the degree of preepiglottic space involvement by tumor may also affect the outcome of definitive radiation therapy in supraglottic squamous cell carcinoma.[80] Both CT and MRI are well suited to demonstrate replacement of the normal fatty tissue by tumor tissue within the preepiglottic space (Fig. 11.**11**). Although sagittal images are best suited to delineate the extent of craniocaudal tumor spread within the preepiglottic space, standard axial images are sufficient to establish the diagnosis.

Tumors arising at the junction of the aryepiglottic fold and infrahyoid epiglottis (ventrolateral supraglottic carcinomas) have a distinctive growth pattern. Typically, they spread to the preepiglottic space and extend around, rather than through, the epiglottis,[75–77,79] and they may invade the upper edge of the thyroid cartilage at the attachment of the thyrohyoid membrane. Ventrolateral supraglottic cancers also tend to involve the infrahyoid strap muscles, the pharyngoepiglottic fold, and the valleculae. Although invasion of the latter structures is best evaluated by means of endoscopic biopsy, it may also be demonstrated with both CT and MRI.

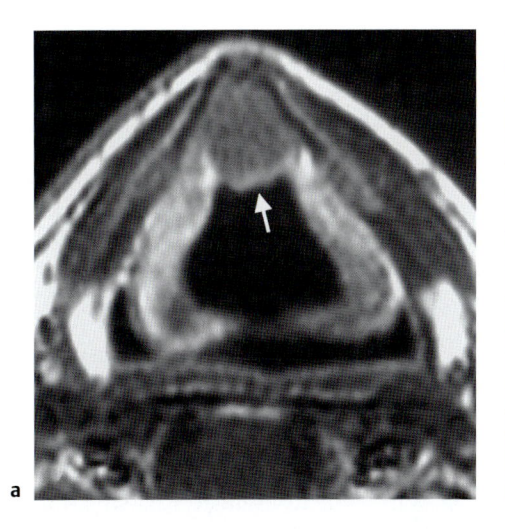

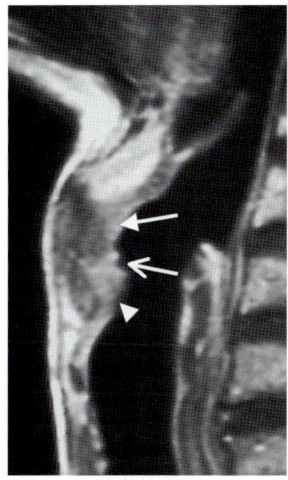

Fig. 11.12 Transglottic spread in a ventral supraglottic cancer underestimated at endoscopy. Patient presenting with a small tumor arising from the mucosa overlying the petiole at endoscopy. **a** Axial and **b** sagittal contrast-enhanced T1W SE images clearly show that the tumor spreads from the supraglottic mucosa into the inferior preepiglottic space (arrows) and downward into the anterior commissure (open arrow) and the anterior subglottic region (arrowhead). Reproduced from Reference 8 with permission.

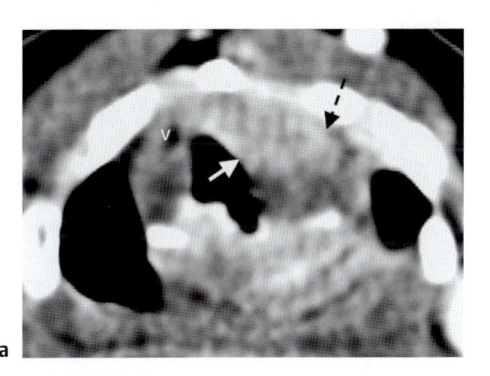

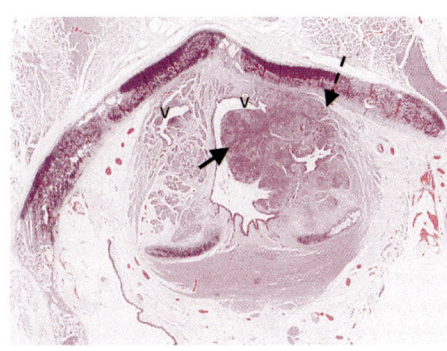

Fig. 11.13 Invasion of the paraglottic space by lateral supraglottic carcinoma detected by CT. Patient presenting with a small tumor arising from the false cord at endoscopy. **a** CT shows a tumor involving the false cord (arrow) and with paraglottic space invasion (dashed arrow). v = laryngeal ventricle. **b** Histology confirmed the CT findings. Tumor originating at the false cord level (arrow) with invasion of the paraglottic space (dashed arrow). v = laryngeal ventricles.

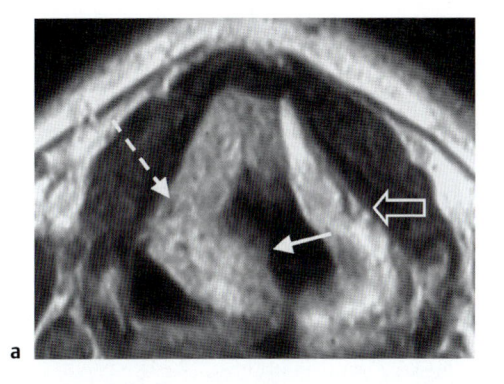

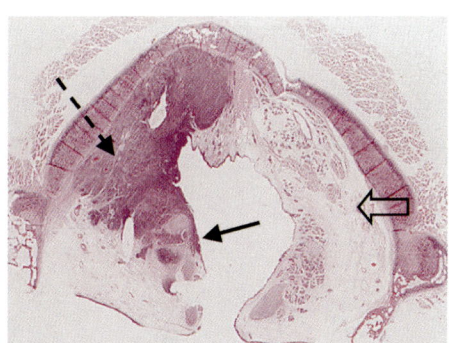

Fig. 11.14 Invasion of the paraglottic space by lateral supraglottic carcinoma detected by MRI. Patient presenting with a large tumor arising from the laryngeal surface of the right aryepiglottic fold at endoscopy. **a** Contrast-enhanced T1W image shows a tumor involving the right aryepiglottic fold (arrow) and with paraglottic space invasion (dashed arrow). Note the normal high signal intensity of the left paraglottic space caused by normal fatty tissue (block arrow). **b** Histology confirmed the MRI findings. Tumor originating from the aryepiglottic fold (arrow) with invasion of the paraglottic space (dashed arrow). Normal left paraglottic space containing fatty tissue and small vessels (block arrow).

Supraglottic tumors originating from the false vocal cord, laryngeal ventricle, or aryepiglottic fold (lateral supraglottic carcinomas) may grow superficially for some time.[9,8,75–77,79] By the time they are diagnosed, however, one half of all lateral supraglottic carcinomas will show substantial infiltration of the paraglottic space. Because these tumors tend to spread submucosally along the paraglottic space to the glottic and subglottic region or other remote areas, sectional images are of particular importance. The primary sign of tumor spread to the paraglottic space on both CT and MRI is replacement of fat by tumor tissue[9,11,75,77] (Figs. 11.**13**–11.**14**).

Tumors arising in the arytenoid or interarytenoid region (posterior supraglottic carcinomas) usually display an aggressive behavior and infiltrate the postcricoid portion of the hypopharynx (Fig. 11.15). Because they tend to spread submucosally, sectional images are the only means to demonstrate the full extent of tumor spread prior to treatment.

The primary lymphatic spread of supraglottic carcinomas is directed toward the superior jugular lymph nodes. Lymph node metastases are common and often bilateral.

Glottic Carcinoma

Glottic carcinoma typically arises from the anterior half of the true vocal cord. While small glottic lesions are readily seen at endoscopy, they may be missed at sectional imaging. Nevertheless, MRI is more sensitive than CT in detecting these early lesions (Fig. 11.**16**). Glottic carcinoma primarily spreads ventrally into the anterior commissure. Evaluation of the anterior commissure can be easily done endoscopically and does not warrant sectional imaging. The anterior commissure consists of the anterior attachment of the true vocal cords. Histologically, it is composed of dense, avascular fibroelastic tissue that acts like a relative barrier to early glottic cancer.[65] Once the tumor has reached the anterior commissure, it may easily spread into the supraglottis or sub-

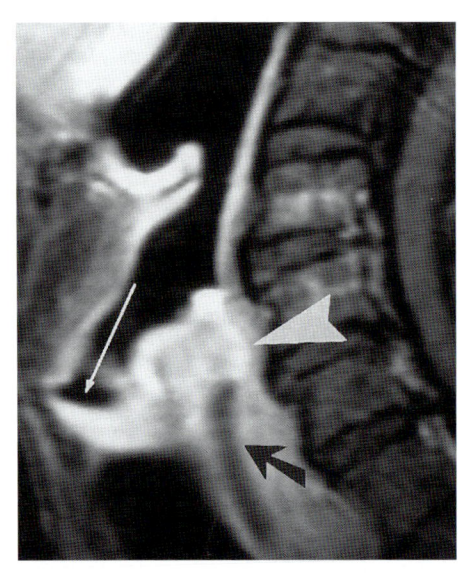

Fig. 11.**15** Posterior laryngeal carcinoma with submucosal involvement of the retrocricoid region. Sagittal contrast-enhanced, fat-saturated T1W SE MR image shows a tumor mass arising from the mucosa overlying the arytenoid with submucosal involvement of the retroarytenoid region (arrowhead). Thin white arrow points to the entrance of the ventricle. Thick black arrow points to the posterior portion of the cricoid cartilage. Reproduced from Reference 8 with permission.

glottis. This type of tumor spread is best evaluated with sectional imaging (Fig. 11.**17**). On axial CT and MR images, neoplastic invasion occurring at the subglottic level below the anterior commissure appears as an irregular thickening of the cricothyroid membrane[8]. The prelaryngeal soft tissues may then become invaded via the natural defects formed by the neurovascular bundles within this membrane, or at the line of its attachment to the undersurface of the thyroid cartilage[81,21]. In the presence of significant anterior subglottic spread, invasion of the thyroid cartilage at the anterior commissure is likely

Posterior extension of early glottic cancer into the vocal process of the arytenoid is relatively uncommon, and initial involvement of the posterior commissure is rare. Nevertheless, advanced glottic carcinomas may spread, along the free edge of the vocal cords, into the posterior commissure (Fig. 11.**18**). Because the posterior commissure can easily be evaluated endoscopically, sectional imaging is not warranted to evaluate this structure alone. Nonetheless, the radiologist should be aware of a potential pitfall at the time of CT examination. Because the mucosa of the posterior commissure bulges during adduction of the true vocal cords, it may simulate pathological thickening due to tumor. CT of the larynx therefore should always be performed during quiet respiration (open glottis, see above). From the posterior commissure, tumor may then spread into the arytenoid and cricoid cartilage or into the cricoarytenoid joint (Fig. 11.**18**). Invasion of the cricoarytenoid joint is difficult to detect with both CT and MRI. Primary posterior glottic tumors may also invade the cricoarytenoid joint as well as the submucosa of the apex of the piriform sinus, thereby gaining access to its lymphatic drainage.

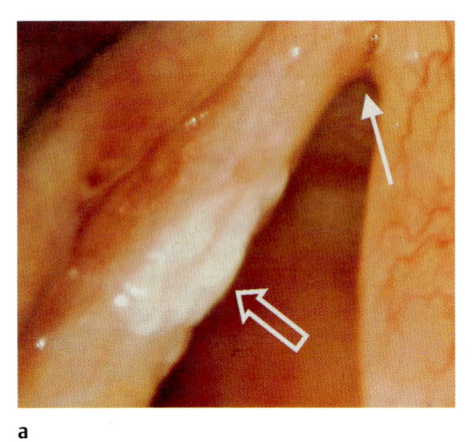

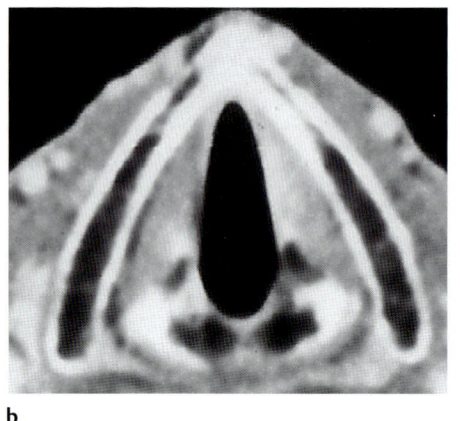

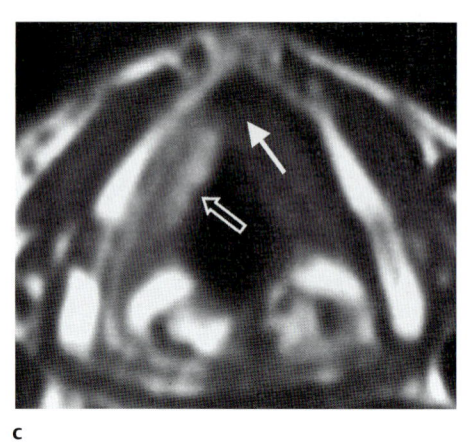

a b c

Fig. 11.**16** Small glottic cancer. **a** Endoscopic image shows a small lesion arising from the anterior half of the right true vocal cord (block arrow). No invasion of the anterior commissure (arrow). **b** CT (2 mm slice) does not demonstrate the tumor. **c** MRI (T2W SE image) nicely demonstrates the small tumor as an area of increased signal intensity (block arrow). No invasion of the anterior commissure (arrow).

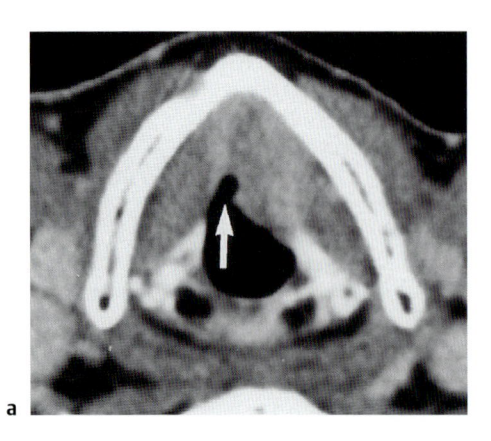

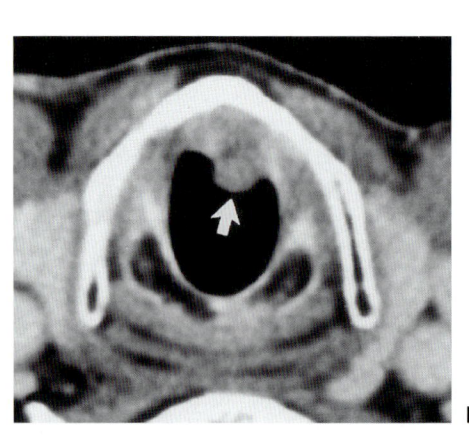

Fig. 11.**17** Glottic cancer with invasion of the anterior commissure and subglottis. **a** Axial contrast-enhanced CT scan at the glottic level shows a left-sided mass invading the anterior commissure (arrow) and the right vocal cord. The tumor mass also abuts the thyroid cartilage. **b** CT scan, obtained at a lower level, shows tumor extension into the anterior subglottic region (arrow). Reproduced from Reference 8 with permission.

a b

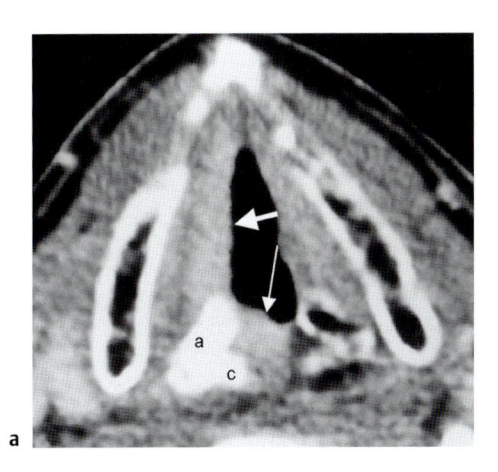

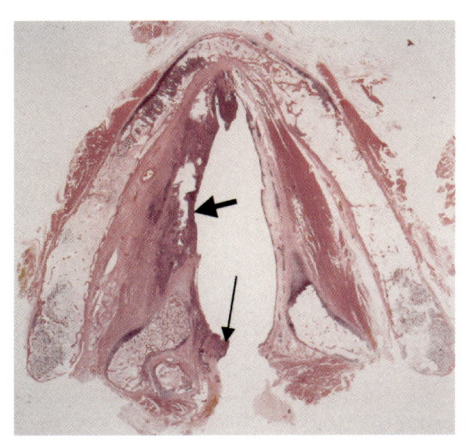

Fig. 11.**18** Glottic cancer with invasion of the posterior commissure. **a** Axial contrast-enhanced CT scan at the glottic level shows a mass invading the posterior commissure (thin arrow) and the right vocal cord (thick arrow). Note major sclerosis of the arytenoid (a) and adjacent cricoid (c) cartilage. **b** Histology confirmed invasion of the posterior commissure (thin arrow) by right-sided vocal cord cancer (thick arrow). There was microscopic invasion of the vocal process of the arytenoid and superoposterior surface of the cricoid cartilage on the right.

When a glottic tumor spreads laterally, it eventually invades the thyroarytenoid muscle, thus leading to vocal cord fixation. If the vocal cord is fixed, the tumor will be staged T3 according to the UICC and AJCC guidelines.[55] Because tumor spread within the paraglottic space is limited by the conus elasticus medially and the perichondrium of the thyroid ala laterally, further spread occurs mainly in a cephalad or caudad direction or, via the cricothyroid membrane, into the infrahyoid strap muscles. Paraglottic tumor spread may be entirely occult clinically and detectable only by means of CT or MR imaging. Although axial images are usually sufficient, coronal images may sometimes provide additional information if the vertical extent of the lesion is not clear.

Subglottic spread is relatively common and may occur either superficially or deep to the elastic cone[64, 125, 126] Deep subglottic spread is very difficult to detect endoscopically, and underestimation of the tumor may occur unless CT or MRI is performed (Fig. 11.**17**). The degree of subglottic spread and the relationship between tumor and the cricoid are best displayed on axial images. Coronal images are of limited help in assessment of subglottic spread, because they are difficult to interpret except in the midcoronal plane.

Lymphatic metastases from glottic carcinoma are uncommon as long as the tumor is confined to the endolarynx. However, once it has traversed the cricothyroid membrane, the frequency of lymph node metastases increases significantly.[10, 11, 77–79]

Transglottic Carcinoma

The term "transglottic carcinoma" generally refers to tumors that involve both the glottis and supraglottis at the time of diagnosis.[8, 75] Opinions differ, however, as to whether this automatically implies that the tumor has crossed the laryngeal ventricle since transglottic growth can occur either anteriorly or posteriorly to the laryngeal ventricle. Some authors restrict the term "transglottic" to tumors that originate from the laryngeal ventricle and grow primarily submucosally into the paraglottic space. In any case, transglottic involvement implies advanced disease and an unfavorable prognosis.[64, 67] The submucosal growth pattern is readily recognized on CT and MR images, although endoscopically it becomes visible only if it bulges the mucosa but remains entirely occult otherwise (Fig. 11.**19**). Invasion of the laryngeal framework and of the cricothyroid membrane is particularly common in transglottic tumors spreading vertically in the anterior midline. Transglottic carcinoma involving the anterior commissure can display a very aggressive behavior, resulting in infiltration of intact layers of perichondrium and replacement of the thyroid cartilage with neoplastic tissue.[62, 64, 68, 75, 76] Such tumors are usually underestimated at endoscopy and CT or MR images are necessary to demonstrate their true extent prior to treatment (Fig. 11.**12**). Posterior spreading carcinomas, whether supraglottic or glottic in origin, may early become transglottic. Transglottic carcinoma is very often accompanied by lymph node metastases.

Subglottic Carcinoma

Involvement of the subglottis by laryngeal cancer usually represents inferior spread of a glottic or supraglottic tumor rather than a primary tumor originating in the subglottis (Fig. 11.**17**). True subglottic tumors are relatively uncommon and are regarded by many investigators as a distinct form of laryngeal carcinoma. According to the literature, 1–8% of all laryngeal tumors are included under this term. Diagnosis of primary subglottic cancers may be delayed as patients present relatively late in the disease process with symptoms such as stridor, hoarseness, dysphagia, or palpable low cervical lymph nodes. In addition, in our experience, these tumors often present as submucosal masses endoscopically, and initial endoscopic biopsy may be negative.

Primary subglottic carcinomas may arise unilaterally but, since midline barriers do not exist at this level, they can easily cross the anterior or posterior midline. A characteristic circular extension of the tumor taking up almost the entire subglottic lumen may be recognized on sectional imaging (Fig. 11.**20**). The conus elasticus plays an important role in directing the growth of small subglottic carcinomas medially into the lumen. Larger tumors, however, rapidly destroy this connective-tissue membrane and tend to invade the cricoid cartilage, spread to the trachea, or grow out of the larynx, thus invading the thyroid gland. Primary subglottic tumors may also spread superiorly and posteriorly into the posterior commissure or cervical esophagus. Invasion of the extralaryngeal structures is seen in about one-half of all subglottic carcinomas at the time of initial diagnosis.[6, 12]

Lymph node metastases are much more common than in glottic carcinoma; the primary drainage is directed toward the paratracheal and pretracheal nodes. These nodes drain to the lower jugular or upper mediastinal nodes.

Hypopharynx

Carcinoma of the Piriform Sinus

Carcinoma of the piriform sinus is readily detected with endoscopy. Early superficial spreading tumors that are limited to the mucosa may be invisible on sectional imaging, although more advanced lesions are readily diagnosed on axial CT or MR images. Because the piriform sinus is usually collapsed during quiet respiration, the exact tumor location may be difficult to determine (Fig. 11.**21**). During a CT study, the piriform sinus can be unfolded

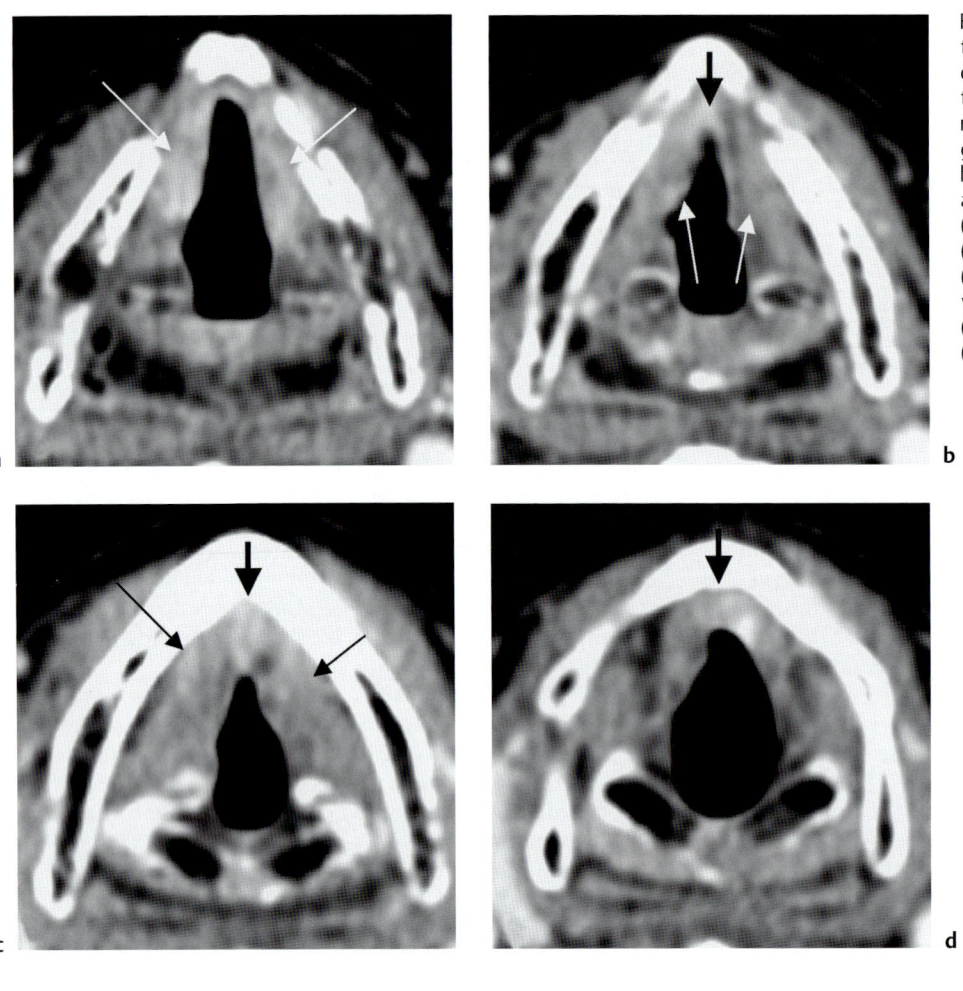

Fig. 11.19 Glottic cancer with submucosal transglottic tumor spread along the anterior commissure. Endoscopically, a bilateral glottic tumor was present with invasion of the anterior commissure. The supraglottis and subglottis were tumor-free. Axial contrast-enhanced CT scans at the supraglottic level (**a** and **b**), glottic level (**c**), and subglottic level (**d**) show a mass involving both vocal cords (thin black arrows), the anterior commissure (thick black arrow in **c**), the false cords (thin white arrows), the low preepiglottic space (thick black arrow in **b**), and the subglottis (thick black arrow in **d**).

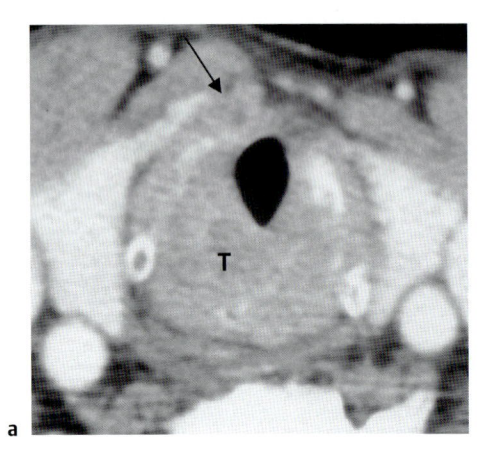

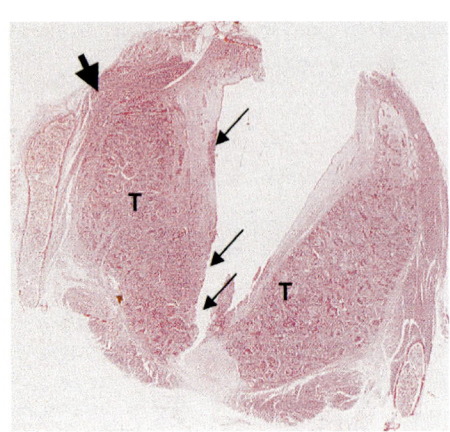

Fig. 11.20 Primary subglottic cancer. Patient presenting with dyspnea. Endoscopy revealed a relatively small mucosal lesion situated below the posterior commissure and in the right subglottis. The rest of the mucosa appeared tumor-free, but diffuse subglottic narrowing was observed endoscopically. **a** Contrast-enhanced CT at the subglottic level shows circumferential subglottic tumor (T) with destruction of the cricoid ring and invasion of paralaryngeal strap muscles (arrow). The rest of the larynx was tumor-free. **b** Corresponding histological slice from specimen confirms circumferential subglottic tumor (T) with massive destruction of the cricoid cartilage. Note the relatively small mucosal component (arrows) as opposed to the extensive submucosal component. Invasion of the paralaryngeal strap muscles (thick arrow). Reproduced from Reference 9 with permission.

during image acquisition by means of a modified Valsalva maneuver.

Depending on the primary location, carcinoma of the piriform sinus can spread into different directions in the axial plane and infiltrate various adjacent structures. Tumors involving primarily the medial wall or the angle of the piriform sinus may infiltrate the larynx by growing anteriorly into the paraglottic space[6, 8–12, 76–79, 117, 128] (Fig. 11.**22**). This tumor growth may be clinically occult. From the paraglottic space, the tumor may spread to the preepiglottic space and into the contralateral hemilarynx beneath intact mucosa. Tumors originating from the lateral wall of the piriform sinus infiltrate toward the common carotid artery. If the tumor encompasses more than 270° of the circumference of the vessel on axial images, it becomes unlikely that it can be removed without resecting the artery[123] (Fig. 11.**23**). Carcinoma of the piriform sinus may also spill over or penetrate the aryepiglottic fold to involve the endolarynx. In this case, the aryepiglottic fold is thickened on axial CT or MR images and it is impossible to decide—based on sectional images alone—whether mucosal spread is present on one side or both. Correlation between the radiological and the endoscopic findings is needed to answer this question. More advanced piriform sinus tumors typi-

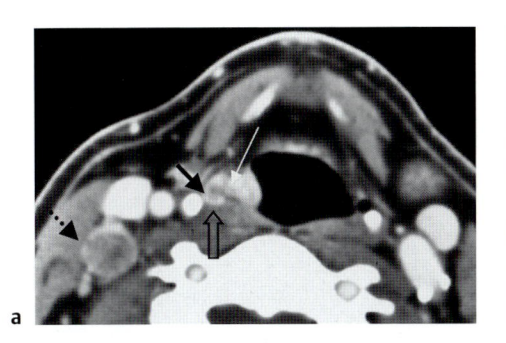

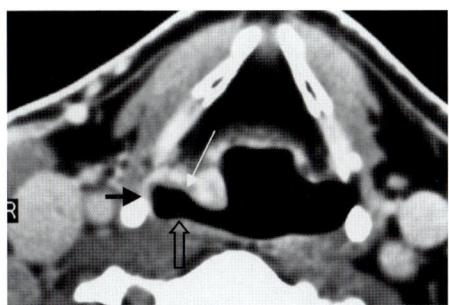

Fig. 11.21 Value of the modified Valsalva maneuver in imaging piriform sinus cancer. **a** Axial contrast-enhanced CT image at the supraglottic level obtained during quiet respiration shows a hypopharyngeal tumor mass involving the medial wall (thin white arrow) and the lateral wall (thick black arrow) of the right piriform sinus. Invasion of the posterior wall may be present (block arrow). Note also invasion of the paraglottic space at the level of the aryepiglottic fold, which is thickened and shows contrast enhancement. Lymph node metastasis (dashed arrow). **b** Image obtained at the same level during a modified Valsalva maneuver. The piriform sinus is unfolded. There is no invasion of the posterior wall (block arrow). However, there is invasion of the medial wall (thin white arrow) and lateral wall (thick black arrow).

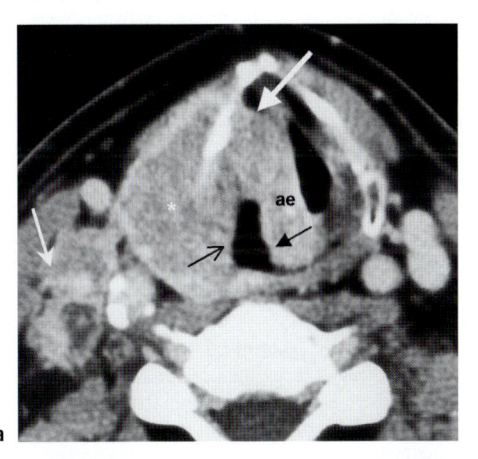

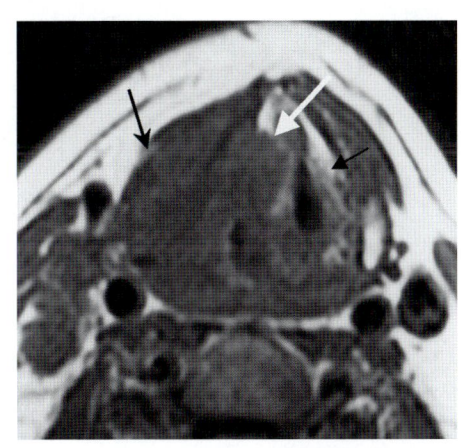

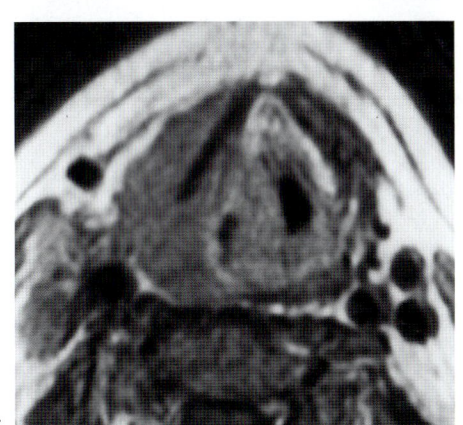

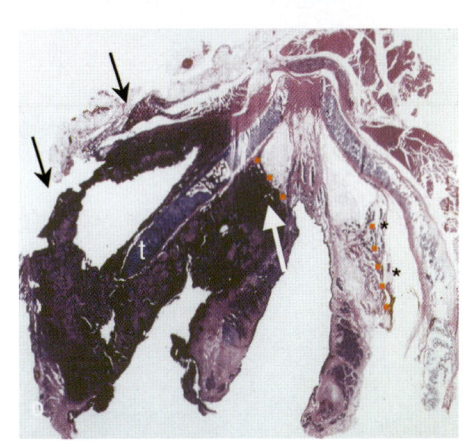

Fig. 11.22 Invasion of the paraglottic space by piriform sinus cancer. **a** Axial contrast-enhanced CT image at the supraglottic level shows a hypopharyngeal tumor mass involving the medial wall (arrow) and the lateral wall (open arrow) of the piriform sinus, and the entire right aryepiglottic fold (ae). Invasion of the paraglottic space (thick white arrow), destruction of the posterior thyroid lamina (asterisk), and invasion of the prelaryngeal muscles. A large lymph node metastasis with central nodal necrosis (stealth arrow) is seen on the right. **b** Axial unenhanced T1W MR image shows a tumor mass with an intermediate signal intensity as it extends into the right paraglottic space (thick white arrow) and into the soft tissues of the neck (stealth arrow). Note the high signal intensity of the noninvaded left paraglottic space due to the high content of fatty tissue (thin black arrow). **c** Axial Gd-enhanced T1W image at the same level shows enhancement of the tumor mass invading the right paraglottic space, the thyroid cartilage, and the soft tissues of the neck. **d** Histological slice from specimen confirms tumor invasion of the right paraglottic space (thick arrow) and of the soft tissues of the neck (stealth arrows). t = thyroid cartilage; asterisks = normal left paraglottic space. The right and left thyroglottic ligaments, which separate the paraglottic from the preepiglottic space, are indicated by red dots. Note massive anterior displacement of the right thyroglottic ligament by the tumor mass. Reproduced from Reference 18 with permission

cally grow caudally into the apex.[128] Once they have reached the apex, they may spread either into the larynx invading the arytenoid, cricoarytenoid joint, and subglottis or they may spread into the postcricoid region of the hypopharynx. Further caudal spread results in invasion of the cricothyroid joint, extralaryngeal soft tissues, upper tracheoesophageal groove, and esophageal verge. Invasion of the esophageal verge may be submucosal and, therefore, undetectable at endoscopy (Fig. 11.24). However, on both axial CT and MR images invasion of the esophageal verge is easy to diagnose. Piriform sinus carcinoma frequently invades the laryngeal framework. Sites of predilection are at the cornua of the thyroid cartilage and at the superior border of the thyroid cartilage (at the transition site with the thyrohyoid membrane). Rarely, tumor may spread through the membrane along the point of penetration of the superior laryngeal neurovascular bundle.

Carcinoma of the Postcricoid Region

Carcinoma of the retrocricoarytenoid region, also called "postcricoid carcinoma," is a particular tumor type, which is uncommon in general but is observed in certain groups at risk, e.g., patients with the Plummer–Vinson (or Paterson–Brown–Kelly) syndrome.[8,69] These tumors spread submucosally, either circumferentially or toward the cervical esophagus. Because tumor growth is mainly submucosal, the true extent only becomes apparent with axial or sagittal CT or MR images (Fig. 11.25). Invasion of the cricoid cartilage is common, and in some cases the tumor may

11 Larynx and Hypopharynx

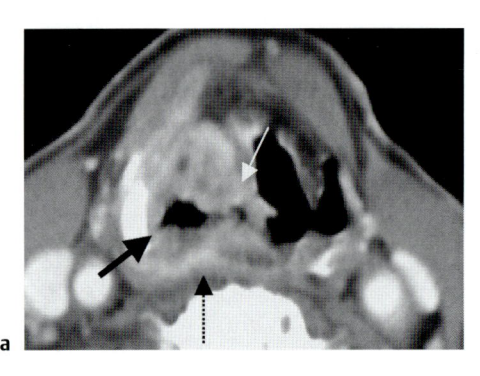

Fig. 11.**23** Invasion of the carotid artery by piriform sinus cancer. Contrast-enhanced CT images at the supraglottic level (**a** and **b**) and oropharynx level (**c**) show a piriform sinus tumor with invasion of the medial wall (thin arrows), lateral wall (thick arrows), and posterior wall (dashed arrows). The tumor extends into the prelaryngeal muscles through the thyrohyoid membrane (arrowhead). There is massive tumor spread along the parapharyngeal and retropharyngeal space (asterisks). The right internal carotid artery is surrounded by tumor (block arrow). **d** MR angiography performed in this patient confirms encasement of the right internal carotid artery by tumor (block arrows). Because surgical resection was not possible, the patient was treated with combined radiation therapy and chemotherapy.

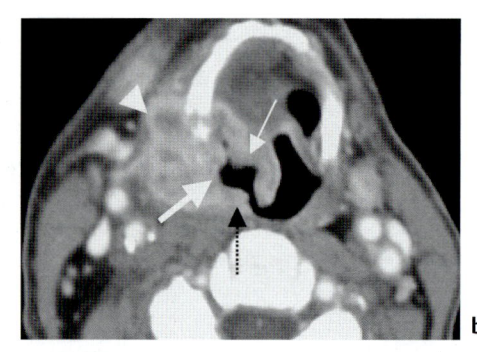

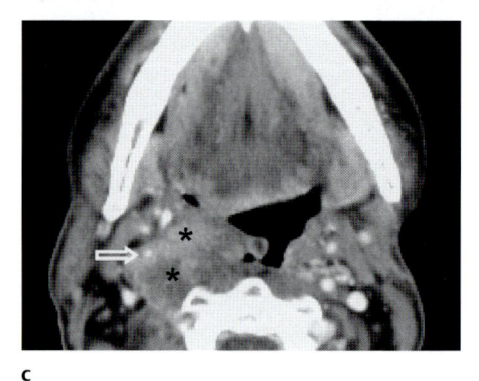

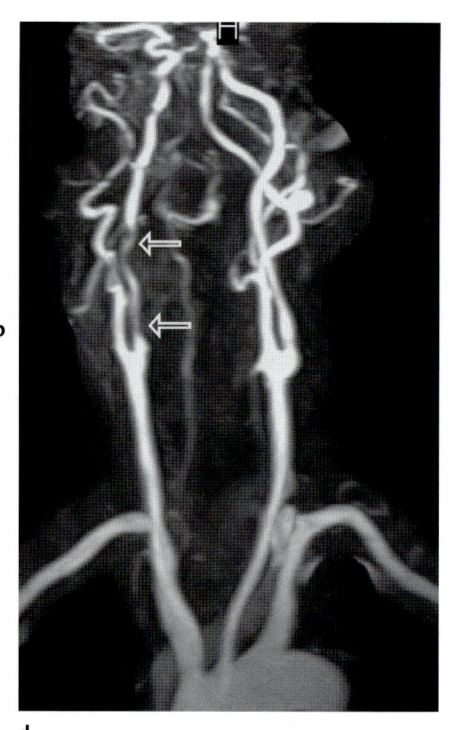

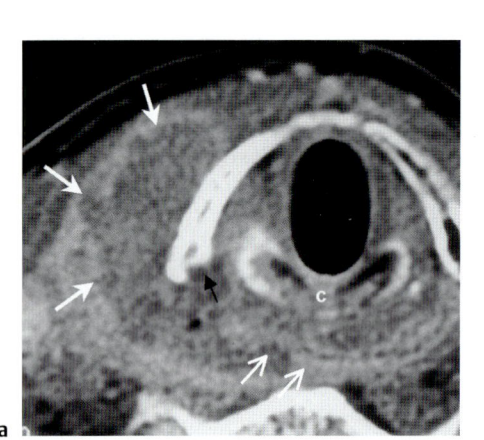

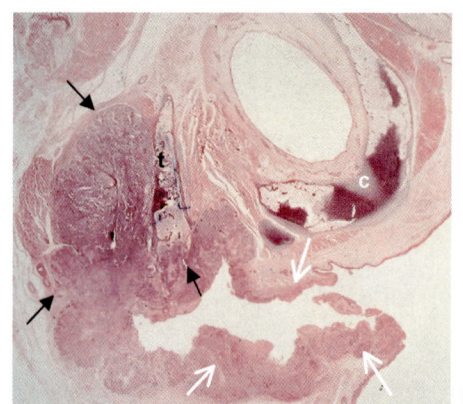

Fig. 11.**24** Invasion of the esophageal verge in a piriform sinus cancer. **a** Axial contrast-enhanced CT image at the subglottic level shows a piriform sinus tumor invading the posterior thyroid lamina (black arrow), the soft tissues of the neck (stealth arrows), and the esophageal verge submucosally (open arrows). c = cricoid cartilage. **b** Axial histological slice from specimen confirms submucosal tumor invasion of the esophageal verge (open arrows) and invasion of the thyroid cartilage and of the soft tissues of the neck (arrows). t = thyroid cartilage; c = cricoid cartilage. Reproduced from Reference 12 with permission.

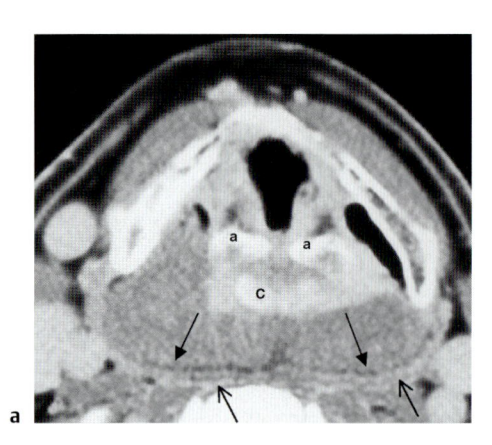

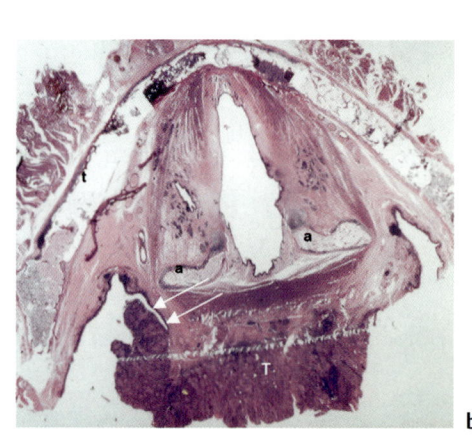

Fig. 11.**25** Postcricoid carcinoma of the hypopharynx. **a** Axial contrast-enhanced CT scan at the glottic level demonstrates a large tumor arising from the postcricoid region and extending into the right piriform sinus. The lumen of the hypopharynx is collapsed (arrows). Note strong enhancement of the normal mucosa over the posterior pharyngeal wall (open arrows). c = cricoid cartilage; a = arytenoid cartilage. **b** Whole-organ, axial histological slice from specimen confirms postcricoid tumor (T) with invasion of the medial wall of the piriform sinus (arrows). t = thyroid cartilage; a = arytenoid cartilage. Hematoxylin–eosin stain. Reproduced from Reference 8 with permission.

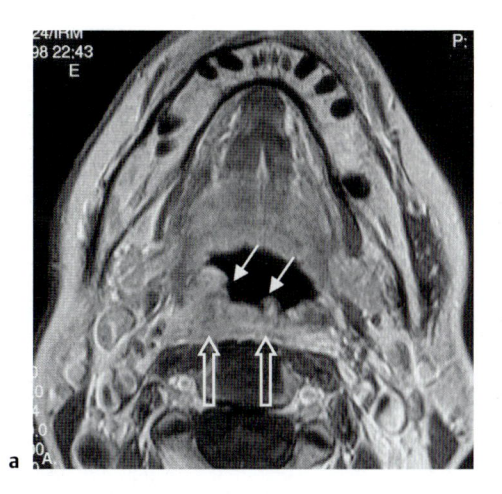

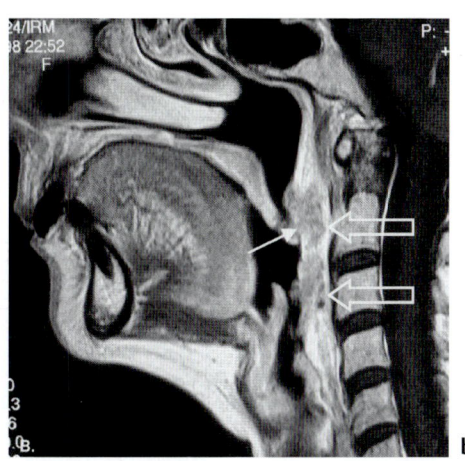

Fig. 11.**26** Posterior wall carcinoma. **a** Axial contrast-enhanced T1W MR image and **b** sagittal contrast-enhanced T1W MR image show a moderately enhancing tumor (arrows) involving the posterior wall of the oropharynx and hypopharynx. Note infiltration of the pharyngeal constrictor muscles and invasion of the retropharyngeal space (block arrows). The prevertebral muscles are not involved.

grow beyond the posterior cricoarytenoid muscle into the thyroid gland and cervical trachea. Perineural infiltration along the branches of the recurrent laryngeal nerve is another common feature of postcricoid carcinoma and results in reduced mobility or fixation of the vocal cord.

Carcinoma of the Posterior Pharyngeal Wall

Carcinoma of the posterior pharyngeal wall commonly presents as a flat, thick tumor spreading at the mucosal surface and often involves both the oropharynx and hypopharynx. These tumors are readily diagnosed at endoscopy, but sectional imaging is needed to evaluate the degree of submucosal spread. On axial CT or MR images, these tumors appear as asymmetrical thickening of the posterior pharyngeal wall (Fig. 11.**26**). Lateral spread of posterior pharyngeal wall cancer will result in invasion of the posterior wall of the piriform sinus followed by circumferential submucosal involvement. Most posterior pharyngeal wall tumors have a tendency to stop at about the level of the arytenoid cartilages. However, cephalad spread to the pharyngoepiglottic fold, glossotonsillar sulcus, and posterior oropharyngeal wall is common. Both spread to the postcricoid region and invasion of laryngeal cartilages are uncommon. Although invasion of the retropharyngeal space may be common initially, involvement of the prevertebral muscles is unusual at initial presentation (Fig. 11.**26**).

Squamous cell carcinoma of the hypopharynx has a relatively poor prognosis. This is because up to 75% of patients have metastases to cervical lymph nodes at initial presentation, and 20–40% of patients will also develop distant metastases.

■ Invasion of the Deep Paralaryngeal Spaces

Invasion of the deep paralaryngeal spaces (preepiglottic and paraglottic space) influences the tumor stage, the surgical approach, and the outcome of radiotherapy.[8, 55, 71, 79, 83, 80, 93, 94] Because endoscopic biopsy cannot detect neoplastic infiltration of the preepiglottic space and paraglottic space, CT and MRI are mandatory for this purpose. Invasion of the deep paralaryngeal spaces by squamous cell carcinoma influences surgical management. For example, invasion of the paraglottic space is a contraindication to vertical hemilaryngectomy. Although invasion of the preepiglottic space per se is not a contraindication to horizontal supraglottic laryngectomy, extensive neoplastic infiltration of the preepiglottic space may result in a more extensive horizontal supraglottic laryngectomy and sometimes supracricoid laryngectomy with cricohyoidopexy or even total laryngectomy (see below). Invasion of the preepiglottic space also influences the tumor stage. If the preepiglottic space is invaded, the tumor will be staged as T3 according to the UICC and AJCC guidelines.[55] Finally, invasion of the deep paralaryngeal spaces may affect prognosis. Most authors agree that invasion of the paraglottic space is often associated with a more aggressive tumor behavior, transglottic spread, a poorer prognosis, and a higher rate of local failure after radiotherapy.[56, 57, 75, 93, 94] Similarly, the degree of preepiglottic space involvement by tumor may also affect the outcome of definitive radiation therapy in supraglottic squamous cell carcinoma.[57, 80, 99]

Contrast-enhanced, thin-slice CT is a sensitive tool for detecting neoplastic invasion of the preepiglottic space and paraglottic space, the respective sensitivity values being from 92% to 100% in the preepiglottic space, and 95% in the paraglottic space.[8, 9, 78, 126] However, the specificity of CT may vary substantially from one space to another. In the preepiglottic space the specificity for tumor invasion is 90–93%, and in the paraglottic space CT is nonspecific (50%), thus indicating a strong tendency toward overestimation of tumor spread in this particular region. Most of the false-positive readings with CT are caused by peritumoral inflammatory reactions.[8, 126]

The sensitivity of MRI to detect neoplastic infiltration of the preepiglottic space is 100% and the specificity is 84–90%; the positive predictive value is 75–80%; and the negative predictive value is 100%.[8, 9, 71, 126] Most false-positive readings with MRI are caused by peritumoral inflammatory reactions within the preepiglottic space. A minority of the false-positive readings are caused by paraglottic space invasion or inflammation, which may be mistaken for preepiglottic tumor spread, as the thyroglottic ligament cannot be identified on current MR images. For the paraglottic space, MRI is not very specific, the reported values ranging from 50% to 76%[8, 126] (Fig. 11.**27**). Most of the false-positive readings are caused by peritumoral inflammatory reactions.

■ Cartilage Invasion

Neoplastic invasion of cartilage or bone is generally believed to diminish the response to radiation therapy, and to increase the risk of tumor recurrence and radiation-induced necrosis.[15, 26, 28, 33, 34] Several recent studies have shown that a variety of CT- and MR-based parameters, such as tumor volume, neoplastic cartilage invasion, and tumor invasion of the preepiglottic space, paraglottic space, and subglottis appear to be powerful predictors of local outcome in laryngeal and hypopharyngeal cancer treated with radiation therapy.[28, 56, 57, 66, 80, 93, 94] The grave prog-

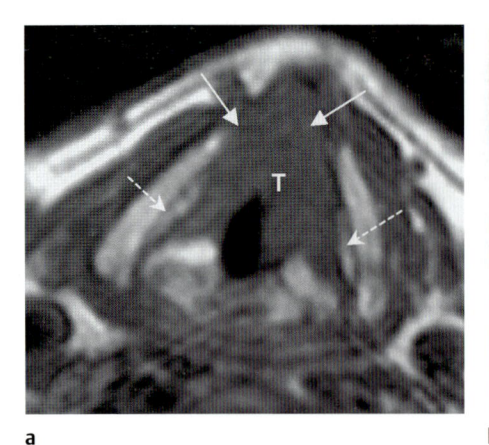

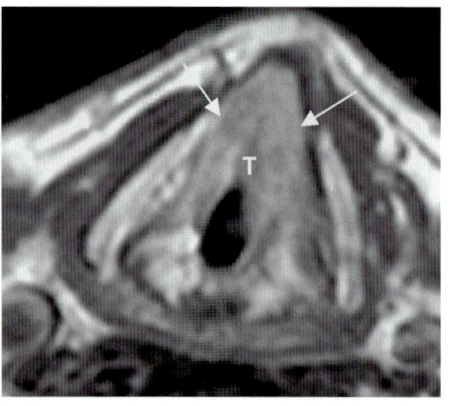

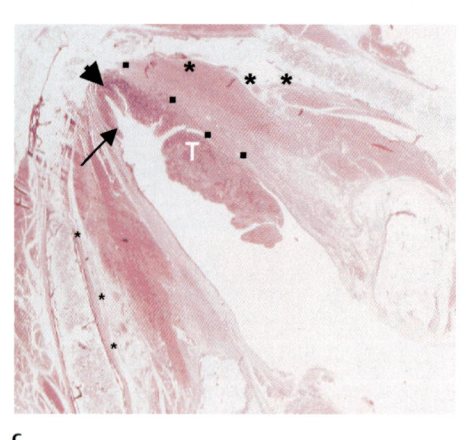

Fig. 11.27 False-positive MR examination for paraglottic space invasion. **a** Axial unenhanced T1W MR image at the glottic level. **b** Axial contrast-enhanced T1W MR image obtained at the same level. A tumor mass that involves both vocal cords (T) is seen. There is apparent extension into the paraglottic space anteriorly (thin white arrows). Note normal aspect of the posterior paraglottic space bilaterally (dashed arrows). **c** Whole-organ axial slice from surgical specimen (hematoxylin stain) shows that the tumor is relatively small (T) and that there are major inflammatory reactions within the vocal cords and paraglottic space anteriorly (asterisks) mimicking neoplastic invasion on MR. Short black arrow points at invasion of the anterior commissure. Thin black arrow points at mucosal involvement of the right vocal cord. The black dots on the left vocal cord delineate the depth of tumor invasion.

Table 11.1 Neoplastic invasion of the laryngeal cartilage: CT versus histology

Author (year)	Patients	Sensitivity	Specificity	Negative predictive value
Castelijns (1988)[27]	16	46%	91%	69%
Sulfaro (1989)[110]	71	47%	88%	—
Becker (1995)[18]	53	66%	94%	86%
Zbären (1996)[125]	40	67%	87%	82%
Becker (1997)[16]	111[a]	61%[a]	92%[a]	85%[a]
	111[b]	91%[b]	68%[b]	95%[b]

Modified with permission from reference 8.
All surgical specimens were evaluated by whole-organ histologic slices.
[a] Results obtained using a combination of the CT criteria extralaryngeal tumor spread and erosion or lysis applied to all cartilages.
[b] Results obtained using a combination of the CT criteria extralaryngeal tumor spread, sclerosis, and erosion or lysis applied to all cartilages.

nostic implication of invasion of cartilage by laryngeal and hypopharyngeal tumors is reflected in the TNM classification, leading automatically to a T4 classification.[55] Many authors believe that invasion of the cartilaginous framework of the larynx by tumor tissue implies that extensive surgery is the only way to offer curative treatment. Although this view has been disputed by some investigators,[28, 34, 87, 113, 117] there is no doubt that pretherapeutic assessment of cartilage invasion deserves particular attention. It is important for the radiologist to correctly diagnose its presence or absence on CT and MR images.

Histological Mechanisms of Cartilage Invasion and Accompanying Inflammatory Phenomena

Cartilage invasion occurs preferentially where the attachments of collagen bundles (Sharpey's fibers) interrupt the perichondrium, thus acting as direct pathways for tumor spread into the cartilaginous tissue. These areas typically include the anterior commissure tendon, the junction of the anterior one-fourth and posterior three-fourths of the lower thyroid lamina, the medial aspect of the posterior border of the thyroid lamina, the cricoarytenoid joint, and the area of attachment of the cricothyroid membrane.[64, 65, 97, 121]

A commonly held notion is that ossified cartilage is much more prone to be invaded by cancer than nonossified cartilage. This has been attributed to the activity of a tumor angiogenic factor (TAF), whereas nonossified cartilage is thought to be resistant to tumor infiltration owing to its capacity to release proteins that inhibit TAF and also collagenases.[24, 25, 46] Recent work has indicated, however, that invasion of nonossified hyaline cartilage may be more common than previously thought by showing that in 11% of invaded cartilages invasion was limited to nonossified portions, leaving ossified portions intact.[16] The suggested mechanism of laryngeal cartilage invasion by neoplastic tissue involves an osteoblastic phase in which hyaline cartilage is transformed into bone, which is followed by an osteoclastic phase in which the newly formed bone is eroded.[16, 20, 45, 46, 51, 52, 97] Osteoclasts are stimulated by prostaglandins and interleukin-1 released by tumor cells. This process is not bound to the direct presence of tumor cells within cartilage but occurs also as a reaction within cartilage in the vicinity of tumor; increased osteoblastic activity and new bone formation are, therefore, seen even before tumor penetrates the perichondrium. In summary, the process of neoplastic invasion of laryngeal cartilage involves three distinct phases: (1) inflammatory changes within cartilage adjacent to tumor, inducing bone remodeling (new bone formation and osteolysis) prior to actual tumor invasion; (2) major osteolysis; and (3) frank invasion by tumor cells.

Detection of Cartilage Invasion with CT

The CT features of the laryngeal cartilages in adults are explained by the different attenuation values of their three tissue components: cortical bone, marrow cavity with high fatty content, and nonossified hyaline cartilage. The ossification pattern of laryngeal cartilage, and particularly the thyroid cartilage, is quite variable. Although tumor tissue by itself has very similar attenuation values to nonossified cartilage, the presence of tumor may also be the cause of new bone formation and osteolysis in the adjacent cartilage. Therefore, patterns of ossification caused by neoplastic growth must thus be clearly distinguished from anatomical variants.

The accuracy of CT for the detection of laryngeal cartilage invasion varies considerably among different reports in the literature (Table 11.1). These discrepancies may in part be explained due to variable technical parameters. For example, older studies have been based on scan times of 4–9 s/slice and 4–6 mm section thickness and thus were more prone to motion and volume averaging artifacts than current standard protocols. Of more influence, however, are the diagnostic criteria used by the different

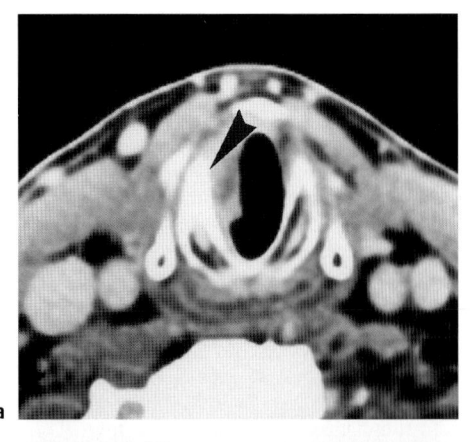

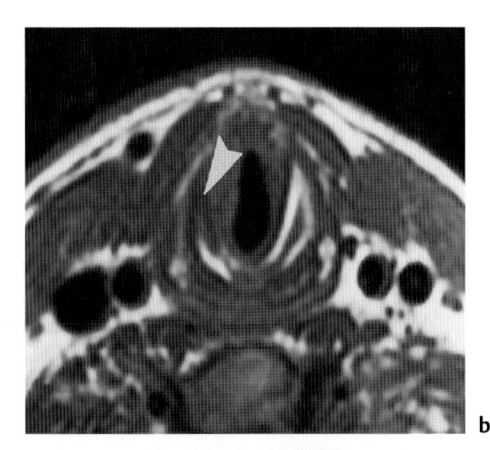

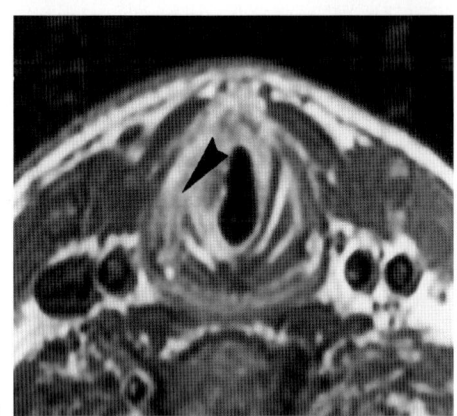

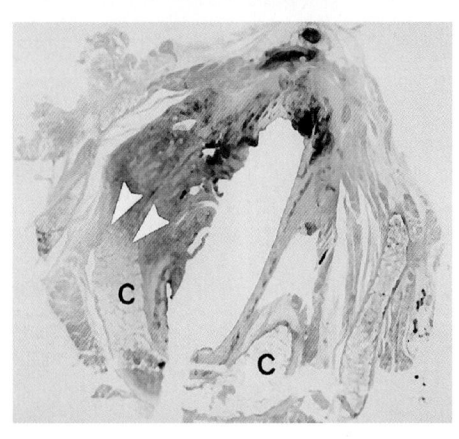

Fig. 11.**28** Neoplastic invasion of the cricoid cartilage detected by both CT and MRI. Glottosubglottic carcinoma of the larynx in a 46-year-old man. **a** Axial contrast-enhanced CT scan at the subglottic level. A mass with homogeneous contrast enhancement is infiltrating the right subglottic region. The cricoid cartilage shows asymmetric sclerosis (arrowhead), indicating cartilage invasion. Note preservation of the inner margin of the cricoid cartilage. **b** Axial T1W SE MR image. A mass with intermediate signal intensity infiltrates the right subglottic region. The right cricoid cartilage shows a decreased signal intensity (arrowhead). **c** Contrast-enhanced axial T1W SE MR image shows extensive contrast enhancement of the right subglottic tumor mass, as well as of the adjacent cricoid cartilage. The extensive enhancement of the right cricoid cartilage (arrowhead) suggests tumor invasion. **d** Axial slice from specimen at the same level shows a large subglottic tumor mass invading the right cricoid cartilage (arrowheads). c = cricoid cartilage. Reproduced from Reference 18 with permission.

investigators to assess invasion of each cartilage (Table 11.**1**). Until recently, the presence of tumor on both sides of a laryngeal cartilage was the only generally accepted diagnostic sign for tumor invasion on CT. Because this sign is positive only in an advanced stage, CT was long considered to be insensitive to cartilage invasion.[3, 27, 70, 110] In order to increase the sensitivity of CT, several other diagnostic signs have been proposed, including changes of the cartilage itself, namely sclerosis, obliteration of the medullary cavity, serpiginous contour, bowing, cartilaginous blow-out and the presence of tumor adjacent to nonossified cartilage.[16, 75, 91, 95, 96] A recent prospective study including 111 patients evaluated the usefulness of each of these criteria using sectional histopathological findings of the resected specimens as the gold standard.[16] Based on this study, four different diagnostic signs and their combinations can be recommended to detect neoplastic invasion of laryngeal cartilage on CT, namely extralaryngeal tumor spread, sclerosis, erosion and lysis. Each of these CT signs corresponds to distinct histological findings and has either a high sensitivity or a high specificity.

Sclerosis is a sensitive sign for the detection of neoplastic cartilage invasion and enables diagnosis of early perichondrial invasion or microscopic intracartilaginous tumor spread (Figs. 11.**18**, 11.**28**).[16, 91] The specificity of this sign varies considerably from one cartilage to another, being lowest in the thyroid cartilage (40%) and higher in the cricoid and arytenoid cartilages (76% and 79%, respectively).[16] Therefore, if a tumor mass is seen adjacent to a sclerotic cartilage, this does not automatically imply that tumor cells are found within the remodeled marrow cavity (Fig. 11.**29**). Conversely, failure at surgery to remove a cartilage that exhibits sclerosis on CT carries a 50–60% risk of leaving tumor behind.

As the process of cartilage invasion progresses, minor and major osteolysis is seen within the areas of new bone formation. Minor areas of osteolysis correspond to the CT criteria of **erosion**, while major areas of osteolysis correspond to the CT criteria of **lysis** (Figs. 11.**30**, 11.**31**). Histologically, erosion and lysis correspond to destruction of bone due to osteoclastic activity, and a direct contact between receding bone and tumor cells is seen within these lytic areas. As a consequence, erosion and lysis can be considered specific criteria for the detection of neoplastic invasion in all cartilages (Figs. 11.**30**, 11.**31**). The overall specificity of erosion and lysis is 93%. However, neither of these criteria is very sensitive as they are bound to the presence of more advanced invasion of laryngeal cartilage.

Extralaryngeal spread occurs due to tumor invasion through a cartilage into the extralaryngeal soft tissues (Figs. 11.**20**, 11.**22**, 11.**32**). This CT criterion is highly specific (overall specificity, 95%) but, because it is only seen very late in the disease process, its sensitivity is as low as 44%. Using the combination of extralaryngeal tumor, sclerosis, and erosion/lysis applied to all cartilages, an overall sensitivity as high as 91% may be obtained (Table 11.**1**). Because the negative predictive value of this combination is 95%, CT may be considered as an excellent test to exclude cartilage invasion prior to treatment. On the other hand, the associated overall specificity of only 68% appears quite low because it is very difficult and impractical to confirm cartilage invasion by means of biopsy. The use of extralaryngeal tumor and erosion/lysis applied to all cartilages yields a specificity of 92%, but the associated sensitivity is only 61% (Table 11.**1**).

Detection of Cartilage Invasion with MRI

The diagnosis of neoplastic cartilage invasion on MRI is mainly based on altered signal behavior of hyaline cartilage and fatty marrow on the different pulse sequences.[16, 18, 27, 28] On T2-weighted MR images, hyaline cartilage invaded by tumor displays

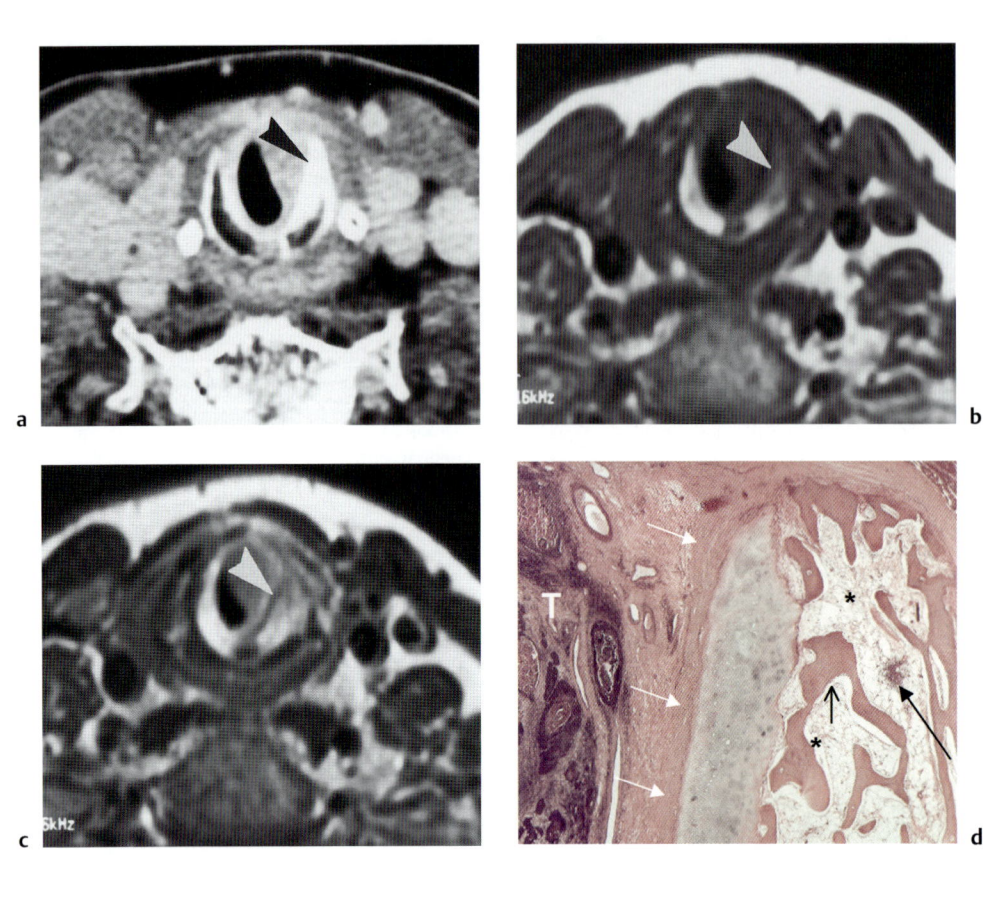

Fig. 11.29 CT and MRI false-positive for neoplastic cartilage invasion due to inflammatory changes in the noninvaded cricoid cartilage. Glottosubglottic carcinoma of the larynx in a 71-year-old woman. **a** Axial contrast-enhanced CT scan at the subglottic level. A mass with homogeneous contrast enhancement is infiltrating the left subglottic region. The left cricoid cartilage shows extensive sclerosis in the tumor's vicinity (arrowhead), suggestive of cartilage invasion. **b** Axial T1W SE MR image. A mass with low signal intensity infiltrates the left subglottic region. The adjacent left cricoid cartilage shows a decreased signal intensity (arrowhead). **c** Contrast-enhanced T1W SE MR image. Contrast enhancement is seen within the left cricoid cartilage (arrowhead) as well as within the subglottic tumor mass. **d** Axial slice from specimen shows a large, left-sided subglottic tumor mass (T) but no evidence of cartilage invasion. The cricoid cartilage shows extensive inflammatory changes with lymph follicles (black arrow), fibrosis (asterisks), and bone resorption (open arrow), but with an intact perichondrium (white arrows). Reproduced from Reference 18 with permission.

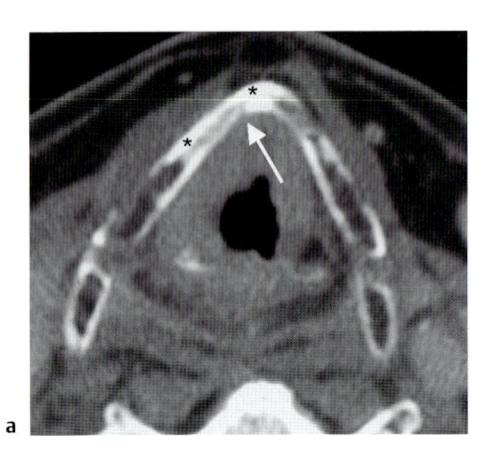

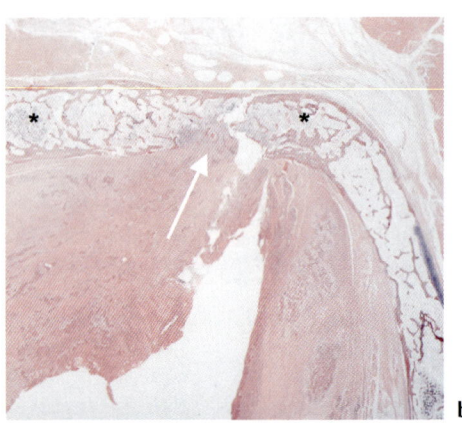

Fig. 11.30 Erosion of the thyroid cartilage in a transglottic cancer. **a** Contrast-enhanced CT scan obtained at the false-cord level shows a tumor mass that abuts the thyroid cartilage. The right thyroid lamina demonstrates a small erosion (arrow) and extensive sclerosis (asterisks). **b** Corresponding axial slice from surgical specimen confirms minor invasion of the thyroid cartilage (arrow) corresponding to the small erosion seen on CT. Note increased density of bone trabeculae (asterisks) surrounding the area of actual invasion and corresponding to sclerosis seen in **a**. Reproduced from Reference 8 with permission.

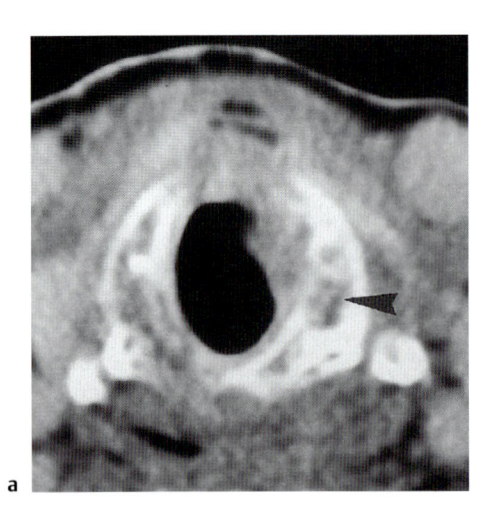

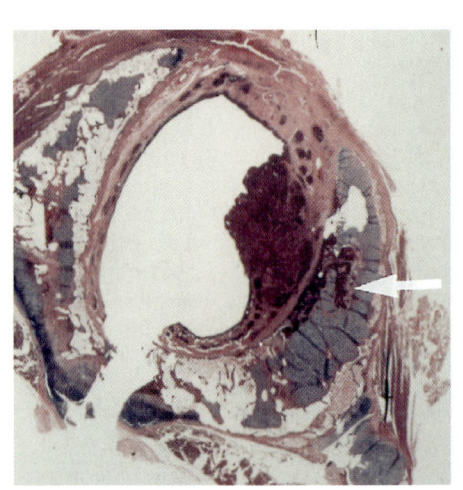

Fig. 11.31 Lysis and sclerosis of the cricoid cartilage in a glottic-subglottic cancer. **a** Contrast-enhanced CT scan obtained at the subglottic level shows a tumor mass that abuts the cricoid cartilage. The left cricoid lamina demonstrates an area of lysis (arrowhead) surrounded by extensive sclerosis. **b** Corresponding axial slice from a surgical specimen at the same level confirms major intracartilaginous tumor spread (arrow) corresponding to lysis seen on CT. Reproduced from Reference 8 with permission.

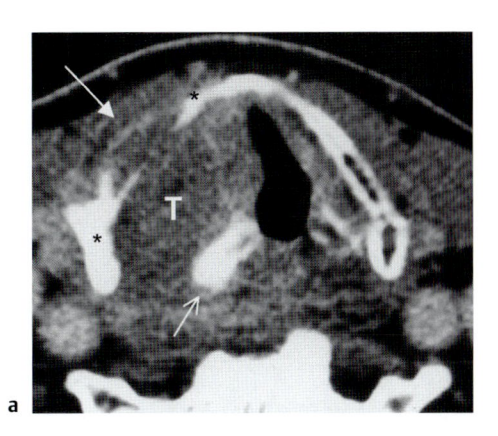

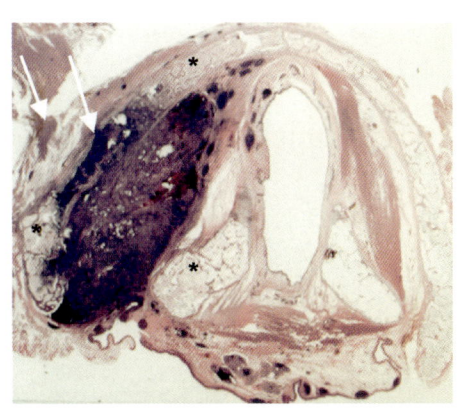

Fig. 11.**32** "Extralaryngeal spread" in a piriform sinus cancer. **a** Contrast-enhanced axial CT scan shows a large tumor mass (T) arising from the right piriform sinus invading the paraglottic space. The right thyroid cartilage displays "extralaryngeal tumor" (arrow) and "sclerosis" (asterisks). The right arytenoid cartilage demonstrates "sclerosis" (open arrow) and an increase in size compared to the contralateral arytenoid cartilage. **b** Axial slice from specimen shows invasion of the thyroid cartilage and of the prelaryngeal muscles (arrows) and no invasion of the arytenoid cartilage. Increased density of bony trabeculae due to new bone formation in the right thyroid cartilage and in the right arytenoid cartilage (asterisks) corresponds to "sclerosis" seen in **a**. Reproduced from Reference 16 with permission.

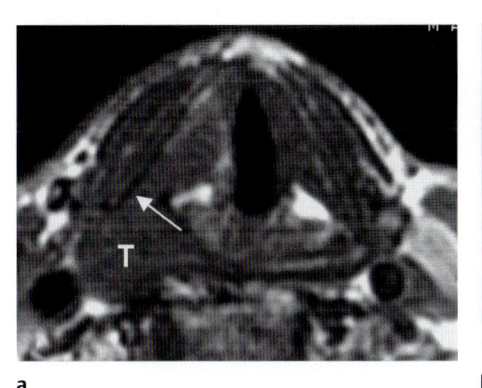

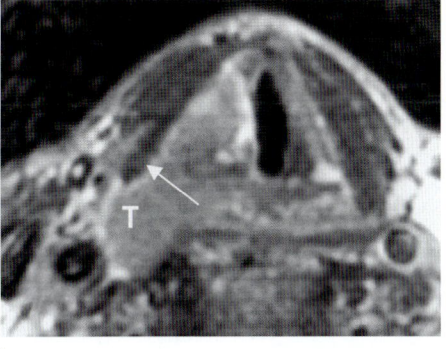

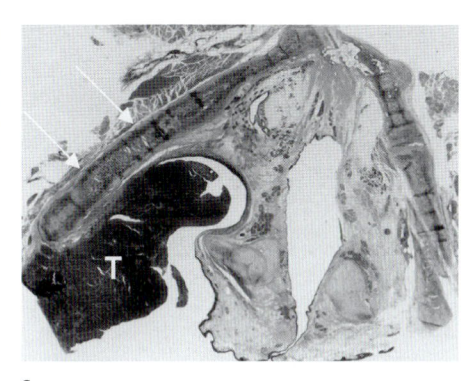

Fig. 11.**33** MRI true negative for neoplastic invasion of the thyroid cartilage. **a** T1W SE image obtained at the supraglottic level shows a right-sided piriform sinus tumor with intermediate to low signal intensity (T). The adjacent right thyroid lamina shows an intermediate to low signal intensity as well (arrow). **b** T1W SE image obtained after intravenous administration of contrast material shows contrast enhancement of the tumor mass (T) but no enhancement of the adjacent thyroid lamina (arrow). This suggests that the thyroid cartilage is composed of non-ossified hyaline cartilage and that no intracartilaginous tumor spread is present. **c** Corresponding axial slice from a surgical specimen at the same level confirms that the right thyroid lamina is composed of nonossified hyaline cartilage (arrows). No cartilage invasion was found at histology. The tumor (T) arises from the lateral wall of the right piriform sinus. Reproduced from Reference 8 with permission.

a higher signal intensity than normal cartilage. On unenhanced T1-weighted MR images, invaded hyaline cartilage and invaded fatty marrow display a low to intermediate signal intensity similar to tumor tissue, whereas areas of enhancement adjacent to the tumor are seen after i.v. injection of gadolinium chelates (Fig. 11.**28**). If these signs are absent, cartilage infiltration can be ruled out with a high level of confidence (Fig. 11.**33**), as indicated by a very high negative predictive value (Table 11.**2**). Unfortunately, the MR findings suggesting neoplastic cartilage invasion are not as specific as expected initially but may be false-positive in a considerable number of instances, as indicated by a positive predictive value of only 68–71%. This is because reactive inflammation, edema, and fibrosis in the vicinity of the tumor may display similar diagnostic features to cartilage infiltrated by tumor (Fig. 11.**29**). Since peritumoral inflammatory changes are most commonly observed in the thyroid cartilage, the specificity of MR imaging to detect neoplastic invasion of the thyroid cartilage is only 56% as opposed to 87% and 95% in the cricoid and arytenoid cartilages.[18] The positive diagnosis of neoplastic invasion of the thyroid cartilage should, therefore, be made with caution on MR imaging. On the other hand, extensive tumor invasion involving both inner and outer aspects of the cartilage (i.e., corresponding to the CT criteria of extralaryngeal tumor) can be diagnosed with a high accuracy with MR imaging (Fig. 11.**22**). The results of MR imaging reported in the literature are summarized in Table 11.**2**. Because all authors have used the same criteria to assess cartilage invasion by means of MRI, the reported overall results do not vary considerably except for minor differences that may be explained by influences of sample size and patient characteristics.

Because of their high sensitivity and high negative predictive value, both CT and MRI are currently considered to be suitable and nearly equivalent imaging methods for pretherapeutic evaluation of cartilage invasion. False-positive results, however, are inevitable with both imaging modalities. Despite the entirely different physical mechanisms by which tissue is interrogated with CT and MRI, the tendency toward "overreading" tumor involvement is strikingly parallel with regard to each individual cartilage (Fig. 11.**29**). This may be because the underlying pathological process leading to overestimation of neoplastic cartilage invasion is the same, namely, reactive inflammation.

Table 11.**2** Neoplastic invasion of the laryngeal cartilage: MRI versus histology

Author (year)	Patients	Sensitivity	Specificity	Negative predictive value
Castelijns (1988)[27]	16	89%	88%	92%
Becker (1995)[18]	53	89%	84%	94%
Zbären (1996)[125]	40	94%	74%	96%

Modified with permission from reference 8.
All surgical specimens were evaluated by whole-organ histological slices.

Table 11.3 Classification of primary tumor (T) for carcinoma of the larynx according to UICC and AJCC[106a]

T Primary tumor
TX	Primary tumor cannot be assessed
T0	No evidence of primary tumor
Tis	Carcinoma in situ

Supraglottis
T1	Tumor limited to one subsite of supraglottis with normal vocal cord mobility
T2	Tumor invades more than one adjacent subsite of supraglottis or glottis or region outside the supraglottis (e.g., mucosa of the base of the tongue, vallecula, medial wall of the piriform sinus), without fixation of the larynx
T3	Tumor limited to larynx with vocal cord fixation and/or invasion of postcricoid area, preepiglottic space, paraglottic space and/or with minor thyroid cartilage erosion (e.g., inner cortex)
T4a	Tumor invades through the thyroid cartilage and/or invades soft tissues beyond the larynx, e.g., trachea, soft tissues of the neck including deep/extrinsic muscle of tongue (genioglossus, hyoglossus, palatoglossus, and styloglossus), strap muscles, thyroid, esophagus
T4b	Tumor invades prevertebral space, mediastinal structures, or encases carotid artery

Glottis
T1	Tumor limited to vocal cord(s) may involve anterior or posterior commissure with normal mobility
T1a	Tumor limited to one vocal cord
T1b	Tumor involves both vocal cords
T2	Tumor extends to supraglottis or subglottis or with impaired vocal cord mobility
T3	Tumor limited to the larynx with vocal cord fixation and/or invades paraglottic space, and/or with minor thyroid cartilage erosion (e.g., inner cortex)
T4a	Tumor invades through the thyroid cartilage and/or invades soft tissues beyond the larynx, e.g., trachea, soft tissues of the neck including deep/extrinsic muscle of tongue (genioglossus, hyoglossus, palatoglossus, and styloglossus), strap muscles, thyroid, esophagus
T4b	Tumor invades prevertebral space, mediastinal structures, or encases carotid artery

Subglottis
T1	Tumor limited to the subglottis
T2	Tumor extends to vocal cord(s) with normal or impaired mobility
T3	Tumor limited to the larynx with vocal cord fixation
T4a	Tumor invades through the thyroid cartilage and/or invades soft tissues beyond the larynx, e.g., trachea, soft tissues of the neck including deep/extrinsic muscle of tongue (genioglossus, hyoglossus, palatoglossus, and styloglossus), strap muscles, thyroid, esophagus
T4b	Tumor invades prevertebral space, mediastinal structures, or encases carotid artery

N Regional lymph nodes
NX	Regional lymph nodes cannot be assessed
N0	No regional lymph node metastasis
N1	Metastasis in a single ipsilateral lymph node, less than 3 cm
N2	Metastasis in a single ipsilateral lymph node between 3 and 6 cm; or in multiple ipsilateral lymph nodes, none more than 6 cm in greatest dimension; or in bilateral or contralateral lymph nodes, none more than 6 cm in greatest dimension
N2a	Metastasis in a single ipsilateral lymph node between 3 and 6 cm
N2b	Metastasis in multiple ipsilateral lymph nodes, none more than 6 cm in greatest dimension
N2c	Metastasis in bilateral or contralateral lymph nodes, none more than 6 cm in greatest dimension
N3	Metastasis in a lymph node greater than 6 cm

M Distant metastasis
MX	Distant metastasis cannot be assessed
M0	No distant metastasis
M1	Distant metastasis

Table 11.4 Classification of primary tumor (T) for carcinoma of the hypopharynx according to UICC and AJCC[106a]

T Primary tumor
TX	Primary tumor cannot be assessed
T0	No evidence of primary tumor
Tis	Carcinoma in situ
T1	Tumor limited to one subsite of the hypopharynx and 2 cm or less in greatest dimension
T2	Tumor invades more than one subsite of hypopharynx or an adjacent site, or measures more than 2 cm but less than 4 cm in greatest dimension without fixation of hemilarynx
T3	Tumor measures more than 4 cm in greatest dimension, or with fixation of hemilarynx
T4a	Tumor invades any of the following: thyroid or cricoid cartilage, hyoid bone, thyroid gland, esophagus, central compartment soft tissue (prelaryngeal strap muscles and subcutaneous fat)
T4b	Tumor invades prevertebral fascia, encases carotid artery, or invades mediastinal structures

N Regional lymph nodes
NX	Regional lymph nodes cannot be assessed
N0	No regional lymph node metastasis
N1	Metastasis in a single ipsilateral lymph node, less than 3 cm
N2	Metastasis in a single ipsilateral lymph node between 3 and 6 cm; or in multiple ipsilateral lymph nodes, none more than 6 cm in greatest dimension; or in bilateral or contralateral lymph nodes, none more than 6 cm in greatest dimension
N2a	Metastasis in a single ipsilateral lymph node between 3 and 6 cm
N2b	Metastasis in multiple ipsilateral lymph nodes, none more than 6 cm in greatest dimension
N2c	Metastasis in bilateral or contralateral lymph nodes, none more than 6 cm in greatest dimension
N3	Metastasis in a lymph node greater than 6 cm

M Distant metastasis
MX	Distant metastasis cannot be assessed
M0	No distant metastasis
M1	Distant metastasis

■ Pretherapeutic T-Classification According to the TNM System

The purpose of tumor staging according to the TNM system is to facilitate clinical research and to help assess the prognosis, both in order to aid the clinician in planning treatment in a given case. The staging criteria for laryngeal and hypopharyngeal carcinoma proposed by the UICC and the AJCC are now almost identical.[55, 106a] The degree of invasion of the primary tumor is most accurately reflected in the *postsurgical* (pT) classification, which is based on histopathological analysis of the resected specimen. The *clinical or pretherapeutic* (T) classification of the primary tumor is used in patients who do not undergo surgery. It is based on all information available prior to treatment, including findings at physical examination, endoscopy, biopsy, and sectional imaging. Local findings affecting the pretherapeutic T-classification of laryngeal and hypopharyngeal cancer vary from one subsite to another and are summarized in Tables 11.3 and 11.4. According to the considerations above, it is obvious that involvement of adjacent subsites often occurs as a result of submucosal spread and can therefore be detected only by sectional imaging.

Although sectional imaging is recommended in the guidelines of the UICC and the AJCC, no recommendations are made regarding the preference of MR imaging or CT. Several studies published in the literature as well as our experience indicate that the use of sectional imaging by either CT or MR imaging may greatly improve the accuracy of pretherapeutic T-classification of laryngeal and hypopharyngeal tumors.[2, 8, 47, 60, 68, 74, 75, 106, 110, 125–127] Al-

Table 11.**5** Overall pretherapeutic staging accuracy for laryngeal and hypopharyngeal cancer, as reported by several study groups

Author (year)	Patients	Tumor origin	CE	CE–CT	CE–MRI
Sulfaro (1989)[110]	71	Larynx and hypopharynx	59%	88%	–
Vogl (1991)[118]	28	Larynx and hypopharynx	64%	–	86%
Zbären (1996)[125]	40	Larynx	57%	80%	87%
Thabet (1996)[116]	98	Larynx and hypopharynx	52%	84%	–
Becker (1997)[8]	111	Larynx and hypopharynx	58%	80%	85%

Modified with permission from reference 8.
The staging accuracy was evaluated considering the pathological stage (pT) as gold standard.
Abbreviations: CE = clinical evaluation including direct laryngoscopy and biopsy; CE–CT = combined information from clinical evaluation, including direct laryngoscopy and biopsy and CT; CE–MRI = combined information from clinical evaluation, including direct laryngoscopy and biopsy and MRI.

Table 11.**6** Atypical forms of squamous cell carcinoma: characteristic radiological features

Atypical forms of squamous cell carcinoma	Tumor location	Enhancement pattern, morphology	Lymph node metastases
Undifferentiated carcinoma of nasopharyngeal type	Supraglottis, hypopharynx, submucosal location	Homogenous enhancement pattern, large tumor mass, no ulceration, no necrosis, no cartilage invasion	Yes
Verrucous carcinoma	Glottis	Inhomogenous enhancement, exophytic mass with a rugged surface, limited deep infiltration, rarely cartilage invasion	No
Spindle cell carcinoma	Supraglottis	Inhomogenous enhancement, bulky, ulcerated lesion, thin stalk	Variable
Basaloid cell carcinoma	Piriform sinus and retrocricoarytenoid region	Inhomogenous, distinct lobulated enhancement pattern on contrast-enhanced T1W SE images	Yes, extranodal spread

Modified with permission from reference 14.

though the staging accuracy of clinical examination with endoscopy alone may be only around 60%, it is increased significantly when combined with either CT or MRI (Table 11.**5**). In addition, the accuracy of clinical staging may vary with regard to the primary tumor site, deteriorating from glottic to supraglottic to transglottic tumors.[60] Conversely, the staging accuracy of sectional imaging is best in transglottic tumors and supraglottic tumors, thus indicating a complementary role for clinical examination/endoscopy and CT/MRI.[110] Regardless of the tumor subsite, several investigators have reported that small mucosal tumors (pT1) were assessed more easily by laryngoscopy, whereas CT/MRI was superior in the evaluation of large (pT3 and pT4) tumors.[60,110,116] In conclusion, data from the literature corroborate the relevance of routine use of either CT or MRI as an adjunct to clinical evaluation and laryngoscopy to improve pretherapeutic staging accuracy.

■ Atypical Forms of Squamous Cell Carcinoma

The term "atypical forms of squamous cell carcinoma" is used for certain distinct histopathological variants of laryngeal and hypopharyngeal carcinoma with different biological behavior, namely, undifferentiated carcinoma of nasopharyngeal type, verrucous carcinoma, spindle cell carcinoma, basaloid cell carcinoma, adenoid squamous cell carcinoma, and giant-cell carcinoma.[1,6,4,14,41,43] According to the literature, 2–7% of all laryngeal and hypopharyngeal tumors are atypical forms of squamous cell carcinoma. These tumors may differ from the common type of squamous cell carcinoma in several aspects regarding diagnosis, prognosis, and therapeutic approach.

Undifferentiated Carcinoma of Nasopharyngeal Type

Undifferentiated carcinoma of nasopharyngeal type is an unusual variant of squamous cell carcinoma with a distinct lymphoid component.[6,14,41,86] Synonyms used in the literature for this tumor include lymphoepithelial carcinoma, undifferentiated carcinoma of nasopharyngeal type, and Schmincke–Regaud lymphoepithelioma. The tumor mainly affects men between 50 and 70 years of age. Infection with the Epstein–Barr virus (EBV) appears to play an important etiological role. The tumor, which is often covered by intact mucosa at endoscopy, most commonly arises in the supraglottic region or in the piriform sinus because these regions are very rich in lymphatic tissue (Table 11.**6**). Since the tumor is rather deep-seated, biopsies must be obtained from beneath the mucosa or the lesion will be missed. Undifferentiated carcinoma of nasopharyngeal type often metastasizes to the cervical lymph nodes and sometimes to the lungs or other organs, and cervical lymph node metastases may be the first presenting symptom. Radiotherapy alone or in combination with chemotherapy appears to be effective in eradicating localized disease. The most striking feature in this particular tumor type is the discrepancy between an intact mucosa at endoscopy and a solid mass having similar imaging features as the common form of squamous cell carcinoma[14] (Fig. 11.**34**). Interestingly, despite the large size of the tumor mass and widespread invasion of the paraglottic space, no cartilage invasion may be seen on sectional imaging. However, CT and MRI may often detect lymph node metastases, typically involving both sides of the neck.

Verrucous Carcinoma

Verrucous carcinoma, or Ackerman tumor, has a reported incidence of 1–4% of all laryngeal cancers.[6,14,43] It must not be confused with the common form of squamous cell carcinoma as it differs both in structural characteristics and in prognosis, which is

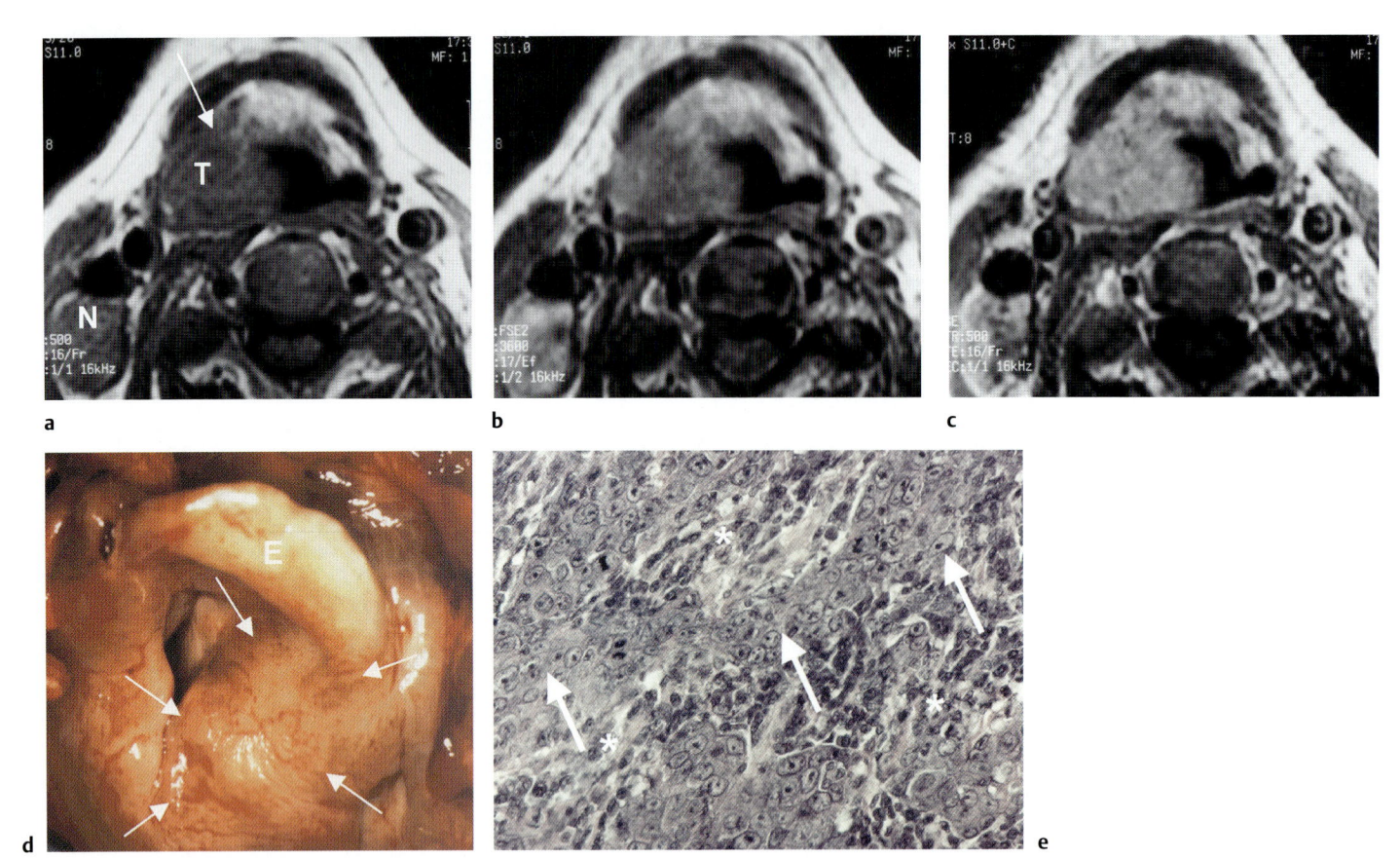

Fig. 11.34 Undifferentiated carcinoma of nasopharyngeal type. MRI appearance in a 76-year-old man with multiple palpable neck masses. Endoscopically, the right aryepiglottic fold was thicker than the left aryepiglottic fold; the mucosa was intact, however. **a** Axial T1W SE image. A tumor mass (T) with low signal intensity invades the right aryepiglottic fold and the paraglottic fat (arrow). N = large metastatic lymph node. **b** Axial T2W FSE image. Slight increase in signal intensity within the tumor mass and within the metastatic lymph node. **c** Contrast-enhanced, axial T1W SE image. Moderate homogeneous enhancement without intratumoral necrosis. Deep submucosal biopsy revealed undifferentiated carcinoma of nasopharyngeal type. The patient underwent total laryngectomy and bilateral neck dissection. **d** Gross surgical specimen viewed from posteriorly and above. The large supraglottic tumor (arrows) is covered by an intact mucosa. E = epiglottis. **e** High-power micrograph showing cords of large, pale epithelial cells with indistinct cell boundaries and vesicular nuclei (arrows) overrun by small lymphocytes (asterisks), characteristic of undifferentiated carcinoma of nasopharyngeal type. Hematoxylin–eosin stain. The patient is free of recurrence six years later. Reproduced from Reference 14 with permission.

excellent when adequate treatment is adopted from the beginning. It occurs predominantly in men in their seventies and eighties and presents clinically as a warty, bulky outgrowth with multiple filiform projections, usually affecting one vocal cord (Fig. 11.35). Viral infection with the human papilloma virus (HPV) type 16 plays an important etiological role.[22] Verrucous carcinoma of the larynx almost never metastizes to the lymph nodes.[6, 14, 43] Considerable controversy exists as to the correct treatment for this tumor. A recurrence rate of 51–71 % after radiation therapy has been reported as opposed to only 7 % recurrence rate after surgery.[43] In addition, several authors have reported a high risk of postirradiation anaplastic or sarcomatoid changes, the latent period for anaplastic transformation being as short as a few months. Surgery alone is, therefore, considered in most centers as the treatment of choice and in most cases the lesion is amenable to conservative surgery (cordectomy, partial voice-preserving laryngectomy). Because cervical and distant metastases have not been reported in verrucous carcinoma, operative treatment typically does not include neck dissection. As suggested by several authors, multiple biopsies may be necessary to establish the diagnosis when a clinically malignant-appearing lesion contradicts a benign histological appearance.[14] The radiological aspect may be of additional help not only in suggesting a diagnosis other than the common form of squamous cell cancer but also in urging additional biopsies so as to obtain the definitive, correct histological diagnosis. Based on the findings of a recent series, verrucous carcinoma may display a characteristic radiological aspect: an exophytic mass with a rugged surface and fingerlike, deep projections; limited deep tumor infiltration; moderate enhancement after administration of contrast material; and absence of lymph node metastases (Table 11.**6**) (Fig. 11.**35**).

Spindle Cell Carcinoma

Spindle cell carcinoma is a rare biphasic variant of squamous cell carcinoma in which a pseudosarcomatous component dominates the microscopic appearance of the tumor. Various synonymous terms have been used to designate this tumor, including spindle cell squamous carcinoma, pseudosarcoma, and pleomorphic carcinoma.[6, 14, 29] The larynx is the most common site, followed by the oral cavity and esophagus.[6, 29] Although these tumors have the same age and sex predilection as the common type of squamous cell carcinoma, most spindle cell carcinomas have been reported to have a highly exophytic, polypoid shape. The tumor arises predominantly from the supraglottic region and two-thirds of the tumors present endoscopically as pedunculated masses attached to the mucosa by a stalk. The treatment of choice is surgery and neck dissection is often indicated. Spindle cell carcinoma may display a characteristic radiological aspect: large, exophytic, pedunculated, masses arising from the supraglottic region or piriform sinus, with inhomogeneous contrast enhancement and with a thin stalk (Table 11.**6**) (Fig. 11.**36**).

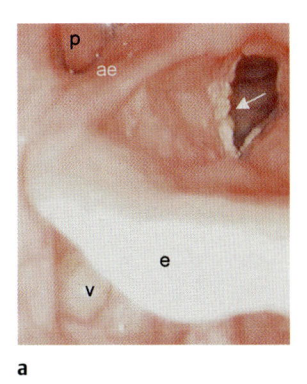

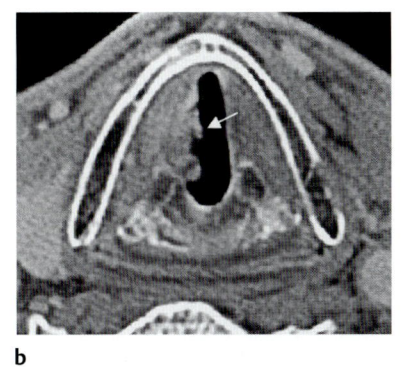

Fig. 11.**35** Verrucous carcinoma. Characteristic endoscopic, CT, and histological appearance in a 73-year-old patient with hoarseness. **a** Image obtained during indirect laryngoscopy shows a white tumor mass (arrow) with characteristic filiform projections arising from the right vocal cord. ae = aryepiglottic folds; e = epiglottis; p = piriform sinus; v = vallecula. **b** Axial CT image (bone window setting) demonstrates the right-sided tumor mass involving the true vocal cord and with a characteristic rugged surface with fingerlike projections (arrow). The patient underwent endoscopic biopsy. **c** Low-power micrograph demonstrates long filiform processes of highly differentiated squamous epithelial cells (asterisks) covered by keratinized cells (arrows). The margins of the tumor are pushing and blunt (open arrows) rather than infiltrating. In advance of the tumor margins a severe inflammatory reaction is seen (thick arrows). Reproduced from Reference 14 with permission.

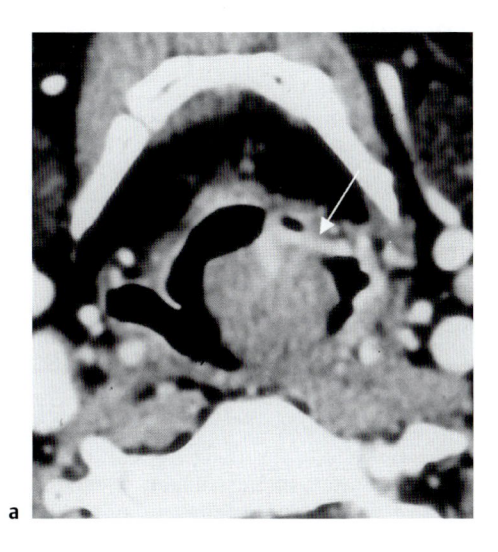

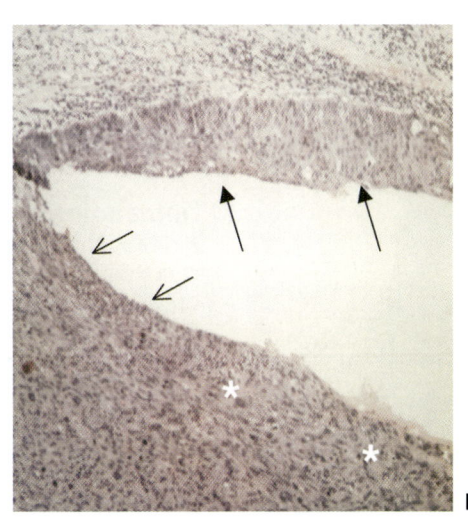

Fig. 11.**36** Spindle cell carcinoma. Characteristic CT and histological appearance in a 67-year-old man presenting with dyspnea. A large pedunculated mass attached to the mucosa of the left aryepiglottic fold by a stalk was seen endoscopically. **a** Axial contrast-enhanced CT image demonstrates a polypoid mass with moderate homogenous enhancement attached to the mucosa by a thin stalk (arrow). **b** Low-power micrograph obtained through the stalk of the tumor demonstrates the transition between intact mucosa (arrows), marked dysplasia (open arrows), and squamous cell carcinoma (asterisks). The patient underwent total laryngectomy followed by radiation therapy and is free of recurrence six years later. Reproduced from Reference 14 with permission.

Basaloid Cell Carcinoma

Basaloid squamous cell carcinoma (also called basaloid cell carcinoma) is a rare tumor with a mixed basaloid and squamous component.[4,6,7,14] It is thought to arise from a pluripotent primitive cell located at the base of the pseudostratified columnar epithelium. The predilection sites are the supraglottic larynx, hypopharynx, and base of the tongue. The prognosis is usually worse than that of the common type of squamous cell carcinoma. The tumor is, therefore, regarded as a high-grade malignancy with a tendency for locally aggressive behavior and early regional and distant metastases. The most common sites of metastatic spread are the cervical lymph nodes followed by the lung, bone, and skin. The treatment of choice is surgery followed by radiation therapy. Because of a high incidence of distant metastases some authors have suggested additional adjuvant chemotherapy.[4,6,14] The tumor may be confused histologically with adenoid cystic carcinoma, adenosquamous carcinoma, or squamous cell carcinoma. Metastases to the lymph nodes may reveal both the squamous and the basaloid component or only one of the two tumor components. The most striking radiological feature observed in this particular tumor type is the distinct lobulated enhancement pattern on enhanced T1-weighted MR images, which is not encountered in the common form of squamous cell cancer[14] (Fig. 11.**37**). This lobulated enhancement pattern corresponds to the macroscopic architecture of the tumor, which consists of tumor lobules dispersed within and surrounded by a fibrovascular stroma (Fig. 11.**37**).

Non-Squamous Cell Neoplasms

Although the vast majority of laryngeal neoplasms are squamous cell carcinomas a variety of benign and malignant tumors of epithelial, neuroectodermal, and mesodermal origin may affect the larynx. These unusual histological types comprise 2–5% of all tumors originating from the larynx.[6,13,17,23,77,35,50] Diagnosis and treatment of these tumors differs from squamous cell carcinoma in several aspects. Squamous cell carcinoma usually presents with obvious mucosal abnormalities and is therefore readily diagnosed with endoscopy, whereas many of the less common his-

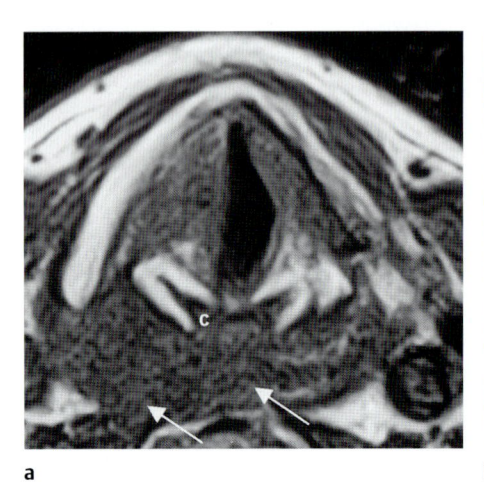

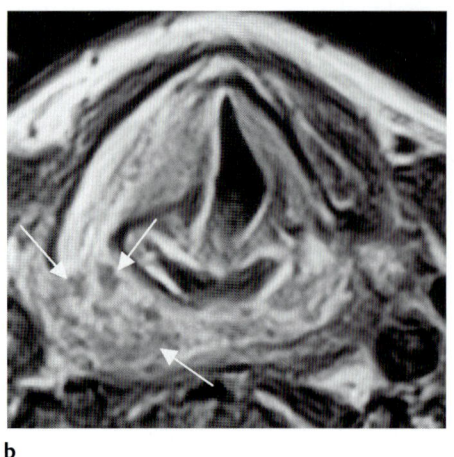

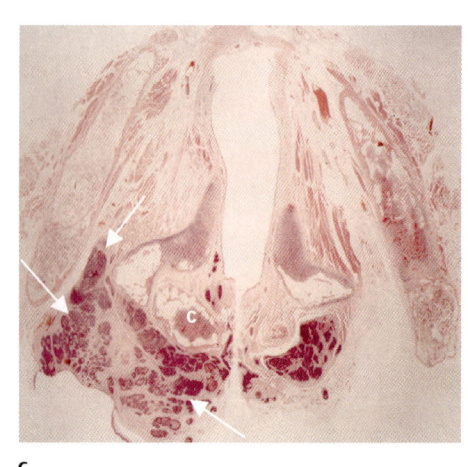

Fig. 11.**37** Basaloid cell carcinoma of the hypopharynx. Characteristic MRI and histological appearance in a 64-year-old patient presenting with pain and dysphagia. **a** T1W SE image. A tumor mass involves the right piriform sinus and the retrocricoarytenoid region (arrows). c = cricoid cartilage. **b** T1W contrast-enhanced SE image. The tumor mass has a distinct lobulated enhancement pattern. The tumor lobules (arrows) display a moderate enhancement, while the stroma surrounding the tumor lobules enhances significantly. The patient underwent total laryngectomy and right-sided neck dissection. **c** Corresponding axial histological slice shows the characteristic tumor lobules (arrows), which are surrounded by a reactive stroma. Hematoxylin–eosin stain. c = cricoid cartilage. None of the laryngeal cartilages was invaded histologically. Reproduced from Reference 14 with permission.

Table 11.**7** Non–squamous cell laryngeal neoplasms categorized by histological type

Type of neoplasm	Percentage
Vasoformative tumors	32.5%
Chondrogenic tumors	20.0%
Hematopoietic tumors	12.5%
Salivary gland tumors	10.0%
Tumors of fatty tissue	7.5%
Metastases	7.5%
Neurogenic tumors	5.0%
Myogenic tumors	2.5%
Fibrohystiocytic tumors	2.5%
Total non–squamous cell tumors	100.0%

Reproduced with permission from reference 13.

tological types of laryngeal tumors do not involve the mucosal surface and therefore require deep, transmucosal biopsies at the site of the tumor mass in order to establish the correct diagnosis. Sectional imaging in these tumors is not only done for delineation of infiltration of the submucosal structures, as with squamous cell carcinoma, but often plays a crucial role in determining the character of the tissue mass and guiding the endoscopist to the most appropriate biopsy site.[102] Because it is usually impossible to differentiate primary mucosal versus submucosal locations with imaging findings alone, the clinical history and the results of endoscopic evaluation should always be taken into consideration when interpreting CT and MR images of the larynx. If endoscopy shows normal mucosa and CT or MRI show a mass, this suggests either the presence of a tumor with an unusual histology or a very rare presentation of a squamous cell carcinoma beneath intact mucosa. Squamous cell carcinoma that arises from the mucosa of the laryngeal ventricle may spread very early into the paraglottic space, invading both the supraglottic and glottic regions, and the small mucosal lesion within the ventricle may be overlooked at endoscopy.[8, 13, 35, 77] Therefore, the tumor may present endoscopically as a submucosal bulge and the true extent may be recognized only by CT or MRI. An additional reason to perform sectional imaging is to search for cervical metastatic adenopathy.

The most common non–squamous cell neoplasms of the larynx and hypopharynx are summarized in Table 11.**7**.

■ Vasoformative Tumors

Vasoformative tumors of the head and neck may be classified as benign tumors (hemangioma) and malignant neoplasms (Kaposi sarcoma and hemangiopericytoma).[6, 90]

Hemangioma

Hemangiomas are neoplastic conditions characterized by an increased proliferation and turnover of endothelial cells, and typically display a rapid proliferation phase during the first year of life followed by an involution phase.[6, 44, 90] As opposed to hemangiomas, **vascular malformations** are not tumors but true congenital vascular anomalies with a normal proliferation rate of endothelial cells (see below). Hemangioma of the larynx occurs in children under the age of 6 months, and is twice as common in females.[6, 13, 17, 44] It is usually located in the subglottic region. Dyspnea and stridor are the most common presenting symptoms. Endoscopy shows a compressible, soft swelling that is dark bluish red or pale red in color and the overlying mucosa is most often intact (Fig. 11.**38**). Treatment in children consists of tracheostomy and the hemangioma is allowed to regress spontaneously.[44]

The radiological features are straightforward. A subglottic mass is typically seen on sectional imaging (Fig. 11.**38**). On CT, hemangiomas display strong enhancement after administration of contrast material. On MRI, hemangiomas display a very high signal intensity on T2-weighted sequences and strong enhancement after administration of gadolinium chelates, allowing a correct diagnosis in most cases.

Kaposi Sarcoma

Kaposi sarcoma is considered as an unusual, multifocal, neoplastic disease of the vascular system.[6, 49] It involves the larynx only very rarely. The disease was rare in Europe and the United States until recently,[49] when it has become more common in association with the acquired immune deficiency syndrome (AIDS). Three forms of Kaposi sarcoma are recognized: classic Kaposi sarcoma affecting men of Mediterranean origin in their seventh decade; Central African Kaposi sarcoma; and AIDS-related Kaposi sarcoma. Currently, the most frequent form of Kaposi sarcoma is associated with AIDS. Most patients with laryngeal

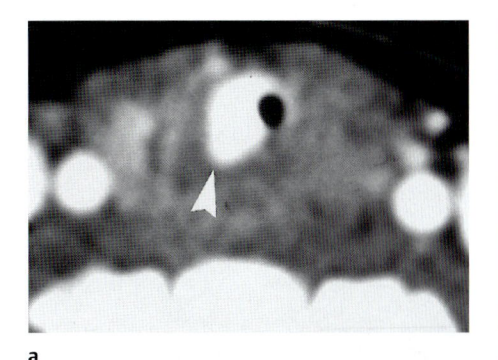

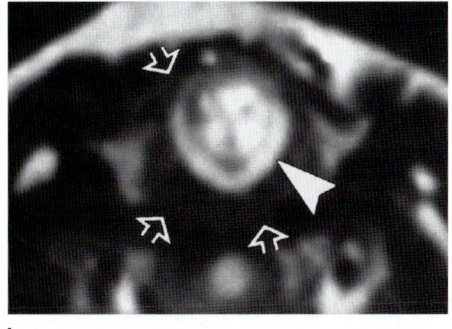

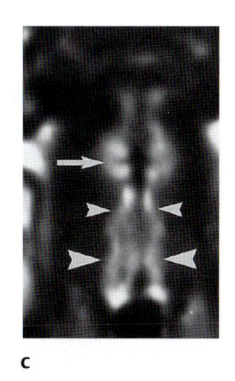

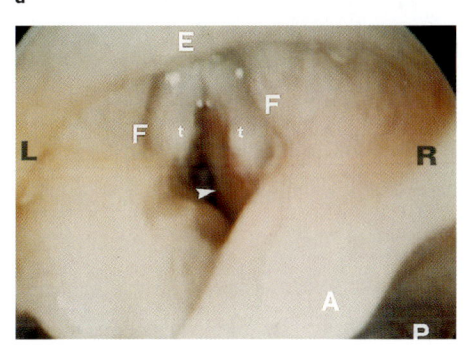

Fig. 11.**38** Infantile hemangioma. Two-month-old girl presenting with dyspnea. **a** Axial contrast-enhanced CT image demonstrates a subglottic soft-tissue mass with very strong enhancement after injection of contrast material (arrowhead), characteristic of an infantile hemangioma. **b** T2W SE MR image obtained in the same patient demonstrates the typical high signal intensity observed in these lesions (arrowhead). The cricoid ring is indicated by open arrows. **c** Coronal T1W contrast-enhanced image demonstrates involvement of the subglottis (small arrowheads) and cervical trachea (large arrowheads). Arrow points to the right laryngeal ventricle. **d** Endoscopic image demonstrates a pale red subglottic mass beneath intact mucosa (arrowhead). t = true vocal cords; F = false cords; E = epiglottis; A = aryepiglottic folds; P = piriform sinuses. Note that—as we are looking from above—the patient's right side (R) is situated to the reader's right side and the patient's left side (L) is situated to the reader's left side. The epiglottis (E), which is located anteriorly, is seen at the top of the image and the piriform sinuses (P), which are located posteriorly, are seen at the bottom of the image. Reproduced from Reference 13 with permission.

Kaposi sarcoma, regardless of whether they are HIV-positive or not, present with multiple classical skin lesions. Involvement of the larynx is, therefore, only to be expected in the late stages when the disease has been diagnosed from the skin lesions. The commonest location of Kaposi sarcoma in the larynx is the epiglottis. The clinical course of Kaposi sarcoma is variable. Elderly patients with classical Kaposi sarcoma may live for many years, and death only rarely occurs as a direct result of the tumor;[49] complete regression of laryngeal involvement has recently been reported with low doses of interferon alfa-2 b[54] in these patients. Central African Kaposi sarcoma involving the larynx is usually rapidly fatal. AIDS-related Kaposi sarcoma usually affects the larynx at a late stage, when lymph nodes and viscera are already involved. In these patients, Kaposi sarcoma is usually associated with a high incidence of lymphomas. The prognosis is usually very poor.

On CT and MRI, Kaposi sarcoma may display a relatively strong enhancement after administration of contrast material. The presence of a relatively hypervascular submucosal laryngeal mass in association with multiple characteristic skin lesions very strongly suggests the diagnosis of Kaposi sarcoma.[13]

■ Tumors of the Laryngeal Skeleton

Cartilaginous and osteogenic neoplasms of the larynx include chondroma, chondrosarcoma, and osteosarcoma. **Chondrosarcoma** is the most frequent sarcoma of the larynx.[6, 13, 17, 42, 108] It predominantly affects males between 50 and 70 years of age. 50–70% of all laryngeal chondrosarcomas originate from the posterior lamina of the cricoid cartilage, whereas 20–35% originate from the thyroid cartilage. Laryngeal chondrosarcoma presents as a lobulated, submucosal mass covered by intact laryngeal mucosa. Laryngeal chondrosarcoma is primarily a local invader and distant metastases of this tumor are unusual. Surgery is regarded as the treatment of choice and is increasingly done in the form of function-preserving laryngeal resection.[115] Tumor recurrence may be seen 10 years or more after local excision or partial laryngectomy. Radiological evaluation is essential for the planning of surgery and to monitor for local recurrence those patients who have had function-preserving surgery.[13, 42, 108, 115, 119]

Coarse or stippled calcifications within the mass are highly suggestive of its chondrogenic nature. CT may not only show very subtle intratumoral calcifications but also defines the exact anatomical origin of the tumor (Fig. 11.**39**). However, there are no reliable CT criteria that enable differentiation between chondrosarcoma and benign chondroma. As in chondrogenic tumors of other locations, the tumor matrix of laryngeal chondrosarcoma has a very high signal intensity on T2-weighted MR images, corresponding to hyaline cartilage with its low cellularity and high water content. Small areas of low signal intensity on T1-weighted and T2-weighted sequences correspond to stippled calcifications; these changes are, however, not as well demonstrated as with CT (Fig. 11.**39**). Although the injection of gadolinium chelates may lead to a diffuse central or peripheral enhancement, these findings are nonspecific in as much as they do not help in differentiating low-grade chondrosarcomas from benign chondroma.[6, 13, 108] The diagnosis of laryngeal chondrosarcoma can be strongly suspected on MRI or CT, although it must be confirmed with deep biopsy.

■ Tumors of the Lymphoreticular System

Tumors of the lymphoreticular system include Hodgkin and non-Hodgkin lymphoma, plasmacytoma, leukemia, and pseudolymphoma. Although about 30% of all malignant lymphomas arise in the head and neck (cervical lymph nodes and Waldeyer's ring), lymphomas of the larynx, either in isolation or as a manifestation of generalized disease, are very uncommon. **Plasmacytoma** of the larynx occurs predominantly in males between 50 and 70 years and involves the epiglottis, the vocal cords, and the false cords.[3, 5, 6, 30] Endoscopically, a pedunculated or slightly prominent mass is seen that bleeds easily and the mucosa above the tumor is usually intact. Approximately 40% of extramedullary plasmacytomas terminate in osseous and soft-tissue dissemination. Treatment may consist of surgical excision or radiotherapy in localized disease or of chemotherapy in the case of dissemi-

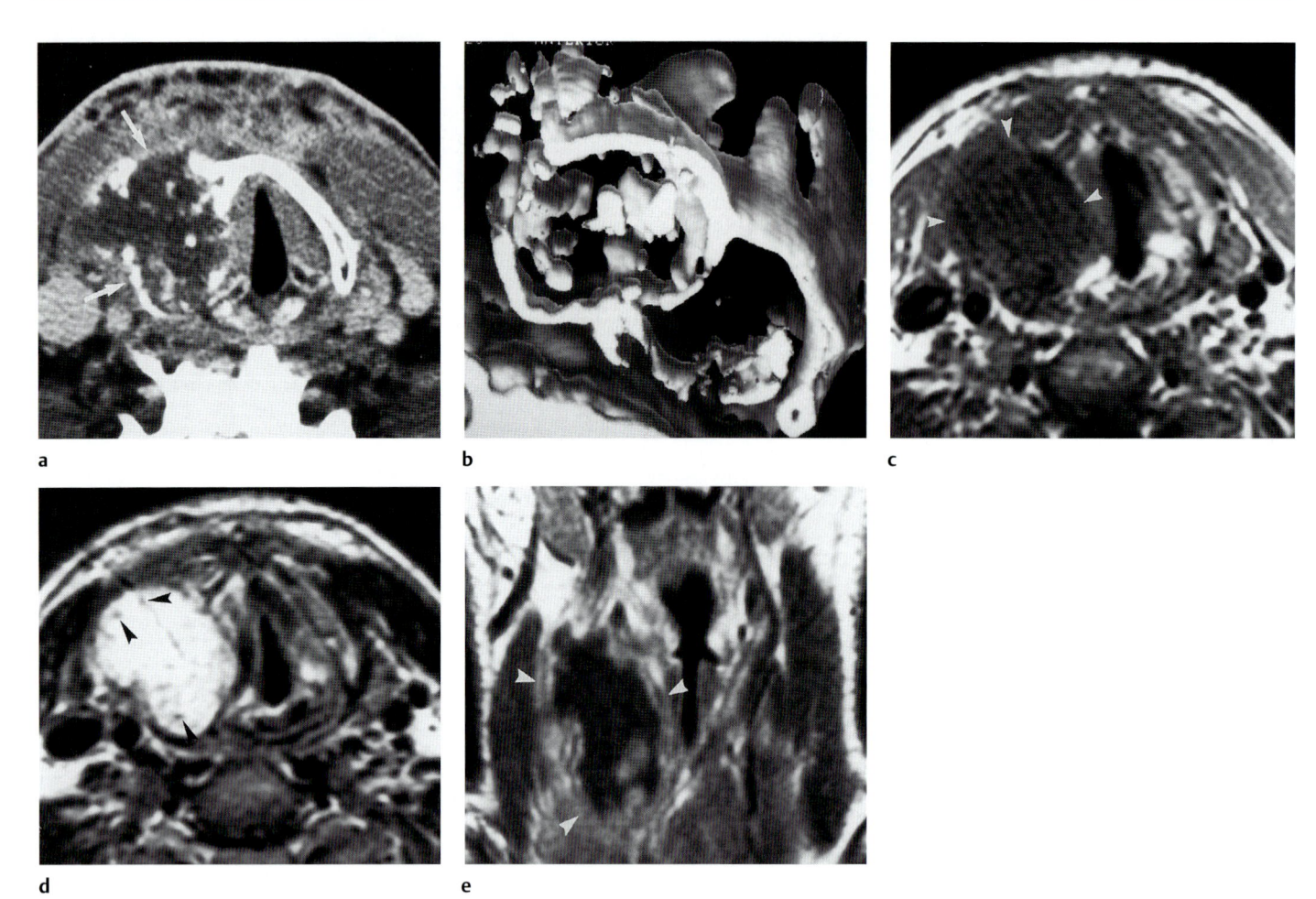

Fig. 11.**39** Chondrosarcoma of the thyroid cartilage. CT and MRI appearance in a 47-year-old man presenting with a hard lump in the neck. **a** Axial contrast-enhanced CT scan shows a large, lobulated mass with coarse and stippled calcifications characteristic of chondrosarcoma (arrows). **b** 3D reconstruction better delineates the lobulated tumor arising from the right thyroid lamina. **c** Axial T1W SE image shows a lobulated mass with low signal intensity that arises from the right thyroid lamina (arrowheads). Normal aspect of the left thyroid lamina. **d** T2W FSE MR image. The tumor mass has a very high signal intensity due to a high water content. The hypointense areas within the tumor correspond to intratumoral calcifications (arrowheads). **e** Coronal contrast-enhanced T1W SE image. Moderate peripheral enhancement (arrowheads). Note extramucosal tumor location. The patient underwent voice-preserving laryngeal resection and is free of recurrence five years later. Reproduced from Reference 13 with permission.

nated disease. The radiological aspect is nonspecific and the major role of CT and MRI consists in demonstrating the submucosal extent of the lesion and following the patients postoperatively.

Tumors of the Minor Salivary Glands

Numerous minor salivary glands are distributed throughout the larynx, particularly in the supraglottic and to a lesser extent in the subglottic region. All known types of benign and malignant salivary gland tumors may arise from the epithelium of these glands, the most common being pleomorphic adenoma, adenoid cystic carcinoma, mucoepidermoid carcinoma, and adenocarcinoma.[6, 13, 17, 58, 105, 38]

Adenoid Cystic Carcinoma

The etiology of **adenoid cystic carcinoma** is unknown, but the tumor is not related to smoking. Unlike most malignant laryngeal tumors, which are seen more commonly in males, there is no significant sex difference in adenoid cystic carcinoma. About 80% of adenoid cystic carcinomas of the larynx lie in the subglottis, typically at the junction with the trachea (Figs. 11.**40**, 11.**41**). The tumor often invades the entire larynx submucosally and infiltrates the thyroid gland and the esophagus. The symptoms of subglottic adenoid cystic carcinoma of the larynx include coughing attacks, wheezing, and occasionally hemoptysis. Pain may be a prominent symptom, owing to the propensity of the tumor to invade nerves. Paralysis of the recurrent laryngeal nerve is a characteristic feature and usually begins unilaterally, but later affects both sides. Survival of patients with adenoid cystic carcinoma is longer than with squamous cell carcinoma, namely, 8 years on average, ranging up to 15–18 years.[6, 13, 38, 105] Regional metastases to the cervical lymph nodes are rare, but metastases to the lungs, bone, and brain almost always occur in the terminal stage. The treatment options in the larynx are surgery and radiation therapy combined with chemotherapy.

Both MRI and CT typically display extensive submucosal tumor spread at the time of diagnosis (Figs. 11.**40** and 11.**41**). The predominantly subglottic tumor has most often already invaded the cricoid cartilage and the thyroid gland, and the radiological features of recurrent laryngeal nerve paralysis may be identified at CT or MRI (see below). Signal intensity at MRI and patterns of contrast enhancement at MRI and CT are not specific in differentiating adenoid cystic carcinoma from other types of tumors. Nevertheless, a low signal intensity on T2-weighted MR images appears to correspond to highly cellular tumors (solid subtype,

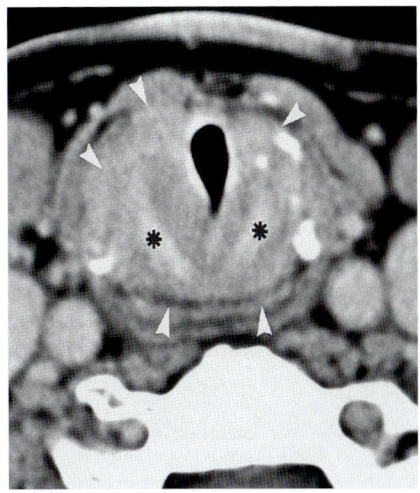

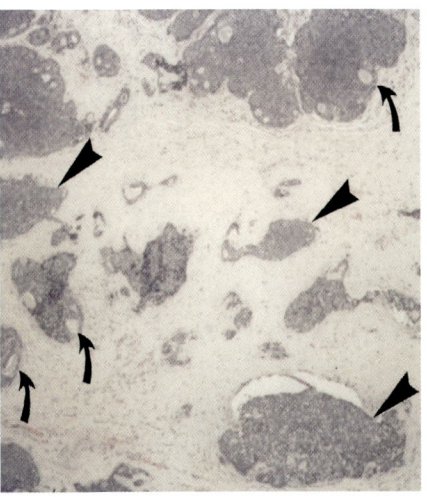

Fig. 11.**40** Adenoid cystic carcinoma. CT and histological appearance in a 51-year-old woman without a history of tobacco or alcohol consumption presenting with increasing dyspnea and stridor over a period of three months. Endoscopy revealed subglottic narrowing with normal-appearing mucosa. Endoscopic biopsy of the subglottis was negative. **a** CT performed prior to endoscopy demonstrates a large primary subglottic tumor that extends beyond the larynx (arrowheads) and invades the cricoid cartilage (asterisks). No cervical lymph node metastases were seen at CT. Because repeat endoscopic biopsies were negative, biopsy using an external surgical approach was performed. **b** Low-power micrograph of a biopsy specimen obtained at the subglottic level demonstrates tumor cells arranged in solid nests (arrowheads) suggesting grade 3 adenoid cystic carcinoma. Further radiological investigations revealed osseous and hepatic metastases. The patient underwent palliative chemotherapy and died one year later of disseminated disease. Reproduced from Reference 13 with permission.

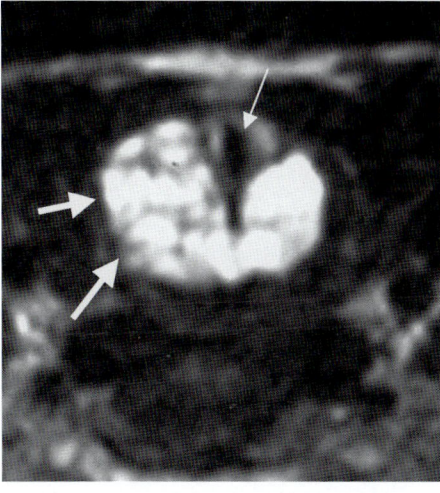

Fig. 11.**41** Adenoid cystic carcinoma. MRI appearance in a 60-year-old woman with dyspnea. Axial T2W image at the subglottic level shows a large mass with invasion of the cricoid cartilage (thick arrows). Note severe airway narrowing (thin arrow). Courtesy of Dr. Guy Moulin, Hôpital La Timone, Marseille, France.

grade 3) with a poor prognosis, while a high signal intensity on T2-weighted images appears to correspond to less cellular tumors (cribriform or tubular subtype, grades 1 and 2) with a better prognosis.[105] Although the imaging findings of laryngeal adenoid cystic carcinoma are nonspecific, the diagnosis may be suspected in Caucasian women without a history of cigarette smoking, with a primary submucosal subglottic tumor, and without cervical lymph node metastases.

Mucoepidermoid Carcinoma

It is believed that mucoepidermoid carcinomas arise from the intercalated ducts of the seromucinous glands. Males are affected six times more often than females, the most commonly affected site being the epiglottis.[6, 13] The biological behavior of mucoepidermoid carcinoma is less aggressive than that of squamous cell carcinoma. As this tumor responds only moderately well to radiotherapy, the treatment of choice is complete surgical removal. The radiological features are nonspecific.

Adenocarcinoma

The tumor is most commonly found in the fifth to seventh decade with a male predominance. Endoscopically, the tumor may present as an entirely submucosal nodule or as a large ulcerated mass.[6, 13, 58] On CT and MRI, extensive submucosal tumor spread may be observed with extensive invasion of the laryngeal skeleton

■ Tumors of Fatty Tissue

Tumors of fatty tissue include lipomas and liposarcomas. Although tumors of fatty tissue are the most frequent of all connective tissue lesions, they are only rarely found in the larynx.[6, 13, 92, 107] Seventy percent of the affected patients are men over the age of 50, and 25% of patients present with multiple lipomas. Lipoma of the larynx most commonly arises in the supraglottic region. Mobile tumors may prolapse into the trachea or esophagus, leading to a foreign body sensation, dyspnea or, occasionally, even death from suffocation.[6, 92] Endoscopically, the tumor may present as a sessile or polypoid submucosal mass. Deep biopsies are mandatory or the lesion will be overlooked at histology. Small lipomas can be removed endoscopically, whereas large lesions require an external surgical approach. The prognosis is excellent with no increased risk for recurrence.

Initial clinical presentation of laryngeal liposarcoma is very similar to lipoma, and surgical therapy with ample excision is the treatment of choice. Elective neck dissection is not indicated, given the absence of cervical metastases. However, local recurrence after surgery and distant hematogenous metastases are common in laryngeal liposarcoma.

The radiological diagnosis of lipoma is straightforward (Fig. 11.**42**). Both CT and MRI provide a definitive diagnosis in virtually all cases. The typical CT characteristics are a homogeneous and nonenhancing lesion with attenuation values from –65 to –125 HU.[13, 17, 107] On MRI, lipoma has the same signal intensity as subcutaneous fat on all pulse sequences (hyperintense on T1-weighted images, decrease in intensity on T2-weighted images, and very low intensity on fat-suppressed T1-weighted images). As in other parts of the body, if portions of the lipoma have the attenuation value or signal intensity characteristics of soft tissue at CT or MRI, and if contrast enhancement is observed within these strands of connective tissue, the diagnosis of a liposarcoma should be considered.

■ Metastases to the Larynx

The most common mechanism of metastatic spread to the larynx is through the systemic circulation: inferior vena cava, right heart, lungs, left heart, aorta, external carotid artery, upper thy-

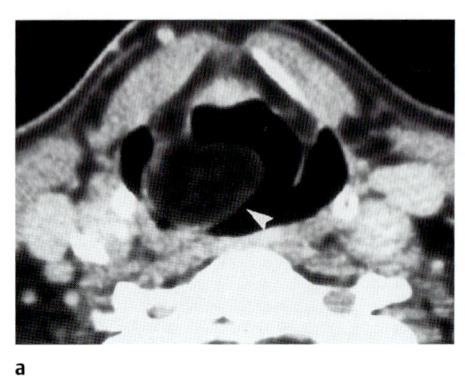

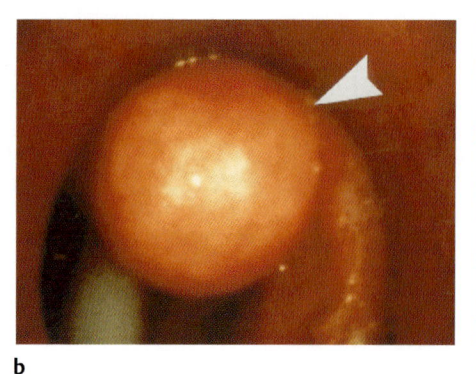

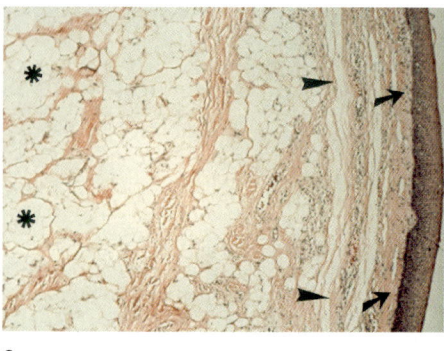

Fig. 11.42 Lipoma in a 77-year-old man with a foreign-body sensation, episodes of suffocation, and change in quality of voice. **a** Axial contrast-enhanced CT scan at the supraglottic level. A homogeneous, nonenhancing lesion with the density of fat is seen at the level of the right aryepiglottic fold (arrowhead). **b** Endoscopic view. A pendunculated mass covered by intact laryngeal mucosa arises from the right aryepiglottic fold (arrowhead). **c** Low-power micrograph showing intact overlying squamous epithelium (arrows). Lobulated laryngeal lipoma composed of mature adipocytes (asterisks) and fibrous pseudocapsule (arrowheads). The patient underwent endoscopic resection and is free of recurrence five years later. Reproduced from Reference 13 with permission.

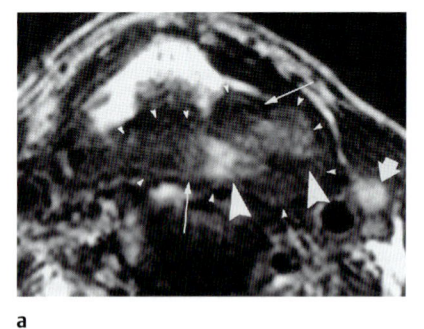

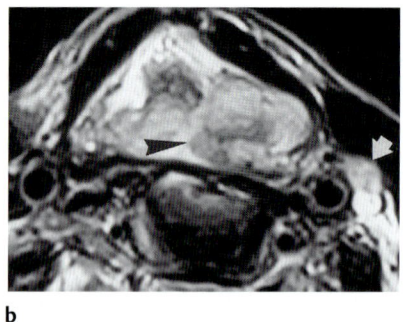

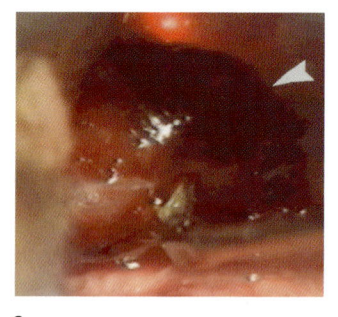

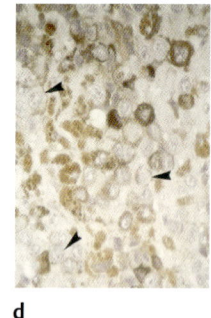

Fig. 11.43 Metastasis from melanotic melanoma in an 81-year-old man with dyspnea and a history of occasional blood in the sputum. **a** Axial unenhanced T1W SE MR image demonstrates a large mass (small arrowheads) involving the left aryepiglottic fold. The mass has areas with low signal intensity (thin arrows) and areas with high signal intensity (large arrowheads). A lymph node with high signal intensity (thick arrow) is seen on the left. **b** T2W FSE MR image at the same level shows that the hyperintense areas on the T1W image become hypointense (arrowhead). The left-sided lymph node maintains a high signal intensity (thick arrow). After administration of contrast material, moderate enhancement of the tumor mass was observed. The signal characteristics suggested a melanotic melanoma of the supraglottic larynx with lymph node metastasis. **c** Endoscopy shows a darkly stained, polypoid, supraglottic tumor involving the left aryepiglottic fold (arrowhead). **d** High-power micrograph demonstrates the typical appearance of melanotic melanoma: large round cells (arrowheads) with hyperchromatic to vesicular nuclei. Large amounts of melanin (brown to black granularity) are seen in the cytoplasm of neoplastic cells. The patient indicated that he had undergone removal of a small "spot" on the scalp at another institution. Inquiry at this institution revealed the diagnosis of melanotic melanoma of the scalp. The laryngeal tumor and the cervical lymph node metastasis were, therefore, considered metastases of the melanotic melanoma of the scalp. Reproduced from Reference 13 with permission.

roid artery, and upper laryngeal artery. However, when no pulmonary involvement is observed, spread via the retrograde circulation of the paravertebral venous plexus and thoracic duct should be considered. The primary sources of metastatic tumor, in order of decreasing frequency, are: skin (melanoma), kidney, breast, lung, prostate, colon, stomach, and ovary.[13,48,99] Laryngeal metastases should be divided into two groups: those metastasizing to the soft tissues, mainly vestibular and aryepiglottic folds, such as melanoma and renal adenocarcinoma; and those metastasizing to the marrow spaces of the ossified thyroid, cricoid, and arytenoid cartilages, such as lung and breast carcinoma.[48] Symptoms of metastatic tumors to the larynx vary according to the affected site. Hemoptysis is an important symptom of laryngeal metastases from renal adenocarcinoma because of the abundant vascularization of these tumors. Treatment of a secondary tumor of the larynx is justified if it is a single metastasis. The type of treatment—partial or total laryngectomy, radiotherapy, and/or chemotherapy—depends on the biological behavior of the primary neoplasm taking into account the quality of life of the patient. The prognosis is usually very poor; however, some well-documented cases of prolonged survival have been reported in the literature.[48]

In most cases, radiological features of laryngeal metastases are nonspecific. However, metastases from renal adenocarcinoma and melanotic melanoma may display typical features at MR imaging (Figs. 11.**43** and 11.**44**). Metastases from renal adenocarcinoma typically display a very strong enhancement after administration of contrast material owing to their hypervascularity and flow voids on MR images, therefore suggesting a diagnosis other than squamous cell carcinoma.[82] Laryngeal metastases from melanotic melanoma display the signal characteristics of melanotic melanoma elsewhere in the body, namely, a high signal intensity on T1-weighted MR images and an intermediate to low signal intensity on T2-weighted MR images due to the paramagnetic properties of melanin. Recently, it has been suggested that the signal intensity characteristics of melanoma may not depend on their classification as melanotic or amelanotic but on how much melanin is present at histopathology.[122]

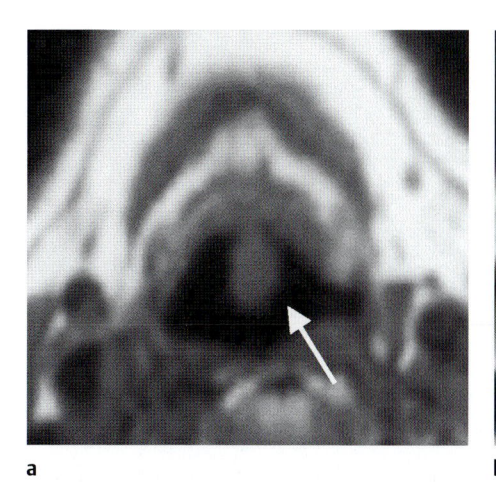

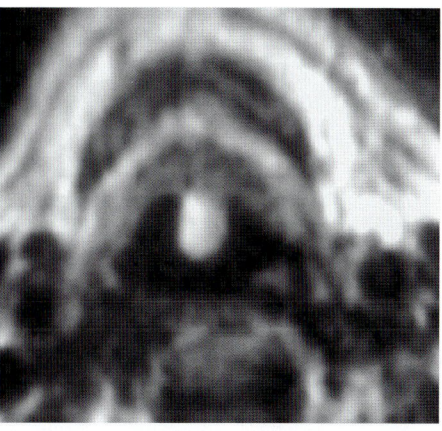

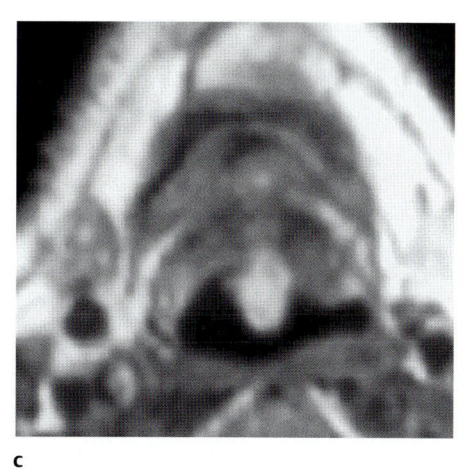

Fig. 11.**44** Metastasis from renal adenocarcinoma in a 65-year-old man with renal adenocarcinoma and metastases to the lungs presenting with dyspnea and a history of occasional blood in the sputum. **a** Axial unenhanced T1W SE MR image demonstrates a small mass (arrow) involving the laryngeal surface of the epiglottis. **b** T2W FSE MR image at the same level shows that the mass is hyperintense. **c** T1W SE MR image after administration of contrast material demonstrates marked enhancement of the tumor suggesting a hypervascular lesion. The lesion was removed endoscopically and histology confirmed a laryngeal metastasis from renal adenocarcinoma.

■ Myogenic Tumors

Laryngeal tumors arising from smooth or striated muscle are rare, and include leiomyoma, angioleiomyoma, leiomyosarcoma, extracardiac rhabdomyoma, and rhabdomyosarcoma. Benign extracardiac **rhabdomyomas** are rare neoplasms of skeletal muscle origin.[6, 13] The predilection sites of rhabdomyoma are in the tongue, pharynx, and larynx. In the larynx, the tumor presents endoscopically as a submucosal, apparently well-circumscribed lesion, most often involving the true vocal cords. As with other submucosal lesions, deep biopsies are mandatory. The treatment of choice is surgery. Because local recurrence is common, even after a period as long as 12 years, ample excision is mandatory.

■ Neurogenic Tumors

Neurogenic tumors include schwannoma, neurofibroma, ganglioneuroma, and granular cell tumors. Peripheral nerve sheath tumors of the larynx are often of the schwannoma type. The symptoms are those associated with any slow-growing tumor of the larynx, such as gradual changes in voice and foreign body sensation during swallowing. Because schwannomas usually arise from the superior laryngeal nerve, they are most often situated in the aryepiglottic fold.[124] Endoscopically, the tumor is covered by a thin mucosa with increased capillaries. Treatment is most often done by an endoscopic approach.

Schwannomas and neurofibromas may display typical features on MRI. Nearly 75% of all nerve sheath tumors have the same signal intensity as the spinal cord on T1-weighted SE sequences, more than 95% have a high signal intensity on T2-weighted SE sequences, and nearly all nerve sheath tumors enhance following intravenous administration of contrast material. The enhancement pattern of neural tumors is highly variable. A target appearance (hyperintense rim and hypointense center) may be seen on contrast-enhanced MR images, and is caused by central areas of cystic or necrotic degeneration.

Morphological Changes Induced by Tumor Treatment and Detection of Tumor Recurrence

The main options for treatment of malignant tumors of the larynx and hypopharynx currently consist of surgery, radiation therapy, surgery followed by radiation therapy, and radiation therapy combined with chemotherapy.[6, 9, 26, 29, 30, 56, 57, 75, 120] The choice is influenced, besides clinical parameters, by the histology, the primary site, the extent of the primary lesion, and the presence or absence of metastases. Some indications are undisputed. For example, it is generally accepted that in situ carcinoma of the glottis (Tis) can be treated endoscopically, and that squamous cell carcinoma of the glottis of categories T1 and T2 responds well to radiation therapy. However, the treatment selected for glottic tumors of categories T3 and T4 and of tumors of other primary sites or non-squamous cell origin may vary among different institutions and countries. A discussion of the controversial issues in this area is beyond the scope of this chapter. Nonetheless, it is appropriate for the radiologist to be familiar with the morphological changes induced by the different forms of treatment.

■ Surgical Procedures, Postoperative Changes, and Tumor Recurrence in the Operated Larynx

Surgical treatment of laryngeal carcinoma has two goals, namely, oncologically adequate excision of tumor tissue and preservation of the essential functions of the larynx as far as possible. Total laryngectomy is a very invasive procedure and considerably impairs the quality of life after surgery. Techniques of "voice-sparing" or "partial laryngectomy" are based on the capability of most patients to retain ability to breathe, swallow, and speak despite the loss of substantial portions of the larynx. Patient selection is the critical determinant for success of voice-sparing laryngectomy and depends, besides general clinical aspects, on local criteria such as extent of deep tumor spread and cartilage invasion.

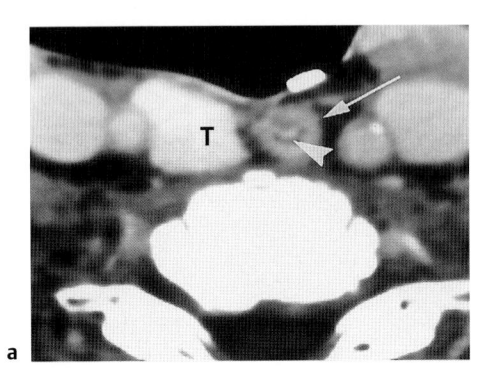

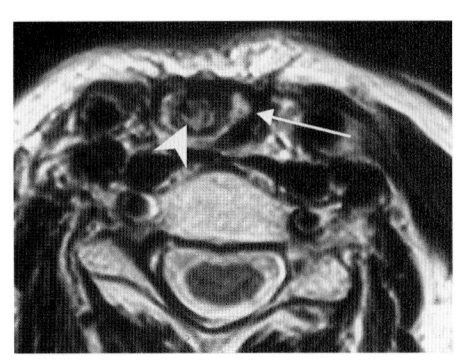

Fig. 11.45 Appearance of the neck after total laryngectomy. **a** Axial contrast-enhanced CT scan shows a normal-appearing neopharynx (arrow) with regular thickness and smooth external margins. Note that the neopharyngeal mucosa enhances significantly (arrowhead). T = right lobe of the thyroid gland. **b** T2W FSE MR image in another patient with total laryngectomy shows a normal-appearing neopharynx (arrow) with regular thickness and smooth external margins. Note that the neopharyngeal mucosa has a high signal intensity (arrowhead).

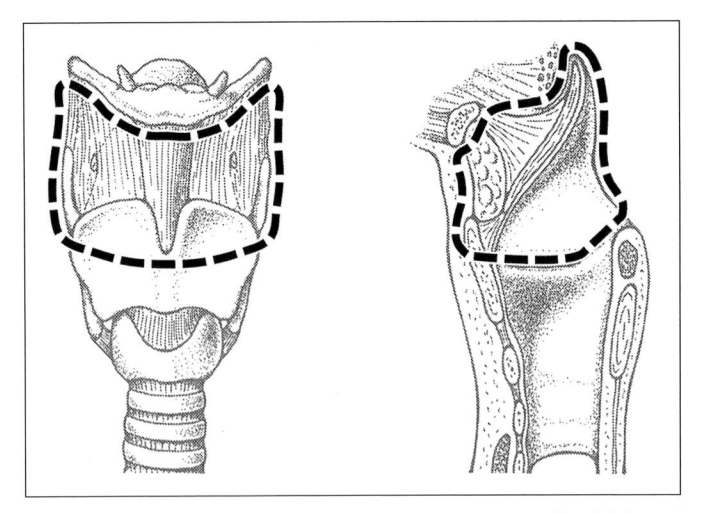

Fig. 11.46 Horizontal supraglottic laryngectomy. **a** Frontal and **b** lateral diagrams of the structures removed during horizontal supraglottic laryngectomy (within dashed lines). Reproduced from Reference 8 with permission.

Total laryngectomy may be necessary in the following four situations: (1) as primary treatment for extensive squamous cell carcinoma or other malignant tumors of the larynx and hypopharynx with invasion of the laryngeal cartilages and the subglottis; (2) for salvage after failed radiotherapy; (3) for local recurrence after partial laryngectomy; and (4) for osteochondroradionecrosis occurring as a complication of radiation therapy.[9,37,83,98] Hematogenous metastases and the presence of synchronous tumors are considered as contraindications to total laryngectomy. With total laryngectomy, the entire larynx, the piriform sinuses, and the strap muscles are removed. The pharyngeal defect is closed in layers (hypopharyngeal mucosa and inferior constrictor muscle), forming a tubular neopharynx from the base of the tongue to the cervical esophagus. On axial CT and MR images obtained after total laryngectomy, absence of the entire larynx and the hyoid bone results in a collapsed and irregular appearance of the mucosa. The so-called neopharynx appears as a round or ovoid tubular structure that extends from the base of the tongue to the esophagus and is surrounded by fat and muscle tissue (Fig. 11.45). The neopharyngeal wall shows a regular thickness and smooth external margins. The normal tracheostoma shows smooth, thin, and regular walls.

The most commonly performed voice-sparing laryngectomy procedures include horizontal supraglottic laryngectomy, vertical hemilaryngectomy, supracricoid laryngectomy with cricohyoidopexy, and supracricoid laryngectomy with cricohyoidoepiglottopexy[29,30,33,36,63,83] **Horizontal supraglottic laryngectomy** is suitable for lesions localized above the ventricle. Involvement of the preepiglottic space does not preclude the operation as long as the tumor does not cross the ventricle. This type of resection includes the upper half of the larynx with the epiglottis, aryepiglottic folds, false cords, preepiglottic space, and a portion of the thyroid cartilage. The lower resection border passes just above the level of the anterior commissure and through the ventricle. Although the arytenoid cartilages are usually spared, one arytenoid cartilage may be removed when it is involved by tumor (Figs. 11.46, 11.47). Contraindications to horizontal supraglottic laryngectomy are neoplastic spread to both arytenoids, the posterior commissure, the postcricoid area, the glottis, the ventricle, and the thyroid cartilage. Sectional imaging studies obtained after horizontal supraglottic laryngectomy reveal absence of the epiglottis, false cords, and preepiglottic fat space, and elevation of the anterior margin of the glottis, which is sutured under the tongue base. The defect created by removal of the false cords is covered by residual pharyngeal mucosa, which is often thickened and redundant. The glottis and subglottis remain unchanged (Fig. 11.47).

Vertical hemilaryngectomy is indicated for selected T1 through T3 glottic carcinomas.[36,83] These lesions can be invasive squamous cell or verrucous carcinomas. Vertical hemilaryngectomy may be employed for primary treatment or for surgical salvage of radiation failures. It is done for tumors that are limited to the true cord and includes removal of the true and false cords on one side, as well as the ventricle and the ipsilateral thyroid ala (Fig. 11.48). If the anterior commissure or the anterior third of the contralateral true cord are invaded by tumor, the resection margins are moved more laterally If the ipsilateral arytenoid is invaded, the arytenoid can be included in the resection. Vertical hemilaryngectomy is contraindicated if there is extension across the ventricle to the false cord or into the subglottis, and if there is invasion of the paraglottic space, thyroid cartilage, and cricoarytenoid joint. Speech preservation and sphincteric airway protection are accomplished by creating a pseudocord using the perichondrium of the resected thyroid cartilage or one of the strap muscles. Postoperative changes observed on CT and MR images after vertical hemilaryngectomy include tilting of the laryngeal axis and shortening of the thyroid cartilage on the side of resection.[36,83] The surgical defect of the thyroid lamina is usually paramedian, and the adjacent cartilage is irregular and sclerotic. A pseudocord (due to scar tissue) extending from the defect in the thyroid cartilage to the arytenoid on the side of the resection distorts glottic symmetry, and is often associated with a laryngocele.

Supracricoid laryngectomy with cricohyoidopexy is currently done to resect advanced supraglottic carcinomas extending to the ventricle, invading the glottis and in selected cases with small areas of thyroid cartilage invasion.[29,30,83] Contraindications to this operation are subglottic spread with invasion of the cricoid cartilage. Supracricoid laryngectomy includes re-

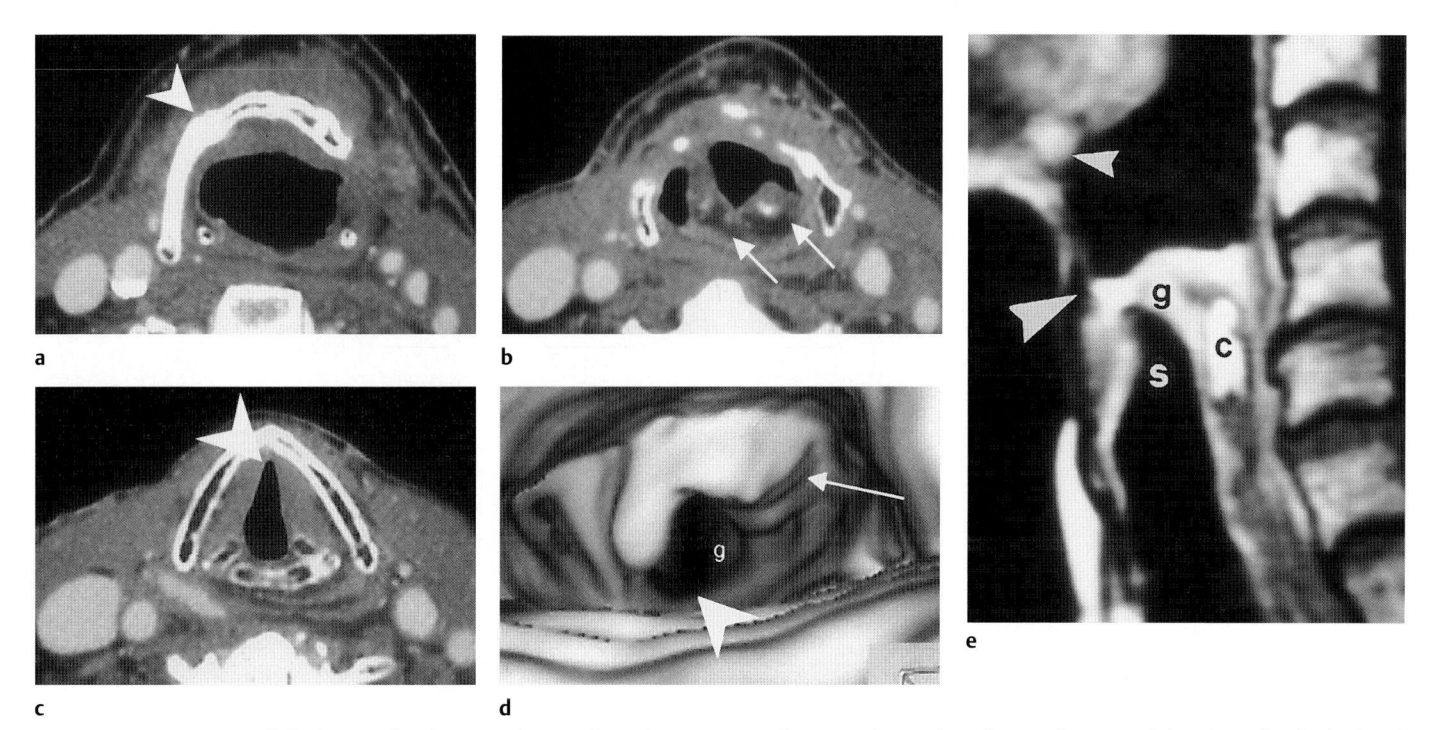

Fig. 11.**47** Appearance of the larynx after horizontal supraglottic laryngectomy. **a–c** Contrast-enhanced CT, axial images. **d** Virtual endoscopy image from spiral CT data set. **e** Sagittal contrast-enhanced T1W MR image. Note absence of the epiglottis and false cords, redundant pharyngeal mucosa (arrows), and normal aspect of the glottic level. The hyoid bone was not resected (small arrowheads). Large arrowhead points to the anterior commissure. g = glottis; c = cricoid cartilage; s = subglottis.

moval of the false and true cords, paraglottic spaces, thyroid cartilage, epiglottis, and preepiglottic space while sparing the cricoid cartilage, the hyoid bone, and at least one arytenoid cartilage (Fig. 11.**49**). The inferior cornu of the thyroid cartilage is also preserved to avoid injury of the adjacent recurrent laryngeal nerve. Cricohyoidopexy is accomplished by moving the cricoid cartilage upward and by approaching the cricoid cartilage and the hyoid bone. After supracricoid laryngectomy with cricohyoidopexy, CT and MRI reveal absence of the epiglottis and thyroid cartilage (with exception of the inferior cornu), and the hyoid bone and the cricoid cartilage become adjacent in the midline. The redundant hypopharyngeal mucosa sutured over one arytenoid is smooth and regular, and the long axis of the neoglottis may become oriented in the transverse plane. A short pseudocord results in asymmetric thickening of the mucosa lining the neovestibule and the subglottis. Formation of pharyngeal pouches of considerable size is commonly observed and they may contain air or liquid contents (Fig. 11.**50**).

Supracricoid laryngectomy with cricohyoidoepiglottopexy is currently used to remove advanced glottic carcinomas. The main difference between supracricoid laryngectomy with cricohyoidopexy and supracricoid laryngectomy with cricohyoidoepiglottopexy concerns the epiglottis, which is entirely resected in the first procedure while it is spared in its suprahyoid part in the latter.

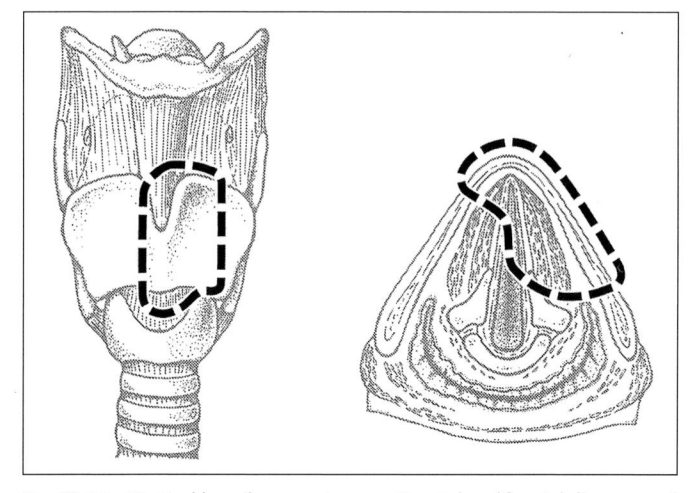

Fig. 11.**48** Vertical hemilaryngectomy. **a** Frontal and **b** axial diagrams of the structures removed during vertical hemilaryngectomy (within dashed lines). Reproduced from Reference 8 with permission.

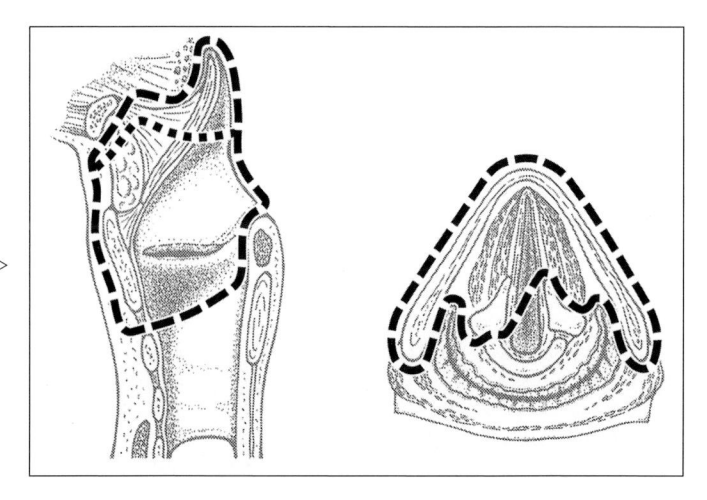

Fig. 11.**49** Supracricoid laryngectomy with cricohyoidopexy and supracricoid laryngectomy with cricohyoidoepiglottopexy. **a** Lateral and **b** axial diagrams of the structures removed during supracricoid laryngectomy with cricohyoidopexy (within long dashes) and during supracricoid laryngectomy with cricohyoidoepiglottopexy (within short and long dashes). The operations differ with respect to the epiglottis, which is resected entirely in the first procedure but is spared in its suprahyoid part in the latter. The inferior resection margins are essentially the same. Reproduced from Reference 8 with permission.

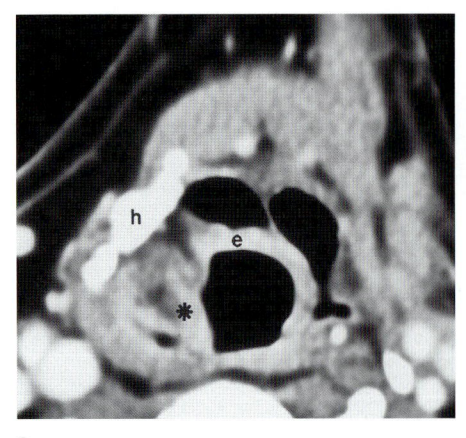

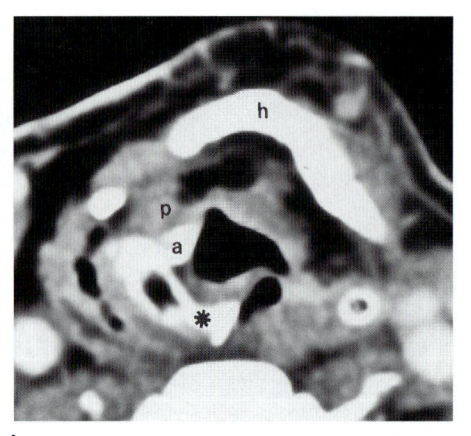

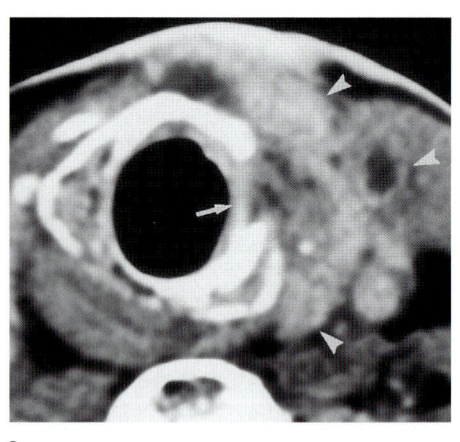

Fig. 11.**50** Tumor recurrence after supracricoid laryngectomy with cricohyoidoepiglottopexy. CT scan obtained three years after supracricoid laryngectomy with cricoepiglottopexy because of suspected tumor recurrence. **a** The neovestibule is divided by the residual epiglottis (e) into an anterior and a posterior half. The mucosa covering the right arytenoid (asterisk) is seen at the level of the hyoid bone (h). **b** The inferior border of the hyoid bone (h) and the cricoid (asterisk) are seen at the same level, and dense scar tissue in front of the residual arytenoid (a) appears as a pseudocord (p). These findings illustrated in **a** and **b** correspond to normal postoperative findings. **c** At the level of the subglottis a large, ill-defined soft-tissue mass is seen with destruction of the cricoid ring (arrow) and extension into the soft tissues of the neck (arrowheads). Note extensive sclerosis of the left cricoid cartilage. Surgery confirmed extensive tumor recurrence. Reproduced from Reference 8 with permission.

Other voice-preserving laryngectomy procedures include **glotto-subglottic laryngectomy**, which is done to resect glottic lesions with subglottic invasion, and **near total laryngectomy**, which may be indicated in transglottic lesions with subglottic invasion. Both techniques allow partial removal of the cricoid cartilage. Hypopharyngeal tumors confined entirely to the pharyngeal wall may be removed without resecting the larynx, whereas more advanced hypopharyngeal lesions may be managed by extended partial laryngectomy.

Only few studies have evaluated the CT appearance of the operated larynx,[36,37,83] and no data are currently available for comparing the relative advantages and drawbacks of CT and MRI. Management of early complications after partial or total laryngectomy, e.g., infection or aspiration, does not usually require preoperative evaluation with CT. Late postoperative complications, e.g., laryngeal stenosis or granuloma formation, present clinically in the form of dyspnea or changes in the quality of voice, and must be distinguished from tumor recurrence. Because the operated larynx may be easily evaluated by indirect inspection or flexible endoscopy, it appears that CT is not warranted as a screening examination in asymptomatic postoperative patients but should rather be used selectively to assess the extent of recurrent tumors that have already been proven with endoscopy.

Although familiarity with the expected anatomical changes after partial or total laryngectomy and their appearance on CT or MRI greatly facilitates radiological interpretation, evaluation of the postoperative larynx remains a challenge. Tumor recurrence in the operated larynx should be suspected in the presence of an irregularly shaped, enhancing soft-tissue mass exceeding 1 cm, a thickened anterior commissure, or lysis of residual cartilages[83] (Fig. 11.**50**).

■ Radiation-Induced Changes and Tumor Recurrence in the Irradiated Larynx

Tumor control with radiation therapy allows the patient to retain a functioning larynx in cases in which surgical cure would require total laryngectomy. Consequently, a growing number of selected patients are treated with radiation therapy alone or radiation therapy combined with chemotherapy. On CT and MR images, a variety of radiation-induced changes may be observed in the head and neck area, and particularly in the larynx and hypopharynx. These may be subdivided into expected changes and complications of radiotherapy. Distinction of radiation-induced changes from recurrent tumor is important, since the majority of radiation-induced changes are self-limited, whereas recurrent or residual tumor alters the therapeutic approach.

Expected Changes

The effects of the relatively high radiation doses ($>60–65$ Gy) that are required for treatment of squamous cell carcinoma of the larynx and hypopharynx are present in all areas of the larynx, hypopharynx, and neck within the radiation port. They affect, to variable degrees, the respiratory epithelium, the deep connective tissues, the laryngeal cartilages, and striated muscle.

Most effects of irradiation on normal endolaryngeal and pharyngeal soft tissues are usually maximal from the end of therapy to 3 months postirradiation. Three months after completion of radiation therapy, these effects are clearly visible on sectional imaging. Radiation-induced edema and fibrosis cause diffuse, symmetric thickening of the laryngeal soft tissues. On contrast-enhanced CT and (fat-suppressed) Gd-enhanced T1-weighted MR images the mucosa and the deeper structures of the larynx exhibit a very strong diffuse or reticulated enhancement, which may either resolve after approximately 12 months or persist indefinitely.[15,88,89] Edema and early fibrosis result in a high signal intensity on T2-weighted MR images, and low signal intensity on T1-weighted MR images; fatty tissue of the preepiglottic and paraglottic space displays low signal intensity, along with a streaky or reticulated pattern on T1-weighted MR images.

Three months after completion of radiation therapy, the characteristic CT and MRI appearances of the larynx and hypopharynx include edema and fibrosis of the epiglottis, aryepiglottic folds and false cords, paraglottic space, anterior and posterior commissure, subglottis, posterior pharyngeal wall, and retropharyngeal space (Fig. 11.**51**). These changes are in part reversible.[88,89]

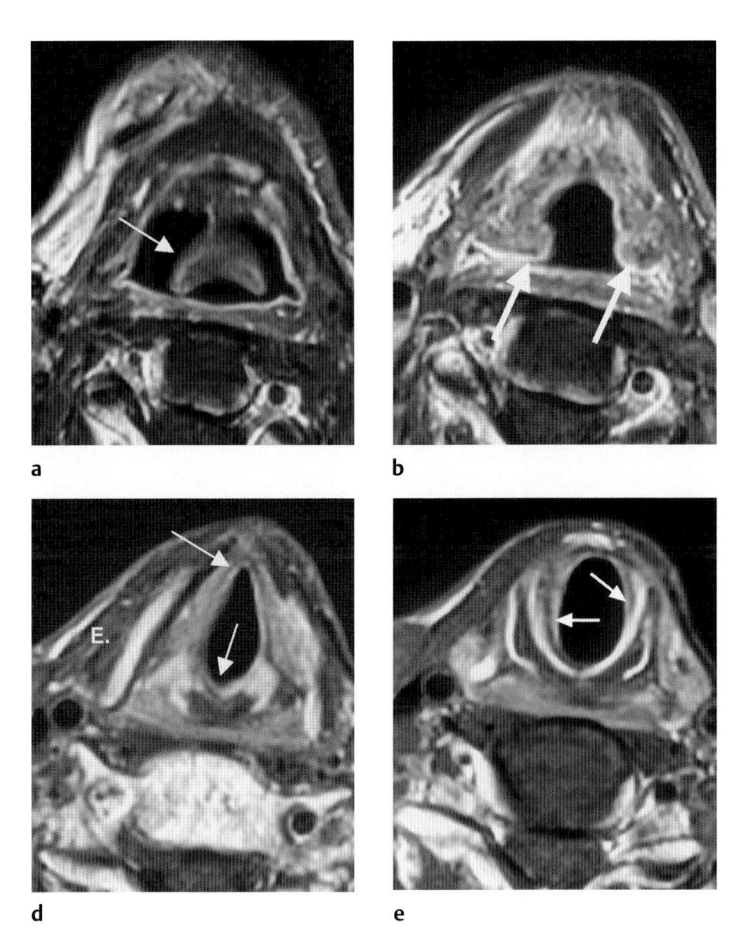

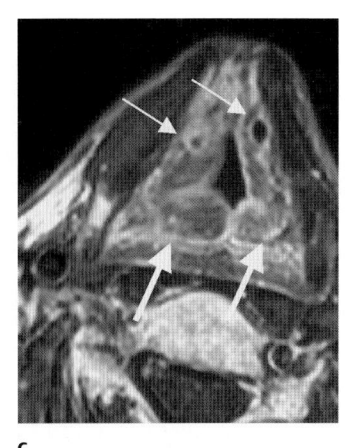

Fig. 11.**51** Radiation-induced edema of the larynx in a 45-year-old patient treated with left radical neck dissection and radiation therapy for carcinoma of the left piriform sinus. Contrast-enhanced T1W MR images obtained 4 months after therapy demonstrate characteristic imaging findings. **a** Edema of the epiglottis in its suprahyoid portion (arrow). **b** and **c** Edema and fibrosis of the aryepiglottic folds (thick arrows) with a characteristic reticulated aspect of the fatty tissue. Note bilateral enlargement of laryngeal ventricles (thin arrows). **d** Slight thickening of the anterior and posterior commissures (arrows). **e** Subglottic thickening corresponding to edematous changes (arrows). Note massive enhancement and thickening of the mucosa overlying the larynx and hypopharynx (**a–e**).

Complications of Radiation Therapy

Complications due to high-dose irradiation of normal tissue may appear immediately after radiotherapy (acute effects), or months or even years after completion of treatment (late effects).[15] Late complications affect mainly tissues with slowly proliferating or nonproliferating cells (bone, cartilage, neural tissue). It is thought that late injuries are caused either by damage of the microvasculature or by stromal cells. Knowledge of the normal imaging findings observed after radiation therapy and of radiation-induced complications reduces the need for biopsy of irradiated tissue, which may lead to poor healing, infection, and fistula formation.[15,88,89]

Radiation-induced complications in the larynx and hypopharynx include soft-tissue necrosis, osteochondronecrosis, pharyngeal motility dysfunction, pharyngeal strictures and fistula formation, and recurrent laryngeal nerve paralysis.[15,21,32,40,72,89]

Soft-tissue Necrosis

Soft-tissue necrosis is most often observed within two years after irradiation and may sometimes occur in large tumors of the larynx and hypopharynx.[8,15] Although spontaneous healing is the rule, this may take more than six months. Surgical treatment may be required in the presence of fistula formation. The CT and MR imaging appearances of soft-tissue necrosis are usually straightforward (Fig. 11.**52**). Coexisting tumor cannot be excluded in the presence of an adjacent soft-tissue mass without follow-up examinations, and biopsy under general anesthesia may even become necessary in some instances in order to clarify the situation.[15] At our institution, we prefer follow-up examinations with either CT or MRI to endoscopic biopsies. If the radiological aspect does not change, a biopsy will not be performed and the patient will be followed carefully with both clinical examination including transnasal fiberoptic laryngoscopy and either CT or MRI. If the radiological aspect changes, biopsy under general anesthesia becomes unavoidable.

Laryngeal Osteochondronecrosis

Radiation-induced osteochondronecrosis is an uncommon complication of radiation therapy for laryngeal carcinoma and has a reported frequency of 1–15%.[15,89] Cartilage covered by intact perichondrium tolerates high doses of irradiation. Because the perichondrium is the sole nutrient source to the underlying cartilage, damage to the perichondrium places the underlying cartilage at considerable risk of perichondritis.[15,26] Viral or bacterial laryngitis, as well as biopsy of the irradiated larynx, may induce irreversible infectious perichondritis and/or osteomyelitis, which may lead to frank necrosis and laryngeal collapse. Destruction of the perichondrium appears to render the cartilage much more susceptible to radiation osteochondronecrosis. Other predisposing factors are short treatment times to achieve a specific dose, large treatment fields, chronic respiratory tract infections, and generalized arteriosclerosis.

The characteristic clinical features are painful swallowing, marked fetor, and occasionally sputum containing pus and cartilaginous sequestra. Chondronecrosis usually develops during radiotherapy, but it may still occur after months or years. In rare cases, chondroradionecrosis develops 20 or even 30 years after radiotherapy. Conservative measures (antibiotics, temporary tracheostomy, and hyperbaric oxygenation) are sometimes successful in resolving the necrotic tissue. Total laryngectomy is recommended if conservative measures are unsuccessful, and if there is a concern that coexistent recurrent tumor may be present. In rare

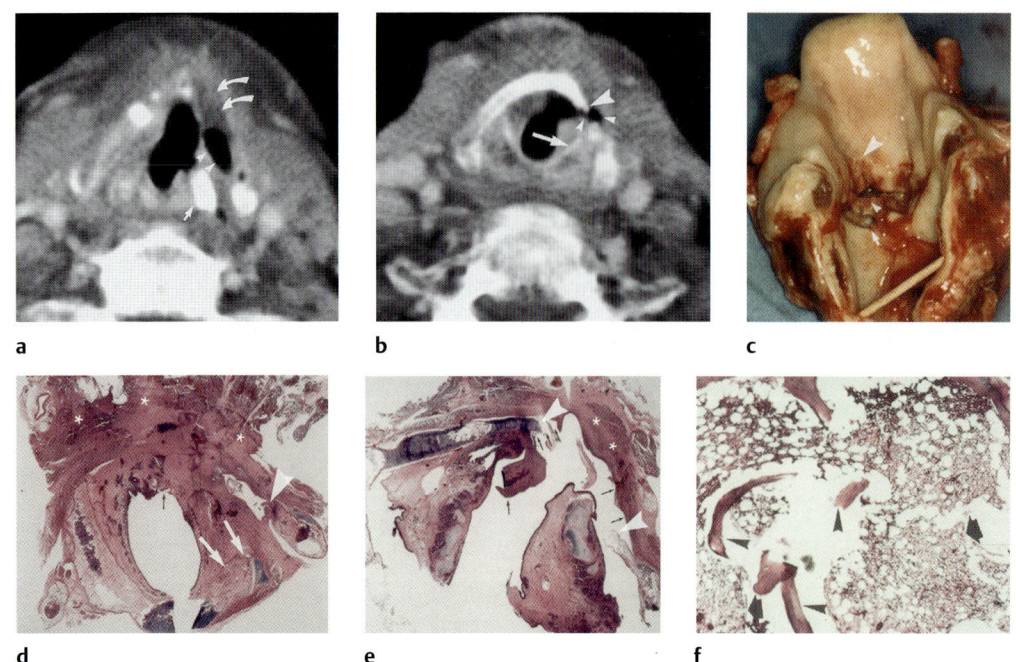

Fig. 11.52 Soft-tissue necrosis and osteochondronecrosis three months after radiation therapy in a 51-year-old patient irradiated for carcinoma of the left vocal cord with invasion of the thyroid cartilage (70 Gy, 2 Gy/fraction). **a** and **b** Contrast-enhanced spiral CT scan obtained 3 months after radiation therapy. Soft-tissue necrosis with deep ulcerations containing gas (small arrowheads) extends from the laryngeal surface into the thyroid cartilage. Fractured cartilage (large arrowhead). Areas of necrosis (curved arrows) extending into the prelaryngeal strap muscles. Note sclerosis of the left arytenoid cartilage (small arrow), and slightly increased density of the left cricoid cartilage (large arrow). Soft-tissue edema throughout the neck. Despite intensive conservative treatment, severe pain, dyspnea, and dysphagia persisted. **c** Total laryngectomy specimen viewed posteriorly shows extensive mucosal ulceration involving the left supraglottic (large arrowhead), glottic (small arrowhead), and subglottic (small arrow) regions. No macroscopic tumor mass is seen. **d**, **e** Whole-organ axial histological slices from specimen obtained at the same levels as **a** (**d**) and **b** (**e**) show mucosal ulceration (small black arrows), necrosis and fragmentation of the left thyroid cartilage (large arrowheads), necrosis of the left cricoid lamina (large arrows), and necrosis of prelaryngeal muscles (asterisks). No tumor tissue was found. Hematoxylin–eosin staining. **f** Detail from the left arytenoid cartilage shows spicules of necrotic bone (arrowheads) within purulent exudate and dense inflammatory infiltrates (thick black arrows). Reproduced from Reference 15 with permission.

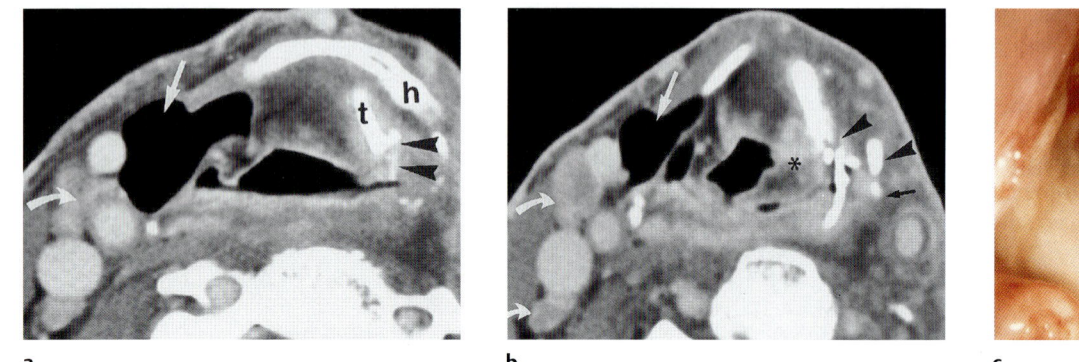

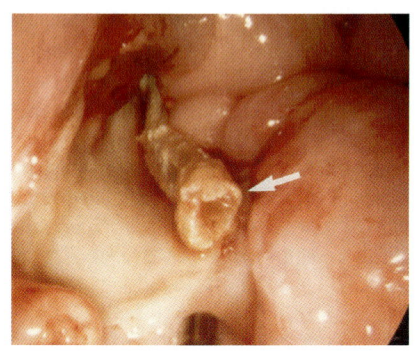

Fig. 11.53 Osteochondronecrosis of the thyroid cartilage in a 68-year-old patient with painful swallowing, hoarseness, and fetor 24 years after left radical neck dissection and radiation therapy for carcinoma of the left piriform sinus. **a**, **b** Contrast-enhanced CT images show craniocaudal collapse of the larynx. **a** The hyoid bone (h) is situated anteriorly to the thyroid cartilage (t). **a** and **b** show fragmentation of the sclerotic left thyroid cartilage (black arrowheads). Fragments of bone are seen in the preepiglottic space and in the soft tissues of the neck (small black arrow). Edema and increased contrast enhancement of the left aryepiglottic fold (asterisk). Incidentally, an external laryngocele is observed on the right (white arrows) and there are several enlarged reactive lymph nodes (curved arrows). **c** Endoscopic view obtained after unfolding of the left piriform sinus shows mucosal edema and denuded, yellowish, and friable thyroid cartilage (arrow). Several deep biopsies showed no tumor cells but only fragments of necrotic bone, suggesting osteoradionecrosis. The patient underwent conservative treatment and repeat follow-up CT studies obtained during a period of three years showed no significant changes of the larynx.

instances, necrosis can be so extensive and fulminant that it reaches the great vessels of the neck, resulting in carotid rupture.

CT and MRI features of osteochondronecrosis include inflammatory swelling adjacent to the area of eventual cartilage necrosis, deep gas-containing ulcerations, sclerotic appearance of the involved cartilages, fragmentation and sloughing of necrotic bone or cartilage, and abscess formation in the strap muscles or along the paraglottic space or fistula formation (Figs. 11.52, 11.53). In rare instances, laryngeal collapse may occur, which can easily be demonstrated on CT or MRI. Progressive sclerosis of the laryngeal cartilages during and after radiotherapy may reflect either tumor recurrence or osteochondronecrosis, or both. In general, progressive cartilage sclerosis must be considered as an indicator of poor prognosis.[88,89] If chondroradionecrosis occurs simultaneously with residual or recurrent tumor,[15,89] the distinction may be impossible by means of a

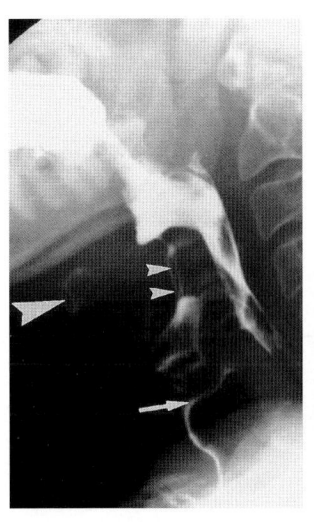

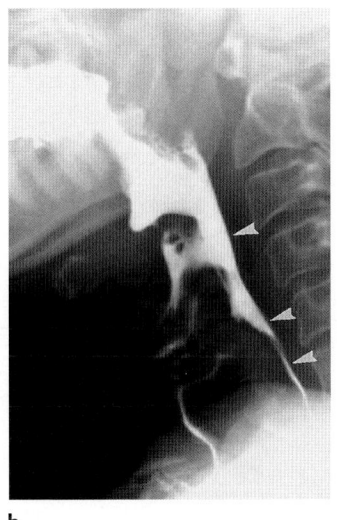

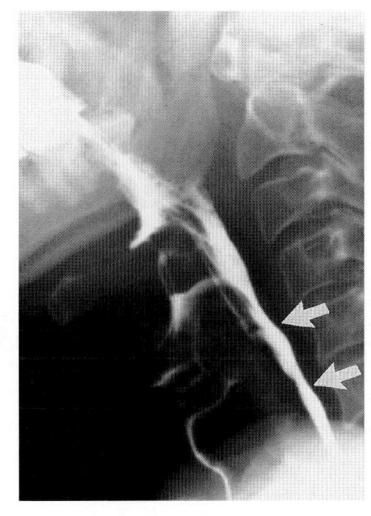

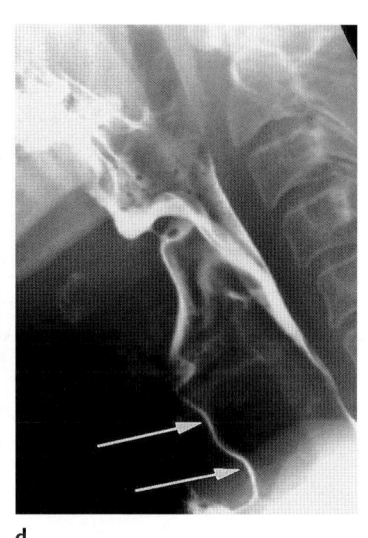

Fig. 11.**54** Pharyngeal stenosis and aspiration. **a–d** Selected stop-frame prints from videopharyngography of a 55-year-old patient with a history of irradiation for carcinoma of the oropharynx and hypopharynx with 79 Gy two years earlier. The patient presented with severe dysphagia, weight loss, and pneumonia. **a** As the bolus is propelled into the oropharynx, no elevation of the hyoid bone is seen (large arrowhead). The epiglottis remains in an upright position (small arrowheads). The bolus then enters the laryngeal vestibule and tracheal aspiration occurs owing to an open glottis (small arrow). **b** A few milliseconds later, the bolus descends into the hypopharynx (small arrowheads). **c** Maximal filling of the hypopharynx shows severe stenosis following radiation therapy (arrows). **d** Emptying of the hypopharynx with markedly diminished peristalsis. Secondary aspiration of residual bolus into the trachea (thin arrows). Note unchanged position of the hyoid bone and epiglottis throughout the entire deglutition due to severe fibrotic scarring of the neck muscles. Placement of a gastrostomy feeding tube was necessary. Reproduced from Reference 15 with permission.

single CT or MRI examination, and even a negative biopsy cannot rule out tumor. In such cases, follow-up imaging studies are the only way to exclude coexistent tumor in the presence of chondroradionecrosis.

Complications of Radiation Therapy in the Hypopharynx

Patients who have undergone radiation therapy for head and neck cancer may develop dysphagia due to tumor recurrence or due to radiation-induced morphological or functional changes.[15, 40, 59, 72] Videopharyngography is the method of choice to evaluate these patients and may reveal pharyngeal and esophageal motility dysfunction and morphological abnormalities such as strictures, ulceration, and fistula formation (Figs. **11.54–11.55**). Extensive neck fibrosis may cause a lack of elevation of the larynx during swallowing, which predisposes to aspiration. In addition, delayed closure of the glottis may lead to severe, life-threatening primary aspiration, while insufficient peristalsis of the pharyngeal constrictor muscles leads to ineffective bolus clearance and secondary aspiration. Radiogenic stenosis most often develops in the reconstructed pharynx after total laryngectomy, and the combination of radiotherapy with chemotherapy appears to predispose to pharyngeal and esophageal stenoses.

Recurrent Laryngeal Nerve Paralysis

Because the cranial nerves are very resistant to irradiation, paralysis is a rather uncommon finding. The suggested mechanism is nerve compression by perineural radiation-induced fibrosis.[21, 109] The hypoglossal nerve is the most commonly affected cranial nerve. Recurrent laryngeal nerve paralysis is uncommon, but it has been reported after external radiotherapy of head and neck cancer or breast tumors and following iodine-131 therapy for hyperthyroidism.[32] The CT and MRI features of recurrent laryngeal nerve paralysis are explained by atrophy of the thyroarytenoid muscle and include an enlarged ventricle, ipsilateral enlargement of the piriform sinus, and atrophy of the true vocal cord (see below).[8, 15] If sectional imaging does not show a tumor mass

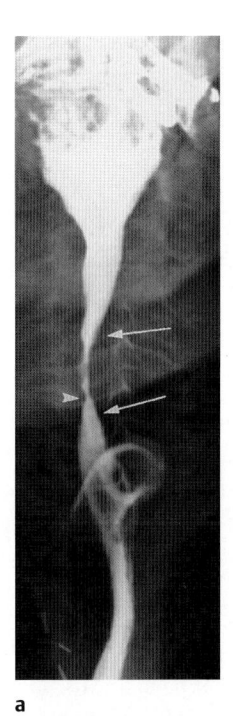

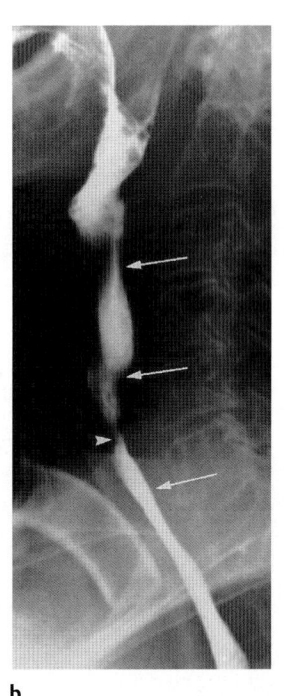

Fig. 11.**55** Pharyngeal stenosis following surgery and radiotherapy. Selected stop-frame prints from videopharyngography of a 55-year-old patient with a history of total laryngectomy followed by radiotherapy for carcinoma of the larynx three years earlier. **a** Frontal and **b** lateral projections. Pharyngeal phase shows a severe, smoothly marginated concentric long-segment stenosis of the reconstructed pharynx (arrows) with an additional short-segment stenotic area (arrowhead). Endoscopy revealed no tumor recurrence. Despite several endoscopic dilations, the patient remained symptomatic, requiring placement of a gastrostomy feeding tube. Reproduced from Reference 15 with permission.

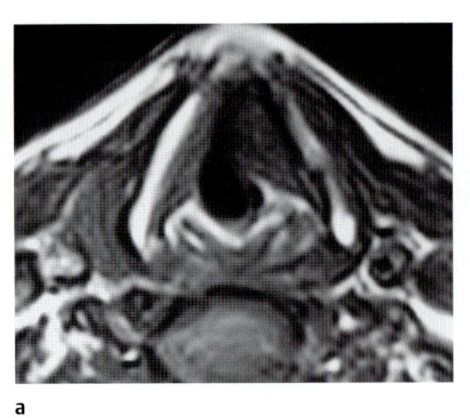

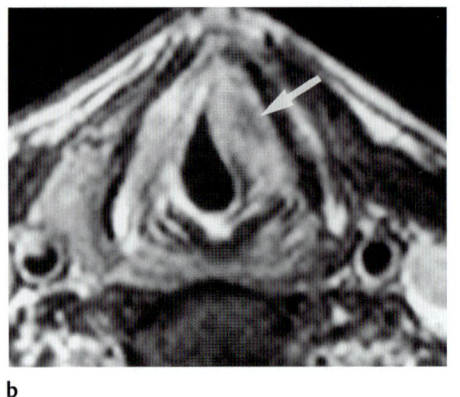

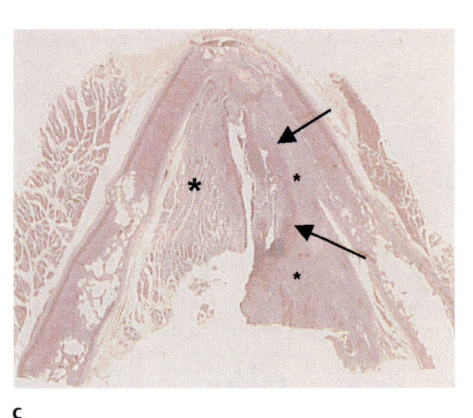

Fig. 11.**56** Detection of tumor recurrence with MRI. Elderly patient with a history of radiation therapy for a small laryngeal squamous cell cancer two years earlier. The patient was complaining of progressive hoarseness. Endoscopy showed an intact mucosa on both vocal cords, but the left vocal cord was fixed. Initial endoscopic biopsy was negative for squamous cell carcinoma. An MRI examination was performed two weeks later. **a, b** T1W SE MR images before (**a**) and after (**b**) injection of contrast material show asymmetry of the vocal cords with an area of inhomogeneous enhancement within the left thyroarytenoid muscle suggesting tumor recurrence. Repeat endoscopic deep biopsy confirmed recurrent tumor. The patient underwent cricohyoidopexy. **c** Whole-organ surgical specimen confirms radiological findings. Black arrows point at the tumor, which is located beneath an intact mucosa. Small asterisks correspond to inflammatory findings within the thyroarytenoid muscle on the left. Large asterisk corresponds to the right thyroarytenoid muscle.

along the entire pathway of the vagus and recurrent laryngeal nerve in a patient with a history of high-dose irradiation of the area, the diagnosis of radiation-induced nerve paralysis should be considered.

Detection of Tumor Recurrence

Tumor recurrence occurring after radiation therapy usually becomes clinically manifest within the first two years. Physical and endoscopic examination is often limited by the changes induced in the mucosa and the underlying soft tissues by radiation therapy, and recurrent carcinoma originating extramucosally may be entirely invisible with endoscopy. The ideal follow-up protocol should therefore include serial sectional imaging with either CT or MRI with a baseline study obtained at 3 months after completion of radiation therapy and repeat studies with the same modality at 3- to 6-month intervals during the first two years. For economic reasons, such a protocol is only rarely feasible, and sectional imaging is usually restricted to patients at high risk for recurrence. The risk of patients treated with definitive radiation therapy may be estimated on the basis of prognostic factors, such as the pretherapeutic TNM stage (based on clinical findings, endoscopy, and imaging), and the pretherapeutic and posttherapeutic sectional imaging findings.[56, 57, 66, 80, 93-95] Imaging studies may thus be limited to patients at high risk for tumor recurrence, whereas patients at low risk may be followed clinically until symptoms or signs of recurrence occur, e.g., changes in the quality of voice, pain, dyspnea, or vocal cord fixation, or a tumor mass is seen on endoscopy. Once recurrence has been proven, the pretherapeutic TNM classification is termed "rTNM," and the pathological TNM classification is termed "prTNM"

CT is most commonly used for the follow-up of patients who have undergone radiation therapy of laryngohypopharyngeal tumors; however, at some institutions, MRI or PET is used to detect tumor recurrence after radiation therapy, surgery, or both.[53]

The tissue characteristics of recurrent tumors are similar to those of primary tumors. Regardless of the imaging technique that is being used, the radiologists must be familiar with the expected morphological changes, as well as with possible early and late complications induced by radiation therapy. Distinction between such nonneoplastic, posttherapeutic changes and signs of recurrent or residual tumor may be difficult, and involves a "learning curve." The diagnostic performance may therefore depend on the radiologist's experience. Successful radiation therapy leads to a substantial reduction of tumor volume within four months, and treatment failure must be suspected if 50% or more of the tumor mass is still visible after this period. Although a subtle or minor focal abnormality should not be considered as evidence of persistent tumor until the third month after treatment, an obvious 2–3 cm mass or a progressively enlarging mass suggests recurrent or residual tumor (Fig. 11.**56**). It has been suggested that it is probably best to avoid imaging at all until three months posttherapy, so that one is not tempted to biopsy the areas of focal CT or MRI abnormality.[75, 80] Biopsy at this stage carries the risk of inducing perichondritis or chondronecrosis.

In summary, diffuse changes in the larynx and hypopharynx should not be regarded as evidence of tumor recurrence. However, focal masses seen on CT or MR images beyond three months after completion of radiation therapy should alert the radiologist to the possibility of residual or recurrent tumor. Fluorodeoxyglucose (FDG-)PET holds promise of facilitating the differentiation between radiation-induced changes and tumor recurrence.[53] A detailed discussion of the latest literature on this subject is beyond the scope of this chapter.

Cystic Lesions, Pouches, Diverticula, and Webs

■ Larynx

Cystic lesions of the larynx include mucosal cysts, laryngoceles, laryngeal mucocele, and thyroglossal duct cysts.[8, 85, 93]

Laryngeal cysts originate from the minor salivary glands within the mucosa of the larynx. They may therefore be seen anywhere within the larynx. Diagnosis of a salivary gland cyst may be suspected clinically and imaging usually confirms the diagnosis. On CT, cysts demonstrate a low attenuation values (0–20 HU) and they show no enhancement after injection of contrast material. On MR, the cysts display a high signal intensity on T2-weighted images and variable signal intensities on T1-weighted images owing to the variable protein content.

Laryngoceles occur as a result of elongation and dilatations of the saccule (laryngeal appendix) of the laryngeal ventricle. A laryngocele often forms due to obstruction of the laryngeal saccule (laryngeal appendix) where it opens into the laryngeal ventricle (Fig. 11.**57**); sometimes a small cancer located near the neck of the saccule may be responsible and thus becomes clinically manifest. Laryngoceles are found in 2% of healthy individuals and in 18% of patients with carcinoma of the larynx. Laryngoceles may contain air or fluid. In the latter case they are also referred to as **saccular cyst** or **laryngeal mucocele**. An **internal laryngocele** extends superiorly in the paraglottic space and appears endoscopically as a submucosal supraglottic mass (Fig. 11.**58**). If the laryngocele extends through the thyrohyoid membrane into the soft tissues of the neck, it is termed an **external laryngocele** (Fig. 11.**59**). An external laryngocele is in fact a combined laryngocele with both internal and external components present. On CT and MRI, a laryngocele presents as a well-circumscribed, air- or fluid-filled structure extending from the laryngeal ventricle into the paraglottic space or through the thyrohyoid membrane into the soft tissues of the neck (Figs. 11.**58**, 11.**59**). Cases of laryngeal mucocele and pyocele is shown in Figs. 11.**58 b**, 11.**59 a**.

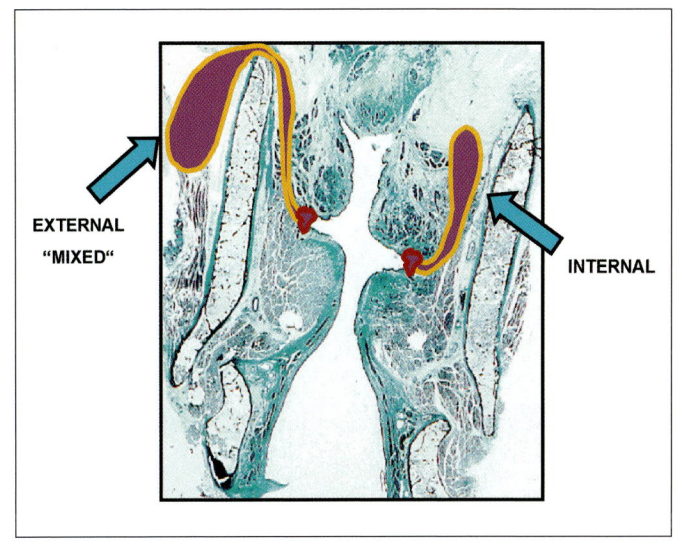

Fig. 11.**57** Schematic representation of the mechanism by which laryngoceles form.

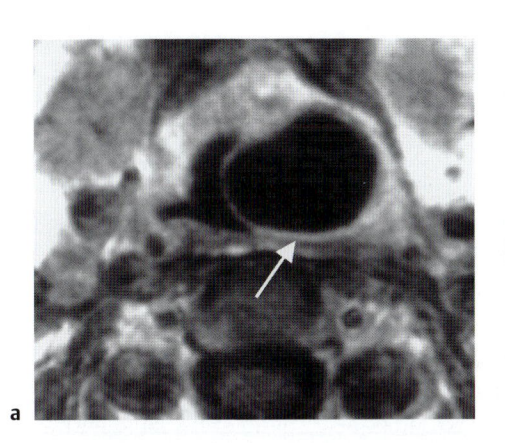

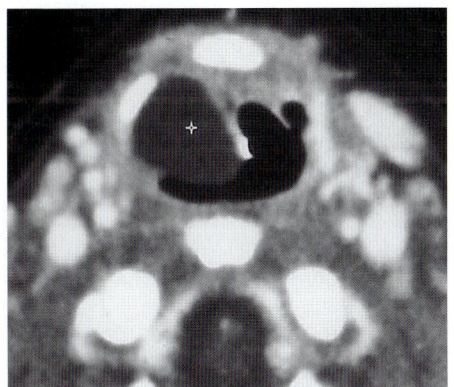

Fig. 11.**58** T1W SE MR image. Two different patients with internal laryngoceles.
a Contrast-enhanced T1W SE MR image in a dyspneic 45-year-old man shows a large, air-filled structure with thin, smooth, enhancing walls (arrow) located in the supraglottic larynx, characteristic of an internal laryngocele. **b** Contrast-enhanced CT image in a severely dyspneic 4-day-old boy shows a large, fluid-filled structure (calipter) with thin, smooth walls located in the supraglottic larynx, characteristic of an internal congenital laryngeal mucocele.

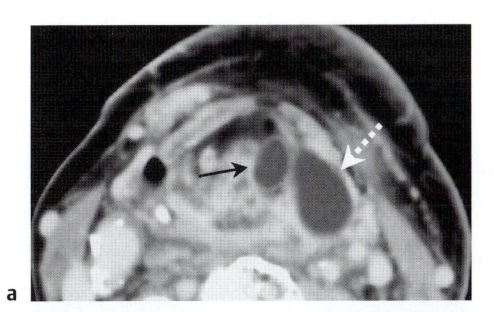

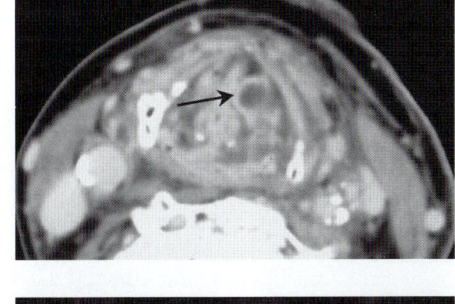

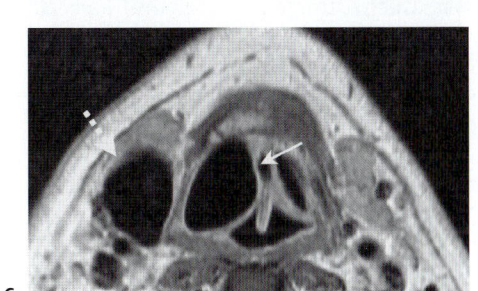

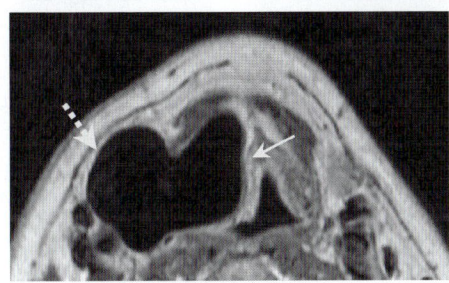

Fig. 11.**59** Two different patients with external laryngoceles. The first patient patient presented with fever, severe dyspnea, and a palpable soft compressible swelling in the left neck. **a, b** Contrast-enhanced CT images at the supraglottic level show a fluid-filled dilated laryngeal saccule (arrow) extending through the thyrohyoid membrane into the soft tissues of the neck (dashed arrow). There is slight enhancement of the walls of the fluid-filled structure (mucocele and pyocele). Note associated inflammatory findings within the neck with marked cellulitis of the anterior soft tissues of the neck. The second patient presented with a palpable swelling of the right neck. **c, d** Contrast-enhanced T1W FSE MR images at the supraglottic level show an air-filled laryngocele (arrows) extending through the thyrohyoid membrane into the soft tissues of the neck (dashed arrows).

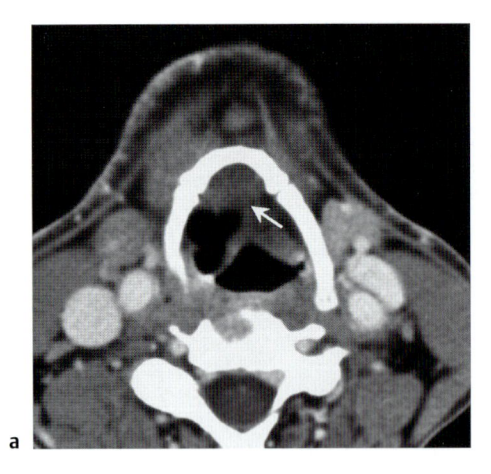

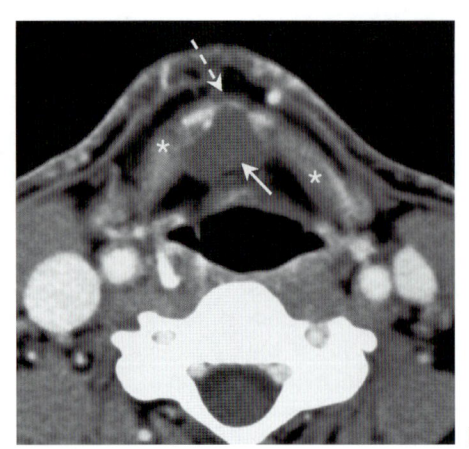

Fig. 11.60 Thyroglossal duct cyst. Contrast-enhanced CT images at the level of the hyoid bone (a) and at the upper supraglottic level (b) showing a midline cystic lesion (arrows), without enhancing walls, extending into the preepiglottic space at the level of the thyroid notch (dashed arrow). Note the close proximity to the hyoid bone, as well as the characteristic location within the strap muscles (asterisks).

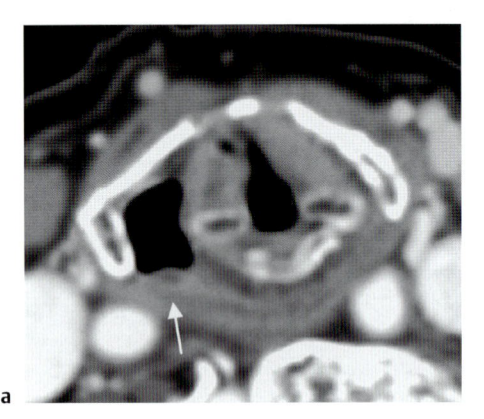

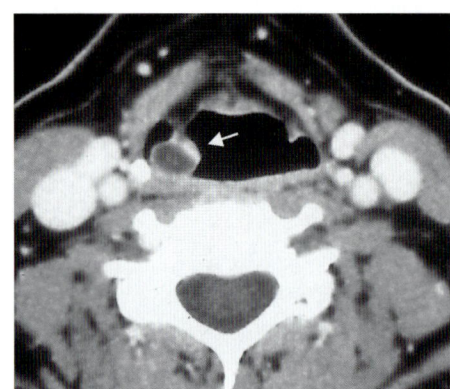

Fig. 11.61 Common carotid arteries. Two different patients with mucous retention cysts of the hypopharynx. a Contrast-enhanced CT image in a 60-year-old woman shows a small cystic lesion (arrow), without enhancing walls, originating from the posterior wall of the hypopharynx, characteristic of a mucous retention cyst. Note as an incidental finding a retropharyngeal course of both common carotid arteries. b Contrast-enhanced CT image in a 45-year-old woman with dyspnea shows a cystic lesion (arrow) with enhancing walls originating from the posterior wall of the aryepiglottic fold (anterior wall of the piriform sinus), characteristic of an infected mucous retention cyst.

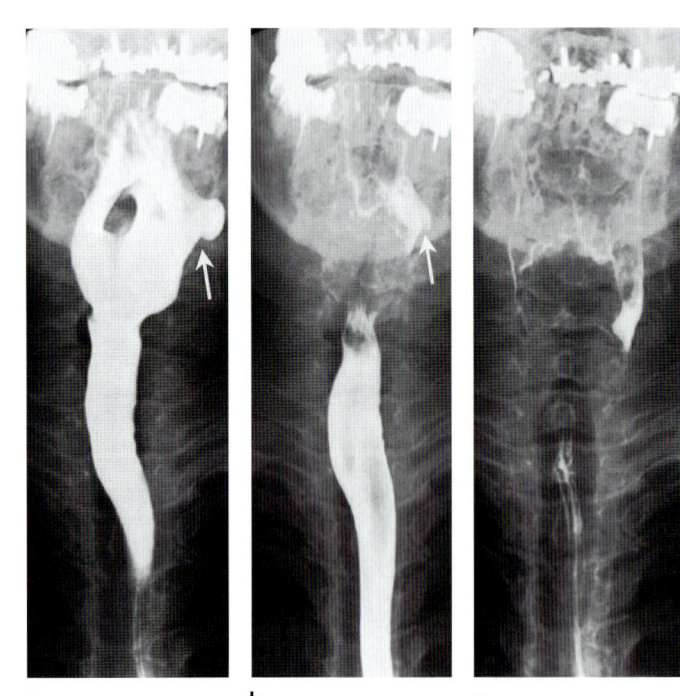

Fig. 11.62 Left-sided inconstant pharyngocele. Videopharyngography sequence nicely shows that early during the pharyngeal phase of deglutition (a) a broad-based pharyngeal pouch forms at the level of the thyrohyoid membrane (arrow). As the pharynx empties (b), the pharyngocele disappears progressively until it is no longer observed at rest (c).

Thyroglossal duct cysts arise from the thyroglossal duct remnant. The infrahyoid thyroglossal duct cyst is typically seen anterior to the larynx within or beneath the strap muscles. It is located in the midline or slightly off the midline (Fig. 11.60). Occasionally, the cyst can bulge over the notch of the thyroid cartilage into the preepiglottic fat space (Fig. 11.60). The paraglottic space is spared, as opposed to the case with laryngoceles, which usually extend into the paraglottic space.

■ Hypopharynx

Cystic lesions of the hypopharynx include **mucosal cysts**, which originate from the minor salivary glands within the mucosa of the hypopharynx. They may be seen anywhere within the hypopharynx and diagnosis is usually straightforward on CT and MRI (Fig. 11.61).

Pharyngoceles, also referred to as "pharyngeal pouches" or "pharyngeal ears," are benign outpouchings of the pharyngeal mucosa of the upper piriform sinus. They are typically seen in the elderly and occur at that portion of the thyrohyoid membrane that receives no support from the inferior and middle pharyngeal constrictors.[59] Pharyngoceles may be subdivided into "inconstant" pharyngoceles, which are seen only during milliseconds while swallowing, and "constant" pharyngoceles, which are also seen at rest after deglutition (Fig. 11.62). Pharyngoceles are caused by an increased pressure in the pharynx, as may be the case in trumpet or saxophone players. An increased pharyngeal pressure may also be caused by mechanical obstruction of the pharynx due to tumors of the hypopharynx and cervical esophagus, strictures, or webs, or by functional pharyngeal obstruction, such as dysfunction of the cricopharyngeus muscle

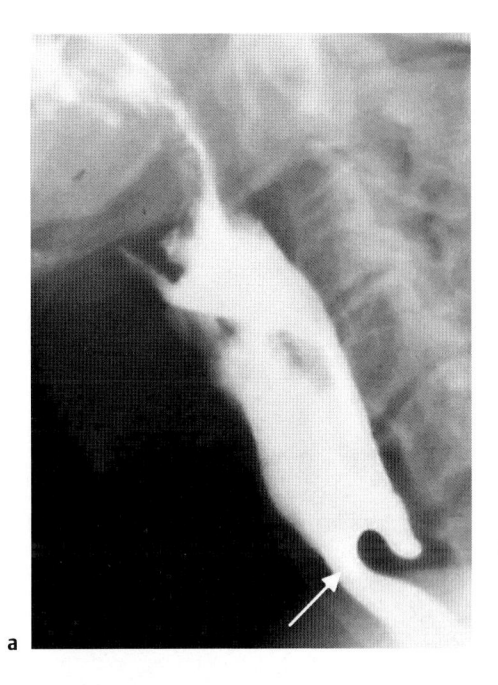

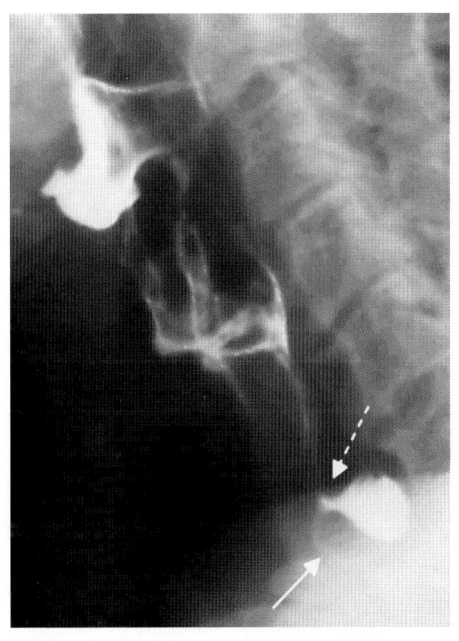

Cystic Lesions, Pouches, Diverticula, and Webs   771

Fig. 11.**63** Zenker's diverticulum in a 54-year-old symptomatic man. Videopharyngography sequence shows that early during the pharyngeal phase of deglutition (**a**) the cricopharyngeus muscle closes prematurely (dysfunction of the cricopharyngeus muscle, arrow). When the peristaltic wave sweeping down the pharynx (**b**) reaches Killian's dehiscence (dashed arrow), the mucosa herniates posteriorly, forming the characteristic pulsion diverticulum, also referred to as "Zenker's diverticulum." Arrow in **b** points at the dysfunction of the cricopharyngeus muscle.

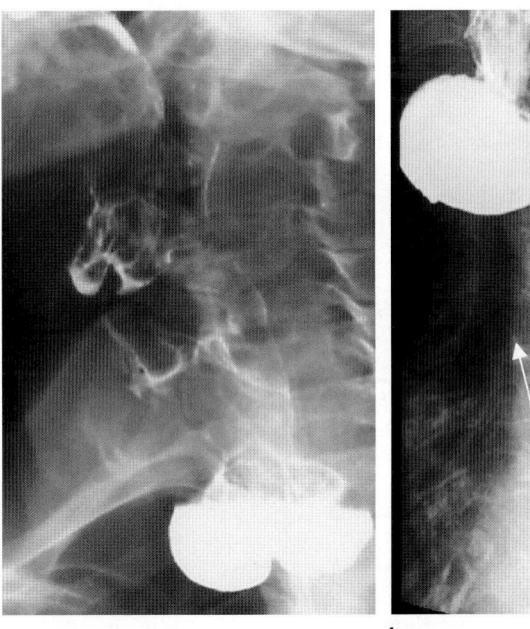

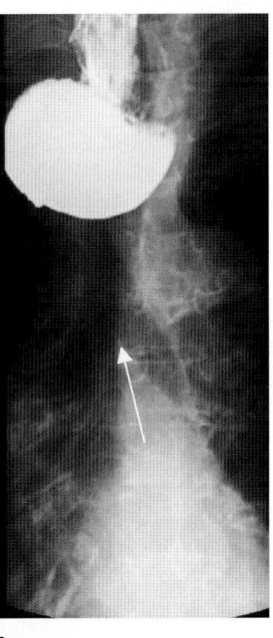

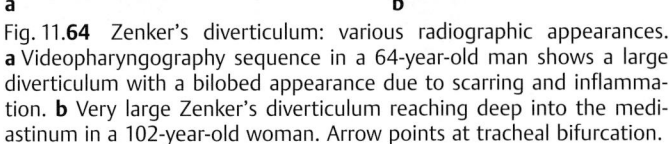

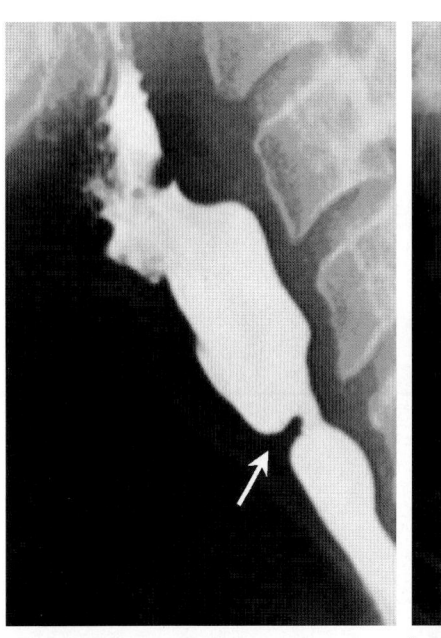

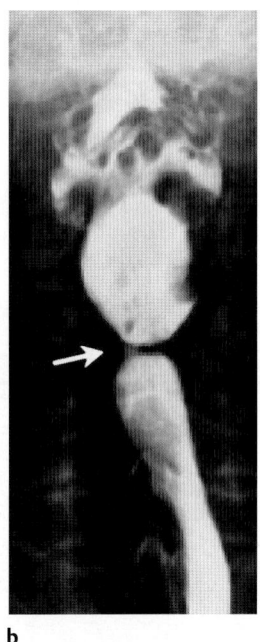

Fig. 11.**64** Zenker's diverticulum: various radiographic appearances. **a** Videopharyngography sequence in a 64-year-old man shows a large diverticulum with a bilobed appearance due to scarring and inflammation. **b** Very large Zenker's diverticulum reaching deep into the mediastinum in a 102-year-old woman. Arrow points at tracheal bifurcation.

Fig. 11.**65** Hypopharyngeal web in a 67-year-old patient with psoriasis. Videopharyngography (**a** lateral view, **b** frontal view) shows a thin membrane arising from the anterior wall of the hypopharynx characteristic of a web.

and pharyngeal hypomotility disorders. The diagnosis of pharyngoceles is usually straightforward. On frontal barium studies, the pharyngoceles appear as broad-based outpouchings filled with barium (Fig. 11.**62**). An air-filled pharyngocele can occasionally be seen on CT as an incidental finding.

Diverticula of the hypopharynx may be subdivided into lateral and posterior diverticula. Lateral pharyngeal diverticula may arise as vestiges of the third and fourth branchial clefts or may be lateral pulsion diverticula. Congenital lateral diverticula present as true branchial cleft cysts and sinuses that connect only with the pharynx internally and end blindly in the neck. Posterior hypopharyngeal diverticula are also known as "Zenker's diverticula." **Zenker's diverticulum** is a mucosa-lined outpouching of the hypopharynx occurring at the anatomical area of weakness known as "Killian's dehiscence" or "Lannier's triangle."[59, 129] Dysfunction of the cricopharyngeus muscle plays a key role in the formation of this pulsion diverticulum.[59, 129] When the cricopharyngeus muscle closes prematurely, the peristaltic wave sweeping down the pharynx raises the intraluminal pressure in the hypopharynx. The resultant increased intraluminal pressure forces the mucosa to herniate through the anatomical weak spot at Killian's dehiscence (Figs. 11.**63**, 11.**64**).

Webs, although more frequent in the upper esophagus, may occur as thin, delicate membranes that typically arise from the anterior wall of the hypopharynx (Fig. 11.**65**). Because many webs can be seen only during a few milliseconds, videopharyn-

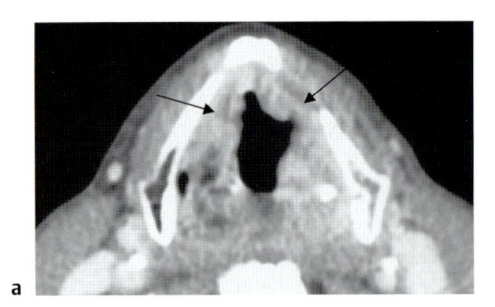

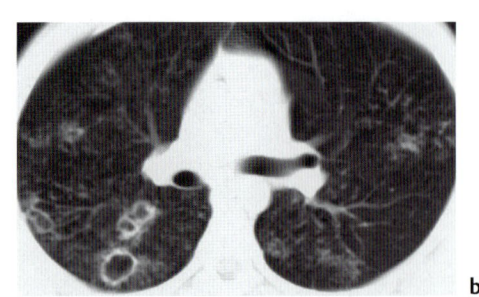

Fig. 11.**66** Tuberculosis with laryngeal involvement in a 37-year-old woman presenting in the emergency room with cough, hemoptysis, and severe dyspnea. **a** CT of the neck reveals a large bilateral laryngeal mass involving both false cords (arrows), ventricles, and paraglottic spaces, radiologically indistinguishable from squamous cell carcinoma. **b** CT image through the chest (lung window setting) shows the characteristic appearance of lung tuberculosis with multiple caverns. On the basis of the characteristic appearance of the lung, the presumed diagnosis was laryngeal tuberculosis. The diagnosis of tuberculosis with laryngeal involvement was confirmed by endoscopic biopsy.

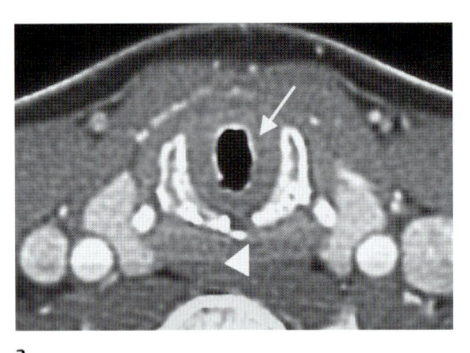

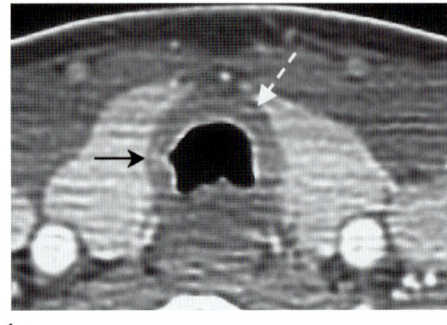

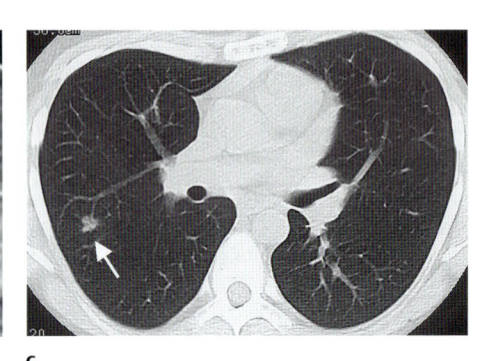

Fig. 11.**67** Wegener's granulomatosis with subglottic, tracheal, and pulmonary involvement in a 35-year-old woman. **a** and **b** Contrast-enhanced CT of the larynx and trachea reveals circumferential, slightly irregular soft-tissue thickening at the subglottic region (arrow), as well as at the level of the cervical trachea (dashed arrow). Note irregular contours of the cricoid posteriorly (arrowhead) and tracheal ring laterally (black stealth arrow). **c** CT image through the chest (lung-window setting) shows a characteristic infiltrate (arrow).

gography in the lateral projection is the examination of choice. Webs are either asymptomatic incidental findings or they may occlude enough of the lumen to cause dysphagia. When they do so, a liquid bolus passing through the hypopharynx will be squirted through the opening of the web in form of a jet ("jet phenomenon"). Webs may be idiopathic or they may be caused by a variety of diseases, such as the Plummer–Vinson syndrome, skin diseases (epidermolysis bullosa, psoriasis, pemphygoid), and graft-versus-host reactions.

Infectious and Inflammatory Conditions

Imaging is rarely done in patients with infectious and inflammatory conditions of the larynx and hypopharynx, as most of these patients are diagnosed clinically.[8, 33, 19] Occasionally, imaging may be done to exclude other etiologies or to look for complications.

Laryngotracheitis, or **croup**, is an infection that occurs in the age group 3 months to 3 years and is caused by a parainfluenza virus. The onset is gradual, with several days of upper and lower respiratory tract symptoms followed by the development of a classic barking cough and stridor. The mucosal swelling is most significant in the subglottic area, where airway narrowing causes the gradual airway tapering described as the "wine bottle" when visualized on plain films. However, plain films should be interpreted with caution and within the clinical context, as the sensitivity and specificity of radiographs in croup has been reported to be low.

Epiglottitis or **supraglottitis** occurs in a slightly older age group and is caused by *Haemophilus influenza* type B. Diffuse thickening of the epiglottis and supraglottic larynx is typically seen on plain films. Because total airway obstruction may occur very rapidly, necessitating emergency tracheotomy, patients with epiglottitis should always be investigated in the emergency room.[33]

A variety of **granulomatous diseases** may affect the larynx and hypopharynx. Although in Europe and North America infections such as tuberculosis, syphilis, or fungal infections rarely affect the laryngo-hypopharyngeal region, these entities have recently gained increasing importance in immunocompromised patients. If granulomatous tissue becomes visible on CT and MRI, it cannot usually be differentiated from neoplasia. Nonetheless, the combination of pulmonary tuberculosis and bilateral diffuse laryngeal soft-tissue lesions without destruction of the laryngeal architecture should raise the suspicion of **laryngeal tuberculosis** (Fig. 11.**66**).

Wegener granulomatosis is a necrotizing vasculitis that causes inflammatory lesions, usually granulomas or areas of necrosis in the respiratory tract and kidney (Fig. 11.**67**). It can involve the larynx. However, usually other areas of the head and neck, such as the orbits and the paranasal sinuses, are involved as well. Nevertheless, laryngeal involvement may be the initial presentation of Wegener granulomatosis. Clinically, the laryngeal lesions may be superficial or may present as submucosal masses, most often in the subglottic region (Fig. 11.**67**). Differential diagnosis includes relapsing polychondritis, amyloidosis, and sarcoidosis (Fig. 11.**68**).

Relapsing polychondritis is a rare connective-tissue disease that causes inflammation of cartilages and may be associated with cardiovascular problems. Relapsing polychondritis may affect the laryngeal cartilages, tracheal cartilages, and cartilages in the nose and ear. Initially, a soft-tissue swelling around the cartilages is seen and then the cartilages are weakened or destroyed. Calcification is seen in the abnormal soft tissues and may be quite extensive.[33]

Laryngeal stenosis and tracheal stenosis may be congenital or may be the sequelae of previous trauma or surgery. Typically, a circumferential narrowing may occur. The length of such a stenosis is best assessed on coronal 2D reconstructions from volumetric data sets (Fig. 11.**69**). Virtual endoscopy images are also very helpful in assessing the degree of stenosis. In addition, CT can often determine whether the stenosis is composed only of soft tissue (in which case laser excision can be performed) or whether the tracheal ring has collapsed inward and the abnormal cartilage is located immediately beneath the mucosa.

Although diagnosis and treatment of pharyngitis is straightforward in general, the situation may be more complex in the **immunocompromised patient with pharyngitis due to opportunistic infection** involving unusual pathogenic organisms. In such situations sectional imaging may be indicated to assess whether the disease is limited to the mucosa or whether abscesses are present. **Necrotizing fasciitis** is a severe, acute, and potentially life-threatening bacterial soft-tissue infection with a very rapid clinical evolution. CT findings include cellulitis, multiple fluid collections with or without gas in various neck compartments, diffuse enhancement of neck fasciae, and myositis of strap muscle. The larynx is often involved, necessitating emergency intubation.[19] **Myositis with or without abscess formation** and, eventually, **myonecrosis** of the pharyngeal constrictor results in dysphagia and severe aspiration (Fig. 11.**70**). If the patient survives, long-term sequelae with persistent scarring may result, especially at the level of the inferior pharyngeal constrictor muscle. In the acute and subacute phase, CT and MRI may demonstrate contrast enhancement of the pharyngeal constrictor muscles or frank disruption of the pharyngeal wall.

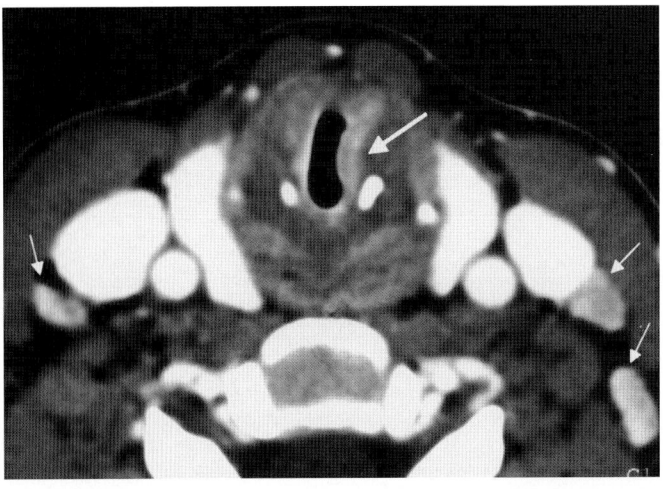

Fig. 11.**68** Amyloidosis with subglottic and nodal involvement in a 35-year-old woman presenting with subglottic narrowing at endoscopy. The mucosa was intact. Contrast-enhanced CT of the neck reveals circumferential soft-tissue thickening at the subglottic region with areas of increased enhancement (arrow). Note the presence of enhancing cervical neck nodes bilaterally (thin arrows). Biopsy revealed amyloid deposits within the subglottic region as well as in the neck. Courtesy of Dr. Guy Moulin, Hôpital La Timone, Marseille, France.

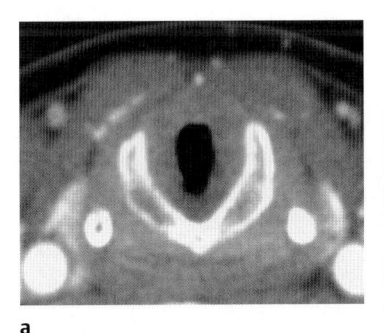

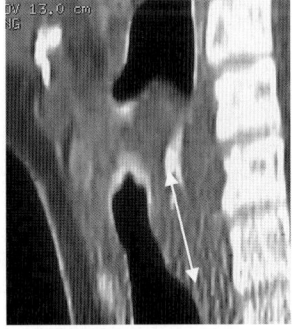

Fig. 11.**69** Subglottic and tracheal stenosis following long intubation. **a** Contrast-enhanced axial image at the subglottic level shows massive circumferential thickening of the subglottic soft tissues. **b** Sagittal 2D reconstruction from the volumetric data set enables better assessment of the craniocaudal extent of the lesion (arrow).

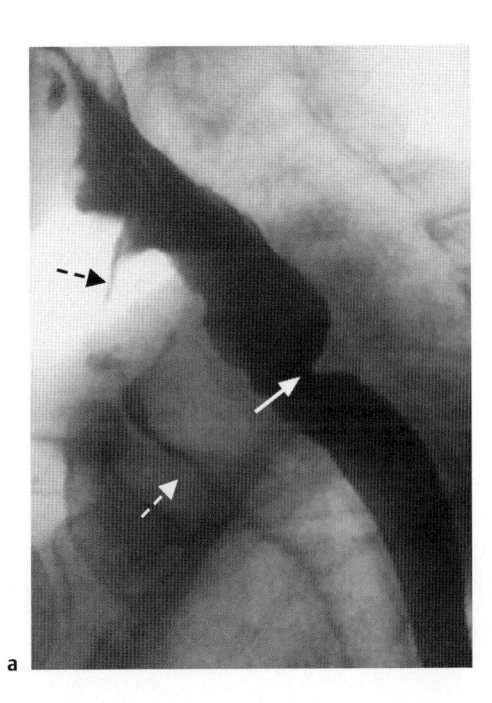

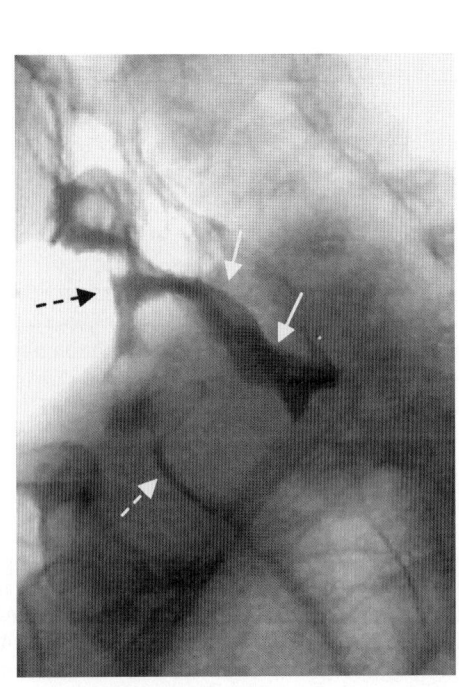

Fig. 11.**70** Necrotizing fasciitis of the neck with involvement of the pharyngeal constrictors and strap muscles. **a** Videopharyngography shows dysfunction of the cricopharyngeus muscle (arrow) and primary aspiration (dashed arrows) early during the pharyngeal phase of deglutition. **b** After deglutition, owing to insufficient peristalsis, contrast material is retained in the hypopharynx (arrows) leading to secondary aspiration (dashed arrows).

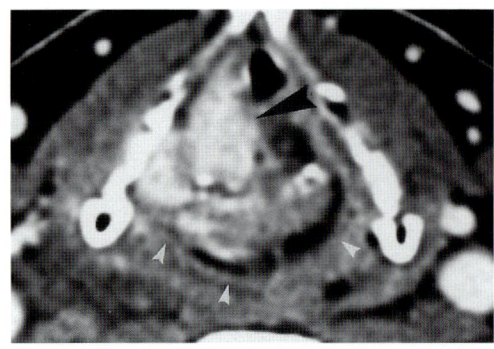

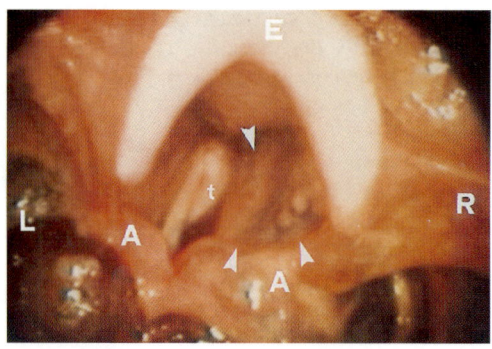

Fig. 11.**71** Venous malformation in a 58-year-old man presenting with hoarseness. **a** CT image at the supraglottic level demonstrates strong enhancement of a large mass involving the right false cord (arrowhead). Small arrowheads point to the aryepiglottic folds. **b** Endoscopic image obtained in the same patient shows a dark red mass (arrowheads) covered by intact mucosa. Note that—as we are looking from above—the patient's right side (R) is situated to the reader's right side and the patient's left side (L) is situated to the reader's left side. The epiglottis (E), which is located anteriorly, is seen at the top of the image and the aryepiglottic folds (A), which are located posteriorly, are seen at the bottom of the image. A = aryepiglottic folds. E = epiglottis. t = left true vocal cord. No treatment was performed. Reproduced from Reference 13 with permission.

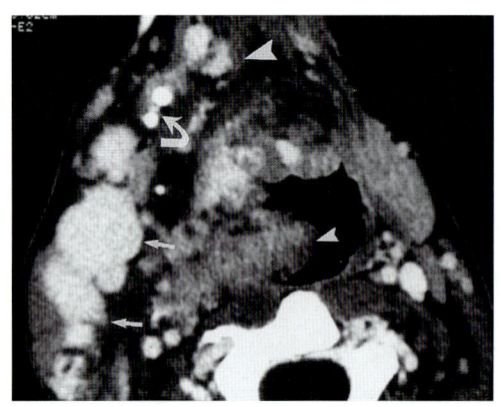

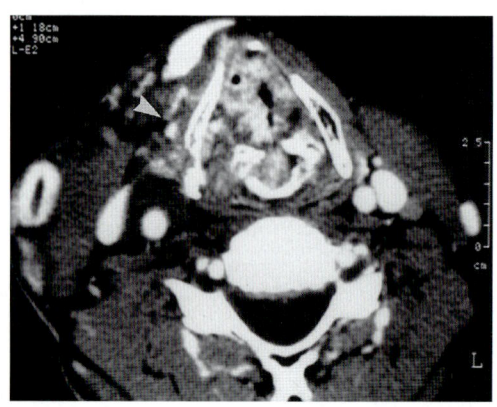

Fig. 11.**72** Laryngeal involvement in extensive cervicofacial angiodysplasia in a 37-year-old man presenting with recurrent episodes of dyspnea. **a** Contrast-enhanced CT image demonstrates cervicofacial angiodysplasia with involvement of the floor of the mouth (large arrowhead), right aryepiglottic fold (small arrowhead), and submandibular space (arrows). Phleboliths are indicated by the curved arrow. **b** Contrast-enhanced CT image obtained at a lower level shows extensive involvement of both vocal cords and strap muscles (arrowhead). Note large tortuous arteries and draining veins characteristic of combined malformations. The patient underwent selective embolization treatment and partial laser excision of the endolaryngeal mass to reduce dyspnea. Reproduced from Reference 13 with permission.

Congenital Lesions

Congenital lesions of the larynx include atresias, clefts, stenoses, webs, laryngomalacia, and vascular malformations. With the exception of vascular malformations, all other congenital lesions of the larynx are extremely rare.

Vascular malformations are classified, on the basis of the predominant type of anomalous vessel, into capillary, venous, and lymphatic malformations.[90] Dyspnea and stridor are the most common presenting symptoms. **Venous** malformations are seen in adults and may present as an isolated, localized lesion in the supraglottic larynx or may be associated with extensive cervicofacial angiodysplasia (Fig. 11.**71**). Males are affected more often than females. Endoscopy shows a compressible swelling that is dark bluish red in color. The overlying mucosa is most often intact. Treatment options include laser excision, cryotherapy, and surgery in localized forms, or selective embolization in diffuse forms.[15,17,90] The radiological features are straightforward. Because venous malformations are low-flow lesions, on CT they may display only moderate enhancement after administration of contrast material, but phleboliths are pathognomonic. On MRI, venous malformations display a very high signal intensity on T2-weighted images and strong enhancement after administration of gadolinium chelates. The identification of venous lakes or the presence of phleboliths allows a correct diagnosis in most cases.

Arterial malformations are high-flow malformations. They include arteriovenous malformations and fistulae. At imaging, enlarged tortuous arteries and draining veins are seen. The arterial components of these lesions appear as flow voids on MR imaging. *Combined* vascular malformations share the features of both high-flow and low-flow lesions. Characteristically, these lesions tend to be highly invasive, they become enormous in size, and they are resistant to all forms of therapy (Fig. 11.**72**).

The differential diagnosis of strongly vascularized lesions in the larynx includes paraganglioma, leiomyoma, and metastases of hypervascular tumors. Laryngeal paragangliomas are neuroendocrine neoplasms arising from the superior or inferior laryngeal paraganglia. These tumors are three times more common in women than in men. However, paragangliomas are very uncommon in the larynx. Paragangliomas typically display multiple curvilinear signal voids on both T1-weighted and T2-weighted images. The conspicuity of these signal void areas increases with tumor size.

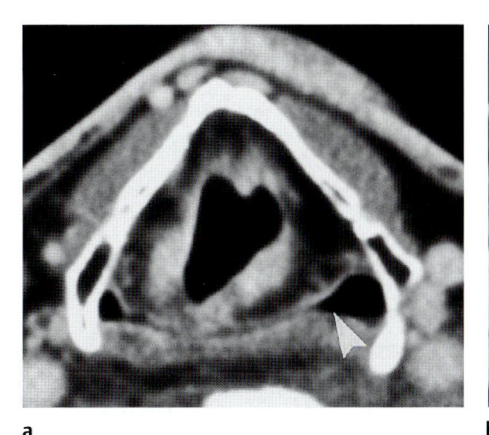

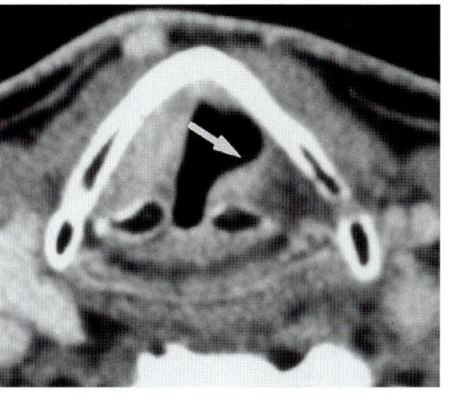

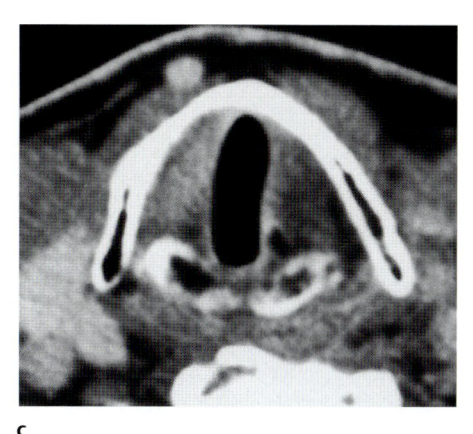

Fig. 11.**73** Recurrent laryngeal nerve paralysis. Contrast-enhanced CT scan at the level of the aryepiglottic folds (**a**), false cords (**b**), and undersurface of the true vocal cords (**c**) demonstrates a wide left piriform sinus (arrowhead), a paramedian position of the left false cord with a widened laryngeal ventricle (arrow), and decreased density of the left vocal cord corresponding to fatty infiltration. These findings indicate paralysis of the left recurrent laryngeal nerve.

Vocal Cord Paralysis

Vocal cord paralysis can be categorized as superior laryngeal nerve deficit, recurrent laryngeal nerve deficit, or total vagal nerve deficit. Paralysis of the recurrent laryngeal nerve is the most common type of vocal cord paralysis.[9, 15, 33] The CT and MRI features of recurrent laryngeal nerve paralysis are explained by atrophy of the thyroarytenoid muscle and include an enlarged ventricle, ipsilateral enlargement of the piriform sinus, paramedian position, and decreased size and/or fatty infiltration of the true vocal cord (Fig. 11.**73**). Although the most common cause of recurrent laryngeal nerve paralysis is iatrogenic, i.e., secondary to thyroid surgery, additional differential diagnostic considerations include mediastinal, thyroid, and esophageal masses and aneurysms. In a patient with recurrent laryngeal nerve paralysis of unknown origin, sectional imaging should be extended to the skull base and the mediastinum to include the entire pathway of the vagus and recurrent laryngeal nerve.

Trauma

■ Larynx

Severe blunt injuries of the larynx are relatively uncommon and are most often due to motor vehicle accidents when the larynx and upper trachea are crushed against the spine. Although emergency tracheotomy or cricothyroidotomy may be required to secure the airway, **laryngeal contusion** usually responds to conservative measures such as voice rest and head elevation, whereas **laryngeal fractures** with dislocation of fragments of cartilage are best repaired surgically within the first 24 hours. Therefore, sectional imaging is indicated in patients in whom laryngeal fractures are suspected clinically in order to determine the presence and extent of damage to the laryngeal framework. CT is now the preferred technique for examining patients with severe trauma and allows excellent delineation of most traumatic lesions. Axial images are sufficient to delineate most types of fractures and dislocations although horizontal fractures are better visualized on coronal 2D reconstructed images.[8, 33, 104] MR imaging is not yet widely used to evaluate patients with acute trauma. In young patients with nonossified cartilage, however, the information provided by MR imaging may be superior to that from CT.

Patterns of laryngeal injury observed on imaging studies include submucosal hematoma, dislocation of joints, fractures of the laryngeal cartilages, and avulsion of the epiglottis (Fig. 11.**74**). Dislocation of the cricoarytenoid joint may occur with minor trauma and is straightforward to diagnose owing to the abnormal position of the arytenoid relative to the cricoid cartilage. Cricothyroid dislocation occurs with severe trauma and CT demonstrates rotation of the cricoid ring relative to the thyroid with widening of the space between the lower thyroid and the cricoid. Fractures of the thyroid cartilage may be vertical or horizontal or may result in shattering of the entire thyroid cartilage[104] (Fig. 11.**74**). Dislocation or avulsion of the epiglottis occurs when the thyroepiglottic ligament is torn or when the superior portion of the thyroid cartilage is dislocated posteriorly.[39] Fractures of the cricoid cartilage tend to occur bilaterally and lead to a collapse of the cricoid ring. In young patients with nonossified hyaline cartilages, MR-imaging is superior to CT in correctly depicting laryngeal fractures (Fig. 11.**75**).

■ Hypopharynx

Perforation of the hypopharynx in adults is caused by ingestion of a chicken bone or fish bone or by instrumentation (endoscopy, biopsy). Such perforation results in soft-tissue emphysema and may lead to the development of a retropharyngeal abscess. Pus and edema can spread throughout the retropharyngeal space and from there into the mediastinum. In the acute setting, lateral plain radiographs may show air in the retropharyngeal space and soft tissues of the neck and pharyngography with water-soluble contrast material easily demonstrates the site of mucosal perforation (Fig. 11.**76**). As most of these patients are treated conservatively, follow-up studies are usually performed in order to monitor the spontaneous closure of the pharyngeal defect. Once the pharyngeal defect is closed, the patients are allowed to eat normally. CT is used routinely to detect complications of pharyngeal perforation, such as retropharyngeal abscess, septic thrombosis of the internal jugular vein, and mediastinitis (see Chapter 12). CT is also very valuable in localizing small or thin foreign bodies, such as fish bones, that have perforated the hypopharynx and are then located entirely within the retropharyngeal space (Fig. 11.**77**). Because these foreign bodies are located outside the

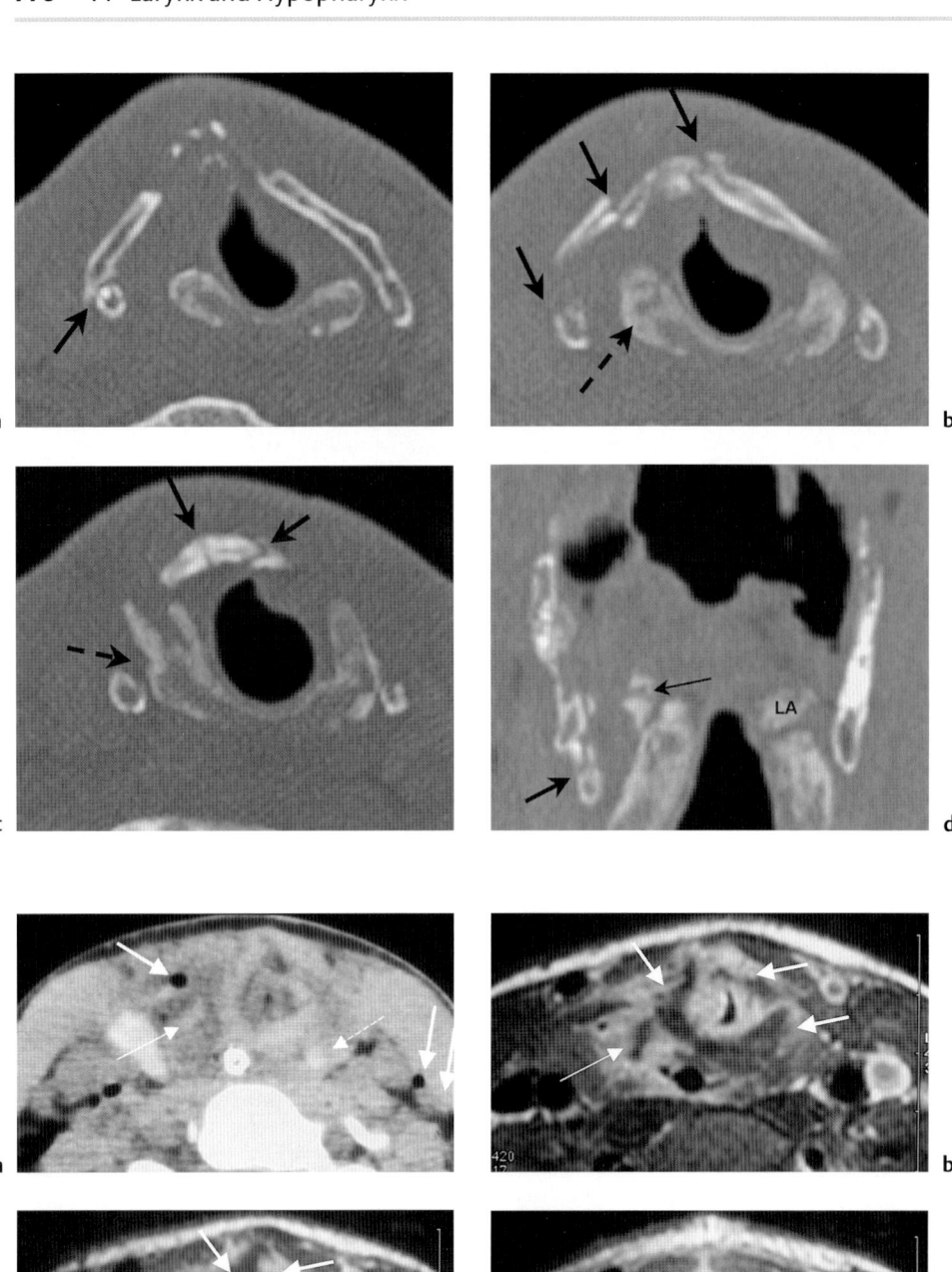

Fig. 11.74 Laryngeal trauma. This patient was involved in a motor vehicle accident and sustained a dashboard injury. Axial thin slice (1 mm) CT images (**a–c**) and coronal 2D reconstruction from volumetric data set (**d**) show a shattered thyroid cartilage (arrows) with posterior displacement of fragments resulting in airway narrowing. The cricoid cartilage is also fractured (dashed arrows) and there is lateral luxation of the fractured right arytenoid cartilage (thin arrow). LA = left arytenoid cartilage in normal position.

Fig. 11.75 Value of contrast-enhanced MR in laryngeal trauma. This 12-year-old boy was involved in a motor vehicle accident. **a** CT performed after emergency intubation revealed minor soft-tissue emphysema with some air bubbles (arrows), as well rotation of the cricoid ring to the left. A fracture of the right inferior cornu of the thyroid cartilage was suspected (thin arrow). The left inferior thyroid cornu is in a normal, undisplaced position (dashed arrow). Because the laryngeal cartilages are not ossified, exact delineation of the fractures is very difficult. **b–d** Contrast-enhanced T1W MR images show a completely shattered cricoid ring (arrows in **b** and **c**) as well as a fracture of the thyroid cartilage involving the inferior right cornu, which is displaced to the right (thin arrow). Note also extensive mucosal laceration (arrow in **d**) and fracture of the first tracheal ring (arrowhead in **d**). The patient underwent surgery, which confirmed the findings.

Fig. 11.76 Perforation of the hypopharynx by a chicken bone in a 75-year-old woman. **a** Plain lateral radiograph of the neck shows extensive soft-tissue emphysema. Note air within the retropharyngeal space (arrows). **b** Pharyngography with low-osmolarity, water-soluble iodinated contrast material shows the perforation site, which is located in the posterior wall of the hypopharynx (arrow). Note accumulation of contrast material within the retropharyngeal space (dashed arrows). The patient was treated conservatively and recovered a few days later.

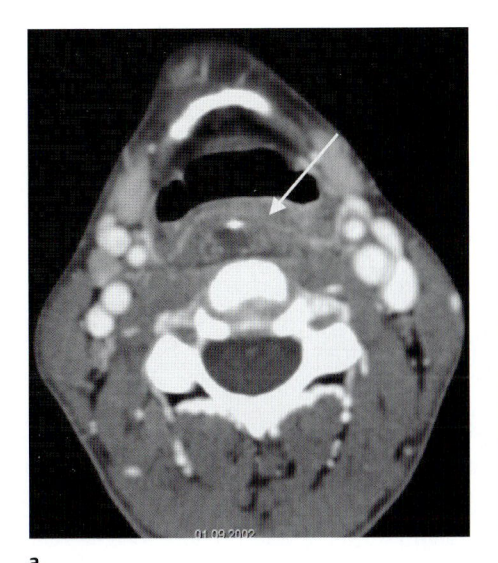

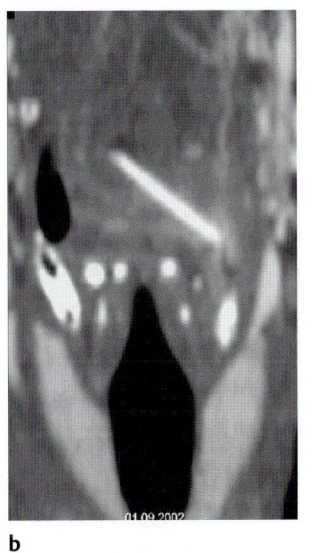

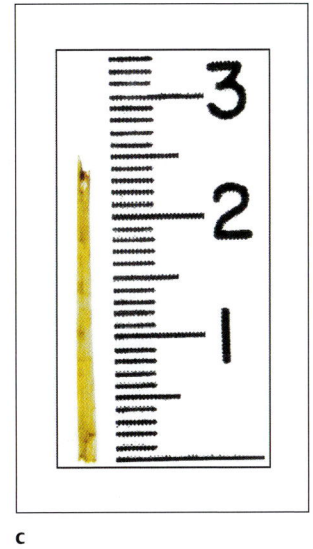

Fig. 11.**77** Perforation of the hypopharynx by a fish bone in a 55-year-old woman. **a** Axial and **b** coronal 2D reconstructions from a contrast-enhanced CT examination show a large retropharyngeal abscess (arrow) with a radiopaque foreign body within the abscess cavity. Endoscopy showed only a small mucosal laceration of the posterior hypopharyngeal wall. Surgical exploration revealed a retropharyngeal space abscess caused by a 2.5 cm long fish bone (shown in **c**), which was retrieved successfully.

hypopharynx, they cannot be seen by the endoscopist. Thus, the imaging may delineate the exact position of the foreign body, which can then be extracted endoscopically after incision of the hypopharyngeal wall at the appropriate site (Fig. 11.**77**).

References

1. Abramson AL, Brandsma J, Steinberg B, Winkler B. Verrucous carcinoma of the larynx. Arch Otolaryngol 1985; 111: 709–715.
2. Archer CR, Yeager VL, Herbold DR. Improved diagnostic accuracy in TNM staging of laryngeal cancer. J Comput Assist Tomogr 1983; 7: 610–617.
3. Archer CR, Yeager VL, Herbold DR. Computed tomography vs. histology of laryngeal cancer: their value in predicting laryngeal cartilage invasion. Laryngoscope 1983; 93: 140–147.
4. Banks ER, Frieson HF Jr, Mills SE, George E, Zarbo RJ, Swanson PE. Basaloid-squamous cell carcinoma of the head and neck. A clinicopathologic and immunohistochemical study of 40 cases. Am J Surg Pathol 1992; 16: 939–946.
5. Barbu RR, Khan A, Port JL, et al. Case report: Extramedullary plasmacytoma of the larynx. Comput Med Imaging Graph 1992; 16: 359.
6. Batsakis JG. Tumors of the Head and Neck. Clinical and Pathologic Considerations, 2 d ed., Baltimore: Williams and Wilkins; 1979.
7. Batsakis JG, El Naggar A. Basaloid–squamous cell carcinomas of the upper aerodigestive tract. Ann Otol Rhinol Laryngol 1989; 98: 919–920.
8. Becker M. Larynx and hypopharynx. Radiol Clin North Am 1998; 36: 891–920.
9. Becker M. Diagnose und Stadieneinteilung von Larynxtumoren mittels CT und MRT. Der Radiologe 1998; 38: 93–100.
10. Becker M. Oral cavity, oropharynx and hypopharynx. Semin Roentgenol 2000; 35: 21–30.
11. Becker M, Hasso AN. Imaging of malignant neoplasms of the pharynx and larynx. In: Taveras JM, Ferruci JT, eds. Radiology: Diagnosis–Imaging–Intervention. Philadelphia: J.B. Lippincott; 1996: 1–16.
12. Becker M, Kurt AM. Infrahyoid neck: CT and MR imaging versus histopathology. Eur Radiol 1999; 9 (Suppl 2): 53–68.
13. Becker M, Moulin G, Kurt AM et al. Non-squamous cell neoplasms of the larynx: radiologic-pathologic correlation. Radiographics 1998; 18: 1189–1209.
14. Becker M, Moulin G, Kurt AM, Zbären P, Dulguerov, Marchal F, Zanaret P, Lehman W, Rüfenacht DA, Terrier F. Atypical squamous cell carcinoma of the larynx and hypopharynx: radiologic features and pathologic correlation. Eur Radiol 1998; 8: 1541–1551.
15. Becker M, Schroth G, Zbären P, et al. Long-term changes induced by high-dose irradiation of the head and neck region: imaging findings. Radiographics 1997; 17: 5–26.
16. Becker M, Zbären P, Delavelle J, et al. Neoplastic invasion of the laryngeal cartilage: reassessment of criteria for diagnosis at CT. Radiology 1997; 203: 521–532.
17. Becker M, Zbären P, Laeng H. MRI and CT of unusual laryngeal neoplasms in adults: radiologic-pathologic correlation. Radiographics, Selected Neuroradiology Scientific Exhibits 1995; 15 (pt 3, CD): 1268.
18. Becker M, Zbären P, Laeng H, Stoupis C, Porcellini B, Vock P. Neoplastic invasion of the laryngeal cartilage: Comparison of MR imaging and CT with histopathologic correlation. Radiology 1995; 194: 661–669.
19. Becker M, Zbären P, Hermans R, Becker CD, Marchal F, Kurt AM, Marré S, Rüfenacht DA, Terrier F. Necrotizing fasciitis of the head and neck: role of CT in diagnosis and management. Radiology 1997; 202: 471–476 .
20. Bennett A, Carter RL, Stamford IF, Tanner NSB. Prostaglandin-like material extracted from squamous cell carcinomas of the head and neck. Br J Cancer 1980; 41: 204–208.
21. Berger PS, Bataini JP. Radiation induced cranial nerve palsy. Cancer 1977; 40: 152–155.
22. Brandsma JL, Steinberg BM, Abramson AL, Winkler B. Presence of human papilloma virus type 16 related sequences in verrucous carcinoma of the larynx. Cancer Res 1986; 46: 2185–2188.
23. Brodsky G. Carcino(pseudo)sarcoma of the larynx: the controversy continues. Otolaryngol Head Neck Surg 1984; 17: 185–197.
24. Carter RL, Tanner NSB. Local invasion by laryngeal carcinoma: Importance of focal ossification within laryngeal cartilage. Clin Otolaryngol 1979; 4: 283–290.
25. Carter RL, Tanner NSB, Clifford P, Shaw HJ. Direct bone invasion in squamous cell carcinoma of the head and neck: Pathological and clinical implications. Clin Otolaryngol 1980; 5: 107–116.
26. Castelijns JA, Becker M, Hermans R. The impact of cartilage invasion on treatment and prognosis of laryngeal cancer. Eur Radiol 1996; 6: 156–169.
27. Castelijns JA, Gerritsen GJ, Kaiser MC, et al. Invasion of laryngeal cartilage by cancer: Comparison of CT and MR imaging. Radiology 1988; 167: 199–206.
28. Castelijns JA, van den Brekel MWM, Tobi H, et al. Laryngeal carcinoma after radiation therapy: correlation of abnormal MR imaging signal patterns in laryngeal cartilage with the risk of recurrence. Radiology 1996; 198: 151–155.
29. Charlin B, Guerrier B, Balmigere G. Subtotal laryngectomy with cricohyoidopexy. Head and Neck Surg 1988; 1: 17–24.
30. Chevalier D, Piquet JJ. Subtotal laryngectomy with cricohyoidopexy for supraglottic carcinoma: review of 61 cases. Am J Surg 1994; 168: 472–473.
31. Clerf LH. The preepiglottic space. Its relation to carcinoma of the epiglottis. Arch Otolaryngol 1944; 40: 177–179.
32. Craswell P W T. Vocal cord paralysis following radioactive iodine therapy. Br J Clin Pract 1972; 26: 571 -572.
33. Curtin HD. Imaging of the larynx: Current concepts. Radiology 1989; 173: 1–11.
34. Curtin HD. The importance of imaging demonstration of neoplastic invasion of laryngeal cartilage. Radiology 1995; 194: 643–644.

35 DeFoer B, Hermans R, Van der Goten A, Delaere PR, Baert AL. Imaging features in cases of submucosal laryngeal mass lesions. Eur Radiol 1997; 6: 913–916.
36 DiSantis DJ, Balfe DM, Hayden RE, et al. The neck after vertical hemilaryngectomy: computed tomographic study. Radiology 1984; 151: 683–687.
37 DiSantis DJ, Balfe DM, Hayden RE, et al. The neck after total laryngectomy: CT study. Radiology 1984; 153: 713–717.
38 Donovan DT, Conley J. Adenoid cystic carcinoma of the subglottic region. Ann Otol (St. Louis)1983; 92: 491–495
39 Duda JJ Jr, Lewin JS, Eliachar I. MR evaluation of epiglottic disruption. AJNR 1996; 17: 563–565.
40 Ekberg O, Nylander G. Pharyngeal dysfunction after treatment of pharyngeal cancer with surgery and radiotherapy. Gastroint Radiol 1983; 8: 97–104.
41 Ferlito A. Primary lymphoepithelial carcinoma of the hypopharynx. J Laryngol Otol 1977; 91: 361–367.
42 Ferlito A, Nicolai P, Montaguti A, Cecchetto A, Pennelli N. Condrosarcoma of the larynx: review of the literature and report of three cases. Am J Otolaryngol 1984; 5: 350–359.
43 Ferlito A, Recher G. Ackerman's tumor (verrucous carcinoma) of the larynx. A clinicopathologic study of 77 cases. Cancer 1980; 46: 1617–1630.
44 Feuerstein SS. Subglottic hemangioma in infants. Laryngoscope 1973; 83: 466–473.
45 Galasko CSB. Mechanism of bone destruction in the development of skeletal metastases. Nature 1976; 263: 507–508.
46 Gallo A, Mocetti P, De Vincentiis M, et al. Neoplastic infiltration of laryngeal cartilages: histocytochemical study. Laryngoscope 1992; 102: 891–895.
47 Gerritsen GJ, Valk J, van Velzen DJ, Snow GB. Computed tomography: a mandatory investigational procedure for T-staging of advanced laryngeal cancer. Clin Otholaryngol 1986; 11: 307–316.
48 Glanz H, Kleinsasser O. Metastasen im Kehlkopf. HNO 1978; 163–167.
49 Gnepp DR, Chandler W, Hyams V. Primary Kaposi sarcoma in the head and neck. Ann Intern Med 1984; 100: 107–114.
50 Gorenstein AG, Neel HB III, Devine KD, Weiland JH. Solitary extramedullary plasmacytoma of the larynx. Arch Otolaryngol 1977; 103: 159–161.
51 Gregor RT, Hammond K. Framework invasion by laryngeal carcinoma. Am J Surg 1987; 154: 452–458.
52 Gregor RT, Lloyd GAS, Michels L. Computed tomography of the larynx: a clinical pathologic study. Head Neck Surg 1981; 3: 284–296.
53 Greven KM, Williams DW III, Keyes JW Jr., et al. Distinguishing tumor recurrence from irradiation sequelae with positron emission tomography in patients treated for larynx cancer. Int J Radiat Oncol Biol Phys 1994; 29: 841.
54 Gridelli C, Palmieri G, Airoma G, Incoronato P, Pepe R, Barra E, Bianco AR. Complete regression of laryngeal involvement by classic Kaposi sarcoma with low dose alpha 2 b interferon. Tumori 1990; 76: 292–293.
55 Hermanek P, Hutter RVP, Sobin LH, Wagner G, Wittekind Ch, eds. TNM Atlas: Illustrated Guide to the TNM/pTNM classification of malignant tumors, 4th ed. Berlin: Springer; 1998; 22–49.
56 Hermans R, Van den Bogaert W, Rijnders A, Baert AL. Value of computed tomography as outcome predictor of supraglottic squamous cell carcinoma treated by definitive radiation therapy. Int J Radiat Oncol Biol Phys 1999; 44: 755–765.
57 Hermans R, Van den Bogaert W, Rijnders A, Doornaert P, Baert AL. Predicting the local outcome of glottic squamous cell carcinoma after definitive radiation therapy: value of computed tomography-determined tumor parameters. Radiother Oncol 1999; 50: 39–46.
58 Houle JA, Joseph P, Batsakis JG. Primary adenocarcinoma of the larynx. J Laryngol Otol 1976; 90: 1159–1163.
59 Jones B, Donner M. Common structural lesions. In: Jones B, Donner M, eds. Normal and Abnormal Swallowing. Imaging in Diagnosis and Therapy. New York: Springer; 1991; 93–108.
60 Katsantonis GP, Archer CR, Rosenblum BN, Yeager VL, Friedman WH. The degree to which accuracy of preoperative staging of laryngeal carcinoma has been enhanced by computer tomography. Arch Otolaryngol Head Neck Surg 1986; 95: 52–62.
61 Keen JA, Wainwright J. Ossification of the thyroid, cricoid and arytenoid cartilages. S Afr J Lab Clin Med 1958; 4: 83–108.
62 Kirchner JA. Invasion of the framework by laryngeal cancer. Acta Otolaryngol (Stockh) 1984; 97: 392–397.
63 Kirchner JA. Pathways and pitfalls in partial laryngectomy. Ann Otorhinolaryngol 1984; 93: 301–305.
64 Kirchner JA, Carter D. Intralaryngeal barriers to the spread of cancer. Acta Otolaryngol (Stockh) 1987; 103: 503–513.
65 Kirchner JA, Fischer J. Anterior commissure cancer—a clinical and laboratory study of 39 cases. Can J Otolaryngol 1975; 4: 637–643.
66 Lee WR, Mancuso AA, Saleh EM, et al. Can pretreatment computed tomography findings predict local control in T3 squamous cell carcinoma of the glottic larynx treated with radiation therapy alone ? Int J Radiat Oncol Biol Physiol 1993; 25: 683–697.
67 Lehmann W, Raymond L, Faggiano F, et al. Cancer of the endolarynx, epilarynx and hypopharynx in south-western Europe: Assessment of tumoral origin and risk factors. Adv Otorhinolaryngol 1991; 46: 145–156.
68 Lenz M, Hypopharynx and larynx. In: Lenz M, ed. CT and MRI in head and neck tumors. Stuttgart: Georg Thieme Verlag; 1992; 107–134.
69 Lindwall N. Hypopharyngeal cancer in sideropenic dysphagia. Acta Radiol (Stockh) 1953; 39: 17–37.
70 Lloyd GAS, Michaels L, Phelps PD. The demonstration of cartilaginous involvement in laryngeal carcinoma by computerized tomography. Clin Otolaryngol 1981; 6: 171–177.
71 Loevner LA, Yousem DM, Montone KT, Weber R, Chalian A, Weinstein G. Can radiologists accurately predict preepiglottic space invasion with MR imaging? AJR 1997; 169: 1681–1687.
72 Logemann J A, Bytell D E. Swallowing disorders in three types of head and neck surgical patients. Cancer 1979; 44: 1095–1105.
73 Mafee MF, Schild JA, Michael AS, Choi KH, Capek V. Cartilage involvement in laryngeal carcinoma: Correlation of CT and pathologic macrosection studies. J Comput Assist Tomogr 1984; 8: 969–973.
74 Mafee MF, Schild JA, Valvassori GE, Capete V. Computed tomography of the larynx: Correlation with anatomical and pathologic studies in cases of laryngeal carcinoma. Radiology 1983; 147: 123–128.
75 Mancuso AA. Evaluation and staging of laryngeal and hypopharyngeal cancer by computed tomography and magnetic resonance imaging. In: Silver CE, ed. Laryngeal Cancer. New York: Thieme; 1991: 46–94.
76 Mancuso AA, Calcaterra TC, Hanafee WN. Computed tomography of the larynx. Radiol Clin North Am 1978; 16: 195–208.
77 Mancuso AA, Tamakawa Y, Hanafee WN. CT of the fixed vocal cord. Am J Radiol 1980; 135: 529–534.
78 Mancuso AA, Hanafee WN. Elusive head and neck carcinomas beneath intact mucosa. Laryngoscope 1983; 93: 133–139.
79 Mancuso AA, Hanafee WN. A comparative evaluation of computed tomography and laryngography. Radiology 1979; 133: 131–138.
80 Mancuso AA, Hanafee WN: Larynx and hypopharynx. In: Mancuso AA, Hanafee WN, eds. Computed Tomography and Magnetic Resonance Imaging of the Head and Neck, 2nd ed. Baltimore: Williams and Wilkins; 1985: 1–503.
81 Mancuso AA, Mukherji SK, Schmalfuss I et al. Preradiotherapy computed tomography as a predictor of local control in supraglottic carcinoma. J Clin Oncol 1999; 17: 631–637.
82 Marlowe SD, Swartz JD, Koenigsberg R, et al. Metastatic hypernephroma to the larynx: unusual presentation. Neuroradiology 1993; 35: 242–246.
83 Maroldi R, Battaglia G, Nicolai P, et al. CT appearance of the larynx after conservative and radical surgery for carcinomas. Eur Radiol 1997; 7: 418–431.
84 Meglin AJ, Biedlingmaier JF, Mirvis SE. Three dimentional computed tomography in the evaluation of laryngeal injury. Laryngoscope 1991; 101: 202–207.
85 Micheau C, Luboinski B, Lanchi P, et al. Relationship between laryngoceles and laryngeal carcinomas. Laryngoscope 1978; 88: 680–688.
86 Micheau C, Luboinski B, Schwaab G, Richard J, Cachin Y. Lymphoepitheliomas of the larynx (undifferentiated carcinomas of nasopharyngeal type). Clin Otolaryngol 1979; 4: 43–48.
87 Million RR. The myth regarding bone or cartilage involvement by cancer and the likehood of cure by radiotherapy. Head Neck 1989; 11: 30–40.
88 Mukherji SK, Mancuso AA, Kotzur IM, et al. Radiologic appearance of the irradiated larynx. Part 1. Expected changes. Radiology 1994; 193: 141–148.
89 Mukherji SK, Mancuso AA, Kotzur IM, et al. Radiologic appearance of the irradiated larynx. Part 2. Primary site response. Radiology 1994; 193: 149–154.
90 Mulliken J B, Glowacki J (1982) Hemangiomas and vascular malformations in infants and children: a classification based on endothelial characteristics. Plast Reconstr Surg 69: 412–420.
91 Muñoz A, Ramos A, Ferrando J, et al. Laryngeal carcinoma: sclerotic appearance of the cricoid and arytenoid cartilage—CT–pathologic correlation. Radiology 1993; 189: 433–437.

92 Ortiz CL, Weber AL. Laryngeal lipoma. Ann Otol Rhinol Laryngol 1991; 100: 783–784.
93 Pameijer FA, Hermans R, Mancuso AA et al. Pre- and post-radiotherapy computed tomography in laryngeal cancer: Imaging-based prediction of local failure. Int J Radiat Oncol Biol Phys 1999; 45: 359–366.
94 Pameijer FA, Mancuso AA, Mendenhall WM, Parsons JT, Kubilis PS. Can pretreatment computed tomography predict local control in T3 squamous cell carcinoma of the glottic larynx treated with definitive radiotherapy ? Int J Radiat Oncol Biol Phys 1997; 37: 1011–1021.
95 Piekarski JD, Heran F, Bosq J, et al. CT imaging of normal and abnormal laryngeal cartilage in adults. Selected Scientific Exhibits: RSNA 1993. Radiographics 1994; 14 (CD): 690.
96 Piekarski JD. Atteinte des cartilages dans les carcinomes pharyngolaryngés. In: Marsot-Dupuch K, ed. Données récentes de l'imagerie en otho-rhino-laryngologie, Collège d'Imagerie pour la Recherche et l'Enseignement en Oto-rhino-Laryngologie (C.I.R.E.O.L.). Paris; 1996; 15: 1–7.
97 Pittam MR, Carter RL. Framework invasion by laryngeal carcinomas. Head Neck Surg 1982; 4: 200–208.
98 Pollak RS. Laryngectomy and radical neck dissection. 1955; 8: 1177–1184.
99 Quinn FB Jr., McCabe BF. Laryngeal metastases from malignant tumors in distant organs. Ann Otol Rhinol Laryngol 1957; 66; 139–143.
100 Reidenbach MM. Borders and topographic relationships of the paraglottic space. Arch Otorhinolaryngol 1997; 254: 193–195.
101 a Reidenbach MM. The preepiglottic space: topographic relations and histological organization. J Anat 1996; 88: 173–182.
101 b Sadler TW, Respiratory system. In: Sadler TW, ed. Langman's Medical Embryology, 5 th ed. Philadelphia: Williams and Wilkins; 1985: 215–223.
102 Saleh EM, Mancuso AA, Stringer SP. CT of submucosal and occult laryngeal masses. JCAT 1992; 16: 87–93.
103 Sato K, Kurita S, Hirano M. Location of the preepiglottic space and its relationship to the paraglottic space. Ann Otol Rhinol Laryngol 1993; 102: 930–934.
104 Schaefer SD. The use of CT scanning in the management of the acutely injured larynx. Otolaryngol Clin North Am 1991; 24: 31–36.
105 Sigal R, Monnet O, de Baere T, Micheau C, Shapeero LG, Julieron M, Bosq J, Vanel D, Piekarski JD, Luboinski B, Masselot J. Adenoid cystic carcinoma of the head and neck: Evaluation with MR imaging and clinical–pathologic correlation in 27 patients. Radiology 1992; 184: 95–101.
106 Silverman PM, Bossen EH, Fisher SR, Cole TB, Korobkin M, Halvorsen RA. Carcinoma of the larynx and hypopharynx: computed tomographic–histopathologic correlations. Radiology 1984; 151: 697–702.
106a Sobin LH, Wittekind C, eds. TNM Classification of Malignant Tumours, 6th ed. Hoboken, NJ: Wiley; 2002:36–43.
107 Som PM, Scherl MP, Rao VM, Biller HF. Rare presentations of ordinary lipomas of the head and neck: a review. AJNR 1986; 7: 657–664.
108 Stiglbauer R, Steurer M, Schimmerl S, Kramer J. MRI of cartilaginous tumors of the larynx. Clin Radiol 1992; 46: 23–27.
109 Stoll B A, Andrews J T. Radiation induced peripheral neuropathy. Br Med J 1966; 1: 834–837.
110 Sulfaro S, Barzan L, Querin F, et al. T-staging of the laryngohypopharyngeal carcinoma; a 7-year multidisciplinary experience. Arch Otolaryngol Head Neck Surg 1989; 115: 613–620.
111 Suojanen JN, Mukherji SK, Wippold FJ. Spiral CT of the larynx. AJNR 1993; 15: 1579–1582.
112 Takashima S, Noguchi Y, Okumura T, Aruga H, Kobayashi T. Dynamic MR imaging in the head and neck. Radiology 1993; 189: 813–821.
113 Tart RP, Mukherji SK, Lee WR, Mancuso AA. Value of laryngeal cartilage sclerosis as a predictor of outcome in patients with stage T3 glottic cancer treated with radiation therapy. Radiology 1994; 192: 567–570.
114 Tien RD, Hesselink JR, Chu PK, Szumowski J. Improved detection and delineation of head and neck lesions with fat-suppression spin-echo MR imaging. AJNR 1991; 12: 19–24.
115 Tirwari RM, Snow GB, Balm AJM, Gerritsen GJ, Vos W, Bosma A. Cartilaginous tumors of the larynx. J Laryngol Otol 1987; 101: 266–275.
116 Thabet HM, Sessions DG, Gado MH, et al. Comparison of clinical evaluation and computed tomographic diagnostic accuracy for tumors of the larynx and hypopharynx. Laryngoscope 1996; 106: 589–594.
117 Vogl TJ, Steger W, Balzer JO, et al. MRI of the hypopharynx, larynx and neck. Eur Radiol 1992; 2: 391.
118 Vogl TJ, Steger W, Grevers G, Schreiner M, Dressel S, Lissner J. MRI with Gd-DTPA in tumors of larynx and hypopharynx. Eur Radiol 1991; 1: 58–64.
119 Wippold FJ, Smirniotopoulos JG, Moran CJ, Glazer HS. Chondrosarcoma of the larynx: CT features. AJNR 1993; 14: 453–459.
120 Wolf GT. Induction chemotherapy plus radiation compared with surgery plus radiation in patients with advanced laryngeal cancer. N Engl J Med 1991; 324: 1685–1690.
121 Yeager VL. Archer CR, Anatomical routes for cancer invasion of laryngeal cartilages. Laryngoscope 1982; 92: 449–452.
122 Yousem DM, Cheng L, Montone KT, Montgomery L, Loevner LA, Rao V, Chung TS, Kimura Y, Hayden RE, Weinstein GS. Primary malignant melanoma of the sinonasal cavity: MR imaging evaluation. Radiographics 1996; 16: 1101–1110.
123 Yousem DM, Hatabu H, Hurst MD, et al. Carotid artery invasion by head and neck masses: Prediction with MR imaging. Radiology 1995; 195: 715–720.
124 Yousem DM, Oberholzer JC. Neurofibroma of the aryepiglottic fold. AJNR 1991; 12: 1176.
125 Zbären P, Becker M, Laeng H. Pretherapeutic staging of laryngeal cancer: clinical findings, computed tomography and magnetic resonance imaging versus histopathology. Cancer 1996; 77: 1263–1273.
126 Zbären P, Becker M, Laeng H. Staging of laryngeal cancer: endoscopy, computed tomography and magnetic resonance imaging versus histopathology. Eur Arch Otolaryngol 1997; 254: 117–122.
127 Zbären P, Becker M, Laeng H. Pretherapeutic staging of hypopharyngeal carcinoma: Clinical findings, computed tomography, and magnetic resonance imaging compared with histopathologic evaluation. Arch Otolaryngol Head Neck Surg 1997; 123: 908–913.
128 Zbaren P, Egger C. Growth patterns of piriform sinus carcinomas. Laryngoscope 1997; 107(4): 511–518.
129 Zbären P, Schar P, Tschopp L, Becker M, Hausler R.Surgical treatment of Zenker's diverticulum: transcutaneous diverticulectomy versus microendoscopic myotomy of the cricopharyngeal muscle with CO_2 laser. Otolaryngol Head Neck Surg 1999; 121(4): 482–487.

12 Other Infrahyoid Neck Lesions

M. Becker

Introduction

Imaging plays an important role in the management of diseases of the neck. It allows differentiation of true masses from pseudomasses, delineation of the exact location and extent of a lesion, and characterization of the lesion. Knowledge of the normal anatomy, as seen on imaging, is the cornerstone for understanding pathological processes. This chapter first reviews the imaging-relevant anatomy and then concentrates on the most common pathological entities affecting the lymph nodes, as well as the nonlymphatic structures of the infrahyoid neck, including the thyroid gland.

Anatomy

The hyoid bone is the landmark structure between the suprahyoid and infrahyoid neck because several fasciae that act as a natural cleavage plane are attached to the hyoid bone. The term *suprahyoid neck* refers to the anatomical region that extends longitudinally from the skull base to the hyoid bone, whereas the term *infrahyoid neck* refers to the anatomical region that extends longitudinally from the hyoid bone to the thoracic inlet.

There are many systems for classifying the structures in the neck. Surgeons divide the superficial structures of the infrahyoid neck into triangles using the superficial musculature, while radiologists and anatomists use the layers of the deep cervical fascia to divide the neck into spaces. This chapter is organized by organ system, with a discussion of the spaces and triangles of the infrahyoid neck at the end.

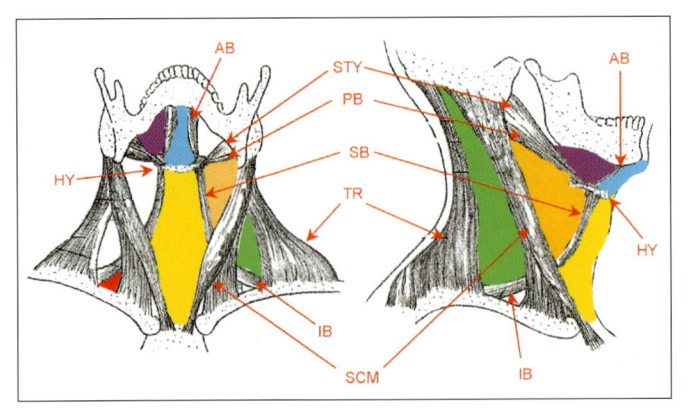

Fig. 12.**1** Muscles and triangles of the neck. Anterior view and lateral view.
Muscles: AB = anterior belly of the digastric muscle; PB = posterior belly of the digastric muscle; STY = stylohyoid muscle; SB = superior belly of the omohyoid muscle; IB = inferior belly of the omohyoid muscle; SCM = sternocleidomstoid muscle; TR = trapezius muscle; HY = hyoid bone.
Suprahyoid triangles: submandibular (purple) and submental (blue).
Infrahyoid triangles: carotid (orange), muscular (yellow), occipital (green), and subclavian (red).

Muscles

The infrahyoid neck is bordered superiorly by the hyoid bone and inferiorly by the sternal angle. The majority of cervical soft tissues of the infrahyoid neck are made up of muscle (Fig. 12.**1**). The *sternocleidomastoid* muscle originates at the mastoid process of the temporal bone behind the ear and runs anteroinferiorly across the lateral aspect of the neck. It then divides into two heads that insert on the sternum and the medial aspect of the clavicle (Figs. 12.**1** and 12.**2**). The sternocleidomastoid muscle is responsible for rotating the head. The *trapezius* muscle originates on the back of the skull and spinous processes of the cervical (seventh) and all thoracic vertebrae and inserts along the acromion and spine of the scapula. It is a broad and flat muscle that is responsible for elevation of the scapula (Figs. 12.**1** and 12.**2**). Both the sternocleidomastoid muscle and the trapezius muscle are innervated by cranial nerve XI (spinal accessory nerve). The *platysma* originates along the mandible and some muscle fibers blend into the muscles of facial expression (Fig. 12.**2**). This very flat muscle covers the anterior portion of the neck and then blends with the fascia of the pectoralis and deltoid muscles. The platysma is innervated by the facial nerve (VII). The *digastric* muscle has two bellies: the anterior belly and the posterior belly, which are connected by a central tendon (Fig. 12.**1**). The anterior belly originates on the internal surface of the mandible and extends to the lateral aspect of the hyoid bone, where it continues as a thick tendon. The posterior belly, which is located in the suprahyoid neck, inserts to the medial surface of the mastoid process. A fibrous pulley from the hyoid bone holds the tendon in place. The anterior belly of the digastric muscle is innervated by the mandibular nerve (V3) and the posterior belly is innervated by the facial nerve (VII). The *omohyoid* muscle has a superior belly and an inferior belly (Fig. 12.**1**). The superior belly originates on the hyoid bone and extends toward the medial aspect of the clavicle, where it continues as a central tendon. The inferior belly runs above the clavicle and inserts on the upper border of the scapula. The tendon between the two bellies of the omohyoid muscle is held in place by a pulley from the medial clavicle. The *strap* muscles, which include the thyrohyoid, sternothyroid, sternohyoid, and superior belly of the omohyoid muscle connect the anterior aspects of the hyoid bone, thyroid cartilage, and sternum (Fig. 12.**2**). They are innervated by C1 to C3. The scalene muscles are the most anterior of the paraspinal muscles. The anterior and middle scalene muscles arise from the transverse processes of the lower cervical vertebrae and insert on the anterior portion of the first rib. The brachial plexus and the subclavian artery run between the anterior and middle scalene muscles at the level of the thoracic inlet (Fig. 12.**2**). The posterior scalene muscle arises from the transverse processes of the sixth and seventh cervical vertebrae and inserts on the second rib.

Blood Vessels

The largest blood vessels in the neck are the common carotid artery and the internal jugular vein (Figs. 12.**2** and 12.**3**). They run vertically in the neck and, therefore, appear as circular structures on axial images. The common carotid artery and the internal jugular vein run medial to the sternocleidomastoid muscle in the upper neck and beneath the sternocleidomastoid muscle in the lower neck. The internal jugular vein lies lateral to the common

Anatomy 781

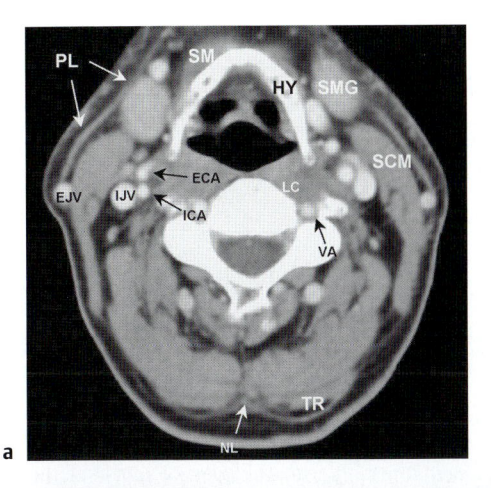

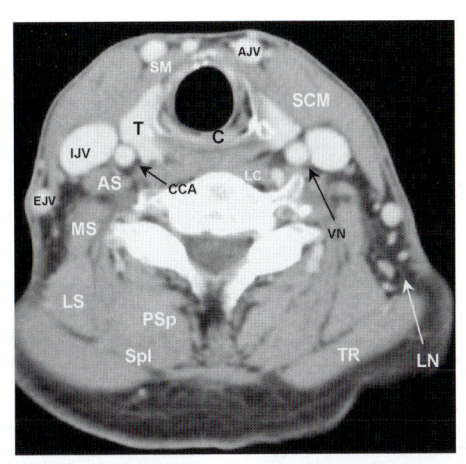

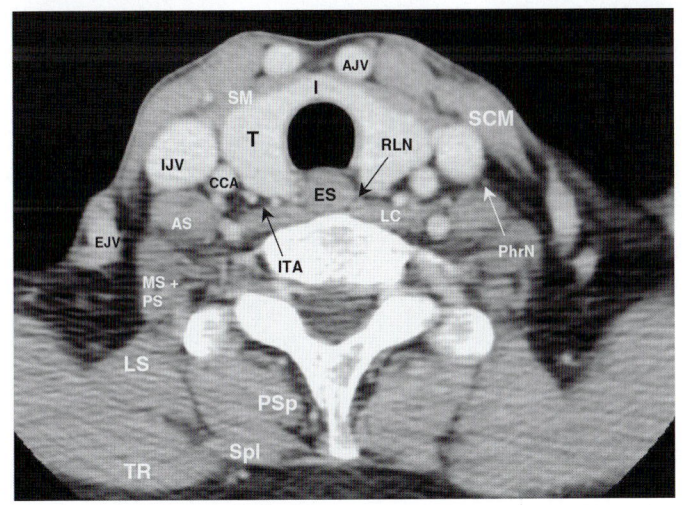

Fig. 12.2 Axial CT anatomy of the neck as seen at the level of the hyoid bone (a), cricoid ring (b), thyroid gland (c), and clavicles (d).
AJV = anterior jugular vein; AS = anterior scalene muscle; BPl brachial plexus; C = cricoid; CCA = common carotid artery; CL = clavicle; ECA = external carotid artery; EJV = external jugular vein; ES = esophagus; HY = hyoid bone; ICA = internal carotid artery; IJV = internal jugular vein; ITA = inferior thyroid artery; LC = longus colli muscle; LN = normal lymph nodes; LS = levator scapulae muscle; NL = nuchal ligament; MS = middle scalene muscle; PhrN = phrenic nerve; PL = platysma; PS = posterior scalene muscle; PSp = paraspinal muscles; RLN = recurrent laryngeal nerve; SCA = subclavian artery; SCLV = subclavian vein; SCM = sternocleidomastoid muscle; SM = strap muscles; SMG = submandibular gland; Spl = splenius capitis muscle; T = thyroid gland; Th1 = first thoracic vertebra; TR = trapezius muscle; VA = vertebral artery; VN = vagus nerve.

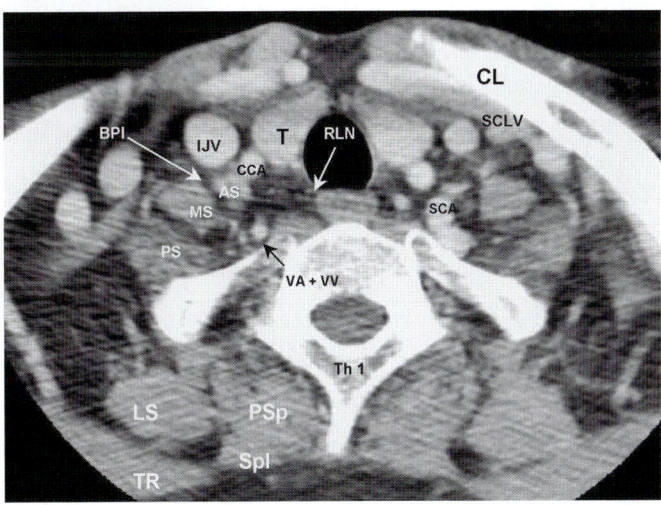

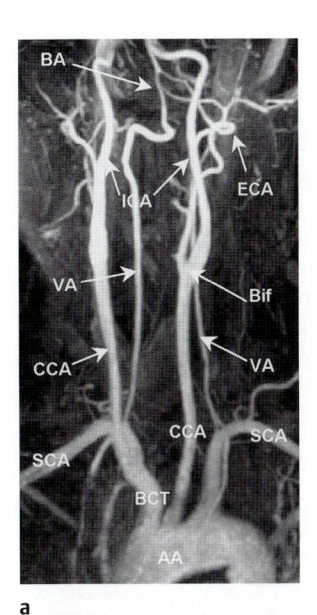

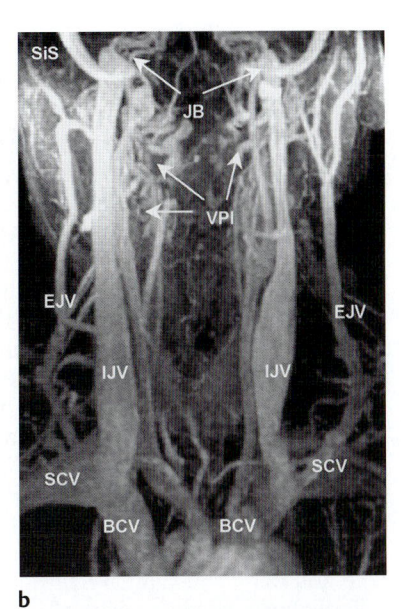

Fig. 12.3 Vascular anatomy of the neck. a MR angiography, coronal projection. b MR phlebography, coronal projection. c 3D reconstruction of cervical vessels from a CT volumetric data set obtained after administration of contrast material.
AA = aortic arch; BA = basilar artery; BCT = brachiocephalic trunk; BCV = brachiocephalic vein; Bif = carotid bifurcation; CCA = common carotid artery; Cl = clavicle; ECA = external carotid artery; EJV = external jugular vein; Hy = hyoid bone; ICA = internal carotid artery; JB = jugular bulb; M = manubrium; OV = occipital vein; S = scapula; SCA = subclavian artery; SCV = subclavian vein; SiS = sigmoid sinus; Thy = thyroid cartilage (ossified portions); VA = vertebral artery; VPl = vertebral venous plexus.

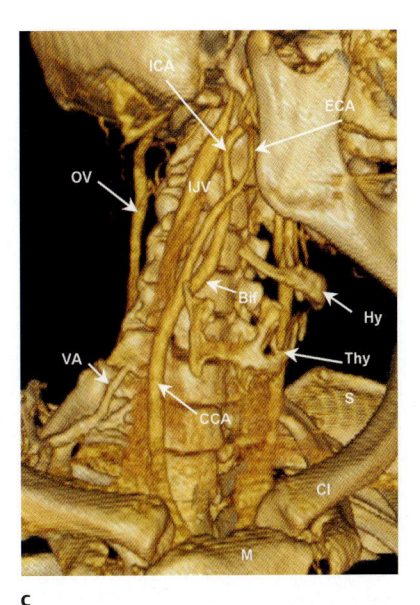

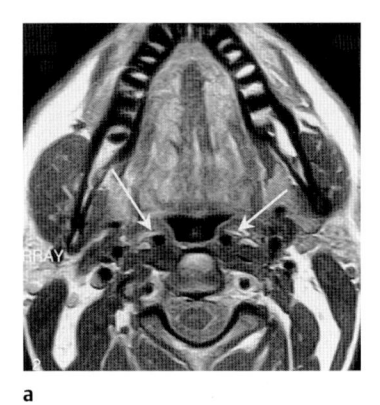

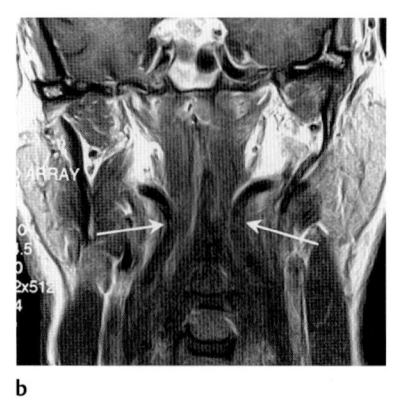

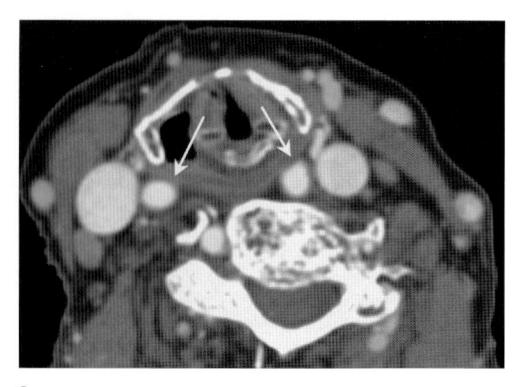

Fig. 12.4 Retropharyngeal course of the carotid arteries. **a** Axial and **b** coronal contrast-enhanced T1W images obtained in a male patient presenting with a bilateral submucosal bulge of the posterior pharyngeal wall. The MR examination was performed to exclude a submucosal tumor. It shows a retropharyngeal course of both internal carotid arteries (arrows) accounting for the submucosal bulge of the posterior oropharyngeal wall. **c** Axial contrast-enhanced CT image in a female patient shows as an incidental finding a retropharyngeal course of the common carotid arteries (arrows).

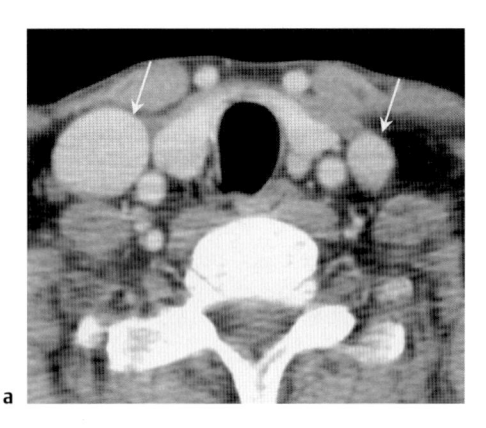

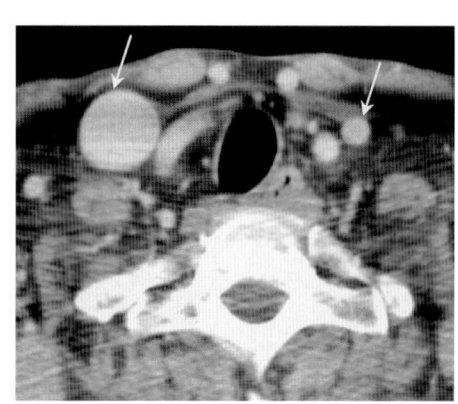

Fig. 12.5a, b Asymmetric internal jugular veins as seen on contrast-enhanced CT images. The right jugular vein is larger than the left. Both jugular veins are indicated by arrows.

carotid artery. The common carotid artery bifurcates into the internal and external carotid arteries at about the level of the hyoid bone. At its bifurcation, the common carotid artery forms the carotid bulb. The internal carotid artery lies posterolateral to the external carotid artery at the level of the carotid bifurcation. It then continues in a cranial direction along the internal jugular vein. The external carotid artery, however, rapidly branches to supply the extracranial head and neck. The vertebral artery arises from the subclavian artery and ascends in the neck along the lateral aspect of the spine. It enters the foramina transversaria at the level of the sixth cervical vertebra and then winds around the lateral mass of the atlas before entering the foramen magnum. The external jugular vein lies between the platysma and the sternocleidomastoid muscles. It empties into the subclavian vein at the level of the anterior scalene muscle.

In some patients the internal and common carotid artery may have a retropharyngeal course (Fig. 12.4). This normal variant may lead to a submucosal bulge of the posterior pharyngeal wall and clinically a submucosal mass may be suspected. Sectional imaging easily clarifies the situation by showing the aberrant course of the carotid artery (Fig. 12.4). The internal jugular vein is usually larger than the common carotid artery and very often the right jugular vein is larger than the left (Fig. 12.5).

Lymph Nodes

The most commonly used classifications for lymph nodes are those of the Union Internationale contre le Cancer (UICC) and the American Joint Committee on Cancer (AJCC). Recently, a new imaging-based nodal classification[131, 132] has been proposed in an effort to standardize descriptions of node location between imaging and physical examination (Figs. 12.6 and 12.7). Level I nodes are located above the hyoid bone, below the mylohyoid muscle, and anterior to a transverse line drawn through the posterior edge of the submandibular glands. Level IA nodes (previously classified as submental nodes) are located between the medial margins of the anterior bellies of the digastric muscles. Level IB nodes (formerly submandibular nodes) represent the nodes that lie lateral to the medial edge of the anterior belly of the digastric muscle. Level II (upper jugular) nodes extend from the skull base to the lower body of the hyoid bone. Level II nodes lie anterior to a transverse line drawn on each axial image through the posterior edge of the sternocleidomastoid muscle and posterior to a transverse line through the posterior edge of the submandibular gland. Level IIA nodes are inseparable from the internal jugular vein or they lie anterior, lateral, or medial to the internal jugular vein. Level IIB nodes (previously classified as upper spinal accessory nodes) lie posterior to the internal jugular vein with a fat plane separating the nodes and the vein. Retropharyngeal nodes lie medial to the internal carotid artery. Level III (middle jugular) nodes lie between the lower body of the hyoid and the lower margin of the cricoid cartilage. These nodes lie anterior to the transverse line drawn on each axial image through the posterior edge of the sternocleidomastoid muscle. Level IV (lower jugular) nodes lie between the lower margin of the cricoid cartilage and the clavicle. Level V (posterior triangle) nodes extend from the skull base to the level of the clavicle. All level V nodes lie anterior to a transverse line drawn on each axial image through the anterior edge of the trapezius muscle. Above the lower margin of the cricoid ring, level V nodes (also named upper level V nodes or VA nodes) lie posterior to a transverse line drawn on each axial image through the posterior edge of the sternocleidomastoid muscle. Below the lower margin of the cricoid ring, level V nodes (also named lower level V nodes or VB nodes) lie posterior and lateral to an oblique line through the posterior edge of the sternocleidomastoid muscle and the lateral edge of the anterior scalene muscle. Level VI (anterior compartment) nodes are located between the hyoid bone and the top of the manubrium, and between the medial margins of the carotid arteries. They include the juxtavisceral, anterior cervical, and external jugular nodes. Level VII nodes are located between the top of the manubrium and the innominate vein. Level VII nodes are superior mediastinal nodes. Supraclavicular nodes are the low level IV or V nodes that are seen on the images that contain a portion of the clavicle. For all levels, if the transverse or oblique lines drawn on the axial images for dividing the levels transect a node, the node is classified into the level in which more of its cross-sectional area is located.[131, 132]

Normal lymph nodes are isodense to muscle on unenhanced CT. They are isointense to muscle on unenhanced T1-weighted MR images and they are slightly hyperintense to muscle on T2-weighted images. Normal lymph nodes enhance slightly more than muscle on both CT and MRI (Fig. 12.2). Normal lymph nodes have well-defined borders and are usually oval. The ratio of the maximum longitudinal length to the maximum transverse length should be greater than 2.[134] They have a fatty hilum, which can often be visualized on CT.

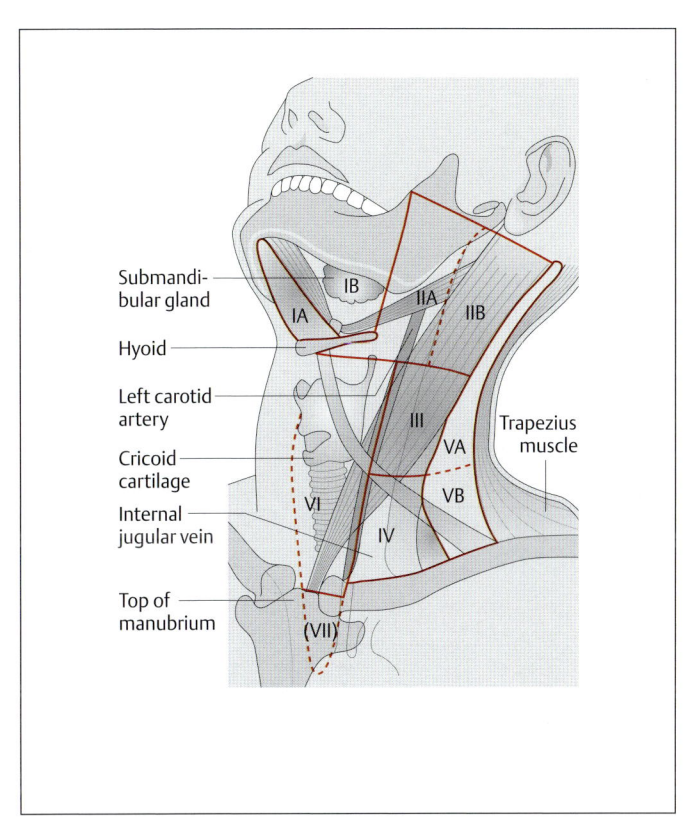

Fig. 12.6 The imaging-based nodal classification. The neck as seen from the left anterior view outlines the levels of the classification. Reproduced from Reference 131 with permission.

Nerves

The vagus nerve (cranial nerve X) accompanies the internal jugular vein through the neck. It lies behind and between the internal jugular vein and the common carotid artery (Fig. 12.2). The vagus nerve innervates mainly the pharynx and the larynx. The spinal accessory nerve (cranial nerve XI) travels obliquely across the lateral neck. superficial to the paraspinal muscles. It innervates the sternocleidomastoid and trapezius muscles. The phrenic nerve, which innervates the diaphragm, descends through the neck along the anteromedial border of the anterior scalene muscle. The recurrent laryngeal nerve, a branch of the vagus nerve, innervates the muscles of the larynx. On the right, the recurrent laryngeal nerve arises from the vagus nerve at the level of the subclavian artery, loops underneath the artery, and ascends in the tracheoesophageal grove (Fig. 12.2). The left recurrent laryngeal nerve arises at the level of the aortic arch, loops beneath the aorta, and ascends in the tracheoesophageal grove to the larynx. The sympathetic nerve chain lies posterior to the internal jugular vein and the internal and common carotid arteries. Finally, the brachial plexus, which forms from the nerve roots of C5–T1, passes between the anterior and middle scalene muscles. Normal nerves are of soft-tissue density on CT and they are hypointense on T1- and T2-weighted MR images. They do not enhance significantly after injection of contrast material.

Viscera

The upper aerodigestive tract located in the infrahyoid neck includes the hypopharynx, the larynx, the trachea, and the esophagus. These organs are discussed in detail in Chapter 11. Surrounding the larynx and trachea are the thyroid and parathyroid glands. The thyroid gland has two lobes connected by an isthmus (Figs. 12.2 and 12.8). A third lobe, the pyramidal lobe, may originate from the superior aspect of the isthmus. The upper border of the thyroid gland is at the level of the mid-thyroid car-

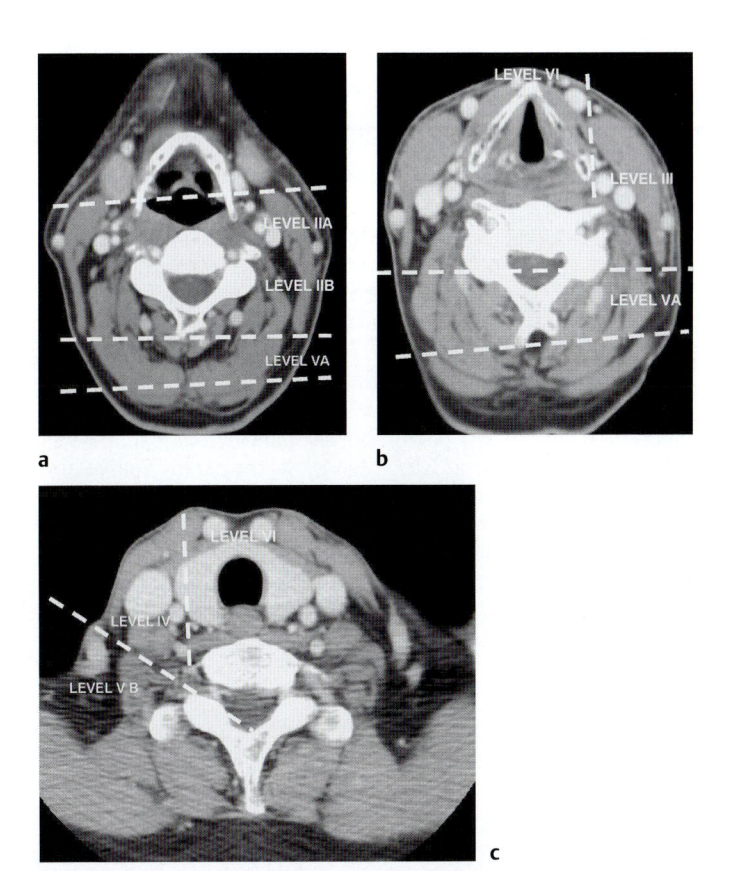

Fig. 12.7 a–c The imaging-based nodal classification to be used on axial CT images.

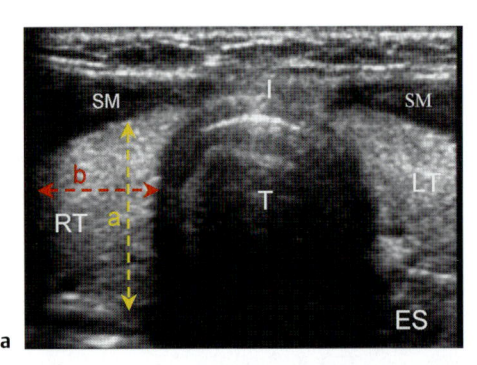

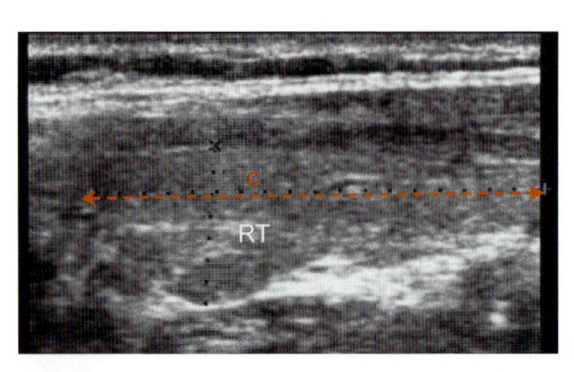

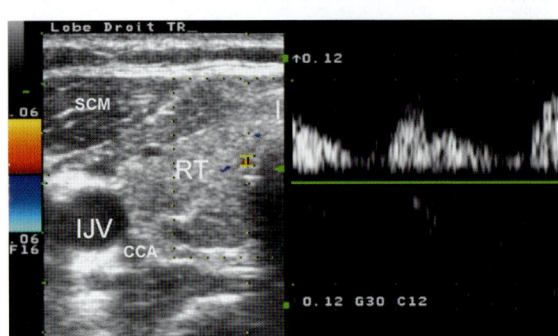

Fig. 12.8 Normal anatomy of the thyroid gland as seen on US. **a** Axial B mode US image, **b** longitudinal B mode US image of the right thyroid lobe, and **c** axial color Doppler US image of the right thyroid lobe. Note the homogeneous relatively hyperechoic parenchymal structure as compared to muscle tissue. The normal vascularization pattern can be appreciated on the color Doppler image.
CCA = common carotid artery; ES = esophagus; I = isthmus; IJV = internal jugular vein; LT = left lobe of the thyroid gland; RT = right lobe of the thyroid gland; SM = strap muscles; SCM = sternocleidomastoid muscle; T = trachea.
Normal US measurements of the thyroid gland: a = 10–17 mm; b = 12–20 mm; c = 40–70 mm.

tilage, whereas the inferior border of the gland is at the fifth or sixth tracheal rings. On unenhanced CT images, the thyroid gland is dense because of its iodine content. On T1-weighted MR images, the thyroid gland is hypointense compared to muscle, and it is slightly hyperintense on T2-weighted MR images. After injection of contrast material, the thyroid gland enhances tremendously. On ultrasound (US), the thyroid gland is hyperechoic as compared to muscle and it shows only a moderate perfusion pattern on color Doppler imaging (Fig. 12.**8**). The blood supply of the thyroid gland consists of the superior thyroid artery (which arises from the external carotid artery) and of the inferior thyroid artery (which arises from the thyrocervical trunk). The superior thyroidal veins drain into the internal jugular vein, and the inferior thyroidal veins drain into the internal jugular and innominate veins. The lymphatic drainage is variable with flow to the internal jugular chain laterally, the retropharyngeal region posteriorly, and the paratracheal region and mediastinum inferiorly.

The four parathyroid glands (two superior and two inferior) are usually not seen on routine CT and MRI examinations. However, the inferior thyroid artery and vein may be used as markers to identify the position of the parathyroid glands on CT and MRI (Fig. 12.**2**). When they are visible, the parathyroid glands display similar signal intensities and contrast enhancement patterns to the thyroid gland. Ectopic parathyroid glands are found between the carotid bifurcation and the anterior mediastinum and occur in 15–20% of the population. In about 8% of cases, parathyroid tissue is located within the thyroid gland.[4]

Fascial Layers and Spaces

There are two main fascia in the extracranial head and neck: the superficial cervical fascia (SCF) and the deep cervical fascia (DCF).[54] The SCF consists of the subcutaneous tissues and envelops the platysma muscle. The DCF has three separate layers: superficial layer (investing), middle layer (visceral or pharyngomucosal), and deep layer (prevertebral). The investing fascia surrounds the sternocleidomastoideus and trapezius muscles (Fig. 12.**9**). The visceral fascia envelops the pharynx, larynx, trachea, esophagus, thyroid, and parathyroid glands. It forms a cylinder oriented in craniocaudal direction in the anterior neck. The prevertebral fascia encircles the paraspinal muscles and spine. The anterior portion of the prevertebral fascia divides into two layers: the alar fascia, which is located anteriorly, and the true prevertebral fascia, which is located posteriorly (Fig. 12.**9**). All three layers of the deep cervical fascia contribute to the carotid sheath. The carotid sheath extends from the skull base to the aortic arch and encircles the internal and common carotid arteries, the internal jugular vein, and the vagus nerve. The sympathetic plexus is located in the medial fascial wall of the carotid space. The strap muscles are surrounded by the infrahyoid fascia, which is made up of layers from the investing and visceral fascia[54] (Fig. 12.**9**).

The cervical fascia divides the neck into distinct compartments or spaces (Fig. 12.**10**). The concept of dividing the extracranial head and neck into different spaces has been widely used by anatomists. With the development of CT and MR imaging, this concept has become increasingly popular among radiologists because, by knowing the spaces and their components, one can generate an anatomically based differential diagnosis (see Tables 12.**1**–12.**5**). The spaces of the extracranial head and neck also play an important role for the pathways of spread of inflammatory and neoplastic disease. They have been compared to vertical elevator shafts that represent natural conduits for tumor or infectious spread. In this chapter, the traditional anatomic nomenclature and also as the nomenclature popularized by Harnsberger, which has become commonly utilized among head and neck radiologists, surgeons, and anatomists, are presented.[54] The suprahyoid neck contains 10 distinct spaces, which are defined by the different layers of the deep cervical fascia (see also Chapter 8). The infrahyoid neck contains six spaces: visceral, retropharyngeal, carotid, prevertebral, posterior cervical, and anterior cervical spaces (Fig. 12.**10**).

Visceral Space

The visceral fascia surrounds the visceral space (Fig. 12.**10**). The contents of the visceral space in the infrahyoid neck include the larynx, hypopharynx, trachea, thyroid gland, and parathyroid glands (Table 12.**1**).

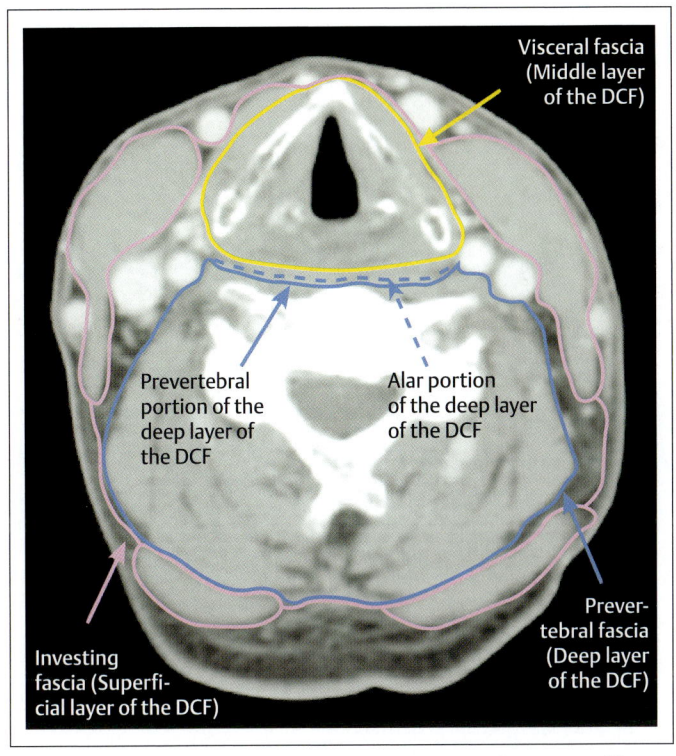

Fig. 12.9 Fascial layers of the infrahyoid neck. DCF = deep cervical fascia.

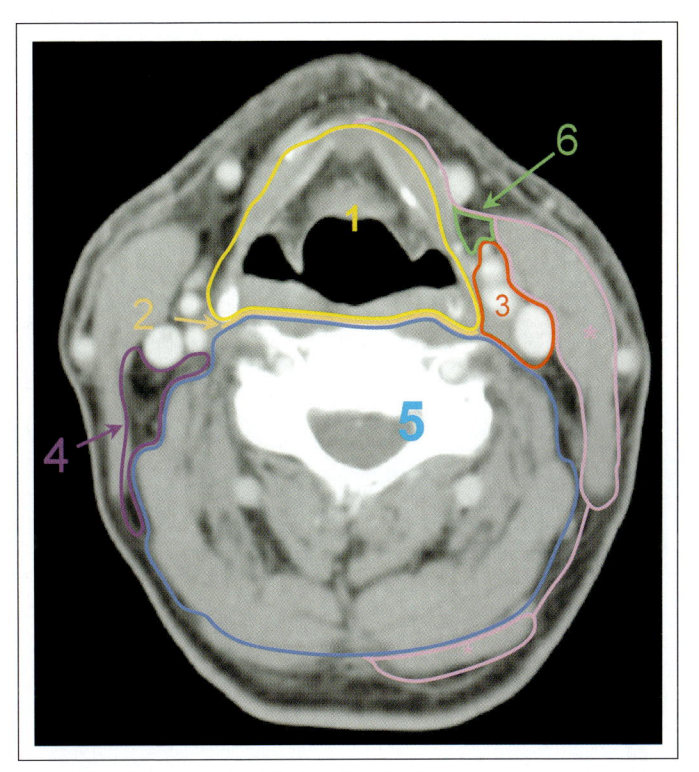

Fig. 12.10 Spaces of the infrahyoid neck. 1 = visceral space; 2 = retropharyngeal space; 3 = carotid space; 4 = posterior cervical space; 5 = prevertebral space; 6 = anterior cervical space; large asterisk = sternocleidomastoid muscle; small asterisk = trapezius muscle.

Table 12.1 Infrahyoid visceral space: extent, contents, and differential diagnosis of the most common pathological conditions

Extent	Contents	Common pathologies
Hyoid bone to mediastinum	Larynx	Squamous cell carcinoma
		Chondrosarcoma
		Laryngocele
	Hypopharynx and cervical esophagus	Squamous cell carcinoma
		Zenker's diverticulum
	Trachea	Carcinoma (squamous cell and adenoid cystic)
		Benign stenosis
	Thyroid gland	Goiter
		Colloid cyst, adenoma
		Carcinoma (papillary, follicular, anaplastic)
		Thyroiditis
	Parathyroid glands	Adenoma
		Hyperplasia
	Remnants of the thyroid/parathyroid anlage	Thyroglossal duct cyst
	Remnants of the 3rd and 4th branchial cleft apparatus	3rd branchial cleft cyst, piriform sinus fistula
	Paratracheal lymph nodes	Metastases (squamous cell carcinoma, thyroid carcinoma, lymphoma)
	Recurrent laryngeal nerves	Paralysis (after surgery, lymph node metastases)

Retropharyngeal Space and Danger Space

The "true" retropharyngeal space is located directly behind the pharynx (Fig. 12.9). It is bordered anteriorly by the visceral fascia and posteriorly by the alar fascia. It continues inferiorly to the level of the T4 vertebral body. The danger space lies between the alar fascia and the true prevertebral fascia. The danger space extends from the skull base to the diaphragm. It contains fatty areolar tissue and cannot be distinguished from the retropharyngeal space on CT and MRI.[35] The danger space is an important pathway for spread of infection into the mediastinum. Because the true retropharyngeal space and the danger space cannot be differentiated from one another by means of sectional imaging, they will be referred together as "retropharyngeal space" in this chapter (Fig. 12.10).

The contents of the retropharyngeal space are retropharyngeal lymph nodes and fatty areolar tissue. Retropharyngeal lymph nodes are found only in the suprahyoid retropharyngeal space, whereas the infrahyoid retropharyngeal space contains only fatty areolar tissue (Table 12.2).

Carotid Space

In the infrahyoid neck, the carotid space is bordered anteriorly by the anterior cervical space, laterally by the sternocleidomastoid muscle, posteriorly by the posterior cervical space and prevertebral space, and medially by the retropharyngeal space and visceral space (Fig. 12.10). The infrahyoid carotid space contains the common carotid artery, internal jugular vein, sympathetic chain, cranial nerve X and lymph nodes (Table 12.3).

Table 12.2 Infrahyoid retropharyngeal space: extent, contents, and differential diagnosis of the most common pathological conditions

Extent	Contents	Key pathologies
Hyoid bone to mediastinum*		Channel for infection and tumor to travel from the neck into the mediastinum: • Inflammatory conditions (cellulitis, abscess, necrotizing fasciitis) • Direct invasion from primary squamous cell carcinoma
	Fatty areolar tissue	Lipoma, liposarcoma
	Remnants of the 3rd branchial apparatus	3rd branchial cleft cysts

* Note that the superior portion of the retropharyngeal space is situated in the suprahyoid neck (skull base to hyoid bone), while the inferior portion is situated in the infrahyoid neck. Lymph nodes are found only in the suprahyoid retropharyngeal space.

Table 12.3 Infrahyoid carotid space: extent, contents, and differential diagnosis of the most common pathological conditions

Extent	Contents	Common pathologies
Hyoid bone to aortic arch*	Common and internal carotid artery	Thrombosis, aneurysm or pseudoaneurysm Dissection
	Internal jugular vein	Thrombosis/thrombophlebitis
	Vagus nerve (X) Sympathetic chain	Schwannoma, neurofibroma
	Carotid body	Paraganglioma
	Lymph nodes	Metastases (squamous cell carcinoma, lymphoma, thyroid carcinoma) Suppurative adenopathy, abscess
	Remnants of the 2nd branchial cleft apparatus	Second branchial cleft cyst

* Note that the superior portion of the carotid space (from the hyoid bone to the foramen jugulare) is situated in the suprahyoid neck.

Table 12.4 Infrahyoid prevertebral space: extent, contents, and differential diagnosis of the most common pathological conditions

Extent	Contents	Key pathologies
Hyoid bone to mediastinum*	Prevertebral, scalene and paraspinal muscles	Abscess
	Vertebral body and pedicle	Osteomyelitis (pyogenic, tuberculous) Metastases Direct invasion of squamous cell carcinoma Chordoma Vertebral body primary tumors
	Brachial plexus roots Phrenic nerve	Schwannoma, neurofibroma, MPNST
	Vertebral artery and vein	Aneurysm or pseudoaneurysm Dissection Thrombosis

* Note that the superior portion of the posterior cervical space is situated in the suprahyoid neck (skull base to mediastinum), while the inferior portion is situated in the infrahyoid neck.

Prevertebral Space

The prevertebral fascia surrounds the prevertebral space. The prevertebral space is located directly posterior to the retropharyngeal space (Fig. 12.**10**). Primary prevertebral space masses typically displace the retropharyngeal space and the posterior wall of the visceral space anteriorly and the carotid space laterally. The contents of the prevertebral space are the prevertebral, scalene, and paraspinal muscles, vertebral body, cervical disk, spinal canal, vertebral artery and vein, phrenic nerve, and brachial plexus roots (Table 12.**4**).

Posterior Cervical Space

The posterior cervical space extends from the skull base to the clavicles (Fig. 12.**10**). It is bordered laterally by the sternocleidomastoid muscle, posteriorly by the trapezius muscle, medially by the posterior cervical space and anteriorly by the carotid space. It contains fat, the spinal accessory nerve (cranial nerve XI), lymph nodes, and the preaxillary brachial plexus (Table 12.**5**).

Anterior Cervical Space

The anterior cervical space is a minor space that is composed entirely of fatty tissue (Fig. 12.**10**). It lies lateral to the visceral space, anterior to the carotid space, and medial to the sternocleidomastoid muscle.

Triangles

The superficial muscles divide the neck into triangles. This traditional anatomical description is still pertinent to physical examination of the neck. The anterior triangle lies anterior to the sternocleidomastoid muscle and mandible (Fig. 12.**1**), and the posterior triangle lies between the trapezius and sternocleidomastoid muscles. The anterior triangle is subdivided into the submental, submandibular, carotid, and muscular triangles. The submental and submandibular triangles lie in the suprahyoid neck, whereas the carotid and muscular triangles lie in the infrahyoid neck. The posterior triangle is subdivided into occipital and subclavian triangles (Fig. 12.**1**).

Table 12.5 Infrahyoid posterior cervical space: extent, contents, and differential diagnosis of the most common pathological conditions

Extent	Contents	Key pathologies
Hyoid bone to clavicle*	Fat	Lipoma/liposarcoma
	Spinal accessory nerve (cranial nerve XI)	Schwannoma, neurofibroma
	Brachial plexus (preaxillary portion)	Direct invasion (apical lung carcinoma, breast carcinoma) Schwannoma, neurofibroma, MPNST
	Lymph nodes	Metastases (squamous cell carcinoma of the nasopharynx, lymphoma)
		Reactive adenopathy, tuberculous adenitis, suppurative adenopathy and abscess
	Sequestrations of primitive embryonic lymph sacs	Congenital lesions (cystic hygroma–lymphangioma spectrum)
	Remnants of the 3rd branchial apparatus	3rd branchial cleft cysts

* Note that the superior portion of the posterior cervical space is situated in the suprahyoid neck (skull base to hyoid bone), while the inferior portion is situated in the infrahyoid neck.

Imaging Techniques

■ CT Scanning

In the infrahyoid neck, CT scan is the examination method of choice. The main advantages of CT in comparison with MRI are rapid image acquisition, availability, and cost. Disadvantages include radiation exposure and the need for iodinated contrast material to obtain adequate soft-tissue contrast. As a rule, the CT examination should completely cover the entire head and neck region, because disease located in the suprahyoid neck can extend or disseminate from the suprahyoid region into the infrahyoid region, or vice versa. Scanning protocols may vary, depending on the technical capabilities of hardware and software. Helical scanning makes it possible to obtain complete data sets from axial acquisitions in less than 20 seconds and to reconstruct overlapping slices at any level. Helical acquisitions with 2–3 mm collimation and 1–1.5 pitch produce images of adequate quality to answer most clinically relevant questions. Since multidetector helical scanning has become available, 2D coronal and sagittal reconstructions of excellent quality may be obtained routinely. Parameters used with 16-row multidetector scanners include 1–2 mm collimated sections overlapped in 0.5–1 mm intervals and a pitch setting of 0.875. Ideally, axial images at the level of the infrahyoid neck should be parallel to the plane of the true vocal cords, which corresponds to the level of the intervertebral disk between C4 and C5, and coronal images should be parallel to the long axis of the great vessels in the neck or should be perpendicular to the hard palate. Contrast enhancement must be performed in such a way that constant opacification of the arteries and veins is obtained and that contrast uptake in a lesion can be seen. Particular attention should also be paid to patient positioning as poor positioning may result in apparent loss of normal symmetry, thus mimicking pathology. Equally important is instruction of the patient so as to reduce breathing and motion artifacts during image acquisition. Because diseases in the infrahyoid neck may extend into the thorax or may be associated with coexisting tumors of the tracheobronchial tree, extended imaging into the thorax may be justified.[13]

■ MR Imaging

Over recent years, MRI has become an important imaging method in the infrahyoid neck. Superior soft-tissue contrast is the most striking advantage of MR imaging in comparison with CT. Inherent drawbacks are the relatively long examination time, limited availability, and cost. MR imaging demands more patient cooperation than CT and cannot be done in patients with claustrophobia, severe dyspnea, or odynophagia, or in the presence of electronic implants. Because the neck is susceptible to motion artifacts from breathing, swallowing, and vascular pulsations, images may be severely degraded on MRI examinations, especially in patients with compromised airways.

MR imaging of the infrahyoid neck is best done at high field strength and requires a head and neck volume coil, thin sections, and at least a set of T1- and T2-weighted images and contrast-enhanced T1-weighted images. Typical image parameters for a standard examination include a slice thickness of 3 or 4 mm with a 0–1 mm intersection gap, a field of view of 16 × 16 cm or less, and two averages. The acquisition matrix should be at least 256 × 256, but 512 × 256 or a 512 × 512 should be used whenever possible. Fat-suppression techniques after intravenous administration of contrast material are extremely useful in delineating tumor extent and necrotic lymph nodes and short tau inversion recovery (STIR) images are particularly sensitive for marrow infiltration or detection of small lesions. Flow compensation techniques, in-plane and out-of-plane saturation, and respiratory and/or ECG gating may often be necessary in order to overcome respiratory, swallowing, and blood motion artifacts. As with CT, the area to be examined should extend from the skull base to the thoracic inlet. Axial images in the infrahyoid neck should be parallel to the plane of the true vocal cords, which corresponds to the level of the intervertebral disk between C4 and C5, and coronal images should be parallel to the long axis of the great vessels in the neck or perpendicular to the hard palate.

■ Ultrasonography

Ultrasonography (US) can be used for the evaluation of a variety of pathological conditions of the infrahyoid neck. It is the examination of choice for the thyroid gland and parathyroid glands, and it is used as a first-line approach to patients presenting with superficial inflammatory conditions of the infrahyoid neck. In addition, in combination with fine-needle aspiration biopsy (FNAB), US allows correct characterization of lymph nodes, nonnodal laterocervical masses, and thyroid masses, making it possible to avoid an open biopsy.[99, 146] US is a dynamic examination technique, which offers the advantage that the investigator is given an immediate impression of the anatomy and functionality of the region of view. For example, in dynamic investigations, applying a Valsalva maneuver allows the examiner to clearly judge whether a cervical mass completely constricts or merely partially compresses the internal jugular vein. Ultrasonography of the infrahyoid is best performed using curved-array or linear-array broadband transducers with a frequency of about 7–12 MHz. As in other parts of the body, the selection of the transducer's frequency depends on the depth of the lesion to be examined and on the attenuation of the interposed tissues. To examine very superficial lesions, a standoff pad made of silicone elastomer may be used. However, this is rarely needed with modern high-frequency transducers, which enable good visualization of the key anatomical structures of this area. Color Doppler and power Doppler imaging are often useful in the examination of the neck, but many diagnoses are made with the standard gray-scale technique. Sonographic documentation of pathological lesions must be carried out in two different planes. Ideally, sonographic imaging sequences should be documented using video recording, because a still image captures only a momentary representation within an overall examination procedure. However, video examination is often not feasible within the framework of routine examinations for various practical and organizational reasons, and documentation is done in the form of still images. Not all radiological teams use sonography because the technique has several drawbacks: it does not explore the deep structures; it is operator-dependent; and documentation is based only on the images selected by the investigator (no standardized reference images for the clinicians).

■ Nuclear Medicine Studies of the Thyroid Gland

Nuclear medicine studies of the thyroid gland are used (1) to assess the functional status of the thyroid gland (hypothyroidism, euthyroidism, and hyperthyroidism); (2) to assess the function of thyroid nodules (increased isotope uptake = hot nodule versus decreased isotope uptake = cold nodule); and (3) to search for metastases of thyroid carcinomas. Nuclear medicine studies of the thyroid gland may be performed with iodine-123 (^{123}I), iodine-131 (^{131}I), and technetium-99 m (^{99m}Tc)-pertechnetate. The preferred agent for imaging the thyroid gland is iodine-123 because of the low radiation dosage and short half-life. Iodine-131, which has a higher radiation dosage and a longer half life than iodine-123, is used for performing whole-body imaging after thyroid ablation and to detect recurrent and metastatic thyroid cancer, mainly papillary and follicular carcinoma. Differentiation between hot nodules (more uptake than the normal thyroid gland) and cold nodules (less uptake than the normal thyroid gland) is important because hot nodules are malignant in only 1–4% of cases, whereas cold nodules may be malignant in up to 25% of cases (see below). Dynamic injection ^{99m}Tc-pertechnetate scintigraphy (also called "radionuclide thyroid angiography") may be used to differentiate malignant from benign thyroid nodules. Angiogenesis, the generation of new vessels, is required for the growth and expansion of a thyroid tumor. It presents with irregularities of vessel endothelium, arteriovenous shunt development, and increased vascularization. If on radionuclide thyroid angiography the nodule is hypoperfused (less vascularity than that of the native thyroid gland), it is likely that the nodule is benign, whereas if the nodule shows normal or increased perfusion it is likely that it is malignant.

■ FDG-PET

Positron-emission tomography (PET) using 2-(^{18}F)fluoro-2-deoxy-D-glucose (FDG) has had a growing impact in neck oncology. As opposed to CT, MRI, and US, which are anatomical imaging techniques, FDG-PET is a technique that is based on the differences in metabolic activity of normal and tumor tissue[16, 111] FDG is a glucose analogue that is trapped preferentially within cells with increased glycolysis, allowing for their detection. Tumor uptake is unrelated to the histological grade. As a metabolic imaging modality, FDG-PET is expected to have an important impact in the management of head and neck malignancies. Currently, FDG-PET is mainly used in assessing lymph node metastases, in searching for unknown primary tumors in the presence of neck metastases, and in the posttherapy setting. This technique has several drawbacks, however. The radiopharmaceuticals have a short half-life (110 minutes for FDG) and must be produced by a cyclotron located close to the imaging site. Investment and running costs are high, and the number of machines is limited. Because spatial resolution is only 3 mm, images are poorly defined and microscopic tumor may be missed.

Neoplastic Lesions

■ Nodal Neoplasms

The most common indication for performing CT or MR imaging of the neck is to look for potential metastasis from a known mucosal malignancy. Less often, imaging may be done for evaluation of an unknown neck mass. The most common neoplasms involving the cervical lymph node groups are metastases from head and neck squamous cell carcinoma, metastases from thyroid cancer, and lymphoma.

Metastatic Squamous Cell Carcinoma

Squamous cell carcinoma is the most common malignancy affecting the upper aerodigestive tract. One of the most important factors affecting survival of patients with squamous cell carcinoma is the presence or absence of lymph node metastases.[66, 126] The incidence of nodal disease in squamous cell carcinoma of the head and neck depends on the primary tumor site. The incidence of metastatic adenopathy at initial presentation varies between less than 10% in glottic cancer and up to 75% in hypopharyngeal cancer. Although there is some variation with tumor site and with the various reports in the literature, the presence of lymph node metastases in patients with squamous cell carcinoma of the head and neck is associated with a 50% reduction in the long-term survival if there is a solitary ipsilateral cervical node, a solitary contralateral node, or extracapsular neoplastic spread in either of these lymph nodes.[66, 126, 132] The presence of lymph node metastases at initial diagnosis is also the greatest prognosticator for recurrent metastatic disease.[66, 128] In some cases, although the primary tumor is controlled, the patients may die of recurrent nodal metastases. In addition, the presence of nodal metastases also directly correlates with the development of distant metastases.

Initially, the assessment of cervical lymph nodes was based purely on clinical evaluation. However, when considering clinically negative (N0) necks, histologically positive lymph nodes have been reported in 20–40% of cases. Accordingly, sectional imaging techniques (CT, MRI, and US) and more recently FDG-PET are widely used to search for lymph node metastases. Anatomically, all lymph nodes in the neck are located within fatty tissue. This fact accounts for the excellent ability of CT to depict lymph nodes as small as a few millimeters. With MRI, fat-suppression techniques after intravenous administration of contrast material may be necessary to best identify small lymph nodes.[11]

The technique of MR lymphography uses ultrasmall superparamagnetic iron oxide (USPIO) particles with a long plasma circulation time that are captured by macrophages in normally functioning lymph nodes. As a result, the signal intensity of normal lymph nodes decreases because of the T2 and susceptibility effect of iron oxide. Iron oxide improves the characterization of the cervical lymph nodes, but the improvement is limited because of technical problems regarding motion and susceptibility artifacts.[7, 124] Because the neck is susceptible to motion artifacts from breathing, swallowing, and vascular pulsations, all images may be degraded on MRI examinations, especially in patients with airway compromise. These artifacts, as well as the poorer resolution compared with CT, are the reason why many radiologists favor CT for investigating for lymph node metastases.[147]

CT and MRI may detect as many as 7.5–19 % clinically negative, tumor-positive nodes.[83–87, 128, 149] If multiple metastases are already noted in the neck, the additional detection of another lymph node metastasis may have only little impact on treatment and outcome. However, if the additional node raises the N stage or is located outside the planned field of treatment, or if imaging depicts a lymph node metastasis in a clinically negative neck, then the impact of imaging is tremendous.

When imaging the neck, size-based criteria, nodal shape criteria, internal nodal architecture criteria, and the criterion of lymph node grouping are applied to CT, MRI, and US.

The size criterion varies considerably among authors. The size criterion is a compromise between sensitivity and specificity.[32] Many authors describe a node as pathological when it is greater than 15 mm in maximum diameter at level II, or greater than 10 mm at all the other levels. Using these criteria, the diagnosis is inaccurate in 20–25 % of cases. Some investigators have suggested that using the minimum axial diameter of the node is a more reliable criterion for detecting nodal metastases.[149] In this system, the minimal axial diameter should not exceed 11 mm for jugulodigastric nodes (level II) and 10 mm in the other regions of the head and neck (Figs. 12.**11** and 12.**12**). These criteria, which yield a sensitivity of 89 % and a specificity of 73 %, have gained wide acceptance in the radiological community. In a recent US study, it has been suggested that a minimal axial diameter of 7 mm in level II nodes and 6 mm for the rest of the neck[146] may represent a reasonable compromise between sensitivity and specificity in necks without palpable lymph node metastases. The clinical implications of using these criteria have not yet been widely evaluated.

In addition, a grouping of three or more nodes with a maximum diameter of 8–15 mm in level II, or 8–9 mm in all other levels, suggests metastatic invasion if they are in the drainage area of the primary tumor site.[146–149]

Normal nodes have an elliptical shape. It has been suggested that the ratio of the maximal longitudinal nodal length to the maximum axial nodal length should be greater than 2 for normal reactive hyperplastic nodes. A value of less than 2 is suggestive of nodal metastasis.[134] This criterion is easily applied with ultrasound because the operator can easily rotate the transducer to obtain a longitudinal and an axial plane through the nodes (Fig. 12.**13**). This criterion may also be applied with 2D coronal and sagittal reconstructions from spiral CT data acquisitions (especially with multidetector scanners, Fig. 12.**14**), as well as with direct coronal or sagittal MRI acquisitions.

All of these criteria apply to homogeneous, sharply delineated nodes. Regardless of the lymph node size, the most reliable imaging finding of metastatic disease is the presence of central nodal necrosis. Central nodal necrosis is seen as an area of low attenuation on contrast-enhanced CT images or low intensity on contrast-enhanced fat-suppressed T1-weighted MR images (Figs. 12.**15**–12.**17**). On T2-weighted images, central nodal necrosis appears as an area of high signal intensity. When comparing CT and MR images in the same patient, the areas of central nodal necrosis appear larger on CT than on MRI. This discrepancy may be explained by the underlying pathological process.[118, 122, 146] Invasion of lymph

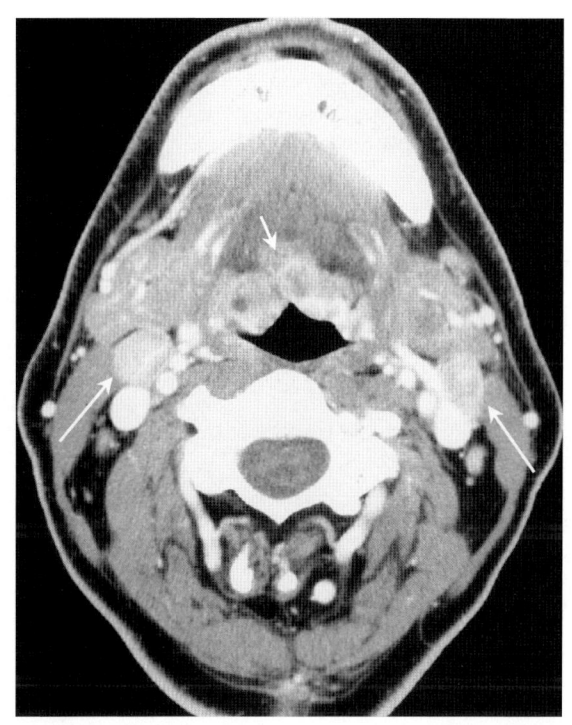

Fig. 12.**11** Homogeneously enhancing enlarged lymph nodes as seen on CT. Contrast-enhanced CT shows a base of the tongue tumor (short arrow) with bilateral enlarged level II lymph nodes (long arrows). The minimal axial diameter was 11 mm on the left and 13 mm on the right. Histology confirmed bilateral lymph node metastases.

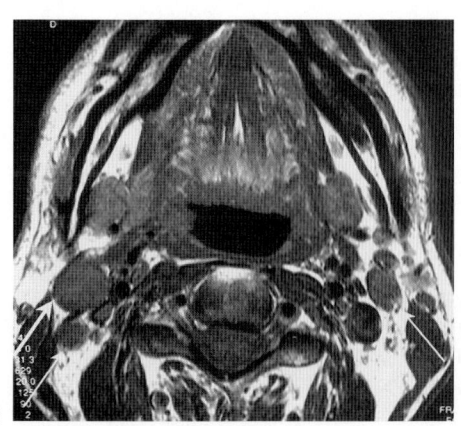

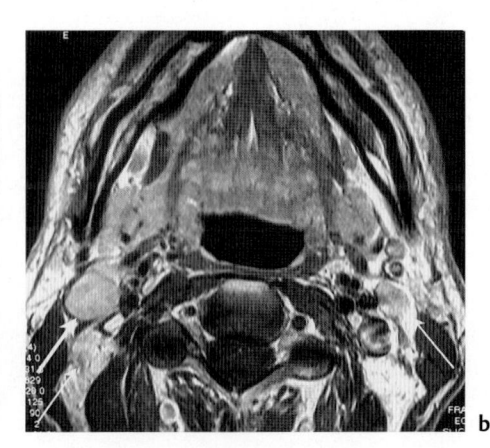

Fig. 12.**12** Homogeneously enhancing and enlarged lymph nodes as seen on MRI. T1W MR images obtained before (**a**) and after (**b**) injection of contrast material in a patient with a supraglottic laryngeal squamous cell carcinoma. Note homogeneously enhancing bilateral level II nodes (thin and thick arrows). Only one lymph node on the right (thick arrows) is enlarged. Histological analysis revealed one lymph node metastasis on the right (thick arrow) and reactive lymph nodes bilaterally (thin arrows).

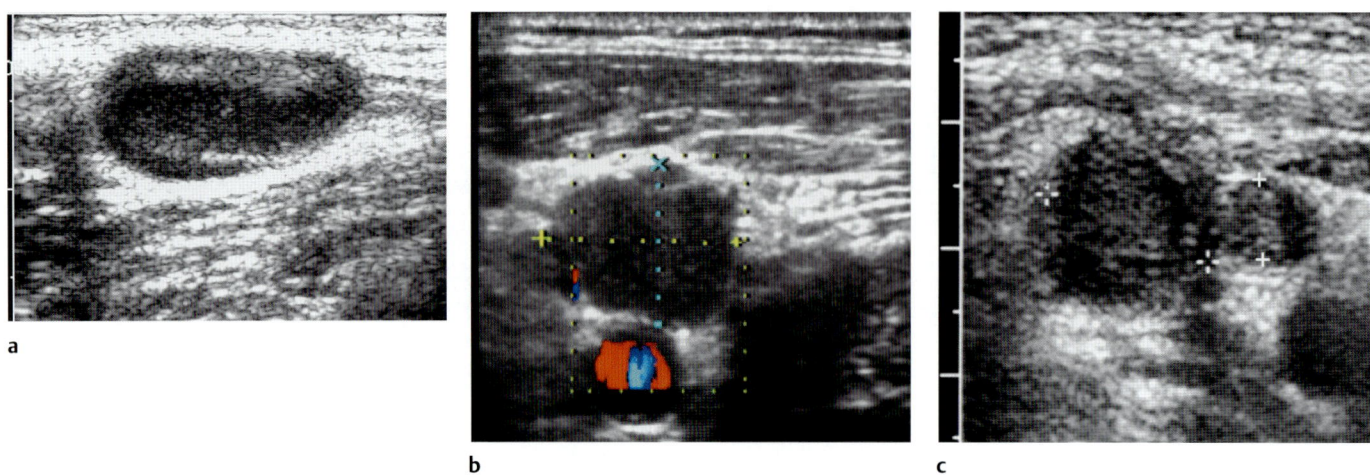

Fig. 12.13 Nodal shape as an indicator of metastatic lymph node involvement as seen on US. **a** Characteristic elliptical shape of a normal hyperplastic lymph node. Note that the ratio of the longitudinal nodal length to the axial nodal length is greater than 2. **b** Fine-needle aspiration biopsy (FNAB)-proven lymph node metastasis of a squamous cell carcinoma of the tonsil. The ratio of the longitudinal nodal length to the axial nodal length is smaller than 2. **c** FNAB-proven lymph node metastases of a squamous cell carcinoma of the hypopharynx. Note spherical shape. None of the lymph nodes shown in **b** and **c** was palpable clinically.

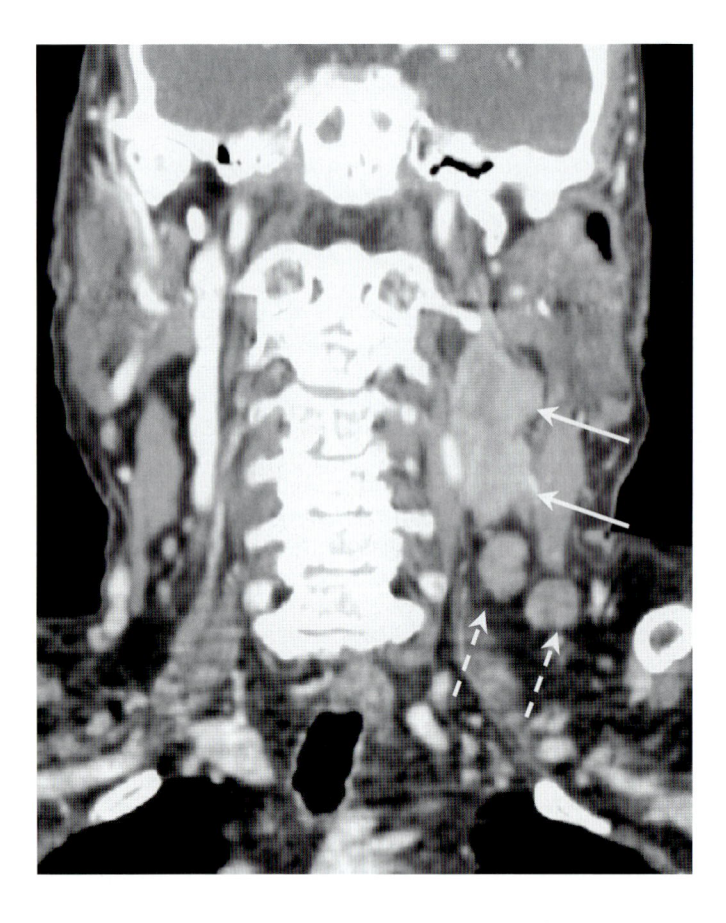

Fig. 12.14 Nodal size and shape as an indicator of metastatic lymph node involvement as seen on CT. Squamous cell carcinoma of the ethmoid sinuses with left-sided level II–IV lymph node metastases. Note enlarged nodes (arrows), as well as nodes with a spherical shape rather than elliptical shape (dashed arrows). In addition, there is inhomogeneous lymph node enhancement of all nodes. Neck dissection confirmed metastatic involvement of all described lymph nodes.

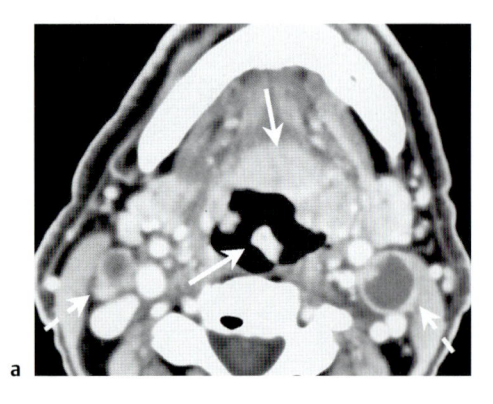

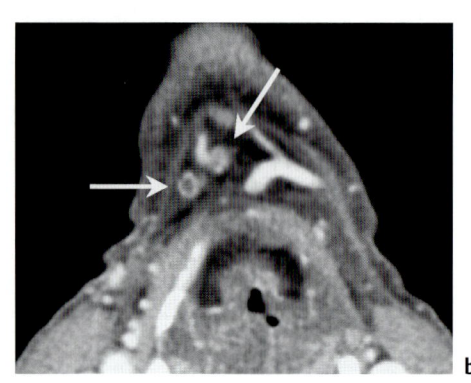

Fig. 12.15 Central nodal necrosis as seen on CT. Contrast-enhanced CT images obtained in four different patients (**a–d**) with squamous cell carcinoma of the upper aerodigestive tract. **a**. Base of the tongue tumor invading the suprahyoid epiglottis (arrows) and with bilateral level II lymph node metastases with central nodal necrosis (dashed arrows). **b** Floor of the mouth cancer with two submental (level I) lymph node metastases with central nodal necrosis (arrows).

Fig. 12.**15 c, d** ▷

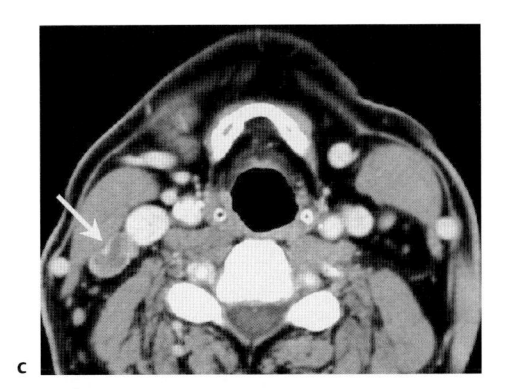

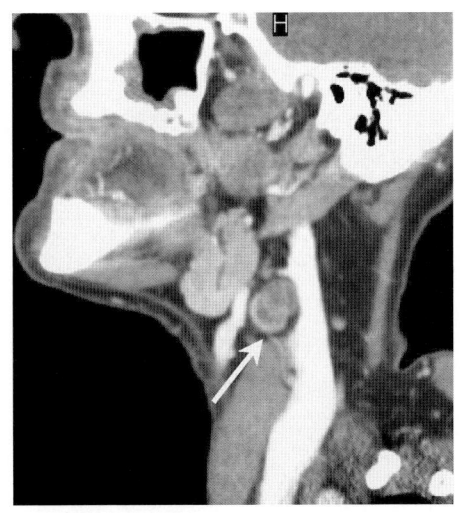

Fig. 12.**15c** Tonsillar cancer with level II lymph node metastasis with central nodal necrosis (arrow). **d** Tongue tumor with level II lymph node metastasis with central nodal necrosis and mass effect on the internal jugular vein (arrow).

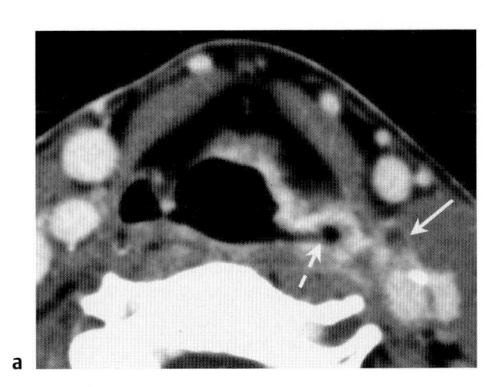

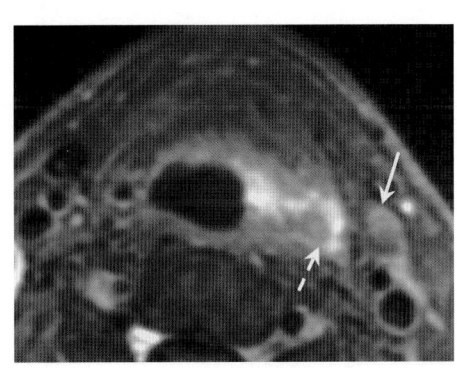

Fig. 12.**16** Central nodal necrosis as seen on CT and MRI. **a** Contrast-enhanced CT image and **b** fat-suppressed, contrast-enhanced T1W image obtained in the same patient at the same level. Squamous cell carcinoma of the left piriform sinus (dashed arrows) with a small level III lymph node with central nodal necrosis (arrows) seen on both examinations. Surgery confirmed metastatic involvement.

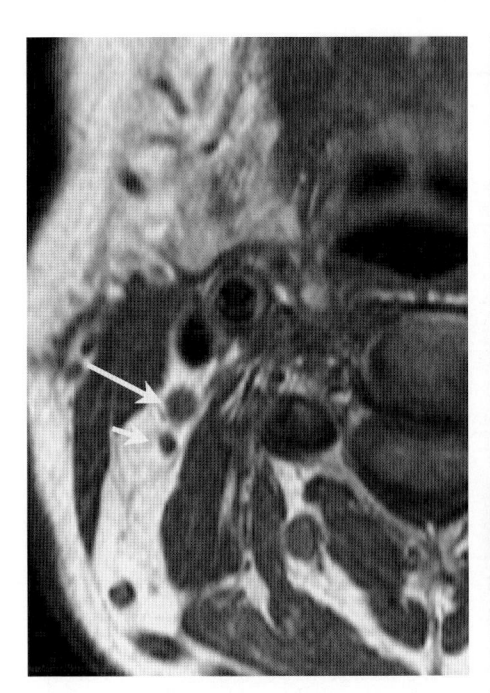

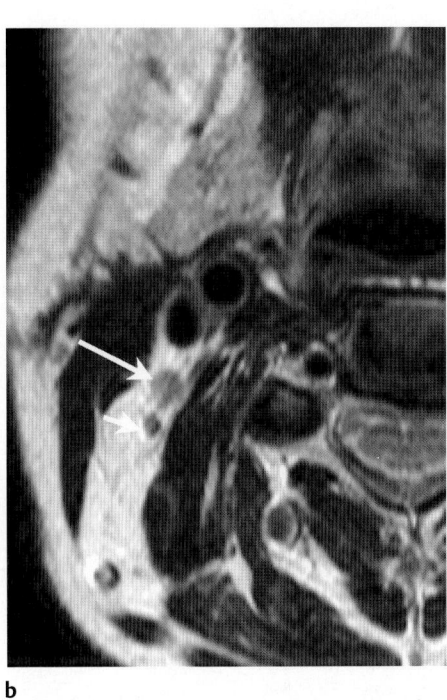

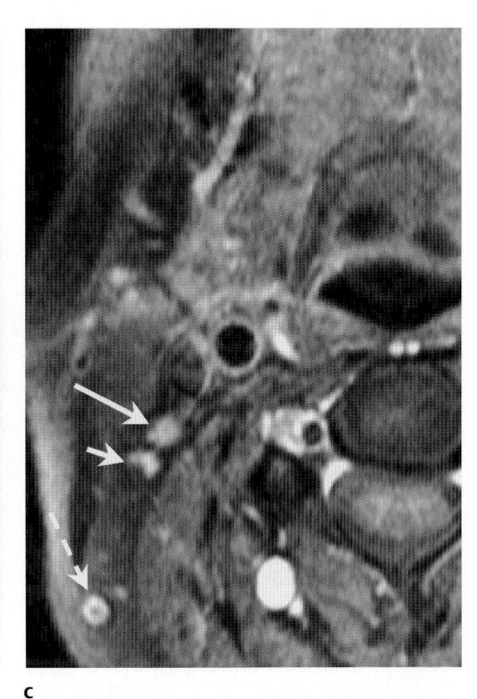

Fig. 12.**17** Small lymph node with central nodal necrosis as seen on a fat-suppressed contrast-enhanced T1W image. Squamous cell carcinoma of the oropharynx. **a** T1W MR image, **b** T2W MR image, and **c** fat-suppressed T1W image obtained at the same level show two small level II lymph nodes. The larger node shows a homogeneous signal intensity on the T1W and T2W images as well as a homogeneous enhancement pattern (arrows). The second lymph node (short arrows) has a nonspecific appearance in **a** and **b**. However, in **c** a fatty hilar metaplasia (short arrow) is observed. In addition, a 3 mm level V lymph node with ring enhancement, suggesting central nodal necrosis (dashed arrow), is seen on the right. Based on imaging findings, the level II lymph nodes were regarded as reactive nodes, whereas the small level V lymph node was regarded as a metastatic node. Surgery confirmed the findings. Note that the small area of central nodal necrosis is seen only on the fat-suppressed, contrast-enhanced T1W MR image.

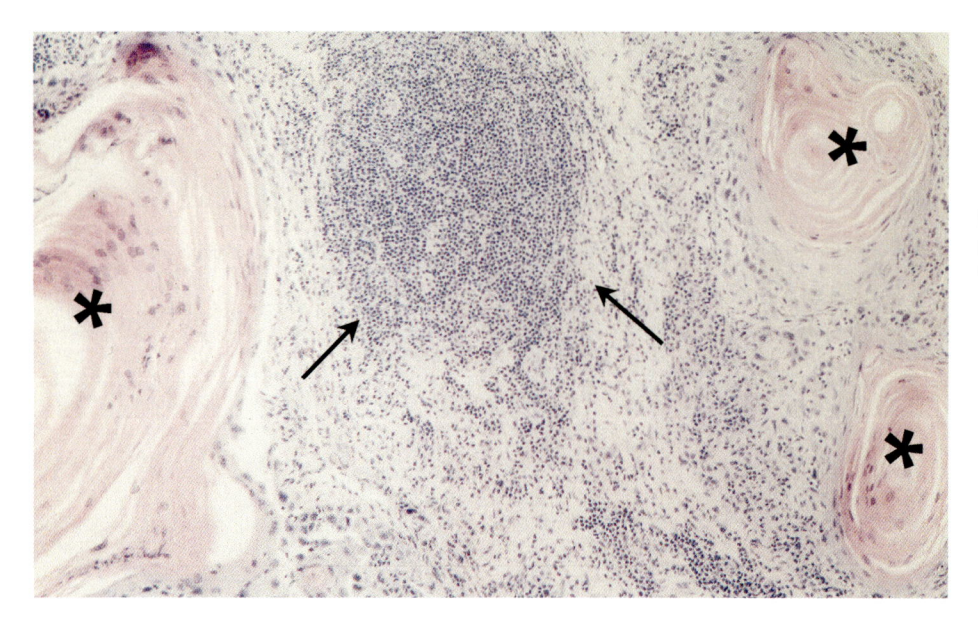

Fig. 12.**18** Photomicrograph of a lymph node metastasis from a well-differentiated squamous cell carcinoma demonstrates invasion of the marginal sinuses of the nodal cortex and nodal medulla by well-differentiated squamous cell carcinoma with keratin pearls (asterisks). Arrows point at a lymph follicle within the nodal cortex.

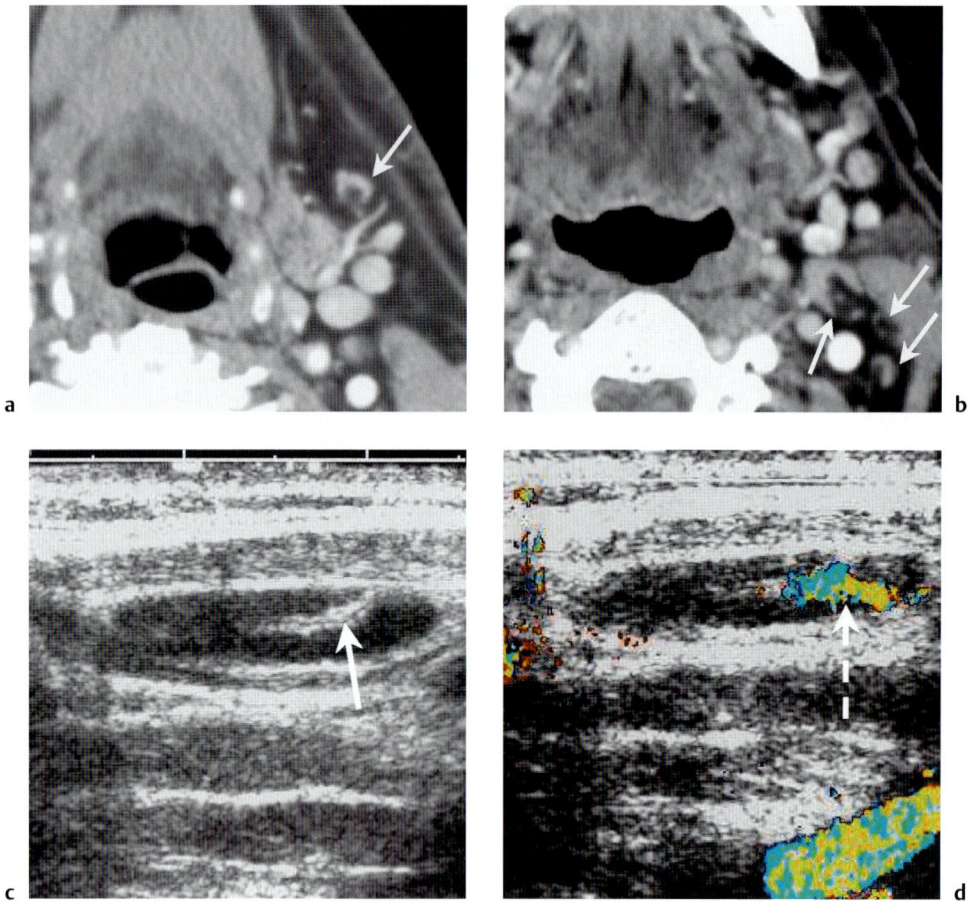

Fig. 12.**19** Fatty hilar metaplasia as seen on CT and US. **a**, **b** Two different patients with lymph nodes with fatty hilar metaplasia (arrows). Note the characteristic U-shape and the fat-containing hilum with a vessel. **c** US of a lymph node with fatty hilar metaplasia and **d** the corresponding Doppler image in another patient show an enlarged elliptic node with a hyperechoic hilum (arrow) and with a hilum vessel (dashed arrow).

nodes by cancer cells first occurs within the marginal sinuses of the nodal cortex (Fig. 12.**18**). Proliferation of the tumor cells then leads to invasion of the nodal medulla, resulting in blockage of the flow of lymph through the node. While the medulla undergoes necrosis, spread of tumor cells to other nodes may occur either via lymphatico-lymphatic or lymphatico-venous pathways. Although it is common practice to refer to such a lymph node as being necrotic, pathologically the nodal medulla contains both tumor cells and interstitial fluid. The necrotic appearance on CT contains both tumor cells and interstitial fluid, whereas on MR only the truly necrotic zones will have signal intensities similar to that of water. Central nodal necrosis has to be differentiated radiologically from fatty hilar metaplasia and an intranodal abscess. Fatty hilar metaplasia is a response to chronic nodal inflammation. Typically, the affected node has a U-shape and the hilum has a lower attenuation value than tumor (Fig. 12.**19**). However, if hilar metaplasia is very small, it may be impossible to differentiate fatty metaplasia from central nodal necrosis. An intranodal abscess

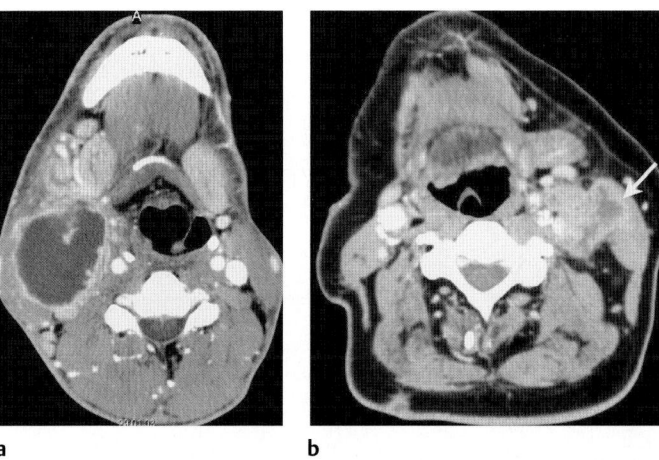

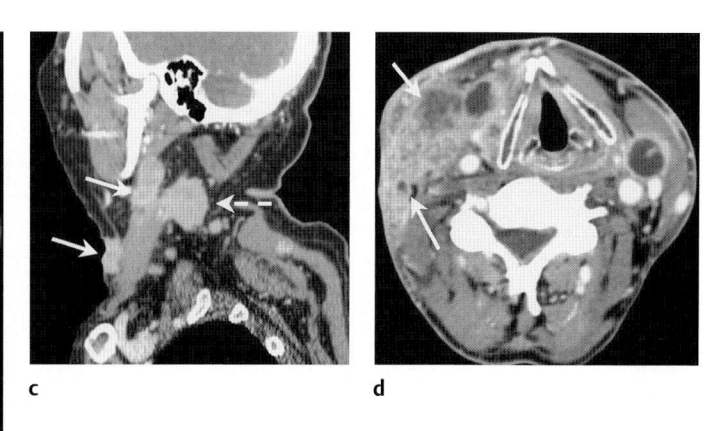

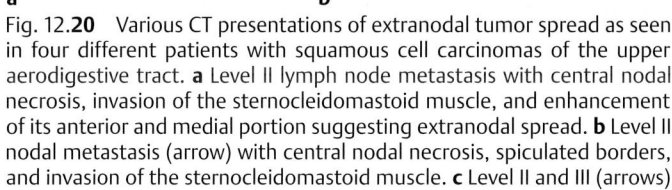

Fig. 12.**20** Various CT presentations of extranodal tumor spread as seen in four different patients with squamous cell carcinomas of the upper aerodigestive tract. **a** Level II lymph node metastasis with central nodal necrosis, invasion of the sternocleidomastoid muscle, and enhancement of its anterior and medial portion suggesting extranodal spread. **b** Level II nodal metastasis (arrow) with central nodal necrosis, spiculated borders, and invasion of the sternocleidomastoid muscle. **c** Level II and III (arrows) and level V (dashed arrow) lymph nodes with spiculated infiltrating borders, suggesting extranodal tumor spread. **d** Bilateral level III lymph node metastases with central nodal necrosis. Note extensive, inhomogeneous enhancement of the right sternocleidomastoid muscle (arrows), which corresponded histologically to diffuse extranodal spread and carcinomatous lymphangitis.

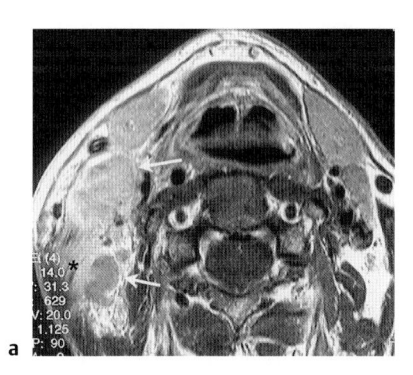

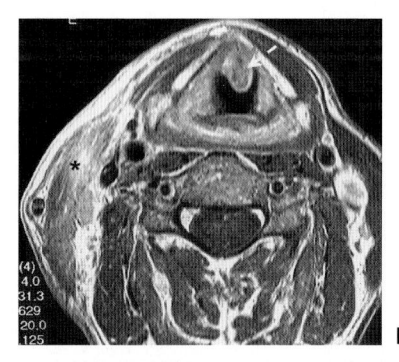

Fig. 12.**21** Extranodal spread with invasion of the sternocleidomastoid muscle in a patient with a tonsillar cancer (not shown) and a supraglottic laryngeal cancer (dashed arrow). Contrast-enhanced T1W MR images (**a** and **b**) show level II lymph node metastases on the right (arrows) with diffuse enhancement of the sternocleidomastoid muscle (asterisks). Histology confirmed extensive muscular invasion.

usually occurs in a patient with an acute infection. Abscessed nodes have a central low density and thick, irregular, and ill-defined margins, all of which may simulate metastatic disease on imaging. Abscessed nodes are usually surrounded by areas of cellulitis. The characteristic clinical findings and the presence of cellulitis may help differentiate abscessed nodes from metastatic nodes at imaging (see below).

Extranodal tumor spread is found at histology in about 25% of nodes less than 1 cm in size, in 40% of nodes less than 2 cm in size, in 50% of nodes 2–3 cm in size, and in 75% of nodes larger than 3 cm.[32, 118, 126] The presence of extranodal extension is seen on contrast-enhanced CT and (fat-suppressed) contrast-enhanced T1-weighted MR images as an enhancing nodal rim, which is irregular and thick with infiltration of the adjacent fat planes[156] (Figs. 12.**20**, 12.**21**). This criterion can be applied only if the patient has not recently had irradiation or surgery of the neck, because these conditions can cause similar imaging findings. Once extracapsular nodal extension has occurred, the tumor may spread to invade the sternocleidomastoid muscle, the carotid artery, the internal jugular vein, and cranial nerves X to XII (Figs. 12.**20**, 12.**21**). Imaging cannot show invasion of the carotid adventitia, but the likelihood of such an event increases with an increasing degree of contact between the tumor and the carotid artery.[155] If the tumor encompasses more than 270° of the circumference of the vessel on axial images, it becomes unlikely that it can be removed without resecting the artery.[155]

Using the above criteria, CT and MRI have a similar performance for the detection of lymph node metastases. The sensitivity of CT and MRI is 67–89% and the specificity is 73–97%.[32, 85, 111, 118, 124, 146, 156] Both techniques have a similar negative predictive value (84% for CT and 79% for MRI), although CT performs slightly better than MRI for all interpretation criteria.[32]

Ultrasound performed for lymph node assessment offers similar or even superior accuracy compared to CT and MR imaging.[146] Ultrasonographic criteria for the detection of lymph node metastases include a rounded shape, hypoechogenicity, and loss of hilar definition (Figs. 12.**13** and 12.**22**). Extracapsular spread is seen on US as poorly defined nodal margins. On power Doppler and color Doppler sonography, malignant nodes may show increased peripheral perfusion, focal absence of perfusion, absence of central vessels, or an irregular pattern of perfusion. A high variation in the resistance index is also indicative of metastatic invasion.[75] However, it should be underlined that these US findings are not specific for metastatic nodes but that there is great overlap with lymphoma and inflammatory nodes. Ultrasound combined with ultrasound-guided fine-needle aspiration biopsy yields a specificity of over 95% and a sensitivity of 42–98%.[139, 146] This technique is not widely available; it is operator-dependent and requires an experienced cytologist.

FDG-PET has shown promising results[16, 41, 78, 111] (Fig. 12.**23**). The sensitivity of FDG-PET is 71–90% and the specificity is 86–99%.[2, 16, 41, 111] In series that have directly compared the perfor-

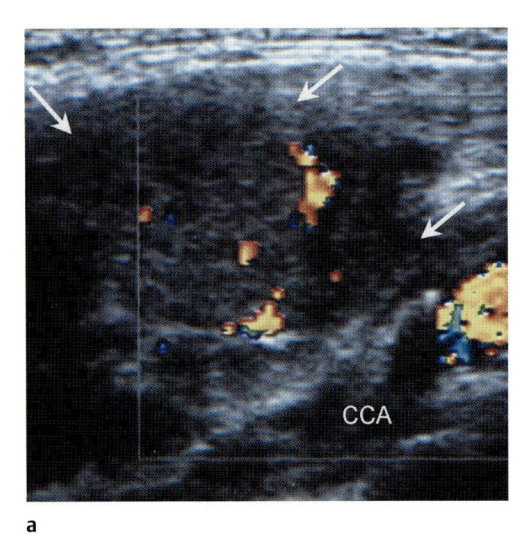

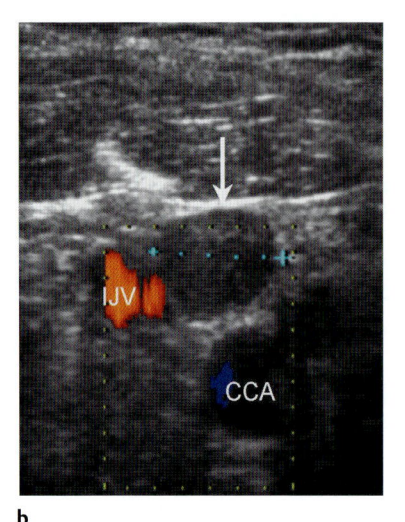

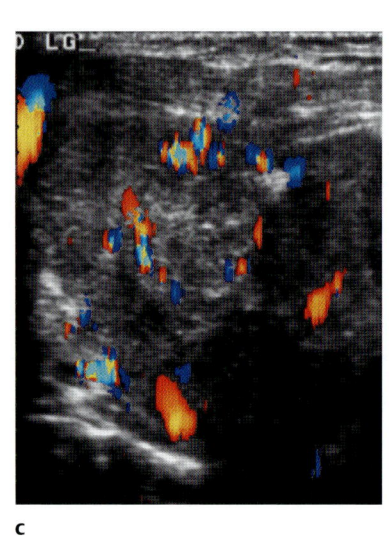

Fig. 12.22 Various presentations of metastatic lymph nodes on color Doppler US. **a** Longitudinal US image of the left neck shows a level III lymph node metastasis with loss of hilar definition, hypoechogenicity, and poorly defined margins (arrows) suggesting extracapsular spread. Note absence of central vessels and focal absence of perfusion. **b** Transverse image of the right neck. 7 mm-large level III lymph node metastasis (arrow) with a rounded shape, hypoechogenicity, loss of hilar vessels, and almost no perfusion. **c** Longitudinal US image shows a large level II lymph node with extracapsular spread and an irregular pattern of perfusion. CCA = common carotid artery; IJV = internal jugular vein.

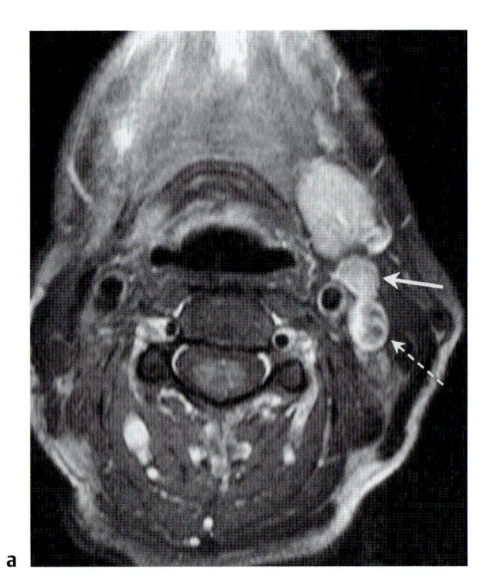

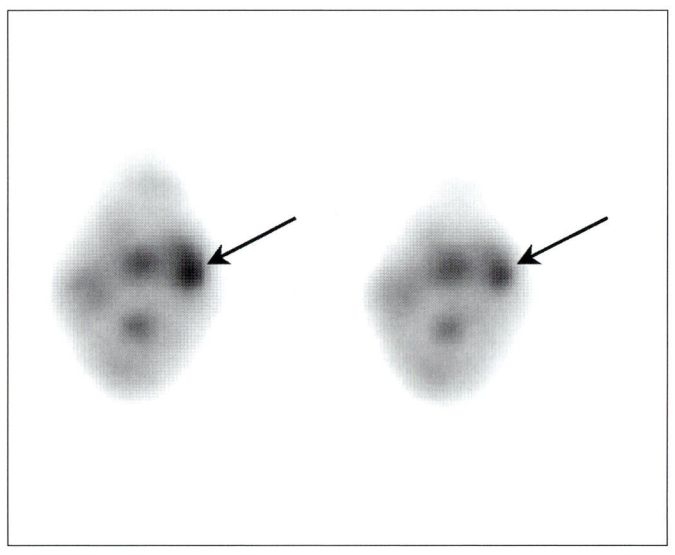

Fig. 12.23 Squamous cell carcinoma metastasis. True positive PET and equivocal MRI. Female patient with a base of the tongue tumor and without palpable lymph nodes. **a** Contrast-enhanced, fat-suppressed T1W MR image shows a level II lymph node on the left with a minimum axial diameter of 10 mm and homogeneous enhancement (arrow). Dashed arrow points at flow artifacts within the internal jugular vein. **b** PET image obtained in the same patient clearly shows a hypermetabolic focus on the left, suggesting metastatic spread. The patient underwent neck dissection and histology confirmed a level II lymph node metastasis.

mance of FDG-PET with CT and/or MRI, FDG-PET performed only slightly better than the anatomical imaging techniques. In a series published a few years ago, which compared the performance of clinical evaluation, FDG-PET, and CT for the detection of lymph node metastases it was shown that, although there was no significant difference between FDG-PET and CT for the detection of lymph node metastases, the combination of both modalities yielded significantly improved results.[16] It appears, therefore, that in the future the use of a new generation of combined CT-PET scanners will increase the performance of this technique. Nevertheless, it should be mentioned that false-positive assessments may occur with FDG-PET because FDG-PET cannot differentiate between malignant nodes and benign reactive nodes. Activated macrophages may, in fact, cause increased FDG uptake.

Lymphoma

Both Hodgkin and non-Hodgkin lymphoma commonly involve the cervical lymph node groups. Involved lymph nodes range in size from 1 cm to 10 cm.[79] Their most striking feature on CT and MRI is their large size, homogeneity, and thin peripheral rim-enhancement[91, 145] (Figs. 12.24–12.27). On US, the involved lymph nodes are most often enlarged, hypoechoic, and well-delineated, and there is loss of the normal elliptical shape (Fig. 12.28). On Doppler US, homogeneous and increased vascularity is the rule, and under treatment this increased vascularization decreases progressively. Nodal necrosis may occur in lymphomatous lymph nodes, but it is much less frequent than with metastatic squamous cell carcinoma or metastatic thyroid cancer. Extrano-

Neoplastic Lesions

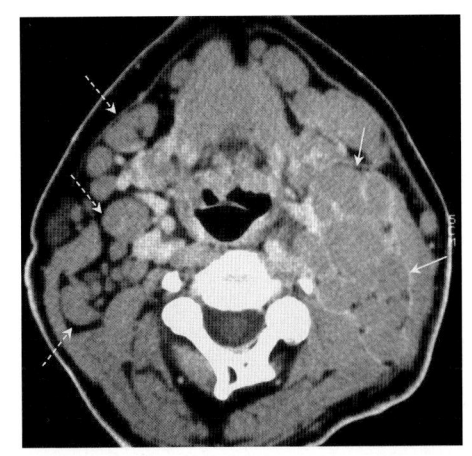

Fig. 12.**24** Non-Hodgkin lymphoma of the neck. Characteristic CT appearance. Contrast-enhanced CT image shows multiple bilateral lymph nodes ranging in size from 1 cm to several centimeters. Involvement of level I and II nodes bilaterally. Note that some of the enlarged lymph nodes show almost no enhancement (dashed arrows), while other involved nodes show a very thin peripheral enhancement (arrows). Absence of central nodal necrosis.

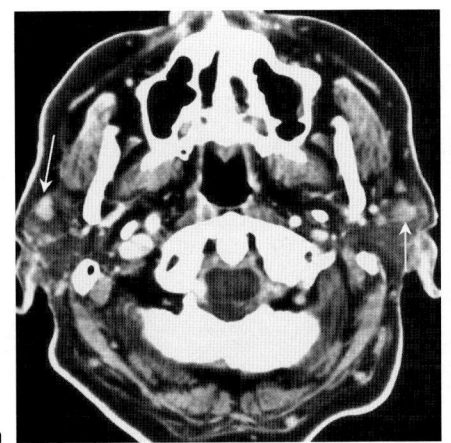

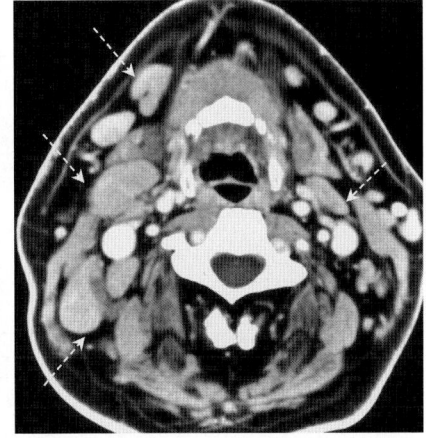

Fig. 12.**25 a, b** Non-Hodgkin lymphoma of the neck with involvement of the parotid glands. Characteristic CT appearance. Contrast-enhanced CT images show multiple enlarged nodes (level I and level II groups, dashed arrows) with homogeneous minor enhancement. Note also enlarged parotid lymph nodes bilaterally (arrows).

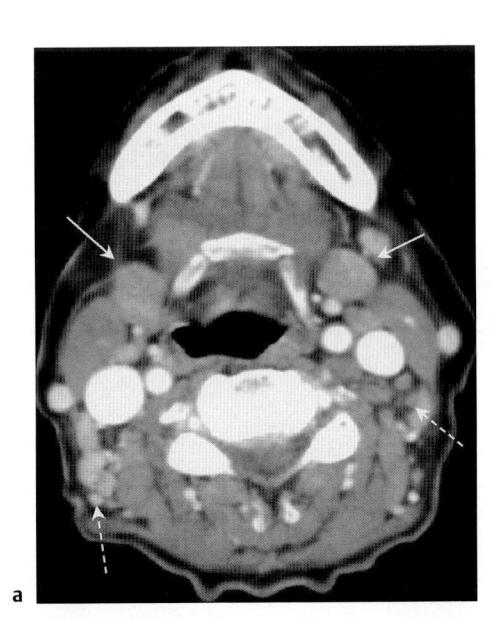

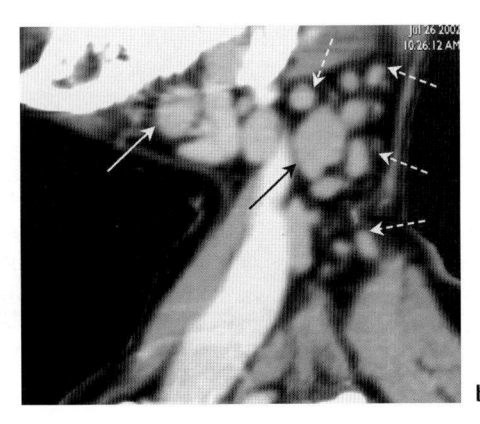

Fig. 12.**26** Non-Hodgkin lymphoma of the neck. Numerous small or moderately enlarged nodes. **a** Contrast-enhanced axial and **b** 2D parasagittal reconstruction from the volumetric data set show some enlarged lymph nodes (arrows) as well as multiple small lymph nodes (dashed arrows) with homogeneous enhancement. Histology confirmed non-Hodgkin lymphoma not only of enlarged nodes but also of small nonenlarged nodes.

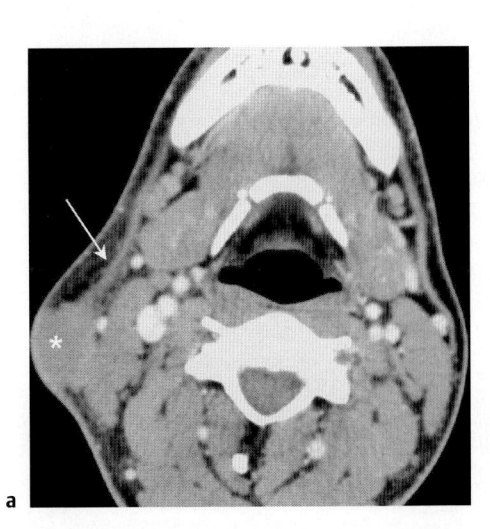

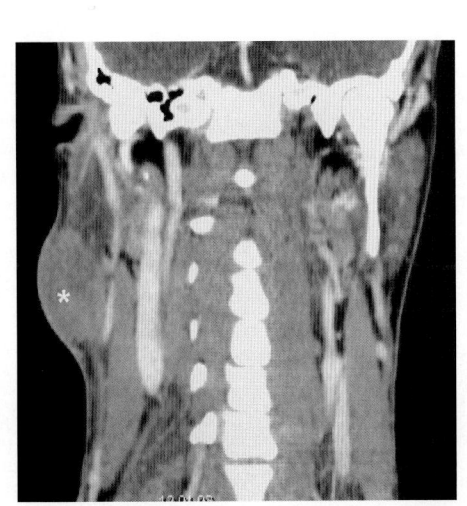

Fig. 12.**27** Non-Hodgkin lymphoma of the neck. Atypical presentation. **a** Contrast-enhanced axial and **b** 2D coronal reconstruction obtained in a young male patient presenting with a rapidly enlarging neck swelling and with inflammatory signs. A large, homogeneously enhancing external jugular mass is seen on the right (asterisk). Note thickening of the platysma and a reticulated enhancement pattern of the surrounding fat, suggesting cellulitis (arrow). Histology revealed non-Hodgkin lymphoma.

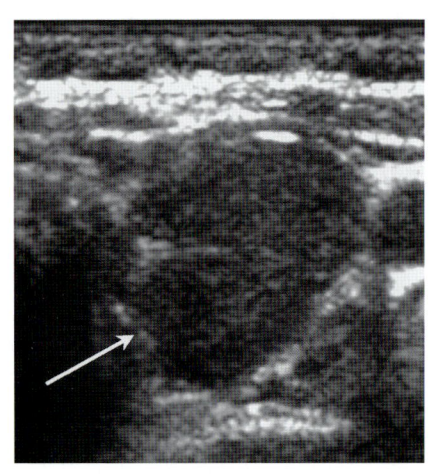

Fig. 12.28 Non-Hodgkin lymphoma of the neck. Characteristic US appearance. Transverse image shows an enlarged lymph node (arrow) with a hypoechoic homogeneous structure and a rounded shape. The borders are well-defined. Multiple lymph nodes with the same imaging characteristics were seen bilaterally.

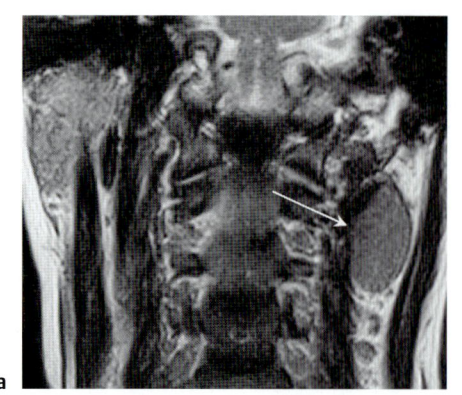

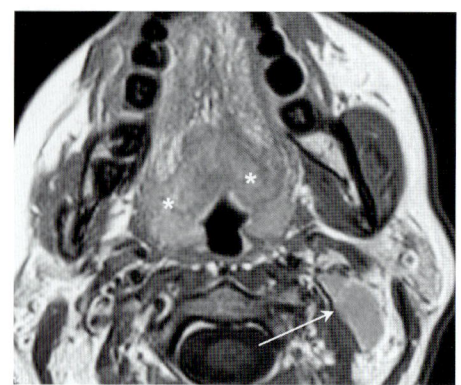

Fig. 12.29 Non-Hodgkin lymphoma of the neck with involvement of Waldeyer's ring. **a** Coronal T2W FSE MR image shows an enlarged level II lymph node with homogeneous signal intensity (arrow). **b** Axial contrast-enhanced T1W image shows homogeneous nodal enhancement (arrow) and involvement of the lingual tonsil (asterisks).

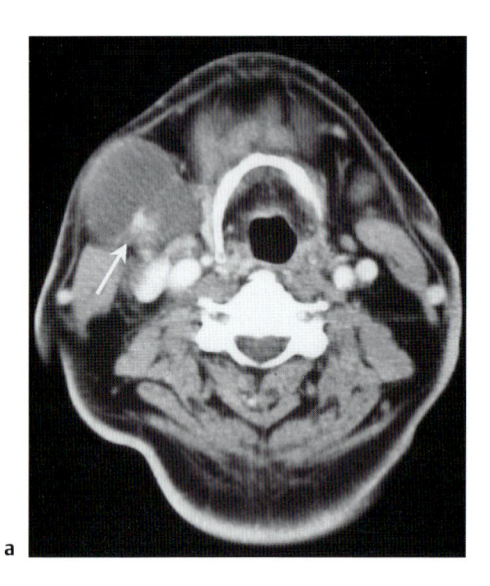

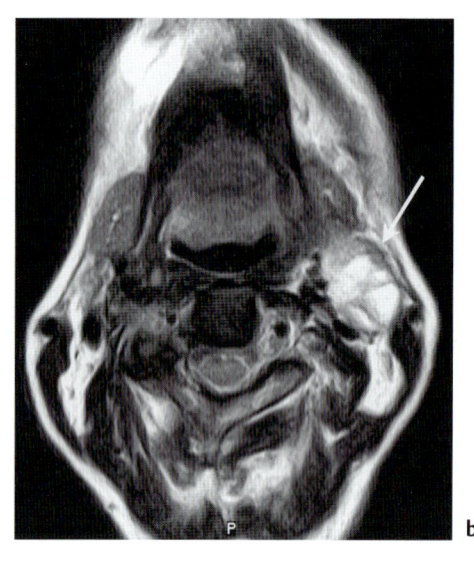

Fig. 12.30 Cystic metastases from papillary thyroid carcinoma. **a** Contrast-enhanced CT in a patient with papillary thyroid carcinoma shows a cystic metastasis (level II) with a small enhancing mural nodule (arrow) on the right. **b** T2W image obtained in another patient with papillary thyroid carcinoma shows a predominantly cystic level II lymph node metastasis with multiple thick septa (arrow).

Table 12.**6** Differential diagnosis of nodes with central nodal necrosis

Malignant
Squamous cell carcinoma
Thyroid cancer
Lymphoma*

Benign
Suppurative adenopathy
Cat-scratch disease
Tuberculosis and nontuberculous mycobacterial infection
Tularemia

* Rare.

dal involvement—most often at the level of Waldeyer's ring—may be seen in up to 23% of patients with non-Hodgkin lymphoma (Fig. 12.**29**); it is, however, unusual in patients with Hodgkin lymphoma (only 4%).[144, 145] Intranodal calcification may be seen after radiation therapy or chemotherapy of both Hodgkin and non-Hodgkin lymphoma. Rarely, it may be seen prior to therapy.

Nodal Metastases from Thyroid Cancer

The appearance of metastatic nodes from papillary thyroid cancer is very variable and includes homogeneously enhancing lymph nodes, hemorrhagic nodes, cystic or necrotic nodes, calcified nodes, and hypervascular nodes (Tables 12.**6**–12.**8**).[130] Because cystic nodes may contain a high concentration of thyroglobulin, they may appear as hypodense on CT and hyperintense on both T1- and T2-weighted MR images (Figs. 12.**30**, 12.**31**). In the presence of intranodal hemorrhage, they have a high density on CT, as well as a high signal intensity on T1- and T2-weighted images. MRI appears to have a high sensitivity for the detection of lymph node metastases from thyroid cancer (95%), but only a limited specificity (51%) and positive predictive value (84%).[53] Papillary thyroid carcinoma is a relatively common cause of intranodal calcification, which may also be seen in metastatic follicular and medullary thyroid cancer. A recent study has shown that metastatic thyroid carcinoma accounts for 42% of cases of malignant nodal calcification with the exception of lymphomatous nodes following radiation therapy or chemotherapy.[44] A differential diagnosis of nodal calcification, central nodal necrosis, and enhancing nodes is given in Tables 12.**6**–12.**8**.

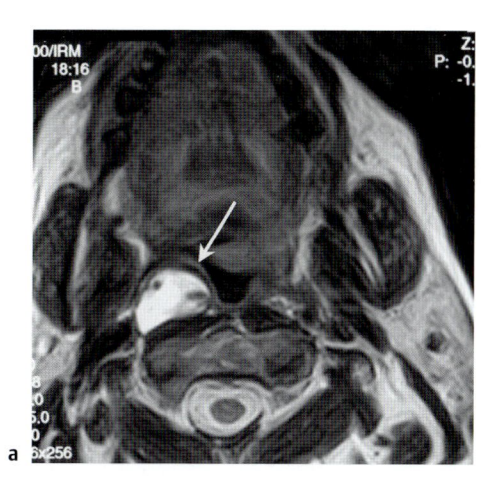

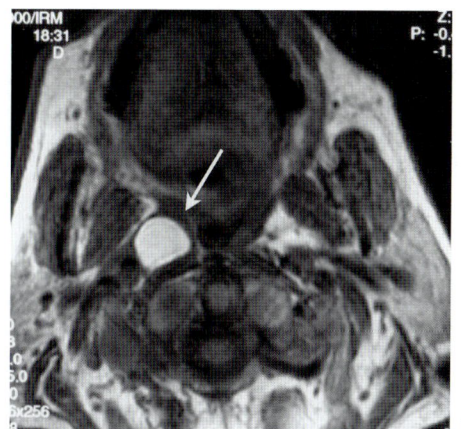

Fig. 12.**31** Retropharyngeal cystic hemorrhagic metastasis from papillary thyroid carcinoma. **a** T2W FSE MR image shows an enlarged hyperintense retropharyngeal lymph node (arrow). **b** Unenhanced T1W image shows that the lymph node has a high signal intensity as well (arrow). Surgical exploration confirmed a cystic metastasis from papillary thyroid carcinoma with intranodal hemorrhage.

Nodal Metastases from Other Tumors

The appearance of nodal metastases from other tumors originating in the extracranial head neck (such as mucoepidermoid carcinoma, adenocarcinoma) or from tumors originating from distant sites (lung, breast, cervical esophagus, abdomen) may be very variable, including solid nodes, necrotic nodes, hypervascular nodes, and calcified nodes. Metastases from renal cell carcinoma and malignant melanoma may show increased vascularity and areas of hemorrhage on CT and MRI. Owing to the paramagnetic properties of melanin, lymph nodes from malignant melanoma may have a characteristic feature on MR imaging. Occasionally, lymph nodes from colon cancer may demonstrate calcifications. Most metastatic neck nodes from distant sites (lung, breast, abdomen, cervical esophagus) occur in the supraclavicular area (low level IV and low level V).

■ Nonnodal Neoplasms

The most common nonnodal neck masses include neurogenic tumors, lipomas, and paragangliomas.

Neurogenic Tumors

Neurogenic tumors include schwannoma, neurofibroma, ganglioneuroma, and granular cell tumors. Schwannomas and neurofibromas are the most common types of neurogenic tumors found in the extracranial head and neck.

Schwannoma

Schwannomas are benign tumors arising from Schwann cells surrounding the peripheral nerves. Schwannomas may be solitary or multiple and they may or may not be associated with neurofibromatosis type 2 (NF2). Schwannomas in the neck typically involve the vagus nerve, the cervical nerve roots, the sympathetic chain, or the brachial plexus[158] (Figs. 12.**32**–12.**35**). Most solitary schwannomas involve the suprahyoid neck, from where they may extend into the infrahyoid neck. The typical age of presentation is between 20 and 50 years of age. Clinical findings are inconstant and include motor dysfunction or pain in the distribution of a sensory nerve. Very often, however, the patients remain asymptomatic until the tumor reaches a considerable size. Schwannomas display typical features on MRI. Nearly 75% of all tumors have the same signal intensity as the spinal cord on T1-weighted MR sequences; more than 95% have a high signal intensity on T2-weighted MR sequences; and nearly all nerve sheath tumors enhance following intravenous administration of gadolinium-based contrast material.[11, 54, 115, 158] The enhancement pattern is highly variable. A target appearance (hyperintense rim and hypointense center) may be seen on contrast-enhanced MR images or contrast-enhanced CT images, and is caused by central areas of cystic or necrotic degeneration (Figs. 12.**33**, 12.**34**). When schwannomas arise within the carotid space (poststyloid compartment of the parapharyngeal space), they typically displace the internal and common carotid artery anteriorly, laterally, or anterolaterally, a feature that is nicely displayed on axial CT and MR images (Figs. 12.**32**–12.**34**). On angiography, schwannomas have been de-

Table 12.**7** Differential diagnosis of nodal calcification

Malignant
Thyroid carcinoma (papillary, medullary, and follicular)
Lymphoma*
Adenocarcinoma (mucin-producing)
Squamous cell carcinoma*
Benign
Tuberculosis
Sarcoidosis
Histoplasmosis
Coccidioidomycosis
Fungal infection: nontuberculous mycobacterial infection
Castleman disease
Rheumatoid arthritis*
Scleroderma
Amyloidosis

* Rare.

Table 12.**8** Differential diagnosis of enhancing nodes

Malignant
Metastatic squamous cell cancer
Metastatic thyroid cancer*
Lymphoma
Metastatic melanoma and renal cell carcinoma*
Benign
Acute viral or bacterial infection
Tuberculosis
Cat-scratch disease
AIDS-related lymphadenopathy
Castleman disease
Kikuchi disease
Kimura disease
Amyloidosis*

* Very strong enhancement.

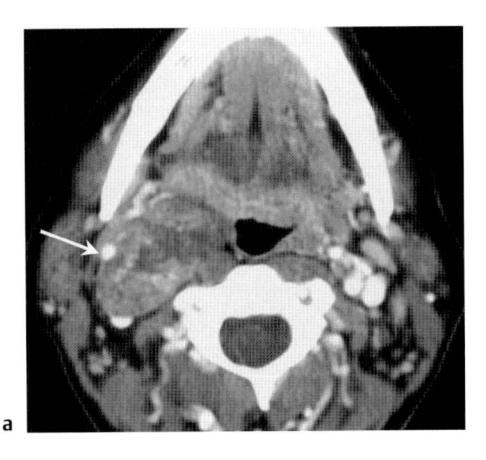

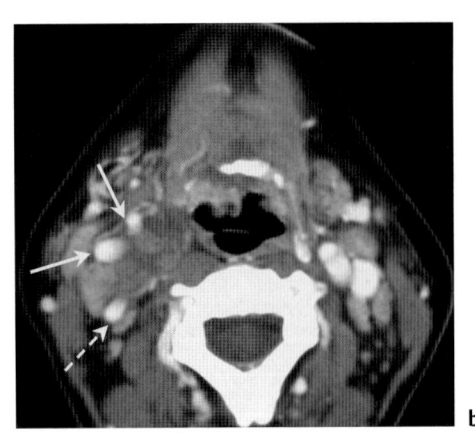

Fig. 12.32 Schwannoma of the sympathetic chain. CT appearance. Young female patient presenting with a palpable mass at the level of the hyoid bone. Contrast-enhanced CT images at the level of the base of the tongue (**a**) and hyoid bone (**b**) show a large hypodense tumor with inhomogeneous enhancement displacing the internal and external carotid arteries (arrows) as well as the internal jugular vein (dashed arrow) laterally. There is marked mass effect on the oropharynx. Surgery revealed schwannoma of the sympathetic chain.

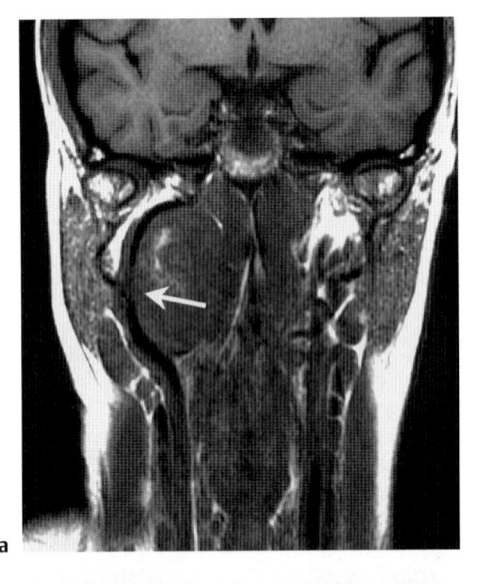

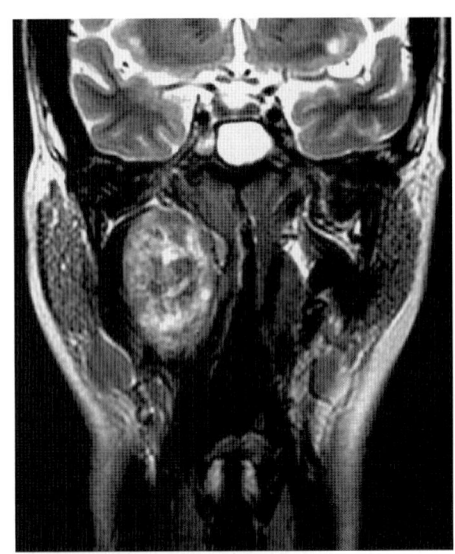

Fig. 12.33 Schwannoma of the sympathetic chain: MR appearance. Young female patient presenting with a palpable soft mass at the level of the hyoid bone. **a** Coronal T1W image shows a large inhomogeneous mass that is isointense to hyperintense to muscle. It is located in the carotid space and displaces the internal carotid artery anterolaterally (arrow). **b** On the T2W FSE image a heterogeneous hypointense and hyperintense signal intensity is seen, suggesting the presence of cystic degeneration and hemorrhage. **c** Axial contrast-enhanced T1W image shows a targetlike appearance with peripheral enhancement and central areas of cystic degeneration. **d** MR angiography shows major lateral displacement of the internal carotid artery and no major vascularity. Surgery confirmed a schwannoma of the sympathetic chain.

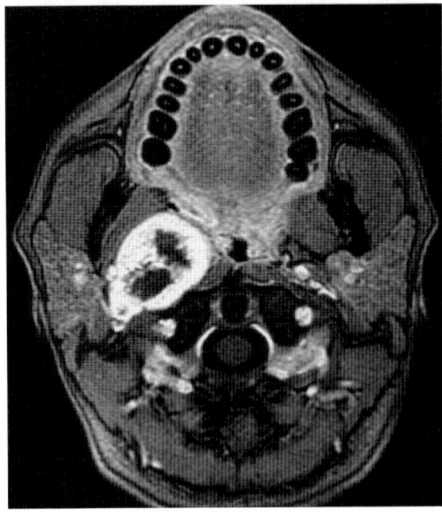

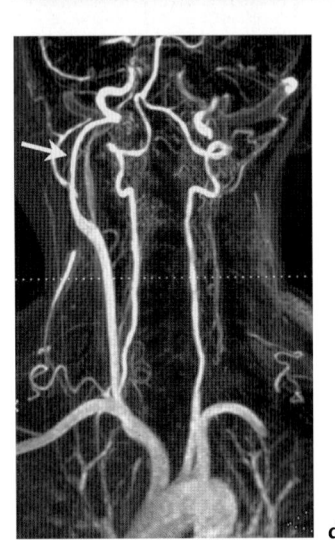

scribed as hypovascular or moderately hypervascular lesions. The hypervascular schwannomas usually show a moderate vascularity and they may reveal puddling of contrast material but no arteriovenous shunting. Surgery is regarded as the treatment of choice, but a 5% recurrence rate has been reported. Very rarely, malignant transformation of schwannomas may occur.[151]

Most schwannomas are a mixture of two histological types of tissue: the cell-rich Antoni type A tissue with chromatin-rich cells arranged in characteristic palisades and in onion rings (Verocay bodies) and the relatively acellular cystic Antoni type B tissue (Fig. 12.34). The Antoni type B pattern is commonly intermixed with the Antoni type A, but an entire tumor may have this arrangement. Regressive changes, including necrosis, cystic degeneration, and lipidization may be prominent and do not bear relation to the size or location of the tumor.[11]

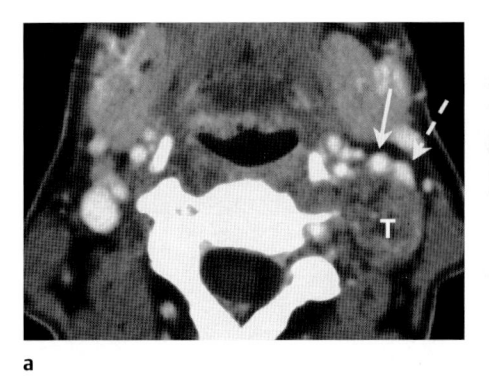

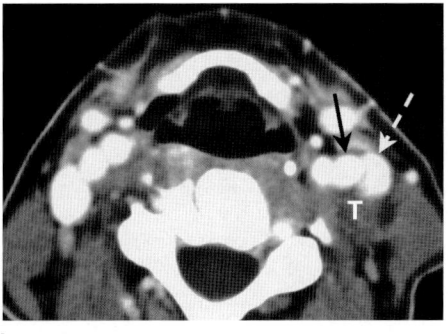

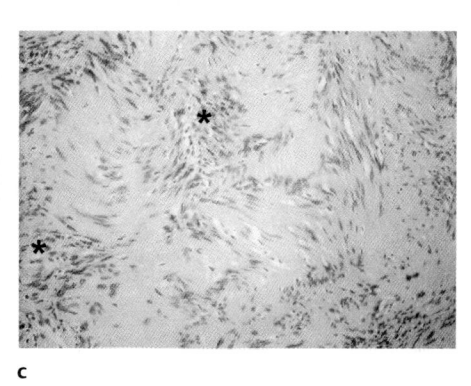

Fig. 12.**34** Schwannoma of the vagus nerve. CT appearance. Young male patient presenting with progressive dysphagia and a palpable mass in the left neck. Contrast-enhanced CT images at the level of the base of the tongue (**a**) and hyoid bone (**b**) show a tumor (T) with inhomogeneous and minor enhancement displacing the internal and external carotid arteries (arrows) as well as the internal jugular vein (dashed arrow) anteriorly. The tumor follows the course of the vagus nerve. Surgery revealed schwannoma of the vagus nerve. **c** Photomicrograph (hematoxylin–eosin stain) shows an Antoni type A pattern with characteristic palisades and onion rings (Verocay bodies, asterisks).

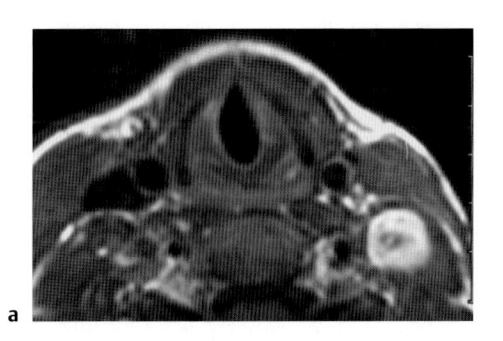

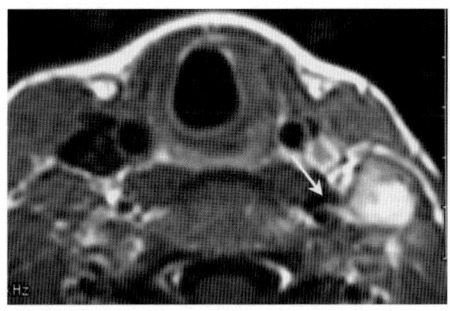

Fig. 12.**35** Schwannoma of the brachial plexus. Young female patient presenting with pain in the distribution of the left C6 dermatome. Contrast-enhanced T1W MR images at the glottic (**a**) and subglottic (**b**) levels show a fusiform mass with extension along the C6 nerve root into the intervertebral foramen (arrow). The tumor mass shows very strong peripheral enhancement and a central nonenhancing zone. Surgery confirmed schwannoma of the C6 nerve root.

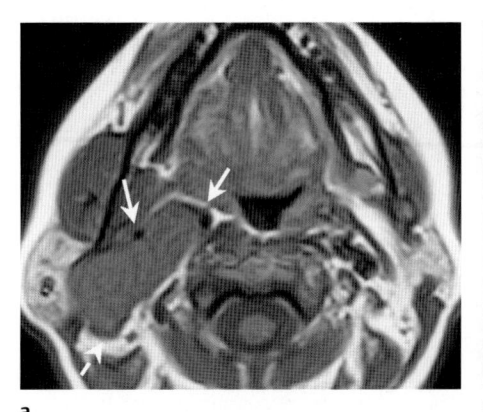

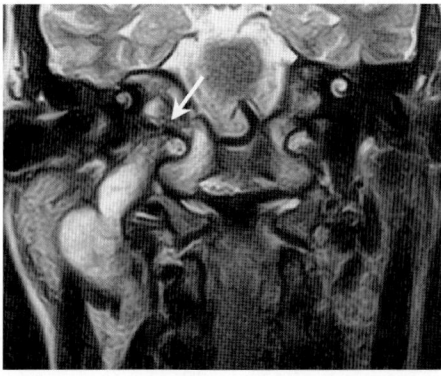

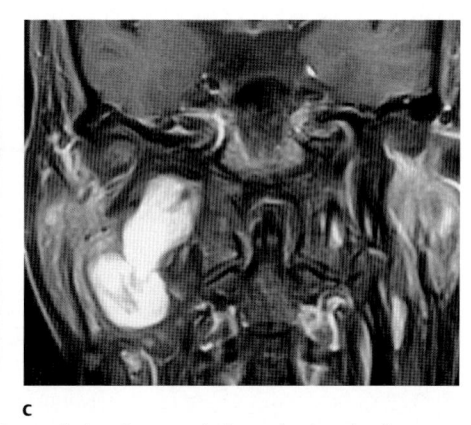

Fig. 12.**36** Solitary neurofibroma of the vagus nerve. Elderly woman presenting with long-standing dysphagia and recurrent laryngeal nerve paralysis. **a** T1W axial MR image shows a mass that is isointense to muscle and displaces the internal carotid artery and the external carotid artery anteriorly (arrows). The internal jugular vein is displaced laterally (dashed arrow). **b** Coronal T2W MR image shows that the fusiform mass has an increased signal intensity and that it extends into the jugular foramen (arrow). **c** Coronal fat-suppressed T1W MR image obtained after injection of contrast material shows major enhancement. MR imaging suggested a tumor arising from the vagus nerve, either a schwannoma or a neurofibroma. Surgery revealed a solitary neurofibroma of the vagus nerve.

Neurofibroma

Neurofibromas arise either from the nerves within the dermis, subcutaneous tissue or other deeper tissues. They are most commonly seen in patients between the ages of 20 and 40 years. Most neurofibromas are slowly growing, painless masses causing no particular symptoms until they reach a considerable size.[11, 54, 151] The nerve of origin is usually incorporated within the neurofibroma and a fusiform configuration is typically seen on gross inspection. Consequently, the nerve has to be sacrificed during surgical extirpation. Histologically, neurofibromas are well-delineated lesions but without a capsule. The tumor is composed of spindle cells and a stroma with large amounts of collagen fibers.

Cervical neurofibromas may be solitary lesions (although rare) or they may be seen in patients with NF1 (von Recklinghausen disease) (Figs. 12.**36**, 12.**37**). NF1 is an autosomal dominant disorder with café au lait spots, peripheral neurofibromas, optic gliomas, and Lisch nodules (pigmented nodules of the iris). The NF1 gene is located on chromosome 17q11.2. The neurofibromas seen in NF1 are either localized or plexiform. Localized neurofibromas are located either within the skin or within the deep soft-tissue structures. They typically develop after the café au lait spots have appeared in childhood or adolescence. The multiple neurofibromas in NF1 are often bilateral along the spinal column (Fig. 12.**37**). Bony abnormalities seen in as many as

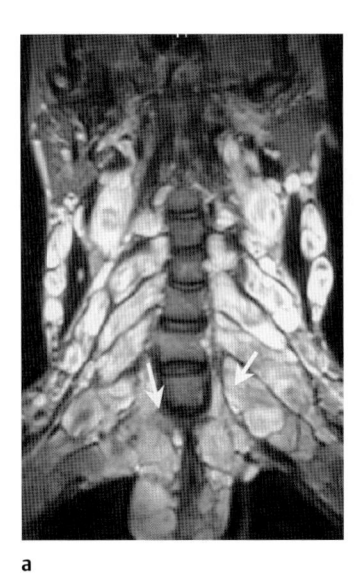

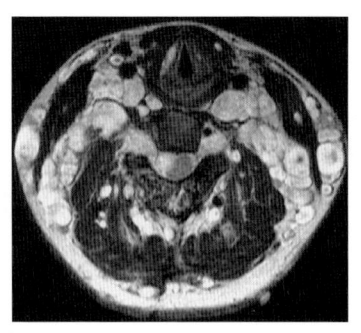

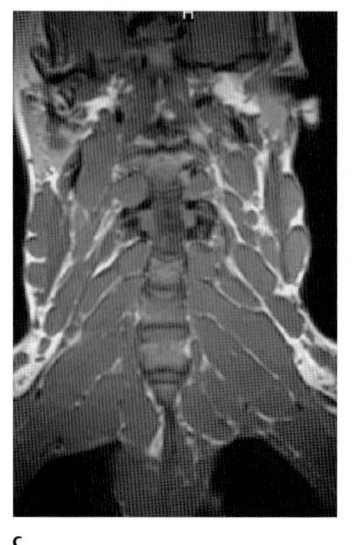

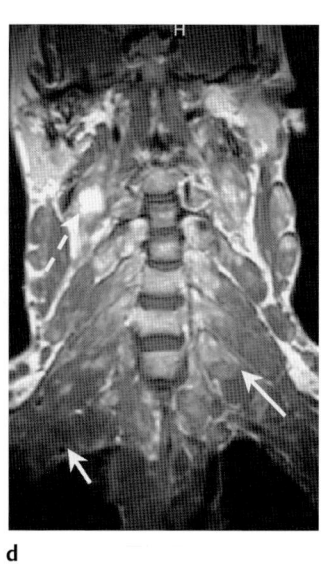

Fig. 12.37 Neurofibromatosis type 1. Characteristic MRI appearance. a Coronal and b axial T2W images demonstrate multiple hyperintense neurofibomas involving virtually all cervical nerve roots, the brachial plexus, the vagus nerves, and peripheral subcutaneous nerve branches. Note also intraforaminal extension (in b) and involvement of the mediastinum (in a). c Coronal T1W image at the same level as a shows that most neurofibromas are isointense to muscle. d Contrast-enhanced T1W image demonstrates variable enhancement patterns ranging from mild (short arrow), moderate (arrow), to intense (dashed arrow).

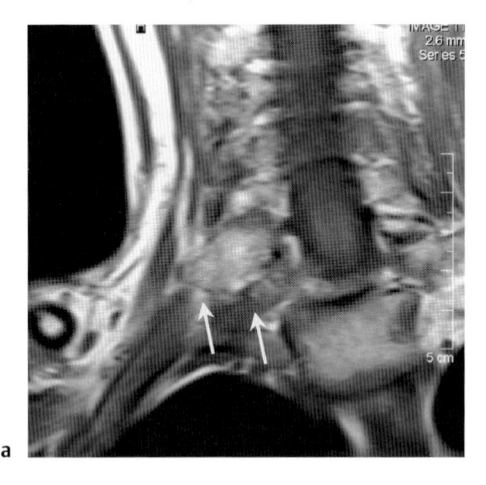

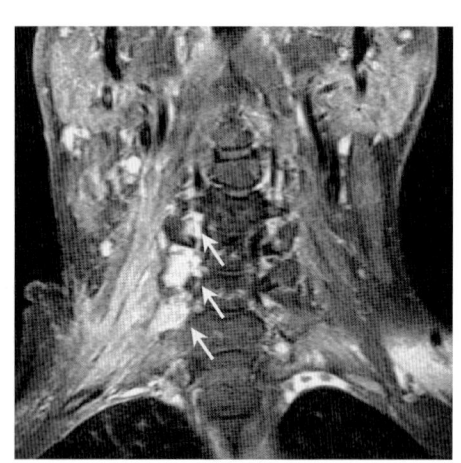

Fig. 12.38 Malignant peripheral nerve sheath tumor (MPNST) in a young male patient without neurofibromatosis type 1. The patient was complaining of pain as well as motor and sensory deficits at the level of C7. a Coronal contrast-enhanced T1W MR image shows a fusiform homogeneously enhancing tumor (arrows) involving the C7 and C8 nerve root and the middle trunk of the brachial plexus on the right. MR imaging suggested the diagnosis of a neurogenic tumor of the brachial plexus. Surgery revealed a MPNST. b Coronal contrast-enhanced fat-suppressed T1W MR image obtained one year after surgery and radiation therapy reveals tumor recurrence at the levels C6–C8 (arrows). Repeat surgery confirmed tumor recurrence. Nine months later the patient showed no local tumor recurrence but he developed multiple lung metastases (not shown).

40% of patients with NF1 include an enlarged spinal canal, scalloping of vertebral bodies, and enlarged intervertebral foramina. The bony abnormalities are caused by meningoceles or by neurofibromas. Malignant degeneration or de novo development of malignant peripheral nerve sheath tumors is seen in 2–6% of cases with NF1.[72] Plexiform neurofibromas manifest as early as early childhood. They are diffuse lesions that typically follow long segments of nerve bundles and invade adjacent muscles and subcutaneous fat.

On CT, solitary neurofibromas may have areas of low attenuation almost approaching the appearance of a cyst. On MRI, solitary neurofibromas have a low signal intensity on T1-weighted MR images, a high signal intensity on T2-weighted MR images, and variable enhancement (Fig. 12.36). Localized neurofibromas in NF1 have similar imaging characteristics to solitary neurofibromas. However, they are often bilateral and follow the cervical nerve roots (Fig. 12.37).

On both CT and MRI, plexiform neurofibromas display a characteristic target appearance. On CT, multiple tumor nodules show a central high-attenuation area that is surrounded by a low-attenuation rim. On T2-weighted MR images, a central low signal intensity area is surrounded by a peripheral high-signal area.[151] This characteristic appearance of plexiform neurofibroma on CT and MRI may be explained by the histological appearance. In plexiform neurofibromas, a central fibrous component is surrounded by peripheral myxomatous tissue.

Malignant Peripheral Nerve Sheath Tumors

Malignant peripheral nerve sheath tumors (MPNST) is the new name adopted by the World Health Organization to unify the previously designated entities of malignant schwannoma, neurofibrosarcoma, and neurogenic sarcoma.[72] These tumors arise de novo (Fig. 12.38) or from malignant transformation of a plexiform neurofibroma. As many as 11% of MPNST are induced by radiation therapy (see below). Most tumors are seen between 30 and 50 years of age, but in a younger age group in patients with NF1.[42] Clinically, the patients complain of a mass that may be painful and they may have motor and sensory deficits. Sudden painful enlargement of a neurofibroma in NF1 should suggest malignant transformation and necessitates biopsy.[150] The imaging findings in MPNST are nonspecific and include a large fusiform and invasive tumor that spreads along nerve trunks and sometimes presents with areas of necrosis and hemorrhage. Prognosis of MNST is affected by a variety of factors, such as age, location of the tumor, margins at initial surgery, and the presence of NF1.[42, 150]

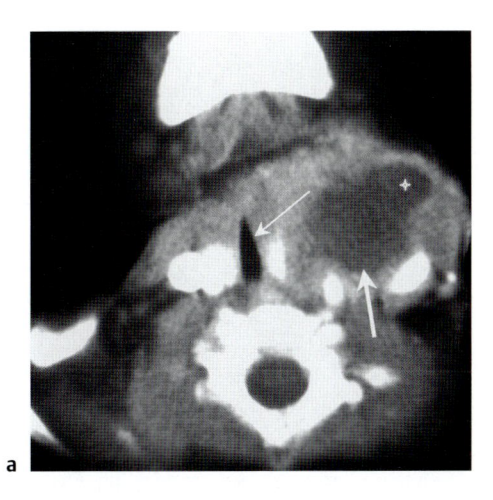

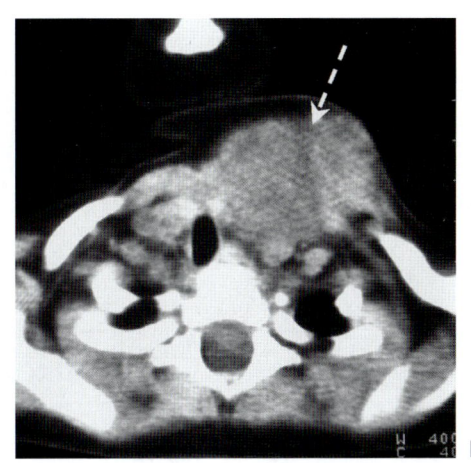

Fig. 12.39 Primary cervical neuroblastoma. Characteristic aspect on CT. Contrast-enhanced CT images (**a** and **b**) obtained in a 2-year-old girl with Horner syndrome and a large palpable cervical mass. A heterogeneous lesion with cystic, necrotic areas (arrow), and solid portions (dashed arrow) is seen on the left. Note invasion of the sternocleidomastoid muscle and thyroid gland and displacement and narrowing of the airway (thin arrow in **a**).

Primitive Neural Tumors

Primitive neural tumors (PNET) arise from primordial neural crest cells that migrate from the developing spinal cord to the sympathetic ganglia, adrenal medulla, or other sites. PNET include neuroblastoma, ganglioneuroblastoma, and ganglioneuroma.

Neuroblastoma typically occurs in children under the age of 5 years. The tumor arises from the sympathetic ganglia along the spinal column. Most neuroblastomas arise in the abdomen. Primary cervical neuroblastoma is rare, with an incidence of 2% (Fig. 12.39). Most neuroblastoma masses seen in the neck are metastases from abdominal neuroblastoma. Primary or metastatic neuroblastoma in the neck very often presents with large masses that encroach on the pharynx and larynx and that may involve cranial nerves IX to XII or the sympathetic ganglia producing dysphagia and dyspnea, and Horner syndrome, respectively. The CT findings are variable and include homogeneous tumors with or without calcifications or heterogeneous lesions with areas of necrosis (Fig. 12.39). On T2-weighted MR images, neuroblastomas display a moderately increased signal intensity and, after injection of contrast material, intense enhancement may be seen. Radionuclide metaiodobenzylguanidine scintigraphy has been used for the assessment of primary and metastatic disease. The sensitivity for the detection of primary neuroblastoma is 94% and the sensitivity for the detection of neuroblastoma metastases is 83%.[151] The prognosis of patients with neuroblastoma depends on age at initial presentation, stage, lymph node metastases, and amplification of the *MYCN* oncogene.

Ganglioneuroma is the fully matured benign counterpart of neuroblastoma. Most ganglioneuromas occur in children older than 10 years of age in the mediastinum and retroperitoneum. Only a minority of cases are seen as paraspinal masses in the neck. Ganglioneuromas present as very large, well-circumscribed tumors that may contain calcifications in up to one-third of cases.

Ganglioneuroblastoma is composed of neuroblastoma cells surrounded by a ganglioneuromatous stroma. The imaging features are nonspecific.

Paraganglioma

Nonchromaffin paragangliomas (also called chemodectomas or glomus complex tumors) arise from neural crest cell derivatives within vessel walls. These glomus body tissues are responsive to changes in pH and blood oxygen and carbon dioxide tensions. In the extracranial head and neck, paragangliomas may arise in the middle ear cavity (glomus tympanicum), in the jugular bulb region (glomus jugulare), in the ganglion nodosum region and cervical portion of the vagus nerve (glomus vagale), and at the carotid bifurcation (carotid body tumor).[11,54,83] In the infrahyoid neck, paragangliomas most commonly occur in the carotid body, which is situated in the carotid bifurcation.[83] Occasionally, a large glomus vagale tumor may extend into the infrahyoid neck and present as a carotid space lesion. Carotid body tumors may affect all age groups but they typically present in women, in the fourth decade of life, and may be multiple in as many as 30% of patients with a family history of paraganglioma. Living in areas of high altitude, such as Peru, Mexico, or Colorado, predisposes to the formation of carotid body tumors. Most head and neck paragangliomas display no functional activity, although functioning active glomus tumors have been reported. Glomus tumors have been reported in association with medullary carcinoma of the thyroid, in familial multiple endocrine neoplasia (MEN) syndromes (especially MEN type I, Table 12.9), in patients with neu-

Table 12.9 Multiple endocrine neoplasia syndromes

Features	MEN I	MEN IIA	MEN IIB
Chromosomal linkage	Chromosome 11	Chromosome 10	Unknown
Thyroid	Goiter Adenoma Thyroiditis	Medullary carcinoma	Medullary carcinoma
Parathyroid	Hyperplasia, adenoma	Hyperplasia	Abnormality very rare
Pheochromocytoma	No	Yes	Yes
Adrenal cortex	Adenoma or carcinoma Glucagonoma VIPoma Carcinoid Zollinger–Ellison syndrome		
Pituitary gland	Adenoma	No	No
Pancreas	Islet cell adenoma Insulinoma Gastrinoma	No	No
Other manifestations	Paraganglioma	No	Café au lait spots Marfanoid facies Mucocutaneous neuromas

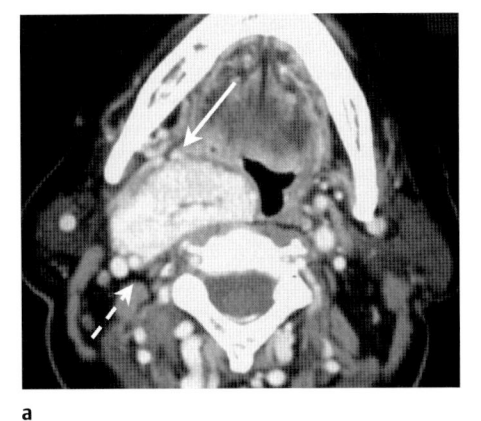

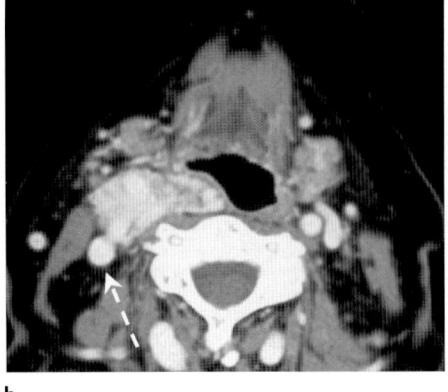

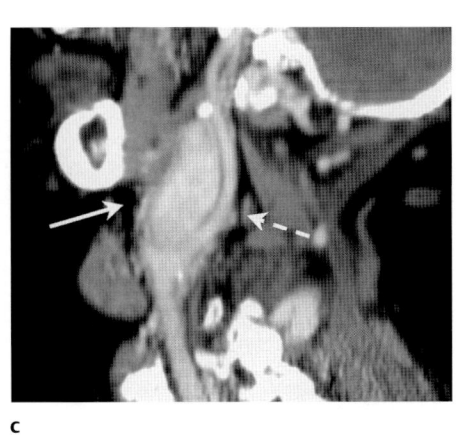

Fig. 12.40 Carotid body paraganglioma. Characteristic CT appearance. **a, b** Contrast-enhanced axial images at the level of the oropharynx and **c** parasagittal 2D reconstruction from a multislice volumetric data set show a hypervascular mass that displaces the external carotid artery anteriorly (arrow) and the internal carotid artery and the internal jugular vein posteriorly (dashed arrows). Note the characteristic splaying of the carotid bifurcation, best appreciated on the 2D parasagittal reconstruction. Arrow in **c** points at the external carotid artery; dashed arrow in **c** points at the internal carotid artery.

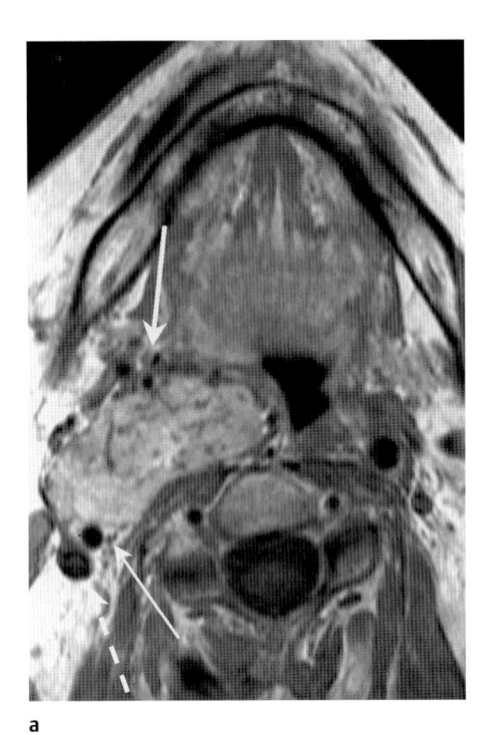

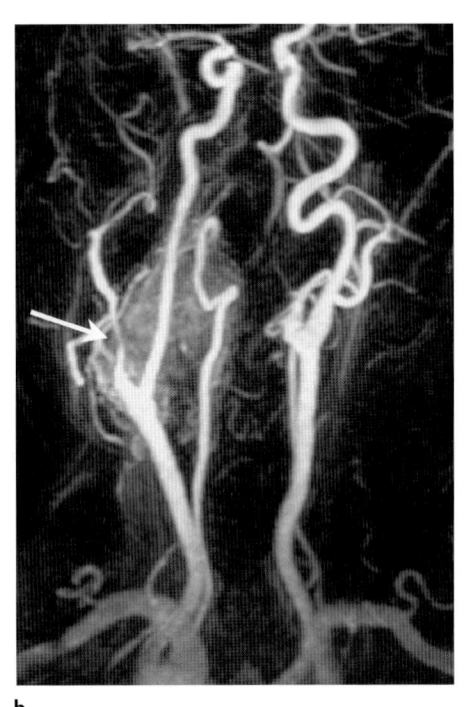

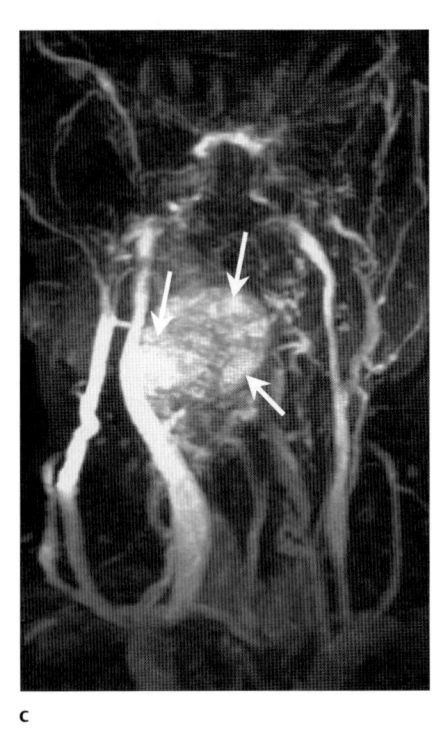

Fig. 12.41 Carotid body paraganglioma. Characteristic MRI and MR angiography appearance. **a** Axial contrast-enhanced T1W image in an elderly woman with a palpable pulsatile mass at the level of the hyoid bone shows a hypervascular mass with characteristic serpiginous flow voids and strong contrast material enhancement. The external carotid artery is displaced anterolaterally (arrow), the internal carotid artery (thin arrow) and the internal jugular vein (dashed arrow) are displaced posterolaterally. **b, c** MR angiography obtained after injection of contrast material: **b** arterial phase and **c** venous phase. The tumor shows early enhancement, which is seen as a hypervascular blush on **b** (note for comparison Fig. 12.33d obtained in a schwannoma). There is also splaying of the carotid bifurcation and narrowing of the external carotid artery (arrow). In the venous phase, large venous lakes are seen with pooling of contrast material (arrows).

rofibromatosis, and in patients with multiple mucocutaneous neuromas. Paragangliomas may metastasize or they may show an aggressive growth pattern causing disabling symptoms and even death by slow, progressive encroachment on vital structures. As many as 10% of all carotid body tumors are malignant. Regional lymph node metastases and metastases to the lung, liver, heart, kidney, and brain have been described.

On contrast-enhanced CT images, paragangliomas appear as highly enhancing lesions found medial to the sternocleidomastoid muscle[11,83,115] (Fig. 12.40). They typically display multiple curvilinear signal voids on both T1- and T2-weighted images (Fig. 12.41). The conspicuity of these signal void areas increases with tumor size and increasing vessel diameter. This MR appearance is not pathognomonic for paragangliomas and it has been reported in other hypervascular lesions, i.e., vascular malformations, hemangiomas, and metastases from renal cell carcinoma.[115] The key to the radiological diagnosis of carotid body paraganglioma is splaying of the proximal internal and external carotid arteries around the mass at the carotid bifurcation (Figs. 12.40, 12.41). Histological analysis of paragangliomas reveals nonencapsulated lesions with ill-defined margins. Chief cells arranged in clusters and round cell nests (*Zellballen*) are surrounded by a delicate stroma containing numerous vascular channels. Invasion of the adventitia of the carotid wall is common (Fig. 12.42). Immunohistochemical studies typically show enolase and neurofilament protein within the chief cells of most

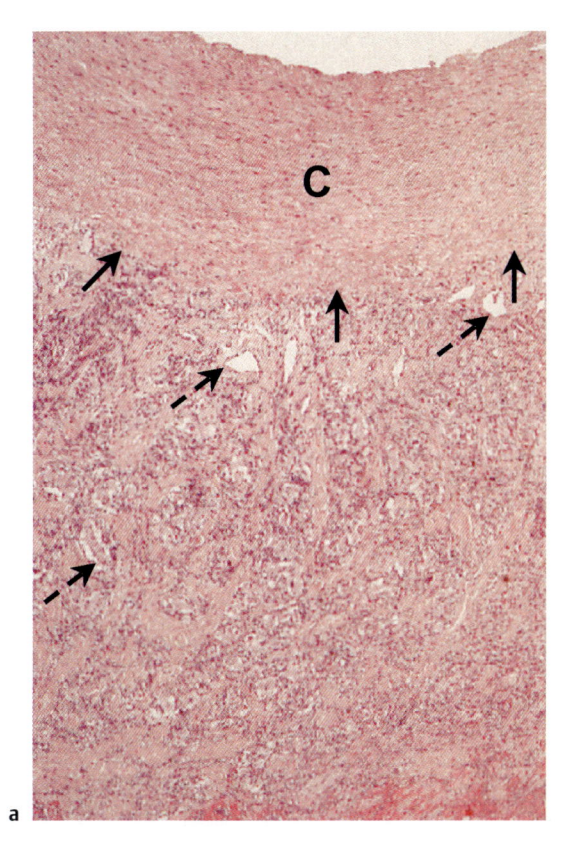

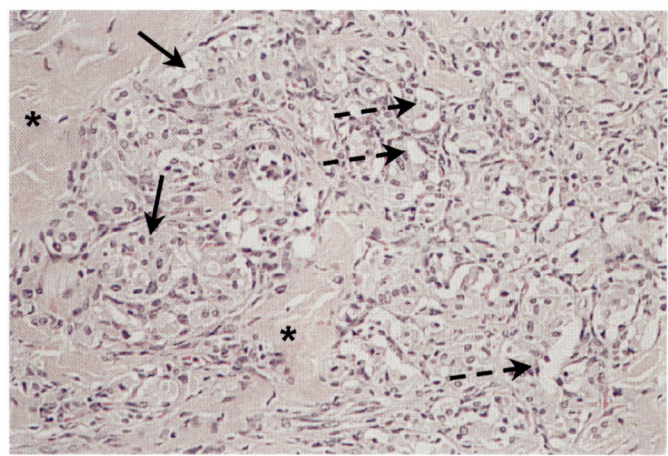

Fig. 12.42 Paraganglioma. Histological appearance. **a** Photomicrograph of a carotid body tumor (hematoxylin–eosin stain) demonstrates its characteristic location relative to the carotid wall (C). The adventitia of the carotid wall (arrows) is invaded by the nonencapsulated tumor mass. Note numerous vascular channels (dashed arrows). **b** Detail from **a** seen at a higher magnification shows the characteristic Zellballen (arrows), a collagen-rich stroma (asterisks), and numerous vascular channels (dashed arrows).

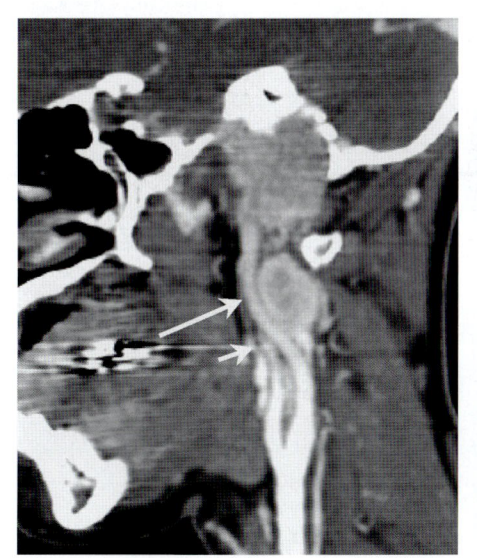

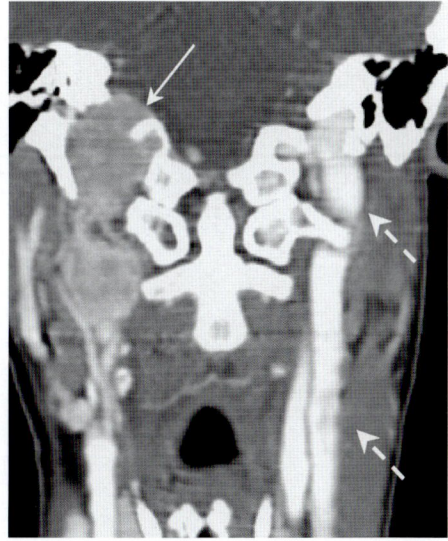

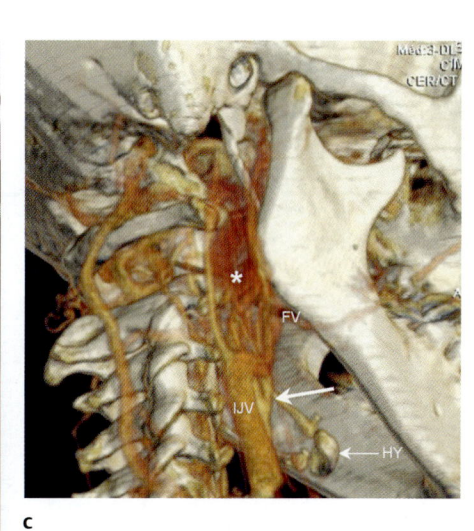

Fig. 12.43 Glomus jugulare tumor in a young female patient presenting with a palpable mass below the angle of the mandible. The patient was otherwise asymptomatic. **a** Parasagittal and **b** coronal 2D reconstructions from a multidetector volumetric data set show a hypervascular carotid space lesion displacing the internal carotid artery (long arrow) and the external carotid artery (short arrow) anteriorly. There is invasion of the internal jugular vein and foramen jugulare (thin arrow). Note the normal appearance of the left internal jugular vein (dashed arrows). **c** 3D vascular reconstruction shows the hypervascular tumor mass (asterisk) located posteriorly to the internal and external carotid arteries. The carotid bifurcation is normal (arrow). IJV = internal jugular vein in its inferior portion; FV = facial vein; HY = hyoid bone.

head and neck paragangliomas as well as a variety of other polypeptides and hormones, such as serotonin, vasopressin, ACTH, and calcitonin.[83]

Both the glomus vagale and glomus jugulare tumors arise around the vagus nerve dorsal to the internal carotid artery. They tend to displace the internal carotid artery and the external carotid artery anteriorly; however, there is no splaying of the carotid bifurcation as in glomus caroticum tumors (Fig. 12.43).

Paragangliomas have to be differentiated from other hypervascular lesions, such as metastases from renal cell carcinoma, thyroid cancer, and melanoma, or amyloid deposition (Fig. 12.44).

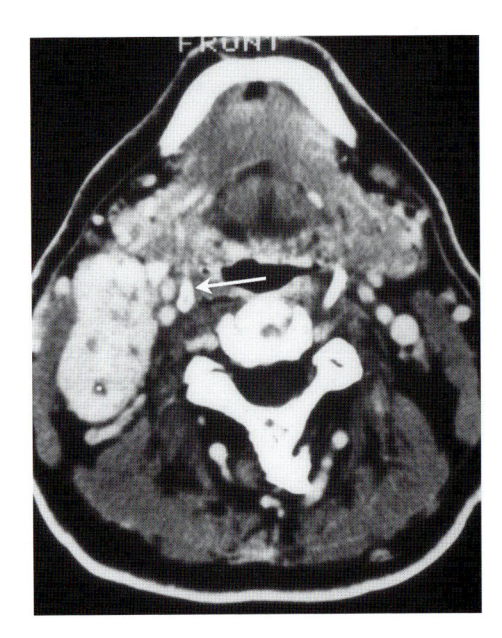

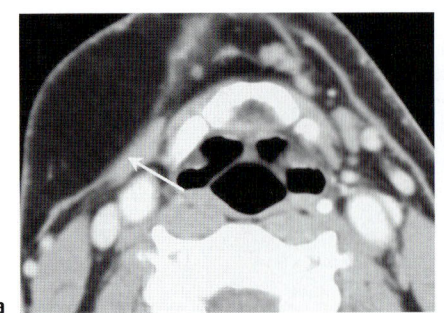

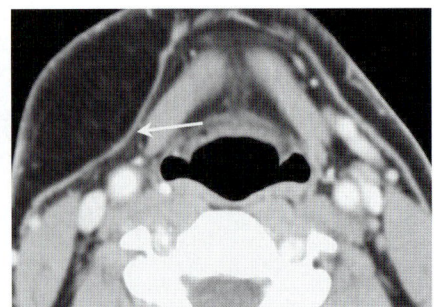

Fig. 12.45 Lipoma. Characteristic CT appearance. Axial contrast-enhanced images at the level of the hyoid bone (**a**) and slightly below it (**b**) show a subcutaneous mass with attenuation values suggesting a lipoma. Note medial displacement of the platysma muscle (arrows). Surgery revealed encapsulated lipoma.

◁ **Fig. 12.44** Amyloidosis. Differential diagnosis of hypervascular neck masses. Contrast-enhanced CT obtained in a patient with a palpable mass on the right shows a hypervascular tumor located laterally and posteriorly to the neurovascular bundle, which is displaced medially (arrow). The diagnosis of a hypervascular lymph node metastasis was suggested radiologically. Surgery revealed amyloid deposition in internal jugular lymph nodes (level II).

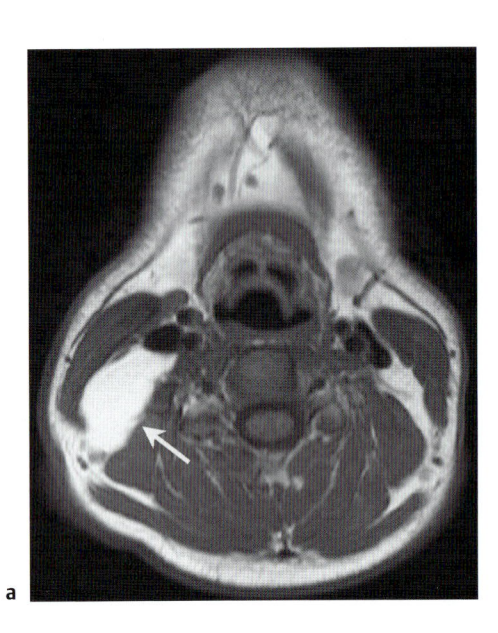

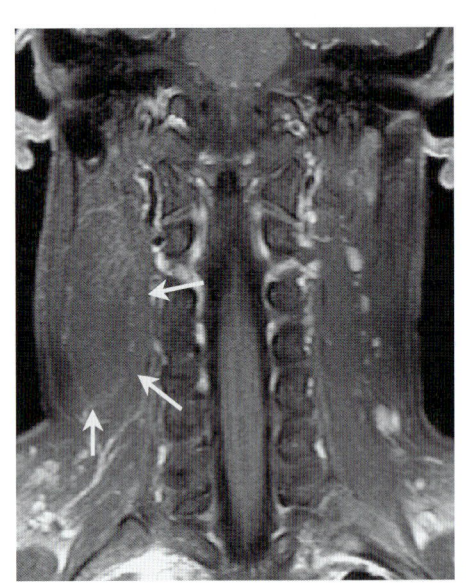

Fig. 12.46 Lipoma. Characteristic MRI appearance. **a** T1W MR axial image shows a hyperintense mass located within the posterior cervical space (arrow). **b** Contrast-enhanced, fat-suppressed coronal MR image shows that the mass is composed of adipose tissue and that it does not enhance (arrows), therefore suggesting the diagnosis of a lipoma. Surgery confirmed the findings.

Lipomatous Neoplasms

Lipoma

Although **lipomas** are the most common tumors of mesenchymal origin in the body, only 13% arise in the extracranial head and neck. Most head and neck lipomas are located subcutaneously (superficial to the superficial layer of the deep cervical fascia) and in the posterior cervical triangle. In rare instances, they may arise in the retropharyngeal space or they may insinuate around the common carotid artery and internal jugular vein. Subcutaneous tumors are most often asymptomatic. They may grow slowly over several years or they may remain stable over time. On palpation, superficial lipomas are usually soft and can therefore be distinguished from other cervical masses. Lipomas arising in the deep spaces of the neck may present with symptoms related to mass effect on the pharynx, larynx, or esophagus, such as dysphagia, snoring, sleep apnea syndrome, and dyspnea. Deep lipomas are more difficult to detect clinically and they are more difficult to resect than superficial lipomas. Therefore, the recurrence rate in deep space lesions is higher. Histologically, lipoma is composed of mature adipose tissue arranged in lobules, separated by fibrous tissue septa. Most tumors are well-circumscribed and encapsulated, although infiltrating nonencapsulated lipomas have been reported.

The radiological diagnosis of lipoma is straightforward. Both CT and MRI provide a definitive diagnosis in virtually all cases (Figs. 12.**45**, 12.**46**). The typical CT characteristics are of a homogeneous and nonenhancing lesion with attenuation values from –65 to –125 HU (Fig. 12.**45**). On MRI, lipoma has the same signal intensity as subcutaneous fat on all pulse sequences (hyperintense on T1-weighted images, a decrease in intensity on T2-weighted images, and very low intensity on fat-suppressed T1-weighted images (Fig. 12.**46**). As in other parts of the body, if portions of the lipoma have the attenuation value or signal intensity characteristics of soft tissue on CT or MRI, and if contrast enhancement is observed within these strands of connective tissue, the diagnosis of a liposarcoma should be considered.

Multiple Symmetric Lipomatosis (Madelung Disease)

Multiple symmetric lipomatosis (MSL), also known as Launois–Bensaude syndrome or Madelung disease, is a rare disorder predominantly seen in middle-aged men. However, the disease has

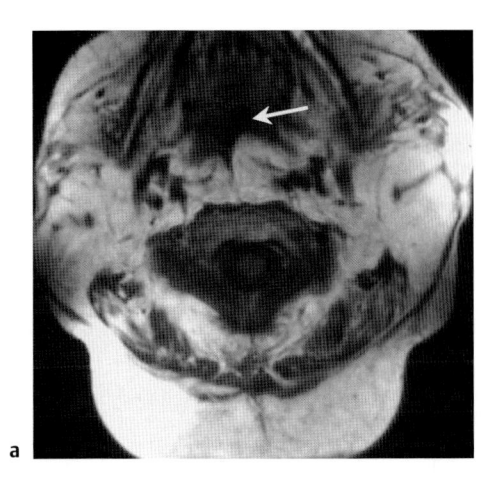

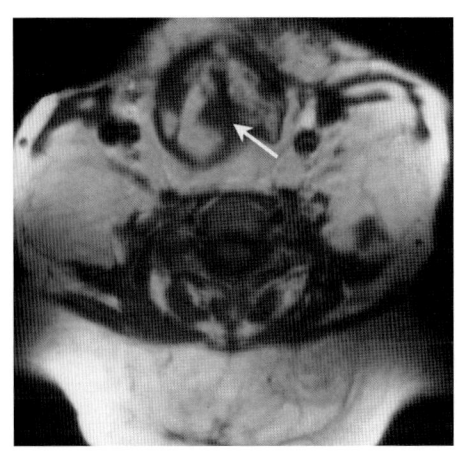

Fig. 12.**47** Madelung disease. Characteristic MRI appearance. Middle-aged man with Madelung disease complaining of severe dyspnea and dysphagia. The MR examination was performed prior to surgical debulking. T1W images at the level of the oropharynx (**a**) and larynx (**b**) show unencapsulated fat masses distributed throughout all neck spaces, leading to major narrowing of the pharynx and larynx (arrows).

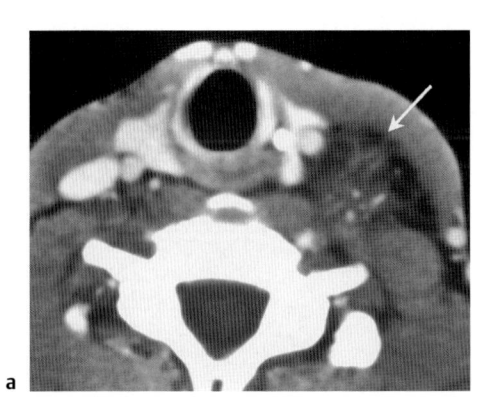

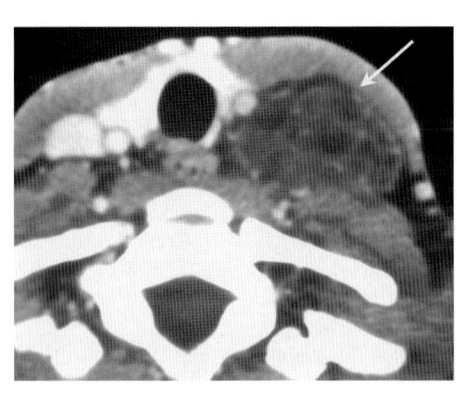

Fig. 12.**48** Liposarcoma of the neck. Characteristic CT appearance. **a**, **b** Contrast-enhanced CT images at the level of the infrahyoid neck obtained in an elderly man show a mass with low attenuation values and with some strands of enhancing tissue (arrows). The tumor is not encapsulated in its superior portion (**a**). Note medial displacement of the internal jugular vein and common carotid artery. Surgery revealed low-grade liposarcoma.

also been described in children. The disorder is characterized by multiple symmetrical deposits of unencapsulated fat masses distributed around the neck, shoulders, and other parts of the trunk, often associated with nervous system abnormalities.[1,3,76] Recently, it has been suggested that MSL may be a neurometabolic disorder with heterogeneous clinical expression whose pathogenesis is still unknown. However, a close relationship to alcoholism, metabolic disturbances, and malignant tumors has been observed.[1,3,76,160] Patients usually complain of their cosmetic appearance, but treatment can be given for decreased neck motion and/or aerodigestive problems. The only effective therapy in cases of dyspnea and dysphagia is surgical debulking, with liposuction reserved for smaller lesions. A standard facelift pattern can be used for skin incisions and removal, with good cosmetic results.

Sectional imaging is used to document the distribution of excess fat in the neck in patients with Madelung disease (Fig. 12.**47**). In addition, imaging is used to assess the course of the major vessels within the fat, the presence of tracheal compression, and nonlipomatous lesions prior to surgery. As a preoperative investigative tool for Madelung disease, both MRI and CT provide the surgeon with adequate information, sonography being less helpful.[3]

Liposarcoma

Liposarcomas are very rare in the head and neck, constituting approximately 2% of all head and neck soft-tissue sarcomas.[95] Unlike ordinary lipomas, liposarcomas are usually deep to the superficial fascia, and they typically involve the visceral, retropharyngeal, and parapharyngeal spaces.[103] Liposarcomas of the neck show no sex predilection and they typically occur in the fifth and sixth decades. They originate de novo from lipoblasts around the fascial planes and not from preexisting lipomas. Histologically, liposarcomas can be subdivided into four types: well-differentiated and myxoid tumors with a good prognosis and pleomorphic and round-cell lesions with a poor prognosis. Wide surgical excision is mandatory. There is some controversy regarding nomenclature and the distinction between atypical lipoma and well-differentiated liposarcoma. These two entities are in fact histologically identical.

Imaging findings in liposarcomas depend upon histological grade. On CT, liposarcomas are inhomogeneous lesions with attenuation values above those of subcutaneous fat. They typically display a mix of fat and soft-tissue elements[43] (Fig. 12.**48**). Very often, unsharp, infiltrating borders are seen, as well as areas of inhomogeneous patchy contrast enhancement. On T1-weighted images, well-differentiated liposarcomas appear as primarily fatty lesions but with signal intensities lower than that of the subcutaneous fat. On fat-saturated, contrast-enhanced images, patchy, inhomogeneous enhancement may be seen. Based on a recent study, it has been suggested that a lesion that has predominantly a fat signal (or fat attenuation value) is, in all probability, an ordinary lipoma. Lesions with less fat, but still mostly fatty, may be either lipoma or well-differentiated liposarcoma. In the absence of a fat signal (or fat-attenuation value), liposarcoma or lipoma cannot be differentiated from other soft-tissue tumors.[43]

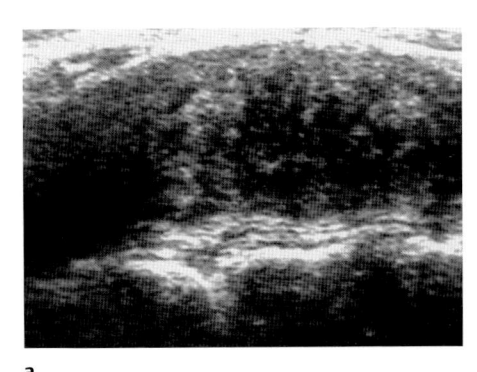

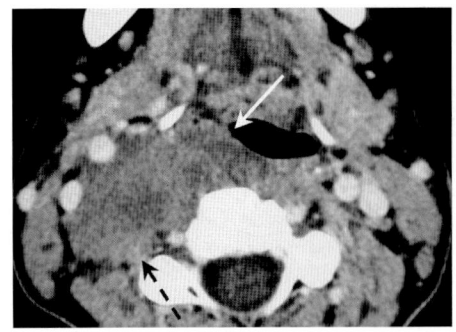

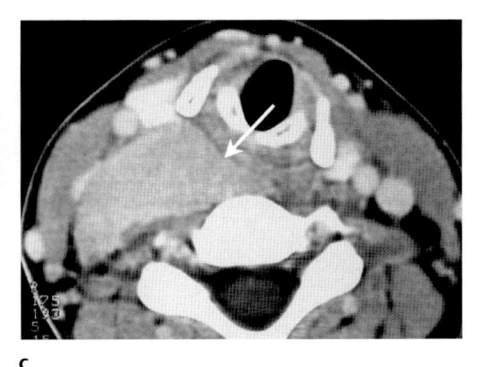

Fig. 12.**49** Aggressive fibromatosis of the neck. **a** US examination of the neck shows a well-delineated hypoechoic mass with some internal echoes. The aspect is nonspecific. **b, c** Contrast-enhanced CT images at the level of the oropharynx (**b**) and larynx (**c**) show a homogeneous tumor mass located mainly in the posterior cervical space. Some parts of the tumor display only minor enhancement (**b**), while other parts display moderate enhancement (**c**). The mass displaces the common carotid artery and internal jugular vein anteriorly. It invades the retropharyngeal space (arrows) and the prevertebral space (dashed arrow). Surgery revealed aggressive fibromatosis. The mass most probably arose from the prevertebral fascia. Courtesy of Dr. Fernando Torrhina and Dr. David Coutinho (Imagens Medicas Integradas, Lisbon, Portugal).

Fibrous Neoplasms

Aggressive Fibromatosis

Aggressive fibromatosis, also called extra-abdominal desmoid tumor, differentiated fibrosarcoma, or fibrosarcoma-like fibromatosis, is a rare, histologically benign but locally aggressive tumor frequently seen in children and young adults.[51] Fibromatosis may occur as a solitary lesion or it may be associated with Gardner syndrome.[113] Gardner syndrome is an autosomal dominant disorder characterized by adenomatous polyps in the colon with a potential for malignant transformation that is virtually 100%. Extracolonic manifestations include biliary involvement, thyroid carcinoma, skeletal and dental manifestations, and mesenteric fibromatosis.[113]

Aggressive fibromatosis lesions arise from the fascial and musculoaponeurotic tissues and are locally infiltrative lesions, resulting in a high rate of local recurrence (20–70%) following surgical resection. They have no metastasizing potential, however. Most fibromatosis lesions are seen in the extremities, and the incidence in the head and neck is estimated at about 7–27%.[107] Most tumors in the neck are located in the supraclavicular fossa or in the muscles. Patients most commonly complain of a painless mass or neurological symptoms including pain or neurological deficit. Complete surgical extirpation is the treatment of choice for primary and recurrent desmoid tumors, although fibromatosis lesions present difficult locoregional control. The location and extent of the tumor, as well as the potential for significant morbidity and mortality, dictate the most appropriate therapeutic option. During surgery, the accessory or phrenic nerve, parts of the brachial plexus, or bony structures may have to be resected, resulting in persistent neurological or functional deficits.[62] Radiotherapy is indicated in incompletely excised or recurrent tumors. Radiation is seldom recommended as a primary treatment.

Histologically, aggressive fibromatosis is composed of well-differentiated, highly cellular fibrous tissue. Aggressive fibromatosis lesions enhance slightly on CT, and are often inseparable from adjacent muscles (Fig. 12.**49**). On MRI, aggressive fibromatosis has variable signal intensity on T1- and T2-weighted images and the contrast enhancement pattern ranges from none, through inhomogeneous, to intense homogeneous enhancement.[70] Neither the signal intensity nor the pattern of contrast enhancement has any significant relationship to the biological behavior of the tumor. Margins may be sharply defined or ill-defined (Fig. 12.**49**).

Fibrosarcoma

Fibrosarcoma is a rare lesion in the head and neck. The most common sites are the mandible, maxilla, face, infrahyoid neck, and larynx. Unlike aggressive fibromatosis, fibrosarcoma has the potential for metastasis (more than 60% of cases). The 5-year survival rate is 39–54%. Histologically, fibrosarcoma differs from aggressive fibromatosis by the presence of cellular atypia and relative paucity of collagen. The imaging findings are nonspecific.

Neoplasms of Fibrohistiocytic and Skeletal Muscle Origin

Malignant Fibrous Histiocytoma

Fibrohistiocytic neoplasms include benign fibrous histiocytoma and malignant fibrous histiocytoma. Malignant fibrous histiocytoma is the most common soft-tissue sarcoma and the most common radiation-induced sarcoma in adults[14, 19, 55] (see below). In the infrahyoid neck, the tumor is usually circumscribed and is found within muscle or along fasciae. The imaging findings are nonspecific.

Rhabdomyoma and Rhabdomyosarcoma

Neoplasms of skeletal muscle origin include rhabdomyoma and rhabdomyosarcoma. **Rhabdomyoma** is an uncommon benign lesion, with the majority of cases arising from cardiac muscle, where it is associated with tuberous sclerosis. While cardiac rhabdomyomas are considered to be hamartomatous lesions, extracardiac rhabdomyomas are considered neoplastic. Seventy to ninety percent of extracardiac rhabdomyomas are found in the head and neck region, usually within the upper aerodigestive tract or—less frequently—within the posterior triangle, carotid space, parapharyngeal space or within muscle tissue[25, 29] Men are most commonly affected. In general, there are no significant symptoms as the tumor grows very slowly. A multilocular occurrence in the head and neck, although rare, has been reported.[152, 159] The treatment of choice is surgery. Because local recurrence is common, even after a period as long as 35 years, ample excision is mandatory. The CT and MR imaging findings are nonspecific (see Chapter 8).

Rhabdomyosarcoma is the most common soft-tissue sarcoma in children. Nearly 40% of all rhabdomyosarcomas are seen in the head and neck. The most common form encountered in the head and neck is embryonal rhabdomyosarcoma. The most common sites are the orbit, nasopharynx, middle ear, and nasal cavity

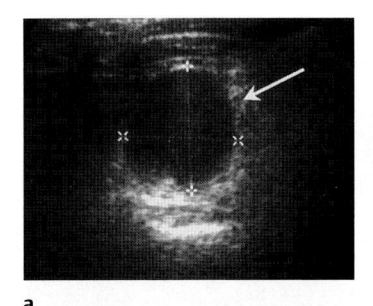

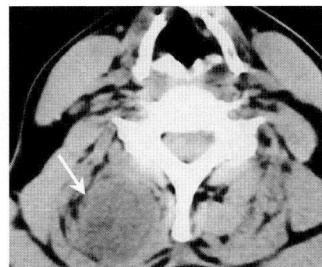

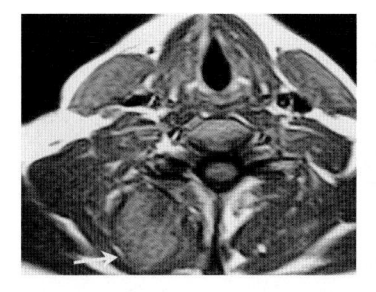

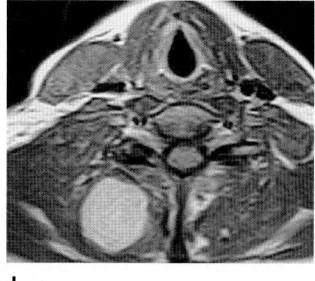

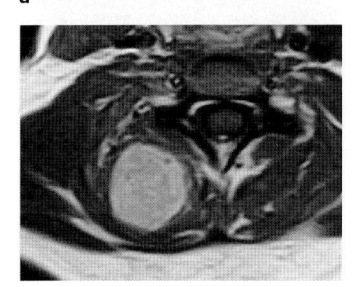

Fig. 12.**50** Pleomorphic hyalinizing angiectatic tumor. **a** US examination of the neck demonstrates a well-delineated, hopoechoic tumor (arrow) located in the paraspinal musculature. **b** Unenhanced CT of the neck shows that the tumor (arrow) has a similar attenuation value to that of muscle. **c** T1W MR image at the glottic level shows that the tumor is well-delineated and that it has a higher signal intensity than normal muscle. The tumor is located within the paraspinal musculature and the splenius muscle is displaced posteriorly (arrow). **d** T2W FSE MR image shows a high signal intensity of the tumor mass. **e** Contrast-enhanced T1W MR image shows homogeneous strong enhancement. The diagnosis of a muscular or fibrohistiocytic tumor was suggested on the basis of imaging findings. Histology revealed a very rare pleomorphic hyalinizing angiectatic tumor. Courtesy of Dr. Fernando Torrhina and Dr. David Coutinho (Imagens Medicas Integradas, Lisbon, Portugal).

(see Chapters 2, 3, and 7). Rhabdomyosarcomas are only rarely seen in the infrahyoid neck. Although the imaging features are nonspecific, CT and MRI most often show an aggressive tumor with bone invasion, perineural spread, and marked contrast enhancement. Treatment consists of chemotherapy and surgery with or without radiotherapy.[105]

Pleomorphic Hyalinizing Angiectatic Tumor

Pleomorphic hyalinizing angiectatic tumor (PHAT) is a rare, recently recognized, low-grade sarcoma most probably derived from stromal fibroblasts.[127] PHAT occurs almost exclusively in adults between 30 and 85 years of age. It is seen in the subcutaneous soft tissues of the lower and upper limbs and trunk and only very rarely in the neck (Fig. 12.**50**). Local recurrences may occur after several years, but distant metastases have not been described so far. Histologically, the tumor is well-circumscribed by a thin fibrous capsule. Variously sized ectatic vessels, which tend to be distributed in clusters, are scattered throughout the lesion. The tumors are composed of plump, spindled, and rounded pleomorphic cells that are arranged in sheets between the ectatic blood vessels.[127] On CT and MRI, the lesions are well-delineated and homogeneous and marked contrast-material enhancement is seen (Fig. 12.**50**).

■ Thyroid and Parathyroid Gland Masses

Thyroid Nodules

Thyroid nodules are common and comprise adenomas, cysts, focal thyroiditis, multinodular goiter, and malignant tumors. Thyroid nodules are estimated to occur in 4–8% of the adult population[89,90] when palpable nodules are involved. The rate reaches values of 20–30% when nonpalpable nodules, detected by means of US, are included[117] Finally, thyroid nodules are seen in as many as 50% of adults over 50 years of age. Thyroid nodules may be either single (one-third) or multiple (two-thirds). The differentiation of a gland with a single nodule from a gland with multiple nodules is essential and can be done with US. The incidence of malignancy in a single nodule is 10–15%, and the incidence of malignancy in a multinodular goiter is 4–7.5%.[89,90] On US, 70% of thyroid nodules are solid, 19% are cystic, and 11% are mixed.[8,9]

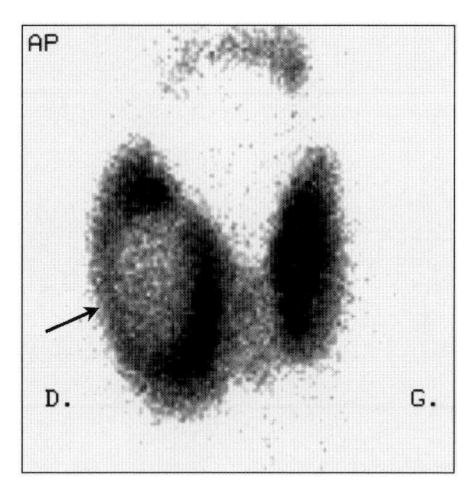

Fig. 12.**51** Anteroposterior view of a ^{99m}Tc-pertechnetate scan shows an area of diminished uptake (cold nodule) in the right thyroid lobe (arrow). US-guided fine-needle aspiration biopsy revealed papillary carcinoma.

Carcinomas are demonstrated in 20% of solid nodules, 12% of mixed lesions, and 7% of cystic lesions.[8,9] It is generally accepted that a ^{99m}Tc-pertechnetate-visualized "hot" thyroid nodule is almost invariably a benign lesion, while the probability of malignancy varies from 10% to 25% in ^{99m}Tc-pertechnetate-visualized "cold" nodules (Fig. 12.**51**). Therefore, fine-needle aspiration biopsy (FNAB) or large-needle aspiration biopsy with or without US guidance is always required to rule out malignancy. FNAB has been found to be a safe and inexpensive procedure, and in several clinical studies this technique has shown high diagnostic accuracy.[99]

Adenoma

Adenomas are benign thyroid neoplasms that may occur in all age groups. They are more common in women than men. Adenomas are usually solitary and are smaller than 3 cm in diameter. Follicular adenomas are composed of glandular epithelium, which is encapsulated by a fibrous stroma. They often display degenerative changes, such as cyst formation, hemorrhage, fibrosis, or calcification.[8,9,84] On CT and MRI, adenomas are either solid and enhancing or reveal cystic degeneration and calcification. On US, differentiation between cystic and solid forms is

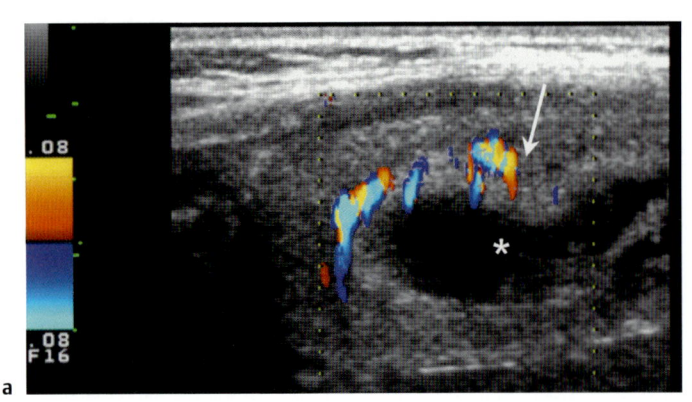

Fig. 12.**52** Follicular adenoma. Cystic versus solid form as seen on US. **a** Color Doppler US image obtained in a young female patient shows a single thyroid nodule within an otherwise normal thyroid gland. The nodule has a central cystic area (asterisk) and a peripheral perfusion pattern. Surgery revealed follicular adenoma. **b** Color Doppler US image obtained in a different patient with hyperthyroidism reveals a single hypoechoic, well-delineated mass (arrow) located within an otherwise normal thyroid gland. Note increased central perfusion. Surgery revealed follicular adenoma.

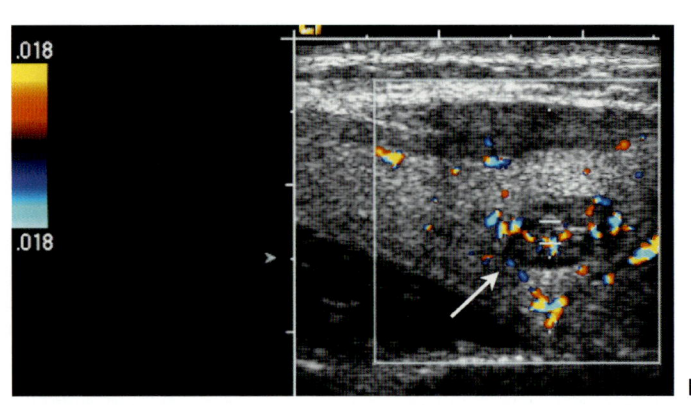

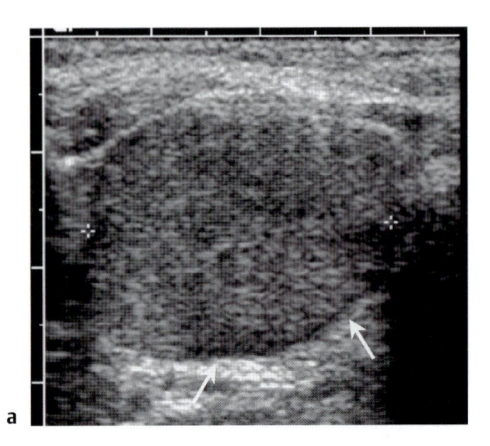

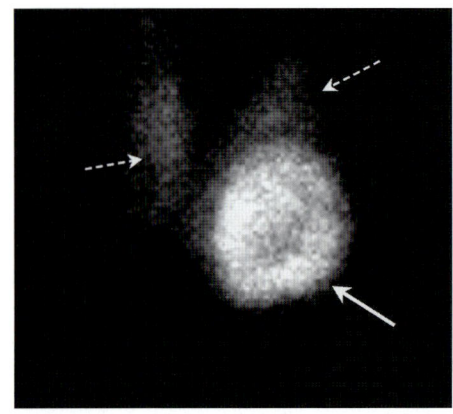

Fig. 12.**53** Follicular adenoma. Characteristic US and scintigraphic appearance. **a** US examination of the thyroid gland in an elderly woman shows a single, homogeneous slightly hypoechoic mass surrounded by a hypoechoic rim (arrow). On Doppler US (not shown) the vascularization pattern was similar to that shown in Fig. 12.**52 b**. **b** Iodine-123 scan (anteroposterior view) obtained in the same patient demonstrates a solitary, radiotracer-avid lesion (hot nodule) in the left lobe of the thyroid gland (arrow). The nodule appears to suppress the remaining right and left lobes (dashed arrows).

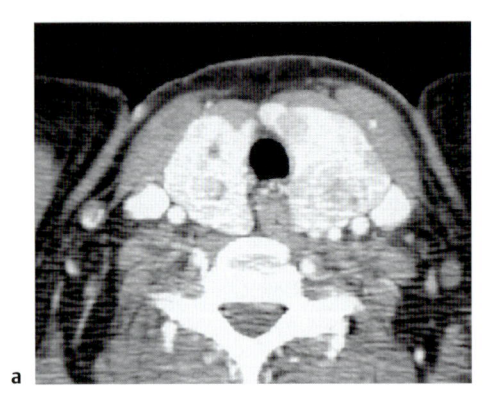

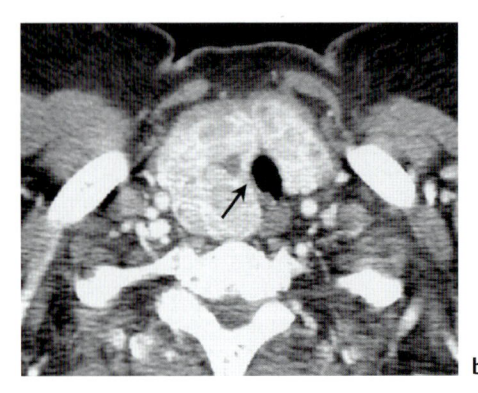

Fig. 12.**54** Multinodular goiter. Characteristic CT appearance. Contrast-enhanced CT images at the level of the cervical trachea (**a** and **b**) demonstrate enlargement of the thyroid gland as well as the presence of multiple thyroid nodules with variable enhancement. Note that the nodules display multiple central low-attenuation areas and there is a slight mass effect on the trachea (arrow).

easily made and color Doppler or power Doppler may nicely display the increased vascularity in the solid forms (Fig. 12.**52**). Thyroid adenomas are either functioning (hot nodule) or nonfunctioning (cold nodule) on radionuclide scans (Fig. 12.**53**).

Multinodular Goiter

Adenomatous or colloid multinodular goiter has an incidence of 3–5% in the general population, with a higher incidence in endemic goiter regions.[89,90,119] Patients usually present with either palpable neck masses or tracheo-esophageal compression and displacement, which is typically seen in substernal goiters. Goiters may be seen with hyperthyroidism, euthyroidism, or hypothyroidism. Histologically, multinodular goiters are composed of either colloid nodules or true adenomas. These nodules are multiple, their size is variable, and they are partly encapsulated. Areas of fibrosis, necrosis, and calcifications are common at histopathology. Accordingly, the findings on CT and MRI are variable, depending on the underlying histology (Figs. 12.**54**, 12.**55**). Calcifications, which are commonly seen in multinodular goiters, are optimally visualized on CT. Colloid has either a low or a high signal intensity on T1-weighted and a high signal intensity on T2-weighted MR images. Blood products have variable signal intensities on T1-weighted and T2-weighted images depending on the stage of blood degradation. Fibrosis has a low signal intensity

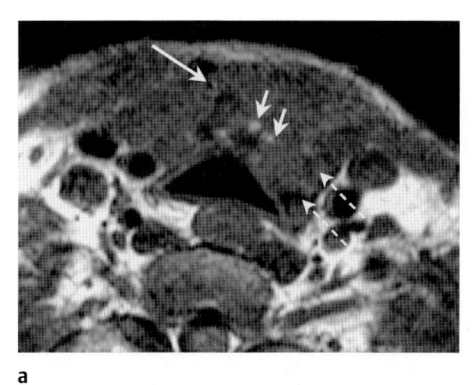

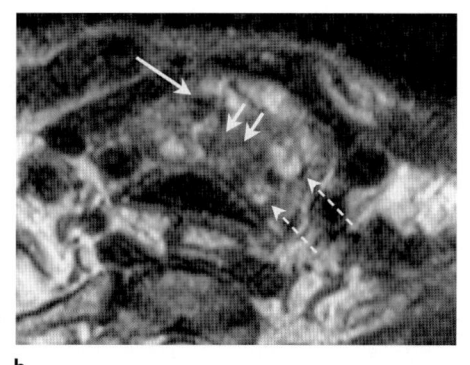

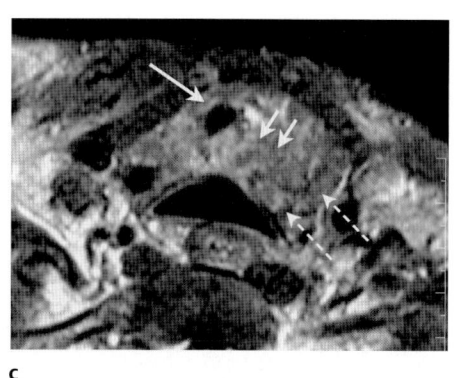

Fig. 12.55 Multinodular goiter. Characteristic MRI appearance. **a** T1W, **b** FSE T2W, and **c** contrast-enhanced T1W MR images at the level of the cervical trachea demonstrate enlargement of the isthmic portion and narrowing and displacement of the trachea. Note that the parenchyma is very heterogeneous with calcifications (anechoic on all pulse sequences; long arrows), adenomas (hypointense on T1, hyperintense on T2, and enhancing after administration of contrast material; dashed arrows), and blood products (hyperintense or hypointense on T1 and hypointense on T2; short arrows).

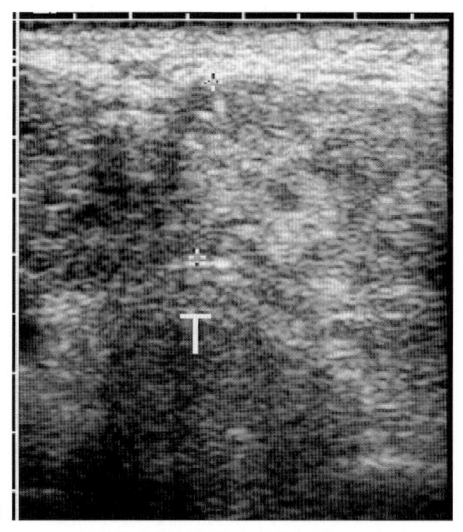

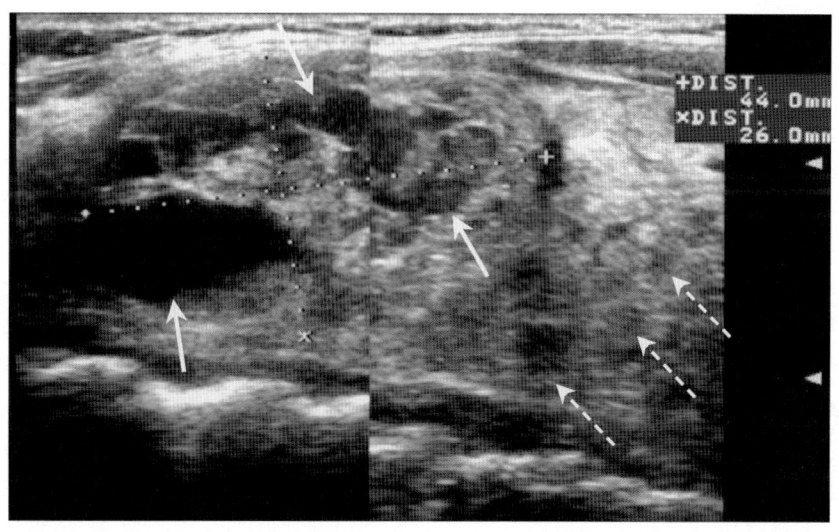

Fig. 12.56 Multinodular goiter. Characteristic US appearance. **a** Axial US image at the level of the isthmus shows an enlarged isthmus (measurement between callipters) with a heterogeneous echostructure. T = trachea. **b** Longitudinal US image through the right thyroid lobe shows a large nodule (measurements between callipters) with areas of cystic degeneration (arrows) as well as numerous other solid hypoechoic areas (dashed arrows).

on both T1-weighted and T2-weighted images, and calcium deposits present as signal voids[56,60] (Fig. 12.55). Tracheal deviation and narrowing may commonly be seen on CT and MR imaging. On US, multinodular goiters present as enlarged nodular glands with a heterogeneous echostructure including solid nodules, cysts, hemorrhagic nodules, and calcified nodules (Fig. 12.56). On ^{99m}Tc-pertechnetate scans, a multinodular goiter appears enlarged and heterogeneous with hot, cold, and spared areas (Fig. 12.57). This characteristic aspect will usually obviate the need for biopsy of a palpable nodule. However, a large, dominant, or growing mass amidst a goiter will most probably be biopsied.

Cysts

Most cysts are the result of degeneration of thyroid adenomas. They are usually hypodense on CT but become isodense when the protein content (including thyroglobulin) is elevated. The MR signal intensities depend on the composition of the cyst. Serous cysts demonstrate a low signal intensity on T1-weighted images and a high signal intensity on T2-weighted images, whereas colloid cysts with high thyroglobulin concentration have a high signal intensity on both T1-weighted and T2-weighted images. On

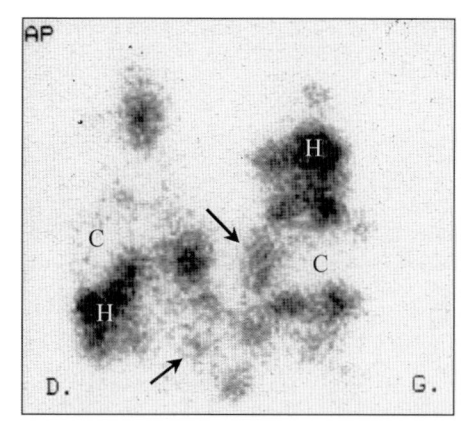

Fig. 12.57 Multinodular goiter. Characteristic scintigraphic appearance. Anteroposterior view of a ^{99m}Tc-pertechnetate scan. The large size of the gland, the presence of cold (C) and hot (H) nodules, and spared areas (arrows) within the heterogeneous gland are characteristic of a multinodular goiter.

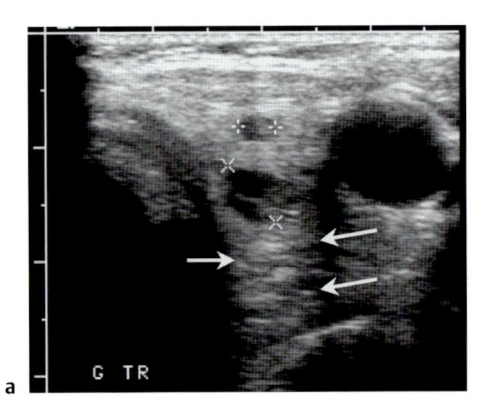

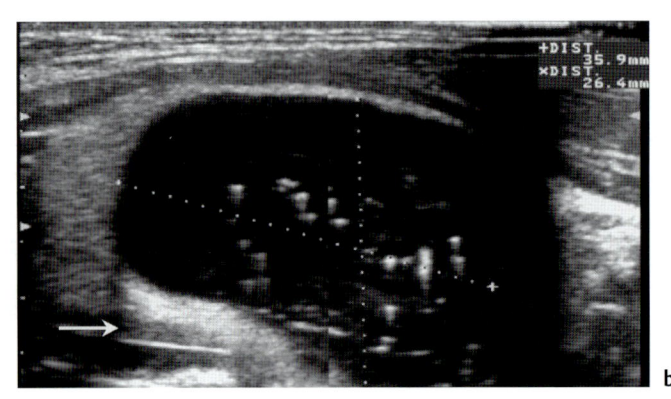

Fig. 12.58 Thyroid cysts. Characteristic US appearance. **a** Axial US image through the left thyroid lobe shows two anechoic lesions (between callipters) with dorsal acoustic enhancement (arrows). **b** Longitudinal US image of the left thyroid lobe in a different patient demonstrates a solitary large cyst with dorsal acoustic enhancement (arrow) and internal echoes suggesting intracystic hemorrhage.

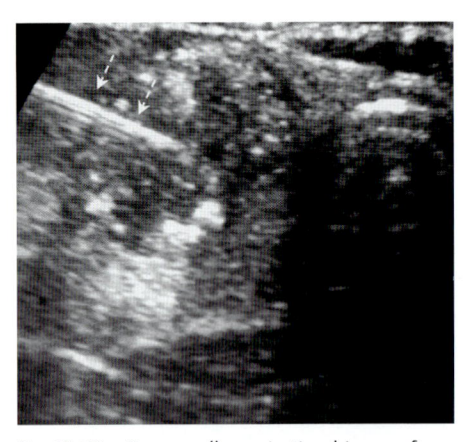

Fig. 12.59 Fine-needle aspiration biopsy of a small, solid, slightly hypoechoic nodule with calcifications (arrows) located in the right thyroid lobe. The tip of the needle (dashed arrows) is in the center of the nodule. Pathology revealed papillary thyroid cancer. Courtesy of Dr. Fernando Torrhina and Dr. David Coutinho (Imagens Medicas Integradas, Lisbon, Portugal).

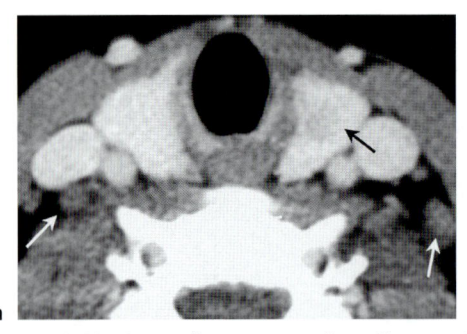

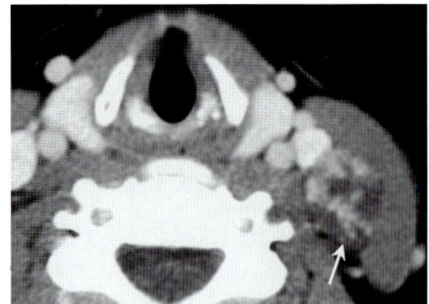

Fig. 12.60 Surgically proven small papillary carcinoma with lymph node metastases. The patient presented with palpable lymph nodes. Contrast-enhanced CT images at the level of the trachea (**a**) and subglottis (**b**) demonstrate a 1 cm nodule in the left thyroid gland (black arrow) with bilateral level IV lymph node metastases (white arrows). Courtesy of Dr. Fernando Torrhina and Dr. David Coutinho (Imagens Medicas Integradas, Lisbon, Portugal).

US, cysts present as anechoic lesions with dorsal acoustic enhancement (Fig. 12.**58**). Hemorrhage may occasionally occur into a cyst, resulting in a sudden increase of the cyst. On CT and MRI, hemorrhagic cysts have the same imaging features as colloid cysts. On US, hemorrhagic cysts have characteristic internal echoes (Fig. 12.**58**).

Thyroid Carcinoma

Malignant thyroid neoplasms include, in descending order of frequency: papillary thyroid cancers (60–80%), follicular carcinoma (15–18%), anaplastic carcinoma (3–10%), medullary carcinoma (4–5%), lymphoma (5%), squamous cell carcinoma (Lindsay tumor), sarcomas, and metastases from tumors arising outside the thyroid gland.[59,60] Finally, the thyroid gland may be invaded by tumors arising from adjacent organs.

Thyroid cancer is uncommon, accounting for around 1.6% of all cancers. The role of imaging in thyroid cancer depends to a large extent on the histology of the tumor. Because the vast majority of thyroid nodules are benign, a major role of imaging is to try to differentiate between benign and malignant lesions. Most thyroid cancers present as cold nodules on radionuclide scans (Fig. 12.**51**). The first-line approach includes nuclear medicine thyroid scans performed with ^{99m}Tc-pertechnetate or radioactive iodine, and ultrasonography combined with fine-needle aspiration biopsy, whereas CT and MRI are used only in selected cases to determine the extent of the tumor preoperatively, as well as the presence or absence of metastases. One must be cautious regarding CT scanning and the administration of contrast-enhanced iodinated compounds, since these agents will interfere with thyroid function tests for up to 6 weeks.

Papillary Carcinoma (Adenocarcinoma)

Papillary carcinoma is the most common thyroid cancer, with a peak incidence in the third and fourth decades. Females are affected more often than males. The prognosis is usually excellent (> 90% at 20 years) provided the size of the lesion does not exceed 5 cm and that the capsule of the thyroid gland is preserved.[23] As many as 20% of papillary carcinomas are multifocal, probably secondary to intrathyroidal lymphatic spread. Most often the tumor is smaller than 1.5 cm in size (Figs. 12.**59**, 12.**60**). However, aggressive forms may invade the larynx and trachea or the cervical esophagus[23,119] (Figs. 12.**61**, 12.**62**). Histology reveals papillae with a fibrovascular core with epithelial lining, nuclear atypia, and psammoma bodies (laminated calcific spherules) in 50% of cases. Follicular elements are common in a papillary carcinoma, and this has led to the histological classification of a "follicular variant" or "mixed papillary–follicular" carcinoma. However, this "mixed cancer" ultimately behaves like a papillary carcinoma. Psammomatous calcifications are easily seen on CT. They are punctate and in some instances appear as "cloudy" calcifications. Amorphous calcifications may also be observed in papillary thyroid carcinoma (Fig. 12.**62**). On CT and MR imaging,

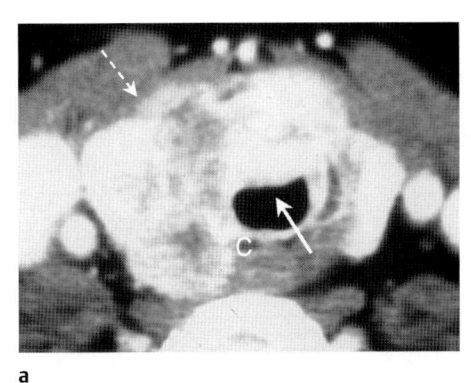

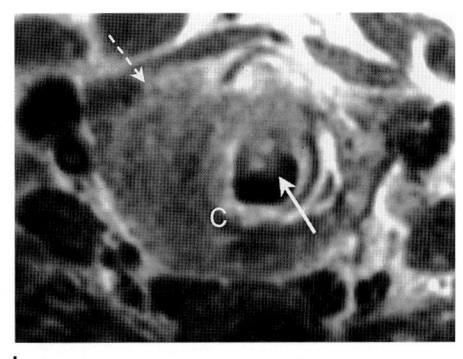

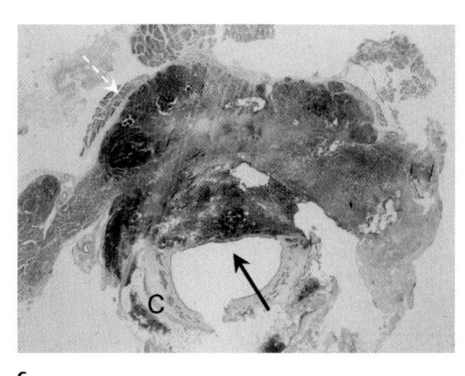

Fig. 12.61 Papillary carcinoma with invasion of the subglottic area. **a** Contrast-enhanced CT image and **b** contrast-enhanced T1W MR image at the level of the subglottis in a patient with progressive dyspnea and stridor show a tumor arising from the thyroid gland invading the right and anterior subglottic region and destroying the cricoid cartilage (C). A tumor nodule is seen in the subglottic airway (arrows). Note also invasion of the prelaryngeal strap muscles (dashed arrows). The patient underwent thyroidectomy and total laryngectomy. **c** Axial whole-organ histological slice from surgical specimen demonstrates a papillary thyroid cancer extending beyond the thyroid gland. Note invasion of the cricoid cartilage (C) and subglottic airway (arrow), as well as invasion of strap muscles (dashed arrow). Hematoxylin–eosin stain.

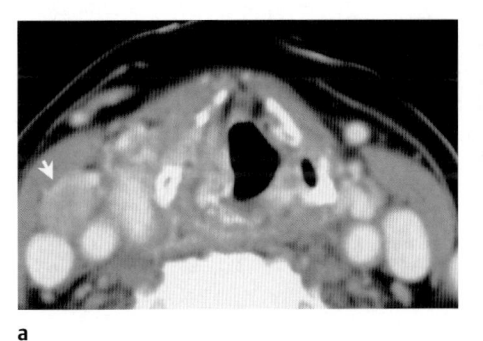

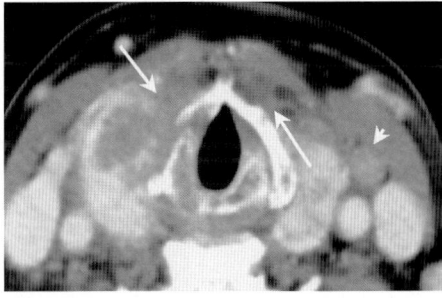

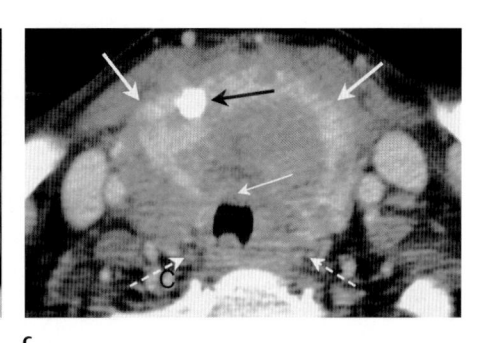

Fig. 12.62 Advanced papillary carcinoma with extraglandular spread and metastatic lymph nodes. Axial contrast-enhanced CT images at the level of the supraglottic larynx (**a**), subglottis (**b**), and cervical trachea (**c**) show a thyroid tumor extending beyond the thyroid gland. Invasion of the prelaryngeal strap muscles (arrows), trachea (thin arrow), and both tracheoesophageal grooves (dashed arrows). Bilateral level III lymph node metastases (short arrows). Note a paramedian position of the left false cord, suggesting recurrent laryngeal nerve paralysis caused by invasion of the left tracheo-esophageal groove. A large amorphous calcification (black arrow) is present within the tumor.

a malignant lesion should be expected when the margins are ill-defined, and when there is extraglandular tumor spread, lymph node involvement, or invasion of the larynx or trachea. However, a well-delineated lesion on CT and MRI does not exclude a malignant tumor. On US, early thyroid carcinomas very often appear as hypoechoic or almost "cystic" anechoic lesions with an incomplete peripheral hypervascular ring and with a central hypervascular zone. This aspect is not specific, so fine-needle aspiration biopsy is mandatory to clarify the histology of the lesion. In more advanced lesions, unsharp margins, extraglandular spread, and lymph node involvement may be seen. However, irregular or ill-defined borders are not specific for malignant lesions as they may occur in 60% of all cancers and in 45% of benign lesions.

In up to 50% of papillary carcinoma cases, lymph node metastases in the neck may precede the clinical recognition of a tumor in the thyroid gland (Fig. 12.**60**). However, as opposed to squamous cell cancer where the prognosis is tremendously influenced by the presence or absence of lymph node metastases, cervical lymph node metastases do not significantly affect the prognosis of patients with papillary carcinoma. Lymph node metastases from papillary carcinoma may occur into the paratracheal and supraclavicular areas (levels IV to VI), and later into the mid-jugular and upper jugular nodes (levels III and II) as well as retropharyngeal nodes (Fig. 12.**31**). Lymph node metastases from papillary carcinoma may have a variable aspect on imaging: solid and hypervascular, solid and cystic, cystic, and cystic and calcified (see above). In general, any lymph node seen in a patient with papillary carcinoma should be suspected of being malignant, irrespective of the size, because of the relatively high rate of lymphatic spread. Postoperatively, thyroid carcinoma recurrences are best detected by ^{131}I scintigrams, which are also the best modality to screen for distant metastases. MRI has been recommended in conjunction with ^{131}I scintigrams in confusing postoperative cases.

Follicular Carcinoma

Follicular carcinomas typically occur in females in their fifth decade. Although macroscopically they may resemble an adenoma, microscopic evaluation clearly shows that these tumors have features of vascular and capsular invasion[8,9,89,90] These aggressive tumors typically invade the surrounding tissue, including the airway. Lymph node metastases are rare (5–13%); but hematogeneous metastases to lung, liver, bone, and brain are common. Differentiated tumor forms and their metastases may take up radioiodine, which can be used to detect and treat metastases. On US, follicular carcinoma is solidly isoechoic in 52% of cases and hypoechoic in 44%. The CT and MRI findings are variable, ranging from a well-delineated nodule to an ill-defined tumor with necrosis and calcification (Figs. 12.**63**, 12.**64**). Advanced tumors may invade the larynx, trachea, esophagus, and tracheoesophageal groove. Patients may then present with dyspnea, dysphagia, and recurrent laryngeal nerve paralysis.

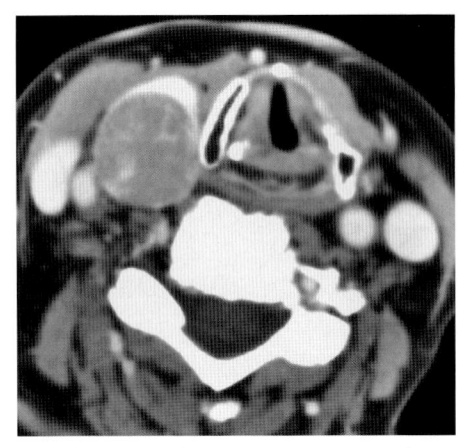

Fig. 12.**63** Follicular carcinoma. Nonspecific CT aspect. Contrast-enhanced CT image obtained in an elderly woman with a palpable neck mass demonstrates a single, well-delineated thyroid nodule on the right. No metastatic lymph nodes were seen on the CT examination. Surgery revealed follicular carcinoma.

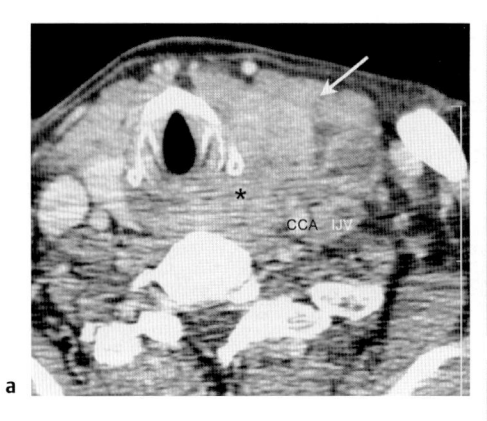

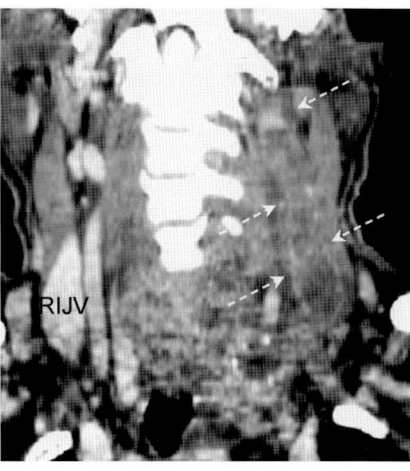

Fig. 12.**64** Advanced follicular carcinoma with internal jugular vein thrombosis. **a** Axial contrast-enhanced CT image and **b** coronal 2D reconstruction from a spiral CT acquisition show a large thyroid tumor originating from the left thyroid lobe, invading the strap muscles (arrow) and the left tracheo-esophageal groove (asterisk), completely surrounding the left common carotid artery (CCA), and invading the internal jugular vein (IJV). Note associated extensive thrombosis of the entire left internal jugular vein (dashed arrows). RIJV = normal right internal jugular vein.

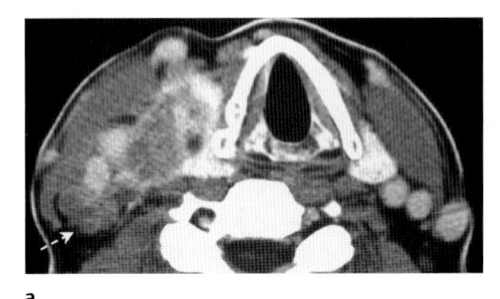

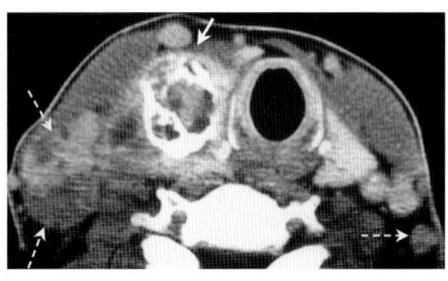

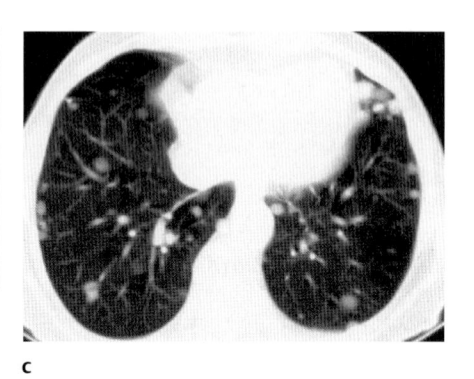

Fig. 12.**65** Anaplastic carcinoma of the thyroid gland. Contrast-enhanced CT images at the level of the glottis (**a**), subglottis (**b**), and lower lung lobes (**c**) demonstrate a large tumor with unsharp borders and calcifications arising within the right thyroid lobe. Diffuse extraglandular spread with invasion of strap muscles (arrow) and carotid space. Level III and level V lymph node metastases (dashed arrows), as well as multiple lung metastases.

Anaplastic Carcinoma

Anaplastic carcinoma is the most aggressive neoplasm in the thyroid gland. It is seen in patients over 50 years of age and the mean survival is 6–12 months. In almost 50% of cases, the anaplastic carcinoma develops within a goiter or may arise from papillary and follicular thyroid cancers.[5] At diagnosis, the tumor is usually large, has areas of hemorrhage and necrosis, and demonstrates invasion into the neighboring soft-tissue structures, larynx, trachea, esophagus, carotid arteries, and internal jugular vein (Fig. 12.**65**). Lymph node metastases, extension into the mediastinum, and distant hematogeneous metastases are common. The imaging features on CT and MRI do not allow differentiation from other advanced thyroid carcinomas.

Medullary Carcinoma

Medullary carcinomas arise from the parafollicular cells, or C cells, of the thyroid. The C cells appear to be derived from neural crest tissue in the ultimobranchial bodies of the branchial pouch system. These cells secrete thyroalcitonin, which decreases serum calcium. Most patients with a medullary carcinoma present with a well-circumscribed solid nodule that is usually nonencapsulated. Histologically, a highly vascularized stroma, amyloid deposition, hemorrhage, and hyalinized collagen may be seen. Seventy percent of medullary carcinomas arise sporadically; the remaining 30% are seen in the familial form without MEN (multiple endocrine neoplasia) and in the familial form associated with MEN (Table 12.**9**). Patients with MEN syndrome may have elevated serum levels of calcitonin, which can be used as a screening test in families with the genetic trait. On CT and MRI, the tumor may be solid; it may demonstrate psammomatous or coarse calcifications, extraglandular spread, and lymph node and distant metastases to the lungs, liver, and bone.

Lymphoma

Thyroid lymphoma is either primary within the gland or may be secondary as part of systemic lymphoma. Eighty percent of thyroid lymphomas arise in patients with Hashimoto thyroiditis[69] (Fig. 12.**66**). Most thyroid lymphomas are non-Hodgkin B-cell lymphomas. Chemotherapy and radiation therapy are the treatment of choice, but the prognosis is, in general, not very good. The radiological aspect is variable and includes an isolated nodule (80%), bilateral nodules (20%) (Fig. 12.**66**), a bulky mass involving the entire gland and with extraglandular extension, a necrotic mass, and involvement of regional lymph nodes. On US,

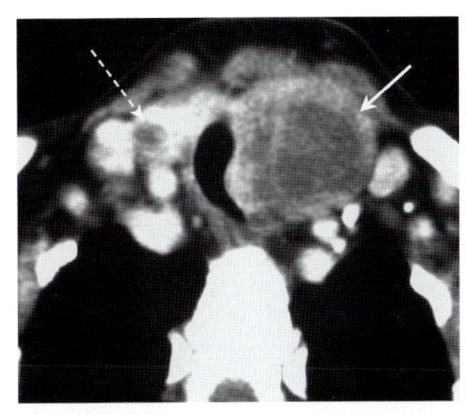

Fig. 12.**66** Primary thyroid non-Hodgkin lymphoma arising in an elderly woman with long-standing Hashimoto thyroiditis. Contrast-enhanced CT image demonstrates a hypoattenuating mass with minor enhancement (arrow) arising in the left thyroid lobe. Note tracheal compression and invasion. An additional small thyroid nodule is seen on the right (dashed arrow), which also proved to be a non-Hodgkin lymphoma.

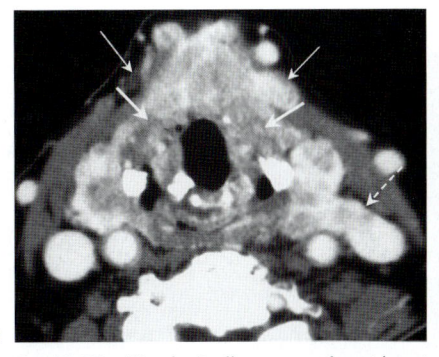

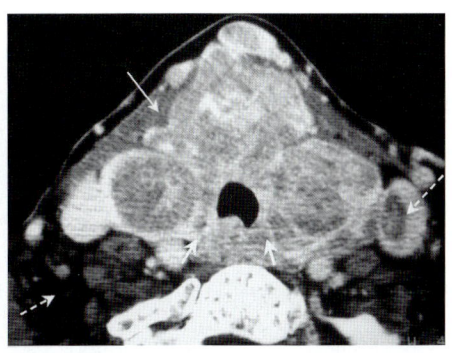

Fig. 12.**67** Histologically proven thyroid metastases from renal cell carcinoma. Contrast-enhanced images at the glottic level (**a**) and at the level of the cervical trachea (**b**) show a multinodular mass invading the entire thyroid gland, the strap muscles (thin arrows), the tracheoesophageal grooves (short arrows), and the thyroid cartilage (arrows), and with a tumor thrombus in the left internal jugular vein (dashed arrows). The imaging findings are indistinguishable from a primary thyroid cancer.

lymphomas are very hypoechoic and the vascularization pattern is quite variable.[118] On CT, the tumor is often hypodense and shows only minor enhancement. On MRI, the tumor is hypointense on both T1- and T2-weighted images and minor enhancement is seen after intravenous injection of contrast material.

Sarcoma

Primary sarcomas of the thyroid gland are very rare. They may arise de novo or following radiation therapy of the neck. Hemangioendothelioma, fibrosarcoma, or liposarcoma are the most common tumors. The prognosis for all sarcomas is poor.

Metastases

The most common sources of thyroid metastases are tumors arising in the breast, lung, kidney, and malignant melanoma. Metastases to the thyroid gland are often clinically occult, although pathologically metastases to the gland may be present in 2–4% of patients dying of malignant disease. Metastases may manifest as single or as multiple masses of variable size within the thyroid gland. Although the imaging findings are not pathognomonic, the presence of multiple thyroid nodules in a patient with a known primary tumor should raise the suspicion of metastatic disease. In advanced forms, the entire thyroid gland may be invaded and differentiation from a primary thyroid tumor may be impossible on CT and MRI images (Fig. 12.**67**).

Parathyroid Masses

Primary hyperparathyroidism (PHPT) occurs in 100–200 people per 100 000. Women are affected 2–3 times more frequently than men. Hyperparathyroidism (HPT) is caused in order of decreasing frequency by a solitary parathyroid adenoma (80–90%), hyperplasia (12–15%), multiple adenomas (2–3%), and parathyroid carcinoma (<1%).[37]

Most parathyroid adenomas are encountered in the normal position of the parathyroid glands and only a minority of cases are found in ectopic parathyroid glands (Fig. 12.**68**). Diagnostic evaluation for PHPT includes nuclear medicine scintigraphy, US, MRI, and CT. Preoperative imaging is rarely done because the operative success rate without preoperative imaging is as high as 95%. However, imaging is usually performed in cases with persistent or recurring HPT requiring reoperation[136] (Fig. 12.**68**). Currently, ^{99m}Tc sestamibi and US are the primary modalities used to assess parathyroid hyperplasia and adenomas located in the normal position of the parathyroid glands. The sensitivity of ^{99m}Tc sestamibi for HPT is 70–100% and the sensitivity of US is 70–80% with a specificity of 90–96%.[50, 108, 112] MRI has sensitivity of 80% and a specificity of 85%.[59, 60] For the evaluation of ectopic adenomas in the mediastinum, MR imaging with fat-suppressed, contrast-enhanced images is the evaluation method of choice. The accuracy rate approaches 90%.[58, 59] Ectopic adenomas in the neck can be assessed with ^{99m}Tc sestamibi, US, CT, or MRI. On US, adenomas are hypoechoic and they may be hypervascular (Fig. 12.**68**). On MRI, adenomas have a low signal intensity on T1-weighted images and variable signal intensities on T2-weighted images and after injection of contrast material (Fig. 12.**68**).

Imaging of the Neck after Treatment

The main options for treatment of malignant tumors of the extracranial head and neck currently consist of surgery, radiation therapy, surgery followed by radiation therapy, and radiation therapy combined with chemotherapy. The choice is influenced by clinical parameters, the extent of the primary lesion, histology, and the presence or absence of nodal or distant metastases.

■ Radiation-Induced Changes in the Neck

Radiation-induced changes in the head and neck area include expected changes and complications of radiotherapy. Distinction of radiation-induced changes from recurrent tumor is important, since the majority of radiation-induced changes are self-limited, whereas recurrent or residual tumor alters the therapeutic approach.[12, 17, 123]

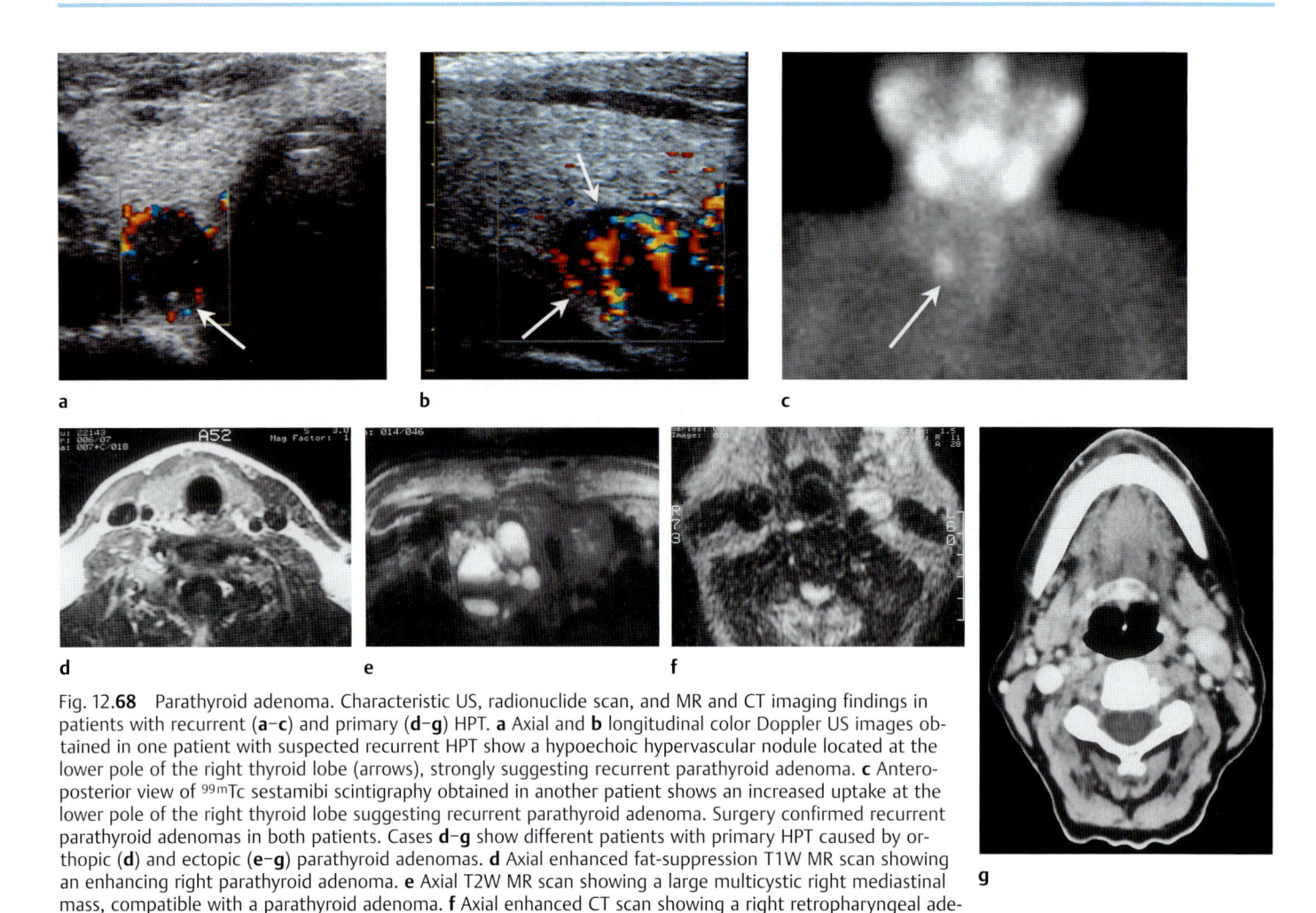

Fig. 12.**68** Parathyroid adenoma. Characteristic US, radionuclide scan, and MR and CT imaging findings in patients with recurrent (**a–c**) and primary (**d–g**) HPT. **a** Axial and **b** longitudinal color Doppler US images obtained in one patient with suspected recurrent HPT show a hypoechoic hypervascular nodule located at the lower pole of the right thyroid lobe (arrows), strongly suggesting recurrent parathyroid adenoma. **c** Anteroposterior view of ^{99m}Tc sestamibi scintigraphy obtained in another patient shows an increased uptake at the lower pole of the right thyroid lobe suggesting recurrent parathyroid adenoma. Surgery confirmed recurrent parathyroid adenomas in both patients. Cases **d–g** show different patients with primary HPT caused by orthopic (**d**) and ectopic (**e–g**) parathyroid adenomas. **d** Axial enhanced fat-suppression T1W MR scan showing an enhancing right parathyroid adenoma. **e** Axial T2W MR scan showing a large multicystic right mediastinal mass, compatible with a parathyroid adenoma. **f** Axial enhanced CT scan showing a right retropharyngeal adenoma, which appears hyperintense. **g** Axial enhanced CT scan showing a large ectopic parathyroid adenoma behind the left submandibular gland. Cases **d–g** courtesy of M.F. Mafee, M.D.

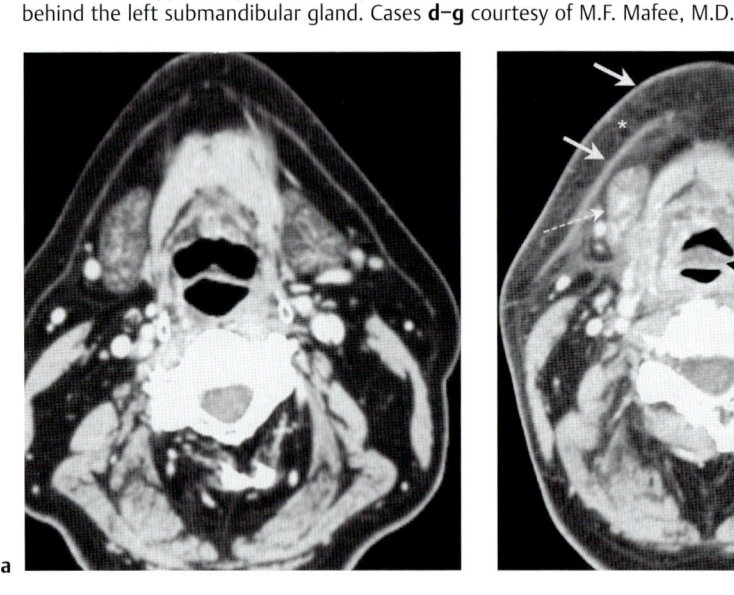

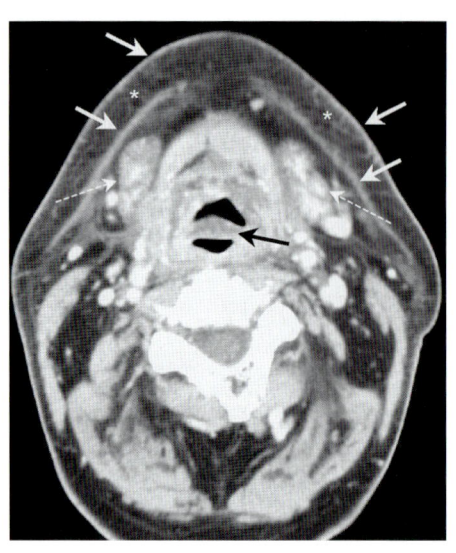

Fig. 12.**69** Characteristic CT features of the neck after radiation therapy. **a** Contrast-enhanced CT image at the level of the suprahyoid epiglottis obtained in an elderly man with a squamous cell carcinoma of the right tonsil prior to radiation therapy. **b** Contrast-enhanced CT image of the same patient at the same level obtained three months after radiation therapy (70 Gy) shows thickening of the anterior neck skin and of the platysma (arrows), a reticulated aspect of the subcutaneous fat within the radiation portals (asterisks), shrinking of the submandibular glands (dashed arrows), and massive thickening of the suprahyoid epiglottis (black arrow).

Expected Changes

Successful radiation therapy leads to a major reduction of tumor volume within three months, and treatment failure must be suspected if 50% or more of the tumor mass is still visible after this period. The relatively high radiation doses (> 60 Gy) that are required for treatment of head and neck tumors lead to marked inflammatory edema and fibrosis of the head and neck region. These changes are observed as early as three months after radiation therapy, and they may persist up to two years later.[12, 17, 73, 104]

Clinically, patients present with a swollen, indurated neck, a "woody" thickening of the skin, loss of anatomical landmarks, and sometimes pain that makes palpation very difficult. The characteristic MR and CT appearances of the neck after radiation therapy include symmetric thickening of the subcutaneous fat of the anterior neck, of the supraglottic laryngeal structures (see Chapter 11), of the posterior pharyngeal wall, and of the retropharyngeal space (Figs. 12.**69**–12.**71**). Edema and fibrosis result in an increased density and a "streaky," reticulated aspect of the

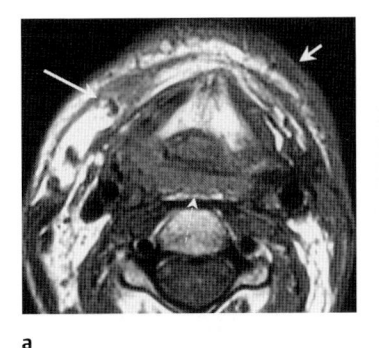

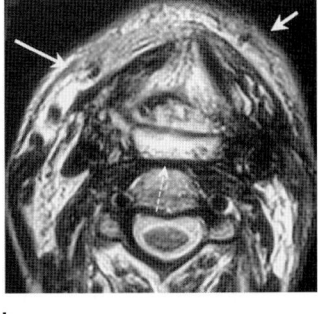

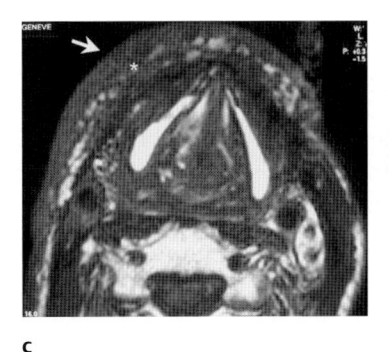

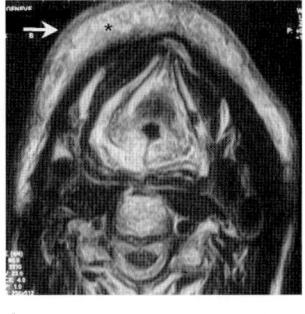

Fig. 12.70 Characteristic MRI features of the neck after radiation therapy for squamous cell carcinoma of the hypopharynx. The images were obtained one year after radiation therapy. **a** T1W and **b** T2W images at the upper supraglottic level and **c** T1W and **d** T2W images at the middle supraglottic level show massive thickening of the skin (short arrows) and of the platysma (long arrows), a reticulated edema of the anterior neck fat (asterisks), massive edema of the supraglottic larynx with near-total airway obstruction, and edema of the retropharyngeal space (dashed arrows).

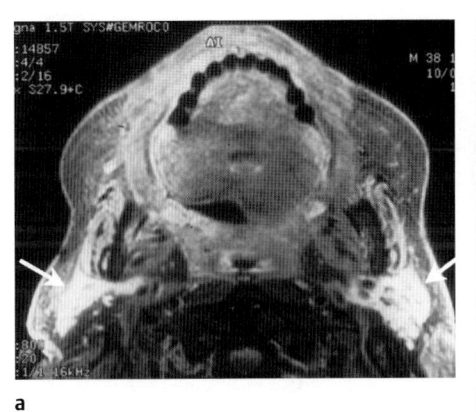

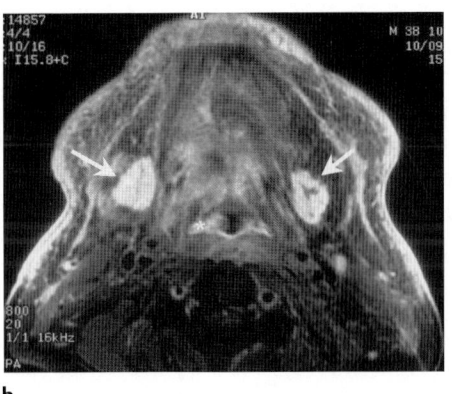

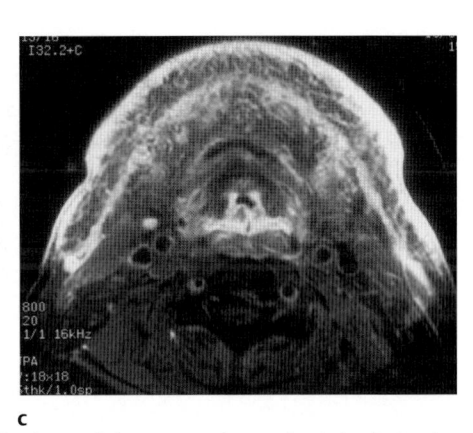

Fig. 12.71 Radiation-induced changes in the neck as seen on contrast-enhanced fat-suppressed MR images (**a–c**). This patient underwent radiation therapy for a tonsillar cancer three months previously. Note massive thickening of the skin and platysma, a reticulated enhancement of the subcutaneous fat corresponding to inflammatory changes, massive enhancement and loss of volume of the major salivary glands (radiation-induced sialadenitis, arrows), and major enhancement of the pharyngeal mucosa (asterisk in **b**). The findings persisted unchanged on follow-up examinations obtained during a period of three years.

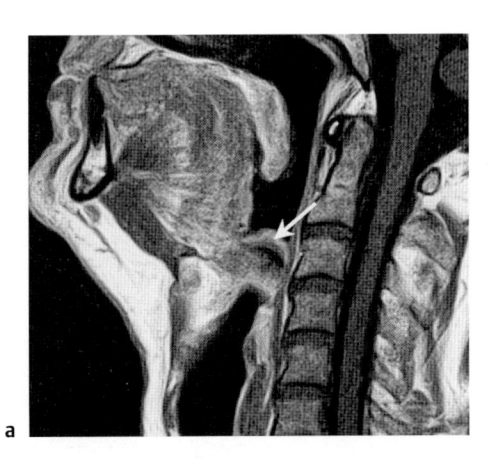

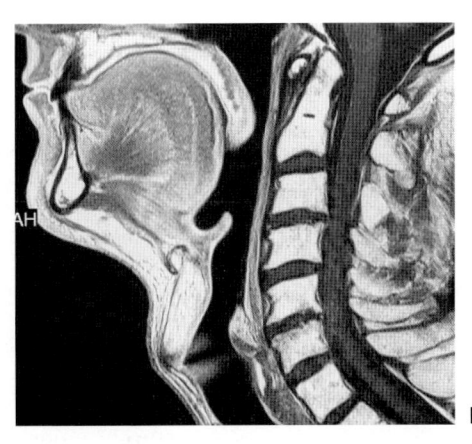

Fig. 12.72 Radiation-induced replacement of erythropoietic marrow by fatty tissue in the cervical vertebral bodies. **a** Contrast-enhanced T1W image obtained in a patient with a base of the tongue tumor (arrow) prior to radiation therapy. **b** Image obtained one year after radiation therapy clearly shows complete regression of the base of the tongue tumor and replacement of erythropoietic marrow by fatty marrow within the cervical vertebral bodies.

fat-containing spaces on CT and a decreased signal intensity with a reticulated pattern on T1-weighted SE MR images. Increased signal intensity is observed on T2-weighted images and STIR images. On both CT and fat-suppressed gadolinium-enhanced T1-weighted SE MR images, the fat-containing spaces that have been included in the radiation portal display a very strong enhancement, which may either resolve after 12 months or persist indefinitely[12, 123] (Fig. 12.71).

Further observed radiation-induced expected changes in the infrahyoid neck include progressive thickening of the carotid wall and replacement of erythropoietic tissue by fatty tissue in the cervical vertebral bodies (Fig. 12.72). Progressive thickening of the carotid wall is caused by accelerated arteriosclerosis.[28] It can easily be appreciated on follow-up examinations of patients who have received radiation therapy of the neck. Replacement of erythropoietic tissue by fatty tissue in the cervical vertebral bodies is seen in virtually all patients who have received radiation nonproliferating cells, e.g., bone, cartilage, and other connective tissues, and neural tissue. The exact mechanism of most late radiation-induced injuries is incompletely understood. It is thought that late injuries are caused by damage of the microvasculature or stromal cells. Late complications depend on several factors, such as total dose and volume of irradiated tissue, homogeneity of dose, daily fraction size, and time interval between fractions.[104] Knowledge of the normal imaging findings observed after radiation therapy as well as the presentation of radiation-induced complications may reduce the need for biopsy of irradiated tissue, which may be complicated by poor healing, infection and fistula formation.

Bone and Cartilage Necrosis

Bone and cartilage necrosis may affect the laryngeal cartilages, the hyoid bone, the mandible, or the temporal bone (see also Chapter 11). The hyoid bone commonly lies in the radiation field in patients with oropharyngeal or laryngohypopharyngeal cancer and it may occasionally undergo osteoradionecrosis and sequestration. Characteristically, the gap between radiation therapy and the development of symptoms is usually 5–10 years. The clinical signs of osteoradionecrosis of the hyoid bone are similar to those of laryngeal chondronecrosis.[12] Histologically, radionecrosis of the hyoid bone usually shows periosteal inflammation with multiple subperiosteal abscesses and sequestra. CT reveals inflammatory swelling adjacent to the hyoid bone, deep gas-containing ulcerations, fragmentation and sloughing of necrotic bone, and fistula formation (Figs. 12.**73**, 12.**74**). Because bone necrosis may be associated with microscopic coexistent tumor in a considerable percentage of cases, follow-up imaging studies with either CT or MRI are mandatory. In those patients where a marked amount of mass effect is seen in conjunction with osteonecrosis, biopsy should be performed to search for tumor recurrence. Treatment of hyoid bone osteoradionecrosis may be lengthy, and healing may take up to several years. Conservative measures (antibiotics, temporary tracheostomy, nasogastric tube, and hyperbaric oxygenation) are sometimes successful in resolving the necrotic tissue. However, surgery is recommended if conservative measures are unsuccessful, and if there is a concern that coexistent recurrent tumor may be present.

Soft-Tissue Necrosis and Pharyngocutaneous Fistula

Soft-tissue necrosis is most often observed within two years after irradiation of oropharyngeal tumors. Atrophy of the mucosa and continued alcohol and tobacco consumption are predisposing factors and preoperative irradiation seems to increase the risk of fistula formation.[12,36] Patients usually present with pain and weight loss because of dysphagia. More than 95% of soft-tissue necroses heal spontaneously, but healing may take more than six months. However, extensive soft-tissue necrosis with fistula formation requires surgical treatment. The radiological aspect of soft-tissue necrosis is usually straightforward (Fig. 12.**73**). However, tumor recurrence must be suspected if a soft-tissue mass is seen in addition to a fistula or area of ulceration. Pharyngography with water-soluble iodinated contrast material is usually used for assessing the extent of a fistula. In addition, CT should be used to look for tumor recurrence and for pretherapeutic planning of the surgical reconstructive procedure.

Carotid Artery Disease

It has been suggested that the incidence of accelerated atherosclerosis from therapeutic radiation in the head and neck area may be greater than expected in nonirradiated patients.[45,65,110] Predisposing factors for radiation angiopathy are high radiation doses, elevated serum cholesterol, and hyperlipidemia. In addi-

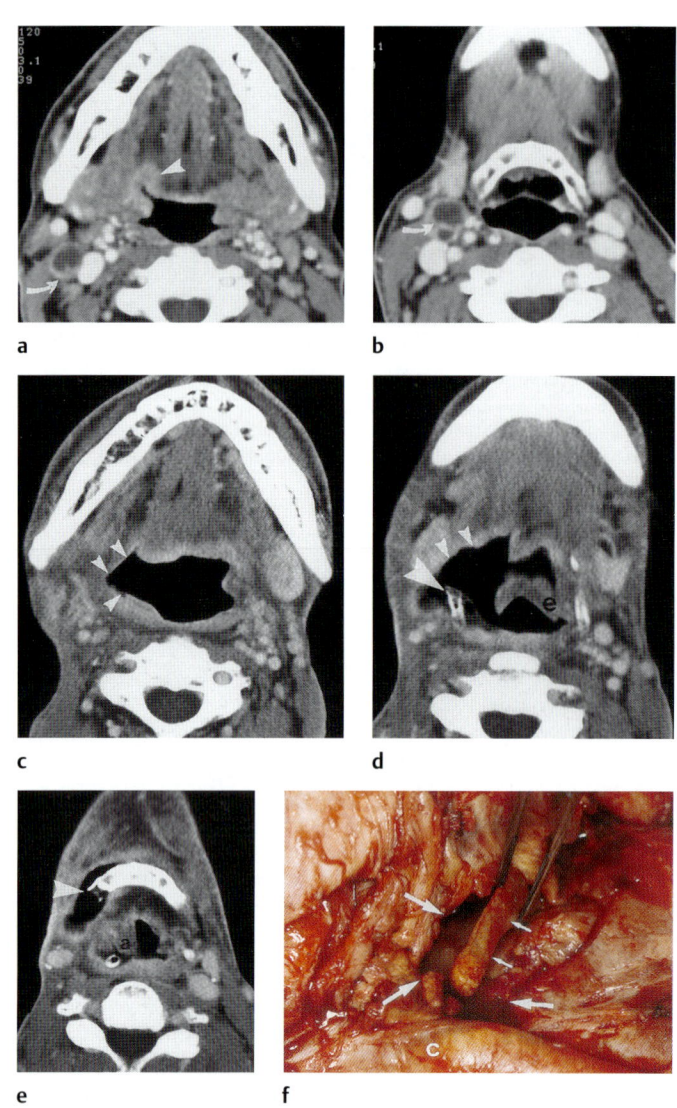

Fig. 12.**73** Osteoradionecrosis of the hyoid bone in a 61-year-old patient presenting with right-sided oropharyngeal carcinoma. **a**, **b** Contrast-enhanced CT images obtained prior to radiation therapy show the inferior border of a right-sided tumor mass invading the glossotonsillar sulcus (arrowhead) and multiple metastatic lymph nodes with central nodal necrosis (curved arrows). Modified radical neck dissection and radiotherapy were performed (70 Gy). Twelve months after surgery and radiotherapy the patient presented with severe pain radiating into the right ear, along with progressive dyspnea and dysphagia. **c–e** Contrast-enhanced CT shows complete regression of the oropharyngeal cancer with residual mucosal ulceration and underlying edema (small arrowheads). A large necrotic cavity is seen and air is present close to the denuded surface of the hyoid bone (large arrowheads). Note severe edema of the epiglottis (e) and aryepiglottic folds (a) following radiation therapy as opposed to the pretherapeutic image (**b**). Since the symptoms of the patient worsened despite conservative treatment, surgical exploration was performed in order to remove all necrotic tissue. **f** Intraoperatively, a large necrotic cavity was found (large arrows). The hyoid bone was very friable and yellowish (small arrows). C = carotid artery. Reproduced from Reference 12 with permission.

therapy of the neck. It is best appreciated on unenhanced T1-weighted images of the neck.

Complications of Radiation Therapy

Side effects due to high-dose irradiation of normal tissue may appear immediately after radiotherapy (acute effects) or months or even years after completion of treatment (late effects).[104] Late complications affect mainly tissues with slowly proliferating or

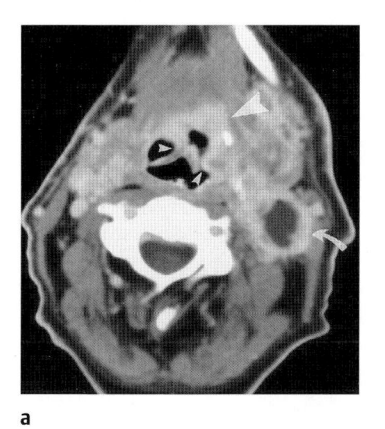

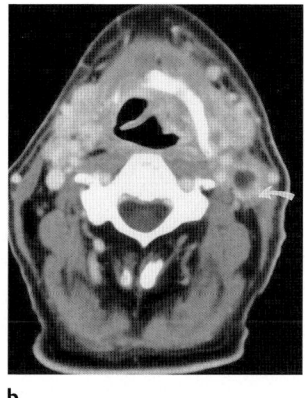

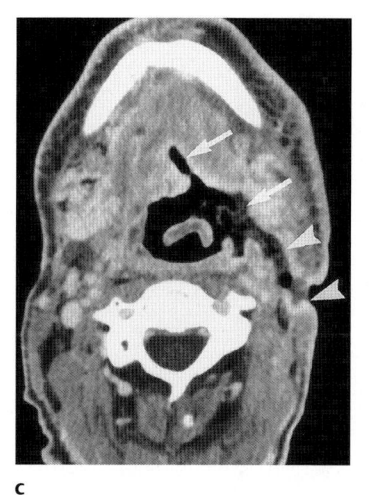

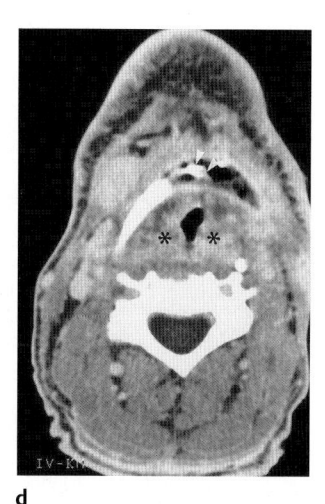

Fig. 12.74 Osteoradionecrosis of the hyoid bone and pharyngocutaneous fistula in a 56-year-old patient presenting with a left-sided oropharyngeal carcinoma. **a, b** Contrast-enhanced CT scans obtained prior to therapy show tumor invading the left vallecula (large arrowhead), the glossoepiglottic fold, and the pharyngoepiglottic fold (small arrowheads). Large necrotic metastatic lymph nodes with signs of extracapsular tumor spread are seen on the left (curved arrows). The patient underwent radiotherapy (86 Gy, 1.8 Gy/fraction) followed by radical neck dissection four months later because of tumor nonsterilization. **c, d** Contrast-enhanced CT images obtained 11 months after surgery show deep soft-tissue ulcerations of the floor of the mouth and of the left pharyngeal wall (arrows). Extensive pharyngocutaneous fistula (large arrowheads) and necrosis of the hyoid bone (small arrowheads) are seen. Note persistent edema of the epiglottis and aryepiglottic folds (asterisks) as well as increased soft-tissue density of the subcutaneous fat following radiation therapy. Reproduced from Reference 12 with permission.

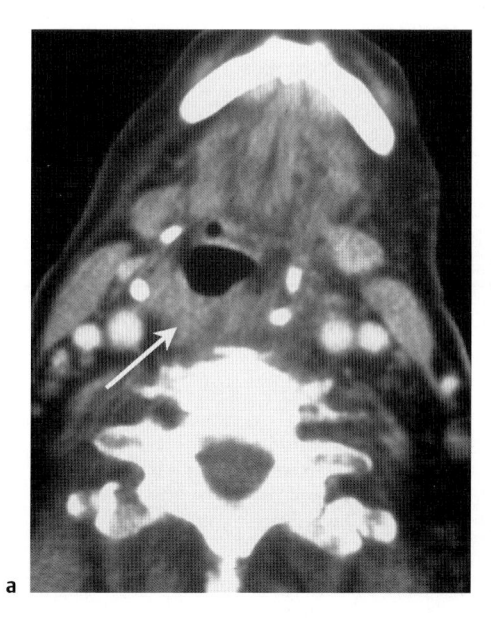

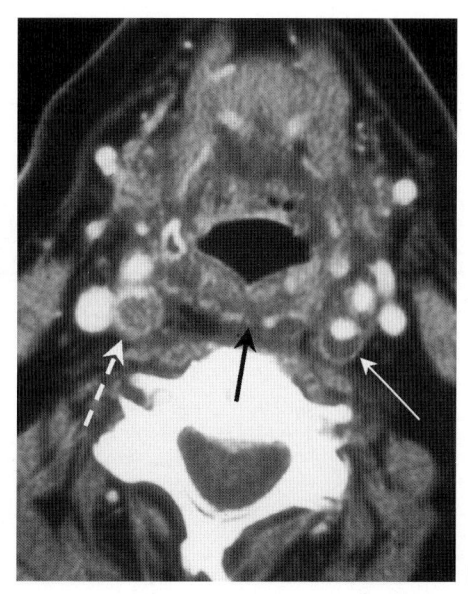

Fig. 12.75 Carotid artery stenosis/occlusion in a 55-year-old woman with a history of oropharyngeal and hypopharyngeal lymphoma. **a** CT scan obtained after completion of radiation therapy shows massive thickening of the posterior pharyngeal wall (arrow) compatible with residual lymphoma or post-irradiation edema. The left and right carotid arteries show normal enhancement. **b** CT scan obtained 12 months later shows persistent thickening of the posterior pharyngeal wall (arrow) corresponding to edema and scarring due to radiation therapy. The right internal carotid artery is occluded (dashed arrow) and the left internal carotid artery shows eccentric stenosis (thin arrow). Since the patient had otherwise no evidence of atherosclerotic disease, the changes were attributed to radiation therapy. Reproduced from Reference 12 with permission.

tion, irradiation of the neck predisposes to radiogenic hypothyroidism, which, in turn, favors degenerative arteriopathy.

Radiation arteriopathy may present as occlusion, subocclusive sclerotic or atheromatous plaque, localized mural thrombus, aneurysm, and, rarely, spontaneous rupture. In the head and neck region, stenoses of the carotid or, less commonly, the vertebral arteries are the most common manifestations. Symptoms usually occur after 1–10 years, but sometimes as late as two to three decades after successful irradiation. Stenoses are often bilateral, involve a long segment, and are related to the treatment field. Occasionally, they may progress to unilateral or bilateral occlusion (Fig. 12.**75**). Although many patients may be asymptomatic initially, appropriate surveillance is recommended, since delayed cerebrovascular consequences are common.[30] The most common symptoms are amaurosis fugax, transient ischemic attacks (TIA), and minor strokes; major strokes are quite uncommon. Acute carotid rupture is a rare complication with life-threatening bleeding, e.g., precipitated by wound complications after operation or by fulminant laryngeal osteoradionecrosis.[12] Transmural necrosis of the vessel wall is rare and may result in formation of a false aneurysm, which presents with acute life-threatening or intermittent hemorrhage (Fig. 12.**76**). Histological examination of the irradiated vessels shows involvement of the intimal, elastic, and muscular layers corresponding exactly to the radiation portals. Typical findings include extensive fibrosis beneath the intima, localized absence of endothelial cells, thinning and fragmentation of the elastic membrane, scars in the muscularis, cleft formation, adventitial fibrosis and thickening, inflammatory ulcers, and intra-arterial thrombi with different degrees of organization.[73, 30, 65, 125]

CT, MRI (including MR angiography), and color Doppler ultrasound are excellent nonivasive modalities for the follow-up of patients who have received high dose irradiation in the head and

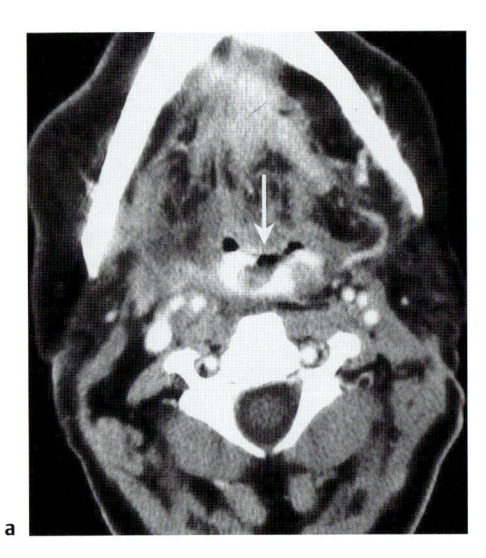

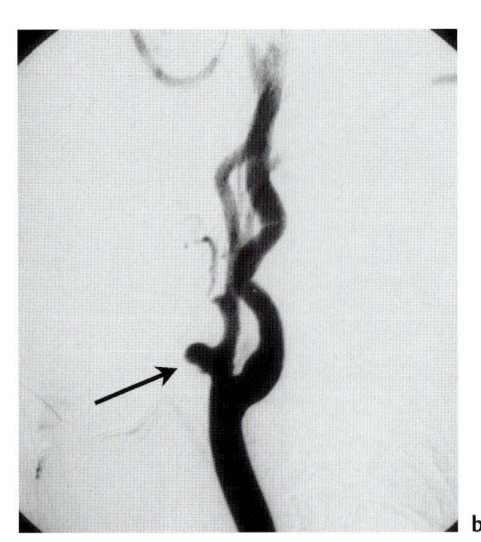

Fig. 12.76 False aneurysm of the external carotid artery in a 59-year-old patient with a history of radiation therapy for laryngeal cancer with 68 Gy followed by salvage laryngectomy and bilateral neck dissection 12 years earlier. The patient presented in the emergency room with massive, intermittent hemorrhagic vomiting and hypovolemic shock. **a** Contrast-enhanced CT image shows active extravasation of contrast material into the neopharynx (arrow). The bleeding source could not be identified. Note bilateral postoperative changes after neck dissection as well as increased attenuation of the subcutaneous fat following radiation therapy. **b** Emergency angiography of the right carotid artery revealed a false aneurysm of the external carotid artery (arrow) without contrast extravasation. Embolization was done to prevent recurrent bleeding, but surgical intervention with carotid bypass grafting became necessary later. Reproduced from Reference 12 with permission.

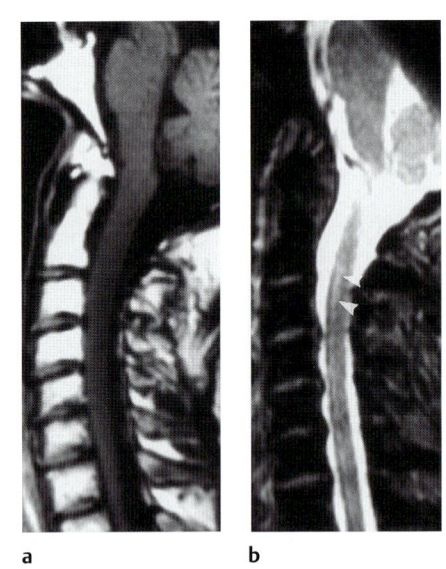

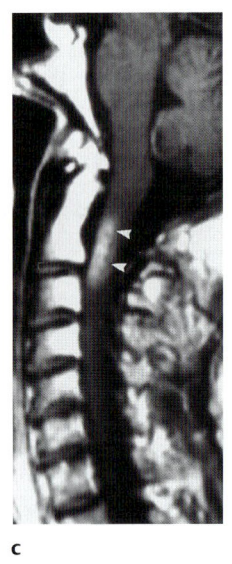

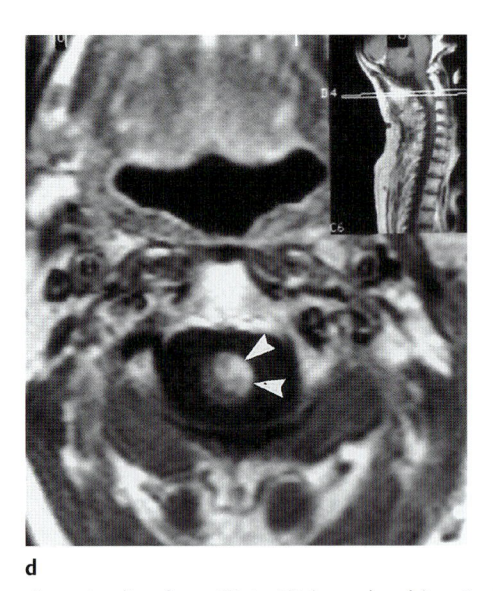

Fig. 12.77 Delayed radiation-induced myelopathy in a 57-year-old patient irradiated for carcinoma of the nasopharynx (76 Gy) two years earlier who presented with left-sided hemisyndrome and right-sided hyperesthesia and pyramidal signs. There was no evidence of tumor recurrence at clinical examination and MRI. The spinal cord had been included in the radiation field. **a** Sagittal T1W SE MR image shows cord swelling with hypointensity, and **b** sagittal T2W SE MR image shows hyperintensity extending from C2 to C3 (arrowheads). **c** Sagittal and **d** axial contrast-enhanced T1W SE MR images show extensive cord enhancement involving mainly the left side (arrowheads), suggesting radiation myelopathy. Note high signal in the vertebral bodies on the unenhanced T1W MR image caused by fatty marrow replacement. Reproduced from reference 12 with permission.

neck. However, angiography remains the gold standard and is reserved for interventional procedures and for those cases where CT, MRI, and US fail to clearly show the vascular pathology (Fig. 12.76). CT and MRI not only demonstrate accurately the vessel wall, allowing an accurate assessment of luminal narrowing, but may also demonstrate obliteration of the carotid space due to adventitial fibrosis.[28]

Radiation Myelopathy

Permanent spinal cord injury is a potentially devastating complication of radiation therapy. Radiation-induced transverse myelitis is an irreversible process with no effective treatment. The incidence of a permanent injury to the spinal cord as a complication of radiation therapy of head and neck cancer has been estimated at 2%.[12] The incidence of radiation myelitis depends on field size, total radiation dosage, and fraction size; low fraction size appears to decrease the incidence of such injuries. Most cases are seen following radiation therapy of nasopharyngeal carcinoma. Symptoms, usually paresthesia, appear 6 months to 2 years after completion of radiation therapy and may progress to total paralysis or may be even lethal. Autopsy findings include generalized distension of the affected segments, extensive demyelination, and coagulation necrosis.

Imaging findings depend on the time interval after onset of symptoms. MR imaging performed within 6–8 months after onset of symptoms shows cord swelling with hypointensity on T1-weighted SE images, hyperintensity on T2-weighted SE images, and strong long-segment enhancement of the cord after injection of contrast material (Fig. 12.77). When MR imaging is obtained more than three years after symptom onset, cord atrophy without abnormal signal intensity is seen.

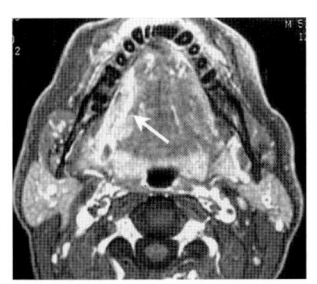

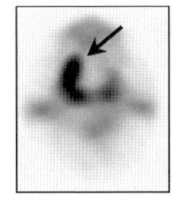

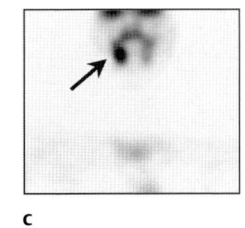

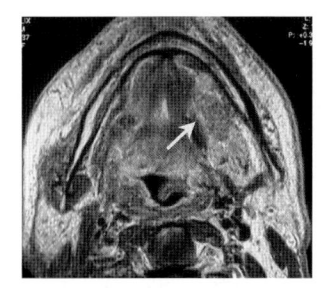

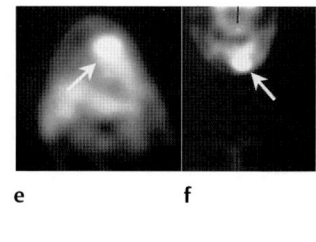

Fig. 12.**78** Detection of tumor recurrence (primary site) after radiation therapy with MRI and PET. **a** Contrast-enhanced, fat-suppressed T1W MR image obtained prior to radiation therapy in a patient with a floor of the mouth tumor on the right (arrow). **b, c** Corresponding axial (**b**) and coronal (**c**) FDG-PET images obtained prior to treatment demonstrate a hypermetabolic focus on the right (arrows). No lymph nodes were seen. The patient underwent radiation therapy for his floor of the mouth tumor. **d, e, f** Four months after completion of radiation therapy, he underwent an MRI examination (**d**) and a PET examination (**e** axial image, **f** coronal image). Both imaging studies clearly show a contralateral recurrent tumor (arrows), although clinical examination was normal. Biopsy confirmed tumor recurrence.

Cranial Nerve Paralysis

Because the cranial nerves are very resistant to irradiation, paralysis is a rather uncommon finding. However, nerve lesions may occur within 2–7 years after completion of radiotherapy.[27] On the basis of surgical and autopsy data, the suggested mechanism is nerve compression by perineural radiation-induced fibrosis.[27] This may occur at any level from the skull base to the infrahyoid neck. The hypoglossal nerve is most commonly affected in the suprahyoid neck, whereas the recurrent laryngeal nerve is the most commonly affected nerve in the infrahyoid neck.[12, 131] Neck dissection after irradiation appears to diminish the risk of hypoglossal nerve palsy.[73] Unilateral involvement may cause no significant symptoms except for slight dysarthria. Lingual atrophy, fasciculations, and deviation can be noted at clinical examination. Recurrent laryngeal nerve paralysis causes the typical clinical finding of dysphonia, and has been reported after external radiotherapy of head and neck or breast tumors and following ^{131}I therapy of hyperthyroidism.[15, 31] The CT and MRI features of hypoglossal and recurrent laryngeal nerve paralysis are described in detail in Chapters 10 and 11, respectively. If sectional imaging does not show a tumor mass along the entire pathway of the hypoglossus, vagus, and recurrent laryngeal nerve in a patient with a history of high-dose irradiation of the area, the diagnosis of radiation-induced nerve paralysis should be considered.

Development of Sarcomas

Previous radiation therapy of the neck is a predisposing factor for the development of sarcomas, the latency period ranging from 5 to 20 years.[92, 106] Postradiation sarcomas in the neck are rare, however. Radiation-induced sarcomas can originate in either the irradiated bone or soft tissues. Most of these tumors are high-grade malignancies. The most common histological subtypes are malignant fibrous histiocytoma (MFH) and osteosarcoma, although other histologies, such as angiosarcoma, rhabdomyosarcoma, fibrosarcoma, and malignant peripheral nerve sheath tumors (MPNST), can occur.

Tumor size and grade are the two most important prognostic factors for all soft-tissue sarcomas associated with radiation therapy. In general, the prognosis of radiation-induced sarcomas is very poor. Treatment includes surgery followed by radiation therapy and chemotherapy in selected cases.[14] The imaging findings in sarcomas of the neck are nonspecific and include a large ovoid or fusiform tumor, areas of necrosis and hemorrhage, a heterogeneous enhancement, and a spiculated, diffusely infiltrating mass, or spread along the epineurium and perineurium of nerve trunks. Although the imaging findings of sarcomas of the neck are not pathognomonic, an appreciation of the expected latency period may help to suggest the diagnosis.

Detection of Tumor Recurrence

Tumor recurrence may occur either at the primary site or in lymph nodes. Recurrent lymph node metastases may be seen with or without associated recurrent primary tumors. In fact, patients may die of recurrent nodal metastases although the primary tumor is controlled. Tumor recurrence at the primary site or in lymph nodes most often becomes clinically manifest within the first two years after radiation therapy. Because physical and endoscopic examination is often limited by the changes induced by radiation therapy, the ideal follow-up protocol should include—in addition to clinical evaluation—serial sectional imaging with either CT or MRI during the first two years. Because of its high cost, however, such a protocol is restricted to patients with an estimated high risk of tumor recurrence, while patients with a low risk of tumor recurrence are followed clinically with imaging studies performed only when tumor recurrence is suspected clinically or endoscopically. The baseline study should not be performed earlier than three months after completion of treatment. Three months after completion of treatment, most of the acute and subacute inflammatory changes should have disappeared.[12, 17, 88, 104, 123] However, in some patients the posttherapeutic changes may not change over a period of two years.

A close communication between clinicians and head and neck radiologists is essential when interpreting CT and MR imaging data.[88] Imaging of the entire head and neck region from the skull base to the thoracic inlet is mandatory, because nodal recurrences may occur in the suprahyoid neck even if the initial tumor was located in the infrahyoid neck. As a general rule, diffuse changes in the head and neck should not be regarded as evidence of tumor recurrence. However, focal masses on CT or MRI, whatever their appearance, should alert the radiologist to the possibility of tumor recurrence (Figs. 12.**78**–12.**80**). They should be regarded as tumor relapse until proven otherwise. In practice, comparison between successive examinations makes diagnosis easier by showing either a new mass and/or reappearance of abnormal contrast enhancement.[57]

Recently, it has been suggested that color Doppler sonography and FDG-PET may be used to reliably assess recurrent tumor in irradiated patients.[40, 46, 111] While color Doppler sonography may reliably detect the presence of recurrent lymph nodes, it cannot assess recurrent tumors at the primary site (located in the visceral space). FDG-PET has been shown to have a sensitivity of 100% at the primary site and 83–93% for nodal disease, and a specificity of 64% at the primary site and 76–97% for nodal disease.[40, 46, 111] These results were similar to or superior to those of CT/MRI depending on the reported series.[40, 46, 11]

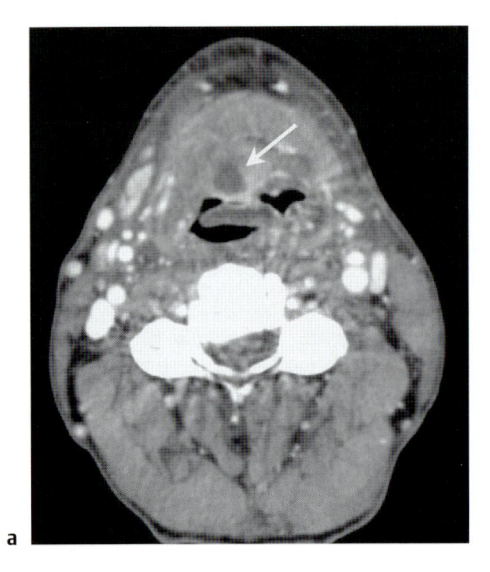

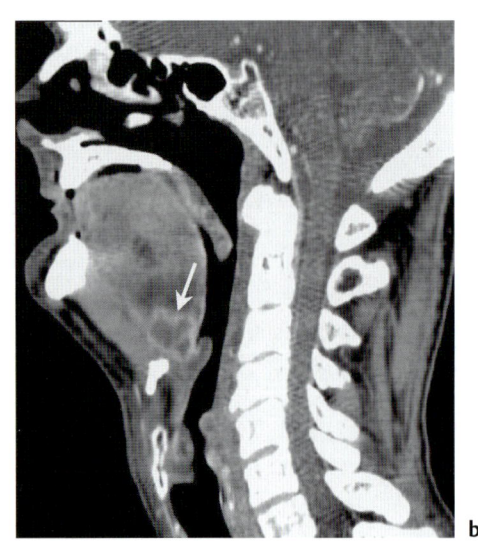

Fig. 12.79 Detection of tumor recurrence (primary site) by means of CT. **a** Axial contrast-enhanced CT image and **b** sagittal 2D reconstruction obtained 18 months after combined radiation therapy and chemotherapy in a patient with a squamous cell carcinoma of both valleculae reveal recurrent tumor involving the base of the tongue and floor of the mouth (arrows). Note associated radiation-induced changes in the neck and larynx. Biopsy confirmed the radiological findings.

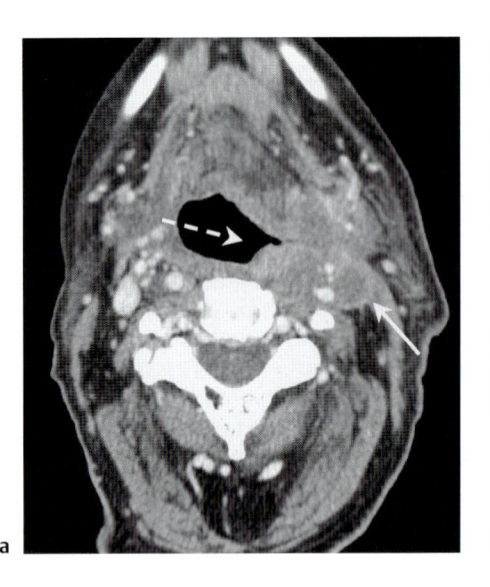

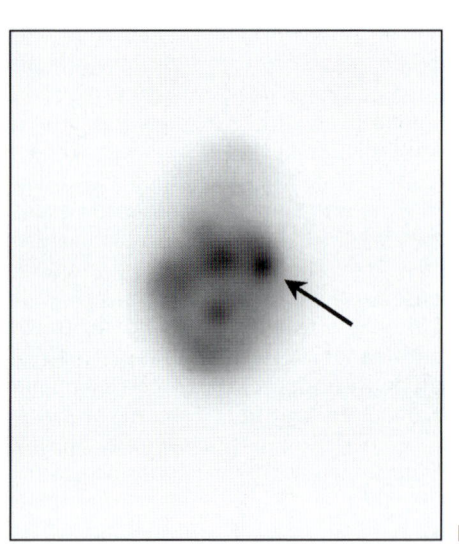

Fig. 12.80 Detection of tumor recurrence (nodal disease) by means of CT and PET. **a** Contrast-enhanced CT image at the level of the base of the tongue obtained 12 months after combined radiation therapy and chemotherapy in a patient with left-sided tonsillar cancer. A level II lymph node metastasis (arrow) is seen on the left. In addition there is asymmetry of the lateral and posterior oropharyngeal wall suggesting recurrent disease also at the primary site. **b** FDG-PET image performed in the same patient reveals a hypermetabolic focus on the left suggesting a lymph node metastasis (arrow). There is no additional hypermetabolic focus. Salvage surgery revealed a level II metastatic lymph node on the left and no recurrence at the primary site.

■ Postoperative Changes after Various Types of Neck Dissection and Reconstruction with Flaps

Postsurgical Changes after Various Types of Neck Dissection

The surgical treatment of cervical lymph node metastases includes radical, extended, modified radical, or selective neck dissection.

The technique of **radical neck dissection** involves removal of all ipsilateral cervical node groups (levels I–V) from the inferior border of the mandible down to the clavicle and from the anterior belly of the digastric muscle to the trapezius muscle. The spinal accessory nerve, ipsilateral submandibular gland, internal jugular vein, and sternocleidomastoid muscle are also removed. Accordingly, CT and MRI performed in patients with radical neck dissection reveal flattening of the ipsilateral neck and absence of the above-mentioned structures (Fig. 12.**81**). As a result of the surgery, the patient develops atrophy of the trapezius muscle (Fig. 12.**82**), progressive shoulder drop, shoulder pain, scapula prominence, and limitation of shoulder abduction.

Extended neck dissection is performed in patients with bulky nodal disease and extensive extranodal spread. Additional lymph node groups and nonlymphatic structures that are not included in the radical neck dissection are removed, such as skin, platysma, strap muscles, and cranial nerves IX and X. Closure of the surgical defect is most often performed with a myocutaneous flap (see below).

Modified neck dissection (also referred to as **functional neck dissection**) includes removal of all ipsilateral lymph node groups with preservation of one or more of the nonlymphatic structures not involved by tumor. Radiographic findings are very subtle, and include minor skin thickening, unsharpness of tissue planes, and flattening of the affected neck side (Fig. 12.**83**).

Selective neck dissection involves preservation of one or more lymph node groups that are routinely removed in radical neck dissection. For example, in the supraomohyoid neck dissection, level I–II lymph node groups are routinely resected, while in the lateral neck dissection, level II–IV nodes are resected.

Postsurgical Changes after Reconstruction with Flaps

Reconstruction of a large soft-tissue defect requires axial, random, or free flaps. **Axial flaps** are taken from adjacent sites, have an arteriovenous system running along the long axis of the tissue to be transferred, and are rotated into place along the vascular

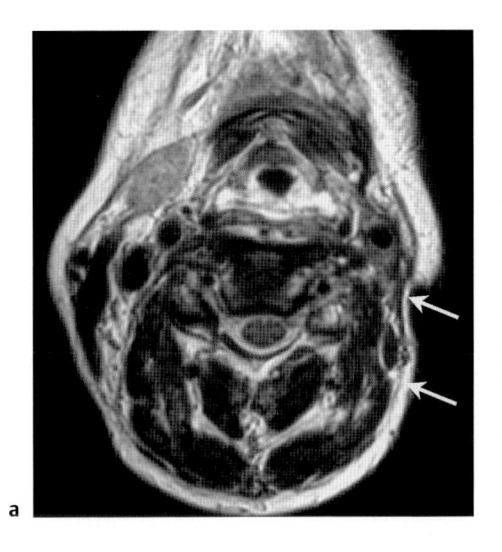

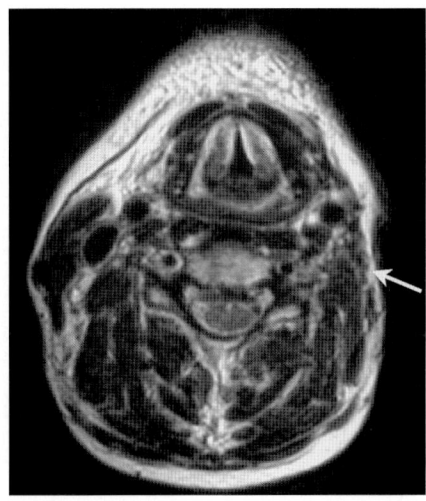

Fig. 12.**81** MRI appearance of the neck after radical neck dissection. T2W FSE images at the level of the hyoid bone (**a**) and supraglottis (**b**) obtained three months after left-sided radical neck dissection show absence of the left submandibular gland, flattening of the ipsilateral neck (arrows), and absence of the left internal jugular vein and left sternocleidomastoid muscle.

pedicle. **Myocutaneous flaps** are one subtype of axial flap that are composed of skin, subcutaneous fat, and muscle. The most commonly used myocutaneous axial flaps are the pectoralis and the trapezius flaps. Because the nerve supply to the flap is often interrupted surgically prior to transfer, fatty infiltration of the muscle tissue within the flap is seen at either CT or MRI (Fig. 12.**84**), whereas the nutrient vascular attachment of the flap can be seen at one margin of the flap.

Free flaps are taken from a distant donor site and transferrend to reconstruct a soft-tissue defect. The reconstruction requires microvascular anastomosis, which may lengthen the operative time significantly. The most commonly used free flaps are the free radial arm flap for intraoral reconstruction and the free fibula flap for mandibular reconstruction. On imaging, no vascular pedicle will be identified as seen in the rotated myocutaneous flaps.

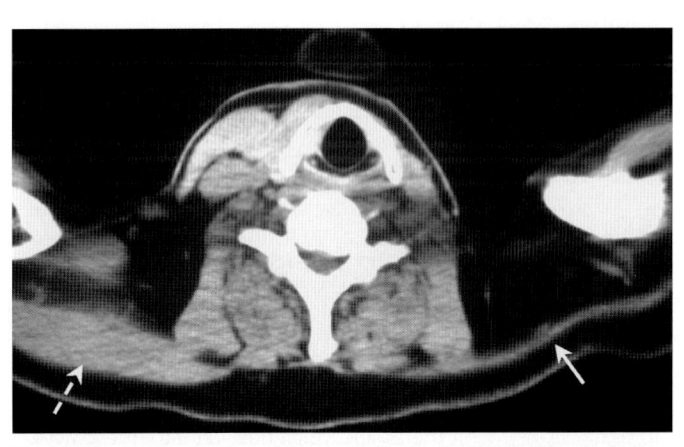

Fig. 12.**82** CT appearance of the neck after radical neck dissection. Contrast-enhanced CT image obtained nine months after left-sided radical neck dissection shows marked atrophy of the trapezius muscle (arrow) and absence of the left sternocleidomastoid muscle. Note for comparison the normal size of the right trapezius muscle (dashed arrow).

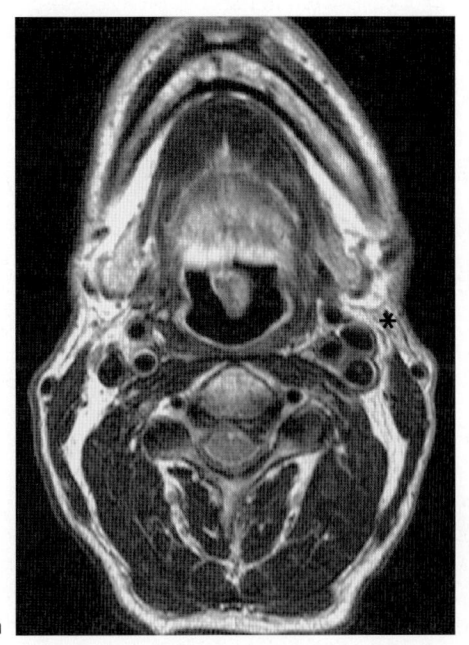

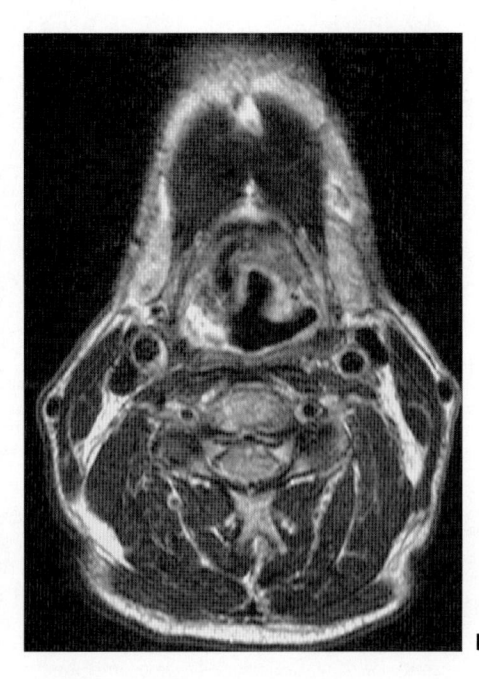

Fig. 12.**83** MRI appearance of the neck after left-sided functional neck dissection. T2W FSE images (**a** and **b**) show only minor skin thickening (asterisk) and subtle flattening of the left side.

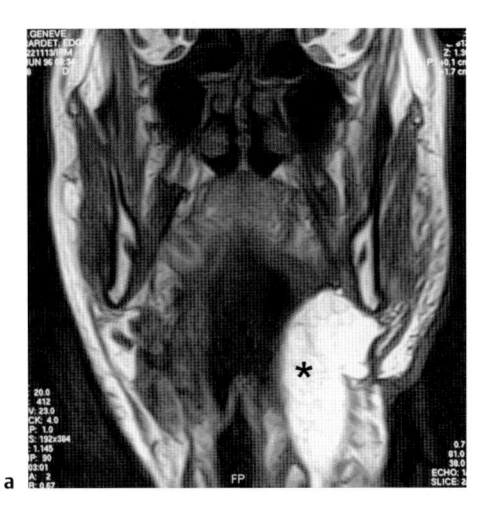

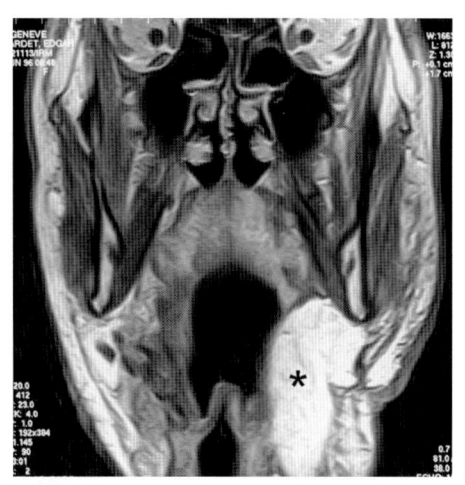

822 12 Other Infrahyoid Neck Lesions

Fig. 12.**84** Normal MRI appearance of the neck after radical neck dissection and reconstruction with a pectoralis flap. Coronal T1W images before (**a**) and after (**b**) injection of contrast material show fatty infiltration of the muscle within the flap (asterisks).

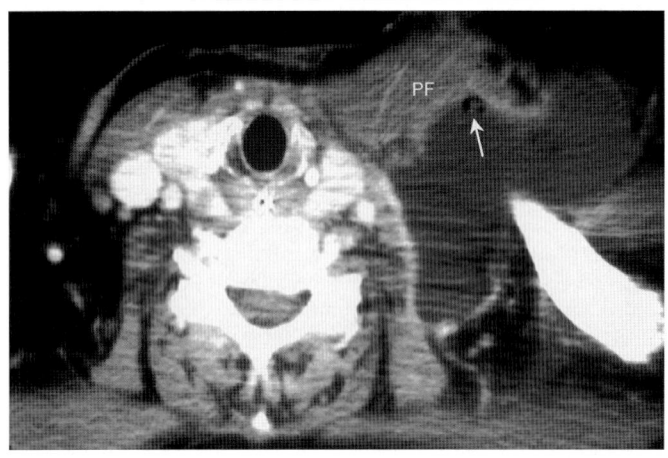

Postoperative Complications and Tumor Recurrence

It has been suggested that a postoperative baseline scan should be obtained 4–8 weeks after surgery. When performed at this time, the baseline scan depicts the altered anatomy of the neck and should have allowed most of the acute postoperative changes to have resolved. On subsequent follow-up examinations, any soft-tissue mass that progressively reduces in size should be considered as resolving hemorrhage and edema. Conversely, any enlarging mass must be considered recurrent disease.

Postoperative complications usually occur within the first month after surgery. Postoperative complications include abscess formation, hematoma, flap ischemia with necrosis, and pharyngocutaneous fistula (Figs. 12.**85**, 12.**86**). Complications of flap ischemia such as necrosis and the formation of pharyngocutaneous fistula are a straightforward diagnosis clinically and radiographically. When abscess formation or hematoma occurs at a later stage, differentiation from recurrent tumor may be very difficult if not impossible by means of imaging

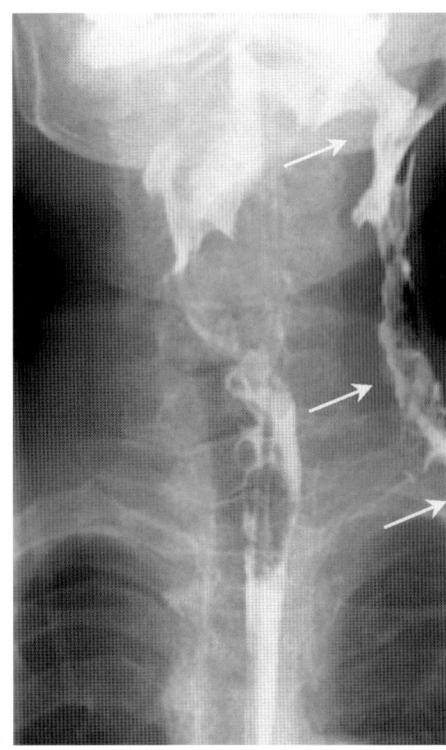

Fig. 12.**85** Postoperative abscess formation two weeks after radical neck dissection and reconstruction with a pectoralis flap. Contrast-enhanced CT at the lower neck level shows a large abscess cavity with air (arrow) deep to the pectoralis flap (PF). Note absence of the internal jugular vein on the left following radical neck dissection.

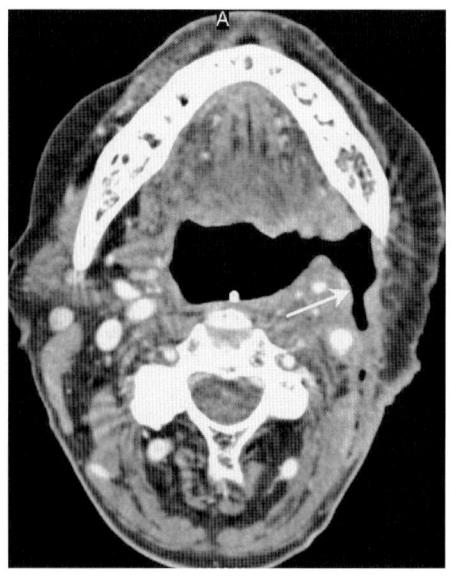

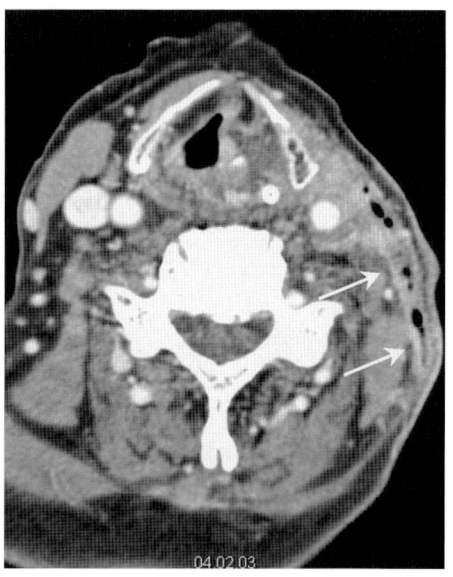

Fig. 12.**86** Postoperative pharyngocutaneous fistula after tonsillectomy and radical neck dissection. **a** Pharyngography performed with water-soluble contrast material 20 days postoperatively shows a large fistula beginning at the level of the left oropharynx and extending along the neck to the supraclavicular fossa (arrows). **b**, **c** Contrast-enhanced CT images obtained in the same patient show a large communication between the oropharynx and the neck dissection site (arrows). Along the neck dissection site a large fluid collection with air inclusions is seen. Note absence of the internal jugular vein on the left, absence of the left sternocleidomastoid muscle, and atrophy of the trapezius muscle following radical neck dissection.

Tumor recurrence in the operated neck is either seen at the site of the primary tumor, within or at the border of a flap or within the neck (within unresected ipsilateral or within contralateral nodes)[142] (Fig. 12.**87**). Most often, however, recurrent tumor is seen at the vascular pedicle. The imaging findings are similar to those of primary tumors with metastatic lymphadenopathy. Tumor recurrence within the flap should be suspected radiologically if a mass with the density or signal intensity characteristics of soft tissue is seen within the flap (Fig. 12.**88**). Tumor recurrence tends to spread along the flap in the craniocaudal direction. Once the altered anatomy has been identified, the diagnosis of tumor recurrence is quite straightforward.

Infectious and Inflammatory Conditions

Infection of the infrahyoid neck is a very common clinical problem occurring in all age groups, especially in children and young adults. The symptoms and signs of neck infections include fever, torticollis, dysphagia, odynophagia, anorexia, dyspnea, a palpable neck mass, diffuse neck swelling, and erythema. Although the clinical symptoms are often suggestive of the diagnosis, CT, MRI, and US (for superficial neck infections) are often used to search for abscesses. Conventional films may still be used as a

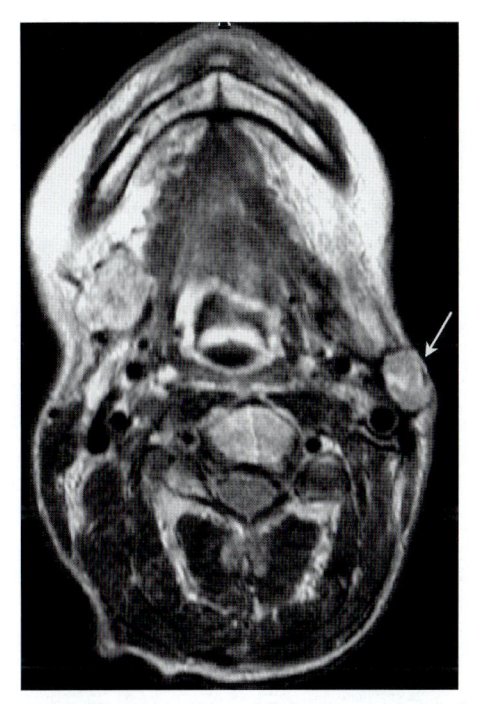

Fig. 12.**87** Recurrent nodal disease one year after radical neck dissection and floor of the mouth surgery in a patient with a floor of the mouth cancer and initial ipsilateral level II and level III lymph node metastases. T2W MR image obtained one year after surgery shows a large metastatic level II lymph node (arrow).

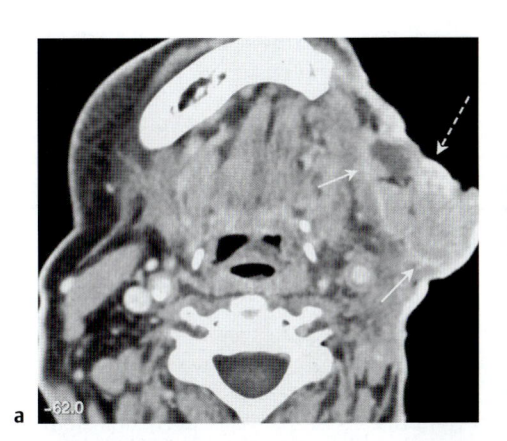

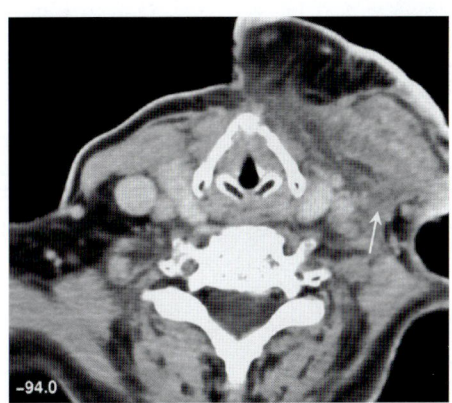

Fig. 12.**88** Tumor recurrence within the pectoralis flap as seen on CT. **a**, **b** Contrast-enhanced CT images obtained two years after buccomandibulectomy, radical neck dissection, and reconstruction with a pectoralis flap in a patient with floor of the mouth tumor and lymph node metastases. A large recurrent tumor is seen within the flap (arrows), extending in craniocaudal direction. The tumor has also invaded the subcutaneous tissue and the skin that covers the flap. Note areas of skin ulceration (dashed arrow).

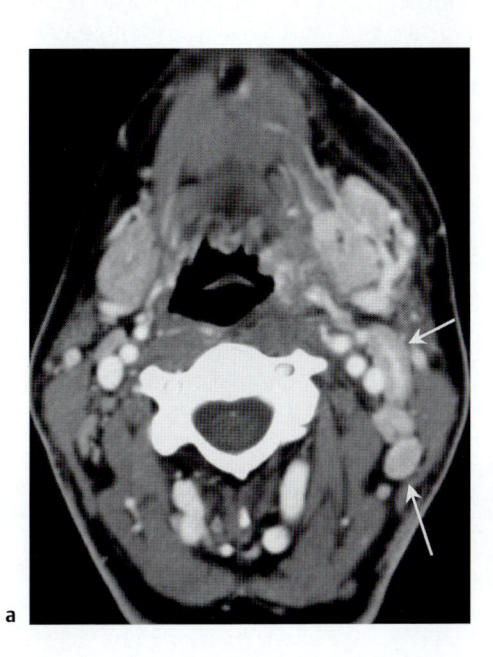

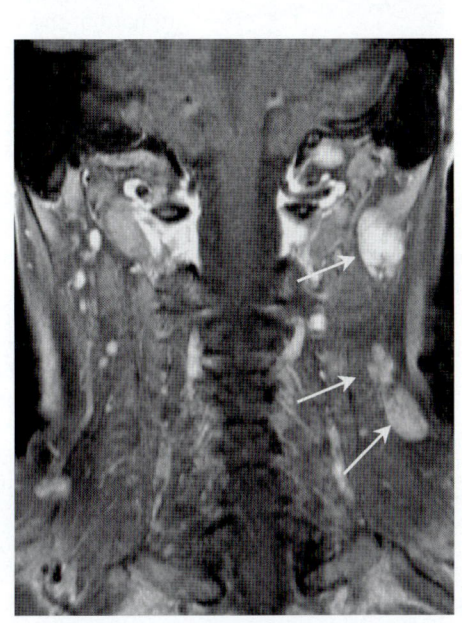

Fig. 12.**89** Reactive lymph nodes as seen on CT and MRI. **a** Axial contrast-enhanced CT through the submandibular glands shows marked enlargement of the left superior internal jugular nodes (level II). The enlarged nodes are homogeneously enhancing and have an elliptical shape.
b Coronal fat-suppressed T1W MR image obtained after injection of contrast material shows marked enlargement of the spinal accessory nodes (level V). The nodes are homogeneously enhancing (arrows) and have an elliptical shape.

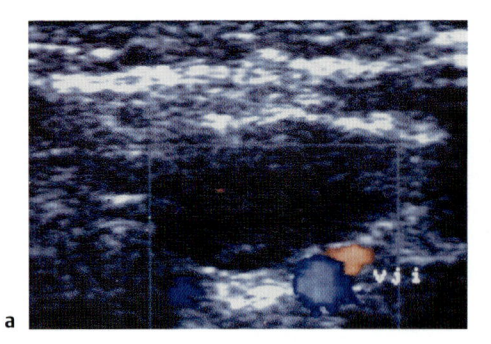

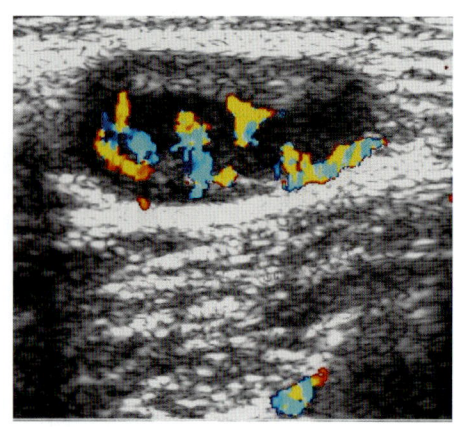

Fig. 12.**90** Reactive nodes as seen on color Doppler US. **a** Longitudinal color Doppler US image shows an oval-shaped enlarged lymph node, with smooth borders, no detectable hilus, and diminished perfusion. **b** Longitudinal color Doppler US image in another patient shows an oval-shaped enlarged lymph node, with smooth borders and increased perfusion running out of the eccentric hilus.

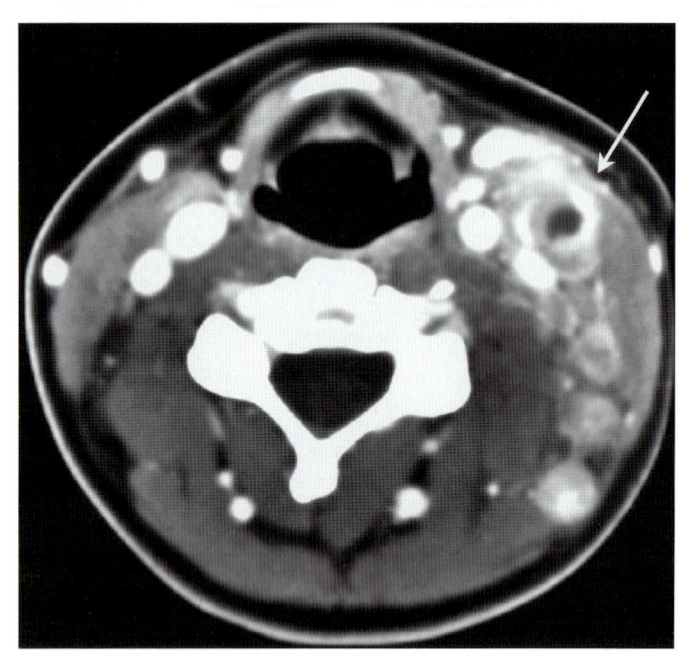

Fig. 12.**91** Suppurative adenopathy seen in a young girl with streptococcal infection. Contrast-enhanced CT shows multiple internal jugular chain nodes (level III) and a spinal accessory (level V) lymph node. An intranodal abscess is seen in one of the nodes (arrow). Note subtle enhancement of the anterior portion of the fascia surrounding the sternocleidomastoid muscle on the left, as well as enhancement of the fatty tissue surrounding the suppurative node.

Inflammatory and infectious lesions of the infrahyoid neck may be classified into three groups: cervical chain nodal inflammation, deep space infection (retropharyngeal), and soft-tissue infections.

Cervical Chain Nodal Inflammation and Infection

Common Viral and Bacterial Diseases

When cervical lymph nodes react to inflammation, they enlarge and are referred to as **reactive adenopathy**. This term is used for nodes less than 1.5 cm in maximum dimension, oval, with homogeneous internal architecture and with variable enhancement on CT or MRI. Nodal enhancement is not a specific finding and it may be seen in a variety of inflammatory and neoplastic diseases (Table 12.**8**). The cause of nonspecific lymphadenitis is often tonsillitis, pharyngitis, and odontogenic infection. The clinical findings reveal a tender neck, fever, elevated white blood cell count, and erythema. The most common bacterial pathogens are streptococcal species, *Staphylococcus aureus*, *Peptostreptococcus*, and *Fusobacterium*.[155] On US, acute nonspecific lymphadenitis presents with enlarged nodes with preserved oval shape and a hypoechoic echostructure. The hilus is not always seen and variable perfusion patterns (diminished to increased perfusion) may be observed on color Doppler US (Fig. 12.**90**). In the subacute inflammation, the nodes tend to become smaller, with preservation of the oval shape, and the internal architecture is less hypoechoic. Finally, in chronic inflammation, the nodes are small, slightly hypoechoic, and with a preserved oval shape.

If there is an acute virulent infection, nodal necrosis may be seen on US, CT or fat-suppressed contrast-enhanced T1-weighted MR images.[11, 54, 86, 118, 127] In this context, nodal necrosis corresponds histologically to an intranodal abscess, and the term **suppurative adenopathy** is used (Fig. 12.**91**). Suppurative adenopathy and malignant adenopathy can be radiologically indistinguishable. Extracapsular spread of infection from the suppurative lymph nodes results in abscess formation. If the internal jugular chain (levels II–IV) is primarily affected, the resulting abscess is located within the carotid space, whereas, if the spinal accessory chain (level V) is primarily involved, the abscess is located within the posterior cervical space. An abscess appears as a single or multiloculated area of fluid density with or without gas collections, usually expands the compartment that is involved, and typically demonstrates a peripheral rim enhancement. The abscess wall is usually thick (Fig. 12.**92**).

preliminary survey in cases with suspected retropharyngeal phlegmon or abscess. For practical reasons (quick availability, high diagnostic performance), CT is still the modality of choice in evaluating inflammatory and infectious diseases of the infrahyoid neck, although it has recently been shown that MRI is superior to CT in the initial evaluation of acute infections of the neck with regard to lesion conspicuity, number of anatomical spaces involved, extension, and source of origin of the infectious process.[98] For practical and logistic reasons, MR imaging is currently still reserved for selected patients with inflammatory lesions in whom the use of iodinated contrast material must be limited or is contraindicated. The role of imaging in neck infections consists in (1) precisely localizing the infectious process, (2) searching for and delineating an abscess, and (3) detecting complications, such as septic internal jugular vein thrombosis with or without distant embolism, arterial rupture, skull base and cervical spine involvement, mediastinitis, and pleural empyema.

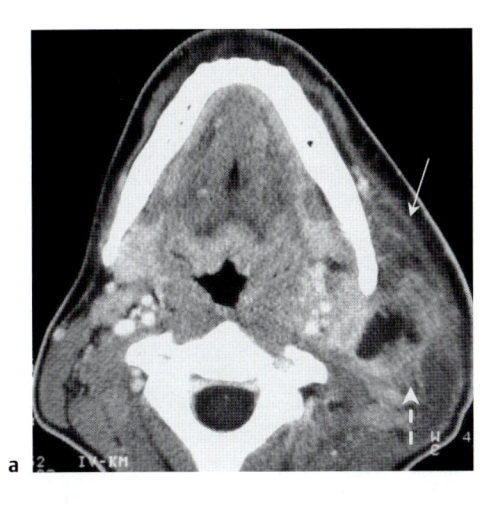

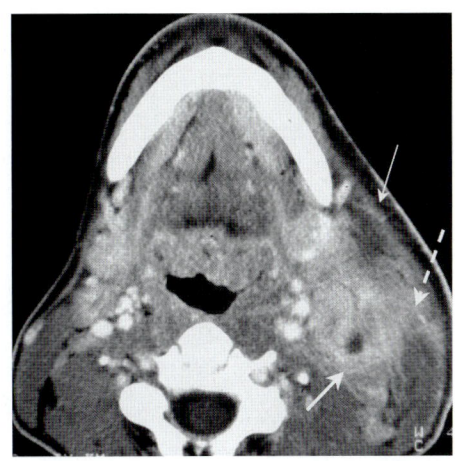

Fig. 12.**92** Lateral neck abscess. Characteristic CT appearance. **a**, **b** Contrast-enhanced CT images show a large abscess with irregular peripheral rim enhancement (arrows), marked enhancement of the sternocleidomastoid muscle (myositis, dashed arrows), and enhancement of the subcutaneous fat (cellulitis, thin arrows). Surgical drainage revealed staphylococci.

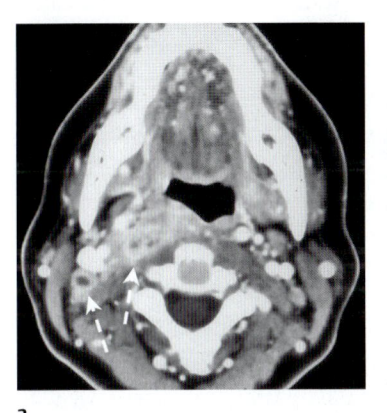

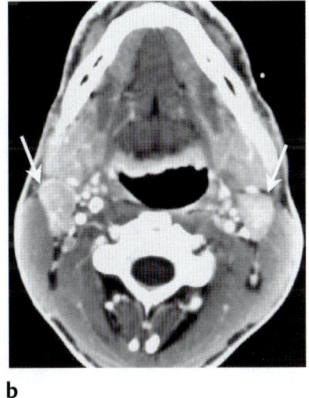

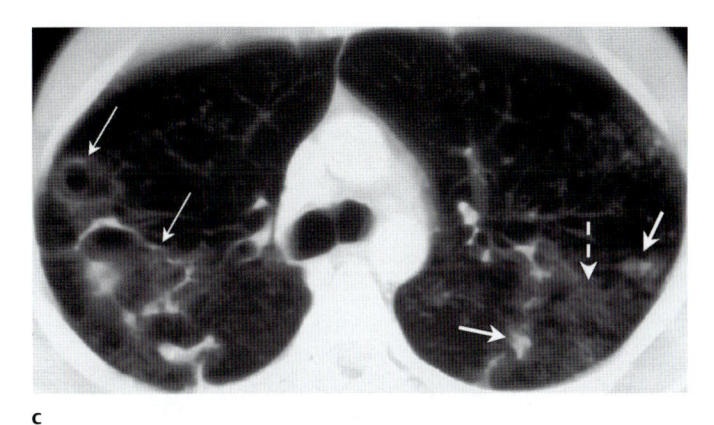

Fig. 12.**93** Tuberculosis with cervical nodal and pulmonary involvement. **a**, **b** Contrast-enhanced CT images obtained in a young female patient show bilateral enlarged jugulodigastric (level II) lymph nodes (arrows) with homogeneous enhancement and right-sided retropharyngeal and upper jugular (level II) lymph nodes with central nodal necrosis (dashed arrows). No nodal calcification was seen in this patient. **c** CT image at the level of the upper lung lobes (lung window setting) shows multiple lung cavities (thin arrows), granulomas (thick arrows), and alveolar opacities (dashed arrow) characteristic of tuberculosis.

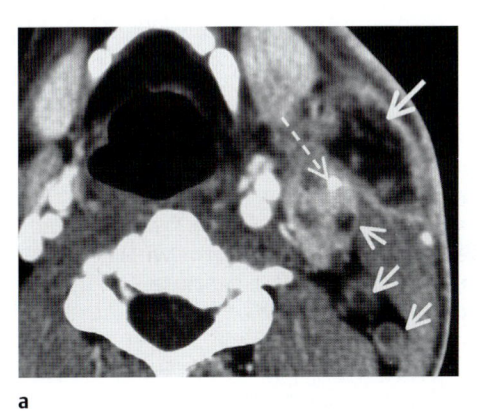

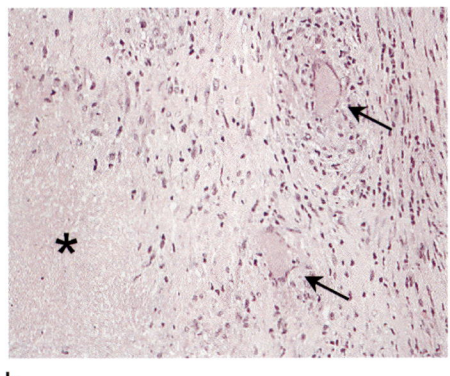

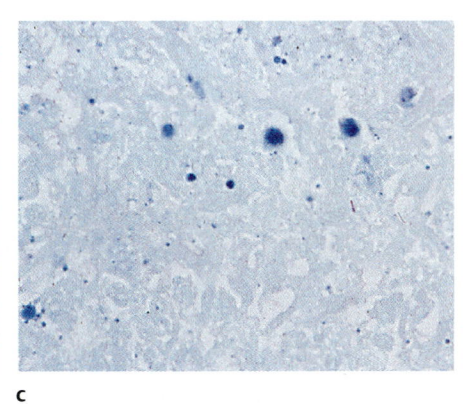

Fig. 12.**94** Tuberculous lymphadenitis. Characteristic CT and histological appearance. **a** Axial contrast-enhanced CT image demonstrates multiple lymph nodes with inhomogeneous contrast enhancement, areas of nodal necrosis (small arrows), and calcifications (dashed arrow). Extracapsular spread of infection from the affected lymph nodes has resulted in abscess formation (large arrow). **b** Photomicrograph (hematoxylin–eosin stain) of a tuberculous lymph node obtained by excisional biopsy demonstrates caseous necrosis (asterisk) surrounded by an inflammatory stroma containing fibrous tissue, epithelioid cells, and Langhans giant cells (arrows). **c** Ziehl–Neelsen stain demonstrates tuberculous mycobacteria. Reproduced with permission from Reference 11.

Tuberculosis and Atypical Mycobacteria

Mycobacterial infections are divided into tuberculosis caused by *Mycobacterium tuberculosis* and nontuberculous infection caused by all mycobacterial species other than *M. tuberculosis*. Tuberculous adenitis occurs when mycobacteria involve the nodes of the infrahyoid neck chains. The internal jugular nodes and the posterior triangle nodes are the most often affected nodes.[48,93,118] In the beginning, the nodes are enlarged and they display homogeneous enhancement. In the subacute phase, a small area of central nodal necrosis is seen, which corresponds to an intranodal abscess. Fibrocalcific changes occur in the chronic phase or after treatment. Tuberculous nodes may, therefore, have a variable but characteristic CT appearance: they are multiple in presentation, with variable enhancement, areas of central nodal necrosis, and globular calcifications (Figs. 12.**93**, 12.**94**). Although

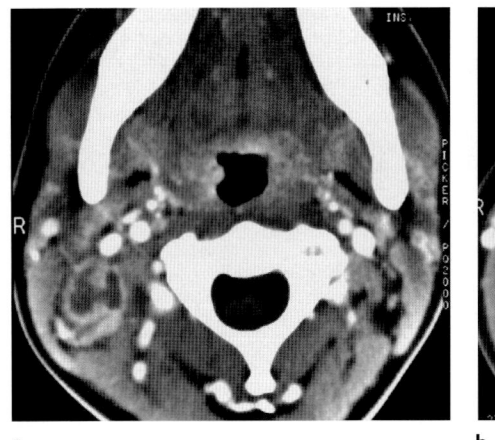

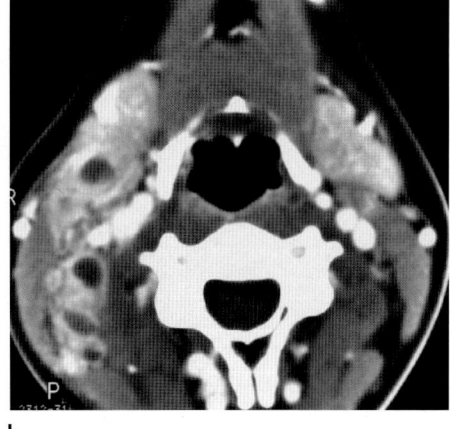

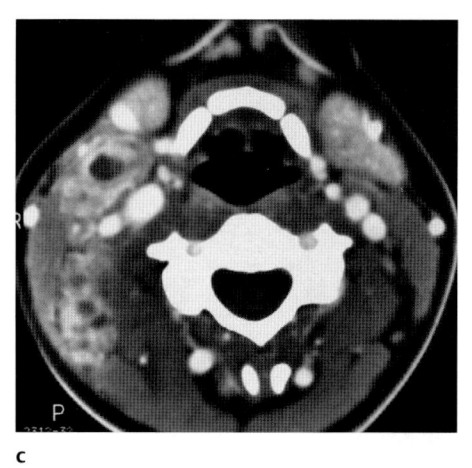

Fig. 12.95 Cat-scratch disease in a young man who had been exposed to a kitten. The bartonella titer was positive for *Bartonella henselae*. Contrast-enhanced CT images at the level of the tonsillar fossae (**a**), anterior belly of the digastric muscles (**b**), and body of the hyoid bone (**c**) show multiple upper internal jugular lymph nodes and spinal accessory lymph nodes (levels II and V) on the right with ring enhancement and areas of central nodal necrosis. Some associated perinodal inflammation is also seen.

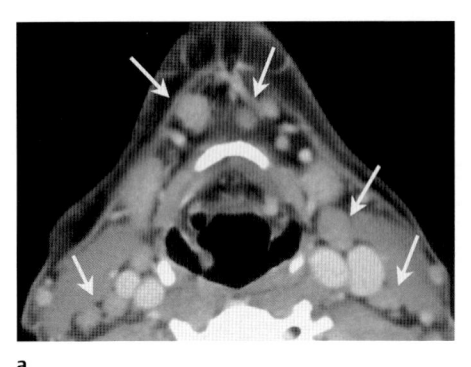

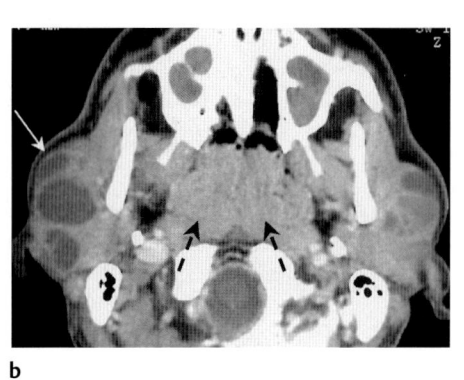

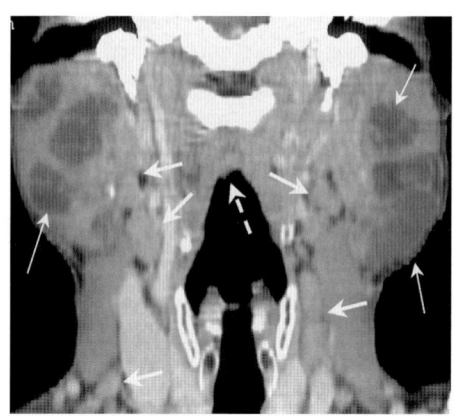

Fig. 12.96 HIV infection with nodal and parotid gland involvement. Characteristic imaging findings. Contrast-enhanced CT images obtained in a young man with enlarged lymph nodes at clinical examination. Axial CT images at the level of the infrahyoid neck (**a**) and suprahyoid neck (**b**), and coronal 2D reconstruction from the volumetric data set (**c**) show multiple enlarged, homogeneously enhancing nodes (arrows), enlarged adenoid tissue (dashed arrows), and bilateral lymphoepithelial cysts in the parotid glands (thin arrows), strongly suggesting HIV infection. Blood tests confirmed HIV infection.

nodal calcifications are most commonly seen in cervical tuberculous adenitis, metastatic thyroid carcinoma, healed irradiated carcinomatous and lymphomatous nodes, and healed necrotic abscessed nodes may also calcify. Egg-shell type calcifications are typically seen in silicosis, sarcoidosis, tuberculosis, and amyloidosis (see Table 12.7).

Nontuberculous mycobacterial infection is the most common cause of a granulomatous disease in children.[116] It is caused by *M. avium intracellulare*, *M. bovis*, *M. scrofulaceum*, and *M. kansasii*. Peak age of presentation is between 2 and 4 years. Clinically, the children present with slowly enlarging nodes and fever, and other signs of infection are usually absent. A delay in diagnosis is common as suppurative bacterial adenitis is suspected and standard antibiotic treatment fails. The nodes typically progress to liquefaction followed by spontaneous drainage into the skin. The imaging findings are similar to those of tuberculosis.[116]

Cat-Scratch Disease

Cat-scratch disease is a relatively common granulomatous disease that may affect children or young adults. It is caused by *Bartonella henselae*, a Gram-negative bacillus. The cat is probably the healthy vector of the disease. The disease may develop after scratches caused by cats, dogs, rabbits, wooden splinters, and fish bones. Following inoculation, an erythematous papule or vesicle forms, which either heals within one week or persists for several months. Several weeks following inoculation, head and neck adenopathy develops in as many as 30% of cases. The enlarged lymph nodes may resolve within a few weeks or may persist up to two years. Some patients develop nodal suppuration that requires surgical treatment. Contrast-enhanced CT and MRI demonstrate enlarged lymph nodes with surrounding edema, as well as areas of central nodal necrosis (Fig. 12.95).

HIV Nodes

In HIV infection, bilateral diffuse lymph node enlargement may be seen on either CT or MRI. This imaging finding is nonspecific and may be observed in a variety of viral infections, such as Epstein–Barr virus and cytomegalovirus.[147] However, in the presence of lymphoepithelial cysts within the parotid glands and large adenoid tissue, HIV infection should be strongly suggested (Fig. 12.96).

Sarcoidosis

Sarcoidosis is a noncaseating granulomatous disease of unknown cause. The most common manifestations in the head and neck include parotid gland involvement, facial nerve palsy, occular involvement, lacrimal gland involvement, and cervical lymph

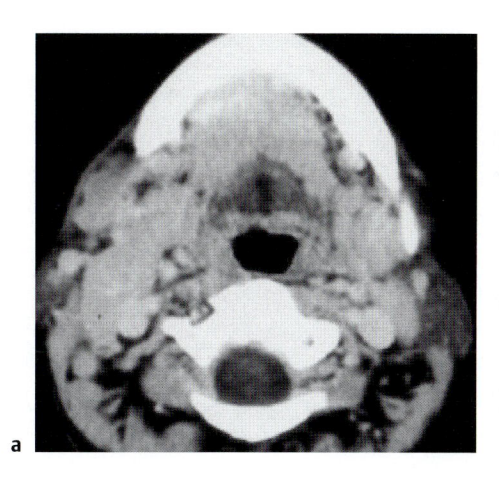

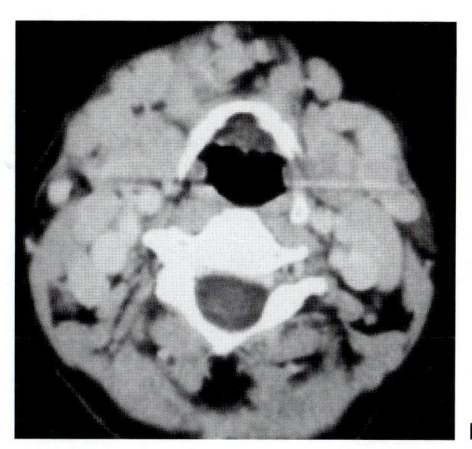

Fig. 12.**97** Castleman disease. **a**, **b** Contrast-enhanced CT images obtained in a young man with multiple palpable lymph nodes show numerous enlarged, homogeneously enhancing lymph nodes. Excisional biopsy of submandibular nodes revealed angiofollicular hyperplasia, or Castleman disease. Courtesy of Dr. Fernando Torrhina (Imagens Medicas Integradas, Lisbon, Portugal).

nodes.[116] Cervical adenopathy is most often bilateral with mobile nontender nodes.[118,127] On CT, enlarged nodes appear homogeneous, with sharp margins and a "foamy" aspect, and calcifications appear to be related to the duration of disease. When the parotid glands are affected, either diffuse enlargement without sialectasis or involvement of the intraparotid nodes may occur. Although the imaging findings are nonspecific, the association between enlarged parotid glands and bilateral enlarged cervical nodes with or without pulmonary involvement should strongly suggest the diagnosis of sarcoidosis.

Other Inflammatory Conditions

Other inflammatory conditions affecting the cervical lymph nodes include Castleman disease, Kawasaki disease, Kimura disease, Kikuchi–Fuchimoto disease, and Rosai–Dorfman disease.

Castleman disease (also called angiofollicular hyperplasia) is a nodal disease that can be seen in the chest (70%) and less commonly in the neck (10%). It typically affects young males less than 30 years old. The patients are usually asymptomatic apart from palpable neck masses. On CT and MRI, the enlarged non-necrotic lymph nodes show massive enhancement after intravenous administration of contrast material[34] (Fig. 12.**97**). Calcifications may be seen occasionally (Tables 12.**7** and 12.**8**).

Kawasaki disease is an acute systemic inflammatory disease that occurs in children less than 10 years of age. The etiology of the disorder is unknown, but the condition probably has an infectious cause. Diagnosis is based upon clinicians' recognition of a symptom pattern that includes high fever, oral cavity changes, polymorphous rash, conjunctival injection, and unilateral or bilateral cervical adenopathy. Most feared are the cardiac manifestations of Kawasaki disease, which result in an overall mortality rate of 2%. On CT and MRI, enlarged reactive lymph nodes may be seen in 50–70% of cases.

Kimura disease is an inflammatory disease that occurs in Asian men in their second to third decades. Cervical lymphadenopathy, peripheral eosinophilia, and elevated serum IgE are characteristic. On CT there is marked enhancement of enlarged lymph nodes and on MRI an increased signal intensity is seen on T1-weighted images associated with variable signal intensities on T2-weighted images (see Chapter 9).[129]

Kikuchi disease is an inflammatory disease characterized by cervical lymphadenopathy, fever, flulike symptoms, and leukopenia. It is typically seen in women in their third decade of life. Generalized adenopathy and hepatosplenomegaly have been reported.

Rosai–Dorfman disease (sinus histiocytosis with massive lymphadenopathy) is a benign histiocytic proliferation occurring most commonly in the first two decades of life. In more than 90% of cases, there is massive, painless enlargement of cervical nodes. Extranodal manifestations are seen in 20–30% of patients and include involvement of the orbit and salivary glands. Large nonspecific lymph nodes are seen on CT and MRI.

■ Infection of the Retropharyngeal Space

As mentioned previously in this chapter, the retropharyngeal space may be divided into a "true" retropharyngeal space (located anteriorly to the alar fascia) and a danger space (located posteriorly to the alar fascia).[54] Because the alar fascia cannot be identified with current imaging, the "true" anterior retropharyngeal space and the danger space will be discussed together in the following. They will be referred to as the "retropharyngeal space."

Retropharyngeal space infection includes cellulitis and abscess. It occurs most commonly in children. Fifty percent of all retropharyngeal space infections are seen in babies 6–12 months of age, and 96% of infections are seen in children younger than 6 years of age. Although less common, retropharyngeal space infection may also be seen in adults.[20,68] Retropharyngeal space infection is most often caused by bacterial infection from the pharynx, nose, and paranasal sinuses. In addition, retropharyngeal space infection is the consequence of suppurative adenitis of the retropharyngeal lymph nodes or it may evolve from direct penetrating trauma (foreign body, endoscopy, intubation). Over the past 15 years, a dramatic increase in retropharyngeal space infection has been observed, this increase being congruent with the increase in culture-positive group A beta-hemolytic streptococcal abscesses.[18,20,135,154] Patients with retropharyngeal space infection typically present with fever, difficulty in breathing and swallowing, drooling, and cervical adenopathy.

Lateral neck films may be used in the initial assessment of a patient with suspected retropharyngeal space infection. The normal prevertebral soft tissues should not exceed 7 mm at the level of C2 for both children and adults, and 22 mm (14 mm for children) at the level of C6.[20,154] Lateral neck films may also demonstrate the presence of air within the retropharyngeal space. Currently, CT is used routinely for the assessment of patients with suspected retropharyngeal space infection. One of the major indications for CT is to differentiate between cellulitis, which may be treated with antibiotics alone, and abscess, which may require surgical intervention.[71] On CT, cellulitis is seen as widening of the retropharyngeal space with low-density areas, "dirty fat" appearance, and no major ring enhancement around the abnormal area (Fig. 12.**98**). An abscess is seen as widening of the retro-

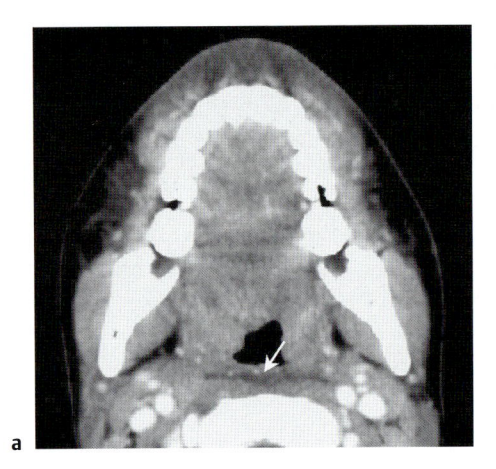

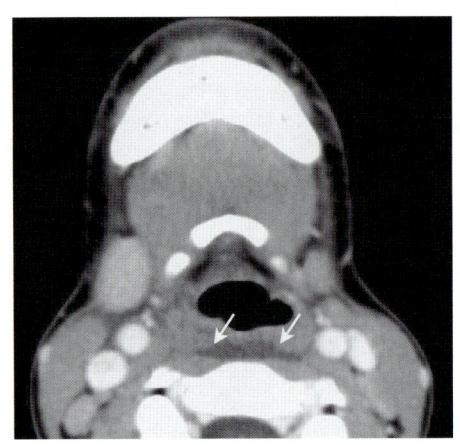

Fig. 12.98 Retropharyngeal cellulitis in a 3-year-old boy with streptococcal angina, dysphagia, and cervical adenopathy. Contrast-enhanced CT images at the level of the oropharynx (**a**) and supraglottic larynx (**b**) show widening of the retropharyngeal space (arrows), increased attenuation of the retropharyngeal fat, and no major irregular ring enhancement. The boy was treated with antibiotics and recovered uneventfully.

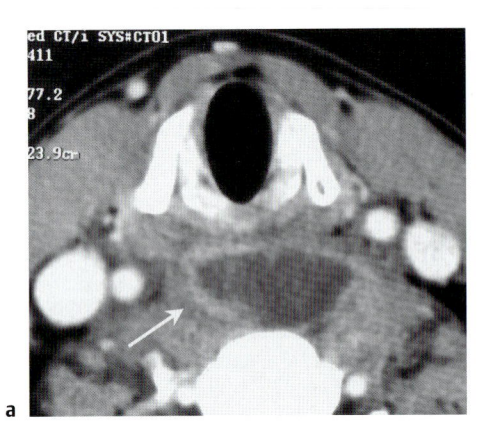

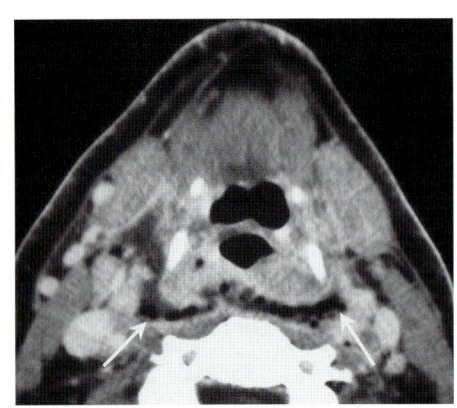

Fig. 12.99 Retropharyngeal abscess. Characteristic CT aspect in two different patients. **a** Contrast-enhanced CT image at the level of the subglottis in a patient with bacterial pharyngitis shows widening of the retropharyngeal space by an abscess with irregular, contrast-enhancing walls. Surgery confirmed a retropharyngeal abscess caused by group A beta-hemolytic streptococci. **b** Contrast-enhanced CT image at the level of the suprahyoid epiglottis obtained in a diabetic patient shows a retropharyngeal abscess with air inclusions suggesting anaerobic pathogens as the causative agents. Surgery confirmed an abscess caused by *Pseudomonas aeruginosa*.

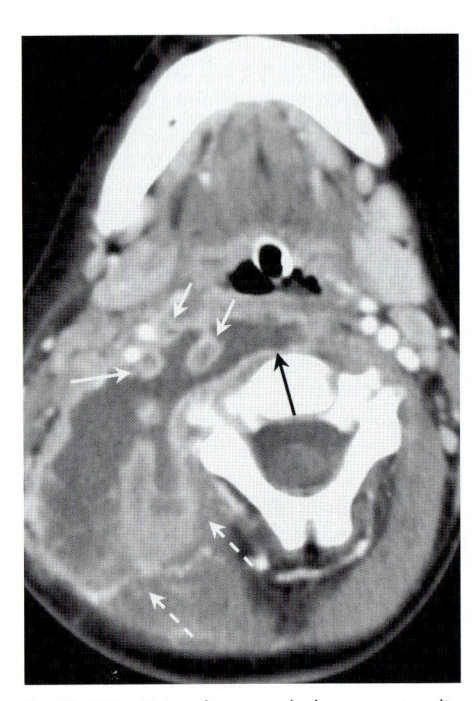

Fig. 12.100 Retropharyngeal abscess extending into adjacent spaces. Axial contrast-enhanced CT image obtained in an intubated 4-year-old boy who presented in the emergency room with major dyspnea, dysphagia, and right-sided neck swelling. A large retropharyngeal abscess (black arrow) is seen extending into the prevertebral space (dashed arrows). White arrows point to enlarged retropharyngeal lymph nodes. Surgery confirmed the findings. The cause of the retropharyngeal abscess was most probably suppurative adenopathy.

pharyngeal space with low-density areas (with or without air-inclusions) and major irregular or ring enhancement around the abnormal area (Fig. 12.**99**). Differentiation between cellulitis and abscess is not always possible on CT. According to recent studies, CT has an accuracy of 74–92% in differentiating between retropharyngeal abscess and cellulitis/phlegmon.[20,137] The reported sensitivity of CT to differentiate between retropharyngeal abscess and cellulitis is 85% and the corresponding specificity is 88%.[137] Irregularity of the abscess wall is a stronger predictor of the presence of pus than the presence of ring enhancement. It has therefore been suggested that clinical findings, as well as radiological findings, should be considered together prior to surgical drainage of a suspected retropharyngeal abscess.[20,137] Most retropharyngeal abscesses are drained by an intraoral approach unless there is lateral spread into the neck.

A common finding in children with retropharyngeal space infection is narrowing of the ipsilateral internal carotid artery (ICA). Despite dramatic narrowing of the ICA ipsilateral to retropharyngeal lymphadenitis and abscess, children do not have neurological deficits, suggesting that such narrowing is a common, benign, and, most likely, incidental imaging finding.

The differential diagnosis of a retropharyngeal abscess is limited and includes: an infected third branchial cleft cyst (see below), Kawasaki disease, tuberculosis, and Epstein–Barr virus infection.[61,63,140]

Complications of retropharyngeal abscesses include spread into adjacent neck spaces, atlantoaxial subluxation, cervical spinal epidural abscesses, septic jugular vein thrombosis, carotid artery rupture, and mediastinitis or osteomyelitis of the cervical bodies (Figs. 12.**100**, 12.**101**). Atlantoaxial subluxation has been well described in children, while it is rare in adults. The mecha-

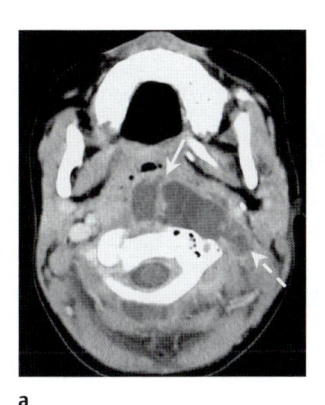

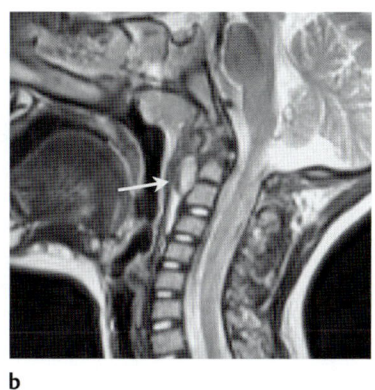

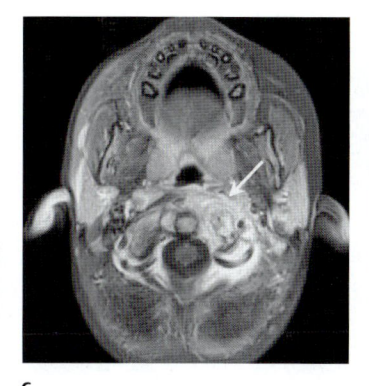

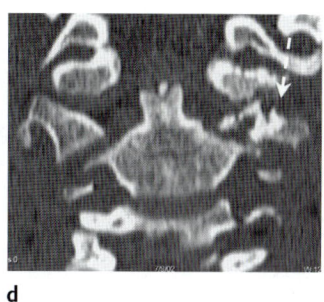

Fig. 12.101 Retropharyngeal abscess complicated by cervical osteomyelitis. **a** Initial axial contrast-enhanced CT and **b** sagittal T2W MR images obtained in an immunocompetent 6-year-old boy presenting with a retropharyngeal abscess (arrows) following pharyngeal infection. The abscess is causing major pharyngeal obstruction and already extends laterally into the posterior cervical space (dashed arrow in **a**). The sagittal MR image shows that at this point the cervical vertebrae are normal. The patient underwent surgical drainage, which confirmed retropharyngeal abscess caused by staphylococci. **c** Axial fat-suppressed contrast-enhanced CT image and **d** coronal 2D reconstruction from volumetric data set obtained two weeks after surgical drainage show enhancement of the left lateral portion of C1 (arrow), as well as fragmentation and osseous collapse (dashed arrow), suggesting osteomyelitis of C1. Repeat surgical exploration confirmed the findings.

nism of subluxation is attributed to softening of the atlantoaxial ligament, allowing greater mobility at the joint.[94] Cervical epidural abscesses are seen as a complication of retropharyngeal abscess in both immunocompetent and immunodeficient patients. *Staphylococcus aureus* is the most common pathogen.[109] Symptoms are caused by sheer mass effect and/or septic thrombophlebitis with cord edema and infarction. MRI is essential for the diagnosis of this complication as well as to monitor therapeutic results. The epidural abscess has a low signal intensity compared to normal spinal cord on T1-weighted images and a high signal intensity on T2-weighted images. After injection of contrast material, three patterns of enhancement may be observed: a homogeneous enhancement pattern, a peripheral enhancement pattern, and a combination of the two. The homogeneous enhancement pattern corresponds to phlegmonous granulation tissue and the peripheral enhancement pattern corresponds to frank abscess formation.

■ Bacterial Soft-Tissue Infections

Bacterial soft-tissue infections may be classified, according to their invasive behavior, as (1) erysipelas (affecting the more superficial layers of the skin and cutaneous lymphatics); (2) cellulitis (extending more deeply into the subcutaneous tissue but sparing fasciae); (3) necrotizing fasciitis (destruction of fasciae and fat, with or without skin necrosis, and with or without myonecrosis); and (4) myositis and myonecrosis.[67, 133, 143] The different forms of infectious soft-tissue inflammation defined above have particular features on CT. Cellulitis is characterized by thickening of the cutis and subcutis and increased density of fatty tissue with streaky, irregular enhancement and without fluid collections (Fig. 12.**102**). Fasciitis appears as thickening or enhancement of fasciae. While the superficial cervical fascia is routinely visible on CT, the three layers of the deep cervical fascia, as well as the fasciae surrounding individual muscle groups, are usually too thin to be visualized on CT and show no significant enhancement after administration of intravenous contrast material. Myositis appears as thickening of cervical muscles or muscle groups with or without inhomogeneous enhancement, and myonecrosis may become visible as a hypodense area within enhancing portions of a muscle or as frank muscle disruption. Any significant enhancement of portions of muscles must be considered pathological on CT because the en-

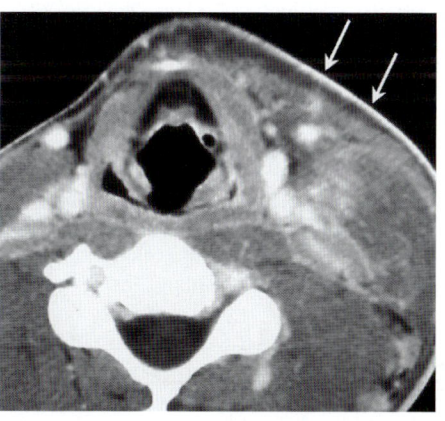

Fig. 12.102 Cellulitis and myositis after minor skin injury. Contrast-enhanced CT shows cellulitis of the left anterolateral neck (arrows), as well as enhancement of the sternocleidomastoid muscle on the left, suggesting myositis. The left platysma muscle is also thickened. Note for comparison the normal right sternocleidomastoid muscle, the normal right platysma, and the normal right anterolateral neck fat. Reactive adenopathies are also present.

hancement of normal muscular tissue does not become visible on postcontrast CT. An abscess appears as a single or multiloculated area of fluid density with or without gas collections, usually expands the compartment that is involved, and typically demonstrates a peripheral rim enhancement.

Necrotizing fasciitis of the head and neck is a severe, acute, and potentially life-threatening streptococcal or mixed bacterial soft tissue infection with a very rapid clinical evolution.[10, 49, 135] It affects both immunocompetent and immunocompromised patients and, unless immediate surgical treatment is given, leads invariably to mediastinitis and fatal sepsis. Among the commonest causes are odontogenic, tonsillar, and pharyngeal infections; less common causes include surgery and radiation therapy.[13, 38, 47, 49, 114] In the past, necrotizing fasciitis has been described by various synonymous terms, each addressing a different aspect of the disease, namely, nonclostridial gangrene, synergistic necrotizing cellulitis, acute hemolytic streptococcal gangrene, and other terms. Since the first description during the American Civil War, necrotizing fasciitis has been reported only sporadically, but a dramatic increase has been observed recently.

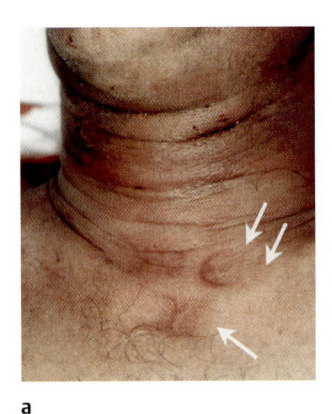

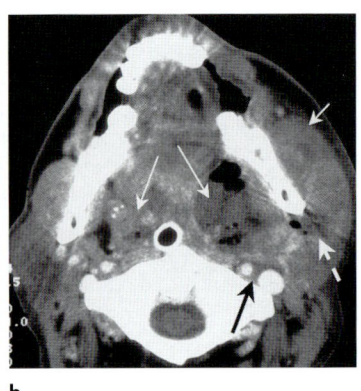

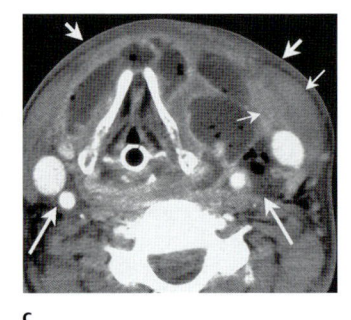

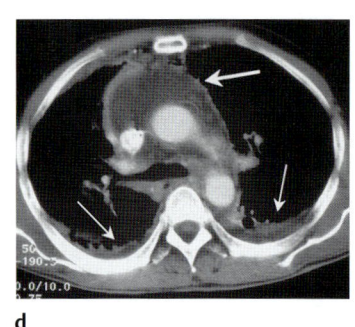

Fig. 12.**103** Necrotizing fasciitis of the neck caused by anaerobes. Characteristic CT appearance in a 58-year-old man with a history of dental treatment seven days earlier, presenting with fever and bilateral erythema of the neck with swelling and induration. Dyspnea necessitated intubation and mechanical ventilation at admission. Photograph of the neck at admission obtained prior to intubation (**a**) shows diffuse neck erythema and edema indicated by thumb prints (arrowheads). Contrast-enhanced CT images at the level of the oropharynx (**b**), supraglottic larynx (**c**), and tracheal bifurcation (**d**) in the intubated patient show diffuse thickening of the cutis and subcutaneous fat, which has increased density (short arrows). There is enhancement of the superficial layer of the deep cervical fascia along the left masticatory space and left sternocleidomastoid muscle (thin short arrows). Enhancement and inflammatory swelling of the left masseter muscle (in **b**) and left sternocleidomastoid muscle (in **c**) indicate myositis. Extensive fluid collections with gas within the strap muscles correspond with myonecrosis (**c**). Multiple fluid collections with gas are seen in both parapharyngeal spaces (long arrows in **b**), left masticator space (dashed arrow in **b**), and both carotid spaces (long thick arrows in **b** and **c**). A large fluid collection is seen in the anterior mediastinum (thick arrows in **d**) and there are bilateral pleural effusions (thin arrows). Cervicotomy and thoracotomy performed immediately after CT revealed necrotizing fasciitis and necrotizing mediastinitis. Reproduced from Reference 13 with permission.

Aerobic microorganisms, especially group A beta-hemolytic *Streptococcus* and *Staphylococcus* were long considered the primary pathogens in necrotizing fasciitis. However, most cases of necrotizing fasciitis represent mixed or synergistic infections involving both aerobes and anaerobes, and the fulminant nature of the process has been attributed to a symbiotic relationship between these organisms. Bacterial enzymes and pyrogenic exotoxins are not only responsible for early systemic toxicity but also favor disintegration of collagenous structures and muscle necrosis. Based on a review of the literature, the cumulative mortality rate of necrotizing fasciitis is estimated at about 25%.[13]

Although the clinical diagnosis of necrotizing fasciitis is straightforward at an advanced stage (diffuse swelling, erythema, vesicle formation, cutaneous gangrene, and systemic symptoms including septic shock and organ failure), it may be very difficult to differentiate cellulitis and necrotizing fasciitis at initial presentation.[13] The distinction is crucial, however, because cellulitis responds to antibiotic treatment alone, whereas survival of patients with necrotizing fasciitis depends on early extensive surgical drainage and debridement in addition to antibiotic therapy, fluid management, and blood pressure support with vasopressors. Owing to this uncertainty in clinical diagnosis, appropriate treatment may be considerably delayed. The use of CT or MRI has therefore been advocated to locate the site and depth of infection.[13]

A combination of cellulitis, fasciitis, myositis, and fluid collections is typically found in necrotizing fasciitis (Figs. 12.**103** and 12.**104**). CT signs of cellulitis are extensive and are usually seen in the entire anterior neck. CT signs of fasciitis are seen both in the superficial and deep cervical fascia. Among the three layers of the deep cervical fascia, the superficial layer is most commonly involved. The common involvement of the deep fascial layers on initial CT may indicate that necrotizing fasciitis is not primarily limited to the superficial musculoaponeurotic system, as suggested by some authors[82,114,133], but shows an infiltrating behavior from the beginning. A possible explanation for primary involvement of the superficial musculoaponeurotic system and deep cervical fascia lies in the lack of vascularity, which may favor the subcutaneous propagation of bacterial infection, particularly due to anaerobes. CT signs of myositis or myonecrosis are most commonly seen in the platysma, the sternocleidomastoid muscles, and the strap muscles. Myositis of these particular muscles may be explained by the predominant involvement of their surrounding fascia, namely, the superficial cervical fascia and the superficial (investing) layer of the deep cervical fascia. Fluid collections seen in necrotizing fasciitis always involve multiple (at least four) neck spaces and do not respect the cervical fascial compartments.[13] Histologically, they most often correspond to liquefied necrotic tissue rather than true abscesses. Additional signs may be found in one-half or fewer of patients with cervical necrotizing fasciitis on the initial CT examination, namely, gas collections, streaky enhancement of mediastinal fat and mediastinal fluid collections, and pleural and pericardial effusions. Extensive gas collections have been considered as a hallmark of necrotizing fasciitis by authors of isolated case reports. However, in a recent series, it has been shown that nearly 40% of patients with necrotizing fasciitis display no gas collections on CT at all.[13] This observation may be explained by the bacteriology, since macroscopic gas collections are found only in the presence of widespread anaerobic infection.

Half of patients with necrotizing fasciitis may present initially with necrotizing mediastinitis, although this may not be suspected clinically (Fig. 12.**103**). In addition, as many as one-third of patients with necrotizing fasciitis present initially with extensive pericardial or pleural effusions. The development of thoracic complications in necrotizing fasciitis may be explained by cervical fascial anatomy. Propagation of pharyngeal infections into the mediastinum occurs predominantly via the carotid space, retropharyngeal space, and prevertebral space.[138] The middle layer of the deep cervical fascia fuses with the parietal pericardium at the level of the tracheal bifurcation, and also closely adheres laterally to the mediastinal pleura. This anatomical relationship may explain not only necrotizing mediastinitis but also involvement of the fascia of the chest wall and of the pericardial and pleural cavity with pleural effusion or empyema.[13,138]

Results of recent studies emphasize the usefulness of follow-up CT scans after initial surgical treatment of necrotizing fasciitis, since further treatment may be guided by means of CT. The identification of persistent fluid collections or progressing infection

Infectious and Inflammatory Conditions

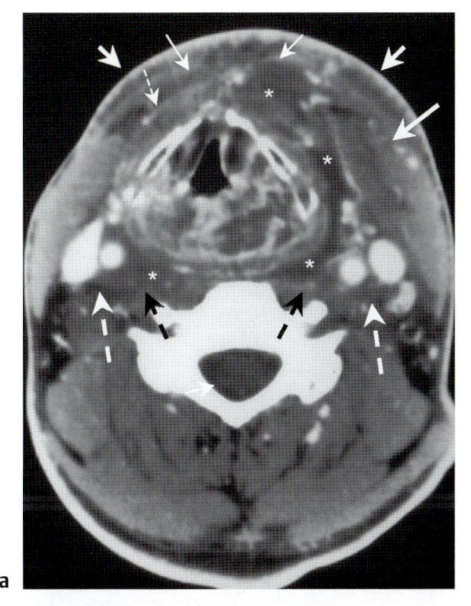

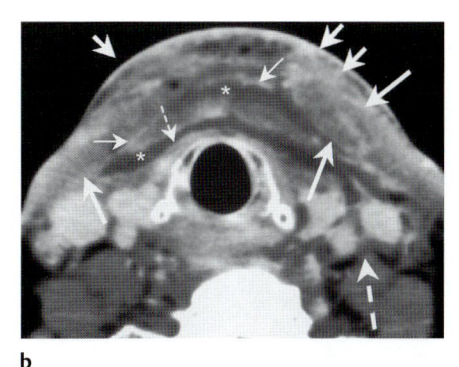

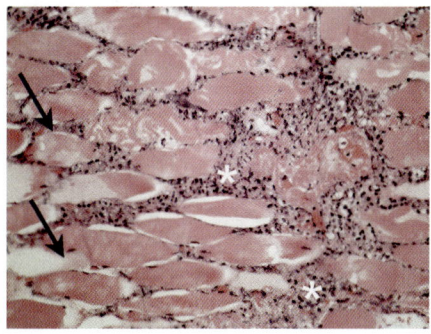

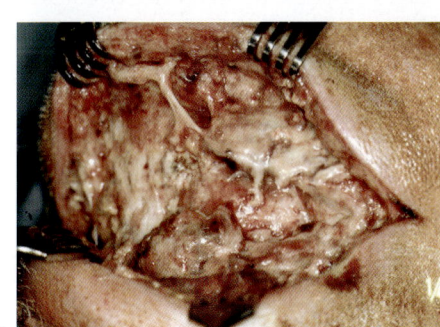

Fig. 12.104 Necrotizing fasciitis of the neck. Characteristic CT, surgical, and histological findings in a 54-year-old man treated for tonsillitis three days earlier, presenting with dysphagia and diffuse, noncrepitant neck swelling without erythema or fever. **a, b** Contrast-enhanced CT images at the level of the supraglottis (**a**) and subglottis (**b**) show diffuse, massive thickening of the skin (short arrows) and there is marked edema and a "dirty" appearance of the subcutaneous fat and platysma. Note enhancement of the investing fascia along the sternocleidomastoid muscles (long white arrows) and strap muscles (short thin white arrows), and enhancement of visceral fascia (short thin dashed arrows) and of the prevertebral fascia (black dashed arrows). Multiple fluid collections are seen along the inner border of the left sternocleidomastoid muscle, within the retropharyngeal space and along the strap muscles (asterisks). Note also inflammatory involvement of the left and right carotid space (long white dashed arrows) and marked myositis of the left sternocleidomastoid muscle with diffuse swelling and irregular contrast enhancement. There is extensive inflammatory edema of the aryepiglottic folds. **c** Photograph of the neck as seen during surgery shows pus covering all fascia and neck muscles, which show diffuse swelling and diminished perfusion. Microscopic evaluation of surgical biopsy specimen of various muscles, subcutaneous fat, and fascial layers revealed cervical necrotizing fasciitis. **d** Microphotograph of a biopsy specimen from the strap muscles (hematoxylin–eosin stain) shows fragmentation of muscle fibers (arrows) and severe inflammatory infiltrates with polymorphonuclear leukocytes and plasma cells between necrotic muscle fibers (asterisks). Reproduced from Reference 13 with permission.

may only be possible with this modality, and findings on cervicothoracic CT often guide further treatment.

The characteristic histological features of cervical necrotizing fasciitis include infiltration of the deep dermis, fasciae, and muscular planes with bacteria and polymorphonuclear cells, and necrosis of fatty and muscular tissue with fragmentation and secondary degeneration of muscle fibers. Necrosis of fasciae is a characteristic feature (Fig. 12.**104**). Vasculitis and thrombosis of small vessels are seen histologically not only in areas that are obviously involved macroscopically on CT but also in apparently healthy tissue adjacent to inflammatory lesions.

Uncommon complications of necrotizing fasciitis seen on follow-up CT scans include perforation of the pharyngeal wall, septic thrombosis of the internal jugular vein, and rupture of the external carotid artery necessitating emergency ligation.[13] Rupture of the carotid artery as a direct complication of adventitial necrosis is rare.

■ Complications of Bacterial Infections

Septic Thrombosis of the Internal Jugular Vein

Septic thrombosis of the internal jugular vein is the most common complication of deep neck infection. Patients typically present with fever, tenderness, and swelling along the course of the internal jugular vein. Septic emboli may settle at distant sites, resulting in thrombosis of the lateral sinus, meningitis, and pulmonary infarcts. Lemierre syndrome is a form of septic internal jugular vein thrombosis that occurs after tonsillitis. This disease was common in the preantibiotic era, often leading to sepsis and death. On CT, septic thrombosis of the internal jugular vein has a characteristic appearance: the low-attenuation luminal thrombus is surrounded by an enhancing wall (Fig. 12.**105**). The remaining lumen has a high attenuation value from the free-flowing contrast material. The perivascular soft tissues of the neck show an inflammatory reaction (cellulitis and myositis) of various intensity. On MRI, the thrombus has different signal intensities on T1- and T2-weighted images depending on the composition of the clot with methemoglobin, whereas flowing blood produces a flow void. On T1-weighted images, old mural thrombi may show enhancement. On Doppler US, the diagnosis of internal jugular vein thrombosis is straightforward owing to the absence of flow and lack of compressibility.

Carotid Artery Rupture

Carotid artery rupture is a serious complication that may be seen in patients with retropharyngeal abscess, parapharyngeal abscess, and necrotizing fasciitis. The site of the hemorrhage is the internal carotid artery in 62% of cases, followed by the external carotid artery (25%) and common carotid artery (13%). Patients typically present a protracted clinical course with recurrent small hemorrhages, soft-tissue hematoma, Horner syndrome, and palsies of cranial nerves IX to XII.

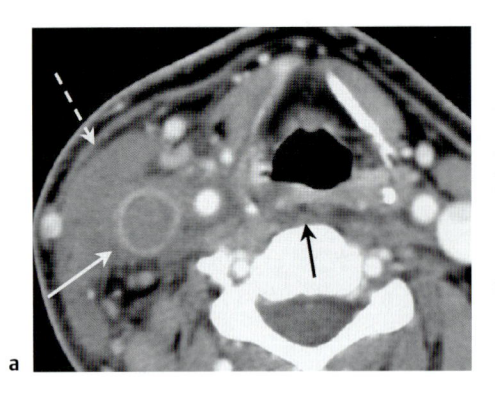

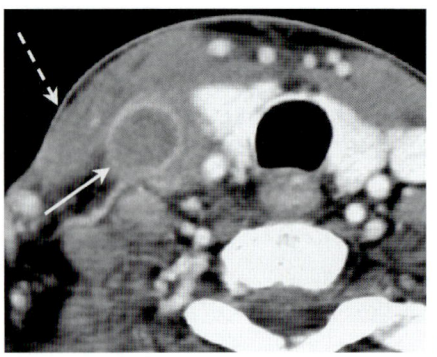

Fig. 12.**105** Septic thrombosis of the internal jugular vein. Characteristic CT appearance. **a, b** Axial contrast-enhanced CT images through the infrahyoid neck show complete thrombosis of the internal jugular vein (white arrows), which is surrounded by inflammatory changes within the posterior cervical space and carotid space (note obliteration of fat). There is marked edema of the right sternocleidomastoid muscle (dashed arrows) and there is some retropharyngeal cellulitis (black arrow).

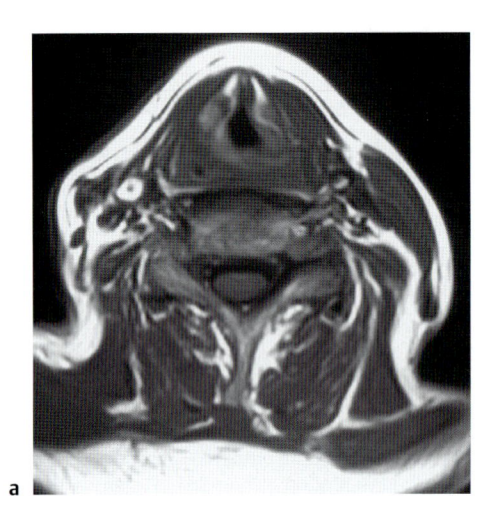

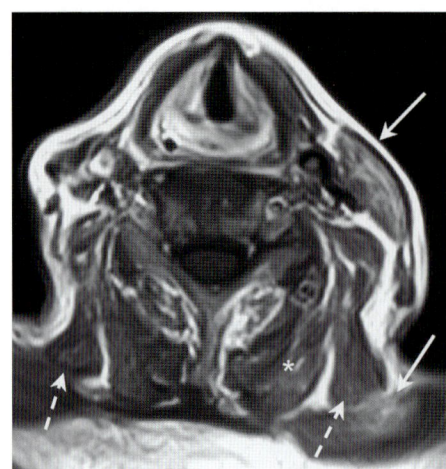

Fig. 12.**106** Dermatomyositis affecting neck muscles in an elderly woman presenting with dysphagia and painful asymmetry of the neck. **a, b** T1W MR images through the infrahyoid neck before (**a**) and after (**b**) injection of contrast material show diffuse enhancement of the left sternocleidomastoid muscle and left trapezius muscle (arrows). There is also some abnormal enhancement in the levator scapulae muscles (dashed arrows) and in the paraspinal muscles (asterisk). Note marked atrophy of the right sternocleidomastoid muscle as a sequela of long-standing disease.

Mediastinitis

Mediastinitis may be caused by esophageal perforation, retropharyngeal and carotid space infection, and cervical necrotizing fasciitis (Fig. 12.**103**). Patients typically present with chest pain and dyspnea. On CT and MRI, widening of the mediastinum, a "dirty" fat appearance, and the presence of fluid collections suggest the diagnosis (Fig. 12.**103**).

■ Vertebral Body Spondylodiskitis

A detailed description of inflammatory and infectious diseases of the cervical spine is beyond the scope of this chapter. However, it is important to realize that pyogenic disk space infections may secondarily involve the retropharyngeal space and carotid space. Spondylodiskitis is usually the result of a blood-borne agent, particularly from the lung or urinary tract. The most common pathogen is *Staphylococcus* followed by *Streptococcus*, *Escherichia coli*, and *Proteus*. In acute spondylodiskitis, patients present with pain and the sedimentation rate is elevated. As the pathogen is usually located in the region of the end plates, destruction of the disk space and the adjacent vertebral bodies takes place. On CT, there is bone sclerosis and a paravertebral soft-tissue mass. On MRI, the disk space displays a low signal intensity on T1-weighted images and a high signal intensity on T2-weighted images. After injection of contrast material, there is marked enhancement of the disk space, the end plates, and paravertebral soft tissues.

■ Inflammatory Diseases of Neck Muscles and Tendons

Focal myositis (of Heffner) is a rare inflammatory condition of skeletal muscles most commonly seen in the extremities. The sternocleidomastoid muscle and the trapezius muscle are rarely affected.[22,24,39] Focal myositis occurs most often in the pediatric age group and is associated with signs of inflammation, torticollis, and fever. On imaging, the affected muscle shows an increased volume, edema, and variable enhancement patterns suggesting inflammation without abscess formation. Occasionally, the aspect may be similar to a muscular tumor. The significance of focal myositis is that it may be mistaken for a neoplasm clinically and radiologically. In these cases, biopsy is necessary to clarify the diagnosis. In general, no treatment is required and resolution takes place within a few months. Occasionally, intravenous steroids and antibiotics are used.

In the neck, **dermatomyositis** typically affects the pharyngeal constrictors and—less often—the trapezius muscles, the strap muscles, and the sternocleidomastoid muscle. On MR imaging, the affected muscles initially show a decreased signal intensity on T1-weighted images, an increased signal intensity on T2-weighted images, and enhancement after administration of contrast material (Fig. 12.**106**). Atrophy is seen in advanced stages of the disease. Evaluation of the pharyngeal constrictors is best done with videopharyngoscopy, which may show functional abnormalities such as dysfunction of the cricopharyngeus muscle, pharyngeal hypomotility, and lack of laryngeal elevation during swallowing, leading to aspiration (see also Chapter 11).

Calcific tendinitis of the longus colli muscle is characterized by the deposition of calcium hydroxyapatite into the longus

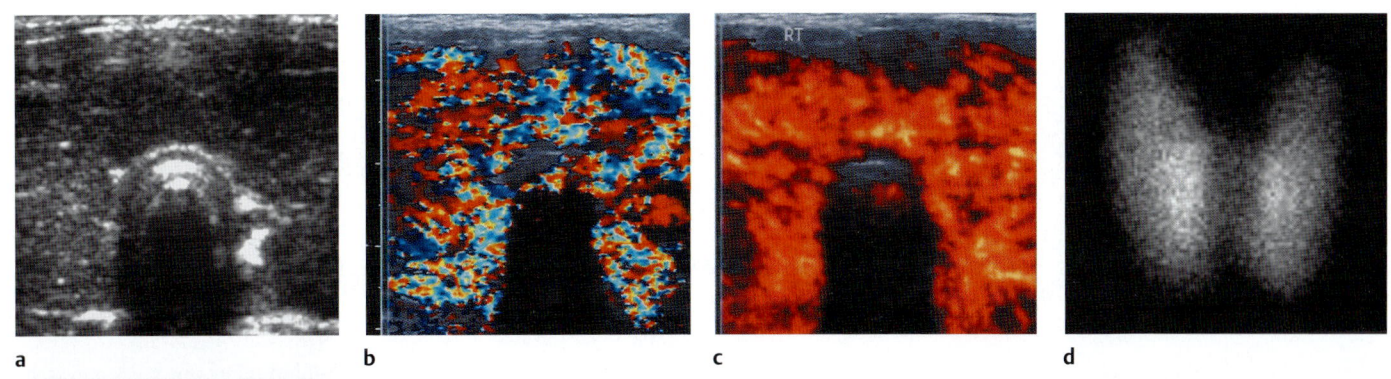

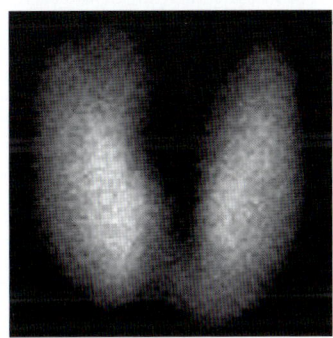

Fig. 12.**107** Graves disease. Characteristic US, color Doppler, and scintigraphic appearance. **a** Axial US image of the thyroid gland shows diffuse enlargement affecting both lobes and the isthmic portion. Note hypoechoic echostructure. **b** Color Doppler and **c** power Doppler images show diffusely increased perfusion ("thyroid inferno pattern"). The peak velocity measured in the inferior thyroid artery was also significantly increased. **d** Anteroposterior view of an ^{123}I scan and **e** anteroposterior view of a ^{99m}Tc-pertechnetate scan show diffuse gland enlargement and increased tracer uptake.

colli tendon. Patients often complain of odynophagia, neck pain with rigidity, and slight fever. On CT, soft-tissue thickening with calcification is seen in the prevertebral area at the level of C1 and C2. The calcifications may resolve when the soft-tissue swelling recedes. On MRI, an increased signal intensity is seen on T2-weighted images and the calcifications may be entirely missed.

■ Inflammatory Lesions of the Thyroid Gland

Inflammatory lesions of the thyroid gland include Graves disease, acute infectious thyroiditis, Hashimoto thyroiditis, Riedel thyroiditis, de Quervain thyroiditis, and amyloidosis.

Graves disease is an autoimmune disorder typically affecting young women and leading to hyperthyroidism.[119] Orbital involvement and pretibial myxedema are among the most common extraglandular manifestations. The diagnosis is confirmed by laboratory tests, which show decreased blood TSH (thyrotropin) levels associated with either a decreased T_3 level or a decreased T_3 and T_4 level. On US, the entire gland (including the isthmus) is diffusely enlarged, "ballooned," and hypoechoic, and there is marked hypervascularity, so-called thyroid inferno pattern (Fig. 12.**107**). Furthermore, the measured peak velocity (in the inferior thyroid artery) is significantly increased. The degree of hypervascularity does not correlate with the degree of hyperthyroidism. However, it is of prognostic value.[119]

Acute infectious thyroiditis is mainly caused by *Streptococcus*, *Staphylococcus* and *Pneumococcus*. Rare causes include actinomycosis, salmonella infections, and tuberculosis. Common symptoms consist of painful swelling of the thyroid gland, odynophagia and dysphagia, and fever. The CT and MRI imaging findings include edema with glandular and neck swelling, and sometimes abscess formation. A special form is recurrent infection caused by a fistula from the apex of the piriform sinus or by a thyroglossal duct fistula (see below).

Hashimoto thyroiditis (also called atrophic lymphocytic thyroiditis or chronic lymphocytic thyroiditis) is an autoimmune

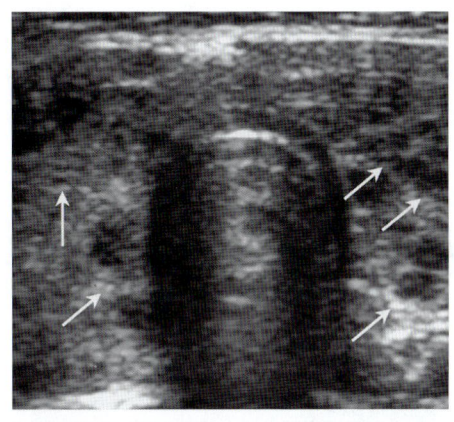

Fig. 12.**108** Hashimoto thyroiditis. US appearance. Axial US image at the level of the isthmic portion shows an atrophic, heterogeneous, predominantly hypoechoic gland with hyperechoic areas (arrows) corresponding to fibrosis. Blood tests were positive for antibodies against thyroid peroxidase.

disorder of unknown origin leading to gland destruction and hypothyroidism. It occurs most often in women over the age of 40 years.[119] The gland may be either moderately enlarged or atrophic, and fibrosis is seen in 12 % of cases. Diagnosis is made based on laboratory tests, which reveal elevated titers of antithyroglobulin antibodies. Hashimoto thyroiditis is associated with an elevated risk of malignant lymphoma and papillary carcinoma. On US, the thyroid gland is often atrophic, hypoechogenic, and with small hyperechoic areas of scar-tissue (Fig. 12.**108**). Because of extensive fibrosis, the surface of the gland may appear polylobulated. On color Doppler imaging, a normal or a decreased vascularization pattern may be observed.[50, 111] The aspect on CT is nonspecific. On T2-weighted MR images, however, an increased signal intensity associated with lower-intensity bands (thought to represent fibrosis) may be seen.[60]

Riedel thyroiditis (also called invasive sclerosing thyroiditis) is a rare disease that belongs to the inflammatory fibrosclero-

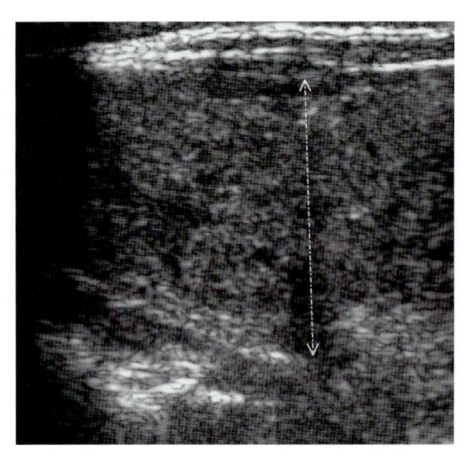

Fig. 12.**109** De Quervain thyroiditis. US appearance. Longitudinal US image of the left thyroid lobe in a patient with de Quervain thyroiditis shows enlargement of the gland (especially of the anteroposterior diameter, between measurements) and marked hypoechogenicity. The isthmic portion was not enlarged.

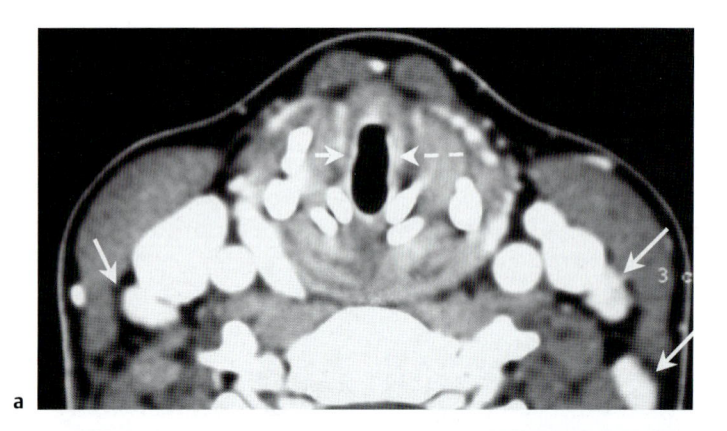

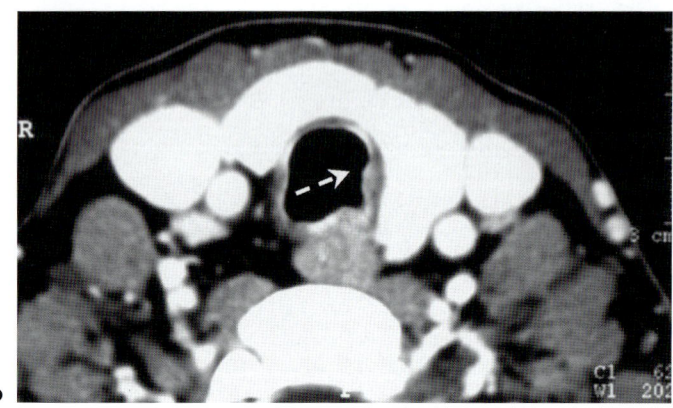

Fig. 12.**110** Biopsy-proven systemic amyloidosis involving the thyroid gland, the larynx, the trachea, and the cervical lymph nodes. Contrast-enhanced CT images at the level of the subglottis (**a**) and cervical trachea (**b**) show asymmetric thyroid gland enlargement, bilateral hypervascular lymph nodes (arrows), and subglottic and tracheal narrowing (dashed arrows) caused by amyloid deposition. Courtesy of Dr. Guy Moulin (Hôpital La Timone, Marseille, France).

images the gland is hypoechoic, and a homogeneous but decreased enhancement pattern has been observed after injection of contrast material.[60] On CT, the aspect is nonspecific.

De Quervain thyroiditis (also called subacute thyroiditis or granulomatous thyroiditis) is thought to be of viral origin, as it often develops after an upper respiratory tract infection (50–90%). The disease typically affects middle-aged women. Common symptoms include fever, malaise, painful gland enlargement, and hyperthyroidism (50% of cases), followed by hypothyroidism with eventual return to a euthyroid stage after 2–3 months.[111] De Quervain thyroiditis may mimic a tumor and biopsy may be necessary to establish the correct diagnosis. US typically depicts enlarged thyroid gland lobes but a normal isthmus (as opposed to Graves disease, where the isthmus is enlarged). The thyroid gland in de Quervain thyroiditis shows either a diffuse or a focal hypoechogenic structure and on Doppler US the vascularization is decreased (as opposed to Graves disease, where there is marked hypervascularity).

Amyloid deposition within the thyroid gland is very rare and leads to diffuse glandular enlargement. Thyroid amyloidosis may be seen both in patients with Hashimoto thyroiditis and in patients with systemic amyloidosis. On US, the gland is diffusely enlarged and hyperechoic. On MRI, the gland is hypointense on both T1- and T2-weighted images and homogeneous enhancement may be seen after injection of contrast material. Amyloid deposition in systemic amyloidosis may also be seen in the cervical lymph nodes.[52, 56, 100] On CT, the enlarged lymph nodes may be hypervascular and/or hemorrhagic (Figs. 12.**44**, 12.**110**). On MRI, the lymph nodes are enlarged and hypointense on both T1- and T2-weighted images.

Congenital/Developmental Lesions

The most common congenital lesions found in the infrahyoid neck include branchial cleft cysts and fistulae, thyroglossal duct cysts, venous malformations, and lymphangiomas.[6, 74, 96, 97, 141, 157] All masses in this group arise from a rest of tissue left behind after formation of the structures in the neck.

■ Branchial Cleft Anomalies

The fetal branchial apparatus develops during the second fetal week and consists of five paired pharyngeal arches separated internally by four endodermal pouches and externally by four ectodermal clefts. During the fourth and fifth weeks of embryonic development, overgrowth of the second through fourth clefts by the second endodermal pharyngeal arch creates the lateral cervical sinus of His, which normally involutes completely. Persistence of the lateral cervical sinus of His may produce cysts, sinus tracts, and fistulae.[6, 141]

First branchial cleft cysts and fistula may occur anywhere from the external auditory canal to the angle of the mandible, including the parotid gland (see also Chapter 9).

Second Branchial Cleft Anomalies

Normally, the second branchial cleft apparatus involutes by the ninth fetal week.[6, 96, 141] When the involution phase is incomplete, the remnant tissue has the potential to grow into a branchial cleft anomaly. **Second branchial cleft anomalies** are located along the embryological tract of the second branchial cleft, which terminates in the primordial sinus of His at the anterior surface of the lower third of the sternocleidomastoid muscle. Second branchial cleft anomalies are the most common branchial cleft anomalies (95%). A history of repeated infections in the region of

sis disease group and may be associated with mediastinal–retroperitoneal fibrosis and sclerosing cholangitis.[120] The etiology is unclear but is thought to be immune-mediated. Riedel thyroiditis occurs preferentially in women around 50 years of age. The hallmarks of the disease are extensive sclerosis of the gland and of the adjacent muscles and fascia, often leading to tracheal and esophageal compression. On palpation, the thyroid gland is very firm ("stony hard"). On US, the gland is hypoechoic and enlarged, similar to goiters in Graves disease.[50, 111] On T1- and T2-weighted

Infectious and Inflammatory Conditions   835

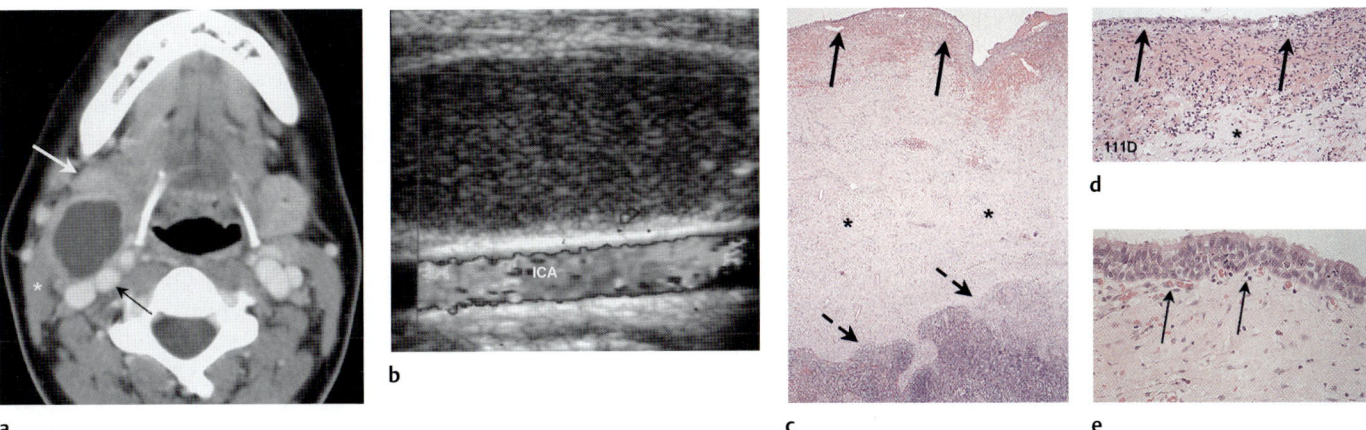

Fig. 12.111 Classic second branchial cleft cyst. Characteristic CT, US, and histological appearance. **a** Axial contrast-enhanced CT image at the level of the hyoid bone demonstrates a cystic lesion with significant capsular enhancement. Thickening of the wall of the cyst is caused by inflammation. Note the embryologically defined location of the cyst. White arrow = submandibular gland; black arrow = internal carotid artery; asterisk = sternocleidomastoid muscle. **b** Longitudinal color Doppler US image shows a mass without internal vessels and with internal echoes suggesting a proteinaceous cyst. The wall of the cyst is slightly thickened. The cyst is located anteriorly from the internal carotid artery (ICA) in its immediate vicinity. The patient underwent surgical excision. **c–e** Photomicrographs from surgical specimen demonstrate the characteristic components of the branchial cleft cyst wall: squamous epithelium (black arrows) surrounded by an inflammatory and fibrotic stroma (asterisks) and lymphoid tissue with germinal centers (dashed arrows). Respiratory epithelium is found in some portions of the cyst wall (thin arrows in **e**).

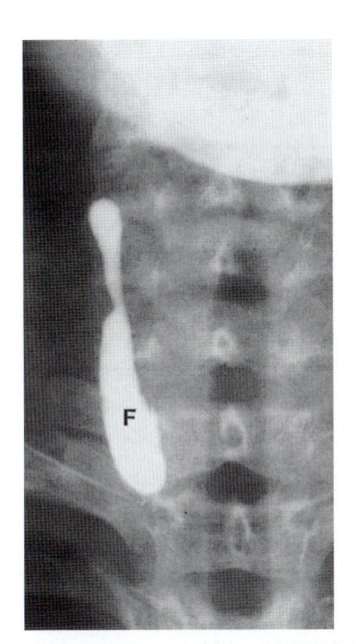

Fig. 12.112 Second branchial cleft fistula as seen on conventional x-ray fistulography. The tract (F), which has been injected with iodinated contrast material, runs down the anterior border of the sternocleidomastoid muscle to the clavicle. Courtesy of Dr. Barbara L. Carter.

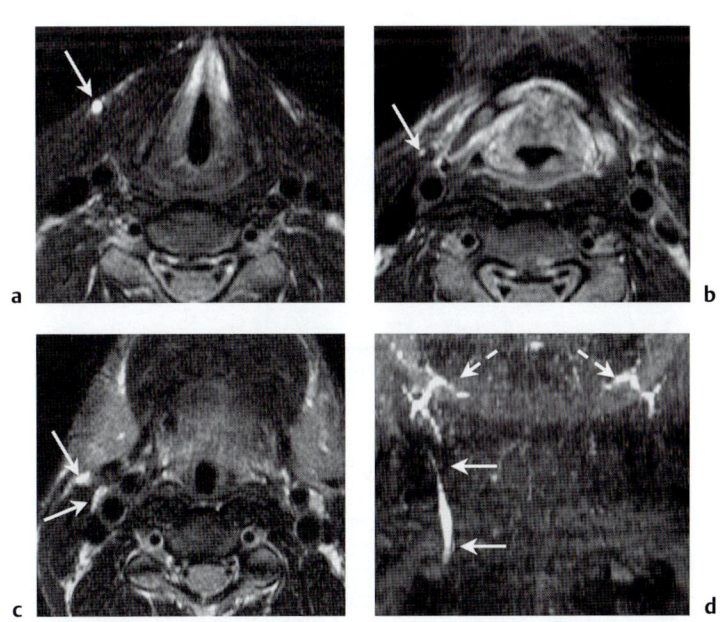

Fig. 12.113 Second branchial cleft fistula as seen on MRI. **a–c** Axial, heavily T2-weighted MR images obtained in a young male patient with a small cutaneous orifice at the lower medial border of the right sternocleidomastoid muscle show a second branchial cleft fistula with a characteristic course (arrows). **d** Coronal MIP reconstruction from the axial images shows the course of the second branchial cleft fistula (arrows). Dashed arrows point to the left and right submandibular ductal systems. Surgery confirmed the findings.

the mandible either in infants or in the young adult often suggests the diagnosis. Second branchial cleft cysts are bilateral in 2–3% of cases and familial tendencies have been noted.[26, 141] Branchial cleft anomalies may be seen in the branchio-oto-renal syndrome, which is an inborn disease of autosomal dominant transmission characterized by ear pits, branchial cleft anomalies, deafness, and renal anomalies heavily compromising prognosis.

The most common form of second branchial cleft anomaly is a cystic mass without sinus or fistula (Fig. 12.**111**). However, any permutation of cyst, sinus, or fistula may be possible. Four types of second branchial cleft anomalies may be distinguished depending on the kind of presentation: fistula, internal sinus, external sinus, and cyst[6, 26, 141] (Figs. 12.**112**, 12.**113**). A *fistula* is a duct-like structure with an external or an internal orifice. The course is pathognomonic. The external (cutaneous) orifice is located along the anterior border of the lower third of the sternocleidomastoid muscle. The tract courses in a caudal direction between the bifurcation of the internal and external carotid arteries and laterally and superiorly to the cranial nerves IX through XII. The internal (pharyngeal) orifice is located in the tonsillar fossa. An *internal sinus* is a blindly ending space near the pharynx opening in the tonsillar fossa (Fig. 12.**112**). An *external sinus* is a blindly ending

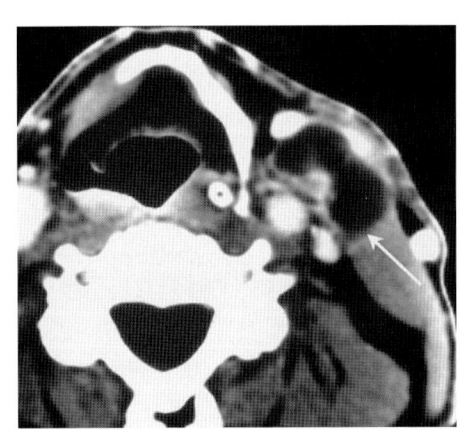

Fig. 12.114 Squamous cell carcinoma arising in a second branchial cleft cyst. This middle-aged man presented with a palpable neck mass on the left. Contrast-enhanced CT at the level of the hyoid bone shows a predominantly cystic lesion with nodular wall thickening (arrow), suggesting a necrotic lymph node metastasis. The remainder of the CT examination was normal. The patient underwent neck dissection and histology revealed squamous cell carcinoma arising in a second branchial cleft cyst.

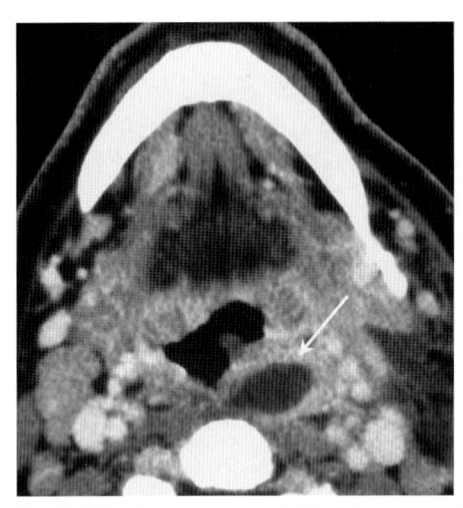

Fig. 12.115 Retropharyngeal third branchial cleft cyst. Contrast-enhanced CT obtained in a young male patient three weeks after surgical drainage of a retropharyngeal abscess reveals a recurrent retropharyngeal fluid collection (arrow) with regular, contrast-enhancing walls. Repeat surgery revealed a branchial cleft cyst, which was completely excised.

space extending inward from a cutaneous opening into the lower third of the neck. A *cyst* is located along the tract described for the fistula. The most common location of a second branchial cleft cyst is in the submandibular space lateral to the carotid bifurcation and anteromedial to the sternocleidomastoid muscle (Fig. 12.**111**). When present on the cyst, a beak that points medially between the internal and external carotid artery is pathognomonic of a second branchial cleft cyst.

In second branchial cleft cysts, US may show a unilocular mass with variable echogenicity ranging from anechoic (fluid in noninfected cysts) to hyperechoic (pus in infected cysts) (Fig. 12.**111**). The wall of the cyst is usually thin and regular. However, in infected cysts, the wall is thickened and marked hypervascularity is noted on the Doppler examination. CT typically reveals a unilocular cystic mass essentially isoattenuating with cerebrospinal fluid (CSF). A uniformly thin peripheral capsular enhancement is characteristic. Infection of the cyst may, however, result in thickening and irregular capsular enhancement (Fig. 12.**111**). Depending on the relative protein concentration within the cyst, second branchial cleft cysts are typically isointense to CSF on T2-weighted MR images, while they have a variable appearance on T1-weighted images. The characteristic histological features of the branchial cleft cyst wall include squamous or respiratory epithelium surrounded by an inflammatory and fibrotic stroma and lymphoid tissue with germinal centers (Fig. 12.**111**). Whenever irregularity of the cyst wall is seen on CT or MRI the possibility of a "cystic" metastasis from a squamous cell cancer (most often from the tonsil) or the possibility of a carcinoma arising within a second branchial cleft cyst should be considered.[21] Although rare, carcinomas may arise in the wall of a second branchial cleft cyst either from squamous epithelium cells found within the wall of the cyst (Fig. 12.**114**) or from ectopic thyroid tissue. Ectopic thyroid tissue may be found not only along the course of the thyroglossal duct tract but also in the larynx, trachea, esophagus, mediastinum, pericardium, and diaphragm, and within second branchial cleft cysts.[21, 81]

In second branchial cleft sinuses and fistulae, diagnosis may be done with fistulography[26] with thin-slice (1 mm) contrast-enhanced CT with 2D coronal and sagittal reconstructions or with very thin heavily T2-weighted MR images (MR "fistulography" with 2D or MIP reconstructions) (Figs. 12.**112**, 12.**113**). The principle of MR "fistulography" is similar to that of MR sialography (see Chapter 9). Fistulography, CT, and MR "fistulography" are very useful in delineating the extension of the lesion, which facilitates complete surgical resection. This complete resection is essential to prevent recurrence.

Third Branchial Cleft Anomalies

Third branchial cleft anomalies are rare. The tract typically courses from the apex of the piriform sinus in a cranial direction posterior to the carotid space and the sternocleidomastoid muscle and superior to cranial nerve XII but inferior to cranial nerve IX to the lower lateroposterior neck. When a cyst is seen in the posterior cervical triangle, the differential diagnosis includes third branchial cleft cyst, lymphangioma, and necrotic level V adenopathy. Rarely, a third branchial cleft cyst may be seen in the retropharyngeal space, simulating a retropharyngeal abscess (Fig. 12.**115**).[63, 102] The clinical history is, however, different inasmuch as patients with retropharyngeal third branchial anomalies will often present with recurrent retropharyngeal infection after previous surgical drainage.[102] Complete surgical excision of the cyst is mandatory to avoid recurrent infection.

Fourth Branchial Cleft Anomalies

Fourth branchial cleft fistulae (also called piriform sinus fistulae) correspond to the persistence of the pharyngobrachialis duct between the upper parathyroid gland and ultimobranchial body on one hand, and the pharynx on the other. The fistulous tract begins at the apex of the piriform sinus and runs in contact with the larynx and trachea. After passing the thyroid cartilage, the tract crosses the lower constrictor muscle of the pharynx and courses behind the body of the thyroid gland. All fourth branchial pouch fistulae run below the superior laryngeal nerve. Theoretically, fourth branchial pouch fistulae may continue inferiorly beneath the aortic arch on the left and beneath the subclavian artery on the right. However, in practice, most tracts do not complete this entire course but are often confined to the perithyroid area.[101] Most fourth branchial pouch anomalies are located on the left and present as suppurative thyroiditis or perithyroid abscess in children and young adults.[121] Misdiagnosis as localized lobar thyroiditis, suppurative thyroiditis, or adenitis has been reported. CT and MRI are essential in demonstrating the communication between the piriform sinus and the

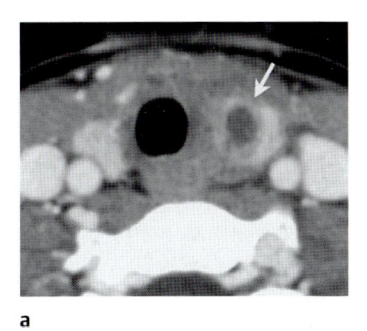

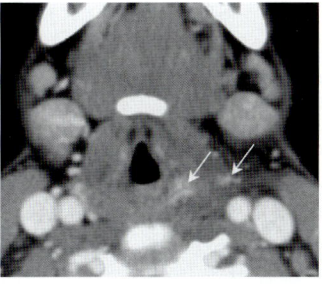

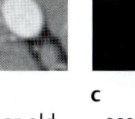

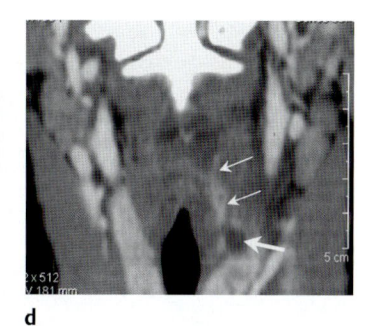

Fig. 12.116 Infected fourth branchial cleft fistula seen in a 6-year-old boy with recurrent swelling of the left lower neck and fever. **a, b** Axial contrast-enhanced CT images from a volumetric acquisition show an abscess located within the left lobe of the thyroid gland (thick arrow). An enhancing tubular structure (thin arrows) is seen that connects the thyroid abscess cavity and the left piriform sinus. **c, d** This fourth branchial cleft fistula is better appreciated on the sagittal and coronal 2D reconstructions. Dashed arrow = piriform sinus; thin arrows = fistula; thick arrow = thyroid abscess. Surgery confirmed the findings.

thyroid gland as the opening of the fistulous tract at the apex of the piriform sinus may not always be visualized endoscopically. Thin slices (1–2 mm) and 2D reconstructions of contrast-enhanced images are very helpful in establishing the diagnosis (Fig. 12.**116**).

■ Thyroglossal Duct Cyst

The thyroid gland develops as an endodermal diverticulum in the midline of the primitive ventral pharynx between the first pharyngeal pouch and second branchial arch. The thyroid gland appears as an endodermal thickening at the diverticulum. This point of origin is later reflected by the foramen cecum. During embryogenesis, the anlage of the thyroid/parathyroid glands descends from the foramen cecum at the tongue base to its final position in the anterior visceral space (Fig. 12.**117**). During this caudal migration, the usually bilobed anlage passes just anterior to the precursor tissue of the hyoid bone, leaving a tract of epithelial tissue called the thyroglossal duct.[74,96,141] The normal thyroglossal duct involutes by the eighth fetal week. Rests of thyroid tissue remaining along the duct may give rise to cysts, fistulae, or solid nodules of thyroid tissue. Ectopic thyroid tissue is most often located at the foramen cecum (see also Chapter 10). In as many as 70% of cases with ectopic thyroid tissue, this is the only functioning thyroid tissue. Ectopic thyroid tissue may also be found in the larynx, trachea, and mediastinum, and within second branchial cleft cysts (see above).

Thyroglossal duct cysts are the most common congenital neck masses and they are usually detected before the age of 20 years, frequently following infection. Thyroglossal duct cysts most commonly occur in the region of the hyoid bone. Fifteen percent of all cysts are located at the level of the hyoid bone, 20% are located in the suprahyoid neck, and 65% are located just below the hyoid bone. Nearly 75% of cysts are located in the midline with paramedian cysts more common on the left. A solid mass within the cyst may indicate either associated ectopic thyroid tissue or carcinoma. Thyroid carcinoma arising within a thyroglossal duct cyst usually occurs in adults. It has been reported in 1% of thyroglossal duct cysts. The vast majority of these tumors are papillary thyroid cancers and a minority are squamous cell carcinomas. Squamous cell carcinomas have a poorer prognosis.[23,96,111]

On US, thyroglossal duct cysts present as hypoechoic lesions with prominent acoustic enhancement. The wall of the cyst may be either thin or thick. In the presence of associated infection, the cyst may contain debris. Nodularity or a soft-tissue mass within the cyst suggests malignancy. CT or MRI typically show a midline or paramedian cystic mass located in the infrahyoid strap muscles at or below the level of the hyoid bone (Figs. 12.**118**–12.**120**). The capsule of the cyst shows a uniformly thin enhancement or—in the case of an infected cyst—a uniformly thick enhancement. The location of the thyroglossal duct cyst within the strap muscles is the key feature that allows differentiation from other adult neck masses that may have a similar CT or MR appearance, i.e., necrotic anterior cervical nodes and thrombosed anterior jugular veins. The latter, however, are located superficial to the strap muscles (Fig. 12.**121**). Histological examination reveals that the wall of the thyroglossal duct cyst is composed of squamous cell mucosa, and thyroid tissue is often present (Fig. 12.**119**). Inflammatory changes may obliterate the mucosa of the thyroglossal duct wall, making the pathological diagnosis difficult.

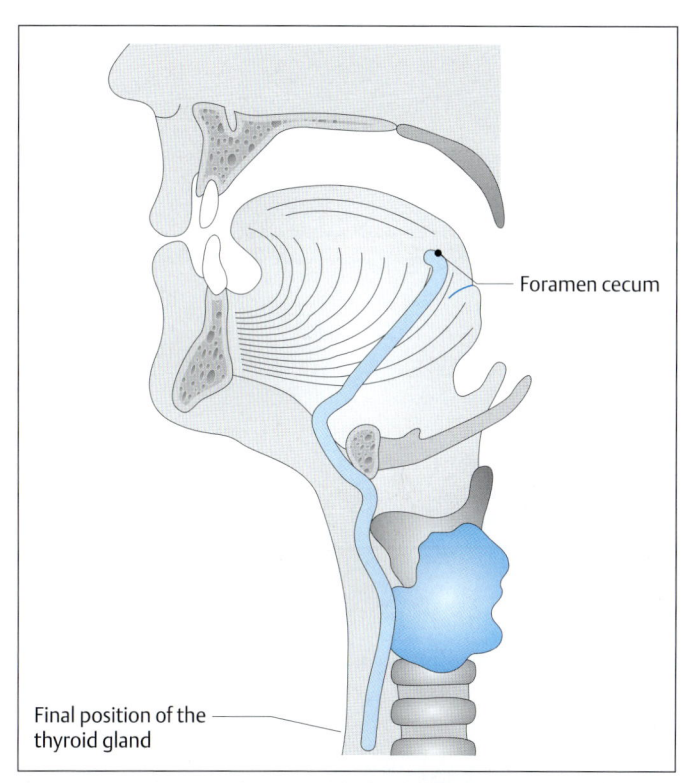

Fig. 12.117 Schematic drawing of the lateral neck shows the path of descent of the thyroid anlage. Thyroid duct cysts, fistulae, and ectopic thyroid tissue can occur anywhere along the course of this duct.

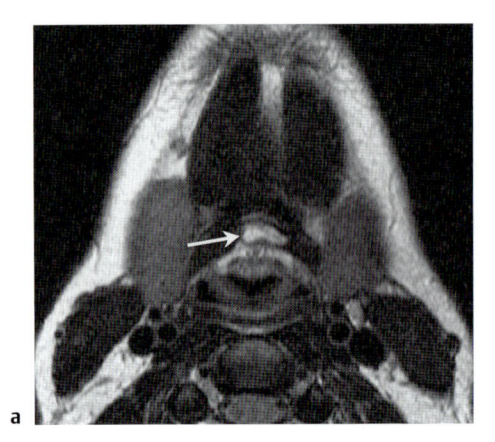

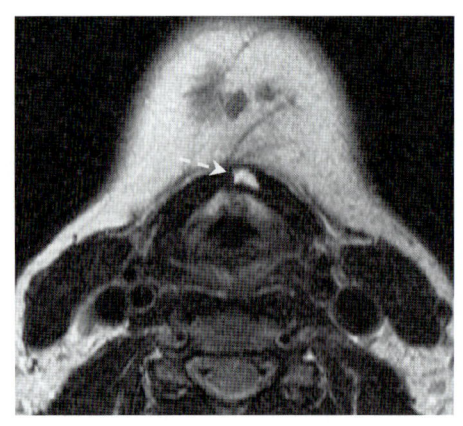

Fig. 12.118 Non-infected thyroglossal duct cyst as seen on MRI. T2W FSE images at the level of the hyoid bone (**a**) and below the hyoid bone (**b**) show a small, median, hyperintense lesion located in immediate vicinity of the hyoid bone partly within the preepiglottic space (arrow) and partly within the strap muscles (dashed arrow). The walls of the cyst are thin and there was no contrast material enhancement on the T1W MR images (not shown).

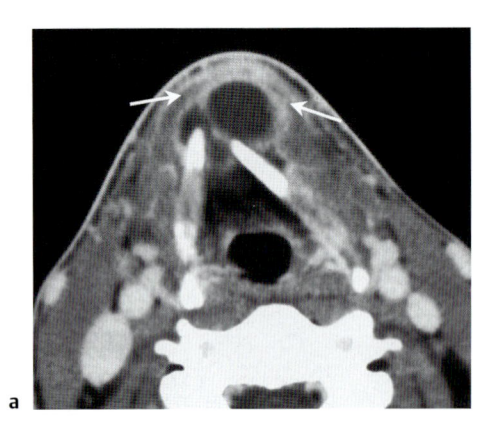

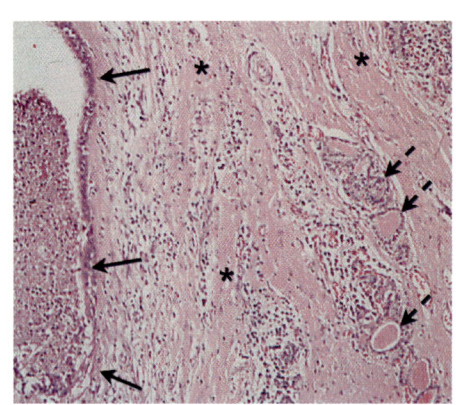

Fig. 12.119 Infected thyroglossal duct cyst. Characteristic CT and histological appearance. **a** Axial contrast-enhanced CT image obtained immediately below the level of the hyoid bone. Key features include midline location and beaking of the strap muscles over the surface of the cyst (arrows). Infection of the cyst has resulted in thickening of the cyst wall and significant capsular enhancement. Associated inflammatory changes within the strap muscles have resulted in muscular and fascial enhancement. **b** Photomicrograph of the excised cyst (hematoxylin–eosin stain) demonstrates the characteristic components of the thyroglossal duct cyst wall: squamous epithelium (arrows) surrounded by an inflammatory and fibrotic stroma (asterisks) and thyroid follicles (dashed arrows). Reproduced from Reference 11 with permission.

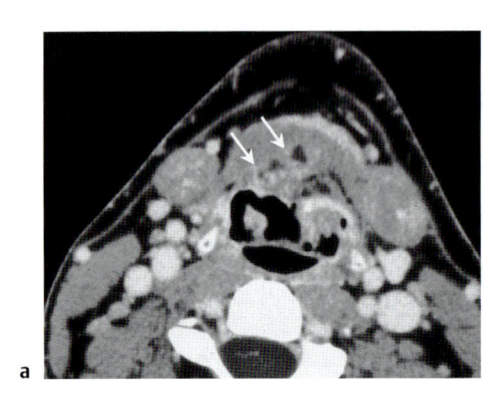

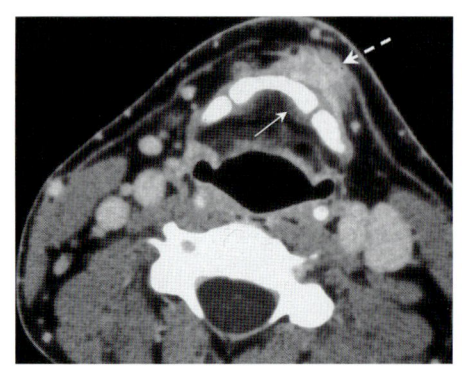

Fig. 12.120 Infected thyroglossal duct fistula. Characteristic CT appearance. Axial contrast-enhanced CT images at the level of the valleculae (**a**) and at the level of the hyoid bone (**b**) show a tubular structure with enhancing walls (arrows) extending superiorly toward the base of the tongue and inferiorly into the region of the hyoid bone. A small left paramedian cystlike structure is seen in the immediate vicinity of the hyoid bone (thin arrow). Note associated inflammatory changes within the strap muscles that have resulted in muscular and fascial enhancement (dashed arrows). Surgery confirmed a thyroglossal duct fistula extending into the base of the tongue.

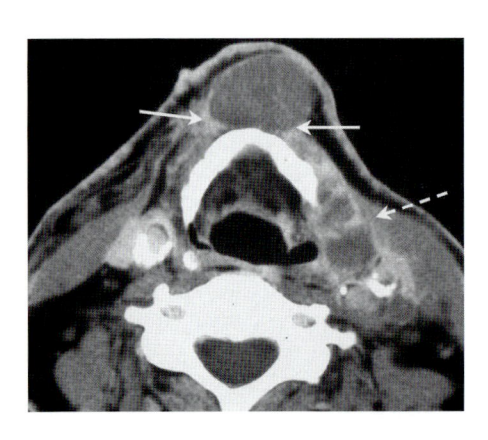

Fig. 12.121 Cystic metastasis from malignant melanoma mimicking a thyroglossal duct cyst. This patient presented with a rapidly enlarging midline mass located at the level of the hyoid bone. Clinically, a thyroglossal duct cyst was suspected. Contrast-enhanced CT image at the level of the hyoid bone shows a cystic mass with thin capsular enhancement located superficially to the strap muscles (arrows), suggesting an anterior cervical lymph node metastasis. Additional metastatic lymph nodes with nodal necrosis are seen on the left (dashed arrow). Surgery revealed nodal metastases from a malignant melanoma. Careful examination of the patient revealed a small malignant melanoma of the left gingiva.

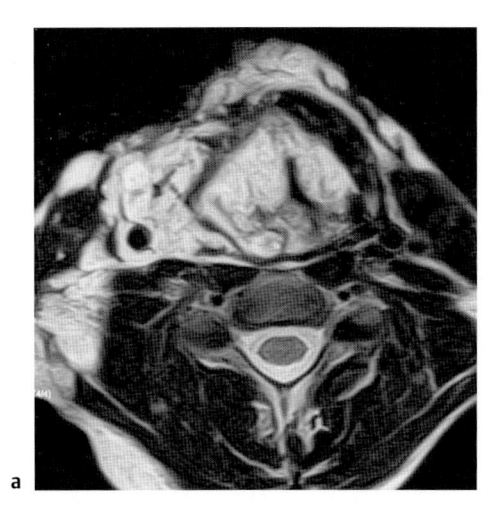

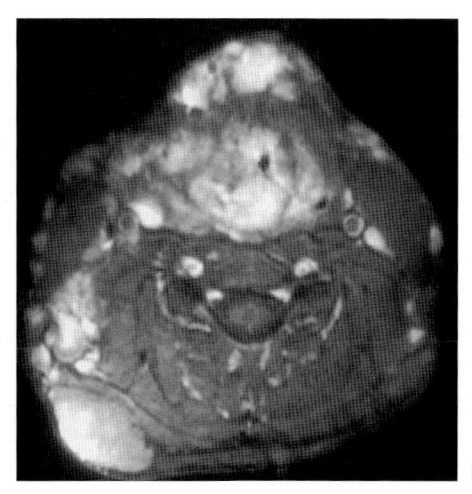

Fig. 12.**122** Extensive venous malformation. Characteristic MRI appearance. **a** Axial T2W MR image at the supraglottic level demonstrates a lesion with very high signal intensity involving the supraglottic larynx, the strap muscles, the carotid space, the posterior cervical space, and the sternocleidomastoid muscle on the right. Absence of flow voids. **b** Contrast-enhanced fat-suppressed T1W image obtained at the same level shows major contrast material enhancement of the lesion, suggesting a venous malformation.

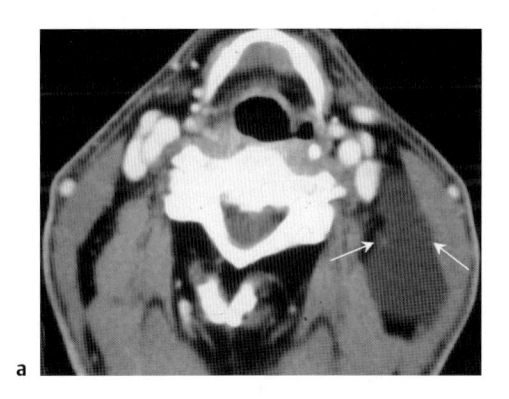

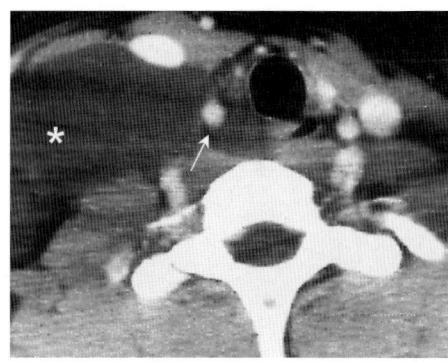

Fig. 12.**123** Cystic hygroma. Characteristic CT appearance. **a** Contrast-enhanced CT image at the level of the hyoid bone shows a cystic lesion in the left posterior cervical space with thin, enhancing septa (arrows), suggesting a cystic hygroma. Surgery confirmed the diagnosis. **b** Contrast-enhanced CT image at the supraclavicular level in a different patient shows a large cystic lesion (asterisk) located in the supraclavicular region. The lesion insinuates around the common carotid artery (arrow) and displaces the internal jugular vein anteriorly. Surgery confirmed **b** cystic hygroma.

■ Vascular Malformations

According to Mulliken and Glowaki,[97] vascular lesions of the head and neck are divided into hemangiomas and vascular malformations. Hemangiomas are neoplastic conditions with an increased proliferation and turnover of endothelial cells. They are the most common tumors of the head and neck in infancy and childhood. Hemangiomas typically display a rapid proliferation phase during the first year of life, followed by an involution phase.

As opposed to hemangiomas, **vascular malformations** are not tumors but true congenital vascular anomalies with a normal proliferation rate of endothelial cells.[97] Typically, they do not regress and may rapidly enlarge in association with trauma or endocrine changes. MRI is the evaluation method of choice for demonstrating the extent and complexity of vascular malformations. Vascular malformations are subdivided into capillary, venous, arterial, and lymphatic malformations. Arterial malformations are high-flow malformations characterized by enlarged, tortuous arteries and draining veins. On MRI serpiginous flow voids are seen on T1- and T2-weighted images owing to the enlarged arterial components. Capillary and venous malformations are low-flow lesions. On CT, venous malformations most often show intense enhancement, and the presence of phleboliths is pathognomonic. On MRI, venous malformations are isointense or hyperintense to muscle on T1-weighted images, become hyperintense on T2-weighted images, and enhance significantly following administration of contrast material (Fig. 12.**122**). Phleboliths may present as round areas of signal void on T1- and T2- weighted images. Areas of thrombosis correspond to high signal intensity areas on T1-weighted images and venous lakes correspond to discrete areas of homogeneous high signal intensity on T2-weighted images.

Lymphangiomas are benign, nonencapsulated lesions that are believed to arise from sequestrations of primitive embryonic lymph sacs.[157] At approximately the sixth gestational week, the jugular lymphatic sacs open and begin to drain into the adjacent jugular veins. If a communication between the jugular sac and the jugular vein fails to develop, the lymph-filled jugular sac dilates.[115, 157] Ninety percent of lymphangiomas become clinically apparent by 2 years of age, while the remaining 10% present as neck masses in the young adult. Lymphangiomas are classified into three histological types on the basis of the size of the abnormal lymphatic spaces. *Capillary lymphangioma* is composed of small, capillary-sized, thin-walled lymphatic channels; *cavernous lymphangioma* is composed of medium-sized dilated lymphatics with a fibrous adventitia; and *cystic lymphangioma* (cystic hygroma) is composed of large dilated lymphatic vessels that range in diameter from a few millimeters to several centimeters[97] (Figs. 12.**123**, 12.**124**). Most cystic hygromas arise in the posterior cervical space (Fig. 12.**123**). The second most common location in the infrahyoid neck is the supraclavicular region. Supraclavicular and posterior cervical space lymphangiomas may also extend into the upper mediastinum (10%). The characteristic CT and MR appearances include a multiseptated cystic mass that may insinuate in and around normal structures, making surgical resection very difficult (Fig. 12.**123**). Occasionally, cystic hygroma may present as a unilocular cystic lesion. On

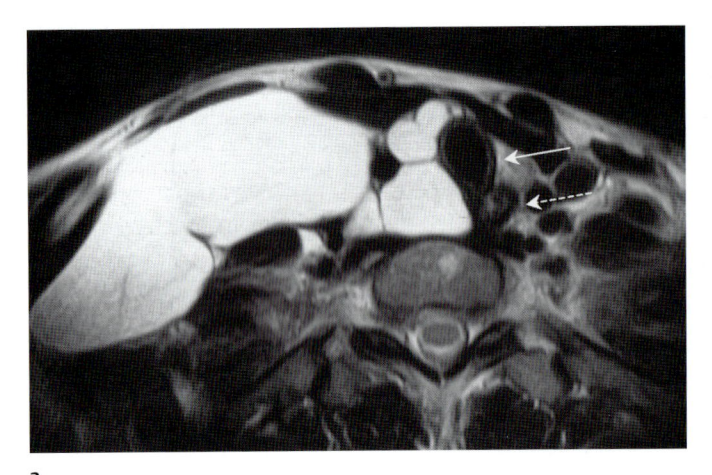

Fig. 12.**124** Cystic hygroma. MRI appearance and microscopic findings. A young man presenting with a soft, compressible swelling of the left neck. **a** Axial T2W FSE image at the level of the cervical trachea demonstrates a multiseptated, cystic lesion originating from the right posterior cervical space. The lesion insinuates between the common carotid artery and the internal jugular vein and displaces the trachea (arrow) and the cervical esophagus (dashed arrow) to the left. **b** Coronal T1W SE image obtained after injection of contrast material shows enhancement of the thin septae (arrow). The cystic spaces have a variable signal intensity (asterisks) due to the variable protein content. Note that the cystic hygroma extends into the mediastinum (dashed arrow) and insinuates around the common carotid and subclavian arteries. CCA = common carotid artery; SCA = subclavian artery; BCT = brachiocephalic trunk. **c** Intraoperative view of the right neck shows a large cystic mass with very thin walls. M = medial; L = lateral; Cr = cranial; Ca = caudal. **d** Photomicrograph (hematoxylin–eosin stain) demonstrates large cystic spaces surrounded by lymphatic channels lined by prominent endothelial cells (arrows). The lymphatic channels are surrounded by a fibrous stroma containing scattered lymph follicles (asterisk).

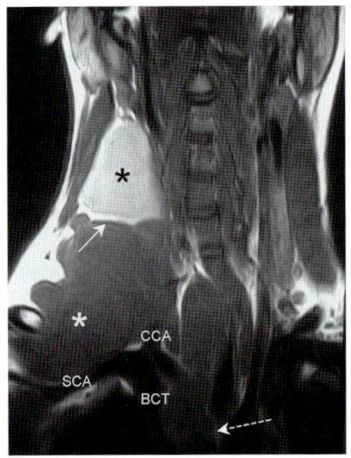

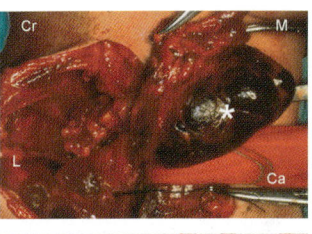

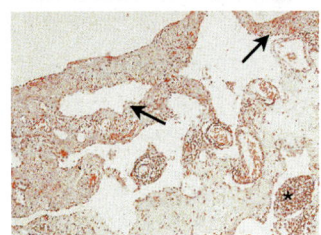

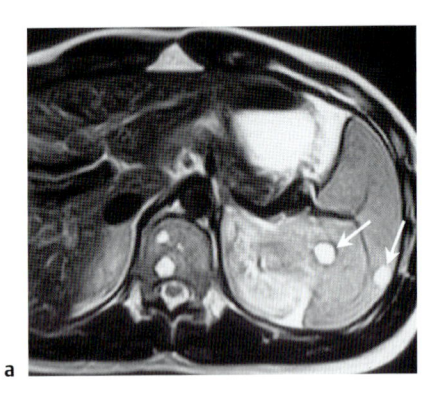

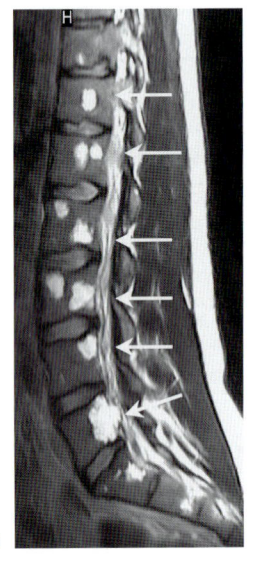

Fig. 12.**125** Cystic angiomatosis. Characteristic MRI appearance. **a** T2W FSE image of the abdomen and **b** sagittal T2W FSE image of the lumbar spine obtained in the patient shown in Fig. 12.**124** show multiple hyperintense lesions in the spleen, lumbar spine, and sacrum (arrows). The lesions did not show any enhancement after injection of contrast material.

T2-weighted MR images, cystic hygromas are typically isointense to cerebrospinal fluid (CSF), while they have a variable signal intensity on T1-weighted images owing to the variable protein content (Fig. 12.**124**). Rapid enlargement of a cervical cystic hygroma is usually due to hemorrhage into the cystic spaces of the mass. Multiple fluid–fluid levels, representing layering of blood and lymph, are characteristic in this clinical setting. Fluid–fluid levels may be identified on CT, but the conspicuity of this finding is more apparent on MR images.[115]

Lymphangiomas may present as isolated lesions or may occasionally be seen in association with cystic angiomatosis.[80] Skeletal–extraskeletal angiomatosis is defined as a benign vascular proliferation involving the medullary cavity of bone and at least one type of tissue. It has also been known as cystic angiomatosis, in which multiple cystic lesions are scattered diffusely throughout the skeleton, often with similar angiomatous changes in other tissues, usually the spleen. The disease is thought to be caused by faulty development of the precursor tissue of the lymphatic system. MR imaging is a very sensitive technique allowing detection of either diffuse or multifocal cystic skeletal lesions with or without visceral involvement (Fig. 12.**125**). Neck lymphangiomas seen in patients with cystic angiomatosis have the same imaging and histological features as isolated lymphangiomas.

Miscellaneous Pathology

Vascular Conditions

A detailed description of vascular conditions affecting the carotid and vertebral arteries as well as the internal jugular veins is beyond the scope of this chapter. However, because some of these conditions may be encountered while imaging the neck for other purposes, such as squamous cell cancer, infectious diseases, or cranial nerve palsy, a brief description of some of these conditions is given below.

Ectatic common or internal carotid artery may present clinically as a pulsatile mass and imaging is performed to exclude a paraganglioma. On CT and standard MRI, a tubular, tortuous, sometimes dilated common carotid artery or internal carotid artery may be seen. If the vessel folds sharply on itself, the appearance of an enhancing carotid space mass may be suggested and MR angiography or CT angiography may clarify the situation.

Dissection of the carotid and vertebral arteries is an often-overlooked cause of stroke, especially in young patients. Most often the dissection is seen in the extracranial vessels at the level of the suprahyoid neck immediately below or at the base of the skull. Dissection involving the infrahyoid portion of the carotid

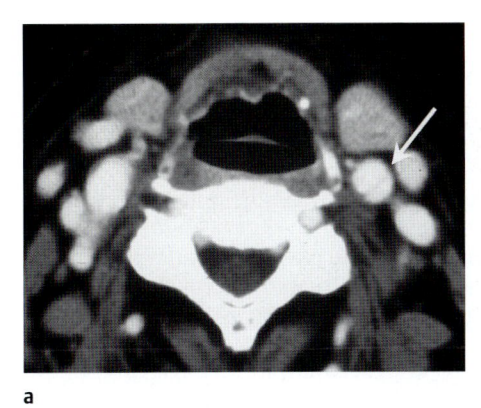

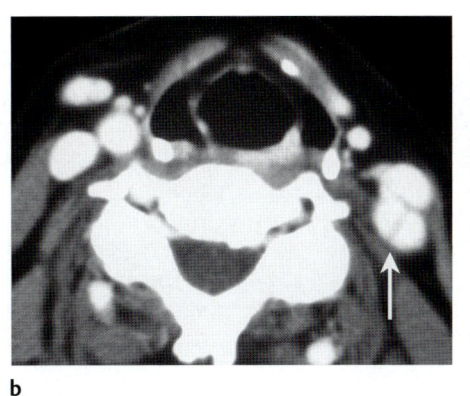

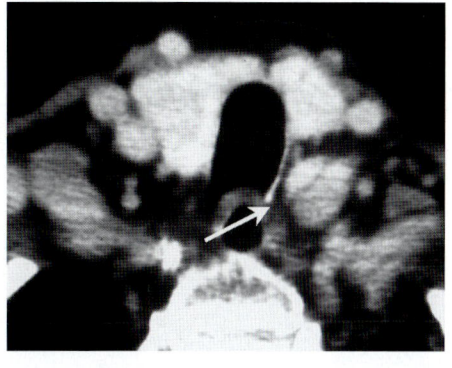

Fig. 12.**126 a–c** Dissection of the common carotid artery in an elderly woman presenting with Horner syndrome two weeks after chiropractic manipulation. Contrast-enhanced CT images of the infrahyoid neck show a tortuous left common carotid artery with an intimal flap and a true and a false lumen (arrows).

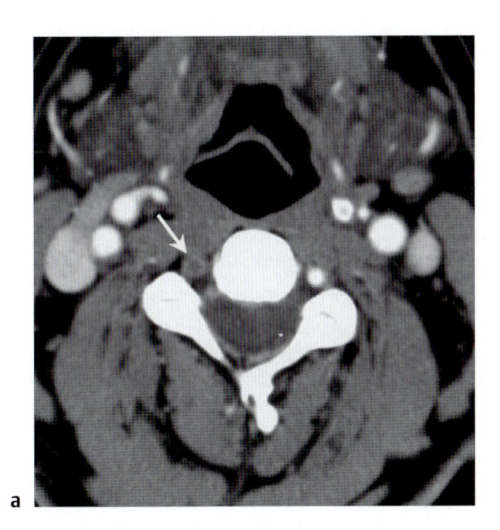

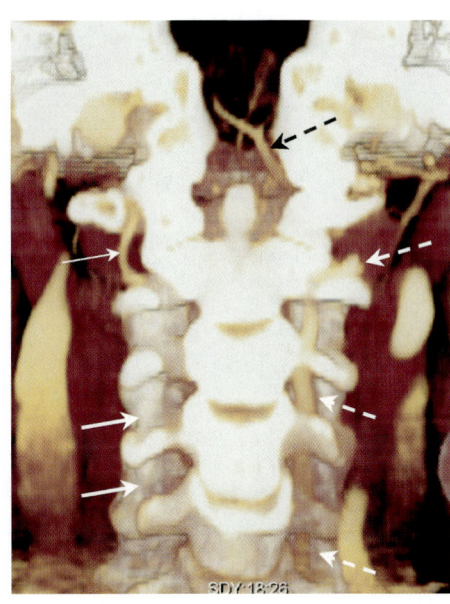

Fig. 12.**127** Dissection of the right vertebral artery in a young male patient presenting with vertigo and nystagmus in the emergency room. There were no sensory or motor deficits. **a** Contrast-enhanced CT image obtained two hours after onset of symptoms reveals occlusion of the right vertebral artery (arrow). **b** Coronal angio-CT reconstruction of the vertebral arteries demonstrates near-total occlusion of the cervical portion of the left vertebral artery (V2 segment, arrows). Thin arrow points to the patent V3 segment. Dashed arrows point to the normal left vertebral artery.

and vertebral arteries is rare, however. In extracranial dissection of the carotid arteries, patients may present with neck and face pain, as well as headache. Weeks to months after the dissection, they may develop Horner syndrome and cranial nerve involvement. In extracranial vertebral artery dissection, vertigo and nystagmus may be the only presenting symptoms. Dissection may occur after blunt trauma, sports injury, chiropractic manipulations, automobile accidents, and coughing (Figs. 12.**126**, 12.**127**). Rarely, direct puncture of the vessel from stab or gunshot wounds may cause vascular dissection. In most cases of extracranial dissection there is a residual lumen and thrombus rapidly fills the false lumen. MR and MR angiography are extremely helpful in detecting vascular dissection (Figs. 12.**128**, 12.**129**). On T1-weighted images, intramural hemorrhage usually has a high signal intensity and the residual patent lumen is seen as an area of flow void (Fig. 12.**128**). Fat-suppressed images may be helpful in distinguishing periadventitial fat from intramural subacute hemorrhage. Although rare, a double lumen (true lumen and intramural dissection) may be seen on CT, MRI, or MR angiography (Figs. 12.**126**, 12.**129**). On MR angiography, segmental tapering by the intramural hematoma, aneurysmal dilatation, and total vascular occlusion may be further observed.

Asymmetric internal jugular vein, an incidental finding on CT or MRI, is without any pathological significance, as a wide

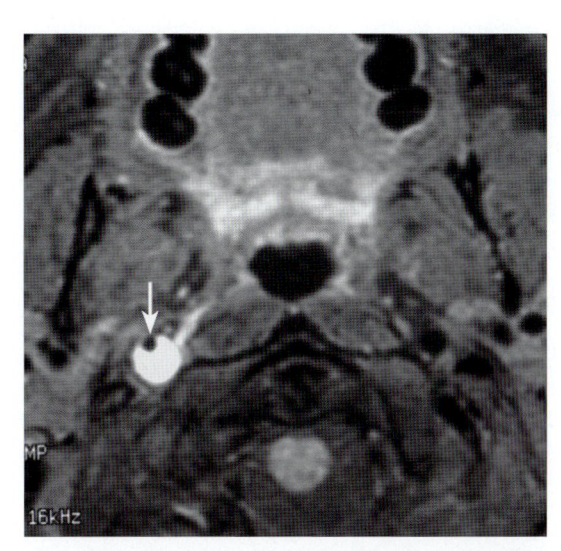

Fig. 12.**128** Dissection of the right internal carotid artery. Characteristic appearance on MRI. Fat-suppressed T1W MR image obtained in a patient with cranial nerve deficits (III, IV) shows the characteristic target appearance of an arterial dissection. The hypointense true lumen (arrow) is patent, while the hyperintense peripheral zone corresponds to thrombus in the false lumen.

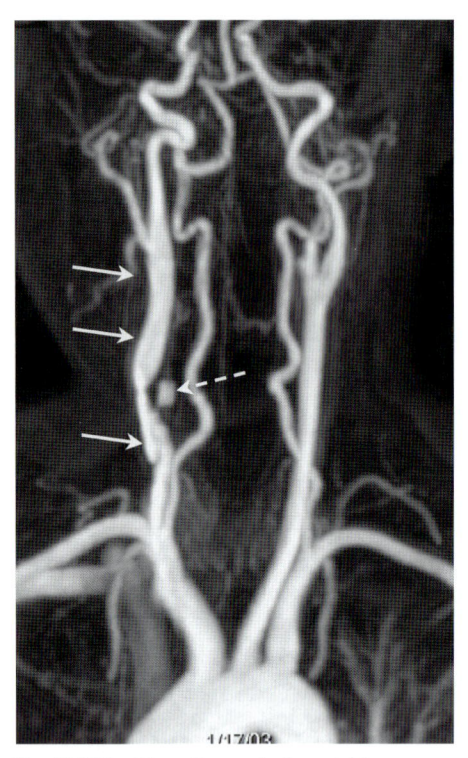

Fig. 12.**129** Dissection of the right common carotid artery with aneurysm formation in a patient with Takayasu arteritis. MR angiography obtained after intravenous injection of contrast material clearly shows the dissection of the common carotid artery on the right. An intimal flap (arrows) separating the true and false lumen is seen. A small aneurysm has formed on the right (dashed arrow).

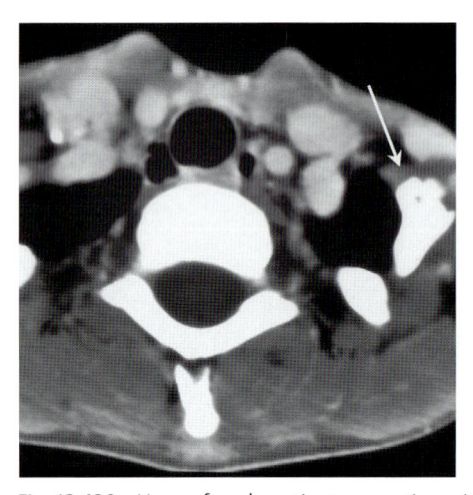

Fig. 12.**130** Young female patient presenting with an indurated supraclavicular mass at clinical examination. Contrast-enhanced CT shows a cervical rib (arrow), which was responsible for the palpable mass.

range of normal variation exists with respect to symmetry of the internal jugular veins. Clinically, patients may be referred to imaging by the referring physician because of a vague fullness of the neck (Fig. 12.**5**).

Jugular vein thrombosis may be caused by a variety of conditions, such as deep space infection (see above), drug abuse, central venous catheterization, and malignant tumors. The findings depend upon the stage of the disease. In the acute phase, there is marked loss of soft-tissue planes surrounding the enlarged, thrombus-filled internal jugular vein (Fig. 12.**105**). In the chronic phase, the internal jugular vein appears as a well-marginated tubular mass with preserved surrounding soft-tissue planes.[54]

Muscular and Osseous Structures That May Be Mistaken for Pathology

The levator scapulae muscle may undergo compensatory hypertrophy in patients with radical neck dissection and sacrifice of the spinal accessory nerve. The hypertrophied muscle should not be interpreted as a posterior neck mass deep to the (atrophic) trapezius muscle (see above).

The levator claviculae muscle is a normal variant seen in 2% of the population. The muscle is situated anterolateral to the levator scapular muscle and should not be mistaken for lymphadenopathy.

Cervical ribs may present clinically as a palpable supraclavicular mass and patients may be referred to CT for a search for lymphadenopathy. The correct diagnosis is easily made, however (Fig. 12.**130**).

Acknowledgments

I thank my colleagues and friends from the Radiology Department of the University Hospital in Geneva, particularly Dr. Jacqueline Delavelle, Dr. Nathalia Dfouni, Dr. Alain Keller, Dr. Romain Kohler, Dr. Haleem Khan, and Dr. Marco Palmesino, as well as Mr. Domingos Orlando and Mr. Philippe Cammarassa from the audiovisual unit, for their contributions.

References

1. Adamo C, Vescio G, Battaglia M, Gallelli G, Musella S. Madelung's disease: case report and discussion of treatment options. Ann Plast Surg 2001; 46(1): 43–45.
2. Adams S, Baum R, Stuckensen T, et al. Prospective comparison of ^{18}F-FDG PET with conventional imaging modalities (CT, MRI, US) in lymph node staging of hesd and neck cancer. Eur J Nucl Med 1998; 25: 1255–1260.
3. Ahuja AT, King AD, Chan ES, Kew J, Lam WW, Sun PM, King W, Metreweli C. Madelung disease: distribution of cervical fat and preoperative findings at sonography, MR, and CT. AJNR 1998; 19(4): 707–710.
4. Akerstrom G, Malmaeus J, Bergstrom R. Surgical anatomy of the human parathyroid glands. Surgery 1984; 95: 14–21.
5. Aldinger KA, Samaan NA, Haney M, et al. Anaplastic carcinoma of the thyroid: a review of 84 cases of spindle and giant cell carcinoma of the thyroid. Cancer 1978; 41: 2267–2275.
6. Ang AH, Pang KP, Tan LK. Complete branchial fistula. Case report and review of the literature. Ann Otol Rhinol Laryngol 2001; 110(11): 1077–1079.
7. Anzai Y, Prince MR. Iron oxide-enhanced MR lymphography: the evaluation of cervical lymph node metastases in head and neck cancer. J Magn Reson Imaging 1997; 75–81.
8. Ashcraft M, VanHerle A. Management of thyroid nodules I. Head and Neck Surg 1981; 216–227.
9. Ashcraft M, VanHerle A. Management of thyroid nodules II. Head and Neck Surg 1981; 297–322.
10. Bahna M, Canalis RF. Necrotizing fasciitis (streptococcal gangrene) of the face. Arch Otolaryngol 1980; 106: 648–651.
11. Becker M, Kurt AM. Infrahyoid neck: CT and MR imaging versus histopathology. Eur Radiol 1999 (9 Pt 2): 53–68.
12. Becker M, Schroth G, Zbären P, et al. Long-term changes induced by high-dose irradiation of the head and neck region: imaging findings. Radiographics 1997; 17: 5–26.
13. Becker M, Zbären P, Hermans R, et al. Necrotizing fasciitis of the head and neck: role of CT in diagnosis and management. Radiology 1997; 202: 471–476.

14. Belal A, Kandil A, Allam A, Khafaga Y, El-Husseiny G, El-Enbaby A, Memon M, Younge D, Moreau P, Gray A, Schultz H. Malignant fibrous histiocytoma: a retrospective study of 109 cases. Am J Clin Oncol 2002; 25(1): 16–22.
15. Berger P S, Bataini J P. Radiation induced cranial nerve palsy. Cancer 1977; 40: 152–155.
16. Benchaou M, Lehmann W, Slosman DO, et al. The role of FDG-PET in the preoperative assessment of N-staging in head and neck cancer. Acta Otolaryngol (Stockh) 1996; 332–335.
17. Bird R J, Bryce D P. Long-term effects of heavy irradiation to the neck. J Otolaryngol 1980; 9: 18–23.
18. Bisno AL, Stevens DL. Streptococcal infections of skin and soft tissues. Current concepts. N Engl J Med 1996; 334(4): 240–245.
19. Bonetta A, Gelli MC, Zini G, Iotti C, Barbieri V, Pedroni C, Armaroli L. Postradiation sarcoma of head and neck: report of two cases. Tumori 1996; 82(3): 270–272.
20. Boucher C, Dorion D, Fisch C. Retropharyngeal abscesses. A clinical and radiologic correlation. J Otolaryngol 1999; 28: 134–137.
21. Briggs RD, Pou AM, Schnadig VJ. Cystic metastasis versus branchial cleft carcinoma: a diagnostic challenge. Laryngoscope 2002; 112(6): 1010–1014.
22. Budde R, Hesse G, Cantemir S, Laubert A. Myositis proliferans. Differential cervical space-occupying lesion diagnosis. HNO 2002; 50(4): 358–361.
23. Cady B. Papillary carcinoma of the thyroid. Semin Surg Oncol 1991; 7: 81–86.
24. Cain AJ, Michie BA, Davis BC, Ram B. Focal myositis of the sternocleidomastoid muscle. J Laryngol Otol 1998; 112(7): 687–689.
25. Carron JD, Darrow DH, Karakla DW. Fetal rhabdomyoma of the posterior cervical triangle. Int J Pediatr Otorhinolaryngol 2001; 61(1): 77–81.
26. Celis I, Bijnens E, Peene P, et al. The use of preoperative fistulography in patients with a second branchial cleft anomaly. Eur Radiol 1998; 8: 1179–1180.
27. Cheng VST, Schulz MD. Unilateral hypoglossal nerve atrophy as a late complication of radiation therapy of head and neck carcinoma. A report of four cases and a review of the literature on peripheral and cranial nerve damages after radiation therapy. Cancer 1975; 35: 1537–1544.
28. Chung TS, Yousem DM, Lexa FJ, Markiewicz DA. MRI of carotid angiopathy after therapeutic radiation. J Comput Assist Tomogr 1994; 18(4): 533–538.
29. Cleveland DB, Chen SY, Allen CM, Ahing SI, Svirsky JA. Adult rhabdomyoma. A light microscopic, ultrastructural, virologic, and immunologic analysis. Oral Surg Oral Med Oral Pathol 1994; 77(2): 147–153.
30. Conomy J P, Kellermeyer R W. Delayed cerebrovascular consequences of therapeutic irradiation. A clinicopathologic study of a stroke associated with radiation-related carotid arteriopathy. Cancer 1975; 36: 1702–1708.
31. Craswell P W T. Vocal cord paralysis following radioactive iodine therapy. Br J Clin Pract 1972; 26: 571–572.
32. Curtin HD, Ishwaran H, Mancuso AA, et al. Comparison of CT and MR imaging in staging of neck metastases. Radiology 1998; 207: 123–130.
33. Datar S, Patanakar T, Armao D, Mukherji SK. Papillary carcinoma in a giant thyroglossal duct cyst. Clin Imaging 2000; 24(2): 75–77.
34. Davis BT, Bagg A, Milmoe Gj. CT and MR appearance of Castleman's disease of the neck. AJNR 1999; 173: 861–862.
35. Davis WL, Harnsberger HR, Smoker WRK, Watanabe AS. Retropharyngeal space: Evaluation of normal anatomy and diseases with CT and MR imaging. Radiology 1990; 174: 59–64.
36. Deland E M. Radiation damage to tissue and its repair. Surg Gynecol Obstet 1941; 72: 372–383.
37. Dellelis RA. Tumors of the parathyroid glands. Atlas of Tumor Pathology, series 3, fascicle 6. Washington DC: Armed Forces Institute of Pathology; 1993.
38. Deroux E. Complications of dental infections. Rev Med Brux 2001; 22(4): A289–295.
39. Dhanasekar G, Rajan MS, Nirmal Kumar B, Watson SD. Focal myositis of the neck with idiopathic orbital myositis. J Laryngol Otol 2002; 116(4): 314–316.
40. Di Martino E, Krombach GA, Nowak B, Sellhaus B, Schmitz-Rode T, Hausmann R, Westhofen M.Color duplex sonography in post-therapeutic neck evaluation. Am J Otolaryngol 2002; 23(3): 153–159.
41. Di Martino E, Nowak B, Hassan HA, Hausmann R, Adam G, Buell U, Westhofen M. Diagnosis and staging of head and neck cancer: a comparison of modern imaging modalities (positron emission tomography, computed tomography, color-coded duplex sonography) with panendoscopic and histopathologic findings. Arch Otolaryngol Head Neck Surg 2000; 126(12): 1457–1461.
42. Ducatman BS, Scheithauer BW, Piepgras DG, Reiman HM, Ilstrup DM. Malignant peripheral nerve sheath tumors. A clinicopathologic study of 120 cases. Cancer 1986; 15(57(10)): 2006–2021.
43. Einarsdittir H, Soderlund V, Larson O, Jenner G, Bauer HC. MR imaging of lipoma and liposarcoma. Acta Radiol 1999; 40(1): 64–68.
44. Eisenkraft BL, Som PM. The spectrum of benign and malignant cervical node calcification. AJR 1999; 172: 1433–1437.
45. Fajardo L F, Berthrong M. Vascular lesions following radiation. In: Rosen PP, Fechner RE, eds. Pathology Annual, Part 1, Vol. 23. Norwalk CT: Appleton and Lange; 1988: 297–330.
46. Fischbein NJ, Assar OS, Caputo GR, et al. Clinical utility of positron emission tomography with ^{18}F-fluorodeoxyglucose in detecting residual/recurrent squamous cell carcinoma of the head and neck. AJNR 1998; 19: 1189–1196.
47. Fliss DM, Tovi F, Zirkin JH. Necrotizing soft tissue infections of dental origin. J Oral Maxillofac Surg 1990; 48: 1104–1108.
48. Fortun C, Barros J Melcon C, Condes E, Cobo E, Perez-Martinez C, Ruiz-Galiana J, Martinez-Vidal A, Alvarez F. Extra-laryngeal head and neck tuberculosis. Clin Microbiol Infect 2000; 6(12): 644–648.
49. Giuliano A, Lewis F, Hadley K, Blaisdell FW. Bacteriology of necrotizing fasciitis. Am J Surg 1977; 134: 52–56.
50. Gooding GA, Sonography of the thyroid and parathyroid. Radiol Clin North Am 1993; 31: 967–989.
51. Graziani M, Logoluso G, Boldrini R, Fasanelli S. Aggressive fibromatosis in childhood. Radiol Med (Torino) 1995; 89(3): 364–367.
52. Gross BH. Radiographic manifestations of lymph node involvement in amyloidosis. Radiology 1981; 138: 11–14.
53. Gross ND, Weissman JL, Talbot JM, et al. MRI detection of cervical metastasis from differentiated thyroid carcinoma. Laryngoscope 2001; 11: 1905–1909.
54. Harnsberger HR. Handbook of Head and Neck Imaging. St. Louis, MO: Mosby-Year Book; 1995.
55. Haberal I, Samim E, Astarci M, Ozeri C. Radiation-induced malignant fibrous histiocytoma of the neck in a patient with laryngeal carcinoma. Am J Otolaryngol 2001; 22(2): 146–149.
56. Hanley JP, MacLean FR, Evans JL, Colls BM, Robinson BA, Patton WN, Heaton DC. Hemorrhagic lymphadenopathy as a presenting feature of primary al amyloidosis. Pathology 2000; 32(1): 21–23.
57. Hermanns R, Pameijer FA, Mancuso AA, et al. Laryngeal or hypopharyngeal squamous cell carcinoma: can followup CT after definitive radiotherapy be used to detect local failure earlier than clinical examination alone? Radiology 2000; 214: 683–687.
58. Higgins CB. Role of magnetic resonance imaging in hyperparathyroidism. Radiol Clin North Am 1993; 31: 1017–1028.
59. Higgins CB, Auffermann W. MR imaging of thyroid and parathyroid glands: a review of current status. AJR 1988; 151(6): 1095–1106.
60. Higgins CB, McNamara MT, Fisher MR, Clark OH. MR imaging of the thyroid. AJR 1986; 147(6): 1255–1261.
61. Homicz MR, Carvalho D, Kearns DB, Edmonds J. An atypical presentation of Kawasaki disease resembling a retropharyngeal abscess. Int J Pediatr Otorhinolaryngol 2000; 11(54(1)): 45–49.
62. Hoos A, Lewis JJ, Urist MJ, Shaha AR, Hawkins WG, Shah JP, Brennan MF. Desmoid tumors of the head and neck–a clinical study of a rare entity. Head Neck 2000; 22(8): 814–821.
63. Huang RY, Damrose EJ, Alavi S, Maceri DR, Shapiro NL. Third branchial cleft anomaly presenting as a retropharyngeal abscess. Int J Pediatr Otorhinolaryngol 2000; 54(2–3): 167–172.
64. Hudgins PA, Dorey JH, Jacobs IN. Internal carotid artery narrowing in children with retropharyngeal lymphadenitis and abscess. AJNR 1998; 19(10): 1841–1843.
65. Huvos AG, Leaming RH, Moore OS. Clinico-pathologic study of the resected carotid artery: analysis of sixty-four cases. Am J Surg 1973; 126: 570–574.
66. Johnson JT. A surgeon looks at cervical lymph nodes. Radiology 1990; 175: 607–610.
67. Kalbacha ME, Stankiewicz JA, Clift SE. Severe soft tissue infection of the face and neck. A classification. Laryngoscope 1982; 92: 1135–1139.
68. Karkanevatos A, Beasley NJP, Swift AC. Acute non-tuberculous retropharyngeal abscess in an adult. A case report and review of the literature. J Laryngol Otol 1997; 111: 169–171.
69. Kasagi K, Hatabu H, Tokuda Y, et al. Lymphoproliferative disorders in the thyroid gland. Radiological appearances. Br J Radiol 1991; 64: 569–575.
70. Kingston CA, Owens CM, Jeanes A, Malone M. Imaging of desmoid fibromatosis in pediatric patients. AJR 2002; 178(1): 191–199.
71. Kirse DJ, Roberson DW. Surgical management of retropharyngeal space infections in children. Laryngoscope 2001; 111(8): 1413–1422.

72. Kleihues P, Louis DN, Scheithauer BW, Rorke LB, Reifenberger G, Burger PC, Cavenee WK. The WHO classification of tumors of the nervous system. J Neuropathol Exp Neurol 2002; 61(3): 215–225.
73. Kleinsasser O. Radiation therapy. In: Kleinsasser O, ed. Tumors of the Larynx and Hypopharynx. New York: Thieme Medical Publishers; 1988: 234–253.
74. Koeller KK, Alamo L, Adair CF, Smirniotopoulos JG. Congenital cystic masses of the neck: radiologic-pathologic correlation. Radiographics 1999; 19(1): 121–146.
75. Koischwitz D, Gritzmann N. Ultrasound of the Neck. Radiol Clin North Am 2000; 38(5): 1029–1045.
76. Kratz C, Lenard HG, Ruzicka T, Gartner J. Multiple symmetric lipomatosis: an unusual cause of childhood obesity and mental retardation. Eur J Paediatr Neurol 2000; 4(2): 63–77.
77. Laiwani AK, Kaplan M J. Mediastinal and thoracic complications of necrotizing fasciitis of the head and neck. Head Neck 1991; 13: 531–539.
78. Laubenbacher C, Saumweber D, Wagner-Manslau C, et al. Comparison of fluorine-18-fluorodeoxyglucose PET, MRI and endoscopy for staging head and neck squamous cell carcinoms. J Nucl Med 1995: 36: 1747–1757.
79. Lee YY, Van Tassel P, Nauert C, et al. Lymphomas of the head and neck: CT findings at initial presentation AJNR 1987; 8: 665–671.
80. Levey DS, MacCormack LM, Sartoris DJ, Haghighi P, Resnick D, Thorne R. Cystic angiomatosis: case report and review of the literature. Skeletal Radiol 1996; 25(3): 287–293.
81. Ljunggren MP, Ebbo D, Koubbi G, Barrault S, Vuong N. How to treat a thyroid adenocarcinoma inside a branchial cyst. Ann Otolaryngol Chir Cervicofac 2002; 119(1): 52–55.
82. Lindner HH. The anatomy of the fasciae of the face and neck with particular reference to the spread and treatment of intraoral infections (Ludwig's) that have progressed into adjacent fascial spaces. Ann Surg 1986; 204: 705–714.
83. Mafee MF, Raofi B, Kumar A, et al. Glomus faciale, glomus jugulare, glomus tympanicum, glomus vagale, carotid body tumors and simulating lesions. Role of MR imaging. Radiol Clin North Am 2000; 38: 1059–1076.
84. Mancuso AA, Dillon WP. The neck. Radiol Clin North Am 1989; 27; 407–434.
85. Mancuso AA, Maceri D, Rice D, et al. CT of cervical lymph node cancer. AJR 1981; 136: 381–385.
86. Mancuso AA, Harnsberger HR, Muraki AS, Stevens MH. Computed tomography of cervical and retropharyngeal lymph nodes: normal anatomy, variants of normal, and applications in staging head and neck cancer. Part II: pathology. Radiology 1983; 148(3): 715–723.
87. Mancuso AA, Harnsberger HR, Muraki AS, Stevens MH. Computed tomography of cervical and retropharyngeal lymph nodes: normal anatomy, variants of normal, and applications in staging head and neck cancer. Part I: normal anatomy. Radiology 1983; 148(3): 709–714.
88. Mancuso AA. Imaging in patients with head and neck cancer In: Million RR, Cassisi NJ, eds. Management of Head and Neck Cancer. A Multidisciplinary Approach, 2 nd ed. Philadelphia: J.B. Lippincott; 1994: 43–59.
89. Mazzaferri EL. Management of a solitary thyroid nodule. N Engl J Med 1993; 328(8): 553–559.
90. Mazzaferri EL. Thyroid cancer in thyroid nodules: finding a needle in the haystack. Am J Med 1992; 93(4): 359–362.
91. Michna G, Ghanem N, Laubenberger J, Schneider B, Kromeier J, Langer M. Relevance of magnetic resonance imaging for the staging and follow up of lymph node pathologies in adults with primary malignant lymphomas. Radiologe 2002; 42(12): 993–999.
92. Modan B, Baidaz D, Mart H et al. Radiation-induced head and neck tumors. Lancet 1974; 1: 277–279.
93. Moon WK, Han MH, Chang KH, et al. CT and MR imaging of head and neck tuberculosis. Radiographics 1997; 17: 391–402.
94. Morita T, Fujiki N, Shiomi Y, Kurata K, Oda N. Atlantoaxial subluxation in an adult secondary to retropharyngeal abscess. Auris Nasus Larynx 2001; 28(2): 177–179.
95. Morse MA, Bossen E, D'Amico TA, Williamson W, Johnson R. Myxoid liposarcoma of the supraclavicular fossa. Chest 2000; 117(5): 1518–1520.
96. Mukherji SK, Fatterpekar G, Castillo M, Stone JA, Chung CJ. Imaging of congenital anomalies of the branchial apparatus. Neuroimaging Clin North Am 2000; 10(1): 75–93.
97. Mulliken JB, Glowacki J (1982) Hemangiomas and vascular malformations in infants and children: a classification based on endothelial characteristics. Plast Reconstr Surg 69: 412–420.
98. Munoz A, Castillo M, Melchor MA, Gutierrez R. Acute neck infections: prospective comparison between CT and MRI in 47 patients. J Comput Assist Tomogr 2001; 25(5): 733–741.
99. Nathan AR, Raines KR, Lee YM, et al. Fine-needle aspiration biopsy of cold thyroid nodules. Cancer 1988; 62: 1337–1342.
100. Newland JR, Linke RP, Kleinsasser O, Lennert K. Lymph node enlargement due to amyloid. Virchows Arch A Pathol Anat Histopathol 1983; 399(2): 233–236.
101. Nicollas R, Ducroz V, Garabedian EN, Triglia JM. Fourth branchial pouch anomalies: a study of six cases and review of the literature. Int J Pediatr Otorhinolaryngol 1998; 44(1): 5–10.
102. Nusbaum AO, Som PM, Rothschild MA, Shugar JM. Recurrence of a deep neck infection: a clinical indication of an underlying congenital lesion. Arch Otolaryngol Head Neck Surg 1999; 125(12): 1379–1382.
103. Otte T, Kleinsasser O. Liposarcoma of the head and neck. Arch Otorhinolaryngol 1981; 232(3): 285–291.
104. Parsons JT. The effect of radiation on normal tissues of the head and neck. In: Million RR, Cassisi NJ, eds. Management of Head and Neck Cancer. A Multidisciplinary Approach, 2 d ed. Philadelphia: J.B. Lippincott; 1994: 245–289.
105. Pappo AS, Meza JL, Donaldson SS, Wharam MD, Wiener ES, Qualman SJ, Maurer HM, Crist WM. Treatment of localized nonorbital, nonparameningeal head and neck rhabdomyosarcoma: lessons learned from intergroup rhabdomyosarcoma studies III and IV. J Clin Oncol 2003; 21(4): 638–645.
106. Patel SR. Radiation-induced sarcoma. Curr Treat Options Oncol 2000; 1(3): 258–261.
107. Perez-Cruet MJ, Burke JM, Weber R, DeMonte F. Aggressive fibromatosis involving the cranial base in children. Neurosurgery 1998; 43(5): 1096–1102.
108. Petti G, Kirk G. Parathyroid imaging. Otolaryngol Clin North Am 1996; 29: 681–691.
109. Piccolo R, Passanisi M, Chiaramonte I, Tropea R, Mancuso P. Cervical spinal epidural abscesses. A report on five cases. J Neurosurg Sci 1999; 43(1): 63–67.
110. Piedbois P, Becquemin JP, Blanc I, Mazeron JJ, Lange F, Melliere D, Le Bourggeois JP. Arterial occlusive disease after radiotherapy: a report of fourteen cases. Radiat Oncol 1990; 17: 133–140.
111. Popperl G, Lang S, Dagdelen O, et al. Correlation of FDG-PET and MRI/CT with histopathology in primary diagnosis, lymph node staging and diagnosis of recurrency of head and neck cancer. Rofo Fortschr 2002; 174: 714–720.
112. Price DC. Radioisotopic evaluation of the thyroid and parathyroids. Radiol Clin North Am 1993; 31: 991–1015.
113. Rai AT, Nguyen TP, Hogg JP, Gabriele FJ. Aggressive fibromatosis of the neck in a patient with Gardner's syndrome. Neuroradiology 2001; 43(8): 650–652.
114. Reed JM, Anaid VK. Odontogenic cervical necrotizing fasciitis with intrathoracic extension. Otolaryngol Head Neck Surg 1992; 107(4): 596–600.
115. Reede DL, Whelan MA, Bergeron RT. Computed Tomography of the infrahyoid neck. Radiology 1982; 145: 397–402.
116. Robson CD, Hazra R, Barnes PD, Robertson RL, Jones D, Husson RN. Nontuberculous mycobacterial infection of the head and neck in immunocompetent children: CT and MR findings. AJNR 1999; 20(10): 1829–1835.
117. Rojeski MT, Gharib H. Nodular thyroid disease: evaluation and management. N Engl J Med 1985; 313: 481–486.
118. Sakai O, Curtin HD, Romo LV, Som PM. Lymph node pathology. Benign proliferative, lymphoma, and metastatic disease. Radiol Clin North Am 2000; 38(5): 979–998.
119. Schmidt G. Schilddrüse. In: Sonographische Differentialdiagnose. Stuttgart: Georg Thieme Verlag; 2002: 431–462.
120. Schwaegerle SM, Bauer TM, Esselstyn C. Riedel's thyroiditis. J Clin Pathol 1988; 90: 515–522.
121. Shimazaki T, Yoshida Y, Umeno H, Nomura Y, Nakashima T. Two cases of piriform sinus fistula which required a long time for diagnosis. Auris Nasus Larynx 1999; 26(4): 501–507.
122. Sigal R. Infrahyoid neck. Radiol Clin North Am 1998; 36(5): 781–799.
123. Sigal R. Post-therapeutic imaging of upper aerodigestive tract tumors. Semin Roentgenol 2000; 35(1): 101–110.
124. Sigal R, Vogl T, Casselman J, et al. Lymph node metastases from head and neck squamous cell carcinoma: MR imaging with ultrasmall superparamagnetic iron oxide particles (Sinerem MR)—results of a phase-III multicenter clinical trial. Eur Radiol 2002; 12(5): 1104–1113.

125 Silverberg GD, Britt RH, Goffinet DR. Radiation-induced carotid artery disease. Cancer 1978; 41: 130–137.
126 Snow GB, Annyas M, Van Slooten EA, et al. Prognostic factors of neck node metastasis. Clin Otolaryngol 1982; 7: 185–192.
127 Smith ME, Fisher C, Weiss SW. Pleomorphic hyalinizing angiectatic tumor of soft parts. A low-grade neoplasm resembling neurilemoma. Am J Surg Pathol 1996; 20: 21–29.
128 Som PM. Update on imaging metastatic cervical lymph nodes: Criteria and differential diagnosis. AJR 1992; 158: 961–969.
129 Som PM, Biller H. Kimura disease involving parotid gland and cervical lymph nodes. CT and MR findings. J Comput Assist Tomogr 1992; 16: 320–322.
130 Som PM, Brandwein M, Lidov M, et al. The varied presentations of papillary thyroid carcinoma cervical nodal disease: CT and MR findings. AJNR 1994; 15: 1123–1128.
131 Som PM, Curtin HD, Mancuso AA. An imaging-based classification for the cervical nodes designated as an adjunct to clinically based nodal classifications. Arch Otolaryngol Head and Neck Surg 1999; 125: 388–396.
132 Som PM, Curtin HD, Mancuso AA. Imaging-based nodal classification for evaluation of neck metastatic adenopathy. AJR 2000; 174(3): 837–844.
133 Stamenkovic I, Lew D. Early recognition of potentially fatal necrotizing fasciitis. N Engl J Med 1984; 310: 1689–1693.
134 Steinkamp HJ, Hosten N, Richter C, et al. Enlarged cervical lymph nodes at helical CT. Radiology 1994; 191: 795–798.
135 Stevens DL. Invasive group A streptococcal infections: the past, present and future. Pediatr Infect Dis J 1994; 13: 561–566.
136 Stevens SK, Chang JM, Clark OH, et al. Detection of abnormal parathyroid glands in postoperative patients with recurrent hyperparathyroidism. Sensitivity of MR imaging. AJR 1993; 160: 607–612.
137 Stone ME, Walner DL, Koch BL, Egelhoff JC, Myer CM. Correlation between computed tomography and surgical findings in retropharyngeal inflammatory processes in children. Int J Pediatr Otorhinolaryngol 1999; 49(2): 121–125.
138 Strauss HR, Tilghman DM, Hankins J. Ludwig's angina, empyema, pulmonary infiltration and pericarditis secondary to extraction of a tooth. J Oral Surg 1980; 38: 223–229.
139 Takes R, Knegt P, Mani J, et al. Regional metastases in head and neck squamous cell carcinoma: revised value of US with US-guided FNAB. Radiology 1996;198: 819–823.
140 Takoudes TG, Haddad J Jr. Retropharyngeal abscess and Epstein–Barr virus infection in children. Ann Otol Rhinol Laryngol 1998; 107(12): 1072–1075
141 Told NW. Common congenital anomalies of the neck. Surg Clin North Am 1993; 73: 599–604.
142 Tomura N, Watanabe O, Hirano Y, Kato K, Takahashi S, Watarai J. MR imaging of recurrent head and neck tumours following flap reconstructive surgery. Clin Radiol 2002; 57(2): 109–113.
143 Tovi F, Fliss DM, Zirkim HJ. Necrotizing soft-tissue infections in the head and neck: a clinicopathologic study. Laryngoscope 1991; 101: 619–625.
144 Urquhart A, Berg R. Hodgkin's and non-Hodgkin's lymphoma of the head and neck. Laryngoscope 2001; 111: 1565–1569.
145 Urquhart AC, Hutchins LG, Berg RL. Distinguishing non-Hodgkin lymphoma from squamous cell carcinoma tumors of the head and neck by computed tomography parameters. Laryngoscope 2002; 112: 1079–1083.
146 Van den Brekel MWM. Lymph node metastases: CT and MRI. Eur J Radiol 2000; 33: 230–238.
147 Van den Brekel MWM, Castelijns JA, Snow GB. Imaging of cervical lymphadenopathy. Neuroimaging Clin North Am 1996; 6: 417–434.
148 Van den Brekel MWM, Castelijns JA, Stel HV, et al. Detection and characterization of metastatic cervical adenopathy by MR imaging: Comparison of different MR techniques. J Comput Assist Tomogr 1990; 14: 581–589.
149 Van den Brekel MWM, Stel HV, Castelijns JA, et al. Cervical lymph node metastasis: Assessment of radiologic criteria. Radiology 1990; 177; 379–384.
150 Wanebo JE, Malik JM, VandenBerg SR, Wanebo HJ, Driesen N, Persing JA. Malignant peripheral nerve sheath tumors. A clinicopathologic study of 28 cases. Cancer 1993; 71(4): 1247–1253.
151 Weber AL, Montandon C, Robson CD. Neurogenic tumors of the neck. Radiol Clin North Am 2000; 38: 1077–1090.
152 Welzel C, Gajda M, Jamali Y, Schrom T, Berghaus A, Holzhausen HJ. Adult multilocular rhabdomyoma as etiology of a space-occupying lesion in the area of the neck. HNO 2001; 49(7): 553–556.
153 Wetmore RF, Mahboubi S, Soyupak SK. Computed tomography in the evaluation of pediatric neck infections. Otolaryngol Head Neck Surg 1998; 119(6): 624–627.
154 Wills PI, Vernon RP. Complications of neck space infections of the head and neck. Laryngoscope 1981; 91: 1129–1136.
155 Yousem DM, Hatabu H, Hurst RW, et al. Carotid artery invasion by head and neck masses: Prediction with MR imaging. Radiology 1995; 195: 715–720.
156 Yousem DM, Som PM, Hackney DB et al. Central nodal necrosis and extracapsular neoplastic spread in cervical lymph nodes: MR imaging versus CT. Radiology 1992; 182: 753–759.
157 Zadvinskis DP (1992) Congenital malformations of the cervicothoracic lymphatic system: embryology and pathogenesis. Radiographics 12: 1175–1189.
158 Zbären P, Becker M. Schwannoma of the brachial plexus. Ann Otol Rhinol Laryngol 1996; 105: 748–750.
159 Zbären P, Lang H, Becker M. Rare benign neoplasms of the larynx: rhabdomyoma and lipoma. ORL J Otorhinolaryngol Relat Spec 1995: 57: 351–355.
160 Zeidler R, Lang S, Rasp G. Giant Madelung's disease. Report of a case and review of the literature. HNO 2002; 50(12): 1075–1078.

Index

A

abducens nerve 203, 212
abscess
　Bezold 318
　brain 391, 394
　carotid space 602–603
　cervical lymph nodes 824, 825
　cervical spinal epidural 828, 829
　choroidal 155
　intracranial 63, 64
　lacrimal glands 278, 279
　lymph nodes 793
　masticator space 610, 611
　odontogenic infections 711, 712
　orbit 226, 229, 391, 392, 394
　otogenic 82
　parapharyngeal space 600
　paratonsillar 562
　parotid gland 643, 644
　parotid space 613, 614
　peritonsillar 594
　postoperative neck 822
　retropharyngeal space 598–599, 618, 827, 828
　retrostyloid parapharyngeal space 602–603
　salivary glands 643, 644
　sinogenic epidural 317, 391, 393
　subdural 391, 393
　subgaleal 395
　submandibular space 616–617
　subperiosteal 64, 392, 394
　　orbital 229–230
　tonsillar 716, 717
　toxocara 174
acinic cell carcinoma
　parapharyngeal space 602
　salivary glands 634, 657, 669, 670, 674, 675
　　minor 704
　sinonasal cavities 431, 433, 434
acoustic nerve 109
　sagittal section 28
acoustic neuroma 117
　pneumocisternography 118
acrocephalosyndactyly type II see Saethre-Chotzen disease
acromegaly 486
actinomycosis, oral cavity/oropharynx 718
adenitis, lacrimal 234, 235
adenocarcinoma
　eye 188
　larynx 759
　low-grade of endolymphatic sac origin 338, 339–340
　minor salivary glands 704, 705
　nasopharyngeal 574
　papillary 574
　renal 760, 761
　sinonasal cavities 433–434
　temporal bone 329, 339, 340
adenoid 553, 557, 558
　hyperplasia 716
　hypertrophy 594

adenoid cystic carcinoma
　jaw 527, 542, 543
　laryngeal 758–759
　masticator space 613
　metastases 433
　parapharyngeal space 602
　perineural extension 318–319, 377, 433
　　hard palate 665
　　masticator space 613
　　salivary glands 655, 670, 673
　　sinonasal cavities 432
　recurrence 433
　salivary gland 634, 657, 659, 671–674
　　minor glands 664, 665, 703–704
　sinonasal cavities 416, 431–433, 434
　survival rate 673
　treatment 434
adenoma
　eye 188
　oxyphilic 668
　parathyroid 813, 814
　pleomorphic 431
　　histology 660
　　malignant transformation 664
　　minor salivary glands 664, 666, 703
　　oral cavity/oropharynx 707
　　parotid 656, 661
　　recurrence 663–664
　　salivary gland 601–602, 634, 656, 659–664, 661
　　sinonasal cavities 431
　sinonasal cavities 416, 431
　temporal bone 96
　thyroid nodules 807–808
　see also pituitary adenoma
adenomatoid odontogenic cyst 518
adenomatoid odontogenic tumor 529
adenopathy
　cervical 827
　reactive 824
　suppurative 824, 825
aditus
　cholesteatoma 79, 80, 82
　coronal oblique 20° sections 20
aerodigestive tract 783–784
agger nasi cells 361, 362, 363
AIDS
　cervical lymph nodes 826
　non-Hodgkin lymphoma 439
　　incidence 340
　ocular lymphoma 186
　parotid lymphoepithelial lesions/cysts 651–654
　salivary glands 651–654
　tuberculosis 74
alae 355
Alagille syndrome 53
Albers-Schonberg disease see osteopetrosis
allergic granulomatosis and angiitis 404
allergy
　nasal cavity 400, 401
　paranasal sinus tumors 412
　paranasal sinuses 400, 401

Alport syndrome 53
alveolar artery, inferior 510–511
alveolar mucosa carcinoma 695
alveolar nerves 511
ameloblastic fibroodontoma 528
ameloblastoma
　mandible 518, 522–523, 524–528, 711
　masticator space 612
　maxilla 518, 522–523, 527
　recurrent 526, 528
　salivary glands 664, 665
　sinonasal cavities 422, 423–424, 426, 427
　skull base 315
　temporomandibular joint 503
amyloid deposition, thyroid gland 834
amyloidosis
　hypervascular neck mass differential diagnosis 803, 804
　lacrimal glands 281
　larynx 772, 773
　orbital 244
　systemic 834
　tongue 724
aneurysmal bone cyst
　giant-cell tumor of maxilla/mandible 532–533, 534
　orbital 226
　sinonasal cavities 425
aneurysms, internal auditory canal 119, 120
angiitis, hypersensitivity orbital 243
angiodysplasia, cervicofacial 774
angiofibroma
　juvenile nasopharyngeal 344, 345, 563–565, 566, 594–595
　sinonasal cavities 416, 418
　skull base involvement 344, 345
angiography, radiotherapy complications 818
angiokeratoma corporis diffusum syndrome 486
angiolymphoid hyperplasia with eosinophilia 646
angiomatosis, cystic 840
angiomatosis retinae 184, 186
angiopathy, radiation 816–818
angiosarcoma, radiation-induced 819
annulus of Zinn 201
annulus tympanicus 19
anophthalmia 146, 370
antinuclear antibodies 243
antrochoanal polyps 565, 567
antrostomy 470, 471, 472
antrum 5
Apert disease
　maxilla anomalies 514
　orbit 216–217
apicitis, petrous 317–318
apocrine hidrocystoma 222
aqueous humor 142
　MRI 145
arachnoid granulations 40
arterial malformations, laryngeal 774
arteriography, glomus tumors 102, 105
arteriopathy, radiation 817

arteriovenous malformations
　facial 540, 541
　oral cavity/oropharynx 721, 722
　orbital 259–262
arteriovenous shunt, orbital varix 259
arthritis
　infectious 486–487
　metabolic 495, 496
　psoriatic 495
　temporomandibular joint 493–499
articular eminence 477
　pneumatization 482, 484
articular tubercle 477
aryepiglottic folds 732, 733, 735
　carcinoma 740
　piriform sinus carcinoma 744
arytenoid cartilage 732, 733
　glottic carcinoma spread 472
　neoplastic invasion 751
aspergillosis
　fungal balls 441
　nasopharyngeal inflammation 561
　orbital 230, 231
　paranasal sinus mucocele 405
　sinusitis 391, 396–397
　skull base 317–318
　Tolosa–Hunt syndrome 236, 237
aspergillosis, sinusitis 400
astrocytic hamartoma, ocular 162, 174, 175
atlantoaxial subluxation 828–829
atlas 300
auditory meatus, internal 28, 29
auditory ossicles 3
　anomalies 44, 45–46
　dislocation 56, 57, 58, 59
　disruption 56
　postoperative imaging 92
auricle deformity 43–44, 45

B

bacterial infection
　cervical lymph nodes 824
　complications 831–832
　eye 154
　retropharyngeal space 827
　sinusitis
　　acute 390–391
　　chronic 400
　soft tissue 829–831
　thyroiditis 833
　see also named conditions and organisms
Bartholin's duct 628
Bartonella henselae 645, 826
basal cell nevus syndrome 419, 422
　mandible 518, 521
　maxilla 518, 520
basiocciput 296
Bell's palsy 66
Bezold abscess 318
blindness
　optic nerve injury 468
　senile macular degeneration 189
blowout fracture 287, 290, 291
bone
　radiation-induced necrosis 816, 817
　remodeling 457
bone cavity, static in mandible 522, 523
bone cyst 455
　hyperparathyroidism 534
　mandible 522
bone disease, renal osteodystrophy 457
bone dysplasia, sinonasal cavities 450

bone marrow
　fibrosis 457
　Paget disease of bone 537
bony labyrinth 3
Boyden procedure 473
brachial plexus 783
　preaxillary 786
　schwannoma 797, 799
brain abscess 391, 394
brainstem 297
branchial apparatus 353
　congenital anomalies 638, 639, 640
branchial arches 731
　development 682
branchial cleft anomalies 834–837
　fourth 836–837
　oral cavity/oropharynx 722–723
　second 834–836
　third 836
branchial cleft cyst 560, 561, 651
　first 613, 614, 638, 639
　infrahyoid neck 834
　parapharyngeal 599–600
　second 613, 615, 722–723
　squamous cell carcinoma 836
　third 836
branchial cleft fistulae 835
　fourth 836–837
　infrahyoid neck 834
branchial cleft sinus, external 835–836
branchio-oto-renal syndrome 53
Brown superior oblique tendon sheath syndrome 285–287
brown tumor 454–457
　diagnostic imaging 455–457
　histopathology 455
　mandible 534
　maxilla 534, 535
　treatment 455
Bruch's membrane 141
bruxism 493
buccal mucosa, carcinoma 693–695
buccal nerve 511
buccopharyngeal fascia 582, 584
bulla ethmoidalis 360, 361, 362–363
buphthalmos 147–148
　persistent hyperplastic primary vitreous 166
Burkitt lymphoma 545–546, 575, 576

C

calcification
　adenocarcinoma of ethmoid sinus 434
　adenoid cystic carcinoma of salivary gland 671
　brown tumor 455, 456
　cervical lymph nodes 796
　chondrosarcoma 333, 334, 337, 757, 758
　chordoma 335, 337
　craniopharyngioma 313
　dermoid cysts 310
　dystrophic postinflammatory 594
　epidermoid cyst 311
　esthesioneuroblastoma 435, 436
　hemangiopericytoma 437
　intraocular 157–158, 159, 160
　　ciliary body medulloepithelioma 189
　　Coats disease 170–171, 172
　　retinopathy of prematurity 169, 170
　lacrimal gland amyloidosis 281
　melanotic neuroectodermal tumor of infancy 436
　meningioma 320, 322, 337, 607

multinodular goiter 808
odontomas 528–529
optic nerve sheath meningioma 269, 270, 271
orbital esthesioneuroblastoma 283
orbital mesenchymal chondrosarcoma 278
papillary thyroid carcinoma 796, 810, 811
parotid duct 651
pleomorphic adenoma 660, 661, 662, 663
recurrent hemangiopericytoma 262, 263
salivary glands 635, 643, 644, 645
schwannoma 337
synovial bodies 498, 499
synovial chondromatosis 678
temporomandibular joint 494, 495, 496
　infectious arthritis 487
teratoma 310
tuberculous lymph nodes 826
Warthin's tumor 667
calcifying epithelial odontogenic tumor (CEOT) 426, 461
　mandible 524, 528
calcifying odontogenic cyst 524–525
calcium hydroxyapatite 832–833
calcium regulation 457
Caldwell–Luc operation 390
　complications 470, 472
　extended 473
Camurati–Engelmann disease 450
canine fossa 510
capillary hemangioma
　orbital 253, 254
　rhabdomyosarcoma 277
capillary malformations, oral cavity/oropharynx 721
carcinoma 110–111
　alveolar mucosa 695
　basaloid 702, 703, 755, 756
　buccal mucosa 693–695
　central epidermal of jaw 542
　clear cell odontogenic
　　mandible 525, 527–528
　　sinonasal cavities 427
　ex-pleomorphic adenoma 670, 674
　extension
　　to retropharyngeal space 599
　　to submandibular/sublingual space 617
　external auditory canal 504
　floor of mouth 690–692
　gingiva 695
　glottic 471–743, 744
　　spread 472, 743
　gums 693–695
　hard palate 695, 701
　lips 689–690
　mandible 542, 543
　masticator space 612–613
　maxilla 472, 542, 543
　metastases 674
　　cystic node 615
　　salivary glands 677, 678
　nasopharyngeal 569–574
　　classification 569, 573
　　clinical presentation 569–571, 572
　　extension 576
　　　patterns 572–573
　　　into retrostyloid parapharyngeal space 608
　　imaging diagnosis 573–574
　　incidence 569
　　metastases 571, 572
　　pharyngeal mucosal space 595
　　spindle cell 575

carcinoma
    submucosal extension 557
    treatment 574
    undifferentiated 702, 703
  oral cavity 617
    perineural spread 701–702
  oropharyngeal 595–597, 791
    extension 596–597
    perineural spread 701–702
    posterior wall 699
  palatine tonsil 695–697
  parotid gland 669, 670
  parotid space 613
  perineural extension 597
  piriform sinus 743–745, 746
  postcricoid region 745, 746, 747
  posterior pharyngeal walls 747
  prevertebral muscle invasion 597
  retromolar trigone 694–695, 701
  skull base involvement 344
  soft palate 596, 699
  spindle cell 702, 754, 755
  squamous cell
    atypical 702–703, 753–755, 756
    branchial cleft cyst 836
    cervical lymph nodes 788–794
    hypopharynx 739–755, 756
    imaging diagnosis 428–431
    larynx 739–755, 756
    metastatic in infrahyoid neck 788–794
    oral cavity/oropharynx 688–703
    papillary 430
    paranasal sinuses 427–431
    perineural spread 431
    salivary glands 674
  subglottic 743, 744
  supraglottic 740–741
  temporal bone 105, 108–109
  thyroid 719, 796, 807, 810–812
  tongue 617
    base 697–699
    oral 692–693
  tonsillar extension into retrostyloid parapharyngeal space 608
  tonsillar pillars 697
  transglottic 473, 744
  undifferentiated of nasopharyngeal type 702, 703
  verrucous 702, 703, 753–754, 755
  see also acinic cell carcinoma; adenocarcinoma; adenoid cystic carcinoma; clear cell odontogenic carcinoma; mucoepidermoid carcinoma; thyroid carcinoma
carotid artery
  aberrant 38
  common 780, 781, 782
    dissection 842
    ectatic 840
  coronal oblique 20° sections 15, 16
  developmental variations 38–40
  dissection 840–841
  ectopic 38, 39, 40
  external 626, 629, 781, 782
  internal 202, 781, 782
    aneurysm 319, 320, 462
    dehiscence 305
    developmental variations 38, 39
    ectatic 840
    foramen lacerum 298, 299
    mycotic aneurysm 229, 230
    thrombosis 618
  radiation-induced wall thickening 815
  radiotherapy-induced disease 816–818

  rupture 817, 828, 831
  sagittal section 28, 29
  tumor invasion 793
carotid body tumors 603, 604, 630
  infrahyoid neck 801, 802
carotid bulb 782
carotid canal 297, 299
  coronal section 10, 11, 12
  fracture 347
carotid space 582, 586, 589
  abscess 602–603
  cellulitis 602–603
  infrahyoid 785, 786
  schwannoma 709, 710
carotid–cavernous fistula 259–262
cartilage, radiation-induced necrosis 816, 817
Castleman disease 827
cat scratch disease 645, 826
cavernous sinus 302, 303
  imaging 212
  nasopharyngeal carcinoma extension 569
  thrombosis 229, 230, 391, 393, 396
cavernous sinus syndrome 572
cellulitis
  carotid space 602–603
  facial 391, 392
  infrahyoid neck 829
  masticator space 610, 611
  necrotizing fasciitis 830
  odontogenic infections 711
  orbital 228–229, 391, 392, 393, 394
  retropharyngeal space 598–599, 827, 828
  retrostyloid parapharyngeal space 602–603
  sublingual space 617
  submandibular space 616–617
cement, dental 510, 511
cemental dysplasia, periapical 529, 531
cementoblastoma 532
  benign 529, 531, 532
cementocytes 510, 511
cementoma 529, 530–531
  gigantiform 529, 531
central epidermal carcinoma of the jaw 542
cerebellar artery, anterior inferior 119, 120
cerebellopontine angle
  cholesteatoma 89
  hemangioma 97
  lymphoma 121, 122
  meningioma 97, 118
  schwannoma 115, 116
cerebellopontine cistern
  aneurysms 119
  epidermoid cysts 121, 212
  vascular loops 119
cerebral atrophy 370
cerebral hemisphere, congenital agenesis 370
cerebral ischemia 618
cerebrospinal fluid (CSF)
  leaks 370, 371
    sinonasal cavities 468–469
    surgical complications 470
  otorrhea 52, 61, 62
    skull base fracture 346, 348
  rhinorrhea 346, 348, 469
cervical fascia
  deep 784, 785
    deep layer 581–584, 586–587, 588
    middle layer 584, 586–587, 588
    superficial layer 581
  superficial 784, 785
cervical lymph nodes
  abscess 824, 825
  cat scratch disease 826

  cervical lymphadenopathy 645
  diagnostic criteria 789, 790
  HIV infection 826
  imaging 793–794
  infection 824–827
  inflammation 824–827
  lymphoma 794–796
  metastatic squamous cell carcinoma 788–794
  necrosis 790, 791, 792, 794
  sarcoidosis 826–827
  shape 789, 790
  size 789, 790
  tuberculosis 825–826
cervical nerve roots, schwannoma 797
cervical ribs 842
cervical space
  anterior 786
  posterior 618, 786, 787
cervical spinal epidural abscess 828, 829
chalazion 222
Charcot–Leyden crystals 398
chemodectoma see glomus tumors
cherubism 443–444
  mandible/maxilla 536, 537
chief cells 802–803
children
  Ewing sarcoma 436
  ganglioneuroma 175, 436
  giant-cell reparative granuloma 454, 455
  hemangioma 756, 757
  juvenile rheumatoid arthritis 495
  juvenile xanthogranuloma 175, 176
  leukemia 251
  melanotic neuroectodermal tumor of infancy 436
  mucoepidermoid carcinoma 668
  nontuberculous mycobacterial disease 826
  ocular disorders 158
  optic nerve glioma 272
  orbital disorders 219
    lymphangioma 257
    metastases 284–285
    pseudotumor 234, 236
  proptosis 275
  recurrent sialadenitis 645, 647
  retropharyngeal space infection 828
  rhabdomyosarcoma 275, 337
    infrahyoid neck 806–807
    masticator space 612
    nasopharyngeal 576–577
    oral cavity/oropharynx 706, 707
    sinonasal cavities 437–438
  salivary gland tumors 659, 660
  suprahyoid neck trauma 618
  temporomandibular joint ankylosis 496
  toxocariasis 172
chloroma
  orbital 252
  sinonasal cavities 442
  skull base 344
choanal atresia (obliteration) 387
choanal cyst 407
choanal polyps 408–410
chocolate cyst, orbital 222, 258
cholangitis, sclerosing 834
cholesteatoma
  acquired 75, 318
  aditus 79, 80, 82
  cerebellopontine angle 89
    congenital 89
  clinical findings 75
  complications 82

congenital
    cerebellopontine angle 89
    middle ear 84–85, 86
    petrous apex 71, 88
    petrous pyramid 87
    skull base 307–312
  diagnosis 76
  epidural 85–89
  extent 79, 80, 82, 83, 84, 86
  external auditory canal 89–90
  facial canal 84, 87
  facial nerve 84
    geniculate ganglion 84, 87
  imaging
    patterns of findings 76–84
    techniques 75–76
  labyrinthine fistula 81, 82–83, 84
  mastoid 75, 81, 82, 83–84
    antrum 82, 83–84, 86
  middle ear 74–90
    congenital 84–85, 86
  pars flaccida 76–77, 79, 80, 81
  pars tensa 78, 79, 80, 81
  petrous apex, congenital 71, 88
  petrous extension 83–84
  petrous pyramid 85–89
    congenital 87
  recurrent 91, 92, 93
  temporomandibular joint 504
  theories 75
cholesterol granuloma 70–73
  inflammatory conditions 318
  nasal 404
  orbital 222–223, 225–226
  paranasal sinuses 404
  skull base 310, 312, 313
chondroblastoma
  mandible/maxilla 537
  metastases 452
  sinonasal cavities 452
  skull base 329, 331, 332
  temporomandibular joint 499, 502
chondroid chordoma 335, 336
chondroma
  mandible/maxilla 537
  sinonasal cavities 451–452
  skull base 329, 333
chondromatosis, synovial 497–499, 677–678
chondromyxoid fibroma, sinonasal cavities 332, 461
chondromyxoid tumors, skull base 329, 332
chondrosarcoma
  craniofacial 458, 460
  diagnostic imaging 460
  grades 459
  imaging diagnosis 334
  larynx 757, 758
  mandible/maxilla 543, 544, 545
  masticator space 612
  sinonasal cavities 458–460
  skull base 329, 333–334, 336
  temporomandibular joint 499, 502
chorda tympani 629
  sagittal section 23
chordoma
  chondroid 335, 336
  imaging diagnosis 336–337
  nasopharyngeal 577, 578
  skull base 329, 333–336
choriocapillaris 141
choristoma
  episcleral 157
  nasopharyngeal 567

orbital 219
choroid
  abscess 155
  anatomy 141–142
  blood supply 142
  cyst 186
  detachment 152–153, 154, 186
  effusion 153, 154, 186
  embryology 137, 138
  hemangioma 152, 177, 184–186, 186
  hematoma 153
  hemorrhage 186
  melanoma 150
  nerve supply 142
  nevi 184
  osteoma 157, 176, 177
  stroma 141–142
  venous drainage 142
choroidal capillaries 143
  permeability 153
Churg–Strauss syndrome, nasal 404
ciliary arteries
  anterior 140, 141
  posterior 202
ciliary body 140, 142
  amelanotic tumor 181
  embryology 137
  leiomyoma 188
  medulloepithelioma 188–189
  metastases 183, 184
  MRI 145–146
ciliary body–choroidal melanoma 181
ciliary ganglion 203
ciliary muscle 142
ciliary nerves 141, 203
  long 141, 202
circle of Willis 35–36
circumvallate papillae 683, 684
claviculae muscle, levator 842
clear cell odontogenic carcinoma
  mandible 525, 527–528
  sinonasal cavities 427
cleft palate 386–387
  DentaScan 547
clivus
  nasopharyngeal carcinoma extension 569
  osteomyelitis 561
cloison sagittale 582, 584
Cloquet's canal 166
Coats disease 150, 169–172, 173–174
  diagnostic imaging 170–172
  intraocular calcification 157, 158
cocaine abuse, sinonasal inflammation 401
cochlea 4, 5, 6, 8
  congenital anomalies 49, 50
  coronal oblique 20° sections 15, 16, 17, 18
  coronal section 11
  double ring effect 125
  MRI 129, 131
  otosclerosis 124–125, 126, 127, 128, 129
  sagittal section 27, 28, 29
cochlear aqueduct
  axial sections 8, 9
  congenital anomalies 52
  coronal oblique 20° sections 20
  coronal section 14, 15
cochlear implantation, imaging assessment 52, 53
cochlear nerve 7
  coronal oblique 20° sections 17
  coronal section 11, 12
cochlear promontory, sagittal section 25
cochleariform process

coronal oblique 20° sections 18
  sagittal section 25
Cogan syndrome, scleritis 156
colloid cyst 316
coloboma 148–149
columella procedure 90–91
computed tomography (CT)
  cholesteatoma 75–76
  densitometry in cochlear otosclerosis 125–126, 127–128
  DentaScan 548
  eye 143
  glomus tumors 102, 103–104
  hypopharynx 737, 738
  infrahyoid neck 787
  larynx 737, 738
    cartilage invasion 748–749, 750, 751
  lymph nodes 793
  malignant tumors 541–542
  mandible 511, 512, 513
  maxilla 511, 512, 513
  nasal cavity 379–380
  nasopharynx 559
  oral cavity/oropharynx 687–688
  orbit 204–205
    normal anatomy 206, 207, 209–215
  paranasal sinuses 379–380
  persistent hyperplastic primary vitreous 167, 168
  pneumocystography 119
  projections 31–32
  retinoblastoma 162, 164
  salivary glands 633–634
    tumors 655–656
  skull base 304
  suprahyoid neck 592–593
  temporal bone 30–32
    trauma 54–55
  temporomandibular joint 481, 482
concha
  bullosa 363, 367, 369
  pneumatized superior 369
condylar agenesis 484–485, 486
condylar canal 301
condylar fossa 301
condylar fractures 504–505
condylar hyperplasia 485, 486
condylar hypoplasia 485–486
condylar process 509
condylodisk 479
congenital abnormalities
  branchial apparatus 638, 639, 640
  cholesteatoma
    cerebellopontine angle 89
    middle ear 84–85, 86
    petrous apex 71, 88
    petrous pyramid 87
  extraocular muscles 287–290
  eye 146–148
  fibrous dysplasia 443–444
  infrahyoid neck 834
  larynx 774
  mandible 513–514
  masticator space 609–610
  maxilla 513–514
  nasal cavity 386–390
  nasopharynx 560–561
  nose 386–390
  oral cavity/oropharynx 719–723
  orbit 215–222
  paranasal sinuses 386–390
  parotid gland 638–642
  parotid space 613, 614

congenital abnormalities
    prestyloid parapharyngeal space 599–600
    retropharyngeal space 597–598
    salivary glands 638–642
    submandibular/sublingual space 613, 615
    temporal bone 41–53
    temporomandibular joint ankylosis 496
conjunctiva
    choristoma 219
    cysts 222
conus elasticus 735
cornea
    anatomy 141
    embryology 137
corniculate cartilage 732, 733
coronal sutures, premature fusion 216, 217
coronoid process 509
    elongated 305, 514, 515
cranial base
    external surface 297–298
    internal surface 298, 299, 301
cranial cavity 295
cranial fossae 295–296
    anterior
        epidermoid cyst 309
        neurenteric cyst 315
    epidermoid cyst 309, 311
    neurenteric cyst 315, 316
    posterior 297, 298, 300, 302–304
cranial nerves
    fifth 345
    neuroma 100
    palsy of sixth 572
    paralysis 819
craniofacial dysostosis 216, 218
craniometaphyseal dysplasia 130, 132
craniopharyngioma 312–315
    extension 314, 315
    extracranial 425–426
        nasopharyngeal 560
craniosynostosis
    orbit 215, 216, 217
    primary congenital isolated 216
cribriform plate 295
    low-lying 305
cricoarytenoid joints 732, 733
    dislocation 775
    glottic carcinoma spread 472
cricoid cartilage 732, 733
    glottic carcinoma spread 472
    neoplastic invasion 751
cricopharyngeus muscle 736–737
    dysfunction 770–771, 771
cricothyroid muscle 732
crista falciformis
    coronal oblique 20° sections 17
    superior 18
croup 772
Crouzon disease
    maxilla anomalies 514
    orbit 216–217
crus commune
    coronal section 14, 15
    sagittal section 26, 27
cryptophthalmos 148
cuneiform cartilage 732, 733
cyclo-oxygenase (COX) 407
cyclo-oxygenase 1 (COX-1) inhibition 408
cysteinyl leukotrienes 408
cystic fibrosis 397–398
    hypoplastic paranasal sinuses 401
cystic hygroma
    cervical 722

infrahyoid neck 839–840
    nasopharyngeal 565, 568
    oral cavity/oropharynx 721, 722
    salivary glands 638, 639, 642
cysticercosis, orbit 226, 227
cytomegalovirus (CMV)
    retinitis 154, 155
    uveitis 156

D

dacryoadenitis 234, 235, 278, 279, 280
dacryocele 222, 223, 288, 289
dacryocystocele, congenital 387–388
dacryocystography 288
dacryocystorhinostomy 288
dacryoliths 288
danger space 584, 785
    retropharyngeal space infection
        extension 599
de Quervain thyroiditis 834
deafness
    conductive after stapedectomy 124
    sensorineural congenital 47
dental anatomy 510–511
dental caries, sinusitis 391
dental development 508–509
dental papilla 508
dental pulp 510, 511
dental radiography 512
DentaScan 542, 546, 547, 548
dentigerous cysts
    mandible/maxilla 516–517, 518
    sinonasal cavities 419, 421
dermal sinus 389
dermatomyositis 243, 832
dermoid cysts 389
    carcinomatous transformation 720
    hairy 568
    nasopharyngeal 564, 565, 567, 568
    oral cavity/oropharynx 720
    orbital 219, 220, 221
    salivary glands 638, 639, 640, 651
    sublingual 720
    sublingual space 617
    submandibular space 615, 617
dermolipoma, conjunctival 219
desmocranium 316
Desmond tumor 461
developmental anomalies
    mandible/maxilla 513–514
    orbit 215–222
    temporal bone 36–41
    temporomandibular joint 484–486
diastematomyelia 316
diffusion-weighted imaging 304
digastric muscle 630, 780, 781
    development 682
    floor of mouth carcinoma spread 691
dilator pupillae muscle 203
ducts of Rivinus 628
dumbbell tumors 659, 663
dura mater 295
dysthyroid orbitopathy 237–239
    myositis differential diagnosis 233
dystrophic calcification, postinflammatory 594

E

ear, inner 3
    congenital anomalies 47–52
    embryology 42–43
    fractures 55

    MRI 33
    trauma 55
ear, middle 3
    adenoma 96
    anomalies 43, 44
    cholesteatoma 74–90
        congenital 84–85, 86
    coronal oblique 20° sections 18, 19, 20, 21
    coronal sections 10, 11, 12, 14
    embryology 41–42
    eosinophilic granuloma 101
    hemangioma 97
    MRI 33
    osteoma 96
    postoperative imaging 91–92
    projectile injuries 58–59, 60
    sagittal section 22, 23, 24, 26, 27, 28, 29
ear, outer 41–42
eccrine hidrocystoma 222
Echinococcus granulosus 226
embryology
    ethmoid sinuses 354, 355
    eye 137–139, 166
    frontal sinuses 355
    hypopharynx 731–732
    larynx 731–732
    mandible/maxilla 508–509, 682
    maxillary sinuses 353–355
    nasal cavity 353, 386
    nasolacrimal duct 139, 386
    nasolacrimal sac 386
    nasopharynx 553
    oral cavity/oropharynx 682–683
    orbit 196
    paranasal sinuses 353–355, 386
    salivary glands 625
    skull base 295
    sphenoid sinus 354, 355
    temporal bone 41–43, 682
    temporomandibular joint 477
emissary vein, prominent 305, 306
emphysema, surgical 618
enamel 510, 511
    development 508–509
enamel organ 508
encephalitis, subdural abscess 393
encephalocele 389
    nasal 386, 388
endolymphatic sac 7
    congenital anomalies 49, 50
    sagittal section 24, 26
    tumor 105, 107, 108
endophthalmitis 155
    sclerosing 172, 174–175
endoscopic sinus surgery, functional 366–367
end-stage renal failure 457
Englemann disease 540
eosinophilic granuloma
    mandible 535, 536
    maxilla 535
    temporal bone 100–101
epidermoid cysts 389
    cerebellopontine cistern 121, 212
    differential diagnosis 310, 312
    imaging 304
    intradural 311
    nasopharyngeal 564, 565, 567
    oral cavity/oropharynx 720
    orbital 219, 220
    salivary glands 638, 639, 640, 651
    submandibular/sublingual space 615, 617
epidural abscess, sinogenic 317, 391, 393

Index 851

epiglottis 732
  carcinoma 740
  dislocation 775
epiglottitis 772
episcleral choristoma 157
episcleritis 156
epithelial odontogenic cysts 419, 421, 422–423
epithelial odontogenic tumors 423–424, 426, 427
epithelial tumors, sinonasal cavities 427
epitympanic retraction pockets 77–78
epitympanum 4, 5
  coronal oblique 20° sections 14, 15, 16, 17, 18, 19
  coronal section 10, 11
  fracture 56
  hypoplasia 46
  sagittal section 22, 23, 26
Epstein–Barr virus (EBV)
  Burkitt lymphoma 545, 546
  infectious mononucleosis 563, 564
  lymphoma 439
  midline destructive granuloma 242–243
  sinonasal lymphoma 402
Erdheim–Chester disease 247
  juvenile xanthogranuloma differential diagnosis 245
erysipelas 829
Escherichia coli 832
esophageal perforation, mediastinitis 832
esthesioneuroblastoma
  metastases 435, 436
  orbital 283
  sinonasal cavities 434–436
  skull base involvement 344, 345
ethmoid bone 295, 296
  anatomy 354, 358, 360–364
ethmoid bulla drainage 367
ethmoid infundibulum 367
ethmoid sinuses
  adenocarcinoma 434
  carcinoma 428, 432
  embryology 354, 355
  esthesioneuroblastoma 435
  infection 394
  innervation 364
  lymphatic drainage 364
  mucocele 406
  mucoepidermoid carcinoma 434
  surgical complications 472–473
ethmoidal air cells
  anterior 367
  middle 362, 367
  posterior 364, 370
ethmoidal complex, posterior 364, 369–370
ethmoidal crest 376
ethmoidal infundibulum 361, 362–363
ethmoidal labyrinth 356
ethmoidal sinuses, anatomy 354, 358, 360–364
ethmoidal uncinate process 360, 361, 362, 363
  variation 363, 367, 369
ethmoidectomy 470, 472
  external 474
eustachian tube 3, 556
  nasopharyngeal opening 554, 556, 557
  sagittal section 29
Ewing sarcoma
  mandible/maxilla 544, 545
  sinonasal cavities 436
exophthalmos 215
exorbitism 215
exostoses, external auditory canal 95
external auditory canal 3
  carcinoma extension 504
  cholesteatoma 89–90
  congenital agenesis 44, 45–46
  coronal oblique 20° sections 16, 17, 18, 20, 21
  coronal section 14, 15
  coronal sections 10, 12, 14
  dysplasia 43
  eosinophilic granuloma 101
  exostoses 95
  first branchial groove 638
  hemangioma 96–97
  osteoma 95
  projectile injuries 58–59, 60
  pyogenic granuloma extension 504
  sagittal section 22, 23, 24, 25
  stenosis 91
  tumor blockage 95
extramedullary hematopoiesis, paranasal sinuses 448–449
extraocular muscles 199, 201
  anomalies in craniosynostosis 217
  congenital anomalies 287–290
  embryology 139
  imaging 206–209, 210–211
  injury during surgery 470, 471
  sheaths 140
eye
  adenocarcinoma 188
  adenoma 188
  anatomy 140–143
  anterior chamber MRI 145
  astrocytic hamartoma 162, 174, 175
  bacterial infections 154
  benign reactive lymphoid hyperplasia 157
  congenital anomalies 146–148
  congenital cystic 147, 221
  embryology 137–139, 166
  foreign bodies 144
  fungal infections 154
  ganglioneuroma 175
  granulomatosis 157, 174, 175
  imaging techniques 143–146
  incontinentia pigmenti 175
  inflammatory disorders 154–157
  intraocular calcifications 157–158, 159, 160
    ciliary body medulloepithelioma 189
    Coats disease 170–171, 172
    retinopathy of prematurity 169, 170
  intraocular hemorrhage 189, 190
  intraocular mass 164
  juvenile xanthogranuloma 175, 176
  leukemia 186, 187
  leukokoria 158–159
  lymphoma 186, 187
  medulloepithelioma 188–189
  MRI 143–146
    artifacts 144, 145
    posterior chamber 145–146
  muscles 201–202
    innervation 202–203
  myelinated nerve fibers 177
  pathology 146–192
  pediatric disorders 158
  potential spaces 146
  schwannoma 187
  subretinal neovascular membranes 177
  trauma 190–191
  vascular system embryology 137, 138, 139
  viral diseases 154–155
  see also orbit; retinoblastoma
eye socket, anophthalmic 191–192

eyeball
  movements 201–202
  venous drainage 204
eyelids 200
  autonomic nerves 203
  cryptophthalmos 148
  cysts 222
  embryology 139
  inflammatory edema 391, 392
  movements 201–202
  muscles 199, 201

F

face
  asymmetry 484–485, 486
  cellulitis 391, 392
  floating 468
  spaces 584–587
facial artery 628, 629
facial canal
  cholesteatoma 84, 87
  CT 32
  dehiscence 305
  postoperative imaging 92, 93
  rotation 46, 47
  schwannoma 98
  trauma 59–61
facial clefting, midline 386, 388
facial nerve 3, 629
  axial sections 4, 5, 6, 9
  cholesteatoma 84
  congenital anomalies 47
  coronal oblique 20° sections 15, 16, 17, 18, 19, 20, 21
  coronal section 11, 12, 14, 15
  extracranial 627
  geniculate ganglion 10, 11, 15, 16, 27
    cholesteatoma 84, 87
    trauma 60
  iatrogenic lesions 61
  internal auditory canal 109
  intraparotid 627
  MRI 635–636
  neurofibroma 100
  neuroma 99, 326
  paralysis 58, 59–61, 61, 68
    adenoid cystic carcinoma 671
    parotid malignancy 659
    pleomorphic adenoma 660, 662
  parotid gland tumor 663
  sagittal section 22, 23, 24, 25, 26, 27, 28
  schwannoma 98–100, 116–117
  traumatic lesions 59–61
facial neuritis 66, 67
facial paralysis, otitis media 62
facial recess 3
  coronal section 12, 14
facial vein, posterior 625, 626–627
falciform crest 109
fasciitis
  necrotizing 773, 829–831
  nodular 461
  odontogenic infections 711
fibroma
  ameloblastic 518
  cementifying 529, 531
  cemento-ossifying 447
  chondromyxoid 332, 461
  ossifying 329, 330
    aggressive psammomatoid 447–448
    juvenile active 447–448
    juvenile aggressive 536, 539

fibroma
    mandible/maxilla 536, 539
        psammomatoid active 536, 539
    sinonasal cavities 445–448
fibromatosis
    aggressive 329, 341, 461, 462
        histology 806
        infrahyoid neck 806
        oral cavity/oropharynx 709
    orbital 275, 277
    sinonasal cavities 461, 462
    skull base 329, 338, 340, 341
fibromyxoma
    odontogenic 529, 530, 531
    sinonasal 460–461
    temporal bone 332
    temporomandibular joint 499, 500
fibrosarcoma
    infrahyoid neck 806
    mandible/maxilla 543, 545
    masticator space 612
    radiation-induced 819
    sinonasal cavities 461, 462
    temporomandibular joint 499, 502
fibrous dysplasia 130, 131
    congenital 443–444
    diagnostic imaging 445, 446
    etiology 444
    histopathology 444
    mandible/maxilla 535–536, 537–539
    monostotic 443, 444, 536
    polyostotic 443, 444, 536, 539
    sinonasal cavities 443–445, 446
    skull base 329, 330
    temporomandibular joint 504
fibrous histiocytoma 329
fistulography 836
FLAIR, skull base 304
flaps
    axial 820–821
    ischemia 822
    myocutaneous 821, 822
    tumor recurrence 823
foramen lacerum 297, 298, 299
foramen magnum 297, 298, 300
foramen of Huschke 483, 484
foramen ovale 298, 299, 300
foramen rotundum 297, 298, 299, 301, 305, 376, 377
foramen spinosum 298, 299, 300
Fordyce's granules 567
foreign bodies
    granuloma 404
    hypopharyngeal 775, 777
    intraocular 144, 190–191
    plastic 190, 191
    rhinoliths 401–402
    wood 190, 191
fossa incudis
    coronal oblique 20° sections 21
    sagittal section 22
fovea centralis 143
fovea ethmoidalis, low position 363, 367, 368, 369
frontal nerve 210, 212
    neurofibroma 266, 267
frontal recess 361, 363
frontal sinuses 363, 364
    anatomy 358, 359
    embryology 355
    lymphoma 440, 441
    obliteration 473
    surgical complications 473–474

frontonasal canal 361
functional endoscopic endonasal sinus surgery (FESS) 470, 471
fungal balls 399, 441
fungal infections
    eye 154
    mycotic sinonasal diseases 396–397
    nasopharyngeal inflammation 561
    orbit 230, 231
    sinusitis 391, 396–397
        chronic 398–400
    skull base 316–317
    Tolosa–Hunt syndrome 236, 237
Fusobacterium 824

G

ganglioneuroblastoma, infrahyoid neck 801
ganglioneuroma 175
    infrahyoid neck 801
    sinonasal cavities 436
Gardner syndrome 450
    mandible/maxilla 532, 533
Garré osteomyelitis 714
gasserian cisterns 221
genioglossus muscle, floor of mouth carcinoma spread 691
geniohyoid muscle 686
ghost cell tumor, odontogenic 524–525
giant-cell reparative granuloma 453–454, 455
    hyperparathyroidism evaluation 457
    mandible/maxilla 532–534
giant-cell tumor
    carcinoma 702
    diagnostic imaging 453, 454
    mandible 532–534
    maxilla 532–534
    pathology 453
    sinonasal cavities 452–453, 454
    skull base 329, 331
    temporomandibular joint 499, 500
gigantism 486
gingiva 510, 511
    carcinoma 695
gingivitis, necrotizing 718
glaucoma
    congenital 147
    persistent hyperplastic primary vitreous 166
    uveal melanoma 177
glenoid fossa 477
    pneumatization 482, 484
glioma, optic nerve 269, 272–273
globulomaxillary cyst 425, 518, 521
glomus faciale 323, 324
glomus jugulare tumor 102, 103–105, 106–107
    differential diagnosis 324, 328
    infrahyoid neck 801, 803
    retrostyloid parapharyngeal space 603
    skull base 323–324
glomus tumors
    infrahyoid neck 801–803
    nasopharyngeal 578
    parapharyngeal 630
    sellar region 324
    temporal bone 101–105
glomus tympanicum tumor 101, 102, 103
    retrostyloid parapharyngeal space 603
glomus vagale tumor
    infrahyoid neck 801, 803
    retrostyloid parapharyngeal space 603, 604, 605
glossectomy 699–700
glossoepiglottic fold 687

glossopharyngeal nerve 682
glycosaminoglycans 479, 481
goiter, multinodular 808–809
Goldenhar's syndrome 53, 218
    deformities 484, 485
    mandibular anomalies 514
Goltz syndrome 147
Gorlin–Goltz syndrome *see* basal cell nevus syndrome
gout 495
granular cell tumor, sinonasal cavities 426
granulocytic sarcoma, orbital 252
granuloma gravidarum, nasal 404
granulomatosis
    allergic and angiitis 404
    eye 157, 174, 175
    see also Wegener granulomatosis
granulomatous disease
    hypopharynx/larynx 772
    orbital 242–243
    sinonasal cavities 402–403
Graves disease 231, 237–239, 833
    myositis differential diagnosis 233
gums, carcinoma 693–695

H

Haemophilus 716
Haemophilus influenzae type b 772
hairy polyp 568
Haller cells 363, 367, 368
hamartoma, nasopharyngeal 564, 565, 568
Hand–Schuller–Christian disease 100, 247
    mandible/maxilla 535
    triad 342
Hashimoto thyroiditis 812, 813, 833
    amyloid deposition 834
hearing loss 53
    see also deafness
Heerfordt syndrome 157, 645
hemangioblastoma, optic nerve 272, 274
hemangioma
    capillary 657
    cavernous
        orbital 253–256
        salivary gland 657
    choroidal 184–186
    histcytoid 646
    hypopharynx 756, 757
    internal auditory canal 120, 121
    intraosseous 329, 330
    larynx 756, 757
    mandible/maxilla 540, 541
    masticator space 609–610
    nasopharyngeal 565, 568
    oral cavity/oropharynx 720
    parotid gland 657
    parotid space 613, 614
    petrous pyramid 120, 121
    retinal 184, 186
    retropharyngeal space 597–598
    salivary gland 634, 657, 658, 674
    sinonasal cavities 416
    temporal bone 96–97
hemangiopericytoma
    mandible/maxilla 540, 541
    orbital 262–263
    recurrent 437
    salivary gland 634
    sinonasal cavities 416, 417, 419, 420, 437
    skull base 329, 333

hematoma
  infrahyoid neck 822
  retropharyngeal 618
hemifacial microsomia 53, 215, 218
hemilaryngectomy, vertical 762, 763
herpes simplex virus, eye infection 154, 155
heterotopia, nasopharyngeal 567
hiatus semilunaris 361, 362, 363
  superior 367
hidrocystoma, apocrine 222
histiocytoma
  benign fibrous 461
  fibrous 329
  malignant fibrous 462, 679
    infrahyoid neck 806
    oral cavity/oropharynx 706–707
    radiation-induced 819
histiocytoses, skull base 342–343
histiocytosis X 100
histiocytoid hemangioma 646
HIV infection
  cervical lymph nodes 826
  see also AIDS
Hodgkin disease 340
  cervical lymph nodes 794, 796
  nasopharyngeal 574–575
  oral cavity/oropharynx 704
Horner syndrome 201, 572
hyaloid membranes 143
  posterior detachment 149–150
hydatid cysts, orbital 226, 227
hydrocephaly, Warburg syndrome 169
hydroxyapatite cement 473–474
hyoglossus muscle 684
  floor of mouth carcinoma spread 691
hyoid bone 682, 780
  radiation-induced necrosis 816, 817
hypercalcemia 457
hyperparathyroid uremic bone disease 457
hyperparathyroidism
  brown tumor 454–455, 534
  giant-cell reparative granuloma 457
  ocular calcification 158, 159
  primary 813
  renal failure 457
hypersensitivity angiitis, orbital 243
hypertelorism 215
  median cleft syndrome 388
hyperthyroidism 808
hypoglossal canal 297, 298, 300
hypoglossal nerve 298, 300, 628
  denervation muscle atrophy 723–724
  neuroma 328
  paralysis 724
  sacrifice 700
hypoparathyroidism, ocular calcification 158, 159
hypopharynx
  anatomy 735–737
  CT 737, 738
  cysts 770–772
  development 731–732
  diverticula 771
  embryology 731–732
  granulomatous disease 772
  imaging techniques 738–739
  inflammatory conditions 772–773
  MRI 737–738, 738–739
  muscles 736–737
  perforation 775, 776, 777
  PET 739
  radiography 739
  regions 735–736
  tissue characteristics on sectional imaging 737–738
  trauma 775, 776, 777
  tumors
    fatty tissue 759, 760
    Kaposi's sarcoma 756–757
    lymphoreticular system 757–758
    myogenic 761
    neurogenic 761
    non-squamous cell 755–761
    pattern of spread 743–747
    radiation therapy complications 767–768
    recurrence 761–768
    sites 743–747
    squamous cell carcinoma 739–755, 756
    supraglottic carcinoma spread 471, 740
    TNM classification 748, 752–753
    treatment 761–768
    vasoformative 756–757
  ultrasonography 739
  vascular abnormalities 756
  wall 736
  webs 771–772
hypophysectomy, transphenoidal 474
hypotelorism 215
hypothyroidism 808
hypotympanum 3
  coronal oblique 20° sections 14, 15, 16, 21
  coronal sections 10
  sagittal section 26

I

image-guided endoscopic surgery of nasal cavity/paranasal sinuses 380
immunocompromised patients, pharyngitis 773
immunosuppressive agents 441
incisive canal 355
  cyst 422, 425
incisive fossa 510
incontinentia pigmenti 175
incus 3, 4, 5, 6
  anomalies 44, 45–46
  cholesteatoma 77, 80
  coronal oblique 20° sections 18, 19, 20, 21
  coronal section 10, 11, 12, 13
  dislocation 56, 57, 58, 59
  otitis media 69, 70
  sagittal section 22, 23, 24
infectious mononucleosis 563, 564
inferior meatal antrostomy 470
inflammatory conditions
  chronic sinusitis 397, 398
  deep neck spaces 594
  eye 154–157
  hypopharynx 772–773
  lacrimal glands 279, 280
  larynx 772–773
  mandible 514, 515
  masticator space 610–611
  maxilla 514, 515
  nasal cavity 390–406
    tumors 412
  nasopharyngeal 561–563
  neck
    infrahyoid 823–840
      muscles/tendons 832–833
  oral cavity/oropharynx 711–718
  orbit 226–230
    idiopathic 230–236
  paranasal sinuses 390–406
    tumors 412
  parapharyngeal space 600
    retrostyloid 602–603
  parotid space 613, 614
  retropharyngeal space 598–599
  salivary glands 642–651, 714–716
  skull base 316–318
  submandibular/sublingual space 616–617
  temporomandibular joint 486–487
  thyroid gland 833–834
infratemporal fossa 554, 559
  rhabdomyosarcoma 277
insulin-like growth factor 1 (IGF-1), nasal polyps 407–408
internal auditory canal 4, 6, 7
  aneurysms 119
  complete study 113
  congenital anomalies 50, 51, 52
  coronal oblique 20° sections 15, 16, 19
  coronal section 12, 13, 14, 15
  hemangioma 97, 120, 121
  heterotopic lesion 120–122
  imaging 112–113
  limited study 112–113
  lipoma 121
  lymphoma 121, 122
  meningioma 97
  metastases 121, 122
  no-contrast FSE study 113
  normal 109, 111, 112–113
  osteoma 96
  pathology 113–118
  sagittal section 27
  varix malformation 120
internal auditory meatus 28, 29
intracranial abscess 63, 64
intracranial bleeding 55
intracranial pressure, increased 157
intravitreal fluid, gravitational 169
iodide mumps 647
iridocorneal angle 142
iris 140, 142
  embryology 137
  MRI 140, 145
iris dilator 203

J

jaw
  central epidermal carcinoma of the jaw 542
  clenching 493
jugular bulb, developmental variations 37–38
jugular foramen 297, 298, 300, 301
jugular fossa 8
  cholesteatoma 86
  coronal oblique 20° sections 20
  coronal section 14, 15
  dehiscence 305, 306
  developmental variations 37–38
  high 305, 306
  sagittal section 29
  schwannoma 327, 329
  tumor differential diagnosis 324, 328
jugular fossa syndrome 572
jugular vein
  external 782
  internal 780, 781
    asymmetric 841–842
    septic thrombosis 831, 832
    tumor invasion 793
  thrombosis 842
    septic 828

juvenile aggressive ossifying fibroma 536, 539
juvenile angiofibroma 418
　nasopharyngeal 344, 345, 563–565, 566, 594–595
juvenile rheumatoid arthritis 495
juvenile xanthogranuloma
　ocular 175, 176
　orbital 245, 247

K

Kaposi's sarcoma 756–757
Kartagener syndrome 401
Kawasaki disease 827
keratoconjunctivitis sicca 241
keratocyst, odontogenic 419, 503
　mandible/maxilla 517–518, 519–520
keratosis
　obliterans 504
　obturans 89
Kikuchi disease 827
Killian's dehiscence 736
Kimura disease 645, 646, 827
　lacrimal glands 281–282
Klebsiella rhinoscleromatis 402–403, 563
Klinefelter syndrome 486
Koerner's septum, erosion 80, 82, 83–84
Kussmaul disease 679
Küttner tumor 646, 716

L

labyrinth, membranous 3
　coronal oblique 20° sections 21
　coronal section 11, 12, 14
labyrinth artery 109
labyrinth–blood barrier disruption 65, 66
labyrinthine concussion/bleeding 55
labyrinthine fistula 81, 82–83, 84
labyrinthine windows
　congenital anomalies 46–47
　CT 123
　pre-/post-operative evaluation 123, 124
　see also oval window; round window
labyrinthitis
　acoustic nerve inflammation 114
　acute 65, 66
　chronic 65–66
　congenital obliterative 52
lacrimal adenitis 234, 235
lacrimal apparatus 204
　congenital anomalies 288
lacrimal canaliculus 289
　obstructions 288
lacrimal duct
　congenital mucocele 387–388
　cyst 222, 223
　injury during surgery 470
lacrimal glands 197, 204
　abscess 278, 279
　amyloid tumor 281
　amyloidosis 244, 281
　autonomic nerves 203
　embryology 138, 139
　epithelial cysts 279
　epithelial tumors 279, 281
　fossa changes 281
　imaging 208, 209
　inflammatory disease 279, 280
　Kimura disease 281–282
　lesions 278–282
　lymphoid tumors 280
　lymphoma 249, 250, 251, 279

malignancy 281
pseudotumor 234, 235, 279, 280
sarcoidosis 280
Sjögren's syndrome 279
tumor involvement in skull base 344
Wegener granulomatosis 279, 280
lacrimal sac
　embryology 139
　fossa 363
　injury during surgery 470
　lymphoma 290
　malignant melanoma 290
　mucocele 288, 289
　　congenital 387–388
　tumors 288, 289–290
lamina cribrosa 140
Langerhans cell histiocytosis 65, 100–101
　mandible 534–535, 536
　maxilla 534–535, 536
　orbital 244–245, 246
　sinonasal cavities 462
　skull base 318, 319, 329, 342–343
　temporomandibular joint 501
Lannier's dehiscence 736
laryngectomy
　glotto-sublottic 764
　near total 764
　supracricoid
　　with cricohyoidoepiglottopexy 763
　　with cricohyoidopexy 762–763, 764
　supraglottic horizontal 762, 763
　total 762
laryngocele 769
laryngotracheal groove 731
laryngotracheitis 772
larynx
　amyloidosis 772, 773
　anatomy 732–735
　arterial malformations 774
　cartilage 732, 733
　　radiation-induced necrosis 816
　　relapsing polychondritis 772–773
　　sclerosis 766
　cartilage invasion 747–748, 748–751
　　CT detection 748–749, 750, 751
　　extralaryngeal spread 744, 745, 749, 751
　　histology 748
　　MRI 749, 751
　　osteolysis 749
　　sclerosis 749
　congenital abnormalities 774
　CT 737, 738
　cysts 768–770
　　saccular 769
　　thyroglossal duct 770
　deep spaces 733–735
　development 731–732
　embryology 731–732
　granulomatous disease 772
　hyaline cartilage 732, 733
　imaging techniques 738–739
　inflammatory conditions 772–773
　MRI 737–738, 738–739
　mucocele 769
　muscles 732, 734, 735, 736
　myositis 773
　necrotizing fasciitis 773
　osteochondronecrosis 765–767
　PET 739
　radiography 739
　regions 732–733, 734
　stenosis 773
　tissue characteristics on sectional imaging 737–738

　trauma 775, 776
　tumors
　　fatty tissue 759, 760
　　Kaposi's sarcoma 756–757
　　laryngeal skeleton 757, 758
　　lymphoreticular system 757–758
　　metastases 759–760, 761
　　myogenic 761
　　neurogenic 761
　　non-squamous cell 755–761
　　patterns of spread 740–743
　　radiation-induced changes 764–768
　　recurrence 761–768
　　sites 740–743
　　squamous cell carcinoma 739–755, 756
　　surgery 761–764
　　TNM classification 748, 752–753
　　treatment 761–768
　　vasoformative 756–757
　ultrasonography 739
　vascular abnormalities 756, 774
　venous malformations 774
　Wegener granulomatosis 772
Le Fort fractures 466, 467–468
leiomyoma
　ciliary body 188
　mesoectodermal 188
　pharyngeal in masticator space 611
Lemierre syndrome 831
lens
　embryology 137, 138
　MRI 140, 145
　suspensory ligaments 137
lenticular process, sagittal section 24
Letterer–Siwe disease 100, 535
leukemia
　acute myelogenous 252
　children 251
　chronic lymphocytic 442
　eye 186, 187
　mandible/maxilla 546
　myelogenous 442
　orbit 251–252
　paranasal sinuses 442
　skull base infiltration 329, 342, 344
leukokoria 158–159
　Coats disease 172
limen nasi 355
lingual artery 629
lingual nerve 511, 629
　atrophy 819
lingual thyroid tissue 719
lingual tonsils 686, 687
lipoma 95
　infrahyoid neck 804
　internal auditory canal 120–121, 121
　larynx 759, 760
　nasopharyngeal 565
　oral cavity/oropharynx 707–708
　parapharyngeal 602
　posterior cervical space 618
　recurrence 804
　retropharyngeal 599, 709, 710
　salivary gland 674, 675
　submandibular/sublingual space 617
lipomatosis, multiple symmetric 804–805
liposarcoma
　infrahyoid neck 805
　larynx 759
　oral cavity/oropharynx 705–706
　salivary gland 675
lips
　carcinoma 689–690
　development 683

Lockwood's ligament 201
longus colli muscle, calcific tendinitis 832–833
loose bodies, temporomandibular joint 497, 498, 499
Ludwig angina 617, 712–713
Lyme disease, temporomandibular joint 495
lymph nodes
  abscess 793
  diagnostic criteria 789, 790
  extranodal tumor spread 793
  fatty hilar metaplasia 792
  infrahyoid neck 782–783
  metastases 792, 793–794
    buccal carcinoma 693
    floor of mouth carcinoma 692
    glottic carcinoma 473
    retropharyngeal 599
    soft palate carcinoma 699
    subglottic carcinoma 743
    thyroid carcinoma 796, 797, 811
    tongue base carcinoma 697
    tonsillar carcinoma 696
  metastatic squamous cell carcinoma 788–794
  necrosis 790, 791, 792, 794
  PET 793–794
  shape 789, 790
  size 789, 790
  ultrasonography 793, 794
  see also cervical lymph nodes
lymphadenitis
  suppurative of retropharyngeal space 598, 599
  tuberculous 825
lymphadenopathy
  cervical 645
  malignant of submandibular/sublingual space 617
  parotid gland 676
  reactive of retropharyngeal space 598
lymphangioma
  capillary 721, 839
  cavernous 721, 839
  cystic 839
  infrahyoid neck 834, 839–840
  masticator space 610
  nasopharyngeal 565, 568
  oral cavity/oropharynx 721–722
  orbital 222, 257–258, 259
  parotid space 613, 614
  posterior cervical space 618
  retropharyngeal space 598
  salivary gland 657, 658
  submandibular space 615
lymphoepithelial lesions, salivary glands 651–654
lymphoepithelioma, nasopharyngeal 571
lymphoid hyperplasia, benign 249
  reactive of eye 157
lymphoma
  cerebellopontine angle 121, 122
  cervical lymph nodes 794–796
  classification 574, 575
  internal auditory canal 121, 122
  lacrimal glands 279
  lacrimal sac 290
  larynx 757
  mandible/maxilla 545–546
  masticator space 612
  nasopharyngeal 574–575, 576–577
  NK/T-cell 438, 439
  ocular 186, 187
  oral cavity/oropharynx 704, 706

orbital 248–251
recurrent 441
retropharyngeal space 599
retrostyloid parapharyngeal space 609
salivary glands 676, 677
sinonasal 402
sinonasal cavities 438–439
Sjögren's syndrome association 654
skull base 329, 341–342
thyroid gland 812–813
see also Hodgkin disease; non-Hodgkin lymphoma
lymphomatoid granuloma, orbital 242–243
lymphoproliferative disorders 340, 341, 342
  orbital 250, 251
lymphoreticular system tumors 757–758
Lynch procedure 473

M

macroglossia 724
macrophthalmia 147–148
macula lutea 142
macular degeneration
  posterior hyaloid detachment 149
  senile 189–190
Madelung disease 804–805
magnetic resonance angiography (MRA)
  skull base 304, 305
  temporal bone 35–36
magnetic resonance imaging (MRI)
  cholesteatoma 76
  cochlea 129, 131
  eye 143–146
  glomus tumors 102, 104–105
  hypopharynx 737–738, 738–739
  inversion recovery pulse sequence 205
  larynx 737–738, 738–739
  larynx cartilage invasion 749, 751
  lymph nodes 793
  malignant tumors 541–542
  mandible 511, 512–513
  maxilla 511, 512–513
  nasal cavity 380, 385
  nasopharynx 559
  neck
    infrahyoid 787
    suprahyoid 592, 593, 619–620
  oral cavity/oropharynx 688
  orbit 205
    normal anatomy 206–215
  paranasal sinuses 380, 385
  persistent hyperplastic primary vitreous 167–168
  retinoblastoma 162
  salivary glands 633–636
    tumors 656–657
  skull base 304
  T1-weighted fat-suppression technique 205
  temporal bone 32–35
    trauma 55
  temporomandibular joint 482, 483
magnetic resonance venography
  jugular bulb 38
  skull base 304
malignant melanoma
  cystic metastasis 838
  lacrimal sac 290
  metastases 442
  parotid space 613
  recurrence 442
  retinal detachment 150, 152

sinonasal cavities 442, 443
uveal 150, 177–183
malignant peripheral nerve sheath tumors (MPNST) 800
  radiation-induced 819
mallear ligament, anterior 24
malleus 3
  anomalies 44, 45–46
  axial sections 4, 5, 6, 8, 9
  cholesteatoma 77, 80
  coronal oblique 20° sections 16, 17, 18
  coronal sections 10, 11
  dislocation 56, 57, 58, 59
  otitis media 69
  sagittal section 23, 24
mandible
  anatomy 509
  condylar agenesis 484–485
  congenital anomalies 513–514
  CT 511, 512, 513
  cysts 514, 516–522
    fissural 518–522
    nonodontogenic 514, 516, 518–522, 523
    odontogenic 514, 516–518, 519–520
  developmental anomalies 513–514
  embryology 477, 508–509, 682
  exostoses 532
  fibromyxoma 460, 461
  hypoplasia 514
  imaging techniques 511–513
  inflammatory disease 514, 515
  MRI 511, 512–513
  myxoma 460, 461
  oral cavity/oropharynx cancer invasion 700–701
  ossification 509
  osteomyelitis 713
  osteoradionecrosis 514, 516
  overgrowth 486
  pathology 513–548
  radiation-induced necrosis 816
  radiography 511–512
  tumors 514, 516, 522–546, 547
    ameloblastoma 711
    benign nonodontogenic 531–535
    benign odontogenic 522–531
    fibro-osseous lesions 535–540
    malignant 541–546, 547
    mixed epithelial odontogenic 528–529, 530
    neurogenic 540–541
    vascular 540, 541
  vascular malformation 540, 541
mandibular arch 508
mandibular canal 509
  neurofibroma 542
mandibular condyle 477
  anatomy 477–479, 480, 481
mandibular denervation, muscle atrophy 723–724
mandibular fossa 297, 300
mandibular ramus 630
mandibulofacial dysostosis 53
  mandibular anomalies 484, 486, 514
  orbit 215, 218
masseter muscle 553, 626, 630
  benign hypertrophy 609
masticator space 554, 555, 559, 591
  abscess 610, 611
  anatomy 580–592
  cellulitis 610, 611
  congenital lesions 609–610
  inflammatory conditions 610–611

masticator space
  lesions 609–613
  mass 583
  muscles 626, 630
  osteomyelitis 610–611
  pathology 593–620
  pseudotumors 609
  tumors
    benign 611
    malignant 612–613, 679
masticatory muscles 553
  denervation atrophy 609
  development 682
  idiopathic atrophy 486
mastoid 3
  cholesteatoma 75, 81, 82, 83–84
  comminuted fractures 56, 58, 59
  developmental variations 36, 37
  hypoplasia 46
  natural radical 82
  pneumatization 44, 45–46, 482, 484
  postoperative imaging 91, 92, 93
  projectile injuries 59
  sagittal section 22
  Schuller projection 30
  Stenvers projection 30, 31
  transorbital projection 30, 31
mastoid air cells
  axial section 3–4, 5, 6
  coronal section 14, 15
  mastoiditis 63, 64
  necrotizing otitis externa 68
mastoid antrum
  coronal oblique 20° sections 20, 21
  coronal section 12, 13, 14
  sagittal section 22
mastoidectomy
  radical 90, 93
  simple 90, 92, 93
mastoiditis
  acute 62–66
    differential diagnosis 65
    imaging 62–65
  chronic 68–74
    clinical findings 68
    imaging 68–74
    otoscopy 68
  extension to temporomandibular joint 496
  subacute 66
maxilla
  anatomy 509–510
  carcinoma 472
  congenital anomalies 513–514
  CT 511, 512, 513
  cysts 514, 516–522
    fissural 518–522
      nonodontogenic 514, 516, 518–522
      odontogenic 514, 516–518, 519–520
  deformities 484–485
  developmental anomalies 513–514
  embryology 508–509, 682
  exostoses 532
  fibromyxoma 460
  floating 468, 469
  fractures 466, 467–468
  hypoplasia 217, 514
  imaging techniques 511–513
  inflammatory disease 514, 515
  MRI 511, 512–513
  myxoma 460
  oral cavity/oropharynx cancer invasion 700–701
  osteoradionecrosis 514, 516

  pathology 513–548
  radiography 511–512
  tumors 514, 516, 522–546, 547
    benign nonodontogenic 531–535
    benign odontogenic 522–531
    fibro-osseous lesions 535–540
    malignant 541–546, 547
    mesodermal odontogenic 529, 530, 531
    mixed epithelial odontogenic 528–529, 530
    neurogenic 540–541
    vascular 540, 541
  vascular malformation 540
maxillary artery 366
maxillary nerve 375
  oral cavity/oropharynx cancer spread 702
maxillary sinus 509, 510
  anatomy 363, 365–366
  blood supply 366
  carcinoma 428
  embryology 353–355
  expansile lesion differential diagnosis 461
  fibromyxoma 460, 461
  innervation 366
  intramural cysts 406–407
  lymphatic drainage 366
  lymphoma 439
  malignant melanoma 442
  mucocele 406
  myxoma 460
  polyps 409
  surgical complications 470, 472
maxillary tuberosity 510
maxillary vein 366
maxillectomy 470, 472
maxillofacial region trauma 466–467
McCune–Albright syndrome 443, 444, 445
  mandible/maxilla 536
meatus, antrostomy
  inferior 470
  middle 470, 471
Meckel syndrome, retinal dysplasia 168
Meckel's cartilage 477, 508, 509
Meckel's cave see trigeminal cavity
median cleft syndrome 388
mediastinitis 828, 830, 832
  necrotizing 830
medulloepithelioma, eye 188–189
megalophthalmos 147–148
melanin 181
melanocytoma, uveal 182–183
melanotic melanoma metastases 760
melanotic neuroectodermal tumor of infancy 436
Ménière type vestibular disorders 49
meninges, pathology 118
meningioma
  en plaque 270, 271
  extension into retrostyloid parapharyngeal space 607
  masticator space 611
  optic nerve sheath 269–271, 272
  orbital 274, 275
  sinonasal cavities 419, 421
  skull base 319–323
  temporal bone 97–98, 118
meningitis 391, 393
meningocele 61
  formation 386
  optic nerve sheath 221
  postoperative imaging 93–94
  skull base 308, 309
meningoencephalocele 61

  postoperative imaging 93–94
  skull base 308
mental foramen 509
Merkel cell carcinoma, sinonasal cavities 436
mesenchyme 295
mesotympanum 3
  coronal oblique 20° sections 14, 15, 16
  sagittal section 26
metaplasia theory of cholesteatoma 75
metastases
  adenoid cystic carcinoma 433
    laryngeal 758
  cervical lymph nodes 788–794
  chondroblastoma 452
  cystic thyroid carcinoma 615
  esthesioneuroblastoma 435, 436
  internal auditory canal 121, 122
  intraocular calcification 160
  larynx 759–760, 761
  lymph nodes 792
    buccal carcinoma 693
    floor of mouth carcinoma 692
    glottic carcinoma 473
    retropharyngeal 599
    soft palate carcinoma 699
    subglottic carcinoma 743
    thyroid carcinoma 796, 797, 811
    tongue base carcinoma 697
    tonsillar carcinoma 696
  malignant melanoma 442, 838
  mandible/maxilla 546, 547
  masticator space 613
  melanotic neuroectodermal tumor of infancy 436
  mucoepidermoid carcinoma 668
  nasopharyngeal 578
  nasopharyngeal carcinoma 571, 572
  neuroblastoma 436
  orbital 212, 213, 284–285
    neuroblastoma 285
  parotid space 613
  retinoblastoma 166
  retrostyloid parapharyngeal space 608–609
  salivary glands 668, 677, 678
    squamous cell carcinoma 674
    tumors 670–671
  sinonasal cavities 463
  skull base 329, 345–346
  submandibular/sublingual space 617
  temporal bone 109, 110–111
  thyroid cancer 796, 797, 811
  thyroid gland 813
  tonsillar carcinoma 696–697
  uveal 183–184
  uveal melanoma 177–178, 179, 181
Michel deformity 48
microphthalmia 146, 147, 215
  Warburg syndrome 169
microsomia, hemifacial 484, 485, 514
microtia 43–44, 45
middle meatal antrostomy 470, 471
midline destructive granuloma 402, 403
  orbital 242–243
migration theory of cholesteatoma 75
Mikulicz syndrome 279, 280
Mondini deformity 48, 49
morning glory disk anomaly 148–149
mouth
  floor 684–685
    carcinoma 690–692
  see also oral cavity; oropharynx
MR sialography 634, 636–638, 648–649, 714–715

MR-guided radiofrequency ablation of tongue base 619
mucocele
　imaging diagnosis 405–406
　inflammatory conditions 318
　lacrimal sac 288, 289
　orbit 283
　paranasal sinuses 405–406
　petrous apex 71
　skull base involvement 344
mucociliary transport 367
mucoepidermoid carcinoma 431, 432, 433, 434
　epiglottis 759
　jaw 527, 542, 543
　parapharyngeal space 602
　salivary gland 634, 668–671
　　minor glands 704, 705
　sinonasal cavities 431, 432, 433, 434
mucormycosis
　nasopharyngeal inflammation 561
　orbital 230
　sinusitis 391, 396, 397
　skull base 317
mucus retention cysts 560, 561
　oral cavity/oropharynx 716–718
Müller cells 142
Müller's muscle 201
　autonomic nerves 203
multiple endocrine neoplasia syndrome, familial 801–802
　thyroid medullary carcinoma 812
multiple myeloma
　following plasmacytoma 440
　mandible/maxilla 545, 546
　orbital 250, 251
　skull base 342
　see also plasmacytoma
mumps 642
　iodide 647
muscle atrophy, denervation 723–724, 725
mycetoma 399
mycobacteria, atypical 825–826
Mycobacterium tuberculosis 825
mycosis fungoides 252
mycotic sinonasal diseases, acute 396–397
myelopathy, radiotherapy-induced 818
mylohyoid line 509
mylohyoid muscle 617, 628, 686
　development 682
　floor of mouth carcinoma spread 691
myocutaneous flaps 821, 822
myonecrosis
　infrahyoid neck 829
　necrotizing fasciitis 830
　pharyngeal constrictor muscle 773
myopia, axial 147
myositis
　focal 832
　infrahyoid neck 829
　larynx 773
　necrotizing fasciitis 830
　odontogenic infections 711
　orbital 232–233, 236
myospherulosis 403
myringoplasty 90–91
myxoma, sinonasal 460–461

N

nasal bones 385
nasal cavity
　allergy 400, 401
　anatomy 355–357
　blood supply 358
　cartilaginous lesions 442–457
　congenital anomalies 386–390
　CT 379–380
　development 353
　embryology 353, 386
　fibro-osseous lesions 442–457
　floor 355, 356
　granuloma gravidarum 404
　image-guided endoscopic surgery 380
　imaging techniques 379–385
　inflammatory diseases 390–406
　innervation 357
　lymphatic drainage 358
　MRI 380, 385
　olfactory region 355
　osseous lesions 442–457
　pathology 386–474
　postoperative changes 470–474
　radiation risk from imaging 385
　respiratory region 355
　roof 355, 356
　standard film radiography 380–385
　trauma 466–468, 469
　tumors 412–442
　　allergic disease 412
　　benign 413–427
　　classification 412, 413
　　inflammatory disease 412
　　malignant 427–442
　　malignant cartilaginous 457–460
　　malignant melanoma 442, 443
　　malignant odontogenic 427–442
　　malignant osseous 457–460
　　metastatic 463
　　miscellaneous 460–463
　　neurogenic 418–427
　walls 355–356, 363
　see also sinonasal cavities
nasal conchae 356
nasal crest 355
nasal cycle 357
nasal dermoid 390
nasal glioma 389, 418
nasal medial processes 386
nasal mucosa
　nasal polyps 408
　pathological changes 366
nasal mucous membrane 357
nasal notch 510
nasal piriform aperture stenosis, congenital 387
nasal polyposis 399, 400
nasal polyps 400, 407–410
　angiomatous 409
　antrochoanal 409, 410
　aspirin-sensitive 408
　choanal 409–410
　fibroblasts 407
　imaging 408, 409
　pituitary adenoma 462
nasal spine 510
nasal vestibule 355
nasoalveolar cyst 425, 518, 520, 522
nasoantral window procedure 470
nasoethmoid region, papillary squamous cell carcinoma 430
nasofrontal duct 361, 362
nasolacrimal canal 363
nasolacrimal duct
　canalization 388
　embryology 139, 386
　mucocele 388
　obstruction 288
nasolacrimal sac embryology 386
nasopalatine duct cyst 422, 425
　maxilla 518, 521
nasopalatine nerve 296, 297, 298
nasopharyngeal angiofibroma, juvenile 344, 345
nasopharyngeal tonsil 553, 557, 558
nasopharynx
　anatomy 553–559, 580, 585, 586–587, 588
　　applied 559
　　regional 558–559
　congenital anomalies 560–561
　cysts 560, 561
　embryology 553
　histology 559
　imaging techniques 559
　inflammation 561–563
　innervation 558
　lymphatics 558
　pathology 560–578
　polyps 565, 567–568
　tumors
　　benign 563–568
　　carcinoma 569–574, 595, 608, 702, 703
　　malignant 568–578
　　teratoma 561
　vascular supply 558
neck
　dissection
　　extended 820
　　modified 820, 821
　　radical 820, 821, 822
　　selective 820, 821
　fascial layers 581–584
　flap reconstruction 820–821, 822
　infrahyoid
　　abscess 822
　　anatomy 780–786, 787
　　blood vessels 780, 781, 782
　　branchial cleft anomalies 834–837
　　congenital lesions 834
　　dissection postoperative changes 820–823
　　fascial layers 784–786
　　fibrohistiocytic neoplasms 806–807
　　fibrous neoplasms 806
　　imaging after treatment 813–823
　　imaging techniques 787–788
　　infections 823–824, 827–832
　　inflammatory conditions 823–840
　　lipomatous neoplasms 804–805
　　lymph nodes 782–783
　　muscles 780, 781
　　neoplasms 788–813
　　nerves 783
　　neurogenic tumors 797–801
　　nodal neoplasms 788–797
　　non-nodal neoplasms 797–807
　　parathyroid gland masses 813
　　postoperative complications 822–823
　　radiation-induced changes 813–820
　　skeletal muscle neoplasms 806–807
　　soft-tissue necrosis 816
　　spaces 784–786
　　thyroid gland masses 807–813
　　tumor recurrence 816, 819, 820, 823
　　vascular malformations 839–840
　　viscera 783–784
　　visceral space 784, 785
　spaces 584–587
　suprahyoid
　　anatomical spaces 590–592

neck
  biopsy 619–620
  imaging techniques 592–593
  interventional MRI 619–620
  pathology 593–620
  spaces 784
  trauma 618
  triangles 780, 786
necrobiotic xanthogranuloma, orbital 247
necrotizing fasciitis 829–831
  clinical diagnosis 830
  complications 831
  histology 831
  larynx 773
  mediastinitis 832
negative pressure theory of cholesteatoma 75
nerve sheath tumors
  masticator space 611
  retrostyloid parapharyngeal space 604–607
  submandibular space 615
nervus intermedius 109
neurenteric cyst 315, 316
  nasopharyngeal 560
neurilemmoma see schwannoma
neuroblastoma
  infrahyoid neck 801
  metastatic potential 436
  olfactory 434–436
  orbital metastases 285
neurocysticercosis 226
neuroepithelioma, peripheral 436
neurofibroma
  facial nerve 100
  frontal nerve 266, 267
  infrahyoid neck 799–800
  larynx 761
  mandible/maxilla 540–541, 542
  nasopharyngeal 565
  oral cavity/oropharynx 708
  orbital 264, 265, 266–267
  plexiform 264, 266, 708, 800
    malignant transformation 800
  retrostyloid parapharyngeal space 606–607
  salivary gland 675
  skull base 323–328
neurofibromatosis 113, 115–116
  macrophthalmia 147
  orbital 218
  plexiform 264, 266
  salivary gland 675
  type I 799–800
    ocular schwannoma 187
    optic nerve glioma 269, 272
    orbital 218, 264, 266
  type II 115
neurofibrosarcoma, malignant 324, 800
neuroma
  acoustic 117
    pneumocisternography 118
  cranial nerve 100
  facial nerve 99, 326
  hypoglossal nerve 328
  multiple mucocutaneous 802
neurosarcoidosis 241, 242
nevi, uveal 184
nodular fasciitis 461
noma, oral cavity/oropharynx 718
non-Hodgkin lymphoma
  cervical lymph nodes 794–796
  classification 575
  mandible/maxilla 545
  masticator space 612
  midline destructive lesions 402

  nasopharyngeal 574–575, 576
  oral cavity/oropharynx 704, 706
  orbital 248
  retropharyngeal space 599
  sinonasal cavities 438
  Sjögren's syndrome association 654
  skull base 340
  thyroid gland 812, 813
nonodontogenic cysts, sinonasal cavities 422, 425
non-steroidal anti-inflammatory drugs (NSAIDs) 408
Norrie disease 168
nose, congenital anomalies 386–390
notch of Rivinus 10, 11
notochordal dysgenesis 316
nuclear medicine
  infrahyoid neck 788
  salivary glands 638
  temporomandibular joint 482

O

oblique muscles 201–202
  Brown superior oblique tendon sheath syndrome 285–287
  imaging 211
  traumatic injury 287
obstructive sleep apnea syndrome 619, 709, 710
occipital condyle 300
ocular detachment 149–154
ocular hypotony 152–153
ocular motility disorders 285–287
  extraocular muscle congenital anomalies 287–290
ocular muscles, traumatic injury 287
oculo-auriculo-vertebral dysplasia 53, 218
oculomotor nerve 202–203
odontogenic cysts
  calcifying 524–525
  sinonasal cavities 419, 421, 422–423
odontogenic ghost cell tumor 524–525
odontogenic infections 711–714
odontogenic keratocyst 419, 503
  mandible/maxilla 517–518, 519–520
odontogenic tumors, sinonasal cavities 423–424, 426, 427
odontoma, mandible/maxilla 528–529, 530
olfactory bulb 357
olfactory nerve fibers 357
olfactory neuroblastoma 434–436
omohyoid muscle 780, 781
oncocytoma 668
Onodi cell 370
ophthalmic artery 202, 203–204
ophthalmic veins 204, 208, 210
  thrombosis 229, 230
ophthalmoplegia, painful external 236
optic canal
  bulging 364, 369–370
  dehiscence 305
  fracture 290, 467
optic disk 143
  blood supply 202
  drusen 157, 176
  leukemia 186
  melanocytoma 182–183
optic nerve 197, 199, 202
  blood supply 202
  compression 290
  damage with orbital fractures 290

  glioma 218, 269, 272–273
  hemangioblastoma 272, 274
  imaging 210, 212
  injury 468
  malformations 167
  medulloepithelioma 188, 189
  melanocytoma 182–183
  metastases 284, 285
  parasitic infections 157, 174, 175
  retinoblastoma 163
  sarcoidosis 241, 242
optic nerve head drusen 176
optic nerve sheath
  enlargement 267–272
  meningeal 202
  meningioma 269–271, 272
  pneumosinus dilatans 268–269
optic nerve sheath meningocele 221
optic neuritis 267–268
optic neuropathy 268–269
oral cavity
  abscess 711, 712
  anatomy 580, 585, 586–587, 588, 683–687
  congenital abnormalities 719–723
  CT 687–688
  denervation muscle atrophy 723–724
  development 682–683
  developmental cysts 720
  embryology 682–683
  imaging techniques 687–688
  infections 718
  inflammatory disease 711–718
  MRI 688
  odontogenic infections 711–714
  tumors 688–711
    benign 707–710
    fibrous tissue 706–707
    lymphoma 704, 706
    malignant 703–707
    muscular tissue 706–707
    non-squamous cell 703–710
    originating in adjacent spaces 709, 710–711
    perineural spread 701–702
    sectional imaging 699–702
    squamous cell carcinoma 688–703
    TNM staging 702
  ultrasonography 688
  vascular malformations 720–722
orbicularis oculi muscle 197, 199, 200
  imaging 211
orbit
  abscess 226, 229, 394
    subperiosteal 229–230, 391, 392
  amyloidosis 244
  anatomy 196–204
  aneurysmal bone cyst 226
  Apert disease 216–217
  apex 198, 199
    fractures 290
    inflammation 234, 235
  arterial supply 203–204
  arteriovenous malformations 259–262
  autonomic nerves 203
  benign lymphoid hyperplasia 249
  blowin fracture 466, 467
  blowout fracture 287, 466, 467
  bony 196–200
    interorbital distance 214–215
  calcifications 212, 213
  carotid–cavernous fistula 259–262
  cellulitis 228–229, 391, 392, 393
  cholesterol granuloma 222–223, 225–226

compartments 197, 209, 212
conal lesions 212
congenital abnormalities 215–222
craniofacial dysostosis 216, 218
craniosynostosis 216, 217
Crouzon disease 216–217
CT 204–205
   normal anatomy 206, 207, 209–215
cystic myositis 226
cystic vascular lesions 222
cysticercosis 226, 227
cysts
   acquired 221–222, 222–226
   aneurysmal bone 226
   appendage 222
   chocolate 222, 258
   dentigerous 222
   developmental 219–221
   enterogenous 221
   epidermal inclusion 222
   epithelial 222
   epithelial implantation 222
   hematic 222–225
   hydatid 226, 227
   microphthalmia 146, 147
defects 218
developmental variations 215–222
embryology 139, 196
Erdheim–Chester disease 245, 247
extraconal peripheral lesions 213
fatty reticulum 197, 199, 200–201
fibromatosis 275, 277
fibro-osseous lesions 282–285
fissure
   fractures 290
   inferior 198, 199
   superior 197, 198
floor 196, 197, 198
   displaced implant 291
fractures 466
fungal infections 230, 231
granulomas 242–243
harlequin appearance 216, 217
hemangioma
   capillary 253, 254
   cavernous 253–256
   intraosseous 283
   sclerosing 254, 257
hypersensitivity angiitis 243
idiopathic midline destructive granuloma 242–243
imaging techniques 204–215
implant 191–192
inflammatory conditions 226–230
   anterior 232
   idiopathic 230–236
innervation 202–203
   imaging 210, 212
intraconal lesions 212, 213
Langerhans cell histiocytosis 244–245, 246
leukemia 251–252
lupus erythematosus 243
lymphomatoid granuloma 242–243
lymphoproliferative disorders 250, 251
mandibulofacial dysostosis 215, 218
motor innervation 202–203
MRI 205
   normal anatomy 206–215
mucocele 283
myositis 232–233, 236
neural lesions 263–267
neurofibromatosis 218
ossification anomalies 215

parasitic infections 226, 227
pathology 215–291
periarteritis nodosa 243
perineuritis 234
peripheral nerves 202–203
periscleritis 234
plagiocephaly 216
pseudorheumatoid nodules 247
pseudotumor 230–236
   classification 231–232
   diagnosis 250
   diffuse 232, 233
   rhabdomyosarcoma 277
roof 196, 197, 198
   fractures 290
Saethre–Chotzen disease 217
sarcoidosis 239–241
sensory innervation 202
septum 199, 200
sinusitis 228
Sjögren's syndrome 241–242
subperiosteal abscess 229–230, 391, 392
subperiosteal hematoma 223–225
   rhabdomyosarcoma 277
subperiosteal lesions 212, 213
subperiosteal phlegmon 229–230, 391, 392
trauma 290–291
tumors 248–252
   brown tumor 455
   chloroma 252
   fibrocystoma 274
   fibroma 275
   fibrosarcoma 275
   fibrous histiocytoma 274–275
   fibrous tissue 272, 274–278
   giant cell tumor 283
   granulocytic sarcoma 252
   hemangioma 253–256, 257, 283
   hemangiopericytoma 262–263
   invasion 283–285
   lymphangioma 222, 257–258, 259
   lymphoplasmacytic 250–251
   meningioma 274, 275
   mesenchymal chondrosarcoma 278
   metastases 212, 213
   multiple myeloma 250, 251
   neurofibroma 264, 265, 266–267
   osteoblastoma 282
   osteoma 282
   osteosarcoma 282, 283
   pilomatrixoma 222
   plasmacytoma 250
   recurrence 284
   rhabdomyosarcoma 275–278
   sarcoma 166, 252
   schwannoma 263–265
   secondary 283–285
   xanthogranuloma 245, 247
varix malformation 222, 258–259, 260
vascular anatomy 203–204
   imaging 208, 209–210
vascular conditions 252–263
vasculitides 242–243
venous drainage 204
wall
   lateral 197, 198
   lateral fractures 291
   medial 196, 197, 198
xanthogranuloma
   juvenile 245, 247
   necrobiotic 247
orbital apex syndrome 405
orbital fissure

inferior 376, 377
superior 297, 298, 299, 301, 305
organ transplantation, posttransplantation lymphoproliferative disorders 441
oropharyngeal isthmus 558
oropharynx
   abscess 711, 712
   anatomy 580, 585, 586–587, 588, 683–687
   congenital abnormalities 719–723
   CT 687–688
   development 682–683
   developmental cysts 720
   embryology 682–683
   imaging techniques 687–688
   infections 718
   inflammatory disease 711–718
   lymphoma 704, 706
   MRI 688
   nasopharyngeal carcinoma extension 571
   odontogenic infections 711–714
   posterior wall carcinoma 699
   tumors 688–711
      benign 707–710
      fibrous tissue 706–707
      malignant 703–707, 791
      muscular tissue 706–707
      non-squamous cell 703–710
      originating in adjacent spaces 709, 710–711
      perineural spread 701–702
      radiotherapy complications 816, 817
      sectional imaging 699–702
      squamous cell carcinoma 688–703
      TNM staging 702
   ultrasonography 688
   vascular malformations 720–722
ossifying fibroma 329, 330
   sinonasal cavities 445–448
   variants 446–447
osteitis deformans 449
osteitis fibrosa 455, 457
   cystica 457, 534
osteoarthritis/osteoarthrosis of temporomandibular joint 493–494, 496, 497
osteoblastoma
   mandible/maxilla 536
   orbital 282
   sinonasal cavities 451, 452
   skull base 329, 331
   temporomandibular joint 499
osteochondritis dissecans 493
osteochondroma
   mandible/maxilla 532
   temporomandibular joint 499
osteochondronecrosis, laryngeal 765–767
osteoclastoma
   sinonasal cavities 452–453
   skull base 329, 331
   temporomandibular joint 499, 500
osteogenesis imperfecta 130, 131
osteogenic sarcoma, skull base 329, 334
osteolysis, larynx cartilage invasion 749
osteoma
   choroid 157, 176, 177
   mandible/maxilla 532, 533
   orbital 282
   paraorbital 450
   sinonasal 413, 414
   sinonasal cavities 450–451
   skull base 329, 331
   temporal bone 95–96
   temporomandibular joint 499
osteomalacia 457

860 Index

osteomyelitis
  cervical vertebral bodies 828, 829
  chronic of jaw 713–714
  clivus 561
  mandible 514, 515, 713
  masticator space 610–611
  necrotizing fungal 317
  odontogenic infections 711
  proliferative periostitis 714
  sclerosing 714
  sinusitis complication 395
  sphenoid bone 561
  suppurative 714
  temporal bone 66
  temporomandibular joint
    extension 496
    infectious arthritis 487
osteopetrosis 130
  mandible/maxilla 540
  sinonasal cavities 449–450
osteophytes, temporomandibular joint 493, 494, 496
osteoradionecrosis 94–95
  fulminant laryngeal 817
  hyoid bone 816, 817
  mandible 514, 516, 816
  maxilla 514, 516
osteosarcoma
  masticator space 612
  orbital 282, 283
  radiation-induced 819
  sinonasal cavities 457–458
ostiomeatal complex 360, 362, 363, 367
  endoscopic surgery 470
  imaging 368
  obstruction 366
otic capsule, congenital anomalies 47–48
otitis externa 496
  malignant necrotizing 66, 67, 68
  nasopharyngeal inflammation 561, 562
  necrotizing 487, 496
otitis media 496
  acute 62–66
  chronic 68–74
    clinical findings 68
    imaging 68–74
    otoscopy 68
    suppurative 68, 69
    tympanosclerosis 74
  serous 65
otomastoiditis 318
otorrhea, cerebrospinal fluid 52, 61, 62
  skull base fracture 346, 348
otosclerosis 122–129
  clinical course 123
  cochlear 124–125, 126, 127, 128, 129
    CT densitometry 125–126, 127–128
  radiography 123–124, 126, 128
oval window 123
  congenital anomalies 46, 47
  coronal oblique 20° sections 19, 20
  coronal section 11
  otosclerosis 123–124
  sagittal section 25, 26

P

Paget disease of bone 129–130, 449
  mandible/maxilla 537, 539, 540
palate
  adenoid cystic carcinoma 431, 432
  floating 468
  hard 683, 684
  carcinoma 695, 701
  soft 683, 684
    anatomy 686
    carcinoma 596, 699
palati muscle
  levator 732
  tensor 682
palatine aponeurosis 554, 556
palatine artery, greater 296, 297, 298
palatine bone 371–375, 376
palatine canal 373, 374, 376
  greater 377
palatine foramen, greater 297, 299, 373, 374, 376
palatine nerves 373, 374, 376
  oral cavity/oropharynx cancer spread 702
palatine tonsil 553, 557, 558, 686, 687
  abscess 716, 717
  carcinoma 695–697
  development 682
  hyperplasia 716
  inflammation 716
palatine velum 554, 556
palatomaxillary suture 297, 299
palatopharyngeal sphincter 556
palatovaginal canal 376, 377
palpebrae superioris muscle, levator 201
papillary cystadenoma lymphomatosum *see* Warthin's tumor
papillary ingrowth theory of cholesteatoma 75
papilledema 157
papillitis 157
papillomas, nasopharyngeal 568
paraffinoma 404
paragangliomas
  histology 802, 803
  infrahyoid neck 801–803
  retrostyloid parapharyngeal space 603, 604–605, 609
  sellar 462–463
  skull base 323–328
paraglottic space 733, 734–735
  cancer invasion 747
  supraglottic carcinoma 740
paralaryngeal space, cancer invasion 747
paranasal sinuses
  allergy 400, 401
  anatomical variations 367–371
  anatomy 358–371
  cartilaginous lesions 442–457
  congenital anomalies 386–390
  CT 379–380
  cystic fibrosis 397
  development 353–355
  embryology 353–355, 386
  extramedullary hematopoiesis 448–449
  fibro-osseous lesions 442–457
  hypoplastic 401
  image-guided endoscopic surgery 380
  imaging techniques 379–385
  inflammatory diseases 390–406
  leukemic manifestations 442
  MRI 380, 385
  mucocele 312, 313, 405–406
  opacification 400
  osseous lesions 442–457
  pathology 386–474
  postoperative changes 470–474
  radiation risk from imaging 385
  retention cysts 406–407
  sarcoidosis 402, 404
  standard film radiography 380–385
  surgery complications 470–474
  trauma 466–468, 469
  tumors 412–442
    allergic disease 412
    benign 413–427
    classification 412, 413
    inflammatory disease 412
    malignant 427–442
    malignant cartilaginous 457–460
    malignant odontogenic 427–442
    malignant osseous 457–460
    metastatic 463
    miscellaneous 460–463
    neurogenic 418–427
  see also sinonasal cavities
paranasal sinusitis, orbital complications 228
parapharyngeal space 554, 555, 558–559
  anatomy 580–592, 589
  extraparotid mass 629
  infection 600
  inflammatory disease 600
  pathology 593–620
  poststyloid 626, 627
    masses 630
  prestyloid compartment 582, 589, 590
    benign tumors 600–602
    congenital lesions 599–600
    lesions 599–602
    malignant tumors 602
    masses 629–630
    neoplasms 627, 629
    parotid gland 625, 626, 627
    pseudotumor 599
  retrostyloid compartment 582, 583, 589, 590
    benign tumors 603–607
    inflammatory disease 602–603
    lesions 602–609
    malignant tumors 608–609
    pseudotumors 602
    vascular abnormalities 602
  tumors 627, 629
    benign 600–602, 603–607, 629, 664, 666
    malignant 602, 608–609
    nasopharyngeal carcinoma spread 572
parasitic infections
  optic nerve head 157, 174, 175
  orbital 226, 227
parathyroid glands 784
  infrahyoid neck masses 813
parathyroid hormone (PTH) 457
paratonsillar abscess 562
parotid artery thrombosis 618
parotid duct 626
  dilated 650
  stones 650, 651
  stricture 679–680
parotid glands
  abscess 643, 644
  absence 638, 639
  accessory 609
  anatomy 625–628
  benign lymphoepithelial lesions 651, 652, 654
  congenital lesions 638–642
  embryology 625
  enlargement differential diagnosis 645, 646
  first branchial cleft cyst 638
  histology 631
  HIV infection 826
  imaging 631–638
  lymphadenopathy 676
  lymphatic drainage 627

lymphoepithelial lesions/cysts 651–654, 826
masses 629
   deep lobe 583
MR sialography 637
multicentric cysts 651, 652
mumps 642
radiography 631, 632
sialography 633
tumors 629, 656, 661
   acinic cell carcinoma 674
   adenoid cystic carcinoma extension 673
   facial nerve 663
   lymphoma 676, 677
   malignant mixed 674
   metastases 677, 678
   neurogenic 674–675
   pleomorphic adenoma 95
   skull base involvement 344, 345
   vascular lesions 657
   Warthin's tumor 664–668
vascular supply 627
see also salivary glands
parotid space 581, 592, 627–628
   abscess 613, 614
   congenital lesions 613, 614
   inflammatory conditions 613, 614
   lesions 613, 614
   malignant tumors 613, 614
   parapharyngeal aspect 628
   synovial chondromatosis 677–678
pars flaccida cholesteatoma 76–77, 79, 80, 81
pars tensa cholesteatoma 78, 79, 80, 81
Passavant's sphincter 556
Paterson-Brown-Kelly syndrome 745
pectoralis flap 822
Pendred syndrome 53
Peptostreptococcus 824
periarteritis nodosa, orbital 243
perineuritis, orbital 234
periodontal disease 546
periodontal ligament 510, 511
periodontal membrane, radicular cysts 422
periorbita 197, 198, 199, 200
peripheral nerves, orbital 202–203
periscleritis, orbital 234
peritonsillar abscess 594
peritonsillar inflammation 716
perivertebral space 584, 592
persistent hyperplastic primary vitreous (PHPV) 149, 164, 166–168
   clinical diagnosis 166
   diagnostic imaging 167–168
   Warburg syndrome 169
petromastoid plate 296
petrosal nerve
   deep 297, 298, 299, 300
   greater 297, 298, 299, 300, 375
petrositis 64
petrosquamous fissure 297, 300
petrotympanic fissure 297, 300
   sagittal section 24
petrous apex
   developmental variations 40–41
   mucocele 71
petrous bone, epidermoid cyst 310
petrous pyramid
   cholesteatoma 85–89
      congenital 87
   cholesterol granuloma 71–72, 72–73
   craniometaphyseal dysplasia 130, 132
   fractures 56
   glomus jugulare tumor 104
   hemangioma 97, 120, 121

osteoma 96
postoperative imaging 93
Stenvers projection 30, 31
transorbital projection 30, 31
petrous temporal 297, 300
pharyngeal aponeurosis 584, 586
pharyngeal arches 731, 732
   development 682
pharyngeal bursa 558
pharyngeal constrictor muscle
   dermatomyositis 832
   myonecrosis 773
pharyngeal constrictor muscles 553, 554, 556, 736, 737
   development 732
pharyngeal isthmus 553, 554, 558
pharyngeal mucosal space 584, 589
   lesions 594–597
   pseudomass 594
   tumors
      benign 594–595
      malignant 595–597
pharyngeal recess *see* Rosenmüller fossa
pharyngeal tonsil 553, 557, 558
   hypertrophy 594
pharyngeal walls
   carcinoma of posterior 747
   obstructive sleep apnea syndrome 619
pharyngitis 716
   immunocompromised patients with opportunistic infection 773
pharyngobasilar fascia 556–558, 582, 584, 586–587, 588
pharyngocele 770–771
pharyngocutaneous fistula 816, 817, 822
pharyngotonsillitis 563
pharynx 553, 580
   hypomotility disorders 771
   obstructive sleep apnea syndrome 619
   perforation 618
   see also hypopharynx; nasopharynx
philtrum 386
phlegmon 394, 395
phrenic nerve 783
phthisis bulbi 156, 158, 159
   persistent hyperplastic primary vitreous 166
Pierre Robin syndrome 514
pigmented villonodular synovitis (PVNS) 499, 502
pilomatrixoma 222, 658
Pindborg tumor *see* calcifying epithelial odontogenic tumor
piriform sinus 735–736
   carcinoma 743–745, 746
   fistulae 836–837
pituitary adenoma
   ectopic nasopharyngeal 565
   extension nasopharyngeal 565, 568
   invasive 319–320
   sinonasal cavities 462–463
plagiocephaly, orbit 216
plasmacytoma
   extramedullary 439–441
   larynx 757–758
   orbital 250
   sinonasal cavities 439–441, 442
   skull base 341, 342
   see also multiple myeloma
platysma muscle 780, 781
   necrotizing fasciitis 830
pleomorphic hyalinizing angiectatic tumor (PHAT) 807

Plummer-Vinson syndrome 692, 745
   hypopharyngeal webs 772
pneumocephalus 469, 470, 471
Pneumococcus 833
pneumoparotitis 679
pneumosinus dilatans 268–269, 370–371
polyarteritis nodosa, orbital 243
polychondritis, relapsing 772–773
positron emission tomography (PET)
   hypopharynx 739
   infrahyoid neck 788
   larynx 739
   lymph nodes 793–794
postcricoid region 736
   carcinoma 745, 746, 747
posttransplantation lymphoproliferative disorders 441
Pott's puffy tumor 395
pouch of Luschka 558
preepiglottic space 733–734, 735
   cancer invasion 740, 747
   oral cavity/oropharynx cancer invasion 700
pregnancy
   nasal granuloma gravidarum 404
   rhinitis 400
   sinonasal cavity hemangioma 416
prenasal space closure anomalies 388–389
prevertebral muscles, oral cavity/oropharynx cancer invasion 702
prevertebral space, infrahyoid 786
primitive neuroectodermal tumor (PNET) 801
   extracranial 436, 437
prognathism 484
prolactinoma 462, 463
proptosis 201, 215
   cavernous hemangioma 254, 257
   children 275
   cholesterol granuloma 225
   rhabdomyosarcoma 275, 276
psammoma bodies 320, 574
psammomatoid active ossifying fibroma 536, 539
psammomatoid bodies 448
pseudogout 495
Pseudomonas, nasopharyngeal inflammation 561, 562
Pseudomonas aeruginosa 487
pseudorheumatoid nodules, orbital 247
pseudotumor
   lacrimal glands 279, 280
   masticator space 609
   orbital 230–236
      classification 231–232
      diagnosis 250
      diffuse 232, 233
      rhabdomyosarcoma 277
   parapharyngeal space
      prestyloid compartment 599
      retrostyloid compartment 602
pterygoid canal 297, 298, 299, 300, 375, 376, 377
pterygoid muscles 553, 626, 630
pterygoid plates 298, 299, 300
pterygoid plexus 366
pterygoid process 298, 299, 300
pterygoid venous plexus, asymmetric 599
pterygomaxillary fissure 371–375, 376, 377
pterygopalatine fossa 199, 200, 356, 371–375, 376
   infections 376
   oral cavity/oropharynx cancer invasion 701–702
   tumors 376

pterygopalatine ganglion 203, 357, 373, 375–376
pyramidal eminence 3, 5, 7
  coronal oblique 20° sections 21
  coronal section 12, 14
  sagittal section 24
pyramidal fracture 468

R

radicular cysts
  mandible/maxilla 516, 517
  periodontal membrane 422
radiofrequency thermal energy 619
radiography
  Caldwell projection 380, 382
  Chamberlain–Town view 384
  conventional
    nasal cavity 380–385
    paranasal sinuses 380–385
    salivary glands 631–632
    Stenvers projection 30, 31
    temporal bone 30, 31
    temporal bone trauma 54, 55
  dental 512
  hypopharynx 739
  intraoral 512
  larynx 739
  lateral view 380, 382, 383
  mandible/maxilla 511–512
  nasal bone views 384, 385
  oblique view 384
  Schuller projection 30, 31
  submentovertical base view 382, 384
  transorbital projection 30, 31
  Waters projection 380, 381
radionecrosis 94–95
radiotherapy
  aggressive fibromatosis 806
  complications 765–768, 816–819
  infrahyoid neck changes 813–820
    complications 816–819
    expected 814–816
  laryngeal cancer 764–768
Ramsey Hunt syndrome 66, 67
ranula
  oral cavity/oropharynx 717, 718
  plunging 560, 561, 718
  salivary glands 639, 640–641
  simple 718
  submandibular/sublingual space 615–616
Rathke's cleft cyst 315, 316, 560
rectus muscles 140, 201, 202
  imaging 211
  injury during surgery 470, 471
  traumatic injury 287
recurrent laryngeal nerve 783
  paralysis 767–768, 775
    radiation-induced 819
Reidel procedure 473
Reiter syndrome, temporomandibular joint 495
renal adenocarcinoma metastases 760, 761
renal disease, chronic 457
renal osteodystrophy 457, 535
retention cysts
  paranasal sinuses 406–407
  postinflammatory 594
  sphenoid sinus 570
retina
  anatomy 140, 142–143
  astrocytoma 162, 174, 175
  blood supply 143
  dysplasia 168–169
  embryology 137, 138
  gliosis 177
  hamartoma combined with retinal pigment epithelial 174
  hemangioma 184, 186
  leukemia 186
  malformations 167
  subretinal neovascular membranes 177
  vascular leakage 150
retinal artery, central 143
retinal detachment 150–152
  choroidal angioma 185, 186
  Coats disease 170, 171, 172
  rhegmatogenous 151–152
  uveal melanoma 179
  Warburg syndrome 169
retinal pigment epithelium 142
  hamartoma combined with retinal 174
  retinal detachment 150
retinal supporting cells 142
retinitis, cytomegalovirus 154, 155
retinoblastoma 140, 141, 159–164, 165, 166
  bilateral 164, 166
  clinical diagnosis 161
  Coats disease differential diagnosis 172
  diagnostic imaging 161–164, 165, 166
  familial 160, 164
  genetics 160
  incidence 160
  leukokoria 158–159
  metastases 166
  recurrent 166, 191
  tetralateral 160–161, 164, 165
  trilateral 160, 164
retinopathy of prematurity 169, 170
  intraocular calcifications 157
retinoschisis, X-linked 148
retrobulbar recess *see* sinus lateralis
retrocricoarytenoid region 736
retrognathia 484
retrograde venography, glomus tumors 102, 105
retrolental fibroplasia *see* retinopathy of prematurity
retromandibular vein 627, 635
retromolar trigone 686–687
  carcinoma 694–695, 701
retropharyngeal lymph node metastases 599
retropharyngeal space 582, 585, 587, 591
  abscess 598–599, 618, 827, 828
    complications 828–829
  cellulitis 827, 828
  congenital lesions 597–598
  hematoma 618
  infections 598–599, 827–829
  inflammatory conditions 598–599
  infrahyoid 785, 786
  lesions 597–599
  pseudotumors 597
  third branchial cleft cyst 836
  tumors
    benign 599
    lipoma 709, 710
    malignant 599
    nasopharyngeal carcinoma extension 572, 573
rhabdomyoma
  infrahyoid neck 806
  laryngeal 761
  oral cavity/oropharynx 709
  parapharyngeal 630
rhabdomyosarcoma
  alveolar 437, 438
  embryonal 438
  infrahyoid neck 806–807
  infratemporal fossa 277
  masticator space 612
  nasopharyngeal 575, 576–577, 578
  oral cavity/oropharynx 706, 707
  orbital 275–278
  radiation-induced 819
  recurrent 277, 278
  sinonasal cavities 437–438
  skull base 329, 337, 338
  treatment 438
rheumatoid arthritis 243
  Sjögren's syndrome association 654
  temporomandibular joint 494–495, 496, 497
rhinitis
  atrophic 402
  medicamentosa 401
  pregnancy 400
  vasomotor 401
rhinoliths 401–402
rhinorrhea, cerebrospinal fluid 346, 348, 469
rhinoscleroma 402–403
  nasopharyngeal 563
rhinosinusitis, chronic 366, 397
  allergic fungal 398–400
rhinosporidiosis 403
Rhinosporidium seeberi 403
ribs, cervical 842
Riedel thyroiditis 833–834
Rosai–Dorfman disease 827
Rosenmüller fossa 553, 554, 556, 557, 558
  asymmetric 594
  nasopharyngeal carcinoma 573
round tumors 659, 666
round window 123
  coronal oblique 20° sections 20
  sagittal section 25, 26

S

saccule 19
Saethre–Chotzen disease
  maxilla anomalies 514
  orbit 217
salivary clear cell carcinoma 527
salivary ducts
  congenital cystic dilatation 638
  stenosis 634
  strictures 634, 679–680
salivary glands
  abscess 643, 644
  AIDS 651–654
  anatomy 625–630
    applied 629–630
  chronic progressive disorders 644–646
  congenital lesions 638–642
  CT 633–634, 656
  cysts 638–640, 642, 651–654
    CT 656
  embryology 625
  endocrine-related disorders 679
  granulomatous lesions 644–646
  histology 630–631
  imaging 631–638
  inflammatory disease 642–651, 714–716
  metabolic disorders 679
  MRI 633–636
    normal appearance 635–636
  neoplasms 654–677
  nuclear medicine 638
  pathology 638–680

sarcoidosis 645
sialography 632–633
Sjögren's syndrome 652, 653, 654, 655
tuberculosis 645
tumors
  benign 658–668
  benign mixed 595, 601–602, 617, 655–656, 659–664
  CT 655–656
  dumbbell 659, 663
  epithelial tissue origin 658–674
  malignant 656, 657, 658–659
  malignant epithelial 668–674
  malignant mixed 670–671, 674
  metastases 668, 670–671, 677, 678
  minor glands 664, 703–704, 758–759
  MRI 656–657
  neurogenic 662, 674–675
  nonepithelial neoplasms 674–676, 677
  round 659, 666
  skin involvement 659
  treatment 659
  vascular lesions 657, 658
ultrasonography 638
see also parotid glands; sublingual glands; submandibular glands
sarcoidosis
  cervical lymph nodes 826–827
  clinical features 240–241
  lacrimal glands 280
  optic nerve 241, 242
  orbital 239–241
    apical inflammation 234, 235
  paranasal sinuses 402, 404
  parotid gland cysts 651
  salivary glands 645
  scleritis 156
  uveitis 157
sarcoma
  mandible/maxilla 542–543, 544
  masticator space 612
  neurogenic 800
  orbital 166
    granulocytic 252
  osteogenic 457–458
    mandible/maxilla 542–543, 544
    nasopharyngeal 578
  radiation-induced 819
  salivary gland 675–676
  temporal bone 109
  thyroid gland 813
scala tympani 8
  coronal oblique 20° sections 19, 20
  coronal section 12, 13
  sagittal section 26, 27
scala vestibuli 8
  coronal oblique 20° sections 19
  coronal section 12, 13
  sagittal section 26, 27
scaphoid fossa 298, 299, 300
scapular levator muscle hypertrophy 842
Schneiderian papillomas 413–416, 568
Schuller projection 30, 31
schwannoma
  acoustic 113, 114–115, 116, 117
    bilateral 116
  acoustic nerve inflammation differential diagnosis 114
  carotid space 709, 710
  eye 187
  facial nerve 98–100
  histology 798, 799
  infrahyoid neck 797–801

jugular fossa 327, 329
larynx 761
malignant 324, 419, 420, 800
mandible/maxilla 540
masticator space 611, 612, 679
nasopharyngeal 565
oral cavity/oropharynx 708, 709, 710
orbital 263–265
parapharyngeal 630
retrostyloid parapharyngeal space 604–606, 607, 609
sinonasal cavities 418–419, 420
skull base 323–328
vagus nerve 100, 327
vestibular 114–115, 116
Schwartze sign 123, 129
scintigraphy of temporomandibular joint 482
sclera
  anatomy 140–141
  embryology 137, 138
  schwannoma 187
scleritis 156
  ocular hypotony 152–153
sclerosing hemangioma
  orbital 254, 257
sebaceous gland cysts 657
  pilomatrixoma 658
sella turcica 295–296
sellar paraganglioma 462–463
semicircular canal 3
  axial sections 4, 5, 7, 8
  congenital anomalies 50, 51
  coronal oblique 20° sections 19, 20, 21
  coronal sections 11, 12, 13, 14, 15
  sagittal sections 23, 24, 25, 26, 27
septal cartilage 355
septoplasty 470, 471
Sharpey's fibers 510, 511, 748
sialadenitis 642
  acute
    submandibular 715
    suppurative 643, 644
  autoimmune 676
  chronic 647–651
    recurrent 643–644, 645, 715–716
    sclerosing 646
  metabolic 679
  postirradiation 647, 648
  recurrent of childhood 645, 647
sialadenopathy, benign lymphoepithelial 652, 654, 655
sialadenosis 678–679
sialectasis, chronic 644, 645
sialodochitis 632, 633, 650, 651
  ductal system dilatation 715
  with Sjögren's syndrome 653
sialodochoplasty 632, 651
sialography 632–633, 680
  contrast materials 633
  techniques 648
sialolithiasis 632, 647–651
  imaging techniques 648, 680
  pathogenesis 648
  salivary gland inflammation 714–715
  symptoms 649
sialolithotripsy, extracorporeal 648, 651
sialoliths, radiopaque 635
sialometaplasia, necrotizing 647
sialopathy 633
sialosis, autoimmune 652, 654, 655
sick mucosa 697
sigmoid sinus, forward-lying plate 305, 306
silent sinus syndrome 401

sinolith 401
sinonasal cavities
  destructive lesion differential diagnosis 403
  epithelial tumors 427
  glandular tumors 431–434
  granulomatous diseases 402–403
  lymphoma 438–439
  plasmacytoma 439–441, 442
sinonasal inflammation, nasal cocaine abuse 401
sinonasal neuroendocrine carcinoma 434
sinonasal papillomas 413–416
sinonasal pathology 386–474
sinonasal polyps 408, 409
sinus lateralis 360, 361, 364
sinus of Morgagni 556, 557
sinus plate erosion 82, 91, 93
sinusitis
  acute 390–396
    radiological diagnosis 391
  allergic 391
  aspergillosis 396–397, 398, 400
  bacterial 400
  chronic 390, 397–398
    fungal 398–400
    hyperplastic 399, 400
    nasal polyps 407
  complications 391–396
  fungal infections 391, 396–397
  intracranial complications 394–396
  maxillary surgery 470
  mucormycosis 396, 397
  orbital 228
Sjögren's syndrome
  lacrimal glands 279
  lymphoma association 676
  MR sialography 632, 636
  orbital 241–242
  parotid gland cysts 651, 652–653
  salivary glands 652, 653, 654, 655
skull base
  anatomy 295–304
    variations 305–306
  anterior lesions 307
  aspergillosis 317
  central lesions 307
  CT 304
  dermoid cysts 307–312
  developmental cysts 307–318
  diagnostic imaging 304
  embryology 295
  epidermoid cysts 307–312
  extracranial lesions 344–345
  fibro-osseous lesions 328–332
  fractures 59, 346–348
  inferior surface 297–298
  inflammatory conditions 316–318
  MRA 304, 305
  MRI 304
  pathology 304, 306–348
  posterior lesions 307
  surgery 304
  trauma 346–348
  tumors 318–342
    ameloblastoma 315
    embolization 305
    metastases 329, 345–346
    nasopharyngeal carcinoma invasion 569, 570–571, 572
sound-conducting system anomalies 43–47
sphenoethmoidal recess 356
sphenoid bone 295, 296
  osteomyelitis 561

spine 298, 299, 300
sphenoid ostium 365
sphenoid sinus
  ameloblastoma 315
  anatomy 362, 364–365
  embryology 354, 355
  encephalocele 389
  esthesioneuroblastoma 435, 436
  mucocele 405, 406
  retention cyst 570
  surgical complications 473, 474
sphenopalatine artery 376
sphenopalatine foramen 356, 376, 377
sphenopalatine ganglion 373
spinal accessory lymph nodes 618
spinal accessory nerve 786
spinal arteries 298, 300
spondylodiskitis, vertebral body 832
squamotympanic fissure 297, 298, 300
Stafne cyst of mandible 522, 523
stapedectomy 123, 124, 125, 126, 128
stapedius muscle
  coronal section 12, 14
  sagittal section 24
stapedius tendon 5, 7
stapes 3
  axial section 5, 7
  congenital anomalies 46
  coronal oblique 20° sections 19, 20
  coronal section 11, 12, 13
  development 682
  dislocation 56, 57, 58, 59
  footplate 123, 124
  sagittal section 25, 26
Staphylococcus 830, 832
  thyroiditis 833
Staphylococcus aureus 643, 824, 829
staphyloma 148
Stensen's duct 649, 650
Stenvers projection 30, 31
sternocleidomastoid muscle 780, 781
  dermatomyositis 832
  necrotizing fasciitis 830
  tumor invasion 793
Stickler syndrome 53
strap muscles 780, 781
  dermatomyositis 832
  necrotizing fasciitis 830
  thyroglossal duct cyst 837
Streptococcus 824, 832
  group A beta-hemolytic 830
  thyroiditis 833
Streptococcus anginosus 396
Streptococcus pneumoniae
  acute sinusitis 390
  tonsillitis 716
Streptococcus viridans 643
Sturge–Weber syndrome 147
  choroidal hemangioma 184
  intraocular calcification 157, 158
styloglossus muscle 684
stylohyoid ligament 682
stylomandibular tunnel 627
stylomastoid foramen 297, 298, 301
stylopharyngeus muscle 554, 556
  development 682
subdural abscess 391, 393
subdural empyema 396
subgaleal abscess 395
subglottic region 735
  cancer invasion 747
sublingual artery 629
sublingual fossa 509

sublingual glands
  anatomy 628–629
  ducts 628
  embryology 625
  histology 631
  imaging 631–638
  innervation 629
  lymphatic drainage 629
  tumors
    acinic cell carcinoma 674
    adenoid cystic carcinoma 672
    floor of mouth spread 704
  vascular supply 629
  see also salivary glands
sublingual nerve 628
sublingual space 581, 628, 684, 685–686
  cellulitis 617
  congenital abnormalities 613, 615
  inflammatory disease 616–617
  lesions 613, 615–618
  Ludwig angina 712–713
  tumors
    benign 617
    floor of mouth carcinoma spread 691
    malignant 617
submandibular duct 628
  calculus 632
  infections 714–715
  stone 632
  stricture 679–680
submandibular fossa 509
submandibular glands
  anatomy 628–629
  cysts 615
  embryology 625
  histology 631
  imaging 631–638
  innervation 629
  lymphatic drainage 629
  MR sialography 637
  mumps 642
  radiography 631
  sialadenitis 715
  sialography 632, 633
  tumors 629, 656, 661
    acinic cell carcinoma 674, 675
    floor of mouth spread 704
    neurogenic 674–675
    Warthin's tumor 664–668
  vascular supply 629
  see also salivary glands
submandibular lymph nodes, malignant tumors 617
submandibular space 581, 686
  abscess 616–617
  cellulitis 616–617
  congenital abnormalities 613, 615
  infections 713
  inflammatory disease 616–617
  lesions 613, 615–618
  Ludwig angina 712–713
  tumors
    benign 617
    floor of mouth carcinoma spread 691
    malignant 617
submental artery 629
submental lymph nodes, malignant tumors 617
subperiosteal abscess 64, 392, 394
  orbital 229–230
subperiosteal edema 391, 392, 393
subperiosteal space, inflammatory edema 391, 392

subretinal hemorrhage, Warburg syndrome 169
suprabulbar recess see sinus lateralis
suprachoroidea 142
supraglottitis 772
suprahyoid space 582
suprasternal spaces 581
sutural ligaments 295
sympathetic nerve chain 783
  schwannoma 797, 798
symphysis menti 509
synovial bodies, calcification 498, 499
synovial chondromatosis, temporomandibular joint 497–499
synovial sarcoma, temporomandibular joint 499
systemic lupus erythematosus (SLE)
  orbital 243
  Sjögren's syndrome association 654
  temporomandibular joint 495

T

Taenia solium 226
tail sign 118
Takayasu arteritis 842
Tangier disease 563
tarsal plates 200
tears
  drainage 204
  Sjögren's syndrome 241
teeth
  anatomy 510–511
  dental caries and sinusitis 391
  development 508–509
  endosseous implantation 546, 548
  histology 510, 511
  innervation 511
  loss 546
  odontoma 529, 530
  replacement 546
tegmen
  developmental variations 36–37
  erosion 82, 83, 84, 91, 93
tegmen antri, low-lying 305
tegmen tympani, low-lying 305
temporal bone
  anatomy 3–29
    axial sections 3–9
  chondroblastoma 452
  congenital abnormalities 41–53
  conventional radiography 30, 31
  coronal oblique 20° sections 14–21
  coronal sections 10–14
  CT 30–32
  developmental variations 36–41
  embryology 41–43, 682
  fractures 347
    classification 54
    clinical findings 54
    imaging findings 54–55
    longitudinal 55–56, 57, 60, 61
    transverse 56, 57, 60
  imaging techniques 30–36
  lateral sinus developmental variations 36, 37
  MRA 35–36
  MRI 32–35
  normal 34, 35
  osteomyelitis 66
  petrous apex infection 561, 562
  posterior cranial fossa 296
  postirradiation changes 94–95
  postirradiation imaging 90–95

postoperative imaging 90–95
projectile injuries 58–59, 60
radiation-induced necrosis 816
sagittal sections 22–29
trauma 54–61
tumors 95–111
   adenocarcinoma 329, 339, 340
   benign 95–105, 106–108
   fibromyxoma 332
   malignant 105, 108–111
   secondary malignancy 109, 110–111
vascular abnormalities 118–120
temporalis muscle 553, 626, 630
temporodisk 479
temporomandibular joint (TMJ)
  ameloblastoma 503
  anatomy 477–481
   normal imaging 478, 479, 480, 482–483
   variations 484–486
  ankylosis 486, 487, 494, 495–497
   congenital 496
   treatment 495–496, 497, 506
  arthritic conditions 493–499
   infectious 486–487
   metabolic 495, 496
   osteoarthritis/osteoarthrosis 493–494, 496, 497
   psoriatic 495
   traumatic 494
  articular disk 478, 479, 480, 483
   derangements 487, 488–492
  articulation 480
  avascular necrosis 489
  cholesteatoma 504
  condylar remodeling 489
  CT 481, 482
  developmental anomalies 484–486
  diagnostic imaging techniques 481–482
  dislocation 505
  displacement 505
  embryology 477
  external auditory canal
   carcinoma extension 504
   herniation into 483, 484
   pyogenic granuloma extension 504
  fibrous dysplasia 504
  fractures 504–505
  gap arthroplasty 506
  hypomobility 495
  inflammation 486–487
  interarticular implants 505–506
  internal derangements 487–493
  joint capsule 479
  joint spaces 479, 481
  keratosis obliterans 504
  ligaments 479
  loose bodies 497, 498, 499
  Lyme disease 495
  meniscal displacement 487–492
  MRI 482, 483
  neoplasms 499–502
  nuclear medicine 482
  odontogenic keratocyst extension 503
  osteoarthritis/osteoarthrosis 493–494, 496, 497
  osteochondritis dissecans 493
  osteophytes 493, 494, 496
  pigmented villonodular synovitis 499, 502
  postoperative conditions 505–506
  pseudodisk 488, 491–492
  Reiter syndrome 495
  retrodiskal tissue 479, 480, 481, 483
   fibrosis 488, 491–492
  tympanic plate defects 484
  rheumatoid arthritis 494–495, 496, 497
  scintigraphy 482
  synovial chondromatosis 497–499
  systemic lupus erythematosus 495
tendinitis, calcific 832–833
tendon of Lockwood, upper 201
tendon of Zinn, lower 201
Tenon's capsule 140, 197, 199, 200
  fasciitis 140, 141
Tenon's space 197, 199, 200
tensor tympani canal
  coronal section 10
  sagittal section 26, 27, 28, 29
tensor tympani muscle 3
  axial sections 5, 6, 7, 9
  coronal oblique 20° sections 14, 15, 16
  development 682
tensor tympani tendon
  coronal oblique 20° sections 17, 18
  coronal section 10, 11
  sagittal section 25
teratoma
  nasopharyngeal 561, 564, 565, 567, 568
  orbital 219
thrombosis, cavernous sinus 229, 230, 391, 393, 396
thyroarytenoid muscle 732, 734, 735, 736
  atrophy 775
  glottic carcinoma spread 473
thyroglossal duct cyst 615, 616, 719, 770
  differential diagnosis 838
  histology 837
  infected 838
  infrahyoid neck 834, 837–838
  non-infected 838
thyroglossal duct remnants 719
thyroid carcinoma 719, 810–812
  anaplastic 812
  cold nodules 807, 810
  cystic metastases 615
  follicular 811, 812
  medullary 812
  nodal metastases 796, 797, 811
  papillary 796, 810–811
thyroid cartilage 732, 733
  fracture 775, 776
  neoplastic invasion 751
thyroid gland 783–784
  amyloid deposition 834
  cysts 809–810
  inflammatory conditions 833–834
  infrahyoid neck masses 807–813
  lymphoma 812–813
  metastases 813
  sarcoma 813
thyroid nodules 807–813
thyroid orbitopathy 233, 237–239
  dacryoadenitis 279
thyroid tissue, lingual 719
thyroiditis 833–834
  acute infectious 833
titanium implants, dental 546
Tolosa–Hunt syndrome 236, 237
tongue
  acute swelling 724
  amyloidosis 724
  anatomy 683–684
  base
   ablation 619
   carcinoma 697–699
   tumor invasion 699–700
  carcinoma 692–693
  denervation muscle atrophy 723
  development 683
  neurovascular bundle tumor invasion 699–700
  oral 692–693
tonsillar pillar carcinoma 697
tonsillitis 716
tonsilloliths 716
Tornwaldt's cyst 560, 594
torus mandibularis 532
torus palatinus 532
torus tubarius 554, 556, 557
Toxocara infection (toxocariasis) 157, 172, 174–175
toxoplasmosis, uveitis 156
trachea, stenosis 773
transforming growth factor b1 (TGF-b1) 564
transverse myelitis, radiation-induced 818
trapezius muscle 780, 781
  dermatomyositis 832
trauma
  bone cyst 522
  carotid artery dissection 841
  complications 468–469
  craniofacial 468–469
  cyst 518
  hypopharynx 775, 776, 777
  intraocular calcification 157, 159
  larynx 775, 776
  maxillofacial 466–467
  ocular 190–191
  ocular muscles 287
  orbital 290–291
  skull base 346–348
  suprahyoid neck 618
  temporal bone 54–61
  temporomandibular joint 504–505
   arthritis 494
Treacher–Collins syndrome *see* mandibulofacial dysostosis
trigeminal cavity 302, 303
trigeminal cistern 302, 303
  dermoid cyst 310
trigeminal ganglion 302, 303
trigeminal nerve 202
  embryology 508
  malignant tumor spread 613
  mandibular division 611
  maxillary branch 357
  nerve sheath tumors in masticator space 611, 612
  ophthalmic division 141, 357
  oral cavity/oropharynx cancer spread 702
tripod fracture 466, 467–468
trochlea, calcification 158, 159
trochlear nerve 203, 212
tuberculosis
  cervical lymph nodes 825–826
  chronic otitis media 71, 74
  laryngeal 772
  nasopharyngeal inflammation 561
  oral cavity/oropharynx 718
  salivary glands 645
  uveitis 156
tumor angiogenic factor 748
turbinate bone
  hypertrophy 400
  inferior 360
  middle 360, 364
   concha bullosa 363, 367
tympanic bone anomalies 43–46
tympanic membrane 3, 8
  coronal oblique 20° sections 16, 17, 18, 19, 20, 21

tympanic membrane
  coronal section 10, 11, 12, 13
  glomus tumors 101–102
  otitis media 69, 70
  sagittal section 22, 23, 24, 25
tympanic plate 477
  developmental defects 483, 484
tympanic ring 477, 484
tympanic sinus 25
tympanoplasty 90–91
tympanosclerosis 71, 73–74
tympanostomy tube, displaced 91, 92

U

ultrasonography
  hypopharynx 739
  infrahyoid neck 787–788
  larynx 739
  lymph nodes 793, 794
  oral cavity/oropharynx 688
  salivary glands 638
  sialolithiasis 648
uncinectomy 470, 471
Usher syndrome 53
utricle 4, 6, 7
  coronal oblique 20° sections 19, 20
  coronal section 12, 13
  sagittal section 26
utricular macula
  coronal oblique 20° sections 19
  sagittal section 26
uvea
  anatomy 141–142
  effusion 154, 186
  function 142
  leukemia 186
  malignant melanoma 150, 177–183
    clinical diagnosis 177–178
    diagnostic imaging 178–183
    differential diagnosis 182
    metastases 177–178, 179, 181
    tumor extension 179, 180, 181, 182
  melanocytoma 182–183
  metastases 183–184
  nevus 184
  schwannoma 187
uveitis 156–157
  ocular hypotony 152–153
uveoparotid fever 157, 645

V

vagus nerve 783
  schwannoma 100, 327, 797, 799
valleculae 687

varix malformation 120
  orbital 222, 258–259, 260
vascular abnormalities
  hypopharynx 756
  larynx 756, 774
  oral cavity/oropharynx 720–722
  parapharyngeal space retrostyloid compartment 602
vascular loops 118–119, 120
vascular malformations
  infrahyoid neck 839–840
  retropharyngeal space 598
vasculitides, orbital 242–243
veli palatini muscle
  levator 556
  tensor 554, 556
    fascia 582, 584
venous malformations
  infrahyoid neck 834
  larynx 774
  oral cavity/oropharynx 721
vertebral artery 782
  dissection 840–841
vertebral bodies
  cervical
    osteomyelitis 828, 829
    radiation-induced changes 815–816
  spondylodiskitis 832
vestibular aqueduct 4, 5, 6
  congenital anomalies 49, 50
  sagittal section 27
vestibular nerve
  inferior 7
    coronal oblique 20° sections 18
    internal auditory canal 109
    sagittal section 27
  schwannoma 114–115, 116
  superior 4, 5
    coronal oblique 20° sections 18
    inferior 27
    sagittal section 26
vestibular neuronitis 114
vestibule, congenital anomalies 49, 50
videopharyngoscopy 832
vidian nerve 375
viral infections
  cervical lymph nodes 824
  de Quervain thyroiditis 834
  eye 154–155
visceral space, infrahyoid 784, 785
vitreous
  anatomy 143
  embryology 137, 138
  hemorrhage in Warburg syndrome 169
  leukemia 186
  MRI 145
  opacities 177

vitreous
  see also persistent hyperplastic primary vitreous (PHPV)
vocal cords 732, 733
  false 732, 740
  paralysis 775
  true 471, 732
Vogt–Koyanagi–Harada syndrome 156
vomer 355
von Hippel–Lindau disease 105, 186
  intraocular calcification 157, 158
  low-grade adenocarcinoma of endolymphatic sac origin 338, 339–340
  retinal hemangioma 184
von Recklinghausen disease *see* neurofibromatosis, type I
vortex veins 141

W

Waardenburgh syndrome 53
Waldenstrom macroglobulinemia 250–251
Waldeyer's ring 558
  lymphoma 574, 575
    non-Hodgkin 796
Warburg syndrome, retinal dysplasia 168–169
Warthin's tumor 651, 652, 664–668
  salivary gland 657
Wegener granulomatosis 242
  lacrimal glands 279, 280
  larynx 772
  nasal cavity 402, 403, 404
  orbital apical inflammation 234
  paranasal sinuses 404
Wharton's duct *see* submandibular duct
Whitnall's ligament 201, 204

X

xanthogranuloma
  juvenile
    ocular 175, 176
    orbital 245, 247
  necrobiotic orbital 247

Z

Zenker's diverticulum 771
zygomatic bone embryology 682
zygomatic process 510